Pediatric Gastrointestinal and Liver Disease

FOURTH EDITION

Pediatric Gastrointestinal and Liver Disease

Editors

Robert Wyllie, MD
Calabrese Chair and Professor, Lerner College of Medicine
Chair, Pediatric Institute
Physician-in-Chief, Children's Hospital
Cleveland Clinic
Vice Chair, Office of Professional Staff Affairs
Cleveland Clinic
Cleveland, Ohio

Jeffrey S. Hyams, MD
Head, Division of Digestive Diseases and Nutrition
Connecticut Children's Medical Center
Hartford, Connecticut
Professor, Department of Pediatrics
University of Connecticut School of Medicine
Farmington, Connecticut

Associate Editor

Marsha Kay, MD
Director, Pediatric Endoscopy
Department of Pediatric Gastroenterology and Nutrition
Children's Hospital
Cleveland Clinic
Cleveland, Ohio

ELSEVIER
SAUNDERS

1600 John F. Kennedy Blvd.
Ste 1800
Philadelphia, PA 19103-2899

PEDIATRIC GASTROINTESTINAL AND LIVER DISEASE, FOURTH EDITION

ISBN: 978-1-4377-0774-8

Notices

Knowledge and best practice in this field are constantly changing. As new research and experience broaden
our understanding, changes in research methods, professional practices, or medical treatment may become
necessary.

   Practitioners and researchers must always rely on their own experience and knowledge in evaluating and
using any information, methods, compounds, or experiments described herein. In using such information
or methods they should be mindful of their own safety and the safety of others, including parties for whom
they have a professional responsibility.

   With respect to any drug or pharmaceutical products identified, readers are advised to check the most
current information provided (i) on procedures featured or (ii) by the manufacturer of each product to be
administered, to verify the recommended dose or formula, the method and duration of administration, and
contraindications. It is the responsibility of practitioners, relying on their own experience and knowledge of
their patients, to make diagnoses, to determine dosages and the best treatment for each individual patient,
and to take all appropriate safety precautions.

   To the fullest extent of the law, neither the Publisher nor the authors, contributors, or editors, assume any
liability for any injury and/or damage to persons or property as a matter of products liability, negligence or
otherwise, or from any use or operation of any methods, products, instructions, or ideas contained in the
material herein.

Library of Congress Cataloging-in-Publication Data

Pediatric gastrointestinal and liver disease/editors, Robert Wyllie, Jeffrey S. Hyams;
associate editor Marsha Kay.—4th ed.
      p. ; cm.
   Includes bibliographical references and index.
   ISBN 978-1-4377-0774-8 (hardcover : alk. paper) 1. Pediatric gastroenterology. 2.
Gastrointestinal system—Diseases. I. Wyllie, R. (Robert) II. Hyams, Jeffrey S. III. Kay,
Marsha.
   [DNLM: 1. Digestive System Diseases. 2. Adolescent. 3. Child. 4. Infant. WS 310]
   RJ446.P44 2011
   618.92'33—dc22

Acquisitions Editor: Kate Dimock
Developmental Editor: Taylor Ball
Publishing Services Manager: Patricia Tannian
Team Manager: Radhika Pallamparthy
Project Managers: Claire Kramer, Jayavel Radhakrishnan
Designer: Ellen Zanolle

To my dance partner and wife, Dr. Elaine Wyllie.
RW

To Eli, Alexander, and Debra.
JH

To my family and dear friends.
MK

Contributors

H. Hesham A-Kader, MD, MSc
Professor of Pediatrics
Chief, Division of Gastroenterology, Hepatology,
  and Nutrition
Department of Pediatrics
University of Arizona
Tucson, Arizona
USA

Sabina Ali, MD
Pediatric Gastroenterology
Children's Hospital and Research Center Oakland
Oakland, California
USA

Naim Alkhouri, MD
Staff Physician
Pediatric Gastroenterology, Hepatology and Nutrition
Cleveland Clinic
Cleveland, Ohio
USA

Estella M. Alonso, MD
Professor of Pediatrics
Northwestern University
Feinberg School of Medicine
Siragusa Transplant Center
Children's Memorial Hospital
Chicago, Illinois
USA

Rana Ammoury, MD
Assistant Professor of Pediatrics
Division of Pediatric Gastroenterology, Hepatology,
  and Nutrition
The University of Arizona Health Sciences Center
Tucson, Arizona
USA

Marjorie J. Arca, MD
Associate Professor of Surgery and Pediatrics
Divisions of Pediatric Surgery and Pediatric Critical Care
Medical College of Wisconsin
Children's Hospital of Wisconsin
Milwaukee, Wisconsin
USA

Arthur B. Atlas, MD
Director
Respiratory Center for Children
Goryeb Children's Hospital
Atlantic Health
Morristown, New Jersey
Assistant Professor
Deptartment of Pediatrics
University of Medicine and Dentistry (UMDNJ)
Newark, New Jersey
USA

Salvatore Auricchio, MD
Professor of Pediatrics
Department of Pediatrics
Faculty of Medicine and Surgery
Universita Degli Studi Di Napoli Federico II
Naples
ITALY

Robert D. Baker, MD, PhD
Professor of Pediatrics
State University of New York at Buffalo
Buffalo, New York
USA

Susan S. Baker, MD, PhD
Professor of Pediatrics
Digestive Diseases and Nutrition Center
State University of New York at Buffalo
Buffalo, New York
USA

Todd H. Baron, MD
Professor of Medicine
Division of Gastroenterology and Hepatology
Mayo Clinic
Rochester, Minnesota
USA

Brad Barth, MD, MPH
Assistant Professor
Department of Pediatrics
University of Texas Southwestern Medical School
Dallas, Texas
USA

Dorsey M. Bass, MD
Associate Professor
Department of Pediatrics
Stanford University School of Medicine
Stanford, California
USA

Phyllis R. Bishop, MD
Professor of Pediatrics
Division of Pediatric Gastroenterology
University of Mississippi Medical Center
Jackson, Mississippi
USA

Samra S. Blanchard, MD
Associate Professor
University of Maryland
School of Medicine
University of Maryland Medical Center
Baltimore, Maryland
USA

Athos Bousvaros, MD, MPH
Associate Professor of Pediatrics
Harvard Medical School
Associate Director
Inflammatory Bowel Disease Center
Children's Hospital
Boston, Massachusetts
USA

John T. Boyle, MD
Attending Physician
Pediatric Gastroenterology, Hepatology, and Nutrition
Children's Hospital of Philadelphia
Academic Clinical Professor of Pediatrics
Department of Pediatrics
The University of Pennsylvania School of Medicine
Philadelphia, Pennsylvania
USA

Steven W. Bruch, MD, MSc
Clinical Assistant Professor
Department of Pediatric Surgery
C.S. Mott Children's Hospital
University of Michigan
Ann Arbor, Michigan
USA

Brendan T. Campbell, MD, MPH
Assistant Professor of Surgery
Department of Pediatric Surgery
Connecticut Children's Medical Center
University of Connecticut School of Medicine
Hartford, Connecticut
USA

Anthony Capizzani, MD
Lecturer
Department of Surgery
University of Michigan
Ann Arbor, Michigan
USA

Christine Carter-Kent, MD
Clinical Assistant Professor of Pediatrics
Associate Staff Physician
Pediatric Gastroenterology and Nutrition
Pediatric Institute and Children's Hospital
Cleveland Clinic
Cleveland, Ohio
USA

Michael G. Caty, MD
John E. Fisher Professor of Pediatric Surgery
Surgeon-in-Chief
Department of Pediatric Surgical Services
Women and Children's Hospital of Buffalo
Professor of Surgery and Pediatrics
Department of Surgery
State University of New York at Buffalo
Buffalo, New York
USA

Louisa W. Chiu, MD
General Surgery Resident
Department of General Surgery
Cleveland Clinic
Cleveland, Ohio
USA

Dennis L. Christie, MD
Professor of Pediatrics
University of Washington
Head
Division of Pediatric Gastroenterology
Children's Regional Hospital and Medical Center
Seattle, Washington
USA

Gail M. Cohen, MD, MS
Assistant Professor of Pediatrics
Wake Forest University School of Medicine
Winston-Salem, North Carolina
USA

Mitchell B. Cohen, MD
Professor and Vice-Chair of Pediatrics
Director, Gastroenterology, Hepatology, and Nutrition
Department of Pediatrics
Cincinnati Children's Hospital Medical Center
Cincinnati, Ohio
USA

Stanley A. Cohen, MD
Pediatric Gastroenterologist
Children's Center for Digestive Health Care
Children's Healthcare of Atlanta
Adjunct Clinical Professor of Pediatrics
Emory University School of Medicine
Atlanta, Georgia
USA

Claudia Conkin, MS, RD, LD
Director, Food and Nutrition Services
Texas Children's Hospital
Houston, Texas
USA

Arnold G. Coran, MD, AB
Professor of Pediatric Surgery
Section of Pediatric Surgery
University of Michigan Medical School
Ann Arbor, Michigan
USA

Laura L. Cushman, BS, MS
Research Associate
Division of Pediatric Clinical Research
University of Miami
Miami, Florida
USA

Steven J. Czinn, MD
Professor and Chair
Department of Pediatrics
University of Maryland School of Medicine
Baltimore, Maryland
USA

David Devadason, MB, BS, MRCP(UK)
Paediatric Gastroenterologist and Honorary Senior Lecturer
Paediatric Gastroenterology, Hepatology, and Nutrition
Royal Hospital for Sick Children, Edinburgh University
Edinburgh
UK

Carlo Di Lorenzo, MD
Professor of Clinical Pediatrics
The Ohio State University
Chief, Division of Pediatric Gastroenterology
Nationwide Children's Hospital
Columbus, Ohio
USA

Ranjan Dohil, MBBCh, MRCP(UK), MRCPCH, DCH(UK)
Professor of Pediatrics
University of California and Rady Children's Hospital
   and Health Center
San Diego, California
USA

Maryanne L. Dokler, MD
Pediatric Surgeon
Nemours Children's Clinic
Courtesy Associate Professor
University of Florida/College of Medicine
Jacksonville, Florida
USA

Marla Dubinsky, MD
Associate Professor of Pediatrics
Cedars-Sinai Medical Center
Los Angeles, California
USA

Bijan Eghtesad, MD
Staff Surgeon
Department of Hepato-Pancreato-Biliary/Liver Transplant
   Surgery
Cleveland Clinic
Cleveland, Ohio
USA

Peter F. Ehrlich, MD, MSC
Associate Professor
Department of Pediatric Surgery
University of Michigan
C.S. Mott Children's Hospital
Ann Arbor, Michigan
USA

Mounif El-Youssef, MD
Associate Professor of Pediatrics
Mayo College of Medicine
Consultant
Gastroenterology and Hepatology
Department of Pediatrics
Mayo Clinic
Rochester, Minnesota
USA

Karan McBride Emerick, MD, MSCI
Associate Professor of Pediatrics
Department of Pediatrics
University of Connecticut School of Medicine
Farmington, Connecticut
Director of the Liver Disease Center
Division of Digestive Disease and Nutrition
Connecticut Children's Medical Center
Hartford, Connecticut
USA

Jonathan Evans, MD
Attending Physician
Division of Pediatric Gastroenterology and Nutrition
Nemours Children's Clinic
Jacksonville, Florida
USA

Rima Fawaz, MD
Instructor in Pediatrics
Division of Pediatric Gastroenterology and Nutrition
Children's Hospital Boston
Harvard Medical School
Boston, Massachusetts
USA

Ariel E. Feldstein, MD
Department of Pediatric Gastroenterology and Nutrition
Cleveland Clinic
Cleveland, Ohio
USA

Laura S. Finn, MD
Associate Professor
Department of Pathology
University of Washington
Seattle Children's Hospital
Seattle, Washington
USA

Douglas S. Fishman, MD
Director of Gastrointestinal Endoscopy
Texas Children's Hospital
Assistant Professor of Pediatrics
Baylor College of Medicine
Houston, Texas
USA

Joseph F. Fitzgerald, MD, BS
Professor of Pediatrics
Division of Pediatric Gastroenterology, Hepatology,
  and Nutrition
Indiana University School of Medicine
Indianapolis, Indiana
USA

David R. Fleisher
Associate Professor of Child Health
Pediatric Gastroenterology
University of Missouri Health Care
Columbia, Missouri
USA

Jacqueline L. Fridge, MD
Northwest Pediatric Gastroenterology, LLC
Portland, Oregon
USA

Joel Friedlander, DO, MBE (MA-Bioethics)
Assistant Professor of Pediatrics and Senior Ethics Scholar
Division of Pediatric Gastroenterology
Department of Pediatrics
Doernbecher Children's Hospital
Oregon Health and Science University
Portland, Oregon
USA

Judy Fuentebella, MD
Pediatric Gastroenterology, Hepatology, and Nutrition
Children's Hospital and Research Center Oakland
Oakland, California
USA

John J. Fung, MD, PhD
Chairman, Department of Surgery, Professor of Surgery
Department of General Surgery and Department of
  HPB/Transplant Surgery
Cleveland Clinic Lerner College of Medicine
Case Western Reserve University
Cleveland, Ohio
USA

Jennifer Garcia, MD
Assistant Professor of Clinical Pediatrics
Division of Gastroenterology, Hepatology, and Nutrition
University of Miami Miller School of Medicine / Holtz
  Children's Hospital
Miami, Florida
USA

Reinaldo Garcia-Naveiro, MD
Assistant Professor
Division of Pediatric Gastroenterology, Hepatology,
  and Nutrition
Rainbow Babies and Children's Hospital
University Hospitals Case Medical Center
Cleveland, Ohio
USA

José M. Garza, MD
Assistant Professor of Pediatrics
Gastroenterology, Hepatology, and Nutrition
Cincinnati Children's Hospital Medical Center
Cincinnati, Ohio
USA

Michael W. L. Gauderer, MD
Professor of Surgery and Pediatrics
Division of Pediatric Surgery
Children's Hospital
Greenville Hospital System University Medical Center
Greenville, South Carolina
USA

Donald E. George, MD
Chief
Division of Gastroenterology and Nutrition
Nemours Children's Clinic
Co-Clinical Associate Professor
Department of Pediatrics
University of Florida
Jacksonville, Florida
USA

Fayez K. Ghishan, MD
Horace W. Steele Endowed Chair in Pediatric Research
Professor and Head
Director
Steele Children's Research Center
Department of Pediatrics
University of Arizona
Tucson, Arizona
USA

Mark A. Gilger, MD
Professor
Department of Pediatrics
Chief
Section of Pediatric Gastroenterology, Hepatology,
  and Nutrition
Baylor College of Medicine
Houston, Texas
USA

Laura Gillespie, MD
Section of Adolescent Medicine
Children's Hospital
Cleveland Clinic
Cleveland, Ohio
USA

Elizabeth Gleghorn, MD
Division Director
Pediatric Gastroenterology, Hepatology, and Nutrition
Children's Hospital and Research Center Oakland
Oakland, California
USA

Glenn R. Gourley, MD
Professor of Pediatrics
Research Director and Fellowship Program Director, Pediatric
    Gastroenterology
University of Minnesota
Minneapolis, Minnesota
USA

Richard J. Grand, MD
Director, Center for Inflammatory Bowel Disease
Professor of Pediatrics
Harvard Medical School
Children's Hospital Boston
Boston, Massachusetts
USA

Reema Gulati, MD
Pediatric Gastrointestinal Fellow
Department of Pediatric Gastroenterology
Cleveland Clinic
Cleveland, Ohio
USA

Sandeep K. Gupta, MD
Professor of Clinical Pediatrics and Clinical Medicine
Adjunct Clinical Professor of Nutrition and Dietitics
Division of Pediatric Gastroenterology, Hepatology,
    and Nutrition
James Whitcomb Riley Hospital for Children
Indiana University School of Medicine
Indianapolis, Indiana
USA

Nedim Hadžić, MD
Consultant and Honorary Reader in Paediatric Hepatology
King's College Hospital
London
UK

Eric Hassall, MBChB, FRCPC, FACG
Professor of Pediatrics
Division of Gastroenterology
BC Children's Hospital
University of British Columbia
Vancouver, British Columbia
CANADA

James E. Heubi, MD
Professor/Associate Chair for Clinical Investigation
    of Pediatrics
Associate Dean for Clinical and Translational Research
Co-Director Center for Clinical and Translational Science
    and Training
University of Cincinnati College of Medicine
Children's Hospital Medical Center
Cincinnati, Ohio
USA

Vera F. Hupertz, MD
Director, Pediatric Hepatology and Transplant Hepatology
Pediatric Gastroenterology and Hepatology
Cleveland Clinic
Cleveland, Ohio
USA

Sohail Z. Husain, MD
Assistant Professor
Pediatrics
Yale University School of Medicine
New Haven, Connecticut
USA

Séamus Hussey, MB, BCh, BAO, BmedSc, MRCPI
Consultant Paediatric Gastroenterologist
National Centre for Paediatric Gastroenterology, Hepatology,
    and Nutrition
Our Lady's Children's Hospital and University College Dublin
Dublin
IRELAND

Jeffrey S. Hyams, MD
Head, Division of Digestive Diseases and Nutrition
Connecticut Children's Medical Center
Hartford, Connecticut
Professor, Department of Pediatrics
University of Connecticut School of Medicine
Farmington, Connecticut
USA

Warren Hyer, MB, ChB, FRCPCH, MRCP
Consultant Paediatric Gastroenterologist
Polyposis Registry
St. Mark's Hospital
Harrow
UK

Paul E. Hyman, MD
Professor of Pediatrics
Louisiana State University
Chief
Pediatric Gastroenterology
Children's Hospital
New Orleans, Louisiana
USA

Sabine Iben, MD
Pediatric Institute/Neonatology
Cleveland Clinic
Cleveland, Ohio
USA

Kishore R. Iyer, MBBS, FRCS, FACS
Surgical Director, Pediatric Liver Program
Director, Adult and Pediatric Intestinal Transplant
    and Rehabilitation Program
Associate Professor of Surgery and Pediatrics
Mount Sinai Medical Center
New York, New York
USA

Maureen M. Jonas, MD
Associate Professor
Department of Pediatrics
Harvard Medical School
Senior Associate in Medicine
Division of Gastroenterology
Children's Hospital Boston
Boston, Massachusetts
USA

Nicola L. Jones, MD, PhD
Staff Gastroenterologist
Division of Gastroenterology, Hepatology, and Nutrition
Hospital for Sick Children
Professor
Departments of Paediatrics and Physiology
University of Toronto
Toronto, Ontario
CANADA

Barbara Kaplan, MD
Staff Pediatric Gastroenterologist
Department of Pediatric Gastroenterology
Cleveland Clinic Foundation
Cleveland, Ohio
USA

Stuart S. Kaufman, MD
Medical Director
Pediatric Liver and Intestinal Transplantation
Georgetown University Hospital
Professor of Pediatrics
Georgetown University School of Medicine
Washington, District of Columbia
USA

Marsha Kay, MD
Director, Pediatric Endoscopy
Department of Pediatric Gastroenterology and Nutrition
Children's Hospital
Cleveland Clinic
Cleveland, Ohio
USA

Deirdre Kelly, MD, FRCP, FRCPI, FRCPH
Professor of Paediatric Hepatology
The Liver Unit
Birmingham Children's Hospital
Birmingham
UK

Samuel A. Kocoshis, MD
Professor of Pediatrics
University of Cincinnati College of Medicine
Director, Nutrition and Intestinal Transplantation
Division of Gastroenterology, Hepatology, and Nutrition
Cincinnati Children's Hospital Medical Center
Cincinnati, Ohio
USA

Benjamin R. Kuhn, DO
Clinical Fellow
Department of Gastroenterology, Hepatology, and Nutrition
Cincinnati Children's Hospital Medical Center
Cincinnati, Ohio
USA

Marc A. Levitt, MD
Associate Professor
Division of Pediatric Surgery
Department of Surgery
University of Cincinnati
Associate Director
Colorectal Center for Children
Cincinnati Children's Hospital Medical Center
Cincinnati, Ohio
USA

Shane D. Lewis, MD
Chief Resident
Department of Surgery
Texas A&M University
Temple, Texas
USA

BU. K. Li, MD
Professor of Pediatrics
Director, Pediatric Fellowship Education
Medical College of Wisconsin
Director
Cyclic Vomiting Program
Division of Gastroenterology, Hepatology, and Nutrition
Children's Hospital of Wisconsin
Milwaukee, Wisconsin
USA

Chris A. Liacouras, MD
Professor of Pediatrics
Attending Gastroenterologist
The Children's Hospital of Philadelphia
The University of Pennsylvania School of Medicine
Philadelphia, Pennsylvania
USA

Danny C. Little, MD
Chief of Pediatric Surgery
Children's Hospital at Scott & White
Department of Surgery
Texas A&M University Health Science Center
College of Medicine
Temple, Texas
USA

Vera Loening-Baucke, MD
Professor Emeritus
Pediatrics
University of Iowa
Iowa City, Iowa
USA
Visiting Professor
Internal Medicine-Gastroenterology
Charite Universitatsmedizin Berlin
Berlin
GERMANY

Kathleen M. Loomes, MD
Associate Professor of Pediatrics
University of Pennsylvania School of Medicine
Attending Physician
Division of Gastroenterology, Hepatology, and Nutrition
The Children's Hospital of Philadelphia
Philadelphia, Pennsylvania
USA

Mark E. Lowe, MD, PhD
Professor of Pediatrics
Director, Division of Gastroenterology, Hepatology,
   and Nutrition
Children's Hospital of Pittsburgh of University of Pittsburgh
   Medical Center
Pittsburgh, Pennsylvania
USA

David K. Magnuson, MD
Chairman
Department of Pediatric Surgery
Cleveland Clinic
Cleveland, Ohio
USA

Lori A. Mahajan, MD
Fellowship Director, Pediatric Gastroenterology
Pediatric Gastroenterology
Cleveland Clinic
Cleveland, Ohio
USA

Petar Mamula, MD
Director, Endoscopy
Division of Gastroenterology, Hepatology, and Nutrition
The Children's Hospital of Philadelphia
Associate Professor of Pediatrics
University of Pennsylvania School of Medicine
Philadelphia, Pennsylvania
USA

James F. Markowitz, MD
Professor of Pediatrics
New York University School of Medicine
New York, New York
Physician
Division of Pediatric Gastroenterology
Schneider Children's Hospital
New Hyde Park, New York
USA

Jonathan E. Markowitz, MD, MSCE
Medical Director
Pediatric Gastroenterology
Greenville Hospital System University Medical Center
Associate Professor
Department of Clinical Pediatrics
University of South Carolina School of Medicine
Greenville, South Carolina
USA

Maria R. Mascarenhas, MBBS
Section Chief
Nutrition
Division of Gastroenterology, Hepatology, and Nutrition
The Children's Hospital of Philadelphia
Associate Professor of Pediatrics
The University of Pennsylvania School of Medicine
Philadelphia, Pennsylvania
USA

Peter Mattei, MD
Assistant Professor of Surgery
The University of Pennsylvania School of Medicine
Attending Surgeon
General, Thoracic, and Fetal Surgery
The Children's Hospital of Philadelphia
Philadelphia, Pennsylvania
USA

Valérie A. McLin, MD
Assistant Professor
Pediatrics
Geneva University Hospital
Geneva
SWITZERLAND

Adam G. Mezoff, MD
Professor
Pediatric Gastroenterology, Hepatology, and Nutrition
Cincinnati Children's Hospital
Cincinnati, Ohio
USA

Giorgina Mieli-Vergani, MD, PhD
Professor of Paediatric Hepatology
Institute of Liver Studies
King's College London School of Medicine at
   King's College Hospital
London
UK

Tracie L. Miller, MD, MS
Professor of Pediatrics and Epidemiology
University of Miami Miller School of Medicine
Miami, Florida
USA

Franziska Mohr, MD, MRCPCH
Staff
Pediatric Gastroenterology
Cleveland Clinic
Cleveland, Ohio
USA

Robert K. Montgomery, PhD
Instructor
Division of Gastroenterology and Nutrition
Children's Hospital Boston
Boston, Massachusetts
USA

Kathleen J. Motil, MD, PhD
Associate Professor of Pediatrics
Baylor College of Medicine
Houston, Texas
USA

Simon Murch, MB, PhD, FRCP, FRCPCH
Professor of Paediatrics and Child Health
Warwick Medical School
University of Warwick
Coventry
UK

Karen F. Murray, MD
Professor of Pediatrics
Pediatric Gastroenterology and Hepatology
Seattle Children's and University of Washington School
    of Medicine
Seattle, Washington
USA

Hillel Naon, MD
Clinical Assistant
Professor of Pediatrics
Keck School of Medicine
University of Southern California
Children's Hospital–Los Angeles
Los Angeles, California
USA

Aruna S. Navathe, MA, RD, LD, CDE, CSP
Clinical Nutritionist
Nutrition and Pharmacy
Children's Healthcare of Atlanta at Scottish Rite
Atlanta, Georgia
USA

Vicky Lee Ng, MD, FRCP(C)
Medical Director, Liver Transplant Program
Staff Gastroenterologist
Gastroenterology, Hepatology, and Nutrition
SickKids Transplant Center
The Hospital for Sick Children
Toronto, Ontario
CANADA

Scott Nightingale, BMed(Hons), MClinEpid, FRACP
Staff Specialist
Paediatric Gastroenterology
John Hunter Children's Hospital
Newcastle, New South Wales
AUSTRALIA

Michael J. Nowicki, MD
Professor of Pediatrics
Division of Pediatric Gastroenterology
Director, Pediatric Endoscopy
Division of Pediatric Gastroenterology
University of Mississippi Medical Center
Jackson, Mississippi
USA

Samuel Nurko, MD, MPH
Director
Center for Motility and Functional Gastrointestinal Disorders
Children's Hospital Boston
Boston, Massachusetts
USA

Keith T. Oldham, MD
Professor and Chief
Division of Pediatrics
Medical College of Wisconsin
Surgeon-in-Chief and Marie Z Uihlein Chair
Children's Hospital of Wisconsin
Milwaukee, Wisconsin
USA

Alberto Peña, MD
Director, Colorectal Center for Children
Division of Surgery
Cincinnati Children's Hospital Medical Center
Cincinnati, Ohio
USA

Robert E. Petras, MD
Associate Clinical Professor of Pathology
Northeastern Ohio Universities College of Medicine
Rootstown, Ohio
National Director for Gastrointestinal Pathology Services
Ameripath Gastrointestinal Institute
Oakwood Village, Ohio
USA

Marian D. Pfefferkorn, MD
Associate Professor of Clinical Pediatrics
Pediatric Gastroenterology, Hepatology, and Nutrition
Indiana University School of Medicine
Riley Hospital for Children
Indianapolis, Indiana
USA

Sarah M. Phillips, MS, RD
Instructor Pediatrics
Gastroenterology, Hepatology, and Nutrition
Baylor College of Medicine
Houston, Texas
USA

Cary Qualia, MD
Pediatric Gastroenterologist
Assistant Professor of Pediatrics
Albany Medical Center
Albany, New York
USA

Shervin Rabizadeh, MD, MBA
Staff Physician
Pediatric Inflammatory Bowel Disease Center
Cedars-Sinai Medical Center
Los Angeles, California
USA

Kadakkal Radhakrishnan, MD, MD (Peds), DCH, MRCP (UK), MRCPCH, FAAP
Pediatric Hepatologist and Gastroenterologist
Medical Director, Nutrition Support and Intestinal
    Rehabilitation
Children's Hospital
Cleveland Clinic
Assistant Professor of Pediatrics
Cleveland Clinic Lerner College of Medicine
Case Western Reserve University
Cleveland, Ohio
USA

Leonel Rodriguez, MD
Children's Hospital Boston
Boston, Massachusetts
USA

Ricardo Rodriguez, MD, FAAP
Chairman, Department of Neonatology
Children's Hospital
Cleveland Clinic
Associate Professor of Pediatrics
Cleveland Clinic Lerner College of Medicine
Case Western Reserve University
Cleveland, Ohio
USA

Ellen S. Rome, MD, MPH
Head
Section of Adolescent Medicine
Department of General Pediatrics
Children's Hospital
Cleveland Clinic
Associate Professor
Department of Pediatrics
Cleveland Clinic Lerner College of Medicine
Case Western Reserve University
Cleveland, Ohio
USA

Joel R. Rosh, MD
Associate Professor of Pediatrics
New Jersey Medical School
Director, Pediatric Gastroenterology
Goryeb Children's Hospital/Atlantic Health
Morristown, New Jersey
USA

Colin D. Rudolph, MD, PhD
Professor and Vice Chair for Clinical Affairs
Department of Pediatrics
Medical College of Wisconsin
Milwaukee, Wisconsin
USA

Daniel F. Saad, MD
Assistant Clinical Professor of Surgery/Pediatrics
Division of Pediatric Surgery
University of South Carolina School of Medicine/Greenville
    Hospital System
Greenville, South Carolina
USA

Shehzad A. Saeed, MD, FAAP, AGAF
Associate Professor
Clinical Director, Shubert Martin Pediatric Inflammatory
    Bowel Disease Center
Division of Gastroenterology, Hepatology, and Nutrition
Cincinnati Children's Hospital Medical Center
Cincinnati, Ohio
USA

Atif Saleem, MD
Internist/Hospitalist
Gastroenterology and Hepatology Department
Mayo Clinic
College of Medicine
Rochester, Minnesota
USA

Bhupinder Sandhu, MD, DSc, MBBS, FRCP, FRCPCH
Consultant Paediatric Gastroenterologist
Professor of Paediatric Gastroenterology and Nutrition
Department of Paediatric Gastroenterology and Nutrition
Bristol Royal Hospital for Children
Bristol
UK

Miguel Saps, MD
Director of Gastrointestinal Motility and Functional Bowel
    Disorders Program
Division of Gastroenterology, Hepatology, and Nutrition
Children's Memorial Hospital
Assistant Professor of Pediatrics
Northwestern University's Feinberg School of Medicine
Chicago, Illinois
USA

Thomas T. Sato, MD, FACS, FAAP
Professor of Surgery
Division of Pediatric Surgery
Children's Hospital of Wisconsin/Medical College of Wisconsin
Milwaukee, Wisconsin
USA

Harohalli Shashidhar, MD, MRCP
Associate Professor and Chief
Division of Pediatric Gastroenterology and Nutrition
Department of Pediatrics
University of Kentucky Medical Center
Lexington, Kentucky
USA

Noah F. Shroyer, PhD
Assistant Professor
Division of Gastroenterology, Hepatology, and Nutrition
Cincinnati Children's Hospital
Cincinnati, Ohio
USA

Joseph Skelton, MD
Assistant Professor
Department of Pediatrics
Wake Forest University School of Medicine
Director
Brenner FIT (Families In Training) Program
Brenner Children's Hospital
Winston-Salem, North Carolina
USA

Lesley Smith, MD, MBA
Division of Pediatric Gastroenterology, Hepatology,
    and Nutrition
Miller School of Medicine
University of Miami
Miami, Florida
USA

Hiroshi Sogawa, MD
Assistant Professor of Surgery
Transplant Surgeon
Mount Sinai Hospital
New York, New York
USA

Oliver S. Soldes, MD, FACS, FAAP
Staff Surgeon
Department of Pediatric Surgery
Cleveland Clinic
Cleveland, Ohio
USA

Manu R. Sood, MD, MBBS, FRCPCH
Associate Professor
Department of Pediatrics
Medical College of Wisconsin
Director of Motility and Functional Bowel Disorders Program
Children's Hospital of Wisconsin
Milwaukee, Wisconsin
USA

Rita Steffen, MD, BA, MA
Staff Physician
Director of Pediatric Gastroenterology Motility Lab
Pediatric Gastroenterology and Nutrition
Children's Hospital
Cleveland Clinic
Cleveland, Ohio
USA

Kara M. Sullivan, MD
Fellow
Pediatric Gastroenterology, Hepatology, and Nutrition
University of Minnesota
Minneapolis, Minnesota
USA

Shikha S. Sundaram, MD, MSCI
Assistant Professor of Pediatrics
The Children's Hospital
University of Colorado Denver School of Medicine
Aurora, Colorado
USA

Bhanu K. Sunku, MD
Assistant Professor of Pediatrics
Director of Clinical Services and Education
Division of Pediatric Gastroenterology and Nutrition
Floating Hospital for Children at Tufts Medical Center
Boston, Massachusetts
USA

Francisco A. Sylvester, MD
Associate Professor of Pediatrics
Division of Digestive Diseases, Hepatology, and Nutrition
Connecticut Children's Medical Center
University of Connecticut School of Medicine
Hartford, Connecticut
USA

Jan Taminiau, MD, PhD
Pediatric Gastroenterology
Emma Children's Hospital/Academic Medical Center
Amsterdam
THE NETHERLANDS
Pediatric Committee
European Medicines Evaluation Agency
London
UK
Committee Member
Dutch Medicines Evaluation Board
Den Haag
THE NETHERLANDS

Jonathan E. Teitelbaum, MD
Director
Pediatric Gastroenterology
The Children's Hospital at Monmouth Medical Center
Long Branch, New Jersey
Associate Professor
Department of Pediatrics
Drexel University School of Medicine
Philadelphia, Pennsylvania
USA

Daniel W. Thomas, MD
Associate Professor
Division of Gastroenterology and Nutrition
Children's Hospital–Los Angeles
Los Angeles, California
USA

Mike A. Thomson, MD, DCH, MBChB, FRCP, FRCPCH
Consultant Paediatric Gastroenterologist and Honorary Reader
    in Paediatric Gastroenterology
Director of International Academy of Paediatric Endoscopy
    Training
Centre for Paediatric Gastroenterology
Sheffield Children's Hospital
Sheffield
UK

Vasundhara Tolia, MD, FAAP, FACG, AGAF
Adjunct Professor of Pediatrics
Michigan State University
Lansing, Michigan
USA

William R. Treem, MD
Vice-Chair, Department of Pediatrics for Clinical Development
Director, Division of Pediatric Gastroenterology, Hepatology, and Nutrition
State University of New York Downstate Medical Center
Brooklyn, New York
USA

Riccardo Troncone, MD
Professor of Pediatrics
Head, European Laboratory for the Investigation of Food-Induced Diseases
University Federico II
Naples
ITALY

Aaron Turkish, MD, BA
Assistant Professor of Pediatrics
New York Hospital Queens
Flushing, New York
USA

John N. Udall, Jr., MD, PhD
Retired Chairman
Department of Pediatrics
West Virginia University Health Sciences Center
Charleston, West Virginia
USA
Visiting Professor
Department of Pediatrics
Kenyatta Hospital
University of Nairobi School of Medicine
Nairobi
KENYA

Yvan Vandenplas, MD, PhD
Professor
Head of Department of Pediatrics
Universitair Ziekenhuis Brussel
Brussels
BELGIUM

Gigi Veereman-Wauters, MD, PhD
Pediatric Gastroenterologist
Universitair Ziekenhuis Brussel Children's Hospital
Free University of Brussels
Brussels
BELGIUM

Ghassan T. Wahbeh, MD
Associate Professor, Pediatrics–Gastroenterology
Director, Inflammatory Bowel Disease Program
Seattle Children's Hospital
University of Washington
Seattle, Washington
USA

Elizabeth C. Wallace, RD, CNSC, LDN
Clinical Dietitian
Clinical Nutrition
Children's Hospital of Philadelphia
Philadelphia, Pennsylvania
USA

R. Matthew Walsh, MD, FACS
Professor of Surgery and Vice-Chairman
Robert Rich Family Chair of Digestive Diseases
Department of Hepatobiliary and Transplant Surgery
Cleveland Clinic
Cleveland, Ohio
USA

Anna Wieckowska, MD
Pediatric Gastroenterologist
Centre Hospitalier Universitaire de Quebec (CHUQ)
Teaching Associate
Laval University of Quebec City
Department of Pediatric Gastroenterology
University of Laval in Quebec City
Quebec City, Quebec
CANADA

Charles G. Winans, MD
Staff Surgeon
Digestive Disease Institute
Department of Hepatobiliary Surgery
Cleveland Clinic
Cleveland, Ohio
USA

Robert Wyllie, MD
Calabrese Chair and Professor, Lerner College of Medicine
Chair, Pediatric Institute
Physician-in-Chief, Children's Hospital
Cleveland Clinic
Vice Chair, Office of Professional Staff Affairs
Cleveland Clinic
Cleveland, Ohio
USA

Sani Z. Yamout, MD
Fellow
Division of Pediatric Surgery
Department of Surgery
State University of New York
Buffalo, New York
USA

Nada Yazigi, MD
Associate Professor of Clinical Pediatrics
Division of Gastroenterology, Hepatology, and Nutrition
Cincinnati Children's Hospital Medical Center
Cincinnati, Ohio
USA

Preface

Since the publication of the First Edition of this book in 1993, the world has changed considerably, and the way medical professionals learn has changed as well. In this new digital age, descriptions of every disease are truly at our fingertips on the keyboards of our computers as we use various search engines. Sitting with a new patient who comes in with an obscure diagnosis is not quite as anxiety provoking as in the past, given our current ability to retrieve a description of his or her disease in seconds. The question then arises: Has a book about pediatric gastroenterology become obsolete? As the editors of the Fourth Edition, we know the answer is a resounding no. Electronic searches, while incredibly valuable, will never take the place of a compendium of knowledge integrated by experts and meant to edify its readers in pathophysiology, disease expression, treatment, and outcome. Moreover, the ability to think, underline, and write notes in the margins of a book (which is yours, of course, and not that of a friend or of the library) will not occur with a fully electronic resource. That is not to say that a book and digital information cannot be complementary. We hope to show with this edition that the two media can work in tandem; most of the references and all board review questions are provided on this edition's companion website—www.expertconsult.com—to complement the book. This saves space and pages and ultimately lowers costs, and these are important features in today's world.

We are proud of the Fourth Edition of Pediatric Gastrointestinal and Liver Disease. We have been able to attract a talented roster of international experts who have ably updated many of the chapters where new information arises at a rapid pace. The book continues to be organized into distinct sections starting with basic aspects of gastrointestinal function, followed by common clinical problems, organ-specific diseases, surgical procedures, and gastrointestinal procedures. The last three sections of the book focus on liver disease, pancreatic disease, and nutritional issues. We have added or expanded chapters in emerging areas such as endoscopic procedures and transplantation, including not only liver transplantation, but also small bowel and pancreatic transplantation, in addition to such topics as polyposis syndromes, liver diseases with a genetic etiology, and nonalcoholic fatty liver diseases.

We continue to be fortunate in receiving expert and unwavering support from the editorial staff at Elsevier. Special thanks to Taylor Ball and Claire Kramer for their assistance during the development and production of this book.

The production of a large book takes many hours of commitment by our authors. We recognize the increasing demands on everyone's time and want to express our gratitude to them for their efforts. They truly are the engine that drives the train over the hills and valleys of the production process. Lastly, we would like to thank our readership over the past 18 years whose feedback and curiosity have inspired us to move forward with this Fourth Edition. We all learn something new every day in the care of children with gastrointestinal and liver disease, and we hope that this book will provide a platform for the attainment of new knowledge.

ROBERT WYLLIE, MD

JEFFREY HYAMS, MD

2011

Contents

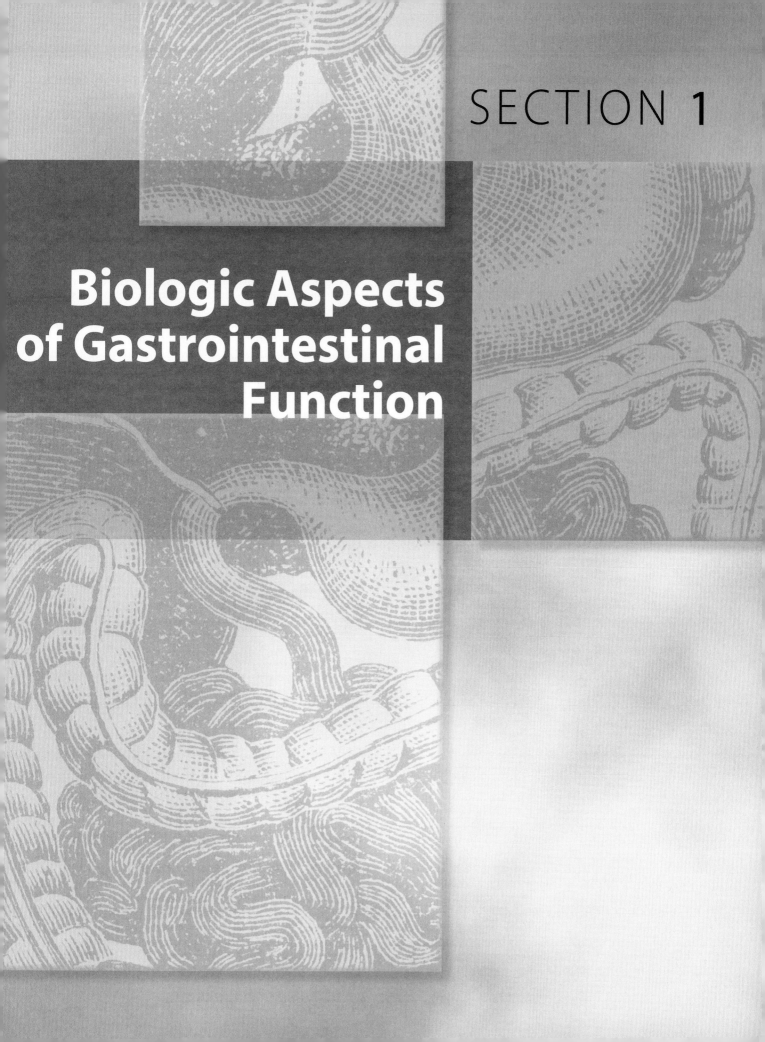

SECTION 1

Biologic Aspects of Gastrointestinal Function

1

DEVELOPMENT OF THE GASTROINTESTINAL TRACT

Robert K. Montgomery • Richard J. Grand

Organogenesis of the human gastrointestinal tract and liver is essentially complete by 12 weeks of gestation. At 4 weeks, the gastrointestinal tract is a straight tube, with identifiable organ primordia. Subsequently, the intestine elongates and begins to form a loop, which protrudes into the umbilical cord. By a process of growth and rotation during the following weeks, the intestine increases in length and turns through 270°, then retracts into the abdominal cavity. The crypt/villus structure is established during this process, as well as the patterns of expression of digestive enzymes and transporters. The intestine elongates approximately 1000-fold from the 5th to the 40th week of gestation, so that at birth, the small intestine is approximately three times the crown–heel length of the infant. A number of the critical genetic regulators of morphogenesis of the gastrointestinal tract have been identified and their mechanisms of action are being elucidated.

MORPHOGENESIS

Proliferation of cells from the fertilized egg gives rise to the blastocyst. The embryo will develop from a compact mass of cells on one side of the blastocyst, called the inner cell mass. It splits into two layers, the epiblast and hypoblast, which form a bilaminar germ disk from which the embryo develops. At the beginning of the third week of gestation, the primitive streak appears as a midline depression in the epiblast near the caudal end of the disk. During gastrulation, epiblast cells detach along the primitive streak and migrate down into the space between the two germ layers.

The process of gastrulation generates the endoderm cells that will form the epithelia lining the gastrointestinal tract. Some of the cells migrating inward through the primitive streak displace the lower germ layer (hypoblast) and form the definitive endoderm. Gastrulation establishes the bilateral symmetry and the dorsal–ventral and craniocaudal axes of the embryo. Formation of the three germ layers brings into proximity groups of cells, which then initiate inductive interactions and give rise to the organs of the embryo. As described later, the molecular mechanisms of many of these processes are now being elucidated.

The gut tube is formed by growth and folding of the embryo. The tissue layers formed during the third week differentiate to form primordia of the major organ systems. A complex process of folding, driven by differential growth of different parts of the embryo, converts the flat germ disk into a three-dimensional structure. As a result, the cephalic, lateral, and caudal edges of the germ disk are brought together along the ventral midline, where the endoderm, mesoderm, and ectoderm layers fuse to the corresponding layer on the opposite side. Thus, the flat endodermal layer is converted into the gut tube (Figure 1-1).

Folding of the embryo forms a closed gut tube at both the cranial and caudal ends. The anterior and posterior ends of the developing gut tube where the infolding occurs are designated the anterior and posterior (or caudal) intestinal portals. Initially, the gut consists of blind-ending cranial and caudal tubes, the foregut and hindgut, separated by the future midgut, which remains open to the yolk sac. As the lateral edges continue to fuse along the ventral midline, the midgut is progressively converted into a tube, while the yolk sac neck is reduced to the vitelline duct (Figure 1-2).

Three pairs of major arteries develop caudal to the diaphragm to supply regions of the developing abdominal gut. The regions of vascularization from these three arteries provide the anatomical basis for dividing the abdominal gastrointestinal tract into foregut, midgut, and hindgut. The celiac artery is the most superior of the three. It develops branches that vascularize the foregut from the abdominal esophagus to the descending segment of the duodenum, as well as the liver, gallbladder, and pancreas, which are derived from the foregut. The superior mesenteric artery supplies the developing midgut, the intestine from the descending segment of the duodenum to the transverse colon. The inferior mesenteric artery vascularizes the hindgut: the distal portion of the transverse colon, the descending and sigmoid colon, and the rectum. The separately derived inferior end of the anorectal canal is supplied by branches of the iliac arteries.

During the early part of the fourth week, the caudal foregut just posterior to the septum transversum expands slightly to initiate formation of the stomach. Continued expansion gives rise to a spindle-shaped or fusiform region. The dorsal wall of this fusiform expansion of the foregut grows more rapidly than the ventral wall, producing the greater curvature of the stomach during the fifth week. The fundus of the stomach is formed by continued differential expansion of the superior portion of the greater curvature. A rotation of 90° around a craniocaudal axis during the seventh and eighth weeks makes the original left side the ventral surface and the original right side the dorsal surface of the fetal stomach. Thus, the left vagus nerve supplies the ventral wall of the adult stomach and the right vagus innervates the dorsal wall. Additional rotation about a dorsal/ventral axis results in the greater curvature facing slightly caudal and the lesser curvature slightly cranial.

By about the third week of gestation, the gut is a relatively straight tube demarcated into three regions: the foregut, which will give rise to the pharynx, esophagus, stomach, and proximal duodenum; the midgut, which is open ventrally into the yolk sac and will produce the remainder of the duodenum, small intestine, and proximal colon; and the hindgut, which

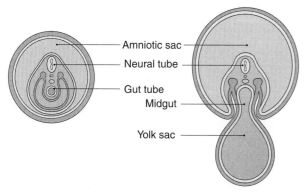

Figure 1-1. Folding forms a closed gut tube at both cranial and caudal ends of the growing embryo. The midgut remains open, but is progressively reduced to the vitelline duct, which remains connected to the yolk sac. Reproduced from Unit 35, Undergraduate Teaching Project of the American Gastroenterological Association, by permission of Milner-Fenwick, Inc.

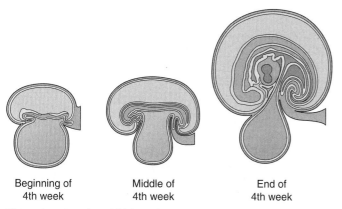

| Beginning of 4th week | Middle of 4th week | End of 4th week |

Figure 1-2. Growth and folding of the embryo form the gut tube–sagittal sections through embryos. Reproduced from Unit 35, Undergraduate Teaching Project of the American Gastroenterological Association, by permission of Milner-Fenwick, Inc.

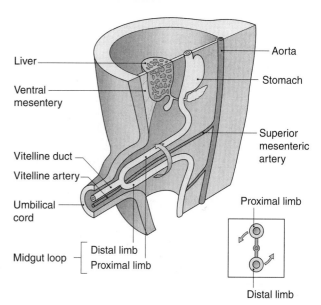

Figure 1-3. Rapid growth of the midgut causes its elongation and rotation. Reproduced from Unit 35, Undergraduate Teaching Project of the American Gastroenterological Association, by permission of Milner-Fenwick, Inc.

will develop into the distal colon and rectum. The hepatic and pancreatic anlagen arise at the junction between the foregut and midgut.

The rapid growth of the midgut causes its elongation and rotation. By 5 weeks, the intestine elongates and begins to form a loop, which protrudes into the umbilical cord. Shortly thereafter, the ventral pancreatic bud rotates and fuses with the dorsal pancreatic bud. Faulty rotation and fusion produces the anomaly known as annular pancreas. At 7 weeks, the small intestine begins to rotate around the axis of the superior mesenteric artery, moving counterclockwise (viewing the embryo from the ventral surface) approximately 90° (Figure 1-3). From 9 weeks onward, growth of the intestine forces it to herniate into the umbilical cord. The midgut continues to rotate as it grows, then returns to the abdominal cavity. By about 10 weeks, rotation has completed approximately 180°. By about 11 weeks, rotation has continued an additional 90° to complete 270°, and then the intestine retracts into the abdominal cavity, which has gained in capacity not only by growth, but by regression of the mesonephros and reduced hepatic growth (Figure 1-4). The control of re-entry has not been elucidated, but it occurs rapidly, with the jejunum returning first and filling the left half of the abdominal cavity, and the ileum filling the right half. The colon enters last, with fixation of the cecum

close to the iliac crest and the upward slanting of the ascending and transverse colon across the abdomen to the splenic flexure. Later growth of the colon leads to elongation and establishment of the hepatic flexure and transverse colon. The position of the abdominal organs is completed as the ascending colon attaches to the posterior abdominal wall. By 12 weeks of gestation, this process is completed (Figure 1-5).

Small intestinal villus and crypt formation occurs through a process of epithelial and mesenchymal reorganization, in a proximal to distal progression. Morphological analysis of human fetal small intestine by scanning electron microscopy demonstrates the first appearance of villi as rounded projections during the eighth week. The stratified epithelium is converted to a single layer of columnar epithelium through a process of secondary lumina formation and mesenchymal upgrowth. By 12 weeks, crypts with a narrow lumen lined with simple columnar cells are present. Between the 10th and 14th weeks, the villi increase in height and develop a more finger-like appearance. The microvilli become more regular and more dense on the apical surface of the enterocytes over this same period. Between 17 and 20 weeks, the first indications of muscularis mucosa develop near the base of the crypts.

Most small intestinal microvillus enzymes begin to appear at 8 weeks. Enzyme analysis of fetal human intestine has detected activities of sucrase, maltase, alkaline phosphatase, and aminopeptidase at 8 weeks of gestation, essentially simultaneously with villus morphogenesis. By 14 weeks, activity levels were comparable to adult intestine. These observations contrast with those in the well-studied rodent models, where enzyme activities are detectable following villus morphogenesis late in gestation, but major changes in levels of activity occur postnatally during weaning. In particular, sucrase in rodents is present only at very low levels until an abrupt upsurge at weaning. In contrast to other hydrolases examined, human lactase activity remains low until nearly the end of gestation (approximately 28 weeks), when it rises abruptly. This has been suggested to be a potential problem for premature infants, but the ability of premature infants to

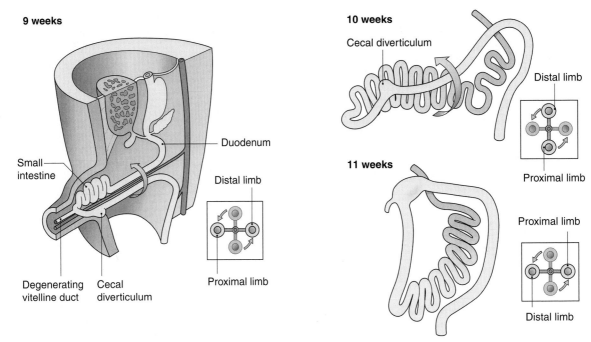

Figure 1-4. The growing midgut continues to rotate and returns to the abdominal cavity. Reproduced from Unit 35, Undergraduate Teaching Project of the American Gastroenterological Association, by permission of Milner-Fenwick, Inc.

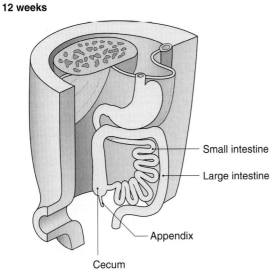

Figure 1-5. The position of the abdominal organs is completed as the ascending colon attaches to the posterior abdominal wall. Reproduced from Unit 35, Undergraduate Teaching Project of the American Gastroenterological Association, by permission of Milner-Fenwick, Inc.

digest milk lactose is potentiated by bacterial fermentation in the colon of unabsorbed lactose and absorption of resultant short-chain fatty acids. Microvillus membrane enzymes demonstrate proximal-to-distal gradients as early as 17 weeks' gestation. The topographical distribution of lactase activity is known to be genetically regulated. In all mammals studied, maximal activity is in the mid-jejunum with activity levels declining proximally and distally. Even at 17 weeks, lactase activity demonstrates this pattern, which is maintained throughout life.

The human fetal colon develops villi and expresses enzymes characteristic of small intestine until late in gestation. A striking characteristic of the developing fetal colon is its initial similarity to the small intestine. The development of the colon is marked by three important cytodifferentiative stages: the appearance (from about 8 to 10 weeks) of a primitive stratified epithelium, similar to that found in the early development of the small intestine; the conversion of this epithelium to a villus architecture with developing crypts (about 12 to 14 weeks); and the remodeling of the epithelium at around 30 weeks of gestation when villi disappear and the adult-type crypt epithelium is established. Consistent with the presence of villus morphology, the colonic epithelial cells express differentiation markers similar to those in small intestinal enterocytes. Thus, sucrase–isomaltase is detectable at 8 weeks in fetal colon, increases 10-fold as villus architecture emerges at 11 to 12 weeks, peaks at 20 to 28 weeks, and then decreases rapidly to barely detectable levels at term. Lactase has not been detected, whereas alkaline phosphatase and aminopeptidase follow a pattern generally similar to that of sucrase–isomaltase.

The cloaca gives rise to the rectum and urogenital sinus. Early in embryogenesis, the distal hindgut expands to form the cloaca. Between the fourth and sixth weeks, the cloaca is divided into a posterior rectum and anterior primitive urogenital sinus by the growth of the urorectal septum. Thus, the upper and lower parts of the anorectal canal have distinct embryological origins. The original cloacal membrane is divided by the urorectal septum into an anterior urogenital membrane and a posterior anal membrane. The anal membrane separates the endodermal and ectodermal portions of the anorectal canal. The former location of the anal membrane, which breaks down during the eighth week, is marked by the pectinate line in the adult. The distal hindgut gives rise to the upper two-thirds of the anorectal canal, whereas the ectodermal invagination called the anal pit represents the source of the inferior one-third of the canal. The pectinate line also marks the separation of the vascular supply of the upper and lower segments of the canal. The upper anorectal canal superior to the pectinate line is served by branches of the inferior mesenteric artery and veins draining the hindgut. By contrast, the region inferior to the pectinate line is supplied by branches of the internal iliac arteries and veins. The innervation of the anorectal canal also reflects the embryologic origins of the upper and lower portions. The superior portion of the canal is innervated by the inferior mesenteric ganglia and pelvic splanchnic nerves, and the inferior canal is supplied from the inferior rectal nerve.

The liver diverticulum arises as a bud from the most caudal portion of the foregut. During embryogenesis, specification of the liver, biliary tract, and pancreas occurs in a temporally regulated pattern. The liver, gallbladder, and pancreas, and their ductal systems develop from endodermal diverticula that bud from the duodenum in the fourth to sixth weeks of gestation.

At about 30 days of embryogenesis, the pancreas consists of dorsal and ventral buds that originate from endoderm on opposite sides of the duodenum. The dorsal bud grows more rapidly, whereas the ventral bud grows away from the duodenum on the elongating common bile duct (Figure 1-6). As the duodenum grows unequally, torsion occurs and the ventral pancreas is brought dorsad so that it lies adjacent to the dorsal pancreas in the dorsal mesentery of the duodenum; the two primordia thus fuse at about the seventh week. The head and uncinate process of the mature pancreas stem from the ventral primordium, whereas the remainder of the body and tail is derived from the dorsal primordium. Subsequently, the ducts originally serving each bud join to form the duct of Wirsung, although the proximal original duct of the dorsal bud often remains as the accessory duct of Santorini.

The prevertebral sympathetic ganglia develop next to the major branches of the descending aorta. The postganglionic sympathetic axons from these ganglia grow out along the arteries and come to innervate the same tissues that the arteries

supply with blood. The postganglionic fibers from the celiac ganglia innervate the distal foregut region from the abdominal esophagus to the entrance of the bile duct into the duodenum. Fibers from the superior mesenteric ganglia innervate the midgut, the remaining duodenum, jejunum, ileum, ascending colon, and two thirds of the transverse colon. The inferior mesenteric ganglia innervate the hindgut, the distal third of the transverse colon, the descending and sigmoid colon, and the upper two thirds of the anorectal canal.

The vagus nerve and the pelvic splanchnic nerves provide preganglionic parasympathetic innervation to ganglia embedded in the walls of visceral organs. Unlike the sympathetic ganglia, parasympathetic ganglia form close to the organs they innervate and produce only short postganglionic fibers. The central neurons of the parasympathetic pathways reside in either the brain or the spinal cord. Preganglionic parasympathetic fibers associated with cranial nerve X form the vagus nerve, which extends into the abdomen where these fibers synapse with the parasympathetic ganglia in target organs including the liver and the gastrointestinal tract proximal to the colon. Parasympathetic preganglionic fibers arising from the spinal cord form the pelvic splanchnic nerves, which innervate ganglia in the walls of the descending and sigmoid colon and rectum. Neural crest cells that migrate into the developing intestinal tract form a critical component of the enteric nervous system. Failure of migration of neural crest cells is the basis of Hirschsprung's disease.

Under normal conditions, the human gastrointestinal tract at term exhibits essential structural and functional maturity, although some functions, such as bile salt conjugation, mature postnatally.

MOLECULAR MECHANISMS

Gastrulation, during which the axes of the embryo are determined and formation of the gastrointestinal tract is initiated, is an essential early step in development of all multicellular organisms. Regionalization and development of specialized organs along the gut tube appear early in evolution, suggesting that the mechanisms regulating gut formation are likely to be early evolutionary developments and similar in most organisms. Current research suggests that the mechanisms governing these processes are indeed highly conserved throughout evolution. Therefore data from model organisms are directly relevant to human development.

There are three major developmental milestones in formation of the gastrointestinal tract. First is the initial specification of the endoderm. Second is formation and patterning of the gut tube that establishes the anterior–posterior axis and the boundaries between different organs. Third is the initiation of formation of organs that are outgrowths of the gut tube, such as liver and pancreas. Experiments in model organisms have identified families of genes involved in endoderm specification that are highly conserved in evolution, whereas other genes may be specific to vertebrate gut development. This overview focuses on current understanding of the molecular basis of these major milestones in gastrointestinal development and the roles of the best understood genes.

Specification of the Endoderm

Specification of the endoderm can be traced to the earliest stages of embryo formation. Classical experiments demonstrated that explants of chick embryos before gastrulation were

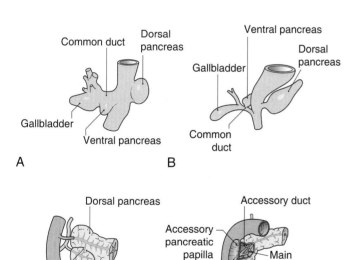

Figure 1-6. Development of the pancreas. (**A**) At 4 weeks, dorsal and ventral buds are formed. (**B**) At 6 weeks, the ventral pancreas extends toward the dorsal pancreas. (**C**) At 7 weeks, fusion of the dorsal and ventral pancreas occurs. (**D**) At 40 weeks, the pancreas is a single organ and ductular anastomosis is complete. From Sleisenger MH, Fordtran JS. Gastrointestinal disease. 4th ed. Philadelphia: WB Saunders, 1989, with permission.

capable of gastrointestinal development, indicating that their fate had already been specified. Evidence is accumulating in support of the hypothesis that the original patterning of the endoderm is cell autonomous, but that full development of the organs requires a reciprocal interaction between the endoderm and mesoderm. Gene families that act to specify endoderm have now been identified in a number of model organisms. One class of genes encodes transcription factors that directly activate target genes. A second class encodes signaling molecules that mediate cellular interactions. At least some of the transcription factors involved in specification of the endoderm continue to be expressed in the gastrointestinal tract throughout development, such as the forkhead-related factors (FOX genes) and GATA factors. Signaling pathways, such as those mediated by members of the transforming growth factor β (TGF-β) superfamily of growth factors, including TGF-β and the bone morphogenetic proteins (BMP), and the hedgehog pathways, act at different times and in different locations to regulate gastrointestinal development.

From its earliest stages, the endoderm is in close apposition to mesoderm throughout the gastrointestinal tract. Tissue recombination experiments have shown that patterning of the endoderm and its differentiation into separate organs results from signaling between the mesoderm and the endoderm. The earliest identified step in anterior–posterior patterning in mouse endoderm requires signaling from mesoderm to endoderm by fibroblast growth factor 4 (FGF-4).[1] Late in gestation, the intestine undergoes an exponential growth in length that is mediated by FGF-9 produced by the epithelium and affecting the mesenchyme.[2] Elongation of the midportion of the small intestine requires signaling by wnt5a through the noncanonical wnt signaling pathway. When this signaling is blocked, in addition to failure of elongation, the vitelline duct fails to close off completely, forming a partial duplication of the intestine, an abnormality reminiscent of Meckel's diverticulum.[3] In both the FGF-9 and wnt5a knockout experiments, cell differentiation in the intestine is normal, indicating that neither is involved in enterocyte differentiation. Other members of the FGF family and their receptors are critical in liver development. Three other important gene families mediating mesoderm/endoderm signaling are sonic hedgehog, the BMPs, and the hox genes.

It remains unclear if a single "master gene" initiates the formation of the endoderm, setting in motion the process of gastrointestinal development. In some of the model systems, genes have been identified that appear to be both necessary and sufficient to specify endoderm, for example the mixer gene in Xenopus.[4] In other model organisms, genes have been identified that are necessary, but may not be sufficient. Deletion of the transcription factor Sox17 eliminates formation of the definitive endoderm in the early mouse embryo, indicating an essential role.[5] Several mouse homeobox genes related to Drosophila caudal are expressed specifically in the intestine. One, Cdx-1, is restricted to the adult intestine, but is expressed widely in the developing embryo. Another, Cdx-2, is expressed in visceral endoderm of the early embryo, but restricted to the intestine at later stages. Forced expression of Cdx-2 will induce differentiation in an intestinal cell line that does not normally differentiate.[6] Cdx-2 is clearly a critical intestine-specific differentiation factor. Conditional ablation in early endoderm demonstrates a key role for Cdx-2 in anterior/posterior patterning, although the mutant intestine retains the primary pattern of hox gene expression.[7] Thus, recent evidence suggests that Cdx-2 may function

as a master gene for the intestine: in mice with Cdx-2 deleted, the large intestine does not form at all and the small intestine does not develop, but forms a simple stratified epithelium.[7]

Two GATA transcription factor genes are essential in specification of the cells that give rise to the intestinal epithelium of Caenorhabditis elegans, whereas a Drosophila GATA factor is encoded by the gene serpent, previously demonstrated to be required for differentiation of gut endoderm. Three members of the GATA family are expressed in vertebrate intestine. Distinct functions for GATA-4, -5, and -6 in intestinal epithelial cell proliferation and differentiation have been suggested, but because of their critical function in formation of other organs such as the heart, their role in early development of the mammalian intestine remains unresolved. In addition to the GATA factors, members of the forkhead-related (Fox) family and members of the wnt/Tcf signaling pathway are critical regulators of endoderm formation. Members of the TGF-β superfamily critical in the initiation of endoderm formation have been identified in vertebrates. One of the effector molecules in this pathway, Smad2, has also been shown to be critical for early endoderm formation.[8] A scaffolding molecule important in the TGF pathway, ELF3, is also required, as null mice lack intestinal endoderm.[9]

Many transcription factors initially identified as liver-specific have key roles in the intestine. When analyzed in mouse development, several of these transcription factors have been found to be expressed in patterns suggesting that they may also regulate intestinal development. For example, hepatic nuclear factor 3β (HNF-3β; now Fox-A2) has been shown to be critical for the earliest differentiation of the gastrointestinal tract and continues to be expressed in the adult progeny of the endoderm.[10] Homozygous null mutants of HNF-3β do not form a normal primitive streak which gives rise to the gut tube and other structures. HNF-3β is critical to formation of the foregut and midgut but not the hindgut.[11] Multiple members of this family have been identified, some of which display intestine enriched or intestine-specific expression. One of the family members (Foxl1), normally expressed in the intestinal mesoderm, is a critical mediator of epithelial–mesenchymal interactions. Its elimination has led to abnormal epithelial cell proliferation and aberrant intestinal development.[12] Thus, it appears likely that during intestinal development, multiple members of the Fox family interact in a complex mechanism that remains to be elucidated.

Formation of the Gut Tube

The gut tube is formed from a layer of endoderm by a process of folding that begins at the anterior and posterior ends of the embryo. Reciprocal signaling between endoderm and mesoderm continues to be critical to the developmental process.

A key mechanism that has emerged as a mediator of endoderm/mesoderm interactions in the organization of the gastrointestinal tract involves the sonic (Shh) and Indian hedgehog (Ihh) signaling proteins. Both Shh and Ihh play critical roles in anterior/posterior patterning and concentric patterning of the developing gastrointestinal tract, at least in part through their role in development of muscle from the mesoderm.[13] One target of this signaling pathway is a second family of signaling molecules, the BMPs, members of the TGF-β superfamily.[14,15]

Shh is first detectable in the primitive endoderm of the embryo, later in the endoderm of the anterior and posterior intestinal portals, and subsequently throughout the gut endoderm and in the adult crypt region. *Bmp4* is expressed in the mesoderm adjacent to the intestinal portals and can be induced ectopically in the visceral mesoderm by Shh protein. The endoderm of the intestinal portals is the source of Shh; the portal regions can act as polarizing centers if transplanted. Shh also induces the expression of *hox* genes. Paracrine signaling by hedgehog produced by the epithelium regulates gastrointestinal patterning and development from antrum to colon.[16,17] Shh is a critical regulator of both foregut and hindgut development, as null mice display foregut anomalies such as esophageal atresia and tracheo-esophageal fistula and hindgut anomalies such as persistent cloaca.[18]

Organ Development

Patterning

In *Drosophila*, the large family of homeotic genes is expressed in the body in a precise anterior to posterior order. The homeotic genes encode transcription factors, incorporating a conserved homeobox sequence, which regulate segmentation and pattern formation. Vertebrates have homologous *hox* genes which play important roles in the formation of distinctly delineated regions of the brain and skeleton. There are four copies of the set of vertebrate genes, *hoxa–d*, which form groups of paralogs, e.g., *hoxa-1*, *hoxb-1*, and *hoxd-1*. Within each group, the genes are expressed in the embryo in an anterior to posterior sequence of regions with overlapping boundaries, e.g., *hoxa-1* in the occipital vertebrae to *hoxa-11* in the caudal vertebrae.

A detailed study of the developing chick hindgut demonstrated a correlation between the boundaries of expression of *hoxa-9, -10, -11,* and *-13* in the mesoderm and the location of morphologic boundaries. Regional differences in expression of homeobox genes in the developing mouse intestine have also been demonstrated.[19] Interference with the expression of specific *hox* genes produces organ-specific gastrointestinal defects. Disruption of *hoxc-4* gives rise to esophageal obstruction due to abnormal epithelial cell proliferation and abnormal muscle development. Alteration of the expression pattern of *hox 3.1* (now *hoxc-8*) to a more anterior location causes distorted development of the gastric epithelium. Loss of mesenchymal *hoxa-5* alters gastric epithelial cell phenotype.[20] Mice with disrupted *hoxd-12* and *hoxd-13* genes display defects in formation of the anal musculature. Expression of the human homologs of a number of homeobox genes has also been shown to be region-specific.[21] These data indicate that the *hox* genes are critical early regulators of proximal-to-distal, organ-specific patterning. Ectopic expression of *hox* genes in chicken leads to altered patterning.[14,15] The *caudal* genes are members of a divergent homeobox gene family and regulate the anterior margins of *hox* gene expression as well as having gastrointestinal-specific roles. Almost all of the *hox* genes analyzed are expressed in mesodermal tissue, likely affecting endodermal development via epithelial–mesenchymal interactions.[22]

Regional Specification

Organs such as the stomach are first identifiable by thickening in the mesodermal layer. Early in the process of patterning, *Bmp4* is expressed throughout the mesoderm. Sonic hedgehog (*Shh*) is expressed in the endoderm and is an upstream regulator of *Bmp4*. The patterning of *Bmp4* expression in the mesoderm regulates growth of the stomach mesoderm and determines the sidedness of the stomach. Location of the pyloric sphincter is dependent on the interaction of *Bmp4* expression and inhibitors of that expression.[23] Patterning of the concentric muscle layer structure is dependent on Shh signaling that induces formation of lamina propria and submucosa, while inhibiting smooth muscle and enteric neuron development near the endoderm.[13,24] Expression of the transcription factor Barx1 in the fetal stomach mesoderm activates two wnt antagonists, inhibiting wnt signaling in the epithelium, which leads to differentiation of the stomach epithelium. Deletion of Barx1 results in reversion of the putative stomach epithelium to an intestinal state.[25] Gastric gland specification and progenitor cell maintenance are controlled by FGF10, which acts in concert with several morphogenetic signaling systems during stomach development.[26]

Stem Cells

Major advances have recently been achieved in understanding intestinal stem cells. Although the presence of stem cells in the small intestine has been generally accepted since the pioneering work of Cheng and Leblond[27] in 1974, studies had stagnated because of the lack of specific markers, although several candidate markers have been under investigation.[28] Knockout of Tcf-4, a component of the wnt signaling pathway, results in a loss of proliferating cells, suggesting that wnt signaling is critical to the maintenance of the stem cell compartment, in addition to regulating cell proliferation[29,30] In pursuing the key role of wnt signaling in regulation of intestinal proliferation, Lgr5(GPR49) has been identified as a downstream wnt target, and Lgr5 expression marks a population of stem cells in small intestine and colon.[31] BMI1 expression also marks intestinal stem cells.[32] Based on radiation and regeneration experiments, intestinal stem cells have been considered to be slowly cycling and located above the Paneth cell zone, predominantly, but not exclusively, at so-called position four above the crypt base. Whereas the BMI1 marked stem cells are consistent with these parameters, the Lgr5 cells are not, as they are located predominantly at the crypt base and are rapidly cycling. These data suggest that there may in fact be two populations of intestinal stem cells, either distinct from one another or partially overlapping, as discussed in detail by Scoville et al.[33] Consistent with this hypothesis, evidence has recently been presented that the putative stem cell marker, DCAMKL1, identifies a slow-cycling intestinal stem cell population.[34]

Isolation and culture of Lgr5 stem cells has been reported. Remarkably, single Lgr5+ cells embedded in Matrigel-generated organoids that contained regions of both proliferating and differentiated small intestinal cells in the absence of any other cell type and requiring only three growth factors (EGF, R-spondin, and jagged) added to a serum-free medium. Although widely assumed to be critical, interaction with mesenchymal cells apparently is not after all an absolute requirement for either proliferation or differentiation of intestinal epithelial cells.[35] Microarray analysis of Lgr5 cells identified Ascl2 as another marker of the Lgr5 intestinal stem cell. In this study, the Ascl2 gene was deleted in the stem cells, significantly depleting the epithelium. After several days, the epithelium regenerated, which the authors attributed to the proliferation of stem cells that had not been killed.[36] The regeneration is also consistent with the presence of a distinct population of stem cells from which the replacement epithelium was derived. The Lgr5, BMI1, and Ascl2 studies used knockin of a reporter gene into the putative stem cell specific gene to demonstrate lineage development from the marked stem cell. Thus, a new standard has been established for identification of stem cell markers, as described for example by Snippert et al.[36a] in their examination of the putative marker prominin or CD133. They found that expression of prominin labeled a larger population than just intestinal stem cells in the stem cell zone, demonstrating that it is not a specific marker. Several other intestinal stem cell markers have been proposed, but until they meet the criterion of lineage tracing from a specifically marked stem cell, they must be regarded with caution.

In the esophagus, a recent report used the "side population" staining phenomenon to isolate and characterize stem cells. These cells could be grown in vitro and regenerate damaged esophagus when transplanted.[37] In the stomach, labeling studies indicate that the stem cells are located in the isthmus region.[38] Consistent with these observations, a villin-cre/rosa mouse model identifies rare putative stem cells mostly located in the isthmus region. Under regenerative conditions, when these cells are marked with lacZ expression, they persist long term and give rise to all of the cell types in the stomach, consistent with their identification as stem cells, although under normal circumstances, they apparently are quiescent and do not contribute to the generation of gastric cells.[39]

In addition to the identification of stem cells, key regulators of the formation of differentiated small intestinal cells from stem cells have been identified. The four cell types of the intestinal epithelium arise in the crypts as two lineages, the absorptive and the secretory, comprising the goblet, enteroendocrine, and Paneth cells. Lineage specification of epithelial cells as secretory cells, rather than absorptive cells, requires expression of the transcription factor Math1.[40] Ngn3 expression guides cells to an enteroendocrine fate,[41] whereas Notch signaling regulates the differentiation of Paneth rather than goblet cells from this lineage.[42] Hes1 represses enteroendocrine cell differentiation in stomach, pancreas, and small intestine, likely through Math1.[43] Downstream of Math1, the transcriptional repressor Gfi1 regulates the allocation of cells to the different secretory lineages.[44] Recent evidence suggests that the location of crypts, likely reflecting the location of the stem cells, is determined by a gradient of BMP.[24]

Development of Organs From Outgrowths

Liver. The liver diverticulum emerges from the most caudal portion of the foregut just distal to the stomach. It is first detectable as a thickening in the endoderm of the ventral duodenum. Hepatogenesis is initiated through an instructive induction of ventral foregut endoderm by cardiac mesoderm. A series of elegant experiments have identified a number of signaling pathways involved in the complex process of development of the liver. The immediate signal is provided by fibroblast growth factors from the cardiac mesoderm that bind to specific receptors in the endoderm.[45] The appearance of mRNA for the liver-specific protein albumin in endodermal cells of the liver diverticulum is one of the earliest indications of hepatocyte induction. Endothelial precursor cells provide another critical factor for hepatogenesis, indicating the importance of interactions between blood vessels and the endoderm.[46] The establishment of competence in the foregut endoderm for initiation of liver development depends on the transcription factors FoxA1 and FoxA2.[47] Expression of the homeobox gene, Hex, is critical for emergence of the liver bud.[48] After formation of the liver bud, hepatocyte growth factor (HGF) is required for continued

hepatocyte proliferation. The hepatic diverticulum grows into the septum transversum and gives rise to the liver cords, which become the hepatocytes. During this process, a combination of signals from the cells of the septum transversum, including BMP, is necessary for liver development.[49] In addition to its role in liver organogenesis, signaling through the wnt/beta-catenin pathway is a critical factor in postnatal liver development.[50]

Pancreas. Development of the pancreas has provided one of the classic examples of epithelial–mesenchymal interactions. Previous investigations showed that growth and differentiation of the pancreas required the presence of mesenchyme, although both endocrine and exocrine cells develop from the foregut endoderm. Analysis of the development of separated endoderm and mesenchyme under different conditions indicated that the "default pathway" of pancreatic differentiation leads to endocrine cells, whereas a combination of extracellular matrix and mesenchymal factors are required for complete organogenesis.[51]

Molecular regulation of pancreas morphogenesis has now been worked out in some detail.[52] The dorsal pancreatic bud arises in an area where Shh expression is repressed by factors from the notochord. Inactivation of Indian hedgehog (Ihh) results in ectopic branching of the ventral pancreas, resulting in an annulus encircling the duodenum, as in the human disorder annular pancreas.[53] Expression of the pdx-1 gene in cells of the pancreatic bud is one of the earliest signs of pancreas development. The protein was found to be expressed in the epithelium of the duodenum immediately surrounding the pancreatic buds, as well as in the epithelium of the buds themselves. Examination of an initial pdx-1 knockout mouse indicated that whereas development of the rest of the gastrointestinal tract and the rest of the animal was normal, the pancreas did not develop. A second group, which independently made a pdx-1 null mouse, found that the dorsal pancreas bud did form, but its development was arrested.[54] The defect due to the pdx knockout was restricted to the epithelium, as the mesenchymal cells maintained normal developmental potential. In addition, the most proximal part of the duodenum in the null mice was abnormal, forming a vesicle-like structure lined with cuboidal epithelium, rather than villi lined by columnar cells, indicating that pdx-1 influences the differentiation of cells in an area larger than that which gives rise to the pancreas, consistent with the earlier delineated domain of expression. A case of human congenital pancreatic agenesis has been demonstrated to result from a single nucleotide deletion in the human pdx-1 gene.[55] Formation of the dorsal, but not the ventral, pancreatic bud requires the homeobox 9 (Hb9) transcription factor.[56] Pancreas transcription factor 1a (Ptf1a) is required for growth of the pancreatic buds.[57] The cell lineages that form exocrine, endocrine islet, and duct progenitors become committed at mid-gestation, with cells expressing the transcription factor Ngn becoming islet cell precursors, distinct from duct progenitors.[58] The staining patterns of these and other regulatory factors in early pancreas development have recently been presented in detail by Jorgensen et al.[59]

Key regulators of gastrointestinal development have been identified. Some of the genes critical in epithelial/mesenchymal interaction, long known to be a fundamental developmental process, are now known. Analysis of the expression pattern of the hox genes suggests that they act to pattern the gastrointestinal tract. The hedgehog proteins mediate several aspects of early development, but inhibition experiments suggest that after organ formation, their role is largely complete. Targeted disruption of several genes that regulate intestinal growth indicates that Bmp secretion has a key developmental role in cell proliferation, villus morphology, and crypt location. Most of the signaling pathways identified are short range, such as the wnt signaling pathway, which plays a key role in development of the gastrointestinal tract and whose malfunctions are a major cause of gastrointestinal cancers. With the exception of EGF, there is little compelling evidence for a critical developmental role for any circulating or luminal growth factor in the development of the intestine.

Increasingly powerful tools of genomic analysis and bioinformatics are providing novel insights into the mechanisms of gastrointestinal development. Microarray analysis of gene expression profiles indicates that the organs of the adult gastrointestinal tract display distinct patterns.[60] Furthermore, the analysis identified some common regulatory elements, including those for HNF1 and GATA factors, in the 5′ flanking sequences of groups of genes expressed in specific regions, suggesting organ-specific regulation. Comprehensive analysis of gene expression is now being used to identify global changes resulting from knockout of key developmental genes such as cdx2.[7] A combination of work on critical individual genes with examination of cell- and organ-specific developmental gene expression profiles should provide a deeper understanding of the regulation of gastrointestinal development.

REFERENCES

27. Cheng H, Leblond CP. Origin, differentiation and renewal of the four main epithelial cell types in the mouse small intestine. V. Unitarian Theory of the origin of the four epithelial cell types. Am J Anat 1974;141:537–561.
31. Barker N, van Es JH, Kuipers J, et al. Identification of stem cells in small intestine and colon by marker gene *Lgr5*. Nature 2007;449:1003–1007.
35. Sato T, Vries RG, Snippert HJ, et al. Single Lgr5 stem cells build crypt–villus structures in vitro without a mesenchymal niche. Nature 2009;459:262–265.

See expertconsult.com for a complete list of references and the review questions for this chapter.

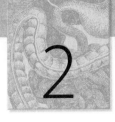

2 BASIC ASPECTS OF DIGESTION AND ABSORPTION

Ghassan T. Wahbeh • Dennis L. Christie

The gastrointestinal tract carries the tasks of receiving nutrient and non-nutrient intake, and through a complex, coordinated system: processing, digesting, absorbing, and expelling the breakdown products. In addition, a huge cumulative volume of fluids from the aerodigestive tract that contain electrolytes, proteins, and bile acids is recycled daily. A minimal fraction of all that traverses through the digestive tract is wasted in feces. The gut is a key center of interaction with ingested and flora microbiota. A complex network of neural and hormonal factors regulates the function of specialized gastrointestinal cells (epithelial, muscular, and glandular). Intestinal folding down to villus and microvillus levels secures an ample surface area for these processes to happen. In the neonatal period, distinct physiologic features seem to allow accommodation to a wider array of nutrients as the infant grows. A significant degree of intestinal adaptation to dietary environmental and anatomic changes exists. Nevertheless, an alteration in the physiology of the gastrointestinal system can result in significant morbidity and mortality. Utilizing some of the known concepts of electrolyte absorption, mortality from acute diarrhea has fallen from 5 million to 1.3 million deaths annually with the use of oral rehydration salts.[1] This chapter provides an overview of the basic aspects of digestion and absorption of the major constituents of our diet, which – besides water – include electrolytes, carbohydrates, proteins, fats, nucleic acids, vitamins, and minerals. Understanding different aspects of digestion and absorption provides a solid base to appreciate how disease states happen and can be managed.

CARBOHYDRATES

Dietary Forms

Carbohydrates (CHO) account for around 50% of the ingested calories in the Western adult diet. The dominant forms of consumed carbohydrates are age variable and include disaccharides (mainly lactose, sucrose, maltose), starch (dominant form of plant carbohydrate storage), and glycogen from animal sources. Some carbohydrates cannot be broken down in the human body (see Nondigestible Carbohydrates).

Lactose, a disaccharide of glucose and galactose, is the main CHO in breast milk and standard cow milk-based infant formula. For many children, cow's milk consumption continues into adolescence and adulthood. Soy-based formulas and hypoallergenic formulas are lactose free and instead contain corn syrup, starch, or sucrose (glucose and fructose). As infant weaning starts, the amount of consumed *starch* (consisting of amylopectin and to a lesser extent amylase) increases to 50% of the total CHO intake in adults. Amylose (molecular weight 10^6) is a linear polymer of glucose molecules linked by $\alpha 1,4$ bonds, whereas amylopectin (molecular weight 10^9) contains additional $\alpha 1,6$ bonds that allow for branching of the polysaccharide units. Starch granules vary in size (e.g., potato > wheat > rice) and shape. The mechanical breakdown of these molecules by chewing affects such variables. Wheat is a unique form of starch; its carbohydrate component is encased in a protein shell. Such differences account for the variable degrees of digestion and absorption among different types of starch.[2] Food processing and preparation may alter the susceptibility of the molecular bonds within starch to enzymatic digestion.[3,4] *Fructose* accounts for the sweet taste of fruit and vegetables as well as soft drinks and processed foods (along with glucose polymers grouped under corn syrup and oligo- and polysaccharides). Table sugar is *sucrose* (glucose and fructose) derived from cane or beet. *Maltose* consists of two glucose molecules. *Glycogen* contains $\alpha 1,4$ linked glucose molecules. It accounts for a small fraction of total carbohydrate intake. Poorly digestible and poorly absorbable saccharides such as lactulose, sorbitol, and sucrulose are frequently consumed, the latter two commonly as sweeteners in sugar-free foods. Other "unavailable" carbohydrates are discussed later.

The breakdown of CHO takes place in the gut lumen as well as at the enterocyte membrane level (Figure 2-1).

Luminal Digestion

Breakdown of starch begins in the oral cavity by salivary α-amylase (mainly from the parotid gland), although limited due to the brief exposure time before swallowing. α-Amylase is inactivated by gastric acid yet some activity may be present within the food bolus. Salivary α-amylase appears in the neonatal period. Amylase is also present in breast milk and plays a more significant role in premature neonates where pancreatic amylase production is low (Figure 2-2).[5]

The majority of starch digestion occurs in the duodenum through the effect of pancreatic amylase. This activity is not restricted to the lumen because amylase may adsorb to the enterocyte luminal surface. α-Amylase is an endoenzyme that cleaves the $\alpha 1,4$ internal links in amylose, leaving oligosaccharides: maltose (two glucose molecules) and maltriose (three glucose molecules). Because α-amylase does not cleave $\alpha 1,6$ bonds or their adjacent $\alpha 1,4$ bonds, digestion of amylopectin also leaves branched oligosaccharides (α-limit dextrins). Amylase activity produces a small amount of free glucose molecules. Only severe pancreatic insufficiency that

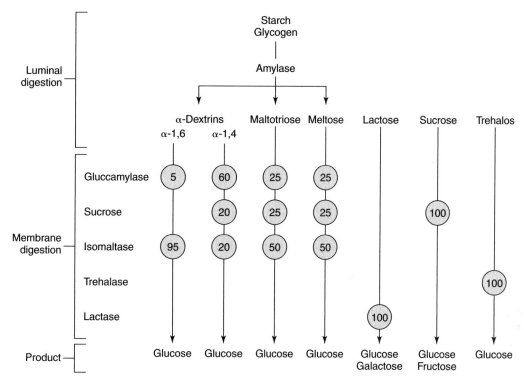

Figure 2-1. Overview of carbohydrate digestion. Numbers in circles indicate percentage of substrate hydrolyzed by brush border enzyme. From Johnson, Gastrointestinal Physiology, 7th ed. 2007, with permission.

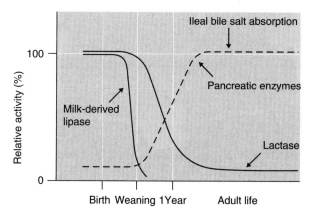

Figure 2-2. Major changes in digestive function in neonates. From Marsh and Riley, 1998, with permission.[15]

leaves less than 10% normal amylase levels affects starch breakdown.[6]

Brush Border Digestion

Only monosaccharides can be absorbed across the enterocyte membrane. Therefore, digestion of disaccharide and the luminal products of starch breakdown must happen by the brush border membrane hydrolases (see Figure 2-1).

Maltase (glucoamylase) breaks the α1,4 links in oligosaccharides 5–9 glucose molecules long. Isomaltase (also called α-dextrinase) breaks α1,6 bonds, acting as a debranching enzyme. It functions in conjunction with sucrase (Figure 2-3), both having their genetic coding on chromosome 3.[7] Sucrase breaks sucrose into glucose and fructose. Sucrase-isomaltase complex cleaves its substrate by a Ping-Pong bibi mechanism

(two substrates, two products, with only one substrate bound to the catalytic site at one time).[2,8]

Lactase breaks lactose into glucose and galactose; its gene is located on chromosome 2.[9] Lactose digestion in the premature neonate may be incomplete in the small intestine but partially salvaged through colonic fermentation. In childhood, lactase level declines from a peak at birth to <10% of the pre-infant weaning level as dietary lactose consumption falls (see Figure 2-2).[10] The decline in lactase in other mammals occurs even if weaning is prolonged.[11] In certain human populations where dairy products are consumed into adulthood (e.g., northern Europe), lactase activity may persist.[12] This phenotype is inherited as an autosomal recessive trait, with intermediate activity levels in heterozygotes. Thus the aberrant allele in the human population is considered to be the one that leads to persistence of the enzyme, not the deficiency.[13] Trehalase breaks down the disaccharide trehalose, which is present in mushrooms. The significance of having a dedicated enzyme to a sugar that is consumed infrequently is unclear.

There is generally an ample supply of disaccharidases; thus the rate of uptake of carbohydrate monomers is the limiting step for their absorption. With the exception of lactase, brush border hydrolases are inducible by presence of the substrate. Disaccharidases are synthesized in the endoplasmic reticulum of the enterocyte, modified in the Golgi apparatus, and integrate into the brush border membrane, anchored by a hydrophobic portion in their structure. Pancreatic enzymes play a role in the modification and turnover of carbohydrases.[14] The half-life of sucrase-iso-maltase drops from 20 h during fasting to 4.5 h after meals.[15] Activity of mucosal carbohydrases is maximal in the duodenum and jejunum, decreasing distally along the small intestine.[16] Most carbohydrate digestion is complete by mid-jejunum.

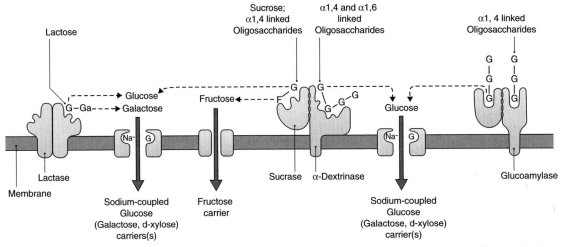

Figure 2-3. Brush border digestion and absorption of carbohydrate. The α1,4 and α1,6 linked oligosaccharides are products of intraluminal amylase digestion of starch. Sucrase-dextrinase and sucrase-isomaltase represent the same enzyme complex. G, glucose; Ga, galactose; F, fructose. Modified from Van Dyke RW. Mechanisms of digestion and absorption of food. In: Wyllie R and Hyams JS, eds., Paediatric Gastrointestinal Disease, 1st ed. 1999: p.18, with permission.

Transport After Digestion

Monosaccharides cross the enterocyte apical membrane via carrier-mediated transport because their size is too large to allow for adequate passive diffusion. There are two families of such transporters that are responsible for the movement of glucose and galactose in the small intestine, kidneys, and brain, and the uptake and release of glucose from all body cells: sodium-coupled co-transporters SGLT (SLC5 gene family) and the GLUT (SLC2 gene family).[17] For glucose and galactose, co-transport with sodium happens down a sodium gradient generated by a Na^+,K^+ ATPase pump in the basolateral membrane (Figure 2-4). Activation of the Na^+ glucose transport protein allows water, electrolytes, and possibly smaller digested molecules (including glucose and oligopeptides) to pass into the intercellular space through relaxation of the tight junctions.[18,19] Fructose is transported by facilitated diffusion handled by GLUT-5 carrier system, which allows a faster rate than simple diffusion down its concentration gradient.[20] All monosaccharides exit the enterocyte by facilitated diffusion across the basolateral membrane in to the portal circulation via the GLUT 2 carrier system. A small amount of hexoses may be utilized within the cell for metabolism.

Nondigestible Carbohydrates

Approximately 10% of ingested starch is not digested in the small intestine. Digestion-resistant starch includes complex molecules that resist amylase activity or are physically inaccessible as in intact grains.[21] Poor chewing of large digestible molecules may compromise enzymatic exposure. Some lactose and fructose may escape complete digestion and pass to the large intestine along with poorly digestible monosaccharides such as lactulose, sorbitol, and sucrulose. Cellulose and hemicellulose are present in fruit and vegetable structure. Cellulose is a polymer of glucose molecules linked by β1,4 bonds that, unlike α1,4 bonds, resist digestion by α-amylase. Hemicellulose is a polymer of pentose and hexose molecules in straight and chained form. Resistant starches constitute dietary "fiber" together with nondigestible noncarbohydrate components present in plant cell wall (e.g., phytates, lignins). Nondigestible carbohydrates are fermented by colonic bacteria, leaving short-chain fatty

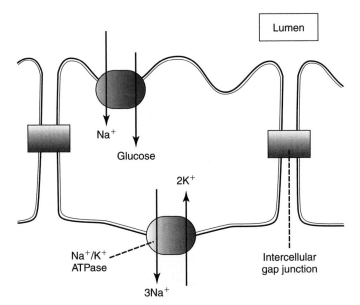

Figure 2-4. Sodium, glucose co-transport.

acids that are readily absorbed and may account for a minute caloric source in the healthy state, in addition to possibly having cellular trophic properties.[22] By-products of this process are lactic, acetic, propionic, and butyric acids, with methane and hydrogen accounting for flatus. Although excessive consumption of nondigestible carbohydrates can result in undesirable gastrointestinal symptoms, dietary fiber offers multiple health benefits.[23]

PROTEINS

Protein Sources

In order to reduce the consumption of amino acids for energy production, the intake of proteins must be accompanied by other calorie sources. In addition to dietary protein, the gastrointestinal tract recycles endogenous proteins in digestive juices and shed epithelial cells amounting up to 65 g daily in adults.[24] The quality of dietary protein relates to its content of essential

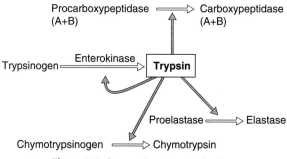

Figure 2-5. Pancreatic enzyme activation.

TABLE 2-1. **Pancreatic Proteases**

Enzyme	Protein Substrate
Endopeptidases	
Trypsin	Basic amino acids (lysine, arginine) Pancreatic proenzymes
Chymotrypsin	Aromatic amino acids (glutamine, leucine, methionine)
Elastase	Aliphatic (nonpolar) amino acids
Exopeptidases	
Carboxypeptidase A	Aromatic, aliphatic amino acids
Carboxypeptidase B	Basic amino acids

amino acids (valine, leucine, isoleucine, phenylalanine, lysine, tyrosine, methionine, tryptophan, and histidine) that cannot be synthesized in humans. An egg, for example, has a high-protein biologic value because it is rich in essential amino acids. Plant proteins are less digestible than animal proteins and contain fewer essential amino acids. Processing of protein (e.g., heat) and co-ingestion with reducing sugars such as fructose can alter its molecular structure and affect digestibility.[25,26] Proteins with high proline content (e.g., casein, gluten, collagen, and keratin) are incompletely digested by pancreatic proteases.[2,27] Other proteins that escape digestion include secretory IgA and intrinsic factor.[28]

Luminal Digestion

Gastric Phase

Digestion of proteins begins in the stomach with exposure to pepsin and hydrochloric acid. In addition to its role in pepsinogen activation, gastric acid denatures protein. Pepsin is secreted by chief cells as pepsinogen and acts as an endopeptidase, breaking peptide bonds within the polypeptide and leaving shorter polypeptides with a small number of free amino acids. Three pepsin isoenzymes have been identified, all optimally active at a pH range of 1–3. The duodenal alkaline medium irreversibly inactivates pepsin. Both pepsin and gastric acid production and secretion are stimulated by gastrin, acetylcholine, and histamine.[29] The gastric phase does not seem critical in protein breakdown, because patients with decreased acid output and/or gastrectomy do not necessarily lose protein.[30]

Intestinal Phase

The main protein digestion site is the proximal small intestine upon exposure to the pancreatic fluid. Unlike amylase and lipase, pancreatic proteases are secreted as proenzymes. The presence of food in the duodenum stimulates the influx of bile with contractions of the gallbladder and secretion of pancreatic fluid. Although mediators of pancreatic stimulation are incompletely understood, the cholinergic intestinal system appears to have greater influence than cholecystokinin for pancreozymes, whereas secretin mainly promotes pancreatic bicarbonate flow. Bicarbonate provides an alkaline pH > 5 required for optimal enzyme function. An over-acidic environment, as seen in Zollinger-Ellison syndrome, deactivates pancreatic enzymes. In response to the presence of bile acids and trypsinogen, enterokinase (enteropeptidase) is released from the brush border cells.[31,32] Enterokinase's only substrate, trypsinogen, is the most abundant proenzyme in pancreatic juices. The subsequent removal of a hexapeptide from the N terminus

of trypsinogen yields the active form, trypsin, which activates the other enzyme precursors as well as its own (Figure 2-5). Pancreatic proteases are either endopeptidases or exopeptidases depending on the site of the peptide bonds each acts upon (Table 2-1). Endopeptidases cleave peptide bonds within the polypeptide chain while exopeptidases remove a single amino acid from the carboxyl terminal. About 30–40% of the products of this process are amino acids, and 60–70% are oligopeptides up to six peptides long.[33] Endogenous proteins (including enzymes) are digested and processed in a similar manner to exogenous proteins.

Pancreatic enzymes also release cobalamin (vitamin B_{12}) from the R protein, allowing the former to bind to intrinsic factor (see later). The enzymes may also play a role in gut immunity against microbials[27] and interact in the modification–regulation of various brush border enzymes such as disaccharidases. Exposure to trypsin changes pro-colipase to colipase, a key player in the assimilation of fat.

Brush Border and Intracellular Digestion

Brush Border

In contrast to carbohydrates, where only monosaccharide units are transported across the enterocyte membrane, small polypeptides can move as such from the lumen (Figure 2-6), possibly through a more efficient mechanism than that for amino acids.[34-36] Because almost all protein that enters the portal vein is in the form of amino acids, further digestion of the oligopeptides must take place either at the brush border level or within the enterocyte cytoplasm. It has been shown in animals with pancreatic insufficiency secondary to pancreatic duct ligation that nearly 40% of ingested proteins were absorbed.[37]

A polypeptide's length determines the rate and the site (brush border versus intracellular) of its assimilation. The brush border peptidases are active at neutral pH and include an array of aminopeptidases, carboxypeptidases, endopeptidases, and dipeptidases. They possess a combined ability to digest hexapeptides or smaller chains into amino acids and dipeptides and tripeptides that are actively transported across the luminal enterocyte membrane. Longer peptides are processed by oligopeptidases, which are predominantly aminopeptidases, removing amino acids from the amino terminus of the peptide. Synthesis of the brush border peptidases occurs in the rough endoplasmic reticulum with little post-translational enzyme modification within the cell or by pancreatic enzymes at the brush border, in contrast to disaccharidases.[38,39] Mucosal enzymes also include folate conjugase needed to hydrolyze ingested folate, and angiotensin converting enzyme.

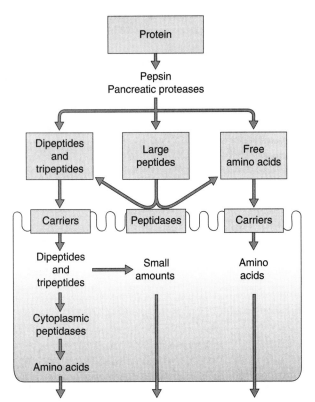

Figure 2-6. Overview of digestion and absorption of protein. From Johnson, 1997, with permission.

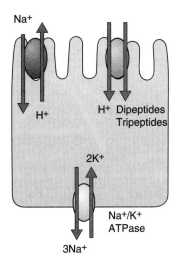

Figure 2-7. Polypeptide-proton co-transport into the enterocyte.

Cytoplasm

Cytosol peptide hydrolases differ in structure and electrophoretic mobility from those in the brush borders and are predominantly dipeptidases and tripeptidases. Further assimilation of small polypeptides into free amino acids takes place in the cytoplasm; however, the capacity to digest peptides more than three amino acids long is lacking. Iminodipeptidase (also called prolidase) is an intracellular hydrolase with specificity to proline-containing dipeptides, which resist luminal digestion but pass into the cytoplasm. In contrast to the brush border enzymes, cytosol peptidases are not exclusive to the intestine and are present in other body tissues.

Transport After Digestion

Amino Acids

Given the rich heterogeneity of amino acid structures, the complex process of transmembrane movement remains incompletely understood. Dipeptides and tripeptides do not compete with amino acids for transport (see Figure 2-6). Amino acid transport proteins are numerous and group specific for neutral, basic, and acidic amino acids with some overlap. A few transport proteins have been extensively studied and characterized.[40,41] Absorption is maximal in the proximal intestine and occurs by active diffusion, Na+-co-transport, and to a lesser extent, simple and facilitated diffusion.[42] The rate of absorption varies for different amino acid groups, being highest for branched chain amino acids.[43] Vasointestinal polypeptide and somatostatin slow these processes down. As noted in glucose transport, activating the co-transport protein may allow paracellular movement of intestinal contents.

Polypeptides

In contrast to amino acids, dipeptides and tripeptides are carried by a single membrane transporter with a broad substrate specificity. This transporter utilizes an H+ gradient and is uniform along the small intestines.[44] The human peptide transporter has been cloned.[45] A brush border Na+, H+ exchange pump, along with Na+, K+ ATPase in the basolateral membrane, maintains this confined acidic milieu (Figure 2-7). Oligopeptide transport into the enterocyte contributes to the lack of specific amino acid deficiency in hereditary disorders of amino acid transport, as seen in Hartnup disease and cystinuria.[46] Both substrates of these carriers are absorbed normally in disease states if presented in the form of small peptides. In the neonatal period, uptake of whole polypeptide macromolecules occurs possibly by pinocytosis or receptor-mediated endocytosis, allowing for passage of such molecules as immunoglobulins in the first 3 months of life.[47]

Exit From the Enterocyte

The movement of amino acids across the basolateral membrane occurs by facilitated and active transport.[48] This is handled by transport proteins different from those in the brush border membrane. In addition to exporting amino acids into the portal circulation, such a transport mechanism takes up amino acids into the enterocyte for use in fasting periods. The basolateral membrane also possesses a peptide transport system similar to the one in the brush border membrane, allowing a small amount of intact peptides to enter the bloodstream.[38]

About 10% of the amino acids absorbed into the mucosa are used for enterocyte protein synthesis in vitro.[49] Luminal protein sources are more readily used than systemic protein, especially in apical villous cells.[50] It has been shown in animals that exclusive parenteral nutrition can lead to mucosal atrophy.[51]

LIPIDS

Dietary Forms

Up to 90% of fat in the average human diet consists of triglycerides; the remainder is phospholipids, plant and animal sterols, and fat-soluble vitamins. In a triglyceride, a backbone of glycerol carries three fatty acids of variable structures. Animal-derived triglycerides generally have long-chain saturated fatty acids (>14 carbon units), the majority being oleate and palmitate. Plant fatty acids are polyunsaturated and include linoleic and linolenic acids that cannot be synthesized *de novo* in humans and are therefore essential. Medium-chain triglycerides have fatty acids with 8–12 carbons. Processing of vegetable fat involves hydrogenation, which increases the melting point, saturates the covalent bonds within the fatty acid, and changes double bonds from *cis* to *trans* isomers.[52] A phospholipid is composed of a backbone of lysophosphatidylcholine and one fatty acid. The average adult diet contains 1–2 g of phospholipids, while 10–20 g are secreted daily in bile.[53,54] Phospholipids are also recycled from cell membranes of shed enterocytes. The main dietary phospholipid is phosphatidylcholine (lecithin), and the predominant fatty acids in phospholipids are linoleate and arachidonate. Cholesterol, in animal fat, is the main dietary sterol in the Western diet. Fat-soluble vitamins are discussed later in this chapter.

Lipids are divided into polar and nonpolar, depending on the nature of their interactions with water. Triglycerides are insoluble in water and form an unstable layer, whereas polar phospholipids can shape into a more stable form. This is key to understanding the dynamics of lipid digestion and absorption across the water phase in the intestinal lumen, the epithelial membrane lipid phase, and later the lymphatic and blood water phase. To provide a better exposed, more stable enzyme substrate, ingested lipids are mechanically and enzymatically broken down to smaller units, then appropriately coated with such hydrophilic molecules as phospholipids and bile salts to help cross through different aqueous phases.

Luminal Digestion (Figure 2-8)

Gastric Phase

The digestion of triglycerides begins in the stomach with action of lingual and gastric lipases, which are stable in acid medium. The degree of relative activity of each is variable among different species. Lingual lipase is secreted from Ebner's glands.[55] Both enzymes break down short- and medium-chain triglycerides more efficiently than longer chain lengths[56] and cannot process phospholipids or sterols. In neonates, pancreatic production of lipase is not fully developed (see Figure 2-2).[57] Breast milk is rich in medium- and short-chain fatty acids that are adequately handled by breast milk–derived lipase (carboxyl ester lipase) and infantile gastric lipase. In adults, it is estimated that 10–30% of ingested lipids is digested before the duodenal stage, yielding diacylglycerols and free fatty acids. Gastric lipase has high activity in patients with cystic fibrosis in the presence of reduced pancreatic lipase and lower pH affecting its activity.[58] There is no absorption of fat in the stomach, except for short-chain fatty acids. Nevertheless, the stomach is the major site of fat emulsification (Figure 2-9). This is achieved in part by the mechanical fragmenting of larger lipid masses. Breast milk fat emulsion droplets are relatively small.[59] In addition, gastric lipase releases some fatty acids together with dietary phospholipids that "coat" intact triglycerides to provide a suspension of emulsified fat droplets. The coordinated gastric propulsion–retropulsion contractions leave lipid droplets smaller than 0.5 μm that are squirted through the pylorus.

Small Intestinal Phase

After meal ingestion, vagal stimulation and cholecystokinin (CCK) release stimulate gallbladder contractions and relaxation of the sphincter of Oddi allowing bile flow into the duodenum. The three main bile acids are cholic, deoxycholic, and chenodeoxycholic acids. Bile acids are secreted almost exclusively in conjugated form, predominantly to glycine and less so taurine.[60] Such modification enhances the water solubility of bile acids, even in slightly acidic medium, by lowering the critical micellar concentration.[61] Conjugation also confers some resistance to pancreatic digestion and prevents calcium–bile salt precipitation.[62] In addition to bile acids, bile is rich in phospholipids; both compounds are amphipathic, having both hydrophilic and lipophilic portions. The concentration of bile acids is usually well above a critical level where micelles (water-soluble aggregates) are formed upon mixing with digested lipids. Micelles are 100–500 times smaller in diameter than emulsion particles, which makes for a water–clear micellar solution in the proximal small intestine. The orientation within a micellar structure is such that the hydrophobic bile acid parts cover the insoluble molecules within, while the hydrophilic portion lines the outer layer, allowing stability in the luminal aqueous phase. However, as a result, the hydrophobic portion of the lipid where lipase acts is contained deep within the emulsion droplet. To allow exposure to lipase, pancreatic phospholipase A_2 is activated by bile acids and calcium to break the phospholipid coat, leaving fatty acids and lysophosphatidylcholine units. The optimal action of phospholipase A_2 requires a bile salt to phosphatidylcholine

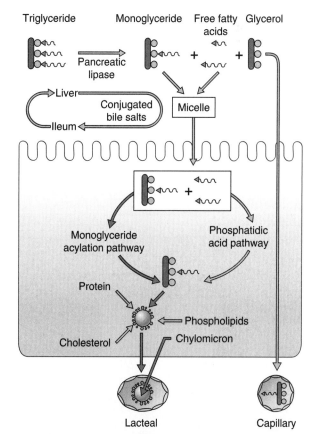

Figure 2-8. Overview of digestion and absorption of triglyceride. From Johnson, 1997, with permission.

molar ratio of 2:1.[63] It has been shown that the presence of bile acids inactivates lipase, which led to the discovery of its cofactor, colipase, in 1963.[64] Colipase is secreted from the pancreas as procolipase at a 1:1 ratio to lipase, which it carries to close proximity to the triglyceride. A by-product of pro-colipase's activation by trypsin is a pentapeptide, enterostatin, thought to play a role in satiety after fat ingestion.[65,66] The products of lipase's activity are 2-monoacylglycerols and free fatty acids. Most ingested cholesterol is in the free sterol form, and a small amount is in cholesterol-ester form, which requires digestion by cholesterol esterase, also called nonspecific lipase. The luminal end products of lipid digestion are fatty acids, 2-monoglycerides, glycerol, lysophosphatidylcholine, and free cholesterol; all are insoluble in water except short- and medium-chain fatty acids and glycerol, which are soluble enough to pass through the unstirred water layer that lines the intestinal epithelium.

Enterohepatic Bile Circulation

Liver cells synthesize and conjugate bile acids starting from cholesterol. Conjugated bile acids are reabsorbed through the enterohepatic circulation. Both processes are in balance to keep an adequate bile acid pool. Because conjugated bile acids are in ionized form in the alkaline intestinal milieu, they cannot be absorbed passively across the enterocyte membrane. It has been shown that active transport of these bile acids takes place in the distal ileum.[67] Ileal bile acid absorption involves Na^+ co-transport down a gradient secured by the basolateral membrane Na^+,K^+ ATPase (Figure 2-10). Within the enterocyte, bile acids are carried by binding proteins that protect the cell against injury from the otherwise free acids.[68,69] Bacterial enzymatic action in the distal small and large intestine leads to deconjugation of bile acids that escape ileal absorption, and removal of the 7-hydroxy group leaving deoxy bile acid forms. A fraction of the unconjugated bile acids are readily absorbed into the gut epithelium, given their lipophilic properties. The acidic environment in the colon results in the change of bile acids to solid form.[61] Only a small amount of bile acids is lost in feces.

Transport of Fat Digestion Products

The lipophilic monoglycerides, fatty acids, cholesterol, and lyophospholipids can pass through the enterocyte membrane by passive diffusion. Because passive diffusion is dependent on the concentration gradient across the membrane, bile acid micellar forms elegantly allow for a high concentration of hydrophobic lipolysis products to be carried into the unstirred aqueous layer (40 μm deep) adjacent to the brush border (Figure 2-11).[70] Once approximated to the brush border membrane, the digested lipids are released from their micellar form in the slightly acid medium maintained at the unstirred water layer on the surface of the epithelium.[71] The presence of a Na^+,H^+ exchange pump keeps a pH of 5–6 in the enterocyte's luminal vicinity (Figure 2-7). Because of their adequate solubility in the unstirred water layer, glycerol, short and medium chain fatty acids diffuse through, independent of micellar formation. In addition to the micellar form, digested lipids may be shuttled

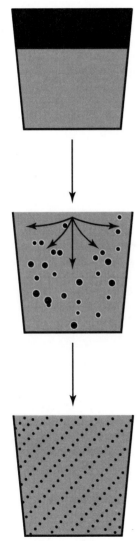

Figure 2-9. Fat emulsification: progressive mechanical breakdown of fat drops with addition of water-soluble coating and progressive reduction in fat droplet size.

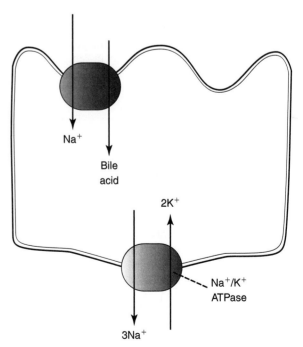

Figure 2-10. Sodium, bile acid co-transport.

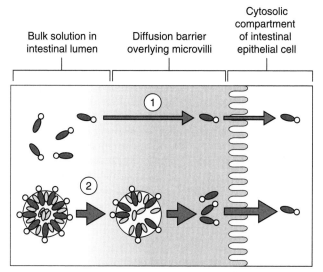

Bulk solution in intestinal lumen | Diffusion barrier overlying microvilli | Cytosolic compartment of intestinal epithelial cell

Figure 2-11. Role of bile acid micelles in optimizing diffusion of lipids into intestinal cells. In the absence of bile acids (arrow 1), individual lipid molecules must diffuse across the unstirred aqueous layer. Therefore their uptake is diffusion limited. In the presence of bile acids (arrow 2), large amounts of the lipid molecules are delivered directly to the aqueous-membrane interface so that the rate of uptake is greatly enhanced. From Westergaard and Dietschy, 1976.[71]

into the enterocyte through other mechanisms.[72,73] The presence of nonmicellar transport structures may explain how, in the absence of bile salts, 50% or more of dietary triglycerides may be absorbed.[15] The adequacy of bile acids usually obviates the need for such soluble forms.[54] There is recent evidence that other carrier-mediated transport exists for cholesterol and other lipids.[74,75]

Intracellular Phase of Fat Assimilation

Once in the enterocyte, triglycerides are resynthesized from 2-monoacylglycrerol and fatty acids as a result of two processes: monoglyceride acylation and phosphatidic acid pathways (see Figure 2-8). In the first, Acyl-CoA synthetase adds an acyl group to a free fatty acid, which is subsequently incorporated into monoglycerides and diglycerides by respective acyltransferases in the smooth endoplasmic reticulum. Long-chain fatty acids are the main substrates for this process because of binding to an intracellular fatty acid binding protein[76] and the fact that short- and medium-chain fatty acids pass through the enterocyte into the portal circulation in free form. The second pathway of triglyceride resynthesis utilizes α-glycerophosphate (synthesized from glucose) as a backbone that is acylated to form phosphatidic acid, which in turn is dephosphorylated, leaving diglyceride. Phosphatidic acid is also important in phospholipid synthesis. When 2-monoglycerides are present in abundance, as in the postprandial stage, the monoglyceride acylation pathway predominates. In the fasting state, the phosphatidic acid part provides triglycerides. Lysophosphatidylcholine is either reacylated to form phosphatidylcholine or hydrolyzed to release a fatty acid and glycerol-3-phosphorylcholine. Endogenous and absorbed cholesterol is re-esterified. Triglycerides, phospholipids, and cholesterol esters are packaged into chylomicrons and very low-density lipoproteins (VLDLs).

Exit From the Enterocyte

Chylomicrons are made only in intestinal cells, whereas VLDLs are also synthesized in the liver. To form a chylomicron, triglycerides, fat-soluble vitamins, and cholesterol are coated with a layer of apolipoprotein (apo A and B types),[77] cholesterol ester, and phospholipids. Chylomicrons are made in the endoplasmic reticulum and later processed in the Golgi complex where glycosylation of the apoprotein takes place. It has been suggested that apo B is involved in the movement of chylomicrons from the endoplasmic reticulum to the Golgi apparatus, as lipids accumulate in the former in patients with abetalipoproteinemia.[78] VLDLs are smaller than chylomicrons. They are synthesized through a different pathway and seem to be predominant in fasting states. Chylomicrons exit the enterocyte by exocytosis. Although they are too large to pass through capillary pores, chylomicrons and VLDL easily cross into the lacteal endothelial gaps that are present in the postprandial phase.[79] Medium-chain triglycerides move directly into the portal circulation.

DIGESTION AND ABSORPTION IN INFANTS

The progressive development of the neonatal gut, to take on new digestive tasks as the nutrient repertoire expands, is a complex process that remains to be further elucidated.

Carbohydrates

Lactose digestion in the premature neonate may be incomplete in the small intestine but partially salvaged from the colon. Lactase level declines from a peak at birth to less than 10% of the preweaning infantile level in childhood (see Figure 2-2). The decline in lactase in other mammals occurs even if weaning is prolonged.[11] Lactase activity may persist in some populations where dairy products are consumed into adulthood.[12] Although nonlactose disaccharides are not abundant in breast milk or standard cow milk-based formulas, other disaccharidases besides lactase are present in the young infant intestinal brush border. The presence of these glucosidases reflects a genetically determined sequence, apparently independent from substrate availability.[80] However, the appearance of pancreatic amylase later in the first year of life as starches are introduced suggests that substrate exposure may play a role in genetic expression of some gastrointestinal enzymes. Amylase is also present in saliva and breast milk.

Proteins

In neonates, pepsin and gastric acid production is lower than that in adults. Acid secretion shows less response to pentagastrin stimulation[81,82] Although this fact belittles the gastric acid role in proteolysis it may allow longer lingual amylase and lipase activity and leave some breast milk antibodies intact.

Pancreatic production of trypsin in the neonate is close to adult level, whereas other pancreatic proteases are low. Pancreatic acinar cells are not as responsive to hormonal stimulation.[83] Enterokinase is present at birth, and mucosal peptidases seem well developed. The role of breast milk proteases remains to be further clarified.

It has been shown that in the neonatal period, uptake of whole polypeptide macromolecules occurs, allowing for passage of such molecules as immunoglobulins.[47]

TABLE 2-2. **Solubility of Vitamins**

	Water-Soluble	Fat-Soluble
A		+
Ascorbic acid	+	
Biotin	+	
Cobalamin (B$_{12}$)	+	
D		+
E		+
Folic acid	+	
K		+
Niacin	+	
Pantothenic acid	+	
Pyridoxine (B$_6$)	+	
Riboflavin (B$_2$)	+	
Thiamine (B$_1$)	+	

Lipids

Several factors facilitate the digestion and absorption of triglycerides in the first few months of life. Aside from pancreatic lipase, production of which is low at birth, some triglyceride assimilation is achieved by breast milk, lingual and gastric lipases (see earlier discussion). Breast milk lipase is stable in stomach acid and requires bile acids to be activated.[84] Triglycerides are uniquely packaged in breast milk, such that they are present in small emulsion droplets. Breast milk is rich in medium- and short-chain fatty acids, which pose less of a digestive challenge. In neonates and young infants, the bile salt pool is smaller than that in adults, possibly because of immature ileal reabsorption.

VITAMINS AND MINERALS

Vitamins are critical for normal human metabolism. They are not manufactured by the human body and can be classified as either water- or fat-soluble (Table 2-2).

Water-Soluble Vitamins

Vitamins that are water soluble are absorbed by passive diffusion. However, vitamin B$_{12}$, folate, ascorbic acid, and thiamine are absorbed by carrier-mediated processes.

Vitamin B$_{12}$

Vitamin B$_{12}$ (cobalamin) is found primarily from animal sources. Gastric acidity releases cobalamin from any associated dietary proteins. At an acidic pH, cyanocobalamin has an extremely high affinity to R proteins produced by salivary glands, gastric parietal cells, and the pancreas. Intrinsic factor, which is produced by the parietal cell, will bind with cobalamin after pancreatic protease hydrolysis of the cobalamin-haptocorrin complex.[85,86] It has been demonstrated that receptors for cobalamin–intrinsic factor complexes exist in the distal ileum. Gastric disease may decrease intrinsic factor production and therefore allow for the loss of ingested vitamin B$_{12}$. Also, pancreatic insufficiency leaves vitamin B$_{12}$–R protein forms unabsorbable. Resection of the terminal ileum or diseases involving the terminal ileum can significantly decrease absorption of vitamin B$_{12}$. Processing the bound cobalamin within the enterocyte is incompletely understood. Vitamin B$_{12}$–intrinsic factor complex

is cleaved and the free form leaves the cell in the plasma, where it binds transcobalamin 2.[38]

Folate

Dietary folate comes mainly from green leafy vegetables, organ meats, and grains. Folic acid is absorbed after hydrolysis of dietary polyglutamates at the brush border membrane by glutamate carboxypeptidase 2 (GCP-2). Malabsorption of folic acid occurs with severe mucosal disease of the proximal small intestine. Patients with inflammatory bowel disease who take sulfasalazine are at risk of folate deficiency because the drug is a competitive inhibitor of several folate-dependent systems. Neural-tube defects in infants are associated with folate deficiency.[87]

Vitamin C

Adequate intake of vitamin C (ascorbic acid) will prevent scurvy. Fresh fruits and juices are abundant sources of vitamin C. Vitamin C is taken up by the enterocyte by active and Na$^+$-dependent processes.[88,89]

Other Water-Soluble Vitamins

Thiamine, riboflavin, pantothenic acid, and biotin have specific active transfer processes. Pyridoxine is absorbed by simple diffusion.

Fat-Soluble Vitamins

Fat-soluble vitamins include vitamins A, D, E, and K. Because these vitamins are not water soluble, they require bile acid micelle formation for adequate absorption. They thus mirror the absorption of dietary fat.

Vitamin A

Vitamin A (retinol) is present in eggs, fish oils, and dairy products. β-Carotene is the most abundant of carotenoids. Cellular uptake of carotenoids occurs by passive diffusion. Cleavage of carotenoids yields apocarotenoids and retinol, subsequently converted to retinol and retinoid acid, respectively. Animal retinol precursors are available as retinyl esters. These retinyl esters are then hydrolyzed to free retinol by pancreatic enzymes and brush border retinyl ester hydrolase.[90] Retinol will then pass into the enterocyte in the micellar form by carrier-mediated passive diffusion. Once in the enterocyte, retinol is re-esterified and packaged together with free carotenoids and apocarotenoids into chylomicrons. Hepatocytes as well as hepatic stellate cells (Ito cells) store vitamin A as retinyl esters.[91]

Vitamin D

Humans get vitamin D from exposure to sunlight, from dietary supplements, and from their general diet. The two main dietary forms of vitamin D are vitamin D$_2$ (ergocalciferol) and vitamin D$_3$ (cholecalciferol). Vitamins D$_2$ and D$_3$ are incorporated into chylomicrons and transported by the lymphatic system into the venous circulation. The assimilation of vitamin D is highly dependent on the bile salts.[92] The absorption of vitamin D occurs primarily in the proximal and mid small intestine and occurs by passive diffusion.[93] Little intracellular metabolism of vitamin D seems to take place once it is in the enterocyte, where it is carried in chylomicrons to the lymphatics. The transfer of vitamin D between lymph chylomicrons and plasma vitamin D binding proteins then takes place. It has been suggested that

TABLE 2-3. **Absorption of Minerals and Trace Elements**

Compound	Proposed Site of Absorption	Probable Mechanism
Calcium	Duodenum	Active
	Remainder small intestine	Passive
Magnesium	Distal small intestine	Active, passive
Iron	Duodenum	Active
Zinc	Small intestine, colon	Active
Copper	Stomach, small intestine	Active

an alternate transport pathway exists, where vitamin D directly passes into the portal circulation.[94] Circulating vitamin D is bound to vitamin D binding protein, which transports it to the liver where vitamin D is converted by vitamin D-25-hydroxylase to 25-hydroxyvitamin D. This form of vitamin D is converted in the kidneys by 25-hydroxyvitamin D-1α-hydroxylase to the active form $1,25(OH)_2$-vitamin D.

Vitamin K, Vitamin E

Vitamin K can be found in two forms: K_1 (phytomenadione) derived from plant sources and K_2 (multiprenyl menaquinones) from intestinal bacteria. Dietary vitamin K also requires micelle formation for adequate absorption. It is absorbed by an active carrier-mediated transport process. Vitamin K_2 absorption is passive.[38] Absorption of vitamin E also occurs by passive diffusion.

MINERALS AND TRACE ELEMENTS

The sites and absorption mechanisms of different minerals and trace elements are displayed in Table 2-3.

Calcium

One-third of total ingested calcium is absorbed. Because calcium will bind strongly to oxalate, phytate, and dietary fiber, decreased absorption occurs when these products are co-ingested. The duodenum is the major site of calcium active uptake, probably through a specific calcium channel. Passive paracellular transport (across tight junctions) also occurs throughout the small intestine.[95] Without vitamin D, only approximately 50% of dietary calcium is absorbed. In the cytoplasm, calcium is carried by a specific binding protein, calbindin D_{28}.[96,97] Exit to the portal circulation occurs against concentration gradient via Ca^{2+} ATPase.[98]

Iron

Iron is more abundant and bioavailable in animal dietary sources than in plant. Lactoferrin, found in breast milk, is an iron binding protein with a specific brush border receptor that increases absorption. Iron is absorbed in the proximal small intestine. Factors enhancing absorption are Fe^{2+} form of iron, gastric acid, ascorbic acid, and co-ingestion with amino acids and sugars. The enterocyte not only handles iron uptake from the intestinal lumen but also exclusively regulates iron balance. Specific iron binding proteins are thought to exist within the brush border membrane. Iron is processed and routed to the circulation as ferritin once it is in cytoplasm. Some iron may bind to nonferritin proteins, which "trap" excess iron and are discarded with shedding of the intestinal epithelium.

Magnesium, Phosphorus, Zinc, Copper

Magnesium is absorbed in the distal small intestine, by both carrier-mediated and paracellular routes. Phosphorus can be taken up more efficiently proximally in the duodenum than the ileum. Zinc is absorbed through passive and carrier-mediated transport in the distal small intestine. There it undergoes an enterohepatic circulation, similar to bile acids. Copper is absorbed by active transport and at high concentrations competes with zinc.[99]

ACKNOWLEDGMENT

The authors wish to thank Brianne Vanderlinden and Blake Agrade for their contributions in this chapter.

REFERENCES

17. Wright BA, Hirayama DF. Loo. Active sugar transport in health and disease. J Intern Med 2007;261:32–43.
20. Douard V, Ronaldo P. Regulation of the fructose transporter GLUT5 in health and disease. Ferraris Am J Physiol Endocrinol Metab 2008;295:E227–E237.
87. Bjorke Monsen AL, Ueland PM. Homocysteine and methyl-malonic acid in diagnosis and risk assessment from infancy to adolescence. Am J Clin Nutr 2003;78:7–21.

See expertconsult.com for a complete list of references and the review questions for this chapter..

FURTHER READINGS

Johnson. Gastrointestinal Physiology. 7th ed. Mosby; 2007.
Johnson, Gerwin. Gastrointestinal Physiology: Mosby; 2001.
Guyton Hall. Textbook of Medical Physiology, 11th ed. Chapter 65: Saunders; 2005.

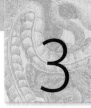

3

BILE ACID PHYSIOLOGY AND ALTERATIONS IN THE ENTEROHEPATIC CIRCULATION

James E. Heubi

Bile acids are important in the processing of dietary lipids and serve three major functions. Bile acids aggregate and form micelles in the upper small intestine, which help solubilize lipolytic products, cholesterol and fat soluble vitamins, thus facilitating absorption across the intestinal epithelium. Bile acids stimulate bile flow during their secretion across the biliary canaliculus. Finally, bile acids are major regulators of sterol metabolism and serve as a major excretory pathway for cholesterol from the body.

Bile acids undergo an enterohepatic circulation within the liver, biliary tract, intestinal tract, and portal and peripheral circulations. This carefully regulated enterohepatic circulation allows for conservation of bile acids. Any alteration in this circulatory pathway can lead to a either a loss of bile acids from the body or displacement from the gastrointestinal tract with associated clinical manifestations. This chapter first reviews the normal bile acid physiology and a discussion of the clinical manifestations of defects of bile acid biosynthesis and clinical conditions associated with alterations in bile acid transport in the liver and gastrointestinal tract.

BIOSYNTHESIS

The two primary bile acids, cholic acid ($3\alpha,7\alpha,12\alpha$-trihydroxy-5β-cholanoic acid) and chenodeoxycholic acid ($3\alpha,7\alpha$-dihydroxy-5β-cholanoic acid), are synthesized in the liver from cholesterol (Figure 3-1). The synthesis of these acids occurs through a tightly regulated enzymatic cascade within hepatocytes involving at least 14 different enzymes.[1] Modifications to the cholesterol nucleus occur via two different biosynthetic pathways: the classic, or neutral, pathway and the alternative, or acidic, pathway. Both pathways work to convert a hydrophobic cholesterol molecule into hydrophilic primary bile acids.

The neutral pathway of bile acid biosynthesis involves the formation of a cholic acid (CA) to chenodeoxycholic acid (CDCA) ratio of approximately 1:1.[2] The initial step of cholesterol synthesis in the neutral pathway involves the 7α-hydroxylation of cholesterol by the rate-limiting enzyme, cholesterol 7α-hydroxylase. Compared with the neutral pathway, the alternative pathway of bile acid biosynthesis predominately yields CDCA with smaller amounts of CA. Although the neutral pathway is felt to be the quantitatively more important pathway of bile acid synthesis, the alternative pathway is likely more functional early in life, and alterations in this pathway may have devastating consequences.[3,4]

Virtually all primary bile acids are conjugated with either glycine or taurine after synthesis by hepatocytes. This conjugation effectively decreases the permeability of bile acids to cholangiocyte cellular membranes, thereby delivering higher concentrations to the intestines.[5] Conjugation also inhibits digestion of bile acids by pancreatic carboxypeptidases and absorption in the proximal small intestine.[6]

ENTEROHEPATIC CIRCULATION

The bile acid pool in humans is typically made up of the primary bile acids, cholic and chenodeoxycholic acid, and the secondary bile acids, deoxycholic and lithocholic acid. Ursodeoxycholic acid accounts for only 1 to 3% of the bile acid pool. This pool of bile acids circulates through the liver, biliary tract, intestine, portal circulation and peripheral serum in response to meal stimuli. Maintenance of a pool of bile acids is essential to normal fat absorption and bile secretion.

For adults and children beyond infancy, newly synthesized bile acids account for approximately 20 to 25% of the total bile acid pool. This percentage can be greatly increased in patients with impaired bile acid reabsorption as found in patients who had ileal resection with Crohn's disease or necrotizing enterocolitis. Once synthesized by hepatocytes, bile acids are excreted into the canalicular lumen. In addition to bile acids, a sodium ion is excreted which creates a gradient to passively draw water into the biliary canaliculi. This flow of bile acids and water serves as the major stimulus for bile flow. While bile acids make up the major solute of bile, other components include phospholipids, organic anions, inorganic anions (especially chloride) and cholesterol.[7]

Most of the bile acids secreted from the liver are stored in the gallbladder as mixed micelles accompanied by phospholipid and cholesterol. On consumption of a meal, the gallbladder contracts and bile acid micelles are delivered to the small intestine (Figure 3-2). In the proximal small bowel, bile acids form mixed micelles with dietary lipolytic products, fatty acids, and monoglycerides. Cholesterol, phospholipids, and fat-soluble vitamins are also solubilized in a similar manner. The lipolytic products are absorbed in the proximal small intestine with reabsorption of bile acids in the distal intestine. Bile acids may be reabsorbed by either passive nonionic diffusion along the length of the gastrointestinal tract or by a sodium-dependent mechanism in the ileum. Reabsorption is limited in the upper small bowel because the pK_a of bile acids tends to be too low for them to be absorbed by nonionic diffusion, although there is some absorption of unconjugated and glycine-conjugated bile acids.

On initial entry into the small intestines, bile acids have a net negative charge. As the bile acids pass through the more distal small intestine, they are deconjugated by the colonized bacteria. This deconjugation confers a neutral charge on the bile

acids and thus permits rapid uptake by intestinal endothelial cells via passive diffusion. The combination of both passive and active reuptake of bile acids provides a very efficient method of recycling bile acids in humans. With each of the 8 to 12 enterohepatic cycles every day, there is a loss of approximately 3 to 5% of the pool of bile acids, with each cycle largely due to an efficient absorption by the combination of passive and active transport systems in the intestine.

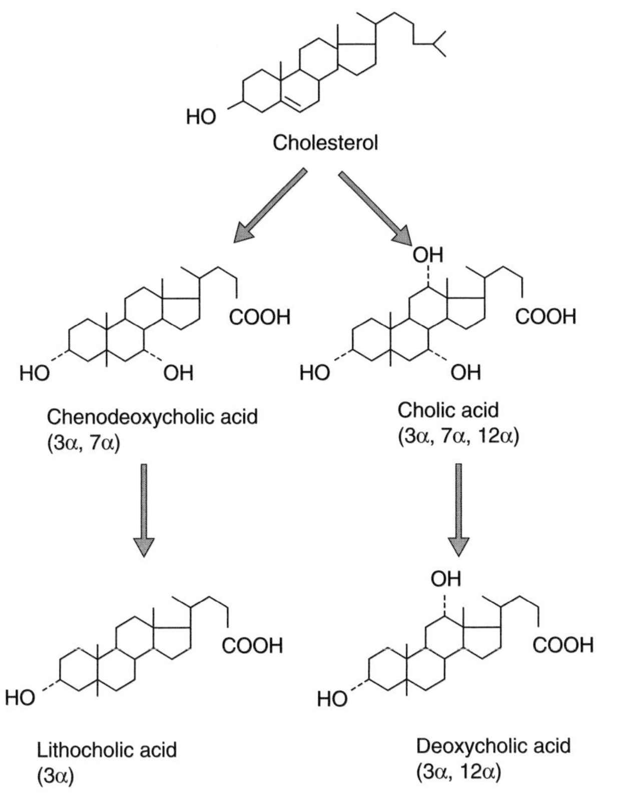

A fraction of bile acids in the pool escape reabsorption in the small intestine and are delivered to the large intestine, where bacterial transformation of the bile acids occurs. After conjugated bile acids are deconjugated, bacterial 7α-dehydroxylation of CA and CDCA may occur, causing formation of the secondary bile acids deoxycholic acid (3α,12α-dihydroxy-5β cholanoic acid) and lithocholic acid (3α-hydroxy-5β cholanoic acid) (see Figure 3-1).

A small amount of bile acids are lost in the stool each day. Although the amount varies by diet and individual, in the adult up to 30 g of bile acids are reabsorbed by the intestines, with 0.2 to 0.6 g being eliminated in the stool daily. The bile acids lost in the stool are replaced by newly synthesized bile acids in the liver through a tightly controlled negative feedback system. The rate-limiting enzyme for bile acid synthesis in the neutral pathway, cholesterol 7α-hydroxylase, is tightly regulated by feedback inhibition from the bile acids returning to the liver through the nuclear receptor, farsenoid X receptor (FXR). This feedback inhibition mechanism ensures that the bile acid pool remains constant in healthy humans, thereby ensuring adequate bile acids to promote bile flow, micelle formation, and cholesterol excretion.

Bile acids enter the portal venous system on absorption by intestinal endothelial cells. These bile acids are bound to albumin and other proteins as they are transported in the portal vein to the liver. Up to 90% of these bile acids are removed by the liver during their first pass. Most of the reuptake is performed by periportal hepatocytes, which then secrete the bile acids into the canalicular space, the rate-limiting step of bile acid transport. A small fraction of the circulating bile acids in the portal

Figure 3-1. Primary bile acids synthesized in liver from cholesterol, and the secondary bile acids produced by bacterial 7α-dehydroxylation.

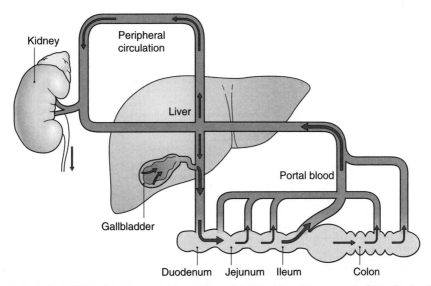

Figure 3-2. The enterohepatic circulation of bile acids. On contraction of the gallbladder, bile acids are expelled into the duodenum. Small arrows indicate passive intestinal absorption, whereas the large arrow in the ileum represents the active uptake of bile acids. The bile acids return to the liver via the portal system. A small fraction of the bile acids spills over into the systemic circulation and is excreted by the kidneys. Adapted from Heubi JE. In: Banks RO, Sperelakis N, eds. Essentials of Basic Science: Physiology. Boston: Little, Brown and Company; 1993, with permission.

blood escape removal by the hepatocytes and spill over into the systemic circulation. Therefore, with each cycling of bile acids, there is a characteristic small spillover of bile acids in the serum that can be measured. The postprandial rise of bile acids serves as a reasonable indicator that the enterohepatic circulation is intact. The serum bile acids undergo filtration by the kidney and can either be excreted in the urine or reabsorbed in the renal tubules for transport back to the liver.

MATURATION OF THE ENTEROHEPATIC CIRCULATION

Neonates are born with an immature enterohepatic circulation of bile acids. A maturation process occurs within the fetal liver and continues throughout the first year of life, which effectively increases the amount of bile acids available for digestion. Bile acid synthesis has been demonstrated as early as the 12th week of gestation.[8] The bile acids produced throughout gestation are different from those produced by infants, children, and adults. Whereas the primary bile acids, CA and CDCA, make up approximately 75 to 80% of the biliary bile acids in adults, they make up less than 50% of the total bile acid pool of the fetus.[9] An immature synthetic pathway of bile acids exists in the developing fetus that not only leads to a decreased rate of bile acid synthesis, but also to the production of "atypical" bile acids not seen in the normal child or adult. These "atypical" bile acids have additional sites of hydroxylation, which may be important in the pathogenesis of cholestatic liver disease in the neonate.[10]

Although newborns initially have a decreased synthesis of bile acids and decreased bile acid pool size, both increase during the first several months of life.[11] The decreased bile acid pool size is accompanied by a reduced concentration of intraluminal bile salts. Both term and preterm normal newborn infants have reduced rates of cholate synthesis and a reduced pool size compared with normal adults when corrected for differences in body surface area.[12] In vitro studies suggest that ileal bile acid transport is decreased in human newborns.[13] In addition to the impaired synthesis and ileal uptake of bile acids in newborns, the pressure generated by contraction of the newborn gallbladder may be insufficient to overcome the choledochal resistance to bile flow. For preterm infants less than 33 weeks' gestation, the gallbladder contraction index may be nonexistent to less than 50%.[14] Impaired gallbladder contraction may explain why 0.5% of normal neonates have gallstones or gallbladder sludge.[15] A decrease in intraluminal bile salt concentration in the neonate contributes to a phenomenon of decreased fat absorption known as "physiologic steatorrhea." Over the first months of life, the bile acid synthetic rate increases and the pool expands with concurrent increase in intraluminal bile acid concentrations.[9]

Despite having a decreased rate of bile acid synthesis and decreased bile acid pool size, the serum bile acid concentration is typically increased in normal preterm and term newborn infants. In fact, the serum bile acid concentration during the first 6 months of life is as high as in adults who have clinical cholestasis.[8] The elevated serum bile acids during this period has been termed "physiologic cholestasis." The early elevation in serum bile acids relates to a poor hepatic extraction of bile salts from the portal circulation. This hepatic uptake is especially impaired in preterm infants. An improvement in the hepatic uptake of bile acids occurs over the first year of life and corresponds to a decrease in the peripheral serum bile acid

concentration. Levels of serum bile acids in infants decrease into the normal range by approximately 10 months of age.[9]

The bile acid composition in neonates is predominately the primary bile acids, CA and CDCA. The secondary bile acids, lithocholic acid and deoxycholic acid, appear in both the serum and bile of infants on intestinal microflora colonization.[9] As the infant matures, primary and secondary bile acids continue to be synthesized and recirculated. The concentration of bile acids in humans eventually approximates the following: cholic acid (36%), chenodeoxycholic acid (36%), deoxycholic acid (24%), and lithocholic acid (1%) (Figure 3-3).[16]

ALTERATIONS IN THE ENTEROHEPATIC CIRCULATION

Disruptions in any part of the enterohepatic circulation of bile acids can lead to the development of clinical manifestations ranging from cholestasis to diarrhea. Alterations may occur at the level of primary bile acid synthesis, in the transport of bile acids across the hepatocyte, at the level of secondary bile acid synthesis, or in ileal transport and the recirculation of bile acids.

Alteration of Primary Bile Acid Biosynthesis

Disorders in bile acid synthesis and metabolism can be broadly classified as primary or secondary. Primary enzyme defects involve congenital deficiencies in enzymes responsible for catalyzing key reactions in the synthesis of cholic and chenodeoxycholic acids. The primary defects include cholesterol 7-hydroxylase (CYP7A1) deficiency, 3β-hydroxy-C_{27}-steroid oxidoreductase deficiency, Δ^4-3-oxosteroid 5β-reductase deficiency, oxysterol 7α-hydroxylase deficiency, 27-hydroxylase deficiency or cerebrotendinous xanthomatosis (CTX), 2-methylacyl-CoA racemase deficiency, trihydroxycholestanoic acid CoA oxidase deficiency, amidation defects involving a deficiency in the bile acid-CoA ligase, and side-chain oxidation defect in the 25-hydroxylation pathway for bile acid resulting in an overproduction of bile alcohols. Secondary metabolic defects that affect primary bile acid synthesis include peroxisomal disorders such as cerebrohepatorenal syndrome of Zellweger and related disorders, and Smith-Lemli-Opitz syndrome. The biochemical presentation of these bile acid synthetic

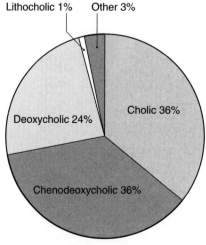

Figure 3-3. Normal distribution of biliary bile acids.

defects includes a markedly reduced or complete lack of cholic and chenodeoxycholic acids in the serum, bile, and urine and greatly elevated concentrations of atypical bile acids and sterols that retain the characteristic structure of the substrates for the deficient enzyme and may have intrinsic hepatotoxicity. These signature metabolites are generally not detected by the routine or classic methods for bile acid measurement, and mass spectrometric techniques presently provide the most appropriate means of characterizing defects in bile acid synthesis. Screening procedures using liquid secondary ionization mass spectrometry (LSIMS), formerly known as fast atom bombardment-mass spectrometry (FAB-MS), indicate that inborn errors in bile acid synthesis probably account for 1 to 2% of the cases of samples sent for analysis from infants, children, and adolescents.

Cerebrotendinous Xanthomatosis

CTX is a rare inherited lipid storage disease with an estimated prevalence of 1 in 70,000. Characteristic features of the disease in adults include progressive neurologic dysfunction, dementia, ataxia, cataracts, and xanthomata in the brain and tendons and in infants with neonatal cholestasis (K. D. R. Setchell, unpublished data, 2003). Biochemically, the disease can be distinguished from other conditions involving xanthomata by (1) significantly reduced primary bile acid synthesis; (2) elevations in biliary, urinary, and fecal excretion of bile alcohol glucuronides; (3) low plasma cholesterol concentration, with deposition of cholesterol and cholestanol in the tissues; and (4) marked elevations in cholestanol. The elevation in 5α-cholestan-3βol (cholestanol) in the nervous system of CTX patients and the high plasma concentrations of this sterol are unique features of the disease.[17,18] Point mutations in the gene located on the long arm of chromosome 2 have been identified that lead to inactivation of the sterol 27-hydroxylase.[19] Neonatal presentation may include elevated serum alanine aminotransferase (ALT), aspartate aminotransferase (AST), and conjugated bilirubin with normal serum gamma glutamyl transpeptidase with biochemical abnormalities normalization by about age 6 months. The liver histopathology findings in these young patients are similar to those observed in idiopathic neonatal hepatitis.

3β-Hydroxy-C$_{27}$-steroid Oxidoreductase Deficiency

This was the first metabolic defect to be described involving an early step in the bile acid biosynthetic pathway; the conversion of 7α-hydroxycholesterol is to 7α-hydroxy-4-cholesten-3-one, a reaction catalyzed by a 3β-hydroxy-C$_{27}$-steroid oxidoreductase. This is the most common of all of the bile acid synthetic defects described to date. Although the clinical presentation of this disorder is somewhat heterogeneous, most patients present as neonates with elevated serum ALT and AST, a conjugated hyperbilirubinemia, and normal serum γ-glutamyl transpeptidase.[20-22] Clinical features include hepatomegaly, with or without splenomegaly, fat-soluble vitamin malabsorption, and mild steatorrhea, and in most instances, pruritus is absent. The liver histologic findings are those of hepatitis, the presence of giant cells, and cholestasis.[20,23,24] The heterogeneity in clinical course of those with early-onset disease is illustrated by some patients who initially resolve their jaundice and are identified later in life, and others with more fulminant disease, eventuating in death or transplantation at an early age. Although the earliest cases were identified in infants, increasingly, idiopathic late-onset chronic cholestasis has been explained by this disorder. In such patients, liver disease is not always evident

initially, and patients may have fat-soluble vitamin malabsorption and rickets, which are corrected with vitamin supplementation. Serum liver enzymes that are often normal in the early stages of the disease later show progressive increases with evidence of progressive hepatic fibrosis. Definitive diagnosis of the 3β-hydroxy-C$_{27}$-steroid oxidoreductase deficiency presently requires mass spectrometric analysis of biologic fluids and is readily accomplished by LSIMS, or by electrospray and tandem mass spectrometry. Molecular techniques that have led to the cloning of the HSD3B7 gene encoding 3β-hydroxy-C$_{27}$-steroid oxidoreductase now permit the accurate genetic basis of the defect.[25] Treatment with cholic acid (available under an IND from the U.S. Food and Drug Administration) leads to gradual resolution of biochemical and histologic abnormalities with an excellent long term prognosis.

Δ^4-3-Oxosteroid 5β-Reductase Deficiency

Application of LSIMS for urine analysis led to the discovery of a defect in the Δ^4-3-oxosteroid 5β-reductase, which catalyzes the conversion of the intermediates 7α-hydroxy-4-cholesten-3-one and 7α,12α-dihydroxy-4-cholesten-3-one to the corresponding 3-oxo-5β (H) intermediates.[26] The clinical presentation of this defect is similar to that of patients with the 3β-hydroxy-C$_{27}$-steroid oxidoreductase deficiency; however, in contrast, the γ-glutamyl transpeptidase is usually elevated, and the average age at diagnosis is lower in patients with Δ^4-3-oxosteroid 5β-reductase deficiency. Infants with Δ^4-3-oxosteorid 5β-reductase deficiency tend to have more severe liver disease with rapid progression to cirrhosis and death without intervention. The Δ^4-3-oxosteroid 5β-reductase deficiency has since been found in a number of patients presenting with neonatal hemochromatosis.[27] Infants with Δ^4-3-oxosteroid 5β-reductase deficiency present with elevations in serum ALT and AST, markedly elevated serum conjugated bilirubin, and coagulopathy. Liver histology and ultrastructural pathology findings include marked lobular disarray as a result of giant cell and pseudoacinar transformation of hepatocytes, hepatocellular and canalicular bile stasis, and extramedullary hematopoiesis with small-bile canaliculi that are sometimes slitlike in appearance and showed few or absent microvilli containing electron-dense material.[26] Increased production of Δ^4-3-oxo bile acids occurs in patients with severe liver disease[28] and in infants during the first few weeks of life.[29] It is important to perform a repeat analysis of urine in the case of a suspected Δ^4-3-oxosteroid 5β-reductase deficiency because on rare occasions, a resolution of the liver disease occurs and the atypical bile acids disappear. The liver injury in this defect is presumed to be the consequence of the diminished primary bile acid synthesis and the hepatotoxicity of the accumulated Δ^4-3-oxo bile acids. The lack of canalicular secretion can be explained by the relative insolubility of oxobile acids and the cholestatic effects of the taurine conjugate of 7α-dihydroxy-3-oxo-4-cholenoic acid.[30] Treatment with ursodeoxycholic acid or cholic acid leads to resolution of histologic and biochemical abnormalities with an excellent long-term prognosis.

Oxysterol 7α-Hydroxylase Deficiency

The recent discovery of a genetic defect in oxysterol 7α-hydroxylase[31] establishes the acidic pathway as a quantitatively important pathway for bile acid synthesis in early life. In the human, the oxysterol 7α-hydroxylase may be more important than cholesterol 7α-hydroxylase for bile acid synthesis in early life. This defect has been reported in a 10-week-old boy, whose parents were first cousins, who presented with severe progressive cholestasis, hepatosplenomegaly, cirrhosis, and liver synthetic failure from early infancy. Serum ALT and AST were markedly elevated and serum γ-glutamyl transpeptidase was normal. Liver biopsy findings included cholestasis, bridging fibrosis, extensive giant cell transformation, and proliferating bile ductules.[31] Oral UDCA therapy led to deterioration in liver function tests, and oral cholic acid was ineffective. The patient subsequently died after orthotopic liver transplant at age 4½ months. The accumulating monohydroxy bile acids with the 3β-hydroxy-Δ^5 structure have been previously shown to be extremely cholestatic.[32] Their hepatotoxicity in this patient is presumed to have been exacerbated by the lack of primary bile acids necessary for the maintenance of bile flow. The patient was homozygous for this nonsense mutation, whereas both parents were heterozygous.[31]

2-Methylacyl-CoA Racemase Deficiency

2-Methylacyl-CoA racemase is a crucial enzyme that is uniquely responsible for the racemization of (25R)THCA-CoA to its (25S) enantiomer, while also performing the same reaction on the branched-chain fatty acid (2R)pristanoyl-CoA. Defects in this enzyme have profound effects on both the bile acid and fatty acid pathways. Mutations in the gene encoding 2-methylacyl-CoA racemase were first reported in three adults who presented with a sensory motor neuropathy[33] and later in a 10-week-old infant who had severe fat-soluble vitamin deficiencies, hematochezia, and mild cholestatic liver disease.[34] Liver histologic findings included cholestasis and giant cell transformation with modest inflammation. The infant had the same missense mutation (S52P) as that described in two of the adult patients, yet was seemingly phenotypically quite different. Two of the adult patients had neurologic symptoms due to tissue accumulation of phytanic and pristanic acids but were asymptomatic until the fourth decade of life, whereas the other adult was described as having the typical features of Niemann-Pick type C disease at 18 months of age and presumably had some liver dysfunction. In the first infant described with the 2-methylacyl-CoA racemase deficiency, the liver from a 5½-month-old sibling, who 2 years previously had died from an intracranial bleed. The mass spectrum and GC profiles in this defect resemble closely those observed in peroxisomal disorders affecting bile acid synthesis, such as Zellweger syndrome. Primary bile acid therapy with cholic acid has proven effective in normalizing liver enzymes and preventing the onset of neurologic symptoms in the infant; in addition, dietary restriction of phytanic acid and pristanic acids is likely to be necessary in the long term for such patients to prevent neurotoxicity from accumulation of these fatty acids in the brain.

THCA-CoA Oxidase Deficiency

A number of patients have been reported to have side-chain oxidation defects involving the THCA-CoA oxidase.[35] The clinical presentation differs among these cases, and although all have an impact on primary bile acid synthesis, neurologic disease was the main clinical feature. Whether these are primary bile acid defects or secondary to single-enzyme defects in peroxisomal β-oxidation is unclear. Two distinct acyl-CoA oxidases have been identified in humans.[36] The human acyl-CoA oxidase active on bile acid C_{27} cholestanoic acid intermediates has been found to be the same enzyme that catalyzes

the oxidation of 2-methyl branched-chain fatty acids. THCA-CoA oxidase deficiency has been shown to be associated with elevated serum phytanic and pristanic acids.[35,36] All had ataxia as a primary feature of the disease, with its onset occurring at about 3½ years of age. None had evidence of liver disease. It is possible, with the exception of the patient described by Clayton and colleagues, that these patients had a 2-methylacyl-CoA racemase deficiency, but the analysis of the cholestanoic acids was not sufficiently detailed to permit the diastereoisomers of THCA and 3α,7α-dihydroxy-5β-cholestanoic acid (DHCA) or pristanic acid to be measured.[35]

Bile Acid CoA Ligase Deficiency and Defective Amidation

The final step in bile acid synthesis involves conjugation with the amino acids glycine and taurine. Two enzymes catalyze the reactions leading to amidation of bile acids. In the first, a CoA thioester is formed by the rate-limiting bile acid-CoA ligase, after which glycine or taurine is coupled in a reaction catalyzed by a cytosolic bile acid-CoA:amino acid N-acyltransferase. A defect in bile acid amidation, presumed to involve the bile acid-CoA ligase, was described in patients presenting with fat and fat-soluble vitamin malabsorption.[37] The index case was a 14-year-old boy of Laotian descent who, in the first 3 months of life, presented with conjugated hyperbilirubinemia, elevated serum transaminases, and normal γ-glutamyl transpeptidase. Subsequently, an additional six patients, who presented as toddlers or older children/adolescents, have been identified who have presented with a history of neonatal cholestasis, growth failure, or fat-soluble vitamin deficiency. The diagnosis is based on the LSIMS analysis of the urine and serum and bile, which reveals a unique spectrum of unconjugated cholic acid and sulfate and glucuronide conjugates of dihydroxy and trihydroxy bile acids. All recently identified patients with this defect have been identified with family specific mutations in the bile acid-CoA ligase gene. Carlton et al. have described a kindred of Amish descent with mutations in the bile acid-CoA: amino acid N-acyltransferase (BAAT).[38] Patients homozygous for the 226G mutation had increased serum bile acids and variable growth failure and coagulopathy without jaundice and normal serum γ-glutamyl transpeptidase concentrations. Homozygotes had only unconjugated bile acids in serum, whereas heterozygotes had increased amounts unconjugated serum bile acids. Administration of conjugates of the primary bile acid, glycocholic acid, under an IND from the U.S. Food and Drug Administration to five recently identified patients has improved their growth and should correct the fat-soluble vitamin malabsorption in this defect.

Cholesterol 7α-Hydroxylase Deficiency

Several patients have recently been identified with a homozygous mutation deletion in the CYP7A1 gene, and when the cDNA of this mutant was expressed in vitro in cultured HEK 293 cells, cholesterol 7α-hydroxylase was found to be inactive.[39] Bile acid synthesis was reduced, and up-regulation of the alternative sterol 27-hydroxylase pathway presumably compensated for the reduced synthesis of bile acids via absent cholesterol 7α-hydroxylase activity. Three patients carrying this mutation were found to have abnormal serum lipids, but, in contrast to an infant identified with a mutation in oxysterol 7α-hydroxylase,[31] there was no liver dysfunction in these patients. Instead, the clinical phenotype was one of markedly elevated total and low-density lipoprotein (LDL) cholesterol and premature gallstones in two patients and premature coronary and peripheral vascular disease in one patient. The elevated serum cholesterol concentration was unresponsive to HMG-CoA reductase inhibitor therapy.

PEROXISOMAL DISORDERS

Peroxisomal biogenesis disorders (PBDs) are multisystem recessively inherited conditions characterized by abnormalities of peroxisome assembly resulting in marked deficiency or absence of peroxisomes. Mutations in the PEX family of genes are the major cause of defective peroxisome biogenesis. Approximately 80% of PBD patients are classified as Zellweger syndrome spectrum (ZSS). These disorders are characterized by an absence of hepatic peroxisomes and can present clinically as seizures, profound developmental delay, blindness, deafness, hypotonia, renal cysts, characteristic facies, and intrahepatic cholestasis.[40] Patients typically present with jaundice and hepatomegaly in the first few weeks of life and progress to death because of central nervous system disease and profound hypotonia or liver failure by 6 to 12 months of age, although survival is variable. Diagnosis can be suggested by the demonstration of very long-chain fatty acids in the serum of these patients by GC-MS.[40] Elevated levels of cholestanoic acids can also be detected in the urine, serum, and bile using LSIMS and gas chromatography–mass spectrometry (GC-MS). Current therapy for these patients is directed toward supportive care. Patients with defects in peroxisomal β-oxidation of hepatotoxic cholestanoic acid intermediates have been treated with cholic acid. Eight patients with peroxisomopathies survived after treatment periods ranging from 4.7 to 11 years.[41] Of these, 4 patients had Refsum disease, whereas the remaining patients had ZSS. An additional 13 patients with peroxisomal disorders have been treated with cholic acid, but 10 died (or are presumed dead) and 3 were lost to follow-up. The treatment failures mostly included those patients with severe ZSS in which multiple organ disease was present. It was concluded that this group will derive minimal benefit from this approach, whereas those patients with single enzyme defects in peroxisomal function causing abnormal bile acid synthesis are likely to show greater responsiveness and benefit from oral cholic acid therapy. In a recent report of a peroxisomal biogenesis disorder due to a *PEX10* deficiency, cholic acid has been successful used in one patient for 10 years.[42]

ALTERATION OF HEPATIC BILE ACID TRANSPORT

Bile acids must be excreted into the canalicular lumen following their synthesis within hepatocytes. It is this excretion of bile acids that serves as the rate-limiting step of bile formation. To maintain a recirculating pool of bile acids, there must also be an efficient uptake of bile acids from portal blood flow. Various bile acid transporters are located within hepatocytes to facilitate flow of bile acids into the canalicular lumen. Defects in any of these bile acid transporters will lead to an impairment of bile flow, interruption of the enterohepatic circulation of bile acids, and subsequent cholestasis.

Two bile acid transporters are located on the basolateral surface of hepatocytes in contact with sinusoidal blood. The Na+-taurocholate cotransporting polypeptide (NTCP) is an

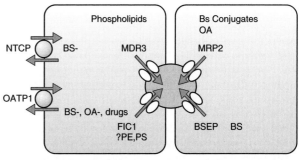

Figure 3-4. Hepatocellular transport of bile acids. The basolateral membranes of hepatocytes express the bile salt (BS) transporters Na+-taurocholate cotransporting polypeptide (NTCP) and organic anion transporting polypeptides (OATP). Bile salts are then transported into the canalicular lumen by the bile salt export pump (BSEP) and multidrug resistance protein 2 (MRP2). In addition, phospholipids are transported across the canalicular membrane by the multidrug-resistant type 3 protein (MDR3) while aminophospholipids are transported by the familial intrahepatic cholestasis type 1 (FIC1) transporter. Not shown is the SGP transporter at the canalicular membrane whose defect is associated with PFIC-2. Adapted with permission from Tomer G, Shneider BL. Gastroenterol Clin North Am 2003; 32:839-855.[59]

ATP-driven, sodium-dependent transporter responsible for the uptake of conjugated bile acids from blood into hepatocytes. A sodium independent bile acid transporter, the organic anion transporting polypeptide (OATP), is also located on the basolateral membrane of hepatocytes and aids in the uptake of bile acids. Excretion of bile acids from hepatocytes into the canalicular membrane is dependent on the bile salt export pump (BSEP) and the multidrug resistance protein 2 (MRP2). Other transporters relevant to the enterohepatic circulation located on the canalicular membrane include the multidrug-resistant type 3 protein (MDR3), the familial intrahepatic cholestasis type 1 (FIC1) transporter, and the SGP transporter. MDR3 is an ATP-dependent transporter responsible for the transport of phospholipids into bile. FIC1 is a P-type ATPase that is part of a family of aminophospholipid transporters (Figure 3-4).[43]

Progressive familial intrahepatic cholestasis (PFIC) represents a group of disorders associated with intrahepatic cholestasis that typically presents in the first year of life. Three different genetic mutations in canalicular transport proteins lead to the development of the three described forms of PFIC (types 1 through 3). All forms of PFIC can present clinically with jaundice, pruritus, failure to thrive, cholelithiasis, and fat-soluble vitamin deficiency. Cirrhosis typically develops in these patients within 5 to 10 years, leading to liver failure. A more complete description of the clinicopathologic and genetic findings in these diseases may be found in Chapter 70.

PFIC-1, also known as Byler's disease (for the Amish descendant first described with the mutation), is an autosomal recessive disorder caused by a mutation in the FIC1 gene. Patients with PFIC-1 will present with intrahepatic cholestasis. Serum bile acid concentration are elevated with an elevated ratio of chenodeoxycholic acid to cholic acid; however, the concentration of biliary bile acids will be low.[44] Other serological markers of this disease will be low or normal γ-glutamyl transpeptidase (GGT) and cholesterol levels. PFIC-1 is a progressive disease that will lead to liver cirrhosis by the second decade of life if left untreated.[44] PFIC-2 is a disease that has a similar clinical and biochemical presentation to PFIC-1. This defect is known to be related to mutations in the SGP transporter at the canalicular membrane. One difference between the two disorders is that patients with PFIC-2 tend to progress to cirrhosis and liver failure more quickly than patients with PFIC-1. Distinction between the two disorders may be accomplished with a liver biopsy. Patients with PFIC-1 tend to have coarse bile visualized on liver biopsy along with blander intracanalicular cholestasis compared with patients with PFIC-2, who show a filamentous or amorphous bile appearance along with giant cell hepatitis.[45]

A third type of PFIC, PFIC-3, is somewhat different from the first two subtypes. In comparison to PFIC-1 and PFIC-2, PFIC-3 is associated with an elevated serum GGT level. Patients with PFIC-3 will present with a severe intrahepatic cholestasis in infancy and will progress to liver failure within the first few years of life. Liver biopsy of these patients will show bile duct proliferation along with periportal fibrosis. This disorder has been associated with lack of a functional MDR3 p-glycoprotein, which results in bile acids exerting a toxic effect on biliary epithelium.[46] This protein is responsible for transporting phospholipids across the canalicular membrane with markedly reduced biliary phospholipids.

No effective medical therapy currently exists for the treatment of PFIC. Ursodeoxycholic acid has been reported to improve liver function in a subset of patients.[47] Medical therapy with antihistamines, bile acid sequestrants, and rifampin may be helpful in the relief of pruritus. Biliary diversion and ileal exclusion are two surgical procedures that may relieve symptoms of pruritus while improving the biochemical markers of cholestasis and liver injury. Liver transplantation is the only effective treatment for patients with PFIC who have progressed to end-stage liver disease.

ALTERATION IN CHOLESTASIS (GENERAL)

Conditions leading to cholestasis, including congenital hepatic transport defects (PFIC 1-3), infection, endocrinopathies, anatomic abnormalities (biliary atresia, choledochol cyst), and metabolic diseases such as galactosemia and tyrosinemia, have a direct impact on the enterohepatic circulation. Cholestasis leads to accumulation of bile acids in the liver and peripheral circulation with reduction in biliary and intestinal luminal concentrations. As a consequence of cholestasis, alterations in the hepatocyte transporters mediated by the nuclear receptor, FXR, work in concert to prevent accumulation of potentially toxic bile acids in the liver. In cholestasis, NTCP activity on the sinusoidal membrane is reduced while BSEP at the canalicular membrane is reduced and cholesterol 7α-hydroxylase, the rate-limiting enzyme in bile acid synthesis, is reduced. In addition, the formation of sulfate and glucuronide conjugates is increased, and bile acid transporters in the kidney may enhance excretion of potentially toxic bile acids.

ALTERATION OF THE ENTEROHEPATIC CIRCULATION OF BILE ACIDS

Intraluminal bile acids are passively transported along the length of the gastrointestinal tract by nonionic diffusion, allowing conservation of some glycine-conjugated and -unconjugated bile acids; however, the ileum with its sodium-dependent active transport system is responsible for the efficient recycling of bile acids in the human. A highly efficient, sodium-dependent transporter, ASBT, is expressed on the apical membrane of the ileal epithelial cells.[48] ASBT is expressed in renal proximal tubular cells. It is also expressed

on cholangiocytes and may be involved in reabsorption of bile acids from bile; however, the importance of this transport process is unknown.[48] Within the ileal enterocyte, bile acids are transported by the intestinal bile acid binding protein (IBABP),[49] and thereafter Ostα and Ostβ facilitate exit from the enterocyte into the portal circulation.[50]

Bile acids can serve as mediators of diarrhea in patients with various clinical conditions that result in bile acid malabsorption. The three types of bile acid malabsorption that have been described include primary, secondary, and tertiary malabsorption. Such alterations in bile acid circulation can be seen in patients with Crohn's disease, ileal resection, radiation injury, or cystic fibrosis and in patients who have undergone a cholecystectomy.[51]

Primary bile acid malabsorption (type 2) is associated with either absent or inefficient ileal bile acid transport.[16] A group of patients with intractable diarrhea of infancy have been shown to have this type of bile acid malabsorption with increased secretion of sodium and water into the intestinal lumen.[51] Infants and children with primary bile acid malabsorption have impaired intestinal absorption of bile acids, a contracted bile acid pool size, decreased intraluminal bile acid concentrations, reduced plasma cholesterol, and malabsorption of water, electrolytes, and lipids.[52] Idiopathic bile acid catharsis in adults has also been associated with a similar type of malabsorption.

Diarrhea has also been associated with secondary bile acid malabsorption (type 1) where terminal ileal dysfunction leads to delivery of increased amounts of bile acids to the colon, which can also induce water and electrolyte secretion.[52] Mild forms of this condition may be seen in cystic fibrosis, radiation-induced injury to the ileum, or Crohn's disease affecting the terminal ileum. One of the most common causes of bile acid–induced diarrhea in older children is ileal resection. The consequence of ileal resection is largely dependent on the liver's ability to compensate for fecal bile acid loss. During times of high fecal losses, the liver can increase synthesis of bile acids up to 10-fold.[53] When excess quantities of bile acids are lost in the stool, fewer bile acids are returned to the liver, leading to upregulation of hepatic synthesis. With relatively short ileal resections, an increased bile acid synthetic rate is able to adequately compensate for fecal losses.[16] Diarrhea will occur in these patients as a direct effect of the bile acids on colonic mucosa.

McJunkin et al. showed that a cholerrheic enteropathy would be induced if dihydroxylated bile acids were present in the fecal aqueous phase in elevated concentrations (>1.5 mM) and stool pH was alkaline.[54] The dihydroxy bile acids, chenodeoxycholic and deoxycholic acid, have hydroxyl groups in the alpha positions on the steroid nucleus and are capable of inducing water and electrolyte secretion. However, this is not the case for ursodeoxycholic acid, whose 7-OH group is in the beta orientation. Patients with small ileal resections tend to have a normal or slightly alkaline fecal pH and higher fecal aqueous dihydroxy bile acid concentrations. The elevated fecal bile acid concentrations can result in colonic water and electrolyte secretion causing diarrhea with modest steatorrhea.[54] Patients with bile acid–induced diarrhea often respond to bile acid binding agents, such as cholestyramine, which act to bind intraluminal bile acids. In young children, the intraluminal concentrations of dihydroxy bile acids may not reach concentrations sufficient to induce water and electrolyte secretion, and bile acid binders may not be helpful; however, with increasing age, the sequestrants may be helpful as the fecal bile acid concentration exceeds the levels associated with diarrhea.

Larger ileal resections in adults can be associated with a bile acid loss of 2.0 to 2.5 g/day. A compensatory increase in the hepatic synthesis of bile acids is unable to compensate for fecal losses.[53] As a result of this bile acid loss, the concentration of intraluminal bile acids falls below the critical micellar concentration (CMC), with associated impaired solubilization of lipolytic products in the upper small intestine. A higher fat concentration will subsequently be delivered to the colon, leading to a significant steatorrhea.[19] Despite such a large loss of bile acids, treatment of diarrhea with binding agents such as cholestyramine is ineffective as the fatty acids and hydroxyl fatty acids delivered to the colon mediate the water and electrolyte secretion responsible for the diarrhea. An improvement in the diarrhea may be seen with dietary substitution of long-chain triglycerides (LCTs) with medium-chain triglycerides (MCTs), which are more easily absorbed with lower concentrations of intraluminal bile acids.[16]

Patients presenting with "tertiary" bile acid malabsorption (type 3) include individuals with a history of previous cholecystectomy or diabetes mellitus, or in association with certain drugs. These individuals typically do not have a severe bile acid malabsorption. As with the other types of bile acid malabsorption, these individuals can develop a diarrhea secondary to nonabsorbed bile acids entering the colon. These bile acids will draw sodium and water into the colon and can enhance colonic motility.

MECHANISM OF BILE ACID-INDUCED DIARRHEA

Bile acids throughout the large and small bowel which may contribute to the development of diarrhea seen in patients with ileal dysfunction. These effects include reduction in fluid and electrolyte absorption, net fluid secretion, altered mucosal structure, increased mucosal permeability, altered motor activity, decreased nonelectrolyte absorption, and increased mucosal cyclic adenosine monophosphate.[16,55-58] All observed effects require that the dihydroxy bile acids must have the 7-OH group in the alpha position (chenodeoxycholic and cholic acid) with no observed effect when it is in the beta orientation (ursodeoxycholic acid).

SUMMARY

Bile acids are vital in the processing and absorption of dietary lipids as well as for the stimulation of bile flow and regulation of sterol metabolism. Multiple enzymatic steps occur in the conversion of cholesterol to the primary and secondary bile acids. A disruption of synthesis in one of the primary bile acids, cholic acid or chenodeoxycholic acid, within the liver will lead to cholestasis as well as fat and fat-soluble vitamin malabsorption. If a disruption in the recycling of bile acids occurs at the level of the intestine, diarrhea or steatorrhea can occur depending on the severity of the interruption. Newborns are particularly susceptible to any disruptions in bile acid synthesis or alterations in the enterohepatic circulation of bile acids because of an immature synthetic pathway of bile acid biosynthesis.

REFERENCES

5. Hofmann AF. The continuing importance of bile acids in liver and intestinal disease. Arch Intern Med 1999;159:2647–2658.
9. Heubi JE. Bile acid metabolism and the enterohepatic circulation of bile acids. In: Gluckman PD, Heymann MA, editors. Pediatrics & Perinatology: The Scientific Basis. 2nd ed. London: Arnold; 1996 p. 663–668.
16. Heubi JE. Bile acid-induced diarrhea. In: Lebenthal E, Duffey M, editors. Textbook of Secretory Diarrhea. New York: Raven Press; 1990 p. 281–290.
22. Heubi JE, Setchell KDR, Bove KE. Inborn errors of bile acid metabolism. Semin Liver Dis 2007;27:282–294.
43. Kosters A, Karpen SJ. Bile acid transporters in health and disease. Xenobiotica 2008;38:1043–1047.
44. Alissa FT, Jaffe R, Shneider BL. Update on progressive intrahepatic cholestasis. J Pediatr Gastroent Nutr 2008;46:2241–2252.

See expertconsult.com for a complete list of references and the review questions for this chapter.

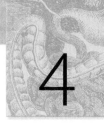

4 INDIGENOUS FLORA

Jonathan E. Teitelbaum

Researchers have estimated that the human body contains 10^{14} cells, only 10% of which are not bacteria and belong to the human body proper.[1] The mammalian intestinal tract represents a complex, dynamic and diverse ecosystem of interacting aerobic and anaerobic, nonpathologic bacteria. This complex yet stable colony includes more than 400 separate species.[2]

Within any segment of the gut, some organisms are adherent to the epithelium, while others exist in suspension in the mucus layer overlying the epithelium.[3] Binding to the epithelial surface is a highly specific process. For example, certain strains of lactobacilli and coagulase-negative staphylococci adhere to the gastric epithelium of the rat, whereas *Escherichia coli* and *Bacteroides* are unable to do so.[4] Bacterial adherence is also modulated by the local environment (i.e., pH), surface charge and presence of fibronectin.[5] Those unbound bacteria within the lumen of the gut represent those organisms shed from the epithelium or swallowed from the oropharynx.

Luminal flora accounts for the majority of organisms within the gut and represents 40% of the weight of feces[1]; however, the fecal flora found in stool samples does not necessarily represent the important host-microbial symbiosis of the mucosal bound flora.[6] Because the majority of indigenous species are obligate anaerobes, their culture, identification, and quantification are technically difficult, and it is estimated that at least half of the indigenous bacteria cannot be cultured by traditional methods.[2,7] Limitations of conventional microbiological techniques have confounded a detailed analysis of the enteric flora and led to a shift from traditional culture and phenotyping to genotyping. Modern techniques of ribotyping, pulsed field electrophoresis, plasmid profiles, specific primers, and probes for polymerase chain reaction (PCR) and nucleic acid hybridization and 16S rRNA sequencing have allowed for identification of bacteria without culturing. Furthermore, specific 16S rRNA-based oligonucleotide probes allow detection of bacterial groups by fluorescent in situ hybridization (FISH). Such techniques are limited only by the number of probes developed to date to identify the bacteria of interest.

Research efforts analyzing the symbiotic relationship that exists within the human gastrointestinal tract have been aided by studies of two well-described systems: the symbiosis between *Rhizobium* bacteria and leguminous plants, and the cooperative interaction between *Vibrio fischeri* and the light-producing organ of the squid. In each host tissue, modifications are made to allow a favorable niche to be established by the symbiont.[8] The use of newer microbiological techniques has helped to further elaborate the ways in which bacteria effect change within the host. For example, the use of laser capture microdissection and gene array analysis of germ-free mice colonized with *Bacteroides thetaiotaomicron* has shown affects on murine genes influencing mucosal barrier function, nutrient absorption, metabolism, angiogenesis, and the development of the enteric nervous system.[9]

Host activities including processing of nutrients and regulation of the immune system are affected by the genetic potential of the indigenous flora, known as the microbiome.[10] The composition of the intestinal microbiome is variable, and its diversity can be affected by alteration in diet and antibiotic use. Genes for specific metabolic pathways, such as amino acid and glycan metabolism, appear to be overrepresented in the microbiome of the distal gut, supporting the notion that human metabolism is an amalgamation of microbial and human processes.[11]

Of the fungi, only yeasts play a major role in the orointestinal tract, with *Candida* being the predominant genus. Various strains are commonly, but not always, present in different locations, suggesting that they may only be transient flora. However, some strains of *C. albicans* can inhabit the gastrointestinal (GI) tract for longer periods of time, as evidenced by the fact that strains isolated from newborns are the same as the mother's.[12] The presence of *Candida* in the GI tract does not indicate candidiasis. The colony counts of *Candida* in normal small and large bowel do not exceed 10^4 colony-forming units (cfu) per milliliter.[12] The introduction of *Candida* into a well-developed fecal flora system under continuous-flow culture did not lead to multiplication of the yeast. Thus, normal bacterial flora appears to provide protection against pathologic colonization by yeast. However, if the fecal flora was destroyed by antibiotics, then the yeast would multiply.[12,13] The addition of a *Lactobacillus* species to the system was able to reduce the colony counts of the *Candida* significantly.[13] It has been found that up to 65% of individuals harbor fungi in the stool.[14] As opposed to the numerous indigenous bacterial flora and yeast forms, there does not appear to be a normal viral flora.[15]

UNDERSTANDING THE INDIGENOUS FLORA BY STUDYING GERM-FREE ANIMALS

Further understanding of the beneficial effects of developing a normal bacterial flora is achieved by the analysis of germ-free animal models (Table 4-1). Germ-free mice have small intestines that weigh less than those of their normal counterparts. Their intestinal wall is thinner and less cellular; the villi are thinner and more pointed at the tip; and the crypts are shallower, resulting in a reduced mucosal surface area.[16] Histologically, the mucosal cells are cuboidal rather than columnar and uniform in size and shape. The stroma has sparse concentrations of inflammatory cells under aseptic conditions with only few lymphocytes and macrophages. Plasma cells are absent, and Peyer's patches are smaller with fewer germinal centers; consequently, there is little or no IgA expression.[17,18] The T-cell component of the lamina propria is largely composed of CD4+ lymphocytes; these

TABLE 4-1. Changes in Intestinal Structure and Function in Germ-Free Animals

Reduced
Mucosal cell turnover
Digestive enzyme activity
Local cytokine production
Mucosa associated lymphoid tissue (MALT)
Lamina propria cellularity
Vascularity
Muscle wall thickness
Motility

Increased
Enterochromaffin cell area
Caloric intake to sustain body weight

Data from Shanahan, F. The host-microbe interface within the gut. Best Pract Res Clin Gastroenterol 2002;16:915–931.

are reduced in numbers in germ-free animals.[19] Furthermore, antigen transport across the intestinal barrier is increased in the absence of intestinal microflora.[20] Cellular turnover is decreased compared with colonized animals, and migration time for ^{3}H-thymidine labeled mucosal cells from crypt to tip is doubled.[17,18] After exposure to enteric bacteria, the intestines of germ-free animals take on a conventional appearance within 28 days, as one notes the infiltration of the lamina propria by lymphocytes, histiocytes, macrophages, and plasma cells.[17,21]

Functional differences have also been noted in the intestines of germ-free animals including a more alkaline intraluminal pH and a more positive reduction potential (E_h).[22] Intestinal transit time and gastric emptying are also decreased in germ-free states.[23] There is also increased absorption of calcium, magnesium, xylose, glucose, and some vitamins and minerals in the germ-free animal.[24] The germ-free animal also has increases in the activity of intestinal cell enzymes, such as alkaline phosphatase, disaccharidases, and α-glucosidase.[24]

Without a microflora, the rate of epithelial cell renewal is reduced in the small intestine, the cecum becomes enlarged, and the GALT is altered.[25] Studies have revealed that colonization of germ-free mice induces GDP-fucose asialo-GM1 α1,2-fucosyltransferase activity in the epithelium, increased neutral glycolipid, fucosyl asialo-GM1, a decrease in asialo-GM1, and the production of Fucα1,2Gal structures.[8] These changes occur selectively based on specific bacterial strains and density.[8] In studying the *Rhizobium*-legume symbiosis, researchers have learned that the soluble factors released by the bacteria signal a release of signaling molecules from the host, resulting in the expression of bacterial genes required for nodulation (*nod* genes).[26] These same genes have now been noted to be abnormal in Crohn's disease and Blau syndrome.[27]

A study evaluating the effect of the microbiome on mouse plasma biochemistry compared serum from germ-free and conventional mice. The study found a large number of chemical species only in the conventional mice. Amino acid metabolites were particularly affected. Multiple organic acids containing phenyl groups were also greatly increased in the presence of gut microbes. Specifically, at least 10% of all detectable endogenous circulating serum metabolites vary in concentration by at least 50% between the germ-free and conventional mice. Several of these molecules were either potentially harmful (e.g., uremic toxins) or beneficial (e.g., antioxidant).[28]

ESTABLISHING THE INDIGENOUS FLORA

Colonization of the newborn's initially sterile gut with bacteria occurs within the first few days after birth. Such colonization appears to be rapid, indeed, bacteria have been found in meconium as early as 4 h after birth.[29] Initial inoculation is with diverse flora including bifidobacteria, enterobacteria, *Bacteroides*, clostridia, and gram-positive cocci.[30,31] *Staphylococcus aureus* has recently been shown to be a major colonizer of the infant gut, perhaps a sign of reduced competition from other microbes.[32] The flora then rapidly changes and is affected by the mode of delivery, gestational age, and diet. Some evidence exists that maternal stress can alter the neonatal intestinal microflora.[33]

The study by Long and Swenson analyzed stools from 196 infants and helped to define intestinal bacterial colonization with anaerobes, including *Bacteroides fragilis*. Among infants born vaginally, 96% were colonized with anaerobic bacteria within 4 to 6 days, with 61% harboring *B. fragilis*.[34] In contrast, at 1 week in infants born full-term via cesarean section, anaerobes were present in only 59% and *B. fragilis* was found in 9%.[34] A study by Gronlund et al. utilizing standard culture techniques could find no permanent colonization with *B. fragilis* before 2 months of age among newborns born via cesarean, with maternal prophylactic antibiotics. At 6 months of age, the colonization rate was 36%, half of that found in a group of vaginally born infants.[35] These studies suggest that the sterile manner in which children are born via cesarean section, as well as the use of perinatal antibiotics, delays intestinal anaerobic colonization. A delay in colonization with aerobic bacteria has also been observed in a study of 70 healthy Swedish newborns, which found that 45% of vaginally delivered versus 12% of cesarean-delivered infants were colonized with *Escherichia coli* by the third day of life.[36]

As to gestational age, significantly fewer vaginally born preterm infants had anaerobes found in their stool at the end of 1 week, as compared with their vaginally born full-term counterparts, suggesting that either local conditions in the preterm infant's intestine, such as lower acidity or the sterile environment of an incubator, affect colonization.[34]

Breast-fed infants born vaginally had similar colonization to vaginally born formula-fed infants at 48 h of age, indicating a similar "inoculum." However, by 7 days, only 22% of breast-fed infants had *B. fragilis*, versus 61% of the formula-fed infants.[34] Harmsen et al. studied the development of fecal flora in six breast-fed and six formula-fed infants during the first 20 days after birth, using newer molecular techniques and comparing them with traditional culturing.[37] The study supported prior studies in demonstrating an initially diverse colonization that became *Bifidobacterium* predominant in the breast-fed group, whereas the formula-fed group had similar amounts of *Bacteroides* and *Bifidobacterium*. Breast-fed infants also had some lactobacilli and streptococci as colonizers,[37] whereas formula-fed infants developed a more diverse flora, which also included Enterobacteriaceae, enterococci, and *Clostridium*.[30,31,37] One study found *Lactobacillus* to be more dominant than *Bifidobacterium* in breast-fed babies.[38] The acquisition of aerobic gram-negative bacilli also varied with feeding type, as 62% of formula-fed infants and 82% of breast-fed infants were colonized by 48 h of life.[34] After weaning, the flora becomes more diverse, with fewer *E. coli* and *Clostridium* and more *Bacteroides* and gram-positive anaerobic cocci, and resembles that of adults.[30,39] The differences in fecal flora observed between breast-fed and formula-fed infants have been proposed to be the result of multiple causes, including the lower iron content and different composition of proteins in human milk, a lower phosphate content, the large variety of oligosaccharides in human milk, and numerous humoral and cellular mediators of immunologic function in breast milk.[40]

Longitudinal studies by Mata et al. of impoverished Guatemalan children born vaginally and breast-fed documented the prevalence of *Bifidobacterium* in this group. Within the first few hours of life, facultative micrococci, streptococci, and gram-negative bacilli were more readily cultured than anaerobes.[39] On day of life 2, almost all infants demonstrated *E. coli* in concentrations of 10^5 to 10^{11} g. Only a few babies had *Bifidobacterium* on the first day of life, while by day 2, 33% were so colonized with concentrations of 10^8 to 10^{10} g.[39] By 1 week all had *Bifidobacterium* at concentrations of 10^{10} to 10^{11} g.[39] By 1 year of age, those that were still breast-fed had bacterial colonization with almost exclusive *Bifidobacterium*.[39]

A study utilizing bacterial enzyme activity as an indirect measure of bacterial colonization found no difference in flora during the first 6 months of life based on the mode of delivery. However, stools collected from formula-fed infants had greater urease activity at 1 to 2 months and higher β-glucuronidase activity at 6 months compared with breast-fed infants.[41] This is in conflict with a study from Finland, in which no differences were found in enzyme activity based on feeding groups.[42] Examples of urease producing fecal bacteria include *Bifidobacterium*, *Clostridium*, *Eubacterium*, and *Fusobacterium*. β-Glucuronidase producers include *Lactobacillus*, *Clostridium*, *Peptostreptococcus*, and *E. coli*.

Despite these differences in colonization with *Bifidobacterium* and *Bacteroides,* as well as differences in the colonization rate with *Clostridium perfringens* (57% in the cesarean group versus 17% in the vaginal group), no differences in gastrointestinal signs such as flatulence, abdominal distention, diarrhea, foul-smelling stool, or bloody stools could be detected.[35]

Infants born vaginally have traditionally thought to acquire their fecal flora from the mother's vaginal and intestinal flora. More recently, this has been called into question, with nosocomial/environmental spread appearing to be significant contributors. Within maternity wards, nosocomial spread of fecal bacteria among healthy newborns has been documented. Murono et al. studied the plasmid profiles of *E. coli* strains isolated from the stool of maternal and infant pairs to determine the degree of vertical versus nosocomial spread. In only 4 of the 29 pairs were shared *Enterobacteriaceae* documented. However, 8 of 10 infants in one hospital did share a single plasmid profile indicating nosocomial acquisition of the fecal flora.[43] Tannock et al. used the same plasmid profiling technique to show that *Lactobacillus* inhabiting the vaginas of mothers did not appear to colonize the infant digestive tract, whereas Enterobacteriaceae and *Bifidobacterium* from the mother's feces could be found to colonize the infant in 4 of 5 cases.[44] The environment appears to play a greater role among infants born via cesarean section and for those separated from their mother for long periods after birth.[43]

As opposed to earlier studies in the 1970s that showed colonization rates with *E. coli* in Western countries of at least 70%[45] and in developing countries of nearly 100%[46] by the first week of life regardless of mode of delivery, a more recent Swedish study found less than 50% colonization.[36] The reduction was attributed to decreased nosocomial spread by the practice of "rooming-in" and early hospital discharge. It took almost 6 months before all infants were colonized with *E. coli*.[36] The turnover rate of individual *E. coli* strains was low, most likely due to a limited circulation of fecal bacteria in the Swedish home. Environmental factors, such as siblings, pets or feeding mode did not affect colonization kinetics.

While some *E. coli* strains appear transient and disappear from the intestine within a few weeks, others become resident for months to years. Resident strains have certain characteristics such as the expression of P fimbriae and a capacity to adhere to colonic epithelial cells. P fimbriae are composed of a fimbrial rod with a tip adhesion that exists in three papG classes. These recognize the Gal α1-4 Gal glycoproteins, with slight differences in binding.[47] Intestinal persistence of *E. coli* has been linked to the class II variety of the adhesin.[48] The resident strains more commonly have other virulence factors, such as the iron-chelating compound aerobactin and capsular types K1 and K5, when compared to the transient strains.[48] Within the Swedish study, the P fimbrial class III adhesion gene associated with urinary tract infections was more common in *E. coli* from children who had cats in their home than among *E. coli* from homes without pets.[36] This raises the question as to whether this *E. coli* could be transferred by close contact with a family cat.

The role of diet on the composition of fecal flora in the older child and adult appears to be minimal, because individuals fed a standard institutional diet had similar fecal flora to those who consumed a random diet.[49] The ingestion of an elemental diet resulted in reduction of stool weight and frequency, but few qualitative changes in the composition of the fecal flora.[50] Furthermore, in analysis of the microorganisms measured in an aliquot of fresh feces, there does not appear to be significant differences in the fecal flora based on a diet's fiber content or meat content.[22] However, studies of the metabolic activity of the flora via measuring of bacterial enzymes have demonstrated marked differences.[22]

BACTERIAL FLORA WITHIN THE VARIOUS SECTIONS OF THE GASTROINTESTINAL TRACT

Oral Flora

Infants with a developing oral ecosystem are amenable to colonization perhaps because specific antibodies capable of inhibiting bacterial adherence are present only in low levels in early infancy.[51] The indigenous microflora of the oral cavity is an integral component of the function of this site. The commensal bacteria help to defend against colonization by pathogens. Secretory immunoglobulin A (S-IgA) represents the main specific defense mechanism of the oral mucosa. The S-IgA of infant saliva and human milk are mainly composed of the IgA1 subclass.[52] IgA proteases are produced by pathogenic bacteria as well as oral commensals. Saliva contains other immunoglobulins and defense factors to inhibit microbial adhesion and growth.[53] After teeth emerge, IgG appears in greater concentrations.[52,53] The early low concentrations of antibodies[52,53] may be beneficial in allowing the invading bacteria to more easily colonize the oral surfaces. Initially only the buccal and palatal mucosa, as well as the crypts of the tongue, allow for colonization, but with the emergence of teeth, new gingival crevices and tooth surfaces become potential niches. Oxygen tension is an important environmental determinant for oral bacteria.

The fastidious anaerobic growth even in edentulous mouths is explained by the formation of biofilms. *Fusobacterium nucleatum*, an obligate anaerobe, appears to play a crucial role in the maturation of oral biofilm communities.[51]

The initial colonization of the oral cavity is dependent on mode of delivery, exposure to antibiotics, feedings, and gestational age.[51] For example, the establishment of the primary bacterial group viridans streptococci is delayed in preterm infants and transiently compensated for by less prevalent inhabitants, such as yeast.[51] The initial colonization by streptococci and *Actinomyces* allows for further colonization by other species. Initial bacteria are acquired through direct and indirect salivary contacts during everyday activities; thus the colonies found within the oral cavity of young children often resemble those of the mother.[54] *Streptococcus viridans* are the first persistent oral colonizers. The principal streptococcal species are *Streptococcus mitis* and *salivarius*. Oral actinomycetes (i.e., *A. odontolyticus*) and various anaerobic species (i.e., *Prevotella melaninogenica, F. nucleatum*) are also found during the first year of life. After the first year of life, the versatility among oral microflora increases remarkably. Among infants, there appears to be no stability among the specific clonal populations, and such instability is noted among adults, but to a lesser degree.[55] This stability, or its lack, appears to be variable based on the bacterial species being studied.[51] Pathologic bacteria such as *Streptococcus mutans*, the main causative bacteria in caries, appear in the oral cavity only after the primary teeth emerge. Children colonized early by this bacterium are more susceptible to caries than those colonized later.[56]

Esophageal Flora

Little is known about the bacterial colonization of the human esophagus. Because of the lack of anatomic or physiologic barriers to colonization, bacteria can be introduced into the esophagus either by swallowing oral flora, or by reflux from a colonized stomach. Early attempts at defining the esophageal flora through samples obtained by luminal washing yielded poor results. Pei et al.[57] used broad-range 16S rDNA PCR to examine biopsy samples from the esophagus of four healthy human adults. They identified 900 16S rDNA clones representing 41 genera of bacteria. Of these, 82.1% were cultivatable bacterial species, and there were about 10^4 bacteria per mm^2 mucosal surface of the distal esophagus. Members of six phyla, *Firmicutes, Bacteroides, Actinobacteria, Proteobacteria, Fusobacteria,* and TM7, were represented. The predominant bacteria was α-hemolytic *Streptococcus* species, and overall the flora was similar to that found in the oropharynx. A subsequent study by the same group defined a second microbiome with a greater proportion of gram-negative anaerobes/microphiles that correlated with disease states such as esophagitis and Barrett's esophagus.[58]

Stomach Flora

The stomach typically contains less than 10^3 cfu/mL. In a limited number of impoverished Guatemalan children, the colony counts ranged from 10^2 to 10^7 cfu/mL.[39] The lower counts are attributed to gastric juices, which destroy most oral bacteria.[22] The microflora of the stomach typically consists of gram-positive and aerobic bacteria with streptococci, staphylococci, *Lactobacillus*, and various fungi being most commonly isolated.[59] Indeed, *Candida* can be isolated from the stomach in up to 30% of healthy people.[14]

Small Bowel Flora

The small intestine represents a transitional zone between the sparsely populated stomach and the exuberant bacterial flora of the colon. Accordingly, the proximal small bowel has bacterial counts similar to that of the stomach, with concentrations ranging between 10^3 and 10^4 cfu/mL in the duodenum[22] and higher concentrations of 10^2 to 10^6 in the Guatemalan childhood study.[39] Jejunal flora is similar to that of the stomach.[5] The predominant species are streptococci, staphylococci, and *Lactobacillus*. In addition, *Veillonella* and *Actinomyces* species are also frequently isolated, but other anaerobic bacteria are present in lower concentrations.[22] Interestingly, small bowel concentrations are variable among animal species. Normal cats were noted to have relatively high numbers of bacteria (10^5 to 10^8 cfu/mL), including many obligate anaerobes in the proximal small intestine. This was thought to be secondary to a strictly carnivorous diet.[60] At the end of the transition, within the distal ileum, the gram-negative organisms outnumber gram-positive organisms.[22] Here, anaerobic bacteria such as *Bacteroides, Bifidobacterium, Fusobacterium,* and *Clostridium* are found at substantial concentrations along with coliforms.[22] The distal ileum has an oxidation-reduction potential (E_h) of −150 mV, which is similar to that of the cecum (−200 mV), thus allowing it to support the growth of anaerobic bacteria.[61]

Colonic Flora

Once in the colon, the bacterial concentrations increase dramatically. Colonic bacterial concentrations are typically 10^{11} to 10^{12} cfu/mL.[22] Here anaerobic bacteria outnumber aerobes by 1000-fold.[22] Predominant species include *Bacteroides, Bifidobacterium,* and *Eubacterium*, with anaerobic gram-positive cocci, *Clostridium*, enterococci, and various Enterobacteriaceae also being common.[22]

CONTROLLING THE GROWTH OF THE INDIGENOUS POPULATION

Various host defenses are responsible for controlling the proliferation of intestinal bacteria, thus limiting the population size (Table 4-2). Such limitation is needed because under optimal conditions in vitro coliform bacteria can divide every 20 min.[22] If this were to occur in vivo the host would quickly become overwhelmed. Within the gastrointestinal tract, bacterial generation time is longer at one to four divisions per day.[62] Within the small intestine, the major defenses against bacterial overgrowth are gastric acid and peristalsis. The ability of the peristaltic wave to propel bacteria is inferred by Dixon's classic study in which he inoculated ^{51}Cr-labeled red blood cells (RBCs) and bacteria into a surgically created subcutaneous loop of rat small intestine. The bacteria and RBCs were noted to be rapidly cleared from the small intestine by the rat's peristaltic activity.[63] The effectiveness of peristalsis in moving bacteria is further emphasized by those circumstances in which one has a loop of intestine with ineffective peristalsis, and bacterial overgrowth is found. Experimental studies show that gastric emptying and intestinal transit are slowed in a germ-free state and restored with recolonization by normal flora.[64]

Gastric acid has also been shown to contribute to the sparse bacterial colonization of the proximal intestine. Gram-negative organisms are particularly susceptible to the effects of a low pH,

No content

TABLE 4-2. Regulation of the Indigenous Microflora

Host Factors
Intestinal motility/peristalsis
Gastric acid
Antibacterial quality of pancreatic and biliary secretions
Intestinal immunity (IgA, Paneth cell products (defensins), lysozyme, bactericidal permeability increasing protein),epithelial cell products
Mucus layer

Microbial Factors
Alteration in redox potential
Substrate depletion
Growth inhibitors (short-chain fatty acids, bacteriocins)
Suppression of bacterial adherence

Data from Batt R, Rutgers G, Sancak A. Enteric bacteria: friend or foe? J Small Animal Prac 1996; 37:261–267.

and a large inoculum of *Serratia* organisms is eradicated within 1 h when in contact with normal gastric acidity.[5] Indeed, patients with achlorhydria harbor coliforms and anaerobic gram-negative bacilli in the proximal small bowel, as well as increased numbers of streptococci, *Lactobacillus*, and fungi.[22] Lowering of gastric acid pharmacologically has been shown to impair host defenses against pathologic bacteria including *Vibrio cholerae*,[65] *Candida*,[66] *Campylocacter*,[67] and *Strongyloides stercoralis*.[68]

Bile duct ligation in experimental animals results in cecal overgrowth with coliforms, suggesting that bile acids or some other component of bile plays a role in the regulation of the bacterial flora.[69] It is suspected that the deconjugation of bile acids by the indigenous flora to create simple bile acids with the ability to inhibit bacterial growth is a possible mechanism.[5]

Microbial interactions constitute a major factor in regulating the indigenous microflora, particularly within the colon. Various interactions can either promote or inhibit growth of organisms. One mechanism would be competition for substrates. An example is the inhibition of the growth of *Shigella flexneri* by coliform organisms that compete for carbon.[70] Another mechanism would be manipulation of the oxygen content of the environment. The maintenance of a reduced environment by facultative bacteria allows the growth of anaerobic bacteria.[22] By-products of bacterial metabolism can create an intraluminal environment that restricts growth. Short-chain fatty acids such as acetic, propionic, and butyric acid can inhibit bacterial proliferation.[22] At sufficiently low pH these acids are undissociated and can enter the bacterial cell to inhibit microbial metabolism.[24] *Lactobacillus* spp., particularly *L. plantarum*, are found throughout the GI tract, and their ability to adhere to mannose-containing receptors on epithelial cells is important in protecting against colonization by pathogens.[71] Finally, some bacteria can produce antibiotic-like substances termed bacteriocins, enocin, and hydrogen peroxide, which can inhibit the growth of other bacterial species or even contribute to self-regulation. Included in this group are colicines produced by strains of *E. coli*.[72]

Mucus provides protection at the mucosal surface with its viscous high-molecular-weight glycoprotein providing a physiochemical barrier that, in concert with secreted immunoglobulins, entraps bacteria.[73] The carbohydrate component of mucin can also compete for receptor-specific binding proteins of microbes.

Host immunity also plays a role in limiting the growth of the indigenous bacterial population. IgA synthesis by B cells of the gut-associated lymphoid tissue is stimulated by the endogenous flora and increased further with pathologic colonization as in *Shigella* infection or bacterial overgrowth.[5] Distinct B-cell populations secrete different types of IgA, which may help control the volume and composition of the flora.[74] Such IgA is thought to prevent bacterial adhesion to epithelial cells.[75] However, isolated IgA deficiency is not associated with alterations in the pattern of colonization.[76] Moreover, the acquisition and composition of T- or B-cell-deficient mice is indistinguishable from that of their immunologically intact littermates.[5] Paneth cells of the small intestine secrete antibacterial peptides called defensins that have antibacterial properties, as well as phospholipase A2, bactericidal permeability-increasing protein, and lysozyme.[5]

The pattern of antibodies directed against fecal bacteria appears to be unique for each individual. People tend to make antibodies against both indigenous bacteria and transient bacteria. The antibodies include polyspecific IgM as well as specific IgG and IgA. Relatively more specific IgA antibodies appear to be directed against transient bacteria as apposed to indigenous bacteria.[77]

SYMBIOSIS BETWEEN HOST AND FECAL FLORA

A microflora-associated characteristic (MAC) is defined as the recording of any anatomical structure or physiological or biochemical function in a microorganism that has been influenced by the microflora. When such changes occur in the absence of microflora, they are designated as a germ-free animal characteristic (GAC).[78] The distinction between MAC and GAC helps to define the symbiotic relationship that exists between human and the microbial host, and elucidates those processes that bacteria perform that are advantageous to the host (Table 4-3). Bacterial β-glucuronidase and sulfatase are responsible for the enterohepatic circulation of numerous substances including bilirubin, bile acids, estrogens, cholesterol, digoxin, rifampin, morphine, colchicine, and diethylstilbestrol.[22] Microflora also play a role in the degradation of intestinal mucin, the conversion of urobilin to urobilinogen and of cholesterol to coprostanol, and the production of short-chain fatty acids (SCFAs).[22,78] Mucin-degrading microbes are evident in all children by age 20 to 21 months.[22] This appears to be a gradual acquisition process starting at about 3 months of age.[78] Bacterial synthesis of vitamins such as biotin, vitamins K and B_{12}, pantothenate, riboflavin, and folate help supplement dietary sources.[24,79] Bacterial enzymatic degradation of urea is probably the only source of ammonia in the animal host.[24]

Scheline stressed that the "gut flora have the ability to act as an organ with a metabolic potential equal to, or sometimes greater than the liver."[80] A broad spectrum of metabolic reactions have been performed by intestinal flora, including hydrolysis, dehydroxylation, decarboxylation, dealkylation, dehalogenation, deamination, heterocyclic ring fission, reduction, aromatization, nitrosamine formation, acetylation, esterification, isomerization, and oxidation.[80,81] Gut flora acts on drugs to result in activation, toxin production, or deactivation. One of the earliest examples of activation by microorganisms is seen with protosil.[82] The bioavailability and pharmacological effect of numerous drugs, such as opiates, digoxin, hormones, and antibiotics, have been demonstrated to be altered by gut flora.[83]

TABLE 4-3. Effects of Enteric Bacteria

Beneficial Effects

Competitive exclusion of pathogens
Production of short-chain fatty acids
Synthesis of vitamins and nutrients
Enterohepatic circulation of numerous substances (e.g., bilirubin, bile acids, estrogens, cholesterol, digoxin, rifampin, morphine, colchicines and diethylstilbestrol)
Degradation of intestinal mucin
Conversion of urobilin to urobilinogen
Conversion of cholesterol to coprostanol
Degradation of urea
Drug metabolism and activation
Development of the immune system
Development of the enteric nervous system

Detrimental Effects

Competition for calories and essential nutrients
Production of harmful metabolites (carcinogens, deconjugated bile acids, hydroxyl fatty acids)
Mucosal damage
Direct effect of bacteria
Exacerbate inflammatory disease

Data from Batt R, Rutgers G, Sancak A. Enteric bacteria: friend or foe? I Small Animal Prac 1996; 37:261–267.

Beta-lyases transform xenobiotic cysteine conjugates to toxic metabolites such as thiols or thiol derivatives.[81] The azoreductase activity of the colonic flora metabolizes the prodrug sulfasalazine to its active aminosalicylate.

SCFA production is thought to occur in the cecum and ascending colon, mainly by the anaerobic flora.[78] It appears that those infants fed breast milk produce fewer SCFAs than those fed formula, in which there is a more varied, adult-like SCFA profile. SCFA produced in the colon may represent up to 70% of the energy available from the ingestion of carbohydrate.[84]

Intestinal microfloral enzymes β-glucuronidase and sulfatase catalyze the deconjugation of estrogens excreted with bile into the intestine to allow for reabsorption as part of the enterohepatic circulation. The presence of estriol-3-glucuronide in the urine is an indicator of estrogen resorption in the intestine.[22] The suppression of the intestinal microflora with antibiotics results in a decrease in the enterohepatic circulation of sex steroids and can thus lower the concentrations of these hormones significantly. Indeed, reports of failed oral contraception have been linked to concomitant use of antibiotics.[85]

Bile acids are derived from cholesterol in the liver. Within the liver, primary bile acids are conjugated and excreted into the bile. Bile acids undergo enterohepatic circulation several times each day. Most of the absorption takes place by active transport in the terminal ileum. In the intestine, conjugated bile acids are acted on by bacterial enzymes and converted to secondary bile acids. These secondary bile acids are either excreted into the feces or absorbed and sometimes further metabolized within the liver into tertiary bile acids. Microbial transformation of bile acids includes deconjugation, desulfation, deglucuronidation, oxidation of hydroxyl groups, and reduction of oxo groups.[86] Because humans are born germ-free, primary bile acids can be found in the meconium of newborn babies. Short-chain bile acids are elevated in children

and adults with cholestasis.[87] In healthy children, the levels of short-chain bile acids are undetectable. The ability to hydrolyze taurine and glycine bile acid conjugates has been detected in *Bifidobacterium*, *Peptostreptococcus*, *Lactobacillus*, and *Clostridium* shortly after birth.[88] The occurrence, substrate specificity, and kinetics of this enzyme activity vary among species and bacterial strain.[88] Jonsson et al. observed a decrease in sulfated conjugates within the stool at approximately 6 months of age. This was the same time that sulfate-rich mucin disappeared, and thus they suspected this was due to the action of microbial desulfanates.[86] Two clostridial strains (*Clostridium* spp. S1 and S2) and *Peptostreptococcus niger* H4 desulfate bile acid 3-sulfates.[86] Jonsson also noted that by 24 months of age, all the children studied had an adult pattern of excreted bile acids in that they were lacking a hydroxyl group at C-7.[86] Bacteria that are known to have 7α-dehydroxylation activity include *Eubacterium*, *Clostridium*, and *Lactobacillus*.[88] Cholesterol elimination is accomplished by two major routes, conversion of cholesterol to coprostanol and 7α-dehydroxylation of bile acids. Infants appear to be unable to perform such elimination during the first several months of life.[86] Thus, during those months, sulfation appears to be a compensatory mechanism for the excretion of breakdown products of cholesterol.[89]

BACTERIAL FLORA IN ILLNESS

Pathologic colonization occurs with the same species that predominate in nosocomial infections, and studies suggest that colonization is a risk factor for infection. This is the theory behind prophylactic decontamination of the digestive tract in the critically ill, which has been shown to reduce mortality.[5] Changes in the composition of the gut flora are common in critical illness due to reduced enteral intake, reduced intestinal motility, use of acid blockade therapy, and broad-spectrum antibiotics.[5] Gram-negative organisms are rarely found in the oropharynx of healthy individuals, yet can be found in up to 75% of hospitalized patients.[90] Similarly, du Moulin et al. documented the effects of antacids on the flora of the stomach. Among 59 critically ill patients, simultaneous colonization of the gastric and respiratory tract was seen with aerobic gram-negative bacteria.[91] This and similar studies have been the basis of the controversy surrounding routine acid blockade therapy for critically ill patients. Overall, it appears as though only in selected patients does the benefit of stress ulcer prophylaxis outweigh the risk of nosocomial pneumonia.[92] Gastric colonization in these patients also appears to be a risk factor for wound infections, urinary tract infections, peritonitis, and bacteremia.[93] Studies aimed at decreasing bacterial overgrowth via selective decontamination of the digestive tract using topical, nonabsorbed antimicrobial agents active against aerobic gram negatives (tobramycin and polymyxin) and fungi (amphotericin), but leaving gram-positive flora to preserve colonization resistance, have been varied. However, a meta-analysis indicates that this strategy is effective in preventing nosocomial respiratory infection and reduces ICU mortality.[94]

Total parenteral nutrition given to experimental animals increased the concentration of aerobic gram-negative organisms in the cecum and bacterial translocation into lymph nodes when compared with enterally fed animals.[95] Indeed, enteral feeding in the critically ill human is associated with fewer nosocomial infections.[96]

BACTERIAL FLORA AND ALLERGY

Although the exact pathophysiology of allergic disease is incompletely understood, it is thought to represent the end result of disordered function of the immune system. The intestinal barrier in the infant is thought to be immature, and thus vulnerable to allergic sensitization during the first few months of life. The intestinal microflora strengthens the immune defense and stimulates the development of the gut immune system.[74] In newborns the type 2 T helper cell (Th2) cytokines, essential mediators in the formation of allergic inflammation, predominate over Th1 cytokines.[74] Th2 cytokines include IL-4, which induces B-cell differentiation into IgE-producing cells, and IL-5, which is important for eosinophil activity. Intestinal bacteria can counterbalance this Th2 activity, promote the development of the Th1 cell lineage, and thus regulate the IgE response.[97] This may be the result of the CpG motif, which can induce polyclonal B cell activation and secretion of Th1 cytokines such as IL-6, IL-12, and interferon (IFN).[98] Intestinal bacteria may also modulate allergic inflammation via modification of antigen uptake,[99] presentation,[100] and degradation.[101,102] Thus, in those children with an aberrant array or insufficient number of intestinal microorganisms, there may be an inability to strengthen the gut barrier or counterbalance a Th2 cytokine profile. This inability to reduce the two major risk factors toward developing allergy may lead to sensitization.

The role of bacteria in the formation of allergy is strengthened by clinical studies demonstrating that there are differences in the microflora between allergic and nonallergic individuals. One study revealed that nonallergic individuals had higher counts of aerobic bacteria during the first week of life, as well as greater numbers of *Lactobacillus* at 1 month and 1 year of age. At age 1 to 2 years, the allergic children have greater prevalence of *Staphylococcus aureus* and Enterobacteriaceae and fewer *Bacteroides* and *Bifidobacterium*.[103] Allergic children also appear to have greater number of *Clostridium* at 3 weeks of age.[103,104] *Bifidobacterium* are known to elicit a Th1 type immune response.[105] In another study, allergic infants were found to have high levels of the adult-type *Bifidobacterium adolescentis* compared with healthy infants who had greater numbers of *B. bifidum*. Comparison of the adhesive properties of these two strains found that *B. bifidum*'s adhesive abilities were significantly greater. These results suggest that the greater adhesive qualities may help to stabilize the mucosal barrier and prevent absorption of antigenic proteins.[106]

Lifestyles that limit antibiotic use and encourage the ingestion of fermented foods appear to result in a decreased risk of developing allergy. Similarly, the early use of antibiotics appears to be a risk factor for developing later atopic disease,[107] although a large Dutch cohort study suggests that such early antibiotic exposure may predispose an individual to wheezing but not to the development of eczema.[108] Inflammation is triggered by toll-like receptors (TLRs), a group of evolutionarily conserved pattern recognition receptors present in intestinal epithelial cells and antigen presenting cells.[107] More than 10 members of the TLR family have been described, each of them possessing specificity toward microbial surface structure elements.[107]

BACTERIAL FLORA AND ANTIBIOTICS

Nearly all antibiotics have an effect on the bacterial flora. The effect is dependent on the intraluminal concentration, as well as the antimicrobial spectrum.[22] Such an effect can be advantageous, and numerous studies have demonstrated the reduction of wound infections following surgery with the use of prophylactic antibiotics.[109,110] Among neutropenic patients, intestinal colonization with gram-negative aerobic bacilli, especially *Pseudomonas aeruginosa*, frequently precedes infection. Prophylactic antibiotics to modify the intestinal flora have been shown to reduce the incidence of infection in this population.[110]

The use of oral ampicillin or penicillin suppresses the normal aerobic and anaerobic flora including *Bifidobacterium*, *Streptococcus*, and *Lactobacillus* spp. and causes overgrowth of *Klebsiella*, *Proteus*, and *Candida* spp.[111,112] However, administration of cefaclor, an oral cephalosporin, and cephalexin appear to cause little change, except for a reduction in Enterobacteriaceae.[112] Erythromycin administration results in fewer marked changes than observed with penicillins; however, there is a significant decrease in Enterobacteriaceae.[112] Oral gentamicin administration results in drastic changes including a marked decline in *E. coli*.[112] However, intravenous gentamicin is excreted into the intestine with bile at lower concentrations and thus alters the flora only slightly.[113] Cefpiramide, a parenteral expanded-spectrum cephalosporin, which is excreted in the bile at high concentrations, suppresses normal flora so markedly that almost all species of organisms are eradicated and the active growth of yeast is promoted.[112] There appears to be a rapid return of the disturbed flora to normal levels within 3 to 6 days after therapy,[112] although a minority of researchers believe recovery time could be longer, on the order of 2 weeks or greater.[114] Suppression of the normal flora results in lowered colonization resistance and promotes overgrowth of resistant organisms,[115] as well as allowing for colonization with pathogens such as *C. difficile*.

Antibiotics may also affect fecal bulk. Volunteers on a constant diet who were administered ampicillin and metronidazole were noted to have a 97% increase in their fecal bulk. This was accompanied by a 69% increase in fecal fiber. The author suggests that the absence of digestion of the fecal fiber by the indigenous flora was the mechanism by which the antibiotics resulted in increased fecal bulk.[116]

BACTERIAL OVERGROWTH

Bacterial overgrowth is the term used when there are excessive amounts of bacteria inhabiting the small intestine. Those disorders that alter small bowel motility appear to predispose individuals to the greatest extent. These include small bowel diverticula, surgically created blind loops, strictures, pseudo-obstruction, scleroderma, diabetic neuropathy, resection of small bowel including the ileocecal valve, cirrhosis, malnutrition, and abdominal radiation.[22] Bacteriologic analysis of the microflora includes aerobic and anaerobic bacteria. Bacterial concentrations can range from 10^7 to 10^9 cfu/mL and rarely to 10.[11,22]

Additional host factors that allow for bacterial overgrowth include defective gastric acid secretion and defective local immunity. The use of acid blockade significantly affects the mean gastric bacterial count, such that as the pH rises above 4, the bacterial count increased from 0 to $10^{6.4}$, and the mean number of bacterial species increased from 0.5 to 4.3.[117]

Clinical manifestations of bacterial overgrowth include diarrhea, steatorrhea, vitamin B_{12} deficiency, protein malnutrition, weight loss, and impaired sugar absorption.[24] There is also evidence that functional disorders such as irritable bowel syndrome may be caused by bacterial overgrowth.[118] These effects are mediated via increased deconjugation of bile salts, volatile fatty acids, alcohols, volatile amines, and hydroxyl fatty acids.[24] These products can result in increasing intraluminal osmolarity and subsequent diarrhea. Malabsorption appears more common when colonization includes anaerobes. Some speculate it is the deconjugation of bile acids, specifically by *Bacteroides* strains, that favors the growth of anaerobes.[119] B_{12} deficiency is thought to be due to uptake of the vitamin by the bacteria; indeed, ingested B_{12} in these patients is found in the feces bound to bacterial cell wall components.[22] Amino acid absorption is also impaired in overgrowth, with increased fecal nitrogen.[22] D-Lactic acidosis has also been linked to bacterial overgrowth and the inability of humans to rapidly metabolize D-lactate.[120]

An increased serum folate or reduced cobalamin provides indirect evidence of bacterial overgrowth. Permeability tests may reflect mucosal damage in overgrowth. Histologically, the intestinal mucosa may lose its villous architecture and most of its absorptive surface. The use of hydrogen breath testing has been shown to be useful. Endoscopic collection of duodenal juice for culture and quantification would be the gold standard. Initial treatment should be directed at the cause of the overgrowth. This is often inapparent, and thus oral broad-spectrum antibiotic therapy is typically employed.

TROPICAL SPRUE

Tropical sprue is characterized by chronic diarrhea, malaise, weight loss, and malabsorption of carbohydrates, fats, vitamin B_{12}, and folate. The disease effects tropical areas, most notably India and the Caribbean area.[22] Onset of symptoms is typically after gastroenteritis; small bowel overgrowth then ensues, and symptoms resolve with treatment including antibiotics.[121] There appears to be significant colonization of the small bowel with Enterobacteriaceae. The fecal flora of affected patients is abnormal in that aerobic organisms outnumber anaerobes.[122] Enterotoxigenic coliforms are thought to colonize the small intestine and contribute to the diarrhea. Histologically, there is villus blunting and infiltration of the lamina propria that are more marked than those found in bacterial overgrowth.[22] Here one also sees delayed small bowel transit.

PROBIOTICS

Documentation of the health benefits of bacteria in food dates back to as early as the Persian version of the Old Testament (Genesis 18:8), which states that Abraham owed his longevity to the consumption of sour milk.[123] In 1908, Nobel prize–winning Russian scientist Elie Metchnikoff suggested that the ingestion of *Lactobacillus* containing yogurt decreases the number of toxin-producing bacteria in the intestine and thus contributes to the longevity of Bulgarian peasants.[124] The term *probiotic* was first used in 1965 in contrast to the word *antibiotic* and defined as "substances secreted by one microorganism, which stimulates the growth of another."[123] A more complete definition would be, "A preparation of or a product containing viable, defined microorganisms in sufficient numbers, which alter the microflora (by implantation or colonization) in a compartment of the host and by that exert beneficial health effects on the host."[123] Current criteria for defining probiotics are found in Table 4-4. Effects of probiotics on improving health have been proclaimed in many areas, including immunomodulation,

TABLE 4-4. Defining Criteria of Microorganisms That Can Be Considered Probiotics

A probiotic should:
1. Be of human origin
2. Be nonpathogenic in nature
3. Be resistant to destruction by technical processing
4. Be resistant to destruction by gastric acid and bile
5. Adhere to intestinal epithelial tissue
6. Be able to colonize the gastrointestinal tract, if even for a short time
7. Produce antimicrobial substances
8. Modulate immune responses
9. Influence human metabolic activities (i.e., cholesterol assimilation, vitamin production, etc.)

cholesterol lowering, cancer prevention, cessation of diarrhea, avoidance of allergy and necrotizing enterocolitis, and treatment of *Helicobacter pylori* infection and inflammatory bowel disease, although for many these claims remain to be proven scientifically.[125] The potential benefits of probiotics have led industry to consider routine addition of these bacteria to infant formulas.[126]

Although typically considered benign and without pathologic potential, there is a report of a 1-year-old immunocompetent patient who was fungemic after being treated with *Saccharomyces boulardii* for gastroenteritis.[127] The Mayo Clinic reported eight patients immunocompromised after liver transplant who were found to have positive blood cultures for *Lactobacillus*.[128] Recently, two infants with short bowel syndrome were found to be bacteremic with probiotic strains of *Lactobacillus GG*.[129] The Food and Drug Administration (FDA) has no authority to establish a formal regulatory category for functional foods that include either probiotics or prebiotics.[130] Thus there is variability among products, and some studies have found that certain preparations contain no viable bacteria.[131]

Various bacteria have been identified as meeting the diagnostic criteria for probiotics, and these include *Bifidobacterium*, a major group of saccharolytic bacteria in the large intestine. It accounts for up to 25% of the bacteria in the adult colon and 95% of that in the breast-fed newborn. They do not form aliphatic amines, hydrogen sulfide, or nitrites. They produce vitamins, mainly B group, as well as digestive enzymes such as casein phosphatase and lysozyme.[132] *Bifidobacterium* produce strong acids as metabolic end products such as acetate and lactate to lower the pH in the local environment, which provides antibacterial effects. One study showed that the supplementation of bottle-fed infants with *Bifidobacterium* successfully lowered the fecal pH to 5.38, which was identical to that of breast-fed infants, yet significantly lower than that of bottle-fed infants, whose fecal pH was 6.38.[133] Determination of survivability found that on average, approximately 30% of ingested *B. bifidum* and 10% of *L. acidophilus* can be recovered from the cecum.[134]

Lactobacillus casei GG (LGG) is another common probiotic. *Lactobacillus* has no plasmids, meaning that antibiotic resistance is stable, and makes only L-lactic acid (not the D-isomer).[135] It inhibits other anaerobic bacteria in vitro including *Clostridium*, *Bacteroides*, *Bifidobacterium*, *Pseudomonas*, *Staphylococcus*, *Streptococcus*, and Enterobacteriaceae.[136] It has also been shown to inhibit the growth of pathogenic bacteria including *Yersinia enterocolitica*, *Bacillus cereus*, *E. coli*, *Listeria monocytogenes*, and *Salmonella*.[137] *Lactobacillus* generates hydrogen peroxide, decreases intraluminal pH and redox potential, and produces bacteriocins that can inhibit the growth of pathologic bacteria.[138] In general, colonization lasts only as long as the supplement is consumed. A study found that when LGG supplementation was stopped, it disappeared from the feces in 67% of volunteers within 7 days.[139]

Saccharomyces boulardii is a patented yeast preparation that has been shown to inhibit the growth of pathogenic bacteria both in vivo and in vitro. It lives at an optimum temperature of 37° C and has been shown to resist digestion, and thus reach the colon in a viable state. It appears to be unaffected by antibiotic therapy. However, once therapy is completed, it is rapidly eliminated.[140]

Probiotics and Promotion of Health

Immunomodulation

The ability of probiotics to affect the host's immune system remains ill defined. Good evidence exists for alterations in the humoral system, most notably IgA. However, effects on the cellular immune system and cytokine production are not as well established. Both human and rodent studies have documented an augmentation of the secretory IgA production during probiotic treatment. Intestinal IgA is a dimer that binds antigens and thus prevents their interaction with the epithelial cell.[141] Studies demonstrate that *L. casei* and *L. acidophilus* enhance the IgA production from plasma cells in a dose-dependent fashion.[142]

Other studies have documented that probiotics can alter cytokine production[143,144] and macrophage phagocytic capacity.[145,146] However, Spanhaak investigated the effects of *Lactobacillus casei* on the immune system in 20 healthy volunteers. In a placebo-controlled trial, the probiotic was found to have no effect on natural killer cell activity, phagocytosis, or cytokine production.[147]

More recent studies have focused on specific strains' ability to affect the immune system, and potential mechanisms by which these changes occur. *Lactobacillus reuteri* was shown to suppress human TNF and MCP, by processes mediated by activation of c-Jun and AP-1.[148,149] This same bacterial species produces reuterin (β-hydroxypropionaldehyde), a potent antipathogenic compound capable of inhibiting a wide spectrum of microorganisms including gram-positive bacteria, gram-negative bacteria, fungi, and protozoa.[149] The probiotic *E. coli* strain M-17 was shown to inhibit TNF-α-induced NF-κB signaling in a dose-dependent fashion.[150]

A direct comparison of the immune regulation of various probiotic strains found that *S. boulardii* could induce higher IgA and IL-10 levels, whereas *B. animalis* and *L. casei* allowed for antagonistic substance production.[151] A better understanding of the strain-specific changes to the immune system may allow us to select specific probiotics, or combinations thereof, for specific disease states.

Cholesterol Levels

Studies of animals randomized to receive yogurt with or without *Bifidobacterium* found that the total cholesterol of all rats fed yogurt was decreased. The probiotic group had a notable increase in high-density lipoprotein (HDL) cholesterol, and a lowering of the low-density lipoprotein (LDL) cholesterol by 21 to 31% compared with those rats fed whole milk.[152,153] The studies of probiotic use among humans appear somewhat mixed, although overall probiotics appeared to have little to no significant cholesterol-lowering effect.[154-159]

The mechanism by which probiotics might lower serum cholesterol levels remains unclear. Observations that 3-hydroxy-3-methylglutaryl coenzyme A reductase in the liver decreased significantly with the consumption of the probiotics point toward a decrease in cholesterol synthesis. Increases in the amounts of fecal bile acids suggest that there is a compensatory increased conversion of cholesterol to bile acids.[160] Others suggest the effect is secondary to precipitation of cholesterol with free bile acids formed by bacterial bile-salt hydrolase.[161] A final mechanism by which probiotics may have an effect is via hydrolysis of bile acids. Those bacteria that hydrolyze efficiently would lead to a faster rate of cholesterol conversion to bile acids and thus lower the serum cholesterol concentration.[162]

Probiotics and Disease

Diarrhea

The mechanism by which probiotics prevent or ameliorate diarrhea can be through stimulation of the immune system, through competition for binding sites on intestinal epithelial cells,[142,163,164] or through the elaboration of bacteriocins such as nisin.[165] These and other mechanisms are thought to be dependent on the type of diarrhea being investigated, and therefore may differ among viral diarrhea, antibiotic-associated diarrhea, and traveler's diarrhea.

The effect of *Lactobacillus GG* on the shortening of rotavirus diarrhea has been well documented. On average, the duration of diarrhea was shortened by 1 day in both hospitalized children[166-173] and those treated at home.[174] As to why LGG appears to be effective for viral diarrhea, but not bacterial, the author speculates that this is due to LGG enhancement of the expression of the elaboration of intestinal mucins. These glycoproteins appear to be protective during intestinal infections. However, the protective qualities are overcome by mucinase-producing bacteria.[175] Probiotics were also proven to increase the number of rotavirus-specific IgA-secreting cells and serum IgA in the convalescent stage,[168-170,176] suggesting that the humoral immune system plays a significant role in the probiotics' effect. Interestingly, a study found equal efficacy of heat-inactivated LGG versus viable bacteria in the treatment of rotavirus; however, the heat-inactivated strains did not result in an elevated IgA response at convalescence.[170] Finally, one study revealed that infants fed formula supplemented with probiotics had a lower risk of acquiring rotavirus-associated gastroenteritis.[177]

The success of probiotics in reducing or preventing antibiotic-associated diarrhea has also been convincing[178-180] and is supported by a Cochrane review.[181] Large studies of hospitalized patients on antibiotics revealed that 13 to 22% of the placebo group and 7 to 9% of the probiotic group developed diarrhea.[182-184] Other studies reveal that probiotics result in firmer stools, and patients have less abdominal pain.[135,185]

The use of probiotics for the treatment of *Clostridium difficile* diarrhea is a logical step, particularly given the historical use of fecal enemas in the treatment of relapsing *C. difficile*.[186,187] Indeed, this is supported by an early case report of four children with relapsing *C. difficile* that responded to supplement with LGG.[188] A study in which *Saccharomyces boulardii* was used in conjunction with standard antimicrobial treatment in 124 adult patients with *C. difficile* found that the probiotic group had no effect on those with their first infection, but the probiotic significantly inhibited further recurrence in those patients with prior

C. difficile disease.[189] Overall, the studies investigating probiotics for use of treatment or prevention of bacterial diarrhea, other than *C. difficile*, appear mixed.[190-196]

Allergy

The use of probiotics in allergic disease is based on their ability to improve gut barrier function and mature the host immune response. Probiotics have been shown to decrease gut permeability in suckling rats exposed to a prolonged cow's-milk challenge. This may be achieved via increase in the secretion of antibodies directed against β-lacto-globulin, a major antigen of the cow milk protein.[99]

Studies by Isolauri investigating cow's-milk-sensitive infants with atopic dermatitis revealed that probiotics greatly improved the extent and intensity of their eczema. Analysis of various inflammatory markers reflected a down-regulation of the T-cell-mediated inflammatory state and eosinophilic inflammatory activity. The author speculated that the probiotic generated enzymes that can act as a suppressor of lymphocyte proliferation and generate protein breakdown products that result in IL-4 down-regulation. Furthermore, an increase in secretory IgA helps in increasing antigen elimination.[197,198] A study by Kalliomaki provided LGG in a double-blind placebo-controlled fashion to pregnant mothers with a first-degree relative who was atopic. The newborn infants were then treated postnatally for 6 months. At 2 years of age, only 23% of the LGG group versus 46% of the placebo group were found to have atopic eczema.[199] However, other studies analyzing the effects of probiotics in the prevention or treatment of eczema have not been as favorable, and the results of a systematic review and a Cochrane analysis do not support their efficacy.[200,201]

Inflammatory Bowel Disease

It has long been conjectured that bacteria or other infectious agents play a role in the pathogenesis of inflammatory bowel disease (IBD). Indeed, it is well accepted that antibiotics are effective in the treatment of Crohn's disease, and certain animal models of colitis have phenotypic manifestations only when exposed to bacteria. Furthermore, anti-neutrophil cytoplasmic antibody (pANCA) associated with ulcerative colitis has been linked to bacteria that express a pANCA-related epitope.[202] Epidemiologic studies have found that *Bifidobacterium* colony counts are decreased in the feces of patients with Crohn's disease.[203,204]

Clinical studies of affected patients have demonstrated the efficacy of probiotics in maintaining remission in ulcerative colitis at rates equivalent or superior to that of mesalamine.[205-207] Among Crohn's patients, the addition of a probiotic to mesalamine resulted in a greater number of patients maintaining remission.[208] Probiotic bacteria have also been shown to be useful in the prevention of acute pouchitis postoperatively.[209] However, a study in children showed no beneficial effect of probiotics in the treatment of Crohn's disease.[210] Thus, according to a Cochrane analysis,[211] the overall efficacy of probiotics for the treatment or maintenance of remission in Crohn disease has not been established and requires further study with larger numbers of patients.

PREBIOTICS

Evidence of the beneficial effects of certain nonpathologic enteric bacteria, probiotics, gave birth to the concept of prebiotics. Gibson defined a prebiotic in 1995 as a "nondigestible food ingredient which beneficially affects the host by selectively

TABLE 4-5. Defining Criteria to Classify a Food Ingredient as a Prebiotic

A prebiotic should:
1. Be neither hydrolyzed nor absorbed in the upper part of the gastrointestinal tract
2. Be a selective substrate for one or more potentially beneficial commensal bacteria in the large intestine; as such, it should stimulate those bacteria to divide, become metabolically active, or both
3. Alter the colonic microenvironment toward a healthier composition
4. Induce luminal or systemic effects that are advantageous to the host

stimulating the growth of and/or activating the metabolism of one or a limited number of health promoting bacteria in the intestinal tract, thus improving the host's intestinal balance."[132] Because this concept has only been recently defined, there are fewer data to support their health-promoting effects. Examples of prebiotics include the fructooligosaccharides and complex oligosaccharides in human milk. Each of these satisfies the defining criteria of prebiotics as outlined in Table 4-5.

Evidence suggests that prebiotics improve the bioavailability of minerals such as calcium,[212-214] magnesium,[212,215,216] and iron for absorption.[217] Increased calcium absorption is hypothesized to be mediated by its increased solubility within the colon due to fermentation of the prebiotic and the subsequent decrease in intraluminal pH, through fermentation of fecal products to SCFAs,[218] or by an increased expression of calcium binding proteins such as calbindin-D9k.[219] This increase has been thought to be clinically relevant in the treatment and or prevention of diseases such as osteoporosis. However, human studies have been of short duration and therefore have not addressed the more important question of effect on bone mineralization.

A meta-analysis of 15 human studies from 1995 to 2005 on the effects of inulin showed that it was associated with a significant decrease in serum triacylglycerides, by 7.5%. Effects on total cholesterol were not as evident.[220] A recent study in which prebiotics were added to infant formula showed no effect on total cholesterol or LDL levels in the study infants as compared to those fed standard formula. Of note, the formula-fed infants did have lower cholesterol and LDL as compared to a group of breast-fed infants.[221] However, animal models do seem to indicate that intake of moderate amounts of inulin or oligofructose affects lipid metabolism.[222,223] The difficulty in demonstrating an equivalent effect in humans may be species or dose related. There does seem to be a greater effect of prebiotics in those individuals with elevated baseline cholesterol levels as opposed to those with normal levels. It is commonly accepted that the principal mechanism by which oligofructose and inulin produce a cholesterol-lowering effect is linked to a decrease in de novo hepatic lipogenesis,[224] although other mechanisms such as via the action of fermentation products (e.g., short-chain fatty acids) or increased cholesterol excretion in feces may play some role. Clearly more research will be needed to further define the role of prebiotics in manipulating lipid metabolism in humans.

Although health benefits are attributed to these compounds, they do have potential side effects. When inulin was given at a dose of 14 g/day, women reported an increase in flatulence, borborygmi, abdominal cramping, and bloating.[225] There also appears to be a laxative effect in which these compounds have been shown to increase the daily stool output from 136 g/day to 154 g/day.[226]

SYNBIOTICS

As Gibson introduced the concept of Prebiotics, he also speculated on the additional benefits one might see if prebiotics were combined with probiotics to form what he called a "synbiotic." He defined this as "a mixture of probiotics and prebiotics that beneficially affects the host by improving the survival and implantation of live microbial dietary supplements in the gastrointestinal tract by selectively stimulating the growth and/or by activating the metabolism of one or a limited number of health-promoting bacteria, and thus improving host welfare."[132] By virtue of the name, it is implied that the prebiotic should offer a selective advantage for the growth of the probiotic it is combined with to provide a synergistic effect. To date, there has been a limited amount of scientific research into this form of supplementation, and it is thus unclear whether this theoretical entity will provide any additional health-promoting effects above those afforded by the prebiotic or probiotic alone.

REFERENCES

22. Simon G, Gorbach S. The human intestine microflora. Dig Dis Sci 1986;31:147S–162S.
34. Long S, Swenson R. Development of anaerobic fecal flora in healthy newborn infants. J Pediatr 1977;91:298–301.
57. Pei Z, Bini EJ, Yang L, Zhou M, et al. Bacterial biota in the human distal esophagus. Proc Natl Acad Sci USA 2004;101:4250–4255.
123. Schrezenenmeir J, deVrese M. Probiotics, prebiotics, and synbiotics–approaching a definition. Am J Clin Nutr 2001;73:361S–364S.
200. Boyle RJ, Bath-Hextall FJ, Leonardi-Bee J, et al. Probiotics for the treatment of eczema: a systematic review. Clin Exp Allergy 2009;39: 1117–1127.
220. Brighenti F. Dietary fructans and serum triacylglycerols: a meta-analysis of randomized controlled trials. J Nutr 2007;137(11 Suppl):2552S–2556S.

See expertconsult.com for a complete list of references and the review questions for this chapter.

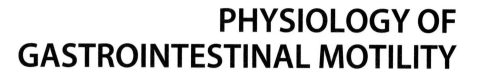

PHYSIOLOGY OF GASTROINTESTINAL MOTILITY

5

Franziska Mohr • Rita Steffen

This chapter discusses gastrointestinal motility – the coordinated motor function of the gastrointestinal tract (GIT) from the mouth down to the anorectal area. Developments in technology have allowed the functional assessment of all areas of the GI tract in both their healthy and diseased states. Normal anatomy and physiology is presented here. The abnormal physiology and specific disease states, which can be characterized by manometric and functional tests, are discussed in the organ-specific sections further on.

The development of the GIT is discussed in detail in Chapter 1.

Motility is the function of the gastrointestinal tract, which has the endowed and controlled power of spontaneous movement. Manometry is the study of this function and measures the pressure of gas or fluids by means of a manometer, which normally registers these changes in mm Hg.[1] Efforts to standardize motility protocols in pediatrics and adults are ongoing and evolving.[1,2]

The basic rule of the gut is that food stimulates contractions above and behind the food bolus and relaxation below or distal to the bolus, forming the peristaltic wave that is probably the most studied phenomenon in the functional assessment of motility in the GI tract. The term "receptive relaxation" describes the opening of the part of the GIT ahead of the bolus to receive the incoming ingested material.

The tubular GIT is functionally separated by specialized sphincters.

The circular and longitudinal layers of smooth muscle of the muscularis externa provide the segmentation for mixing and peristalsis. Manometry measures the timely contraction and relaxation of these muscles in the fasting and the fed state. The outer longitudinal layer is an intact sheath until it separates into three bands of muscle (taeniae coli) extending for the length of the colon. A syncytium of ganglion cells (or Meissner's plexus) occupies the submucosal layer of the gut, and another is situated anatomically between the two muscle layers (the myenteric or Auerbach's plexus). In recent years increasing attention has been devoted to refocusing on the role that interstitial cells of Cajal play on local electrical pacing of bowel contractions.

Smooth muscle contractions are controlled by three things:
- The enteric nervous system (ENS)[3]
- Peptide hormones
- The inherent timing of the myocytes themselves

Smooth muscle of the intestine is excitable tissue with three different potential states, resting, slow-wave, or action or spike potential. Spike potentials are a result of depolarization of the membrane potential due to intracellular accumulation of calcium ions, which causes coupling of smooth muscle

excitation-contraction. Local distention or stretching with activation of myenteric neurons and release of acetylcholinesterase results in depolarization of the membrane, which may cause slow waves to convert to action potentials in the myocytes. Bursts of action potentials are associated with muscle contractions, which are the basis of peristaltic movement of intestinal content from oral to caudal. Neurohumoral modulators influence this activity to span a segment of bowel.[4] The frequency of slow waves varies according to location in the GIT. Intricate control mechanisms are evident in the bowel during the fasting and the fed states. Motility measures these events in their temporal and spatial relationships.

The central nervous system receives and sends limited sympathetic and parasympathetic information into the GI tract. The ENS itself is composed of a stunning number of neurons, equal in magnitude to the number present in the spinal cord. The ENS controls the motility and secretion and responds to neuroendocrine peptides as well as autocrine, paracrine, and other transmitters.[5]

The development of normal GI motor activity is partly driven by the predetermined gestational timetable during fetal development and is also nurtured by suckling, swallow-induced esophageal peristalsis, and cyclic, triphasic small intestinal motor activity fronts.[6] Segmentation and local retention are necessary for optimal contact with brush border enzymes located on the microscopic intestinal villi. These functions are made possible by specialized motor activity that has evolved to sustain nutritional status and growth.

Assessment of motility in pediatric patients is challenging because of frequently suboptimal cooperation compared to adult patients. A spectrum of catheter sizes, spacing between pressure sensors, balloon sizes, and other modifications, plus a great deal of patience and interest, are all needed in order to gather reliable information on pediatric patients referred for motility tests.[7]

ESOPHAGEAL MOTILITY

Anatomical Considerations

The upper third of the esophagus contains striated muscle, followed by a zone of overlap with smooth muscle, whereas the distal two thirds of the hollow tube are formed by smooth muscle alone. The organization of the muscle layers is constant throughout the GIT, with an inner circular muscle layer surrounding the hollow viscus, wrapped by the outer longitudinal muscle layer. Neural control of the striated muscle of the upper esophagus originates in the nucleus ambiguus, whereas the ganglia that control the smooth muscle and lower esophageal sphincter (LES) arise in the dorsal motor nucleus. The central nervous system input to esophageal muscle is carried down via the vagus nerve from cell bodies located in the swallowing center of the medulla. Esophageal lengths have been studied from newborns to adult size and can be estimated by the Strobel formula.[8] Unlike other hollow viscera of the GIT, the esophagus lacks a serosal lining as it courses through the thoracic cavity.

The upper esophageal sphincter (UES) is the barrier keeping inspired air out of the GI tract and preventing ingesta from being aspirated into the trachea. The UES is tonically contracted between swallows. It relaxes for swallows, for releasing gases during eructation, and for vomiting. The pressures in the UES are not symmetric, as posterior pressures are higher than those in the anterior plane. The UES is coordinated with pharyngeal propulsive forces and opens normally to accept the food bolus. Multiple afferent cranial nerves (cranial nerves V, IX, and X) transmit information to the swallowing center in the medulla, and then efferent nerves (cranial nerves V, VII, IX, X, and XII) send control information to the oropharynx and upper esophagus to effect a swallow.

The development of the esophagus and disease-specific alterations of development are discussed in detail in Chapter 20 and 21, respectively.

Physiology of Esophageal Motility

Primary peristalsis is stimulated by swallowing a bolus, and primary peristaltic waves travel at a velocity of 2 to 4 cm/s. Secondary peristaltic waves are seen following distention of the esophagus by a balloon, refluxate, or retained food and resemble primary peristaltic waves in amplitude and duration. Tertiary peristaltic waves are lower amplitude, spontaneous, and nonperistaltic. They may be seen on barium roentgenography and result from independent depolarization of esophageal smooth muscle, not directed by the swallowing center of the brain. The presence of some "dropped" peristaltic waves, which begin in the upper esophagus and are not transmitted all the way to the distal esophagus, is also found in normals. Some double-peaked waves may be encountered in normals, but the presence of triple-peaked waves is only seen in association with spasm of the esophagus.

In a study of 95 normal adults, Richter et al.[9] concluded that

1. Distal esophageal contractile amplitude and duration after wet swallows increases with age.
2. Triple-peaked waves and wet-swallow-induced simultaneous contractions should suggest an esophageal motility disorder. Double-peaked waves are a common normal variant.
3. Dry swallows have little use in the current evaluation of esophageal peristalsis.[9] This landmark study provided the basis for current practice of giving water to the patient to swallow while recording the peristaltic response. When the amplitude of esophageal waves drops below 40 mm Hg, the effectiveness of the stripping wave also diminishes. In adults, amplitudes less than 35 mm Hg are hypotensive, and those greater than 180 mm Hg are hypertensive,[10] but accumulation of comparable data in normal children has been slower.

Manometric evaluation combined with prolonged 24-hour pH testing has shown that low basal LES pressure and transient inappropriate relaxations of the LES have a role in the pathophysiology of gastroesophageal reflux in children.[11,12] When 49 esophageal manometry (EM) studies were done in 27 premature babies, nonperistaltic pressure waves were speculated to contribute to poor clearance of refluxed material.[13]

Corroborating evidence from 42 children with gastroesophageal reflux disease (GERD) came from a study with paired EM and pH testing that replicated the findings of increased esophageal acid exposure, reduced basal LES pressure and peristalsis, and more drift of basal LES tone compared to healed patients. Drift in basal LES pressure had the highest predictive value for GERD refractory to therapy.[14] The topic of reflux as a motility disorder in itself and its treatment and complications is covered in more detail in Chapters 20 and 22.

Figures 5-1 and 5-2 demonstrate normal esophageal motor propagation from the pharynx to the LES. Normal relaxation of the LES is shown in Figure 5-1, and normal relaxation of the UES is shown in Figure 5-2.

LES pressure remains largely unchanged from birth through adulthood, although variable basal pressures have been reported in different study cohorts. As the esophageal length grows with age, so do the UES and LES lengthen from infancy to adulthood. The circular muscle component of the LES is responsible for the tonic end-expiratory pressure. The diaphragmatic component of the LES is responsible for the phasic changes in pressure that occur with respiratory excursions of the chest. The LES measures close to 1 cm in the newborn and grows to a length of 2 to 5 cm in the adult.[15] There is an increase in LES pressure that develops in premature infants studied from 27 to 41 weeks' gestational age.[16] Although esophageal peristalsis appears to take longer to mature, LES basal pressure and relaxation have been noted to be well developed even at early postconceptual age. LES pressures averaged 20.5 ± 1.7 mm Hg in the fasting state compared with 13 ± 1.3 mm Hg in the fed state in healthy premature infants.[13] Many factors have been identified to have an influence on LES pressure, including medications, hormones, and certain types of food.

Tracking the neuromuscular development of the GI tract in the preterm infant has led to increased understanding of feeding difficulties in this age group. The ontogeny of this maturation process leads to arrival of normal pattern of innervation and contractile activity that can be measured in near-term infants.[17] There are significant differences in performing and analyzing the spectrum of motility disorders in pediatric patients compared to adults. An appreciation of developmental stages of GI function and age-related expression of motility disorders is required to diagnose and treat infants, children, and adolescents.

Phasic contractions are isolated peaks of pressure above the baseline that are seen from the pharynx to the rectum. Phasic contractions represent the activity front of the muscle. Sequential phasic contractions in the esophagus and GIT are visually recognized as a peristaltic event, leading to aboral transport of intestinal secretions and ingested food through the GIT. Computer software is available to scan manometric tracings for peristaltic sequences and quantitatively measure the amplitude, velocity, and duration of the contractions. Thus, phasic contractions are readily recognizable motor events that occur throughout the GIT and occur in organized patterns that are characteristic to the segment of digestive tract under investigation. It is the regular occurrence of these patterns that has allowed gastrointestinal manometry to map out normal and, hence, abnormal motility in patients.

Characteristics of normal and abnormal esophageal motility are presented in Table 5-1 and Table 5-2, respectively.

The neural control of deglutition and the esophagus is discussed in more detail in Chapter 20.

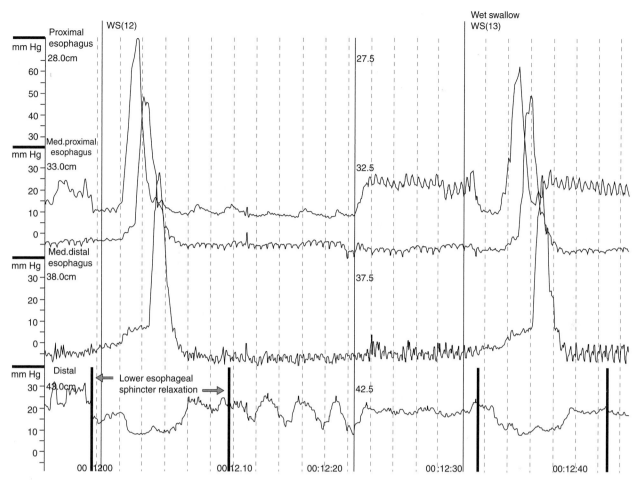

Figure 5-1. Normal esophageal manometry demonstrating sequential peristaltic waves in the first three rows in the esophagus. The tracing at the bottom is from the lower esophageal sphincter, which relaxes from baseline, then returns to baseline, effectively closing the sphincter. A second wet swallow approximately 30 seconds later provides an almost identical repeated pattern of the waveforms to the right.

GASTRIC MOTILITY

Designed for optimal digestion and absorption, the stomach provides a combination of mixing and forward propulsion of food. The fundus of the stomach dilates to accommodate liquid and gas, and the antrum grinds and triturates food particles before they are propelled into the duodenum. Particles greater than 5 mm are retrojected into the fundus for further milling into smaller pieces. Control of the stomach is diverse in origin and is partly governed by its own inherent electrical control activity.

Gastric function can be measured with radionuclide gastric emptying studies, electrogastrography (EGG), antroduodenal manometry (ADM), and other studies. Normal and abnormal gastric function and its assessment are discussed in more detail in Chapters 5 and 29, respectively.

MOTILITY OF THE SMALL INTESTINE AND COLON

Anatomical Considerations

In the neonate, the small intestinal length is about 270 cm, and it grows and develops to a final length of 400 to 500 cm in the adult. It extends to the ileocecal junction (ICJ), and its motor function dictates the rate of nutrient absorption by regulation

of the contact time between the absorptive surface area and the ingested food bolus. The ICJ prevents reflux of the colonic content into the small intestine and represents a sphincteric structure. Of the two muscular layers of the small intestine, the function of the muscularis mucosa is poorly defined at this point, whereas the muscularis externa seems to play the predominant role in the process of food propulsion and digestion. Contractions of the inner, circular layer of the muscularis externa lead to luminal occlusion and displacement of gut contents. Inhibition and disinhibition of adjacent circular muscle leads to segmentation, an important function during digestion. Bolus transit is facilitated by contractions of the outer, longitudinal layer of the muscularis externa, which will lead to shortening of the gut and widening of the lumen.

The saclike structure of the cecum serves a storage function. In the colon, three longitudinal muscle strips (taeniae coli) are overlying a circumferential circular muscle layer in the ascending, transverse, and descending colon and spread to envelop the rectosigmoid colon. Contractions of these two muscle layers facilitate the prominent mixing pattern of the colon through narrowing of the lumen and shortening of the colon. Colonic motility shows dominant mixing and less coordinated aboral propulsion to achieve sufficient time for the slow process of fecal desiccation. In the rectum, transverse mucosal folds extend past the midline to slow fecal passage and to help retain stool in the rectosigmoid region.

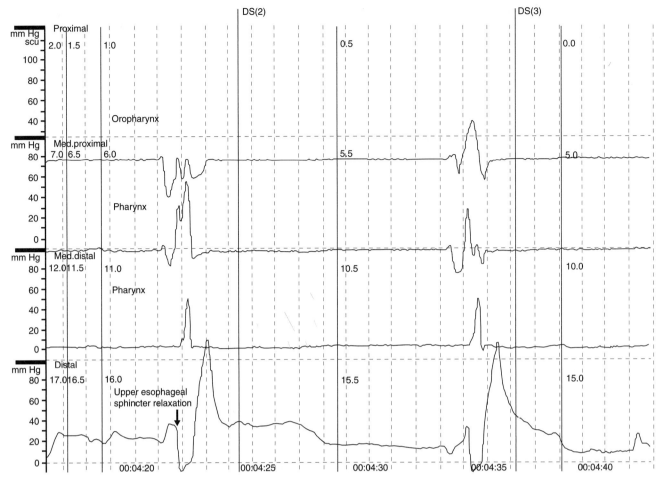

Figure 5-2. Normal esophageal manometry demonstrating oropharyngeal pressure waves in the upper three rows with a swallow. The lowest tracing shows a pressure sensor in the upper esophageal sphincter with baseline tonic pressure approximately 20 to 40 mm Hg. The UES relaxes to open, coordinated in timing to receive the bolus from the hypopharynx, then closes by returning the pressure back up to the baseline. Two sequential swallows are shown, separated in time by about 30 seconds.

The anus comprises smooth muscle, which forms the internal anal sphincter (IAS) as a thickened extension of the circular muscle layer, as well as the three strands of striated muscle of the external anal sphincter (EAS). Through tonic contractions, the levator ani muscles (puborectalis, pubococcygeus, and iliococcygeus) maintain continence.

Small Intestinal and Colonic Transit

Small intestinal transit shows great variability in humans and ranges from 78 to 392 minutes in healthy adults. Slower transit times have been reported in the obese or postmenopausal women,[20,21] although in general the transit times seem to be unaffected by the aging process.[22] During digestion, liquids and solids are leaving the stomach at different speeds; however, in the small intestine both are propelled equally, and the caloric density and nutrient class dictate the transit time. Protein and fat solutions have a relatively slower transit in proportion to the number of calories. This process allows for optimal absorption for all ingested nutrients.[23]

Colonic transit is a slow process and lasts for 1 to 2 days in healthy individuals. As observed for the small-intestinal transit times, colonic transit is slower in women than in men.[21] It is affected by the menstrual cycle and slows during the follicular phase.[24] The colonic microflora can affect colonic transit, as

TABLE 5-1. Esophagus: Normal Values

LES	Basal pressure: <1 year, 40-45 mm Hg; >1 year, 28-33 mm Hg Other studies: infant to 2 years vary from 13 to 27 mm Hg 22.4 ± 4.7 mm Hg [18] 29.1 ± 2.4 mm Hg [15] Relaxation at the time of the swallow almost completely to baseline Relaxation timed to relaxation of UES
Body	Resting pressure: varies with respiration, lower than gastric baseline pressure Amplitude > 30-40 mm Hg, < 180 mm Hg; duration 2-4 cm/s Need more data on normal children.
UES	Resting pressures: 30-150 mm Hg, 18-44 cm H20 in infants (19) Relaxation at the time of the swallow almost completely to baseline, relaxes at same time as LES

LES, lower esophageal sphincter; UES, upper esophageal sphincter.

observed in a study in which ingestion of the probiotic *Bifidobacterium animalis* shortened colonic transit time in women.[25] Recently, data on normal values for segmental and total colonic transit time (CTT) have been contributed to the relatively small volume of literature available in pediatric patients. Transit was measured in 22 healthy children (median age, 10 years; range, 4 to 15 years) after they ingested markers daily for 6 consecutive days. Using Abrahamsson's method, a single abdominal

TABLE 5-2. **Abnormal Esophageal Manometry**

Abnormal Esophageal Manometry	
Cricopharyngeal achalasia	Dysfunctional, incomplete relaxation of the UES
	May be suspected by a prominence of CP muscle radiologically
	The UES spasm is often not corroborated manometrically
CP/UES low pressures	With neuromuscular disorders, places child at risk for recurrent aspiration
Achalasia	Absence of peristaltic waves in the body (required for diagnosis)
	Elevated resting pressure in the body may be seen with a "water balloon" or "common cavity" type of appearance with simultaneous waves
	Incomplete LES relaxation, but this is variable
	Elevated LES resting pressure
	Dilated esophagus will have higher baseline pressure than gastric baseline pressure
	May have variable abnormalities in UES, such as elevated resting pressure
Vigorous achalasia	Subgroup of achalasia patients who have the above findings, plus tertiary esophageal contractions of high amplitude
Chagas disease	Some tertiary care centers may see patients from Latin America, or parents may have an adopted child with achalasia secondary to infection with *Trypanosoma cruzi*
Spasm or Disorders Characterized by Elevated Pressure:	
Nutcracker esophagus	High-amplitude, usually >180 mm Hg, peristaltic waves
	High-amplitude nonperistaltic contractions in distal esophagus
	Common to see increased duration of waves
Nonspecific spasm	More common than nutcracker or DES in childhood
	Multiple contractions of varying amplitude and duration may follow a single swallow
	Baseline pressure may be elevated
	Contractions may be simultaneous and nonperistaltic
	Occasionally pressures exceeding 300 mm Hg are seen in spastic disorders
Diffuse esophageal spasm	Distal esophageal amplitudes > 140 mm Hg, duration prolonged >7 seconds; multiple contractions with these characteristics follow one swallow
	At least 10% of wet swallows are repetitive, simultaneous (nonperistaltic) contractions
	Sequences of normal peristalsis
	Increased duration and amplitude of contractions, but some will have normal amplitude
	Most have normal LES; however some demonstrate incomplete LES relaxation or hypertensive LES
Hypertensive LES	Elevated LES pressure, >45 mm Hg
	LES relaxes normally and esophageal peristalsis is normal
Other Disorders	
Nonspecific motor disorders	May see dropped peristalsis in patients with esophagitis
	Simultaneous contractions, double-peaked contractions, tertiary contractions, or decreased-amplitude ineffective contractions (ineffective esophageal motility) <30 mm Hg in the distal esophagus
Gastroesophageal reflux	Normal peristalsis, but may show TLESRs
	Mean LES pressure may be significantly lower than normal
Dermatomyositis	Decreased proximal esophageal pressure
	Distal esophagus remains normal
Scleroderma	Decreased LES resting pressure
	Incomplete LES relaxation
	Absence of peristaltic wave or diminished waves in distal esophagus
	Proximal esophagus remains normal until later in the disease when striated muscle in the proximal third begins to appear

CP, cricopharyngeal; DES, diffuse esophageal spasm; LES, lower esophageal sphincter; TLESR, transient lower esophageal sphincter relaxation; UES, upper esophageal sphincter.

x-ray set at low radiation was taken on day 7. The mean total CTT was 40 hours with the upper limit of normal established at the 95th percentile at 84 hours. Each segment was found to have the following upper limits: ascending colon: 14 hours, transverse colon: 33 hours, descending colon: 21 hours, and rectosigmoid: 41 hours.[26]

Specialized Cells of the Small Intestine and Colon

The normal motor activity of the small intestine and colon relies on the intricate combination of functions delivered by different specialized cell types of the intestine. Smooth muscle, nervous tissue and the interstitial cells of Cajal (ICCs) each serve specific functions and have to work in unison to achieve normal digestion.

Smooth Muscle

The myocytes of the small intestine and colon are electrically active cells. They contain a single nucleus in their spindle-shaped bodies and maintain a resting potential between −40 and −80 mV through Na^+, K^+-ATPase activity. In the small intestine, slow waves of spontaneous membrane potential fluctuations have been documented at a speed of 11 to 12 cycles per minute (cpm). In the colon, these slow waves have been observed at frequencies ranging between 2 and 6 cpm as well as between 9 and 13 cpm. These slow waves control frequency and direction of phasic contractions. Intracellularly rapid depolarization is followed by partial repolarization to a prolonged plateau phase of depolarization with subsequent full repolarization. Slow waves alone are insufficient to achieve contractions. Additional intestinal stimulants increase amplitude and duration of the slow wave plateau potential or induce rapid high-amplitude spike potentials leading to intestinal contractions.[27-29]

Nervous Tissue

The innervation of the small intestine and colon is directed through two distinct systems, intrinsic and extrinsic innervation. Intrinsic innervation is regulated predominantly through the myenteric plexus in the gut wall and for some motor reflexes through the submucosal plexus. It exceeds the extrinsic system greatly in the number of neurons and plays the dominant role in normal GI motility with the external innervation providing modulatory function. Extrinsic nerves connect to the extraintestinal ganglia, the spinal cord and the central nervous system (CNS). The vagus and splanchnic nerves innervate the small intestine all the way to the proximal colon. The innervation of the remainder of the colon and IAS is carried through the pelvic nerves and the EAS and pelvic floor muscles receive their input through the pudendal nerves.

Intrinsic Innervation. The enteric nervous system (ENS) has the ability to initiate physiological motor activity even when no extrinsic input is received. As in the CNS, no blood vessels and connective tissue are present in the myenteric ganglia, which consist of neurons and glial cells only. Nutrition is provided through diffusion in the interstitial fluid. Most myenteric neurons contain either tachykinins (40 to 45% of neurons) or vasoactive intestinal polypeptide (VIP) (40 to 45% of neurons) with no overlap between the two. Tachykinin neurons mediate excitatory function through release of substance P, neurokinin A, and acetylcholine, whereas the inhibitory functions are provided through the VIP and nitric oxide (NO) containing myenteric neurons.[30,31] In addition, serotonin 5-HT$_4$ receptors have been found on enteric neurons. Activation of the presynaptic receptor through 5-HT$_4$ agonists as well as inhibition of serotonin reuptake with citalopram leads to increased phasic contractions in healthy humans.[32,33] Cholinergic effect on colonic motility has been shown through cyclooxygenase 1 (COX-1) and COX-2 in myenteric ganglia.[34]

Extrinsic Innervation. The parasympathetic and sympathetic nerve systems carry efferent extrinsic fibers that connect to the enteric ganglia in the myenteric plexus. The efferent vagus nerves contain a combination of preganglionic parasympathetic excitatory as well as inhibitory fibers and sympathetic fibers from the cervical ganglia. The cell bodies of these nerves are found in the dorsal motor nucleus of the brainstem. Excitatory effects are mediated through activation of nicotinic receptors, whereas inhibition of motor activity is achieved through NO and VIP release. Stimulation of the pelvic nerves will lead to subsequent contraction of the colon, shortens colonic transit time, and facilitates anal relaxation. When stimulated the hypogastric nerve increases anal pressure through effects on the IAS. The EAS, however, shows increased activity after stimulation of the pudendal nerve.[35] Experimental review has shown that the distal GIT seems to be under tonic inhibitory control mediated through the sympathetic nervous system.[36]

The afferent fibers of the vagal nerve receive information from the small intestine and colon through the splanchnic nerves by way of second-order neurons from the dorsal horn of the spinal cord. Theses afferent nerve fibers terminate in the brainstem nucleus solitarius. The sensory fibers of the anus arise from the pudendal nerve. Sensory information is gathered through a variety of pathways. Free nerve endings respond to chemical stimuli, and mechanoreceptors are activated by passive distention or active contraction. Mesenteric and serosal receptors are thought to mediate visceral pain perception in response to tension or forceful contraction.[37-39]

Interstitial Cells of Cajal

The interstitial cells of Cajal are cells equipped for high metabolic activity and active ion transport. They contain a single nucleus, large numbers of mitochondria, and endoplasmic reticulum, as well as many surface membrane caveoli. At this point at least six distinct populations of ICCs have been identified in the small intestine. ICCs have been found within the myenteric plexus (ICC-MY), intramuscularly, as well as in the deep muscular plexus.[40] The colon shows prominent distribution of ICCs in the submucosal region. In the rectum and IAS, a high number of ICCs have been identified at the submucosal and myenteric borders and along the muscle bundles of the IAS.[41] Even In the EAS, a somatic muscle structure, ICCs can be found.[42]

ICCs in the small intestine express a variety of receptors including VIP$_1$, muscarinic receptor (M$_2$ and M$_3$), and neurokinin receptors (NK$_1$ and NK$_3$), which suggests modulation by neuronal pathways.[43] They are found in close proximity to excitatory muscarinic tachykinin neurons as well as inhibitory nitrinergic neurons in the deep muscular plexus and seem to play a significant role in neurotransmission.[44]

Another important role of the interstitial cells of Cajal is induction of slow-wave potentials through their inherent electrical pacemaker activity. In animal models, the absence of ICCs in the myenteric plexus as well as administration of monoclonal antibodies that diminish ICCs, abolishes any measurable slow-wave pattern.[45,46] The observed pacemaker pattern of small intestinal ICC-MY has been described as initial upstroke depolarization followed by a plateau phase.[47] In the colon, the ICCs at the submucosal border drive the slow-wave pattern and gradually diminish in the myenteric region. The pacemaker function of the ICCs is driven by cyclic ion fluctuations and is reduced when extracellular calcium is depleted or high potassium solutions for depolarization are used. However, L-type calcium channel blockers seem to have no effect on the electrical rhythm that depends on the release of calcium from intracellular stores as well as the rate of sarcoplasmic reticulum calcium refilling.[47-49] In addition, high-conductance chloride channels as well as potassium channels regulate membrane potential in ICCs and may help facilitate rhythmic intestinal pacemaking activities.[50-52]

Physiological Patterns in Small Intestinal Motility

In the fasting state, the migrating motor complex (MMC) occurs in three phases in the small bowel. Phase I is characterized by motor quiescence. In phase II, random, intermittent contractions similar to those in the fed state are seen. Phase III is characterized by high-amplitude, high-frequency contractions that sweep the intestinal contents toward the ileum. The peristaltic wave of the MMC may start anywhere from the lower esophagus to the small bowel. The antrum contracts at a frequency of 3 cpm and the small intestine at 11 to 12 cpm in phase III. This interdigestive pattern cleans the bowel of undigested residual food, bacteria, and sloughed enterocytes, all of which move ahead of the advancing front of intestinal contraction. In younger children the MMC occurs more frequently, and

TABLE 5-3. Antroduodenal Manometry

Normal – MMC Appears in Fasting State

Phase I – inactivity or quiescence
Phase II – intermittent contraction activity with random periodicity and amplitude
Phase III – Regular contractions in the antrum at 3 per minute, and in the small bowel at 11-13 per min complete the migrating motor complex
An MMC cycle lasts about 100 min, but depending on age may be more frequent in young children
Then a meal is given, and provocative medications if needed.
Fed state – Contractions occur irregularly and they vary in amplitude
Meal composition affects quality and amplitude of contractions.

Abnormal

In CIPO – retrograde contractions, low-amplitude contractions, absence of phase III, nonpropagated bursts of duodenal activity
Myopathic process – low-amplitude contractions, no phase III seen
Neuropathic process – abnormal wave form and propagation

CIPO, chronic intestinal pseudo-obstruction; MMC, migrating motor complex.

for older adolescents the interval between MMCs is about 100 minutes, similar to adults.

When the normal housekeeping function of the MMC is altered, stasis of intestinal contents promotes dilation of the small intestine and bacterial overgrowth. Disorders of gastric emptying such as gastroparesis are also evaluated with ADM, although radionuclide gastric emptying for solids and liquids should precede ADM for the evaluation of gastroparesis (Table 5-3). Feeding will abolish the MMC pattern, rendering the pattern back to phase II, which is optimal for mixing and absorption.

The pattern of normal ADM has been established in children with no upper GI or small bowel symptoms and was found to be similar to that of adults.[53] In a study by Ittmann et al. comparing ADM in 19 preterm infants to that in 9 term infants, fasting antral activity was found to be comparable in both groups. The data also suggested that the temporal association of antral duodenal motor activity develops in association with progressive changes in duodenal motor activity.[54] Data are available from a group of 95 children with signs and symptoms of motility disorder in contrast to 20 control children. The authors concluded that there are some manometric features that have a clear association with motility disorders in children:

- Absent, abnormal migration of or short interval between phase III of the MMC
- Persistent low-amplitude contractions
- Sustained tonic contractions[55]

In addition, when controlled for meal composition with standardized upright awake and recumbent sleep periods, circadian variation in ADM is known to occur in normal subjects.[56] The experience with ADM was felt to be best left to the referral center in one study, inasmuch as the authors encountered a frustratingly large number of nonspecific abnormalities in 72% of older patients. However, ADM was helpful in recommending a new therapy (medication, surgery, feeding, or referral) in 28.7% of patients.[57]

It is possible to measure GIT motility wherever the catheter can be reasonably and safely positioned. An example of this is ileal manometry in children following ileostomies and pull-through operations. In a group of 23 children who had ileal manometry studies (mean age, 7 years, range, 2 months to 17 years), some of the patterns were found to be different from those in adults, whereas contractions in infants and toddlers were similar to those in adults.[58] Functioning ileostomies were

cannulated and random phasic contractions were the most common feature recorded. Phase III of the MMC was found in only two of the 23 children. The ileum was found to have some characteristics in common with the proximal small bowel and the colon. In fact, the origin of the colonic high-amplitude propagating contraction (HAPC) was in the ileum in the form of propagating or clustered contractions in some of the patients.

Figure 5-3 demonstrates the pattern seen in normal ADM recording.

Physiological Motor Patterns in Colonic Motility

In contrast to small bowel motility in which fasting produces the MMC pattern, colonic manometry (CM) will demonstrate HAPCs with the stimulus of a meal. Food stimulates phasic and tonic motor activity in the colon, called the gastrocolonic reflex, and this can be seen within 10 minutes of ingestion. The amplitude of an HAPC varies widely from 50 mm Hg to more than 180 mm Hg and is defined as extending at least 30 cm of colon as detected by the pressure sensors. Pressures higher than this are associated with mass movement of colonic contents and defecation. Some definitions will vary in amplitude and distance of the colon traversed by the peristaltic sequence. The HAPC has consensus as being rapidly migrating, high-amplitude, long-duration contractions that move the contents of the colon toward the rectum. Low-amplitude peristaltic contractions are also seen, and these are also propagated sequences with lower amplitudes in the range of 5 to 40 mm Hg. Rectal motor complexes (RMCs) are a local phenomenon, occurring more frequently at night, at a frequency of 2 to 4 per minute and amplitude greater than 5 mm Hg and lasting about 10 minutes. RMCs are postulated to play a role in fecal continence.[59]

The circular muscle layer produces phasic contractions that are analyzed by their appearance as single pressure waves, the timing of groups of peristaltic waves, and the timing of phases or recurring motility patterns.[60] Colonic motor response has been shown to vary according to meal composition: carbohydrate meals will induce a response, but the response is shorter than with fatty meals. Fatty meals will induce prolonged, segmental, and retrograde phasic activity that may delay colon transit.[61] Antegrade propagation of sequenced phasic contractions is aboral propagation of the wave front. In the colon, retrograde or orally directed contractions function to mix fecal contents and facilitate absorption. Figure 5-4 demonstrates normal HAPC activity on CM. During sleep, colonic activity quiets considerably. By contrast, morning awakening is a stimulus to colonic motility, which may contribute to the regularity some individuals experience in the timing of bowel actions. Also recognized are low-amplitude propagated phasic contractions, which occur more frequently in a 24-hour cycle than HAPCs. Although the significance of these awaits further elucidation, it is speculated that LAPCs play a role in preserving nocturnal fecal continence. The sigmoid colon may have a role in protecting continence, as it is here that the flow of fecal contents is considerably slowed before reaching the rectum. In the rectum, RMCs have been identified on prolonged colonic manometry and are also speculated to play a role in preserving nocturnal continence.[59] The infant will defecate spontaneously by reflex, and the older developing child learns to withhold bowel movements until a convenient or appropriate time for emptying the colon. Manometric findings in colonic motor studies are presented in Table 5-4.

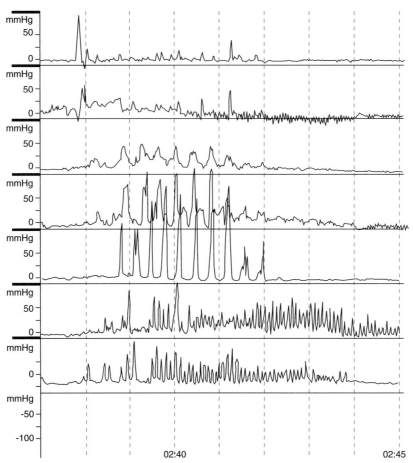

Figure 5-3. Normal antroduodenal manometry. The recording is taken as the catheter migrates upward. The top row is pharyngeal, the second row is in the UES, and the third and fourth rows are in the esophagus. The fifth row is recording strong phasic antral contractions at a frequency of 3 cpm, and the last rows are picking up the migrating motor complex in the duodenum. The frequency of contractions in the duodenum is 11-14 cpm.

Colonic distention appears to be a stimulus for contraction to propel stool in a caudad direction, although some retrograde contractions will occur and result in mixing and segmentation of stool. In a study combining CM and urodynamic studies in children with constipation and voiding difficulties, CM was found to be abnormal in all subjects. In the subgroup in whom neuropathy affecting both the colon and urinary bladder was present, successful treatment of the constipation did not result in resolution of urinary symptoms.[62] This is in contrast to the improvement expected in children with frequent urinary tract infections and vesicoureteral reflux secondary to chronic functional fecal retention with megarectum, fecal impaction, and encopresis.

Similar findings and natural history would be expected in children with spinal cord dysfunction, such as myelomeningocele or trauma. In a review of 32 CM studies in children who were not found to have colonic disease, it was found that HAPCs are more frequent in younger children before and after a meal, and that colonic contractions that are different in morphology from the HAPC occur more commonly with increased age.[63]

ADDITIONAL MOTOR FUNCTIONS

Ileocolonic Junction

The ICJ plays a significant role in the prevention of coloileal fecal reflux. The acute angle at the insertion of the ICJ into the colon likely plays a dominant role in this function. If the tissue sustaining this acute angle is destroyed or the ICJ is excised, the safeguard function of the ICJ against fecal reflux is no longer effective[64] and ileal fecal bacterial count increases.[65] Cecal delivery of ileal content alternates between bolus movements and periods of stasis, implying that the ICJ helps to regulate colonic filling.[66] The ICJ resembles a sphincteric structure and shows phasic contractions within a localized high-pressure zone; however, only a small proportion of MMC cycles seem to traverse the ICJ into the colon in humans.[67] Ingestion of food increases both ICJ tone and phasic activity, which is controlled through extrinsic and intrinsic pathways. Distention of the colon will lead to reflex ICJ contractions that are not abolished even when the vagal or pelvic nerves are blocked.[68] However, transection of the splanchnic nerve blocks this reflex. In a similar fashion, when the extrinsic pathways are interrupted, the phasic ICJ contractions increase as a result of muscarinic receptor activity.[69]

Anus and Pelvic Floor

The anal canal averages 2.8 cm in adults and exhibits gender differences with larger diameters in men than in women.[70] An additional high-pressure zone extends upward into the rectum for as much as 6 cm in adults and aids in achieving fecal continence. At baseline resting anal canal pressure is reflective of IAS tone, because 75 to 85% of the tone is contributed from its

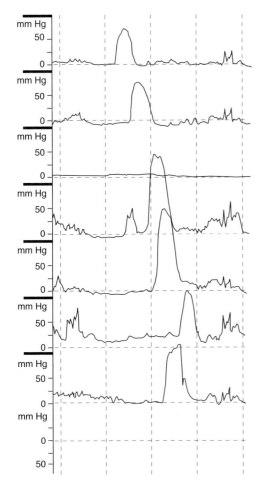

Figure 5-4. Normal colonic manometry. This recording demonstrates normal postprandial high-amplitude propagating contractions (HAPCs). These contractions are phasic, or isolated peaks from baseline, and usually more than 100 mm Hg. The recording sensors are located 10 cm apart, and the top tracing represents the most proximal port located in the cecum. The lowest tracing represents a pressure port recording from the rectosigmoid junction. On the left a contraction starts in the fourth row down, corresponding to the distal transverse colon near the splenic flexure, and propagates over 30 cm to the rectosigmoid. About 2 min later another HAPC is recorded to the right, this time starting at the ascending colon and propagating down to the rectosigmoid region.

tonic contraction. The remaining 15 to 25% is contributed by the overlap with part of the EAS. Squeeze pressure indicates the voluntary augmentation of pressure achieved by the EAS. Maximal voluntary squeeze pressures are measured and are normally expected to double the amount of baseline pressure, but often can exceed this. Voluntary recruitment of the squeeze exercise is represented graphically as an upsurge in baseline pressure and represents the phasic EAS contraction, which is important in preserving continence during cough, sneezing, lifting, and exercise[71] (Figure 5-5).

Again, data in children are limited. In a study by Benninga et al. of 13 normal children (age range, 8 to 16 years), resting anal tone was 33 to 90 mm Hg, maximum squeeze pressure was 81 to 276 mm Hg, threshold for rectal sensation (volume first sensed) was 5 to 50 mL, the threshold for eliciting the rectoanal inhibitory reflex (RAIR) was 5 to 40 mL, and the critical volume (volume of first urge or "call to stool") was 90 to 180 mL.[72]

The transitional zone above the pectinate line, the anal crypt region, and the anal canal are rich in free and organized nerve

TABLE 5-4. Colonic Manometry

Normal Values

Some are available, more information on normal children needed
HAPCs – 80-100 mm Hg, with meal and/or bisacodyl. HAPCs last for 10 s and travel at least 30 cm of the colon.
LAPCS – 5-40 mm Hg, speculated to have role in nocturnal continence
Rectal motor complex – seen more frequently at night, also thought to have a role in nocturnal continence. Amplitude >5 mm Hg, frequency 2-4 per min[59]

Abnormal Values

No gastrocolic reflex or augmentation of contractions after a high-fat, high-calorie-density meal
Absent HAPCs

HAPC, high-amplitude propagating contraction; LAPC, low-amplitude propagating contraction.

endings that differentiate among solid, liquid, and gaseous anal content and promote fecal continence. In the sitting position, the anorectal angle tightens, which contributes to fecal continence. In contrast, a squatting position or hip flexion facilitates opening of the anorectal angle, which leads to easier defecation that requires less straining.[73] During voluntary defecation, relaxation of the puborectalis facilitates IAS relaxation and opens the anorectal angle further; in addition, rectal contractions elicit propulsion of fecal content through increased rectal pressure. In contrast, flatus passage is not associated with any change in the anorectal angle. Rapid pressure increase in the rectum with simultaneous colonic contractions forces the gas past the acute angle without allowing solids or liquids to pass at the same time.[74]

Figure 5-6 demonstrates the appearance of the normal RAIR.

Fewer data on normal values in children are available compared to adults. The information from Nurko et al.[75] is summarized in Table 5-5.

SUMMARY

Manometry of the digestive tract from the mouth to the anorectal area, together with the other laboratory techniques such as gastric emptying, marker studies for colon transit time, impedance monitoring, and other tests of functional gastrointestinal tract information, is still evolving as a diagnostic tool for digestive motility disorders. Nevertheless, all of these tools have already become indispensable for the pediatric gastroenterologist.

Because the design of the catheter is related to its application, a range of catheter lengths and spacing between sensors is needed for children. In older children, spacing is consequently farther apart to cover more of the intestine. There is a lack of standardization for some of the motility protocols and contraction characteristics; the diversity of sizes and spacing of recording sites contributes to this problem when comparing multiple authors' manuscripts in the literature. Most of these studies receive a combination of qualitative and quantitative analysis. Recognition of artifacts is essential to interpreting all motility studies, because artifacts must always be excluded from analysis. Artifacts are most often secondary to motion of the child, coughing and movement of the catheter out of the desired zone of interest. Caution is advised in interpreting motility studies to avoid overreading and to exclude artifacts from the analysis.

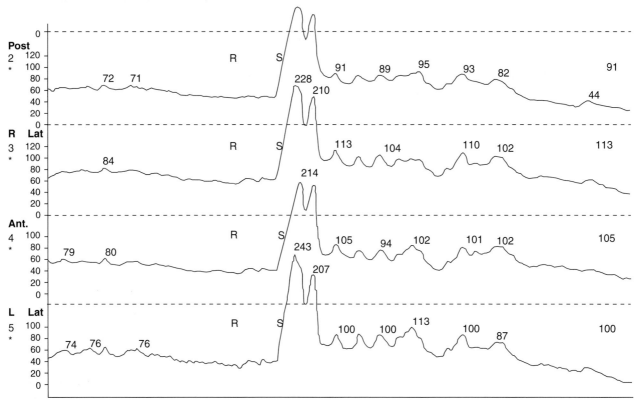

Figure 5-5. Anorectal manometry. Normal voluntary squeeze pattern in the anal canal is demonstrated in all four quadrants as an abrupt rise from resting baseline pressure to form a double-peaked or M-shaped pattern.

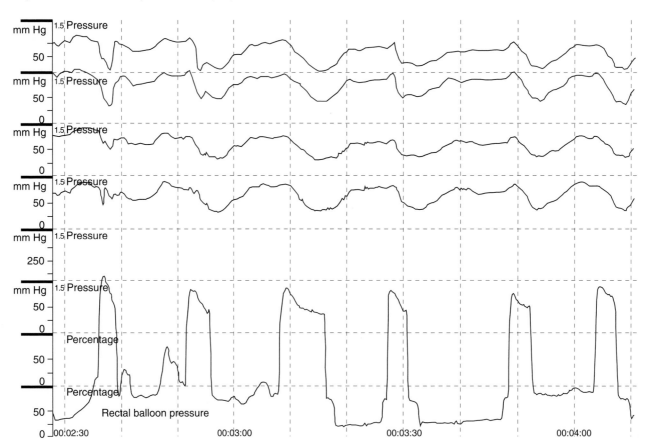

Figure 5-6. Normal anorectal manometry in a 17-month old-child: no sedation was used, and the patient sucked on a bottle during the test. The top four tracings measure pressure in four quadrants of the anal sphincter, and the lowest tracing indicates the pressure of air instilled into the rectal balloon. Corresponding reflex drops in the baseline smooth muscle of the internal anal sphincter appear in the tracings immediately above the inflation stimulus. Serial inflations show the reflex drop to be easily reproduced with volumes of air ranging from 20 to 40 mL. The tracing demonstrates a well-developed rectoanal inhibitory reflex, ruling out Hirschsprung's disease. At the far left, an abrupt drop in pressure is considered to be artifact caused by catheter migration out of the sphincter zone. Artifactual drops in pressure are distinguished from the third reflex relaxation in this series, which is a smooth decline in pressure followed by a smooth recovery to baseline pressure.

TABLE 5-5. **Normal Anorectal Manometry**

Normal (Limited Data)

IAS (smooth muscle) and EAS (striated muscle) are in a state of tonic contraction

75-85% of basal anal canal tone is from the IAS, remaining 15-25% from the EAS

Length of the sphincter may be only 5 mm in a small infant and vary from 2 to 4 cm in older children. Anal canal length (varies with age): 3.3 ± 0.8 cm

Basal pressure varies from 25 to 85 cm water.

Squeeze pressures resulting from voluntary contraction of the EAS should normally double or triple from baseline resting pressure.

Rectal pressure: rises with filling with stool, balloon distention, and straining (Valsalva maneuver)

IAS shows RAIR with drop in pressure in response to rectal distention, and the amplitude of the reflex relaxation increases with increasing balloon distention volumes.

Threshold volume is the minimum amount of air that will cause the RAIR

Sensory Volumes

Volume first sensed (VFS) – threshold of rectal sensation: 5 ± 2 mL to 14 ± 7 mL air

Volume of first urge ("critical volume," VFU) – minimum volume sensed creating a sensation of urge or call to stool; critical volume: 101 ± 39 mL

Maximum volume tolerated (MVT) – volume of constant relaxation: 104 ±49 mL

Defecation Dynamics

Resting anal pressure: 57 ± 10 mm Hg to 67 ± 12 mm Hg

Maximum squeeze pressure: 118 ± 32 to 140 ± 52 mm Hg

Strain

Cough

Modification

Modification with biofeedback, coaching maneuvers identified as needing improvement, Such as: recognition of rectal sensation, relaxation of the EAS upon straining (corrects PPC), and increasing intra-abdominal and intrarectal pressures upon straining.

EAS, external anal sphincter; IAS, internal anal sphincter; PPC, paradoxical puborectalis contraction; RAIR, rectoanal inhibitory reflex.

REFERENCES

16. Newell SJ, Sarkar PK, Durbin GM, et al. Maturation of the lower oesophageal sphincter in the preterm baby. Gut 1988;29:167–172.
19. Sondheimer JM. Upper esophageal sphincter and pharyngoesophageal motor function in infants with and without gastroesophageal reflux. Gastroenterology 1983;85:301–305.
26. Wagener S, Shankar KR, Turnock RR, et al. Colonic transit time–what is normal?. J Pediatr Surg 2004;39:166–169.
28. Rae MG, Fleming N, McGregor DB, et al. Control of motility patterns in the human colonic circular muscle layer by pacemaker activity. J Physiol 1998;510(Pt 1):309–320.
54. Ittmann PI, Amarnath R, Berseth CL. Maturation of antroduodenal motor activity in preterm and term infants. Dig Dis Sci 1992;37:14–19.
55. Tomomasa T, DiLorenzo C, Morikawa A, et al. Analysis of fasting antroduodenal manometry in children. Dig Dis Sci 1996;41:2195–2203.
63. Di LC, Flores AF, Hyman PE. Age-related changes in colon motility. J Pediatr 1995;127:593–596.
72. Benninga MA, Wijers OB, van der Hoeven CW, et al. Manometry, profilometry, and endosonography: normal physiology and anatomy of the anal canal in healthy children. J Pediatr Gastroenterol Nutr 1994;18:68–77.

See expertconsult.com for a complete list of references and the review questions for this chapter.

6

GASTROINTESTINAL MUCOSAL IMMUNOLOGY AND MECHANISMS OF INFLAMMATION

Simon Murch

The portion of the immune system resident within the intestine faces significant challenges. A single layer of epithelium separates the largest population of immune cells in the body from a massive number of bacteria. It is therefore probably not surprising that the mediation and control of intestinal immunity follows rules quite distinct from those governing systemic immune reactivity.

The overall challenges faced by the intestine include not only achieving efficient nutrient absorption, but also maintaining tolerance toward dietary antigens and the enteric microbiota, while retaining the ability to react vigorously to intestinal pathogens.[1,2] Such balance of immunological response is made possible by the depth of interaction between the ancient innate immune system and the evolutionarily more recent adaptive immune system.[3] The footprints of evolution are clearly seen within the immune system of the intestine, and different cells that first arose in completely distinct evolutionary eras work together within the human intestine. This has led to addition of control mechanisms over time, rather than simple replacement of more archaic cell types by evolutionarily more modern successors – in much the same way that a present-day car uses the same basic mechanistic underpinnings of the Ford Model T, but with a much more sophisticated array of modern regulatory and effector equipment. Such improved functioning may come at a price—1930s cars were never sidelined by faulty engine-monitoring software chips. Similarly, dysfunction of regulating cell types that have arisen relatively late in evolutionary history may lead to profound disturbance of intestinal immune homeostasis, although the effector mechanisms of the more ancient elements of the mucosal immune system function perfectly well.

The important question is why intestinal inflammation isn't more common. The intestinal lumen contains 10 times as many bacterial cells as there are human cells in the entire body (10^{14} vs. 10^{13}).[2] About 80% of the body's entire immune system resides in the intestine. All that separates them is a single epithelial layer. We ingest large amounts of complex dietary antigens, which would invoke severe systemic reactions if injected parenterally. This has required establishment of mechanisms that inhibit potential reactivity to both dietary antigens and the gut flora. Inflammation often occurs as a consequence of breakdown of these mechanisms.

There has been a huge amount of study attempting to dissect such mechanisms. Many of the proof-of-principle studies have been in mice, and relatively less is known of human mucosal immunology. The same broad principles do, however, apply, as evidenced by diseases occurring in people with genetic mutations affecting immune function. The mucosal immune system is undoubtedly highly complex, with multiple cell types and mechanisms involved. This review attempts to steer a path between unhelpful oversimplification and bewildering overcomplexity. References are, however, given to review articles that will provide more in-depth detail. First, it may be helpful to provide an overview of important components of the intestinal environment that contribute to the maintenance of immune tolerance in such a potentially inflammatory environment. Later in the chapter, more detail is given about individual elements and mechanisms.

HIERARCHY OF GUT IMMUNE RESPONSES

Many of the cell populations that cause tissue damage and inflammation are of innate immune origin (e.g., macrophages, neutrophils, eosinophils, mast cells). Their products may cause epithelial disruption, tissue breakdown, and vascular thrombosis. Some may respond directly to invading bacteria without prior involvement of adaptive immune cells. However, these effector cell types are most commonly recruited by induced chemotactic cytokine (chemokine) expression and may be activated by secreted T cell products and/or immune complexes. This represents the downstream effector response.

Immediately upstream are the B and T cells. B cells undergo shift in isotype from the default IgM state dependent on the local cytokine environment and cell-cell contact with T cells.[4,5] In general, IgA responses protect against inflammation, whereas IgG is more proinflammatory. IgE responses may also promote inflammation by disrupting epithelial barrier and neural function. Among T cells, there are CD4-expressing helper cells (T_H) that produce cytokines to alter function of other cells and CD8-expressing cytotoxic cells (T_C) that are capable of directly killing other cells. There are three major groups of T helper cells that can drive different forms of intestinal inflammation: T_H1 cells (producing interferon-γ and IL-2), T_H2 cells (producing the interleukins IL-4, IL-5, and IL-13) and T_H17 cells (producing IL-17).[6,7] These are discussed in more detail later in the chapter.

The lineage commitment and functional state of T cells depends critically on input from antigen-presenting cells. These are thus the most upstream part of the gut immune hierarchy.[8] Sensing of bacterial luminal contents by dendritic cells is critical in this process (Figure 6-1), as is the local cytokine environment that shapes dendritic cell-lymphocyte interactions.[9] Thus, T_H1 cells are generated by dendritic cells producing IL-12, T_H2 cells in response to IL-4, T_H17 in response to transforming growth factor (TGF)-β, IL-23 and IL-6, and T_{REG} cells in response to TGF-β or IL-10.[6-9] Consequently sensitization, rather than tolerance, may occur if pathogens induce local cytokine production at the time of initial priming.

GENERATION OF INFLAMMATION

Pathogens may break immune tolerance by disrupting the epithelial barrier and/or inducing secretion of proinflammatory cytokines by resident subepithelial macrophages. They may also induce expression of chemokines, leading to recruitment of other inflammatory cells. These may react to other antigens penetrating the breached epithelial barrier, or self-antigens liberated from tissues as a consequence of tissue damage. Providing there is adequate repair of the epithelial barrier and clearance of the initiating pathogen or antigen, such inflammatory responses are normally damped down by regulatory immune responses, which are discussed in more detail later. The triggering of chronic inflammatory disorders by pathogens represents a failure of regulatory responses, or of epithelial barrier repair.

MECHANISMS THAT PREVENT INFLAMMATORY REACTIONS TO GUT LUMINAL CONTENTS

Epithelial Integrity

The epithelium plays a very important role in mucosal immune responses. Epithelial barrier function is utterly critical in preventing immune reactions to the gut flora and antigen.[10] First, bacterial ingress is minimized by secretion of mucus by goblet cells and antibacterial peptides (such as α and β defensins) by Paneth cells.[11] Paneth cell α-defensin production in fact shapes the composition of the bacterial flora, thus indirectly regulating mucosal T cell responses.[12] Two mechanisms may disrupt this

coordinated Paneth-cell response to the normal flora – defects in either bacterial autophagy (a process of intracellular bacterial digestion and consequent immune presentation) or intracellular bacterial response (through loss-of-function polymorphism in the NOD2 pattern recognition receptor) will lead to suboptimal immune response to bacteria and are strongly associated with the development of Crohn's disease.[11,13]

Second, tight junction integrity limits penetration of antigens via the paracellular route, where they may be taken up by antigen-presenting cells. Studies suggest that peptide chains longer than 11 amino acids are normally excluded – these are too short to invoke effective T cell activation.[14] Experimental studies of animals with leaky intestinal epithelium (mutated cell adhesion genes) confirm that such leakiness alone is sufficient to drive transmural inflammation in response to the normal flora.[15] Human genetic disorders with impaired gut epithelial adhesion (e.g., epidermolysis bullosa) are also characterized by inflammation.[16] At a population level among developing-world children, increase in paracellular permeability is associated with nutritional failure, intestinal inflammation, and overall mortality.[17,18] Such paracellular leakiness may be induced by pathogens, or by local production of cytokines, notably tumor necrosis factor (TNF)-α and interferon-γ,[19,20] but is opposed by local production of the cytokine TGF-β,[21] a multifunctional regulatory mediator that plays numerous roles in maintaining intestinal immune tolerance.[7-10,22] Thus infections or local inflammatory reactions may impair epithelial barrier function, thereby increasing the chance of secondary inflammatory or sensitizing events.

The epithelium also functions as a regulator of mucosal lymphocyte populations, through constitutive secretion of chemokines such as CCL25 (TECK) in the small intestine and CCL28 (MEC) in the colon.[23] This induces retention of B and T cells that have been primed within mucosal lymphoid follicles, following their circulation via the thoracic duct and subsequent homing to the mucosa.[5,7] The epithelium also produces mediators that induce local adaptation of retained cells toward a regulatory,

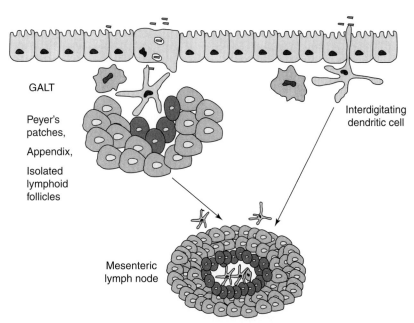

Figure 6-1. Uptake of bacteria or dietary antigens by dendritic cells. This can occur (see left) through M cells (large irregular epithelial cell in diagram) above organized GALT follicles. Dendritic cells may participate in local immune reactions and/or migrate in efferent lymphatics to the mesenteric lymph nodes. Dendritic cells may also sample luminal antigen directly (see right) by extending processes between enterocytes.

noninflammatory type.[10] However, when epithelium is stressed or activated, it produces other chemokines that attract ingress of polymorph neutrophils (IL-8), monocytes (MIP-1α), T cells (CCL20), or eosinophils (eotaxins), dependent on the initiating stimulus.[24] One important and consistent feature of intestinal immune regulation is the different responses made by such newly recruited cells compared to the locally adapted populations.[25] Thus the epithelium may play a critical role in determining the overall status of mucosal immune responses.[10]

Finally, epithelial cells may play a role in antigen presentation that may promote tolerance, by presenting absorbed antigens to lymphocytes in an inherently nonsensitizing manner, because these cells do not express the co-stimulatory ligands required for full T cell activation.[26,27]

IgA Production

IgA is generated in response to the gut flora and other luminal antigens – probably after their uptake by antigen-presenting cells and transport to lymph nodes within the gut wall.[28] These mesenteric lymph nodes appear to be highly important in segregating mucosal from systemic immune responses and regulating intestinal tolerance mechanisms.[5,28,29] IgA-producing plasma cells generated in the mesenteric lymph nodes then home back to the gut from the circulation and go on to secrete specific IgA beneath the epithelium.[4,5] This secreted IgA is taken up and transported through the epithelial cells into the lumen (Figure 6-2). This has two effects: adhering to bacteria and minimizing their invasiveness, and down-regulating transcellular absorption of antigen through the epithelial cell (enterocyte). By contrast, IgE accelerates antigen uptake by the enterocyte (and may also induce tight junction leakiness through triggering of subepithelial mast cells).[30,31] Thus there appears

to be dynamic balance between IgA and IgE with respect to sensitization potential.

Regulatory Lymphocytes

These are a critical component of the gut's anti-inflammatory repertoire.[22,32] They are discussed in more detail later in the chapter. Broadly, there are several types of regulatory lymphocytes, recognized by their pattern of surface molecule expression (e.g., CD4+CD25+ T cells) or cytokine production (e.g., TGF-β producing T_H3 cells, IL-10 producing TR1 cells). One molecule is critical in generation of these regulatory cell types: the transcription factor Forkhead Box P3 (FOXP3).[22,32,33] Mutations in FOXP3 cause a severe inflammatory autoimmune disorder, affecting the intestine and other organs (IPEX syndrome), confirming the importance of regulatory lymphocytes in preventing gut inflammation.[34,35] Recent data suggest that mucosal IgA production and regulatory T cell generation may function as a coordinated system, with regulatory T cells providing the major help for IgA responses, ensuring immunological tolerance to the enteric flora.[36]

Coordinated Immune Responses

It is not only the ability to make regulatory responses that inhibits inflammation. Animals deficient in a wide variety of immunological molecules or cell types will spontaneously develop inflammation in response to the normal gut flora. This may relate to an inability to regulate the composition of the flora, allowing overgrowth of pathogens, or because the immunodeficiency predisposes to making a pathologically skewed response to normal bacteria.[32] A balanced immune response thus appears critical in preventing skewed and damaging intestinal inflammation.

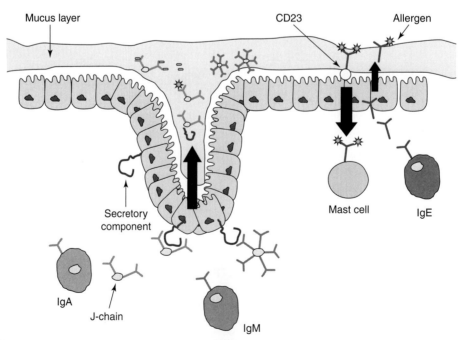

Figure 6-2. Bacteria and antigens need to penetrate a mucus layer, secreted by goblet cells and containing Paneth cell-secreted defensins. Polymeric IgA and IgM are transported across the epithelium in association with secretory component and may bind to bacteria and antigens in the lumen. This both modifies uptake of antigens and minimizes bacterial penetration. By contrast (see right), following sensitization, antigen-specific IgE may also be transported into the lumen where it binds antigen, and is then taken back through the enterocyte by luminal expression of the IgE receptor CD23. When the antigen is presented to subepithelial mast cells, their activation increases epithelial permeability, allowing nonspecific antigen ingress.

Infants with a variety of inborn immunodeficiency disorders develop intestinal inflammation, often only remitting after correction of the underlying disorder (e.g., by bone marrow transplant).[35]

Gut Flora

Normal mucosal tolerance cannot be established in the absence of a gut flora: animals maintained germ-free do not tolerize effectively.[37,38] However, different bacteria have different effects on this process. Thus it is unclear how much the changes in gut bacterial composition in human children that have occurred in the past 50 years have contributed to the increased incidence of allergic and inflammatory diseases.[39,40]

Generation of regulatory lymphocytes within the gut is at least partly dependent on the gut flora.[41] This is mediated both by signals from the epithelium and directly through dendritic cells, which require input from gut bacteria via pattern recognition molecules such as Toll-like receptors in order to provide appropriate inductive signals to the T cells.[10,32] The other molecule critical in induction of regulatory T cells (T_{REG}) is TGF-β, which is also important in developing IgA responses.[4,32]

It is becoming clear that specific components of the flora, rather than the overall bacterial load, may be critical in the development of normal mucosal immune responses. Although much of the literature on probiotics has focused on the properties of lactobacilli and bifidobacteria species, other bacterial types appear much more important in maturing the mucosal and systemic immune systems. A carbohydrate produced by *Bacteroides fragilis* induced both mucosal and systemic immune shift away from T_H2 toward T_H1 responses.[37] Segmented filamentous bacteria are critical, at least in mice, in maturing mucosal T helper cell and IgA responses.[42-44] It thus appears that, among the myriad bacterial species found in the gut, only relatively few have shaped host mucosal immune responses during evolution.[44]

Micronutrients

Generation and function of regulatory T cells is dependent on specific micronutrients—specifically zinc, vitamin A, and vitamin D.[45-48] Vitamin A is also important in maintenance of epithelial integrity[49,50] and generation of gut homing plasma cells within gut-associated lymphoid tissue (GALT).[51] The consequence of micronutrient deficiency in intestinal inflammatory or allergic states may therefore be an inability to restore normal regulatory responses, and thus an exaggerated inflammatory response.

ORGANIZATION OF THE MUCOSAL IMMUNE SYSTEM

The gut-associated lymphoid tissue (GALT) is organized within three compartments: diffusely scattered through the lamina propria beneath the intestinal epithelium, within the epithelial compartment itself, and in organized lymphoid follicles such as Peyer's patches (Figure 6-3).

The diffuse lymphoid tissue of the intestinal lamina propria is dominated by plasma cells, most of which (in health) are IgA-producing, although in early infancy IgM-producing cells are more common. T lymphocytes within this compartment are more commonly CD4+ rather than CD8+. These CD4+ cells

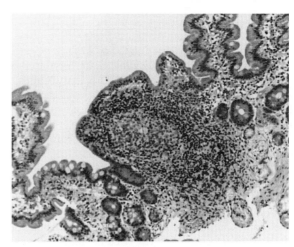

Figure 6-3. An organized lymphoid follicle in the duodenum. Large numbers of dark-staining intraepithelial lymphocytes may be seen in the epithelium overlying the follicle. *(See plate section for color.)*

may be subdivided functionally into T effector (T helper – T_H) and T regulatory (T_{REG}) cells. The T_{REG} cells are particularly important in maintaining immune homeostasis within the intestine. In addition, the mucosal lamina propria contains numerous dendritic cells and macrophages, most of which are locally adapted to their antigen-rich environment. During inflammatory responses, increased expression of chemotactic cytokines (chemokines) and other proinflammatory mediators leads to recruitment of additional T and B cells, monocyte/macrophages, and other cell types such as polymorphonuclear neutrophils, eosinophils, and mast cells.[23,24] The pattern of cellular recruitment will depend on the polarity of T cell responses induced following antigen presentation to the T cells by dendritic cells or macrophages.[6,9,52] These cells from the innate immune system are finely attuned to local microbiological influences, and therefore components of the gut flora may have a profound effect on overall immune responses within the intestine.

The intraepithelial compartment contains populations of lymphocytes that are uncommon elsewhere in the immune system.[7,53] Among T cells, around three quarters of the intraepithelial lymphocytes (IELs) are CD8+ (i.e., cytotoxic T cells). Minority T cell populations (type b IELs), whose true function in man is uncertain, include cells expressing neither CD4 nor CD8 (CD4-CD8- T cells), cells expressing CD8 with two α chains rather than the usual αβ combination, and cells with the T cell receptor composed of γ and δ chains (γδ cells) rather than the α and β chains usually found in circulating T cells (αβ cells). There is also a significant population of natural killer (NK) cells and natural killer T cells (NKTs) in this compartment. They may be involved in distinct mechanisms of antigen presentation based on enterocyte expression of nonclassical major histocompatibility complex (MHC) molecules.[7,53] Both T cells and NK cells jointly provide a surveillance role for the intestinal epithelium and may be induced to cause cell death of enterocytes in circumstances of infection or local production of the cytokine IL-15.

Organized lymphoid follicles occur throughout the intestine. They are most numerous in the terminal ileum, where they cluster to form macroscopically visible aggregates known as Peyer's patches. The follicles do not have afferent lymphatics and are notable for unusually permeable overlying epithelium, due to the presence of M cells (so called because of their ultrastructural appearance of microfolds).[54] This permeability ensures penetration of luminal antigens to a subepithelial pocket containing large numbers of antigen-presenting dendritic cells. These lymphoid follicles are therefore able to sample and respond to a wide variety of luminal antigens, both bacteriological and dietary. Efferent lymphatics from the Peyer's patches drain to the mesenteric lymph nodes, where immune responses are further amplified.

The appendix is a specialized intestinal region with dense aggregation of lymphoid follicles. It appears to be important in mucosal immune priming, as appendectomy protects against later development of ulcerative colitis, and neonatal appendectomy prevented later development of colitis in mutant mice.[55,56] The appendix is now thought to function as a immune-mediated reservoir for the indigenous host flora, allowing repopulation of the colon after infection.[57,58] The bacteria adhere to biofilms, enriched in mucus and defensins from the innate immune system and IgA from the adaptive immune system. The similarity of such biofilms in mammals and nonmammalian vertebrates, including frogs, suggests an ancient origin for immune support of indigenous bacterial species.[57] The biofilm is capable of excluding bacteria from the colonic epithelial surface in health, although this barrier becomes defective in intestinal inflammation.[59] Blind outpockets of the distal gut, similar to the appendix, have arisen by convergent evolution across many unrelated species, suggesting a more important function than had previously been ascribed to the appendix.[57]

Bacterial translocation into organized mucosal lymphoid follicles has been studied in resected appendix tissues from human infants.[60] This gives an insight into the initial reactions to early colonizing bacteria within mucosal lymphoid tissue. Bacterial translocation within the appendiceal mucosa was identified in all specimens from infants aged over 2 weeks, with whole bacteria identified beneath follicular epithelium, within follicles, and in efferent lymphatics. Few lymphoid follicles were present at birth, but they increased rapidly on colonization, with germinal centers identifiable by 4 weeks. IgM plasma cells increased rapidly from 2 weeks, declining from 6 weeks as IgA plasma cells began to dominate, reaching their peak at around 10 weeks.

COMPONENTS OF THE MUCOSAL IMMUNE SYSTEM

Innate Immunity Within the Intestine

It is particularly important to recognize that the gut is an organ of huge evolutionary longevity: indeed, well-developed gastrointestinal tracts can be identified in fossils of organisms from the Cambrian period. Thus immunological tolerance of gut luminal contents must have been established before the development of any adaptive immune responses. Many products of innate immunity, in addition to defensins, including C-type lectins, surfactants, and cathelicidins, contribute to shape the host's immune response to the flora and indeed the composition of the flora itself.[61,62]

There are a number of cells of innate immune lineage that play roles in presenting antigens to lymphocytes of the adaptive immune system, and their own responses help to shape subsequent adaptive immune responses.[61] So-called professional antigen-presenting cells, such as dendritic cells, macrophages, and B cells, can efficiently take up antigen (by phagocytosis or specific receptor-mediated uptake) and then present to naive

T cells fragments of that antigen bound to class II MHC molecules.[63,64] The consequent T cell response will be shaped by both expression of co-stimulatory molecules and secretion of cytokines by the antigen-presenting cell. Dendritic cells are the most efficient activators of T cells because of their constitutive expression of co-stimulatory molecules such as B7. There is important functional heterogeneity within populations of professional antigen-presenting cells; thus both dendritic cells and macrophages may function as locally adapted resident populations or as recently recruited more proinflammatory cells. Such local adaptation is one of the key mechanisms underpinning the maintenance of immune tolerance within the intestine.

The intestinal epithelium can contribute to antigen presentation, processing ingested antigen and presenting using both classical and nonclassical MHC molecules. However, the enterocyte does not express co-stimulatory molecules, so this form of antigen presentation does not activate lymphocytes but may render them anergic – incapable of proliferation and activation.

Other cell types in the intestinal mucosa may act as nonprofessional antigen-presenting cells, including fibroblasts and vascular endothelial cells. Such interactions with lymphocytes may become functionally important in inflammatory states, but are unlikely to play a role in the normal maintenance of immune tolerance. This review thus focuses first on the primary interactions between innate and adaptive immune cells in establishing and maintaining tolerance to dietary antigens and the enteric flora (Table 6-1).

Dendritic Cells Within the Intestine

Dendritic cells play a central role in the maintenance of immunological tolerance within the intestine, through their primary role of taking up antigens and presenting them to lymphocytes. They provide an important means of sampling luminal contents – both

TABLE 6-1. Some Interactions Between Innate and Adaptive Immune Responses to the Enteric Flora

Recognition Element	Microbial Component	Effect Transduced
TLR-2	Peptidoglycans	NF-κB response
TLR-4	Lipopolysaccharides	NF-κB response
TLR-5	Flagellins	NF-κB response
TLR-9	Bacterial DNA	NF-κB response
Nod-1, Nod-2	Bacterial molecules	NF-κB response
Mannose receptor	Bacterial carbohydrates	↑Ag presentation
Complement components	O- and N-linked glycans	Opsonization, possible regulatory response
Mannan-binding lectin	Bacterial carbohydrates	Complement activation
Surfactant proteins A and D	O- and N-linked glycans	↑Phagocytosis, regulate T cell and macrophage activation

Exposure to bacterial determinants, sensed by receptors expressed on or within innate immune cells, alters their function during cross-talk with cells of the adaptive immune system (T and B cells). Secreted molecules (e.g., complement, surfactant proteins) bind to bacterial determinants and in turn modulate innate-adaptive immune interactions. Many of these interactions are carbohydrate based.
NF-κB, nuclear transcription factor-κB; TLR, Toll-like receptor.

microbial and dietary in origin. Three distinct mechanisms have been identified by which such sampling may be effected.

First, dendritic cells cluster in the subepithelial region of organized lymphoid follicles, such as Peyer's patches. Specialized epithelial cells in the surface epithelium, so-called microfold or M-cells, are much more permeable to luminal antigens than are normal epithelial cells. Such focal epithelial leakiness allows ingress of luminal antigens of all kinds. However, recent evidence suggests that there may be some specificity in uptake, as M cells express the lectin glycoprotein-2, which allows selective adherence and uptake of fimbriated bacteria.[65] Bacterial or dietary components crossing the M cells are then taken up in turn by dendritic cells. These may function in turn by presenting processed antigen to T cells within the local area of the lymphoid follicle (see Figure 6-1). In addition, it has been demonstrated that dendritic cells in Peyer's patches may phagocytose live bacteria that have penetrated through M cells and may then migrate to the regional draining mesenteric lymph nodes.[28] It is in this site that fundamental adaptive immune responses may occur, including generation of antigen-specific IgA.[28,29]

Second, it is now known that subepithelial dendritic cells, situated in isolated fashion away from organized lymphoid follicles, may insinuate processes between adjacent enterocytes to sample luminal contents.[66,67] This appears to be a coordinated mechanism, involving induced focal breakdown of the mechanisms that normally maintain tight junction integrity.

Third, antigen may be transported through the enterocyte following uptake either by IgG, which is shuttled back and forth across the epithelium by the neonatal Fc receptor for IgG,[68] or by IgE, which is taken up by induced luminal expression of the low-affinity IgE receptor CD23[30,31] (see Figure 6-2). This antibody-mediated uptake will thus be antigen specific, rather than the less selective uptake across Peyer's patches or following periepithelial dendritic cell sampling.

Conserved Pattern-Recognition Receptors and Dendritic Cell Function

Dendritic cells do not present antigen in isolation from the massive numbers of enteric bacteria situated so close to them, across the epithelial barrier.[67] Indeed, these bacteria induce profound changes in the behavior of the entire enteric immune system, and indeed may even shape systemic immune responses away from the intestine.[37] The effects of the enteric flora on the behavior of dendritic cells are mediated through a number highly conserved pattern recognition molecules.[69] These may be situated on the cell surface or may be expressed intracellularly. Pattern recognition molecules in both extracellular and intracellular sites signal through shared pro-inflammatory pathways, converging on nuclear transcription factor-κB (NF-κB). On the cell surface, various Toll-like receptors (TLRs) recognize conserved sequences in bacteria, viruses, fungi, and protozoa. Similarly, within the cell, Nod1 and Nod2 recognize sequences in bacterial cell walls. Binding of the conserved microbial sequence by these pattern recognition receptor transmits a signal through NF-κB that induces nuclear transcription of cytokines such as TNF-α. This has the effect of altering the interaction between the antigen-presenting cell and any lymphocytes with which it interacts.

Subgroups of Dendritic Cells

Dendritic cells may be subdivided functionally into myeloid (monocyte-like) or plasmacytoid (plasma cell-like). Myeloid dendritic cells produce predominantly the cytokine interleukin-12

(IL-12) and plasmacytoid cells interferon-α (IFN-α), which may affect the behavior of cells in their vicinity and the subsequent polarization of lymphocytes to which they present antigen.[9,10]

In comparison with dendritic cells from the spleen, intestinal dendritic cells tend to produce more of the regulatory cytokine IL-10, which may contribute to the maintenance of immune tolerance in such a highly antigen-challenged site.[9,32] Within Peyer's patches, a subset of dendritic cells expressing the CD11b molecule promote a more T$_H$2 skewed response among T cells, whereas subgroups that do not express this molecule (CD11b⁻) induce a more T$_H$1 skewed response. Similarly, expression of CD103 (αE integrin) by Peyer's patch dendritic cells is associated with a tendency to T$_H$2 or regulatory cell polarization.[70] The factors determining expression of markers such as CD11b and CD103 are not well understood in humans, and there appear to be a number of other subsets with different surface marker expression and function (Table 6-2).

Although the field is complex and evolving, the overall pattern is that cells that are locally adapted to the lamina propria generally inhibit the development of delayed-type hypersensitive reactions, in a manner that is not seen among splenic or Peyer's patch lymphocytes, to promote immune tolerance.[70] In contrast, newly arrived dendritic cells, recently derived from the bone marrow, exhibit unrestricted responses to antigens and bacterial products in the intestinal microenvironment.

The gut flora may play an important role in the conditioning of dendritic cells within the intestine to such local adaptation. This important change in their functional properties depends in part on molecules released by intestinal epithelial cells upon bacterial exposure, including thymic stromal lymphopoietin (TSLP) and retinoic acid (a vitamin A derivative).[10,71] Other cytokines that contribute to this process include IL-10 and TGF-β, which may be produced by

TABLE 6-2. Functionally Important Subgroups of Innate Immune Cells

Cell Type	Identifying Markers	Effects
Peyer's patch dendritic cells	CD11b+	T$_H$2 skewed response, T$_{REG}$ response
	CD11b–	T$_H$1 skewed response
	CD103+	T$_H$2 skewed response, T$_{REG}$ response
	CD103–	T$_H$1 skewed response
Lamina propria dendritic cells	CD103+ resident cells	T$_H$2 skewed response, T$_{REG}$ response
	CD103– newly recruited	T$_H$1 skewed response
Resident macrophages	CD14–	Reduced LPS response
Newly recruited macrophages	CD14+	Full LPS response (TNF-α, etc.)
Polymorph neutrophils	CD11b/CD18, CD66b (activated)	Release proteases, free radicals, G-CSF, IL-8, etc.
Mast cells	Mast cell tryptase, c-kit	Release tryptase, histamine, 5-HT, TNF-α
Eosinophils	Eosinophil peroxidase, CD66b (activated)	Release ECP, IL-4, histamine, leukotrienes
Basophils	CD63 (activated), CCR3	Release IL-4, histamine, leukotrienes
Natural killer cells	CD16, CD56	Induced apoptosis

a number of cells within the microenvironment, including other locally adapted dendritic cells.

Dendritic Cells and Induction of Immune Tolerance Within the Intestine

A central mechanism for maintenance of tolerance within the intestinal environment is the induction of a regulatory phenotype in T cells that interact with the locally conditioned dendritic cells. As discussed, the transcription factor FOXP3 and the cytokine TGF-β are critical components in the transition of a naive T cell to a regulatory phenotype (T_{REG}).[22,32,72,73] Subgroups of locally adapted Peyer's patch and lamina propria dendritic cells (expressing CD103) and lamina propria macrophages are particularly effective in inducing FOXP3 expression in naive T cells.

In addition, dendritic cells may alter the homing potential of T cells with which they interact, by inducing expression of specific integrins that favor homing back to the gut, following passage from efferent lymphatics to the thoracic duct and back into the circulation.[72,73] Finally, Peyer's patch and mesenteric lymph node dendritic cells play a role in the isotype shift of B cells toward IgA, which dominates intestinal immunoglobulin production in health and contributes to maintenance of intestinal homeostasis.[4,5,29]

Dendritic Cells and Effector Immune Responses to Pathogens

Dendritic cell function can clearly not be restricted to the induction of tolerance in all circumstances. This would be quite inappropriate in the case of pathogens, which require prompt responses from the mucosal immune system. This response may follow recruitment of new dendritic cells and macrophages, which have not undergone local conditioning. The response of epithelial cells to pathogen-induced damage includes expression of both chemokines such as IL-8 and MIP-3α, which induce cell recruitment, and cytokines such as IL-1, IL-15, and TNF-α, which may activate or prime locally recruited cells. The consequences will be an appropriate proinflammatory response and the generation of effector and memory T cells, polarized toward appropriate immune responses on future challenge.

As mentioned previously, micronutrient status is particularly important in dendritic cell function, and thus the establishment and maintenance of immune tolerance. In particular, vitamins A and D and zinc are essential factors in the ability of intestinal dendritic cells to induce regulatory T cells[45-47] and IgA responses.[51] Thus, treatment of established micronutrient deficiency in enteropathy or other inflammatory states may be clinically important.

Intestinal Macrophages

Macrophages are highly important effector cells, capable of producing over 100 mediators upon activation.[25] Among these mediators, the molecules TNF-α, IL-1β, and IL-6 have very important pro-inflammatory effects. Excess production of TNF-α and IL-1β have been particularly associated with intestinal inflammatory conditions,[74] and therapeutic inhibition of these molecules by biological therapies has had profound effects on complex inflammatory responses in vivo. As with dendritic cells, macrophages express an extensive range of bacterial pattern recognition receptors, notably TLRs. Their response to TLR ligation is a much more potent proinflammatory response than seen in dendritic cells, mediated through NF-κB, in which

cytokines such as TNF-α, free oxygen radicals, proteases, and nitric oxide are released.[25] In addition, secretion of enzymes such as matrix metalloproteases may have important effects on extracellular matrix integrity, release of endothelins may affect vascular supply,[74] and reactive oxygen and nitrogen radicals have proinflammatory as well as antibacterial effects.

Similarly to dendritic cells, there is evidence of important local adaptation among macrophages.[75] Intestinal macrophages do not proliferate, and their numbers are continually replenished by blood-derived monocytes, which in turn become locally adapted. As with other regulatory mucosal responses, the cytokine TGF-β plays a critical role in the transformation from newly recruited monocyte to locally adapted macrophage.[25] Locally conditioned intestinal macrophages do not make a full reaction to bacterial lipopolysaccharides (LPS), as they have down-regulated expression of CD14, a molecule critical in function of TLR-4 in its inflammatory response to bacterial LPS.[25,76] In addition, resident lamina propria macrophages show down-regulated expression of receptors for IgG and IgA, although retaining strong phagocytic and bactericidal activity.[77] Furthermore, resident macrophages contribute significantly to normal tolerance to the flora by depleting the lamina propria environment of tryptophan, which is necessary for full T cell activation, through expression of the enzyme indoleamine 2,3-dioxygenase (IDO).[78] Recent data suggest that such locally adapted macrophages may also play an important immunomodulatory role during gut inflammation, by secreting IL-10 that in turn induces a local regulatory T cell response.[79]

Lamina propria macrophages have important effector roles in host defense against invading microorganisms. They kill most ingested bacteria, more efficiently than unadapted monocytes, despite their relative lack of proinflammatory response. They are also able to neutralize viruses of many kinds, thus functioning as effective gatekeepers to the lamina propria. However, when large-scale influx of newly recruited monocytes occur in response to chemokine expression during inflammatory responses, these newly recruited former monocytes produce large amounts of proinflammatory cytokines and may thus potently amplify mucosal inflammation. Within the inflamed mucosa in Crohn's disease, around a third of mucosal macrophages express CD14 and are thus recently recruited cells able to make an uninhibited response to bacterial LPS.[76] Important in this influx are a subgroup of cells that show characteristics of both macrophages and dendritic cells, which both present antigen and promote both T_H1 and T_H17 responses.[80,81]

Polymorphonuclear Neutrophils

Polymorph neutrophils do not play a significant role in intestinal antigen presentation, and their most important contribution is in the proinflammatory response to pathogens. Activation of intestinal epithelial cells by pathogens induces secretion of the chemokine IL-8, which leads to enhanced neutrophil recruitment.[82] Neutrophils then become involved in immediate responses to invading pathogens and may damage tissue through release of proteases, cytokines, and reactive oxygen and nitrogen radicals.[83]

Although their best-recognized role in host defense is in immediate proinflammatory responses, the role of neutrophils within the intestinal microenvironment is more complex and nuanced. This is demonstrated by the development of intestinal inflammation in disorders of neutrophil function, such as chronic granulomatous disease or glycogen storage disease-1b.[84] Impaired neutrophil function has been linked more generally to the development of inflammatory bowel disease (IBD), and enhancement of neutrophil function by stimulatory factors such as granulocyte colony-stimulating factor (G-CSF) may have an anti-inflammatory effect in Crohn's disease.[85]

Eosinophils, Basophils, and Mast Cells

There is overlap of function among these cell types, all of which are involved in T_H2 type immune responses within the intestine. All appear important in host defense against helminth infection and may have effects on intestinal motility.[86-88] On activation, which frequently occurs in the context of IgE-mediated intestinal reactions, these cell types produce an overlapping array of cytokines and proinflammatory mediators. These have the effects of inducing vascular permeability and promoting antigen penetration. Activation of these cell types may also directly affect intestinal neural function.[89,90] Mast cells are closely situated by enteric nerves – indeed, the c-kit ligand involved in mast cell generation is also critical in generation of the interstitial cells of Cajal that function as pacemaker cells within the myenteric plexus.[90] Eosinophil and mast cell dominated gut disorders are characterized by dysmotility and enhanced pain sensation (visceral hyperalgesia).[91]

Recruitment of eosinophils is particularly dependent on the T_H2 group cytokine IL-5 and the eotaxin subfamily of cytokines. Commitment of precursor cells within the bone marrow to the eosinophil lineage is dependent on the transcription factor GATA-1.[87] Eosinophils are constitutively present at low density in most of the gastrointestinal tract, with the exception of the esophagus. In addition to effector functions during inflammatory reactions, eosinophils can also function as antigen-presenting cells, inducing antigen-specific T cell stimulation. For reasons that are currently unclear, there has been rapid temporal increase in eosinophilic gut disorders, in particular eosinophilic esophagitis.[92,93] In such disorders, there is frequently an increase in tissue mast cell and basophil density, pointing toward a coordinated immune response. This is likely to represent a conserved mechanism for combating intestinal helminth infection, which has been almost ubiquitous throughout evolutionary history. Whether the relative absence of helminth infection in privileged modern societies actually contributes to dysregulation of this coordinated response, through lack of normal induction and priming, is the subject of much interest.[94]

Adaptive Immunity Within the Intestine

Adaptive immune responses in the gut are mediated by cells of both T cell and B cell lineage. The earlier rather simple differentiation of T cell populations, into CD4 (helper) and CD8 (cytotoxic) cell types and functional subdifferentiation into $T_H1/Tc1$ and $T_H2/Tc2$ cells based on cytokine secretion patterns,[6,52] now appears to represent a gross underestimate of a highly varied grouping of many cell types, each capable of modulating anti-infective or inflammatory responses. Much of the data on such subpopulations comes from murine study and must be interpreted with some caution. However, there is no doubt that the intestinal mucosa hosts a large array of different lymphocyte subpopulations and that there may be very complex levels of control that are only partly understood.

Archaic Lymphocyte Populations

The intestine is unusual in that it maintains relatively high expression of cells that arose much earlier in evolution than classical T and B cells. Some of these function on the borderline between innate and adaptive immunity, maintaining the ability to provide rapid response to newly encountered pathogens, while also demonstrating some elements of immune adaptation. It may not be coincidental that these cells are highly represented in the epithelial compartment, where exposure to luminal organisms and pathogens may he highest. They are known as Type b IELs.[7,53]

NKT cells show some overlap of function with NK cells of the innate immune system, but differ in their ability to produce high levels of cytokines such as IL-2 and IFN-γ. All are restricted by the nonclassical MHC molecule CD1d, whereas some possess an invariant T cell receptor α chain (Vα24 NKT cells), which recognizes lipid antigens presented by the nonclassical MHC molecule CD1d expressed by the epithelium.[95] This is important in host defense against mycobacterial glycolipids but may be subverted in allergy, and allergic responses to dietary lipid antigens may be mediated in this manner.[96,97]

Most $\gamma\delta$ T cells within the intestine are of a type (Vδ1) that is uncommon in peripheral blood. They express receptors that are more akin to NKT cells than conventional $\alpha\beta$ T cells.[7,53] They particularly recognize stress-induced molecules (MICA, MICB) on epithelium and are thus thought to play a particular role in surveillance of epithelial integrity. Overall, $\gamma\delta$ cells thus appear to protect the epithelium, possibly by elimination of stressed or infected cells. Although best recognized for their increase within the epithelium in celiac disease, there is experimental evidence to suggest that lack of $\gamma\delta$ cells may cause an amplification of tissue damage in intestinal infection or inflammation.[98,99] However, in other circumstances, $\gamma\delta$ cells may contribute to inflammatory damage.

B Lymphocyte Populations

Intestinal B cells also show important differences from circulating B cell populations. There is overrepresentation of an archaic cell type unusual in the circulation (B1 cells). B1 cells arose earlier in evolution than conventional B cells (B2 cells). Although they can produce antibody and present antigen, they do not mature into memory cells.[100] Most intestinal B1 cells express CD5, a molecule involved in B-B cell interaction. They predominantly produce IgM of broad specificity (natural antibody), binding particularly to bacterial carbohydrates. B1 cells migrate to the intestine from the peritoneal cavity and may undergo isotype shift to IgA within the mucosa,[101,102] although this remains controversial.[4] B1 cells form a first line of defense against bacterial invasion from the gut lumen, by contributing to immunoglobulin coating of bacteria within the lumen.[100]

The isotype of conventional B2 cells is also skewed compared to elsewhere in the body, with great predominance of IgA-producing cells generated within Peyer's patches and mesenteric lymph nodes.[29,102] It has been estimated that 80% of a human's plasma cells are located in the gut, with 80 to 90% of them producing secretory IgA, leading to production by an adult of approximately 3 g of secretory IgA daily.[4] Within the small intestine, as in plasma, IgA1 (specific for protein antigens) is the dominant secretory isoform, whereas in the colon IgA2 (specific for bacterial LPS and lipoteichoic acid) dominates.[103]

Shift in immunoglobulin isotype from the default IgM occurs under the influence of local cytokines, but is also dependent on direct cell-cell contact with T cells, through the CD40-CD40 ligand interaction.[5] As required for induction of a regulatory phenotype in T cells, the generation of IgA-producing plasma cells appears to be dependent on the normal flora and the cytokine TGF-β.[28,29]

Whereas most circulating IgA is monomeric, most intestinal luminal IgA is of secretory type, consisting largely of dimers and tetramers, joined by a polypeptide J-chain and stabilized by a molecule called secretory component that provides resistance to proteolysis.[103] The complex is taken up by the polymeric Ig receptor on enterocytes, and then shuttled across the enterocyte to be secreted into the lumen. In addition to protecting secretory IgA from proteolysis, this receptor may itself play a role in immune responses by direct antimicrobial effects and by inhibiting pathogen and antigen ingress through the epithelium.[104]

Luminally secreted IgA performs a number of functions that tend to diminish inflammation, including reducing uptake of particulate antigens, neutralizing biologically active molecules, inhibiting bacterial adherence, and enhancing activity of innate immune factors such as lactoferrin. Within the enterocyte, IgA can retard transfer of pathogens including human immunodeficiency virus (HIV) and can aid elimination of immune complexes, whereas within the mucosa IgA has anti-inflammatory activities including complement inhibition, while contributing to bacterial opsonization.[103] Thus IgA-deficient individuals show increased uptake of food antigens and may demonstrate low-grade enteropathy.[105]

Homing and Recruitment of B Lymphocytes

Common to both B1 cells and conventional (B2) cells is the ability to home to the mucosal surface.[4] This is mediated in the high endothelial venules of GALT and mesenteric lymph nodes by expression of mucosal addressin cell adhesion molecule-1 (MadCAM-1), which interacts with L-selectin on lymphocytes, followed by specific binding of those expressing the mucosal integrin α4β7. Following recruitment of lymphocytes by this mechanism, they are held within the intestine by local chemokine expression. Within the small intestine, epithelial production of the chemokine CCL25 (TECK) induces retention in the lamina propria of both T and B cells expressing the chemokine receptor CCR9.[23] Regional variation within the intestine of chemokine production by the epithelium induces homing of specific subgroups of T and B cells, so that colonic tropism is mediated by interaction between epithelial CCL28 (MEC) and lymphocyte CCR10.[23,24]

Induction of Mucosal IgG and IgE Responses

Immunoglobulin class-switching within the intestine is not always or entirely directed toward IgA. In the presence of cytokines other than TGF-β, isotype shift toward IgG or IgE may occur. Thus, during inflammatory or pathogen-induced reactions, the production of T_H1 or T_H2 cytokines by T cells within the lymphoid follicle may ensure that naive B cells are committed toward IgG2 (IFN-γ) or IgE (IL-4), so that they mature into gut-homing IgG2 or IgE producing plasma cells.[52] These would be retained within the lamina propria by chemokine interactions, as before. However, their interaction with antigens would induce a quite distinct immunological consequence compared to IgA.

T Cell Populations in the Intestine

As discussed, intraepithelial T cells are usually of the CD8+ (cytotoxic) type, whereas lamina propria T cells are more commonly CD4+ (helper) cells. There is functional subdivision of

T cell responses, based on the pattern of cytokines that these cells produce on activation (Table 6-3). In contrast to previous dogma, there is emerging evidence that some T helper cells are able to alter lineage commitment within the gut, particularly between T_H17 and T_{REG} phenotype, depending on local environmental inputs.[106] Long-lived populations of both CD4+ and CD8+ cells provide important immunological memory within the lamina propria.[107,108]

T Helper Cells (CD4+ Cells)

T_H1 cells produce predominantly IL-2 and IFN-γ.[6] These cytokines promote the classic cell-mediated response, including macrophage activation, matrix breakdown and tissue remodeling, while inhibiting production of most immunoglobulin classes. This is an effective immune response to intracellular pathogens, limiting bacterial dissemination at the price of tissue scarring and granuloma formation. naïve T cells are directed to the T_H1 lineage by exposure to IL-12 from innate immune cells or IFN-γ from other T cells, via the transcription factor T-bet.

T_H2 cells produce predominantly IL-4, IL-5, IL-6, IL-10, and IL-13.[6] These cytokines produce the classic humoral response, inhibiting macrophage activation but promoting IgE antibody production and allergic responses. This is an effective immune response to helminth infestation, but less effective against bacterial infections. Cells commit to the T_H2 lineage via exposure to IL-4, acting via the transcription factor GATA-3.

TABLE 6-3. Functionally Important Groups of Adaptive Immune Cells

Cell Type	Identifying Markers	Effects
T helper cells	CD3+CD4+	Subgroup-dependent (T_H1,2 or 17 – as below)
T_H1 cells	CXCR3+, CCR5+, Tbet+	Produce IL-2, IFN-γ
T_H17 cells	IL-17+, IL-21+, ROR-γT+,	Produce IL-17, IL-21, IL-22
T_H2 cells	CCR4+, CCR3+, GATA-3+	Produce IL-4, IL-5, IL-13
Cytotoxic T cells	CD3+, CD8+	Cell lysis. Also produce cytokines (T_C1, T_C2 – as for T_H1, T_H2)
T regulatory cells	FOXP3+Subtypes include CD4+,CD25+ cells, T_H3 cells (TGF-β producing), TR1 cells (IL-10 producing)	Produce regulatory cytokines (IL-10, TGF-β), induce "bystander suppression" in T cells of all specificities. Critical in mucosal tolerance.
γδ T cells	T cell receptor γδ	Surveillance of damaged epithelium
Natural killer T (NKT) cells	CD3+, CD56+CD1d-restricted	Produce IL-2, IFN-γ, lipid ag response
B1 cells	CD5+	Produce natural antibody (IgM)
B2 cells	CD20+, CD5-	Mature into antibody producing plasma cells (IgM, IgA, IgG, or IgE depending on priming environment)

T_H17 cells produce predominantly IL-17 and IL-22 and are generated through exposure to IL-23,[109,110] TGF-β, and IL-6, acting via the transcription factor ROR-γT.[110] This represents an important axis of host defense against extracellular bacterial and fungal infections, because of the effects of these cytokine on neutrophil recruitment. However, overproduction of T_H17-associated cytokines has been implicated in autoimmunity and inflammatory bowel disease. In mice, IL-17 cells are induced within the mucosa by segmented filamentous bacteria but not other members of the indigenous flora and may mediate protection against intestinal pathogens.[111] ATP generated by bacteria within the lumen may be important in this process.[112] Treatment with vancomycin or ampicillin, but not metronidazole/neomycin, has disrupted the flora-induced generation of T_H17 cells, which mediate host responses to fungi, potentially explaining the effects of antibiotic treatment in causing intestinal candidiasis.[111,112]

T Cytotoxic Cells (CD8+ Cells)

Although the area of the intraepithelial compartment is smaller than the lamina propria, the density of T cells is higher (around 20 per 100 epithelial cells). Thus around 70% of intestinal T cells are CD8+.[53] As mentioned, many CD8+ IELs are conventional CD3+CD8αβ+ (type a IELs), functioning much like circulating CD8 cells, whereas others express the otherwise uncommon CD8αα homodimer (type B IELs) and function similarly to the other archaic lineages (γδ cells, NKT cells) found in this compartment.[7] Type a IELs provide immunological memory and function in a primarily cytolytic manner, inducing cell death by production of granzymes or inducing apoptosis by engagement of Fas.[7] In addition they may produce T_H1 type cytokines. These cells have been primed to antigen in GALT and then home back to the intestine before crossing into the epithelial compartment.[53] Type b IELs may develop within the intestine rather than the thymus and show a more autoreactive immune response, recognizing self molecules exhibited by infected or transformed cells.[53] Overall, CD8 cells play an important role in maintaining epithelial health and integrity – critical because the epithelium is a dominant regulator of overall intestinal immune homeostasis.

During viral infections, CD8 cells within both the epithelium and lamina propria will be important in host defense. Following infection with several viruses, mice maintained enhanced CD8 effector and memory responses within the intestinal mucosa for substantially longer than in occurred in the spleen.[108] This was particularly marked among lamina propria CD8 cells rather than IELs, suggesting that this represents a long-lived memory population that plays a protective role against pathogen invasion.

T Regulatory Cells

One of the most fundamental insights in recent years has been the recognition of the importance of regulatory T (T_{REG}) cells within the intestine. Much of this review has focused on the generation of these intestinal cells, which are critically important to prevent immune reaction to the gut flora and dietary or self antigens.

The development of severe autoimmune enteropathy in apparently immunocompetent infants remained unexplained until discovery that a number had mutations in an X-chromosome encoded transcription factor (FOXP3) that was also mutated in mice with a multifocal autoimmune disease.[34,35] FOXP3 was subsequently shown to be pivotal in generating T_{REG} cells,[33] and FOXP3+ cells are the only currently known cells whose primary function is to mediate dominant immune tolerance (recessive tolerance is cell specific, due to deletion in the thymus or to apoptosis or anergy in the periphery). These cells inhibit immunological reactivity through several mechanisms, including direct cell-cell contact (via CTLA-4), secreting immunoregulatory cytokines (TGF-β or IL-10) and modifying the functions of antigen-presenting cells.[32,72,73] Blockade of either TGF-β or CTLA-4 is sufficient to induce spontaneous intestinal inflammation.[32]

T_{REG} may be either naturally occurring cells generated within the thymus (nT_{REG}), characterized by their CD4+CD25+ phenotype,[32,113] or induced within tissues in response to TGF-β (iT_{REG}).[72] Within the intestine, epithelial responses to the flora and to vitamin A promote a dendritic cell phenotype that favors iT_{REG} generation.[10,71] By contrast, in response to mucosal inflammation, production of IL-10 by locally adapted macrophages induces formation of T_{REG} and thus acts to damp down inflammation.[79]

Because the field has developed so fast, the literature contains references to a number of cell types (e.g., TGF-β producing T_H3 cells, IL-10 producing Tr1 cells) that may not represent true discrete lineages of T_{REG}, or that may overlap with other regulatory cell types. In general, FOXP3 expression is taken as the hallmark of the T_{REG} phenotype. However, some FOXP3 cells with regulatory properties have also been reported, and it is unclear whether they may represent chronically stimulated effector T cells that have finally down-regulated their proinflammatory cytokine production but persist in IL-10 production.[32]

Regulatory function has been reported among subgroups of CD8 cells, including both type a and type b IELs. Again, this may related to secretion of the regulatory cytokines TGF-β and IL-10 by these cells.[32] Similarly, production of TGF-β has been reported in some γδ cells, which may contribute to their recognized ability to support epithelial integrity.[99] The presence of so many distinct cell types with regulatory properties underlines the importance of limiting immune reactivity in the gut, in the face of its massive antigenic and bacterial exposures.

ESTABLISHMENT AND MAINTENANCE OF ORAL TOLERANCE TO ANTIGENS AND THE FLORA

Mechanisms of Oral Tolerance

Antigen exposure in the intestine may have both local and systemic consequences. A local secretory IgA response may occur, or systemic immune responses may ensue, including circulating antigen-specific IgG, IgE, or IgA, and/or a state of immunological tolerance may be invoked.[114] As discussed, tolerance induction within the intestine for foodstuffs and commensal bacteria is critical to normal physiology.

Oral tolerance is a specific suppression of immune responses to an antigen following its oral ingestion. It represents an extension of peripheral tolerance to self antigens and uses essentially similar mechanisms, including lymphocyte deletion, anergy, and suppression.

There are two essential mechanisms of induction of oral tolerance. High-dose oral tolerance is mediated by T cell anergy (in some circumstances deletion) after ingestion of antigen at high doses. Low-dose oral tolerance is mediated by induction of regulatory cells, following presentation by intestinal APCs after ingesting low doses of antigen. This is T cell activation dependent and may thus be more difficult to induce around birth, when T cell reactivity may be lower. Antigen-specific iT_{REG}, induced in this manner, migrate to mesenteric lymph nodes, suppressing local immune responses, and then migrate from the bloodstream back to the intestine or other organs, where they suppress reactivity of surrounding lymphocytes of various specificities by secreting immunosuppressive cytokines such as TGF-β and IL-10. This phenomenon is known as bystander suppression.[9,22,114]

Of potentially clinical importance, low-dose oral tolerance is indeed more difficult to establish in infancy than high-dose tolerance.[115] Feeding of low-dose myelin basic protein to neonatal mice induced a paradoxical sensitization to antigen and worsened autoimmune neurological disease, rather than invoking protective oral tolerance as seen in adults.[116] In view of the obligatory role of bacterial exposures in inducing the iT_{REG} that mediate low-dose tolerance,[41] this phenomenon may occur particularly in circumstances of inappropriate bacterial exposures from the flora or of reduced innate immune responsiveness (loss-of-function TLR polymorphisms are associated with allergy). Evidence of impaired low-dose oral tolerance in atopic human infants is seen among those who sensitize to maternally ingested dietary antigen despite exclusive breast feeding,[117] who frequently manifest intolerance of hydrolysate feeds and require amino acid formulas.[118] Such infants often present with multiple food allergies and indeed show a paucity of TGF-β producing lymphocytes in the duodenal mucosa.[119] This represents a failure to primarily establish oral tolerance mechanisms. The outgrowing of food allergic sensitization is indeed associated with development of T_{REG} populations.[120]

By contrast, classical cow's milk enteropathy (CMSE) occurred in infants who had been formula fed from birth (thus attaining high-dose oral tolerance), often after suffering rotavirus or other pathogens – indeed, CMSE was often known as postenteritis syndrome. In such circumstances, sensitization followed loss of epithelial barrier function and was usually restricted to a single or very few antigens. This represents a transient loss of primarily acquired oral tolerance.

The clinical use of high-dose oral tolerance is employed in the emerging stratagem of specific oral tolerance induction, in which allergens are fed at increasing dosage.[121]

Importance of Early Life Exposures

The period after birth in which the gut is first colonized and nutrition first ingested is one of the most critical for the entire immune system. Within minutes of the entry of bacteria to the gut lumen, NF-κB responses are switched on within intestinal epithelium, and immune cellular recruitment to the gut is stepped up.[122] This epithelial NF-κB response is down-regulated quickly, and the epithelium becomes endotoxin tolerant.[122] In human infants during the first week of life, cytokine levels are transiently elevated to levels similar to those seen in IBD.[123] Numbers of IELs increase and stabilize, while organized lymphoid follicles develop in terminal ileum and appendix during the first weeks of life.[60] In normal circumstances, immunological reactivity to the bacterial flora and dietary antigens follows a coordinated tolerogenic manner, with development of mucosal IgA responses and a regulatory lymphocyte network.

If events do not follow this ideal – if the infant has constitutive immunological defects, or there is inadequate or inappropriate bacterial input to the epithelium and innate immune

system to allow such a coordinated tolerogenic response – then mucosal lymphocytes may develop an effector rather than regulatory phenotype, or they may fail to be deleted appropriately or rendered anergic. The high frequency of elective cesarean section or perinatal broad-spectrum antibiotic prescription among developed-world infants, together with the high prevalence of loss-of-function polymorphisms in TLRs and NOD receptors (presumably of previous evolutionary benefit or neutrality), means that large numbers of infants may not now receive adequate input to establish primary immune tolerance.[39,40] This may contribute significantly toward the rising incidence and broadening presentation of childhood allergic disease, and possibly also inflammatory bowel diseases.

Proof-of-principle studies have of course been in animals and may not entirely recapitulate human responses. The transient epithelial NF-κB response seen at birth in vaginally delivered mice was not seen in those delivered by cesarean section.[122] The development of effective oral tolerance mechanisms does not occur in the absence of gut colonization – indeed, absence of flora has systemic effects, including a skewing toward a T_H2 response and failure to develop normal splenic architecture.[37] Abnormalities of colonization may be specific, because individual species rather than total bacterial numbers determine the immunological imprinting process.

The development of an effector response toward elements of the gut flora will take place within intestinal lymphoid follicles. In one immunodeficient mouse model (TCR mutant), which develops colitis only if colonized, it was found that removal of such lymphoid follicles by appendectomy completely prevented the development of colitis, even when colonized.[56] However there was a narrow time window, of 3 weeks after birth, when removal of the appendix was effective. This finding has potentially important implications for human intestinal inflammatory disease, in that the consequences of aberrant early-life induction of tolerance to the flora were initially silent, and that an inevitable colitis developed a long time after the initial sensitization event. It remains possible that events determining the development of IBD in children may occur some years before the disease ever manifests, possibly even in infancy.

PATTERNS OF INFLAMMATORY RESPONSE WITHIN THE INTESTINE

There are relatively few and somewhat stereotyped mechanisms of intestinal inflammation. The resultant outcome will depend first on whether the initiating stimulus can be dealt with adequately (i.e., pathogens cleared, dietary allergens excluded, etc.), second on whether any structural damage to nerves, blood vessels, or tissue interstitium has occurred during the acute episode, and third on whether adequate repair mechanisms and regulatory immune responses are invoked to heal the epithelial barrier and dampen inflammatory responses. Failure in any of these three processes may lead to an ongoing chronic inflammatory response.

Acute Inflammation Induced by Pathogens

Many pathogens induce breakdown of the epithelial barrier. Not only do they gain access to the host tissues, but this allows allowing nonspecific ingress of other bacterial types. In the absence of bacterial production of immunomodulatory toxins, the initial inflammatory response will come from the epithelium, which will display stress molecules, thus activating

IELs, and secrete chemokines that attract populations of circulating, uninhibited monocytes, dendritic cells, polymorph neutrophils, and lymphocytes. The initial response from newly-recruited monocytes will include production of proinflammatory cytokines (notably TNF-α, IL-1β), reactive oxygen and nitrogen radicals, and proteases. This is entirely similar to processes in acute IBD. The effects of such a macrophage response will be to activate vascular endothelium, thereby promoting ingress of more acute inflammatory cells. Additional early responses from NK cells, resident mast cells, and archaic lymphocyte populations within the epithelium (type b IELs) include release of T$_H$1 type cytokines. Both macrophages and dendritic cells will respond through their pattern recognition receptors (TLRs, NOD molecules) and alter their activation state and pattern of cytokine production. Additional innate immune responses including complement activation and production of leukotrienes may further promote nonspecific recruitment of all kinds of leukocytes. Breakdown of extracellular matrix further modulates monocyte/macrophage activation and function.

At this early stage, resident memory lymphocytes will respond to previously encountered antigens (e.g., commensals, dietary antigens) that enter nonspecifically as a consequence of epithelial breakdown. Providing that antigen-specific tolerance has previously been established, these should be T$_{REG}$ and should act to limit secondary immune responses. If, however, the initial priming event had generated effector T cells, previously silenced by bystander tolerance mechanisms, these cells too may become activated and may augment the local inflammatory response and even perpetuate it after the pathogen has been cleared (as seen in CMSE/postenteropathy syndrome, or the triggering of ulcerative colitis by pathogens).

Unless there are pathogen-specific memory T and B cells within the mucosa from prior exposure to the pathogen, these will now be generated within Peyer's patches and mesenteric lymphoid follicles, as for other antigens. However, the priming circumstances now differ, and the dominant local cytokine may not be TGF-β but a more proinflammatory cytokine, as a consequence of the inflammatory activation. Production of IL-12 will induce a T$_H$1 phenotype in naive T cells, appropriate for intracellular pathogens. Production of IL-6, TGF-β, and IL-23 induce a T$_H$17 phenotype, appropriate for extracellular pathogens. Conversely, production of IL-4 induces a T$_H$2 phenotype, appropriate for helminth responses. The memory cells generated in this way will home back to the gut and ensure early production of the appropriate cytokine response should initial innate immune responses fail to clear the pathogen or if the pathogen should be encountered again. If a pathogen has previously been encountered, early production of cytokines or release of antibody by appropriately primed memory cells will speed this process in the acute stage of infection. This priming has been confirmed in humans: mucosal T cells activated in vitro, by astrovirus infection of biopsies taken from adults, showed clear HLA-DR restricted T$_H$1 responses.[124]

This initial scenario may be modified by bacterial toxins, some of which act as superantigens, and may thus activate resident effector lymphocytes of various specificities.[125,126] Some organisms such as mycobacteria may persist intracellularly and induce a chronic immunopathology, as seen in intestinal tuberculosis. However, if the local immune response is sufficient to control and clear the invading pathogen, regulatory and repair mechanisms are invoked. Once again it is the innate

immune and archaic lymphocyte populations that dominate. Epithelial integrity is restored, with processes including killing of stressed or infected enterocytes by NK cells and type b IELs, production of trophic cytokines such as keratinocyte growth factor by $\gamma\delta$ cells, and production of TGF-β by many cell types. There is up-regulated local production of TGF-β and IL-10 from dendritic cells and macrophages as a response to the inflammation,[79] and the regulatory environment restores as many of the acutely recruited cells die by apoptosis or become locally adapted.

Following an acute infectious insult, inflammation will thus persist if the pathogen cannot be cleared, epithelial repair mechanisms are defective,[127] or there is an inadequate regulatory response. Malnutrition, particularly where there is deficiency of vitamins A and D or zinc, may contribute to all three predispositions. It is thus notable that the severity of malnutrition in Gambian children is reflected by dominance of T$_H$1 over T$_{REG}$ cytokines within the mucosa.[19]

Chronic Immune-Mediated Inflammation

This is usually driven by T cell clones, although tissue damage may be mediated by induced recruitment and activation of macrophages, neutrophils, mast cells, or eosinophils. In some circumstances autoantibody-induced damage may occur, but this is usually a T cell-dependent specific response, as seen in celiac disease or autoimmune enteropathy.[35]

Depending on the pattern of induced cytokines, chronic T cell responses may be T$_H$1-dominated (inducing a macrophage-mediated Crohn's disease-like lesion), T$_H$2-dominated (inducing an antibody-dominated UC-like response or an eosinophil-mediated pathology), or T$_H$17-dominated (inducing either a neutrophil-dominated lesion or an autoimmune response). Such a lesion may be partly attenuated by compensatory increase in T$_{REG}$ cells or cytokines.

T$_H$1- or T$_H$17-Dominated Responses

These show some overlap.[109] Cytokines produced by these cells, in response to their triggering activator (bacterial or dietary antigens, bacterial superantigens), drive various innate effector cell types. Macrophages are activated by secreted T$_H$1 or T$_H$17 cytokines, and in turn secrete potent proinflammatory cytokines such as TNF-α, IL-1β, and IL-6 and a variety of other radicals, mediators, and enzymes. These cytokines in turn affect other cell types, including epithelial cells, fibroblasts, and vascular endothelium. There is consequent tissue remodeling, including extracellular matrix degradation, vascular thrombosis, neovascularization, neural damage, increased collagen production, and often formation of new inflammatory lymphoid follicles (Figure 6-4). In certain circumstances, particularly if there is persistence of organisms or foreign material within macrophages, these cells aggregate and transform into granulomas. This is induced by T$_H$1 cytokines and is characteristic of a T$_H$1 response.

T$_H$2-Dominated Responses

There are two major patterns of induced inflammatory response.

First, excess IL-4 or IL-13 production by T$_H$2 cells induces a predominantly humoral response, with mucosal production of IgG and/or IgE. Tissue-bound secreted IgG may fix complement and thus trigger complement-mediated tissue damage, as seen in the epithelium in ulcerative colitis. Secreted IgE may

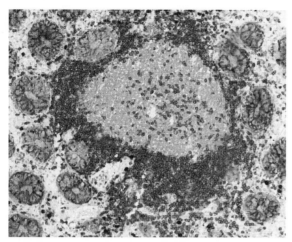

Figure 6-4. CD3+ T cells (showing dark [brown in color plate] surface staining) clustered in the cortex of an inflammatory colonic follicle). Individual T cells may also be seen within the medulla. *(See plate section for color.)*

bind via its Fc receptor to tissue mast cells, triggering degranulation and release of proinflammatory mediators on exposure to its antigen. Consequent responses may include recruitment of large numbers of effector innate immune cells such as polymorph neutrophils. These cells may act jointly to induce matrix degradation vascular disruption. Mast cells and eosinophils in particular may contribute to tissue remodeling, through promoting neovascularization and fibrosis.[128-130]

Where a T_H2 response is dominated by IL-5 rather than IL-4, the inflammatory response is characterized by increased mucosal recruitment of eosinophils, and there is usually marked up-regulation of the eotaxin subfamily of chemokines. Such eosinophil-dominated mucosal inflammation is associated with allergic responses and is characterized by induced dysmotility as well as tissue damage. Extensive tissue remodeling occurs, as is seen in eosinophilic esophagitis, and there is a marked predisposition to fibrosis.[87,92,129]

Inflammation Induced by Vascular or Neural Damage

As discussed throughout this chapter, the integrity of the epithelial barrier is critical in maintaining immunological harmony within the gut. Transient breakdown of epithelial integrity, whether induced by pathogens, chemicals, toxins, or adhesion defects, leads rapidly to mucosal inflammation because of the vast driving force to the mucosal immune system. The constitutive regulatory environment, where continuous low-grade inflammation is held actively in check, is overcome as chemokines, adhesion molecules, and cytokines are up-regulated and a phalanx of unadapted effector cells are recruited. Factors that can chronically disrupt epithelial integrity can thus induce chronic inflammatory change. It is therefore predictable that significant abnormalities in blood supply or innervation in the intestine may promote inflammation.

Mesenteric ischemia may occur for many reasons and may be focal or more generalized. Acute generalized tissue ischemia prejudices epithelial integrity, inducing a state of low-grade inflammation marked by up-regulated chemokine production. However, the very factor causing the epithelial distress is itself protective against the full inflammatory consequences,

as recruitment of inflammatory cells from the blood is limited because of lack of vascular supply. If the supply is restored, there is a rapid influx of inflammatory cells, and tissue damage is greatly magnified. Thus a sequence of ischemia followed by reperfusion is more damaging than chronic ischemia alone. Such a sequence may contribute to inflammation in disorders such as neonatal necrotizing enterocolitis, where mesenteric blood flow abnormalities predispose to disease. Blockade of chemokines induced by ischemia, reducing the recruitment of the unadapted effector cells, ameliorates such large vessel disease.[131,132] More severe chronic inflammation occurs when multiple small vessels are damaged by vasculitis, leaving effector cell recruitment still possible through unaffected nearby vessels: this can cause life-threatening intestinal inflammation that may be misdiagnosed as IBD.[133]

Intact neural function is also important in the maintenance of epithelial integrity and reduction of inflammation. Cholinergic signaling alters transepithelial passage of macromolecules, and psychological stress may promote intestinal inflammation by impairing epithelial barrier function.[134,135] There is also a descending inhibitory neural influence on intestinal inflammatory responses through the sympathetic nervous system.[136] Finally, the function of glial cells within the myenteric plexus appears critical for maintaining intestinal homeostasis, and targeted disruption of enteric glia in mice induced a profound necrotizing enterocolitis-like inflammatory ileitis.[137,138] This severe inflammation was induced, at least in part, by the direct regulation of epithelial integrity by *S*-nitrosoglutathione.[139]

CONCLUSIONS

This review thus ends where it began: by recognition that the intestine is an organ that faces huge challenges from its contents. There is an exquisitely coordinated response, involving nerves, blood vessels, epithelium, and fibroblasts as well as evolutionarily ancient and rather newer immune cells, in which all function together to protect the epithelium and the barrier it provides. There are numerous disparate mechanisms in place, all of which damp down potential inflammation. However, the normal flora is not the invader at the gate, but an essential player in the establishment of these mechanisms of such tolerance – providing, of course, that its composition is appropriate for the host. That composition is one thing we have managed to alter beyond recognition for infants in the developed world during the past century.[39] Just how much this has contributed to the rising incidence of allergic and inflammatory diseases of the intestine and beyond is a matter for speculation. Such a change is, however, very rapid in evolutionary terms. The sudden emergence of celiac disease in the Neolithic Revolution[140] and of hay fever with the pollution of the Industrial Revolution[141,142] suggests that the immune system does not adapt easily to abrupt revolutionary changes in the environment. The impact of the Technological Revolution on ancient flora-induced priming mechanisms within the gut may have had effects much greater than so far recognized.[39,40] Immune tolerance centers on the gut and affects the immune system throughout the body. The consequences of impaired imprinting of tolerance within the gut are usually inflammatory, and a relatively small number of inflammatory mechanisms, driven for the most part by newly recruited unadapted cells, underpin the whole panoply of intestinal inflammatory disorders. Once those new cells get in, there goes the neighborhood.

REFERENCES

1. Turner JR. Intestinal mucosal barrier function in health and disease. Nat Rev Immunol 2009;9:799–809.
3. Duerkop BA, Vaishnava S, Hooper LV. Immune responses to the microbiota at the intestinal mucosal surface. Immunity 2009;31:368–376.
22. Barnes MJ, Powrie F. Regulatory T cells reinforce intestinal homeostasis. Immunity 2009;31:401–411.
32. Izcue A, Coombes JL, Powrie F. Regulatory lymphocytes and intestinal inflammation. Annu Rev Immunol 2009;27:313–338.
69. Strober W. The multifaceted influence of the mucosal microflora on mucosal dendritic cell responses. Immunity 2009;31:377–388.
92. De Brosse CW, Rothenberg ME. Allergy and eosinophil-associated gastrointestinal disorders (EGID). Curr Opin Immunol 2008;20:703–708.

See expertconsult.com for a complete list of references and the review questions for this chapter.

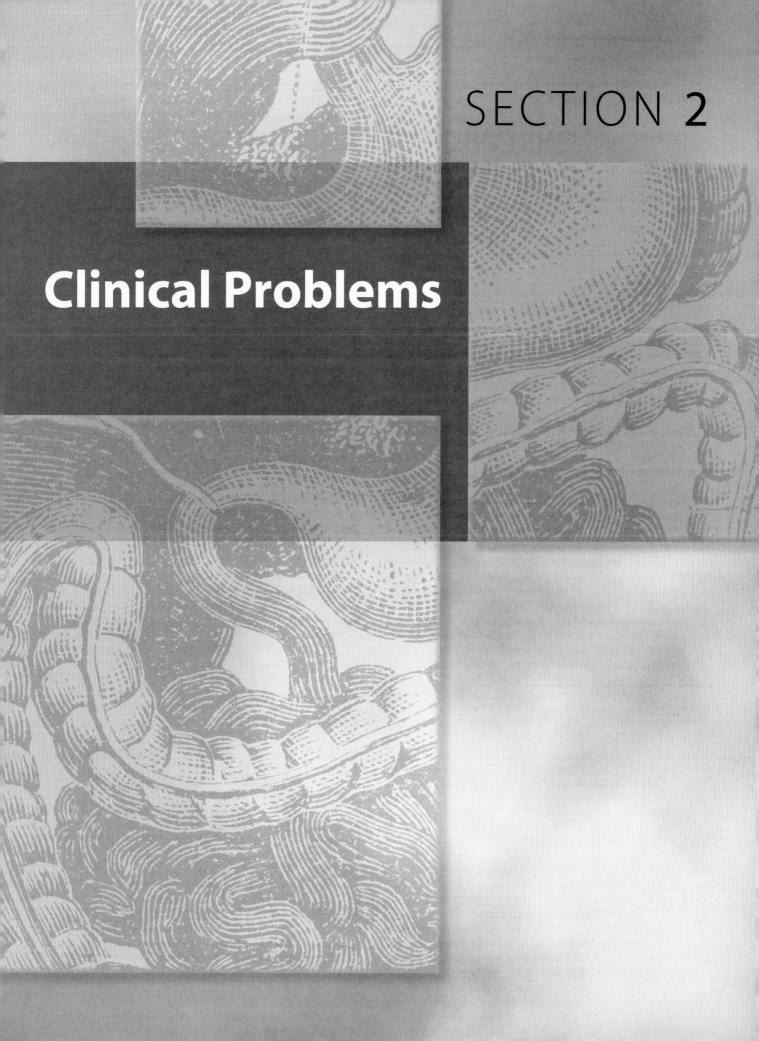

SECTION 2

Clinical Problems

7

CHRONIC ABDOMINAL PAIN OF CHILDHOOD AND ADOLESCENCE

Lori A. Mahajan • Barbara Kaplan

Despite almost six decades of research, chronic abdominal pain of childhood and adolescence remains a common and often-times challenging affliction for patients, their families, and health care providers. The term *recurrent abdominal pain* (RAP) was derived from the British pediatrician John Apley's pioneering study of 1000 school children in 1958.[1] He characterized abdominal pain as chronic or recurrent if at least one episode of pain occurs per month for three consecutive months and is severe enough to interfere with routine functioning. Initial studies indicated that chronic abdominal pain affects 10 to 15% of school-age children; however, more recent community-based data suggest that as many as 46% experience RAP during childhood.[2-4]

Many classification schemes for recurrent abdominal pain have been proposed over the past several decades. For practical purposes, the pain is often classified as either organic or nonorganic, depending on whether a discrete cause is identified. Nonorganic RAP or "functional" gastrointestinal disorder (FGID) refers to abdominal pain that cannot be explained on the basis of inflammatory, anatomic, metabolic, or neoplastic processes. FGID is not synonymous with psychogenic or imaginary abdominal pain, and it is generally accepted as representing genuine pain. Efforts have recently been made to update the symptom-based diagnostic classification system for functional gastrointestinal disorders in children and adults, leading experts to establish the Rome III criteria.[5] Using these criteria, a positive diagnosis of a functional gastrointestinal disorder is made as opposed to the former method of diagnosis in which a functional disorder was only considered as a diagnosis of exclusion. These criteria are detailed later in this chapter.

Early investigators found an organic cause for RAP in only 5 to 10% of patients.[1] Progressive refinement of endoscopic techniques and radiologic imaging modalities as well as the advent of newer technologies such as breath hydrogen testing, motility studies, and wireless capsule endoscopy have greatly enhanced our ability to identify organic causes of RAP. As a result, the percentage of patients with FGIDs appears to be decreasing. A study by Hyams and associates examined 227 children with RAP. A total of 76 patients (33%) were found to have definable causes of RAP such as inflammatory bowel disease, carbohydrate malabsorption, peptic inflammation, or celiac disease.[6] El-Matary et al, also identified organic abnormalities in 30% of children with RAP.[7]

The possibility of overlooking a serious organic condition is of foremost concern to the physician and family, often-times making the formulation of a credible diagnostic and management strategy quite taxing. In the search for the etiology of the abdominal pain, the pediatric patient is at risk for extensive, possibly invasive and expensive diagnostic testing as well as therapeutic interventions that may not be without side effects or long-term complications. This chapter offers an approach to the diagnosis and care of pediatric patients with recurrent abdominal pain that emphasizes a basic screening evaluation for possible organic etiologies, the use of new diagnostic strategies that incorporate symptom-based criteria for functional gastrointestinal disorders, and options for symptom monitoring and management.

Epidemiology

Because the precise pathogenesis of recurrent abdominal pain in pediatric patients has remained unclear for decades, many researchers have turned to epidemiology for insight. In Apley's original survey of 1000 unselected children in primary and secondary schools, 10.8% of children were found to have recurrent abdominal pain.[1] There was a slight female predominance with a female-to-male ratio of those affected of 1.3:1. Of note, there were no complaints of pain in children younger than 5 years of age. Between 10% and 12% of males ages 5 to 10 years had recurrent abdominal pain, followed by a decline in incidence with a later peak at age 14 years. In contrast, however, females had a sharp rise in the incidence of recurrent abdominal pain after age 8 years, with more than 25% of all females affected at age 9 years, followed by a steady decline. More recent population-based studies have shown a similar prevalence. Hyams and colleagues studied 507 adolescents in a suburban area in the United States.[2] The researchers found that abdominal pain occurred at least weekly in 13 to 17% of adolescents, but that only half of these individuals had sought medical attention within the preceding year.

Thus, the incidence of RAP is likely higher than clinical experience would lead us to believe. Sociocultural, familial, and cognitive-behavioral factors help determine the response of the child and family to the pain and affect the likelihood of seeking medical attention.

Family History

Several studies have suggested an interplay between genetic predisposition and particular social influences in the development of FGIDs. Five studies of monozygotic twins with FGIDs have been conducted. A large study that applied the Rome II criteria for the diagnosis of irritable bowel syndrome (IBS) failed to show an increased concordance rate in monozygotic twins.[8] The remaining four studies showed an increased concordance of IBS in monozygotic twins.[9-12] In the Norwegian twin study, the presence of restricted fetal growth with birth weight less than 1500 g was a significant risk factor for the development of IBS. In this subset of patients, IBS developed an average of 7.7 years earlier. The authors noted significantly lower birth weights in monozygotic twins with IBS versus those without.[12] It has subsequently been suggested that impaired maturation of the nervous system interacts with specific genes to induce IBS.

A significantly higher proportion of children with FGID have relatives with alcoholism, conduct or antisocial disorder, attention deficit disorder, or somatization disorder when compared with children with organically based abdominal pain.[13] The patient often comes from a "painful family" (i.e., family members have a high frequency of medical complaints).[1,14] The parents and siblings of patients with FGID have an increased incidence of recurrent abdominal complaints, mental health disorders, and migraine headaches when compared with controls. Stone and Barbero found that 44% of fathers and 56% of mothers of patients with FGID had been diagnosed with medical illnesses.[14] Approximately 46% of these fathers with medical conditions had gastrointestinal illness and 10% had migraines. Similarly, half of the mothers had gastrointestinal complaints diagnosed as "functional" by their physician, and 10% carried the diagnosis of migraine headaches. In addition, approximately 25% of the mothers with a child with FGID had a mild level of psychiatric depression. It is unclear whether the mother's feelings result from having a child with FGID or whether the mother's emotional state contributes to the child's development of pain.[15]

Perinatal and Medical History

The mothers of patients with FGIDs report that their pregnancies were characterized by excessive nausea, emesis, fatigue, or headaches. Difficult labor and delivery with breech presentation or cesarean section is reported in 20 to 31%. Neonatal difficulty, including respiratory distress, infection, or colic, is reported in 20%. The child's past history may also reveal recurrent nightmares, toilet training difficulties and enuresis.[14,16] Current research strongly suggests that psychosocial factors are also closely associated with recurrent abdominal pain without necessarily manifesting as overt psychological illness.

Pathophysiology of Functional Recurrent Abdominal Pain

Chronic abdominal pain is a multifactorial experience currently believed to result from a complex interaction between psychosocial and physiologic factors via the brain-gut axis. Functional recurrent abdominal pain is thought to result from alterations in the neurophysiologic functioning at the level of the gut, spinal afferents, central autonomic relay system, and/or brain. Alterations along this pain axis are thought to result in central nervous system amplification of incoming visceral afferent signals resulting in hyperresponsiveness to both physiologic and noxious stimuli. This failure of down-regulation and concomitant pain amplification has come to be known as visceral hypersensitivity.[17] The precise cause of visceral hypersensitivity in patients with functional recurrent abdominal pain is not yet

clear. Researchers currently believe that transient noxious stimuli, such as mucosal infection or injury, can alter the synaptic efficiency of peripheral and central neurons.[18] This may occur through altered release of serotonin (5-HT) from the enteroenteric cells in the myenteric plexus and/or the release of inflammatory cytokines from activated immune/inflammatory cells following exposure. Through a process known as the *wind-up*, neurons can develop a pain memory than can persist long after the removal of the noxious stimulus.

For many years, functional abdominal pain was considered a motility disorder. Pineiro-Carrero and colleagues demonstrated that patients with FGIDs had more frequent migrating motor complexes with slower propagation velocities compared with healthy controls on antroduodenal motility studies.[19] In addition, these patients also had high-pressure duodenal contractions that were associated with abdominal pain during the study period. Subsequently, Hyman and coworkers identified manometric abnormalities in 89% of pediatric patients with FGIDs undergoing antroduodenal manometry.[20] Years of subsequent research in adult and pediatric patients, however, have led to the conclusion that although patients with functional abdominal pain have motility abnormalities, no specific pattern of motility disturbance is diagnostic for any subgroup of patients.

Psychosocial factors have also been extensively studied with regard to the development and perpetuation of functional recurrent abdominal pain. Early life factors such as family attitude toward illness, abuse history and major loss may significantly influence a person's psychosocial development and thereby their coping skills, social support systems and susceptibility to life stress. Particular personality traits and family psychosocial dynamics have been identified in association with functional recurrent abdominal pain of childhood. Children with RAP are frequently timid, nervous, or anxious and are often described as perfectionists or overachievers.[16] Measures of intelligence in these children have not been found to differ significantly from those of controls. Birth order has been thought to possibly contribute to the development of symptoms, because children with RAP are typically the first- or last-born in the family.[14,16]

Research shows that children with FGIDs, like behaviorally disordered children, experience more life stressors than do healthy controls.[21] Mother, teacher, and child self-report questionnaires indicate that children with FGIDs have higher levels of emotional distress and internalize problems more often than asymptomatic children.[22] Children with RAP, however, have not been found to have an increased incidence of depression or other psychological disorders when compared with children with chronic abdominal pain of organic etiology.[15,23] Raymer and colleagues found that psychological distress accompanies both organic and nonorganic abdominal pain in pediatric patients and that psychological evaluation does not readily distinguish organic from functional pain.[23]

The child's home environment has also been found to greatly influence the child's FGID. Parents relate the onset of pain to significant events such as family disturbance, excitement, or punishment approximately 70% of the time. Marital discord with excessive arguing and/or violence, separation, or divorce is found in almost 40% of affected families. Also, extreme parenting techniques such as excessive punishment or parental oversubmissiveness have been commonly identified in these families.[14]

Specific psychiatric disorders associated with FGIDs in children include generalized anxiety disorder, obsessive-compulsive disorder, attention deficit hyperactivity disorder, and major depressive disorder.[24] Compared to well children, children with chronic abdominal pain are less confident of their ability to change or adapt to a stress and are less likely to use accommodative coping strategy.[25] Increased child affluence appears to be associated with an increased rate of adult IBS. One hypothesis to explain this association is that crowded living conditions at an early age may protect against development of postinfectious IBS. This hygiene hypothesis has also been proposed as an explanation of the different rates of inflammatory bowel disease (IBD) in different countries.[26]

EVALUATION OF THE CHILD WITH CHRONIC ABDOMINAL PAIN

The initial evaluation of the child with chronic abdominal pain should include a comprehensive interview with the child and parents, a thorough physical examination, and specific screening laboratory studies. In addition to performing the evaluation, the physician must also convey genuine concern and establish a trusting and supportive environment. The clinician must ensure that adequate time is allotted for this process.

History

As with any other medical condition, a thorough and detailed history is the most important component of the patient's assessment and often leads to the correct diagnosis. Initial questions should be directed at the patient, using a developmentally appropriate technique. It is important to hear the patient's complaints in his or her own words and to minimize parental influence on the patient response to questions. Examiners should ask the patient to indicate with his or her own hand the location of the pain. It is not helpful when the entire hand is swept diffusely across the abdomen, but it may be helpful when one finger is used to localize an area of pain.

Information should be sought regarding the quality, intensity, duration and timing of the pain. Sharp pain suggests a cutaneous or more superficial structural origin; poorly localized pain is more characteristic of a visceral or functional etiology. The examiner should inquire how well the patient sleeps at night. Pain that awakens the patient from sleep usually indicates organic disease. Temporal correlation of the abdominal pain and other symptoms such as emesis, diarrhea, constipation, or fever is also suggestive of organic disease. In addition, physicians should ask whether there is any relationship between the pain and food consumption, activity, posture, or psychosocial stressors.

Medications, including prescription, over-the-counter, and herbal products, should be accurately recorded. Questions should include whether the child started taking such products before the onset of the abdominal pain. This is of particular importance in patients with conditions such as juvenile rheumatoid arthritis or recurrent headaches who regularly use nonsteroidal anti-inflammatory medications (NSAIDs) for pain relief, because these medications are known to cause both gastritis and mucosal ulceration. The examiner should ask whether medications have been taken in an attempt to relieve the child's abdominal pain, and if so, how efficacious they were. Transient improvement following a laxative may indicate chronic constipation as the cause of the recurrent pain. Temporary relief following acid suppression therapy may indicate peptic inflammation as the etiology.

Physical Examination

The physical examination should begin during the history-gathering process. The physician should carefully note the patient's facial expressions, respiratory pattern, body positioning, and movements. Also, it is imperative to carefully note how the child interacts with family members during the interview and how he or she climbs onto and down from the examination table. It is usually reassuring when the patient energetically jumps from the table following the examination.

The importance of performing a meticulous physical examination cannot be overemphasized. To facilitate a thorough examination, all clothing should be removed and the patient placed in a gown. It is important for the examiner to carefully cover the patient to maintain modesty and prevent embarrassment. The physical examination should be performed with the parents present. This often makes the child more comfortable and allows the parents to appreciate the thoroughness of the examination. The older child or adolescent may prefer that only the same-sex parent remain in the room during the examination. It is usually best to ask the patient what would make him or her the most comfortable.

The clinician should carefully review the child's growth parameters using standard charts. Normal growth is reassuring and is a consistent finding in children with functional recurrent abdominal pain. In contrast, growth failure or weight loss is suggestive of an organic etiology. Typically, patients with functional abdominal pain do not exhibit significant autonomic arousal. The presence of diaphoresis, tachycardia, or elevated systolic blood pressure may actually suggest an acute organic etiology of the abdominal complaints.

Particular attention should be given to the abdominal examination. It is essential to an adequate examination that the patient is as relaxed as possible, room lighting is adequate, and the abdomen is fully exposed from the xiphoid to the symphysis pubis. Before laying hands on the abdomen, carefully inspect the abdomen for the presence of distention, peristaltic waves, striae, dilated vessels, or scars indicative of previous surgery. Next, the character of the bowel sounds should be assessed. High-pitched, frequent bowel sounds may indicate a partial bowel obstruction; hypoactive bowel sounds are consistent with an ileus. While auscultating the abdomen, slight compression with the stethoscope should be applied over the area of complaint to help grade the severity of the pain.

Detailed palpation of the entire abdomen should then be performed to evaluate organ size, presence or absence of masses, or any areas of tenderness. Carnett's test can be performed to aid in distinguishing visceral or somatic pain from central hypervigilance.[27] Once the region of maximal abdominal pain is identified, the patient is asked to assume a partial sitting position, thereby flexing the abdominal wall musculature. Increased abdominal pain (a positive test) is suggestive of a muscle wall etiology (a hernia or cutaneous nerve entrapment) or a central nervous system contribution to the pain, whereas a negative test is consistent with a visceral contribution to the pain. Because frequently identified organic causes of chronic abdominal pain in children are localized to the urinary tract, careful attention must be given to each flank in an attempt to detect tenderness.

Areas where hernias may occur including the umbilicus and inguinal area should carefully be examined. The perianal region must be thoroughly inspected for fissures, fistulas, or skin tags. Digital rectal examination is mandatory to assess external anal sphincter tone, the size of the rectal vault, the volume and consistency of stool present in the rectal vault, and the hemoccult status of the stool. Because the child is often free of abdominal pain at the time of the initial examination, it is important to reexamine the child during an episode of abdominal pain.

Laboratory and Imaging Studies

Laboratory, radiologic, endoscopic, and ancillary evaluation of the patient with chronic abdominal pain should be individualized according to the information obtained during the history and physical examination. Most clinicians recommend the following studies as an initial screen for all patients with recurrent abdominal pain: complete blood count with differential, urinalysis with culture, serum aminotransferases, erythrocyte sedimentation rate, and fecal examination for ova and parasites. It has been suggested that these screening studies, if normal, in combination with a normal physical examination, effectively

TABLE 7-1. Organic Causes of Chronic Abdominal Pain

Gastrointestinal
  Esophagitis (peptic, eosinophilic, infectious)
  Gastritis (peptic, eosinophilic, infectious)
  Peptic ulcer
  Celiac disease
  Malrotation (with Ladd's bands or intermittent volvulus)
  Duplications
  Polyps
  Hernias (diaphragmatic, internal, umbilical, inguinal)
  Inflammatory bowel disease
  Chronic constipation
  Parasitic infection
  Bezoar or foreign body
  Carbohydrate malabsorption
  Intussusception
  Tumor (e.g., lymphoma)
Hepatobiliary/pancreatic
  Biliary dyskinesia
  Sphincter of Oddi dysfunction
  Chronic hepatitis
  Cholelithiasis
  Cholecystitis
  Choledochal cyst
  Chronic pancreatitis
  Pancreatic pseudocyst
Respiratory
  Infection, inflammation, or tumor near diaphragm
Genitourinary
  Ureteropelvic junction obstruction/hydronephrosis
  Nephrolithiasis
  Recurrent pyelonephritis/cystitis
  Hematocolpos
  Mittelschmerz
  Endometriosis
Metabolic/hematologic
  Porphyria
  Hereditary angioedema
  Diabetes mellitus
  Lead poisoning
  Sickle cell disease
  Collagen vascular disease
Musculoskeletal
  Trauma, tumor, infection of vertebral column (e.g., leukemia, herpes zoster, diskitis)

rule out an organic cause in 95% of cases.[28] Other noninvasive studies such as lactose breath hydrogen testing and abdominal ultrasound should be performed if indicated. Ultrasound has gained a prominent role over the past decade because it is painless and does not involve radiation. Three separate studies to investigate the diagnostic value of routine abdominal ultrasound in children with recurrent abdominal pain, however, have failed to demonstrate its utility in this clinical setting.[29-31] In these studies, a total of 217 patients were evaluated. A total of 16 patients were found to have abnormalities identified by abdominal ultrasound, but in no case could the pain be attributed to the abnormality. Thus, the ultrasound did not influence management. In addition, one author suggested that the ultrasound may have even been detrimental when findings such as accessory uterine horn, a uterus that was small for age, and absence of an ovary were identified, because these caused anxiety and prompted further unnecessary consultation.[31]

DIFFERENTIAL DIAGNOSIS

More than 100 causes of abdominal pain have been identified in children and adolescents. Table 7-1 lists many of these causes by organ system. The following discussion briefly reviews the more commonly identified organic causes of recurrent abdominal pain of childhood as well as more recent diagnostic considerations, including eosinophilic esophagitis and biliary dyskinesia. Table 7-2 lists "alarm features" that are suggestive of an organic etiology of symptoms in children with RAP.

Acid Peptic Disease

Acid peptic disease refers not only to ulcer formation in the stomach and duodenum, but also to gastroesophageal reflux disease, gastritis, and duodenitis. The vast majority of pediatric patients with peptic disease present with RAP. Abdominal pain secondary to peptic ulceration in adult patients is considered classic if it is located in the epigastric region, occurs following meals, and awakens the patient in the early morning

TABLE 7-2. Alarm Features Suggestive of Organic Etiology in Child With RAP

History
  Patient age < 5 years
  Constitutional symptoms: fever, weight loss, joint symptoms, recurrent oral ulcers
  Dysphagia
  Emesis, particularly if bile- or blood-stained
  Nocturnal symptoms that awaken child from sleep
  Persistent right upper or right lower abdominal pain
  Referred pain to the back, shoulders, or extremities
  Dysuria, hematuria, or flank pain
  Chronic medication use: NSAIDs, herbals
  Family medical history of IBD, peptic ulcer disease, celiac disease, atopy
Physical examination
  Growth deceleration, delayed puberty
  Scleral icterus/jaundice, pale conjunctivae/pallor
  Rebound, guarding, organomegaly
  Perianal disease (tags, fissures, fistulas)
  Occult or gross blood in stool
Screening laboratory studies
  Elevated WBC or ESR
  Anemia
  Hypoalbuminemia

ESR, erythrocyte sedimentation rate; WBC, white blood cell count.

hours. Pain experienced by children younger than age 12 years may be atypical and occurs anywhere in the middle to upper abdomen, may or may not be unrelated to meals, and has no periodicity. The presenting complaints in children older than age 12 years with peptic disease are similar to the classic adult pattern.[32] Endoscopy is the procedure of choice when mucosal abnormalities are suspected, because contrast radiography of the upper gastrointestinal tract has been found to be unreliable for establishing the diagnosis of peptic ulcer disease in children.

Ulcers are typically associated with underlying systemic illness in children younger than age 10 years. Gastric ulcers may occur in association with extensive burn injuries, head trauma and ingestion of nonsteroidal anti-inflammatory medications, selective COX 2 inhibitors, or corticosteroids. Such ulcers usually do not recur, and there is typically no family history of ulcer disease. In contrast, ulcers in older children usually occur in the absence of underlying illness or medication usage. A positive family history can often be elicited. Such ulcers are often recurrent and have been associated with antral colonization with *Helicobacter pylori*. Epidemiologic studies show that the rate of acquisition of *H. pylori* increases with age, is higher in blacks than whites and is inversely proportional to socioeconomic status.[33] Intrafamilial clustering of *H. pylori* infection has been found, suggesting person-to-person spread of the bacteria.[34]

Because *H. pylori* IgG seropositivity has a sensitivity and specificity of only 45 to 50% in children, it is not recommended as first line testing for the diagnosis of *H. pylori* infection.[35] The ^{13}C-urea breath test (UBT) is a noninvasive method for diagnosis of *H. pylori*. A recent prospective, multicenter study of 176 children in the United States showed the sensitivity and specificity of the UBT to be 95.8% and 99.2%, respectively, when a urea hydrolysis rate above 10 μg/min was considered positive. Even in young children between the ages of 2 and 5 years old, the sensitivity and specificity were both 100%.[36] Another noninvasive diagnostic test, the monoclonal immunoassay for detection of *H. pylori* in stool, has been developed and studied in children. In 118 children ages 0.3 to 18.8 years, this assay showed excellent sensitivity and specificity both before (98% and 100%, respectively) and after therapy (100% and 96.2%).[37] Although these noninvasive tests have high diagnostic accuracy in children, they do not confirm the presence of an ulcer or gastritis. For this reason, endoscopy with antral biopsy remains the preferred method of diagnosis of *H. pylori* infection in pediatric patients.[38] The breath test and monoclonal stool immunoassay remain valuable tools to monitor eradication of the organism following therapy.

Carbohydrate Intolerance

Dietary carbohydrates that are malabsorbed serve as substrates for bacterial fermentation in the colon. By-products of bacterial fermentation include hydrogen, carbon dioxide, and volatile fatty acids such as acetate, propionate, and butyrate. The resultant clinical symptoms of carbohydrate intolerance include abdominal cramping, bloating with abdominal distention, diarrhea, and excessive flatulence.[39]

Malabsorption of lactose is widely recognized as a cause of gastrointestinal distress. The prevalence of lactose malabsorption varies widely among different races, with the lowest prevalence found in Scandinavia and Northwestern Europe. In sharp contrast, between 70% and 100% of North American Indians, Australian aboriginal populations, and inhabitants of Southeast Asia are lactose intolerant. There is also a high prevalence in those of Italian, Turkish, and African descent.[40] Historical information regarding the temporal relationship of lactose consumption to clinical symptoms has been found to be a poor predictor of the presence of lactose intolerance.[41] The least invasive means to establish the diagnosis of lactose malabsorption is breath hydrogen testing. If the test is positive, a strict lactose elimination diet for 2 weeks and maintenance of an abdominal pain diary is advised. Complete resolution of abdominal complaints confirms lactase deficiency as the cause. Subsequently, lactose can be reintroduced into the diet and the patient supplemented with lactase during periods of lactose consumption to minimize symptoms.

Fructose and sorbitol are also common dietary carbohydrates that may be malabsorbed. Fructose-containing foods include honey, fruits, fruit juices, and many commercially available fruit-flavored and/or carbonated beverages. The fruits highest in fructose include apples (5 g/100 g of apple) and pears (5 to 6.5g/100 g of pear). The fructose contents of apple and pear juice are comparable (6 g/100 mL of juice). Excessive intake of these products may lead to abdominal pain in susceptible individuals and should be discouraged. Sorbitol is a polyalcohol sugar commonly found in "sugar-free" gums and confections. It is poorly absorbed by the small intestinal mucosa and has been shown to cause chronic abdominal pain in children.[42]

Celiac Disease

Celiac disease or gluten-sensitive enteropathy is becoming an increasingly recognized cause of chronic abdominal pain in both the pediatric and adult populations. It is a chronic inflammatory disorder of the small intestine caused by exposure to dietary gluten in genetically susceptible individuals. Although the typical presentation involves diarrhea, steatorrhea, iron deficiency anemia, abdominal distention, and failure to thrive, latent or atypical forms of the disease are becoming more commonplace. Patients may present at any age with nonspecific abdominal complaints. With improved recognition of the clinical complexity of this condition and the availability of more sensitive and specific screening tests, celiac disease is now considered a worldwide public health problem. It affects as much as 0.5% to 1% of Europeans or those of European ancestry; however, the majority of cases remain undiagnosed.[43] Known predisposing factors in the pediatric population include autoimmune thyroid disease, trisomy 21, Turner's syndrome, IgA deficiency, and type 1 diabetes mellitus.

Serologic tests currently available serve as excellent screening tools. The tissue transglutaminase (tTG) antibody enzyme-linked immunoassay has emerged as the universally recommended screening test for celiac disease.[44,45] Because between 2% and 10% of individuals with celiac sprue have selective IgA deficiency, IgA levels should be measured at the time of celiac screening. In the IgA-deficient individual, less specific antigliadin IgG antibodies or tissue transglutaminase IgG antibodies are ordered. Unfortunately, the positive predictive value of gliadin antibodies is relatively poor. In one series, the positive predictive value of gliadin IgG corrected for its expected prevalence in the general population was less than 2%.[46] Routine use of antigliadin assays is no longer recommended. The gold standard for diagnosis remains upper endoscopy with biopsy of the distal duodenum/proximal jejunum. Diagnostic histologic findings include total or subtotal villous atrophy, lowering of the ratio of villous height to crypt depth (normal, 3 to 5:1), an increase in intraepithelial lymphocytes (normal, 10 to 30 per 100 epithelial cells), and extensive surface cell damage and infiltration of the lamina propria with inflammatory cells.

Inflammatory Bowel Disease

Studies from the United States and Europe have confirmed a definite increase in the overall incidence rates of pediatric and adult IBD over the past 4 decades.[47-50] A recently published retrospective epidemiological investigation showed that the rate of IBD in children in the United States has doubled over the past decade.[50] The overall incidence rates among white children was significantly higher than among African American and Hispanic children. Crohn's disease was diagnosed more often in all ethnic groups as compared to ulcerative or indeterminate colitis, and African American children were found to be predominantly affected by Crohn's disease. These increased rates are likely in part due to recent advances in diagnostic technology.

Chronic abdominal pain is a common complaint of children with IBD. More than 80% of children with ulcerative colitis present with abdominal pain, hematochezia, and diarrhea.[51] The onset of Crohn's disease is oftentimes more insidious, and presenting complaints are more variable. Symptoms may include chronic abdominal pain, anorexia, weight loss, growth failure, and diarrhea. Associated abdominal pain may be intense and frequently awakens the child from sleep. Perianal disease may develop in up to 30 to 50% of children with Crohn's disease, emphasizing the importance of careful inspection of the perianal region during physical examination.[52]

Laboratory findings suggestive of IBD include anemia, elevated erythrocyte sedimentation rate, thrombocytosis, hypoalbuminemia and heme-positive stool. Elevated fecal markers of inflammation, calprotectin and lactoferrin, have also been found to strongly correlate with mucosal intestinal inflammation.[53,54] Serologic markers, including antibodies against the yeast *Saccharomyces cerevisiae* (ASCA), perinuclear anti-neutrophil cytoplasmic autoantibodies (pANCA), and antibodies to outer membrane porin of *Escherichia coli* (anti-OmpC), have also been found over the past decade to be potentially valuable biologic markers for IBD. Studies, however, have shown the sensitivity of these tests to range from 47 to 84% and the specificity to range from 84 to 100% in high-prevalence populations. The positive predictive value (PPV) has recently been shown to be as low as 60%, and false positive tests are possible.[55-58] A study of 227 pediatric patients showed that the measurement of the combination of erythrocyte sedimentation rate and hemoglobin has a higher positive predictive value and is more sensitive, more specific, and less costly than the commercially available serologic antibody testing.[58]

Wireless capsule endoscopy is another recent medical innovation that enables clinicians to directly visualize the mucosa of the upper gastrointestinal tract and small bowel. This innovative technology is progressively gaining favor and enabling clinicians to determine the health of the small bowel. Capsule endoscopy is detailed elsewhere in the text. Despite these technologic advances, accurate diagnosis of IBD relies on a combination of clinical, laboratory, radiologic, endoscopic, and histologic findings.

Intestinal Parasites

Giardiasis is an infection of the small intestines with the protozoan parasite *Giardia lamblia*. This organism is found throughout temperate and tropical regions worldwide and is the most common human protozoal enteropathogen.[59] Infection typically follows ingestions of fresh water contaminated with the cysts. Although infection is self-limited in the majority of cases, 30% of patients develop chronic symptoms of abdominal pain, nausea, flatulence, diarrhea, and weight loss secondary to malabsorption. Diagnosis is made through identification of the cysts or trophozoites on light microscopy of fresh stool specimens or the more sensitive enzyme-linked immunosorbent assay for *Giardia* antigen.

Individuals infected with parasitic helminths such as *Ascaris lumbricoides* (roundworm) and *Trichuris trichiura* (whipworm) are often asymptomatic. Heavy infestation, however, may lead to chronic abdominal pain, anorexia, diarrhea, rectal prolapse, or even bowel obstruction.[60] Ova and parasite screening of the stool should be performed when infection is suspected.

Chronic Constipation

Chronic constipation is a common cause of RAP in children and accounts for up to 25% of all referrals to the pediatric gastroenterologist.[61] This condition leads to colonic distention, gas formation and painful defecation. There are both functional and organic (myogenic, neurologic, mechanical) forms of chronic constipation.[62] In patients with functional constipation, there is typically voluntary withholding of stool. This may be secondary to such factors as the previous painful passage of stool or refusal to use a public restroom. Such withholding behavior, if prolonged, results in rectal and colonic accumulation of stool, overstretching of anal sphincters, and resultant fecal soiling. Thus, both physical and psychological factors perpetuate this cycle. Diagnosis is often readily made through history and physical examination. A flat-plate radiograph of the abdomen is sometimes helpful, especially if the patient's body habitus precludes deep palpation of the abdomen.

Congenital Anomalies

Intestinal malrotation occurs when there is incomplete or abnormal rotation of the intestines about the superior mesenteric artery.[63] The majority of symptomatic cases present in infancy, and the diagnosis is readily made by the presence of the "double bubble" on plain radiograph of the abdomen or malpositioned bowel on upper gastrointestinal series or barium enema.[64] In the older child, the diagnosis may not be readily apparent, as the presentation is not typically duodenal obstruction. Some 50% of older children with intestinal malrotation present with chronic abdominal pain with or without emesis. The associated abdominal pain is usually transient and poorly localized. There are typically no associated abnormal physical or laboratory findings. The pain is most often postprandial and may be accompanied by bilious emesis, diarrhea, or evidence of malabsorption.[65]

Gastrointestinal tract duplications are tubular or cystic structures, attached to the intestine, often sharing a common muscular wall and vascular supply. The most commonly involved site is the ileum. Chronic abdominal pain, gastrointestinal hemorrhage, and obstruction due to mass effect have been identified as the most common presenting signs and symptoms of duplications in children. When identified, surgery is recommended.[66]

Genitourinary Disorders

Ureteropelvic junction (UPJ) obstruction is an established cause of renal damage in the pediatric population. Early diagnosis allows salvage of renal tissue as well as renal function. UPJ obstruction is more common in males and is most often left-sided.[67] Nonspecific RAP may be the only presenting complaint in a child with this condition. Of note, it has been shown that a normal urinalysis and physical examination do not always exclude a genitourinary abnormality as the cause of the recurrent pain, and ultrasound is necessary if the diagnosis is suspected.[68] In infancy, the diagnosis of UPJ obstruction is rarely delayed, because the patient usually presents with a palpable abdominal mass or urinary tract infection that prompts imaging studies. As children become older, the diagnosis becomes more difficult because the presenting complaint is often nonspecific RAP. Studies show that approximately 70% of patients older than age 6 years with UPJ obstruction present with RAP.[67] It is especially important to consider this diagnosis when the pain is referred to the groin or flank region, and when it is paroxysmal in nature. Additional diagnostic clues include palpation of an abdominal mass to the left or right of midline or hematuria on urinalysis.

Nephrolithiasis is another diagnostic consideration in the child with RAP. In a recent study of 1440 children with nephrolithiasis, the most common presenting complaint was recurrent abdominal pain, reported in 51%.[69] Dysuria was reported in only 13% of these patients, and only 26.7% were found to have hematuria. This condition is more common in males, with a 3:1 ratio. When evaluating a patient with RAP, genitourinary disorders must be kept in mind and further imaging studies performed if clinically indicated.

Eosinophilic Esophagitis

Eosinophilic esophagitis (EE) is becoming an increasingly recognized entity in both pediatric and adult patients. The esophagus, which is normally devoid of eosinophils, has been found over the past decade to be an immunologically active organ capable of recruiting eosinophils in response to a variety of stimuli.[70] Eosinophilic esophagitis is characterized by eosinophilic infiltration of the esophagus presumably due to allergic or idiopathic causes. Common presenting symptoms include epigastric pain, nausea, vomiting, growth failure, dysphagia, and pill or solid food impaction. The disorder has a slight male predominance. A common finding in children is a history of food or environmental allergies and peripheral eosinophilia.[71]

This disorder may have a similar endoscopic appearance to reflux esophagitis with circumferential rings and vertical grooves noted.[72] The rings appear to be caused by lamina propria and dermal papillary fibrosis due to mediators that stimulate the tissue eosinophils or from the eosinophils themselves. An association with Schatzki ring formation has also been described.[73] Strictures are typically located in the proximal or mid-esophagus, as opposed to reflux-induced strictures, which are located in the distal esophagus.[71] The presence of white specks adherent to the esophageal mucosa has recently been found to be highly specific for EE. The specks microscopically are composed of eosinophils.[74] The diagnosis of EE is based

on finding more than 20 eosinophils per high-power field on esophageal biopsies or finding eosinophilic microabscesses on biopsies as opposed to reflux esophagitis, in which fewer than 7 eosinophils per high-power field are seen. Patients with EE have normal 24-h pH probe studies and often do not benefit from acid-suppressive therapy. Many patients with EE benefit from food allergy testing with subsequent elimination diets and topical corticosteroid therapy such as swallowed fluticasone.[75,76]

Biliary Dyskinesia

Biliary dyskinesia or hypokinetic gallbladder disease refers to decreased contractility and poor emptying of the gallbladder that leads to symptomatology. In children, the presentation may include right upper quadrant or epigastric pain, nausea, vomiting, and fatty food intolerance. The diagnosis is made utilizing functional gallbladder emptying studies. Ultrasonography is typically normal. If the diagnosis is suspected, scintigraphy should be performed to measure gallbladder volume before and 30 min after intravenous cholecystokinin (CCK) is injected to stimulate gallbladder emptying. In most centers, a gallbladder ejection fraction of greater than or equal to 35% is considered normal. In a recent pediatric study, 41 of 42 patients diagnosed with biliary dyskinesia became pain-free following laparoscopic cholecystectomy.[77]

DIAGNOSIS OF CHILDHOOD FUNCTIONAL ABDOMINAL PAIN DISORDERS

The diagnosis of functional pediatric disorders has evolved since the turn of the millennium from the exclusion of organic disease to the utilization of positive symptom criteria in combination with a conservative diagnostic approach. This paradigm shift has most recently resulted in the Rome III criteria, published in April 2006.[5] An international team of pediatric gastroenterologists met in Rome and arrived at a consensus for the symptom-based diagnosis of pediatric functional gastrointestinal disorders. Table 7-3 lists these functional pediatric gastrointestinal disorders. A positive diagnosis of a functional gastrointestinal disorder can be made using symptom-based criteria, thereby reducing the tendency to order studies to rule out other potential disease processes.

Functional Dyspepsia

The prevalence of functional dyspepsia ranges between 3.5% and 27% in children.[78,79] A diagnosis of functional dyspepsia can be made in children mature enough to provide an accurate history of pain that is present at least once per week for at least 2 months before diagnosis. The persistent or recurrent discomfort is typically centered in the upper abdomen (above the umbilicus) and there is no evidence of an inflammatory, anatomic, metabolic, or neoplastic process that explain the subject's symptoms. In addition, there is no evidence that dyspepsia is relieved by defecation or is associated with the onset of a change in stool frequency or stool form. The mandatory use of upper endoscopy before making this diagnosis was eliminated in the new Rome III criteria to decrease the use of an invasive investigation that has a low diagnostic yield for significant pathology in the pediatric population. In adults, there are two presentations of functional dyspepsia. In ulcer-like dyspepsia, the most bothersome symptom is pain centered in the

TABLE 7-3. ROME III Classification of Childhood Functional Abdominal Pain Disorders

H1. Vomiting and aerophagia
H1a. Adolescent rumination syndrome
H1b. Cyclic vomiting syndrome
H1c. Aerophagia
H2. Abdominal pain-related FGIDs
H2a. Functional dyspepsia
H2b. Irritable bowel syndrome
H2c. Abdominal migraine
H2d. Childhood functional abdominal pain
H3. Constipation and incontinence
H3a. Functional constipation
H3b. Nonretentive fecal incontinence

Drossman D, Corazziari E, Talley N, et al. The Functional Gastrointestinal Disorders: Diagnosis, Pathophysiology and Treatment. A Multinational Consensus, 3rd ed. McLean, VA: Degnon Associates; 2006.

upper abdomen. In dysmotility-like dyspepsia, the predominant symptom is the sensation of early satiety, upper abdominal fullness, bloating, or nausea centered in the upper abdomen. Under the new Rome criteria, committee members found insufficient evidence to adopt these criteria for children.

Irritable Bowel Syndrome

Before the diagnosis of irritable bowel syndrome in pediatric patients, the diagnostic criteria must be fulfilled at least once per week for at least 2 months. The abdominal discomfort or pain must be associated with two or more of the following at least 25% of the time: improvement with defecation, onset associated with a change in frequency of stool, or onset associated with a change in form/appearance of stool. Also for the diagnosis of IBS, there must be no evidence of an inflammatory, anatomic, metabolic, or neoplastic process that would explain the patient's symptoms. Other symptoms that have been found to support the diagnosis of IBS include abnormal stool frequency (more than three bowel movements per day or fewer than three bowel movements per week), abnormal stool form (lumpy, hard, loose, or watery), abnormal stool passage (straining, fecal urgency, or the sensation of incomplete evacuation), passage of mucus, or abdominal bloating.[5] As with other functional disorders, the diagnosis should be made only following a detailed history and physical examination as outlined previously in this chapter. In the absence of alarm features suggestive of an organic etiology of abdominal pain, the child who meets Rome III criteria for IBS should be given a positive diagnosis.

Childhood Functional Abdominal Pain

Functional abdominal pain can be diagnosed when all of the following criteria are fulfilled at least once per week for at least 2 months: episodic or continuous abdominal pain, insufficient criteria for other functional gastrointestinal disorders that would explain the pain, and no evidence of an inflammatory, anatomic, metabolic, or neoplastic process that would explain the patient's symptoms.[5]

Abdominal Migraine

Abdominal migraine is a paroxysmal disorder reported to affect 1 to 4% of children and is more common in girls. The average age of onset is 7 years with a peak at 10 to 12 years.[80,81]

Children with at least two paroxysmal episodes, of intense abdominal pain within the past 12 months lasting 1 hour or more, with intervening symptom-free intervals lasting weeks to months, may have abdominal migraines. Occasionally, these episodes awaken the child or occur upon rising. The pain interferes with normal activities. In order for this diagnosis to be made, there must also be two or more of the following symptoms: anorexia, nausea, vomiting, headache, photophobia, or pallor. In addition there must be no evidence of inflammatory, anatomic, metabolic, or neoplastic process that explains the child's symptoms. Some children do not meet classic criteria but respond well to antimigraine therapy.

THERAPEUTIC STRATEGY DEVELOPMENT

Reassurance

Functional abdominal pain in a child or adolescent often affects the entire family. The therapeutic approach must, therefore, be directed at the entire family as a unit, and an effective physician-family relationship must be established. Successful therapy depends on education, reassurance, and ongoing support for the patient and family members. It is of utmost importance, therefore, for the physician to gain the trust of the child and parents and to establish a supportive and caring environment.

Once the diagnosis of functional abdominal pain has been made, it is important to clearly review with the child and parents how the diagnosis was established and address any lingering concerns they may have. It is often helpful to show the child's growth parameters on the growth chart to emphasize that normal growth and development are present. Physicians should detail how the constellation of symptoms fits the diagnostic criteria of a functional condition. It is important to reassure the family further by reviewing the normal physical examination and screening laboratory studies and stress to the family that this is a common condition affecting up to 20% of all school-age children.[2] Knowing that other families are similarly afflicted and are successfully coping with the condition may provide reassurance and a sense of confidence for the family.

Central to the initiation of a therapeutic relationship with the patient and family is to acknowledge that the pain the child is experiencing is genuine and not imagined. It is often helpful to explain the pain and the term *functional*, so the patient and parents have a better understanding of the situation. Using an analogy such as the almost universally experienced headache may be helpful. Most will understand that headaches cause genuine pain and do not necessarily represent underlying organic pathology. It is also helpful to explain that research indicates that abdominal pain may result from specific visceral hypersensitivity and that the contractions of the gastrointestinal tract are often related to our emotional states through hormonal and neural pathways. Thus, emotional upset or stress may result in such symptoms as nausea, abdominal cramping, constipation, diarrhea, diaphoresis, or pallor in susceptible individuals.

Set Realistic Therapeutic Goals

The goal of therapy is to decrease stress or tension for the child while promoting normal patterns of activity and school attendance. Focus should be placed on improvement of daily symptoms and quality of life, while not guaranteeing complete resolution of symptoms. This should be explained in detail to the patient and family early in the course of management.

Identify and Address Specific Obstacles Related to School Attendance

Absence from school is relatively common among children with FGIDs. Liebman observed school absenteeism of more than 10% of school days in 28% of these children. Regular school attendance was observed in only 9%.[16] Rapid return to school with alteration of specifically aversive elements should be advised. The importance of acknowledging the abdominal pain without encouraging it should be emphasized to the parents. If the pain is not acknowledged, the child may exhibit extreme pain behavior in order to convince the parent that the pain exists. Therefore some authors recommend designating a certain time of the day for the child to discuss the pain with the parent.[82] Also, discuss with the parents the possibility that secondary gain may play a role in the continued pain behavior of the child. Assess how often pain behavior has resulted in the child remaining home from school or being exempt from participation in physical education class at school or performance of household duties. If pain appears to be maintained by secondary gain, specific rules need to be established. For example, if the child is in enough distress to stay home from school, he or she is then considered ill enough to remain in bed without any television, videogames, toys, or other special privileges.

In many cases, helping the child with recurrent abdominal pain (either organic or functional) is a challenging task for many reasons. Even if the underlying pain is adequately controlled, children may feel overwhelmed by the amount of make-up schoolwork that confronts them, and this may perpetuate school absenteeism. For this reason, at the initial evaluation, it is imperative to ask how much school has been missed and determine whether the family has devised a way to complete missed school assignments. If no such plan exists, advise the parents to contact the school to find out exactly what make-up work is necessary and negotiate with school officials a reasonable timeline for completion of the work. Occasionally, a reduction in the workload may be necessary if it seems overly burdensome. In addition, it has been suggested that children will find make-up work more manageable if it is broken into small components, with a schedule that emphasizes steady progress rather than final products.[83]

School restroom facilities represent another obstacle to regular school attendance, because many children simply refuse to use them. Children seem to avoid school restrooms for a variety of reasons including poor sanitation, lack of privacy, and lack of adequate time to use the facilities. Such concerns present particular problems for children with gastrointestinal disorders that lead to the urge to defecate frequently or with short notice. Children with significant anxiety related to the use of public restrooms need to learn in stages how to use these facilities. Experts recommend that children should first learn to use the restroom at the homes of friends and relatives and then proceed to bathrooms located at public locations such as the mall, department stores, or the movies.[83] It is oftentimes helpful for the physician to write a letter to school officials outlining that for medical reasons, the patient should be granted liberal bathroom privileges and be permitted to leave the classroom whenever necessary. This allows the patient to have more control to prevent accidents and may permit the child to use the bathroom when other children are not present.

Another obstacle to school attendance may be the fear of a significant episode of abdominal pain that the patient cannot manage. Children with FGIDs tend to have poor coping skills with regard to their pain and may exhibit such exaggerated distress that they are rushed for medical evaluation or an ambulance is called. Children with functional abdominal pain are often caught in a vicious cycle of anticipation of pain, increased anxiety, concomitant physiological arousal, lowered pain threshold, and increased distress.[84] All therapeutic strategies should be designed to teach the pediatric patient that he or she can cope with the pain. After prolonged school absenteeism, it is advisable to encourage abbreviated attendance at school initially to help the patient build confidence that he or she can manage an episode of pain while at school.[83] It is best to advise initial return to school for several hours per day with gradual escalation of the time in the classroom. Should a pain episode occur while at school, it is advisable that the patient be permitted to lie down in the nurse's office for a brief period until able to return to class rather than call home or leave school early. The child may also benefit from referral to a specialist for training in relaxation techniques.

Abdominal Pain Diary: The Patient and Family Take Responsibility

The patient and family need to take an active role with a chronic disorder such as recurrent abdominal pain. The patient and family should be encouraged to maintain a symptom diary at the initial medical visit and at anytime a therapeutic measure is initiated. The diary often empowers them with observational skills and insight they would not have had otherwise. As in clinical studies, prospective observations are more reliable than those made retrospectively. Abdominal pain diaries should be customized according to the patient and clinical scenario. At a minimum, the diary should include the following entry columns[1]: date and time when the symptom exacerbation occurred,[2] the location of the pain,[3] the character, severity (on a scale of 1 to 10) and duration of the pain,[4] factors preceding onset of symptoms (food, activity, psychosocial stressors, school attendance, interactions with friends or family, menses),[5] description of daily stooling pattern,[6] and identified relieving factors.[85] Many times, patients and their families are surprised when they identify exacerbating factors such as psychological stressors, excess fat in the diet, or stooling irregularities that are amenable to therapy.

Negotiate Therapy

To maximize the potential for compliance, the physician, the patient, and the family must agree on the plan of therapy. This is done after adequate evaluation and education regarding the patient's condition has taken place. The physician should make inquiries regarding the family's understanding of, personal experience with, and interest in a variety of treatments. The physician should then provide choices consistent with the family's wishes and beliefs, rather than mandate a particular course of therapy.[85]

Patients with mild symptoms with little impact on psychosocial functioning usually respond well to reassurance, education, and applicable dietary or lifestyle modifications. Those patients with moderately severe symptoms typically require pharmacotherapy and/or behavioral therapy. If abdominal symptoms are severe, continuous, and unrelated to changes in gastrointestinal functioning, psychoactive medications for central analgesia (such as tricyclic antidepressants or serotonin reuptake inhibitors) are indicated in addition to a "team approach" including psychiatrists, behavioral specialists, dietitians, and social workers working in combination with the primary care physician and gastroenterologist.

DIET

Dietary recommendations have been found in clinical practice to be helpful for some patients with FGIDs of childhood. If specific dietary triggers are identified such as lactose, fructose, caffeine, spicy foods, fatty foods, carbonated beverages, large meals, or gas-forming vegetables, they should be reduced or eliminated from the diet. Excess consumption of artificial sweeteners such as mannitol or sorbitol should also be avoided as this may lead to increased flatus production with concomitant abdominal discomfort and distention.[42] The increased popularity and consumption of sports drinks and flavored waters is due to the perception by the public that they are "healthy alternatives" to soda. However, they may result in considerable abdominal pain and excess flatus in some patients. This is due to the high content of nonabsorbable disaccharides, especially in the case of low-calorie beverages. The excess nonabsorbed carbohydrate undergoes bacterial fermentation in the colon with resultant gas, bloating, and loose stools, similar to the symptoms of lactose intolerance. Thus, changing to regular nonflavored, noncarbonated water is a simple and inexpensive strategy in the management of some patients with recurrent abdominal pain.

The role of increased dietary fiber in patients with FGIDs remains controversial. A Cochrane analysis reviewing randomized or "quasi-randomized" pediatric trials of dietary therapy versus placebo in school-aged children with RAP based on Rome II criteria failed to demonstrate a benefit to either lactose elimination or fiber supplementation in the pediatric age group.[86] However, a total of only four trials that included a total of 173 patients formed the entire study group. There is a significant need for controlled and randomized trials of dietary therapy in pediatric patients, especially given the lack of anticipated potential adverse effects compared to pharmacologic therapy.

Most studies of dietary fiber intake and irritable bowel syndrome in adults have shown that although dietary fiber does improve constipation, it does not appear to consistently improve abdominal pain. A meta-analysis concluded that only three previously performed studies in adults were of "high quality." The authors determined that even the positive studies showed no significant improvement in stool frequency, abdominal pain, and bloating.[87] As a general rule, the number of grams of fiber consumed daily should be at least the age of the patient in years plus five up to the adult recommendation of 30 g/day. The patient should be advised to increase dietary fiber gradually, as a rapid increase may lead to increased colonic gas production, abdominal distention, and pain. The importance of regular, well-balanced meals consumed in calm surroundings with minimal distractions should also be emphasized. Potentially dangerous restrictive or fad diets should be discouraged.

PHARMACOTHERAPY

The placebo response rate can be very high in functional gastrointestinal disorders, making it difficult to establish superiority of a new treatment over placebo. In functional dyspepsia, the placebo response has varied from 13 to 73%, whereas for IBS,

the reported range has been up to 88%.[88] There have been limited placebo-controlled trials evaluating the therapeutic effect of pharmacologic agents in pediatric patients with FGIDs. As with many disorders, data from adult studies are, therefore, extrapolated and medications judiciously prescribed to the pediatric population. Patients symptoms that are severe enough to disrupt daily activities will likely benefit from pharmacologic therapy. Such therapy should be individualized and directed toward the predominant symptom.

Histamine Receptor Antagonist Therapy

For patients with predominant dyspepsia (discomfort centered in the epigastrium, nausea, early satiety, postprandial fullness, recurrent emesis), a short course of empiric therapy with an H2-histamine receptor antagonist is acceptable. In clinical practice, failure to respond to such medication or a recurrence of symptoms following discontinuation of the therapy should prompt further evaluation. Review of the literature identified only one study performed in the pediatric population to evaluate the effects of acid suppression therapy on FGIDs. See et al. conducted a double-blinded, placebo-controlled trial of famotidine in a small group of children with dyspepsia and abdominal pain.[89] The investigators found that famotidine only subjectively improved symptoms, but placebo was equally effective when the authors applied an objective score. There are currently no pediatric data to support the long-term benefit of antisecretory therapy in patients with FGIDs.

Cyproheptadine, a central and peripheral H1 nonselective histamine receptor antagonist with antiserotonergic properties, was recently studied for the treatment of functional abdominal pain in childhood. A double-blind, randomized, placebo-controlled trial was performed in 29 children ages 4 to 12 years with FAP. Patients were randomized for 2 weeks to placebo or cyproheptadine. Eighty-six percent of children in the cyproheptadine group and 36% of those in the placebo group had improvement or resolution of abdominal pain at the end of the study.[90]

Peppermint Oil

Peppermint oil has been used to soothe the gastrointestinal tract for hundreds of years. It relaxes intestinal smooth muscle by decreasing calcium influx into the smooth muscle cells. A meta-analysis of five randomized, double-blinded, placebo-controlled trials performed in adult patients supported the efficacy of peppermint oil in the treatment of irritable bowel syndrome.[91] One randomized, double-blind, controlled trial in pediatric patients with IBS demonstrated the efficacy of enteric-coated peppermint oil capsules (Colpermin, Pfizer Consumer Healthcare) in the reduction of pain during the acute phase of IBS.[92] Children weighing 30 to 45 kg received one capsule (187 mg peppermint oil) and those over 45 kg received two capsules, three times daily. Use of enteric-coated products reduces side effects such as nausea and heartburn. Unfortunately, this product is usually not covered by insurance companies in the United States and is relatively expensive.

Anticholinergic Agents

Anticholinergic agents such as dicyclomine (Bentyl, Axcan Scandipharm) and hyoscyamine (Levsin, Levbid, NuLev, all by Schwarz Pharma) are commonly used in the United States to treat pain associated with functional intestinal disorders. These agents are smooth muscle relaxants that block the muscarinic effects of acetylcholine on the gastrointestinal tract, thereby relaxing smooth muscle and potentially reducing spasm and abdominal pain, slowing intestinal motility, and decreasing diarrhea. Although commonly prescribed, the efficacy of these agents has not been clearly established in adult trials, nor have any randomized, double-blind, placebo-controlled trials been conducted in the pediatric population. Potential side effects if used in high dosages include drowsiness, blurred vision, dry mouth, tachycardia, constipation, and urinary retention. In clinical practice, anticholinergic agents are best utilized on an as-needed or episodic basis given up to four times daily. When postprandial symptoms are predominant, they can be most helpful if given before meals. With chronic use, dicyclomine and hyoscyamine become less effective, and a low-dose tricyclic antidepressant should be considered should the patient's pain be constant and/or disruptive to daily functioning.

In addition, hyoscyamine is also available in combination with atropine, scopolamine, and phenobarbital (Donnatal, PBM Pharmaceuticals). Another combination medication available in the United States is Librax (Valeant Pharmaceuticals International), which is an antispasmodic medication with anticholinergic properties (clidinium bromide) combined with chlordiazepoxide hydrochloride. These combination medications have gained popularity over the years, but have not been well evaluated in clinical trials. They cannot currently be recommended for use in pediatric patients, because they have the potential for unwanted sedative and addictive side effects.

Tricyclic Antidepressants

Tricyclic antidepressants (TCAs) may offer some relief to patients with FGID. The neuromodulatory and analgesic effects of these agents result from a combined anticholinergic effect on the gastrointestinal tract, mood elevation and central analgesia. Unfortunately, data from placebo-controlled trials of the usefulness of these agents for patients with FGID are limited. Because antidepressants are used on a continuous basis rather than on an episodic basis when symptoms arise, they should be reserved for those with frequent or continuous abdominal complaints.

Tricyclic antidepressants have been in use for more than 50 years. They have a "quinidine-like" effect, are arrhythmogenic, and can lower the seizure threshold. This class of antidepressants has been the most widely studied for the treatment of irritable bowel syndrome in adults and is relatively inexpensive. In a meta-analysis, TCA medications in adults were shown to result in significant improvement in global gastrointestinal symptoms as compared with placebo.[93] The dosage needed to produce relief of recurrent abdominal pain is typically considerably less than that routinely used for the treatment of primary depression, and therefore, potentially serious cardiovascular side effects are less likely. Well-defined dosing guidelines are not available. Many clinicians start with very low doses of 0.2 mg/kg/day and slowly titrate up to 0.5 mg/kg/day for medications such as amitriptyline. The medication is usually given as a single bedtime dose. Because of the potential for development of serious cardiac arrhythmias in patients with prolonged QT syndrome, some advocate obtaining an electrocardiogram before initiation of TCA therapy. Also important to note is that the timing of onset of pain relief may occur almost immediately

or take as long as 10 weeks.[94] Amitriptyline may promote sleep, whereas desipramine and nortriptyline may be preferred when less anticholinergic and sedative effects are desired.

Two recent clinical trials have evaluated the efficacy of TCA therapy in the treatment of functional abdominal pain in children. A single-center study in a suburban pediatric gastroenterology practice in California conducted in 33 adolescents with IBS found a beneficial effect of amitriptyline in comparison to placebo in terms of quality of life and pain relief.[95] A larger, multicenter randomized double-blinded trial on the efficacy of amitriptyline in the treatment of FGID was performed on 90 children. Patients weighing under 35 kg received 10 mg per day, whereas those over 35 kg were given 20 mg per day. The authors showed improvement in 59% of the children receiving amitriptyline in the intention-to-treat analysis. Of note, 75% of children in the placebo group also reported fair to excellent pain relief. Both groups of children had a similar significant improvement in pain, disability, depression, and somatization scores during the 4 weeks of the trial. The safety of the low-dose amitriptyline in addition to clinical improvement led the authors to conclude that the use of this medication may be justified in children with FGIDs.[96]

Serotonergic Agents

Serotonin is found in high concentrations in the enterochromaffin cells located in the epithelial layer of the gastrointestinal tract. At least 14 serotonin receptor subtypes with varying actions in the peripheral and central nervous systems exist. Of these receptors, 5-HT3 and 5-HT4 receptors appear to play a role in the pathophysiology of IBS, and recent studies suggest that pharmacologic agents directed toward these receptors improve symptoms in these patients.

Selective serotonin reuptake inhibitors (SSRIs) may be helpful for some patients with unremitting pain and impaired daily functioning, even if no depressive symptoms are present. The highly selective serotonin reuptake inhibitor citalopram (Celexa, Teva Pharmaceuticals USA) has recently been studied in children with FGIDs.[97] The authors conducted a 12-week open-label flexible-dose trial. Children were given 10 mg daily initially with progressive dose escalation to 40 mg per day by week 4 if no clinical improvement occurred. By week 12, half the children rated their symptoms as very much improved. The study also showed improvement in comorbid depression and anxiety. There are no published controlled studies of the use of SSRIs for FGIDs in children; however, studies in adults do suggest that they can be effective in functional abdominal pain syndromes. These agents are often prescribed because of their lower side-effect profile as compared to TCAs. In addition, as noted in the earlier pediatric study, they are regarded as superior for treatment of comorbid psychiatric conditions such as anxiety or panic disorders, obsessive disorders, or depression.

The most commonly prescribed 5-HT3 receptor antagonists are ondansetron (Zofran, GSK Pharma) and granisetron (Kytril, Roche Laboratories). In the upper gastrointestinal tract, some chemotherapeutic and radiotherapeutic agents cause the release of 5-HT from enterochromaffin cells. Serotonin then activates vagal afferents via 5-HT3 receptors, triggering emesis by stimulation of the area postrema and chemoreceptor trigger zone. Ondansetron and granisetron are very effective in reducing postchemotherapy nausea, but do not consistently alleviate the pain associated with FGIDs or alter stooling pattern. These agents, therefore, are not routinely recommended for functional gastrointestinal pain syndromes unless nausea is a predominant symptom.

Another 5-HT3 antagonist, alosetron (Lotronex, Prometheus Laboratories Inc.), was approved in 2000 for the treatment of women with diarrhea-predominant IBS. It appears to decrease visceral sensation, prolong and reduce postprandial motility, increase colonic compliance, enhance jejunal water and sodium absorption, and induce constipation by slowing left colon transit time.[98] Four large, randomized, placebo-controlled, double-blind trials have been conducted to assess the efficacy of alosetron in adult women with diarrhea-predominant IBS. All studies showed improvement in measured outcomes including fecal urgency and abdominal pain.[99-102] The most common side effect is constipation, occurring in 22 to 39% of patients. A significant adverse event with an unclear association with alosetron is acute ischemic colitis, with an estimated incidence of 0.1 to 1%. The drug was temporarily removed from the market, but was reapproved by the FDA in the spring of 2002 with certain restrictions including a risk management program and enrollment of prescribing physicians. The efficacy of this medication in men is unclear, as few male subjects were enrolled in the trials. No pediatric studies have been performed.

Probiotics

Probiotics are living microorganisms that when ingested in adequate amounts may confer a health benefit to the host. Many food supplements containing probiotic microorganisms are commercialized; however, only 10% of these have the composition claimed on the label. Therefore, it is challenging for the consumer as well as the health care professional to know which products are of good quality.

It has been postulated, as in small bowel bacterial overgrowth, that alterations in gut flora are associated with gastrointestinal dysfunction. Investigators have studied the use of probiotics in patients with IBS. In a double-blind randomized controlled trial, 50 children with IBS were treated with either *Lactobacillus* GG (3×10^{10} colony-forming units twice daily) or placebo for 6 weeks.[103] The authors did not identify any significant differences between the treatment and placebo groups on any stated outcome measure with the exception of abdominal distention. *Lactobacillus* GG (3×10^9 colony-forming units twice daily) was again studied more recently in a larger, 4-week placebo-controlled study of 104 patients ages 6 to 16 years who fulfilled the Rome II criteria for functional dyspepsia, IBS, or FAP.[104] Twenty-five percent of the children in the *Lactobacillus* GG group compared to 9.6% in the placebo group responded to therapy. Children with IBS were more likely to respond to the probiotic therapy when compared to the placebo or FAP groups. Although these findings suggested efficacy, the confidence intervals were wide and the sample sizes in the individual groups were small.

Despite their increasing popularity and lack of FDA monitoring, few adverse side effects have been linked to probiotic consumption. The clinician must be mindful that probiotics are over-the-counter supplements and are, therefore, not covered under standard health insurance plans. Further studies are needed to better define the role of probiotic use in children with FGIDs before they can be routinely recommended.

PSYCHOLOGICAL THERAPIES

In recent years, there has been increased emphasis on specific psychological therapies for FGIDs of childhood. Because functional gastrointestinal disorders are so complex, a multidisciplinary approach is oftentimes beneficial. The physician with a busy practice schedule must set reasonable appointment time limitations with these patients and their family members and must recognize when management is best shared with mental health professionals. Currently, there are no comparative data in the pediatric patient population to determine which psychological therapies are superior or which are better for a particular patient group or gastrointestinal complaint. The physician should be familiar with available therapies and should identify and establish a therapeutic working relationship with a local behavioral specialist.

Cognitive-Behavioral Therapy

Cognitive-behavioral therapy (CBT) involves identifying maladaptive thoughts, perceptions, and behaviors and using this information to teach the patient coping skills and how to gain control of their symptoms. Six studies (including 167 children) of cognitive-behavioral therapy in children with RAP have been conducted.[105-110] Finney et al. administered a brief multicomponent CBT to 16 children ages 6 to 13 years with RAP. Eighty-one percent of patients reported significant reductions in pain, school absences, and medical utilization.[105] Robins et al. reported the results of a randomized controlled trial of 40 children with RAP who received CBT compared with a control group of 29 children with RAP who were given standard medical care. Both groups had reduced abdominal pain, somatization, and significantly less functional disability at 3 and 6-12 month follow-up visits. Children who received CBT reported significantly lower abdominal pain at post-therapy and follow-up visits than controls. They also had less functional disability than controls; however, the differences were not statistically significant.[106] Sanders and colleagues conducted two randomized controlled multicomponent CBT trials studying the treatment of FGID in children. In the first trial, 16 children ages 6 to 12 years were randomly assigned to an 8-week wait-list control group versus CBT consisting of parent training and relaxation training. Parents in the CBT group were trained to ignore nonverbal pain behaviors, redirect children to an activity following verbal pain complaints, and provide praise and positive reinforcement following compliance. The number of pain-free children in the CBT group following therapy was significantly higher than the control group at posttreatment (75% versus 25%) and at the 3 month follow-up visit (87.5% versus 37.5%).[107] The authors later conducted a larger study of 44 children with RAP and use of shorter CBT consisting of only six sessions. The authors found the CBT group to have more pain-free children and lower relapse rates at follow-up.[108] Humphreys and Gervirtz conducted a randomized trial with four therapy groups: fiber; fiber and relaxation; fiber, relaxation and CBT; and fiber, relaxation, CBT, and parent training. All treatment groups reported pain reduction; however, the three treatment groups with a psychological therapy component reported greater reduction in pain, sick behaviors, school absences, and medication use. Pain elimination was reported in 72% of psychological treatment participants versus 7% of the fiber-only group. No significant difference was identified among the three psychological treatment groups.[109] More recently, a nonrandomized clinical trial of children ages 5 to 13 years with FGID using CBT versus standard medical therapy was performed. Both therapies were administered by two pediatricians. CBT consisted of relaxation, psychoeducation, and parent training. Over a 3-month period, those in the CBT group reported a significant reduction in pain as compared to those in the control group (86.6% versus 33.3%).[110]

These six studies recently underwent Cochrane review.[111] The trials were deemed to be relatively small and had some weaknesses in design and reporting. Because each of the included studies reported a statistically significant benefit to participants in the intervention group, the Cochrane reviewers thought CBT is, therefore, worth considering for some children with RAP, but pointed out the need for further, better-quality research using CBT. The American Academy of Pediatrics subcommittee on chronic abdominal pain in children recently rated CBT as an "efficacious treatment."[112]

Relaxation (Arousal Reduction) Training

Relaxation or arousal reduction training includes a variety of techniques to teach patients to counteract the physiological sequelae of stress or anxiety. The most commonly used techniques include progressive muscle relaxation training; biofeedback for striated muscle tension, skin temperature, or electrodermal activity; and transcendental or yoga meditation. Most techniques incorporate a quiet environment, a relaxed and comfortable body position, and a mental image to focus attention away from distracting thoughts or body perceptions. Audiotapes may be used to guide practice at home. Relaxation training has been shown in adults to significantly reduce gastrointestinal symptoms as compared with controls.[113] There is little information on the effectiveness of biofeedback and none on the effectiveness of other forms of arousal reduction training in children with FGIDs.

Hypnotherapy

Hypnosis involves the use of body relaxation and helps the child focus on imaginative, comforting, and safe experiences to overcome symptomatology. The induction phase involves eye fixation and hand levitation techniques to increase the patient's openness to suggestion. Subsequently, the hypnotherapist uses progressive muscular relaxation and "gut-directed" hypnotherapy. For example, the patient is asked to place his or her hands on the area of most abdominal pain, to feel the warmth radiating from the hands into the abdomen, and to associate the warmth with the relief of pain and spasm. Hypnosis has been reported to be beneficial in adult patients with IBS and even to reduce colonic contractile activity and to normalize thresholds for pain from distention of a rectal balloon.[114] In a small series of pediatric patients, a single session of instruction in self-hypnosis was found to result in resolution of functional abdominal pain within 3 weeks.[113] A recent randomized controlled trial of 53 pediatric patients with either functional abdominal pain or irritable bowel syndrome compared hypnotherapy over a 3-month period to standard therapy. Hypnotherapy was conducted by an experienced hypnotherapy nurse and occurred outside the medical session. It consisted of six 50-minute sessions. Standard care was conducted by study physicians in a tertiary medical center and consisted of education, dietary advice, fiber, and

pain medication. In addition, six 30-minute sessions of "supportive therapy" were conducted. Although pain scores in both groups decreased significantly at 1-year follow-up compared to baseline, hypnotherapy was statistically superior in both reduction of pain intensity and pain frequency. At 1-year follow-up, treatment was successful in 85% of the hypnotherapy group versus 25% of the standard therapy group.[115] One center in Israel reported having implemented hypnosis for the past 3 years as the preferred treatment for patients with functional chronic abdominal pain following laparoscopy and appendectomy without organic pathology identified. The authors recently studied 17 patients ages 11 to 18 years who met the criteria for functional chronic recurrent abdominal pain (FCRAP) based on Rome III criteria. Hypnosis was not effective in three patients. In the other 14 adolescents, all clinical symptoms resolved after a single session of hypnosis.[116] Clearly, further studies need to be performed.

PROGNOSIS

Long-term follow-up of individuals who had been admitted to the hospital as children for RAP indicates that between 35% and 50% will have complete resolution of their symptoms.[117-119] Abdominal pain continues into adulthood in approximately 25%, and the remaining individuals may develop other complaints such as headaches. Apley and Hale demonstrated that those patients who received therapy consisting of an explanation of the RAP and reassurance developed fewer nonabdominal complaints in later life and were less likely to relapse than individuals who had received no such therapy.[117] In a recent pediatric meta-analysis of 18 studies that included 1331 children with RAP followed for a median of 5 years, 415 (29.1%) of the children had abdominal pain at follow-up. In the same analysis, a subgroup of 278 patients was compared to 2901 formerly well patients. The authors found that 41.3% of the patients with RAP had abdominal pain at 12-year follow-up compared to 10.1% of the formerly well patients.[120] Chitkara et al. demonstrated that approximately 8% of children experience functional recurrent abdominal pain and that 18 to 61% of these children will continue to report symptoms of abdominal pain 5 to 30 years later.[121]

Prognostic indicators of RAP have also been identified and are summarized in Table 7-4. Apley found that factors predictive of a good outcome included female sex, age of onset after 6 years, treatment started within 6 months of symptom onset, and a "normal family." Poor prognostic indicators included male sex, onset of symptoms before age 6 years, symptoms of greater than 6 months duration before therapy, and a "painful family."[117] In addition, Magni and colleagues identified a painful family, many surgical procedures, a low educational level, and low socioeconomic status as poor prognostic indicators in children with RAP.[119] Long-term studies also indicate that once the diagnosis of FGIDs is made, an organic disorder is rarely identified.[118] Mulvaney et al. identified three trajectories in 132 pediatric patients ages 6 to 18 years with FGID by administering the Children's Somatization Inventory and the Functional Disability Inventory four times over a period of 5 years. A model with three unique trajectories was identified that fit both the symptom and impairment data. Two trajectories indicated relatively long-term improvement, and one indicated continued high levels of symptoms and impairment. Although they did not have the most severe pain at

TABLE 7-4. **Factors Influencing Long-Term Prognosis of Functional Abdominal Pain**

Factor	Prognosis Better	Prognosis Worse
Sex	Female	Male
Age of onset	>6 years	<6 years
Family	Normal	"Painful"
Duration of symptoms	<6 months	>6 months
Education level completed	≥High school	<High school
Socioeconomic class	Middle-upper	Lower
Operation (appendectomy, tonsillectomy)	Infrequent	Frequent
Psychologic characteristics at baseline*	Absent	Present

Data from Apley J, Hale B. Children with recurrent abdominal pain: how do they grow up? BMJ 1973; 3:7-9; Magni G, Pierri M, Donzelli F. Recurrent abdominal pain in children: a long term follow-up. Eur J Pediatr 1987; 146:72-74; Mulvaney S, Lambert W, Garber J, Walker L. Trajectories of symptoms and impairment for pediatric patients with functional abdominal pain: a 5-year longitudinal study. J Am Acad Child Adolesc Psychiatry 2006; 45:737-744.
*Psychologic characteristics: anxiety, depression, lower perceived self-worth, negative life events.

baseline, the group of patients with high levels of symptoms and impairment at 5-year follow-up were found to have had significantly more anxiety, depression, lower perceived self-worth, and more negative life events at baseline.[122] These variables, therefore, may be considered red flags of a poor long-term outcome and may be useful for treatment planning when identified. Long-term follow-up studies of patients with FGID as defined by the newly established Rome III criteria are not yet available.

PREVENTION

Prevention of FGIDs begins with the primary care physician at the well-child visits. Parents should be advised against demonstrating excessive anxiety about minor illnesses and avoid providing secondary gain to children with minor injuries and illnesses. Parents should also be advised against oversubmissiveness or rigid parenting styles with excessive use of punishment.[123] Open communication between family members as the child grows should be encouraged. Physicians should stress the importance of a supportive, loving environment and recommend that the family members work together to find solutions early for stressful situations the child encounters.

CONCLUSION

Chronic abdominal pain of childhood and adolescence is one of the most common yet challenging conditions encountered in clinical practice. Although the differential diagnosis is broad, a comprehensive history and physical examination in combination with routine screening laboratory evaluation should lead to an accurate diagnosis. The newly established Rome III criteria now provide for a positive diagnosis of a functional gastrointestinal disorder in the pediatric patient using symptom-based criteria, thereby reducing the tendency to order expensive diagnostic testing as well as therapeutic interventions that may not be without side effects or long-term complications. Establishment of a therapeutic relationship with the family, reassurance, and realistic goal-setting are central to therapy. The goal of therapy is to decrease stress or tension for the child while promoting normal patterns of activity and school attendance. Dietary, pharmacologic, and psychologic therapies are available. Long-term follow-up to assist medically in symptom control as well as provision of reassurance and support may be necessary.

REFERENCES

5. Drossman D, Corazziari E, Talley N, et al. The Functional Gastrointestinal Disorders: Diagnosis, Pathophysiology and Treatment. A Multinational Consensus. 3rd ed. McLean, VA: Degnon Associates; 2006.
83. Walker L. Helping the child with recurrent abdominal pain return to school. Pediatr Ann 2004;33:128–136.
86. Huertas-Ceballos A, Logan S, Bennett C, et al. Dietary interventions for recurrent abdominal pain (RAP) and irritable bowel syndrome (IBS) in childhood. Cochrane Database Syst Rev 2008:CD003019.
96. Saps M, Youssef N, Miranda A, et al. Multicenter, randomized, placebo-controlled trial of amitriptyline in children with functional gastrointestinal disorders. Gastroenterology 2009;137:1261–1269.
111. Huertas-Ceballos AA, Logan S, Bennett C, Macarthur C. Psychosocial interventions for recurrent abdominal pain (RAP) and irritable bowel syndrome (IBS) in childhood (Review). Cochrane Library 2009:Issue 4.

See expertconsult.com for a complete list of references and the review questions for this chapter.

8

APPROACH TO THE CHILD WITH A FUNCTIONAL GASTROINTESTINAL DISORDER

Paul E. Hyman • David R. Fleisher

About half the patients attending pediatric gastroenterology clinics have symptoms that do not have a readily discernible cause. Knowing how to relieve the physical and emotional suffering in patients without disease is a necessity for every clinician.[1,2] The purpose of this chapter is to offer conceptual groundwork and concrete suggestions about how to recognize and manage these patients.

BIOMEDICAL MODEL

In Western civilization, the traditional and dominant model for understanding disease has been the biomedical model.[1] The biomedical model makes two assumptions: (1) any symptom can be traced back to a single cause, and (2) every symptom is either "organic," meaning there is an identifiable, objectively defined pathophysiology, or "functional," meaning without identifiable, objectively defined pathophysiology. This dualistic approach implicitly places "organic disease" in high esteem. Functional disorders are considered less serious, psychological, or often without etiology or treatment. The biomedical model works for a broken bone or a kidney stone, but not so well when there are chronic problems such as headaches, abdominal pain, or chronic fatigue.

What Are the Defining Characteristics of Functional Disorders?

Symptoms of disease are caused by objectively demonstrable tissue damage causing organ malfunction. By contrast, functional symptoms are caused by events that are in the repertoire of responses inherent in disease-free organs.[3] This definition of "functional" purposely avoids the implication of psychological origins because organ dysfunction may be caused by factors that are not psychological. Moreover, "psychogenic" is often interpreted as "psychopathologic" and may offend patients by implying that functional symptoms are caused by wrong thoughts and are not real.[4] Some parents may interpret a psychological diagnosis in their child as blaming them for being bad parents.

Children with functional disorders may have biomarkers that provide insight into the pathophysiology behind the symptoms. In children with irritable bowel syndrome, 80 to 100% were found to have rectal hypersensitivity, "an exaggerated perception to events, such as controlled rectal distension, compared to control subjects." Rectal hypersensitivity is a biomarker for irritable bowel syndrome, an abnormality in pain

physiology that is not present in healthy children[5,6] or in children with disease.[7] A biomarker was defined as a "characteristic that is objectively measured and evaluated as an indicator of normal biologic processes, pathogenic processes, or pharmacologic responses to a therapeutic intervention."[8] Another example of a biomarker occurs in functional diarrhea. There was no fed pattern after eating, but instead there was a pattern of repeated phase 3 episodes of the fasting migrating motor complex.[9] Thus, in several pediatric functional disorders, investigators have discovered pathophysiologic biomarkers for functional disorders.

The simplest example of a functional symptom is the runner's leg cramp. It is caused by fatigue-induced spasm in a healthy muscle. The pain may be severe, but not due to disease or delusion. Diagnostic tests, other than observation, and treatments, other than rest, are not indicated.

There are negative consequences of failure to recognize functional conditions. There are also therapeutic opportunities afforded by recognition of the functional component of illness. The following case vignette exemplifies what can happen if a functional illness is ignored.

A 17-year-old female noted the insidious onset of crampy abdominal pain and loose stools without blood during her first semester in premedical education in a city far away from home. Midsemester she was upset by a separation initiated by a high school boyfriend. She skipped breakfast and lunch to avoid having to interrupt her classes to use the rest room. She lost weight. Her physician ordered screening laboratory tests and a GI consult. Inflammatory bowel disease (IBD) and celiac serologies and screening labs were normal. The consultant performed upper and lower endoscopy and 24-h pHmetry. All were normal. She complained of sharp pains under the ribcage after meals, and the frequency and severity of the abdominal pain worsened. She was unable to return to class because of worsening pain intensity. Her physician ordered a surgical consult. The surgeon ordered a hepatobiliary iminodiacetic acid (HIDA) scan. The ejection fraction was 33% (adult normal 35 to 90%). The gastroenterologist performed an endoscopic retrograde pancreatogram and cholecystogram that showed no dilation and no stones. The surgeon removed the gallbladder. The patient had prolonged pain after surgery and was discharged on nasojejunal tube feedings, narcotics for abdominal pain, and polyethylene glycol for constipation. She remained out of school for many months, disabled by pain and unable to eat.

This case involved a previously healthy adolescent with irritable bowel syndrome and unrecognized comorbid anxiety and depression due to several adolescent environmental stressors. Her physicians and family approached the problem from the biomedical point of view with the presumption that her illness must have an organic etiology. A clinician trained in the biopsychosocial model would have recognized and treated irritable bowel syndrome (IBS) as well as the concurrent stress and physiological responses to it. Instead, this patient underwent extensive testing for diseases to explain her symptoms. Each negative test result reinforced the parents' worries that something important was being missed and caused the patient to focus more on her mystery disease and avoid recognition of the emotional impacts of separations from her family, her ex-boyfriend, and her failure to adjust to college. The clinician, family, and patient were upset and frustrated by the failure to find organic pathology to explain the "daily vomiting and abdominal discomfort." Finally, a surgeon removed her gallbladder, which caused more pain. A psychiatric consultant found no eating or thought disorder and criticized the gastroenterologists for requesting the consultation, stating that the request might have been motivated by the physicians' failure to find what was wrong.[4] The patient, family, and clinicians inadvertently cocreated disability by considering only organic etiologies and avoiding the reality of the patient's stressful experiences and functional, physiologic responses to stress, namely, IBS and functional nausea and vomiting.

This adolescent's illness fell into the gap between conventional medicine and conventional mental health. There was opinion shared by clinicians and family that a disease was to blame for the patient's symptoms. The psychiatrist found no evidence of psychiatric disease. The surgeon believed the HIDA scan was abnormal, resulting in a diagnosis of biliary dyskinesia, although there are no normal values in children. Maladaptive thinking was compounded by the patient's passive coping style and the effects of narcotics on digestive physiology. Physicians and family viewed psychosocial factors as separate from, and less important than, medical disease.

BIOPSYCHOSOCIAL MODEL

The biopsychosocial model, proposed by Engel in 1977,[3] is an alternative to the biomedical model. In the biopsychosocial model, the goal is to understand and treat *illness*, the patient's subjective sense of suffering, rather than confining the diagnostic effort to no more than finding disease. Biopsychosocial clinicians recognize that symptoms may develop from several different influences, not just disease. Symptoms may stem from normal development (for example, infant regurgitation), psychiatric disease (examples include pain disorder, conversion disorder, factitious disorder by proxy), impact of culture and society (for example, a man with chest pain ignores the signals because he carries no health insurance), and functional disorders, in which symptoms are real, but there is no easily discerned disease. Examples include tension headache, irritable bowel syndrome, and functional dyspepsia. Several influences may converge to form a clinical syndrome. For examples, a disease, Crohn's disease, may occur together with a functional disorder, irritable bowel syndrome, so that the patient may suffer intolerable abdominal pain and diarrhea even when Crohn's disease is in remission.[10] Rumination syndrome (a functional disorder) may coexist with social anxiety (a psychiatric

disorder), resulting in a person who cannot leave the house because of "vomiting."

Rather than reducing a cluster of symptoms to a single pathophysiology (reductionism), the biopsychosocial model expands the potential for understanding a problem from simultaneously interacting systems at subcellular, cellular, tissue, organ, interpersonal, and environmental levels. For example, an event such as changing schools may be a psychological stressor that in turn alters cellular immunity and disease susceptibility. Or, change at a subcellular level, such as hepatitis C infection, may influence organ function, the person, the family, and society. There is an interactive relationship between psychosocial and biomedical factors in the clinical expression of illness and disease.

EARLY LEARNING-DEVELOPMENTAL ASPECTS OF FUNCTIONAL GASTROINTESTINAL DISORDERS

To understand many of the pediatric functional disorders, it is necessary to consider the child's point of view. For example, neonates are born with reflexes that ensure defecation. About the time that other neonatal reflexes disappear, so do the reflexes for defecation. As a consequence, the 6- to 8-week-old infant must learn to defecate by contracting the abdominal muscles to increase intra-abdominal pressure, while relaxing the sphincter and pelvic floor muscles. In a few healthy infants, learning to coordinate two muscle groups simultaneously does not come easily. These infants may scream for 20 minutes or more to increase intra-abdominal pressure. Finally, they relax their pelvic floors simultaneously with a Valsalva maneuver and defecate. This clinical presentation is called *functional dyschesia*.[11]

The infant who perceives pain with passing a large hard stool will learn to avoid defecation. Next, anticipation of pain with the urge to defecate results in an inability to relax the pelvic floor. The maladaptive response to fear of painful defecation, contracting the pelvic floor with the perceived need to defecate, becomes internalized and results in *functional constipation*. For about the first 5 years of life, functional constipation persists unless adults ensure that the child enjoys painless defecation. When asked in language that they understand, toddlers and preschool children endorse that they are afraid of hard, painful stool. School-aged children use denial to defend themselves against those who would like to help them. Their feigned nonchalance and apparent indifference are because they are ashamed and unaware of the cause or natural history of functional constipation. They state that they do not feel the urge to defecate. Careful observation contradicts the child's explanation for refusing to defecate. Each day the child has episodes of stiffening the legs, facial expression turning blank or grimacing, and complaining of a bellyache. These episodes last about 90 seconds. These behaviors are external manifestations of the child's perception of high-amplitude propagating colonic contractions, signaling that it is time to defecate. Unfortunately, the child with functional constipation interprets the crampy pain from the stretching of the rectal wall as abdominal pain rather than a urge to defecate. At this age, educating the children and parents about functional constipation and motivating behavior change in the child are keys to successful resolution.

Functional symptoms during childhood are sometimes accompaniments to normal development (e.g., infant regurgitation), or they may arise from maladaptive behavioral responses to internal or external stimuli (e.g., in functional constipation, fecal retention is a behavioral consequence of painful defecation). The expression of a functional gastrointestinal disorder depends on an individual's autonomic, affective, and intellectual development, as well as on concomitant organic and psychological disturbances.

For example, infant regurgitation is a problem for months during the first year. Functional diarrhea affects infants and toddlers, but the outcome is unknown because stools are no longer checked after the child is toilet trained. Through the first years of life, children cannot accurately report symptoms such as nausea or pain. The infant and preschool child cannot discriminate between emotional and physical distress. With our current limitations, irritable bowel syndrome and functional dyspepsia are diagnosed only after the child becomes a reliable reporter for pain in the early school years.

First Visit

The biopsychosocial clinician recognizes that half the patients in clinic will have functional disorders. In functional disorders, few diagnostic tests are necessary or desirable. The clinician must be prepared to diagnose and treat functional disorders by communicating the relevant information to a patient and parents who are receptive. Therefore, developing rapport is most important during the initial stages of the diagnostic interview.

Depending on the age and experience of the child, the doctor's white coat may be a nocebo, the antonym for placebo.[12] Toddlers fear the white coat because of negative past associations with gagging sticks and needle pokes. Adolescents may despise the white coat because it is a symbol of authority. The white coat may be a barrier to effective communication. If the family is already in the examination room, it is appropriate to knock and then open the door slowly. Take a moment to scan the room, and smile when you introduce yourself. Then go around the room shaking hands to acknowledge each individual, including siblings. If you acknowledge siblings early and often, they will be less competitive for their parent's attention during the interview.

There are three goals for the interview: (1) gather information, (2) develop a therapeutic alliance with the family, and (3) communicate information and initiate a treatment plan. The interviewer sits and listens as the child or parent narrates the chief complaint and history. The interviewer does not interrupt. The parent expects to be interrupted and begins with a high-pressure stream of details. Pressured speech is a measure of the historian's anxiety. Pressured speech gradually fades to normal, and eventually the historian stops talking. Next the clinician repeats the salient features of the narrative, to prove that he was listening. At this point the patient and family are pleasantly surprised that the doctor listened without interruption and remembered the story.

In the early phase of the interview, the clinician asks open-ended questions. The clinician usually knows at this point whether he is working with organic disease or a functional disorder because the history included signs and symptoms of disease or not. See Table 8-1 for signs and symptoms of disease. If the patient has not volunteered the information, the clinician should ask. If "red flags" are absent, than the clinician asks questions that focus in on the functional disorders. "Are you saying that 3 or 4 days a week for the past 2 months you had bellyaches that felt better after defecation, and the stool

TABLE 8-1. Signs and Symptoms Associated With Chronic Abdominal Pain

Disease	Unhelpful Signs and Symptoms	FGID
Blood in emesis or stool	Waking with abdominal pain	Pain at the umbilicus
Fevers		Pain is only symptom
Weight loss		Pain lasts <10 min
Waking with diarrhea		

FGID, functional gastrointestinal disorder.

came out too hard, and it felt like you could not get it all out? Then you have irritable bowel syndrome." "Are you telling me that you get bellyaches after every meal? You feel bloated and nauseated? Why, you have dyspepsia! We can begin treating it today as functional dyspepsia because 85% of adolescents with dyspepsia have no endoscopic disease.[13] Or we can scope and be sure about the cause for symptoms. Which style would be better for you?"

EFFECTIVE REASSURANCE

There are several components to effective reassurance. First, the clinician develops rapport with the patient and caretakers by being attentive and empathetic. The second component requires an answer to the four questions that concern most parents: (1) *What is wrong?* It's cyclic vomiting. (2) *Is it dangerous?* No. (3) *Will it go away?* Probably, but we do not know when. (4) *What can we do about it?* First we educate you all about cyclic vomiting. Then we describe the drugs we use to prevent episodes and the drugs we use to treat episodes, and weigh the risks and benefits of all the management possibilities. The third component for effective reassurance is a promise of continuing availability.

The following case vignette exemplifies how recognition of functional symptoms can help in clinical management.

A bright 9-year-old girl was brought for evaluation for recurrent abdominal pain that had caused her to miss 3 weeks of school. Her symptoms became disabling some time after the onset of her mother's untreated episode of anxious depression. The child expressed worries about her parents' safety when they traveled. She insisted on sleeping on the couch nearer to her parents' bedroom, rather than in her own room. At the time of the consultation, the mother stated that she was sure there was an organic cause for her daughter's abdominal pain. Moreover, she was certain that the pains were severe because of the child's stoic behavior after an accidental fracture of her forearm in the past. ("She has a high pain threshold, so when she actually complains, I know she's really hurting!"). The mother said she was told by previous physicians that none of many diagnostic procedures found anything physically wrong. A mental health assessment was suggested. The mother said she didn't have much faith in psychologists and could not see the purpose of such a recommendation. (Doing so would have made her feel as though she was abandoning her role as protector of her child's health and concurring with the insulting implication that her daughter was faking illness.)

In fact, this child had a real illness. It did not involve disease, but it had three identifiable elements: (1) a functional disorder, functional abdominal pain,[14,15] prevalent in girls her age; (2) separation anxiety[15]; and (3) somatizing, that is, the conscious or unconscious use of symptoms to avoid recognition of her anxiety and remain in the comforting presence of her concerned mother and at home in the mothering environment.[16]

The diagnosis offered to the mother was functional abdominal pain syndrome.[15] The clinician described the child's condition, including its high prevalence in healthy schoolchildren, and explained that the symptoms were due to heightened activation of healthy sensory and motor nerves in the gastrointestinal tract. Like a runner's leg cramp or a swimmer's shiver after a cold dip, functional symptoms are part of how the healthy body works. Although her child's pains could be severe at times, they neither resulted from nor caused disease. The functional nature of her child's pains explained why diagnostic tests for diseases had been unrevealing. Skillful communication, which addressed the worries and concerns elicited from the mother during the history, permitted her and the clinician to avoid the "physical-versus-emotional" controversy. She was relieved to learn that her daughter's pains, although sometimes severe, were not dangerous. She abandoned her insistence on more invasive, stressful diagnostic tests. The doctor's unhurried, painstaking efforts at obtaining an extended history and her gentle but thorough physical exam convinced the mother that her daughter's symptoms were being taken seriously. Making use of their rapport, the physician then reflected, in a nonjudgmental, concerned manner, on all of the emotional stress they had suffered as a family and how any normal child might have reacted to it with anxiousness. At that point, the mother was ready to hear the doctor's thoughts about emotional issues. She was also ready to shift her concerns away from the hidden malignancy that she feared was causing her child's pains, toward concern about the developmental damage accruing as a result of missed school. Once reassured, she became ready to place the expectation on her child to return to school, even though her girl still had some complaints. The change in the mother's attitude did not "cure" her child's anxiety, but the mother's new confidence in her daughter's health ended the vicious cycle of symptoms and fear that dominated their relationship. The physician made herself available to the parents, the child, and the school nurse to support efforts at getting her back into school.[3]

In this case, the concept of functional disorders was used to avoid adversarial interaction in which the parent could, at first, only accept an organic diagnosis. The physician recognized the child's anxiety[16] and its possible causes. The concept of functional disorders allowed the physician to avoid having to make the choice of either ordering more diagnostic tests (against her better judgment) in order to preserve the doctor-patient relationship, at least temporarily, or stating what was unacceptable to the mother, thereby breaking off the relationship and any opportunities for further help.

Acceptance of the nondangerous nature of a child's abdominal symptoms and the unwavering support of the physician enabled the mother to place an expectation on her daughter to do what she had to do, namely, return to school. This is a stressful juncture at which the mother, on one hand, is made to feel heartless by increasing displays of suffering by her child on hearing that she will go to school and, on the other hand, recognition that her child's *use* of genuine abdominal pain for psychological gain was leading to abnormal codependency and invalidism. Proof of the effectiveness of management was that the magnitude of pain issue diminished within a few days and excessive school absences ceased.

When a child becomes dependent on the uncritically accepting, comforting nearness of the parent, and the parent is unable to bear the guilt created by the accusatory tantrums of her child, the parent-child relationship becomes inimical to normal development of both. The clinician who succeeds in managing the functional disorder complicated by anxiety-induced somatizing and helps remove the patient's "need to be sick" has accomplished a triumph of clinical management.[4]

BIOMEDICAL VERSUS BIOPSYCHOSOCIAL MODELS

It is likely that the majority of clinicians include elements of both the biomedical and biopsychosocial models in their practice. It can be argued, however, that all illnesses, organic and functional, are best managed within the framework of the biopsychosocial rather than the biomedical model of practice.

The biomedical and biopsychosocial models of practice share the same goals, namely, improving patients' well-being. However, the scope of what is considered to be impairment and the extent to which the clinician considers the origin and remedies to that impairment differ.[2] The biomedical model limits the role of the physician to the diagnosis and treatment of disease and assumes that doing so restores well-being. The biopsychosocial model expands the meaning of the goal and the clinical process by which it is achieved. Illness is defined as the patient's subjective sense of suffering.[13] The goal of management is to identify the patient's disease as well as other factors contributing to suffering. The biopsychosocial model includes an analysis of the relationship and contributions of each factor in the patient's illness. Such was *not* done in the case of the 18 year old pre-medical student but was attempted with some success in the 9 year old girl with abdominal pain and school absence.

A schematic summary by which the biomedical and biopsychosocial models can be contrasted is presented in Figure 8-1.[3] The large circle represents *Illness*. The six smaller circles within it represent six constituent categories, one or more of which may contribute to a patient's illness. Category one represents *disease*. This category is the principal focus of the biomedical model. Category two represents *psychological disorders*, that is, behavior or psychological syndrome or pattern causing distress and disability.[16] Excluded from this category are normal emotional responses to stressful events such as grief at the loss of a loved one. The third category represents *functional symptoms*, such as IBS. The fourth category represents *somatizing*, the conscious or unconscious use of physical symptoms of any etiology for psychological purposes or personal advantage.[4,17] The fifth category represents symptoms that are *manifestations of normal development* and are neither organic nor functional, but prompt patients to seek medical evaluation (e.g., adolescent gynecomastia). The sixth circle represents *failure in the relationship between the patient and society*, such as no access to treatment. Each of these categories has an approach to management that any interested physician can use productively.[3,4,15]

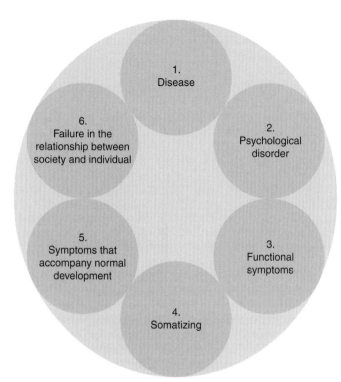

Figure 8-1. A schematic summary by which the biomedical and biopsychosocial models can be contrasted.

This scheme helps the clinician explore areas of illness that are often neglected in the biomedical model of care. The illness of the 17-year-old premedical student reported earlier involved at least three of the six possible categories: anxious depression (psychological disorder); irritable bowel syndrome and functional nausea and vomiting (functional); and intensifying quest for an organic etiology, the unconscious purpose of which was to avoid emotionally painful issues (somatizing).

TREATMENT

Once the clinician is sure that the problem meets symptom-based diagnostic criteria, it is helpful to read aloud to the family the criteria from the Rome III classification.[15,18,19] Reading from a Rome III document is a strong argument for parents who are not convinced by the clinician's words alone. Next, it is helpful to provide the patient with a plausible explanation for the problem. Following the education piece, there may or may not be a need for further treatment. Effective reassurance may be all that is needed in many situations. To reinforce the educational lessons, and to assist one parent describing the disorder to other family members, it is a good idea to hand a parent a pamphlet about the disorder obtained from the International Foundation for Functional Gastrointestinal Disorders at www.IFFGD.org.

Treatment of chronic neuropathic pain caused by local sensory hypersensitivity and/or amplification of nonspecific central arousal systems may focus on the central nervous system or on afferent neurons from the hollow viscus. Pain perception occurs in the cortex, on the cingulate gyrus. It is influenced by past experiences, catastrophization, and expectation for pain as well as afferent signals. Cognitive behavioral therapy[20-22] and hypnosis[23] are effective for treating chronic abdominal pain in receptive children and adolescents. Several classes of drugs have effects on either afferent nerves and/or central arousal systems.

The tricyclic antidepressants have been helpful for many forms of chronic neuropathic pain. In addition, amitriptyline is effective in suppressing episodes of cyclic vomiting syndrome or abdominal migraine, preventing migraine headaches. Two recent controlled trials yielded equivocal results with amitriptyline in children with IBS.[24,25] Both trials used low doses of amitriptyline, a factor that may have been the cause of the response not different from placebo. Alternatively, an exceptional placebo response of 80% may reflect the biopsychosocial approach of the investigators, who provided effective reassurance and an expectation that the medicine would be effective.[25]

APPROACH TO THE CHILD OR ADOLESCENT WITH PAIN-ASSOCIATED DISABILITY SYNDROME

The term *pain-associated disability syndrome (PADS)* describes a downward spiral of increasing disability and pain (or other symptom, such as nausea) for which acute pain treatments do not eliminate pain or disability – the inability to engage in activities of daily life.[26] PADS pain may be due to tissue pathology, but is more often associated with one or more functional gastrointestinal disorders. The suffering seems out of proportion to objective evidence of disease. PADS is limited to preteens and teens. It is associated with a passive coping style, and nearly always with a sleep disorder. PADS patients have overt or undiagnosed cognitive or emotional stressors that must be addressed to relieve underlying autonomic arousal.

PADS patients fall into a gap between biomedical medicine and conventional mental health, as central and enteric nervous systems interact. Pain activates nonspecific central nervous system arousal. Pain memories create an expectation for more pain; a maladaptive coping style is associated with patients who feel helpless to control their pain, and hopeless about symptom reduction. Symptoms are proportional to the patient's perception of his or her own academic or social competence. Although brief interventions may improve symptoms, no patient stays better without the family understanding the diagnosis and participating in treatment.

If the patient and family accept the diagnosis, treatment is partially or totally successful in relieving suffering and returning the patient to normal daily activities. A multidisciplinary, biopsychosocial team approach is optimal, because clinicians, patient, and family must communicate frequently and honestly. The burden of healing shifts from a medical model, in which the patient is passive and the clinicians test and treat, to a rehabilitation model, in which the patient is responsible for learning to help herself, with clinicians as guides. The team is usually led by a physician and a child health psychologist. Other team members may include a physical therapist, dietitian, occupational therapist or child life specialist, teacher, and family therapist. We have the patient and family sign a contract with us on the first day, promising to participate in all treatment to the best of their ability. Next we make a schedule designed to fill every day with activities to prevent the patient from ruminating about troubles, but instead exercise her body and her mind so that she is tired at day's end and sleeps well each night. The physician prescribes medicine to ensure restful sleep: amitriptyline, trazodone, mirtazapine (7.5 mg dose), or eszopiclone. The physician may add other chronic pain medications, such as gabapentin or clonidine. The psychologist finds one or more forms of relaxation that the patient enjoys, such as relaxation breathing, yoga, hypnosis, guided imagery, or biofeedback games.

The psychologist applies cognitive-behavioral therapy (CBT) to introduce the patient to an active coping style and problem solving. The family asks why a psychological treatment for abdominal pain. It is helpful for them if the clinician explains that the pain is not under the PADS patient's control because pain is coming from pain nerve signals that arise from pressure or stretching of the gastrointestinal tract walls and amplified by arousal centers deep in the brain. It seems as if the brain modulates many body activities that are not under conscious control, such as pain, blood pressure, pulse, and respirations. However, with training, the thinking part of the brain can learn to control these. "Take respirations: please hold your breath! Now the thinking part of the brain is controlling your respirations, overriding the unconscious control. OK. Breathe again." With CBT, catastrophic thinking is replaced by hope for successful treatment. Passive behaviors are replaced by active coping. The physical therapist provides an exercise program enjoyable for the patient, guaranteed for success each day, such as walking the mall or running with the family dog. The patient receives instructions to exercise because exercise releases endorphin painkillers from the patient's own body.

If the psychologist diagnoses a comorbid psychological disorder amenable to drug therapy, such as panic disorder, anxiety disorder, depression, or attention deficit disorder, there may be cause to add psychotropic medications to treat them. The team physician may prescribe psychotropic drugs and/or ask for a psychiatry consultant to assist. We explain to the patient and family that psychotropic drugs reduce suffering to help the patient focus on learning the skill set she will need to avoid a recurrence, and that we plan to taper the drugs as soon as the patient acquires confidence in the necessary skills.

The PADS patient misses school for 2 months or more because of symptoms and repeated hospitalizations. Returning to school often requires that a treatment team member advise the school about PADS and the patient's impending return. Sometimes it is best to begin with just a few hours a day, for the patient's favorite subjects. As with daily exercise, the idea is to choose incremental steps with expectations for success.

PADS has not been described in adults or in young children. There must be some developmental vulnerability to PADS, perhaps related to the identity uncertainty and confusion that is the developmental focus at that age.

WHAT SHOULD A PEDIATRIC GASTROENTEROLOGY CONSULTATION ACCOMPLISH?

The clinician explains that brain and the gastrointestinal tract are connected. Nerve circuits run in both directions, and both brain and gut influence each other. It is not helpful to separate illness into one or the other.

Management consists of communication that satisfies the parents' and child's cognitive and emotional needs caused by the child's symptoms. How can their particular needs be known? This can be accomplished by asking four open-ended questions of parents.[4] (This might best be done in the absence of the child.)

1. What have you been told about your child's symptoms?
2. What are your concerns now?
3. What is your worst fear?
4. What are your spouse's concerns?

If doctor-parent rapport is good (i.e., if they feel that the physician has listened to them with respect and empathy[15]), the parent may reveal, in depth, exactly what is needed from the clinician in order for them to feel that the illness or symptoms are under control. This can be accomplished by conveying *three essential communications*.[4] The first is an understanding of the symptoms, including (a) the diagnosis (which implies that their child's symptoms are not unique and that the physician isn't at a loss); (b) the mechanisms of symptom production, that is, what goes on physiologically that creates the symptom; (c) the physically benign nature of the functional symptoms; (d) what to do about the symptoms when the child seems to be in severe discomfort; and (e) the outlook regarding the course of the symptoms over time, that is, will recovery take days, months, or years?

The second essential communication is *effective reassurance*. Information alone may not enable parents to change their focus from the child's symptoms to the goal of pursuing normal development, such as returning to regular school. In order to change their behavior, the clinician must try to discover the parents' unstated and perhaps unrecognized fears. The unhurried clinician discerns clues that may seem unimportant, but are deeply painful, such as a parent who lost a sibling or parent during childhood. Once these emotional burdens are uncovered, the displacement of emotional pain from the parent's past onto the child's current symptoms may be relieved by telling the parent that, notwithstanding the tragedy of their own parent's colon cancer, in general, colon cancer in children is extremely rare. The moment reassurance becomes effective, it is signaled by a change in the parent's mood from worry and frustration to perceptible relief.

The third essential communication is based on the recognition that physicians make mistakes. Diseases can be missed or new ones supervene. Therefore, the physicians' *offer of continuing availability by telephone or email* is a warranty for the diagnosis, the management plan, and the doctor's unfailing open-mindedness toward any future concern. Time becomes a diagnostic and therapeutic tool. Functional symptoms are not easily "cured" and may recur intermittently for years. Continuity of care by a physician who is willing to "own the problem" together with the parents and child is a powerful antidote to obsessive worry and overutilization of medical resources.

PEDIATRIC FUNCTIONAL GASTROINTESTINAL DISORDERS

What follows is the compendium of pediatric functional gastrointestinal disorders and their diagnostic criteria as defined by the infant/toddler and child/adolescent committees of the Rome III proceedings.[18,19] The value of Rome criteria is better viewed with two caveats in mind.

First, the Rome process was inaugurated for research purposes, to organize the confusion of diagnostic terms applied to functional GI symptoms before the latter 20th century. The development of clear terminology allowed for research in these disorders to be performed around the world based on a standard nomenclature.

Second, evidence-based medicine is a movement to put medical care on a more scientific footing using data from clinical trials rather than anecdotal reports. To be sure, this shift to science is welcomed, but the "evidence" from clinical trials is often limited in its application to individual patients. Subjects in clinical trials are typically "cherry-picked," meaning that they have a single disease; they are excluded if they have multiple conditions or are receiving other medications or treatments that might mar the purity of the population under study. People are also excluded who are too young or too old to fit into the rigid criteria of the scientific protocol. Yet these excluded patients are the people who populate doctors' clinics. It is about these patients that a physician must think deeply, taking on the task of developing an empirical approach, melding statistics from clinical trials with personal experience and even anecdotal reports.[17] Therefore, modern practitioners need to understand the distinction between research criteria (as exemplified by Rome III) and clinical criteria (as exemplified by the practitioner who considers evidence presented in the literature along with his or her clinical judgment.) Current Rome III criteria for pediatric functional disorders are provided next.

Infant Regurgitation

Must include *both* of the following in otherwise healthy infants 3 weeks to 12 months of age:
- Regurgitation two or more times per day for 3 or more weeks
- No retching, hematemesis, aspiration, apnea, failure to thrive, feeding or swallowing difficulties, or abnormal posturing

Infant Rumination Syndrome

Must include *all* of the following for at least 3 months:
- Repetitive contractions of the abdominal muscles, diaphragm, and tongue
- Regurgitation of gastric content into the mouth, which is either expectorated or rechewed and reswallowed, and three or more of these: onset between 3 and 8 months, does not improve after treatment for gastroesophageal reflux disease, to anticholinergic drugs, hand restraints, formula changes, gavage, or gastrostomy feedings. It is unaccompanied by signs of nausea or distress. It does not occur during sleep or when the infant interacts with individuals.

Cyclic Vomiting Syndrome

Must include *both* of the following:
- Two or more periods of intense nausea and unremitting vomiting or retching lasting hours to days, and return to usual state of health lasting weeks to months

Infant Colic

Must include *all* of the following in infants from birth to 4 months of age:
- Paroxysms of irritability, fussing, or crying that start and stop without obvious cause
- Episodes lasting 3 or more hours per day and occurring at least 3 days per week for at least 1 week
- No failure to thrive

Functional Diarrhea

Must include *all* of the following:
- Daily painless, recurrent passage of three or more large, unformed stools
- Symptoms that last more than 4 weeks
- Onset of symptoms that begins between 6 and 36 months of age. Passage of stools that occurs during waking hours
- There is no failure-to-thrive if caloric intake is adequate

Infant Dyschezia

In a child less than 6 months old, must include:
- At least 10 minutes of straining and crying before successful passage of soft stools
- No other health problems

Functional Constipation

Must include *1 month* of at least *two* of the following in infants up to 4 years of age:
- Two or fewer defecations per week
- At least one episode per week of incontinence after the acquisition of toileting skills
- History of excessive stool retention
- History of painful or hard bowel movements
- Presence of a large fecal mass in the rectum
- History of large-diameter stools that may obstruct the toilet

Adolescent Rumination Syndrome

Must include *all* of the following:
- Repeated painless regurgitation and rechewing or expulsion of food that:
  1. Begins soon after ingestion of a meal;
  2. Does not occur during sleep;
  3. Does not respond to treatment for gastroesophageal reflux;
  4. Does not involve retching;
  5. Provides no evidence of an inflammatory, anatomic, metabolic, or neoplastic process that explains the subject's symptoms.
- Criteria fulfilled at least once per week for at least 2 months before diagnosis

Aerophagia

Must include *at least two* of the following:
  1. Air swallowing;
  2. Abdominal distention due to intraluminal air;
  3. Repetitive belching and/or increased flatus.
- Criteria fulfilled at least once per week for at least 2 months before diagnosis

Functional Dyspepsia

Must include *all* of the following:
- Persistent or recurrent pain or discomfort centered in the upper abdomen (above the umbilicus)
- Not relieved by defecation or associated with the onset of a change in stool frequency or stool form (i.e., not irritable bowel syndrome)
- No evidence of an inflammatory, anatomic, metabolic, or neoplastic process that explains the subject's symptoms
- Criteria fulfilled at least once per week for at least 2 months before diagnosis

Irritable Bowel Syndrome

Must include *both* of the following:
- Abdominal discomfort (an uncomfortable sensation not described as pain) or pain associated with two or more of the following at least 25% of the time:
  1. Improvement with defecation
  2. Onset associated with a change in frequency of stool
  3. Onset associated with a change in form (appearance) of stool

- No evidence of an inflammatory, anatomic, metabolic, or neoplastic process that explains the subject's symptoms
- Criteria fulfilled at least once per week for at least 2 months before diagnosis

Abdominal Migraine

Must include *all* of the following:
- Paroxysmal episodes of intense, acute periumbilical pain that lasts for 1 hour or more
- Intervening periods of usual health lasting weeks to months
- The pain interferes with normal activities
- The pain is associated with two or more of the following:
  1. Anorexia
  2. Nausea
  3. Vomiting
  4. Headache
  5. Photophobia
  6. Pallor
- No evidence of inflammatory, anatomic, metabolic, or neoplastic processes that explain the subject's symptoms
- Criteria fulfilled two or more times in the preceding 12 months

Childhood Functional Abdominal Pain

Must include *all* of the following:
- Episodic or continuous abdominal pain
- Insufficient criteria for other FGIDs
- No evidence of an inflammatory, anatomic, metabolic, or neoplastic process that explains the subject's symptoms
- Criteria fulfilled at least once per week for at least 2 months before diagnosis

Childhood Functional Abdominal Pain Syndrome

Must satisfy criteria for childhood functional abdominal pain and have at least 25% of the time *one or more* of the following:
- Some loss of daily functioning
- Additional somatic symptoms such as headache, limb pain, or difficulty sleeping
- Criteria fulfilled at least once per week for at least 2 months before diagnosis

Functional Constipation

Must include *two or more* of the following in a child with a developmental age of at least 4 years with insufficient criteria for diagnosis of IBS:
- Two or fewer defecations in the toilet per week
- At least one episode of fecal incontinence per week

- History of retentive posturing or excessive volitional stool retention
- History of painful or hard bowel movements
- Presence of a large fecal mass in the rectum
- History of large diameter stools which may obstruct the toilet
- Criteria fulfilled at least once per week for at least 2 months before diagnosis

Nonretentive Fecal Incontinence

Must include *all* of the following in a child with a developmental age at least 4 years:
- Defecation into places inappropriate to the social context at least once per month
- No evidence of an inflammatory, anatomic, metabolic, or neoplastic process that explains the subject's symptoms
- No evidence of fecal retention
- Criteria fulfilled for at least 2 months before diagnosis

CONCLUSION

"The decision to seek medical care for a symptom arises from a parent's or caretaker's concern for the child. The caretakers' threshold for concern varies with their own experiences and expectations, coping style, and perception of their child's illness. For this reason, the office visit is not only about the child's symptom, but also about the family's conscious and unconscious fears. The clinician must not only make a diagnosis, but also recognize the impact of the symptom on the family's emotional tone and ability to function. Therefore, any intervention must attend to both the child and the family. Effective management depends on securing a therapeutic alliance with the parents. The clinician depends on the reports and interpretations of the parents, who know their child best, and the observations of the clinician, who is trained to differentiate between health and illness."[27] It is unlikely that functional disorders will be missed or mistreated by clinicians practicing the biopsychosocial model of medical care.

REFERENCES

15. Drossman DA, senior editor. The Functional Gastrointestinal Disorders — Rome III. McLean, VA: Degnon Associates; 2006 p. 749-751.
18. Hyman PE, Milla PJ, Davidson G, et al. Infant and toddler functional gastrointestinal disorders. Gastroenterology 2006;130:1519–1526.
19. Rasquin A, Di Lorenzo C, Forbes D, et al. Childhood functional gastrointestinal disorders: child/adolescent. Gastroenterology 2006;130:1527–1537.

See expertconsult.com for a complete list of references and the review questions for this chapter.

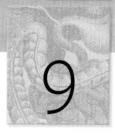

9 VOMITING AND NAUSEA

BU. K. Li • Bhanu K. Sunku

It is accepted that the ability to vomit developed as a protective mechanism to rid the body of ingested toxins.[1] Unfortunately, vomiting also frequently occurs unrelated to the ingestion of noxious agents, a circumstance that produces several clinical challenges. First, vomiting is a sign of many diseases that affect different organ systems. Therefore, determining the cause of a vomiting episode can be difficult. Second, vomiting can produce several complications (e.g., electrolyte derangement, prolapse gastropathy, Mallory-Weiss syndrome) that demand diagnosis and treatment. Third, vomiting is a frequent complication of medical therapy (surgical procedures, cancer chemotherapy). Fourth, selection of appropriate therapy for this distressing problem is essential to improve patient comfort and avoid additional medical complications of the vomiting.

VOMITING EVENT

Definition

Vomiting (emesis) is a complex reflex behavioral response to a variety of stimuli (see later discussion). The emetic reflex has three phases: (1) a prodromal period consisting of the sensation of nausea and signs of autonomic nervous system stimulation, (2) retching and (3) vomiting or forceful expulsion of the stomach contents through the oral cavity.[2-5] Although the overall sequence of these three phases is stereotypical, each can occur independently of the others. For example, nausea does not always progress to vomiting, and pharyngeal stimulation can induce vomiting without a prodrome of nausea. It is important to note that *vomiting* and *regurgitation* (defined as effortless reflux of the intragastric contents into the esophagus) are not synonymous. Clinically, vomiting can be distinguished from regurgitation, because regurgitation is not preceded by prodromal events, retching does not occur, and gastric contents are not forcibly expelled. The differentiation between vomiting and regurgitation is critical, as each has different causes and is produced by distinctive physiologic mechanisms.

Physical Description

The events that herald the onset of the act of vomiting are nausea and several autonomic manifestations.[2,5-6] *Nausea* is a subjective experience that is difficult to define. It is usually described as an unpleasant, but painless, sensation localized to the epigastrium associated with the feeling that vomiting is imminent. The autonomic signs include cutaneous vasoconstriction, sweating, dilation of pupils, increased salivation, and tachycardia. Several gastrointestinal (GI) motor events characterize the emetic prodrome.[6-9] There is inhibition of spontaneous contractions within the GI tract and dilation of the proximal stomach. The esophageal skeletal muscle shortens longitudinally, pulling the relaxed proximal stomach (hiatus and cardia) into the thoracic cavity, with loss of the abdominal segment of the esophagus. These changes result in an anatomy that allows the free flow of gastric contents into the esophagus.[10] Soon after, a single large-amplitude contraction is initiated in the jejunum and propagates toward the stomach at 8 to 10 cm/s.[8,11] This retropulsive event is termed the *retrograde giant contraction* (RGC). It propels the duodenal contents into the stomach before the onset of retching.[10,12] The RGC is followed by a brief period of moderate-amplitude contractions in the distal small intestine and a second period of inhibition lasting several minutes.[7]

The two major somatic motor components of vomiting (retching and expulsion) are produced by the coordinated action of the respiratory, pharyngeal, and abdominal muscles resulting in rhythmic changes in intrathoracic and intraabdominal pressures.[4,13] During each cycle of retching, the glottis closes and the diaphragm, external intercostal muscles, and abdominal muscles contract,[14,15] producing large negative intrathoracic and positive intraabdominal pressure spikes. The esophagus dilates and the atonic proximal stomach continues to be displaced into the thoracic cavity. The antireflux mechanisms are overcome, and the gastric contents move to and fro into the esophagus with each cycle of retching.[10]

Sometime after the onset of retching, expulsion or vomiting occurs. During this event the external intercostal muscles and the hiatal region of the diaphragm relax and the abdominal muscles and costal diaphragm contract violently,[14,15] producing positive pressures in both abdomen and thorax, resulting in oral propulsion of the gastric contents. Retrograde contraction of the cervical esophagus assists in oral expulsion.[9] After expulsion, antegrade peristalsis in the esophagus clears the lumen of residual material[3]; the proximal stomach returns to its normal intra-abdominal position, restoring the normal antireflux anatomy.

Gastrointestinal Motor Activity During Nausea and Vomiting

GI motor activity during the emetic reflex is mediated by the vagus nerve.[7-9] Vagal preganglionic parasympathetic fibers can activate both inhibitory and excitatory pathways in the enteric nervous system. A wide range of stimuli induce nausea and vomiting[8]; however, these GI motor events do not appear to be the cause of the sensation of nausea. Moreover, the stereotypical somatic pattern of retching and vomiting continues even when the GI motor correlates of vomiting are prevented by disruption of the vagal efferents.[8,9]

Although GI motor activity is not necessary for retching and vomiting, the motor changes that do occur may serve a significant role. As a defense against noxious ingested agents,[1] relaxation of the stomach can confine a toxin before it is expelled, and the RGC can move toxins and alkaline duodenal secretions to the stomach to buffer and dilute gastric irritants (e.g., vinegar, hypertonic saline) in preparation for expulsion. The buffering of the gastric contents can also serve to protect the esophagus from acid injury. Finally, changes in the position of the stomach can place it in an advantageous position for compression by the abdominal musculature.[10]

A different pattern of GI motor activity is observed in circumstances in which nausea is induced by motion.[16,17] Before the onset of nausea, an increase occurs in the gastric slow wave from 3 to 9 cycles/min.[18] This phenomenon, known as *tachygastria*, is controlled by central cholinergic and α-adrenergic pathways.[19] In motion-induced nausea, the GI motor activity appears to play a role in the induction of symptoms.[18]

Emetic Reflex

The emetic reflex consists of an afferent limb (receptor and pathway), central integration and control, and an efferent limb (pathway and effector) (Figure 9-1).[20,21] This reflex can be induced by visceral pain and inflammation, toxins, motion, pregnancy, radiation exposure, postoperative states, and unpleasant emotions. The diverse afferent receptors and pathways may originate within the gut, oropharynx, heart, vestibular system, or central nervous system (e.g., area postrema, hypothalamus, and cortical regions). These multiple afferent pathways are integrated within the brainstem, and the emetic reflex is completed through a common integrated efferent limb consisting of multiple pathways and effectors.

Within the GI tract, multiple receptors are capable of initiating the emetic reflex.[5,22] Mechanoreceptors present within the muscularis are activated by changes in tension and may be stimulated by passive distention or active contraction of the

bowel wall. These conditions are present in bowel obstruction, a clinical state in which vomiting is prominent. Chemoreceptors within the mucosa of the stomach and proximal small bowel respond to a wide range of chemical irritants (hydrochloric acid (HCl), copper sulfate, vinegar, hypertonic saline, syrup of ipecac) and are involved in the emetic reflex induced by radiation and chemotherapeutic agents. The afferent pathways from the GI tract are mediated principally via the vagus nerves; the splanchnic nerves play a minor role.[22] Vagal afferent fibers project centrad principally to the dorsomedial portion of the nucleus of the solitary tract (NTS) and to a lesser extent to the area postrema and the dorsal motor vagal nucleus.[22-24]

Circulating toxins can trigger the emetic reflex. The major detector of blood-borne noxious agents is the chemoreceptor trigger zone (CTZ),[25-27] which is located within the area postrema on the floor of the fourth ventricle, outside of the blood-brain barrier. Substances in the cerebrospinal fluid and blood stream can be detected by the cells of this region. Several types of receptors for endogenous neurotransmitters and neuropeptides have been localized to the CTZ.[26,28] Intravenous infusion or direct application of these neuroactive agents (dopamine, acetylcholine, enkephalin, peptide YY, substance P) to the CTZ can induce vomiting.[29,30] Stimulation of the CTZ is essential for the induction of vomiting by these and other agents (apomorphine, cisplatin), but not for that induced by the stimulation of abdominal vagal afferents or motion. In addition to playing a role in vomiting, the area postrema is involved in taste aversion, the control of food intake, and fluid homeostasis.[27]

Activation of the afferent limb of the vomiting reflex may also occur through real or apparent motion of the body. Motion-induced vomiting is the result of a sensory mismatch involving the visual, vestibular, and proprioceptive systems,[31] although an intact vestibular system is a necessary component.[32] Histamine (H_1) and cholinergic muscarinic receptors are involved in the afferent limb of this pathway.[33] In addition to the foregoing afferent pathways, stimulated by unpleasant situations or in instances of conditioned vomiting (e.g., anticipatory vomiting in chemotherapy), higher cortical centers can activate the emetic reflex.

After activation, the afferent systems project centrad. Although no single central locus has been identified as a "vomiting center," two models of central coordination of the emetic reflex have been proposed: (1) a group of nuclei (paraventricular system of nuclei, defined by their connection to the area postrema) form a linked neural system whose activation can account for all of the phenomena associated with vomiting[34,35]; and (2) vomiting is produced by the sequential activation of a series of discrete effector (motor) nuclei[1] as opposed to being activated in parallel by a single locus. Furthermore, the concept of a localized "vomiting center" has been refuted by recent anatomic studies implicating a widely distributed area within the medulla as being involved in the organization and control of the emetic reflex.[36,37]

Neurochemical Basis

A wide variety of neurotransmitters, neuroactive peptides, and hormones are involved in the emetic reflex. As investigations proceed into the physiology of vomiting and the pharmacology of antiemetic agents, the role of these and other mediators will continue to be defined.

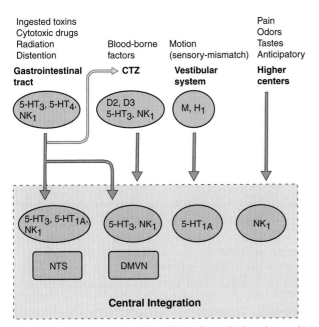

Figure 9-1. Schematic representation of the afferent limb and central integration of the emetic reflex. Receptors known to be involved in each pathway are listed within ovals. The region of central integration is designated by a dashed box to indicate that no single central locus exists as a "vomiting center." The nucleus of the solitary tract (NTS) and the dorsal motor vagal nucleus (DMVN) may each play a role in central integration. Receptor abbreviations: 5-HT, 5-hydroxytryptamine (serotonin); D, dopamine; M, acetylcholine muscarinic; H, histamine; NK, neurokinin.

Dopaminergic pathways have long been known to participate in the emetic reflex. Apomorphine, a commonly used experimental emetic agent, acts through the dopamine (D_2 subtype) receptor.[38] Furthermore, several clinically effective antiemetic agents (e.g., metoclopramide) are D_2 receptor antagonists. The site of action of these agents (agonists and antagonists) is the CTZ,[25,27] where a high density of D_2 receptors is present.[28] These receptors participate in the emetic reflex induced by several, but not all, noxious agents acting through the CTZ. In addition to this subclass of receptors, recent evidence has implicated D_3 receptors within the area postrema as having a role in the emetic reflex.[39]

The importance of serotonin (5-hydroxytryptamine or 5-HT) and serotonin receptors[40] in the emetic reflex has been demonstrated by the observation that cisplatin-induced vomiting can be prevented by blockade of $5-HT_3$ receptors.[41,42] In addition to its involvement in mediating the emetic response to several chemotherapeutic agents, $5-HT_3$ receptors play an important role in vomiting induced by radiation therapy[43] and noxious substances in the GI tract.[44,45] The $5-HT_3$ receptors are present on vagal afferent fibers in the GI tract and the presynaptic vagal afferent terminals within the central nervous system, specifically in the NTS and CTZ in the area postrema.[46,47] Current evidence indicates that chemotherapeutic agents, irradiation, and various noxious substances act directly on the GI mucosa, inducing release of serotonin from enterochromaffin cells.[42,48] Vagal afferents terminating near these cells are stimulated, producing afferent activation of the emetic reflex. The precise role of the $5-HT_3$ receptors on the presynaptic vagal afferents within the central nervous system has not been fully elucidated, but they appear to facilitate the emetic reflex induced by some afferent pathways (e.g., cranial irradiation, chemotherapeutic agents within the cerebrospinal fluid).[43,49] Other members of the 5-HT receptor family also may be involved in the emetic reflex. The $5-HT_4$ receptor has been shown to be necessary in the afferent limb of the emetic reflex induced by at least one GI irritant.[50] Blockade of central $5-HT_{1A}$ receptors, located primarily in the NTS, prevents emesis induced by a broad range of stimuli.[51,52]

Animal studies have convincingly linked physical and psychological stress to gastric stasis via central corticotropin-releasing factor (CRF) acting on CRF-R2 at the dorsomotor nucleus of the vagus.[53] During exposure to stress, CRF initiates the hypothalamic-pituitary-adrenal (HPA) axis and could play an initiating role in emesis. The role of CRF in humans remains to be established, but its effects can produce the behavioral, neuroendocrine, autonomic, immunologic, and visceral responses to stress.

Substance P (a member of the neurokinin family of peptides) and its receptor neurokinin NK_1 (tachykinin) are widely distributed in the central nervous system and peripheral neural and extraneural tissues.[54,55] Evidence in animal models of vomiting has demonstrated that this ligand and receptor are critical to the emetic response produced by a wide range of stimuli.[56-58] NK_1 receptor antagonists prevent vomiting produced by intravenous (morphine) and intragastric toxins (ipecac, copper sulfate), chemotherapeutic agents (cisplatin), and motion. The site of action of these antagonists is believed to be NK_1 receptors located in the central nervous system (NTS, dorsal motor vagal nucleus).[57-59] Because blockade of this receptor prevents emesis induced by both peripheral and central acting agents, it has been suggested that NK_1 receptors are critical elements in the central integration or effector pathway common to all emesis-inducing stimuli.[57] The first of the tachykinin receptor

antagonists has been approved for treatment of chemotherapy-induced vomiting. Given its link between stress and GI motility, CRF may also be responsible for stress-induced nausea and dyspepsia.

CLINICAL ASPECTS OF VOMITING

Temporal Patterns

There are three temporal patterns of vomiting: one *acute* and two recurrent, *chronic* and *cyclic* (Figure 9-2). Because of its frequent association with infections of childhood such as viral gastroenteritis, the *acute* form is the most common and is characterized by an episode of vomiting of moderate to high intensity. Recurrent vomiting is also a common problem encountered by pediatric gastroenterologists. Over a 5-year period, we evaluated 106 consecutive cases that could be further subclassified: two-thirds as *chronic*, a low-grade, daily pattern, and one-third as *cyclic*, an intensive but intermittent one (Table 9-1).[60] Those with the chronic pattern were mildly ill, whereas those with the cyclic pattern tended to have severe bouts associated with stereotypic pallor, listlessness, and dehydration. Because both the acute and cyclic patterns can produce intense vomiting, until the repetitive nature (more than three episodes) becomes evident, the cyclic pattern is understandably misclassified as an acute one and thus is typically misdiagnosed as a viral gastroenteritis or food poisoning.

Differential Diagnosis

The diagnostic profile varies by the temporal pattern of vomiting (Table 9-2).[60-62] The *acute* pattern is dominated by infections both in and outside the GI tract. Other causes include food poisoning, obstruction of the GI tract, and increased intracranial pressure resulting from neurological injury. Among those with the *chronic* pattern, GI disorders outnumbered extraintestinal ones by a ratio of 7:1; the most common were peptic and infectious (*Helicobacter pylori*–induced) inflammation of the upper GI tract.[60] In contrast, the diagnostic profile in those with the *cyclic* pattern was reversed; extraintestinal disorders exceeded GI ones by a ratio of 5:1. Although the hallmark of idiopathic

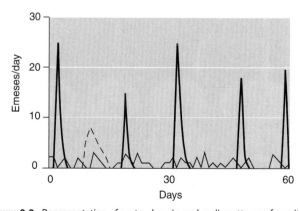

Figure 9-2. Representation of acute, chronic, and cyclic patterns of vomiting. Three temporal patterns of vomiting are depicted: *acute*—, *chronic* - - -, and *cyclic*—. The number of emeses per day is plotted on the vertical axis over a 2-month period. The *acute* pattern is represented by a single episode of moderate vomiting intensity; the *chronic* pattern by a recurrent low-grade vomiting pattern that occurs on a daily basis; and the *cyclic* pattern by recurrent, discrete episodes of high-intensity vomiting that occur once every several weeks with normal health in between.

TABLE 9-1. **Differentiating Acute, Chronic, and Cyclic Patterns of Vomiting**[60]

Clinical Feature	Acute	Chronic Recurrent	Cyclic Recurrent
Epidemiology	Most common	Two thirds of recurrent vomiting cohort	One third of recurrent vomiting cohort
Acuity	Moderate-severe, ± dehydration	Not acutely ill or dehydrated	Severe, dehydrated
Vomiting intensity	Moderate to high	Low, 1–2 emeses per hour at the peak	High, ~6 emeses per hour at peak
Recurrence, rate	No	Frequent, >2 episodes per week	Infrequent, ≤2 episodes per week
Stereotypy	Unique – *if child has had three similar episodes, consider cyclic pattern*	No	Yes
Onset	Variable	Daytime	Early morning
Symptoms	Fever, diarrhea	Abdominal pain, diarrhea	Pallor, lethargy, nausea, abdominal pain
Household contacts affected	Usually	No	No
Family history of migraine headache		14% positive	82% positive
Causes	Viral infections	Ratio of *GI* to extra-GI causes 7:1; upper GI tract mucosal injury most common (esophagitis, gastritis)	Ratio of *extra-GI* to GI causes 5:1; cyclic vomiting syndrome most common (also hydronephrosis, metabolic)

TABLE 9-2. **Causes of Vomiting by Temporal Pattern**[60–62]

Category	Acute	Chronic	Cyclic
Infectious	Gastroenteritis* Otitis media* Streptococcal pharyngitis Acute sinusitis Hepatitis Pyelonephritis Meningitis	*Helicobacter pylori** Giardiasis Chronic sinusitis*	Chronic sinusitis*
Gastrointestinal	Inguinal hernia Intussusception Malrotation with volvulus Appendicitis Cholecystitis Pancreatitis Distal intestinal obstruction syndrome	Anatomic obstruction GERD ± esophagitis* Eosinophilic esophagitis* Gastritis* Peptic ulcer or duodenitis* Achalasia SMA syndrome Gallbladder dyskinesia	Malrotation with volvulus
Genitourinary	Pyelonephritis UPJ obstruction	Pyelonephritis Pregnancy Uremia	Acute hydronephrosis secondary to UPJ obstruction
Endocrine, metabolic	Diabetic ketoacidosis	Adrenal hyperplasia	Diabetic ketoacidosis Addison's disease MCAD deficiency Partial OTC deficiency MELAS syndrome Acute intermittent porphyria
Neurologic	Concussion Subdural hematoma Reye's syndrome	Arnold-Chiari malformation Subtentorial neoplasm	Abdominal migraine* Migraine headaches* Arnold-Chiari malformation Subtentorial neoplasm Reye's syndrome
Other	Toxic ingestion Food poisoning	Rumination Functional Bulimia Pregnancy	Cyclic vomiting syndrome* Munchausen-by-proxy (e.g., ipecac poisoning)

*Most common disorders. GERD, gastroesophageal reflux disease; MCAD, medium chain acyl-CoA dehydrogenase deficiency; MELAS, mitochondrial myopathy, encephalopathy, lactic acidosis, and strokelike episodes; OTC, ornithine transcarbamylase deficiency; SMA, superior mesenteric artery; UPJ, ureteropelvic junction.

cyclic vomiting syndrome is the cyclic pattern of vomiting, episodic vomiting is also the central manifestation of a number of renal (e.g., acute hydronephrosis from ureteral-pelvic junction obstruction), endocrine (e.g., Addison's disease), and metabolic disorders (e.g., disorders of fatty acid oxidation).

Causes of vomiting also vary with the age of the child (Table 9-3).[63-95] Although most congenital anomalies of the GI tract present in the neonatal period, webs and duplications can be discovered throughout childhood.[64,65] Malrotation or nonfixation of the small intestine complicated by intermittent volvulus can cause

TABLE 9-3. **Etiology of Vomiting by Organ System and Age at Presentation**

Cause	Neonate (≤1 month)	Infant (1-12 months)	Child (1-11 years)	Adolescent (>11 years)	Reference
Extra-GI Infections					
Otitis media		+	+	−	
Acute or chronic sinusitis			+	+	
Streptococcal pharyngitis			+	+	
Pneumonitis		+	+	−	
Pyelonephritis	+	+	+	+	
Meningitis	+	+	+	+	
GI Infections					
Gastroenteritis		+	+	+	
Infectious colitis		−	+	+	
Parasitic infections			+	+	
H. pylori gastritis			+	+	
Giardiasis			+	+	
Hepatitis			+	+	
Hepatitic abscess			+	−	
Anatomic Insults					
Congenital atresias and stenoses, tracheoesophageal fistula, webs, duplications, imperforate anus	+	+	−	−	63-65
Distal intestinal obstruction syndrome	+	+	+	+	66
Inguinal hernia	+	+	+	+	
Malrotation with volvulus	+	+	+	+	67,68
Intussusception		+	+	−	69
Appendicitis			+	+	70
SMA syndrome			+		71
Bezoar			+	+	
Duodenal hematoma			+	+	
Surgical adhesions			+	+	
Mucosal Injuries					
GERD ± esophagitis, stricture	+	+	+	+	
Eosinophilic esophagitis			+	+	
Gastritis ± H. pylori			+	+	
Eosinophilic gastroenteropathy			+	+	
Peptic ulcer or duodenitis			+	+	
Cow or soy protein sensitivity	+	+	+		
Celiac disease		−	+	+	
Chronic granulomatous disease		−	+	−	72
Ménétrier's disease			+	−	73
Crohn's disease		−	+	+	
Ulcerative colitis			+	+	
Typhlitis			+	−	74
GI Motility Disorders					
Oropharyngeal discoordination	+	+	+	−	
Achalasia			−	+	
Gastroparesis			−	+	75
Paralytic ileus	+	+	+	+	
Hirschsprung's disease	+	+	−		
Pseudoobstruction	+	+	−		76
Familial dysautonomia		+	+	−	77
Visceral GI Disorders					
Cholecystitis			−	+	
Cholelithiasis			−	+	
Gallbladder dyskinesia				+	78
Choledochal cyst	+	+	−		
Pancreatitis			+	+	

+, Typically presents in this age group; −, occasionally or rarely presents in this age group. GERD, gastroesophageal reflux disease; SMA, superior mesenteric artery.

TABLE 9-3. **Etiology of Vomiting by Organ System and Age at Presentation—cont'd**

Cause	Neonate (≤1 month)	Infant (1-12 months)	Child (1-11 years)	Adolescent (>11 years)	Reference
Endocrine Derangements					
Adrenal hyperplasia	+	+			
Addison's disease	+	+	+	+	79
Diabetic ketoacidosis		–	+	+	
Pheochromocytoma			–	–	80
Carcinoid syndrome			–	–	81
Zollinger-Ellison syndrome				–	82
Metabolic Derangements					
Organic acidemias	+	+	–		
Disorders of fatty acid oxidation	–	+	+		83
Amino acidemias	+	+	–		
Urea cycle defects	+	+	–		84
Hereditary fructose intolerance	–	+			
Mitochondriopathies	–	+	+		85
Storage diseases	+	+	–		
Acute intermittent porphyria			–	+	86
Genitourinary Disorders					
Hydronephrosis secondary to uteropelvic obstruction		+	+	–	87
Renal stones			+	+	
Uremia			+	+	
Hydrometrocolpos	–	+	+	+	
Pregnancy				+	
Neurologic Disorders					
Hydrocephalus with shunt dysfunction	+	+	+	+	
Arnold-Chiari malformation		+	+	+	
Pseudotumor cerebri		–	+	+	88
Concussion	–	–	+	+	89
Subdural hematoma	+	+	+	+	
Subarachnoid hemorrhage			+	+	
Subtentorial neoplasm			+	+	90
Reye's syndrome			+	–	
Migraine headaches			+	+	
Abdominal migraine			+	+	91,92
Epilepsy			+		93
Other Causes					
Overfeeding		+			
Rumination			+	+	
Toxic ingestion			+	–	
Lead poisoning			+	–	
Food poisoning			+	+	
Functional vomiting			+	+	
Bulimia				+	
Cyclic vomiting syndrome		+	+	+	60,62,94
Munchausen-by-proxy (ipecac poisoning)		–	+		95

+, Typically presents in this age group; –, occasionally or rarely presents in this age group. GERD, gastroesophageal reflux disease; SMA, superior mesenteric artery.

episodic vomiting at any age and result in catastrophic necrosis, short bowel syndrome, and extended parenteral alimentation.[67,68] Duodenal obstruction from superior mesenteric artery syndrome is associated with acute weight loss from anorexia nervosa, extensive burns, and immobilization in a body cast.[71] Duodenal hematoma typically follows accidental trauma to the abdomen in bicycling children but can result from abuse of toddlers.

Although peptic and infectious injuries of the upper GI tract are most common, allergic (eosinophilic esophagitis) and inflammatory (Crohn's disease) ones also occur. Two unusual forms that affect toddlers include chronic granulomatous disease-induced antral obstruction[72] and cytomegalovirus-associated Ménétrier gastropathy associated with hypoalbuminemia and anasarca.[73] Typhlitis, a necrotizing inflammation of the cecum, principally affects children with acute lymphocytic leukemia during chemotherapy-induced neutropenia.[74] Besides a congenital form of intestinal dysmotility (chronic idiopathic intestinal pseudoobstruction), acquired viral and diabetes-induced gastroparesis can begin during adolescence.[75] Gallbladder dyskinesia, a cause of nausea, vomiting, and right upper quadrant pain, is a newly recognized entity in adolescents.[78]

Addison's disease can mimic cyclic vomiting syndrome at all ages, manifesting itself with recurring bouts of vomiting and hyponatremic dehydration even before hyperpigmentation appears.[79] Pheochromocytoma, as part of a multiple endocrine neoplasia type 2b,[80] carcinoid syndrome,[81] and gastrinoma[82] are rare in children and adolescents. Although metabolic disorders usually present in infancy with vomiting and failure to thrive, medium-chain acyl-CoA dehydrogenase deficiency,[83] partial ornithine transcarbamylase deficiency,[84] and acute intermittent porphyria[86] can present with episodic vomiting in older children and adolescents.

Acute hydronephrosis resulting from ureteral pelvic junction obstruction can present as a cyclic vomiting pattern, so called Dietl's crisis.[87] Increased intracranial pressure can result not only from structural subtentorial lesions (brainstem glioma, cerebellar medulloblastoma, and Chiari malformation) but also from pseudotumor cerebri associated with obesity, corticosteroid taper, vitamin A deficit or excess, tetracycline usage, and hypophosphatasia.[88] Both migraine headache and abdominal migraine are associated with vomiting in 40% of affected patients.[96] Epilepsy as a cause of recurrent abdominal pain and vomiting without evident seizure activity remains a controversial entity.[97]

Functional vomiting and Munchausen by proxy (ipecac poisoning) have to be considered when the clinical pattern does not fit known disorders, the laboratory testing is negative, and psychosocial stresses are evident (see the later section on functional vomiting). Because of its lipid solubility, ipecac can be detected on a toxicology screen as late as 2 months after administration.[95]

Clinical Clues to Diagnosis

Clinical clues to aid in differential diagnosis are presented in Table 9-4. Hematemesis more commonly results from peptic esophagitis, prolapse gastropathy, and Mallory-Weiss injury, and less often from allergic injury, Crohn's disease, and vasculitis involving the upper GI tract. In the face of nonspecific gastric petechiae, vomiting occasionally originates from a bleeding diathesis such as that of von Willebrand disease. Of the causes of morning vomiting upon wakening, the most worrisome is a neoplasm of the posterior fossa. More common causes of early morning nausea and vomiting associated with a history of congestion, postnasal drainage, cough-and-vomit sequence include environmental allergies and chronic sinusitis, and cyclic vomiting syndrome. Vertigo is commonly associated with a migraine headache or middle ear dysfunction (e.g., Ménière syndrome).

Unlike adults, for whom eating often provides pain relief, children more often experience postprandial exacerbation of their abdominal pain and vomiting. Malodorous breath may be associated with chronic sinusitis, H. pylori gastritis, giardiasis, and small bowel bacterial overgrowth. Although seen infrequently, visible peristalsis in infants and a succussion splash in children are indications of a gastric outlet obstruction that

is causing gastric distention and retention of fluid. Abdominal masses can be seen in congenital (e.g., mesenteric cyst) or acquired nonneoplastic (e.g., ovarian cysts) and neoplastic (e.g., Burkitt's lymphoma) lesions. In a sexually active female adolescent, pregnancy should always be considered as a cause of an abdominal mass and excluded by a human chorionic gonadotropin level.

Repetitive, stereotypical, intense bouts of vomiting that begin abruptly in the early morning hours and resolve rapidly are characteristic of cyclic vomiting syndrome (see the later sections on cyclic vomiting syndrome and abdominal migraine). Chronic vomiting can be associated with neurological injury such as cerebral palsy or a metabolic disorder that affects muscle tone (e.g., mitochondriopathy).[85] Neurological impairment can be associated with either oropharyngeal discoordination with aspiration or gastroesophageal reflux disease that often does not improve with time.

Evaluation

Evaluation of the child with acute vomiting is usually the purview of the primary care or emergency room physician. The clinical assessment of hydration without laboratory confirmation is usually sufficient basis to begin intravenous rehydration (Table 9-5).[61,98] Viral testing and bacterial cultures in stool in presumed gastroenteritis or colitis can identify the infectious risk to others. If the physical examination reveals acute abdominal signs, abdominal radiographs and surgical consultation are indicated. When the emesis is voluminous and frequent, empiric antiemetic therapy (e.g., promethazine suppositories) may forestall progression to dehydration and the need for intravenous therapy.

In a child presenting with chronic vomiting, screening laboratory tests (e.g., amylase, lipase) and empiric treatment with H_2 receptor antagonists or proton pump inhibitors can precede more definitive testing. If the condition does not improve on therapy, definitive tests may be considered: an esophagogastroduodenoscopy to detect suspected peptic, allergic, infectious, and inflammatory mucosal injuries; small bowel radiography to identify possible anatomic lesions and Crohn's disease; an abdominal ultrasound to assess potential cholelithiasis, pancreatic pseudocyst, or hydronephrosis, and sinus computed tomography (CT) to document chronic sinusitis. Sinus evaluation has a 10% yield in chronic vomiting.[60]

In evaluating a child with cyclic or episodic vomiting, laboratory test results are typically abnormal only during the symptomatic attack; therefore blood and urine screening for metabolic disorders must be obtained *during the episode*.[61] The serum chemistry profile can detect hyperglycemia in diabetes mellitus or hypoglycemia in disorders of fatty acid oxidation, hyponatremia in Addison's disease, an anion gap and low bicarbonate in organic acidemias, elevated hepatic transaminases in hepatic and biliary disorders, and elevated lipase in pancreatic disorders. Blood is analyzed for elevations of ammonia in urea cycle defects, lactic acid in mitochondriopathies, amino acids in aminoacidemias, and deficiency of carnitine in disorders of fatty acid oxidation. After screening children for pyuria (infection) and hematuria (stones), the urine is analyzed for elevations in organic acids, carnitine esters, δ-aminolevulinic acid, and porphobilinogen in organic acidurias, disorders of fatty acid oxidation, and acute intermittent porphyria, respectively. Positive results on screening

TABLE 9-4. **Clinical Clues to Diagnosis**

Associated Symptom or Sign	Diagnostic Consideration
Systemic Manifestations	
Acute illness, dehydration	Infection, ingestion, cyclic vomiting, possible surgical emergency
Chronic malnutrition	Malabsorption syndrome
Temporal Pattern	
Low-grade, daily	Chronic vomiting pattern, e.g., upper GI tract disease
Postprandial	Upper GI tract disease (e.g., gastritis), biliary and pancreatic disorders
Relationship to diet	Fat, cholecystitis, pancreatitis; protein allergy; fructose, hereditary fructose intolerance
Early morning onset	Sinusitis, cyclic vomiting syndrome, subtentorial neoplasm
High intensity	Cyclic vomiting syndrome, food poisoning
Stereotypical (well between episodes)	Cyclic vomiting syndrome (see Differential Diagnosis in Table 9-2)
Rapid onset and subsidence	Cyclic vomiting syndrome
Character of Emesis	
Effortless	Gastroesophageal reflux, rumination
Projectile	Upper GI tract obstruction
Mucous	Allergy, chronic sinusitis
Bilious	Postampullary obstruction, cyclic vomiting syndrome
Bloody	Esophagitis, prolapse gastropathy, Mallory-Weiss injury, allergic gastroenteropathy, bleeding diathesis
Undigested food	Achalasia
Clear, large volume	Ménétrier's disease, Zollinger-Ellison syndrome
Malodorous	*H. pylori*, giardiasis, sinusitis, small bowel bacterial overgrowth, colonic obstruction
Gastrointestinal Symptoms	
Nausea	Absence of nausea can suggest increased intracranial pressure
Abdominal pain	Substernal, esophagitis; epigastric, upper GI tract, pancreatic; right upper quadrant, cholelithiasis
Diarrhea	Gastroenteritis, bacterial colitis
Constipation	Hirschsprung's disease, pseudoobstruction, hypercalcemia
Dysphagia	Eosinophilic esophagitis, achalasia, esophageal stricture
Visible peristalsis	Gastric outlet obstruction
Surgical scars	Surgical adhesions, surgical vagotomy
Succussion splash	Gastric outlet obstruction with gastric distention
Bowel sounds	Decreased: paralytic ileus; increased: mechanical obstruction
Severe abdominal tenderness with rebound	Perforated viscera and peritonitis
Abdominal mass	Pyloric stenosis, congenital malformations, Crohn's, ovarian cyst, pregnancy, abdominal neoplasm
Neurologic Symptoms	
Headache	Allergy, chronic sinusitis, migraine, increased intracranial pressure
Postnasal drip, congestion	Allergy, chronic sinusitis
Vertigo	Migraine, Ménière's disease
Seizures	Epilepsy
Abnormal muscle tone	Cerebral palsy, metabolic disorder, mitochondriopathy
Abnormal funduscopic exam or bulging fontanelle	Increased intracranial pressure, pseudotumor cerebri
Family History and Epidemiology	
Peptic ulcer disease	Peptic ulcer disease, *H. pylori* gastritis
Migraine headaches	Abdominal migraine, cyclic vomiting syndrome
Contaminated water	*Giardia*, *Cryptosporidium*, other parasites
Travel	Traveler's (*Escherichia coli*) diarrhea, giardiasis

tests necessitate appropriate definitive testing. For example, the absence of ketones, presence of dicarboxylic aciduria, and elevated urinary esterified free carnitine ratio of greater than 4:1 implicate a disorder of fatty acid oxidation and diagnosis entails definitive plasma acylcarnitine and urinary acylglycine profiles. Definitive evaluation of GI tract involvement includes small bowel radiography for anatomic lesions, an esophagogastroduodenoscopy for mucosal inflammation, and an abdominal ultrasound for renal, gallbladder, pancreatic and ovarian lesions. With a history suggestive of increased intracranial pressure (e.g., headache, onset upon wakening), magnetic resonance imaging (MRI) of the brain is the best test to visualize the subtentorial region. In the absence of laboratory radiographic or endoscopic findings, if cyclic vomiting syndrome is suspected, an empiric trial of prophylactic antimigraine may be initiated.

TABLE 9-5. Initial Diagnostic Evaluation by Temporal Pattern of Vomiting[61,98]

	Acute	Chronic	Cyclic (*Test During the Episode!*)
	Studies		
Screening testing	Electrolytes BUN Creatinine	CBC, ESR ALT, AST, GGTP, amylase Urinalysis Stool *Giardia* ELISA	Blood CBC Glucose, electrolytes, ALT, AST, GGTP amylase lipase Ammonia Lactate Carnitine Amino acids Urine Urinalysis Organic acids δ-ALA, porphobilinogen Carnitine
Definitive testing	Rotazyme Stool *Giardia* ELISA Abdominal radiographs Surgical consult	Endoscopy with biopsies Sinus CT UGI/SBFT series Abdominal ultrasound	UGI/SBFT series Endoscopy with biopsies Sinus CT Head MRI Abdominal ultrasound Definitive metabolic testing

ALA, aminolevulinic acid; ALT, alanine transaminase; AST, aspartate aminotransferase; BUN, blood urea nitrogen; CBC, complete blood count; CT, computerized tomography; ELISA, enzyme-linked immunosorbent assay; ESR, erythrocyte sedimentation rate; GGTP, γ-glutamyl transpeptidase (gamma); MRI, magnetic resonance imaging; UGI/SBFT, upper gastrointestinal with small bowel follow-through.

Complications

The two principal complications of acute or cyclic vomiting (during the episode) include dehydration with electrolyte derangement and hematemesis from prolapse gastropathy or Mallory-Weiss injury. The electrolyte disturbance resulting from varying losses of gastric HCl, pancreatic HCO_3, and GI NaCl is generally corrected with standard intravenous replacement. Hypochloremic, hypokalemic alkalosis results from high-grade gastric outlet obstruction and predominant loss of gastric H^+ and Cl^- ions. Risk factors for development of alkalosis in pyloric stenosis include female gender, African American race, longer duration of illness, and more severe dehydration.[99] Preoperative restoration of electrolyte balance reduces the perioperative morbidity.

Prolapse gastropathy occurs more commonly than the Mallory-Weiss injury at the gastroesophageal junction. The former injury presumably results from repeated severe trauma resulting from herniation of the cardia through the gastroesophageal junction. No therapy or short-term acid suppression suffices.

Complications of persistent peptic injury to the esophagus (e.g., stricture formation and Barrett's metaplasia) and bronchopulmonary aspiration are more likely to occur with long-standing chronic vomiting associated with gastroesophageal reflux disease in which the esophageal mucosa undergoes prolonged acid exposure. Growth failure as a complication of chronic vomiting can be caused by loss of calories, inflammatory burden, or protein-losing enteropathy. Aggressive nutritional rehabilitation may require continuous nasogastric or transpyloric feedings.

Pharmacologic Treatment

Although the therapy should be directed toward the cause, empiric therapy of the vomiting symptom may be indicated when the severity of the acute or cyclic vomiting places the child at risk of dehydration and other complications. Although laboratory confirmation of cyclic vomiting syndrome is not possible, a positive response to the antimigraine therapy can support the diagnosis. A comprehensive listing of therapeutic agents by pharmacologic category is presented in Table 9-6.[100-102]

Antihistamines (e.g., meclizine) are minimally active antiemetics but have efficacy in motion sickness because of their effects on vestibular function of the middle ear. As a result of D_2 receptor antagonist activity, phenothiazines (e.g., promethazine) have mild to moderate activity in chemotherapy-induced vomiting but carry a substantial risk of extrapyramidal reactions. Butyrophenones (e.g., droperidol) have mild to moderate efficacy when used in chemotherapy and postoperative settings. Their use is limited by extrapyramidal reactions. Benzodiazepines have minimal antiemetic efficacy but are useful adjuncts to other antiemetics. Cannabinoids have mild to moderate potency but can be associated with dependence.

The newer serotonergic agonists and antagonists have demonstrated marked antiemetic efficacy. The 5-HT_3 antagonists have demonstrated greater antiemetic efficacy in postoperative and chemotherapy settings than did previous regimens. $5\text{-HT}_{1B/1D}$ agonists (e.g., triptans) have recently shown promise for aborting pediatric migraine headaches[103] and cyclic vomiting.[104,105] Because 5-HT_3 and $5\text{-HT}_{1B/1D}$ agents have both central and peripheral actions, the antiemetic effects may result from a combination of both.

CLINICAL ASPECTS OF NAUSEA

Nausea, a uniquely unpleasant sensation that typically precedes the act of vomiting, is difficult to precisely define. A variety of stimuli, including labyrinth stimulation, visceral pain, and unpleasant memories, may induce nausea. Although the precise mechanism of nausea is unknown, evidence suggests that the neural pathways responsible for nausea and vomiting are the same. Nausea may result from less intense activation, whereas more intense activation of the same neural pathways triggers vomiting. During nausea, gastric tone and peristalsis are

TABLE 9-6. Antinausea and Antiemetic Medications[100-102]

Drug Class/Generic	Brand Name	Dosages*	Mechanisms	Side Effects	Indications	Potential Applications
Antihistamines (Minimal Antiemetic Activity)						
Diphenhydramine	Benadryl, Benylin	~1.25 mg/kg q 6 h PO or IV	Vestibular suppression, anti-ACh effect, and H_1 antagonist	Sedation, anticholinergic effects[†]	Motion sickness, mild chemotherapy-induced vomiting	Contraindicated with MAO inhibitors, GI obstruction
Hydroxyzine	Atarax, Vistaril	0.5-0.6 mg/kg q 6 h PO				
Dimenhydrinate	Dramamine	1.25 mg/kg q 6 h PO or IM				
Cyclizine	Marezine	1 mg/kg q 8 h PO or IM; >10 years of age: 50 mg q 4-6 h PO or IM		Sedation		
Meclizine	Antivert	>12 years of age; 25-100 mg/24 h PO divided tid-qid	Vestibular suppression, anti-ACh effect			
Phenothiazines (Mild to Moderate Antiemetic Activity)						
Promethazine	Phenergan	0.25-0.5 mg/kg per dose q 4-6 h PR or IM	D_2 receptor antagonist at CTZ and H_1 antagonist	Anticholinergic effects,[†] extrapyramidal reactions	Chemotherapy-induced vomiting	
Prochlorperazine	Compazine	>10 kg: 0.1-0.15 mg/kg per dose IM >10 kg: 0.4 mg/kg per 24 h divided tid-qid PO or PR Maximum 10 mg/dose	D_2 receptor antagonist at CTZ			
Chlorpromazine	Thorazine	>6 months of age: 0.5-1 mg/kg per dose IV or PO q 6-8 h				
Substituted Benzamides (High Antiemetic Activity)						
Cisapride	Propulsid	0.2-0.3 mg/kg tid-qid PO Adults: 10 mg tid-qid PO	$5-HT_4$ agonist with ACh release in gut	Diarrhea, abdominal pain, headache	GER, gastroparesis	Arrhythmias with antifungal and macrolide antibiotics, cyclic vomiting
Metoclopramide	Reglan	0.1 mg/kg per dose IM, IV, or PO up to qid. The total daily dose should not exceed 0.5 mg/kg. Adults: 10 mg IM, IV, or PO 30 min before each meal and at bedtime	D_2 antagonist at CTZ and gut, $5-HT_4$ agonist in gut	Irritability and extrapyramidal reactions	GER, gastroparesis, chemotherapy-induced vomiting	
Trimethobenzamide	Tigan	Children <14 kg: 100 mg/dose PR tid-qid Children 14-40 kg: 100-200 mg/dose PO or PR tid-qid Not recommended for neonates or premature infants.	D_2 antagonist at CTZ			
5-HT3 Receptor Antagonists (High Antiemetic Activity)						
Ondansetron	Zofran	0.15 mg/kg IV q 8 h or 0.15-0.40 mg/kg Surface area <0.3 m²: 1 mg/dose PO Surface area 0.3-0.6 m²: 2 mg/dose PO Surface area 0.6-1.0 m²: 3 mg/dose PO Surface area >1 m²: 4 mg/dose PO	$5-HT_3$ antagonist at CTZ and vagal afferents in gut	Headache	Chemotherapy, postoperative	Cyclic vomiting
Granisetron	Kytril	Age 2-16 years: 10 µg/kg IV q 6 h				
Tropisetron	Navoban	8-12 mg/m² qd				
Palonosetron	Aloxi	3 µg/kg/dose IV max dose 0.5 mg × 1		QT prolongation		Cyclic vomiting

*Note that these are doses used for antiemetic effects rather than other indications.
†Anticholinergic effects – blurred vision, dry mouth, hypotension, palpitations, urinary retention. Within the same drug class, in the blank space, the same attributes apply from the medication above.
ACh, acetylcholine; CTZ, chemotrigger zone; D, dopamine; H, histamine; 5-HT, 5-hydroxytryptamine; GABA, γ-aminobutyric acid; GER, gastroesophageal reflux; MAO, monoamine oxidase.

Continued

TABLE 9-6. Antinausea and Antiemetic Medications—cont'd

Drug Class/Generic	Brand Name	Dosages*	Mechanisms	Side Effects	Indications	Potential Applications
Tachykinin Receptor Antagonists						
Aprepitant	Emend	Adult 3 day regimen: 1st dose 125 mg 1 h before chemotherapy and 80 mg qd. Casopitant days 2-3	NK₁ receptor antagonist in CTZ	Fatigue, dizziness, diarrhea	Chemotherapy-induced nausea and vomiting	
Casopitant	Rezonic	PO × 1 or 3-day IV + PO (90 mg IV day 1 + 50 mg PO qd days 2-3)		Neutropenia		
Anticholinergics (Minimal Antiemetic Activity)						
Scopolamine	Transderm Scop	Not recommended for pediatric use. 1 patch is 1 mg scopolamine q 3 days	Vestibular suppression, anti-ACh effect on central pattern generator	Sedation, anticholinergic effects†	Prophylaxis of motion sickness	
Benzimidazole Derivative (Mild to Moderate Antiemetic Activity)						
Domperidone	Motilium	0.6 mg/kg per dose tid-qid PO or <2 years: 10 mg PR bid-qid 2-4 years: 15 mg PR qid 4-6 years: 23 mg PR qid >6 years: 30 mg PR qid	D₂ antagonist in gut	Headaches	Gastroparesis, chemotherapy	Not available in the United States
Butyrophenone (Mild to Moderate Antiemetic Activity)						
Droperidol	Inapsine	0.05-0.075 mg/kg per dose IM or IV for one dose	D₂ antagonist at CTZ, anxiolytic action and sedation	Hypotension, sedation, extrapyramidal effects	Chemotherapy, postoperative	
Benzodiazepines (Minimal Antiemetic Activity)						
Lorazepam	Ativan	0.05-0.1 mg/kg per dose IV	Enhanced central GABA-ergic inhibition inducing anxiolysis, sedation, and amnesia	Sedation, respiratory depression	Chemotherapy adjunct	Cyclic vomiting adjunct
Diazepam	Valium	0.1-0.3 mg/kg IV prn Maximum: <0.6 mg/kg per 24 h				
Corticosteroids (Mild to Moderate Antiemetic Activity)						
Dexamethasone	Decadron	Initial dose: 5-10 mg/m² IV, maximum 20 mg, then 5 mg/m² q 12 h IV	Unknown	Unknown	Adrenal suppression	Chemotherapy
Cannabinoids (Mild to Moderate Antiemetic Activity)						
Dronabinol	Marinol	>12 years: 5 mg/m² per dose q 4-6 h PO	Unknown	Disorientation, vertigo, hallucinations	Chemotherapy	
Nabilone	Cesamet	<18 kg: 0.5 mg PO bid 18-30 kg: 1 mg PO bid >30 kg: 1 mg PO tid				

*Note that these are doses used for antiemetic effects rather than other indications.
†Anticholinergic effects – blurred vision, dry mouth, hypotension, palpitations, urinary retention. Within the same drug class, in the blank space, the same attributes apply from the medication above.
ACh, acetylcholine; CTZ, chemotrigger zone; D, dopamine; H, histamine; 5-HT, 5-hydroxytryptamine; GABA, γ-aminobutyric acid; GER, gastroesophageal reflux; MAO, monoamine oxidase.

TABLE 9-7. **Differential Diagnosis of Nausea**

Gastrointestinal

Gastroesophageal reflux disease

Allergic bowel disease, e.g., eosinophilic esophagitis

Delayed gastric emptying, e.g., postinfectious gastroparesis

Intestinal pseudoobstruction and other dysmotility syndromes

Biliary dysfunction, e.g., biliary dyskinesia

Food poisoning, e.g., *Bacillus cereus*

Gastric outlet obstruction, malrotation

Nongastrointestinal

Brain and ear, nose and throat

    Migraine headaches

    Migraine variants, e.g., abdominal migraines, cyclic vomiting syndrome

    Chronic sinusitis, allergic rhinitis

    Motion sickness, e.g., vertigo

    Autonomic dysfunction, e.g., postural orthostatic tachycardia syndrome

    Eustachian tube dysfunction, e.g., middle ear infection or Ménière's

    Arnold-Chiari malformation

    Brainstem tumor, e.g., brainstem glioma, cerebellar medulloblastoma

Systemic and behavioral

    Eating disorders (e.g., anorexia nervosa, bulimia)

    Thyroid dysfunction

    Pregnancy and hyperemesis gravidarum

    Drug-induced (e.g., chemotherapy, ingestion)

    Postoperative state

diminished, whereas duodenal and proximal jejunal tone tend to be increased.

The major nausea pathways can be activated with chemical, visceral, vestibular, and central nervous system stimulation. Chemical stimulation results from the action of blood-borne toxins (e.g., chemotherapy) on the CTZ in the area postrema where the blood-brain barrier is virtually nonexistent.[106] The visceral pathway is activated directly by stomach irritation caused by ingested agents (drugs and toxins) or indirectly by enhanced gastric acid secretion resulting from physical and emotional stressors.[107] The vagus and sympathetic nerves, via the nucleus tractus solitarius and nodosum ganglion, respectively, mediate the nausea arising from gastric irritants. Antral balloon distention stretching the gastric walls is another mechanism that can evoke nausea.[108] The vestibular pathway involves afferent nerves that project to the vestibular nuclei and lead to activation of the brainstem mediated via histamine H_1 and muscarinic cholinergic pathways. This pathway is most commonly activated when a person is subjected to a novel motion environment.[109] Onset of nausea during motion correlates with gastric dysrhythmias including tachygastria and the release of vasopressin from the posterior pituitary.[108] Nausea can arise in the central nervous system during anticipatory nausea that often precedes recurring chemotherapy. Previous studies have identified motion sickness, trait anxiety, depression, female sex, and young age of subject to be predictors of anticipatory nausea and vomiting.[110]

Another area of ongoing investigation is the proposed involvement of neuroendocrine response to stress. In extensive animals studies by Taché's group, secretion of corticotropin-releasing factor atop the hypothalamic-pituitary adrenal axis in response to physical or psychological stress, cytokines, or

TABLE 9-8. **Evaluation of Nausea**

GI Anatomic	Mucosal	Motility
Contrast UGI/SBFT Abdominal ultrasound Gastric barostat	EGD with biopsies	Solid-phase GE scan GB HIDA scan

Non-GI Autonomic	Organic (Other)	Migraine
Orthostatic pulse increase Tilt-table testing Stress-induced	CT sinuses MRI subtentorial	Historical criteria Trial of medication

EGD, esophagogastroduodenoscopy; GB, gallbladder; GE, gastric emptying; HIDA, cholescintigraphy; UGI/SBFT, upper gastrointestinal series with small bowel follow-through.

ingested noxious substances can cause gastroparesis via sympathetic outflow.[53] Hypothalamic antidiuretic hormone (ADH) release may also help mediate gastric stasis and symptomatic nausea.[111]

Clinical Clues and Differential Diagnosis

There are distinct autonomic signs that often accompany the symptoms of nausea. Hypersalivation is due to activation of salivary centers that are in close proximity to the medullary vomiting center. Pallor, listlessness, and tachycardia often accompany nausea. Several lines of research implicate the autonomic nervous system (ANS) in the expression of chemotherapy-induced nausea.[112] Bellg measured peak values of heart rate, pulse, pallor, and skin temperature to assess autonomic reactivity over time. These autonomic measures varied in relation to time of emesis, but were all associated with the development of nausea.[113] The list of potential causes of nausea is extensive and overlaps known etiologies of vomiting (Table 9-7).

Evaluation

The evaluation of the symptom of chronic nausea usually involves an investigation that overlaps that of vomiting (Table 9-8). If one suspects an anatomical cause of nausea that is associated with projectile vomiting or bilious emesis, contrast radiography of the stomach and small bowel is indicated. An abdominal ultrasound can be useful in the initial evaluation of symptoms of meal-related nausea with or without right upper-quadrant (RUQ) and left upper-quadrant (LUQ) pain for detecting gallstones or pancreatic pseudocyst, respectively. If no gallstones are found but the nausea and RUQ pain persists, a finding on cholecystokinin-stimulated gallbladder hepatobiliary iminodiacetic acid (HIDA) scan of less than 30% emptying is compatible with gallbladder dyskinesia.[114]

If mucosal injury is suspected from meal-induced nausea, pain, and/or vomiting, an esophagogastroduodenoscopy will detect peptic or allergic esophagitis and gastritis with or without *H. pylori*, as well as eosinophilic gastroenteritis. Crohn's disease and celiac disease are unusual organic causes of nausea. If nausea, early satiety, and bloating are noted, disordered gastric motility should be suspected. Although a solid-phase gastric emptying scan can be useful in this scenario, it unfortunately is a relatively insensitive test. More distal intestinal dysmotility can be suggested by chronically dilated intestinal loops on flat plates and delayed small bowel transit on contrast radiography.

Additional specialized motility tests performed in a few pediatric GI centers include the gastric barostat, antroduodenal motility, and electrogastrography (EGG). The gastric barostat is useful in detecting impaired gastric compliance and visceral hypersensitivity in the stomach. Antroduodenal manometry can demonstrate myopathic, neuropathic, or obstructive contraction patterns.[108] EGG can demonstrate dysrhythmias (e.g., tachygastria) both in the presence and the absence of altered gastric emptying.[109] The combination of these tests has been used in adults to delineate a full-blown gastric neuromuscular disorder with abnormal gastric emptying and EGG results to be treated with prokinetic agents to a visceral hypersensitivity associated with normal results to be tried on tricyclic antidepressants.[108] An important nongastrointestinal cause of nausea to evaluate includes autonomic dysfunction. In the clinic, one can screen for postural orthostatic tachycardia syndrome (POTS) by looking for a 30 beat/min rise in heart rate following a change in position from supine to upright. A more definitive evaluation includes a tilt-table test to more precisely confirm the postural orthostatic tachycardia response.

There are several important, less appreciated causes of early morning nausea. If postnasal drip or congestion occurs in the morning, chronic sinusitis or allergic rhinitis should be suspected and if no response to antihistamines, a sinus CT performed. Other common causes include cyclic vomiting syndrome (CVS), abdominal migraines, or migraine headaches and should be suspected based on the stereotypical pattern, pallor, and listlessness; a positive response to a trial of antimigraine medication can serve as a supporting evidence. However, if the nausea becomes persistent and intractable, an MRI would be indicated to exclude a subtentorial neoplasm or Chiari malformation.

Nausea that results from gastric retention from gastroparesis, pseudoobstruction, or mechanical obstruction is typically reduced by the action of vomiting. If abdominal pain or altered bowel function are accompanied by nausea, irritable bowel syndrome should be considered.[108] In contrast, nausea of central origin, such as that accompanying a migraine, is typically poorly relieved by vomiting. Many patients complain of chronic nausea without full-blown retching or vomiting.

In some cases, nausea can persist for months or even years despite an exhaustive evaluation that has excluded numerous organic disorders. On the basis of laboratory exclusion, this can be classified as functional nausea and/or included under the broader umbrella of functional dyspepsia. As with many incapacitating functional gastrointestinal disorders, it is often difficult to convince the parents that such intractable nausea does not have an organic basis. This concern often compels the parents to seek out more experts and additional laboratory, radiographic, and endoscopic testing on behalf of the affected child.

Pharmacologic Treatment

Nausea, in part because of the abundance of incapacitating accompanying autonomic symptoms, can become extremely disabling for the child and adolescent. Treatment of chronic nausea requires a multidisciplinary approach. One must take into account that many of those affected are school-aged children with various stressors related to school, family, and friends. For example, prolonged school absenteeism can be self-perpetuating and may require the help of a psychologist to acknowledge the validity of the symptoms, modify stress awareness, and devise a graded program of reintroducing the child back to school.[111] Stress reduction through a structured program of biofeedback or relaxation therapy can be an essential aid.[111]

A trial of medication can be useful in ameliorating symptoms of nausea and narrowing the possible causes. A positive response to acid suppression or gastric prokinetics can support the possibilities of a peptic disorder or gastric dysmotility. If migraine or migraine equivalent is suspected based on the historical criteria, a trial of β-blockers or tricyclic antidepressants such as amitriptyline may prevent the attacks. Suspected allergies or chronic sinusitis with nighttime postnasal drip may respond to a course of antihistamines and/or antibiotics. When no specific cause is discerned, a series of trials of D_2 antagonists, H_1 antagonists, and $5-HT_3$ antagonists may provide some relief of nausea (see Table 9-6).

Dietary modification can be useful when gastric neuromuscular dysfunction is present and the ability of the stomach to triturate and empty meals is compromised.[108] Because liquids require less neuromuscular effort than solids to empty, a staged approach to advance the diet from liquids to soups to starches can be beneficial. Other nondrug treatments include the complementary medicine approaches. Ginger given 1 h before motion sickness has been shown to decrease nausea associated with gastric dysrhythmias in adults.[108] Also, acustimulation via a transcutaneous electrode has been shown to reduce nausea due to pregnancy, chemotherapy, and the postoperative state.[108] Although gastric electrical stimulation to the neuromuscular circuitry can reduce the refractory nausea and vomiting by 70 to 80% in patients with gastroparesis, the mechanism of action appears to be other than one of improved motility.[108]

Chronic Idiopathic Nausea

Nausea can present as the predominant symptom in certain children where no specific organic cause can be found. When this occurs several times weekly unassociated with vomiting, the term *chronic idiopathic nausea* may be applied. Distinct from functional dyspepsia, where postprandial timing and epigastric discomfort are predominant, *chronic idiopathic nausea* is defined by Rome III criteria in adults when weekly nausea occurs for at least 3 months' duration and no specific organic cause can be identified.

The most typical case is an adolescent female who has daily nausea that is most intense during the morning and improves by the afternoon. Oftentimes, an extensive radiographic and endoscopic evaluation fails to reveal a cause in the sinuses, brainstem, upper GI tract anatomy and mucosa, gastric motility, gallbladder motility, and autonomic nervous system (postural orthostatic tachycardia syndrome). The nausea may be disabling and cause substantial school absences.

Evaluation by esophagogastroduodenoscopy and/or pH probe testing may be necessary as the nausea can be caused by mucosal injury from peptic, allergic, and inflammatory conditions affecting the upper GI tract in adults.[115] Nausea can also be a symptom of delayed gastric emptying from either gastroparesis or pyloric outlet obstruction. Evaluation by gastric scintigraphy and/or antroduodenal manometry may help identify a gastric dysmotility. Therapeutic intervention may include prokinetic agents or pyloric balloon dilation with pre-pyloric botulinum toxin injection.

As with many functional gastrointestinal disorders in children, a standard approach to evaluation and treatment of chronic nausea has not been established. The nausea may be intractable and the adolescent fully bedridden and absent from school for months, similar to those affected by pain-associated disability syndromes. Management of the unpleasant sensation and the return to normal functioning is difficult. Similar to that used to treat other functional gastrointestinal pain disorders, the initial approach involves: (1) acknowledgement that the adolescent's symptoms are real and will be taken seriously, (2) reassurance that the medical evaluation will be thorough to exclude treatable conditions, (3) a series of empiric therapies to treat potential underlying conditions (e.g., acid reflux) and to relieve the child's discomfort, and (4) identification that the principal goal is to rehabilitate the adolescent to normal function even as the nausea persists. Because each treatment may take several weeks (e.g., to achieve therapeutic levels), it is critical to set realistic expectations for the parents that this evaluative, therapeutic, and rehabilitative approach is unlikely to lead to an immediate cure and is more likely to lead to incremental improvement over several months.[111] The return to school after a prolonged absence may require the medical psychologist to diagnose and treat the accompanying separation anxiety and plan a graduated return to school.[116]

The large number of antiemetic agents have limited efficacy for relief of nausea. For example, 5-HT$_3$ antagonists or promethazine provide limited benefit. Ginger may be used and can help the nausea.[117] A trial of a prokinetic D$_2$ agent such as metoclopramide or domperidone can help determine if enhancing gastric emptying helps the nausea, but the central side effects limit their usefulness. Low-dose tricyclic antidepressant therapy has been shown to benefit affected adults and has been used to help affected adolescents in our experience.[118]

SPECIFIC VOMITING DISORDERS

Cyclic Vomiting Syndrome and Abdominal Migraine

Although cyclic vomiting syndrome is now increasingly recognized, it remains a disorder of unknown etiology and pathogenesis characterized by recurrent episodes of vomiting separated by periods of symptom-free or baseline health.[60-62]

Although its exact prevalence is unknown, estimates of two studies of Caucasian children aged 5 to 15 years and Turkish children aged 6 to 17 years reported a prevalence of approximately 2%.[119,120] CVS was initially described in English by Samuel Gee in 1882,[121] and a strong association with migraine headaches noted as early as 1898 by Whitney.[122] Similar to the gender profile in migraine headaches, there is a slight predominance of girls over boys (57:43).

CVS is an idiopathic disorder with an acute clinical presentation with vomiting that is typically misdiagnosed as viral gastroenteritis or food poisoning resulting in a 2.6-year delay in diagnosis. Recently, consensus guidelines for diagnostic criteria and treatment were established by a task force of experts through the North American Society for Pediatric Gastroenterology, Hepatology, and Nutrition[123] as shown in Table 9-9.

The older terminology used *abdominal migraine* to identify those with GI symptoms, both abdominal pain and vomiting.[91,92] The current consensus differentiates *cyclic vomiting syndrome* from *abdominal migraine* based on the vomiting being the predominant symptom over pain. In reality, these populations overlap and patients can be classified either way, as 80% of children with CVS have abdominal pain and 46% of those with

TABLE 9-9. Diagnostic Criteria for Cyclic Vomiting Syndrome

- At least 5 episodes overall or a minimum of 3 episodes noted in a 6-month period
- Recurrent episodes of vomiting and nausea lasting 1 hour to 10 days and occurring at least 1 week apart
- Stereotypical pattern and symptoms in the individual patient
- Vomiting during episodes occurring at least 4 times per hour for at least 1 hour
- Returning to baseline health between episodes
- Not attributable to another disorder

Data from Li BUK, et al, 2008.[123]

abdominal migraine have some vomiting.[124-126] Many of the secondary features of pallor, listlessness, and nausea are found in both.[127] Electroencephalographic and autonomic function data also support a pathophysiologic overlap between the two entities.[128,129]

In our series of children who were diagnosed with cyclic vomiting syndrome, the typical patient is a 5- to 8-year-old girl who has stereotypical, severe (median 15 emeses per episode) episodes once every 2 to 4 weeks, yet returns to normal or baseline health between episodes. Although the term *cyclic* is used, because only 49% have regular intervals, *episodic* would be a more precise term. The attacks most frequently begin in the early morning hours or on awakening, are preceded by a short prodrome (0.5 to 1.5 h), last 24 to 48 h, require intravenous (IV) hydration (58%), and cause 24 days (median) of school absence per year. Because most episodes result in dehydration, acute episodes of CVS are often treated in the emergency department and are often misdiagnosed as acute gastroenteritis. Common symptoms (in more than 75% of the children) include pallor, lethargy, anorexia, nausea, retching, and abdominal pain. Nausea is often identified by patients as the most persistent and distressing symptom unrelieved by vomiting and evacuating the stomach. The parents can usually (72%) identify a proximate event, most often excitement stress (e.g., birthday, holiday), an infection (e.g., upper respiratory infection), or a food (e.g., chocolate, cheese). However, typical migraine *symptoms* of headaches and photophobia affect only 30 to 40% of children. The natural history is for the recurrent vomiting to resolve during the teenage years only to be replaced by migraine headaches.

Some adolescent patients with increasing frequency of episodes deteriorate to a "coalescent" form of CVS, characterized by interictal daily nausea, less intense vomiting, and disability that can linger for weeks to months.[130] This coalescent pattern, more typical of adolescents and adults, can exacerbate underlying stress and anxiety, which can have an adverse effect on daily function and result in nutritional and functional debilitation.

Although no etiopathogenesis has been identified, several tenable hypotheses have been proposed. Recent investigations have identified mitochondrial gene mutations (single-nucleotide polymorphisms in the control region), autonomic dysfunction (sympathetic over parasympathetic predominance), and hypothalamic-pituitary-adrenal axis activation. A strong matrilineal inheritance pattern, evidence of impaired mitochondrial energy production and single nucleotide polymorphisms have been identified by Boles and Williams.[131] Chelimsky has described a sympathetic hyperreactivity on autonomic nervous system testing and an association with postural orthostatic tachycardia.[132] Sato and Wolff[133,134] described a subset of CVS children who have marked activation of the hypothalamic-pituitary-adrenal axis, and Taché[135] and Li have proposed that corticotropin-releasing factor may serve as a trigger of vomiting in CVS.

Coexisting neurologic findings of developmental delay, generalized seizures, and hypotonia as well as neuromuscular disease manifestations have been found in up to 25% of CVS patients.[136] Labeled as CVS+, these patients have a three- to eightfold higher prevalence of dysautonomia-related disorders and constitutional abnormalities (e.g., hypothyroidism).

Although the cyclic *pattern* (high intensity, on or off) of vomiting is the key diagnostic feature of CVS, the pattern represents a starting point for diagnostic testing and the syndrome refers to those idiopathic cases in whom the diagnostic testing is negative.[137] Recent consensus guidelines suggest a targeted diagnostic approach for testing.[123] Evaluation for surgical causes of vomiting, including malrotation/volvulus and renal hydronephrosis, can be screened via upper gastrointestinal radiograph and renal ultrasound. Alarm symptoms include abdominal signs (bilious vomiting, tenderness, severe pain), triggering events suggestive of a metabolic disorder (fasting, high-protein meal), abnormal neurological examination (altered mental status, papilledema), and progressive worsening or a conversion to a chronic pattern of vomiting episodes.[123] In the absence of abnormal screening lab work, an initial trial of empiric therapy can be considered in children with a cyclic pattern of vomiting. In *abdominal migraine*, the pain is the primary symptom and is often severe causing the child to writhe and/or remain a fetal position. Similar to those in CVS, episodes of abdominal migraine are stereotypical (similar time of onset, duration, and associated symptoms) and similarly associated with autonomic pallor, listlessness, and a family history of migraine headaches.[91,92]

Treatment for CVS can be divided into *lifestyle modifications*, *supportive therapy* (antiemetic and sedative therapy during episodes), *prophylactic therapy* (daily treatment to prevent episodes), and *abortive therapy* (to prevent progression from prodromal symptoms to the vomiting). Avoidance of identified triggers, lifestyle changes (frequent caloric intake, full fluid intake, regimented sleep), and psychological interventions (stress reduction) can help during the interepisodic period. Supportive measures include intravenous fluids containing 10% dextrose to diminish catabolism and a less stimulating environment with a combination of antiemetics and sedation to lessen nausea and vomiting. High-dose 5-HT$_3$ antagonist antiemetics (e.g., ondansetron 0.3 to 0.4 mg/kg) have been used to attenuate episodes with encouraging results.[138] Sedation in the form of diphenhydramine, lorazepam, or chlorpromazine when combined with antiemetics can help alleviate the unrelenting nausea during an episode and may in some cases shorten the episode by inducing sleep.

Daily prophylaxis should be considered in children with frequent episodes (more than one per month) or severe episodes (prolonged for more than 2 to 3 days), or for those who fail a trial of abortive and supportive therapy. Most of the prophylactic medications are borrowed from treatment of migraine (antimigraine, anticonvulsant, and low-estrogen birth control) (Table 9-10).[138-140] Recent consensus recommendations include cyproheptadine as a first-line agent in children 5 years or younger and amitriptyline as first line for those older than 5.[123] Abortive therapy should be considered for those who have sporadic episodes that occur less than once per month, short episodes (less than 24 hours in duration), or those who

have breakthrough episodes while on prophylaxis. Use of nasal 5-HT$_{1B/1D}$ (e.g., sumatriptan, zolmitriptan) antimigraine agents can abort episodes in the early stages.[141] With its unpredictable disruptive, occurrence, high level of morbidity, common misdiagnosis, and lack of well-established therapy, parental support from the physician and from support groups may help alleviate some family stress and reduce frequency of episodes.[98]

Postoperative Nausea and Vomiting

The prevalence of postoperative nausea and vomiting (PONV) in children is 20 to 24% after elective operations including strabismus repair, tonsillectomy, dental surgery, and inguinal herniorraphy.[142,143] Although the mechanisms have not been elucidated, there appear to be a number of risk factors for the development of PONV. These include age greater than 2 years, female gender, certain operations (tonsillectomies, strabismus repair, otoplasties, and ureter surgery), anesthetic used (cyclopropane has greater risk than isoflurane, enflurane, and halothane), postoperative opioid analgesia, prior PONV, and a history of motion sickness.[142,144] Factors that improve PONV in adults include better perioperative hydration, use of propofol anesthesia, decreased opioid use, shorter operations, laparoscopic surgery, and decompression of the GI tract.

Randomized, double-blind, placebo-controlled trials have established that 5-HT$_3$ antagonists reduce postoperative emesis following general anesthesia in preadolescent children undergoing strabismus correction,[145] tonsillectomy,[146] and other elective operations,[147] with the exception of craniotomy.[148] Head-to-head comparisons have established the superior efficacy of 5-HT$_3$ antagonists to droperidol[146,149,150] and metoclopramide.[146] Although single intravenous intraoperative doses of either ondansetron (0.15 mg/kg)[151] or granisetron (0.4 µg/kg) appear equally effective during the first 4 h,[145,152] some studies detect a prolonged effect lasting 24 h.[145,153] Recently available single-dose intravenous palonosetron is also effective in preventing PONV in the first 24 hours following surgery.[154] A recent randomized, double-blind placebo-controlled trial also demonstrated the efficacy of intraoperative prophylactic use of ondansetron on postoperative nausea and vomiting.[155] Most but not all recent controlled trials using perioperative electroacupuncture point P6 demonstrate significantly reduced postoperative nausea and vomiting as judged by the number of episodes of emesis or the use of rescue antiemetics.[156] Ketorolac used for postoperative analgesia provided equivalent pain relief to morphine but with significantly less vomiting.[157] Well tolerated either alone or in combination with a corticosteroid and 5-HT$_3$ antagonist, tachykinin receptor (NK$_1$) antagonist aprepitant is now approved and effective in adults for PONV.[158,159]

Chemotherapy-Induced Emesis

The current theories by which chemotherapy induces emesis include injury to the GI tract with release of serotonin and learned (anticipatory) responses.[160] Factors known to increase the incidence of vomiting in response to chemotherapy include young age (toddlers), female gender, emetogenicity of the agent (high, cisplatin; moderate, cyclophosphamide; mild, methotrexate), dose, and higher rate of administration. In one study in children, chemotherapy increased urinary 5-HT and 5-hydroxyindoleacetic acid (5-HIAA) excretion, whereas 5-HT

TABLE 9-10. Medications Used to Treat Cyclic Vomiting Syndrome and Abdominal Migraine[60-62,100-102,131-133]

Drug Class	Brand Name	Dosages	Mechanism of Action	Side Effects	Comments
Abortive					
Supportive					
IV hydration		D_{10} 0.45 normal saline	Stops ketosis, replaces Na^+, K^+, and lost volume		Glucose may be most effective component by terminating ketosis
Sedatives					
Diphenhydramine	Benadryl	1.0-1.25 mg/kg IV q 6 h	H1 receptor antagonist	Vestibular suppression, hypotension, sedation, dizziness anticholinergic	Useful adjunct to chlorpromazine
Lorazepam	Ativan	0.05-0.1 mg/kg IV q 6 h	Central enhanced GABA-ergic inhibition inducing sedation, anxiolysis, and amnesia	Sedation, respiratory depression	Adjunct to allow child to sleep
Chlorpromazine	Thorazine	0.5-1 mg/kg IV q 6 h	D_2 receptor antagonist	Hypotension, seizures, dystonic reactions when given alone	Use with diphenhydramine
Antimigraine					
Isometheptene	Midrin	Age >12 years, 1 capsule/h PO but ≤5 capsules q 24 h	Sympathomimetic vasoconstrictor	Dizziness	Not effective in vomiting child
Sumatriptan	Imitrex	Age >12 years, 6 mg SQ, may repeat in 1 h (maximum dose: 2 injections/24 h), 20 mg intranasally at episode onset	$5\text{-}HT_{1D}$ agonist induces cerebral vasoconstriction, relaxes gastric fundus	Transient burning in neck and chest, headache	Use SQ form if child is vomiting. Contraindicated with coronary vasospasm or hemiplegic or basilar artery migraine
Ketorolac	Toradol	0.5-1.0 mg/kg IV/IM × 1, then 0.2-0.5 mg/kg q 6-8 h ≤ 30 mg/dose	Cyclooxygenase inhibitor of prostaglandin synthesis	GI bleeding, contraindicated in ASA sensitivity	Can be given intravenously. Contraindicated with ASA sensitivity
Antiemetic					
Ondansetron	Zofran	0.15-0.4 mg/kg IV q 6-8 h	$5\text{-}HT_3$ antagonist in CTZ and vagal afferents in gut	Headache	Use IV form if child is vomiting
Granisetron	Kytril	0.10 µg/kg q 6-8 h			
Prophylactic					
Antimigraine					
Propranolol	Inderal	0.25-1 mg/kg per day maximum PO divided bid or tid 10-20 mg tid	β_1, β_2 adrenergic antagonist	Hypotension, bradycardia, fatigability	Use in small doses. Contraindicated in asthma, heart block. Withdraw gradually, monitor pulse
Atenolol	Tenormin	0.7-1.4 mg/kg per day PO divided bid or tid	β_1 adrenergic antagonist H_1 antagonist and $5\text{-}HT_2$ antagonist	Sedation, anticholinergic effects,* weight gain due to appetite stimulation	Contraindicated with asthma MAO inhibitors, GI obstruction
Cyproheptadine	Periactin	0.25-0.5 mg/kg per day PO divided bid or tid			1st choice <5 y old

*Anticholinergic effects include blurred vision, dry mouth, hypotension, palpitations, urinary retention.
Ach, acetylcholine; ASA, acetylsalicylic acid; CTZ, chemotrigger zone; GABA, γ-aminobutyric acid; H, histamine; 5-HT, 5-hydroxytryptamine; MAO, monamine oxidase; SST, supraventricular tachycardia.

Continued

Table 9-10. Medications Used to Treat Cyclic Vomiting Syndrome and Abdominal Migraine[60-62,100-102,131-133]—cont'd

Drug Class	Brand Name	Dosages	Mechanism of Action	Side Effects	Comments
Pizotyline	Sandomigran	1.5 mg/day divided qd or tid			Not available in the United States
Amitriptyline	Elavil	Begin at 0.25-0.5 mg/kg/day qhs and advance to 1-2 mg/kg qhs	Tricyclic antidepressant, increases synaptic norepinephrine and $5-HT_2$ antagonist	Sedation, anticholinergic effects* constipation	Contraindicated with SVT, MAO inhibitor, GI obstruction. Monitor EKG QTc interval before starting. 1st choice >5 yrs old. Monitor therapeutic levels
Nortriptyline	Pamelor	0.5-1 mg/kg/day qhs			
Neuroleptic					
Phenobarbital	Luminal	2 mg/kg per day PO qhs	$GABA_A$ potentiation of synaptic inhibition	Sedation, cognitive impairment	Contraindicated with acute intermittent porphyria, abdominal epilepsy
Carbamazepine	Tegretol	Age <6 years, 10-20 mg/kg per day PO divided bid or tid 6-12 years, 400-800 mg/day PO divided bid or tid >12 years, 600-1200 mg/day PO divided bid or tid	Slows Na^+ channel activation	Sedation, anticholinergic effects*	Contraindicated with MAO inhibitors
Alternatives: valproic acid, topiramate, gabapentin, levetiracetam					Neurology specialty consultation suggested before administration
Prokinetic					
Erythromycin	Erythrocin, Pediamycin, E-mycin	20 mg/kg per day PO divided qid	Motilin agonist stimulates gastric motility	Gastric cramps in larger doses	Use in small, prokinetic doses 5-20 mg/kg per day, gastroparesis
Cisapride	Propulsid	0.2-0.3 mg/kg dose PO tid or qid	$5-HT_4$ agonist with ACh release in gut	Diarrhea, abdominal pain, headache	Can cause arrhythmias with imidazole antifungals and macrolide antibiotics, gastroparesis
Birth control					
Norethindrone/ ethinyl estradiol	Loestrin 1.5/30		Attenuates estrogen drop before onset of menses	Estrogen effects	Catamenial migraines
Supplements					
l-Carnitine	Carnitor	50-100 mg/kg per day divided bid or tid	Energy metabolism	Diarrhea, fishy body odor	
Coenzyme Q10	CoQ 10	10 mg/kg per day divided bid or tid	Energy metabolism antioxidant	Dizziness, elevated transaminases	

*Anticholinergic effects include blurred vision, dry mouth, hypotension, palpitations, urinary retention.
Ach, acetylcholine; ASA, acetylsalicylic acid; CTZ, chemotrigger zone; GABA, γ-aminobutyric acid; H, histamine; 5-HT, 5-hydroxytryptamine; MAO, monamine oxidase; SST, supraventricular tachycardia.

antagonists diminished the vomiting and 5-HIAA excretion, thus implicating serotonin in the pathophysiologic cascade.[161]

The new 5-HT$_3$ antagonists are more efficacious than former regimens that included metoclopramide-dexamethasone and chlorpromazine-dexamethasone combinations.[162,163] All three 5-HT$_3$ antagonists – ondansetron 3 mg/m^2,[164] granisetron 10 μg/kg,[165,166] and tropisetron 0.2 mg/kg[167] – have similar rates (75 to 96%) of complete or major control of chemotherapy-induced vomiting.[168] Few side effects were noted except for headache (ondansetron) and constipation (tropisetron). These 5-HT$_3$ agents appear to be more effective on the early emesis (within the first 24 h) than late (1 to 2 weeks after chemotherapy).[162] These 5-HT$_3$ agents were effective on repeated cycles of chemotherapy without loss of efficacy, could be potentiated by dexamethasone,[169] and were more effective in larger than standard doses with no additional adverse effects.[170] The 5-HT$_3$ agents also appear effective in controlling radiotherapy-induced emesis.[171] Lorazepam has been suggested as an adjunctive agent for the treatment of acute chemotherapy-induced nausea and vomiting.[172] New tachykinin receptor antagonists (NK$_1$) (aprepitant) have just been approved in chemotherapy-induced emesis and may be more effective in the late phase of nausea and vomiting.

Functional Vomiting

The term *psychogenic vomiting* is now rendered obsolete, because the Rome II-III criteria for functional GI disorders have been used in the past decade to define chronic unexplained symptoms for which no organic cause can be found. In the past, both pediatricians and psychologists presumed a psychogenic origin when no organic cause and no DSM-IV psychiatric diagnosis is found to explain the vomiting. Currently, it has become evident that comorbid anxiety and depression commonly accompany functional GI disorders rather than cause them.

Currently, the classification *functional vomiting* has been defined by the Rome III criteria in adults to describe recurrent chronic vomiting of unknown cause that is not cyclical and that persists for a minimum of once weekly. Although not yet similarly defined in children, we would apply the analogous term to denote noncyclic vomiting in children and adolescents as well. One example would be a child who vomits once or twice before each soccer game or other stress events but is able to continue after the emesis. Clinicians often refer to this ill-defined entity as a "nervous stomach." Careful consideration must be given to exclude organic causes of vomiting such as peptic, allergic, and inflammatory disorders (e.g., eosinophilic esophagitis), mechanical obstruction (e.g., malrotation), and psychological disorders (e.g., bulimia, rumination, chronic cannabinoid use) before applying the label of functional vomiting.

There are limited data on the effective management of *functional vomiting*. If the vomiting results in significant medical complications such as hematemesis or weight loss, or loss of functioning at school or in activities, diagnostic testing and treatment are warranted. Although uncommon in functional vomiting, frequent vomiting can lead to dehydration, electrolyte imbalance, impaired nutrition, and dental erosions. Treatment should be directed toward restoring the adolescent to full activity despite persistence of vomiting as outlined in *chronic idiopathic nausea*. If there is significant disability, concomitant separation anxiety should be considered and, if found, treated by a medical psychologist. There may be a therapeutic role for cognitive-behavioral therapy, stress reduction techniques and hypnotherapy, and a graduated plan to return the child to school.

Although there are few studies on pharmacotherapy in this newly defined functional disorder, 5-HT$_3$ antagonists and phenothiazine antiemetics have been used but are usually ineffective. Unless the vomiting is frequent and alters the child's activities, the cost and side effects may not warrant the taking of daily medication. Anecdotal experience in children and adolescents indicates that moderate daily doses of tricyclic antidepressants, similar to their effects on functional abdominal pain, may be of benefit.

REFERENCES

53. Taché Y. Cyclic vomiting syndrome: the corticotropin-releasing-factor hypothesis. Dig Dis Sci 1999;44:79S–86S.
123. Li BUK, Lefevre F, Chelimsky GG, et al. North American Society for Pediatric Gastroenterology, Hepatology, and Nutrition Consensus Statement on the Diagnosis and Management of Cyclic Vomiting Syndrome. J Pediatr Gastroenterol Nutr 2008;47:379–393.
133. Sato T, Igarashi M, Minami S, et al. Recurrent attacks of vomiting, hypertension, and psychotic depression: a syndrome of periodic catecholamine and prostaglandin discharge. Acta Endocrinol 1988;117:189.
136. Boles RG, Powers AL, Adams K. Cyclic vomiting syndrome plus. J Child Neurol 2006;21:182–188.
172. Dupuis LL. Options for the prevention and management of acute chemotherapy-induced nausea and vomiting in children. Paediatr Drugs 2003;5:597–613.

See expertconsult.com for a complete list of references and the review questions for this chapter.

DIARRHEA

Gigi Veereman-Wauters • Jan Taminiau

Parents often consult a pediatric gastroenterologist with questions about their child's stool pattern. Personal and cultural beliefs influence their perception of what may be a problem. Precise questions about the aspect of the child's defecation pattern and the visual appreciation of a stool sample are important on the first encounter. Normal stool consistency and frequency evolve during childhood. It is commonly accepted that the evacuation of liquid or semiformed stools from 7 times a day to once every 7 days is normal in breast-fed babies. Formula-fed babies have more formed or even harder stools. Colic and cramping are eagerly attributed to difficult defecation. The latest innovations in infant formula are the addition of pre- or probiotics that are intended to favor a bifido-predominant intestinal flora and therefore softer stools.[1] Defecation frequency and stool volume decrease from birth to 3 years of age when an "adult" pattern is reached. Infants pass 5 to 10 g/kg/day and adults an average of 100 g/day.[2,3] There is an individual variation in what can be considered a normal stool pattern. Healthy toddlers may open their bowels more than three times a day,[4] and stool consistency may be loose with identifiable undigested particles.[5,6] However, in normal circumstances, intestinal nutrient and water absorption should be sufficient for homeostasis and growth of the organism. If such is not the case, fecal losses cause deficits and disease.

In this chapter we discuss the clinical approach to pediatric patients with diarrhea and the differential diagnosis for different age groups. Specific etiologic conditions are discussed in other chapters.

PHYSIOLOGY OF INTESTINAL CONTENT HANDLING

In adults, 8 to 10 L of fluid containing 800 mmol sodium, 700 mmol chloride, and 100 mmol potassium enters the proximal small intestine daily.[7] Two liters comes from the daily diet, and the remainder from secretions of the salivary glands, stomach, biliary and pancreatic ducts, and proximal small intestine. The small intestine absorbs all but 1.5 L of this amount of fluid containing 200 mmol sodium/L; the colon absorbs all but 100 mL containing approximately 3 mmol sodium of the remaining fluid. Regardless whether a subject ingests a hypotonic meal, such as a steak with an osmolality of 230 mOsm/kg water, or a hypertonic meal, such as milk with a doughnut with an osmolality of 630 mOsm/kg water, the very permeable proximal small intestine allows movement of water and electrolytes into the lumen, rendering the meal isotonic with plasma as it reaches the proximal jejunum. The aforementioned secretions augment the volume of the 300-mL milk-doughnut meal to 1200 mL and the steak-meal from 600 to 2000 mL in the duodenum, and further increases the volume of the milk-doughnut meal to 2000 mL when starches and lactose are digested. In the jejunum, fluids and electrolytes are in equilibrium with plasma, allowing optimal absorption.[8,9]

Water absorption is only possible together with solutes. In the absence of food, all water is absorbed through the neutral NaCl carrier, located mainly in the ileum. This is the so-called sodium-hydrogen exchanger, as the negatively charged anions chloride and bicarbonate are exchanged. With the NaCl carrier a single molecule of sodium co-transports 50 molecules of water. After a meal, the glucose-galactose-sodium carrier (SGLT1), located mainly in the jejunum, transports most sodium and water. One molecule of sodium then co-transports 250 molecules of water.[10] All macronutrient transport through the small intestinal epithelium is driven by Na^+ transport: amino acids, dipeptides, and fatty acids. The maximal absorption for both the NaCl carrier and the SGLT1 is estimated at 5 to 7 L. After 2 m of small intestinal absorption by the nutrient sodium carriers, the chloride content diminishes, probably suggesting substantial postprandial use of the NaCl carrier.[11]

In the human colon water absorption is again dependent on Na^+ absorption. Na^+ is absorbed through an electrogenic process at the apical membrane and maintained by the basolateral Na,K-ATPase, which in each cycle extrudes three Na^+ ions for two K^+ ions. Another proportionally larger Na^+ absorptive mechanism is the electrical neutral Na-Cl absorption in which Na^+ is exchanged for H^+ and Cl^- for bicarbonate. This Na^+ absorption is coupled with short-chain fatty acids (SCFAs). The proximal colon contains high luminal concentrations of organic nutrients (nonstarch polysaccharides from plant walls and proteins not absorbed by the small intestine) and high bacterial growth rates parallel high fermentation rates. Of the three SCFAs (acetate, propionate, and butyrate), butyrate is the most abundant and physiologically important. Butyrate serves as a major energy source for colonocytes and plays a crucial role in their growth and differentiation. The butyrate-bicarbonate exchange is the main driving force for Na-Cl absorption, each molecule co-transporting 50 molecules of water. Maximal absorption amounts to 3 to 5 L daily.[12]

The Na^+ absorptive processes are restricted to small intestinal villous cells, whereas Cl^- secretory processes are located in the small intestinal crypts. In the colon, Na^+ absorption occurs in the crypts; consequently, additional hydraulic forces due to a small neck enlarge Na^+ and water absorption enormously.[13]

This Na^+ absorptive state is reversed to a Cl^- secretory state under the influence of cAMP or calcium secretagogues. In the small intestine Cl^- secretion induced by these secretagogues occurs mainly in the crypts.

DEFINITIONS OF DIARRHEA

Feces contain up to 75% water. A relatively small increase in water losses will cause liquid stools. In infants, stool volume in excess of 10 g/kg/day is considered abnormal.[3] Diarrhea is the frequent (more than three times a day) evacuation of liquid feces. Fecal composition is abnormal and will often be malodorous and acid due to colonic fermentation and putrefaction of nutrients. Stools may contain blood, mucus, fat, or undigested food particles. The urge to evacuate stools may cause incontinence and nocturnal defecation in toilet-trained children.

Acute diarrhea is often self-limiting and lasts for a few days. When persisting for over 3 weeks, this condition is considered chronic.

CLINICAL OBSERVATIONS OF TYPES OF DIARRHEA

Diarrheal stools may be watery, acid, or greasy and may contain blood, mucus, or undigested food particles. Parents often worry about the color of their child's feces. Red (blood) and white (cholestasis) are alarming, but all shades of yellow, brown, and green should be tolerated.

Various pathophysiological mechanisms causing diarrhea have been clarified. Often several mechanisms act simultaneously.

Watery Diarrhea

Mechanisms of intestinal fluid and electrolytes absorption and secretion have been studied extensively. Oral intake and intestinal secretions account for about 9 L of fluid per day at the level of the Treitz ligament in older children and adults.[9] Fluid reabsorption in the small intestine is determined by osmotic gradients. Sodium, potassium, chloride, bicarbonate, and glucose play key roles. Primarily sodium creates an osmotic gradient allowing passive water diffusion. The sodium pump, sodium potassium adenosinetriphosphatase (ATPase), located in the basolateral enterocyte membrane, maintains a low intracellular sodium concentration.[14] In adults, the fluid content at the level of the ileocecal valve has decreased to 1 L.[15] Colonic water reabsorption will determine the water content of the stools.

In the case of *osmotic diarrhea*, undigested nutrients (e.g., mono- or disaccharides) increase the osmotic load in the distal small intestine and colon, leading to decreased water reabsorption.[16,17] The intestinal electrolyte content becomes lower than the serum content. Therefore an "osmotic gap" can be calculated. The fecal osmotic gap is (290 − 2 × (sodium + potassium concentration). In the presence of osmotic molecules, the osmotic gap will be at least 50 units. In *osmotic diarrhea* associated with carbohydrate malabsorption, stools are acid with pH under 5, and fasting will improve the symptoms. Milk of magnesia, used as a laxative, causes osmotic diarrhea without pH drop.

In the case of *secretory diarrhea*, a noxious agent causes the intestinal epithelium to secrete excessive water and electrolytes into the lumen.[17-19] There is no osmotic gap (less than 50) and food intake does not affect symptoms. Examples are bacterial toxins that turn on adenylate cyclase activity, as well as certain gastrointestinal peptides, bile acids, fatty acids, and laxatives.

Steatorrhea

In the case of fat malabsorption, stools may be greasy and stain the toilet bowl. Steatorrhea occurs when fecal fat in a 72-h stool collection exceeds 7% of oral fat intake over 24 h. Isolated fat malabsorption strongly suggests exocrine pancreatic insufficiency due to absence of lipase or colipase.[20] More generalized exocrine pancreatic insufficiencies such as cystic fibrosis and Shwachman's syndrome cause multiple nutrient malabsorption. Small intestinal damage and villous atrophy lead to malabsorption of all nutrients including fat.

Creatorrhea/Azotorrhea

Creatorrhea (azotorrhea) or the excretion of proteins also occurs in pancreatic insufficiency and in protein-losing enteropathy.[21] Fecal albumin losses can be demonstrated using intravenously injected ^{51}Cr-labeled albumin[22] or indirectly by the amount of fecal α1-antitrypsin.[23] In pancreatic insufficiency or subtotal villous atrophy, creatorrhea or azotorrhea is always accompanied by other obvious clinical signs caused by generalized malabsorption.

Mucus and Blood

Intestinal inflammation is an important cause of diarrhea. The mucosa is invaded and destroyed by a cellular inflammatory infiltrate secreting numerous cytokines. Normal absorptive processes are impaired, exudative materials (mucus, blood) are excreted, and intestinal motility is altered. Intestinal inflammation may be caused by allergic reactions, by infections, or by idiopathic autoimmune-type reactions as seen in inflammatory bowel disease (IBD).

Undigested Food Particles

In toddlers, undigested food particles are often visible in looser stools. Usually the child thrives and is otherwise free of symptoms. This condition is called chronic nonspecific diarrhea of childhood (CNSD) and is considered a functional problem.[24] An accelerated intestinal transit in this age group may be caused by the failure of nutrients to interrupt the migrating motor complexes and to induce a fed pattern.[25]

Overflow Incontinence (Paradoxical Diarrhea)

Some children present with foul-smelling diarrhea but a careful physical evaluation, including a digital rectal examination, will reveal constipation and rectal impaction. Patients with fecal overflow and often incontinence or encopresis need treatment for chronic constipation. It is important to explain the pathophysiology of the situation to the family. Treatment starts with disimpaction, preferably without rectal treatments. Thereafter more frequent defecation is promoted and the child's behavior is modified by a training program.

PATHOPHYSIOLOGY OF SECRETORY DIARRHEA

Diarrhea is mainly caused by abnormal fluid and electrolyte transport by decreased absorption or increased secretion. The human colon is capable of absorbing 3 to 5 L per 24 h, but decreased small intestinal absorption of 8 to 10 L of daily fluid can exceed this colonic capacity. Decrease of small intestinal absorption by more than 50% will lead to diarrhea in this setting. If colonic absorption is diminished as a result of colonic disease, the normal amount of 1.5 L arriving in the cecum might not be absorbed and then also lead to diarrhea. After the initial discovery that bacterial enterotoxins stimulate chloride and water secretion, it was later found that more than 50% of intestinal secretion is controlled by enterochromaffin cells releasing 5-hydroxytryptamine that activates the enteric nervous system, secondarily enhancing enterocyte chloride secretion also by signal transport to distant areas of the nervous system. Also, inflammatory mediators (histamine, serotonin, prostaglandins) produced by immune cells, intestinal mast cells, eosinophils, macrophages, neutrophils, and mesenchymal cells in the lamina propria and submucosa are capable of initiating and enhancing intestinal secretion. These mediators may stimulate enterocytes directly and also activate the enteric nervous system. Moreover, this process of electrogenic chloride and bicarbonate secretion inhibits electrically neutral sodium chloride absorption in the small intestine and the colon through intercellular messengers. Because of the net fluid movement into the lumen, this is a combined cause of malabsorption of water and electrolytes and enhanced secretion, seen as diarrhea. From a pathophysiological perspective, solitary secretion is rare.

PATHOPHYSIOLOGY OF OSMOTIC DIARRHEA

In osmotic diarrhea a meal has the same, normal dilution in the duodenum, but thereafter water content of the intestinal lumen will increase. For instance, lactase-deficient subjects are unable to reabsorb adequate fluid because lactose is not metabolized to galactose and glucose, which act to help transport water and electrolytes.

Osmotic diarrhea can be induced to alleviate constipation. Healthy normal adults receiving increasing doses of polyethylene glycol 3350 (PEG) or lactulose have been studied. PEG 3350 (lower molecular weights do not bind water as well) is poorly absorbed, not digested by human or bacterial enzymes, carries no electrical charge, and causes pure osmotic diarrhea. With daily doses of 50 to 250 g/day, stool weight increases gradually from 364 to 1539 g/day. Stool water content does not rise above 80% because of high fecal concentration of PEG. PEG attracts water: stool weight, water output, and fecal PEG output correlate in a linear fashion.

With lactulose doses increasing from 45 to 125 g/day, stool weight increases from 254 to 1307 g/day. Water content percentage increases from 79% to 90%. With increasing lactulose doses, fecal organic acid content decrease while carbohydrate content increases. This means that with lower dosages up to 95 g/day, organic acids are absorbed and water absorption is co-transported. Only in higher dosages is lactulose no longer fermented so that it contributes directly to diarrhea. Interestingly, electrolyte concentrations in diarrheal stools are higher with lactulose than PEG, and a linear correlation between organic acid output and electrolyte output is obvious. However, conservation of electrolytes is excellent even with water output over 1200 g/day. Diarrhea in lower dosages is mainly caused by unabsorbed organic acids and with higher dosages by a combination of organic acids and undigested carbohydrate. Because there is no correlation between organic acid concentration and rate of individual bowel movements, the argument of rapid colonic emptying or effects on colonic motility is probably not justified.[26]

In lactose-intolerant patients with diarrhea, the introduction of 50 g lactose for 14 days was compared with the same amount of sucrose. Interestingly, the fecal weight in both groups did not change and was around 350 g per 24 h. On the other hand, the number of stools decreased in both groups, as did symptom score; there was less pain, less flatulence, less bloating, and fewer borborygmi. Only in the lactose groups did pH and breath hydrogen excretion drop. This suggests that clinical symptoms in lactose intolerance can be subject to psychogenic factors.[27]

In the short bowel syndrome, lactulose feeding of 60 g/daily showed lower carbohydrate and organic acid excretion in the stools, carried out in comparison with volunteers fed lactulose for 2 weeks. This experiment demonstrates a spontaneous adaptation of the gut flora in short bowel syndrome patients with intact colon.[28]

The contribution of fat to osmotic diarrhea is still under debate. Triglycerides do not directly contribute to diarrhea, but their fatty acids might. Medium-chain fatty acids are absorbed in the colon like short-chain fatty acids, or are lost in the feces like long-chain fatty acids. In carbohydrate malabsorption, sodium and water remain in the lumen until the colon is reached, where up to 90 g sugars can be metabolized daily by intestinal microbiota. A considerable amount of short-chain fatty acids contribute substantially to energy absorption as well as co-absorption of sodium and water.[29]

PATHOPHYSIOLOGY OF INFLAMMATORY DIARRHEA

Inflammatory diarrhea can be caused by infection, allergy, Crohn's disease or ulcerative colitis (IBD), or other causes. Multiple pathways may be involved in producing diarrhea. After the initial adherence or invasion of infectious agents, various immune cells release inflammatory mediators. Cytokines (such as IL-1, TNF-α), chemokines (such as IL-8, which attracts eosinophils), and prostaglandins induce intestinal secretion by enterocytes and activate enteric nerves. Secondly, subepithelial myofibroblasts destroy the basement membrane by metalloproteinases, damaged enterocytes are extruded, and villous atrophy develops followed by regenerative crypt hyperplasia in the small intestine and colon. These surfaces are covered with immature enterocytes, with insufficient disaccharidase and peptide hydrolase activity. Na$^+$ coupled glucose, NaCl, and amino acid transporters are reduced, but these crypt cells maintain their Cl$^-$ secretory abilities.

In this damage and repair phase, capillaries may leak substantial amounts of protein and calcium, magnesium, and phosphate. For instance, in inflammatory bowel disease, malabsorption only occurs after extended resections, but these protein and mineral losses are frequently encountered and contribute to bone demineralization.[30]

In IBD with colitis, the main electrolyte transport abnormalities are decreased Na$^+$ and Cl$^-$ absorption leading to impaired water absorption and secretion. The inflamed colonic mucosa loses its transepithelial resistance with subsequent increased electrical conductance and enhanced permeability. The transmucosal potential difference is decreased or lost, and electrogenic Na$^+$ transport is impossible. Also Na,K-ATPase activity is decreased and passive Cl$^-$ absorption and electroneutral Na$^+$ and Cl$^-$ absorption are decreased. Thus, the major pathogenic factor in the diarrhea of colitis is this impaired NaCl and water absorption instead of increased Cl$^-$ secretion.

In microscopic colitis with minimal inflammation, electroneutral NaCl absorption is decreased while a normal potential difference is maintained, as is electrogenic Na$^+$ absorption.

Corticosteroids stimulate the transmucosal potential difference and stimulate electrogenic Na$^+$ absorption and hence Cl$^-$ and water absorption in addition to a general anti-inflammatory effect. This explains the immediate beneficial effects of corticosteroids in IBD prior to mucosal healing.

Minor intestinal damage is caused by enterotoxin producing–bacteria such as *Vibrio cholerae*, enterotoxigenic *Escherichia coli*, *Campylobacter*, *Yersinia*, *Salmonella*, and *Shigella*. Small bowel morphology remains unaltered in many bacterial diarrhea. Diarrhea is caused by two mechanisms: enterotoxins and a rise in c-AMP in villus and crypt cells. c-AMP blocks NaCl uptake in villus cells, causing NaCl malabsorption and diarrhea. Heat-stable toxin has similar effects by raising c-GMP in villus cells. Bacterial toxins induce 5-hydroxytryptamine release by enterochromaffin cells and stimulate the enteric nervous system both locally and distally. An increased calcium concentration in the crypt cells enhances Cl secretion to a variable degree. The wide range of water excretion in cholera, between 1 and 10 L diarrhea per day, is thought to be related to this nervous stimulatory effect. The secretory effect on c-AMP is less pronounced. This mineral malabsorptive secretory diarrhea is related to risks of dehydration. As the bacteria arrive at the distal ileum and colon, they penetrate the mucosa and cause inflammation. This produces bloody diarrhea with tenesmus. The secretory phase has then diminished.

Minor inflammation is noticed with parasites (*Giardia*, cryptosporidiosis), bacteria (enteroadherent or enteropathogenic *E. coli*), viruses (rotavirus, astrovirus, and Norwalk agent) and idiopathic lymphocytic colitis. The pathogenesis of rotavirus diarrhea is complex. The small bowel distal to the duodenum is affected over a variable length. Mature villous enterocytes are infected, and the virus replicates, shuts down cell function (production of disaccharidases), and induces cell lysis and villous atrophy after 2 to 3 days. Rotavirus causes short-term malabsorption with steatorrhea. The increased mitotic index and migration of crypt enterocytes generate immature cells with limited glucose-Na transport, neutral NaCl transport, low disaccharidase activity, and increased Cl secretion, but the life-threatening dehydrating diarrhea is not easily explained by this mechanism, also because of its patchy distribution. These pathophysiologic changes are identical in other villus atrophies such as celiac disease. An explanation may be the substantial production of nonstructural protein 4 (NSP4) by rotavirus. It is secreted into the intestine and reabsorbed by other enterocytes carrying specific surface receptors. NSP4 has been shown to be an enterotoxin, which enhances Cl secretion through raised intracellular calcium. This mechanism is capable of augmenting secretion by the enteric nervous system locally and more distally.[31]

In the proximal small intestine, *Salmonella*, *Shigella*, *Campylobacter jejuni*, *Yersinia enterocolitica*, and enteroinvasive *E. coli* do not damage enterocytes, but cause diarrhea through enterotoxins. In the terminal ileum and the large intestine, enterocytes are destroyed and the submucosa invaded, causing inflammation. In ulcerative colitis and Crohn's disease, the inflammation is moderate to severe. In celiac disease, the degree of inflammation is usually severe. In food allergy, the inflammation might be minor in the small intestine to severe in the large bowel in infants with cow's milk, soy, or chicken hypersensitivity. The severity of diarrhea is not directly related to the severity of intestinal inflammation because the effect by the immune system and secretion-inducing mediators is variable.

CLINICAL RELEVANCE OF ACUTE INFECTIOUS DIARRHEA

In children, acute diarrhea is almost entirely caused by infectious agents and lasts 5 to 10 days. Bacterial diarrhea tends to decline from the start because toxins are irreversibly attached to enterocytes and disappear with movement of new enterocytes from crypt to villus tip, whereas viral diarrheas augment during a few days because of the development of villous atrophy and last longer until its recovery. The only important issue is the assessment of dehydration as a life-threatening risk factor. The other rare risk is septicemia, which if suspected should be treated presumptively with antibiotics. Pseudomembranous enterocolitis (caused by *Clostridium difficile*) is suspected when bloody diarrhea occurs after antibiotic use. Diarrheal fluid has a lower sodium content than plasma, cholera (90 mmol/L), bacteria, and viruses (40 to 60 mmol/L) and is always hypotonic compared to plasma. Thus the extracellular space becomes hypertonic, and more water is lost than sodium. Depending on the volume of diarrhea, rapidity of onset, and duration, the resulting dehydration is generally normotonic, sometimes hypertonic or hypotonic in plasma sodium concentration. Even in hypertonic dehydration, substantial amounts of sodium have been lost and need to be replaced.[32]

Assessment of Dehydration

In children some symptoms are more prominent, correctly observed by junior and senior physicians, whereas others are missed or overdiagnosed.

Signs of dehydration are thirst, decreased skin turgor, acidotic breathing, delayed capillary refill, sunken fontanelle, deep sunken eyes, dry mucosal membranes, lack of tears, and oliguria.[33] At 2% dehydration, with already raised plasma aldosterone, antidiuretic hormone, and renin, thirst is the only symptom; at 4% dehydration, all of the foregoing are present. At 5% dehydration, the pulse rate increases, and at 10%, shock occurs.[32]

DIFFERENTIAL DIAGNOSIS

In this section the differential diagnostic categories of acute and chronic diarrhea in children are listed (Tables 10-1 and 10-2); the approach to a clinical problem is discussed in the next section. Although exhaustive, tables are never final, as new entities will be recognized. Specific gastrointestinal conditions are discussed in other chapters. The clinician should document the problem and actually see fecal samples. Important determinants are whether the problem is acute or chronic, whether the diarrhea has been present since birth, whether the child is healthy and thriving, and what the findings are on history and clinical examination. Nongastrointestinal problems may cause diarrhea in infants and young children (otitis media, urinary tract infection). Acute diarrhea is usually caused by infectious gastroenteritis. Most conditions are self-limiting. The *E. coli* count four types of pathogens: enterotoxigenic, enteroinvasive, enteropathogenic, and enterohemorrhagic *E. coli*.[34]

Some bacterial infections demand antibiotic treatment: *Shigella*, *Yersinia*, *Campylobacter*, and *Clostridium*. Probiotics are promising agents for restoring the intestinal flora and prevention as well as treatment of enteric infections.[35]

TABLE 10-1. Acute Diarrhea (< 3 weeks)

Infectious
Viral
  Rotavirus
  Norwalk Agent
  Enterovirus
  Calicivirus
Bacterial
  Enteroinvasive *E. coli*
  Enterohemorrhagic *E. coli*
  Enterotoxigenic *E. coli*
  Enteropathogenic *E. coli*
  Shigella
  Salmonella
  Yersinia
  Campylobacter
  Clostridium difficile
  Vibrio cholerae
  Aeromonas
Protozoa
  Giardia
  Cryptosporidium
  Entamoeba histolytica

Allergy
Short exposure to allergen
Challenge to known allergen

Toxic
Drug side effects
Acute abdomen with diarrhea as presenting symptom
Intussusception

Extraintestinal Infections
Respiratory
Urinary
Sepsis

All disease entities that commence abruptly but last more than 3 weeks if untreated are listed under chronic conditions (see Table 10-2[17]). The most frequent cause of protracted diarrhea of infancy is *villous atrophy secondary to mucosal injury* by an infectious agent[36] or an allergen.[37] These conditions cause watery diarrhea due to electrolyte and nutrient (carbohydrate and fat) malabsorption as well as enhanced secretion in some. Intolerance to cow's milk, soy protein, or another protein causes allergic enterocolitis in infants. Vomiting and diarrhea, usually with bloody stools, is immediate or within weeks of exposure to the allergen.[38]

It is well recognized that enteral nutrition is essential for mucosal healing and that prolonged exclusive intravenous support leads into a vicious cycle. Hydrolyzed and elemental formulas allow early refeeding of the damaged intestine. The most severe forms of protracted diarrhea necessitate long-term parenteral nutrition or intestinal transplantation. A clinicopathologic analysis of a group of these truly intractable forms of infantile diarrhea reveals underlying autoimmune and histological abnormalities such as tufting enteropathy or congenital microvillous inclusion disease. This latter condition is often fatal (45%).[39,40] Infants with microvillus inclusion disease develop severe watery diarrhea soon after birth (250 to 300 mL/kg) due to a variable degree of villus atrophy and severe brush border abnormalities, without an inflammatory infiltrate. The glucose-Na carrier has a function up to 30% of controls, basal NaCl uptake is 20% of normal controls, and NaCl secretion is slightly enlarged. Stools contain small intestinal concentrations of electrolytes. Oral rehydration solution (ORS) in a dose of 40 mL/kg is absorbed well without enhancing diarrhea, but most infants dehydrate and need intravenous rehydration.[41] Some infants have a delayed onset until the second or third month of life and go unnoticed with some failure to thrive. They have loose stools and metabolic acidosis due to fecal bicarbonate losses. In mild forms, hydrolysates are tolerated, but most infants are dependent on parenteral nutrition.[42]

Tufting enteropathy or intestinal epithelial dysplasia has a less severe but identical presentation with some tolerance to hydrolysates. Diarrhea usually starts in the early infant period but may be delayed, villus atrophy is variable, and the histological diagnosis is difficult because of the lack of specific markers.[43]

Syndromatic diarrhea consists of a combination of congenital diarrhea with variable villus atrophy and facial and hair dysmorphism. Depending on the degree of villus atrophy, diarrhea is severe with substantial losses of sodium and a limited life span to mild forms with normal villi and sodium diarrhea with acceptable growth and body weight.[44]

Furthermore, *infectious* diarrhea can be long-lasting in the case of some bacteria (*Salmonella, Clostridium*) or parasites (*Giardia, Cryptosporidium*). *Giardia* and *Cryptosporidium* can cause malabsorption through damage of the brush border. Steatorrhea in giardiasis is also caused by parasitic consumption of bile salts. *Giardia lamblia* infection causes epithelial barrier dysfunction owing to down-regulation of the tight junction protein claudin 1 and increased epithelial apoptosis. Na+-dependent D-glucose absorption is impaired, and active electrogenic anion secretion is activated. The mechanisms of diarrhea in human giardiasis comprise leak flux, malabsorptive, and secretory components.[45]

Inborn errors of metabolism can present with early persisting diarrhea as one of the presenting symptoms: e.g., galactosemia, tyrosinemia, and familial chloride diarrhea. Congenital chloride diarrhea is a defect in the small intestinal Cl/HCO$_3$ exchanger leading to malabsorption of chloride. In the proximal small intestine, its function is to secrete bicarbonate in exchange for absorption of chloride to neutralize gastric acid and more distally to reabsorb the secreted chloride by the Cl/HCO$_3$ exchanger. Infants present with severe watery diarrhea in the first week of life; serum electrolytes are unique in showing metabolic acidosis, hypochloremia, hypokalemia, and hyponatremia. Fecal chloride concentration exceeds the concentration of cations (sodium and potassium). Delivery of chloride to the duodenum can be achieved with proton pump inhibitors. Recently oral butyrate therapy was used in doses of 50 to 100 mg/kg/day to stimulate the SCFA sodium pump in the colon and drive sodium and chloride over the mucosal membrane, normalizing serum electrolyte concentrations and fecal excretion.[46,47]

Congenital sodium diarrhea is a disorder of impaired Na-H exchanger function. All genes of these exchangers are mapped, but no abnormality could be detected in any of them. Children have watery diarrhea with high sodium concentrations; stools are alkaline because of the lack of hydrogen exchange for sodium, whereas in all other congenital diarrheas stools are acidic.[48]

Abetalipoproteinemia and hypobetalipoproteinemia are rare defects in postmucosal transport of fat. In the enterocyte, chylomicron formation and attachment of the microsomal triglyceride transfer proteins to fatty acids defaults its assembly, causing fat congestion in the enterocyte with subsequent steatorrhea. In frozen biopsies, fat accumulation is seen with Sudan fat staining; in a blood smear, acanthocytes are distinguished because

TABLE 10-2. **Differential Diagnosis of Chronic Diarrhea (> 3 weeks)**

Infantile Protracted Diarrhea With Villous Atrophy
  Postinfectious
  Food allergy
  Malnutrition
  Congenital histological dysmorphism
    Microvillus inclusion disease
    Tufting enteropathy
  Syndromatic diarrhea
 	
Infectious
  Bacterial
  Parasitic
 	
Inborn Errors of Metabolism
  Familial chloride diarrhea
  Sodium-hydrogen exchange defect
  Abetalipoproteinemia and hypobetalipoproteinemia
  Folic acid malabsorption
  Selective vitamin B_{12} malabsorption
  Galactosemia
  Tyrosinemia
  Wolman's disease
  Acrodermatitis enteropathica
 	
Carbohydrate Malabsorption
  Congenital
    Lactase deficiency
    Glucose-galactose malabsorption
    Sucrase-isomaltase deficiency
    Glucoamylase deficiency
    Fructose malabsorption
  Secondary
    Lactase deficiency
    Secondary disaccharidase deficiencies
    Acquired monosaccharide malabsorption
 	
GI Organ Pathology
  Small intestine
    Celiac disease
    Tropical sprue
    Whipple's disease
    Intestinal lymphangiectasia
    Eosinophilic gastroenteropathy
    Enterokinase deficiency
	Short bowel syndrome
	  Ischemia
	  Lymphoma
	  Motility disorders
	    Small bowel overgrowth
	    Intestinal pseudoobstruction
	    Congenital absence of ileal bile receptor
	Pancreas
	    Cystic fibrosis
	    All conditions leading to exocrine insufficiency, e.g., Shwachman's
	Liver
	    All conditions leading to cholestasis, bile salt deficiency
	
	Immune Defects
	  $\alpha\gamma$-Globulinemia
	  Isolated IgA deficiency
	  Defective cellular immunity
	  SCIDS
	  AIDS
	  Autoimmune enteropathy
	
	IBD
	  Crohn's disease
	  Ulcerative colitis
	
	Fecal Impaction With Overflow Incontinence
	  Hirschsprung's disease
	  Anorectal malfunction
	  Functional constipation
	
	Dietary
	  Overfeeding
	  Nondigestible carbohydrates
	
	Toxic Diarrhea
	
	Toddler's Diarrhea
	
	Polle Syndrome or Munchhausen by Proxy
	
	Factitious Diarrhea
	
	Nongastrointestinal
	  Hyperthyroidism
	  Tumors
	    APUDoma
	    Ganglioneuroma
	    Neuroblastoma

AIDS, acquired immunodeficiency syndrome; SCIDs, severe combined immunodeficiency syndrome.

the cytoskeleton of erythrocytes needs betalipoproteins for its structure.

Carbohydrate malabsorption leads to colonic fermentation and diarrhea. Severe congenital forms such as glucose-galactose malabsorption or sucrose-isomaltase deficiency are rare but necessitate a prompt diagnosis and adequate dietary treatment. Glucose galactose malabsorption manifests itself the first days of life. Lactose is hydrolyzed to glucose and galactose. The glucose-galactose sodium carrier dysfunctions at a level of 30% of normal capacity, trapping water and electrolytes in the intestinal lumen at isotonic concentrations. In the ileum, the NaCl carrier salvages some electrolytes and water and in the colon and bacterial degradation product SCFAs stimulate sodium absorption, but this remains insufficient to prevent severe dehydrating diarrhea. A diet without lactose, sugar, and glucose polymers, but with protein and fructose is well tolerated since amino acid-sodium carriers are unaffected and fructose, is absorbed passively. Within years some adaptation of glucose transport allows addition of sugar to the diet. The diagnosis is based on a positive glucose hydrogen breath test, positive urinary glucose, and positive Clinitest on stools while on a carbohydrate diet or

glucose uptake testing on small intestinal biopsies. The genetic defect can be identified in a few centers.[49]

Fructose malabsorption has been implicated in toddler diarrhea and in isolated fructose malabsorption, a rare autosomal recessive disorder. Fructose absorption occurs probably in the small intestine via facilitated transport through the carrier GLUT5. A defect has not been established, and inadequate expression in toddler diarrhea has not been shown. The fructose hydrogen breath test is positive in all hydrogen producers, and malabsorption can only be tested clinically with fructose challenge. Fructose is present in fruits and fruit juices, which also contain high amounts of the nonabsorbable carbohydrate sorbitol. Malabsorption is dose dependent, with diarrhea developing if the daily dose exceeds 15 mL/kg body weight, although this has still to be proven.[50]

Disaccharidase deficiencies cause persistence of the undigested carbohydrate along with an isotonic luminal content into the colon, where bacteria ferment up to 90 g of undigested sugar into SCFAs, stimulating sodium and water absorption. This results in small-volume diarrhea with low quantities of fecal electrolytes. Complaints of borborygmi, abdominal cramps, bloating, and flatulence suggest disaccharide intolerance. Clinically, lactase deficiency occurs after small bowel injury, such as viral and parasitic infections. Constitutional lactase deficiency manifests itself after the age of 5 to 6 years in white populations and somewhat earlier in nonwhites. Congenital lactase deficiency has been described but is rare,[51] and a locus (2q21) has been identified.[52] Sucrase-isomaltase deficiency shows after the first fruit or vegetable feeding to an infant. Maltase-glucoamylase deficiency presents with diarrhea after starch ingestion. The diagnosis can be made using the appropriate carbohydrate breath hydrogen test or Clinitest estimation of reducing sugars in the liquid stools (sucrose has to be hydrolyzed before testing with boiling).[53]

Secondary carbohydrate malabsorption is common post enteritis and needs temporary treatment. Lactase is the most commonly affected disaccharidase.

Specific *organ pathology* of the small intestine, the liver, and the pancreas affects stool consistency. In the case of the *small intestine*, mucosal damage due to various offenders results in diarrhea and malabsorption, e.g., celiac disease, eosinophilic gastroenteritis, and short bowel syndrome.

Celiac disease, gluten-sensitive enteropathy, presents with diarrhea, anorexia, weight loss, failure to thrive, or abdominal distention. Overt malnutrition is now less commonly encountered because diagnosis is often facilitated by anti-transglutaminase antibody screening. Patients are often detected in the phase with milder symptoms. Villus atrophy leads to malabsorption of fat, carbohydrates, and proteins. Steatorrhea is present in 70% of children. The absence of steatorrhea in the remainder is unexplained but not simply due to anorexia with insufficient fat intake. When in the past the diagnosis was made through laparotomy and surgical biopsies were obtained at several small-intestinal levels, villus atrophy could be present through the whole small intestine without causing steatorrhea. This experience challenged the assumption of a gluten dosage-related extent of villus atrophy over a variable length distal to the duodenum. Still, the usual presentation of diarrhea is fatty stools with an egg odor. Depending on the severity of the inflammatory infiltrate, chloride secretion might be enhanced, and diarrhea presents with a more watery aspect. In rare cases secretion is abundant, leading to dehydration at presentation: the so-called celiac crisis.

Eosinophilic gastroenteritis occurs in children; complaints are in keeping with mild and severe forms of inflammatory bowel disease within 75% peripheral eosinophilia. Symptoms are abdominal pain, nausea, vomiting, and weight loss with diarrhea. An eosinophilic infiltrate is present in the mucosa, sometimes extending to muscle layer and serosa of the gut. Depending on the degree of mucosal inflammation, protein-losing enteropathy ensues, and depending on the degree of villus atrophy, steatorrhea occurs. The treatment is comparable with inflammatory bowel disease.[54]

In short bowel syndrome, the intestinal absorptive capacity is insufficient for growth as a consequence of congenital short length of the intestine, surgical resection, or dysfunction. Intermittent and more generalized intestinal motility disorders called intestinal pseudoobstruction lead to small bowel overgrowth and maldigestion. Bacterial overgrowth in the small intestine occurs due to regurgitation of bacteria from the colon or stasis. Bile salts are precipitated or deconjugated and hydroxylated, become less amphiphilic, and no longer participate in micelle formation. In pseudoobstruction syndromes, bacterial overgrowth frequently occurs and children benefit from antibiotics.

In short bowel syndrome, steatorrhea is caused by a diminished absorptive surface area, decreased transit time, and diminished bile salt pool due to fecal losses. Steatorrhea is aggravated by bacterial overgrowth, as mentioned, and postoperative temporary gastric hypersecretion. Most children have sufficient small bowel adaptation in a few years to sustain normal growth and development despite persistent diarrhea and steatorrhea.

All conditions causing *exocrine pancreatic insufficiency* cause steatorrhea. The most frequent entity is cystic fibrosis; others are Shwachman's syndrome or chronic pancreatitis. In cystic fibrosis, pancreatic insufficiency develops after more than 90% of exocrine pancreatic secretory capacity has been lost. This explains why a substantial number of infants with CF due to ongoing obstruction of pancreatic ducts become gradually pancreatic insufficient during the first year of life. The high variability of pancreatic insufficiency (10 to 80% steatorrhea) at the time of diagnosis is in keeping with this diminishing function. With pancreatic enzyme replacement therapy, steatorrhea disappears in 50% and improves in the remainder. Malabsorption of medium-chain triglycerides (MCTs) improves with pancreatic enzyme supplements.[55] Insufficient bile salt secretion contributes to steatorrhea and might explain the ongoing malabsorption in 50% of patients. Pancreatic and biliary secretions have a severely diminished bicarbonate content, leading to an acidic duodenum and proximal jejunum with less efficient enzyme release from acid-resistant coated granules and precipitation of some bile salts, also contributing to steatorrhea. Despite normalization of steatorrhea with optimal enzyme replacement lean body-mass development lags behind because of chronic anorexia in permanent chronic lung infection and inflammation. Up to the age of 8 years, body weight improves with pancreatic enzyme replacement therapy. Afterwards it declines; in all cystic fibrosis patients, growth is stunted, suggesting insufficient intake. Nutritional support, including additional tube feeding, improves body weight.

Shwachman's syndrome is another cause of exocrine pancreatic insufficiency in childhood. In this condition, bile salt and bicarbonate secretion are normal, whereas pancreatic enzyme output is low. Steatorrhea normalizes in many patients after the age of 5 years.[56] Isolated lipase and colipase deficiency has been reported.[57,58] Enterokinase deficiency causes lack of activation of pancreatic proenzymes, leading to steatorrhea and creatorrhea. Besides malnutrition, these infants have edema due to low serum proteins. Recently, mutations in the proenteropeptidase gene have been identified as the cause of congenital enterokinase (or enteropeptidase) deficiency.[59]

All *cholestatic hepatic* conditions cause deficient intestinal fat absorption because of bile salt deficiency. In biliary atresia, congenital biliary stenosis, choledochal cyst, and cystic fibrosis, bile salt secretion becomes insufficient to reach the critical micellar concentration in the duodenal lumen (3 mmol/L).[60] Below this concentration, micelles cannot be formed to trap fatty acids and fat-soluble vitamins.[61] Within micelles, penetration of the unstirred layer of the mucosa is facilitated and fat absorption is 120 times more efficient. MCTs are less dependent on micelles for digestion and absorption. Steatorrhea still occurs to a variable extent in operated biliary atresias. Addition of MCT to the diet as an energy source is advised, but elongation to long-chain fatty acids does not occur in the human body, because of inefficient energy wasting in this elongation process. MCT cannot therefore replace long-chain fatty acids as a fat source in the diet of infants and children with bile salt deficiency. Because long-chain fatty acid malabsorption without any bile salt secretion is about 50%, this justifies keeping long-chain fats in the children's diet.[62]

Congenital absence of the ileal receptor for bile acid uptake (the apical sodium co-dependent bile acid transporter) leads to bile acid losses with a diminished bile acid pool. Affected infants have steatorrhea, failure to thrive, and low plasma levels of low-density lipoprotein cholesterol. They lack the postprandial rise in serum bile acids; the gallbladder has not accumulated bile in the fasting periods.[63]

In Zellweger's syndrome, abnormal bile acids are not amphiphilic enough to contribute to micelle formation. The resulting steatorrhea can be somewhat improved with oral bile acid supplementation.[64]

Immune active cells are scattered in the intestinal wall. In the case of congenital *immune deficiencies*, such as severe combined immunodeficiency syndrome (SCIDS) or acquired immunodeficiency syndrome (AIDS), diarrhea is often an early warning sign. Poorly understood autoimmune derangements lead to generalized enteropathy. Autoimmune enteropathy in infants and children presents as steatorrhea to watery diarrhea with failure to thrive. Histology of the small intestine shows villus atrophy and an inflammatory infiltrate indistinguishable from celiac disease. A gluten-free diet has no effect, but in some infants a hypoallergenic formula controls symptoms. Other children require immunosuppressive therapy with mixed results. In addition to villus atrophy, these children have other autoimmune diseases such as diabetes mellitus type 1, thyroiditis, autoimmune anemia, and glomerulonephritis. The onset of diarrhea is within the first 3 months of life, the volume of diarrhea is around 125 mL/kg, and sodium content 100 mmol/L, suggesting a combination of malabsorption and inflammation-mediated increased secretion of electrolytes.[40]

Inflammatory conditions of the small intestinal or colonic wall manifest themselves by blood and mucus in loose stools. The most frequent chronic IBDs are Crohn's disease and ulcerative colitis. The incidence of Crohn's disease is rising and the age at presentation decreasing. A population study of the incidence in the UK and Ireland yielded an alarming incidence of 5.2 per 100,000 children under age 16 years per year.[65] In inflammatory bowel disease, diarrhea is caused by decreased sodium, chloride, and water absorption; the inflamed mucosa is less tight and more permeable with diminished water absorption and secretion. Diarrhea is not voluminous. Important features are protein loss and, with it, loss of calcium and magnesium. Malabsorption does not occur until more than 1 m of distal small bowel is resected; steatorrhea is an uncommon feature of inflammatory bowel disease. Inflammatory mediators may induce chloride secretion in proximal unaffected small bowel.[66] It becomes increasingly clear that IBD is caused by a multitude of single immunological defects, most strikingly detected in (young) children. In diseases with defects of innate immunity such as chronic granulomatous disease of childhood, 17% acquire IBD[67]; in glycogen storage disease type 1b it is 9%.[68] In diseases with defects of adaptive immunity such as SCIDS, IBD develops in 30%, and 28% of children with Wiskott-Aldrich syndrome acquire IBD.[69] The pathophysiology of diarrhea is not solved for all those defects, but the development of inflammation is a sufficient explanation for diarrhea. A scrutinizing approach to isolated immune defects in children with IBD will help elucidate the pathophysiology.

Overflow incontinence is often misinterpreted as diarrhea. The differential diagnosis for fecal impaction includes Hirschsprung's disease, congenital anorectal malformations, and functional constipation depending on the clinical features and the age of the child.

Dietary mistakes are a frequent cause of diarrhea is a thriving child. Overfeeding or the ingestion of large quantities of indigestible carbohydrates such as sorbitol in fruit juice can easily be corrected.

Toddler's diarrhea or chronic nonspecific diarrhea is benign condition in a thriving, healthy child. Stools are loose and reveal identifiable remains of recent food intake. Rapid intestinal transit may be the cause of this benign condition. It has been shown in small intestinal motility studies that fasting activity was normal, but postprandial motility was abnormal. The initiation of postprandial activity is accompanied by disruption of MMCs. In toddler's diarrhea, the MMCs continue and go along with increased intestinal transit.[70] Another mechanism may be the dumping of bile acids and hydroxy fatty acids into the colon, leading to cholerrheic diarrhea. This was substantiated by stool examination.[71] The precipitating event of chronic nonspecific diarrhea is often an acute episode of gastroenteritis with watery diarrhea. Study of intestinal biopsies revealed normal morphology, but increased adenyl cyclase activity and Na,K-ATPase activity, in keeping with the assumption of recovering mucosa.[72] It was also claimed that correction of a low fat intake leads to resumption of symptoms.[73] Clinically these children have a nonspecific diarrheal pattern, grow normally, and are obviously well. Some might have their symptoms reduced by diminishing their consumption of fructose, sorbitol, and other sugars dependent on facilitated mucosal transport.[24,50,74]

This might hold for an irritable bowel syndrome–like picture with predominant diarrhea and without pain in older children, but as in adults, distinct mild abnormalities or forms of diseases are found in increasing numbers, such as lactose intolerance, microscopic colitis, fructose malabsorption, food hypersensitivities, and celiac disease.

Symptoms improve with dietary modifications: increased fat and fiber intake, limited fluid intake, and avoidance of fruit juices.[75]

Irritable bowel syndrome (IBS) can be diagnosed in older children and adolescents with alternating stool patterns. By definition, organic disease is absent, but one should not feel compelled to rule out every possible organic diagnosis using invasive tests. Psychosocial stressors need to be identified and deserve attention.[76] Often IBS is preceded by an infectious episode.[77] The pathways leading to IBS and the relationship between hormonal or mucosal markers and mood remain largely unidentified. Both mucosal changes (increased enterochromaffin cells) and depression have been identified as predictors for postinfectious IBS.[78]

Medications or toxic substances may cause diarrhea as a primary or as a side effect. Some are taken by prescription, some accidentally, some intentionally. Melanosis coli, or the presence of pigmented colonocytes on sigmoid biopsy, strongly suggests laxative abuse.[79]

In the case of contradictory findings and severe persistent diarrhea of unclear etiology, suspicion of *Polle syndrome* or *Munchausen by proxy* may arise. Observation of the child in isolation is useful in such cases.[80]

Finally, a number of nongastrointestinal conditions cause diarrhea by hormonal or neurosecretory pathways (e.g., hyperthyroidism). Rare *tumors* cause true secretory diarrheas. The gastrinoma syndrome has been reported from the age of 7 years. In children the presentation is with abdominal pain, rarely with typical ulcer pain, hematemesis, vomiting, and melena. A small intestinal biopsy showing goblet cell transformation in a patient with persistent diarrhea and unexplained steatorrhea should lead to investigation of gastrinoma. High acid output into the proximal small bowel leads to precipitation of bile salts with a diminished critical micellar concentration, causing steatorrhea. Calcium binding to malabsorbed fatty acids leads to free oxalate absorption and kidney stone formation. Vipoma syndrome presents at all ages as profuse watery diarrhea with fecal losses between 20 and 50 mL/kg/day. The culprit usually is a ganglioneuroblastoma-producing vasoactive intestinal peptide (VIP), although the exact mechanism causing diarrhea is unknown.[81] Hypokalemia is often present and may be a clue to the presence of a tumor-based diarrhea.

APPROACH TO THE CHILD WITH DIARRHEA

The approach to a child presenting with diarrhea will first consist of a careful history and physical examination (Table 10-3). Diagnostic work-up will be performed depending on this first evaluation, on the age of the child, and on the duration of diarrhea. One should favor noninvasive tests and keep in mind that a diagnosis of functional or factitious diarrhea is not necessarily an exclusion diagnosis.

History taking includes perinatal course (constipation, cystic fibrosis), previous surgery (short bowel, terminal ileum), and family history (celiac disease, IBD). The severity of the diarrhea, the type of stools, and the presence of associated symptoms should be assessed. The physician should examine a stool sample. A dietary history should be obtained at the first visit. Prior weight and the child's growth chart are of great importance to evaluate the presence of weight loss or failure to thrive.

The *physical examination* should include all systems with specific attention for growth and development, head and neck region, and obviously abdomen and rectum. The assessment of pubertal stage is useful to assess malnutrition with delayed puberty (Table 10-4).

Based on history and clinical examination, one should attempt to establish the likelihood that symptoms are organic (as opposed to functional), to distinguish malabsorptive from colonic or inflammatory forms of diarrhea, and to assess the need for further examinations[82] (Table 10-5).

TABLE 10-3. **Investigations**

Noninvasive	
Observe, document	
Historical food intake	
Laboratory parameters	
Inflammation	ESR, CRP, liver function
Allergy	IgE, RAST
Nutrition	CBC, urea and electrolytes, PT, vitamins A, E, D, B$_{12}$, Ca, ferritin, folate, triglycerides, cholesterol
Immunity	IgA, anti-endomysium IgA, human tissue transglutaminase
Toxicology	
Thyroid function	
Stool	
Cultures	
Steatocrit	
Sudan III stain	
Elastase	
72-h fecal fat collection	
α1-Antitrypsin	
Osmotic gap	
Breath tests evaluating absorption	
^{13}C-lactose breath test	
^{2}H-lactose breath test	
^{13}C mixed triglyceride breath test	
Sweat Cl test	
Plain abdominal x-ray	
Small bowel follow-through	
White blood cell scan	
Invasive	
Esophagogastroduodenoscopy with small bowel biopsy	To rule out villous atrophy, celiac disease, histological abnormalities To perform enzyme assays
Sigmoidoscopy with biopsy	To rule out allergic or inflammatory colitis
Ileocolonoscopy with biopsy	To rule out IBD
Duodenal intubation	To rule out exocrine pancreatic insufficiency
Anorectal manometry/deep rectal biopsy	To rule out Hirschsprung's disease

CBC, complete blood cell count; CRP, C-reactive protein; ESR, erythrocyte sedimentation rate; IBD, inflammatory bowel disease; PT, prothrombin time; RAST, radioallergosorbent test.

TABLE 10-4. Essential Elements of the Physical Examination of the Child With Diarrhea

Growth chart
Vital signs
Muscle mass
Subcutaneous fat
Pubertal stage
Psychomotor development
Skin (perianal)
ENT region
Abdomen
Organomegaly
Tenderness
Rectal exam
Stool sample
Color
Consistency
? Occult blood → Hemoccult
? pH → Indicator
? Fermentation → Clinitest

ENT, ear, nose, and throat.

TABLE 10-5. Initial Assessment of Chronic Diarrhea

Data Collection	Differential
Step 1: History	
Duration > 3 weeks	
Defecation frequency – pattern (? nocturnal)	Hypersecretion – inflammation
Fecal aspect: watery – foamy – floating – mucus – blood – undigested particles	Congenital absorption defects – steatorrhea – inflammation – Toddler's diarrhea
Associated symptoms: abdominal cramping – flatulence – fever – extraintestinal symptoms	Carbohydrate malabsorption – IBD
Dietary history	Toddler's diarrhea – undigestible carbohydrates
Step 2: Physical Examination	
Biometry: normal growth	Functional, dietary
Biometry: failure to thrive	Malabsorption
Mucous membranes (oral sores)	IBD
Distended abdomen	Fermentation (carbohydrate malabsorption), fecal impaction, inflammation
Abdominal mass	IBD – tumor – fecal impaction
Rectal anomalies	IBD
Extraintestinal symptoms: pulmonary, joints, eye, skin	CF, IBD, celiac disease
Step 3: Laboratory Tests	
Rise in inflammatory parameters	IBD
Electrolyte disturbances	Hypersecretive state
Anemia	Mixed malabsorption: celiac disease, IBD
Low fat-soluble vitamins	Steatorrhea: CF, abetalipoproteinemia Mixed malabsorption: celiac disease, IBD
Elevated transaminases	IBD
Elevated bilirubin, bile acids	Cholestasis, CF
Elevated pancreatic enzymes	IBD
Low albumin	Protein-losing enteropathy: IBD
Low cholesterol, triglycerides	Abetalipoproteinemia
Elevated human tissue transglutaminase or IgA anti-endomysium	Celiac disease
Stool cultures	Rule out bacterial or parasitic infection

CF, cystic fibrosis; IBD, inflammatory bowel disease.

Red flags (Table 10-6) such as severe continuous and nocturnal diarrhea, blood and mucus in the stools, very acid stools, weight loss, or failure to thrive and associated symptoms strongly suggest a specific organic cause.

Some typical descriptions of the different types of diarrhea are given next.

Watery and inflammatory diarrheas are characterized by nocturnal diarrhea and occasionally incontinence. With carbohydrate malabsorption, the dietary connection may be present in the medical history. In true *secretory* diarrhea, fasting may cause some degree of amelioration because food also stimulates secretion, but diarrhea persists, including nocturnal diarrhea, incontinence, and sometimes dehydration. In the case of *malabsorptive* diarrhea, signs of steatorrhea with flatulence, bulky greasy foul-smelling stools, and weight loss may be discrete or even absent. Steatorrhea is much more frequent in exocrine pancreatic insufficiency (10 to 80%) than in mucosal disease such as celiac disease (12 to 15%). In *inflammatory* diarrheas, children usually have long-standing anorexia, stunted growth, and weight loss. Inflammation causes diarrhea and fecal protein losses. Stools are usually not abundant, but contain mucus and sometimes blood. Dehydration is lacking. Abdominal pain is localized with a palpable infiltrate, diffuse pain, and tenderness. Systemic manifestations of inflammatory disease such as aphthous ulcers in the buccal mucosa, uveitis and arthralgia or erythema nodosum need to be sought.

Investigations are frequently needed to better direct the differential diagnosis or to confirm the suspicion of a specific disease (see Table 10-3). Initial investigations are *laboratory tests* and stool cultures. The blood tests can indicate the presence of inflammation, allergy, nutritional deficiencies, or immune or endocrine disorders.

A meaningful screening test for celiac disease is IgA anti-endomysium antibody or human transglutaminase assay.[83] Note that the patient may be IgA deficient and that a firm diagnosis of celiac disease is still based on small bowel biopsy.[84] However, an excellent correlation of a new serological marker, anti-actin filament antibody IgA, with the degree of intestinal villous atrophy was recently reported.[85]

Stool cultures are not needed in benign acute diarrhea as most cases are viral and self-limiting. In the presence of "red flags" or protracted diarrhea, cultures including microscopic examination for ova, cysts, and parasites of at least three fresh stool samples are in order. Malabsorption is usually generalized, meaning that (fermented) carbohydrates, fat, and protein are excreted. Carbohydrate fermentation lowers fecal pH below 5.

Stool fat can be identified with various methods. Single stool samples can be analyzed for fat using the Sudan III stain[86] or the acid steatocrit.[87]

Qualitative examinations for fat content in stools consist of heating a mixture of feces, alcohol, and water. The Sudan stain reveals neutral fat and triglycerides but not the fatty acid soaps; these are remaining dietary triglycerides and phospholipids from endogenous sources (bile, enterocytes, bacteria).

TABLE 10-6. Red Flags or Warning Signals in the Patient With Chronic Diarrhea Suggesting More Serious Pathology

Stools
    Blood
    Mucus
    Acid (perianal excoriation)
    Nocturnal
Weight loss or failure to thrive
Associated symptoms
    Fever
    Rash
    Arthritis

The quantitative 72-hour fecal fat collection is cumbersome but widely used. Stool collection has to be done for 3 days, because bowel movements vary from day to day in children. Fat intake needs to be constant prior to and during the collection. Because of the lack of standardization between laboratories and the limited diagnostic value of a positive result, the relevance of this method is being questioned, at least in adults.[88,89] Normal values up to the age of 6 months are a mean of 7.5 g fat per 100 g of stool and afterwards of 5 g fat per 100 g of stool. The upper limits are up to the age of 6 months: 15 g per 100 g of stool; up to the age of 4 years: 9 g; and afterwards 7 g. This translates into 15% of ingested fat up to the age of 6 months, 10% up to the age of 3 years, and 5% afterwards.[90,91] A useful and sensitive test is the fecal elastase 1[92] in a single stool. Be aware of normal fat excretion in celiac disease in 30% of children despite severity of the disease and that in Shwachman's syndrome steatorrhea disappears after the age of 5 years for unknown reasons.

The presence of protein in stools due to intestinal losses or *creatorrhea* can be reflected by fecal α1-antitrypsin.[23]

Fecal calprotectin, a neutrophil product, is a promising marker for gastrointestinal inflammation, but the test has not yet been widely introduced.[93,94]

Measurement of stool volumes is meaningful in severe congenital diarrheas. Very high volumes are only seen in structural defects of the epithelium such as microvillus inclusion disease (MVID) and intestinal epithelial dysplasia (IED, previously named tufting enteropathy). In MVID, stool volumes at birth range from 120 to 150 mL/kg/day and increase over time to 250 to 300 mL/kg/day. In IED, stool volumes remain in the same range at birth (60 to 180 mL/kg/day) and later on (80 to 120 mL/kg/day) but may also increase to over 200 mL/kg/day. In congenital chloride diarrhea (CCD), stool volume amounts to 1 L per day. In congenital sodium diarrhea (CSD), the volume fluctuates around 105 to 130 mL/kg/day. In glucose-galactose malabsorption (GGM), stool volumes between 70 and 100 mL/kg/day are reported. High diarrheal volumes are an indication for congenital morphological abnormalities. Fasting abolishes diarrhea in GGM, but in MVID and IED, diarrhea diminishes only slightly due to some villus atrophy and lower capacity of transporters; in CSD and CCD diarrhea continues unabated.[41,43,48]

Measurement of stool electrolytes for calculation of the *osmotic gap* is useful as a guideline for classification of watery diarrhea. The normal plasma osmolality of 290 mOsm/kg H_2O is essentially isotonic with plasma. Na^+ and K^+ concentration must be measured in stool and multiplied by 2 to account for the obligate (mainly organic) anions in the stool. The osmotic gap or the difference between stool osmolality (290 mOsm) and ($Na + K$ times 2) concentrations should normally be less than

125 and is usually less than 50. In secretory diarrhea, twice the sum of stool Na^+K^+ approximates stool osmolality; stool weight is minimally or moderately reduced during fasting and remains above 200 g per 24 hours. In general, if stool Na^+ concentrations are greater than 90 mmol and the osmotic gap is less than 50, secretory diarrhea is present. Conversely, if stool Na^+ is less than 60 mOsm and the osmotic gap is greater than 125, osmotic diarrhea is likely. Nonabsorbable luminal constituents that displace Na^+ cause osmotic diarrhea. Osmotic diarrhea improves during fasting, and stool weight returns to values under 200 g per 24 hours. In most cases, stool sodium concentration is between 60 and 90 mmol and the calculated osmotic gap between 50 and 100 mOsm, indicating that both secretory and malabsorptive pathophysiological elements are present.

In congenital diarrheas, measurement of electrolytes is useful for disease differentiation. In MVID, fecal sodium is 79 mmol/L, potassium 19 mmol/L, chloride 70 mmol/L, and osmotic gap less than 84 mOsm/L. In IED stool sodium is usually 70 to 120 mmol/L,[100-110] potassium 22 mmol/L, and chloride 33 mmol/L. In CCD, fecal chloride is 158 mmol/L ± 16 mmol/L (normal 5 to 25), sodium 55 ± 27 mmol/L (normal 20 to 50), potassium 56 ± 20 mmol/L (normal 83 to 95), and fecal Na + K less than Cl. In CSD, sodium is 98 to 190 mmol/L, chloride 84 to 109 mmol/L, and potassium has not been reported; urine values for sodium are less than 10 mmol/L, and fecal Na is greater than K + Cl. It is clear that in clinical practice fecal electrolytes do not differentiate among diseases, except for CCD. Currently genetic testing is available for all mentioned congenital diarrheas and should be initiated early.[41,43,48] In MVID, the defect is a MYO5B mutation in the myosin promoter,[95] in CCD SCL26A3 gene mutations were found,[96] and in CSD the mutations are SPINT2.[97] IED or tufting enteropathy is caused by a mutation in epithelial cell adhesion molecule on chromosome 2p21.[98]

Hydrogen breath tests are widely used to assess carbohydrate maldigestion. The lactose hydrogen breath test is easily performed and is as sensitive and specific as the mucosal lactase assay.[99] A dose of lactose (2 g/kg) is given after overnight fast, and hydrogen exhalation is monitored. In the absence or reduced presence of lactase, intestinal microbiota ferment lactose and a hydrogen peak appears. A rise of 10 ppm above baseline is considered positive by some,[100] but most require a rise of 20 ppm. Symptoms are also monitored during the test. However, some children harbor a flora that does not produce hydrogen, yielding false negative tests (up to 25%). Therefore a trial of lactose-free diet should be considered when the diagnosis is suspected.[82] A high baseline or a double peaked curve may be caused by bacterial overgrowth. The ^{13}C-xylose breath test has also been proposed to diagnose small bowel overgrowth in children.[101]

^{13}C-carbohydrate breath tests indicate the absorption of the tested ^{13}C-labeled carbohydrate. The ^{13}C-lactose breath test can be used in children to asses lactose absorption.[102] The ^{13}C-sucrose similarly tests sucrase activity. Stable isotope breath tests are harmless, noninvasive, and child-friendly but require more specialized laboratory equipment for analysis.

Another useful ^{13}C-breath test is the ^{13}C-mixed triglyceride breath test to measure lipase activity.[103] In addition to being an excellent alternative to duodenal aspirate for pancreatic enzyme analysis, this test can assess the efficacy of exogenous lipase supplementation in cystic fibrosis.[104]

The *sweat chloride* test is indicated in any case of infantile chronic diarrhea and suspicion of cystic fibrosis. It is the first step in the differential diagnosis of steatorrhea (Table 10-7).

TABLE 10-7. **Differential Diagnosis of Steatorrhea**

Situation:	Chronic, foul smelling, foamy stools in a child with failure to thrive
	↓
	Laboratory tests: fat-soluble vitamins, triglycerides, cholesterol
	Hb, albumin, inflammatory parameters
	↓
	Rule out cystic fibrosis: Cl sweat test
	If dubious results: genetic analysis of D508 and alleles
	↓
	72-h fecal fat collection with stable fat intake:

Normal	→	Reconsider diagnosis		
Elevated	→	Small bowel biopsy	→	Rule out celiac disease
		Special fat staining	→	Rule out abetalipoproteinemia

	↓
	If normal: assess pancreatic secretion fecal elastase 1
	^{13}C mixed triglyceride breath test
	Or secretin test with duodenal fluid collection

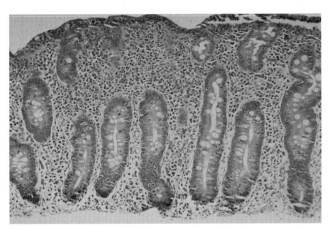

Figure 10-1. Small bowel biopsy from patient with celiac disease demonstrating villous atrophy and increased number of intraepithelial lymphocytes (*see plate section for color*).

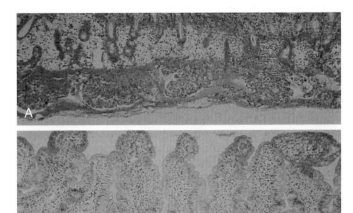

Figure 10-2. Small bowel biopsy before (**A**) and after (**B**) soy challenge in child with soy allergy. After the challenge, the epithelium is damaged: villi are destroyed and the mucosa is invaded by a dense cellular infiltrate (*see plate section for color*).

Radiological examinations are contributive to rule out subobstruction (plain x-ray in the upright position) and fecal impaction and to document small intestinal lesions (enteroclysis). Sonography, when performed by an experienced radiologist, is helpful to document intestinal wall thickening.[105] White blood cell scanning[106] and magnetic resonance imaging techniques[107] have been proposed as noninvasive methods to evaluate intestinal inflammation, especially in Crohn's disease. These methods do not allow a diagnosis but a follow-up of documented lesions.

In the case of chronic diarrhea and a strong suspicion of intestinal damage or inflammation, *endoscopic* and *histological examinations* are warranted. Except for flexible rectosigmoidoscopy, endoscopic procedures are performed under propofol or general anesthesia or with conscious sedation.[108] A small bowel biopsy is essential for the diagnosis of celiac disease (Figure 10-1). Other causes of villus atrophy can be demonstrated such as allergic enteropathy (Figure 10-2). Ileocolonoscopy with biopsies is diagnostic for various types of colitis and Crohn's disease.[109,110]

Duodenal tubage and analysis of pancreatic secretions before and after stimulation with secretin is the classical test to document pancreatic exocrine deficiency.[111] A somewhat simplified technique was described in which duodenal fluid is aspirated through an endoscope after stimulation with pancreozymin and secretin.[112] Valuable indirect tests that might replace the secretin test are the ^{13}C mixed triglyceride breath test and fecal chymotrypsin and elastase 1. The ^{13}C mixed triglyceride breath test is very sensitive in severe cases of pancreatic insufficiency but fails to detect mild cases, whereas the fecal elastase 1 test has a high sensitivity and specificity and a lower cost.[113]

In the case of fecal impaction with fecal incontinence, a history of early constipation and a suggestive digital rectal examination, *anorectal manometry*, and *deep rectal biopsies* are indicated to rule out Hirschsprung's disease.

CLINICAL MANAGEMENT

The diagnosis will obviously guide therapeutic management of a patient with diarrhea.[114] Acute self-limiting diarrhea necessitates little intervention besides some dietary adjustments.

Treatment of Acute Infectious Diarrhea

Profuse diarrhea with signs of or risk for dehydration necessitates oral rehydration with the adapted ORS. Despite its proven efficacy and widespread use in developing countries, oral rehydration therapy is insufficiently applied in the United States.[115]

Current recommendations are to refeed early on after a short period of rehydration.[116,117]

In bacterial diarrheas, the glucose-sodium transporter and the basolateral Na,K-ATPase are always preserved and functional. Using this pathway, equimolar luminal glucose and sodium can transport sodium to the extracellular space. ORS with sodium in a range between 50 and 90 mmol/L can rehydrate children in 3 to 4 hours. This was also proven in viral diarrheas where the glucose sodium transporter is not fully expressed on immature enterocytes on partially atrophic villi. The patchy nature of villus atrophy and preservation of sufficient normal villi explain the efficacy of ORS in this condition. The recommended quantity of ORS if offered on demand is 10 to 45 mL per kg bodyweight. Thirst is an important guide to limit rehydration time. The degree of dehydration or the child's age does not influence the efficacy of rehydration. Parenteral rehydration is equally effective but is only indicated when the child has such abundant quantities of diarrhea that he or she cannot drink enough ORS and becomes too tired, which is rare. The child might have enormous thirst and drink forcefully enough to cause vomiting initially, but subsequently vomiting tends to disappear. In difficult cases, a nasogastric tube can be used to rehydrate. The advantage of immediate maximal rehydration is that after 3 to 4 hours the child might start to eat his normal food (breast feeding, bottle feeding, or toddler feeding) with maintenance of ORS at 10 mL/kg body weight after each watery stool produced.

The addition of soluble fiber to ORS has benefits for the treatment of cholera. Fiber is digested to SCFAs, which transport additional Na over the colonic mucosa into the extracellular space. In milder diarrheas, a benefit could not be demonstrated.

Drugs are generally not used for acute diarrhea. Loperamide is not recommended for infants and young children. A newer agent, racecadotril, an enkephalinase inhibitor with antisecretory and antidiarrheal actions, appears safe and well tolerated in the treatment for acute diarrhea in children.[117a] This is a promising drug, but its effectiveness in children is unproven.[117b,117c]

The composition and function of intestinal microbiota have been the focus of recent scientific interest. Probiotics and prebiotics are therefore the subject of multiple studies on intestinal physiology and pathophysiology, including acute diarrhea. Probiotics are live, nonpathogenic microorganisms that have a beneficial effect on their host. They include bacteria, especially bifidobacteria and lactobacilli, and yeasts such as *Saccharomyces boulardii*.[118] Prebiotics are nondigestible food ingredients that selectively stimulate the growth of beneficial microbiota.[119]

The addition of a probiotic, *Lactobacillus GG*, to ORS in a European multicenter trial resulted in shorter duration of diarrhea, less chance of a protracted course, and faster hospital discharge.[120] Meta-analyses conclude that selected probiotics such as lactobacilli[121] and *Saccharomyces boulardii*[122] have a favorable effect on acute gastroenteritis and can shorten the diarrheic period within 24 hours. It was shown only to work in children with rotavirus diarrhea with reducing substances in the stools. The effect was diminishment of reducing substances in the stools, probably due to sugar digestive enzymes in probiotics, which has been shown for lactobacillus and *Saccharomyces*. In fact it might therefore not be a strict probiotic effect.[122a]

Prevention of Acute Infectious Diarrhea

Prebiotics have not demonstrated an effect in children suffering from acute gastroenteritis.[119] However, the administration of prebiotics to toddlers who attend day care may be protective against febrile episodes[123] and acute gastroenteritis.[124]

It is expected that the recent worldwide introduction of rotavirus vaccination will positively affect morbidity and mortality. Large national vaccination programs are probably cost-effective.[125,126]

Treatment of Chronic Diarrhea

Chronic diarrhea is caused by malabsorption (as in osmotic diarrhea), or by secretory or inflammatory diarrhea. Luminal nutrients, such as protein, trigger mucosal mediators, inducing increased secretion.[127] Fasting therefore diminishes secretory diarrhea somewhat, as it does in malabsorptive osmotic and inflammatory diarrheas. In diseases, all three mechanisms are frequently involved; consequently, for pathophysiologic, diagnostic, and therapeutic purposes a separation is not clear-cut. Hydrolyzed formulas cause less secretion and are therefore indicated in mucosal disease.[128] Long-chain triglycerides should be tried in most chronic diarrheas because they are osmotically inert, calorie dense, and absorbed to a variable extent in biliary obstruction, pancreatic insufficiency with enzyme supplements, and mucosal disease. MCTs are absorbed in the small and large bowel, constitute an excellent energy source but do not replace long chain fat. Poly- and disaccharides may increase diarrhea and should be titrated, monitoring fecal reducing substances and stool frequency. This supports the approach of an oral regimen with normal constituents and caloric density and with limited place for special ingredients. There are no data on probiotics and chronic diarrhea. Treatment of specific disease entities is discussed in related chapters.

Other Measures

Oral or enteral feeding is essential to stimulate mucosal recovery and avoid protracted diarrhea. Elemental and semielemental formulas and modular diets[129] allow early refeeding despite a damaged mucosa with impaired digestive capacity.

Parents should be encouraged to normalize their child's diet as soon as possible, because restricted diets lead to chronic nonspecific diarrhea.[130] Parenteral nutrition should be avoided and, if needed, combined with minimal enteral feeding.

In unusual and unclear situations, the possibility of factitious diarrhea or Munchausen by proxy should be considered. Observing the child in isolation should be preferred to a useless escalation of diagnostic tests and therapeutic interventions.

REFERENCES

33. Mackenzie A, Barnes G, Shann F. Clinical signs of dehydration in children. Lancet 1989;28:1038.
45. Troeger H, Epple HJ, Schneider T, et al. Effect of chronic *Giardia lamblia* infection on epithelial transport and barrier function in human duodenum. Gut 2007;56:328–335.
122. Szajewska H, Skorka A, Dylag M. Meta-analysis: *Saccharomyces boulardii* for treating acute diarrhoea in children. Aliment Pharmacol Ther 2007;25:257–264.
127. Heyman M, Desjeux J. Significance of intestinal food protein transport. J Pediatr Gastroenterol Nutr 15:48-57.

See expertconsult.com for a complete list of references and the review questions for this chapter.

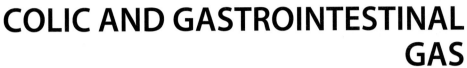

COLIC AND GASTROINTESTINAL GAS

11

Rana Ammoury • Sandeep K. Gupta

GASTROINTESTINAL GAS

Excessive gastrointestinal gas is a frequent presenting complaint to both primary care and specialty physicians. Although 10 to 30% of the general adult population report symptoms related to excessive gastrointestinal gas, its prevalence in children remains unknown.[1,2] The investigation of gas-related complaints is challenging because of the difficulty of measuring the volume or composition of gastrointestinal gas and verifying its relation to symptoms. In addition, it has been suggested that the perception of gassiness and bloating in some patients with abdominal pain is more likely a manifestation of irritable bowel syndrome than true excessive gastrointestinal gas.[3]

Patients with complaints of excessive gastrointestinal gas are at risk of being subjected to expensive and unnecessary diagnostic tests in an effort to "cure" a nonexistent problem, and it is important to appreciate the physiology of gastrointestinal gas in order to understand its relationship to disease. The vast majority of unscientific notions and home remedies available for gassiness further challenge effective and efficient management of such patients. In this chapter, the physiology of gastrointestinal gas is reviewed, along with a discussion of the clinical manifestations of excessive gastrointestinal gas and infantile colic.

Composition of Gastrointestinal Gas

Gastrointestinal gas may originate from three sources: (1) swallowed air, (2) intraluminal production, i.e., bacterial production and reaction of acid and bicarbonate, and (3) diffusion from the blood (Figure 11-1). Gas may be lost from the gastrointestinal tract via eructation or belching, passage of flatus, bacterial consumption, and diffusion into the blood stream. Although there are no published data on the gas content of the gastrointestinal tract of an infant or a child, studies in healthy adults indicate that the normal gastrointestinal tract contains less than 200 mL of gas.[4]

More than 99% of gastrointestinal gas is made up of five gases, namely carbon dioxide (CO_2), hydrogen (H_2), methane (CH_4), nitrogen (N_2), and oxygen (O_2), in varying percentages (Table 11-1). Two of these, H_2 and CH_4, are combustible and can be explosive in a proper mixture with O_2. All these gases are odorless. Odoriferous gases are present in trace amounts, i.e., less than 1% of flatus, and are sulfur based. Most of the symptoms from excessive gastrointestinal gas are attributable to the five odorless gases, though socially, the odoriferous gases are the most unacceptable.

Sources and Relative Distribution of Gastrointestinal Gases

The main source of N_2 is swallowed air. An adult ingests more than half an ounce (15 mL) of air with each swallow, the main components of which are N_2 and O_2, and as such, these are the main components of gastric luminal gas. CO_2, H_2, and CH_4 are mainly produced within the gastrointestinal lumen. CO_2 is generated through the interaction of hydrogen ion and bicarbonate and found in large volumes in the duodenum following the chemical reaction between gastric hydrochloric acid and alkaline intestinal fluid. The distal small intestine gas composition is not well defined. In patients with pathologic conditions such as small bowel bacterial overgrowth, significant amounts of H_2 are generated in the small intestine.[5]

Both H_2 and CH_4 are generated in the colonic lumen. H_2 is mainly a product of bacterial fermentation; germ-free rats and newborn infants do not produce H_2.[4] Carbohydrates, e.g., lactose, and proteins to a much lesser significance, are substrates for bacterial production of H_2. Colonic microbiota, mainly *Methanobrevibacter smithii*, generate CH_4 using H_2 and CO_2.[6] About one-third of adults carry sufficient numbers of methanogenic bacteria to produce appreciable CH_4.[7] The tendency to produce CH_4 appears to be familial and determined by early environmental factors rather than genetic causes. CH_4 tends to be trapped within stool, and large CH_4 producers have stools that float in water.

Generation of H_2 and CH_4 are also enhanced by carbohydrate overload, as in excessive intake of fruit juices; ingestion of poorly absorbed carbohydrates such as cauliflower, cabbage, broccoli, Brussels sprouts, and beans; or disaccharidase deficiency. Disaccharidase deficiency may be primary, as noted in primary lactose intolerance, or secondary, as in a variety of maladies including celiac disease, allergic enteropathy, inflammatory bowel disease, giardiasis, and viral gastroenteritis.

Symptoms Attributable to Gastrointestinal Gas

Excessive gastrointestinal gas may contribute to a number of symptoms including eructation, abdominal distention and bloating, excessive flatulence, and infantile colic.

Eructation

This behavior, also referred to as belching or burping, is often considered normal in infants. In fact, infants are encouraged to burp during and after feeds in the hope of minimizing gastroesophageal reflux and feeding intolerance. As in infants, who are liable to swallow air during normal periods of crying

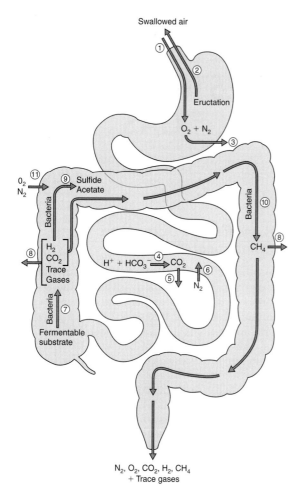

Figure 11-1. Physiology of gastrointestinal gas production. From Feldman M, Friedman L Sleisenger M. Sleisenger & Fordtran's Gastrointestinal and Liver Disease, 7th ed. Philadelphia: Saunders; 2002, with permission.[4]

TABLE 11-1. Composition of Intestinal Gas

Odorless gases (99%)
Carbon dioxide
Hydrogen*
Methane*
Nitrogen
Oxygen
Odoriferous gases (<1%)
Dimethylsulfide
Hydrogen sulfide
Methanethiol

*Combustible.

study reported that patients with a history of abdominal bloating had significantly delayed transit of small intestinal gas compared to a healthy control population.[11]

Abdominal distention may result from excessive aerophagia and increased gastrointestinal gas production, as in malabsorption syndromes. Children with aerophagia often have a nondistended abdomen upon rising, which progressively distends over the day and may be accompanied by crampy abdominal pain. The physical examination may be impressive for abdominal distention and tympany. Plain abdominal films reveal gaseous distention of the bowel. Symptoms and signs may be so intense as to mimic intestinal obstruction[8] or celiac disease. Fatal tension pneumoperitoneum has been reported secondary to aerophagia.[12]

Abdominal distention is also part of the symptom constellation of irritable bowel syndrome.[13] The discomfort associated with bloating in patients with irritable bowel syndrome is more due to dysmotility and heightened perception.[14] No appreciable differences were found in the volume of gastrointestinal gas in adults with complaints of bloating versus controls, although there was an increased symptomatic response to gas infusion in patients with bloating.[9]

Flatulence

An adult passes flatus an average of 10 times per day with an upper limit of 20 times a day. The frequency of flatus does not correlate with age or gender, though data on children are lacking.[4] Although flatulence can be a social embarrassment, comfort should be derived from the fact that over 99% of the flatus consists of odorless gases. Increased gastrointestinal gas production, rather than aerophagia, is usually responsible for flatulence in adults, though it is not known if the same can be extrapolated to children.[8] The source of the flatus may be assessed by gas chromatographic analysis of flatus collected via a rectal tube. Aerophagia should be considered the main contributor if N_2 is the leading component; predominance of H_2, CO_2, and CH_4 would suggest increased intraluminal production, e.g., secondary to bacterial fermentation of malabsorbed carbohydrates.

An extensive radiological and endoscopic evaluation of a patient with excessive flatulence alone is generally fruitless and should be avoided.[15] Efforts should instead be directed at eliciting a detailed history (Table 11-2). Appropriate investigation should be considered if the flatulence is accompanied by other symptoms such as diarrhea, hematochezia/melena, abdominal pain, or weight loss. Otherwise, dietary modifications directed toward limiting intake of fruit juices and poorly absorbed

and feeding, excessive eructation in older children and adults is almost always secondary to aerophagia.[8] Undue aerophagia may result from excessive gum chewing, use of a straw, imbibing of carbonated beverages, clenching on a pencil, or oral breathing as in adenotonsillar hypertrophy or unrecognized H-type tracheoesophageal fistula; patients should be counseled on chewing the food slowly and not gulping. Rare patients with excessive belching have been found to have eosinophilic esophagitis (personal observation). In adults, chronic eructation is generally thought to be a functional disorder.[4]

Gas-bloat syndrome, seen in children following gastric surgery such as Nissen fundoplication, results from an inability of the patient to belch/eructate effectively. Although this can be a source of significant patient discomfort and family distress, the condition is generally transient and self-resolves.

Abdominal Distention

Bloating refers to a person's sensation of abdominal fullness, whereas distention connotes visible or measurable increase in abdominal girth. Patients often attribute the feeling of abdominal bloating to excessive gas burden. The relationship between the amount of intestinal gas and symptoms, however, is not linear. Studies of adult patients with complaints of excessive gas have revealed that the quantity of intestinal gas is usually not different between "gassy" and "nongassy" subjects.[9,10] One

TABLE 11-2. Symptoms and Signs Suggesting Air Swallowing or Bacterial Fermentation as the Cause of Excessive Flatulence

Symptom or Sign	Air Swallowing	Bacterial Fermentation
Increased eructation	Yes	No
Increased salivation	Yes	No
Gas is stress related	Yes	No
Gas is meal related	No	Yes
Abdominal bloating	Yes	No
Malodorous gas	No	Yes
Nocturnal gas	No	Yes

Adapted from Suarez and Levitt (2000).[15] Reproduced with permission.

TABLE 11-3. Summary of Conditions That Present With Symptoms Similar to Infantile Colic

Neurological abnormalities, including Arnold-Chiari malformation
Congenital glaucoma
Ocular foreign body or abrasions
Infections, including otitis media
Gastroesophageal reflux disease
Dietary protein allergy
Disaccharidase deficiency
Constipation
Anal fissures
Rashes, including candidal dermatitis
Urinary tract infection
Renal pathology, including ureteropelvic obstruction
Biliary tree pathology, including stones
Acute abdominal pathologies, including intussusception and volvulus
Incarcerated hernia
Hair tourniquet syndrome
Occult fracture
Maternal drug effect, including illicit and prescription drugs

Adapted from Gupta (2007).[123] Reproduced with permission.

carbohydrates, such as cabbage and legumes, may need to be enforced. Excessive consumption of high-carbohydrate-containing beverages is more apt to be a culprit in children than high intake of cruciferous vegetables such as cabbage. A detailed inquiry into intake of liquid medications and sugar-free drinks should be undertaken, because these products contain sorbitol. Sorbitol is an artificial sweetener that is poorly absorbed and readily fermented by colonic bacteria.

If the patient is bothered by odoriferous flatus, commercially available charcoal-lined seat cushions and undergarments (GasBGon Flatulence Filter; Dairiair, Greenville, NC) have been shown to effectively absorb sulfur gases.

COLIC

The word *colic*, which stems from the Greek "kolikos," the adjective of "kolon," refers to acute and unexpected abdominal pain, independent of age. Infantile colic is a widespread clinical condition affecting between 5 and 28% of infants in the first 3 months of life.[16-19] It refers to paroxysms of excessive, high-pitched, inconsolable crying that is frequently accompanied by flushing of the face, tensing of the abdomen, clenching of the fists, drawing up of the legs, and passing of gas in an otherwise healthy infant.[20] In order to appreciate excessive crying, it becomes important to understand the normal crying pattern of an infant. In 1962, Brazelton[21] delineated this pattern based on prospective data from 80 infants from birth through 12 weeks of age. He noted that infants cried and fussed for a median of 1.75 hours per day at 2 weeks of age, which increased to a peak of 2.75 hours per day at 6 weeks of life and gradually declined to less than 1 hour per day by the 12th week of life. The classical and most often cited definition of infantile colic emerged from a study by Wessel and colleagues[22] in 1954 and is based on the rule of threes: "periods of crying that last for 3 hours or more per day for 3 or more days per week for a minimum of 3 weeks." This condition generally resolves spontaneously by the age of 3 months.[23,17] The episodes tend to peak at 6 weeks of age and are most common in the late afternoon and evening hours.[21] The acoustic characteristics of the crying in colic are different from normal crying episodes: colicky crying is louder, higher, and more variable in pitch and has more turbulence or disphonation than does noncolicky crying.[24] The mothers of colicky infants rate their infants' cries as more urgent, piercing, grating, arousing, aversive, distressing, discomforting, and irritating than do the mothers of noncolicky infants.[25] Together, these characteristics help differentiate colic, which affects approximately 700,000 infants in the United States each year, from other more serious conditions (Table 11-3). Colic affects infants of all socioeconomic strata equally, and there are no reported differences in prevalence between boys and girls, breast- and formula-fed babies, and presence or absence of a family history of atopy.[26] Infantile colic may be graded as mild, moderate, or severe, but there currently are no set definitions for clinicians.[23]

Proposed Etiologies of Infantile Colic

Despite the advances made over the decades in recognizing infantile colic as a clinical entity, it remains poorly defined and understood. Parents often assume that the cause of excessive crying is of gastrointestinal origin, though there is lack of definitive proof establishing this relationship.[27] Several causative factors have been suggested (Table 11-4),[28] although a unifying theory of its pathogenesis is still lacking.

Excessive Gastrointestinal Gas

Excessive gastrointestinal gas load may result from aerophagia secondary to the inconsolable crying exhibited by the colicky infant or from increased gas generation from colonic fermentation. There is paucity of data to support the hypothesis that excessive gastrointestinal gas precipitates a colicky episode. Harley,[29] in 1969, demonstrated radiographically normal gastric outlines at the beginning of a crying episode, and excess gas was only found after the infant stopped crying, indicating that the abdominal distention seen in colicky babies is mostly due to the large amount of air swallowed while crying. In addition, measures to prevent aerophagia, such as upright position, are of little benefit in the management or prevention of infantile colic.[30,31] Despite these data, simethicone, a defoaming agent, has been proposed for the treatment of infantile colic. A randomized, placebo-controlled, multicenter trial of simethicone versus placebo in colicky infants failed to detect a significant difference between the two treatment modalities, thereby refuting, albeit indirectly, this hypothesis.[32]

TABLE 11-4. **Proposed Etiologies of Infantile Colic**

Gastrointestinal
Nutritive
Excessive gastrointestinal gas
Carbohydrate malabsorption
Mode of feeding
Protein allergy/intolerance
Nonnutritive:
Motility
Gastroesophageal reflux
Gut hormones
Altered intestinal flora
Psychosocial

Adapted from Gupta (2002).[28] Reproduced with permission.

Carbohydrate Malabsorption

Malabsorption of dietary carbohydrates has been proposed as a possible cause of colic through the production of excess colonic gas with resultant abdominal cramping and discomfort. Investigations aimed at uncovering evidence of malabsorption such as stool α1-antitrypsin levels, pH, reducing substances, and occult blood have been unrewarding, and no significant differences have been found between colicky and noncolicky infants.[30]

In the first year of life, a number of infants may display partial malabsorption of dietary carbohydrate present in human milk or formula.[33-35] This phenomenon of "physiological malabsorption" due to enzyme insufficiency may be a cause of colic, especially given that enzyme insufficiency generally resolves at approximately 3 months of age, which coincides with when colicky behavior usually subsides.[33,34] Studies measuring breath H_2 levels in colicky infants have produced inconsistent results.[36-39] Two studies showed an association between elevated breath H_2 levels and infantile colic, though there was a considerable overlap in the H_2 excretion values between colicky infants and controls.[36,37] On the other hand, Hyams and colleagues[38] reported no difference in breath H_2 levels between colicky and noncolicky infants fed standardized nonabsorbable carbohydrate. Duro and colleagues[39] demonstrated carbohydrate malabsorption through increased breath H_2 excretion from fruit juices containing sorbitol and a high fructose-to-glucose ratio in infants with colic.

The role of lactose consumption in infantile colic is controversial. Lack of symptom improvement was demonstrated by two studies that examined the effects of lactase supplementation in infants with colic[40,41] and in one study that used low-lactose containing formula in infants with colic.[42] Kanabar et al.,[43] however, found symptomatic improvement in a subset of colicky infants following pretreatment of feeds with lactase. Although the available data on the role of malabsorption in infantile colic are limited and contradictory, carbohydrate malabsorption may be the pathogenic factor in a subset of infants with colic.

Mode of Feeding

The prevalence, pattern, and amount of crying associated with infantile colic are reportedly similar in both human milk- and formula-fed infants,[26,44-46] though one study reported an earlier peak of colicky behavior in formula-fed infants compared with human milk-fed infants (age 2 weeks versus 6 weeks).[47] Evans et al.[48] compared the effect of two modes of nursing on infantile colic, namely prolonged emptying of one breast versus equal drainage of both breasts at each feed. The former group had a lower incidence of colic over the first 6 months of life, but the majority of mothers in this group felt it necessary to offer the second breast at the end of a feed to satisfy their infant's hunger. Based on this study, prolonged nursing from one breast may reduce colic in infants.

Protein Allergy/Intolerance

The immunological model of colic focuses on possible allergens such as cow's-milk proteins in human milk or infant formula as an underlying cause, though convincing, reproducible evidence is lacking, or controversial at best.[42,49-52] An early study by Jakobsson and Lindberg[49] reported that the exclusion of cow's-milk protein from the diet of mothers of nursed infants with colic resulted in symptom resolution. Campbell[50] also suggested a role for cow milk-protein in the pathogenesis of infantile colic. In his study, 68% (13/19) of infants exhibited resolution of colic with dietary modifications that consisted of switching from a cow's-milk protein-based formula to soy protein-based formula, or switching from the latter to a protein-hydrolysate formula. Oggero and colleagues[53] found similar results with resolution of symptoms in 95.5% (42/44) of formula-fed colicky infants with soy protein-based or protein-hydrolyzed formula. In addition, Lucassen et al.[54] randomized colicky infants to either a whey-hydrolysate or a standard formula, with the former demonstrating decreased crying duration of 63 min/day (95% confidence interval = 1 to 127 min/day). Forsyth,[51] in contrast, found that the resolution of symptoms witnessed early on was not sustained. He alternated the feedings of 17 colicky infants between a casein-hydrolysate formula and a cow's-milk protein-containing formula. Infants fed the hydrolysate formula had less crying and colic initially, but the effects diminished over time. Although Lindberg[55] reported that approximately 25% of infants with moderate or severe colic responded favorably to a diet free of cow's-milk protein, and Estep and Kulczycki[56] found free amino-acid based formula to be beneficial in infantile colic, their approach has been described as controversial.[57] Hill and colleagues[58] took protein intolerance further and performed a randomized, controlled trial to investigate the effects of a low-allergen maternal diet on colic among nursed infants. Broad maternal dietary modifications that included the exclusion of cow milk, eggs, peanuts, tree nuts, wheat, soy, and fish were associated with an objective reduction in colic-like distress among 6-week-old infants.

Conversely, Thomas et al.[44] noted that the prevalence of colic was similar between infants fed human milk, formula, and formula-supplemented human milk, and they concluded that dietary protein hypersensitivity may not be the cause of colic in otherwise healthy infants. These results were supported by a questionnaire-based study of the prevalence of colic among nursed, formula-fed, and formula-supplemented nursed infants where no associations were shown between the source of infant nutrition and development of colic.[59] Leibman[60] also failed to uncover objective evidence of protein allergy in his study of 56 infants with colic. In spite of these results, one study supported the use of pancreatic enzyme supplements in lactating mothers for the treatment of infantile colic.[61] The authors theorized that hydrolysis of human milk-protein by pancreatic enzyme supplements would benefit colicky infants with cow's-milk allergy; no further studies have been reported to support this theory.

Motility

Transient dysregulation of the nervous system during development may cause intestinal hypermotility in infants with colic, particularly during the first few weeks of life. Jorup[62] stated that most cases of infantile colic can be explained by colonic hyperperistalsis and increased rectal pressure, and this hypothesis has been supported by studies reporting the beneficial effects of antispasmodics, such as dicyclomine, on infantile colic.[63,64] Whether dicyclomine exerts its effect via the relief of gastrointestinal spasms by a direct relaxant effect on the colonic smooth muscle, or through sedative central nervous system effects, is unclear; however, its utility in infants has been limited because of its central effects and potential for respiratory depression. In a controlled trial, an herbal tea preparation containing chamomile, fennel, and balm mint as antispasmodics was shown to benefit colicky infants.[65] It should be noted that fennel tea was recently reported to have mutagenic effects on bacteria and carcinogenic effects in mice.[66] Savino and his group[67] suggested that a phytotherapeutic agent with *Matricaria recutita*, *Foeniculum vulgare*, and *Melissa officinalis* improved colic in infants through its antispasmodic activity.

A double-blind, placebo-controlled clinical trial investigated the use of cimetropium bromide, a quaternary ammonium semisynthetic derivative of the belladonna alkaloid scopolamine, in 86 colicky infants.[68] In this study, cimetropium bromide reduced the duration of crying in the treated group compared with controls, and although treated infants did have more sleepiness, neither respiratory distress nor apnea was observed.

Gastroesophageal Reflux

It is appealing to explore a cause-effect relationship between gastroesophageal reflux (GER) and infantile colic, especially in view of the prevalence of GER during infancy. Similar to infantile colic, GER may present with excessive crying, but the crying is generally less intense in GER.[31] GER often displays other symptoms such as regurgitation and emesis that are not associated with colic.[30,69]

Few studies have examined the role of pathologic GER in colicky infants, and the results are mixed. In a study of 26 infants with persistent, excessive crying of more than 4 weeks' duration, who had been labeled colicky, Berkowitz and colleagues[70] detected pathologic GER in 61% (16/23) of the infants using a 24-hour continuous intraesophageal pH monitoring study. Although the data appeared compelling, cause-effect relationship could not be established because these infants did not exhibit classic symptoms of GER, such as regurgitation and emesis. Moreover, 12 of the 16 (75%) infants with pathologic GER were aged 4 months or older, by which age infantile colic has generally resolved. In another study of 24 infants under the age of 3 months, who had excessive crying and presumed GER, only one infant had pathologic GER by pH study.[69] Therefore, the question remains whether pathologic GER is indeed a causative factor of infantile colic. Although some data suggest that GER is implicated in a small subset of infants with severe colicky symptoms, in the absence of regurgitation and vomiting, GER is not a common cause of infantile irritability.[71,72]

Gut Hormones

The gastrointestinal tract contains a repertoire of hormones, transmitters, and other biologically active proteins, such as prostaglandins, that are involved in the regulation of intestinal motility. Of these, motilin is the most investigated as a player in the etiopathogenesis of infantile colic. Basal motilin levels have been shown to be raised in colicky infants independent of their diet and are higher at birth in infants who later develop colic.[73,74] It is speculated that motilin promotes gastric emptying, which increases small bowel peristalsis and decreases transit time. These could contribute to perceived intestinal pain and lend substance to the hyperperistalsis theory.[75] A recent study showed that colicky infants have higher serum levels of ghrelin, which is thought to be implicated in promoting abnormal hyperperistalsis and increased appetite, compared to their healthy counterparts.[76] Random urinary concentrations of 5-hydroxy-3-indoleacetic acid (5-OH IAA), a serotonin metabolite, were measured in infants with and without colic; 5-OH IAA levels were elevated in colicky infants, suggesting that elevated serotonin concentrations may participate in the pathogenesis of infantile colic.[77]

Altered Intestinal Flora

The intestinal microbiota plays an important role in human health by producing nutrients and preventing gut colonization by potentially pathogenic microorganisms. Increasing attention has been directed to the role of intestinal microflora in the pathogenesis of various gastrointestinal processes including infantile colic. According to Lehtonen et al.,[78] an aberrant gut microbial composition, such as inadequate lactobacilli level in the first months of life, may affect the intestinal fatty acid profile, thereby favoring the development of colic. However, his study failed to show any detectable differences in the intestinal microflora between colicky and noncolicky infants.[78] A subsequent study by Savino and colleagues[79] demonstrated lower counts of intestinal lactobacilli in colicky infants compared with healthy infants. In a separate study, these investigators reported that *Lactobacillus brevis* and *Lactobacillus lactis* were found only in colicky infants, whereas *Lactobacillus acidophilus* was cultured only from healthy infants.[80] In an additional study by Savino and colleagues,[81] modulation of the intestinal microflora of colicky infants using probiotics was investigated. In this prospective study, a cohort of 90 exclusively nursed colicky infants was equally and randomly assigned to probiotic *Lactobacillus reuteri* or simethicone treatment. Infants in the *L. reuteri*-treated group displayed an improvement in crying behavior within 1 week of treatment compared with the simethicone-treated group. Addition of prebiotics to the formula of infants with colic also demonstrated a reduction in crying episodes.[82]

A recent study that evaluated the colonization pattern of gas-forming coliforms in colicky infants and healthy controls by molecular methods found coliform bacteria, particularly *Escherichia coli*, to be more abundant in colicky infants.[83] Rhoads and his colleagues[84] explored whether gut inflammation could provide a pathophysiological mechanism for colic. In their study, infants with colic had fecal calprotectin levels twofold higher than in healthy controls, with values in a range comparable to those in children with inflammatory bowel disease.

Psychosocial Factors

This aspect of infantile colic has long been proposed, widely studied, and passionately debated. In 1944, Spock[85] had suggested that infantile colic could be due to transmission of anxiety and tension from the mother to the infant. Stewart et al.[86] reported, in a prospective study in 1954, that mothers of excessive criers experienced more psychological conflicts regarding their maternal role and displayed more hostility toward their child. In contrast, two other studies found that maternal emotional factors did not play a role in excessive infant crying; however, an association was found between infantile colic and a history of emotional tension or depression early in the pregnancy.[26,87] Interestingly, Zwart and colleagues[88] in 2007 demonstrated that infants with severe excessive crying show normalization of their behavior during hospitalization and are unlikely to have a medical cause for their colic. The most important risk factor for their crying was a complicated pregnancy or birth, suggesting that these experiences might predispose parents to regard normal crying behavior as excessive.

Various studies have also examined the relationship between maternal smoking and infantile colic.[89-91] Prevalence of colic was twofold higher in infants of mothers who smoke.[89] Moreover, a Canadian study found increased likelihood of colic with maternal alcohol consumption at 6 weeks of gestation and shift-work during pregnancy.[59] However, being married or having a common-law partner and being employed full-time during the pregnancy were associated with a reduced risk of infantile colic. A recent study by Canivet and colleagues[92] showed psychological and psychosocial factors to be significantly related to an increased risk of infantile colic and that these factors interacted with age, parity, social support, and educational level in a complex manner. The authors suggested lending support and special attention to very young women and single mothers. On the other hand, Rautava et al.[93] demonstrated that socioeconomic factors do not play a role in the cause of colic in Finnish infants. Instead, superior maternal intelligence and higher education were found to be associated with higher incidences of infantile colic.[26]

Management of Infantile Colic

The management of infantile colic can be challenging and frustrating because definitive or curative therapies are currently unavailable. Over the years, various remedies have been investigated and proposed as treatments for colic; however, few have been confirmed through rigorous scientific evaluation in the form of randomized controlled trials (Table 11-5). Despite the often favorable clinical outcome of infantile colic, crying and irritability remain among the most common reasons why parents seek medical care.

Limiting Aerophagia

Suggestions on limiting aerophagia, including frequent burping and the use of bottles with an appropriate teat aperture size, should be presented to the caregiver. Infant feeding bottles with collapsible bags may also help reduce aerophagia.

Dietary Management

Based on some of the studies that have addressed the efficacy of a low-allergen diet in mothers of breast-fed infants, a strict cow's-milk-free diet for the mother may be suggested. Another dietary option is to broaden the maternal diet modification by excluding dairy products, eggs, wheat, nuts (peanuts and tree nuts), and fish while advising them to ensure adequate calcium intake.[58] It should be cautioned that these dietary interventions can be challenging and may generate additional stress in an already anxious environment. Hence, these interventions should only be continued if they are effective.

For formula-fed infants, the use of hypoallergenic formulas including casein- and whey- hydrolysate formulas may be

TABLE 11-5. Management Options for Infantile Colic

Limiting aerophagia
  Frequent burps
  Use of appropriate teat aperture size for bottles
Dietary management
  Cow's-milk protein-free diet for mothers
  Use of hypoallergenic formulas
Pharmacological therapy
  Simethicone
  Sucrose solution
  Lactase enzyme
  Probiotics
Alternative therapy
  Herbal tea
  Gripe water
  Minimal acupuncture
  Chiropractic spinal manipulation
  Cranial osteopathic manipulation
Behavioral intervention
  Promoting physical contact
  Parent education

beneficial, although their effects may diminish over time. As for soy protein-based formulas, the European Society for Pediatric Gastroenterology, Hepatology and Nutrition (ESPGHAN) Committee on Nutrition reported that their use in infants with colic lacked adequate supporting data and remains controversial.[94] In addition, extensively hydrolyzed formulas should be reserved for infants with true cow's-milk protein allergy and may not be considered as a first dietary approach.

Pharmacological Therapy

Pharmacotherapy for infantile colic is limited, and the data are mixed. Simethicone is a defoaming agent that reduces the surface tension of mucus, allows entrapped air bubbles to coalesce and disperse, and promotes the expulsion of intestinal air.[95] A systemic review that included three randomized controlled trials found that only one showed possible benefit, but noted that the authors did not elucidate their definition of colic in that study.[52] A second review found that although the use of simethicone was not supported by good-quality trials, it had no reported adverse effects and it was widely used based on common consensus.[96]

Although dicyclomine was shown to be more effective than placebo in a number of randomized controlled trials, it is contraindicated for infants less than 6 months of age based on a number of serious adverse effects. These adverse events, including shortness of breath, apnea, syncope, seizures, hypotonia, and coma, were mostly seen in infants younger than 7 weeks of age.[63,64,97]

Sucrose has been thought to cause the release of endogenous opioids, providing an analgesic effect in infants with colic.[98] Two randomized trials demonstrated a positive response with sucrose, but the effect was short lived.[99,100] Akcam and Yilmaz[101] observed that 30% glucose solution caused improvement in 64% (16/25) of colicky infants and suggested its use as a safe, effective, easily achievable, and well tolerated alternative therapy. It should be noted, however, that the placebo response in that study was 48% (12/25 patients).

Several studies in which lactase enzyme was added to the milk feeds of infants with colic have not shown significant reductions in crying.[102,103] A recent review that included four randomized controlled trials determined that the available evidence precluded firm conclusions.[96]

The study by Savino and colleagues[81] was the first to evaluate the efficacy of probiotic supplementation on infant colic. At the end of the study, 95% (39/41) of the *Lactobacillus reuteri* treatment group were considered "responders" and no significant adverse effects were reported. The mechanism by which *L. reuteri* reduces colic should be the subject of future clinical investigation to allow screening for even more effective therapies. The use of probiotics is generally safe, but incidents of bacteremia/septicemia, pneumonia, and meningitis have been reported in the literature, especially in immune-compromised patients.[104]

Alternative Therapies

A number of homeopathic remedies, such as herbal tea and gripe water, have been used in the treatment of colic. Although no significant adverse events have been reported with their use, the quantity of tea containing chamomile, vervain, licorice, fennel, and lemon balm that needed to be consumed (32 mL/kg/day) in order to deliver relief is concerning, especially if it displaces milk or formula intake.[65] Gripe water, although not as popular in the United States, is widely used in Europe, Asia, and Africa. Among other ingredients, it can contain anise, angelica, caraway, cardamom, catnip, chamomile, cinnamon bark, dill, fennel, ginger, and sodium bicarbonate (baking soda). Various companies manufacture gripe water, and the family must be informed that some brands may contain alcohol.

Other complementary interventions have been explored for the treatment of colic. Minimal acupuncture or light needling was tested in a group of infants with colic in a quasirandomized study. Four treatments with light needling on one point in the hand significantly decreased crying intensity in the treatment group compared to controls.[105] As for chiropractic spinal manipulation, a number of studies may suggest a positive effect,[106,107] but the only blinded trial, by Olafsdottir et al.,[108] showed no statistical difference between spinal manipulation and placebo treatment groups. In another open, controlled, prospective study, 28 infants were randomized to receive either cranial osteopathic manipulation once weekly for 4 weeks or no treatment.[109] The osteopathic group had reduced crying and improved sleeping. However, confirmatory, larger clinical trials are needed before recommendations about complementary treatments for colic can be made.

Behavioral Interventions

Promoting physical contact, by holding or swaddling the crying infant while limiting overstimulation, can be beneficial. For example, gentle movement in a rocking chair with lights dimmed out may promote soothing. These behaviors can be difficult to implement in the evening hours when colic generally peaks, as several family activities occur during this time of the day. As such, devices to provide a vibration sensation to the infant are widely available, although their clinical utility has not been extensively studied. One study did not find crib vibrators to be more effective than infant massage in treatment of infants with colic.[110] The caregiver, in his/her continued search for possible comfort measures, may also consider "white noise" – a combination of multiple frequencies of sound often used to mask other sounds. It is thought to soothe infants with colic as it emulates intrauterine sounds. Some common household sources of white noise include the vacuum cleaner, fan, or hair dryer.

Parent education and behavioral management have been evaluated for treatment of infantile colic. Keefe et al.[111] demonstrated that a 4-week home-based behavioral intervention was more effective than routine care in reducing parenting stress. Dihigo[112] evaluated behavior modification in treating colicky infants. Among infants whose parents received individualized counseling and education interventions, crying was reduced significantly from nearly 4 hours to slightly more than 1 hour per infant. Appropriate and timely anticipatory guidance regarding infant colic should be implemented to increase the caregiver's awareness of the condition and prepare them for interactions with a newborn with colic before the condition manifests.

Complications and Long-Term Outcomes

Although the majority of infants with colic recover uneventfully by 3 to 4 months of age, this may not always be the case. Colic in infants can negatively affect the entire family. Infantile colic may lead to earlier discontinuation of breast feeding and the introduction of infant solids, frequent formula changes, maternal distress and irritability, disturbed maternal-infant interaction, suboptimal father-infant interaction, an increased risk for physical abuse, and preschool behavioral problems.[113-116] Vik and colleagues[117] showed that infantile colic and prolonged crying at 2 months were associated with high maternal depression scores 4 months later. In addition, excessive infant crying can increase the risk of shaken baby syndrome.[118] In one prospective study of more than 1000 Finnish children (3 months to 3 years old) with and without infantile colic, families with previously colicky infants exhibited more dissatisfaction with their daily family functioning 3 years following resolution of the disease compared with families without colicky infants.[119] In addition, 64 children in the UK who presented with persistent crying in early infancy (but not necessarily infantile colic) were reevaluated at 8 to 10 years of age.[120] Children with a history of persistent crying were more likely to develop hyperactivity and academic difficulties later in childhood compared with age-matched classroom controls (18.9% versus 1.6%). Another prospective 10-year study reported a significant increase in the susceptibility to recurrent abdominal pain, allergic diseases, and psychological disorders in childhood in subjects who suffered from infantile colic.[121] Ellett et al.[122] reported that the majority of parents of colicky infants described negative feelings about their experience, and although they reported no further problems with their previously colicky children, they believed that family relationships were affected and that communication and support were impaired.

CONCLUSIONS

Gastrointestinal gas and infantile colic continue to be enigmas and cause distress in many patients and their families. However, most often patients do not have an actual increase in gastrointestinal gas volume, but rather their complaints are derived from a misunderstanding of normal physiology, a misinterpretation of symptoms, or an increase in intestinal sensitivity. Symptoms from actual increases in gastrointestinal gas volume can be seen in children with aerophagia, dysmotility, or malabsorption from poorly absorbed carbohydrates.

Although a general consensus regarding the exact etiology of infantile colic is lacking, it is most likely to be multifactorial in genesis. Its self-limiting nature has precluded the use of invasive investigations to establish a pathophysiological model in vivo. Nevertheless, there are a variety of potential interventions, including dietary modifications, pharmacological therapies, and behavioral options, that can assist in the positive management of infantile colic until causative factors can be fully elucidated and efficacious therapies developed.

REFERENCES

8. Hyams JS. Editorial review – Intestinal gas in children. Curr Opin Pediatr 1996;8:467–470.

32. Metcalf TJ, Irons TG, Sher LD, et al. Simethicone in the treatment of infant colic: a randomized, placebo-controlled, multicenter trial. Pediatrics 1994;94:29–34.

67. Savino F, Cresi F, Castagno E, et al. A randomized double-blind placebo controlled trial of a standardized extract of *Matricaria recutita, Foeniculum vulgare* and *Melissa officinalis* (ColiMil) in the treatment of breastfed colicky infants. Phytother Res 2005;19:335–340.

81. Savino F, Pelle E, Palumeri E, et al. *Lactobacillus reuteri* (American type culture collection strain 55730) versus simethicone in the treatment of infantile colic: a prospective randomized study. Pediatrics 2007;119: 124–130.

120. Wolke D, Rizzo P, Woods S. Persistent infant crying and hyperactivity problems in middle childhood. Pediatrics 2002;109:1054–1060.

See expertconsult.com for a complete list of references and the review questions for this chapter.

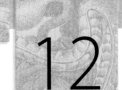

CONSTIPATION AND FECAL INCONTINENCE

12

Vera Loening-Baucke

Constipation and functional fecal incontinence (formerly called encopresis) represent common problems in children. Constipation can be caused by many different disorders. Constipation is most commonly due to functional constipation, which is constipation not due to organic or anatomical cause or intake of medication.

In a primary care clinic in North America, 3% of infants suffered from constipation in the first and 10% in the second year of life.[1] Issenman et al. reported that 16% of 22-month-olds were thought by their parents to be constipated.[2] Yong and Beattie[3] reported that 5% of otherwise healthy 4- to 11-year-old British schoolchildren had constipation lasting more than 6 months. In a primary care clinic in the United States, 18% of 4- to 17-year-old children had functional constipation.[4] Publications from Brazil report that 18% to 37% of children suffer from constipation.[5-7]

Fecal incontinence is the involuntary loss of formed, semi-formed, or liquid stool into the child's underwear, most often associated with functional constipation after the child has reached a developmental age of 4 years. In a primary care clinic, the prevalence rate for functional fecal incontinence (once per week) was 4.4%.[4] The fecal incontinence was associated with constipation in 95%. The fecal incontinence was not associated with constipation or underlying disease in 5% (functional nonretentive fecal incontinence). Rare organic conditions for fecal incontinence should be considered and ruled out.

The aims of this chapter are to describe defecation disorders in children: functional constipation, functional constipation with fecal incontinence, and nonretentive fecal incontinence; to discuss their evaluation and treatment; and to report on short-term and long-term treatment outcome.

PATHOPHYSIOLOGY

As with many pediatric gastrointestinal disorders, the etiology and course of functional constipation and fecal incontinence are increasingly conceptualized from a broad biopsychosocial perspective that assumes that a child's condition is a function of multiple interacting determinants, such as genetic predisposition, environmental factors, life stress, psychologic state, coping, social support, and interactions between physiologic and psychological factors via the central and enteric nervous systems.[7]

FUNCTIONAL CONSTIPATION IN INFANTS AND TODDLERS

Stool frequency depends on the age of the child. A number of studies revealed a decline in stool frequency from more than four stools per day during the first week of life to 1.2 per day at

4 years of age, with a corresponding increase in stool size. Fontana et al.[8] showed that in the first 3 years of life, 97% of healthy children had at least one bowel movement every other day. By 4 years of age, 98% of normal children were toilet trained.

The Rome III Committee suggested diagnostic criteria for constipation in *infants and toddlers* up to 4 years of age.[9] The criteria are mostly symptom-based (Table 12-1).

Constipation in the newborn and in early infancy is a special situation because of the possibility of a serious congenital disorder. If meconium passage is delayed for more than 24 hours, several diseases need to be considered. Hirschsprung's disease is rare but must be considered. Evaluation for Hirschsprung's disease may include a barium enema, anorectal manometry, and rectal suction biopsy. The diagnosis is confirmed by the absence of ganglion cells in the submucosal and myenteric plexus in the rectal biopsy. Anatomical defects of the spinal cord, such as myelomeningocele, or anorectal anomalies, such as anal atresia and anal stenosis, must also be ruled out by examination and, if necessary, by appropriate imaging studies. Meconium plugs may cause neonatal constipation and may be associated with either Hirschsprung's disease or cystic fibrosis. Other organic causes of constipation are endocrine, metabolic, and neuromuscular diseases.

During a 42-month period, 4157 infants and toddlers between 0 and 24 months of age were seen in our General Pediatric Clinics for health maintenance and acute care visits.[1] The prevalence rate for constipation in children in the first year of life was 3%, and 10% during the second year of life, with 97% having functional constipation.[1] The ratio of constipated boys to girls was 1.1:1.[1]

The onset of constipation frequently occurs with hard stools after the change from breast milk to commercial formula or introduction of solids, and in toddlers during toilet training. The most common cause of constipation in infants and toddlers is an acquired behavior after experiencing painful defecation. This notion is supported by 93% of parents of infants and toddlers with functional constipation reporting hard to rock-hard stools, 27% reporting having seen blood around their child's stool, and 42% reporting that children were crying and screaming when passing stools.[1] Fear of defecation leads to voluntary withholding of stool, called retentive posturing. Instead of relaxing the pelvic floor for defecation, the retentive infant will contract the pelvic floor and gluteal muscles in an attempt to avoid defecation. Infants will often grunt, arch their back, and stiffen their legs, whereas toddlers often rise on their toes and rock back and forth while squeezing the buttocks together and stiffening their legs, or assume other unusual postures. These maneuvers are often misinterpreted by the parents as straining for defecation. Forty-five percent of our constipated infants

TABLE 12-1. The Rome III Criteria for Functional Constipation in Neonates and Toddlers

Diagnostic Criteria for Functional Constipation in Neonates and Toddlers[9]

At least 2 of the following symptoms must occur for at least 1 month:
<2 defecations per week
>1 episode per week of incontinence after the acquisition of toileting skills
History of excessive stool retention
History of painful or hard bowel movements
Presence of a large fecal mass in the rectum, and
History of large-diameter stools that may obstruct the toilet

TABLE 12-2. The Rome III Criteria for Functional Constipation in Children and Adolescents

Diagnostic Criteria for Functional Constipation in Children and Adolescents[10]

Symptom must occur at least once per week for at least 2 months and include 2 or more of the following in a child with a developmental age of >4 years with insufficient criteria for diagnosis of irritable bowel syndrome:
Two or fewer defecations in the toilet per week
At least 1 episode of fecal incontinence per week
History of retentive posturing or excessive volitional stool retention
History of painful or hard bowel movements
Presence of a large fecal mass in the rectum
History of large diameter stools that may obstruct the toilet

and toddlers exhibited stool withholding behavior.[1] Only 10% had an abdominal fecal mass present, and 53% of those with a rectal examination had a rectal impaction.[1] Incontinence may be mistaken for diarrhea by some parents. Other accompanying symptoms may include irritability, decreased appetite, or early satiety. The accompanying symptoms disappear immediately following passage of a large stool.

The physical examination should be complete with special attention to the size of the rectal fecal mass during abdominal examination and, if not felt, during the rectal examination.

Some otherwise healthy infants less than 6 months of age appear to have significant discomfort and excessive straining associated with defecation and crying for over 10 minutes, followed by successful passage of soft to liquid stools. These infants do not have constipation but have infant dyschezia. This defecation disorder is seen in the first few months of life and can occur several times a day. It is speculated that this disorder occurs when neonates fail to coordinate increased intra-abdominal pressure with relaxation of the pelvic floor. Symptoms improve and then resolve without intervention in most cases. Parents need to be reassured that this phenomenon is part of the child's learning process and that there is no intervention necessary. The parents should be advised not to use rectal stimulation. Laxatives are unnecessary.

Breast-fed infants may defecate after each feeding, and other exclusively breast-fed infants may have infrequent soft bowel movements. In our review of 4157 infants and toddlers, we found that 18 well-nourished infants, who were exclusively breast-fed, had long intervals between soft to loose bowel movements (2 to 14 days, mean 5.4 ± 3.0 days).[1] This bowel pattern is considered normal for breast-fed infants.

FUNCTIONAL CONSTIPATION IN CHILDREN AND ADOLESCENTS

The Rome III Committee suggested diagnostic criteria for constipation in children and adolescents. The criteria are mostly symptom-based (Table 12-2).[10]

Estimates of constipation have varied between 0.3% and 8% in the pediatric population. In primary care, 18% of 4- to 17-year-old children were treated for functional constipation.[4] A positive family history has been found in 28% to 50% of constipated children, and a higher incidence has been reported in monozygotic than dizygotic twins.[11]

Often the onset of functional constipation in children more than 4 years of age occurs when a child begins to attend school, when toilet use is regulated to special times and toilets may not

be clean and private. Children who have been constipated for years may have had withholding behavior long before the visit to the physician, and by the time they are evaluated, the rectum has become dilated and has accommodated to the point that withholding is no longer necessary in order to delay the passage of stools. The term *excessive volitional stool retention* is used to describe older children who still withhold their stools without necessarily displaying retentive posturing.

Constipation is also present in some children with irritable bowel syndrome. These children have functional abdominal pain or abdominal discomfort as their main complaint.

COMPLICATIONS OF CONSTIPATION

Functional fecal incontinence is the most obvious complication of constipation. Other complications are also frequently seen (Table 12-3). Chronic abdominal pain and anal and rectal pain are reported by approximately half of the children. Severe attacks of abdominal pain can occur just before a bowel movement, for several days before a large bowel movement, or daily. Many children suffer from vague chronic abdominal pain. Some patients with large stool masses throughout the entire colon may not experience any abdominal pain. Other complications of constipation are urinary symptoms such as daytime and/or nighttime urinary incontinence and urinary tract infections. Daytime urinary incontinence was present in 29% of our constipated and fecal incontinent children, bedwetting in 34%, and one or more urinary tract infections in 33% of girls and 3% of boys.[12] The social stigma that goes along with increased flatulence and the odor of fecal incontinence can be devastating to the child's self-esteem and to his/her acceptance by siblings, parents, peers, and teachers. Children with constipation report a lower quality of life than a healthy control group, children with inflammatory bowel disease, or those with gastroesophageal reflux.[13]

FUNCTIONAL FECAL INCONTINENCE

Functional fecal incontinence is the involuntary loss of formed, semiformed, or liquid stool into the child's underwear. The fecal incontinence is involuntary, although it can be prevented for short periods of time if the child concentrates carefully on closing the external anal sphincter and uses the toilet frequently. Functional fecal incontinence can be associated with functional constipation (constipation-associated fecal incontinence) or can occur without constipation (functional nonretentive fecal incontinence). Distinguishing between constipation-associated

TABLE 12-3. **Complications of Constipation**

Fecal incontinence
Pain:
    Abdominal pain
    Anal or rectal pain
Anorexia
Urinary complications:
    Daytime urinary incontinence
    Nighttime urinary incontinence
    Urinary tract infection
    Vesicoureteral reflux
    Urinary retention
    Megacystis
    Ureteral obstruction
Rarely, life-threatening events such as shock or toxic megacolon
Social exclusion by siblings, parents, peers, and teachers

TABLE 12-4. **Clinical Features of Constipation With Fecal Incontinence**

Difficulties with defecation began early in life, in 50% of children before 1 year of age
Passage of enormous stools
Obstruction of the toilet by stool
Symptoms due to the increasing accumulation of stool:
    Retentive posturing
    Fecal incontinence
    Abdominal pain and irritability, anal or rectal pain
    Anorexia
    Urinary symptoms:
        Daytime urinary incontinence
        Nighttime urinary incontinence
        Urinary tract infection
Unusual behaviors in an effort to cope with the fecal incontinence:
    Nonchalant attitude regarding the fecal incontinence
    Hiding of dirty underwear
    Lack of awareness of an incontinence episode
Dramatic disappearance of most symptoms following the passage of a huge stool

and nonretentive fecal incontinence is necessary for treatment planning.

In the United States, only 25% to 30% of children are reliably toilet trained by 2 years of age, and 80% by 3 years. Of normal children, 97% were toilet trained by 4 years of age. The relatively wide range in age for achieving bowel control among normal children influences the definition of fecal incontinence to children who are at least 4 years of age.[14] It is reported to affect 2.8% of 4-year-old children, 1.5% of 7- to 8-year-old children, and 1.6% of 10- to 11-year-old children. The male to female ratio ranges from 2.5:1 to 6:1.

Although functional constipation and fecal incontinence are no longer seen as indicative of serious psychological disturbance, these children experience more emotional and behavior problems than do children who do not have fecal incontinence.

Constipation-Associated Fecal Incontinence

Eighty-five percent of constipated children more than 4 years of age had fecal incontinence at presentation.[15] Loening-Baucke[4] showed a 4% prevalence rate for functional fecal incontinence in a retrospective review in 482 children, 4 to 17 years of age, attending a primary care clinic in the United States. In this study fecal incontinence was coupled with constipation in 95% of the children.[4] The clinical features of constipation with fecal incontinence are listed in Table 12-4. Some children will have intermittent fecal incontinence. A period free of fecal incontinence may occur after a huge bowel movement, which may obstruct the toilet, and fecal incontinence will resume only after several days of stool retention. Usually, the consistency of stool found in the underwear is loose or clay-like. Sometimes the core of the impaction breaks off and is found as a firm stool in the underwear. Occasionally, what appears to be a full bowel movement is passed into the underwear. Children with functional fecal incontinence often deny the presence of stool in their underwear and the accompanying foul and penetrant odor, many children hide their dirty underwear, and most have a nonchalant attitude regarding the incontinence. Parents usually find this situation very frustrating, and fecal incontinence becomes a major issue of contention between the parent and the child.

Seventy-nine percent of children with functional constipation and fecal incontinence had a history of retentive posturing.[16] Successively greater amounts of stool are built up in the rectum with longer exposure to its drying action, and a vicious cycle is started. Stool retention results when stool expulsion has not occurred for several days. When stool retention remains untreated for a prolonged period of time, the rectal wall becomes stretched and a megarectum develops. The intervals between bowel movements become longer, and the rectum becomes so large that the stored stool can be felt as an abdominal mass that sometimes reaches up to the umbilicus or higher. A large fecal mass on abdominal examination was present in 59% and a large fecal mass in the rectum in 95% of constipated children more than 4 years of age.[16] In addition, the sensation of fullness disappears after chronic stool retention and the need for retentive behavior disappears. The progressive fecal accumulation in the rectum eventually leads to pelvic floor muscle fatigue and poor anal sphincter competence, leading to leakage of formed, soft, or semiliquid stools.

Functional Nonretentive Fecal Incontinence

It has been recognized that not all patients with functional fecal incontinence have constipation.[17-19] They have functional nonretentive fecal incontinence. The diagnostic criteria suggested by the Rome III team[10] are listed in Table 12-5.

Most children with nonretentive fecal incontinence have daily bowel movements, and many have complete stool evacuations of normal consistency in their undergarments, which often occur in the afternoon. The diagnosis is made on the basis of a history of normal bowel movement frequency and no evidence of constipation by history and physical examination.

In the United States, functional nonretentive fecal incontinence is an infrequent cause of fecal incontinence in children. In our tertiary patient population at the University of Iowa Hospitals and Clinics, 6% of 323 consecutive children with fecal incontinence had functional nonretentive fecal incontinence, whereas 94% had underlying constipation.[20] In a primary care clinic, functional nonretentive fecal incontinence was present in 5% of the fecally incontinent children.[4] A recent study evaluating the applicability of the new PACCT criteria (similar to the Rome III criteria) reported functional nonretentive fecal incontinence in 9% of the patients referred to a tertiary Italian hospital with complaints of chronic constipation of at least 2 months' duration.[21] Burgers and Benninga[22] from the

TABLE 12-5. The Rome III Criteria for Functional Nonretentive Fecal Incontinence

Diagnostic Criteria for Functional Non-Retentive Fecal Incontinence[10]
Once a week or more for the preceding 2 months in a child of a developmental age > 4 years, a history of:
Defecation into places inappropriate to the social context
No evidence of an inflammatory, anatomic, metabolic or neoplastic process considered likely to be an explanation for the subject's symptoms
No evidence of fecal retention

TABLE 12-6. Important Information to Elicit by History and Physical Examination

History	Physical Examination
Complete with special attention to:	Complete with special attention to:
Stooling habits:	Abdominal examination
Character of stools in toilet	Anal inspection
Character of stools in underwear	Rectal digital examination
Stool withholding maneuvers	Neurologic examination, including perianal sensation testing
Age of onset of constipation/fecal incontinence	
Abdominal pain	
Urinary symptoms:	
Day wetting	
Bed wetting	
Urinary tract infections	
Dietary habits	

Netherlands reported that up to 20% of their children with fecal incontinence had nonretentive fecal incontinence. Functional nonretentive fecal incontinence is more common in boys; male to female ratios ranged from 3:1 to 6:1.

The underlying mechanism is largely unknown. It has been suggested that children with nonretentive fecal incontinence have a higher incidence of psychological problems. Van der Plas et al.[23] showed behavior problems in 35% of these children, but after treatment the abnormal scores improved significantly, supporting the notion that the fecal incontinence plays an etiologic role in the occurrence and maintenance of behavior problems in these children. It has been observed that the frequency of daytime and nighttime urinary incontinence is higher compared with constipated children, suggesting an overall delay in the achievement of toilet training or the neglect for normal physiological stimuli to go to the toilet. Anorectal manometry, rectal barostat, and colonic transit studies are normal. A complex multifactorial disorder has been suggested.[22]

INVESTIGATIONS

History

The history should include information regarding the general health of the child and the presenting signs and symptoms (Table 12-6). A careful history needs to elicit the intervals, amount, diameter, and consistency of bowel movements deposited into the toilet and of stools deposited into the underwear at the present time. The amount, intervals, diameter, and consistency of bowel movements are important because some children may have daily bowel movements but evacuate incompletely, as evidenced by periodic passage of very large amounts of stool of hard to loose consistency. Do the stools clog the toilet? Is or was stool withholding/retentive behavior present? What was the age at onset of constipation and/or fecal incontinence? Was there a problem with the timing of passage of meconium? The character of the stools is reviewed from birth for consistency, caliber, and frequency. Is abdominal pain present? Are urinary incontinence or urinary tract infection present? What are the dietary habits?

Physical Examination

The physical examination should be thorough in order to rule out an underlying disorder (see Table 12-6) and should include a rectal examination. Weight and height should be plotted. An abdominal fecal mass can be palpated in approximately half of these children during abdominal examination. Sometimes the mass extends throughout the entire colon, but more commonly the mass is felt suprapubically and midline, sometimes filling the left or the right lower quadrant. In many cases, inspection of the perineum shows fecal material. The anal size and location

need to be assessed. A low anal pressure during digital rectal examination suggests either fecal retention with inhibition of the anal resting pressure or a disease involving the external or internal anal sphincter, or both. The neurological examination should include perineal sensation testing in cooperative children using a Q-tip. Loss of perianal skin sensation can be associated with various neurologic diseases of the spinal cord.

In most cases, a carefully performed rectal examination causes a minimal degree of physical or emotional trauma to the child. Often the rectum is packed with stool, which may be of hard consistency or, more commonly, the outside of the fecal impaction feels like clay and the core of the fecal retention is rock hard. Sometimes the retained stool is soft to loose. No rectal fecal impaction is felt in children with a recent large bowel movement and in children with nonretentive fecal incontinence. Occasionally, the rectal examination will reveal an organic cause for the constipation, such as a large anal fissure, anal stenosis, anal atresia with perineal fistula, or a tight rectal ampulla, suggestive of Hirschsprung's disease. Rarely, a sacral tumor obstructing the rectum has been found. Failure to appreciate the degree of fecal retention in these children can lead to erroneous treatments, can further delay effective treatment, or can lead to misdirected psychotherapy.

Laboratory Investigation

Most children with functional constipation with or without fecal incontinence need no or minimal laboratory work-up apart from a careful history and physical examination. Rarely, blood studies (deficiency or excess of thyroid or adrenal hormones, electrolyte imbalances, and calcium level, antigliadin, anti-tissue transglutaminase (TTG) and endomysial antibodies), urine culture, x-ray studies, anorectal manometric studies, or rectal biopsy will be necessary. Special investigations are indicated in the presence of any child with failure to thrive, symptoms suggestive of Hirschsprung's disease, and when anorectal malformation or postoperative state are complicating factors.

Occult Blood Testing

It is recommended that a test for occult blood be performed on the stool of all infants with constipation, as well as in any child who has abdominal pain, failure to thrive, intermittent diarrhea, or a family history of colon cancer or colonic polyps.

Abdominal Radiographs

Radiologic studies usually are not indicated in uncomplicated constipation. A plain abdominal film can be very useful in assessing the presence or absence of retained stool, its extent, and whether or not the lower spine is normal, in a child with fecal incontinence and absence of a fecal mass on abdominal and rectal examination, in children who vehemently refuse the rectal examination, in children who are markedly obese, and in children who are still symptomatic while on laxatives.

Barium Enema Study

A barium enema is unnecessary in uncomplicated cases of constipation; however, an unprepped barium enema is helpful in the assessment of Hirschsprung's disease in which a transition zone between aganglionic and ganglionic bowel may be observed, in other neuronal disorders in which extensive bowel dilatation may be seen, and in the evaluation of the postsurgical patient operated for anal atresia or Hirschsprung's disease.

Colonic Transit Study

A colonic transit study provides an objective measure of the severity of constipation in children, but is unnecessary in most children with functional constipation with or without fecal incontinence.[24] It does not influence the initial decision as to how to treat the child.

Anorectal Manometry

Anorectal manometry is unnecessary in children with functional constipation with or without functional fecal incontinence. The main clinical role of anorectal manometry is in the evaluation of children with severe constipation, where the diagnosis of Hirschsprung's disease needs to be excluded. It may also be helpful in evaluating other conditions, such as spinal defects and anal achalasia.

We have performed numerous manometric studies in children with functional constipation and fecal incontinence and have documented many abnormalities, including increased threshold to rectal distention and decreased rectal contractility as compared to controls.[25] In follow-up, after 3 years of therapy, many children will show continued abnormalities of anorectal function, leaving them at risk for recurrent problems.[26,27] Another abnormality is the contraction of the external anal sphincter and pelvic floor muscles instead of relaxation of these muscles during defecation attempts.[25,28,29]

Colonic Motility Study

A colonic motility study is unnecessary in most children with functional constipation. A colonic motility study may be helpful in children with suspected dysmotility of the colon or the total gastrointestinal tract.

TREATMENT

Functional Constipation in Infants and Toddlers

After assessment of the constipated infant/toddler, all parents receive education, including explanation about the hard and painful defecations that are the primary precipitants of constipation during infancy and the toddler years.[1,30-32]

Diet and Fiber

Acute, simple constipation in infants and toddlers is usually treated first with sorbitol-containing juices, such as prune, pear, and apple juice; addition of pureed fruits and vegetables; formula changes; or medication with high sugar content, such as barley malt extract or corn syrup. Dietary changes can include decreasing excessive milk intake.

Several studies have claimed a causal relationship between cow's milk exposure and constipation in children,[33-37] but this could not be confirmed by Simeone et al.,[38] Loening-Baucke,[1] and Benninga et al.[39]

Laxative

If despite dietary changes, the stool is still hard and painful to evacuate, then osmotic laxatives are given, such as polyethylene glycol, lactulose, sorbitol, or milk of magnesia (Table 12-7). The key to effective maintenance is ensuring painless defecation until the child is comfortable and acquisition of toilet learning is complete. Behavior modification using rewards for successes in toilet learning is helpful.

Functional Constipation With and Without Fecal Incontinence in Children and Adolescents

Most children with functional constipation with or without fecal incontinence benefit from a precise, well-organized plan. The treatment is comprehensive and has four phases: education, disimpaction, prevention of reaccumulation of stools, and withdrawal of treatment.

Education

Effective education is an important first step in the treatment and includes developmentally appropriate explanation to parents and child of the anatomy and physiology of defecation and its associated disorders, explanation of the prevalence of constipation and fecal incontinence and discussion of the related shame, embarrassment, and social issues.

The physician must explain to the family that the rock-hard stools are difficult and painful for the child to pass. The child therefore associates bowel movements with pain, which leads to stool withholding, which leads to rock-hard stools. Thus a vicious cycle is started that leads to chronic fecal retention and eventually to functional fecal incontinence. We point out that constipation existed long before incontinence first was noted. The child and parent are told that many children are troubled with this condition. We stress that the stooling problem is not caused by a disturbance in the psychological behavior of the child and is not the parents' fault. It occurs involuntarily and usually without the knowledge of the child, although the child may be able to prevent the incontinence for short periods of time if the child concentrates carefully on closing the external anal sphincter and uses the toilet frequently. The parents need to understand that there is no quick solution for this condition and that months to years of treatment will be necessary.

In most cases, a detailed plan eliminates the parents' and the children's frustration and improves compliance for the prolonged treatment necessary. Some of the parents do not possess the skills necessary to follow a demanding regimen or to effectively manage their child's behavior. These parents need to be identified so that the educational efforts can be optimized. A caring relationship is established, because the treatment of

TABLE 12-7. **Suggested Medications and Dosages for Maintenance Therapy of Constipation**

Medication	Age	Dose
For Long-Term Treatment (Years):		
Polyethylene glycol		
3350 (MiraLax)	>1 month	0.7 g/kg body weight/day[16,30] or 0.4 g/kg body weight/day[54]
3350+electrolytes (Movicol)		13.8-40 g/day[40,41]
4000 (Forlax)	>6 months	0.5 g/kg body weight/day[43]
Lactulose or sorbitol	>1 months	1-3 mL/kg body weight/day, divide in 1-2 doses
Milk of magnesia	>1 month	1-3 mL/kg body weight/day, divide in 1-2 doses
Mineral oil	>12 months	1-3 mL/kg body weight/d, divided in 1-2 doses
For Short-Term Treatment (Months):		
Senna (Senokot) syrup/tablets	1-5 years	5 mL (1 tab) with breakfast, max. 15 mL/d
	5-15 years	2 tablets with breakfast, maximum 3 tablets/d
Glycerin enemas	> 10 years	20-30 mL/day (1/2 glycerin and ½ normal saline)
Bisacodyl suppositories	>10 years	10 mg daily

TABLE 12-8. **Suggested Medications for Fecal Disimpaction**

Medication	Age	Dose
Slow Oral Disimpaction		
Polyethylene 3350 without electrolytes (for 3 days)[42]		1.5 g/kg body weight/day
Polyethylene 3350 with electrolytes (for 6 days)[41]	2- to 4-year-olds	52 g/day
	5- to 11-year-olds	78 g/day
Milk of magnesia (for 7 days)		2 mL/kg body weight twice/day
Mineral oil (for 7 days)		3 mL/kg body weight twice/day
Lactulose or sorbitol (7 days)		2 mL/kg body weight twice/day
Rapid Rectal Disimpaction		
Glycerin suppositories	Infants and toddlers	
Phosphate enema	<1 year	60 mL
	>1 year	6 mL/kg body weight, up to 135 mL twice

functional constipation with or without fecal incontinence is a long-term process. Without the family's and the child's compliance, the recommended therapy will not be successful.

Disimpaction

Suggested medications and dosages for disimpaction are given in Table 12-8. Disimpaction can be achieved comfortably, without the use of enemas, with oral laxatives, such as polyethylene glycol with electrolytes[40,41] and without electrolytes.[42,43] A study by Youssef et al.[42] demonstrated that 1.5 g/kg body weight/day of electrolyte-free polyethylene glycol for 3 days was efficient in removing the rectal fecal impaction within five days. In a study by Candy et al.,[41] 92% of the children were disimpacted using an escalating dose of up to 78 g of polyethylene glycol 3350 plus electrolytes for 6 days. The fecal impaction can also be softened and liquefied with large quantities of oral mineral oil or other osmotic laxatives with the oral administration continued daily until the fecal mass is passed. Fecal incontinence, abdominal pain, and cramping may increase during oral disimpaction.

The rapid removal of the fecal retention with hypertonic phosphate enema (135 mL) is now rarely used. Severe vomiting with hypernatremia, hyperphosphatemia, hypocalcemia, hypokalemia, dehydration, seizures, coma, and death have been reported after the first phosphate enema in a few children with functional constipation who were less than 5 years of age.[44]

Therefore, the hypertonic enema should be given in the clinic or doctor's office to those children who have never received a phosphate enema before. Normal (isotonic) saline enemas may be used but are often not effective. Cleansing soap-suds enemas should be avoided, because they can result in bowel necrosis, perforation, and death. Tap-water enemas are often not effective and should not be used because they can cause water intoxication by dilution of serum electrolytes, seizures, or death.

Manual disimpaction is an extreme technique and should be performed rarely, if necessary, under anesthesia.

Prevention of Reaccumulation of Stools (Maintenance Therapy)

Behavior Modification. The child needs to be reconditioned to normal bowel habits by regular toilet use. The child is encouraged to sit on the toilet for up to 5 minutes, three to four times a day following meals. The gastrocolic reflex, which goes into effect during and shortly after a meal, should be used to his or her advantage. The children and their parents need to be instructed to keep a daily record of bowel movements, fecal and urinary incontinence, and medication use. This helps to monitor compliance and helps to make appropriate adjustments in the treatment program by parents and physician. If necessary, positive reinforcement and rewards for compliant behavior are given for effort and later for success, using star charts, little presents, or television viewing or computer game time as rewards.

Fiber. Dietary fiber increases water retention and provides substrate for bacterial growth with increase of colonic flora and gas production during colonic fermentation of fiber. Several studies reported that the fiber intake is lower[45,46] or similar[24] in constipated children as compared to controls. The dietary recommendation for children older than 2 years of age is to consume an amount of dietary fiber equivalent to age in years plus 5 g/day.[47] Recommended are several servings daily from a variety of fiber-rich foods such as whole-grain breads and cereals, fruits, vegetables, and legumes. Synthetic preparations are available, such as guar gum and pectin fiber, glucomannan,[48,49] cocoa husk,[50] or a yogurt drink with a fiber mixture.[51] Treatment programs for the majority of children with functional constipation have included increase in dietary fiber, in addition to scheduled toilet sittings and daily laxatives.[19,25-28]

Laxatives. In most constipated patients, daily defecation is maintained by the daily administration of laxatives beginning in the evening of the clinic visit. Suggested dosages of commonly used laxatives are given in Table 12-7.

Polyethylene glycol (PEG) without added electrolytes (PEG 3350, MiraLax, Braintree Laboratories, Inc., Braintree, MA; PEG 4000, Forlax, Ipsen, Paris, France) and polyethylene glycol 3350 with electrolytes (Movicol, Norgine Pharmaceuticals Ltd., United Kingdom) have been developed and now tested for long-term daily use as a laxative in infants, toddlers, and older children.[40,41,43,52-58] PEG is tasteless, odorless, and colorless and has no grit when stirred in juice, Kool-aid or water for several minutes. PEG is not degraded by bacteria; is not readily absorbed and thus acts as an excellent osmotic agent; and is safe.[41,52,56]

Lactulose and sorbitol are nonabsorbable carbohydrates. They cause increased water content by the osmotic effects of lactulose, sorbitol, and their metabolites. They are fermented by colonic bacteria, thereby producing gas and sometimes causing abdominal discomfort. Both are easily taken by children when mixed in soft drinks.

The mechanism of action of milk of magnesia is the relative nonabsorption of magnesium and the resultant increase in luminal osmolality.

Mineral oil is converted into hydroxy fatty acids, which induce fluid and electrolyte accumulation. Mineral oil should never be force-fed or given to patients with dysphagia or vomiting because of the danger of aspiration pneumonia. Anal seepage of the mineral oil, often causing an orange stain, is an undesirable side effect, especially in children going to school.

Senna has an effect on intestinal motility as well as on fluid and electrolyte transport and will stimulate defecation. We use senna when liquid stools produced by osmotic laxatives are retained and in children with fecal incontinence and constipation due to organic or anatomic causes. The North American Society for Pediatric Gastroenterology, Hepatology and Nutrition has recommended senna products for short-term therapy.[59]

Occasionally, I advise the use of a 10-mg bisacodyl suppository or either a phosphate or a glycerin enema daily as initial treatment for several months in an older child who would like immediate control of the functional fecal incontinence.

The most commonly used laxatives today are polyethylene glycol and lactulose. Magnesium hydroxide (milk of magnesia), mineral oil, and sorbitol have also been used for long-term treatment. Laxatives should be used according to body weight and severity of the constipation. The choice of medication for functional constipation does not seem as important as the child's and parents' compliance with the treatment regimen. There is no set dosage for any laxative. There is only a starting dosage for each child (see Table 12-7) that must be adjusted to induce one to two bowel movements per day that are loose enough to ensure complete daily emptying of the lower bowel and to prevent fecal incontinence and abdominal pain.

Psychological Treatment. Functional constipation and in particularly fecal incontinence affect the lives of these children and families in several areas: physically, psychologically, educationally, socially, and in terms of self-esteem. If a coexisting behavior problem is secondary to constipation and/or functional fecal incontinence, then it will improve with treatment. The presence of coexisting behavioral problems often is associated with poor treatment outcome. Children who do not improve should be referred for further evaluation, because continued problems can be due to noncompliance or control issues by the child and/or the parent.

Follow-up Visits and Weaning From Medication

Because the management of functional constipation with or without fecal incontinence requires considerable patience and effort on the part of the child and parents, it is important to provide necessary support and encouragement through regularly scheduled office visits. Progress should be initially assessed periodically by reviewing the stool records and repeating the abdominal and rectal examination to ensure that the problem is adequately managed. If necessary, dosage adjustment is made and the child and parents are encouraged to continue with the regimen. After regular bowel habits are established, the frequency of toilet sitting is reduced and the medication dosage is gradually decreased to a dosage that maintains one bowel movement daily and prevents the fecal incontinence. Once the child feels the urge to defecate and initiates toilet use on his/her own, then the scheduled toilet times are discontinued. After 6 to 12 months, reduction with discontinuation of the medication is attempted. Treatment (laxatives and/or toilet sitting) needs to resume if constipation, fecal incontinence, or abdominal pain recur.

What Can Go Wrong in the Treatment?

Physician as well as the parents and children make frequent mistakes. Frequent mistakes by physicians are treating with stool softeners and laxatives, but not removing the fecal impaction; removing the fecal impaction, but failing to start maintenance therapy; giving too low a laxative dose; not controlling the adequacy and success of therapy with follow-up visits and a rectal examination; stopping the laxative too soon; and not providing education, anticipatory guidance, continuing support, and regular follow-up. Frequent mistakes by the parents and children are not insisting that the child use the toilet at regular times for defecation trials; not giving the medication daily, or worse, discontinuing the laxatives as soon as the fecal incontinence has disappeared; and not restarting the laxative after the child had a relapse.

Treatment of Nonretentive Fecal Incontinence

The treatment of children with nonretentive fecal incontinence has not been well defined. The treatment approach consists of education, filling out a bowel diary, and strict toilet training (three times daily, 5 minutes after meals without any distractions). An additional reward system, such as praise and small gifts, can enhance motivation. An appropriate diagnosis of functional nonretentive fecal incontinence is significant because these patients do not benefit from laxatives. It has been suggested that some children with nonretentive fecal incontinence may benefit from psychological intervention.[59,60]

OUTCOME

Constipation in Infants and Toddlers

Dietary changes resolved all symptoms of constipation in 25%.[1] With laxative treatment, 92% of constipated infants and toddlers responded.[1]

Functional Constipation With and Without Fecal Incontinence in Children and Adolescents

Outcome in most publications of functional constipated children (more than 4 years of age) with or without fecal incontinence was assessed by rates of successful treatment and recovery. The constipation was rated as successfully treated if the child had in the last month more than three bowel movements per week, fewer than two fecal incontinence episodes per month, and suffered no abdominal pain, independent of laxative use.[12,62] Recovery was defined by the same criteria, except that the child was off laxatives for at least 1 month.[17,25-28,63-65] Both clinical experience and data from the literature suggest that the longer functional constipation goes unrecognized and untreated, the less successful is the treatment.

Behavior Modification

The only study to examine behavior modification as monotherapy for children with functional constipation and fecal incontinence was by Nolan et al.[64] from Australia. In this randomized study, they found that 1 year after start of behavior modification, 36% had recovered, and more children, 51%, had recovered with behavior modification and additional laxative treatment ($p < 0.08$).

Fiber

Three randomized double-blind controlled studies to evaluate fiber in constipated children are available and show benefits.[49-51] Glucomannan, 100 mg/kg body weight daily (maximal 5 g/day) with 50 mL fluid/500 mg and placebo for 4 weeks each were evaluated in 31 constipated children, in a crossover design.[49] While on fiber, significantly fewer children complained of abdominal pain as compared to placebo (10% versus 42%) and significantly more children were relieved from constipation (45% versus 13%). In another study, a significantly higher number of parents and children reported subjective improvement in stool consistency while on cocoa husk.[50] Kokke el al.[51] reported that, in an 8-week trial, a mixture of dietary fiber was similar to lactulose in regard to stool frequency, fecal incontinence frequency, abdominal pain, and flatulence.

The recommendation to increase fiber in the diet of constipated children should be continued.

Laxatives and Behavior Modification

One-Year Outcome. At least nine well-designed studies have evaluated 1-year outcome (Table 12-9). Laxative treatment with behavior modification dramatically improved constipation, abdominal pain, and functional fecal incontinence. Four of these studies looked at children who had constipation with or without functional fecal incontinence.[62,63,66,67] They showed that 47% of these children in the United States,[66] 47% in Italy,[67] and 31% to 59% in the Netherlands[62,63] had recovered 1 year after start of treatment (see Table 12-9). The largest study by van Ginkel et al.[62] involved 399 Dutch children; 83% were successfully treated with lactulose and 59% had recovered 1 year after start of treatment.

Five of the nine studies evaluated children with functional constipation with fecal incontinence. The 1-year recovery rates ranged from 33% to 51%.[16,25,64,68,69] They showed that 33% to 51% of the children in the United States[16,25,68,69] and 51% of the children in Australia[64] had recovered 1 year after start of therapy with milk of magnesia, Lactulose, or polyethylene glycol.

Long-Term Outcome. Long-term outcome studies (4- to 10-year follow-up) report recovery rates between 48% and 69% (Table 12-10).[62,67,70-73] One study specifically targeted younger children (less than 4 years of age) to examine whether early intervention might improve outcome.[70] Of 90 children who were followed for a mean of 7 years after beginning treatment, 63% recovered. Staiano et al.[67] followed 62 children, 1 to 11 years of age, and found that 48% had recovered after 5 years. Early age of onset of constipation and family history of constipation were predictive of persistence, they found. The largest follow-up study is by van Ginkel et al.[62] They initially enrolled 418 children with functional constipation, two thirds with and one third without fecal incontinence. All were older than 5 years of age at initiation of therapy. Some of the children were followed for as long as 8 years, with a median follow-up of 5 years. Fifty-nine percent had recovered at the 1-year follow-up. Three-year data showed a decline in the recovery rate, to about 50%, as some children relapsed and were not restarted on laxative therapy. The recovery rate of 193 children was 63% after 5 years, 69% of 120 children had recovered after 7 years, and 68% of 48 children had recovered after 8 years.[62] However, 50% of recovered children had at least one relapse, and approximately 30% of children who had reached adolescence were still having problems with constipation or fecal incontinence. These findings suggest that this is not a problem all children will eventually outgrow.

Other Treatments

Biofeedback Treatment as Adjunct Therapy. The concept of applying biofeedback to certain anorectal functions is logical because anorectal function is regulated by physiologic processes, some of which are under cortical influence, such as the ability to sense rectal distention and impending defecation and the ability to relax and contract the striated muscles of the pelvic floor. Patients can be taught these functions. Previous research has shown that from 25% to 56% of constipated children have an abnormal contraction of the external anal sphincter and pelvic floor muscles during attempted defecation. One small randomized study did show statistically significant benefit of additional biofeedback treatment[74]; however, four other

TABLE 12-9. **One-Year Recovery Rates in Constipated Children With or Without Fecal Incontinence**

Author	Subject Number	Laxative	Recovery Rate
Constipation With or Without Fecal Incontinence			
Abrahamian and Lloyd-Still[66]	68	Multiple laxatives	47%
Staiano et al.[67]	31	Lactulose	47%
van Ginkel et al.[63]	212	Lactulose	31%
van Ginkel et al.[62]	399	Lactulose	59%
Constipation With Fecal Incontinence			
Levine and Bakow[68]	110	Mineral oil	51%
Loening-Baucke[25]	97	Milk of magnesia	43%
Nolan et al.[64]	83	Multiple laxatives	51%
Loening-Baucke[69]	181	Milk of magnesia	39%
Loening-Baucke and Pashankar[16]	39	Polyethylene glycol 3350	33%

TABLE 12-10. **Long-Term Recovery Rates in Constipated Children With and Without Fecal Incontinence**

Author	Subject Number	Age (Years)	Laxative	Years of Follow-up	Recovery Rate
Constipation Only					
Loening-Baucke[70]	90	1-4	Milk of magnesia	Mean 7	63%
Michaud et al.[73]	45	0.5-14	Lactulose	10	54%
Constipation With and Without Fecal Incontinence					
Staiano et al.[67]	62	1-11	Lactulose	5	48%
van Ginkel et al.[62]	193	>5	Lactulose	5	69%
Constipation With Fecal Incontinence					
Loening-Baucke[71]	129	>4	Milk of magnesia	Mean 4	53%
Procter and Loader[72]	76	0.3-16	Laxative	6	64%

randomized studies found no statistically significant benefit of biofeedback treatment with conventional treatment when compared to conventional treatment alone, on 6-month, 1-year, and long-term follow-up.[29,65,71,75]

Cisapride. Cisapride induces gastrointestinal peristalsis by stimulation of $5-HT_4$ receptors in the myenteric plexus and antagonizing $5-HT_3$ receptors. It appears that cisapride does not contribute significantly to the recovery from childhood constipation, and it has been taken off the market because of serious cardiac side effects.

Functional Nonretentive Fecal Incontinence

A study of children with functional nonretentive fecal incontinence in which laxative treatment with and without biofeedback treatment was compared showed poor clinical outcome in both groups (39% versus 19%).[23] Another study raised the possibility that there may be a negative impact of oral laxatives treatment in these children.[19]

Voskuijl et al.[76] studied 114 children with functional nonretentive fecal incontinence for approximately 10 years. Recovery was defined as having less than one episode of fecal incontinence in 2 weeks while not using medication, such as loperamide, for at least 1 month. After 2 years of intensive medical and behavioral treatment, only 29% had recovered. Thereafter, a steady increase in recovery percentage was seen, 65% at 5 years and 90% at 10 years follow-up. At the age of 12 years, 49% of patients still had not recovered, and at age 18 years,

15% had not recovered. No prognostic factors for success were found.[76]

Because the etiology of functional nonretentive fecal incontinence is not known, further studies and evaluation of different treatments will be necessary before better treatment recommendations can be made.

REFERENCES

9. Hyman PE, Milla PJ, Benninga MA, et al. Childhood functional gastrointestinal disorders: neonate/toddler. Gastroenterology 2006;130:1519–1526.
10. Rasquin A, Di Lorenzo C, Forber D, et al. Childhood functional gastrointestinal disorders: child/adolescent. Gastroenterology 2006;130:1527–1537.
16. Loening-Baucke V, Pashankar DS. A randomized, prospective, comparison study of polyethylene glycol 3350 without electrolytes and milk of magnesia in children with constipation and fecal incontinence. Pediatrics 2006;118:528–535.
40. Candy D, Belsey J. Macrogol (polyethylene glycol) laxatives in children with functional constipation and faecal impaction: a systemic review. Arch Dis Child 2009;94:156–160.
62. van Ginkel R, Reitsma JB, Büller HA, et al. Childhood constipation: longitudinal follow-up beyond puberty. Gastroenterology 2003;125:357–363.
76. Voskuijl WP, Reitsma JB, van Ginkel R, et al. Longitudinal follow-up of children with functional nonretentive fecal incontinence. Clin Gastroenterol Hepatol 2006;4:67–72.

See expertconsult.com for a complete list of references and the review questions for this chapter.

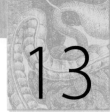

13 FAILURE TO THRIVE

Harohalli Shashidhar • Vasundhara Tolia

As an integral component of childhood, growth is an important indicator of a child's well-being. The growth pattern is the result of the complex interaction between genetic and environmental factors.[1] When children do not grow and meet the expectations that their families and society hold, there are implications for both the child and family. Growth monitoring, an essential tool of pediatric health assessment, aids in diagnosis of growth deviations from the expected norm and gives early clues to the presence of an underlying illness.

EPIDEMIOLOGY

Failure to thrive (FTT) describes inadequate growth in childhood and implies significant deviation from expected or established growth patterns. Failure to thrive is attributable to a set of heterogeneous factors that affect growth. In the influential textbook of the late 19th century, Emmett Holt described an infant who "ceased to thrive" in 1897. The term *failure to thrive* may not have been used in print until 1933.[2] *Growth* or *weight faltering* is preferred by some to avoid the pejorative "failure."[3]

The prevalence of FTT has been reported as 1 to 5% of all referrals to pediatric hospitals and from 10 to 20% of all children who are treated in ambulatory care settings.[4] In one of the authors' personal series (V. Tolia), the frequency of the diagnosis of FTT in the gastroenterology outpatient clinic at a tertiary care institution varied between 2.7% and 6.6% annually during the years 1998 to 2003 in neurologically normal children, with an average incidence of approximately 4% during these 6 years.

The UNICEF report in 2006 highlights the prevalence of failure to thrive or underweight status, especially in the developing world. An estimated 148 million children under 5 years (23%) are underweight, more than half of them being in Southern Asia. Approximately 17% of infants born annually in the developing world and 7% in industrialized countries weigh less than 2500 grams (5.5 pounds). The underweight prevalence in rural areas is almost double that for their urban counterparts, whereas it is similar in boys and girls.[5]

In the United States, 2% of children under 5 years, are underweight and 8% of infants are born with a birth weight less than 2500 g.[5,6] Results from the 2003-2006 NHANES indicate that an estimated 3.3% of children and adolescents aged 2 to 19 years are underweight. Trends from 1971-1974 to 2003-2006 show an overall decrease in underweight among children and adolescents from 5.1% to 3.3%.[7]

FTT has crucial implications for the child, including physical and developmental retardation as well as emotional and behavioral problems.[8] In the late 1960s, the "medical" etiology such as metabolic, infectious, and nutritionally derived conditions was made distinct from the environmental aspects when evaluating poor growth during infancy and childhood, differentiating "organic" from "nonorganic" failure to thrive.[9] However, this dichotomy in diagnosis is inadequate to explain a significant overlap in the spectrum of growth failure and has a limited usefulness because multiple factors may contribute to FTT in a patient. There are three basic mechanisms for occurrence of FTT: (1) insufficient nutritional intake because of the child's inability to feed properly, e.g., neurological disabilities, oropharyngeal malformations, feeding aversion, anorexia; (2) proper amount of nutrition consumed but inadequately absorbed and/or utilized, e.g., malabsorption syndromes; and (3) abnormal utilization of calories, or increased metabolic requirements as in chronic diseases or hypermetabolic states. It may appear that children with genetic or chromosomal abnormalities do not belong to any of these groups. A majority of these are programmed to have low growth parameters, and although they remain at special risk for developing FTT, use of specific growth charts will plot their growth appropriately. FTT occurs when deviation from their established growth patterns is present.

DEFINITION

There is no consensus regarding the definition and criteria of FTT.[10] *Failure to thrive* is a term used by pediatricians to describe infants and toddlers, under 3 years of age, with an abnormally low weight for age and gender. In older children, it is commonly referred to as growth failure. Identification of FTT and an assessment of the severity of the nutritional state are important to identify children at risk and to provide appropriate intervention. It is surprising, therefore, that such a common and important problem lacks a consistent definition.[11]

Although there is consensus that the definition of failure to thrive should be based on anthropometric parameters, there are no universally accepted anthropometric criteria.[12]

The usual indicators in identifying growth deviation are weight or height for age, or weight for height and, in some instances, body mass index. The measures employed to identify growth deviation are:

1. Major percentile line on the growth charts (3rd or 5th percentile)
2. Standard deviation from the mean weight/height
3. Percentage of median ({(actual weight − median weight)/median weight} × 100)
4. *Z* scores, or standard deviation scores, that express anthropometric data normalized for age and sex {(observed weight − median weight)/standard deviation of reference population}

Commonly utilized cutoff values for diagnosis of failure to thrive are included in Table 13-1.[13] Z scores calculated with software available from the Centers for Disease Control and Prevention are more often employed in research studies to allow more precise description of anthropometric status than percentile curves.

Other tools employed in defining failure to thrive include conditional growth charts, wherein deviation from growth is interpreted in terms of previously established growth patterns.[14] A recent prospective study comparing five anthropometric methods of classifying failure to thrive validated weight for age as a simple and reasonable marker for FTT.[15]

The importance of utilizing identical criteria to assess and compare prevalence of undernutrition for research and clinical purposes cannot be overemphasized. It has been shown that different criteria of growth failure identify children with different risk profiles and yield a wide-ranging prevalence. A Danish study of birth cohorts investigated three of the criteria for FTT: slow weight gain conditional on birth weight, thinness based on low body mass index, and downward crossing of two or more percentiles from birth. The criterion of conditional weight gain was associated with lower birth weight, small-for-gestational-age, and deviant overall development. In contrast, downward crossing of percentiles on an ordinary weight-for-age chart was associated with a low risk of adverse physical and mental development.[16] An earlier study also found that crossing of two weight percentile lines suggested only borderline failure to thrive, although this included a subgroup of children who suffer adverse long-term cognitive outcomes.[17]

The World Health Organization (WHO) undertook a comprehensive review of the uses and interpretation of anthropometric references in the early 1990s. Subsequently, an international study was conducted to collect primary growth data and related information from 8440 healthy breast-fed infants and young children from diverse ethnic backgrounds and cultural settings (Brazil, Ghana, India, Norway, Oman, and the United States) to establish the new 2006 WHO child growth charts. The use of different growth charts also classifies children with FTT differently. Using the CDC 2000, NCHS 1978, and WHO 2006 charts, the incidence of failure to thrive varied from 0.7 to 4.0% in the same cohort of infants younger than 3 months. Traditional terminology used to describe failure to thrive includes "wasting" (underweight for height) and "stunting" (below normal height for age).[18]

Wasting or a weight deficit is suggested as a marker for acute undernutrition, whereas stunting is an indicator for chronic malnutrition. An anthropometric classification of FTT using all three growth parameters for practical use (weight, height, and head circumference) is shown in Table 13-2. This divides the diagnosis into three major categories with the disease groups associated with each type.

NORMAL GROWTH PATTERNS

Diagnosis and definition of failure to thrive depends on recognition of normal or expected growth pattern and the physiological variations from the norm.

The pattern of growth may vary in specific circumstances. Breast-fed infants follow a different growth trajectory than bottle-fed babies. They display a faster growth rate in the first 2 or 3 months, after which the growth slows down in comparison to bottle-fed infants. Despite their slower growth rate, breast-fed infants eventually reach the same final height by 2 years of age.[19] The new child growth standards are based on the premise that the breast-fed baby is the norm for healthy growth among infants.[20] Differential growth patterns and growth velocity in premature or low-birth-weight infants require corrected age to be used to plot the growth percentiles. Separate growth charts are available for children with Down syndrome and for children with cerebral palsy. Altered growth patterns are observed in almost all the autosomal chromosomal anomalies.

Growth from birth to maturity has been described as occurring in three additive phases: infancy, childhood, and adolescence.[21] Each stage is characterized by early rapid growth that later reaches a plateau before the next stage of growth begins, until adult stature is reached at the end of adolescence. There are periods of saltation and stasis despite the widely held belief that growth is a continuous process.[22]

The growth velocity slows at about 8 years of age. In fact, no measurable growth may be observed in normal healthy children between 7 and 10 years of age for up to 3 months.[23] This second phase ends as rapid growth is once more introduced at 10 to 12 years of age in the phase known as the adolescent growth spurt, which lasts through to adulthood. It reaches a peak about 2 years after it begins, at a point of "peak velocity," and moves gradually toward the adult stature at 16 to 18 years. This postnatal somatic growth variation is thus genetically determined but modified by the environment.[24]

Many children demonstrate physiological shifts to ascend or descend through the growth centiles to be closer to the 50th percentile, a phenomenon described as "regression to mean."[24]

TABLE 13-1. Commonly Used Criteria for Defining Failure to Thrive

A. Percentiles
   Weight or weight for height less than 3rd or 5th percentile[13] or
B. Percent of median
   Weight expressed as a percentage of median weight for age[13] or
   Weight expressed as a percentage of median weight for height (<80 being abnormal)[13]
   Height expressed as a percentage of median height for age (<90% being abnormal)[13]
C. Standard deviation or Z scores
   Weight (or) <2 standard deviations below the mean for sex and age
   Weight for height < 2 standard deviations below the mean for sex and age
   Z scores of −2.0 or less for weight for age, height for age, or weight for height[13]
D. Crossing of percentiles
   Downward crossing of more than two *major* percentile lines after having achieved a previously stable pattern

TABLE 13-2. Three Major Anthropologic Categories of Failure to Thrive

	Weight	Height	Head Circumference	Associated Diseases
Type I	Decreased	Decreased/normal	Normal	Malnutrition of organic or nonorganic etiology usually secondary to intestinal, pancreatic, liver diseases or systemic illness or psychosocial factors
Type II	Decreased	Decreased	Normal	Endocrinopathies, bony dystrophy, constitutional short stature
Type III	Decreased	Decreased	Decreased	Chromosomal, metabolic disease, intrauterine and perinatal insults, severe malnutrition

Infants may also demonstrate shifts consistent with their genetic potential such as "catch-down" and "catch-up" growth. Seasonal variation in growth has been described.[25] Many of these growth deviations can only be distinguished in retrospect and highlight the difficulty in separating pathological growth failure from physiological variation in growth. A longitudinal study of children in California demonstrated that up to 62% of children between birth and 6 months of age, 20% to 27% of children between 6 and 24 months of age, and 6% to 15% of children between 24 and 60 months of age crossed two major percentiles in weight for height. Significant shifts were also demonstrated in body mass index for children between 24 and 60 months of age.[26] Pediatricians must consider the prevalence of growth rate shifts during infancy and early childhood while they counsel parents regarding growth or prior to additional evaluations of deviant growth.

Other entities such as familial short stature and constitutional leanness or thinness highlight the genetic variations that underpin physiologic growth variants. Constitutional leanness denotes a nonpathologic state of decreased body mass index that has been described to occur both in children and in adults.[27,28]

Among preterm newborns, the term *small for gestational age* (SGA) usually refers to infants born with a birth weight below the 10th percentile, based on population curves. Preterm SGA newborns comprise a heterogeneous group. The majority of these SGA infants have intrauterine growth retardation (IUGR).[29] Symmetrical SGA refers to both body weight and head circumference below the 10th percentile for gestational age in relation to standard curves and is considered to begin in early pregnancy. Asymmetrical SGA refers to birth weight below the 10th percentile for gestational age.[30]

The value of any index of FTT lies in its usefulness in identifying the child at risk and in predicting the severity of other coexisting nutrition-related problems. Attention to the percentile curves of length, weight, and head circumference gives valuable clues to the etiology of FTT. When all measurements are decreased, the incidence of organic disease is about 70%. Gastrointestinal and nutritional disorders are more common when only the weight is below the 5th percentile.[31] Table 13-3 shows a partial list of various diseases in which FTT can occur.

PATHOGENESIS

FTT affects growing children in many important ways regardless of its etiology. FTT is associated with persistently small stature. Severe malnutrition has been shown to cause permanent structural aberrations in the central nervous system.[32] Even mild malnutrition in the absence of significant growth failure has been associated with developmental impairment and disability.[33] Moreover, undernourished children with FTT are more likely to have infectious diseases.[34,35] They are more prone to changes in cell-mediated immunity, complement levels, and opsonization that increase susceptibility to various infections.[36] Severe FTT can be associated with secondary changes in cardiovascular and gastrointestinal functioning.[37]

Failure to thrive in infancy has been shown to be associated with persisting deficits in intelligence quotient (IQ) in later childhood.[3]

Physiological growth variants such as constitutional leanness have been shown to have altered resting energy expenditure in relation to fat-free mass, and recently a mitochondrial gene variant has been described in mothers and their offspring who are lean.[38,28]

CAUSES AND CONTRIBUTORY FACTORS

FTT is most commonly caused by inadequate calorie intake, which can arise when food is not available or from insufficient food intake due to feeding and behavioral problems. Table 13-4 depicts potential risk factors for the development of this type of FTT.

Psychosocial factors contributing to FTT are the emotional neglect of the child or a lack of appropriate attachment, a lack of education and knowledge about parenting, poverty, and abuse of the child. Poverty by itself is the single greatest risk factor for undernutrition.[39]

Parents may make accidental errors in food preparation or may not know basic child-care practices.[40] Many mothers

TABLE 13-3. Major Causes of Failure to Thrive

Decreased Caloric Intake

Aversive feeding disorders
Impaired swallowing
    Neurological (e.g., brainstem lesions, Arnold-Chiari malformation)
    Dysphagia (e.g., eosinophilic esophagitis)
Injury to mouth and esophagus
    Trauma and burns – physical, chemical, or radiation
    Oropharyngeal or esophageal inflammation
Congenital anomalies affecting oropharyngeal and upper gastrointestinal tract
Chromosomal abnormalities
Genetic diseases
Diseases leading to anorexia (e.g., systemic illness, psychological, acquired immunodeficiency syndrome, neglect or abuse, chemotherapy or radiation therapy)
Accidental or inadvertent
    Difficult lactation
    Improper formula preparation or feeding technique
    Poor diet/bizarre diet
Psychosocial
    Maternal and/or infant related factors
Iatrogenic
    Restrictive or elimination diets
    Special diets from misdiagnosis

Increased Requirements

Sepsis/febrile states
Trauma
Burns
Acquired or congenital chronic cardiorespiratory disease
Hyperthyroidism
Diencephalic syndrome
Excessive involuntary movement or poorly controlled seizure
Chronic systemic diseases including chronic infections

Impaired Utilization

Inborn errors of metabolism

Excessive Caloric Losses

Persistent vomiting (e.g., gastric outlet obstruction, gastroesophageal reflux)
Malabsorptive states due to mucosal or luminal etiology (e.g., celiac disease, protein-losing enteropathy, enzyme deficiency, inflammatory or allergic enteropathy)
Pancreatic insufficiency (e.g., cystic fibrosis, Shwachman-Diamond syndrome)
Congenital gut lesions or short gut syndrome leading to intestinal failure
Chronic immunodeficiency
Chronic enteric infections or parasitic infestations
Postenteritis syndrome
Chronic liver disease with cholestasis

TABLE 13-4. Risk Factors for FTT Associated With Inadequate Caloric Intake

Infant Related
IUGR
Prematurity
In utero toxin exposure (e.g., alcohol, tobacco, cocaine)
Postnatal toxin exposure (e.g., lead, prematurity)
Acute illnesses
Neurologic diseases and autistic spectrum of disorders
Anatomic abnormalities including oromotor dysfunction
Chromosomal or genetic diseases
Developmental delay
Maternal/Caregiver
Depression
Lack of education
Single parent
Abuse/neglect
Improper feeding techniques
Family
Poverty
Family dysfunction or lack of social support
Aberrant beliefs or factitious disorders
Abuse/neglect
Domestic violence
Substance abuse

of children with FTT have been reported to have aberrant responses to show appropriate physical or emotional concern or care because their parental role models often were inappropriate and faulty.[41] An extreme example of maternal deprivation and the effect was described by Philip Van Ingen in 1915. Children admitted without maternal supervision and care registered a mortality of 51% as compared to 27% in those whose mothers provided care and nursing for at least part of the time in institutions for foundlings or abandoned infants in New York at the turn of the century.[42] Krieger and Sargent described growth failure associated with sensory deprivation in infants and toddlers whose mothers were "passive or openly rejecting." Even in the absence of neuropathology, these children displayed features akin to brain-damaged children, but effects were reversible when children were placed in a positive environment and given adequate nutrition.[43]

A recent example of growth stunting in institutionalized children has been reported in a study of children at adoption. Up to 44% of the previously institutionalized children showed growth stunting at adoption. Relative to nonadopted children and children adopted early from foster care, children who spent time in an institution performed more poorly on cognitive and language screens with increased time in institution related to lower performance. These children were more likely to fall behind academically and access intervention services, although family environment did not differ between postinstitutionalized and nonadopted children.[44]

Deliberate starvation and food restriction is a contributing factor to cases of FTT. Although these severe cases are few, they do occur and, according to the law, all cases of FTT resulting from underfeeding or neglect by caregivers must be reported to child protective services (CPS).[45] Earlier reports on mothers of infants with FTT having been more deprived, abused, and neglected than controls have not been substantiated in later studies.[46]

Although undernutrition may result from failure to offer adequate calories, it may also occur because of inadequate ingestion of food by the infant. Recent studies suggest that the role of deprivation and neglect has been overstated and that undemanding behavior, low appetite, and poor feeding skills in infants themselves may contribute to the onset and persistence of FTT.[47] The origin of FTT can be complex, and the most common time for FTT problems to emerge is at the time of weaning.[48]

Feeding disorders are now commonly recognized in the pediatric population, with prevalence estimates ranging from 25 to 35% in developmentally normal children with no obvious disease. Food acceptance patterns develop early in life, and the progression through weaning and the acceptance of more solid textures can be difficult for some young children. Many parents of children who fail to thrive report feeding difficulties in their child such as spitting food out, vomiting, and refusal of solid food.[49] Food refusal may occur with or without obvious reasons such as excessive food temperature, inappropriate-sized pieces, and insensitive or forceful feeding techniques. In some cases where this does occur, a child can later refuse new textures and/or solids, leading to an overdependence on milk with resultant insufficient calorie intake for normal growth.[50]

Diagnosis of infantile feeding disorder is typically delayed, resulting in late intervention. In one study of children with feeding disorders, the mean age at presentation was 21 months, whereas symptoms had occurred since a mean age of 5.6 months. This study emphasized the difficulty primary care physicians face in recognizing infantile feeding disorders and the prolonged work-ups performed by subspecialists.[51] Feeding plays a major role in infancy, and onset of feeding problems thus typically occurs in infants. These include predominant orosensory and -motor dysfunction leading to difficult sucking and pharyngeal dysphagia.[52] Features common to infants with feeding difficulty include avoidant feeding behavior and intrusive feeding practices in combination with a "trigger" that predates the onset of behavior.[51] Examples of such triggers include forceful or mechanistic feeding by parental anxiety about the size or the growth rate of the infant. A significant proportion of children with poor feeding may not meet criteria for FTT. Moreover, parental response to difficult feeding may relate more closely to weight gain or loss than to infant feeding behavior.[53]

An organic disorder may lead to an infantile feeding disorder that may in turn be responsible for the symptoms even if the original medical condition is corrected. In this biological-psychological-social model, a disease process, such as gastroesophageal reflux, causes gagging, choking, and emesis. The child develops incompatible feeding behaviors by refusing food to avoid the negative consequences. The parent may resort to several means to feed the child. This in turn strengthens the child's resolve to avoid the food, or the pain and discomfort associated with feeding. Parent-child relationship becomes conflictual with a struggle for control.[54] Presence of certain clinical clues during the observation of a feeding session are valuable in distinguishing predominant feeding disorder from failure to thrive with secondary feeding issues. This is discussed further in the section on evaluation.

Newborn and infant feeding problems may also arise from lack of coordinated swallowing, breathing, and sucking. Low birth weight and prematurity appear to be risk factors in the development of eating problems.[55] Severe feeding problems are more prevalent (40 to 70%) in children with developmental disabilities and chronic disease.[56] Other etiologies for feeding disorders include neurodevelopmental disorders, disorders of appetite regulation, metabolic diseases, sensory defects, conditioned dysphagia, and anatomic abnormalities.

The presence of oromotor dysfunction (OMD) may prevent some children from achieving a satisfactory nutritional intake.[57] Some children with FTT have been suggested to have an eating disorder, which has been termed infantile anorexia nervosa.[58] Food refusal in this category typically occurs at the time of transition from spoon to self-feeding. The child does not communicate hunger, lacks interest in food, and shows a significant growth deficiency in absence of an antecedent traumatic event or an underlying illness. FTT may also involve an underlying appetite regulation problem in the child. Children who fail to thrive take insufficient energy to gain weight normally, in contrast to controls. In the same randomized study, affected children also did not decrease their intake at a meal subsequent to consuming a high-calorie drink, suggesting abnormal appetite regulation.[59,60]

Children with growth failure caused by emotional deprivation often exhibit apathy and developmental delay, whereas infants with FTT because of feeding disorders are likely to be willful and communicative, are appropriately developed, and display vivacity.[61] A recent study has shown increased IL-6 level as an attributable factor for anorexia in children with failure to thrive.[62]

Despite long-standing clinical experience of unusual feeding difficulties in children with autism, published literature describing their association with FTT is scarce. Children with autism may experience growth failure accompanied by severe feeding problems starting in the first year of life. Presence of severe or atypical feeding problems and FTT in infancy should alert to possible underlying autistic spectrum of disorders.[63] Food selectivity and feeding issues were identified in up to a quarter of children with autism in a population-based study.[64]

Infants with extremely low birth weight (ELBW) and short gut syndrome are at increased risk of FTT.[65] "Diencephalic syndrome" is characterized by euphoria, a hyperalert state, hyperactivity, tremor, irritability, optic atrophy, and pallor, without anemia, and typically failure to thrive with no history of inadequate food intake. This syndrome is typically caused by a tumor in the brainstem but has also been described to occur with a posterior fossa tumor.[66]

EVALUATION OF FAILURE TO THRIVE

A thorough physical examination including height, weight, and head circumference, especially in young children, should be performed. Accurate assessment of the child's height, weight, and head circumference is essential. These should be plotted on the growth charts and related to previous measurements. A single assessment of height and weight may have limited usefulness because it does not provide any indication of whether the child's growth pattern is deviating from the previous percentile. Another anthropometric measure is triceps skinfold thickness, which gives a useful validated indicator of total body fat and consequently of the body energy stores. Routinely collected child health record height/length and weight data are compatible with no systematic bias, at least in children over 8 months old, supporting their use in clinical practice and research.[67]

Despite the common emphasis on the search for an underlying pathology, major organic causes are unusual. Exhaustive investigations for organic causes and prolonged hospitalizations to evaluate family dynamics and poor infant weight gain are costly and frequently fail to yield a definitive diagnosis. A full detailed pediatric assessment including physical examination and psychosocial evaluation will usually exclude organic disease. The medical history and review of systems can provide important clues. Table 13-4 depicts some of these factors that aid in such assessment.

Some of the organic diseases that may cause FTT are listed in Table 13-3.[68] Some disorders typically result in failure to thrive at presentation. For example, in children with eosinophilic esophagitis disorder, failure to thrive was the most common symptom at onset of disease, particularly in young children with a median age of 2.8 years.[69] In addition, neurological difficulties that manifest as oral motor delay or dysfunction affect how able the child is to cope with changing textures of foods.[52,57] Indeed, a complex interaction exists among behavioral, oral, and medical etiology in children with feeding problems.[52]

Special situations associated with failure to thrive include chromosomal anomalies, cerebral palsy, syndromic disorders, and children with prenatal exposure to toxins. These groups of disorders typically have characteristic physical findings. A complete developmental assessment including careful evaluation should be made for dysmorphic features and for signs of neurologic, pulmonary, cardiac, and gastrointestinal disorders and nutritional deficiency. Submucosal cleft palate is often missed and, when present, may indicate a feeding problem. In some infants, presenting symptoms and signs of regurgitation, vomiting, poor feeding, diarrhea, dysphagia, coughing, abdominal distention, and wasting and those of primary pathology contributing to FTT may be obvious. However, eosinophilic esophagitis and celiac disease may have subtle presentations. When there is a clear medical explanation for the growth deficit, the diagnosis is not difficult.

Depending on the age of the child, and the severity and length of the condition at diagnosis with FTT, children may present with a range of physical symptoms from mild weight loss and diminished height to weakness and gluteal muscle wasting so severe that folds of skin hang loose. Signs of neglect may be indicated by a diaper rash, impetigo, flat occiput, poor hygiene, protuberant abdomen, lack of appropriate behavior, and inappropriate infantile postures.[70] Some children with nonorganic FTT may exhibit listlessness, expressionless facies, hypervigilance, and/or self-stimulatory stereotypical movements of their bodies and hands.[67,71] Observation of the child for drooling and assessment of bowel habits is essential.

A combination of history taking and observation of a feeding session provides strong clinical clues to the presence of a behavioral cause for food refusal. This will provide important information about parent-child interaction and the emotions surrounding feeding and how the baby feeds. Integration of a few structured questions regarding infant behavior, parental feeding practices, infant symptoms, and triggers for the onset of symptoms may help clinicians distinguish between organic and nonorganic causes for food refusal or low intake. Observing a mealtime, together with information from the diaries, allows discussion with the parents on appropriate interventions.[72] These also help differentiate organic disorders with disordered feeding from a predominant feeding disorder. The presence of a nonorganic trigger for the subsequent feeding difficulty can be identified at an initial interview. Examples include onset of refusal or decrease in intake during a transition in feeding method, a traumatic event, or the presence of abnormal and intrusive feeding practices such as nocturnal feeding

TABLE 13-5. Assessment of a Feeding Session

Observe the Child for	Observe the Parents for
Interest in own and others' food	Aware of child's needs and demands
Portion size, type, and texture of food	Portion size, type, and texture of food offered
Child's posture	Proper positioning and use of appropriate utensils, pacing of feeding (too fast or too slow)
Is the child able or unable to eat?	Management style, e.g., verbal or physical force, focusing on negative behaviors, and ignoring appropriate behavior
Is the child willing or unwilling to eat?	Emotional style, e.g., frustration, anxiety, distraction
Ability to communicate needs	
Reaction to parents' behavior	Control over child's behavior
Desire to self-feed	Ability to tolerate mess

TABLE 13-6. Clinical Clues to Differentiate Predominant Organic From Predominant Nonorganic Failure to Thrive

Predominant Organic Disease Not Present	Predominant Organic Disease Present
Spoon or bottle refusal	Accepts spoon or bottle at first
Presence of anticipatory gagging and "pocketing of food in mouth"	Absent
Picky about texture or type of food	Acceptance of a variety of foods
Presence of abnormal feeding practices (nocturnal feeding, force feeding, prolonged meals)	Absent
Onset after a trigger or traumatic event (choking episodes, prolonged nasogastric feeding, etc.)	Usually absent
Vivacious infant	Lethargy
Poor appetite	Interested in eating
Absence of organic symptoms	Diarrhea or abdominal distention

Adapted and modified from Levy et al. (2009)[51] and Panetta et al. (2008).[73]

or prolonged mealtimes. Examples of aversive infant behavior during mealtime include anticipatory gagging at the sight of food or as soon as the child is fed and/or turning face away from food. These offer particularly helpful clues to the presence of a feeding disorder (Table 13-5).[51]

Infant vivacity, food restriction, and/or feeding rituals along with poor appetite show an association with nonorganic FTT, whereas vomiting, irregular bowel movements, and abdominal distention point toward an organic etiology.[73] Other factors indicating the presence of a behavioral cause include food refusal, food fixation, and abnormal parental feeding practices; onset after a traumatic trigger; and presence of anticipatory gagging.[51] Poor intake or poor weight gain does not discriminate between organic and nonorganic causes. Clinical features that differentiate predominant nonorganic failure to thrive from organic failure to thrive are summarized in Table 13-6.

A comprehensive nutritional assessment has five components: dietary history, medical and medication history, physical examination, growth and anthropometric measurements, and laboratory tests.

INVESTIGATIONS

Necessary laboratory testing to search for an organic disease should be guided by the history and physical examination. Laboratory studies not suggested on the basis of the initial examination are rarely helpful. Fewer than 2% of the laboratory studies performed in evaluating children with FTT were of diagnostic value.[74] A few routine screening tests, such as a complete blood count, blood urea nitrogen (BUN), creatinine, serum electrolytes, albumin, calcium, phosphorus, alkaline phosphatase, urinalysis, and urine culture, help in excluding systemic diseases. Estimation of bone age offers clues to presence of pathological growth failure. Delayed bone age in relation to chronological age occurs with growth failure secondary to malnutrition, chronic illness, and endocrine causes such as growth hormone deficiency. However, delayed bone age also occurs with physiological growth variants such as constitutional growth delay. Some of the special investigations needed for further testing in selected patients are shown in Table 13-7. It is important to construct a complete picture of all aspects of and influences on the child's feeding. Dietary assessment

is complex and involves taking a dietary recall, completion of a food diary, and, if possible, feeding observation. A 24-hour recall may not reflect the "normal" eating pattern and cannot be used for accurate calculation of nutrient intake, so a 3-day diet diary is used to assess the calorie intake. Any use of alternative or complementary medications should always be asked about. Some investigations may emerge as potential tools for nutritional rehabilitation. For example, a strong correlation between insulinlike growth factor 1 (IGF-1) and height, weight, and protein catabolism may emphasize the need to normalize IGF-1 levels in children with cystic fibrosis.[75] Mutations in the IGF-1 receptor are also recognized as a genetic defect causing IUGR that persists to the postnatal period.[76]

MANAGEMENT

The physician must be an advocate for the child and his/her family without becoming an adversary of the parents. Appropriate drug and/or dietary intervention are instituted for organic disease. In addition, counseling of parents about the disease, its outcomes, and any available support groups is recommended. Close follow-up with growth monitoring will help to restore the child's well-being. A multidisciplinary team approach requires close liaisons among the pediatrician, pediatric gastroenterologist, psychologist, and speech and language therapists as well as dietitians.[77,78] Home-based intervention has been shown to be effective in management of failure to thrive.[79] Hospital admission is only justified when the child is seriously ill or is at risk of physical or sexual abuse or in the face of severe parental concern and anxiety. Some experts have advocated inpatient treatment to enhance growth recovery in nonorganic failure to thrive.[80] However, this may also promote anxiety.[81] Helping parents can be difficult and must be done in a sensitive way without blaming or criticizing parenting skills. Only in rare instances of suspected neglect or abuse does the child need to be removed from the home environment. The possibility that calorie deprivation in infancy will produce severe, irreversible developmental deficits is the reason that treatment should begin expeditiously. The overall aims of intervention are to increase nutritional intake, to induce catch-up growth, to resolve feeding difficulties

TABLE 13-7. Guide to Optional Investigations in Failure to Thrive

A. Decreased Intake or Inadequate Calories

Calorie counts and dietary recall

B. Increased Caloric Loss or Malabsorption

Celiac antibodies
Stool α1-antitrypsin, fecal elastase
Upper and lower endoscopy with tissue biopsy, disaccharidase assay
Pancreatic stimulation tests
Breath hydrogen test
Sweat chloride test

C. Presence of Systemic Disease

Karyotype
Quantitative immunoglobulins
HIV antibodies
Urine pH with simultaneous serum bicarbonate
Urine amino acids, organic acids, catecholamines
Liver function tests including prothrombin time
Electrolytes, BUN, and creatinine
Chest x-ray, echocardiogram, ECG
Head MRI
Abdominal ultrasound
Bone age, skeletal survey

D. Nutritional Assessment

Serum albumin, Prealbumin, and retinol binding protein
Serum zinc, iron studies
Vitamin A and D level (retinol and 25(OH) vitamin D_3)

E. Miscellaneous

Heavy metal screening (lead, arsenic)
Gastrointestinal hormones such as vasoactive intestinal peptide (VIP)

BUN, blood urea nitrogen; ECG, electrocardiogram; HIV, human immunodeficiency virus; MRI, magnetic resonance imaging.

TABLE 13-8. Some Commercially Available Products for Caloric Supplementation

Product	Calorie Concentration	Description
Baby rice/ oatmeal cereal	60 kcal per 15 g (¼ cup)	Carbohydrate
Corn oil	8 kcal/mL	Mixture of saturated and unsaturated fats
Microlipid	4.5 kcal/mL	50% safflower oil emulsion
MCT Oil	8 kcal/mL	100% MCT oil
Moducal	3.8 kcal/g	Glucose polymers
Polycose	4 kcal/g	Glucose polymers
Caloreen	3.9 kcal/g	Glucose polymers
Polycal	3.9 kcal/g	Maltodextrins
Resource Benecalorie	7 kcal/mL (1.5-oz serving gives 330 kcal plus 7 g protein)	High oleic sunflower oil, calcium caseinate, mono- and diglycerides

MCT, medium-chain triglyceride.

and improve feeding style, and to create positive interactions between the mother and child, the special focus being to promote a positive feeding environment.[82]

The main goal of dietary intervention in the management of undernutrition is to increase calorie intake to enable "catch-up" weight gain at a rate that is greater than average for age so that the weight deficit is repaired or overcome. A healthy infant at birth requires 110 kcal/kg/day, decreasing at 1 year of age to approximately 100 kcal/kg/day. A child who fails to gain weight normally and whose weight is below the 5th percentile will not experience "catch-up" unless calorie intake is higher than basal requirement for age. A common regimen is to increase caloric intake by 50% greater than basal requirement (e.g., 150/ kcal/kg/day in a 1-year-old child).[82] Another way to determine caloric requirements for infants with poor growth is to determine the calories required by using the following formula:

RDA for age (kcal / kg)
~ideal weight for height (kg) / actual weight (kg)

where ideal weight for height is the median weight for the patient's height (as read from the NCHS weight for height curves). Indirect calorimetry and equations for resting energy expenditure help assessment of energy requirements but are not routinely available or utilized.[83]

High calorie intake is difficult to achieve, because many toddlers eat small food portions and are not able to consume large quantities at any one time. Energy intake can be increased by frequent meals, use of energy-dense foods, and adding extra calories to foods. Strategies to improve caloric intake in infants include frequent feeds and addition of calorie-rich additives such as baby rice cereal or baby oatmeal. In older children with poor appetite and early satiety, consumption of calorie- and protein-rich foods such as dairy, soy products, and peanut butter is encouraged while avoiding low-calorie foods and beverages. Addition of fats and oils such as safflower, canola, or margarine to consumed foods may increase caloric density while preserving smaller portion sizes. A few of the commercially available calorie supplements are listed in Table 13-8. Use of such supplements is best achieved under the guidance of a nutritionist and close monitoring. It should be noted that high-calorie, balanced, complete dietary supplements or replacements are also commercially available for drinking and/or tube feeding.

Appetite stimulants such as cyproheptadine (Periactin), a serotonin and histamine antagonist, and megestrol (Megace), an antineoplastic progestational compound, have been utilized in an attempt to enhance caloric intake. Particularly useful situations include anorexia complicating chemotherapy, cystic fibrosis patients, and during transition from tube to oral feeds in children.[84-86] Most of the reported experience is anecdotal. A small randomized, placebo-controlled study demonstrated significant gains in weight and height velocities and serum IGF-1 in a group of underweight, otherwise healthy children receiving cyproheptadine therapy for a period of 4 months compared to the placebo group. Cases of precocious pseudopuberty and adrenal insufficiency have been reported with off-label "appetite stimulant" syrup (containing cyproheptadine and methandienone), as well as excessive virilization with use beyond age 1 or 2 years. Further studies will be required to assess the long-term outcome of treated children.[87]

During the catch-up growth phase, existing stores of vitamins may not be sufficient. A multivitamin preparation including iron and zinc is recommended. Close follow-up and frequent contact with the health care team are essential for reinforcing nutritional recommendations and psychosocial support. Involvement with the family by community social service workers, visiting nurses, and nutritionists is important to ensure a nurturing environment for the children.[78]

During nutritional recovery, some malnourished children experience the symptoms of a nutritional recovery syndrome, including excessive sweating, hepatomegaly (caused by increased glycogen deposition in the liver), widening of the sutures (the brain growth is greater than the growth of the skull in infants with open sutures), and irritability or mild hyperactivity.[88] If weight gain does not occur in 4 to 6 weeks, oral feedings should be supplemented with feeding by a nasogastric tube. Feeding assessment by an occupational therapist to improve sucking and swallowing may be needed. If weight gain is inadequate after nasogastric tube feeding or if prolonged nasogastric tube feeding will be required (more than 2 months), gastrostomy tube placement may be appropriate.[60] The use of tube feeding as part of the medical management of many children's illnesses can create some problems as well as ameliorate others.[89] The psychological management of long-term tube feeding is an important element in reducing the anxiety and concern about a child who cannot or will not eat. In most children with neurologic compromise, it is required on a long-term basis, especially in those at risk for aspiration with swallowing. Despite preplacement concerns, caregivers report being pleased with the gastrostomy tube following placement, especially when it meets the expectation of improved nutrition.[90]

Refeeding syndrome is a potentially fatal complication that occurs with administration of high-calorie feeds during nutritional rehabilitation of severely malnourished children. Refeeding syndrome may occur within hours or days of initiating parenteral or enteral nutrition. Fluid and electrolyte derangements occur including hypokalemia, hypomagnesemia, and, notably, hypophosphatemia. The pathophysiology of refeeding syndrome is poorly understood, although hypophosphatemia is a typical and diagnostic feature that has been well described.[91] An increase in caloric intake stimulates insulin production, which in turn leads to intracellular uptake of phosphorus, glucose, and water, decreasing serum phosphate. Phosphate depletion leads to myocardial dysfunction and arrhythmias. Concurrent hypokalemia and hypomagnesemia amplify the risk of fatal cardiac arrhythmias and sudden death.[92] In addition, hypokalemia may cause muscle weakness and ileus, whereas hypomagnesemia may result in hyperactive reflexes, tetany, and muscle cramps.[93] Hemolysis, rhabdomyolysis, seizures, delirium, and acute renal tubular necrosis are other features of refeeding syndrome. Recognition that refeeding syndrome may occur in any child recovering from a period of suboptimal nutrition and a careful attention to hydration, serum electrolytes, and cardiac status in the initial 3 to 5 days are essential to prevention of the syndrome. A suggested strategy is starting with iso-osmolar/isocaloric feeds at 75% of required caloric intake with a gradual increase over 3 to 5 days. Protein intake is also gradually increased from 0.6-1 g/kg/day to 1.2-1.5 g/kg/day over several days. Oral supplementation of sodium, potassium, magnesium, and phosphorus is sufficient and appropriate to correct electrolyte abnormalities. These must be given intravenously when severe symptoms are present.[91]

When feeding disorders are present, accurate diagnosis and effective treatment depend on the collaboration of an interdisciplinary team of experts. Successful behavioral intervention and therapeutic approach in treating medically caused feeding difficulties address all aspects of biological-psychological-social interactional model.[54] The etiology of feeding disorders in autism appears to involve an unusually complex model of dysfunction in sensory, cognitive, and emotional response interacting with dysfunctional attachment and learned behaviors. Effective treatment therefore requires a multifaceted approach.[63]

Figure 13-1 provides an algorithm for management of calorie intake in a child with FTT.

OUTCOME

Neurodevelopmental Outcome

Development of the brain and cognitive processes takes place during the first 3 years of a child's life,[94] and brain growth during infancy and early childhood may determine cognitive ability.[95,96] FTT in this age carries a high risk for negative effects on intellectual development later in life. Cognitive development appears associated not only with birth weight but also with early neonatal weight gain and subsequent head circumference increase. Improving early neonatal growth may improve long-term outcome in extremely preterm infants to some extent.[97] Growth faltering during the critical period from birth to 8 weeks is noted to be associated with persisting deficits in IQ at 8 years. In this study, the relationship between infant growth from birth to 8 weeks and later intellectual development was linear over the range of weight velocities.[3]

Although previous data from long-term studies in children with poor nutrition suggest lower mean IQ scores and a high incidence of attention deficit disorder in comparison to a control group, more recent studies show better results with increases in cognitive development that appear to be related to growth recovery.[98] Prolonged hospital admission in FTT infants appears to have an adverse effect, with intellectual delays persisting at 3 years of age despite maintenance of weight gain. However, a large percentage of the infants in this study had been removed from parental custody at the time of follow-up. Infants who achieve more optimal growth tended to be full-term at birth and without a history of abuse.[99] A study of children with a significant FTT followed at school age found that half the children had IQs below 80 with increased adversive aggression and poor attention scores.[100] Intellectual functioning was related only to parental and caretaker socioeconomic status or maternal education in both the studies, suggesting that a cognitively enriched environment may be important to subsequent intellectual performance in these children.

Evidence from meta-analysis of studies shows an IQ deficit of 3 to 4 points in children with failure to thrive in infancy when subsequently tested at 3 years to school age. Whether this makes for a significant difference for practical functioning is debatable.[8,101,102]

GROWTH OUTCOME

Failure to thrive can be associated with some reduction in childhood weight and height. However, this effect may be less obvious when adjusted for confounding factors such as parental height. Follow-up studies have also shown that cumulative impact of social and behavioral risk factors affect long-term growth more than failure to thrive alone.[102,103] Failure to thrive coupled with SGA birth weight has a particularly severe effect on long-term growth outcome.[104]

SGA infants show reduced catch-up growth potential as evident in later childhood and as young adults. Infants born with IUGR enrolled in the national Collaborative Perinatal Project at 7 years of age remained smaller than infants born without IUGR in both weight and height for age. The differences were significant and largely independent of genetic and postnatal environmental influences.[105] The growth deficits persist until

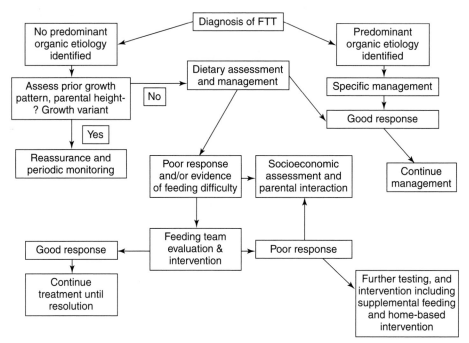

Figure 13-1. Algorithm for management of a child with failure to thrive (FTT).

young adulthood, although at this age, factors such as maternal age affect final growth. There also appears to be a gender predisposition, with males being more affected than females by young adulthood.[106]

Initial growth restriction in infancy and early childhood has long-term health implications in being overweight and development of metabolic syndrome. Children who are severely stunted have an increased risk of being relatively overweight.[107] Adolescents who were low birth weight (less than 2500 g) are likely to have increased serum triglycerides and be either overweight or overtly obese.[108] A birth cohort study of men aged 18 years found an increase in mean Hgb A_1C with decreasing birth weight for the gestational age.[109] Prospective, epidemiological, and observational studies have also shown increased rates of feeding difficulties in children with FTT, with additional nonspecified "neurologic" findings in some of them.[57] Slow feeding and delayed acquisition of age-appropriate feeding skills are commonly observed.

CONCLUSION

There is persuasive evidence pointing to the potential adverse effects of infant growth faltering for subsequent child development.[39,110] Although early failure to thrive may predispose to poor neurocognitive outcome, early intervention and an enriching social environment are important mitigating factors. Growth restriction in the fetal and early neonatal period has been associated with an increased risk of being overweight, of metabolic syndrome, and cardiovascular disease in adult life.[111]

Recent studies have led to a radical shift in our understanding of the condition. FTT is now seen as a form of growth deviation and undernutrition whose etiology and evolution lies in a complex interaction of biological, psychological, and socioenvironmental influences rather than social factors alone. Children may deviate from expected or established growth patterns as part of physiological phenomena or as a result of genetic factors. Early recognition of these variants avoids inaccurate

labeling, unwarranted investigations, and unnecessary anxiety. Future research should develop useful screening tools that can distinguish physiological growth variants from true failure to thrive requiring proper identification and intervention. Development of markers that are reliable and easy to use may include measures of resting energy expenditure, genetic markers, or hormonal profiles. Some of the traditional anthropometric criteria such as crossing of a major percentile line may overestimate the presence of failure to thrive, underscoring the necessity for adopting universal criteria to reliably predict pathological growth failure. Successful and early intervention to address feeding problems may mitigate or even prevent failure to thrive and improve family interaction. Removal of blame from the family, their close involvement as part of management team, and respect are an integral part of this long-term process.

ACKNOWLEDGMENTS

We acknowledge the services of Mrs. Jan Wilkins for technical help with the preparation of the manuscript.

REFERENCES

16. Olsen EM, Skovgaard AM, Weile B, Jorgensen T. Risk factors for failure to thrive in infancy depend on the anthropometric definitions used: the Copenhagen County Child Cohort. Paediatr Perinat Epidemiol 2007;21:418–431.
17. Corbett SS, Drewett RF, Wright CM. Does a fall down a centile chart matter? The growth and developmental sequelae of mild failure to thrive. Acta Paediatr 1996;85:1278–1283.
26. Mei Z, Grummer-Strawn LM, Thompson D, Dietz WH. Shifts in percentiles of growth during early childhood: analysis of longitudinal data from the California Child Health and Development Study. Pediatrics 2004;113:e617–e627.
38. Parker E, Phillips DI, Cockington RA, et al. A common mitochondrial DNA variant is associated with thinness in mothers and their 20-yr-old offspring. Am J Physiol Endocrinol Metab 2005;289:E1110–E1114.

44. Loman MM, Wiik KL, Frenn KA, et al. Postinstitutionalized children's development: growth, cognitive, and language outcomes. J Dev Behav Pediatr 2009;30:426–434.

51. Levy Y, Levy A, Zangen T, et al. Diagnostic clues for identification of nonorganic vs organic causes of food refusal and poor feeding. J Pediatr Gastroenterol Nutr 2009;48:355–362.

54. Manikam R, Perman JA. Pediatric feeding disorders. J Clin Gastroenterol 2000;30:34–46.

83. Fung EB. Estimating energy expenditure in critically ill adults and children. AACN Clin Issues 2000;11:480–497.

101. Corbett SS, Drewett RF. To what extent is failure to thrive in infancy associated with poorer cognitive development? A review and meta-analysis. J Child Psychol Psychiatry 2004;45:641–654.

104. Casey PH, Whiteside-Mansell L, Barrett K, et al. Impact of prenatal and/or postnatal growth problems in low birth weight preterm infants on school-age outcomes: an 8-year longitudinal evaluation. Pediatrics 2006;118:1078–1086.

106. Hack M, Schluchter M, Cartar L, et al. Growth of very low birth weight infants to age 20 years. Pediatrics 2003;112:e30–e38.

108. Nair MK, Nair L, Chacko DS, et al. Markers of fetal onset adult diseases: a comparison among low birthweight and normal birthweight adolescents. Indian Pediatr 2009;46(Suppl):s43–s47.

See expertconsult.com for a complete list of references and the review questions for this chapter.

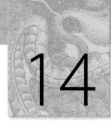

14

GASTROINTESTINAL HEMORRHAGE

Joel Friedlander • Petar Mamula

Gastrointestinal hemorrhage is one of the most serious presenting complaints a pediatric gastroenterologist may need to diagnose and treat. A proper understanding of the various etiologies and available treatment modalities is necessary to ensure successful outcome. Multiple review articles have examined these in detail; however, very little is known about the true epidemiology of pediatric gastrointestinal bleeding.[1-7] The only studies examining this topic were performed in an intensive care setting where the incidence of upper gastrointestinal bleeding was found to range from 6 to 25%.[8]

There are many causes of gastrointestinal bleeding, ranging from the ones requiring urgent treatment to those that resolve without any therapy.[9] Determining which is occurring is the art of medicine, and this chapter attempts to convey the practice of this art by discussing a diagnostic approach and therapeutic options available to pediatric practitioners.

Definitions

1. Melena is the passage of dark, black, tar-colored stool usually associated with esophageal, gastric, or upper small bowel gastrointestinal hemorrhage.
2. Hematochezia is the passage of bright red blood or maroon-colored material from the rectum usually associated with distal small bowel or colonic gastrointestinal bleeding.
3. Hematemesis is the passage of bloody or dark brown ("coffee grounds) appearing material from the mouth usually associated with bleeding in the gastrointestinal tract proximal to the ligament of Treitz.[9]

Initial Presentation and Assessment

The child or adolescent with gastrointestinal (GI) bleeding may present to medical attention in a wide variety of ways and locations including a local emergency room, a pediatrician's office, a phone call from a parent, or an inpatient hospital ward. Regardless of the location, by asking several brief and pointed questions, the medical provider will be able to assess the need for immediate intervention and subsequently establish a specific diagnosis. Initial open-ended questions are indicated in Table 14-1.

Based on the answers to these questions, one could approximate the severity of bleeding, where the patient needs to be sent, and what services need to be readied for therapy. For example, large-volume bleeding, history of portal hypertension or coagulopathy, ill appearance, or unstable vital signs would prompt emergent care with rapid medical transport. On the other hand, if the answers do not suggest a need for emergent care or if the care plan has already started, further questions will help assess a possible cause. Specific historical areas that should be addressed are indicated in Table 14-1.

The answers to the open-ended and historical questions must be taken in appropriate context with the understanding that in times of emergency, parents and children may overestimate the amount of blood, duration of the event, or frequency. A good estimate of the amount of blood is the appearance of blood in the toilet. If the water is opacified (not transparent), it is likely significant.[9] If the child is old enough to provide a reliable history, additional questions should be asked of him/her and if needed without parental presence. One should also remember that having one positive historical event does not forgo the possibility of another one that could be more serious. For example, a child who ingests blueberries that cause a melanotic type stool could also have a bleeding duodenal ulcer that could cause melena.

Along with a directed history of the current events, a directed social and family history should be performed (see Table 14-1). These may direct the physician to specific conditions that could be presenting for the first time. In addition, various foods and medications can cause stool or vomitus to falsely appear to contain blood (Table 14-2).

Physical Examination and Laboratory Evaluation

Once the practitioner takes an appropriate history he/she should be able to place the child into one of two pathways: emergent and nonemergent. This should subsequently be substantiated by a physical examination and laboratory evaluation. The physical examination should also be similarly focused to direct the possible sick patient to appropriate care quickly. It should primarily assess a directed ABC approach of general **A**ssessment for well or ill, evidence of brisk **B**leeding (blood in the oral cavity or on rectal examination), and vital signs directed at **C**irculatory adequacy (heart rate, orthostatic vital signs, pulse pressure, blood pressure, urine output). The balance of the physical examination will analyze possible causes of bleeding such as splenomegaly as evidence of or portal hypertension, lip and buccal hyperpigmentation in cases of Peutz-Jeghers syndrome, emaciation and perianal disease suggestive of Crohn disease, or abdominal distention and ill appearance in patients with intussusception. A directed physical examination with appropriate areas of interest is outlined later. Once the physical examination is complete, a targeted set of diagnostic laboratory studies should be requested. Similar to the history with a primary and secondary assessment, the laboratory studies should be ordered in a proper sequence. Unless the bleeding is obvious, the presence of blood should usually be confirmed with the appropriate test kit. Except in cases where upper GI bleeding appears to be minor, it should almost always be investigated with nasogastric (NG) lavage to assess the volume and for evidence of continued bleeding.[10,11] This is performed with a double-lumen vented

TABLE 14-1. **Historical Information**

Open-ended Questions

Describe the location, quantity, and appearance of the bleeding.
What is the physical appearance and vital signs of the patient (if available)?
What medical conditions does the child have? (Liver disease, inflammatory bowel disease, etc.)
What medication is the child on? (Anticoagulants, nonsteroidal anti-inflammatory drugs, etc.)

History

Description of onset, location, duration, occurrence
Exposure to raw food, reptiles, travel, or toxins
Foreign body ingestion
Exposure to others with similar symptoms
Ingestion of specific foods or medications (Table 14-2)[110-112]
Other associated symptoms (mouth sores, pain, rashes, vomiting, swelling, headaches, neck pain, chest pain, diarrhea, fevers, bruising, infections)
Medications (nonsteroidal anti-inflammatory drugs [NSAIDS], warfarin, hepatotoxins, antibiotic use)

Review of Systems

GI disorders
Liver disease
Bleeding diatheses
Anesthesia reactions

Family History

Gastrointestinal disorders (polyps, ulcers, colitis)
Liver disease
Bleeding diatheses
Anesthesia reactions

TABLE 14-2. **Substances That Color Stool or Emesis**

Red: candy, fruit punch, beets, laxatives, phenytoin, rifampin
Black: bismuth, activated charcoal, iron, spinach, blueberry, licorice

TABLE 14-3. **Targeted Physical Examination**

Vital signs: orthostasis, pulse pressure, instability, urine output
General: appearance (well or ill), fever, mental status
Head, eyes, ears, nose, and throat: trauma, scleral injection, petechiae, lip and buccal pigmentation, epistaxis, erythema or burns to posterior pharynx, bleeding
Chest/cardiovascular: tachycardia, murmur, capillary refill
Abdomen: tenderness, splenomegaly, hepatomegaly, caput medusa, distention, ascites
Genitourinary: fistula, swelling
Rectal: gross blood, melena, tags, tenderness, fissure, fistula, swelling, inflammation
Dermatological: pallor, jaundice, rash, arteriovenous malformation (AVM), bruising, petechiae

TABLE 14-4. **Possible Laboratory Studies**

Complete blood count
Prothrombin time/international normalized ratio/partial thromboplastin time
Complete metabolic profile (electrolytes, liver function tests)
Type and screen
If significant loss: type and cross and fibrinogen level
Stool culture including assay for *Escherichia coli* O157:H7, *Shigella*, *Salmonella*, *Yersinia*, *Campylobacter*; *C. difficile* toxins A and B; *Cryptococcus* and *Giardia* assays; and ova and parasite smear if indicated by history
Erythrocyte sedimentation rate, C-reactive protein, γ-glutamyl transpeptidase if indicated by history
Hemoccult and Gastroccult testing

pediatric-sized NG tube. The tube is placed nasally, after adequate lubrication and topical anesthesia, and advanced into the stomach. Placement confirmation may differ from institution to institution, but commonly used methods include pH testing or air bubble technique. After the placement, the tube is irrigated with 50-mL aliquots of room-temperature sterile water until the irrigant is clear. If one is unable to lavage, the tube might be positioned against the stomach wall or clogged by the presence of a clot or gastric contents. Repositioning of the tube and/or flushing it should resolve this. The lavage is usually reported as amount of fluid necessary until the tube aspirate is clear. Confirmation of the material as blood should be performed with appropriate gastric testing equipment.[9,12] Presence of dark ("coffee-grounds") material suggests blood that has been exposed to oxygen for some time and indicates that the acute bleeding may have ceased, whereas bright red blood that does not readily clear indicates active bleeding. The absence of blood suggests bleeding distal to the ligament of Treitz or lack of bleeding. Some prefer not to place the NG tube because of a theoretical risk of dislodging a clot in the stomach or varix, although this is unlikely.[9] NG lavage is often very helpful to the practitioner when making clinical decisions about the necessity of urgent medical interventions and the severity and location of bleeding, as well as ongoing monitoring of bleeding, and in ensuring good visualization during endoscopy.[10,11]

Laboratory studies directed to assess blood volume status include ordering of a complete blood count (CBC), ability to clot by performing international normalized ratio (INR), and a blood type and screen in case a transfusion is indicated. These are usually the first line of tests obtained. The CBC should be interpreted using the mean corpuscular volume (MCV) and mean corpuscular hemoglobin (MCH) to assess the chronicity of the condition, or with appropriate medical history for hemoglobinopathy. Low MCV/MCH levels (microcytic, hypochromic) suggests chronic bleeding or an "acute on chronic" condition, whereas normal levels indicate an acute blood loss. If the patient has folate or B_{12} deficiency, the values may vary from the expected. These deficiencies often create a macrocytic process with an elevated MCV and MCH. Blood urea nitrogen (BUN) to creatinine ratio may also be helpful in determining the source of bleeding. A ratio greater than 30 has 98% sensitivity and 68% specificity for upper GI bleeding.[13,14] This occurs because of the rise in serum urea level as a by-product of amino acid catabolism secondary to digestion of blood in the GI tract. To assess the severity of bleeding, serial CBCs can be obtained. If the history is suggestive of a nonemergent cause of bleeding, such as anal fissure, rectal polyp, or a simple nosebleed, limited laboratory studies would be required and a CBC may suffice.

Lower GI bleeding is usually assessed through a combination of the foregoing laboratory studies and the appearance of the rectal effluent or rectal examination.[15] Although hematochezia is usually representative of lower GI bleeding, brisk upper GI bleeding may cause this, too. Important components of the physical examination are indicated in Table 14-3. Laboratory studies that should be obtained at the time of GI bleeding are indicated in Table 14-4.

Initial Interventions

The child with gastrointestinal hemorrhage may present in stable condition or with various degrees of circulatory compromise including shock. While performing an initial assessment the

TABLE 14-5. **Imaging Studies and Associated Indications**

Test	Indication
Abdominal x-ray	Constipation Foreign body Vomiting
Upper gastrointestinal series	Dysphagia Odynophagia Drooling Obstruction Vomiting
Barium enema	Suspected stricture Intussusception Hirschsprung's disease (late)
Ultrasound (Doppler recommended for liver disease)	Portal hypertension Intussusception Possible inflammatory bowel disease
Meckel's scan	Meckel's diverticulum
Tagged RBC scan	Obscure gastrointestinal bleeding
MR/CT/direct angiography	Obscure gastrointestinal bleeding Suspected arteriovenous malformation

TABLE 14-6. **Endoscopy and Associated Indications**

Test	Indication
Esophagogastroduodenoscopy	Hematemesis, melena, hematochezia
Flexible sigmoidoscopy	Hematochezia
Colonoscopy	Hematochezia
Small bowel enteroscopy Capsule endoscopy Balloon enteroscopy Spiral enteroscopy	Obscure gastrointestinal blood loss

patient should be kept NPO (nil per os) in order to decrease the risk of further aggravating the bleeding and in anticipation of diagnostic tests or endoscopy that will require sedation, and have intravenous (IV) access obtained. If the child appears ill, two large-bore IV lines should be placed. Depending on the need for initial fluid resuscitation, aliquots of 10 to 20 mL/kg of normal saline should be infused quickly (30 to 60 minutes) as per recent practice parameters from the American College of Critical Care Medicine for shock.[16-19] If blood loss is rapid, this volume may need to be replaced with packed red blood cells and appropriate clotting factors/fibrinogen depending on the condition. In case of a planned urgent endoscopic procedure, patients should have ample reserves to tolerate anesthesia. A serum hemoglobin level above 8 g/dL is usually adequate as long as the heart rate and blood pressure are appropriate. Attempting to intervene with unstable vital signs and a low blood volume may cause more harm than benefit to the patient. Along with volume repletion, all equipment and support staff necessary for successful completion of the procedure should be readily available, and when indicated, surgical backup should be considered.

Secondary Interventions and Further Testing

Once the child is stabilized and initial testing results return, the practitioner needs to determine the source of bleeding. If it appears that the source of bleeding originated from outside of GI tract such as pulmonary or nasopharyngeal, the appropriate specialist should be consulted. Advanced imaging modalities such as computerized tomography (CT) or magnetic resonance imaging (MRI) could be ordered to assist in diagnosing these conditions (Table 14-5).[20,21] There are multiple causes of bleeding and no single algorithm will cover all of them; thus, a careful individualized approach utilizing variety of tests is needed. For example, a large-volume esophageal or gastric bleed may be easier to identify and necessitate fewer studies than a slow, indolent small bowel hemorrhage. Etiologies relating to specific bleeding lesions of the GI tract are discussed here in more detail, including a discussion of various imaging techniques. Infectious and autoimmune causes are covered elsewhere in this volume.

Pediatric gastroenterologists should be skilled in a variety of endoscopic techniques described next and listed in Table 14-6.

Some of these may require advanced skills for which additional endoscopic training may be required. It is advisable to have an experienced endoscopist available for assistance. The North American Society for Pediatric Gastroenterology, Hepatology, and Nutrition (NASPGHAN) and the American Society for Gastrointestinal Endoscopy (ASGE) have issued guidelines and competence requirements for individuals performing these procedures.[22,23] In addition, a discussion between the endoscopist and family or legal guardian should occur regarding the risks, benefits, alternatives, methods, and indications/purpose for the procedure. One should also consider limited ethical or legal capacity for a parent to refuse care for a life-threatening condition.[24] If a parent refuses intervention during the need for life-saving therapy, legal assistance, court intervention, or a social work consult should be obtained immediately.

Esophageal/Gastric/Proximal Duodenum

Bleeding from the upper GI tract can often be readily discovered by NG lavage and further located by endoscopy.[10,11] NG lavage has good positive predictive value for high-risk endoscopic lesions in patients with acute upper GI bleeding.[10] The purpose of the esophagogastroduodenoscopy (EGD) is to confirm the diagnosis and possibly treat the bleeding lesion. If a patient presents with hematemesis or has blood or heme-positive content found on NG lavage, radiographic testing is rarely indicated unless the EGD is negative.[25,26] Possible imaging modalities before performing EGD include an abdominal x-ray to localize a foreign body, ultrasound with Doppler to evaluate the liver and abdominal vasculature, or CT scan to evaluate organomegaly, masses, or vasculature.[27]

Small Bowel

Small bowel bleeding is often suspected based on the absence of upper endoscopic or lavage findings and the appearance of a dark melanotic or maroon-colored stool. The color of stool will depend on the location of bleeding and the bowel transit time. In rare cases of very brisk proximal small bowel bleeding with rapid transit time, hematochezia might be encountered. In addition to endoscopic techniques, various imaging studies can be utilized to diagnose small bowel bleeding including upper GI small bowel follow through, nuclear scintigraphy, CT enterography and angiography (CTA), ultrasound with Doppler, direct angiography, and MR angiography or venography (MRA/MRV). Nuclear radionucleotide scan may be used to diagnose a rapidly bleeding small bowel lesion. In general, brisk bleeding is needed for a red blood cell nucleotide scan to be successful with a rate of bleeding of more than 0.05 to 0.5 mL per minute.[27-31] Some authors suggest 24-hour delayed images be obtained in order to increase its sensitivity.[32] Alternatively, if Meckel's diverticulum is suspected, a Meckel's scan using technetium-99 pertechnetate that is taken up by the ectopic gastric tissue can be useful. Administration of IV ranitidine for 24 to 48 hours before the study, thus up-regulating the H_2 receptor in the ectopic gastric tissue, may optimize chance of success.[33] In case of persistent bleeding in which the preceding studies are negative, a CTA or MRA/MRV may offer visualization of a vascular malformation. The yield of such testing is relatively low, but in the correct clinical setting, it can be helpful.[34] Finally, direct angiography by a trained pediatric interventional radiologist offers a way to visualize and embolize the bleeding vessel.[27,35]

Newer endoscopic modalities can also be useful to image and intervene in the small bowel. Techniques that have become more recently available include single and double balloon enteroscopy, spiral enteroscopy, and capsule endoscopy (CE). These techniques are discussed in more detail in Chapter 64. Each of the modalities has its risks and benefits. Capsule endoscopy is more widely implemented and is approved by the FDA for patients 2 years of age and older, although the youngest patients reported children who were 18 months old.[36,37] A majority of patients older than 8 years are able to swallow the capsule; younger patients and those unable to swallow it need the capsule to be placed endoscopically.[25] The capsule endoscopy may visualize the bleeding lesions, but with its current design, it offers no therapeutic options. Studies have shown that the diagnostic efficacy of CE for obscure small bowel bleeding ranges between 55 and 81%.[36] During the past 5 years, balloon enteroscopy has become available, whereas spiral endoscopy is still considered experimental. The pediatric literature on the use of these techniques is very sparse, with no reports as of this writing of single balloon and spiral endoscopy and a very limited number of children reported to have undergone double balloon endoscopy. A recent study, the largest to date, described safety and feasibility of small bowel examination using double balloon enteroscopy technique in 48 pediatric patients who had 92 procedures performed for indications ranging from post liver transplant biliary obstruction in the setting of Roux-en-Y anastomosis and obscure gastrointestinal bleeding, to surveillance of polyposis syndromes.[38] This technique requires special training and is time consuming, but offers the opportunity for direct visualization of the entire small bowel in select cases, and therapy. Panendoscopy at the time of surgical exploration is another possible modality, but with the advent of the foregoing technologies, it has become less commonly utilized.[39]

Colonic Lesions

Hematochezia almost always originates in the colon, except in a very rare case of brisk upper GI bleeding. To evaluate the source of bleeding, and after ruling out infectious causes in the appropriate setting, colonoscopic examination is the best initial diagnostic choice. If the bleeding lesion is not detected during colonoscopic examination, EGD may be needed. If inflammatory bowel disease is suspected, both EGD and colonoscopy are recommended to evaluate the full extent of the disease.[40] When polyps are suspected, colonoscopy is the ideal choice because of its diagnostic ability, and also its ability to provide definitive treatment.[41] Radiological techniques as discussed previously may also be used.

Preparation for Procedure

Depending on the procedure of choice, there are a variety of preparations that need to be made. The first is to ensure that the patient is medically stable, especially for tests requiring

sedation, and in the setting of anticipated ongoing and potentially severe bleeding. The second is to make sure that the support staff and all the necessary equipment are available for the procedure. If this is not possible, patient transfer to an appropriately equipped facility should be considered. The choice of transfer modality (i.e., ground versus air) depends on the patient's condition and distance to be traveled and is best made in conjunction with the transport team.

The preparation for EGD mostly consists of adequate NPO time. This may differ depending on the institution's sedation policy, but is approximately 2 to 3 hours for liquids and 6 hours for solids[42,43] depending on the type of fluids ingested and the patient's age. The NG lavage can be very helpful in assisting with evacuation of gastric contents to ensure adequate endoscopic visualization of the mucosa. In the great majority of cases of acute GI bleeding in pediatric patients, general anesthesia is administered by a dedicated anesthesia team providing necessary level of sedation and analgesia, thus allowing the endoscopist to focus solely on the procedure at hand, especially for prolonged procedures. Endotracheal intubation is frequently utilized to prevent aspiration.

The preparation for colonoscopic examination requires not only the appropriate NPO time, but also a bowel purgative, which is of the utmost importance to ensure proper mucosal visualization. If the endoscopist attempts to perform a colonoscopy without proper cleansing, this will make a thorough examination very difficult and increase the chance of complications. The bowel preparation for colonoscopy may need to be adjusted depending on the type of bleeding encountered and the endoscopist's preference. For example, for patients with a history of hematochezia and diarrhea secondary to presumed colitis, standard bowel preparation should suffice, whereas a patient with melena or maroon-colored stool may require a more aggressive approach with large-volume (40 mL/kg/hr) colon lavage, or until the rectal effluent is clear. A variety of bowel preparations are available, and a detailed review is available in Chapter 62 and elsewhere.[44,45]

There is an ongoing debate regarding video capsule endoscopy preparation. Some advocate colonoscopy-type preparation with or without simethicone, whereas others elect a prep similar to that for an EGD.[46] Video capsule endoscopy is discussed in greater detail in Chapter 64.

THERAPY

In order to determine the best approach for treatment of GI bleeding one needs to gather information from all available sources including thorough history and physical examination, as well as appropriate interpretation of results from various diagnostic tests. Once the diagnosis is suspected or made, the choice of therapy with the best possible chance of success and the least possibility of adverse events is determined (see Table 14-7).[47,48]

In patients with upper GI bleeding, proton pump inhibitor (PPI) therapy is frequently utilized. Several adult studies recommend intravenous PPI therapy in such settings.[49] However, no studies exist in the pediatric literature that address this practice. Theoretically, the nonacidic gastric pH can help stabilize clot formation, and IV use can achieve this faster than oral PPI administration.

For patients with variceal bleeding, pediatric literature review suggests octreotide to be a safe agent, although it can

TABLE 14-7. Therapy

Supportive Care
IV fluids (isotonic)
Blood products (packed red blood cells, fresh frozen plasma)
Pressors (dopamine, etc.)

Specific Care
Proton pump inhibitors (omeprazole, lansoprazole, pantoprazole)
Somatostatin analogue (octreotide)

Endoscopic Therapy
Injection (sclerosant, epinephrine, normal saline, hypertonic saline)
Coagulation (bipolar, monopolar, heater probe, laser, argon plasma)
Variceal injection and ligation
Band ligation
Polypectomy
Endoscopic clip
Endoscopic loop

also be used for nonvariceal bleeding.[50] Octreotide should be used with caution, especially in patients with known cardiac disease, because it affects not only splanchnic circulation, but other vasculature as well. In addition, there is a risk of bowel ischemia, and close monitoring for signs of bowel injury are necessary. The dose of octreotide starts at 1 μg/kg followed by 1 to 2 μg/kg/h as a continuous infusion, with slow 25% titration to dose and then tapering off once bleeding is stabilized.[51,52]

Once the patient is stabilized, medical therapies are instituted, and necessary diagnostic tests are obtained. EGD or colonoscopy is often necessary. It is advisable to choose the largest age-appropriate instrument size possible, which will optimize the use of various instruments that might be necessary for therapy, as well as enable proper flushing of blood and debris when needed. The endoscopists should be familiar with the size of available endoscopes and accessories. In some cases the size of the endoscope's working channel may dictate the therapeutic approach. For example, not all equipment will fit through a neonatal-size endoscope.

Endoscopic tools to achieve hemostasis include modalities such as heat, electricity, argon plasma, injectable vasopressors, laser, and mechanical tamponade.[53] The more common and readily available modalities include electrical, heat, and tamponade agents.[54] An electrical current applied with a bipolar probe causes coagulation of the bleeding site, which may be used in conjunction with pressure, known as captive coagulation. The settings of the electrical generating unit for cautery varies by manufacturer and should be set according to its instructions.[55] Usual settings for the bipolar probe range from 15 to 25 W.[25] With small lesions, the probe is placed directly on the blood vessel or lesion. Otherwise, cautery is performed around the bleeding site in pulses of 2 to 3 seconds until hemostasis is achieved.[25,55] A final cautery at the center of the lesion is then performed. This technique can also be performed to prevent further bleeding in a high-risk lesion such as a visible vessel, a sentinel clot, or a cherry-red spot.[25,55] A large bleeding artery may require three to six applications of cautery using similar circumferential application followed by center application.[55] Contraindications to performing these techniques include hemodynamically unstable patient, significant arterial bleeding that obscures the visual field, esophageal variceal bleeding, and arteriovenous malformations larger than 1 cm in size.

Another technique that can be used alone or in conjunction with the foregoing is injection therapy. Various agents, when injected at the bleeding site, will cause vasoconstriction or sclerosis. An example is 1:10,000 epinephrine solution injected into the bleeding lesion in 0.5- to 1-mL aliquots. Hypertonic saline/epinephrine, thrombin, and ethanol can also be used.[25] Each agent has specific doses, formulations, and methods of administration, and the endoscopist should be familiar with those before their use. Endoscopic therapy for GI bleeding is discussed in more detail in Chapters 61 and 62.

A technique that is becoming more frequently used in pediatrics is endoscopic clips. They offer the ability to stop bleeding quickly using continuous tamponade on areas where the bleeding site is readily seen. In nonvariceal bleeding, their efficacy in hemostasis has been described to range from 84 to 100%.[25] Finally, monopolar probes, argon plasma coagulation, hot biopsy forceps, and heater probes can also be used.[56-58] If bleeding cannot be stopped or is very significant, surgery to repair the lesion should be considered.[55]

Esophageal variceal bleeding is treated either with injection of a sclerosing agent or by band ligation.[59] Because of its large size, the banding apparatus may be difficult to use in patients 2 years of age and younger. Several studies have shown the increased safety of banding compared to sclerotherapy as method of choice for treatment of esophageal varices.[60-62] This technique involves sucking the varix into the banding channel and then releasing the band over the varix. The bands are placed in a distal-to-proximal fashion up to 5 cm from the gastroesophageal junction.[55] A potential advantage of sclerotherapy compared to band ligation may be the ability to inject multiple vessels, whereas placement of bands could obscure the view and prevent treatment of all the bleeding vessels. In a randomized trial of 49 children with esophageal varices, banding was found to achieve eradication of varices faster when compared to sclerotherapy, with a lower rebleeding rate and fewer complications.[63] Various agents for sclerotherapy are available including sodium morrhuate, ethanolamine, sodium tetradecyl sulfate, polidocanol, 99.5% ethanol, 3% phenol, and D50.[64,65] Bleeding during sclerotherapy can be encountered in up to 25% of cases, but it is effective 90% of the time.[66] Gastric varices may require additional techniques such as the use of tissue glue or adhesives.[55] These lesions are more difficult to treat and it is harder to achieve adequate long-term hemostasis when compared to esophageal varices. If all the foregoing modalities are ineffective, emergent surgical consult or use of the Sengstaken-Blakemore or Minnesota tube might be necessary. One should be readily familiar with placement before use, although the tubes are not sized for smaller pediatric patients.[67]

With lower GI bleeding, the same principles of initial patient stabilization should be applied. Once the preparation is completed, colonoscopy can identify the bleeding lesion, and similar choices as with upper GI bleeding regarding hemostasis options are available. A colonic polyp is a common etiology of bleeding, and therapy involves polypectomy. A technician familiar and experienced with polypectomy technique should be available for assistance. The polyp can be removed by a variety of techniques depending on its size and type. The colonoscope should be oriented so that the polyp is in the 5 o'clock position. A polyp less than 7 mm in size can be removed with a cold snare, and those less than 3 mm in size with a cold forceps. Hot biopsy forceps are not always necessary for lesions 5 mm or smaller and may be associated with a higher risk of bleeding in some circumstances.[68,69] With larger polyps, a polypectomy snare with cauterization is used, and the setting is adjusted depending on the

TABLE 14-8. Neonatal Differential Diagnosis

Hematemesis
Swallowed maternal blood
Stress ulcer
Gastritis
Duplication cyst
Vascular malformation
Vitamin K deficiency
Hemophilia
Maternal idiopathic thrombocytopenic purpura
Maternal NSAID
Trauma (NG tube, nasal suction)
Hematochezia
Swallowed maternal blood
Dietary protein intolerance
Infectious colitis
Necrotizing enterocolitis
Hirschsprung's disease and enterocolitis
Malrotation with volvulus
Duplication cyst
Vascular malformation
Hemophilia
Maternal idiopathic thrombocytopenic purpura
Maternal NSAID
Anal fissure
Intussusception

TABLE 14-9. Infant Differential Diagnosis

Hematemesis/Melena
Esophagitis
Gastritis
Stress ulcer
Duplication cyst
Vascular malformation
Vitamin K deficiency
Hemophilia
Varices
Hematochezia
Anal fissure
Intussusception
Infectious colitis
Dietary protein intolerance
Meckel's diverticulum
Duplication cyst
Vascular malformation

type of cautery unit, the manufacturer's recommendation, and the location of the polyp. Polyps on the right side of the colon, which has a thinner wall, should be removed using lower settings as compared to the left colon. Adult literature on electrocautery settings for polypectomy recommends ranges from 15 to 40 W depending on the device, with the most common setting of approximately 20 W.[70] The specific settings in regards to use of cutting, blended, or coagulation modality vary throughout the literature, with the most commonly used being blended current.[68,71,72] Nylon loops, wire snare, and clips can be used to stop bleeding if postpolypectomy bleeding occurs.[25,70] The clips and loops can also be placed on the polyp stalk before polypectomy in order to reduce chance of bleeding, especially in case of large polyps or piecemeal polypectomy. Further discussion of polypectomy technique is covered in Chapter 62.

Causes and Differential Diagnosis

Newborns and Infants

Upper and lower GI bleeding in the very small child (Tables 14-8 and 14-9) can be challenging not only because the differential is varied and the infant has a limited blood supply, but because there is also a relatively limited ability to intervene through a pediatric neonatal endoscope.[73]

The most common causes of bleeding include swallowed maternal blood in breast-fed babies and rectal or anal fissure. This is readily diagnosed with a good history and physical examination. An Apt test can be used to differentiate maternal from infant blood, with a positive result indicating infant blood. The test is based on the fact that infant fetal hemoglobin resists denaturation with alkali better than does adult hemoglobin. Therefore, exposure of adult blood to sodium hydroxide will result in a brown color, whereas infant blood will be pink.[74-76]

More severe causes of upper tract bleeding in an infant include stress ulcerations, with gastric lesions occurring four times more frequently than duodenal lesions.[73,77] Approximately one third of patients may have a coinciding esophageal

lesion. These usually occur secondary to significant events around delivery including asphyxia, trauma, sepsis, intracranial bleeding, or heart disease, but they can occur in 1 to 1.5% of healthy infants, as well.[73,77] Regardless of the cause, most cases can be diagnosed with upper endoscopy and rarely recur. Bleeding can also be associated with vitamin K deficiency, milk protein allergy, blood dyscrasias such as hemophilia and von Willebrand's disease, maternal immune thrombocytopenia, and nonsteroidal anti-inflammatory drug use.[78] Infants older than 1 month may also have erosive disease related to peptic or acid injury of the esophagus or gastric mucosa. This is usually associated with irritability, vomiting, or regurgitation.[79]

Aside from anal fissure, the most common cause of lower GI bleeding is milk or soy protein allergy. Milk protein allergy usually presents with hematochezia and will often have a low associated serum albumin level.[80] Flexible sigmoidoscopy can be helpful to confirm the allergy, but most often the diagnosis is made based on clinical signs and symptoms as well as history. Other causes of lower GI bleeding include necrotizing enterocolitis, infectious colitis, volvulus, intussusception, Hirschsprung's disease, and very rarely Meckel's diverticulum. Necrotizing enterocolitis usually presents in the premature infant and is preceded by feeding intolerance. Severity can range from mild to severe with intestinal perforation and peritonitis.[81] Hirschsprung's enterocolitis may also present with hematochezia, diarrhea, and severe illness. The child may have a history of delayed passage of meconium. Infectious colitis must always be suspected especially with a family history of exposure to animals such as reptiles. *Clostridium difficile* toxin positivity under the age of 1 year must be interpreted cautiously because many children are carriers without clinical disease.[82-84] Volvulus and intussusception can present with hematochezia in addition to abdominal distention and/or bilious vomiting and should prompt an immediate surgical evaluation.[27] In intussusception, colicky pain and abdominal mass on physical examination are often found. The classic description of "currant jelly" stool is not always present and might be a late sign of bowel necrosis. In cases of recurrent intussusception or outside of the common age range, the possibility of a lead point should be investigated.[85] Although it may stem from a transient process such as mesenteric adenitis, it may also occur from a polyp, duplication cyst, or lymphoma or other masses. A lead point is more likely to be found in an infant or older child than in a toddler.[86] The most sensitive test for diagnosis of intussusception is ultrasound.[87] A symptomatic Meckel's diverticulum may present with painless rectal bleeding of significant quantity.[88] The blood is classically described as maroon colored, but could also be red or melanotic.

GI Bleeding in Toddlers and School-Aged Children

The close proximity of this age group to infancy suggests that many of the causes are similar to those described previously. Additional causes include mechanical or burn mucosal injury secondary to a foreign body, pill or caustic ingestion, food allergy, vasculitis (Henoch-Schönlein purpura), systemic disease, or head trauma.[89,90] *Helicobacter pylori* infection may be a cause of gastritis and gastric or duodenal ulceration. Infectious illnesses may result in persistent vomiting leading to an esophageal Mallory Weiss mucosal tear (Table 14-10).

More severe causes of upper GI bleeding in this age group include Dieulafoy lesion, esophageal varices secondary to chronic liver disease, and NSAID-induced ulceration. A Dieulafoy lesion is a relatively rare isolated submucosal vascular anomaly without ulceration that protrudes through the mucosa and may cause serious and recurrent bleeding.[91,92] It can occur anywhere in the GI tract, but is usually found in the stomach. Esophageal varices occur as mentioned earlier with associated stigmata of chronic liver disease, but may also occur in the setting of extrahepatic portal hypertension. A Mallory-Weiss tear is associated with a history of recurrent retching from a variety of conditions.[93] Each of the foregoing conditions usually prompts a need for an upper endoscopy. Depending on the cause and bleeding severity, endoscopic therapy may or may not be needed.

Lower GI bleeding due to Meckel's diverticulum or juvenile polyp are more likely to present in this age group. Bleeding from both of these is usually painless. Meckel's diverticulum bleeding occurs due to the presence of ectopic gastric mucosa causing acid-induced erosion on the opposite, antimesenteric side of the small bowel. The lesions can function as a lead point for intussusception in up to 60% of patients 5 to 14 years old. In recurrent intussusception, the likelihood of finding a lead point increases from 4% to 14-19%.[86] A polyp may present as an isolated lesion or, in the case of multiple polyps, be associated with a polyposis syndrome (i.e., juvenile polyposis, Peutz-Jeghers syndrome, familial adenomatous polyposis, and others).[94,95] These conditions are discussed in more detail in Chapter 43. Other causes of lower GI bleeding include duplication cysts, lymphonodular hyperplasia, and extensive gastric heterotopia.[96] Duplication cysts may also cause bleeding when related to obstruction or intussusception.[27,97]

There are other infectious, vascular and inflammatory conditions that may present in this age group with hematochezia including Henoch-Schönlein purpura (HSP), hemolytic-uremic syndrome (HUS), inflammatory bowel disease (IBD), vascular malformations, and bleeding secondary to typhlitis/chemotherapy. HSP usually presents with a lower extremity and buttock rash with abdominal pain. Seventy percent of patients have the abdominal pain component with a third of those having melena or hematemesis.[98-100] A variety of bacterial infections including *Clostridium difficile* and Shiga-toxin-producing organisms can cause bleeding. Often this is accompanied by significant diarrhea and abdominal pain. Inflammatory bowel disease may present as chronic colitis resulting in hematochezia, but also as occult blood loss in the setting of poor growth, anemia, and hypoalbuminemia. Vascular malformations may occur

TABLE 14-10. Child Differential Diagnosis

Hematemesis/Melena

Esophagitis
Gastritis
Peptic ulcer disease
Mallory-Weiss tear
Esophageal varices/gastric varices
Portal hypertensive gastropathy
Pill ulcerations
Foreign body ingestion
NSAID use

Hematochezia

Anal fissure
Infectious colitis
Polyp
Lymphoid nodular hyperplasia
Inflammatory bowel disease
Henoch-Schönlein purpura
Intussusception
Meckel's diverticulum
Hemolytic uremic syndrome
Vascular malformation
Ischemic colitis
Typhlitis/neutropenic colitis
Duplication cyst
Dieulafoy lesion

as isolated lesions or as a part of various syndromes and may present at any age. Some of these include Osler-Weber-Rendu disease, Klippel-Trénaunay syndrome, blue rubber bleb nevus syndrome, hereditary or familial colonic varices, progressive systemic sclerosis with telangiectasias, and Turner syndrome with intestinal telangiectasias.[101-103] These can be investigated with colonoscopy, angiography, CTA, video capsule endoscopy, or balloon enteroscopy. Therapy of such vascular lesions is difficult, and although some may be amenable to an endoscopic approach, they are often treated surgically.

GI Bleeding in Adolescents and Young Adults

Older children and adolescents may present with variety of conditions including manifestations of congenital disorders, but also those similar to their adult counterparts. The common causes of upper GI bleeding include ulcerations of the gastric and duodenal mucosa, esophagitis, and gastritis (Table 14-11). This may present as melena or hematemesis depending on the severity of the bleeding. The presentation of bleeding from the foregoing causes usually is late in the course of illness. They may have a described history of acid brash, halitosis, dysphagia, periprandial pain, or NSAID use.[104,105] *Helicobacter pylori* infection should be ruled out, and fecal antigen is highly sensitive and specific for this purpose. Hematemesis can occur secondary to a Mallory-Weiss tear with a history of GI illness or retching.[106] With physical examination findings of portal hypertension (splenomegaly, caput medusae, asterixis, jaundice), variceal bleeding is the likely source. Patients taking medications can have pill-induced esophagitis with severe odynophagia. Common culprits include NSAIDs, aspirin, tetracycline (doxycycline), potassium, quinidine, iron, and alendronate.[107]

Causes of lower GI bleeding in this age group are similar to those previously described and include infectious and inflammatory colitis, or polyps. The most common causes of infectious colitis include *Salmonella, Shigella, Yersinia, Campylobacter, E. coli* O157:H7, and *Clostridium difficile*.[9] A recent new

TABLE 14-11. **Adolescent Differential Diagnosis**

Hematemesis/Melena

Esophagitis
Gastritis
Peptic ulcer disease
Mallory-Weiss tear
Esophageal varices/gastric varices
Portal hypertensive gastropathy
Pill ulcerations
Foreign body ingestion
NSAID use

Hematochezia

Anal fissure
Infectious colitis
Polyp
Lymphoid nodular hyperplasia
Inflammatory bowel disease
Henoch-Schönlein purpura
Intussusception
Meckel's diverticulum
Hemolytic uremic syndrome
Vascular malformation
Ischemic colitis
Typhlitis/neutropenic colitis
Duplication cyst
Dieulafoy lesion

subtype of *Clostridium difficile* (BI/NAP1/027) may cause severe life-threatening illness.[84] Other causes of colitis include virus and parasites such as cytomegalovirus (CMV), adenovirus, and *Entamoeba histolytica*. To rule out infectious colitis, stool studies including all the foregoing infectious agents are often necessary. If the child is immunocompromised, further testing is indicated for viral sources such as CMV or adenovirus and *Cryptosporidium*. Juvenile polyposis syndrome can present in late childhood or adolescence, as opposed to isolated juvenile polyps, which typically present at a younger age. If polyps are found, they should be removed and sent to pathology for diagnosis, because this condition is associated with an increased risk of cancer, similar to the other polyposis syndromes including familial adenomatous polyposis, Peutz-Jeghers syndrome, and hereditary nonpolyposis colorectal cancer (HNPCC). Each of the foregoing syndromes requires careful monitoring, and specific guidelines

for surveillance are available.[94,95,108,109] Additional information on these can be found in Chapter 43 or at www.genetests.org.

CONCLUSIONS

Gastrointestinal bleeding is a very important and relatively common presenting complaint to the pediatric gastroenterologist. The causes can range from false bleeding due to food ingestion that resembles blood, or bleeding from a simple anal fissure, to the other extreme of life-threatening esophageal variceal bleeding secondary to chronic liver disease and portal hypertension. Regardless of the source, diagnostic work-up requires diligence and skill in obtaining detailed and targeted history and physical examination that will help the practitioner develop a carefully thought-out plan for proper intervention. Among other resources, endoscopy is an invaluable tool in both investigation and treatment of GI bleeding.

REFERENCES

5. Boyle JT. Gastrointestinal bleeding in infants and children. Pediatr Rev 2008;29:39–52.
6. Fox VL. Gastrointestinal bleeding in infancy and childhood. Gastroenterol Clin North Am 2000;29:37–66.
9. Wyllie R, Hyams JS, Kay. M. Pediatric Gastrointestinal and Liver Disease: Pathophysiology, Diagnosis, Management. 3rd ed. Philadelphia: Saunders Elsevier; 2006.
10. Aljebreen AM, Fallone CA, Barkun AN. Nasogastric aspirate predicts high-risk endoscopic lesions in patients with acute upper-GI bleeding. Gastrointest Endosc 2004;59:172–178.
25. Kay MH, Wyllie R. Therapeutic endoscopy for nonvariceal gastrointestinal bleeding. J Pediatr Gastroenterol Nutr 2007;45:157–171.
61. Saeed ZA, Stiegmann GV, Ramirez FC, et al. Endoscopic variceal ligation is superior to combined ligation and sclerotherapy for esophageal varices: a multicenter prospective randomized trial. Hepatology 1997;25:71–74.
70. Morris ML, et al. Electrosurgery in gastrointestinal endoscopy: principles to practice. Am J Gastroenterol 2009;104:1563–1574.
95. Haidle JL, Howe JR. Juvenile polyposis syndrome. In: Gene Reviews 2008. Retrieved Oct 9, 2009, from: www.ncbi.nlm.nih.gov/bookshelf/br.fcgi?book=gene&;part=jps#jps.Chapter_Notes

See expertconsult.com for a complete list of references and the review questions for this chapter.

15 OBESITY

Joseph Skelton • Gail M. Cohen

The Surgeon General,[1] the Institutes of Medicine,[2] and the World Health Organization[3] have classified childhood obesity as an epidemic in need of immediate and wide-reaching attention. The prevalence of childhood obesity has nearly tripled over the past 20 years with 17% of children now considered obese.[4] Pediatric health care providers have focused on prevention of the long-term sequelae of obesity, but now find themselves screening for and treating diseases previously found only in adults. Of children with newly diagnosed diabetes, nearly half have type 2.[5,6] Childhood obesity is significantly associated with increasing health care costs,[7,8] with an estimated $14 billion spent yearly in caring for obese children and their weight-related comorbidities.[9] Improvements in cardiovascular mortality in young adults are leveling off or worsening,[10] and life expectancy may be shortened in this next generation.[11] There is a paucity of "gold standards" for treatment, but many approaches are effective, and new approaches, such as bariatric surgery, are increasingly used and studied.

DEFINITIONS

Any definition of obesity must take into account two important criteria: diagnosis of increased body fat, and identification of an increased risk of adverse health outcomes. Currently there are no accepted standards for body fatness for either adults or children.[12] As a result, body mass index (BMI), which is calculated as weight (in kilograms) divided by the square of height (in meters), is used as a screening tool for both adult and childhood obesity. Although BMI cannot determine body fat content, it has been shown to accurately identify children with increased adiposity in a population with fairly high specificity and moderate sensitivity.[13,14] Alternative methods of determining body fat content include skinfold thickness or waist circumference, but are difficult to reliably perform in a clinical setting. Even though skinfold thickness measurement is predictive of total body fat in children,[15] it is not recommended for routine use because of the lack of readily available reference data, the training involved in performing it, and measurement error between operators.[16] Waist circumference is useful in predicting insulin resistance and other comorbidities in children,[17,18] but not as useful in predicting total adiposity.[19] As with skinfold thickness, there is difficulty in performing it reliably, especially in obese populations; it does not have readily available standards in children and is therefore not recommended for routine clinical use.[16] Other more precise and sensitive methods of determining adiposity are too expensive (ultrasound, computed tomography, magnetic resonance imaging, dual-energy x-ray absorptiometry, air displacement plethysmography) or are lacking normative data in children (bioelectric impedance analysis).

In adults, overweight is defined as a BMI at or above 25 kg/m², and obesity as a BMI at or above 30. These cutoff points were determined based on short-term and long-term health risks in adults.[20] In children, such cutoffs have not been conclusively determined. The length of time before many adverse health outcomes are evident and the relatively small sample sizes of early studies of cardiovascular risks have made such a determination problematic. Statistically derived cutoff points define overweight in children as BMI at or above the 85th percentile for age and gender compared with nationally representative populations, and obesity as BMI at or above the 95th percentile. These cutoffs were originally created arbitrarily and for clinically practical reasons. However, more recent studies have found that for several short- and long-term outcomes, children with BMI percentiles above these levels have a higher risk of morbidity than their peers with lower BMI percentiles. Definitive BMI cutoffs that can accurately predict the risks of adverse consequences have not been determined, but they are likely to depend not only on the outcome of interest, but on the ethnicity/race or other characteristics of the individual and population as well. An international definition of overweight and obesity, derived from nationally representative cross-sectional growth studies in six countries, has not been found to be of practical use in the United States. Use of these cutoffs proposed by the International Obesity Task Force (IOTF) has led to vast underidentification of obesity, although the identification of overweight was more accurate.[21] Recent expert recommendations recognize that a BMI at or above the 95th percentile in older teens is higher than a BMI of 30 kg/m.² Therefore, the committee recommended that obesity be defined as a BMI of 95th percentile or at or above 30 kg/m², whichever is lower. For children younger than 2 years of age, BMI is not used, and use of weight-for-height is recommended (weight-for-height above the 95th percentile is considered overweight).[16]

There is a need to establish nomenclature for higher levels of obesity for children under consideration for bariatric surgery or other aggressive forms of treatment.[22] A BMI at or above 40 kg/m² is the level of morbid obesity in adults, and a starting point for bariatric surgery consideration. This has also been proposed for children, but it is not pertinent to younger children or even in early adolescents, for whom a BMI of 40 or more is extremely high. A BMI above the 97th percentile is found on growth charts, but has not been extensively studied in relation to future comorbidity risk. As part of the 2007 Expert Recommendations to identify children at an extreme level of obesity, a BMI ≥ 99th percentile for age and gender was proposed as severe childhood obesity.[23] Recent analysis of NHANES data demonstrates significant cardiometabolic differences between those at this level of obesity (≥ 99th percentile) and lower levels (95th-97th percentile).[24] Compared to older NHANES data, the prevalence of severe childhood obesity has increased over

300% in the past 25 years to a present level of 3.8%.[24] More than 400,000 children have a BMI of 40 kg/m^2 or more, which is the adult classification of morbid obesity.[24] During the period 1971-1974, obese children were on average 12% above the obese threshold, but by 1999-2000 obese children were 14% above this threshold.[25] Over time more children are becoming obese, and those that are obese are heavier on average.

The growth charts that are currently in use in the United States were published by the Centers for Disease Control and Prevention in 2000.[26] They were developed using data from five nationally representative survey data sets: the National Health Examination Surveys II and III in the 1960s; NHANES I and II in the 1970s; and NHANES III from 1988-1994. The data from these surveys were pooled, with the exception of weight data for children at least 6 years old in NHANES III because of the apparent increase of weight in this group of children. The purpose of these charts, which is primarily clinical, is to follow a child's growth over time; use of the charts to define overweight and obesity in a given population is a secondary purpose.

Despite the evident shortcomings in using BMI and BMI percentiles to screen for overweight and obesity in children, it is the current standard of care for all children. The American Academy of Pediatrics (AAP) recommends calculating BMI as the preferred measure for evaluation of childhood overweight and obesity.[16,23] This recommendation includes the calculation and plotting of BMIs for all children over the age of 2 years, at least yearly. The tracking of BMI and weight status can be of use to identify early onset obesity. A child's BMI reaches a natural nadir between 5 and 6 years of age and then rises again, a phenomenon called the adiposity rebound. An early nadir and increase, occurring before 5 years of age, is associated with increased risk of hypertension and obesity in adulthood, primarily due to increased fat, rather than lean muscle, deposition.[27] However, it has not been clearly determined whether intervening with early adiposity rebound prevents later obesity.

EPIDEMIOLOGY

The epidemiology of overweight and obesity, in both children and adults, in the United States has changed dramatically over the past several decades. In 1980 the prevalence of obesity among adults was 15%; in 2004 it was 32.9%.[28] There is an indication that levels of obesity among adults may be leveling off, as no statistically significant increases in the prevalence were found between the periods of 2003-2004 and 2005-2006.[29] Similar trends have been found for children and adolescents. During the period 1971-1974, the prevalence of overweight among children and adolescents age 2 to 19 years was 15.3%, and the prevalence of obesity in the same group was 5.1%.[25] For the period 2003-2006, the corresponding prevalence rates were 31.9% and 16.3%, respectively.[30] These trends may be leveling off as well; no statistically significant changes were observed among overweight and obesity prevalence rates in children from the periods 2003-2004 and 2005-2006.

Each age group of children and adolescents has experienced alarming trends (Table 15-1).[30-32] Similar increases were seen in both boys and girls, as well as among children of different racial/ethnic groups.[4] During this time period, there is increasing disparity between racial/ethnic groups, with Mexican Americans and African Americans showing marked increases in obesity prevalence, particularly in teen-aged boys.[30-32]

ETIOLOGY AND PATHOGENESIS

At the most basic level, obesity is a result of an imbalance between energy intake and expenditure. The acute rise in obesity prevalence, cardiovascular disease, and other chronic illnesses suggests that changes in human environment and lifestyles are behind this epidemic. Bouchard elegantly outlined a model of this epidemic and its main contributors, grouped into four areas: built environment, social environment, behavior, and biology.[33] In this model, the built and social environment combine to create an "obesogenic" environment, leading to "obesogenic" behaviors. Biological predisposition then has a profound influence on an individual's energy balance, and therefore risk of obesity.

Obesogenic Environment

From the convenience of fast food to the increasing use of cars instead of walking, changes in the built and social environment over the past 50 years have significantly contributed to childhood obesity. Attempts are frequently made to isolate a small number of significant contributors to the obesity epidemic, but much like the biologic control of appetite (see later discussion), this is a complex problem. Changes in the social environment are represented by the increase in energy-dense foods and drinks, easily available in large portions and at low prices. Changes in family structure, including single-parent households and dual-career couples, have led to increased use of high-calorie, high-fat convenience foods.[34] Higher socioeconomic status is a risk factor for obesity in developing countries, and protective in already developed countries.[35] In developing countries, the wealthy are able to afford higher calorie foods and mechanized transportation and are less likely to have jobs that require manual labor. In developed or industrialized countries, much of the obesity epidemic is thought to be due to food insecurity, where a person or family is at risk of being unable to provide food.[36] This can lead to the purchase of bulk, energy-dense foods, which are often less expensive and engineered to be highly palatable, thereby increasing overall caloric intake and decreasing nutrient quality.[37] A larger proportion of the calories in these foods are in the form of inexpensive sweeteners (high-fructose corn syrup) and fat, theorized to increase appetite and lead to addictive behaviors, but there is little proof of these qualities in the foods.

Systematic examinations of built environments reveal few consistent findings.[38] Children are less susceptible to the decreased caloric expenditure of motorized travel and

TABLE 15-1. Increased Prevalence of Obesity Among U.S. Children and Adolescents, Based on Age and Gender-Specific Body Mass Index (BMI) Growth Charts

Ages (years)	Prevalence of Obesity (BMI ≥ 95th Percentile)			
	NHANES II 1976-1980	NHANES III 1988-1994	NHANES 1999-2002	NHANES 2003-2006
2-5	5%	7.2%	10.3%	12.4%
6-11	6.5%	11.3%	15.8%	17%
12-19	5%	10.5%	16.1%	17.6%

Adapted from Ogden et al.,[4] Hedley et al.,[32] and Ogden et al.[30]

sedentary jobs, but electronic entertainment plays a large role. Video games, television, computers/Internet, and even cell phone use have led to increasing hours of sedentary activity in children (averaging more than 21 hours a week), which has been clearly associated with obesity.[39] There is evidence that "screen time" use over the AAP's recommended limit of 2 hours a day increases child and later adult risk of obesity.[40,41] Finally, investigation of the environment of children, including the safety of local roads, proximity of schools and playgrounds, hazards, walkability and safety of neighborhoods, and population density all affect a child's weight status and risk of future obesity.[38] In summary, obvious changes in the nutritional and activity (sedentary and physical) environments of children, possibly mediated by changes in families and socioeconomic status, have contributed significantly to this epidemic.

Behavior

Much research has centered on various eating and activity behaviors and the potential impact each has on childhood obesity risk and prevalence. Little direct evidence exists for the importance of a single eating pattern to an individual's weight status; rather it is more likely that several eating behaviors exist concurrently and interrelatedly, and the impact each has is modified by the individual's genetics, ethnicity, and gender. Eating behaviors such as those described next are thought to contribute more to excess energy consumption than to absolute weight status.[16,23,42]

The specific eating behaviors that have been targeted as potential mediators of obesity include restaurant food consumption; sugar-sweetened beverage consumption; fruit juice consumption; increasing portion sizes; energy-dense food consumption; decreased fruit and vegetable consumption; irregular or no breakfast consumption; and frequent snacking. Although these behaviors would seem to have a large impact on weight status, studies have generally been inconclusive for this specific relationship. Because these behaviors have been found to be associated with excessive energy intake, however, assessing and addressing these behaviors may encourage decreased energy consumption.

Various activities have been suggested as either attenuating or increasing BMIs in children. Physical activity or exercise is thought to be beneficial for prevention of obesity as well as weight loss. A recent systematic review of the literature[43] concluded that, whereas some of the more recent studies have found an inverse relationship between physical activity and weight status, many studies found no relationship between the two. Additionally, sedentary activity, specifically television viewing, is associated with higher weight status[44]; however, a dose-response relationship between the two has not been determined. Despite this uncertainty, the AAP recommends no more than 2 hours of screen time per day for children older than 2 years of age.[40]

Parenting and parenting style has become a new focus of intervention and prevention of obesity. A popular theory of parenting style developed over time categorizes by expectations for self-control and sensitivity.[45,46] The application of this theory to parental feeding approaches has determined risks for childhood obesity, with overly controlling practices (authoritarian) having the highest risk (Table 15-2).[47] Although the mechanism of this has not been fully delineated, it does present opportunities for treatment and prevention at early ages.

Biology

There have been great strides in understanding the control of appetite, energy expenditure, and overall weight control in the past two decades, most notably in the discovery of the leptin gene in 1994.[48] Although leptin did not turn out to be the "smoking gun," it unveiled a complex regulatory system of energy intake and expenditure, using short-term and long-term feedback mechanisms to balance appetite and metabolism. Further, a paradigm shift occurred in how adiposity, and more specifically the adipocyte, is viewed. No longer seen as a storage cell for excess calories, visceral adipose cells are categorized as independent endocrine cells with important roles in metabolism, inflammation, and cardiovascular disease (Table 15-3).[49]

Figure 15-1 and Table 15-4 summarize key hormones and signaling agents involved in the control of energy intake (usually manifested in appetite and meal initiation and termination) and energy expenditure (through physical activity and metabolism). The gastrointestinal, central nervous, and adipose/storage systems are the primary areas involved in the short- and long-term balance of energy and weight. Despite the elegance of this network, it is still influenced greatly by environmental stimuli. As an example, initiation of meals is influenced to a greater degree by environmental signals, whereas meal size and termination may be influenced to a greater degree by biologic signals.[50] As of 2005, only 176 cases of human obesity have been identified as caused by a single-gene mutation, surprisingly low given the number of biologic determinants of appetite and weight.[51] All chromosomes except Y have areas associated with obesity phenotypes, with 135 different candidate genes having been identified. In all, more than 600 genes have been associated with human and animal models of obesity.

Leptin deficiency or leptin receptor abnormalities are exceedingly rare. Although it was described in two severely obese cousins with undetectable serum leptin levels, leptin deficiency has been identified in very few individuals.[52] Within a high-risk group (individuals with hyperphagia, severe early-onset obesity, and some from consanguineous families), only 3% had mutations in the leptin receptor gene.[53] In a population of individuals severely obese since childhood, nearly 6% had a mutation in

TABLE 15-2. **Parenting Styles and Prevalence of Obesity, from the Study of Early Child Care and Youth Development**

Parenting Style	Expectations for Self-control	Sensitivity	Prevalence of Parenting Style in Study (N)	Prevalence of Obesity
Authoritative	High	High	20.5% (179)	3.9%
Authoritarian	High	Low	34.2% (298)	17.1%
Permissive	Low	High	15.1% (132)	9.8%
Neglectful	Low	Low	30.2% (263)	9.9%

Adapted from Rhee KE et al. (2006).[47]

TABLE 15-3. **Adipose-Derived Hormones and Cytokines (Adipokines)**

Name	Function/Effects	Effect
Adiponectin	Inhibits inflammatory and other metabolic processes	Increases insulin sensitivity, decreases atherosclerosis; independent risk factor of metabolic syndrome; linked to nonalcoholic fatty liver disease risk
Interleukin (IL)-6	Stimulates hepatic production of C-reactive protein (proinflammatory)	Decreases insulin sensitivity; increases atherosclerosis
Tumor necrosis factor (TNF)-α	Stimulates acute-phase reactants	Decreases insulin sensitivity; increases atherosclerosis
Plasminogen activator inhibitor (PAI)-1	Inhibits plasminogen and fibrinolysis	Increases risk of thromboembolic events
Leptin	Satiety signal via AgRP/NPY neurons; multiple other effects in body	Leptin resistance linked to obesity
Resistin	Highest concentration in mononuclear cells, but found in adipocytes; stimulates inflammatory cytokines	Role in insulin resistance unclear
Visfatin	Inhibits apoptosis of neutrophils; promotes B cell maturation	Decreases insulin resistance
Omentin	Function not clear	Levels decreased with obesity, increased with increases in high-density lipoprotein (HDL) cholesterol and adiponectin

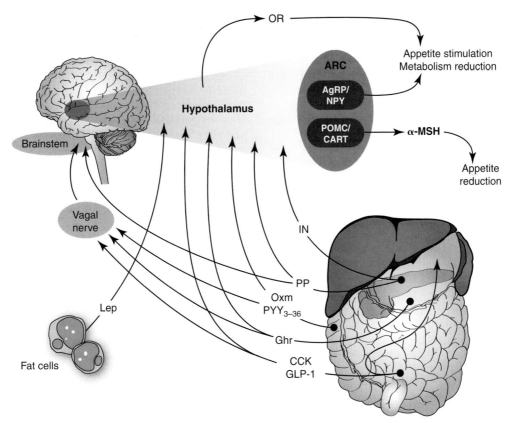

Figure 15-1. Key hormones and signaling agents involved in the control of energy intake (usually manifested in appetite and meal initiation and termination) and energy expenditure (through physical activity and metabolism).

the melanocortin 4 receptor gene (MC4R, the target of α-MSH, a centrally released appetite-reducing signal), making it one of the most common monogenic forms of obesity. However, there are no available therapies for this mutation.[54]

There are other exciting discoveries, aside from the neuroendocrine control of appetite, which present potential targets for intervention. Endocannabinoids are anabolic regulators of metabolism, increasing energy intake, promoting energy storage, and decreasing energy expenditure.[55] Antagonists to this receptor have been shown to improve obesity as well as other aspects

of the metabolic syndrome (insulin resistance, hyperlipidemia), but concerns about depression and other side effects have limited its use.[56,57] There is increasing interest in gut microbiota and its possible regulation of obesity. Predominance of specific groups of bacteria (Bacteroidetes, Firmicutes) has been associated with obesity in mouse models, with increasing evidence of an association in humans.[58,59] There appears to be bacterial control of metabolic process that could affect energy regulation, but clear pathways have not been fully determined. Even more interesting is the possible role of infection in adipogenesis.

TABLE 15-4. **Hormones and Other Signals Involved in Weight Control**

Short Name	Full Name	Origin	Function/Role in Weight Homeostasis
AgRP	Agouti-related peptide	Arcuate nucleus (hypothalamus)	Increases appetite; decreases metabolism
ARC	Arcuate nucleus	Hypothalamus	Area of energy regulation; location of CART, POMC, AgRP, NPY
CART	Cocaine-amphetamine-regulated transcript neurons	Arcuate nucleus (hypothalamus)	Reduces energy intake
CCK	Cholecystokinin	Intestines	Reduces appetite (short term); slows gastric emptying; stimulates gallbladder contractions
Ghr	Ghrelin	Stomach	Increases appetite (short term)
GLP-1	Glucagon-like peptide 1	Intestines – L cell	Stimulates insulin release; reduces appetite
In	Insulin	Pancreas	Reduces energy intake
Lep	Leptin	Adipose tissue	Reduces energy intake
α-MSH	α-Melanocyte-stimulating hormone	POMC (ARC, hypothalamus)	Reduces energy intake
NPY	Neuropeptide Y	Arcuate Nucleus	Increases appetite; decreases metabolism
OR	Orexin	Hypothalamus	Increases appetite
Oxm	Oxyntomodulin	Colon	Reduces appetite
POMC	Pro-opiomelanocortin	Arcuate nucleus (hypothalamus)	Releases α-MSH; reduces energy intake
PP	Pancreatic polypeptide	Pancreas	Reduces appetite
PVC	Periventricular nucleus	Hypothalamus	Appetite and autonomic regulation
PYY$_{3-36}$	Peptide YY	Ileum, colon	Reduces appetite; slows gastric emptying

Animal models have demonstrated that adenoviral and other viral inoculations increased adipogenesis.[60-62] Further studies demonstrated a higher percentage of obese humans had adenovirus-36 antibodies than did nonobese subjects.[63] Again, these findings are interesting, but far from conclusive.

The influence of genetics on obesity is unmistakable, with studies estimating the heritability of BMI to be between 20 and 60%.[64] Twin studies have found that genes account for nearly 80% of variation in body fat and BMI.[65] It is impossible to tease out the environmental influences of body weight when investigating its genetic origins. Although it appears that individuals may be predisposed to weight gain, it is within the context of an obesogenic environment, with many modifiers, both known (parenting style) and unknown (infections), which further complicate the dissection of human obesity.

ASSESSMENT OF THE OBESE CHILD

The assessment of the obese child requires investigation of his or her personal history, including a dietary and physical activity assessment, a focused family history, review of systems, and a physical examination.[16,23,66] In addition, laboratory, radiographic and/or subspecialty evaluation may become necessary. Each of these components will be discussed in turn.

Taking the medical history of an obese child should focus on three main goals: identification of modifiable risk factors; identification of risks for medical comorbidities; and assessment of the patient's and family's readiness to change their behavior.

Modifiable Risk Factors

Nutrition

Dietary assessment can take various forms and may be a difficult endeavor. A 24-hour recall, intake diary, or food frequency questionnaire can be helpful; each has its own advantages and disadvantages. For example, 24-hour dietary recall involves significant recall bias, and intake diaries require precise amounts and recipes to be clinically useful. Although there is no standard

in-office assessment of eating behaviors, attempts should be made to assess certain eating behaviors for which there are some data to support their roles in overconsumption of energy (fast food or other restaurants, sugar-sweetened beverages, portion sizes, energy-dense foods, few fruits and vegetables, skipping breakfast, frequent snacking).

Physical Activity

Because the development of obesity is invariably an imbalance in energy intake and expenditure, assessment of the child's physical activity is also critical. As with a dietary history, assessing physical activity is also difficult. A self-report or self-administered checklist to determine frequency, amount of time, and intensity of activity is commonly used for older children and adolescents. Children less than 10 years old are generally not able to accurately report this type of history; in these cases, parental recall is substituted. Although adolescents have the ability to participate in activities similar to adults, younger children have very different patterns of activity. Asking questions regarding the amount of time spent outside or involvement in sports programs outside of school can be a good proxy for activity in younger children.

Sedentary Activity

The amount of time spent in sedentary activity, specifically television viewing, has been found to be associated with higher BMI percentiles.[41,67] Although this relationship is not as strong for other sedentary behaviors, such as playing computer or video games, these pastimes can replace more active pursuits and must be balanced. A thorough activity history includes time spent engaging in sedentary activity as well.

Medical Comorbidity Risk

Family History

The family history is crucial for assessment of the risk for persistence of obesity into adulthood, as well as the risk of current and future comorbidities. Family history should be assessed specifically for three important conditions among first- and second-degree relatives: obesity, type 2 diabetes mellitus (T2DM), and cardiovascular disease, including hyperlipidemia and hypertension.

Although weight status is generally determined by multifactorial influences, a child's weight status is also strongly influenced by parental weight status. The risk of persistent obesity is higher if one or both parents are obese,[68-70] regardless of the child's current age or weight status. Both maternal and paternal weight status have been shown to independently and significantly influence the child's BMI, even after adjusting for lifestyle, environment, and presence of comorbidities.[71]

The development of T2DM has a strong genetic component. A positive family history for T2DM is a risk factor for insulin resistance in children. Certain racial/ethnic groups (American Indian) are at particularly high risk because of the high prevalence rates found in adults and children.[72] Family history should also be assessed for cardiovascular disease; this should encompass myocardial infarction, stroke, hyperlipidemia, and recognized risk factors for cardiovascular disease, including obesity, hypertension, and diabetes. Obesity and family history of hypertension are independent risk factors for the development of hypertension in children.[16]

Physical Examination

The physical examination should include all of the components of a standard pediatric examination, with particular attention paid to certain aspects. Anthropometry is crucial in this evaluation; height and weight should be measured at each clinic visit, and a BMI should be calculated. The BMI should then be plotted yearly on a standard growth chart to determine the BMI percentile for age and sex. Special attention should be paid to measurement of blood pressure. It should be measured manually using an appropriately sized cuff; blood pressure measurements can then be interpreted with the aid of reference tables.[73]

The fundi should be visualized, looking specifically for signs of increased intracranial pressure, especially if there is a history of headaches. This can be an indication of the presence of pseudotumor cerebri. The thyroid should be examined for goiter in the context of signs of hypothyroidism; the oropharynx should be examined for redundant tissue or enlarged tonsils for concerns of sleep disturbances.

The skin examination is very important in the evaluation of obesity. Acanthosis nigricans, which is a hyperpigmented, hyperkeratotic velvety plaque most often found on the back of the neck, in the axillae, or other body folds and over joints, may be associated with insulin resistance. Keratosis pilaris, skin tags, intertrigo, and furunculosis are all potential findings; violaceous striae characteristic of Cushing syndrome are found less often.

Although cardiac, pulmonary, and abdominal examinations may be difficult in the obese child, they remain important components of the evaluation. Irregular sounds, murmurs, wheezing, and organomegaly, specifically hepatomegaly, are all significant findings on examination. Secondary sexual development should also be assessed. Obesity is associated with premature pubarche and stigmata of polycystic ovary syndrome, including hirsutism, in girls; it is also associated with gynecomastia in boys. The genitals of an obese male may appear small and be concerning for micropenis, but retraction of the pubic fat pad and palpation of the penis and testicles will most often reveal normal genitalia.

The lower extremities are important to examine carefully. Limitation of movement or pain can be signs of underlying disease, specifically slipped capital femoral epiphyses (hips) or Blount disease (knees). Additionally, the lower back and the feet and ankles should be examined as sources of pain, with particular attention to fallen or flat arches (pes planus).

Syndromes or genetic abnormalities causing obesity may also be of concern. These are extremely rare and usually are identified through common presentations. Prader-Willi may be identified at a young age characterized by short stature, small hands and feet, almond-shaped eyes with round face, hypogonadism, and significant developmental delay. POMC mutations (see Figure 15-1 and Table 15-4) are associated with adrenal insufficiency and present with red hair and pale skin. Retinitis pigmentosa in the setting of obesity, polydactyly, short stature, and developmental delay should lead to consideration of Laurence-Moon or Bardet-Biedl syndromes. Fragile X syndrome should be considered with the presentation of hyperactive behavior, large forehead, prominent jaw, large ears, and mental retardation, but macroorchidism should raise suspicion in an obese child. Mutations in the melanocortin receptor of the hypothalamus (MC4R4), which is involved with inhibiting appetite, are associated with tall stature and advanced bone age. In summary, short stature (with the exception of MC4R4), developmental delay, hypotonia, and abnormal facies found in an obese child should prompt a consultation with a geneticist.

Comorbidities

As the obesity epidemic worsens, pediatric care providers must transition from assessing for future risk of weight-related comorbidities to the detection and treatment of them. Although not comprehensive, Table 15-5 provides a focused Review of Systems, and Table 15-6 summarizes the comorbidities associated with pediatric obesity and testing to assist in their identification.[66,74] The review of systems should focus on symptoms of potential comorbidities. The degree of obesity does not reliably predict the presence of comorbidities, and many of the symptoms may be unrecognized as related to weight status by the family. Some of the problems most commonly identified during the review of systems are disordered sleep and obstructive sleep apnea; menstrual disorders and polycystic ovary syndrome; and abdominal pain, signaling nonalcoholic fatty liver disease, gastroesophageal reflux, gallbladder disease, or constipation.

Although the risks associated with obesity in children are not as well studied as they are in adults, there is convincing evidence that the risks of many conditions are increased with early-onset obesity. Cardiovascular disease risk factors (hypertension, hypertriglyceridemia) are markedly higher in obese youth.[75] The incidence of elevated blood pressure has increased in recent years and has been primarily attributed to the parallel increase in childhood obesity.[76] Blood pressure tends to track in an individual over time; thus, elevated blood pressure readings during childhood or adolescence are predictive of the development of adult hypertension, and elevated BMI increases the risk that high blood pressure will persist into adulthood. Although the end-organ effects of elevated blood pressure are rarely seen among pediatric patients, because of blood pressure tracking, it is clear that adult effects of hypertension have their origins in childhood.

Nonalcoholic fatty liver disease is of growing concern, as obesity and insulin resistance are risk factors for this problem.

TABLE 15-5. **Review of Systems**

System	Symptom	Explanation
Respiratory	Shortness of breath, exercise intolerance, wheezing, cough	Asthma, aerobic deconditioning
Gastrointestinal	Vague recurrent abdominal pain	Nonalcoholic fatty liver disease
	Heartburn, dysphagia, regurgitation, chest or epigastric pain	Gastroesophageal reflux
	Abdominal pain or distension, flatulence, fecal incontinence, anorexia, enuresis	Constipation
	Right upper quadrant or epigastric pain, vomiting, colicky pain	Gallbladder disease, gallstones
Endocrine	Polyuria, polydipsia	Type 2 Diabetes Mellitus
	Amenorrhea, oligomenorrhea, or menorrhagia	Polycystic ovary syndrome
Orthopedic	Hip, knee, groin, or thigh pain, painful gait	Slipped capital femoral epiphysis
	Knee pain	Slipped capital femoral epiphysis or Blount disease
	Foot pain	Increased weight bearing, pes planus
Sleep problems	Loud snoring, apnea, daytime sleepiness, restlessness, short attention span, behavioral problems	Obstructive sleep apnea, disordered sleep
Mental health	Flat affect, sad mood, loss of interest, worries	Depression, anxiety
	Body dissatisfaction, school avoidance, poor self-esteem	Depression, anxiety
	Hyperphagia, binge eating, bulimia	Disordered eating
Genitourinary	Nocturia, nocturnal enuresis	Disordered sleep
Dermatology	Rash, irritated skin	Intertrigo
	Darkened skin around neck and axilla	Acanthosis nigricans

Adapted from Barlow[23] and Krebs.[16]

TABLE 15-6. **Weight-Related Comorbidity Assessment**

Condition	Tests	Reason	Note
Cardiac disease	Lipid profile	Hyperlipidemia, hypertriglyceridemia, heart disease risk	
Hypertension	24-hour ambulatory BP monitoring	Rule out "white coat hypertension"	Use appropriately sized cuffs and age appropriate norms
	CBC, metabolic panel, renin assay, urinalysis, renal ultrasound	Determine if other causes of hypertension	
Fatty liver disease	Liver ultrasound; α1-antitrypsin, ceruloplasm, ANA, hepatitis antibodies	Determine cause of elevated transaminases	Persistent elevation of AST, ALT for >6 months warrants further investigation
	Liver biopsy	Determine cause of elevated transaminases, assess degree of hepatitis	Imaging cannot accurately determine inflammation and fibrosis
Type 2 diabetes mellitus	Fasting glucose, glucose tolerance test, urinary microalbumin	Assess for insulin resistance, renal involvement	Fasting glucose > 125 mg/dL indicative of diabetes; 100-125 considered prediabetes
Sleep apnea	Polysomnogram	Evaluate sleep	Can also indicate disordered sleep pattern
Orthopedic disease	Hip x-rays	Evaluate for SCFE	Frog-leg positioning
	Knee x-rays	Evaluate for Blount disease	
Polycystic ovary syndrome	17-OH progesterone, DHEAS, androstenedione, testosterone, LH, FSH, possibly pelvic ultrasound		
Precocious puberty	LH, FSH, testosterone or estradiol, DHEAS	Early onset of obesity	Physical examination often sufficient to evaluate
Pseudotumor cerebri	Fundoscopic examination, lumbar puncture	Papilledema indicative of increased intracranial pressure; elevated opening pressure on puncture	

Adapted from Barlow[23] and Krebs.[16]

ALT, alanine transaminase; ANA, antinuclear antibodies; AST, aspartate aminotransferase; BP, blood pressure; CBC, complete blood count; DHEAS, dehydroepiandrosterone sulfate; FSH, follicle-stimulating hormone; LH, luteinizing hormone; SCFE, slipped capital femoral epiphysis.

Fatty liver is a general term for fat infiltration of the liver, with simple steatosis representing infiltration without inflammation. Nonalcoholic steatohepatitis indicates inflammation with or without fibrosis and cirrhosis. The use of transaminases and imaging, particularly ultrasound, is of some use, but may miss mild inflammation and scarring. Liver biopsy is the only method to reliably diagnose fatty liver and determine the degree of fibrosis and cirrhosis. No guidelines have been established to guide evaluation and treatment, but studies are underway. Other gastrointestinal problems, such as gallstones and constipation, can often go undiagnosed and are important to evaluate in obese children.

There has been a sharp rise in the incidence of type 2 diabetes mellitus (T2DM) among children and adolescents in recent years that has paralleled the increase in incidence of obesity over the same time period.[77-79] Many more obese children have insulin resistance without evidence of overt DM than have been diagnosed with T2DM. Obesity causes insulin resistance through a variety of mechanisms, including impaired insulin signaling, interfering with glucose transport, and decreased insulin clearance; hyperglycemia only occurs when the body is unable to secrete sufficient compensatory insulin. Increased risks are also found with the development of diabetes, especially among certain ethnic/racial groups, with Hispanics and African Americans having lower insulin sensitivity than whites.[80] Findings such as acanthosis nigricans, or symptoms such as polydipsia and polyuria, should prompt evaluations (see Table 15-6). A fasting glucose between 100 and 125 indicates possible impaired glucose tolerance and is often referred to as prediabetes, and subsequent oral glucose tolerance testing may be indicated. There is little agreement as to the correct treatment of impaired glucose tolerance aside from weight management. Assessment of glucose tolerance is of unknown clinical use.

Sleep apnea and other sleep disorders can cause significant morbidity in children, both physically (right ventricular hypertrophy and pulmonary hypertension) and behaviorally (diminished attention and poor school performance). Prevalence is high in severely obese children, perhaps as high as 50%.[81] Symptoms can be obvious, such as witnessed apneas and loud snoring, or subtle, as found in younger children with symptoms of attention deficit hyperactivity disorder. Overnight polysomnography is necessary for diagnosis.

Orthopedic complications of obesity are common.[82] Slipped capital femoral epiphysis (SCFE) involves displacement of the proximal femoral epiphysis from the metaphysis and occurs most commonly in adolescents aged 12 to 15 years, during the adolescent growth spurt. SCFE has been associated with higher BMI; in one study, 81% of children diagnosed with SCFE had BMI above the 95th percentile. The incidence of SCFE is rising, in correlation with the rising incidence of childhood obesity. Blount disease results from an abnormal growth of the proximal tibial physis and primarily results in a nonphysiologic varus deformity of the tibia. It is also associated with childhood obesity; the magnitude of deformity is strongly correlated with increased weight.

Other orthopedic conditions are also associated with obesity. These include valgus deformity; musculoskeletal pain, including back, knee and foot pain; increased risk of fracture; and abnormal gait and overall function. Although obesity is not the only sole predisposing cause of any of these conditions, treating obesity may help decrease the overall incidence of each.

Polycystic ovary syndrome (PCOS) is characterized by hyperandrogenism, hyperinsulinism, menstrual dysfunction, and associated metabolic and cardiovascular complications.[83] Clinically, PCOS manifests as oligomenorrhea, hirsutism, and polycystic ovaries on ultrasound. Although it can occur in both normal-weight and obese women and girls, obesity often precedes the development of PCOS and contributes to its pathogenesis mainly through increased insulin levels and insulin resistance. PCOS is a risk factor for future development of T2DM. The incidence of PCOS among obese adolescents is not well defined; however, among adolescents diagnosed with PCOS, 55 to 73% are obese as well. Weight loss in obese girls with PCOS should be the initial treatment modality, as it has been shown to decrease both androgen and insulin levels in this population. Although radiologic abnormalities are not necessary for diagnosis, elevations of testosterone and an increase in LH:FSH ratio of 2-4:1 are indicative of PCOS in light of symptoms.

Pseudotumor cerebri, also known as idiopathic intracranial hypertension, is a condition characterized by increased intracranial pressure in the absence of intracranial pathology.[84] Obesity is a known risk factor for pseudotumor in adults, particularly among females, and is an increasingly identified risk factor among children as well. One case series of 27 pediatric patients found that 59% of the patients diagnosed with pseudotumor cerebri were either overweight or obese.[85] The etiology of pseudotumor cerebri is largely unknown; therefore, there is no consensus on treatment. Among obese patients, however, weight loss can lead to an improvement in symptoms. Weight loss of as little as 10% of body weight has been found to be curative in some patients.[86]

Metabolic syndrome as a distinct entity in children is somewhat controversial. The metabolic syndrome refers to a constellation of cardiovascular risk factors long studied in adults.[87,88] In children there are no clearly established guidelines for the diagnosis metabolic syndrome; most pediatric guidelines are extrapolations of adult criteria. The risk factors include increased waist circumference, low high-density lipoprotein (HDL) cholesterol, elevated triglycerides, insulin resistance, and hypertension. The diagnosis can be made when three or more of the five risk factors are present. Clinical utility, aside from estimating cardiovascular disease risk in obese children, is limited.

Laboratory Evaluation

The extent of the laboratory evaluation of childhood obesity depends on the BMI, presence of risk factors, and concerns arising from the history. Risk factors include a family history of obesity-related diseases, comorbidities in the patient, and smoking. The initial evaluation includes:

- BMI of 85th to less than 95th percentile and no risk factors: fasting lipid levels
- BMI of 85th to less than 95th percentile, with risk factors: fasting lipid levels, AST and ALT levels, and fasting glucose level
- BMI of 95th percentile or higher: fasting lipid levels, AST and ALT, levels and fasting glucose level

Lipid evaluation is recommended beginning at 2 years of age, with additional testing as outlined earlier starting at 10 years of age, and thereafter repeated every 2 years. Further testing is based on the history and physical examination, and age-appropriate norms should be utilized. Table 15-6 outlines testing to consider for many potential comorbid conditions. In most cases, if a condition is highly suspected or confirmed, referral to or consultation with the appropriate subspecialist is warranted.

Family and Patient Readiness to Change

Treatment is likely to be more successful if the family is in agreement that changes in behaviors regarding diet and activity are warranted. The transtheoretical model of change, usually understood as stages of change, helps the care provider and family understand the natural progression of behavior change.[89] This process is not linear, and individuals progress and regress through the stages at different times and speeds: stage 1, precontemplation; stage 2, contemplation; stage 3, preparation; stage 4, action; stage 5, maintenance. Adaptations of this theory can be found in motivational interviewing, a "client-centered" style that recognizes ambivalence to change and works to resolve that ambivalence in an effort to successfully motivate individuals to change.[90] There are no standardized approaches to reliably assess willingness to change behaviors, but it is recommended that some assessment of the family's willingness to discuss weight-related issues is important. Treatment should be approached in a collaborative, family-centered manner.[16,23,66]

TREATMENT

The AAP Recommendations for Treatment of Child and Adolescent Overweight and Obesity, published in 2007,[16,23,42,66] recommend a staged approach for pediatric weight management. Which stage of treatment to initiate for a particular patient is based on that child's age, BMI percentile, and history of success in previous stages of treatment. The stages of treatment are summarized in Table 15-7 and are discussed in more detail next.

For children 2 to 18 years of age with BMI percentiles between the 5th and 85th (i.e., normal-weight children), primary care physicians are recommended to counsel patients and their families about obesity prevention. This should include counseling regarding nutrition, activity, and screen time. Younger children with BMI percentiles in the 50th to 85th range are at risk for becoming overweight during adolescence.

Stage 1: Prevention Plus

The initial stage of treatment for all children with BMIs at or above 85th percentile is called Prevention Plus and should take place in the primary care physician's office. Stage 1 intervention differs from primary prevention in that it is provided by either the primary care physician or an allied health care provider who has had some additional training in weight management or behavioral counseling and is based on the patient's and family's readiness to change their behavior. This intervention focuses more intensely on the recommendations and includes closer follow-up, generally on a monthly basis.

Stage 1 interventions include the following: encouragement to consume five or more servings of fruit or vegetables/day; minimization of sugared beverage consumption; screen time limitation of no more than 2 hours/day; and encouragement to participate in 1 hour/day or more of physical activity. Eating behaviors are also stressed in Stage 1. Specifically, the family is counseled regarding eating breakfast every day, eating more meals at home, eating more meals as a family, and avoiding overly strict eating restrictions.

Weight goals for Stage 1 treatment are generally maintenance of weight, with an expected decrease in BMI with linear growth. This stage should be continued for a 3- to 6-month period, at which time progress should be assessed. If there is no improvement during this period, progression to Stage 2 treatment is indicated. Children whose BMIs fall between the 85th and 95th percentiles, have tracked consistently in this range over time, and have no medical comorbidities may have a relatively low risk for increased body fat. In that case, they may be continued in the prevention or Prevention Plus stage and not advanced to higher stages of treatment.

TABLE 15-7. Stage of Obesity Treatment

Stage	Components	Implemented	Staff and Skills	Frequency	Advance to Next Stage of Treatment
1. Prevention Plus	Increased intensity of healthy lifestyle recommendations	Primary care office	Primary care physician or trained provider	Varies, but consider monthly weights	No improvement in weight status over 3-6 months
2. Structured Weight Management	Stage 1 components with increased structure (meal planning) and support (monitoring); Medical screening as indicated	Primary care office, consider use of dietitian	Primary care physician/ secondary provider; dietitian; additional training (behavioral counseling, parenting skills, nutrition)	Monthly	No improvement in weight status over 3-6 months
3. Comprehensive Multidisciplinary Intervention	Stage 2 components with increased intensity of behavior change strategies, frequency of contact, and specialists involved	Primary care office coordination; community-based weight management program; pediatric weight management center; or appropriate commercial program	Multidisciplinary team with childhood obesity expertise; primary care-based program with counselor, dietitian, and use of outside activity program	Ideally weekly visits for 8-12 weeks, then monthly	Varies based on available programs and family/patient preference and understanding
4. Tertiary Care Intervention	Stage 3 components with advanced treatment, including meal replacement, very low calorie diet, medication, and bariatric surgery	Pediatric weight management center; residential program; access to subspecialty care	Multidisciplinary team with childhood obesity expertise, including experienced physician/secondary provider to assess comorbidities	Per established protocols	Per established protocols

Adapted from Spear et al.[66]

Stage 2: Structured Weight Management

Stage 2 treatment can also be provided in the primary care office. It is provided ideally by a registered dietitian with additional training in childhood obesity, in conjunction with the primary care provider. Stage 2 provides the patient and family with more structure and continued close follow-up at monthly intervals.

Structured Weight Management incorporates the same counseling as Prevention Plus; in addition, other techniques and topics are included. A well-balanced diet with structured meals and snacks, at least 1 hour/day of supervised activity, no more than 1 hour/day of screen time, closer supervision of behaviors by the patient and the family, and behavior (as opposed to weight) goal targets are all included in Stage 2. For children under 12 years old, parental involvement in behavioral changes is crucial; this involvement can be gradually decreased as the child gets older.

Weight goals for Stage 2 are similar to those for Stage 1: weight maintenance and therefore subsequent decrease in BMI with continued linear growth of the child. In addition, if weight loss is achieved, it should be limited to 1 pound per month or less for children 2 to 11 years of age, and 2 pounds per week or less for older children and adolescents. Patients should be followed for 3 to 6 months; if no or insufficient progress is made during that period, they should be advanced to Stage 3.

Stage 3: Comprehensive Multidisciplinary Intervention

Stage 3 treatment generally exceeds what can be accomplished in a primary care office; however, several offices might coordinate to provide this treatment locally. The multidisciplinary team should consist of a behavioral counselor, a registered dietitian, and an exercise specialist. A physician (potentially the primary care provider) should oversee and monitor any medical issues. A Comprehensive Multidisciplinary Intervention includes more intensive behavioral change counseling and encompasses frequent follow-up for an extended period. Weekly visits for 8 to 12 weeks at a minimum are recommended.

The nutritional and activity goals for Stage 3 treatment include those for Stage 2 treatment. The addition of a multidisciplinary team at this stage allows for more intense treatment. In addition to the Stage 2 goals, Stage 3 also includes a structured diet and activity plan to provide for negative energy balance; a structured behavioral modification program incorporating food and activity monitoring and short- and long-term goals; inclusion of close family members in the treatment plan, especially for children 2 to 11 years of age; and modification of the home environment to facilitate weight loss. Anthropometric measurements and assessments of dietary intake and physical activity should be conducted at regular intervals during Stage 3 treatment.

Weight loss goals for Stage 3 are similar to those at previous stages. Weight maintenance or slow weight loss should be encouraged, until BMI is below 85th percentile. For children 2 to 5 years of age, weight loss should not exceed 1 pound per month; for older children and adolescents, weight loss should not exceed 2 pounds per week. Lack of success with treatment at Stage 3 should prompt consideration of advancement to Stage 4 treatment; it is not, however, the sole criterion for

advancement. Maturity and motivation should both be considered in transitioning to Stage 4 treatment.

Stage 4: Tertiary Care Intervention

Stage 4 treatment is called Tertiary Care Intervention. There is only limited experience with it in the pediatric population, but it may be appropriate for a subset of obese children and adolescents. Stage 4 is by definition a tertiary care weight management multidisciplinary team that operates within an established protocol. The team should have extensive experience and training with pediatric obesity and associated comorbidities, and should consist of a physician, a nurse practitioner, a registered dietitian, a behavioral counselor, and an exercise specialist. Components of Stage 4 treatment vary, but may include such modalities as restrictive diets, medications, and bariatric surgery (see later discussion).

Nutrition and Physical Activity Interventions

There are few clinical trials that adequately control for the complexity of behaviors, environment, and families demonstrating efficacy of specific dietary approaches for long-term weight loss in children. There are some approaches that have demonstrated effectiveness and have been used in the treatment of obese children. Early studies utilized the Traffic Light or Stoplight Diet, which groups foods based on nutrient quality and caloric density[91,92] and is a practical tool for monitoring food intake. Low-glycemic-index diets, based on the body's insulin response to a particular carbohydrate, have been found to be effective in some studies of weight loss in adolescents. These diets have the benefits of being able to curb overeating and are highly palatable. However, other studies have not proven the same benefit, and there is some disagreement over the most accurate measure of glycemic index. Glycemic index is based on measurements of a single food, whereas most meals are of mixed foods, in which the glycemic load has not been determined.[93]

Low-carbohydrate diets have been very popular in recent history. They were used in very-low-calorie and protein-sparing modified fast diets in the 1980s in children. More recent manifestations, in line with popular culture and fad diets, were ketogenic diets, where ketosis is induced by low carbohydrate intake, thereby curbing appetite. Although early studies demonstrated efficacy in children,[94] these approaches are difficult to follow over the long term, and their safety in children is unproven. Adult studies have found that the superior weight loss at 6 months of treatment (versus low-fat diet) is lost at 1 year.[95]

At present, there are no definitive dietary approaches recommended for all overweight and obese children. Instead, clinicians should focus on the quality and quantity of dietary carbohydrates and fats. A focus on food behaviors is likely to carry the greatest efficacy. Examples include breakfast skipping, snacking, meals away from home (fast food), and sweetened beverage intake.[66]

Similarly, specific exercise or physical activity recommendations for weight loss are lacking in the literature. Common sense interventions would encourage children to increase general physical activity through play or exercise. However, several trials have demonstrated that decreasing sedentary activity can be a means to improving child weight status. An early study showed a greater, sustainable weight loss in children by reinforcing a decrease in sedentary activity[96] versus reinforcement of increasing physical activity. This has been demonstrated in other studies and cultures.[97-99] Many organizations, including the AAP, recommend that children participate in at least 1 hour per day of physical activity, with approximately 30 minutes of that occurring during the school day. There are no recommendations for specific structured or unstructured (play) physical activity, but clinicians should recognize the barriers to physical activity encountered by children and families, including unsafe neighborhoods, lack of transportation to sports, and loss of physical education in schools.[66]

Behavioral Approaches

The core tenets of pediatric obesity treatment come from pioneering work of Epstein and colleagues. Distinct from low-calorie dietary interventions, Epstein's work employed a behavior change model, including reinforcement, monitoring, and most important, inclusion of primary caregivers.[91,92,96,100,101] This last component, inclusion of the family, has transitioned into a family-based approach, where adult caregivers are vital to the success of the program. This aspect, however, may lose some importance in older teens.[102] There is some evidence in younger children that a parent-only approach may be as effective as including the child in treatment.[103,104]

Also clear from classic studies is the need for frequent contact with the treatment team to establish behavior change, usually with weekly visits for a period of time, as well as long-term follow-up.[66,102] Another consideration in behavioral approaches is the cost, as frequent contact and multidisciplinary team components increase cost. This has led to group programming, where care can be delivered to larger numbers of families while utilizing the support of peers. Cost analysis has shown this to be less expensive than individual treatment,[105] but there is not sufficient data showing efficacy compared to individual treatment approaches. Although much remains to be determined, recommendations advocate for a family-based approach featuring behavior modification techniques.

Behavior modification is often misunderstood among physicians and other health care providers. The components of behavior change, as it pertains to the treatment of pediatric obesity, are self-monitoring, stimulus control, and goal setting.[102,106]

- Self-monitoring: This technique is used to help patients gain awareness of habits. This is usually done through record keeping, diaries, and logs. Through this, they can identify areas contributing to their weight gain of which they were previously unaware. This is best accomplished through feedback from a clinician, i.e., a dietitian reviewing food records and providing specific feedback. Simple food logs and records are often expanded to encompass other behavioral components of eating, such as level of hunger, boredom, and mealtime environment. This can provide valuable information for stimulus control (see later discussion).
- Stimulus control: Changing environmental cues that lead to increased caloric intake and sedentary activity is a component of many treatment regimens. This is applied in two forms: establishing new routines and changing access. Again, these can apply to both physical activity (changing work schedules to facilitate going to a gym) and nutritional intake (removing high-calorie foods from the home).
- Goal setting and contracting: This approach is one of the more widely used in behavior change. Caution must be exercised because it can often be applied in detrimental ways, such as setting a goal of losing 5 pounds. Successful goal setting can

be implemented using the acronym SMART, making goals Specific, Measurable, Attainable, Realistic, and Timely. In obesity treatment, it is important to have the goal pertain to a behavior, such as walking or snacking, versus a health- or weight-related goal. SMART especially pertains to short-term goals, even though setting long-term goals can also be useful. For children, contracting can be useful, helping to maintain focus and provide structure to a reward. Rewarding success in reaching a goal is important for all children and should be negotiated between parent and child. It is also helpful to make the goal an activity or privilege, instead of food or money. Rewards should also be small so they can be used frequently.

An approach being increasingly utilized in the treatment of pediatric obesity is motivational interviewing. Originally developed to treat various addictions in adults in the 1980s,[107] and later adapted to other behaviors,[108,109] motivational interviewing is a patient-centered counseling approach that utilizes specific techniques. The goal is to elicit intrinsic motivation for changing a behavior, recognizing that ambivalence to change is normal. Through this approach, the patient is guided to understand and resolve this ambivalence to change by expressing reasons for and against changing. It is considered patient-centered because the clinician is to remain nonjudgmental, empathic, and supportive and should ask permission before sharing information or advice. Although the approach is now being studied intensively, only two published studies have utilized motivational interviewing in a pediatric obesity treatment setting. While neither study identified significant differences in weight loss between intervention and control groups, results appear promising. Families appeared to appreciate the approach, and motivational interviewing was successful in instigating families to think about changing eating habits.[110-112] Training of providers in these techniques can be completed in relatively short periods of time (2 to 5 days), and motivational interviewing can be applicable to many different areas of pediatric practice.

Pharmacotherapy

Although there has been great interest in medications for weight loss, very few have been studied in children, and even fewer approved for use. Traditionally, appetite inhibition has been the focus of therapy, with stimulants being most often employed. However, side effects, risk of addiction, and other complications have limited their usefulness. Presently, only two medications are approved for limited use for weight loss in children, with neither approved for long-term use.

Sibutramine is a serotonin reuptake inhibitor that acts centrally to decrease appetite. It is approved for use in children 16 years of age and older, for use for up to 2 years.[113] It has been shown to increase weight loss over placebo in patients (including children) in structured programs.[66] Reported side effects are increased heart rate and blood pressure. Orlistat, an intestinal lipase inhibitor, has also been shown to be effective in providing additional weight loss safely in children and is approved for use in children 12 years of age and older.[66] By inducing malabsorption of upward of 30% of ingested fats, energy intake is lowered. Safety and efficacy beyond 4 years of use has not been determined. The most frequent side effects are understandably gastrointestinal, such as cramping, flatus, and oily stools. Orlistat is also now available in an over-the-counter formulation for patients 18 years of age or older.

With both medications, effective weight loss always occurs in conjunction with a diet and exercise plan geared toward weight loss, and in the case of orlistat, with a low-fat diet. Weight loss in comparison to diet and exercise interventions alone is modest,[66] and weight regain after cessation of treatment is common and expected.

Bariatric Surgery

Although there is increasing evidence to support the use of bariatric surgery in adolescents, overall, there is still much to study with respect to safety of this in children. An expert committee of pediatricians, scientists, and pediatric surgeons developed recommendations for the consideration of bariatric surgery in adolescents.[22] Criteria were purposely conservative, reserving this option for children who have failed to improve their health and weight via standard mechanisms, including a multidisciplinary pediatric obesity treatment program for at least 6 months. Further, it is recommended this procedure only be performed at centers experienced in the care of obese children. Surgery is considered in children who have reached full physical maturity, determined through Tanner Staging and bone age (typically girls at least 13 years of age, boys at least 15 years of age). Adolescents and their parents must agree on having the procedure and commit to lifelong follow-up. This precludes offering the surgery to those without the mental capacity to consent to surgery (i.e., mental retardation). Surgery is considered in those with a BMI at or above 40 kg/m^2 with a weight-related comorbidity, or a BMI at or above 50 kg/m^2 with a serious or severe comorbidity (type 2 diabetes, pseudotumor cerebri, sleep apnea). It is recommended that a thorough preoperative evaluation be conducted at a pediatric center with expertise in obesity treatment and surgery, and close, lifelong medical follow-up continue postoperatively.

The surgical procedures that are considered for adolescents are Roux-en-Y gastric bypass and adjustable gastric banding. Presently, there is greater experience with gastric bypass, but there is increasing evidence of the safety and effectiveness of adjustable gastric banding.[114,115] Gastric bypass induces weight loss by two mechanisms: malabsorption of calories by the bypass of significant portions of the small intestine (50 to 100 cm of duodenum and jejunum), and by gastric restriction. Both data extrapolated from adults as well as increasing amounts of data in children show safety and efficacy of this procedure. There remain concerns, however, primarily with the malabsorption of nutrients in children, and the irreversible nature of the procedure. There has been a case report of dry beriberi in a child, thought to be from noncompliance with vitamin supplementation and from stricture formation.[116]

Adjustable gastric banding works by gastric restriction, with the placement of a silicone band around the fundus of the stomach, which is connected to a port placed beneath the skin. This port is accessed via needle to inflate and deflate the band as needed, which decreases and increases the lumen of the stomach. The surgery is less invasive and reversible, though surgeons recommend the procedure be considered permanent. Although vitamin and mineral supplementation is still considered important, malabsorption is not experienced with this surgery.

Long-term follow-up is vital to the success of these procedures. This follow-up can be problematic when adolescents leave their primary caregiver's home. There is no consensus about which surgery is best for adolescents, nor is there consensus about who the ideal candidate for surgery should be.[117] There is still much research and evaluation needed on long-term outcomes of bariatric surgery in adolescents.

CONCLUSIONS

Childhood obesity is a complex problem that has become a priority for pediatric health care providers across the globe in recent decades. A careful and thorough approach is necessary when assessing the causes and complications of a child's obesity, as well as in planning interventions. Treatment requires diverse approaches and disciplines; including the family of an obese child is crucial to successful treatment. New recommendations outline a systematic approach to evaluation and treatment. Novel interventions, such as bariatric surgery, hold promise for morbidly obese teens.

REFERENCES

16. Krebs NF, Himes JH, Jacobson D, et al. Assessment of child and adolescent overweight and obesity. Pediatrics 2007;120(Suppl. 4):S193–S228.
22. Inge TH, Krebs NF, Garcia VF, et al. Bariatric surgery for severely overweight adolescents: concerns and recommendations. Pediatrics 2004;114:217–223.
23. Barlow SE. Expert committee recommendations regarding the prevention, assessment, and treatment of child and adolescent overweight and obesity: summary report. Pediatrics 2007;120(Suppl. 4):S164–S192.
42. Davis MM, Gance-Cleveland B, Hassink S, et al. Recommendations for prevention of childhood obesity. Pediatrics 2007;120(Suppl. 4):S229–S253.
47. Rhee KE, Lumeng JC, Appugliese DP, et al. Parenting styles and overweight status in first grade. Pediatrics 2006;117:2047–2054.
66. Spear BA, Barlow SE, Ervin C, et al. Recommendations for treatment of child and adolescent overweight and obesity. Pediatrics 2007;120(Suppl. 4):S254–S288.
101. Epstein LH, Valoski A, Wing RR, McCurley J. Ten-year outcomes of behavioral family-based treatment for childhood obesity. Health Psychol 1994;13:373–383.

See expertconsult.com for a complete list of references and the review questions for this chapter.

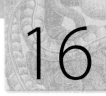

16 EATING DISORDERS IN CHILDREN AND ADOLESCENTS

Ellen S. Rome • Laura Gillespie

Eating disorders represent a diverse group of diseases that occur in increasingly younger children, adolescents, and young adults. Anorexia nervosa has been described as "the relentless pursuit of thinness,"[1] whereas bulimia nervosa literally is derived from the Greek phrase "appetite like a bull," highlighting the binges rather than the purges. Eating disorder not otherwise specified refers to everything that isn't anorexia nervosa or bulimia nervosa by strict definition; in other words, it represents a diverse group ranging from those who have binge eating disorder, or binges without the purges/compensatory behaviors, to those who restrict but have not yet lost the weight or failed to grow. Definitions have recently been challenged, because of recognition of presentation in younger children and other factors.[2] Of note, anorexia nervosa involves either weight loss leading to maintenance of body weight less than 85% of that expected for age, or a failure to gain the expected amount of weight during a period of growth; in other words, a child does not need to have lost weight, but just fail to grow, for concern of an eating disorder to be raised. Typically, the adolescent or young adult who is either overweight or otherwise dissatisfied with his or her body goes from initial dieting efforts to an intense preoccupation with weight loss, eating, and/or exercise. With increasing severity, food-related activities interfere with family and school functions, affecting school performance last if at all. Definitions for anorexia nervosa, bulimia nervosa, and eating disorder not otherwise specified can be found in Table 16-1.

A working group of multidisciplinary experts in the field of eating disorders recently recommended changes to existing cognitive criteria in anorexia nervosa and bulimia nervosa, including changing or adding wording to help alert health care professionals to the developmental limitations of children that may keep them from "sounding" like a patient with an eating disorder when they have already began to slide down that slippery slope.[2] Younger children do not start with the same vocabulary for their illness; they may not state that they are afraid of getting fat, that they hate their bodies, that they are afraid of certain foods. These words may come out weeks or months after refeeding has begun, with a few even voicing earlier fears of growing up or getting bigger, or having their bodies change with puberty. Their actions still push them along a path that leads to food refusal, compensatory behaviors, with resultant failure to grow along expected parameters if allowed to persist or undetected by parents and care providers. One strong concept remains clear: when a parent or other caring adult voices concern about an eating disorder, the pediatrician needs to remain vigilant to prevent its appearance, as a large percentage of families who voice the concern could have earlier intervention than currently occurs, perhaps with better outcomes.[3]

CHANGING FACE OF THE EPIDEMIOLOGY

Eating Disorders as an Equal Opportunity Disease

Anorexia nervosa and bulimia nervosa have been estimated to affect 1% and 4%, respectively, of young adolescent girls,[4-7] with an increasing number of boys recognized at earlier ages.[8,9] Eating disorders not otherwise specified (EDNOS) has an estimated prevalence of 10%.[10-12] Certain populations have been traditionally seen as at risk, including athletes in the "visual sports," such as ballet, gymnastics, and figure skating, those teens engaging in "visual activities" such as modeling, and transition times such as the physical shifts that occur at 11 to 14 years of age, and at 17 to 19 years of age at the time of transition from high school to college. Of note, only 5 to 10% of the general adult population has been found to have disordered eating in older studies, contrasting with the 15 to 62% of female college athletes found to have disordered eating.[13-15] More recently, a study of the prevalence of the female athlete triad among high school athletes found that 18.2% of girls met the criteria for disordered eating, 23.5% for menstrual irregularity, and 21.8% for low bone mass, with 5.9% meeting two of the three criteria, and 1.2% meeting criteria for all three components of the triad.[16] Almost half of the girls (47%) had engaged in pathogenic behaviors at least four times in the month before the survey, with 24% using two or more different pathogenic behaviors in the month before the survey. Girls using these abnormal behaviors were more likely to have oligomenorrhea or amenorrhea and were more likely to have lower bone density, as would be expected. The main message is that children and adolescents may not walk in the door with the label "eating disorder" or "female athlete triad," but if anything in the history, clinical examination, or laboratory findings raises a red flag, the astute clinician should pursue a set of easy questions to elicit abnormal eating attitudes and behaviors early rather than when those behaviors have become firmly entrenched. Those questions are outlined in Table 16-2 with further elaboration in this chapter. Age barriers have also been crossed in the detection of eating disorders. Traditionally, bulimia nervosa has been seen as occurring slightly later than anorexia nervosa, with few cases found and documented before the age of 14 years.[17,18] Anecdotally, younger patients with bulimia nervosa can be found; in our practice, our youngest presenting patient was 5 years old, with binges and purges occurring daily since age 3 1/2 years, triggered by sexual abuse perpetrated by multiple care providers since she was 2 years old. Maladaptive coping strategies can emerge at any age and stage, with disordered eating a particularly common one.

TABLE 16-1. Diagnostic Criteria for Anorexia Nervosa, Bulimia Nervosa, and Eating Disorders Not Otherwise Specified

Anorexia Nervosa

1. Intense fear of becoming fat or gaining weight, even when underweight
2. Refusal to maintain body weight at or above a minimally normal weight for age and height (e.g., weight loss leading to maintenance of body weight < 85% of that expected, or failure to gain weight during a period of growth leading to body weight < 85% of weight expected)
3. Disturbed body image, undue influence of weight or shape on self-evaluation, or denial of the seriousness of the current low body weight
4. Amenorrhea or absence of at least three consecutive menstrual periods for postmenarchal females (also considered amenorrheic if periods only inducible after estrogen therapy)

Types

Restricting type: No regular binges or purges (self-induced vomiting or use of laxatives or diuretics)
Binge eating/purging type: Regular binges or purges in patient who also meets the foregoing criteria for anorexia nervosa

Bulimia Nervosa

1. Recurrent episodes of binge eating, characterized by:
   a. Eating a substantially larger amount of food in a discrete period of time (e.g., in 2 hours) than would be eaten by most people in similar circumstances during that same time period
   b. A sense of lack of control over eating during the binge
2. Recurrent inappropriate compensatory behavior in order to prevent weight gain (e.g., self-induced vomiting, use of laxatives, diuretics, fasting, or hyperexercising)
3. Binges or inappropriate compensatory behaviors occurring, on average, at least twice weekly for at least 3 months
4. Self-evaluation unduly influenced by body shape or weight
5. The disturbance does not occur exclusively during periods of anorexia nervosa

Types

Purging type: Regularly engages in self-induced vomiting or use of laxatives/diuretics
Nonpurging type: Uses other inappropriate compensatory behaviors (e.g., fasting, hyperexercising, without regular use of vomiting or medicines to purge)

Eating Disorder Not Otherwise Specified (those that do not meet criteria for AN or BN by DSM-IV)

1. All criteria for AN except has regular menses
2. All criteria for AN except weight still in normal range
3. All criteria for BN except binges < twice/week or < 3 months
4. A patient with normal body weight who regularly engages in inappropriate compensatory behavior after eating small amounts of food (e.g., self-induced vomiting after eating two cookies)
5. A patient who repeatedly chews and spits out large amounts of food without swallowing
6. Binge eating disorder: recurrent binges without the compensatory behaviors associated with BN

Adapted from the American Psychiatric Association, Diagnostic and Statistical Manual of Mental Disorders, 4th ed. (DSM-IV). Washington, DC: American Psychiatric Association; 1994.

One study by Peebles, Wilson, and Lock[8] compared children 12 years and younger (n = 120) with anorexia nervosa with older adolescent patients (n = 850 13- to 19-year-olds). A higher incidence of males was found than in prior studies, 16.5% of the younger patients versus 7.8% of the older group, slightly lower but consistent with our findings of 22.1% versus 10.1% boys in the younger versus older groups, respectively.[9] Children were also more likely to present with a lower percentage of ideal body weight (p < .05), a shorter duration of illness (p < .001), with more precipitous weight loss than seen in adolescents with eating disorders (p < .001). Older adolescents

TABLE 16-2. Useful Questions in Eliciting a History of Eating Disorders

What is the most you ever weighed? At what height? When was that?
What is the least you ever weighed? At what height? When was that?
Do you have a weight above which you would feel really uncomfortable? What weight is that?
Do you have a weight below which you do not want to get? What weight is that?
What do you think you should weigh? *How much time/energy do you put into that?*
Vomiting, diet pills, laxatives, diuretics, other methods? If yes, how often, which kinds, over what time period?
What do you do for exercise? Level of intensity? *How stressed are you if you miss a workout?*
What did you eat yesterday? (quantity as well as quality, breakfast, lunch, dinner, snacks, fluids)
What foods do you avoid? Any fear foods (ones you used to eat that are no longer "safe")?
Do you count calories and/or fat grams? If so, how many do you allow yourself?
When was your last period? The one before that? Have you missed any periods? What weight were you at your last period?
Have you ever had sex? With guys, girls, or both? If heterosexual and has had sex, what do you use for your two methods of contraception? Do you use condoms sometimes, most of the time, or all the time? Has anyone ever done anything to you sexually that made you uncomfortable?
Cigarettes? Drugs? Alcohol?
Has anyone ever bullied or teased you? About weight/body, or other teasing?

were more likely to engage in purging, bingeing, diet pill use, or laxative use (p < .001 for each). The timing of weight loss may result in more damaging effects in periods of critical growth, including bone deposition.[19] Similarly, an Australian nationally representative sample of 5- to 13-year-olds characterized the expression of early-onset eating disorders, finding that only 51% met current weight criteria as defined by current diagnostic criteria, with 61% having life-threatening complications of malnutrition.[20] The prepubescent child may have lower fat stores than an adult, magnifying the effects of a milder percentage of weight loss.[8,19] Lower thresholds for eating disorder detection have been recommended to prevent the medical and psychologic sequelae that may be greater at these key periods of growth.[3,19]

Eating disorders affect girls and boys now from all socioeconomic strata and ethnic groups, no longer remaining the sole perceived domain of upper-middle-class white girls. The challenge appears to be failure to recognize disordered eating, combined with lack of access to care in our more indigent populations. Media, or our "SuperPeer," can play a role in bringing eating disorders to diverse populations: in Fiji after the introduction of television featuring pop American shows such as Beverly Hills 90210 in the 1990's, a sharp increase in the prevalence of disordered eating attitudes and behaviors was noted. Eating disorders have been found in developed and developing countries, with higher detection in areas that have been "modernized."

Predictive Factors

In an Australian population-based sample, factors most strongly predictive of the development of eating disorders included being female and being perceived as overweight by one's parent.[21] Other predictive factors included mother's elevated body mass

TABLE 16-3. Risk Factors for Eating Disorders

Maternal/Parenting Factors
Pregnancy with birth complications
Weight-related teasing of the child
Parental obesity
Low degree of parental contact
High parental expectation
Overanxious parenting
Parental alcoholism or drug use
Family discord
Individual Factors
Childhood obesity
Being perceived as overweight
Anxiety
Perfectionism
Obsessive-compulsive disorder
Abuse (sexual, physical, emotional)
Low self-esteem
Chronic dieting

index, child's social problems, low social-related self-efficacy, and neurocognitive difficulties. Possible risk factors, identified retrospectively, can be found in Table 16-3. Of note, parental concern about their own weight, shape, or eating habits can have considerable impact on a child's eating disorder behaviors, with "monkey see, monkey do" fairly operative.[22]

ASPECTS OF THE HISTORY AND PHYSICAL EXAMINATION

Through a careful history and physical examination, much information can be revealed about the chronicity of the child's illness, abnormal eating attitudes and behaviors, and potential strategies for management depending on the findings. The history can start with both parent and child together, asking the teen/child first why he/she thinks she is there today. How the parent and child respond can set a tone; the child may look to the parent to prompt a response, or may avoid eye contact with body language stating that she does not want to be there. Or, the parent may not let the child get a word in edgewise (giving a useful Rorschach test and causing the astute clinician to limit who gets to respond when). Hidden agendas or discrepancies in perspective between parent(s) and child can be clarified through skillful interviewing. The child can be asked if she feels overweight, underweight, or just right? Has he or she ever tried to change her weight or body shape, and for what purpose? Does she have any "trouble spots," or areas of the body that she finds truly uncomfortable emotionally or physically? Asking the child how hard he or she struggles to maintain, gain, or lose weight simultaneously assesses his or her efforts directed to abnormal eating attitudes and behaviors while acknowledging the stress the child may feel over weight issues. Table 16-2 reviews other useful questions to ask on that initial interview.

Asking a dietary history with both parent and child together can provide a useful reality check; the child may say she has cereal for breakfast, and the mother rolls her eyes and says, "Only three bites!" Conversely, an afternoon small snack per the teen may actually be half a box of cereal, several portions' worth of leftover dinner, and various other items minimized by a teen not wishing to reveal the scope of a binge due to shame, guilt, anger, or other emotion. Are family meals stressful? Can the teen eat at friends' houses comfortably? Is she avoiding situations where food will be part of the experience? Who prepares the food, and how often do family meals occur? Many children and adolescents engage in a gradual switch from "healthy eating," cutting out junk food, red meat, or other items after an educational session at school, home, via media, or from the family, then move to strict avoidance of an entire food group such as fat grams or protein. An initial drive for health gets usurped by a drive to diet and be thin as the only goal; in the athlete, this shift from a drive to improve performance to a drive to be thin as the main/only goal can actually detract from athletic performance. This shift may be initially heralded as a positive by the family, but when a carnivorous family is faced with a new lacto-ovo vegetarian, who then moves to being vegan (abstaining from all meat, fish, fowl, dairy, and eggs), the parent may not realize how little the child is actually eating.[23] Although vegetarian diets may be pursued in a healthy fashion, the adolescent may use it as a means of further restriction invisible to the parent.

The clinician should ask whether the teen has any "taboo" foods, or foods that she simply cannot or will not eat. Some patients may conscientiously label read, keeping a running tally per meal of what they are "allowed," eliminating not just trans fats, but all fats, with the misguided belief that if less fat is good, *no* fat is better. Parents and children may not realize that children's brains require at a minimum 30 to 50 grams of fat for proper myelination or "hard-wiring" of memory; this fact may present family mealtime challenges when Dad is on the Ornish diet or other no-fat/low-fat diet to manage his heart disease, or Mom is on a low-cholesterol diet for her health. Magical thinking can occur; for instance, one adolescent boy needed to be told repeatedly that the act of watching TV would not make him fat – that calories would not magically move from the TV to his body, causing him to swell up like a giant loofah sponge. He had clearly heard an antiobesity message, and his starved brain had put its own spin on it; with obsessive-compulsive tendencies getting it to stick there. Other patients may avoid looking in a certain mirror that always puts weight on their hips, literally from their perspective. This extreme delusional thinking often resolves with refeeding.[24] Other obsessions or compulsions can include unusual use of utensils in eating, cutting food into tiny pieces, chewing each bite multiple times, or not allowing different foods ever to touch before consumption. The parent may also note that the child engages in restless/repetitive movements used intentionally or unconsciously by the child to purge calories.

Level of school and family functioning should be ascertained, as the teen with an eating disorder may have narrowed interests or avoid situations where food is involved. More sensitive questions about sex and drugs and rock and roll (cigarette use, drug use, alcohol use, sexual activity, and past sexual abuse) should be asked privately, after establishing confidentiality, with the explicitly stated caveat that the provider will break confidentiality if anything life threatening or dangerous is revealed by either parent or child. Once confidentiality has been established, the clinician should specifically ask how the teen controls weight, as these behaviors may be embarrassing to the child, or he may not wish to have the parents know the extent of his habits. Is the teen vomiting to control weight? If so, with what methods – finger, spoon, or spontaneously? Do they brush, gargle, or rinse after? Vomiting patients should be taught to gargle with mouthwash, or with water with or without baking soda after purging, as brushing can bring acid to crevices it may otherwise

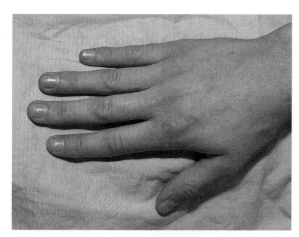

Figure 16-1. Russell sign in an adolescent girl who uses her finger to induce vomiting to control weight.

not have reached. Does the teen vomit only after a binge, and what qualifies as a binge? This last question becomes relevant as many children with eating disorders will label a normal meal a "binge." What are the other methods of purging, including diet pills, laxatives, and diuretics (which brands of each, how much, how often)? How much caffeine per day, and in what forms? Mood, obsessive-compulsive symptoms, depression, and suicidal ideation should be assessed. Review of systems should include questions about early satiety, bloating, and reflux; stool frequency, and loose or formed, diarrhea or constipation; other signs of chronic disease, including thyroid symptoms, unintentional weight loss or gain, signs of suggestive of celiac disease or inflammatory bowel disease (IBD) and signs of malignancy. Syncope or "grayouts" (near-syncope), weakness and fatigue, easy bruising, pallor, and other physical signs and symptoms should be elicited. Exercise can be used as a means of purging; type of exercise, intensity, and hours per day should be assessed. The amount of perceived stress associated with missing a workout can serve as a marker of exercise compulsion.

Physical Findings

The physical examination should include height, weight after voiding in a gown facing backwards on the scale, and orthostatic blood pressure and pulse measurements. Some centers do not weigh patients backwards, preferring "open weights" for all, but for those individuals limited cognitively by brain starvation, the numbers can trigger increasing dieting or disordered eating attitudes and behaviors. Those clinicians who know by experience which of their patients do well with that knowledge and which will find the numbers triggering can use their individual judgment case by case; but nursing staff may support care better by making it a universal procedure to be discreet with all patients, using words such as, "It is our policy to weigh all new patients backwards on the scale after voiding, and you may discuss this further with Dr. __," clearly and respectfully. Clinicians should also be alert to the possibility of weight manipulations, either via water loading to falsely elevate weight, use of weights in underwear or various orifices, or other strategies. For these reasons, many centers insist on the weight in a gown, often after a "pat down" with patients known or suspected of hiding weights, after voiding, with urinalysis checking for specific gravity, protein, and ketosis. Dehydration may result in an accelerated heart rate, masking a sinus bradycardia as a result of a feeding disorder.

TABLE 16-4. Physical Findings in Patients With Eating Disorders

Organ System	Finding
Skin	Dry; atrophic with restricting; Russell sign with purging using a finger; easy bruising
Mouth	Dental erosions on lingual and occlusal surfaces from vomiting
Face	Parotitis in those who purge
Thyroid	Not enlarged; but euthyroid sick syndrome notable with dry skin, cold intolerance, constipation
Cardiac	Bradycardia; orthostatic hypotension; mitral valve prolapse in a third
GI	Palpable loops of stools when constipated, diffuse abdominal discomfort,
Temperature	Hypothermic
Extremities	Acrocyanosis, Raynaud syndrome, edema with third spacing
Hair	Loss of shine or thickness; hair loss on head; lanugo on trunk/extremities
CNS	Nerve compression/sciatica from lack of padding
Musculoskeletal	Stress fractures, osteopenia
Breast	Atrophy
GU	Atrophic vaginitis; loss of libido

CNS, central nervous system; GI, gastrointestinal; GU, genitourinary.

Other aspects of the physical examination include a thorough head-to-toe examination, with attention to the parotid glands (looking for parotitis from vomiting), dental erosions on the lingual and occlusal surfaces, Russell sign (callus of the knuckle from hitting it with teeth during purging; see Figure 16-1), bradycardia, hypothermia, and orthostatic hypotension by pulse (an increase in heart rate greater than or equal to 20 when going from horizontal to vertical) or by blood pressure (diastolic dropping by 10 points from lying to standing), Tanner staging of breasts and pubic hair (genitals and pubic hair in boys), noting atrophy of breasts, abdominal masses (including palpable loops of stool from constipation), scaphoid appearance, swelling of extremities, acrocyanosis, and edema in dependent areas. Examination of optic disks can also help to rule out blurred disk margins, with a full neurologic examination necessary to elicit any positive findings requiring brain imaging to identify a brain tumor, low in likelihood but a concern in boys in whom the prevalence of eating disorders is less likely than in girls and in any girl with positive neurologic findings. A summary of physical findings can be found in Table 16-4.

MEDICAL COMPLICATIONS OF EATING DISORDERS

Adolescents with eating disorders at all ends of the spectrum may be remarkably normal on physical examination. However, medical complications of eating disorders may invisibly occur, caused directly or indirectly by three processes: (1) caloric restriction, (2) purging behaviors, and (3) binges. Almost every organ system can be affected by these behaviors.[25-27]

Medical Complications of Caloric Restriction

Medical sequelae of starvation include major effects on brain, bone, and heart, but all organ systems are affected. Cardiac effects are the most life threatening, with prolonged starvation

TABLE 16-5. Medical Criteria for Admission

Bradycardia (heart rate < 50)
Orthostatic hypotension
Hypothermia
Precipitous weight loss
Hypokalemia or other electrolyte imbalance
Refeeding syndrome
Failure of outpatient management

increasing the risk of myocardial wasting, arrhythmias, and risk of sudden cardiac death. In anorexia nervosa, decreased cardiac chamber size and thinning of the left ventricle have been reported,[28,29] as well as decreased blood pressure and reduced cardiac output.[30] Increased peripheral vascular tone combined with decreased cardiac output may decrease peripheral circulation, leading to noticeably cold hands and feet, Raynaud syndrome, and cyanosis, with added edema due to third spacing. Sinus bradycardia, sinus arrhythmias, and hypotension may be seen as protective adaptations to prolonged starvation, occurring gradually over time. Alone, these changes are not life threatening, but in combination with hypokalemia, addition of caffeine or other form of cardiac stimulation, and other factors, they may be fatal. Direct myocardial damage occurs with use of emetine, the active ingredient in ipecac, which binds irreversibly to cardiac muscle. Fortunately, ipecac is no longer recommended by poison control centers for induced purging after childhood ingestions. Many pharmacies have taken it off the shelves, but this is not true in all countries. Other examples of direct myocardial impairment include prolonged corrected QT interval, ventricular dysrhythmias, and reduced myocardial contractility, all of which can be lethal but are correctible with refeeding. Bradycardia, hypotension, and hypothermia should be appropriately used as cues indicating medical compromise and the need for intervention. Medical criteria for admission to the hospital for acute medical stabilization can be found in Table 16-5.

Refeeding syndrome refers to the congestive heart failure that occurs from the combination of total body depletion of phosphorus stores during catabolic starvation faced with increased cellular influx of phosphorus during anabolic refeeding.[31,32] Rapid refeeding has also been associated with congestive heart failure, probably caused by the large increase in afterload in patients with cardiac wasting.[33] To avoid refeeding syndrome, many centers will proactively give a phosphorus replacement product such as Nutraphos (250 mg phosphorus, 164 mg sodium phosphate, 278 mg potassium phosphate; Willen), at a dose of 500 mg orally twice a day for 5 days, to provide the recommended daily allowance of 1000 mg phosphorus per day during acute refeeding for the hospitalized patient.

Endocrine complications of starvation include euthyroid sick syndrome, where peripheral conversion of thyroxine to triiodothyronine is decreased, with a high or high-normal level of reverse triiodothyronine.[27,30] The decrease in triiodothyronine may represent another adaptive response to starvation by helping to reduce the metabolic rate in the face of decreased energy stores. Suggestive symptoms include cold intolerance, dry skin, coarse hair, bradycardia, slowed relaxation of reflexes, and hypercarotenemia. Adolescents with anorexia nervosa should not be given thyroid hormone solely on the basis of a low T_4 level. Growth hormone and cortisol levels may be elevated in anorexia nervosa. Hypercortisolemia has been associated with the osteopenia found in patients with eating disorders.[34]

Elevated levels of growth hormone likely reflect the associated decrease in insulinlike growth factor 1 (IGF-1), which normally inhibits growth hormone secretion at the level of the hypothalamus and the pituitary. With refeeding, growth hormone levels fall to normal within a few days.

Starved patients may manifest hematologic changes including pancytopenia, neutropenia without an apparent increased susceptibility to infection, and a normochromic or hypochromic anemia, all of which resolve with refeeding.[27] The bone marrow often becomes hypocellular. Some patients with a microcytic anemia also require supplemental iron, although most anemia secondary to anorexia nervosa is not associated with iron deficiency. Despite pancytopenia, most of these children and adolescents do not get sick more often than children without eating disorders. In a recent review article, Hütter et al. noted that anemia and mild neutropenia were detectable in almost one third of patients with anorexia nervosa and up to 10% show evidence of thrombocytopenia. Interestingly, peripheral blood cell counts do not predict bone marrow atrophy or gelatinous transformation, which occurs in as many of 50% of patients with anorexia nervosa.[35]

Gastrointestinal findings include delayed gastric emptying and slowed motility, with patients often describing feelings of early satiety, bloating, postprandial discomfort, and constipation.[27,36] Abnormal liver function tests may reflect fatty infiltration of the liver and tend to normalize with weight gain. Children and adolescents with anorexia nervosa may also have transient hypercholesterolemia, also reversible with weight gain; in general, checking cholesterol levels during chronic starvation should be avoided, as the teen tends to use an elevated level as an excuse to restrict his or her daily fat intake further.

Renal effects include elevated blood urea nitrogen (BUN), reflecting dehydration and a decreased glomerular filtration rate.[37] Starvation can also cause total body sodium and potassium depletion; 25% of patients with anorexia nervosa will have peripheral edema with refeeding. This effect is likely caused by increased renal sensitivity to aldosterone and the action of increased insulin secretion on the renal tubules. A minority of patients may present with mild polyuria, displaying impaired or erratic release of vasopressin in response to osmotic challenge.[38] Children and adolescents may display increased BUN from dehydration and decreased glomerular filtration rates, with increased risk of renal stones. Even in the face of severe malnutrition, many of these patients have remarkably normal laboratory values.

Amenorrhea, hypoestrogenism, and osteopenia occur commonly in girls with low weight as well as in patients with bulimia; a later section addresses these issues specifically.

Medical Complications From Purging

Chronic, self-induced vomiting has been associated with hypokalemic, hypochloremic, metabolic alkalosis.[27,39] Loss of hydrogen, chloride, and water from gastric fluid results in chloride and volume depletion, which triggers a secondary hyperaldosteronism. Tubular reabsorption of sodium and excretion of potassium increase; the loss of hydrogen ions, both from tubular excretion and from gastric fluid, causes an exchange of hydrogen and potassium at the cellular level, with worsening hypokalemia. Sodium levels tend to be low or normal, but can also be high in the face of acute dehydration. Remarkably, some teens who report vomiting more than 20 times per day can have normal electrolytes, whereas others purging only three to four times per week may present with values that are markedly abnormal. In one series of 37 patients followed with anorexia nervosa, 24% had prolonged corrected QT, with all but one case associated with hypokalemia, hypomagnesemia, or medications.[40]

As noted earlier, teens who use ipecac to purge are at risk for irreversible myocardial damage along with a diffuse myositis secondary to emetine toxicity.[37] Diuretic abuse as a form of purging can result in electrolyte abnormalities through tubular excretion of potassium and hydrogen; low levels of calcium, magnesium, and zinc can also be found. Urine in these patients may take on a greenish or fluorescent hue, alerting the astute clinician to ask about and test for these substances. Laxative abuse can cause loss of fluids and electrolytes via the stool with subsequent metabolic acidosis, increased BUN, and risk for renal stones due to dehydration. When used in combination with diuretics, the combination can produce severe electrolyte imbalances. Acute laxative withdrawal can result in fluid shifts of 10 to 20 lb acutely with peripheral edema, which tends to panic the individual.

Chronic vomiting can also lead to a classic set of dental erosions on the lingual and occlusal surfaces; the astute dental hygienist may pick this up even before a pediatrician notices. Teeth may have sensitivity to heat or cold from this perimolysis (dental enamel erosion). Chronic vomiting may also result in a looser lower esophageal sphincter, with a resultant increase in gastroesophageal reflux. Chronic esophagitis may put the patient at risk for the development of Barrett's esophagus after years of reflux/purging. Forced emesis can also result in Mallory-Weiss tears, or rarely gastric or esophageal rupture. Rarely, aspiration pneumonia can result from forced emesis with coughing or from vomiting in a decreased state of consciousness, as may occur after a binge on alcohol or drugs. Parotid enlargement can occur, which acutely worsens when the teen quits vomiting, much as smoker's cough worsens after smoking cessation. Serum amylase levels may be elevated, from salivary amylase, with normal lipase levels accordingly.

Medical Complications of Binges

Bingeing on sugary foods may increase dental caries. Acute binges of high volume may cause acute gastric dilatation and rupture.[41] Binge-purges have also been shown to be a risk factor for secondary amenorrhea, with an odds ratio of 4.17.[42] Binges also can cause emotional havoc, with guilt/shame interfering with day-to-day life of those individuals.

AMENORRHEA AND OSTEOPENIA

Delayed puberty is usually defined by no secondary sexual characteristics by age 14 years, and primary amenorrhea can be defined as no menarche by age 15 years; clinicians should be concerned if menarche has not occurred by 3 years from onset of puberty (adrenarche and/or thelarche). In fact, most girls achieve menarche within 2 years of occurrence of both thelarche and adrenarche, with 3 years representing more than 2 standard deviations from normal. Secondary amenorrhea means the absence of menstruation after cycles have been previously established, usually defined as no periods in at least 3 months. Amenorrhea has been associated with hypothalamic dysfunction, weight loss, decreased body fat, hyperexercising, and stress

in individuals with eating disorders.[27] The mechanism involves suppression of gonadotropin releasing hormone (GnRH) secretion by the hypothalamus. Amenorrhea can precede weight loss in 50 to 75% of patients with eating disorders.[43,44]

Bone requires three components for health: adequate calcium intake, defined as 1300 to 1500 mg per day in peripubertal children and all adolescents; weight-bearing exercise; and sex steroids (testosterone in boys, estrogen in girls). Osteopenia results from a negative net balance between bone deposition and bone resorption. Unlike the osteopenia occurring in postmenopausal women, caused mainly by an increase in bone resorption, in children and adolescents with eating disorders, osteopenia results from a failure to deposit bone at key times in development, combined with increased resorption. For girls, a critical time of bone deposition should occur between ages 11 and 14 years, with 40 to 60% of peak bone mass deposited in healthy girls at that time; for boys, peak growth spurt with increased bone deposition occurs slightly later (Table 16-6). Increased bone loss through resorption occurs with hypoestrogenism (seen with amenorrhea) and hypercortisolemia (associated with chronic stress). An additional 5% accrues in the third decade, with even that low amount accounting for a significant decrease in fracture risk.[45] Even a 10% decrease in adult bone mineral density is associated with a two- to threefold increase in fracture risk.[46] Net gains in bone positively correlate with physical activity, weight gain, and calcium and protein intake; net loss correlates with age.[45] Inadequate calcium and protein intake lead to decreased bone formation, as well. Excess glucocorticoids decrease calcium absorption from the gut and inhibit bone formation through direct, receptor-mediated osteoblast effects.[47,48] Acquisition of bone mineral normally continues through the second decade, with peak bone mass reached in late adolescence or early adulthood.[49,50]

Even brief periods of amenorrhea can have significant effects on bone. Osteopenia may occur relatively quickly, or else children and adolescents may have had unrecognized illness for a prolonged period of time.[49] Longer duration of illness and younger age of onset correlate with osteopenia, emphasizing again the need for early recognition and treatment. Exercise that is not excessive may offer some protection against bone loss in anorexia nervosa,[51] but there is a fine line between exercise balance and "too much of a good thing," as occurs with hyperexercising. Eumenorrhea, without hormonal help, can be a useful marker for balanced levels of exercise; but for those girls who need contraception or who are extremely low weight, the benefits of oral contraceptives may outweigh the lack of "cue" that hormonally regulated cycles provide. Many girls and their mothers add hormonal therapy under the presumption that all is well with weight if they just have their periods. Klibanski et al. found that in exceptionally low weight women with anorexia nervosa (body weight less than 70%), the addition

TABLE 16-6. Determinants of Peak Bone Mass in Adolescents

Inheritance and race (African Americans with greater bone density than whites)
Muscle strength
Physical activity
Circulating estrogens and androgens
Dietary calcium
Weight, height
Smoking (negative correlation)

of hormonal therapy (oral contraceptives, or OCs) acted like a "bone Band-Aid" preventing further bone loss.[52] The underweight group prospectively treated with estrogen showed a 4.0% increase in mean bone mineral density, whereas underweight non–estrogen supplemented women had a further 20.2% decrease in bone mineral density. Women in the control group who spontaneously resumed menses showed a 19.3% increase in bone mass; each woman in this group had an initial body weight above 70% of expected. Estrogen replacement in the less extremely underweight group was not associated with improved bone density.[52] Only weight gain with reestablishment of normal estrogenization was associated with bone gain in the very underweight female with anorexia nervosa, with increased bone mineral seen even before the return of menses.[53,54]

Myths and misconceptions arise frequently for adolescents, their mothers, and even care providers with respect to oral contraceptives and periods. Many mistakenly believe it will make them gain weight – clearly a deal breaker for the teen with an eating disorder! Since the advent of extended-use contraceptives such as Seasonale (levonorgestrel and ethinyl estradiol, Bar/Duramed Pharmaceuticals Inc.), teens may also be under the mistaken belief that having three consecutive periods (e.g., in January, February, and March) is adequate for estrogenization for the entire year. A number of teens with eating disorders also have no desire to regain menses, serving as an emotional barricade to starting OCs.

In explaining the medical consequences of their eating disorder to children and adolescents, it is often useful to frame it in terms of brain, bones, heart, and gastrointestinal (GI) tract, where the clinician can help them link symptom with cause. For instance, in the face of starvation, the body is relatively clever – it tries to slow movement from the mouth to the anus in order to capture any bit of nutrition and fluids it may see, knowing that it has not been recently provided with what it needs to grow (or maintain functions for the postpubertal child). So, there is more time for water to be drawn off from the bowel (hence the constipation), and more time for gut flora to break food down into gas (causing the bloating). The slowed GI movement will correct only when the body feels confident that it will see food in the right amounts for a long enough period of time. For some children this takes weeks, for others, months. In terms of heart, insufficient food intake breaks down heart mass as well as other muscle mass, and unlike an athlete's heart, with a big, juicy heart muscle depolarizing and repolarizing, on electrocardiogram (ECG) a wasted heart muscle will only have a little bit of mass to depolarize and repolarize, making for a very low-voltage ECG. The treatment for each of these conditions is to provide the appropriate amount of food, in the right balance, including two to three servings of protein each day, 30 to 50 grams of fat minimum for brain health, and a minimum of 1500 calories to start refeeding.[55] Bones also weigh something, and bone density requires weight gain in order to have bone gain. If a teen has a bone density 1.5 to 2 standard deviations below normal, they can be told that their osteopenia, or thinning bones, will not correct without weight gain, and that the body is clever and will preferentially use calories for the areas most needed, such as brain, bone, and heart. "Love handles" and padding are luxuries that the child will not gain until the basics are covered. On the other hand, it is useful to acknowledge that the teen may perceive weight gain in all the wrong places, but that bloating is air, not weight, and their perceptions may not shift for a long while, making this process stressful.

A pitch for a therapist versed in eating disorders to serve as a coach for stress management and building other skills can be useful at this time.

Treatment

The role of parents has evolved over the past few decades. In the 1980s, "parentectomy," or removal of the parents from the recovery equation, just as an appendectomy removes a vestigial appendix, was the norm. Prolonged admissions were also common, leading insurance companies to rein in treatment centers and swing the pendulum to shorter stays, without objective data that patients were served better when the stay was exceptionally brief (yet more "cost effective"). In the mid-1990s, parents were deemed to be an integral part of the solution; ignoring them in the equation doomed families unnecessarily to years of stressful holiday suppers and family vacations. More recent data suggest that parents should and can play a role in their children's recovery. In a study of 54 girls with eating disorders (mean age 15.8 ± 1.6 years), Zaitsoff and Taylor found greater motivation for change to be associated with less body dissatisfaction, more adaptive parent-adolescent relationships, and fewer depressive symptoms.[56] This study suggests that involvement of families in treatment for adolescents with disordered eating may serve to enhance motivation to recover.

Use of parents as part of the solution has been best documented and studied in pursuit of the Maudsley model of family-based treatment for eating disorders. In a small study of 20 families, half receiving standard treatment and half also participating in a parent-to-parent consultation, the latter group described feeling less alone, more empowered to help their child, and more able to reflect on changes in family interactions.[57] Where possible, this peer network of parent-to-parent support can add value. Historically, this method was described as early as the 1970s by Dr. Alexandra Elliott, among the first documenting the benefits of parent support in their children's recovery from an eating disorder. Adolescents who have never had family meals may give noticeable "pushback" during treatment when parents are placed in a position of "monitoring" them; the pediatrician should strongly recommend family dinners from conception onward to help prevent both obesity and eating disorders!

Nutritional rehabilitation, combined with parent coaching to help learn the basics of refeeding during Maudsley usage, represents the cornerstone of treatment. Supportive psychological services and use of medicines can provide the tools with which to enact these changes and help children, adolescents, and families survive the process and learn better coping strategies. Body image distortions may last far longer than nutritional depletion, with those individuals severe enough to require hospitalization still showing evidence of body image distress long after weight restoration. For individuals with amenorrhea and eating disorders, the best course of action involves improvement of eating habits and nutritional status. Menses will often resume at the weight at which they turned off, giving a relative weight goal for many of these women. A gain in percent body fat may not be necessary for the resumption of menses[58]; however, increases in dietary intake in order to provide sufficient caloric intake to meet energy expenditure should be pursued even in women of normal weight. Calcium intake should be at least 1200 mg/day (four dairy or calcium-containing servings, or a 500-mg calcium supplement with 400 mg vitamin D, twice a day); some data suggest calcium intake should be increased to 1500 mg/day.[59,60] Adequate iron and protein consumption must also be encouraged, especially because many eating-disorder patients assiduously avoid red meat and other forms of animal protein in an effort to "eat healthy."

While bradycardic, children and adolescents with eating disorders should not engage in any forms of exercise or ingest any caffeine. In treating the nonbradycardic child or adolescent with disordered eating, exercise can be modified, serving as a stress management strategy using appropriate intake to keep the patient in positive energy balance. Better prognosis is associated with younger age, less weight loss, and shorter duration of illness, whereas a worse prognosis is associated with vomiting, a history of extreme or precipitous weight loss, and depression.

Modern Dilemmas: Media as a Trigger or Solution?

Adolescents are media-savvy and high-frequency users on the whole, raising the question about whether their media usage might trigger eating disorders. In a prospective study of nearly 3000 girls ages 12 to 21 years, Field et al.[61] found that reading "teen magazines" was significantly associated with the development of an eating disorder. Visiting "pro-ana" (sites promoting anorexia nervosa) and "pro-mia" (sites promoting bulimia nervosa) can be a red flag for disordered eating behaviors. In a sample of 711 secondary school children in Belgium from 7th, 9th, and 11th grades, Custers and Van den Bulck[62] found that 12.6% of the girls and 5.9% of boys had visited pro-anorexia websites. For girls in the study, visiting pro-ana sites was associated with a higher drive for thinness, worse body image, and more perfectionism. The chicken-and-egg issue remains – do these sites reinforce already negative self-images, or actually create them?

Wilson et al. looked at responses from 76 patients in an eating disorder program, ages 10 to 22 years, and 106 parents, of a total of 698 families surveyed about pro–eating disorder site usage versus pro-recovery site usage.[63] Although 52.8% of parents were aware of pro–eating disorder sites, only 27.6% had discussed them with their child. Almost two thirds (62.5%) of parents were unaware of pro-recovery sites. Among the children, adolescents, and young adults surveyed, 41% had visited pro-recovery sites, 35.5% had visited pro–eating disorder sites, 25.0% visited both, and 48.7% had not visited either pro–eating disorder or pro-recovery sites. New and improved techniques for weight loss or purging (negative behaviors) were learned by 96.0% visiting pro–eating disorder sites and 46.4% visiting pro-recovery sites; thus, both kinds of sites shared the potential for aiding and abetting eating disorder behaviors. Those patients visiting these sites were similar in health outcomes to non–website users, but website frequenters had a longer duration of illness, had more hospitalizations, and had spent less time on homework. The ambivalence associated with recovery is suggested, with a coexistent drive to seek information and medical help to recover in a subset of patients, but with the siren's pull of that eating disorder voice serving to find ways to learn new behaviors and reinforce old ones. Of note, recovery sites may have started with good intent, but users can find equally triggering content with medically unsafe dieting techniques on these sites as well as on the pro–eating disorder sites. Also, parents may have awareness of risk behaviors including Internet sites that would not be "parent-approved" material, but just as

with other risk behaviors, they may underestimate prevalence in their own households. Parents need to be schooled in media literacy, to help immunize their children against its effect and to better monitor site visits as points for intervention.

PROGNOSIS: BONE, BRAINS, AND BABIES (OR FUTURE FERTILITY)

Long-term prognosis for individuals with eating disorders can be generalized for parents into the rule of thirds: one third of patients get better, moving on to normal lives, normal careers, normal relationships, walking away from their eating disorder relatively unscathed. Another third of patients recover, but when stressed, revert back to abnormal eating attitudes and behaviors as a maladaptive coping strategy or default coping mechanism. The bottom third of patients have a chronic and relapsing course, with a significant percentage dying prematurely of their illness.

Steinhausen narrowed this data further in a review of all the follow up studies in the latter half of the 20th century for patients specifically with anorexia nervosa, finding that 1 of 5 individuals with anorexia nervosa experienced chronic symptoms and medical complications.[64] In a recent study, adult women with anorexia nervosa had a sixfold increased mortality as compared with the general population, an excess of mortality two to three times higher than that found with mental disorders in general, and specifically schizophrenia, bipolar disorder, and depression.[65-68] Of note, these higher mortality rates held even 20 or more years after a first admission for the illness. In a Swedish study of 51 individuals with anorexia nervosa with a mean age of onset of 14 years compared with 51 age-matched controls studied 18 years after patients' disease onset (mean age 32 years at time of study), 12% continued to have persistent eating disorder symptoms, 39% of the study group had at least one psychiatric disorder, and 1 of 4 was unemployed because of psychiatric problems, with poor general outcome overall in 12%.[69] Poor outcome was predicted by premorbid obsessive-compulsive personality disorder, low age of onset, and autistic traits. The good news was that none had died. Of note, Sweden's mortality rate for individuals with chronic anorexia nervosa has been found to be lower (1.2% versus nearly 20%) than the mortality rates found in other countries, perhaps reflective of better treatment strategies in recent years.[69,70] Earlier data had found that in long-term follow-up of individuals with chronic and relapsing disease, those identified via referral to a tertiary care center for their eating disorder or inpatient facility, high mortality rates (17, 18, and 16%, respectively) corresponded to a standardized mortality ratio of 9.8.[71-73]

Fertility is preserved in individuals with eating disorder recovery. In a study of 66 patients in an infertility clinic, 16.7% had diagnosable eating disorders.[74] In 50% of these previously amenorrheic patients, oligomenorrhea recurred when their eating disorder flared. A common concern voiced by these women was that their eating disorder had damaged their bodies. In another study of 29 women with unexplained infertility evaluated for weight control practices, 19 of 26 women were able to conceive once they reached 98% of predicted ideal body weight.[75] At study's end, 5 more women had conceived, or 92% of the study cohort. Of note, when their body weight reached between 85 and 95% of their ideal body weight, their LH:FSH ratio reached a maximum (above 3.5), normalizing with further weight gain. Thus, even though menses may return, a higher weight may be required to achieve fertility. In another study of 83 adolescents, menses returned when weight averaged 92.1 + 7.4 SD%; all patients who wanted to conceive on longer follow-up were able to do within a year of trying to get pregnant.[76]

Once pregnant, recovering eating disorder patients tend to gain less weight, have more complications of pregnancy, have smaller babies with lower 5-minute Apgar scores, have more problems with breast feeding, and have more difficulties with postpartum adjustment.[74] Those women who manage to bring their symptoms into remission during pregnancy may escalate symptoms again postdelivery.[77] Another worrisome finding is that some mothers with eating disorders underfeed their children. A Dutch longitudinal study of 50 anorectic mothers found failure to thrive in 17% of their children in the first 4 years of life, with seven children showing stunted growth and a low weight for height.[78] In a few cases, the children showed a dramatic growth spurt when the mother was admitted into a treatment center for eating disorders. In a study of five mothers with bulimia, Stein and Fairburn noted inadequate feeding practices for their infants, with undue concern expressed about their child's weight and shape.[79] One child was severely underweight, whereas another was obese. Obstetricians and fertility specialists need to keep a high vigilance for disordered eating in their patients presenting with oligomenorrhea, amenorrhea, and infertility. Delay in pregnancy should be advised until after they have addressed eating disorder symptomatology, and early diagnosis and treatment may reduce maternal and fetal complications. Pediatricians and obstetricians can partner in the care of the affected mother and child dyad.

NEXT STEP

Several questions remain with respect to eating disorders. With respect to girls with amenorrhea, how often should bone density be followed, and which technologies are recommended? DEXA scans annually remain the current standard of care, started on all girls with at least 6 months of amenorrhea by most specialists in the medical care of eating disorders. How should we treat bone loss? The role of oral contraceptives remains controversial, but potentially necessary in those adolescents and young adults who are sexually active or in the exceptionally low-weight individual as a bone "Band-Aid." How much vitamin D is recommended, and should we test all children and adolescents? Finally, and most challenging, how can we best motivate adolescents and young adults with disordered eating to change lifestyle habits to promote bone, brain, and heart health?

The use of carepaths for acute inpatient stabilization has been a recent focus. Different standards of care for treatment currently exist worldwide, without published protocol outcomes. Quality improvement data via use of a standardized protocol can help evaluate quality of care issues, enhancing care while working to decrease costs of care. At our center, data on 52 patients hospitalized for acute medical stabilization using our nutritional insufficiency carepath showed an average length of stay of 6.81 days, average age of patients 17 years, with resolution of bradycardia, orthostasis, ECG abnormalities, and electrolyte imbalances at time of discharge. Length of hospitalization was influenced by time to resolution of orthostatic hypotension, normalization of potassium levels was not based on weight gain but on potassium supplementation, as expected.[80] An ongoing QI project serving as a national collaborative will further tease out other aspects of care relevant to recovery in children, adolescents, and young adults.

PREVENTION: HOW CAN WE DO BETTER?

An integrated approach to both eating disorders and obesity prevention in childhood and adolescence has great promise as a means of promoting positive parenting and minimizing disease risk at both ends of the spectrum.[81-83] In a study using semistructured interviews with content analysis to identify recurrent themes from 27 individuals receiving treatment for eating disorders, Loth et al.[84] found eight recurrent themes to help families prevent the onset of eating disorders. These themes included:

- Enhance parental support
- Decrease weight and body talk in the home and elsewhere
- Provide a supportive home food environment
- Model healthy eating habits and physical activity patterns
- Help children build self-esteem beyond looks and physical appearance
- Encourage appropriate expression of feelings and use of coping mechanisms
- Increase parents' own understanding of eating disorder signs and symptoms
- Gain support in dealing appropriately with parents' own struggles

In other words, "Do as I say, not as I do" will not prevent eating disorders, just as it does not work for a smoker to raise a nonsmoking teenager. Encouraging family dinners starting from infancy onward is far easier than trying to institute them at age 15 years, and helping parents remember to praise actions, rather than just appearance, can improve their children's functioning. Many children struggle with learning delayed gratification, especially in a media world where everything is a mouse click away, or a switch of the remote; helping children learn to fail gracefully as well as to succeed can start young, with learning processes reinforced at different developmental stages. Parental chronic dieting should be neither seen or heard, but instituting family wellness patterns, such as Friday night bowling rather than popcorn and a movie, can get families engaged in activities that decrease the incidence of both eating disorders and obesity.

Prevention remains of paramount importance, with mounting pressure to avoid triggering eating disorders while fostering increasing athletic participation and decreasing national and international rates of obesity. Clarification on best programs to prevent both obesity and eating disorders deserves future attention. Imaging modalities such as DEXA scans involve low radiation risk but only two-dimensional data; future technology may be able to give more accurate three-dimensional readings. Finally, the role of specific treatment modalities, including medicines such as the anabolic steroid DHEA, currently not FDA approved and under study, and the bisphosphonates, which have implications for future fetal bones and lifelong bone of young women for whom they are prescribed, requires further study in the treatment of osteopenia and osteoporosis.

REFERENCES

2. Workgroup for Classification of Eating Disorders in Children and Adolescents, Bravender T, Bryant-Waugh R, Herzog D, et al. Classification of child and adolescent eating disturbances. Int J Eat Disord 2007;40(S3): S117–S122.
4. Fairburn CG, Harrison PJ. Eating disorders. Lancet 2003;361:407–416.
8. Peebles R, Wilson JL, Lock JD. How do children with eating disorders differ from adolescents with eating disorders at initial evaluation? J Adolesc Health 2006;39:800–805.

52. Klibanski A, Biller BMK, Schoenfeld DA, et al. The effects of estrogen administration on trabecular bone loss in young women with anorexia nervosa. J Clin Endocrinol Metab 1995;80:898–904.
61. Field A, Camargo C, Taylor C. Peer, parent, and media influences on the development of weight concerns and frequent dieting among pre-adolescent and adolescent girls and boys. Pediatrics 2001;107:54–60.
81. Haines J, Neumark-Sztainer D. Prevention of obesity and eating disorders: a consideration of shared risk factors. Health Educ Res 2006;21:770–782.

83. Irving LM, Neumark-Sztainer D. Integrating the prevention of eating disorders and obesity: feasible or futile? Prev Med 2002;34:299–309.

See expertconsult.com for a complete list of references and the review questions for this chapter.

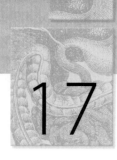

17 JAUNDICE

Kara M. Sullivan • Glenn R. Gourley

The term *jaundice* originated from the French *jaune,* which means "yellow." Jaundice, or icterus (from the Greek *ikteros*), refers to the yellow discoloration of the skin, sclerae, and other tissues caused by deposition of the bile pigment bilirubin. Jaundice is a sign that the serum bilirubin concentration has risen above normal levels (approximately 1.4 mg/dL after 6 months of age; 1 mg/dL = 17 μmol/L). The intensity of the yellow color is directly related to the level of serum bilirubin and the related degree of deposition of bilirubin into the extravascular tissues. The yellow skin of hypercarotenemia is not associated with yellow sclerae.

BILIRUBIN METABOLISM

The term *bilirubin* is derived from Latin (*bilis*, bile; *ruber*, red) and was used in 1864 by Städeler[1] to describe the red-colored bile pigment. Bilirubin is formed from the degradation of heme-containing compounds (Figure 17-1). The largest source for the production of bilirubin is hemoglobin. However, other heme-containing proteins are also degraded to bilirubin, including the cytochromes, catalases, tryptophan pyrrolase, and muscle myoglobin.

The formation of bilirubin is accomplished by cleavage of the tetrapyrrole ring of protoheme (protoporphyrin IX), which results in a linear tetrapyrrole. The first enzyme system involved in the formation of bilirubin is microsomal heme oxygenase.[2] It is located primarily in the reticuloendothelial tissues and to a lesser degree in tissue macrophages and intestinal epithelium. This enzyme system results in reduction of the porphyrin iron (Fe^{3+} to Fe^{2+}) and hydroxylation of the α methine (=C–) carbon. This α-carbon is then oxidatively excised from the tetrapyrrole ring, yielding carbon monoxide. This excision opens the ring structure and is associated with oxygenation of the two carbons adjacent to the site of cleavage. The cleaved α-carbon is excreted as carbon monoxide, and the released iron can be reused by the body. The resultant linear tetrapyrrole is biliverdin IXα. The *IX* designation is a result of Fischer's grouping of the protoporphyrin isomers, group IX being the physiologic source of bilirubin.

The stereospecificity of the enzyme produces cleavage almost exclusively at the α-carbon of the tetrapyrrole. This is unlike in vitro chemical oxidation, which results in cleavage at any of the four carbons (α, β, γ, and δ) linking the four pyrrole rings and produces equimolar amounts of the α, β, γ, and δ isomers. The central (C10) carbon on biliverdin IXα is then reduced from a methine to a methylene group ($-CH_2-$), thus forming bilirubin IXα. This is accomplished by the cytosolic enzyme biliverdin reductase.[3] The ubiquity of this enzyme results in very little biliverdin ever being present in the circulation.

Bilirubin formation can be assessed by measurement of carbon monoxide production. Such assessments indicate that the daily production rate of bilirubin is 6 to 8 mg/kg per 24 hours in healthy, full-term infants and 3 to 4 mg/kg per 24 hours in healthy adults.[4,5] In mammals, approximately 80% of bilirubin produced daily originates from hemoglobin.[6] Degradation of hepatic and renal heme appears to account for most of the remaining 20%, reflecting the very rapid turnover of certain of these heme proteins. Although the precise fate of myoglobin heme is unknown, its turnover appears to be so slow as to be relatively insignificant.

Catabolism of hemoglobin occurs very largely from the sequestration of erythrocytes at the end of their life span (120 days in adult humans, 90 days in newborns, 50 to 60 days in rats). A small fraction of newly synthesized hemoglobin is degraded in the bone marrow. This process, termed *ineffective erythropoiesis*, normally represents less than 3% of daily bilirubin production but may be substantially increased in persons with hemoglobinopathies, vitamin deficiencies, or heavy metal intoxication. Infants produce more bilirubin per unit body weight because their red blood cell (RBC) mass is greater and their RBC life span is shorter. In addition, hepatic heme proteins represent a larger fraction of total body weight in infants.

Bilirubin requires biotransformation to more water-soluble derivatives before excretion from the body.[7] Bilirubin is not linear but rather has extensive internal hydrogen bonding, as shown in Figure 17-2. The internal hydrogen bonding of bilirubin makes the molecule extremely hydrophobic and insoluble in aqueous media. Knowledge of this stereochemistry is important for understanding phototherapy.

When bilirubin is transported from its sites of production to the liver for excretion, a carrier molecule is necessary. Albumin serves this purpose and has very high affinity for bilirubin (affinity constant $\sim 10^8$).[8]

Bilirubin is taken up into the hepatocyte from the hepatic sinusoids by either passive diffusion or a high affinity transport protein in the basolateral plasma membrane known as organic anion transporting polypeptide 2 (human OATP2, recently named OATP1B1, under new nomenclature[9]; transporter symbol SLC21A6) which also transports other bilirubin glucuronides and bromsulfophthalein.[10,11] This carrier protein is competitively inhibited by simultaneous exposure to bromsulfophthalein or indocyanine green.

Once within the aqueous environment of the hepatocyte, bilirubin is again bound by a protein carrier, glutathione-S-transferase, traditionally referred to as ligandin. This is a family of cytosolic proteins that have enzymatic activity and also bind nonsubstrate ligands. Although the affinity of purified glutathione-S-transferase for bilirubin (acid dissociation constant $= 10^6$) is less than that of albumin, this compound is believed to be of importance in preventing bilirubin and its conjugates from refluxing back into the circulation.[12]

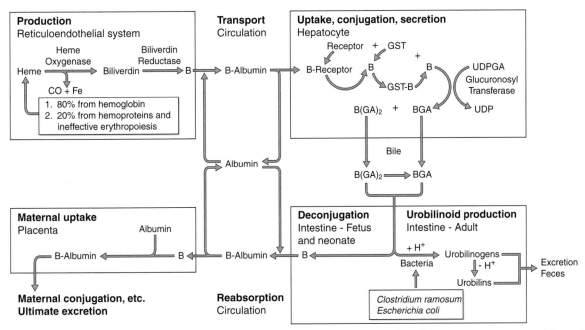

Figure 17-1. Metabolism of bilirubin (B) in the fetus, neonate, and adult. GA, glucuronic acid; UDP, uridine diphosphate; GST, glutathione-S-transferase.

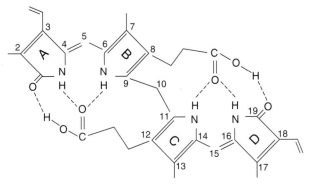

Figure 17-2. 4Z,15Z-Bilirubin IXα. The internal hydrogen bonding that shields the polar propionic acid groups is responsible for the hydrophobic nature of bilirubin.

Bilirubin is conjugated with glucuronic acid in the hepatocyte. The glucuronic acid donor is uridine diphosphate glucuronic acid (UDP-glucuronic acid). The enzyme responsible for this conjugation is bilirubin glucuronosyltransferase (BGT). Several different classes of glucuronosyltransferases, with different substrate specificity (e.g. thyroxine, steroids, bile acids, and xenobiotics), have been described. Catalysis of bilirubin by BGT results in both monoglucuronides and diglucuronides of bilirubin (BMGs and BDGs, respectively). This conjugation disrupts the internal hydrogen bonding of bilirubin, and the resulting glucuronide conjugates are more water soluble. Depletion of hepatic UDP-glucuronic acid results in decreased BDGs and increased BMGs. BGT activity for bilirubin can be induced by narcotics, anticonvulsants, contraceptive steroids, and bilirubin itself. Alternatively, BGT activity can be decreased by caloric and protein restriction. The specific isoform responsible for bilirubin conjugation is UGT1A1 (EC 2.4.1.17), which is part of the UDP glycosyltransferase superfamily of enzymes encoded by the *UGT1* gene complex on chromosome 2.[13] More than 30 different mutations in the *UGT1* gene have been described that cause

Gilbert's syndrome and Crigler Najjar syndromes I and II. After bilirubin conjugation, the BMGs and BDGs are excreted through the hepatocyte canalicular membrane into the bile canaliculi. This is accomplished by the ATP-dependent transporter known as canalicular multispecific organic anion transporter (cMOAT) or multidrug resistance-associated protein (MRP2).[14] Mutations in the cMOAT/MRP2 gene cause Dubin-Johnson syndrome.[15] In normal adult duodenal bile, 70% to 90% of the bile pigments are BDGs, and 7% to 27% are BMGs. Smaller amounts of other bilirubin conjugates are also seen. However, in normal infants there is decreased BGT activity in the liver,[16] and duodenal bile contains less BDG and more BMG than in the adult.[17] After the first week of life, the rate-limiting step in bilirubin clearance is secretion of bilirubin conjugates by the hepatocyte.[18] Canalicular secretion of bilirubin conjugates can be increased by choleretic agents (e.g., phenobarbital, ursodeoxycholic acid[19]) and decreased by cholestatic agents (e.g., estrogens, anabolic steroids) or pathologic conditions (e.g., liver disease, sepsis).

Under normal conditions, there is evidence that bilirubin conjugates equilibrate across the sinusoidal membrane of hepatocytes. This results in the presence of small amounts of bilirubin conjugates in the systemic circulation. If there is diminished hepatic glucuronidation of bilirubin (e.g., in the neonate), there will be a decreased amount of bilirubin conjugates present in the serum.[20]

In many pathologic circumstances, BMGs and BDGs are not excreted from the hepatocyte fast enough to prevent reflux back into the circulation. The increased serum levels of bilirubin conjugates result in the spontaneous (nonenzymatic) transesterification of bilirubin glucuronide with an amino group on albumin, producing a covalent bond between albumin and bilirubin. This product is known as delta bilirubin or bilirubin-albumin.[21] Delta bilirubin is not formed in hyperbilirubinemic conditions unless there is elevation of the conjugated bilirubin fraction. Delta bilirubin is direct-reacting (Van den Bergh's test) and is cleared from the circulation slowly owing to the long (~20-day[22]) half-life of albumin.

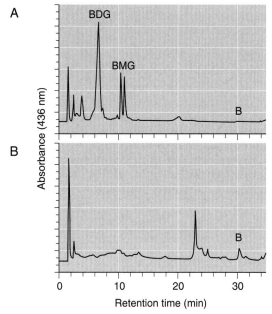

Figure 17-3. Bile pigment excretion in an adult as assessed by HPLC. (**A**) Duodenal bile (20 μL) from a normal man (GG). (**B**) Fecal extract equivalent to 50 mg of wet stool from the same normal man (GG). The BDGs and BMGs that predominate in adult bile are not present in adult stool because they are converted to urobilinoids by intestinal bacteria. Small amounts of bilirubin (B) are present in adult feces. From Gourley (1997),[79] with permission.

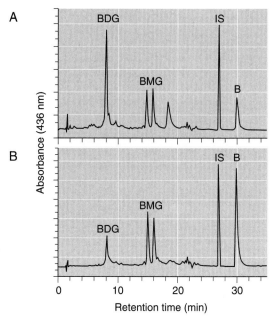

Figure 17-4. (**A**) The analysis of a sample of duodenal bile (20 μL) from a full-term, jaundiced, 6-day-old infant. (**B**) The analysis of a sample of fecal extract equivalent to 4 mg wet stool from the same infant. Neonates lack an intestinal bacterial flora, and hence large quantities of BDGs, BMGs, and bilirubin (B) are present in feces. The deglucuronidation action of intestinal β-glucuronidase is evident from the relatively decreased amounts of BDG and the increased amounts of BMG and B. IS, internal standard. From Gourley (1997),[79] with permission.

When bilirubin conjugates enter the intestinal lumen, several possibilities for further metabolism arise. In adults, the normal bacterial flora hydrogenate various carbon double bonds in bilirubin to produce assorted urobilinogens.[23] Subsequent oxidation produces the related urobilins. The large number of unsaturated bonds in bilirubin results in a large family of related reduction-oxidation products known as urobilinoids, which are excreted in the feces. The conversion of bilirubin conjugates to urobilinoids is important because it blocks the intestinal absorption of bilirubin, known as the enterohepatic circulation.[24] Neonates lack an intestinal bacterial flora and are more likely to absorb bilirubin from the intestine. This difference in bile pigment excretion between adults and neonates is demonstrated in Figures 17-3 and 17-4. Bilirubin conjugates in the intestine can also act as substrate for either bacterial or endogenous tissue β-glucuronidase. This enzyme hydrolyzes glucuronic acid from bilirubin glucuronides. The unconjugated bilirubin produced is more rapidly absorbed from the intestine.[25] After birth, increased intestinal β-glucuronidase can increase the neonate's likelihood of experiencing higher serum bilirubin levels.[26] In a prospective randomized double-blind study, β-glucuronidase inhibition was shown to be associated with increased fecal bilirubin excretion and less jaundice in breast-fed neonates.[27]

Neonates are at risk for the intestinal absorption of bilirubin because (1) their bile contains increased levels of BMG, which allows easier conversion to bilirubin; (2) they have within the intestinal lumen significant amounts of β-glucuronidase, which hydrolyzes bilirubin conjugates to more easily absorbed bilirubin; (3) they lack an intestinal flora to convert bilirubin conjugates to urobilinoids; and (4) meconium, the intestinal contents accumulated during gestation, contains significant amounts of bilirubin and β-glucuronidase.[28] Conditions that prolong meconium passage (e.g., Hirschsprung's disease, meconium

ileus, meconium plug syndrome) are associated with hyperbilirubinemia. Earlier passage of meconium has been shown to be associated with lower serum bilirubin levels. The enterohepatic circulation of bilirubin can be blocked by the enteral administration of compounds that bind bilirubin, such as agar, charcoal, and cholestyramine.

ASSESSMENT OF JAUNDICE

Measurements of serum bilirubin are very common in the newborn nursery and in one study were made at least once in 61% of full-term newborn infants.[29] Two components of total serum bilirubin can be measured routinely in the clinical laboratory: conjugated bilirubin (direct fraction in Van den Bergh's test because the color change takes place directly, without the addition of methanol) and unconjugated bilirubin (indirect fraction). Although the terms *direct* and *indirect* are used equivalently with conjugated and unconjugated bilirubin, this is not quantitatively correct, because the direct fraction includes both conjugated bilirubin and delta bilirubin. Elevation of either of these fractions can result in jaundice. There is a long history of undesirable variability in the measurement of serum bilirubin fractions.[30,31] Of the various laboratory methods, the Jendrassik-Grof procedure is the method of choice for total bilirubin measurement, although this method also has problems.[32] When the total serum bilirubin level is high, factitious elevation of the direct fraction has been reported. Experimental evidence indicates that the minute fraction of bilirubin that is not bound to albumin, referred to as the unbound or "free" bilirubin concentration, correlates more strongly with bilirubin toxicity than does total bilirubin concentration.[33] However, there are no clinically established methods of measuring free bilirubin.

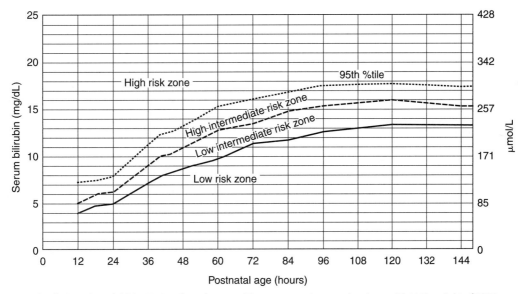

Figure 17-5. Nomogram for designation of risk in 2840 well newborns at 36 or more weeks gestational age with birth weight of 2000 g or more or 35 or more weeks gestational age and birth weight of 2500 g or more, based on the hour-specific serum bilirubin values. The serum bilirubin level was obtained before discharge, and the zone in which the value fell predicted the likelihood of a subsequent bilirubin level exceeding the 95th percentile (high-risk zone) Used with permission from Bhutani et al. (1999).[41]

Two newer methods have been developed that can more accurately determine the various bilirubin fractions (unconjugated, monoconjugated, diconjugated, and albumin-bound or delta): high-performance liquid chromatography (HPLC)[34] and multilayered slides (Ektachem).[35] HPLC analysis is superior but too expensive and time-consuming for the clinical laboratory. HPLC analysis of serum from normal human neonates in the first 4 days of life[36] showed that unconjugated and conjugated bilirubin levels rise in parallel, with the conjugated fraction making up only 1.2% to 1.6% of total pigment (compared with 3.6% in adults). Because of the long half-life of delta bilirubin, the conjugated bilirubin measurement indicates relief from biliary cholestasis earlier than the direct bilirubin measurement does.

There are conflicting data regarding the relative accuracy of measurements of capillary and venous serum bilirubin. However, as Maisels[37] pointed out, the literature regarding kernicterus, phototherapy, and exchange transfusion is based on bilirubin measurements in capillary samples.

Noninvasive transcutaneous methods to assess jaundice at the point of care are available and include Bilichek (Respironics, Murrysville, PA)[38,39] and Jaundice Meter (Konica Minolta Sensing Americas, Inc. Ramsey, NJ).[40] A neonatal hour-specific total serum bilirubin nomogram has been developed that can predict the risk of subsequent hyperbilirubinemia based on total serum bilirubin[41] (Figure 17-5) or transcutaneous bilirubin,[38] thus facilitating follow-up and intervention for infants.

NEONATAL JAUNDICE

Infants usually are not jaundiced at the moment of birth, because the placenta has the ability to clear bilirubin from the fetal circulation. However, during the first week of life, most if not all infants have elevated serum bilirubin concentrations (above 1.4 mg/dL). As the serum bilirubin rises, the skin becomes more jaundiced in a cephalopedal manner. Icterus is first appreciated in the head and progresses caudally to the palms and soles. Kramer[42] found the following serum indirect bilirubin levels as jaundice progressed: head and neck, 4 to 8 mg/dL; upper trunk, 5 to 12 mg/dL; lower trunk and thighs, 8 to 16 mg/dL; arms and lower legs, 11 to 18 mg/dL; palms and soles, more than 15 mg/dL. When the bilirubin was higher than 15 mg/dL, the entire body was icteric. Jaundice is best appreciated by blanching the skin with gentle digital pressure under well-illuminated (white light) conditions. Visual assessment has been shown to be unreliable as a screening tool to detect significant neonatal hyperbilirubinemia.[43,44]

Moderate jaundice (above 12 mg/dL) occurs in at least 12% of breast-fed infants and 4% of formula-fed infants, and severe jaundice (above 15 mg/dL) occurs in 2% and 0.3% of these respective feeding groups.[45]

Fundamentally, jaundice has only two causes: increased production or decreased excretion of bilirubin. These mechanisms are not mutually exclusive; specific examples are listed in Table 17-1. One possible clinical approach to arrive at these diagnoses is presented in Figure 17-6.

The high incidence of jaundice in otherwise completely normal neonates has resulted in the term *physiologic jaundice*. However, physiologic jaundice is merely the result of a number of factors involving increased bilirubin production and decreased excretion. Jaundice should always be considered to be a sign of possible disease and not routinely explained as physiologic. Specific characteristics of neonatal jaundice to be considered abnormal until proved otherwise include (1) development of jaundice before 36 hours of age, (2) persistence of jaundice beyond 10 days of age, (3) a serum bilirubin concentration higher than 12 mg/dL at any time, and (4) elevation of the direct-reacting fraction of bilirubin to more than 2 mg/dL at any time.

Factors associated with increased neonatal bilirubin levels are prematurity; low birth weight; certain races (East Asian, Native American, Greek); maternal medications (e.g., oxytocin); premature rupture of the membranes; increased weight loss after birth; delayed meconium passage; breast-feeding; and neonatal infection. Factors associated with decreased neonatal

TABLE 17-1. Causes of Neonatal Hyperbilirubinemia

Increased production of bilirubin
  Fetal-maternal blood group incompatibilities
  Extravascular blood in body tissues
  Polycythemia
  Red blood cell abnormalities (hemoglobinopathies, membrane and
    enzyme defects)
  Induction of labor
Decreased excretion of bilirubin
  Increased enterohepatic circulation of bilirubin
  Breast feeding
  Inborn errors of metabolism
  Hormones and drugs
  Prematurity
  Hepatic hypoperfusion
  Cholestatic syndromes
  Obstruction of the biliary tree
Combined increased production and decreased excretion of bilirubin
  Sepsis
  Intrauterine infection
  Congenital cirrhosis

bilirubin levels include maternal smoking, black race, and certain drugs given to the mother (e.g., phenobarbital).

Neonatal Jaundice Caused by Increased Production of Bilirubin

The most common cause of severe early jaundice is fetal-maternal blood group incompatibility with resulting isoimmunization. Maternal sensitization develops because of leakage of erythrocytes from the fetal to the maternal circulation. When the fetal erythrocytes carry different antigens, they are recognized as foreign by the maternal immune system, which forms antibodies against them. These antibodies (immunoglobulin G) cross the placental barrier into the fetal circulation and bind to fetal erythrocytes. In Rh incompatibility, sequestration and destruction of the antibody-coated erythrocytes takes place in the reticuloendothelial system of the fetus. In ABO incompatibility, hemolysis is intravascular, complement-mediated, and usually not as severe as in Rh disease. Significant hemolysis can also result from incompatibilities between minor blood group antigens (e.g., Kell). These conditions are associated predominately with elevation of unconjugated bilirubin, but occasionally the conjugated fraction is also increased.

Rh incompatibility usually does not develop until the second pregnancy. Therefore, prenatal blood typing and serial testing of Rh-negative mothers for the development of Rh antibodies provide important information to guide possible intrauterine care. If maternal Rh antibodies develop during pregnancy, potentially helpful measures include serial amniocentesis (with bilirubin measurement),[46] ultrasound assessment of the fetus, intrauterine transfusion, and premature delivery. The prophylactic administration of anti-D γ-globulin has been most helpful in preventing Rh sensitization. The newborn infant with Rh incompatibility presents with pallor, hepatosplenomegaly, and a rapidly developing jaundice in the first hours of life. If the problem is severe, the infant may be born with generalized edema (fetal hydrops). Laboratory findings in the neonate's blood include reticulocytosis, anemia, a positive direct Coombs' test, and a rapidly rising serum bilirubin level. Intravenous γ-globulin has been shown to reduce the need for exchange transfusions in Rh and ABO hemolytic disease and is recommended if the total

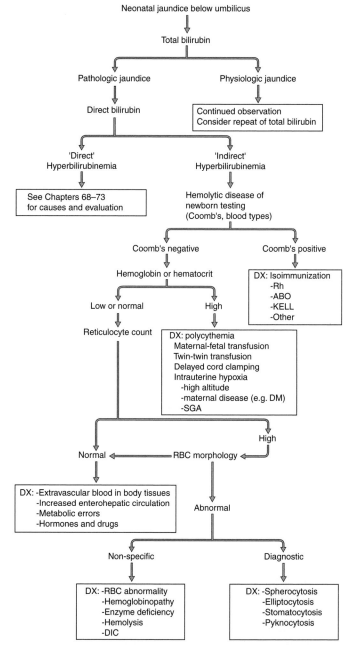

Figure 17-6. A clinical approach to the diagnosis of neonatal jaundice.

serum bilirubin (TSB) is rising despite intensive phototherapy or the TSB level is within 2 to 3 mg/dL (34 to 51 μmol/L) of the exchange level.[47] Exchange transfusion continues to be an important therapy for seriously affected infants.[47,48]

ABO incompatibility usually manifests clinically with the first pregnancy. ABO hemolytic disease is largely limited to infants with blood group A or B who are born to group O mothers. ABO hemolytic disease is relatively rare in type A or B mothers. Development of jaundice is not as rapid as with Rh disease; a serum bilirubin concentration higher than 12 mg/dL on day 3 of life would be typical. Laboratory abnormalities include reticulocytosis (above 10%) and a weakly positive direct Coombs' test, although this is sometimes negative. Spherocytes are the most prominent feature seen in the peripheral blood smear of neonates with ABO incompatibility.

When extravascular blood is present within the body, the hemoglobin can be rapidly converted to bilirubin by tissue macrophages. Examples of this type of increased bilirubin production include cephalohematoma; ecchymoses; petechiae; occult intracranial, intestinal, or pulmonary hemorrhage; and swallowed maternal blood. The Apt test can be used to distinguish blood of maternal or infant origin because of differences in alkali resistance between fetal and adult hemoglobin.[49]

Polycythemia (venipuncture hematocrit above 65%) can cause hyperbilirubinemia because the absolute increase in RBC mass results in elevated bilirubin production through normal rates of erythrocyte breakdown. A number of mechanisms can result in neonatal polycythemia, including maternal-fetal transfusion, a delay in cord clamping, twin-twin transfusions, intrauterine hypoxia, and maternal diseases (e.g., diabetes mellitus). Therapy for symptomatic polycythemia is partial exchange transfusion (PET); therapy for asymptomatic polycythemia remains controversial. Crystalloids are as effective as colloids in PET and are cheaper, more readily available, and confer less risk of infection or anaphylaxis.[50]

A number of specific abnormalities related to the RBC can result in neonatal jaundice, including hemoglobinopathies and RBC membrane or enzyme defects. Hereditary spherocytosis is not usually a neonatal problem, but hemolytic crises can occur and can manifest with a rising bilirubin level and a falling hematocrit. The characteristic spherocytes seen in the peripheral blood smear may be impossible to distinguish from those seen with ABO hemolytic disease. Other hemolytic anemias associated with neonatal jaundice include drug-induced hemolysis, deficiencies of the erythrocyte enzymes (e.g., glucose-6-phosphate dehydrogenase [G6PD] deficiency, pyruvate kinase deficiency), and hemolysis induced by vitamin K or bacteria. α-Thalassemia can result in severe hemolysis and lethal hydrops fetalis. γβ-Thalassemia may also occur, with hemolysis and severe neonatal hyperbilirubinemia. Drugs or other substances responsible for hemolysis can be passed to the fetus or neonate across the placenta or via the breast milk. Co-inheritance of Gilbert's syndrome along with the foregoing hematologic abnormalities is associated with an increased incidence of hyperbilirubinemia in neonates and older individuals.[51]

Induction of labor with oxytocin has been shown to be associated with neonatal jaundice. There is a significant association between hyponatremia and jaundice in infants of mothers who received oxytocin to induce labor. The explanation for this observation is not clear.

Neonatal Jaundice Caused by Decreased Excretion of Bilirubin

Increased enterohepatic circulation of bilirubin is an important factor in neonatal jaundice. Conditions that prolong meconium passage (e.g., Hirschsprung's disease, meconium ileus, meconium plug syndrome) are associated with hyperbilirubinemia, presumably by allowing more time for intestinal bilirubin absorption. Earlier passage of meconium is associated with lower serum bilirubin levels. The enterohepatic circulation of bilirubin can be blocked by enteral administration of compounds that bind bilirubin, such as agar, charcoal, and cholestyramine.

Breast feeding has been identified as a significant factor related to neonatal jaundice.[45,52,53] Breast-fed infants have significantly higher serum bilirubin levels than formula-fed infants on each of the first 5 days of life, and this unconjugated hyperbilirubinemia can persist for weeks to months. Research has shown that bilirubin is a significant antioxidant that is possibly of physiologic benefit in protecting against cellular damage by free radicals. During the first week of life, some distinguish this early jaundice as "breast-feeding jaundice" to differentiate it from the later breast milk jaundice syndrome, which occurs after the first week of life and in which the breast milk supply is well established. There is probably overlap between these conditions and physiologic jaundice. Early reports linking breast milk and jaundice with a steroid (pregnane-3α,20β-diol) in some milk samples[54] have not been confirmed by subsequent, larger studies employing more sensitive methods.[55] There are conflicting data regarding the association of this jaundice with increased lipase activity in the breast milk, which results in increased levels of free fatty acids that could inhibit hepatic BGT. The enterohepatic circulation of bilirubin might be facilitated by the presence of β-glucuronidase[26] or some other substance in human milk. Other factors possibly related to jaundice in breast-fed infants include caloric intake, fluid intake, weight loss, delayed meconium passage, intestinal bacterial flora, and inhibition of BGT by an unidentified factor in the milk. It has been suggested that a healthy, breast-fed infant with unconjugated hyperbilirubinemia, normal hemoglobin concentration, normal reticulocyte count, normal blood smear, no blood group incompatibility, and no other abnormality on physical examination may be presumed to have early breast-feeding jaundice.[56]

Because there is no specific laboratory test to confirm a diagnosis of breast milk jaundice, it is important to rule out treatable causes of jaundice before ascribing the hyperbilirubinemia to breast milk. The American Academy of Pediatrics provides recommendations for the evaluation and treatment of neonatal jaundice.[47] The age of the infant is important in assessing the risk of hyperbilirubinemia (Figure 17-7) and the need for evaluation and treatment with either phototherapy (see Figure 17-5) or exchange transfusion (Figure 17-8). If the bilirubin level is rising, published recommendations support encouraging mothers to breast feed more frequently, with an average suggested interval between feeds of 2 hours and no feeding supplements. More frequent nursing may not increase intake, but it has been suggested to increase peristalsis and stool frequency, thus promoting bilirubin excretion. However, one study comparing "frequent" (9 feedings per day) versus "demand" (6.5 feedings per day) feeding schedules during the first 3 days of life showed no significant relation between the frequency of breast feeding and infant serum bilirubin levels in 275 infants.[57] The point at which breast feeding should be discontinued is controversial; recommendations include total bilirubin levels of 14,[58] 15,[59] 16 to 17,[60] and 18 to 20 mg/dL.[61] When breast feeding is interrupted, formula feeding may be initiated for 24 to 48 hours, or breast and formula feeding can be alternated with each feeding. A fall in the serum bilirubin level of 2 to 5 mg/dL[62] is consistent with a diagnosis of breast milk jaundice. Breast feeding may then be resumed; although the serum bilirubin levels may rise for several days, they will gradually level off and decline.[56,59] In one study, interruption of breast feeding for approximately 50 hours (during which time a formula was given) was shown to have the same bilirubin-lowering effect as a similar duration of phototherapy.[63] If formula is substituted for breast milk for several days, it is not clear which formula would be most cost effective in lowering serum bilirubin. However, it has been

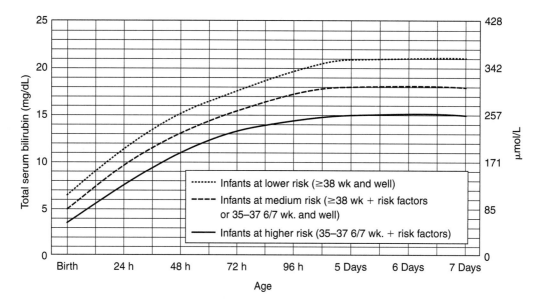

- Use total bilirubin. Do not subtract direct reacting or conjugated bilirubin.
- Risk factors = isommune hemolytic disease. G6PD deficiency, asphyxia, significant lethargy, temperature instability, sepsis, acidosis, or albumin < 3.0 g/dL (if measured)
- For well infants 35–37 6/7 wk can adjust TSB levels for intervention around the medium risk line. It is an option to intervene at lower TSB levels for infants closer to 35 wks and at higher TSB levels for those closer to 37 6/7 wk.
- It is an option to provide conventional phototherapy in hospital or at home at TSB levels 2–3 mg/dL (35–50 μmol/L) below those shown but home phototherapy should not be used in any infant with risk factors.

Figure 17-7. Guidelines for phototherapy in hospitalized infants of 35 or more weeks' gestation. These guidelines are based on limited evidence and the levels shown are approximations. The guidelines refer to the use of intensive phototherapy, which should be used when the total serum bilirubin (TSB) exceeds the line indicated for each category. Infants are designated as "higher risk" because of the potential negative effects of the conditions listed on albumin binding of bilirubin, the blood-brain barrier, and the susceptibility of the brain cells to damage by bilirubin.

shown that neonates fed a casein hydrolysate have less jaundice than neonates fed a routine formula,[64,65] that casein hydrolysate formula inhibits β-glucuronidase,[66] and that the majority of the β-glucuronidase inhibition in hydrolyzed casein is due to L-aspartic acid.[67] A controlled randomized double-blind study showed that feedings of minimal aliquots of L-aspartic acid or enzymatically hydrolyzed casein for β-glucuronidase inhibition resulted in increased fecal bilirubin excretion and less jaundice, without disruption of the breast-feeding experience.[27]

There is much controversy about the potential dangers of hyperbilirubinemia in full-term and near-term newborns who do not have hemolytic disease. Regardless of whether hyperbilirubinemia in these infants causes mild neurodevelopmental or intellectual handicaps, there is no doubt that frank kernicterus in this population is rare. However, it appears that in the United States we are currently experiencing a reemergence of classic kernicterus,[68,69] and warnings from the Centers for Disease Control and Prevention, the American Academy of Pediatrics, and the Joint Commission on Accreditation of Healthcare Organizations indicate that otherwise healthy full-term and near-term infants are at risk. Since 1992 there has been a voluntary kernicterus registry in the United States that, as of April 2004, contained 176 individuals.[70,71] Although G6PD deficiency is present in approximately one third of these individuals with kernicterus, another third had no obvious etiology and appeared to be healthy breast-feeding infants.

Several inborn errors of metabolism can cause neonatal hyperbilirubinemia. Crigler-Najjar syndrome (CN), or congenital nonhemolytic jaundice,[72] is characterized by a hereditary deficiency of hepatic BGT. This syndrome may be divided into CN1 and CN2 (Arias' syndrome) according to the response to phenobarbital – a significant decrease of serum bilirubin in CN2 and no response in CN1. In CN1, serum bilirubin levels typically range from approximately 15 to 45 mg/dL, and there is a risk of both neonatal and later kernicterus. Hyperbilirubinemia is less severe in CN2 patients, varying from approximately 8 to 25 mg/dL. CN2 is associated with a much lower incidence of kernicterus, although such damage has been documented. Bile pigment analysis has been reported to aid in the differentiation of CN1 from CN2 and in the differential diagnosis of unconjugated hyperbilirubinemia. In both forms of CN, traces of monoconjugates can be detected in serum and bile, but no diconjugates are present. Whereas phenobarbital can increase the level of serum monoconjugated bilirubin even in patients with CN1, the diagnosis of CN1 versus CN2 is based on finding a substantial decrease of unconjugated bilirubin in the serum after administration of phenobarbital in CN2. In the first months of life, a phenobarbital trial can still be unsuccessful in the presence of CN2. Therapy for CN1 hyperbilirubinemia can be safe and effective to prevent kernicterus[73] and has included lifelong phototherapy, bilirubin binders (agar, cholestyramine, calcium phosphate) to interrupt the enterohepatic circulation, plasmapheresis for acute episodes of severe hyperbilirubinemia related to intercurrent illness, and, rarely, heme oxygenase inhibition to prevent bilirubin production. In CN1, orthotopic liver transplantation has been performed, even though liver function

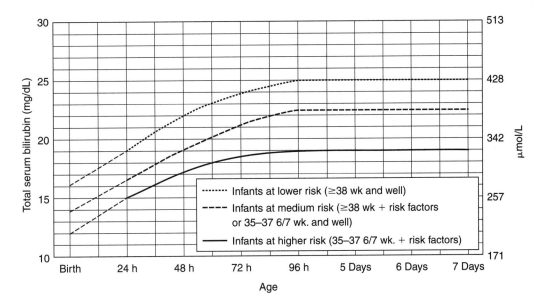

- The dashed lines for the first 24 hours indicate uncertainty due to a wide range of clinical circumstances and a range of responses to phototherapy.
- Immediate exchange transfusion is recommended if infant shows signs of acute bilirubin encephalopathy (hypertonia, arching, retrocolitis, opistholonos, fever, high pitched cry) or if TSB is 2.5 mg/dL (85 μmol/L) above those lines.
- Risk factors - isoimmune hemolytic disease, GEPD deficiency, asphyxia, significant lethargy, temperature instability, sepsis, acidosis.
- Measure serum albumin and calculate B/A ration (see legend).
- Use total bilirubin. Do not subtract direct reacting or conjugated bilirubin.
- If infant is well and 35–37 6/7 wk (median risk) can individualize TSB levels for exchange based on actual gestational age.

Figure 17-8. Guidelines for exchange transfusion in infants 35 or more weeks' gestation. Note that these guidelines represent a consensus of most of the committee but are based on limited evidence, and the levels shown are approximations. During birth hospitalization, exchange transfusion is recommended if the TSB rises to these levels despite intensive phototherapy. For readmitted infants, if the TSB level is above the exchange level, repeat TSB measurement every 2 to 3 hours and consider exchange if the TSB remains above the levels indicated after intensive phototherapy for 6 hours. Used with permission from American Academy of Pediatrics Subcommittee on Hyperbilirubinemia. Management of hyperbilirubinemia in the newborn infant 35 or more weeks of gestation. Pedatrics 2004;114;297–316, fig. 4.

is otherwise normal, because of concern about kernicterus. Gene therapy for CN1 is appealing but remains experimental.[74] Several mutations in the bilirubin UDP-glucuronosyltransferase (UGT 1) gene of CN1 and CN2 patients have been identified which result in complete inactivation of this enzyme in CN1 patients and markedly reduced glucuronidation in CN2 patients. A third type of CN has also been reported; it resembles CN1 in that there is no biliary excretion of bilirubin glucuronide. However, patients with CN3 do excrete monoglucoside and diglucoside conjugates of bilirubin. It has been speculated that CN3 patients lack the long-proposed permease, which has been hypothesized to transport UDP-glucuronic acid to the luminal side of the endoplasmic reticulum, where glucuronosyltransferase is located. This absence forces utilization of a very inefficient substrate for conjugation to bilirubin, UDP-glucose.

Various hormones and drugs may cause development of neonatal unconjugated hyperbilirubinemia. Congenital hypothyroidism can manifest with serum bilirubin higher than 12 mg/dL before the development of other clinical findings. Similarly, hypopituitarism and anencephaly may be associated with jaundice caused by inadequate thyroxine, which is necessary for hepatic clearance of bilirubin.

Infants of diabetic mothers have prolonged and higher serum bilirubin levels than control patients. Explanations include prematurity, polycythemia, substrate deficiency for glucuronidation (secondary to hypoglycemia), and poor hepatic perfusion (secondary to respiratory distress, persistent fetal circulation, or cardiomyopathy).

The Lucey-Driscoll syndrome[75] consists of neonatal hyperbilirubinemia within families in whom there is in vitro inhibition of BGT by both maternal and infant serum. It is presumed that this is caused by gestational hormones.

Drugs may interfere with the metabolism of bilirubin and result in hyperbilirubinemia or displacement of bilirubin from albumin.[76] Such displacement increases the risk of kernicterus and can be caused by sulfonamides, moxalactam, or ceftriaxone (independent of its sludge-producing effect). The popular Chinese herb Chuen-Lin, given to 28 to 51% of Chinese newborn infants, has been shown to have a significant effect in displacing bilirubin from albumin. Pancuronium bromide, chloral hydrate, and ibuprofen have been suggested as causes of neonatal hyperbilirubinemia. Jaundice may result from drug-induced liver disease.

Prematurity is frequently associated with unconjugated hyperbilirubinemia in the neonatal period. Hepatic UDP-glucuronosyltransferase activity is markedly decreased in premature infants and rises steadily from 30 weeks' gestation until reaching adult levels at 14 weeks after birth.[16] In addition there may be deficiencies for both uptake and secretion. Bilirubin clearance improves rapidly after birth. Intralipid has been suggested to decrease bilirubin binding affinity for plasma proteins and increase free bilirubin in infants up to 28 weeks gestational age.[77]

Metabolic diseases including galactosemia, hereditary fructose intolerance, tyrosinemia, α1-antitrypsin deficiency, and others can manifest with jaundice and are described elsewhere in this text.

Hepatic hypoperfusion can result in neonatal jaundice. Inadequate perfusion of the hepatic sinusoids may not allow sufficient hepatocyte uptake and metabolism of bilirubin. Causes include patent ductus venosus (e.g., with respiratory distress syndrome), congestive heart failure, and portal venous thrombosis. Obstruction of the biliary tree can cause neonatal jaundice; its causes, including such entities as biliary atresia, choledochal cyst, cholelithiasis, and cholangitis, are discussed elsewhere in this text. Gallbladder sludge produced by ceftriaxone, total parenteral nutrition, or postsurgical fasting can potentially develop into symptomatic gallstones.

Other cholestatic syndromes can result in jaundice owing to decreased excretion of bilirubin. These syndromes manifest with elevation of the direct (conjugated) bilirubin fraction and are reviewed elsewhere in this text.

Neonatal Jaundice Caused by Both Increased Production and Decreased Excretion of Bilirubin

In neonatal diseases with jaundice caused by decreased excretion and increased production of bilirubin, both conjugated and unconjugated bilirubin fractions can be elevated. Bacterial sepsis increases bilirubin production by producing erythrocyte hemolysis as a result of hemolysins released by bacteria. Endotoxins released by bacteria can also decrease canalicular bile formation.

Intrauterine infection is an important cause of neonatal hepatitis and jaundice and is reviewed elsewhere in this text. Congenital cirrhosis and hepatic fibrosis have also been reported as causes of jaundice in newborn infants. Abnormal erythrocytes may contribute to bilirubin production.

Toxicity of Neonatal Jaundice

Reviews of neonatal bilirubin toxicity[76,78,79] and the mechanisms of bilirubin cytotoxicity[80] have been published elsewhere. Yellow staining of brain nuclei in a severely jaundiced baby was first reported by Hervieux[81] in 1847. The term *kernikterus* (from the German *kern*, "nuclei," and the Greek *ikterus*, "jaundice" or "yellow") was first used by Schmorl[82] in 1903, when he described similar yellow staining of certain brain nuclei in six infants who died with severe neonatal jaundice. It has been suggested that the term *kernicterus* should be reserved for cases exhibiting classic symptoms and findings (Table 17-2), with *bilirubin encephalopathy* used for all the other conditions of brain damage thought to be related to jaundice, though often these terms are used interchangeably. Although kernicterus was originally a pathologic term, it has also been used to describe the acute and chronic clinical conditions shown in Table 17-2. Historically, the most common setting in which kernicterus has occurred is maternal-infant Rh blood group incompatibility. Infants with hemolytic jaundice are more vulnerable to bilirubin toxicity than are newborns with nonhemolytic uncomplicated jaundice.[83,84] However, hemolysis is not necessary for kernicterus. This is strikingly exemplified by CN,[72] a disorder

TABLE 17-2. Clinical Features of Bilirubin Encephalopathy (Kernicterus)

Acute	Chronic
Poor feeding with feeble suck	Motor delay
Lethargy	Choreoathetosis
High-pitched cry	Asymmetric spasticity
Hypertonia/hypotonia	Paresis of upward gaze
Decerebrate/opisthotonic posturing	Dental enamel dysplasia
Seizures	Mental retardation
Sensorineural hearing loss	Cognitive dysfunction
Incomplete Moro reflex	Sensorineural hearing loss
Thermal instability (hypothermia/ hyperthermia)	
Eye findings (setting sun, oculogyric crises)	
Fever	
Death	

From Gourley (1997),[79] with permission.

in which deficient hepatic bilirubin glucuronidation results in decreased bilirubin excretion with severe hyperbilirubinemia and, potentially, kernicterus. Kernicterus also has been identified in otherwise healthy breast-fed, full-term newborn infants with no evidence of hemolysis.[70,85] Though the neonatal period is the most common time for bilirubin-related brain damage, the neurotoxicity of bilirubin has also been documented in adults with CN.[86]

The acute and chronic clinical findings associated with kernicterus (see Table 17-2) are seen in severely jaundiced infants after the first 48 hours of life. Early in the course, the symptoms may be subtle, mimicking those of sepsis, asphyxia, or hypoglycemia. Bilirubin encephalopathy can manifest in a more subtle fashion, with lowered IQ and abnormal cognitive function,[87,88] yet no associated spasticity or athetosis.

Pathologic findings in kernicterus have classically been described as preferential bilirubin (icteric) discoloration of the basal ganglia, with relative sparing of the cerebral cortex and white matter. Brainstem involvement affects mainly cranial nerve nuclei of the tegmentum, particularly the oculomotor and dentate nuclei, and the cerebellar flocculi. Associated destructive lesions in the white matter, such as periventricular infarcts, have also been reported. The staining of specific brain nuclei (kernicterus) must be distinguished from the nonspecific staining that results from damage to the blood-brain barrier and is associated with diffuse staining of the brain. Magnetic resonance imaging demonstrates characteristic findings in the globus pallidus and subthalamic nuclei.[79,89]

The absolute level of serum bilirubin has not been a good predictor of the risk of severe neonatal jaundice. However, it has long been known that kernicterus is likely when serum unconjugated bilirubin levels are higher than 30 mg/dL and unlikely when they are lower than 20 mg/dL.[83,84] In one study, 90% of the patients with bilirubin levels greater than 35 mg/dL either died or had cerebral palsy or physical retardation.[90] On the other hand, no developmental retardation was found in infants with bilirubin levels lower than 20 mg/dL. Albumin concentration is an important variable because of its high affinity for binding with bilirubin. Drugs and organic anions also bind to albumin and can displace bilirubin, thereby increasing the level of free bilirubin, which can diffuse into cells and cause toxicity.[91] The most notable example of this is the kernicterus that occurred with low bilirubin levels when sulfisoxazole was given to premature infants.[92]

Management of Neonatal Jaundice

The management of neonatal jaundice has been reviewed elsewhere, including a practice parameter developed by the American Academy of Pediatrics[47] (see Figures 17-6 to 17-8). In both conjugated and unconjugated hyperbilirubinemia, initial therapy should be directed at the primary cause of the jaundice. In addition, elevation of the unconjugated bilirubin fraction should prompt concern about possible kernicterus independent of the cause of the jaundice. Medication usage must be monitored. Drugs such as ceftriaxone are also strong bilirubin displacers with a potential for inducing bilirubin encephalopathy. Therapeutic options to lower the unconjugated bilirubin concentration include phototherapy, exchange transfusion, enzyme induction, interruption of the enterohepatic circulation, and interruption of breast feeding. In addition, intravenous γ-globulin is recommended to reduce the need for exchange transfusions in Rh and ABO hemolytic disease.

Phototherapy consists of irradiation of the jaundiced infant with light and has been reviewed elsewhere.[93] The photon energy of light changes the structure of the bilirubin molecule in two ways, both of which interrupt the internal hydrogen bonding and make the bilirubin more water-soluble, so that it can be excreted into bile or urine without glucuronidation. One change involves a 180° rotation around the double bonds between either the A and B or the C and D rings, converting the normal Z configuration to the E configuration. $4Z,15E$-Bilirubin is preferentially formed and can spontaneously reisomerize to native bilirubin. More importantly, a new, seven-membered ring structure can be formed between rings A and B, resulting in "lumirubin" or "cyclobilirubin." Lumirubin appears to be the major route to explain the success of phototherapy. Phototherapy devices employing woven fiberoptic pads are now available. In general, phototherapy is used to prevent serum bilirubin concentrations from reaching levels that would necessitate exchange transfusion. Phototherapy is now frequently done at home, as endorsed by the American Academy of Pediatrics. Despite documented complications, phototherapy is widely used and is generally safe. Phototherapy should not be employed without prior diagnostic evaluation of the cause of the jaundice. Optimal positioning and irradiance are important.

Exchange transfusion is the most rapid method to acutely lower the serum bilirubin concentration. Indications for exchange transfusion vary (see Figure 17-8). Although there are many well-described risks with exchange transfusion, mortality should be low (less than 0.6%) if it is performed properly.

There are a number of pharmacologic approaches to the prevention and treatment of neonatal hyperbilirubinemia.[94] The enterohepatic circulation can be interrupted by enteral administration of agents that bind bilirubin in the intestine and prevent reabsorption, such as agar, cholestyramine, and activated charcoal. Increased intestinal peristalsis would be expected to allow less time for bilirubin absorption. Frequent feedings and rectal stimulation are associated with lower serum bilirubin levels. Enteral feedings of bilirubin oxidase, an enzyme that degrades bilirubin, is another approach that remains experimental at present. Another experimental approach utilized intravenous bilirubin oxidase.

Because neonatal hepatic UDP-glucuronosyltransferase activity is low, it is not surprising that induction of hepatic UDP-glucuronosyltransferase results in lower serum bilirubin levels. Such induction in the neonate can be accomplished with prenatal maternal use of phenobarbital or diphenylhydantoin. In the postnatal period, use of phenobarbital by the neonate has the same bilirubin-lowering effect. Clofibrate has been shown to induce BGT and decrease both neonatal total serum bilirubin levels and duration of phototherapy.[95]

An alternative approach to treat neonatal hyperbilirubinemia is to block the first enzyme responsible for the production of bilirubin, heme oxygenase. This can be accomplished by several different metalloporphyrins. Tin-protoporphyrin has been used successfully in the experimental management of jaundice in neonates with ABO incompatibility. In addition to inhibiting bilirubin production, metalloporphyrins are photosensitizers that can accelerate the destruction of bilirubin by light but can cause unwanted side effects. Kappas and colleagues[96] compared tin-mesoporphyrin (SnMP, Stannsoporfin, Stanate, 6 μmol per kilogram of birth weight) versus phototherapy given to paired infants according to strict criteria determined by plasma bilirubin levels and age and concluded that a single dose of SnMP entirely supplanted the need for phototherapy and significantly reduced medical resources used to monitor hyperbilirubinemia. Other clinical trials showed that one dose of SnMP given shortly after birth decreased the development of jaundice in preterm Greek newborns and reduced the need for phototherapy.[97] Despite these results, SnMP is not approved for use and a phase II clinical trial is currently in progress.

Another experimental therapy for neonatal hyperbilirubinemia is hemoperfusion. Research into this method has employed hemoperfusion with ion exchange, bilirubin oxidase, and sorbents.

JAUNDICE IN INFANTS AND OLDER CHILDREN

A brief list of the causes of jaundice in infants and older children is presented in Table 17-3. Several hereditary hyperbilirubinemia syndromes may manifest in infants or older children.[98] These include Gilbert's syndrome, Dubin-Johnson syndrome, and Rotor's syndrome.

Gilbert's syndrome usually is not recognized until after puberty. It is characterized by a hereditary, chronic, mild, unconjugated hyperbilirubinemia with otherwise normal liver function test results. Gilbert's syndrome appears to be a heterogeneous group of disorders that share a decrease in hepatic BGT activity of at least 50%. Based on plasma clearance of other organic anions (bromsulfophthalein and indocyanine green), there appear to be at least four subtypes of Gilbert's syndrome. Mild hemolysis can be seen. Patients with this disorder show a pronounced increase of serum bilirubin concentration in response to fasting. The clinical manifestations of Gilbert's syndrome in whites are commonly associated with a DNA polymorphism involving an extra TA in the TATA promoter region of *UGT1A*, the gene that encodes bilirubin UDP-glucuronosyltransferase, although more rare heterozygous missense mutations in the coding region of *UGT1A* have also been reported.[99] Asians with Gilbert's syndrome rarely demonstrate this TATA polymorphism but instead, most commonly have a Gly71Arg mutation in exon 1 of *UGT1A*.[100] Odell[101] speculated that some infants with neonatal jaundice are manifesting Gilbert's syndrome because of the transient hormonal milieu

TABLE 17-3. Causes of Jaundice in Infants and Older Children

Metabolic disorders
  Hereditary hyperbilirubinemias
    Gilbert's syndrome; Dubin-Johnson syndrome; Rotor's syndrome;
      Crigler-Najjar syndrome
  α1-antitrypsin deficiency
  Cystic fibrosis
  Hemochromatosis
  Wilson's disease
Viral hepatitis
  Hepatitis A, B, C, D, E; Epstein-Barr virus; cytomegalovirus
Autoimmune hepatitis
Biliary tract disease
  Cholecystitis; cholelithiasis; Caroli's disease; choledochal cyst
Tumor
  Hepatic; biliary; pancreatic; peritoneal; duodenal
Red blood cell abnormalities
  Sickle cell disease
  Thalassemia
  Hemolysis
Drugs/toxins
  Acetaminophen; valproate; chlorpromazine; *Amanita* toxin; sepsis;
    others
Sclerosing cholangitis
  Primary; secondary to inflammatory bowel disease
Veno-occlusive disease
  Pyrrolidizine alkaloids; bone marrow transplantation; chemotherapy
Impaired delivery of bilirubin to liver
  Congestive heart failure; cirrhosis

(estrogenization) of the fetus. Data shows that infants homozygous for this DNA polymorphism have a more rapid rise in jaundice during the first 2 days of life.[102] Individuals carrying the TATA polymorphism have increased jaundice if they have hematologic diseases such as G6PD deficiency, β-thalassemia, or hereditary spherocytosis.[103] Although some individuals with Gilbert's syndrome complain of fatigue or abdominal pain, rigorous study suggests that symptoms do not differ significantly from controls,[104] and in general there are no negative implications for health or longevity. Limited data raise concern about metabolism of xenobiotics metabolized by BGT that might be impaired in Gilbert's syndrome.[99]

Dubin-Johnson syndrome[105] and Rotor's syndrome[106] are two distinct but similar hyperbilirubinemia syndromes with autosomal recessive inheritance. In both syndromes the direct and indirect fractions of bilirubin are elevated but the results of other liver function tests, including serum bile acid concentrations, are normal. Rotor's syndrome can be seen in early childhood, whereas Dubin-Johnson syndrome manifests from birth to 40 years of age. In both conditions total serum bilirubin levels usually range from approximately 2 to 7 mg/dL, with at least half present as conjugated bilirubin, but can reach 20 mg/dL under certain conditions (e.g., intercurrent illness).

Dubin-Johnson syndrome is more common than Rotor's syndrome, and the hyperbilirubinemia is often exacerbated by pregnancy and the use of oral contraceptives. Liver histology is completely normal in Rotor's syndrome. In Dubin-Johnson syndrome, liver examination may reveal a distinctive brown-black pigmentation that is visible grossly, with storage located in the lysosomes microscopically. This pigment is believed to originate from melanin or from metabolites of epinephrine. Dubin-Johnson syndrome is more common in males, but there is no male predominance in Rotor's syndrome. Oral

cholecystography is normal in Rotor's syndrome but often fails to visualize the gallbladder in Dubin-Johnson syndrome.

An important pathophysiologic finding in Rotor's syndrome is the marked reduction in hepatic anion storage. This is consistent with the finding of deficient glutathione S-transferase activity in a patient with Rotor's syndrome.[107] Decreased storage allows both direct and indirect bilirubin fractions to reflux back into the circulation, explaining the elevation of both in serum. Hepatic anion storage is normal in Dubin-Johnson syndrome, but there is a marked decrease in secretion by the biliary canaliculus, allowing reflux of conjugated bilirubin back into the circulation. This is due to a defect in the ATP-binding cassette (ABC) transporter located in the apical canalicular membrane. This transporter, originally known as canalicular multispecific organic anion transporter (cMOAT), also called multidrug resistance-associated protein 2 (MRP2), is encoded by the gene *ABCC2*, located on chromosome 10q24. Mutations of this gene can produce a defective, nonfunctional, or absent cMOAT/MRP2 resulting in Dubin-Johnson syndrome.[108]

Also useful in differentiating these two syndromes is the difference in total urinary excretion of coproporphyrins I and III. Urinary coproporphyrin excretion is 2.5 to 5 times higher than normal in Rotor's syndrome but is usually normal or slightly elevated in Dubin-Johnson syndrome. Further, there are significant differences in the distribution of total urinary coproporphyrins I and III, with isomer I less than 80% of the total in Rotor's syndrome[109] and more than 80% of the total in Dubin-Johnson syndrome (normal, 25%).[110]

Patients with Rotor's syndrome are asymptomatic and require no therapy. Although jaundice is lifelong, there is no associated morbidity or mortality. Although Dubin-Johnson syndrome is also associated with normal health and longevity, a significant number of patients have nonspecific abdominal complaints and hepatomegaly. Diagnosis can be made by confirming conjugated hyperbilirubinemia and otherwise normal liver function tests. Coproporphyrin excretion in the urine or hepatic scintigraphy[111] allows differentiation of the two syndromes.

The other causes of jaundice listed in Table 17-3 are described elsewhere in this textbook.

REFERENCES

24. Poland RL, Odell GB. Physiologic jaundice: the enterohepatic circulation of bilirubin. N Engl J Med 1971;284:1–6.
41. Bhutani VK, Johnson L, Sivieri EM. Predictive ability of a predischarge hour-specific serum bilirubin for subsequent significant hyperbilirubinemia in healthy term and near-term newborns. Pediatrics 1999;103:6–14.
47. American Academy of Pediatrics Subcommittee on Hyperbilirubinemia. Management of Hyperbilirubinemia in the Newborn Infant 35 or More Weeks of Gestation. Pediatrics 2004;114:297–316.
70. Johnson LH, Bhutani VK, Brown AK. System-based approach to management of neonatal jaundice and prevention of kernicterus. J Pediatr 2002;140:396–403.
99. Bosma PJ. Inherited disorders of bilirubin metabolism. J Hepatol 2003;38:107–117.
103. Bergeron MJ, Gourley GR. Disorders of bilirubin metabolism. In: Orkin SH, Look AT, Nathan DG, editors. Nathan and Oski's Hematology of Infancy and Childhood. Philadelphia: Saunders Elsevier; 2009 p. 103–145.

See expertconsult.com for a complete list of references and the review questions for this chapter.

ASCITES 18

Michael J. Nowicki • Phyllis R. Bishop

Ascites is defined as the pathologic accumulation of fluid within the peritoneal cavity. The word ascites is derived from the Greek *askites* and *askos*, meaning "bag," "bladder," or "belly." Ascites is found in patients of all age groups and has even been described in utero. The major causes of ascites in the pediatric age group are related to diseases of the liver and kidneys. However, ascites can result from heart disease, malignancy, pancreatitis, disruption of the urinary or biliary tract, and abdominal trauma.

ETIOLOGY

The etiology of ascites differs considerably according to the age of the patient. Similarly, the composition of the ascitic fluid varies dependent on the cause. In addition, there are certain intraabdominal processes that mimic ascites, including omental cysts, intestinal duplications, fluid-filled intestinal loops, and large ovarian cysts.[1-3]

Fetal Ascites

Fetal ascites has been associated with a myriad of conditions and may occur with hydrops, both immune and nonimmune. In the fetus, isolated ascites – fluid accumulation in the peritoneal cavity without fluid accumulation in other body cavities or subcutaneous tissue – is less commonly described (Figure 18-1). The majority of reports are of single cases or small case series. In one large series, isolated ascites accounted for nearly one third of all fetal ascites.[4] Regardless of the underlying associated disease, the pathogenesis of fetal ascites is the same as that for the postterm infant.

Isolated fetal ascites can be due to gastrointestinal abnormalities, genitourinary abnormalities, cardiovascular abnormalities, congenital infections, metabolic disease, and genetic abnormalities. In addition, isolated ascites may be a harbinger of impending hydrops fetalis. The use of high-resolution ultrasonography and a structured investigative protocol has led to a decrease in the proportion of fetal ascites defined as idiopathic to 4%, from rates in previous series of 15 to 45%.[4-8] A list of some causes of fetal ascites is presented in Tables 18-1 and 18-2.

The causes of gastrointestinal abnormalities associated with isolated fetal ascites may be intestinal or hepatic. Intrauterine bowel perforation with subsequent meconium peritonitis is the cause most commonly reported.[4,5] Bowel obstruction without perforation has also been implicated, including obstruction due to intrauterine intussusception, malrotation, and jejunal atresia.[4,5,9,10] Primary intestinal lymphangiectasia and omphalocele have been reported as causes of isolated fetal ascites.[5] Rare hepatic causes include biliary atresia, ductal plate malformation, neonatal iron storage disease, and Niemann-Pick disease type C.[5,11-13]

Genitourinary causes of fetal ascites include hydronephrosis, multicystic kidney, cloacal dysgenesis, hydrometrocolpos, and urinary obstruction with subsequent perforation.[4,5,14,15] Cardiac anomalies that lead to cardiac failure and resultant increased hepatic pressure can cause isolated ascites, including structural abnormalities (tetralogy of Fallot, coarctation of the aorta and atrioventricular [AV] canal) and dysrhythmias.[4,5]

Congenital infections that lead to hydrops have also been reported to cause isolated fetal ascites, probably related to hepatic injury. However, as a group, congenital infection accounts for a small proportion (8 to 11.5%) of fetal ascites.[4,5] The list of infections includes cytomegalovirus, toxoplasmosis, syphilis, enterovirus, varicella, hepatitis A virus, and parvovirus B19. In one series, parvovirus B19 accounted for nearly 50% of all congenital infections causing ascites.[5] It can lead to ascites by causing intestinal perforation or by inducing anemia, and resulting high-output cardiac failure.

The list of metabolic causes of fetal ascites includes Wolman disease, sialic acid storage disease, Niemann-Pick disease type C, Gaucher's disease, infantile galactosialidosis, Sly disease, and infantile GM gangliosidosis.[5,16-18] Chromosomal abnormalities that have been associated with fetal ascites include Turner syndrome, Down syndrome, and trisomy-18. Other causes include pulmonary (laryngeal atresia, cystic adenomatosis malformation), hematologic (anemia), neoplastic, and ovarian causes, as well as fetal abuse.[19-23]

The prognosis of fetal ascites varies widely, reflecting the underlying etiology. Fetuses with isolated ascites have a higher rate of survival (52%) than those with ascites associated with other anomalies (43%) or hydrops (33%).[5] Age at diagnosis of ascites appears to be a reasonable prognostic indicator. In one series, diagnosis of ascites at less than 24 weeks' gestation had a higher fetal loss (79%) than diagnosis at more than 24 weeks' gestation (45%).[5] In another series, diagnosis in the second trimester was associated with a higher mortality rate (63%) than diagnosis in the third trimester (10%), even when elective termination of pregnancy was excluded.[4]

Treatment of fetal ascites has been accomplished with intrauterine paracentesis and abdomino-amniotic shunting. Paracentesis typically leads to short-term improvement in ascites, often requiring repeated procedures. It has been used to improve neonatal pulmonary function[24] and to avoid dystocia if performed just before vaginal delivery.[25] Abdomino-amniotic shunting is not used for isolated uncomplicated fetal ascites alone because of the risk of preterm labor. However, it has been successfully used for ascites associated with polyhydramnios and hydrops.[26,27] The risk of treatment must be balanced against the risk of fetal loss and preterm labor, keeping in mind that fetal ascites may resolve spontaneously.[8,15,28-30]

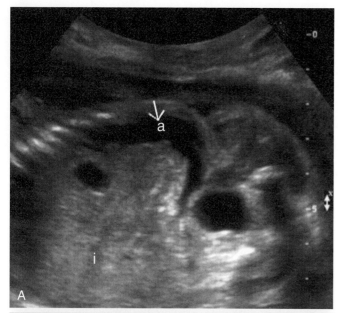

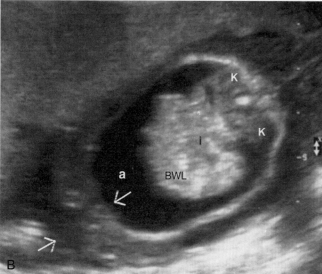

Figure 18-1. Fetal ascites can be seen by ultrasonography as an isolated finding (**A**) or complicating hydrops (**B**). In isolated fetal ascites no other fluid collections or edema is demonstrable; ascites (a) is seen surrounding the intestines (i). When accompanying hydrops, fetal ascites is associated with body wall edema (the area between the arrows). BWL, bowel; K, kidney.

Neonatal Ascites

Ascites in the neonate is caused by many of the same disorders that cause fetal ascites, often simply reflecting persistence of fetal ascites (see Tables 18-1 and 18-2).[13,14,16,31] Similar to fetal ascites, neonatal ascites has been associated with a number of conditions, most reported as single cases. Neonatal liver diseases, such as α1-antitrypsin deficiency, biliary atresia, congenital hepatic fibrosis, and hepatitis, infrequently produce ascites in the first month of life.[32-34] However, severe hepatic injury due to metabolic liver disease is frequently accompanied by ascites. Ascites can be a presenting sign of Budd-Chiari syndrome.[35,36] A well-described cause of neonatal ascites is perforation of the common bile duct. Usually reported as "spontaneous," perforation of the common bile duct can result from abuse (Figure 18-2). Most cases of spontaneous bile duct perforation occur in the

TABLE 18-1. Hepatobiliary Causes of Ascites

Fetal	Neonatal	Infant and Child
Biliary atresia	α1-Antitrypsin	α1-Antitrypsin
Cytomegalovirus	deficiency	deficiency
Niemann-Pick	Budd-Chiari	Budd-Chiari syndrome
disease type C	syndrome	Cirrhosis
Neonatal	Cirrhosis	Congenital hepatic
hemochromatosis	Hepatitis	fibrosis
	Perforated common	Hepatitis
	bile duct	Perforated common
		bile duct

neonatal period, most frequently between the ages of 4 and 12 weeks.[37] Clinically these infants have ascites and hyperbilirubinemia, without significant increase in aminotransferase levels[38]; ultrasonography may demonstrate ascites or fluid around the gallbladder without bile duct dilation, suggesting perforation.[39] Biliary leakage can be demonstrated by hepatobiliary iminodiacetic acid (HIDA) scanning, but definitive diagnosis is made by laparotomy[38] Treatment consists of prompt surgical intervention with intraoperative cholangiography, drainage of the spilled bile, and surgical correction with cholecystostomy or T-tube drainage.[38,40] The typical location for spontaneous bile duct perforation is the junction of the cystic and common bile ducts.[41] Hypotheses for this condition include embryologic weakness of the wall of the bile duct with resulting diverticulum, focal ischemia, and perforation.[42,43]

Uroascites accounts for nearly 30% of all cases of neonatal ascites.[44] Most cases of neonatal uroascites result from obstructive uropathy due to posterior urethral valves[45]; however, ureterocele, lower ureteral stenosis, and ureteral atresia have also been implicated. Rarely, neonatal rupture of the bladder occurs without a demonstrable anatomic urinary obstruction.[46] In the face of obstructive uropathy, rupture of the urinary system and resulting uroascites provides decompression and better renal function.[47] With uroascites, the intraperitoneal urine is "autodialyzed" by the peritoneal membrane, resulting in a characteristic serum biochemical profile including marked hyponatremia, hyperkalemia, and raised serum creatinine levels.[48] The presence of these serum findings and a low protein content of the ascitic fluid strongly support the diagnosis of uroascites.

Iatrogenic causes of ascites have been reported, particularly with placement of umbilical vein catheters. These catheters may erode through the liver or perforate the peritoneum and result in total parenteral nutrition (TPN) ascites or lead to uroascites by eroding through the bladder or causing rupture of a patent urachus.[48-53] Rupture of the urinary bladder following catheterization has also been associated with uroascites.[54] The use of an intravenous vitamin E preparation, E-Ferol, caused outbreaks of liver injury with ascites in premature infants.[55]

Gastrointestinal causes of neonatal ascites include intestinal malrotation with malposition of the portal vein, intestinal perforation, gastroschisis, and acute appendicitis.[56,57] Neonatal ascites has been reported in cases of a ruptured corpus luteum cyst and hydrometrocolpos.[58,59] Neoplastic processes that have presented with neonatal ascites include transient myeloproliferative disorder associated with Down syndrome, ruptured hepatic mesenchymal hamartoma, and myofibromatosis of the ovary.[60-62] Metabolic conditions that have been described in association with neonatal ascites include GM1 gangliosidosis,

TABLE 18-2. **Nonhepatic Causes of Ascites**

Fetal	Neonatal	Infant and Child
Gastrointestinal disorders	Gastrointestinal disorders	Pancreatitis
Meconium peritonitis	Malrotation of the intestines	Chylous ascites
Malrotation of the intestines	Intestinal perforation	Posttraumatic
Intussusception	Jejunal atresia	Nontraumatic
Jejunal atresia	Cystic fibrosis	Urinary tract
Cystic fibrosis	Acute appendicitis	Nephrotic syndrome
Infection	Uroascites	Peritoneal dialysis
Parvovirus	Obstructive uropathy	Heart failure
Syphilis	Bladder rupture	Ventriculoperitoneal shunts
Cytomegalovirus	Renal rupture	Liver transplantation
Toxoplasmosis	Renal extravasation	Neoplasm
Genitourinary tract disorders	Bladder rupture	Serositis
Hydronephrosis	Spontaneous	Henoch-Schönlein purpura
Multicystic kidney	Umbilical artery catheter	Eosinophilic gastroenteritis
Urinary tract obstruction	Urinary catheter	Other
Ovarian cyst	Nephrotic syndrome	Vitamin A intoxication
Chylous ascites	Chylous ascites	Central hyperalimentation
Cardiac disorders	Cardiac disorders	Chronic granulomatous disease
Dysrhythmias	Dysrhythmias	
Heart failure	Heart failure	
Neoplasm	Pancreatitis	
Other	Other	
Inborn error of metabolism	Metabolic storage diseases	
Trisomy	Lysosomal storage disease	
Turner's syndrome	Wolman's disease	
Hemolytic anemia	Central hyperalimentation	
Idiopathic	Intravenous vitamin E	

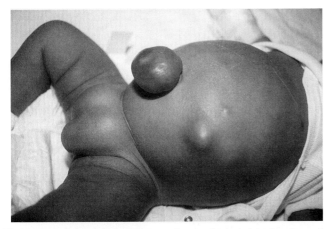

Figure 18-2. Ruptured bile duct secondary to physical abuse in a 4-month-old baby. Tense ascites is seen with resulting marked umbilical hernia and bilateral inguinal hernias. A ventral wall hernia is also present, providing an important clue to abuse.

Salla disease, Gaucher disease, mucopolysaccharidosis type VII, infantile galactosialidosis, and free sialic acid storage disease.[16,17,63-66]

Ascites in Infants and Children

Hepatobiliary

Cirrhosis is the most common cause of hepatic ascites in infants and children; it may be caused by a number of underlying conditions (see Table 18-1). Acute onset of ascites and hepatomegaly may result from obstruction of hepatic vein outflow, the Budd-Chiari syndrome. As in the neonate, spontaneous perforation of the bile duct can lead to bile peritonitis and subsequent ascites.

Pancreatic

Ascites in acute pancreatitis is uncommon in adults and occurs only rarely in children, typically as a result of abdominal trauma or congenital obstruction of the pancreatic duct.[67,68] Amylase concentration may be normal or only slightly raised in the infant with pancreatitis, negating an important serum marker for the diagnosis of acute pancreatitis.[68,69] This may be partially explained by the delay in pancreatic isoamylase production. Negligible at birth, serum amylase reaches adult levels by 2 to 3 years of age.[70] Various mechanisms for ascites in patients with acute pancreatitis have been proposed. One cause is disruption of the pancreatic duct leading to spillage of pancreatic juice into the peritoneum, resulting in chemical peritonitis. There may be a capillary leak syndrome without ductal disruption. Alternatively, there may be the coincidental occurrence of pancreatitis in an individual with another reason for ascites. Finally, the increased amylase concentration may be related to renal failure and decreased renal clearance, not pancreatic injury.[71] Paracentesis is a valuable tool in the diagnosis of pancreatic ascites. Findings supportive of pancreatic ascites include high concentrations of amylase (greater than 1000 IU/L) and protein (3 g/dL) in the ascitic fluid, a high ascites: serum amylase ratio, and a low serum:ascites albumin concentration gradient (below 1.1 g/L).[67,72,73] Ascites appears to be an accurate and independent predictor of severity of pancreatitis and pseudocyst formation.[74] In acute pancreatitis, ascites is predictive of a poor outcome. In one study the mortality rate for individuals with acute pancreatitis and ascites was 40%; the ascites:serum amylase ratio (greater than 1) was 83% sensitive and 92% specific as a predictor of death.[71]

Chylous

Chylous ascites is an uncommon finding in children, arising from obstruction of lymphatic drainage or secondary to trauma. Obstruction may lead to direct leakage of chyle through a

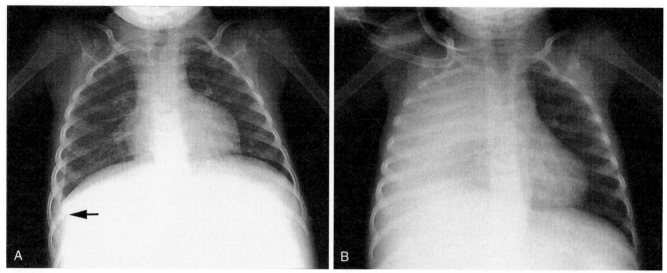

Figure 18-3. (A) A small hydrothorax is seen as a rim of pleural fluid (arrow) on chest radiography in a child with ascites due to α1-antitrypsin deficiency. (B) Massive hydrothorax with complete obscuration of the right lung field developed later in the same child, despite diuretic therapy. Note the paucity of gas in the fluid-filled abdomen on both radiographs.

lymphoperitoneal fistula or by exudation of chyle through lymphatics without evidence of fistula.[75] Trauma results in the disruption of lymphatic vessels; it has been estimated that 10% of all chylous ascites is related to child abuse.[76] Overall, chylous ascites occurs with equal frequency in adults and children; in one large series of individuals with chylous ascites, 51% were less than 15 years old.[75] Characteristics of chylous ascites include a "milky" appearance, a specific gravity greater than 1.012, an alkaline pH, a negative culture, and the presence of fat globules.[77]

Miscellaneous

Ascites can develop as a result of right heart failure and constrictive pericarditis. Ventriculoperitoneal shunts can cause ascites as a result of subclinical bacterial peritonitis,[78] immune reaction,[78] high protein content,[79] and seeding of the peritoneum by tumor.[80] Intra-abdominal neoplasms associated with ascites include Wilms' tumor, renal clear cell sarcoma, germ cell tumors, malignant peritoneal mesothelioma, and peritoneal seeding of neuroblastoma.[81-83] Other miscellaneous causes of ascites in children include chronic eosinophilic ascites,[84] hemorrhagic ascites due to Henoch-Schönlein purpura,[85] and vitamin A intoxication.[86]

Complications of Ascites and Conditions That Mimic Ascites

Hydrothorax

An uncommon, although significant, complication of cirrhotic ascites is hepatic hydrothorax, defined as the presence of a significant pleural effusion in the absence of a primary cardiac or pulmonary cause.[87,88] The overall incidence of hepatic hydrothorax in cirrhosis has been estimated to be 5%.[89] The effusion most commonly occurs on the right (85.4%), being found less commonly on the left (12.5%) or bilaterally (2%).[89] Clinical presentation varies widely, ranging from an asymptomatic finding to severe respiratory embarrassment (Figure 18-3). The mechanism of hepatic hydrothorax remains unclear; the most accepted hypothesis is the transdiaphragmatic flow of ascites

into the pleural space.[89] A negative intrathoracic pressure exacerbates the flow into the pleural space, possibly explaining why hepatic hydrothorax is sometimes seen without obvious abdominal ascites.[90] The fluid composition is similar to that found in cirrhotic ascites.[89] As hepatic hydrothorax is simply ascites that has entered the chest, treatment is the same as for ascites. Initially sodium and fluid restriction in combination with diuretics should be used. Therapeutic thoracentesis can provide symptomatic relief but often needs to be repeated frequently. Attempts at controlling recurrence with pleurodesis, peritoneovenous shunt, chest tube insertion, and repair of the diaphragm have met with limited success. Decreasing portal pressure has been successful in controlling the production of ascites, and thus the development of hydrothorax. Transjugular intrahepatic portosystemic shunting has given good results.[91] Octreotide has also been used successfully to treat hydrothorax; the mechanism of action is presumed to be an increase in renal blood flow, glomerular filtration rate, and urinary sodium secretion.[92] Liver transplantation is the definitive treatment.[93]

Pancreatic Pleural Effusion

Acute pancreatitis is complicated by pleural effusion as commonly as ascites. In a prospective study, pleural effusion was found in 20% of adults with pancreatitis, and ascites was found in 18%. In this study pleural effusion was symptomatic in 15% and ascites was symptomatic in only 6% of patients.[74] Pleural effusion is a sensitive predictor of the severity of acute pancreatitis, being found in 24 to 84% of severe cases and 4 to 9% of mild cases. Pleural effusion is also a predictor for the development of a pancreatic pseudocyst. Pleural effusion may arise due to intra-abdominal pancreatic pseudocyst, intrathoracic pancreatic pseudocyst, and pancreaticopleural fistula. A high percentage of pancreatitis-induced pleural effusions are not associated with pseudocyst or fistulas, but rather arise from the transdiaphragmatic lymphatic channels. Pancreatic lymphatics are juxtaposed to the left hemidiaphragm, explaining in part the predilection for left-sided pleural effusion (54 to 60%) with pancreatitis. Thoracentesis may be helpful when the diagnosis of pleural effusion is in question; the finding of a high amylase level supports a pancreatic origin. Treatment is typically not required, because most pleural effusions due to acute pancreatitis resolve spontaneously.

PATHOPHYSIOLOGY

Anatomy and Physiology

Ascites arises when the hydrostatic and osmotic pressures within the hepatic and mesenteric capillaries result in a net transfer of fluid from blood vessels to lymphatics at a rate that overcomes the drainage capacity of the lymphatics. The liver is supplied by the portal vein and hepatic artery, which perfuse the hepatic sinusoids; the whole of the hepatic blood flow exits via the hepatic veins, entering the inferior vena cava (Figure 18-4). In the liver, precapillary resistance is greater than postcapillary resistance, resulting in a low sinusoidal pressure (2 mm Hg). Under normal conditions, lymph produced at the sinusoidal level enters the space of Disse, eventually exiting the liver via the transdiaphragmatic lymphatic vessels and entering the thoracic duct, which empties into the left subclavian vein. The sinusoidal membrane is highly permeable to albumin; thus the protein concentrations of hepatic lymph and plasma are nearly the same, limiting any significant osmotic gradient.

Blood from the intestinal mesenteric capillaries drains into the portal vein via the mesenteric veins (see Figure 18-4).

The mean mesenteric capillary pressure is around 20 mm Hg. The mesenteric capillary membrane is relatively impermeable to albumin such that the protein concentration of mesenteric lymph is one-fifth that of plasma. This resulting osmotic gradient favors the return of interstitial fluid into the capillary. The lymph that is produced drains from regional lymphatics into the thoracic duct; the rate is 800 to 1000 mL per day in the adult.[94]

Cirrhotic Ascites

The development of cirrhotic ascites is preceded by portal hypertension. The scarring that defines cirrhosis leads to an increased sinusoid pressure, resulting in an increase in the hydrostatic pressure gradient across the sinusoidal membrane, which in turn results in increased lymph formation. Once the hepatic lymph production exceeds the drainage, lymph seeps through the hepatic capsule, entering the peritoneal cavity. In severe cirrhosis, changes may occur in the sinusoidal membrane, including the formation of a basement membrane, defenestration, and collagen deposition in the space of Disse (see Figure 18-4). This results in decreased permeability of the sinusoidal membrane to protein and thus a decrease in lymph protein content and a decrease in the osmotic gradient. The permeability to protein of the hepatic capsule also decreases, which further inhibits ascites formation.[94,95]

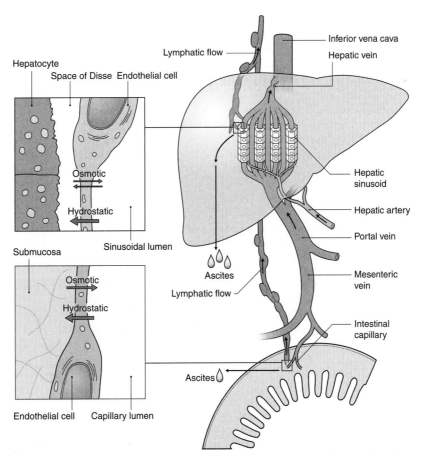

Figure 18-4. Hepatic lymph is formed by filtration of sinusoidal plasma into the space of Disse; it drains from the liver via the transdiaphragmatic lymphatic vessels to the thoracic duct. The sinusoidal endothelium is highly permeable to albumin; there is normally no significant osmotic gradient across the sinusoidal membrane. Intestinal lymph drains from regional lymphatics into the thoracic duct. The mesenteric capillary membrane is relatively impermeable to albumin; there is a significant osmotic gradient that promotes the return of interstitial fluid into the capillary lumen. Ascites occurs when the net transfer of fluid from blood vessels to lymphatic vessels exceeds the drainage capacity of the lymphatics; fluid leaks through the hepatic capsule and, to a lesser extent, the intestine. IVC, inferior vena cava; a., artery, v., vein. Adapted from Dudley (1992), with permission.[94]

Sinusoidal and portal hypertension lead to responsive changes in the mesenteric capillaries to decrease mesenteric lymph production. Arteriolar contraction leads to increased precapillary resistance and resulting decreased hydrostatic pressure in the capillaries. The surface area for transudation is decreased. Capillary membrane permeability is reduced, slowing the movement of protein and fluid in the vessel. The interstitial hydrostatic pressure increases as fluid accumulates, opposing further fluid loss.[94]

Pathogenesis of Cirrhotic Ascites

Cirrhotic ascites is characterized not only by portal hypertension, but also by retention of sodium and water. Three major hypotheses have been proposed to explain the sequence of events that result in the development of ascites, as well as the sodium and water retention. The first hypothesis (underfill) suggests that ascites, due to portal hypertension, results in a contracted blood volume, decreased renal perfusion, and secondary renal retention of sodium and water. If this were true, affected patients would have intravascular hypovolemia and low cardiac output. Yet, cirrhotic ascites is typically characterized by an expanded blood volume and high cardiac output. An alternative hypothesis (overfill) is that sodium and water retention occurs, leading to increased blood volume. The increased blood volume in combination with portal hypertension results in ascites.

More recent data have led to a third hypothesis in which the primary mechanism is peripheral vasodilation.[96] Cirrhosis leads to increased resistance to portal flow and the development of portal hypertension, collateral vein formation, and shunting of blood to the systemic circulation. Hepatic endothelin-1, a potent vasoconstrictor, modulates intrahepatic resistance in portal hypertension due to cirrhosis.[97] With the development of portal hypertension, there is increased local production of vasodilators, mainly nitric oxide, leading to splanchnic arterial vasodilation.[98] Early in cirrhosis there is moderate splanchnic arterial vasodilation that has a limited effect on the effective arterial blood volume, which is maintained within the normal range by increases in plasma volume and cardiac output. With advanced cirrhosis, splanchnic vasodilation is so pronounced that the arterial pressure falls owing to a marked decrease in effective arterial blood volume. As a result, there is homeostatic activation of vasoconstrictor and antinatriuretic factors, resulting in retention of sodium and water so that arterial pressure is maintained. Ascites results from the combination of portal hypertension and splanchnic arterial vasodilation.[99]

In decompensated cirrhosis, a hyperdynamic circulatory state exists, with an expanded blood volume, increased cardiac output, tachycardia, wide pulse pressure, and peripheral dilation. Hypoalbuminemia decreases the osmotic gradient and worsens lymph formation, drawing interstitial fluid into the vascular space. Peripheral edema occurs when increased abdominal pressure from ascites increases inferior vena cava pressure, producing an increase in hydrostatic pressure in the capillaries of the lower extremities.

Noncirrhotic Ascites

Evidence suggests that ascites caused by heart failure or nephrotic syndrome results from decreased effective arterial blood volume with secondary activation of the central nervous sympathetic adrenergic system, the renin-angiotensin-aldosterone system and vasopressin, leading to renal sodium and water retention.[100] In heart failure, hepatic congestion increases portal venous pressure. In nephrotic syndrome, hypoalbuminemia increases the movement of plasma into the interstitium. In chylous ascites, there is direct leakage of chyle into the peritoneal cavity. Pancreatic and bile-induced ascites result from a chemical peritonitis.

DIAGNOSIS

History and Physical Examination

Patients who develop ascites often have a history of increased abdominal girth and recent weight gain. In cirrhotic ascites, there may be a history of chronic liver disease or hepatitis. In noncirrhotic ascites, there may be a history of cardiac anomalies and heart failure, abdominal trauma, ventriculoperitoneal (VP) shunt, or renal disease. Significant ascites may present as a protuberant abdomen, bulging flanks, or dullness to percussion in the flanks. The etiology of ascites can be ascertained by historic clues. Physical findings of chronic liver disease include the presence of jaundice, palmar erythema, xanthomas, spider angiomas, caput medusa, and muscle wasting.

The two most helpful techniques for determining ascites by physical examination are shifting dullness and a fluid wave. Shifting dullness has a sensitivity of 60 to 88% and a specificity of 56 to 90%.[101] The minimum volume needed to detect shifting dullness is about 1.5 to 3.0 L.[102] The test for a fluid wave has a sensitivity of 50 to 80% and a specificity of 82 to 92%.[101]

Body-Imaging Studies

Plain abdominal radiography is not used routinely to determine the presence of ascites, although it may detect ascites indirectly; findings include changes in the hepatic angle or the presence of a flank stripe sign. The most sensitive technique for the detection of ascites is ultrasonography, which can detect as little as 100 mL of free abdominal fluid in the adult. In patients with minimal ascites, fluid collects in the most dependent spaces, the hepatorenal recess (Morison's pouch) and the pelvic cul-de-sac, allowing the detection of less than 10 mL of fluid (Figure 18-5).[101] In infants, ultrasonography can detect as little as 10 to 20 mL of fluid in the perivesical area.[103] In addition to the presence

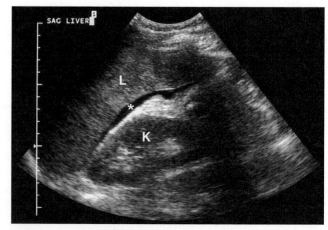

Figure 18-5. Ascites is seen in Morison's pouch (*) between the liver (L) and kidney (K) of a 6-year-old child with cirrhosis.

of ascitic fluid, ultrasonography can also show other findings that may assist in determining the underlying etiology, such as particulate material in patients with necrotizing enterocolitis or bowel wall edema in lymphangiectasia. Ascites can also be detected by computed tomography (CT) or magnetic resonance imaging (MRI). Of interest, chylous ascites can sometimes be differentiated from other types by the unique finding of a biphasic fat-fluid level by ultrasonography or CT.[104]

Diagnostic Abdominal Paracentesis

Paracentesis is a useful tool in determining the cause of new-onset ascites. In addition, in long-standing ascites, paracentesis is recommended to detect bacterial peritonitis when there is clinical deterioration, particularly abdominal pain or fever. Analysis of ascitic fluid should address the likely potential causes, based on history. The presence of raised amylase levels in ascitic fluid indicates pancreatitis or intestinal perforation; the additional finding of polymicrobial infection indicates intestinal perforation. Urea and creatinine concentrations that are higher in ascitic fluid than those in serum indicate uroascites. Raised bilirubin levels in ascitic fluid suggest disruption of the biliary tree or intestinal perforation. Triglyceride concentration that is higher in ascitic fluid than in serum indicates chylous ascites.

A useful measurement is the serum:ascites albumin concentration gradient, which in simplest terms is the difference in albumin concentration between serum and ascitic fluid. Ascites can be divided into two categories, high gradient (above 1.1 g/dL) and low gradient (below 1.1 g/dL). High-gradient ascites is present when there is portal hypertension, in conditions such as cirrhosis, alcoholic cirrhosis, heart failure, massive liver metastases, fulminant hepatic failure, Budd-Chiari syndrome, portal vein thrombosis, veno-occlusive disease, and myxedema. Low-gradient ascites occurs in the absence of portal hypertension in conditions such as pancreatic ascites, biliary ascites, nephrotic syndrome, connective tissue–induced serositis, tuberculous ascites, and peritoneal carcinomatosis.[105,106] The serum:ascites albumin concentration gradient is superior to measurement of ascitic total protein concentration in determining the cause of ascites. In a head-to-head comparison, the serum:ascites albumin gradient was able to differentiate the cause of ascites resulting from portal hypertension 97% of the time, compared with 56% for total protein concentration.[107]

Fluid obtained at paracentesis should at a minimum be sent for cell count and differential, Gram stain and culture, and albumin concentration (serum albumin should also be obtained). These studies will determine whether peritonitis or portal hypertension is the cause of the ascites. Other studies on the ascitic fluid should be directed by historic and clinical features in an attempt to confirm clinical suspicion as to the cause of ascites.

Complications from paracentesis are uncommon, although bleeding is seen occasionally. With the exception of frank disseminated intravascular coagulopathy, paracentesis can be performed despite a prolonged prothrombin time.

TREATMENT

Most, but not all, patients with ascites require treatment. Small quantities of ascites that do not produce symptoms or have no clinical sequelae may require little or no therapy. Tense ascites

TABLE 18-3. Goal of Diuretic Therapy

Pretreatment Weight (kg)	Desired Daily Weight Loss (g)*
5-10	25-100
11-20	50-200
21-30	100-300
31-40	150-400
41-50	200-500
>50	250-500

*0.5-1.0% of body weight per day.

typically requires prompt treatment because of symptoms such as severe abdominal pain and respiratory embarrassment. The etiology of ascites should also be considered when a treatment plan is being developed. For example, in the majority of patients, pancreatic ascites is self-limiting and needs no specific therapeutic intervention, whereas cirrhotic ascites requires treatment in the majority of cases. The treatment options for cirrhotic ascites are outlined next.

Sodium and Fluid Restriction

Because of the significant role of sodium homeostasis in the development of ascites, a major goal of treatment is to limit sodium intake. Restriction of sodium to 2 mEq per kg bodyweight is usually suggested, although a "no added sodium" diet has also been used. Sodium restriction is sufficient as a lone therapy in a minority of patients; most require a combination of sodium restriction and diuretic therapy. Water restriction is typically initiated when the serum sodium level decreases to 125 or 130 mEq/L or less.

Diuretics

The goal of diuretic therapy is to reduce body weight by about 0.5 to 1% (up to 300 to 500 g) each day until ascites is resolved and then to prevent reaccumulation (Table 18-3). The cornerstone of treatment for cirrhotic ascites is diuretic therapy, in particular agents that combat the hyperaldosteronism characteristic of this form of ascites. Spironolactone has proved to be the most effective diuretic because of its ability to block the binding of aldosterone to specific receptors in the cortical and medullary collecting tubules (Figure 18-6). Because of its action distally spironolactone inhibits the resorption of only 2% of filtered sodium. In patients with ascites, the bioactive metabolites of spironolactone have prolonged half-lives, ranging from 24 to 58 hours; as a result, more than 5 days is required to achieve steady state. Administration of medication more than once daily is unnecessary; adjustment of dose should take into account the prolonged half-life.

In nonazotemic cirrhotic patients with avid sodium retention, head-to-head comparison showed a superior response in those treated with spironolactone (95%) compared with patients receiving furosemide (52%). Patients who did not respond to furosemide had higher plasma levels of renin and aldosterone; when subsequently treated with spironolactone, 90% of these patients responded.[108] Failure of patients with cirrhotic ascites to respond to spironolactone can be tied to enhanced sodium resorption in the proximal tubule and resulting decreased fractional sodium delivery to the distal renal tubule.

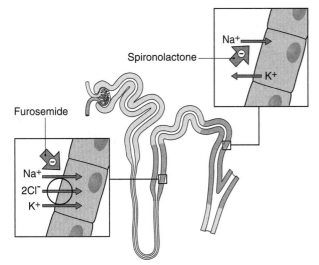

Figure 18-6. Metabolites of spironolactone act on the cortical and medullary collecting tubule by inhibiting the binding of aldosterone to a specific receptor protein there, resulting in impairment of sodium absorption and potassium excretion. Furosemide acts on the renal epithelial cells of the thick ascending loop of Henle by inhibiting the sodium chloride–potassium carrier co-transport system.

Furosemide is the other commonly used diuretic for cirrhotic ascites. It exerts its effect on the thick ascending limb of the loop of Henle (see Figure 18-6), increasing the fractional excretion of sodium by as much as 30% of filtered sodium. Furosemide has no effect on the distal and collecting tubules. In contrast to spironolactone, furosemide is absorbed rapidly and has a fast onset of activity; peak activity is seen at 1 to 2 hours and duration of activity is 3 to 4 hours.[109]

Diuretic therapy should be guided by the severity of the ascites. In less severe ascites a stepwise approach can be used, whereas in severe ascites combination therapy should be started from the beginning. When a stepwise approach is used, spironolactone is started as a single morning dose of 2 to 3 mg per kg bodyweight (up to 100 mg; Table 18-4). In the absence of response, the dose is increased by 2 mg/kg (up to 100 mg) every 5 to 7 days up to a maximum of 4 to 6 mg/kg/day (up to 200 to 400 mg). If there is still not an adequate response, furosemide is added, the initial dose being 1 mg/kg (up to 40 mg). The dose of furosemide can be increased every 5 to 7 days by 1 mg/kg (up to 40 mg) until a response is seen or a maximum dose of 4 mg/kg (up to 160 mg) is reached. In severe ascites, combination therapy with both spironolactone and furosemide can be initiated. The starting dose is similar to that for the medications when used sequentially; spironolactone at 2 mg/kg (up to 100 mg) and furosemide at 1 mg/kg (up to 40 mg) each morning.

The doses are increased every 5 to 7 days by 2 mg/kg (up to 100 mg) for spironolactone and 1 mg/kg (up to 40 mg) for furosemide until a response is seen or maximum doses are reached.

Diuretic therapy is not without complications. Treatment with spironolactone can lead to hyperkalemic acidosis, and furosemide therapy can lead to hypokalemic alkalosis. When used in combination, disturbances of potassium and pH occur less commonly. Overaggressive diuretic therapy, particularly intravascular furosemide, can lead to intravascular volume depletion and resulting renal failure. Other complications include hyponatremia, hepatic encephalopathy, antiandrogenic effects, and muscle cramps.

TABLE 18-4. Diuretic Treatment

	Spironolactone	Furosemide
Starting dose	2-3 mg/kg, up to 100 mg	1 mg/kg, up to 40 mg
Incremental dose	2 mg/kg, up to 100 mg	1 mg/kg, up to 40 mg
Maximum dose	4-6 mg/kg, up to 400 mg	2-4 mg/kg, up to 160 mg

Therapeutic Paracentesis

Paracentesis is used to treat ascites that has not responded to medical therapy, to give rapid relief from large-volume ascites and periodically to treat refractory ascites. Therapeutic paracentesis of medically resistant tense ascites is safe, rapid, and effective. Paracentesis is superior to diuretics in eliminating ascites, shortening the duration of hospitalization, and reducing the complication rate.[110] Total large-volume paracentesis is as safe as repeated partial paracentesis. Removal of large volumes of ascitic fluid is accompanied by increased cardiac output and decreased systemic vascular resistance, leading to a decrease in blood pressure. Resulting effective hypovolemia potentiates the neurohumoral and renal abnormalities as evidenced by increased serum norepinephrine, plasma renin activity and aldosterone levels, elevation of serum creatinine and blood urea nitrogen levels, and a reduction in serum sodium concentration. These physiologic changes, although not clinically apparent, can be prevented by the administration of albumin as a volume expander at the time of paracentesis. In the only reported experience of large-volume paracentesis in children, albumin was administered to provide hemodynamic stability and as a replacement for removed ascitic albumin. Albumin infusion was begun at the beginning of paracentesis; 0.5 to 1.0 g 5% albumin per kg dry bodyweight was infused over 1 to 2 hours. In this report all procedures were well tolerated, with only a single episode of decreased urine output that responded to volume expansion; no bleeding or infectious complications were seen.[111]

The use of albumin in conjunction with large-volume paracentesis has potential drawbacks including down-regulation of the albumin synthesis gene, cost, and risk of infection.[110] Synthetic plasma expanders, such as dextran and polygeline, are as effective as albumin in preventing clinical complications of paracentesis (i.e., hyponatremia and renal impairment). However, albumin is more effective than synthetic plasma expanders in preventing postparacentesis hypovolemia, defined by an increase in plasma renin activity or aldosterone concentration.[112] Patients receiving albumin after total paracentesis have a longer time before rehospitalization and a longer survival time than those receiving synthetic plasma expanders.[112] Albumin infusion, in conjunction with adequate oral protein intake, may counter the depletion of protein associated with repeated large-volume paracenteses.

An alternative to volume expansion for prevention of circulatory dysfunction following large-volume therapeutic paracentesis is the use of vasoconstrictors. In head-to-head comparisons, both noradrenaline and terlipressin (a vasopressin analog) were as effective as albumin infusion in ameliorating circulatory dysfunction following therapeutic paracentesis in cirrhotic patients.[113,114]

Even though total paracentesis is superior to diuretics in eliminating ascites, it does not negate the need for diuretics.

Recurrence of ascites after paracentesis is much higher (93%) in patients receiving placebo than in those receiving diuretics (18%).[115]

A major drawback of paracentesis is early recurrence of ascites, because paracentesis does not address the mechanisms resulting in formation of ascites.[99]

Transjugular Intrahepatic Portosystemic Stent Shunting

Transjugular intrahepatic portosystemic stent (TIPS) shunting was developed in order to provide a means to lower portal pressure, without the need for invasive vascular surgery. A TIPS provides a direct, intrahepatic connection between the portal and systemic circulations, resulting in a decrease in sinusoidal pressure and hepatic lymph production. As such, TIPS placement has been shown to prevent rebleeding from varices and to alleviate cirrhotic ascites. In adults, a TIPS is indicated when there is a need for large-volume paracentesis more than three times per month.[110] There are no such guidelines for children; however, for the child with cirrhosis and refractory ascites, a TIPS can be useful as a treatment bridge to transplantation. A TIPS can reverse some of the renal abnormalities arising from cirrhosis, leading to increased urinary sodium excretion and free water clearance, and an improved glomerular filtration rate. The renal response to diuretics also improves. Compared with adults, a TIPS procedure can be technically more difficult in children, in part because of the small vessel size. Another major contributing factor may be the underlying cause; biliary atresia is a major cause of cirrhosis in children. The periportal fibrosis characteristic of biliary atresia has been associated with a reduced size of the portal veins and a higher resistance during portal vein puncture.[116] In biliary atresia, the hepatic veins tend to be on the periphery and follow a tortuous course. Although technically difficult, a 94% "technical success" rate has been reported.[116] Complications associated with the TIPS procedure include bleeding (due to puncture of the hepatic capsule, inferior vena cava, and portal veins), perforation of a local organ (kidney, gallbladder, or colon) and problems with the contrast material (allergic reactions and renal failure). The most common postprocedure complication is restenosis or reocclusion of the stent. Early (less than 30 days) restenosis is reported in nearly 25% of children having a TIPS placed. Shunt obstruction can arise from intimal hyperplasia or by stent migration due to growth. It has been suggested that periodic sonography be performed every 3 to 6 months to follow stent patency.[117] Hepatic encephalopathy can follow TIPS placement, although it is less common in children than in adults. Worsening liver failure due to inadequate hepatic perfusion is reported even less frequently. In reported children with TIPS placement, nearly 60% have had liver transplantation; no failed attempts at transplantation following a TIPS have been reported.[116,117]

Other Treatments

Peritoneovenous shunts were developed to shunt ascitic fluid back into the central circulation. Although superior to diuretics in relieving ascites, peritoneovenous shunts are fraught with complications, including shunt obstruction, coagulopathy, superior vena caval thrombosis and obstruction, pulmonary embolization, and sepsis. These shunts have been all but abandoned, being replaced by large-volume paracentesis[118];

peritoneovenous shunting may be useful in patients who are not candidates for liver transplantation, TIPS placement, or repeated large-volume paracentesis.[110] Attempts at ultrafiltration of ascitic fluid and reinfusion into the blood have not been successful in supplanting other treatments. Liver transplantation may be the only effective treatment for some patients.

SPONTANEOUS BACTERIAL PERITONITIS

Spontaneous bacterial peritonitis (SBP) is defined as an infection of ascitic fluid without evidence of an intra-abdominal source. Secondary bacterial peritonitis is defined as an intraabdominal infection caused by a problem that requires surgical treatment.

The true incidence of SBP in children is unknown, but is thought to be similar to that in adults. In adult patients with cirrhosis and ascites, the incidence of SBP per hospital admission is 8 to 27%. About half of the infections are community acquired and the other half nosocomial. The incidence of SBP in patients with fulminant hepatic failure and ascites is significantly higher (40%). Presenting signs and symptoms of SBP may be subtle and variable; in some cases the patient is asymptomatic. Findings in SBP include abdominal pain, abdominal distention, fever, vomiting, worsening liver disease, worsening encephalopathy, or renal failure. Diffuse abdominal pain is the rule, with rebound tenderness present less often.

The pathogenesis of SBP is not definitely known but is most likely multifactorial. The typical patient has cirrhosis and ascites, although ascites alone for any reason predisposes to SBP. SBP has been reported with nephrotic syndrome, fulminant hepatic failure, and cardiac ascites. Translocation of bacteria from the intestine to peritoneal fluid via peritoneal lymph nodes is thought to be the most common source of the infection. Other implicated sites are the pulmonary tract, urinary tract, and skin. Factors contributing to successful infection of the peritoneal fluid are depressed reticuloendothelial phagocytic activity and decreased antibacterial opsonization. Low complement levels and low protein levels in ascitic fluid further increase the risk of SBP. Patients with ascites fluid protein concentration of less than 1 g/dL are 10 times more likely to develop SBP than those with protein levels greater than 1 g/dL. Cirrhotics with SBP are more likely to have defective opsonization (100%) than cirrhotics without SBP (14%). Similarly, cirrhotics with SBP are more likely to have decreased complement levels (89 to 100%) than those without SBP (14 to 59%).

The most common cause of SBP in adult patients is gram-negative aerobic organisms; *Escherichia coli* and *Klebsiella pneumoniae* are most often isolated. In children, the causative organisms differ somewhat different, with *Streptococcus pneumoniae* being most commonly cultured; other common organisms include *E. coli*, *K. pneumoniae* and *Staphylococcus aureus*. *Neisseria meningitidis* (serogroup Z) has also been reported as the etiology of SBP in children.

Diagnosis of SBP is made with a high degree of clinical suspicion and analysis of ascitic fluid. A polymorphonuclear leukocyte (PMN) count of 250 cells/mL is the threshold considered diagnostic of ascitic fluid infection. Lactate levels, pH, and total protein levels are less reliable in determining whether or not infection exists. Gram stain is usually negative because of the low concentration of organisms, but may be helpful in discriminating between SBP and secondary peritonitis. Bedside inoculation of blood culture bottles with ascitic fluid is superior to delayed inoculation in the lab. Culture of 2 to 10 mL ascitic fluid detects 80 to 93% of organisms. Based on cell count and culture results, SBP is classified as: (1) culture-positive neutrocytic (PMN count 250 cells/mL with positive culture); (2) culture-negative neutrocytic (PMN 250 cells/mL with negative culture); or (3) monomicrobial nonneutrocytic bacterascites (PMN count < 250 cells/mL and positive culture for a single organism). Some data suggest that culture-negative neutrocytic ascites could resolve spontaneously and may be less severe than culture-positive neutrocytic SBP. Other studies have found similar short-term outcomes in culture-negative compared with culture-positive cases, including a mortality rate of 16 to 50%. Therefore, culture-negative neutrocytic ascites must be considered a true infection and treated aggressively. Monomicrobial nonneutrocytic bacterascites resolves spontaneously in 62 to 86% of cases. Patients with symptoms at the time of paracentesis are more likely to go on to develop SBP and should receive antibiotic treatment. Empiric antibiotic therapy should be instituted if the ascitic fluid PMN count is 250 cells/mL; a complete antibiotic course should be completed even if culture results are negative.

In adults, third-generation cephalosporins are the recommended first-line therapy for SBP, having been found to be superior to ampicillin-tobramycin combination. Cefotaxime (2 g every 8 to 12 hours) and ceftriaxone (2 g daily) yielded a cure rate of 80 to 90% and 95 to 100% respectively. In a randomized trial of 100 adults with SBP, a 5-day course of cefotaxime (2 g every 8 hours) was as effective as a 10-day course. In a multicenter randomized study of cirrhotic adults with SBP, oral ofloxacin (400 mg every 12 hours) resulted in the same 84% cure rate as intravenous cefotaxime. However, more recent data suggest that empiric use of cefotaxime for SBP may need to be reevaluated.[119,120] Failure rates for cefotaxime range from 29% to 44%, particularly among patients with nosocomial infections. In these studies, failure was attributed to organisms that were either resistant or with inherent insufficient susceptibility to cefotaxime.[119,120]

When clinical response is good, repeat paracentesis is not necessary. If response is suboptimal or secondary peritonitis is suspected, follow-up paracentesis is recommended 48 hours after the first.

Attempts at prophylaxis against spontaneous bacterial peritonitis have focused on avoiding exposure to pathogens by selective bowel decontamination. Short-term selective bowel decontamination with oral antibiotics has been effective in adults. Norfloxin (400 mg daily) has been shown to lower the incidence of SBP in cirrhotic patients with ascites and gastrointestinal bleeding from 37% to 10%. Daily norfloxin has also been shown to decrease the recurrence rate of SBP from 35% to 12%. Ciprofloxacin (750 mg once weekly) has been shown to decrease the incidence of SBP from 22% to 3.6%. Trimethoprim-sulfamethoxazole has also been effective in decreasing the incidence of SBP and bacteremia from 27% to 3%. Side effects of antibiotic therapy include candidal esophagitis and selection of resistant organisms. For these reasons, long-term prophylaxis with antibiotics is debatable. Diuretics, a mainstay of ascites treatment, have been shown to increase opsonic activity and complement levels in ascitic fluid, making it less susceptible to infection. The mechanism is thought to be simple concentration.

REFERENCES

73. Akriviadis EA, Kapnias D, Hadjigavriel M, et al. Serum/ascites albumin gradient: its value as a rational approach to the differential diagnosis of ascites. Scand J Gastroenterol 1996;31:814–817.
94. Dudley F. Pathophysiology of ascites formation. Gastroenterol Clin North Am 1992;21:216–236.
99. Ginès P, Cárdenas A, Arroyo V, Rodés J. Management of cirrhosis and ascites. N Engl J Med 2004;350:1646–1654.

See expertconsult.com for a complete list of references and the review questions for this chapter.

CAUSTIC INGESTION AND FOREIGN BODIES

19

Christine Carter-Kent

The ingestion of caustic substances and foreign body ingestion rank among the most common potential medical emergencies in the pediatric age group. Once a caustic or foreign body ingestion occurs, it is the responsibility of the physician and other medical personnel involved to determine whether these are minor occurrences and the child can be monitored at home, or whether the event is a true emergency and the child requires intervention immediately. It is widely accepted that the more accessible an item is in the environment, especially that of a young toddler to child, the more likely it is that the item will be found and subsequently swallowed. It is the responsibility of the parent to minimize exposure to potentially harmful agents, but it is also the responsibility of pediatric physicians to provide education to families regarding the types of household items that carry potential risk to children. This chapter will focus on the types of items that are typically implicated in caustic and foreign body ingestions, the expected result of such exposure, intervention required based on severity of the exposure, and long-term outcome.

INGESTION OF CAUSTIC AGENTS

Types of Caustic Agents and Prevention

The ingestion of caustic agents is a common problem encountered in pediatrics. Many exposures are negligible and require minimal intervention; however, there are substances that have consistently been associated with severe esophageal injury, including chemical burns, necrotic esophageal mucosa, esophageal perforation, and esophageal strictures. Over time, household bleach has been the most common agent reported worldwide in association with accidental caustic ingestion in children.[1] Bleaches, usually sodium hypochlorite, but including sodium perborate, hydrosulfite, and hydrogen peroxide, cause tissue damage by oxidation.[2]

According to the 2007 Annual Report from the American Association of Poison Control Centers, the most frequently ingested substances in children under 5 years of age in the United States were cosmetics/personal care products, household cleaning substances, and analgesics.[3] "Hair relaxer" is another common household liquid. Ingestion of hair relaxers, which are alkali products, does not typically result in significant injury, although pain and minor erythema in the mouth may occur.[4,5] The herbicide glyphosate surfactant (Roundup) is a mild acid, but ingestion of large volumes (usually in suicide attempts) has resulted in severe esophageal damage. The systemic toxicity and pulmonary complications following ingestion of this agent are generally of greater consequence to survival.[6] The types of agents ingested may also differ by

the child's home environment. For example, Edmonson et al. reported that children who reside on a farm were more likely to ingest alkaline farm products including dairy pipeline cleaners.[7] Ingested agents that have most often been associated with fatalities in all age groups include sedatives, antipsychotics, opioids, and antidepressants.[3]

Caustic ingestions in the pediatric age group show a bimodal distribution, with the first peak occurring in very young children under the age of 5 years and the second peak occurring in teenagers. The majority of caustic ingestions in toddlers and young children are accidental; however, in teenagers and young adults, ingestions are most often purposeful with self-harm or suicide being the ultimate goal. Studies have shown that in the 13- to 19-year-old age group, unintentional ingestions outnumber intentional ingestions.[3]

The method by which known caustic agents are stored and handled may have a significant impact on the accessibility of these products by young children. Countries that have established national prevention programs targeted at parents of young children have experienced a decline in accidental exposures and esophageal injuries.[8] For example, the Poison Prevention Packaging Act of 1970 stated that caustic agents should have "special packaging" that is designed to be difficult for children under 5 years of age to open, and that the amount of the caustic agent should be limited to 10% of the product.[9] In third-world countries where prevention campaigns are not as widespread, children continue to have high rates of caustic ingestion and may come to medical attention later with more severe injuries.[10] One of the mechanisms that leads to caustic exposure in developing countries is the use of secondary containers. Secondary containers that are unlabeled may be used to store household products or even sold in open marketplaces with serious consequences when consumed.

MECHANISMS OF DAMAGE TO THE GASTROINTESTINAL TRACT

The type of injury sustained after a caustic ingestion is influenced by multiple factors. The most important factors are the type and amount of agent ingested, as well as the length of time since the ingestion took place. These determinations can be difficult if the ingestion is unwitnessed. When evaluating young children as opposed to teenagers, it is important to note that children need to take in only a small amount of a corrosive substance for damage to occur, whereas teenagers require significantly larger quantities to sustain the same damage.[1] Agents can be divided into acids (pH 2 to 6), alkalis (pH 7 to 12), and bleaching substances (pH 7). It is important to determine the nature of the agent ingested, because acidic substances and alkaline substances produce different esophageal injuries. Alkaline substances tend to be more palatable, thereby allowing the patient to ingest more of the agent, whereas acidic products are quite distasteful and smaller quantities are typically consumed. Alkaline substances produce liquefaction necrosis with severe submucosal damage and deep tissue penetration. Acidic substances produce coagulative necrosis leading to eschar formation with limited further tissue damage.[11]

Table 19-1 lists many of the common acidic and alkaline household agents that are implicated in caustic ingestions. In a published series evaluating 473 pediatric caustic ingestions, the most common agents consumed were household bleach (36.6% of patients) and oven cleaner (23% of patients).[12] Other common agents include dishwashing liquids, drain cleaners, and cosmetic products. Table 19-2 lists the classification for injury to the gastrointestinal tract as outlined by Zargar et al.[13] Several other classifications have been proposed as well. In particular, the classification by Estrera et al. details a Grade 4 injury that involves eschar, full-thickness mucosal changes, and true perforation.[14]

Pill Esophagitis

It is important to mention that the pill, tablet, or capsule forms of a variety of medications have been associated with what is now termed *pill esophagitis*. These injuries can be different from other caustic ingestions. Pill esophagitis bridges the gap between caustic ingestions and foreign body ingestions. Once a tablet becomes lodged in the esophagus, it causes location irritation to the mucosa and often the release of the contents from the tablet can cause even more injury (Figure 19-1). Medications that have been most commonly implicated in reported cases of pill esophagitis include antibiotic and antiviral medications, with tetracycline being the most reported offender.[15] Other frequently reported medications include alendronate, nonsteroidal anti-inflammatory drugs (NSAIDs), potassium chloride, and quinidine. Risk factors for pill esophagitis include decreased salivary flow, esophageal motility abnormalities, medications formulation (pill size and shape), ingestion of medication in the supine position, anatomical abnormalities (atrial enlargement), and medications that alter the tone of the lower esophageal sphincter.[16] When an endoscopy is performed in patients with suspected pill esophagitis, abnormal findings are almost always discovered, including discrete ulcers and erythematous mucosa; however, hemorrhage, mediastinitis, and penetration of the great vessels has been reported as well.[15]

LOCATION OF INJURY

The lips, mouth, and oropharynx may be damaged by caustic liquids. Caustic material may pool in the hypopharynx because of upper esophageal sphincter spasm. Granulated caustic materials such as dishwasher detergent, denture cleaner, or caustic soda may stick onto the mucosa in the oropharynx and upper esophagus. Profound damage then occurs to periglottic tissues. This can cause severe contraction and scarring, leading to partial or complete obstruction of the airway and upper esophageal sphincter.[17]

In adults, stenosis of the esophagus is directly related to the amount of caustic material ingested: 2 to 3 ingested tablespoons of caustic soda (44 to 66 g) is associated with a high risk of

TABLE 19-1. Ingestible Caustic Materials Around the House

Type	Most Damaging Agents	Other Agents
Alkaline drain cleaners	Sodium hydroxide, potassium hydroxide	Ammonia, sodium hypochlorite, aluminum particles
Acidic drain openers	Hydrochloric acid, sulfuric acid	
Toilet cleaners	Hydrochloric acid, sulfuric acid, phosphoric acid	Ammonium chloride, sodium hypochlorite
Oven and grill cleaners	Sodium hydroxide	Borax (perborate)
Denture cleaners	Persulfate, hypochlorite (bleach)	
Dishwasher detergent	Sodium hydroxide	
Household bleach	5% sodium hypochlorite (approximate pH 11)	Ammonia salt
Swimming pool cleaner	Calcium carbonate, calcium chlorate, calcium hypochlorite, calcium hydroxide	
Battery acid (liquid)	Sulfuric acid	
Rust remover	Hydrofluoric acid, phosphoric acid, oxalic acid	
Household delimers	Phosphoric acid, hydrochloric acid, hydroxyacetic acid	
Barbeque cleaners	Sodium hydroxide, potassium hydroxide	
Hair relaxer	Sodium hydroxide	
Weed killer	Dichlorophenoxyacetic acid, ammonium phosphate, propionic acid	
Glyphosate and surfactant (Roundup)	Glyphosate herbicide	Surfactants
Automatic dishwashing	Sodium carbonate, sodium phosphate	

Source: National Library of Medicine. Health and Safety Information on Household Products. Available at: http://householdproducts.nlm.nih.gov/.

stenosis and perforation.[18] The amount of material swallowed that causes severe damage in young children is likely significantly less. Perforation of the esophagus due to damage from caustic material is possible and can result in profound illness due to mediastinitis. In addition, the ulceration may extend into the tracheobronchial tree, resulting in an esophagobronchial fistula, or into a major blood vessel, resulting in life-threatening hemorrhage. Perforation of the stomach results in damage to the surrounding tissues including the pancreas and bowel.

A large-volume ingestion, at least 1 tablespoon (15 mL) of granulated lye in an adult, is required to produce serious damage to the duodenum.[19] Caustic material passing into the stomach can often result in pylorospasm, in which case the duodenum is spared; however, pylorospasm will result in more severe damage to gastric antrum and may cause profound scarring, contraction of the antrum, and gastric obstructive symptoms in the future.

TABLE 19-2. **Classification of Caustic Injury**

Grade	Visible Appearance	Clinical Significance
Grade 0	History of ingestion, but no visible damage or symptoms	Able to take fluids immediately
Grade 1	Edema, loss of normal vascular pattern, hyperemia, no transmucosal injury	Temporary dysphagia, able to swallow within 0-2 days, no long-term sequelae
Grade 2a	Transmucosal injury with friability, hemorrhage, blistering, exudate, scattered superficial ulceration	Scarring, no circumferential damage (no stenosis), no long-term sequelae
Grade 2b	Grade 2a plus discrete ulceration and/or circumferential ulceration	Small risk of perforation, scarring that may result in later stenosis
Grade 3a	Scattered deep ulceration with necrosis of the tissue	Risk of perforation, high risk of later stenosis
Grade 3b	Extensive necrotic tissue	High risk of perforation and death, high risk of stenosis

Source: Zargar et al., 1991.[13]

MANAGEMENT OF CAUSTIC INGESTION

Acute Management

Common features on presentation after caustic ingestion include drooling, vomiting, and refusal of intake by mouth (PO). The patient may also experience visible mouth lesions such as erythema of the lips and oral mucosa. A careful history of the ingested material is essential. The most important initial factors in management include determining whether the patient is at risk for respiratory compromise or impending shock. If either is a concern, proper emergency measures should be taken. Tracheal intubation may be required with severe respiratory symptoms. An indwelling catheter should be placed to provide fluids and broad-spectrum antibiotic coverage, with total parenteral nutrition given until enteral feeds are possible.

When concerns regarding severe esophageal and gastric necrosis are raised, emergency esophagogastrectomy may be required to avoid extension of corrosion to nearby organs.[20] The presence of shock, fever, or prostration indicates profound tissue damage and requires immediate surgical consultation. Gastric perforation is almost invariably fatal as a result of toxic and septic effects of acute hemorrhagic pancreatitis, multiple bowel perforations, and peritonitis. Urgent and aggressive surgical debridement of all necrotic tissue in the chest and abdomen has been shown to significantly improve survival.[21] Endoscopy in the setting of a suspected perforation should only be performed in concert with the surgeon, and only if required for planning the surgical approach.

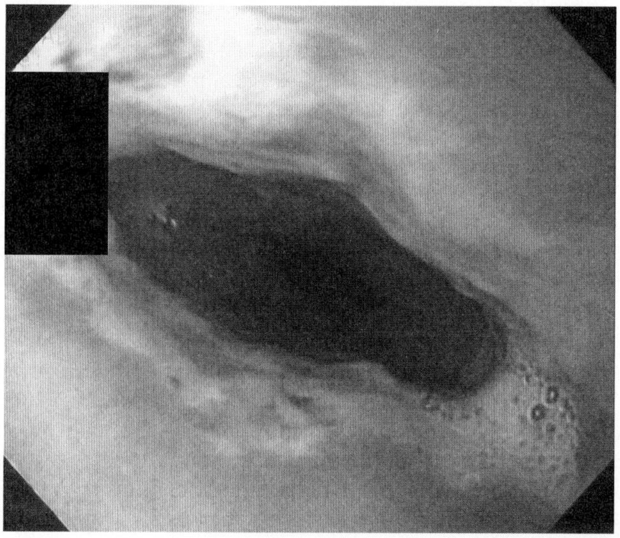

Role of Endoscopy

If a patient is symptomatic with a known or suspected caustic ingestion, has experienced an intentional ingestion, or has ingested certain types of caustic agents, an upper endoscopy is indicated. If the patient is asymptomatic, a watch and observe approach can be taken after ingestion of certain products.[22,23] If the child is discharged after observation only, it is the physician's responsibility to ensure that follow-up will be undertaken and that preventive teaching is provided. It is important to note that the patient's presenting signs and symptoms do not necessarily correlate with the extent of oropharyngeal and esophageal injury.[24-26] In a recent study of 50 consecutive cases of caustic ingestions, 70% of patients with oral injury did not have esophageal injury, whereas 12% of patients without oral injury did have evidence of esophageal injury on endoscopy.[11]

In most cases, if required, an upper endoscopy should be performed immediately and can be diagnostic. In a large study of 473 patients who underwent endoscopy after caustic ingestion, 379 patients sustained esophageal lesions (80%), whereas 81 children sustained gastric damage (17%).[12] The majority of children were diagnosed with mild lesions, Zargar's stage 1 to 2a. Endoscopy in the setting of caustic ingestion should be performed with anesthesia present to provide adequate airway protection via orotracheal or nasotracheal intubation. The object of endoscopy is to categorize the extent and grade of injury according to Zargar's classification (see Table 19-2). Once the degree of injury is known, treatment and prognosis can be determined. Endoscopes with a diameter as small as 36 mm can be passed safely through a severely inflamed and narrowed lumen to identify the extent of injury. In the past, endoscopy usually stopped at the first evidence of severe injury, but some centers now consider it appropriate to identify the full extent of injury, at least to the level of the duodenum. The procedure should be terminated if a perforation is suspected or encountered. Air insufflation is minimized to decrease the risk of a "blowout" through a deeply ulcerated area. In the case of severe ulceration in a viscus, computed tomography is useful to examine the deeper tissues. Although endoscopic ultrasonography has been proposed, before it can be generally recommended, further evidence is required of both its practicality and usefulness in this situation.[27,28]

Figure 19-1. "Pill esophagitis" in a teenage girl on doxycycline. *(See plate section for color.)*

Management Based on Endoscopic Findings

In the face of extensive damage, Zargar's grade 2b or higher in the esophagus, a nasogastric or nasointestinal tube should be left in place. This can be passed over a guidewire left in the esophagus as the endoscope is removed. A tube with the largest diameter possible should then be placed over the guidewire. The tube will act as a route for feeding and, if necessary, a stent.[29,30] As the swelling decreases, the child can feed around the tube, and when the child is able to swallow saliva adequately, oral feeding can be started. Total parenteral nutrition will be required if enteral feeding is not possible initially. Antibiotics should be used only if there is fever or evidence of deep ulceration on endoscopy. Corticosteroids have used by several groups in an attempt to decrease the amount of stricturing that takes place. It has been determined that steroids have no beneficial effect in decreasing scar formation or strictures, and steroids may increase the incidence of complications.[31,32]

If the damage is of grade 2a or less, management consists of adequate nutrition by mouth and observation. Repeat endoscopy should take place in 2 to 3 weeks to ensure that there is no evidence of a developing stricture and that healing is progressing well. Normal acid reflux can impair healing and intensify damage.[33] All patients with Zargar's grade 2 or higher damage should be maintained on acid reduction therapy, ideally a proton pump inhibitor twice daily, until ulcerations have completely healed. A pH probe test should be performed to identify the quantity of acid reflux. If it is excessive or there is abnormally slow clearance of acid, long-term prophylactic acid suppression therapy should be considered.

FOLLOW-UP AND LONG-TERM MANAGEMENT

Long-term management of gastrointestinal complications after caustic injury, including prolonged stricture and cancerous or precancerous lesions, has been varied. It is widely accepted that every child who has suffered Zargar's grade 2 damage or greater should undergo endoscopy 3 weeks after the ingestion to assess healing and the development of a stricture. If a stricture is present, dilation should be started at this time using Savary-Gilliard bougies or balloons of graduated size (Figure 19-2).

Often when strictures develop after caustic ingestion, repeated dilations over a period of several years are required to maintain adequate esophageal diameter. Symptoms that indicate the need for stricture dilation include odynophagia, dysphagia, or decreased oral intake with weight loss. Kukkady and Pease described a case series of 10 patients with known esophageal strictures after caustic injuries that were followed over time. They reported that a total of 424 dilations were performed in these patients over the course of 9 months to 4 years, with esophageal perforation occurring in two patients.[34] In developing countries, children may present later with caustic injury and esophageal strictures, which leads to the development of more severe, fibrotic esophageal stenotic lesions. Esophageal perforation rates at the time of endoscopy in these regions have been reported to be as high as 18%.[10] Other severe complications such as mediastinitis, pneumothorax, peritoneal soiling, and brain abscess have been reported at the time of stricture dilation.[35,36]

Once any deep ulcerations have healed over, there is empirical evidence that dilation followed immediately by the application of mitomycin C solution to the scarred area may impede scar tissue regeneration and decrease the number of dilations

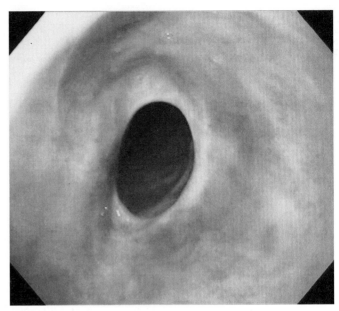

Figure 19-2. Esophageal stenosis in a toddler resulting from ingestion of oven cleaner. *(See plate section for color.)*

required.[37,38] Figure 19-3 details mitomycin C application. Laser-assisted remodeling of stenotic areas has been reported with good to excellent results.[39] Steroid injection, self-expanding stents, and NG intubation have also been used as techniques for the treatment of caustic strictures.

In the case of strictures that require frequent dilation or when esophageal perforation occurs with dilation, surgical intervention is also a consideration. Surgical techniques typically performed include partial esophagectomy and local resection of the stenotic lesion with esophageal reconstruction. In the adult literature, esophageal reconstruction utilizing a portion of the colon as an intervening segment during the reconstructive procedure has been reported. In a study of 336 adult patients who underwent esophageal reconstruction with colonic interposition, 76% of the patients with long-term results available had excellent functional results.[40]

It is important to note that motility in the injured tissue is affected permanently after deep injury to the esophagus. Alkaline injury appears to cause a serious and long-term change in motility more frequently than acid-derived injury. The initial injury leads to delayed esophageal clearance with low-caliber and simultaneous waves.[41] Depending on the depth of the scar, the myenteric plexus may be damaged and the normal syncytium of smooth muscle cells may be interrupted. More than 70% of patients will suffer from dysphagia as a result of the motility disorder with delayed esophageal clearance of both ingested food and gastric refluxate.[42] Peptic esophagitis with the background of the caustic injury itself increases the risk of esophageal cancer, both squamous cell and adenocarcinoma.[19] Careful lifetime follow-up is required for all children who have experienced Zargar's grade 2 or greater damage and with visible scarring. If there is profound scarring, an excellent case can be made to resect this area to eliminate the risk of future adenocarcinoma.

INGESTION OF FOREIGN BODIES
Types of Common Foreign Bodies

Approximately 80% of foreign body ingestions occur in the pediatric age group.[43] It is estimated that 98% of foreign body ingestions in children are accidental.[44] The most common foreign

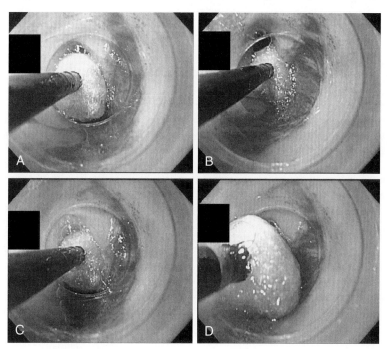

Figure 19-3. Application of mitomycin C to dilated, stenotic lesion in the esophagus. **(A)** Dry pledget is advanced from clear plastic hood on endoscope. **(B)** Mitomycin C is injected down forceps sheath onto pledget. **(C)** Pledget is held on mucosa at site of dilation. **(D)** Pledget is withdrawn into hood for safe removal. *(See plate section for color.)*

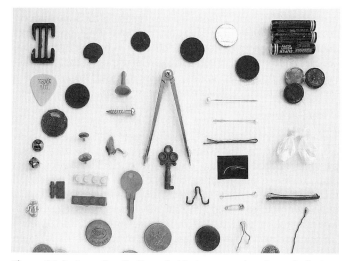

Figure 19-4. A small collection of objects removed endoscopically in a single practice.

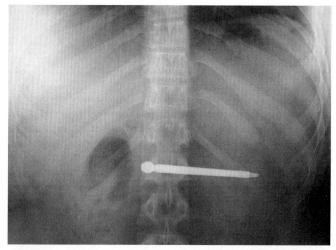

Figure 19-5. Trigonometry compass in the stomach of a teenage boy, swallowed while daydreaming in class. The compass was removed endoscopically.

body ingested by children in the United States is a coin. Other common objects ingested by American children include small toys, game pieces, batteries, marbles, and small earrings (Figures 19-4 and 19-5). In other countries, the types of foreign bodies ingested by children may differ based on cultural practices. For example, in Asian countries where fish (without removal of bones) is a dietary staple, fish bones are the most common type of foreign body identified.[45,46] Pork bones and chicken bones are also frequent offending agents in these cultures.

In adolescents and adults, the most common type of foreign body reported has been esophageal food impaction, with meat being the most likely item found at endoscopy. Often, underlying pathology exists that predisposes these patients to impaction. These occurrences are most often accidental; however,

unlike children, intentional ingestions occur often in adolescents and adults. Intentional ingestions are most often performed by patients with psychiatric problems or impairment by alcohol or drugs. It is not unusual to find repeated episodes of multiple objects ingested by these patients.

Whether the foreign body ingestion is witnessed or unwitnessed may also play a role in the outcome for the patient. Several large, retrospective pediatric series of children presenting to the emergency setting with esophageal foreign body have reported that between 16 and 25% of patients have unwitnessed ingestions.[47,48] For unwitnessed patients under the age of 2 years, wheeze and fever are more commonly found than in patients with witnessed foreign body aspirations.[47]

Common Locations of Foreign Bodies

Oropharynx and Esophagus

In a study of 1338 Chinese patients in which 84% of the patients experienced impaction due to fish bones, the area of the cricopharyngeus or higher was the most common location for foreign body impaction.[45] The most common esophageal location for foreign bodies to become impacted is at the level of the thoracic inlet. It has been estimated that 60 to 70% of items impacted in the esophagus are located in this area, as this is the most narrow portion of the esophagus. The two other common esophageal locations for foreign bodies to become impacted include the level of the aortic notch (in 10 to 20% of patients) and just above the lower esophageal sphincter (in 20% of patients).[43]

Stomach and Intestines

The majority of foreign bodies that reach the stomach will pass uneventfully through the rest of the gastrointestinal tract. Size of the object is one of the most important factors in determining whether retrieval is necessary from the stomach. Objects longer than 5 cm or wider than 2 cm will likely be unable to traverse the pylorus and will require endoscopic retrieval.[49] The duodenal C loop and terminal ileum/ileocecal valve are other areas where long, sharp, or oddly shaped objects may become impacted. Sharp-ended objects, such as toothpicks or nails, can become jammed across the lumen of the bowel, resulting in a walled-off perforation and small abscess, presenting as an acute abdomen. Any foreign body impacted beyond the duodenum requires surgical consultation.

Preexisting Conditions Associated With Foreign Body Complications

It is now widely accepted that several preexisting esophageal disorders place patients at risk for foreign body impaction in the esophagus, as well as significant mucosal damage. In a published series of 484 occurrences of pediatric esophageal foreign body impaction, 14% of patients had an underlying esophageal abnormality, with many patients experiencing more than one ingestion over the period of 15 years.[48] It has been reported that the relative risk for complications related to esophageal foreign body aspiration exceeds 8 when patients have a preexisting esophageal condition.[50] Preexisting conditions that place patients at risk for esophageal impaction include Schatzki's ring, eosinophilic esophagitis, severe gastroesophageal reflux disease with peptic stricture, tracheoesophageal fistula with previous surgical intervention, esophageal motility disorders, and previous caustic ingestion with subsequent esophageal narrowing.

Eosinophilic Esophagitis

Eosinophilic esophagitis is associated with symptoms of abdominal pain, chest pain, nausea, and dysphagia. Eosinophilic esophagitis has also been associated with foreign body impaction in the esophagus, particularly food impaction. In adults it has been reported that approximately 60% of patients are diagnosed with eosinophilic esophagitis after presenting with food impaction.[51, 52] In children, presentation with food impaction is less common. The Swiss Esophageal Esophagitis Database documented that of 251 confirmed cases of eosinophilic esophagitis, 87 patients (35%) experienced at least one case of food impaction requiring endoscopic removal with 2% of patients experiencing esophageal perforation at the time of the endoscopic procedure.[53]

Unusual Foreign Bodies

Bezoars

A bezoar is defined as a mass or concretion of foreign material located within the gastrointestinal tract. Several types of bezoars have been described, and specific categories have been defined, which include lactobezoars, phytobezoars, trichobezoars, and pharmacobezoars.[54] A lactobezoar is defined as a mass mainly composed of undigested milk matter and is the most common form of bezoar occurring in infants and toddlers. Thus far, more than 60 cases have been reported with ages ranging from the first few days of life to 3 years of age.[55] Phytobezoars are the most commonly occurring bezoars in all age groups and are defined as a masses of undigested fiber matter that are typically associated with fibrous fruits and vegetables. Among the most common phytobezoars described in the literature are persimmon bezoars or diospyrobezorars. This is due to properties of the skin of the fruit, including the presence of phlobotannin, which make it especially prone to concretion formation.[56] The formation of a trichobezoar, a mass of hair, string, or other nonfood fibers, has also been associated with the "Rapunzel syndrome." Rapunzel syndrome describes trichobezoars with a long tail extending from the stomach to the small intestine and has been associated with several cases of ileal and jejunal intussusception.[57] Pharmacobezoars have been formed after ingestion of several types of medication, with oral fiber supplements identified as the most common offender. The management of bezoars can be medical (utilizing several types of chemical dissolution or prokinetic agents), endoscopic, or surgical (when the object is too large for endoscopic removal).

Body Packing

The intentional ingestion of illegal drugs such as cocaine, hashish, or heroin for purposes of concealment is termed "body packing" or "body stuffing." Packaging for the illegal substances may consist of plastic wrap, or condoms or other latex-based materials. The concealment may be performed as part of a deliberate plan to smuggle illegal substances or as a last resort when arrest or detection is imminent. Although the "mules" (individuals who have ingested the drugs) are most often adults, in recent years several case reports have been published in which children have been used as "mules." The first case series, reported by Traub et al., describes two teenage boys both presenting with active symptoms including opioid intoxication and rectal bleeding.[58] The second case described a 6-year-old male administered opioids for concealment by his grandfather who presented to the emergency room with symptoms of opioid intoxication.[59] If body packing is suspected, plain abdominal x-ray should be performed, as it has been reported to have a detection sensitivity of 85 to 90%. Typical findings on x-ray include multiple, small radiodense foreign bodies or the "double condom sign," air trapped between the latex layers of the condom packaging material.[60] Although the successful endoscopic removal of an intact condom containing heroin via a snare has been described, it is now widely accepted that endoscopic removal of packages containing illegal drugs from the gastrointestinal tract is absolutely contraindicated.[61] This is due to the high risk of perforation of the packaging leading to severe drug toxicity, seizure, cardiac arrhythmia, and possible death. If the patient is asymptomatic, conservative management with whole bowel irrigation can be attempted. If this approach is unsuccessful or the patient is symptomatic, surgical intervention and removal of the substance may be required.

Rectal Foreign Bodies

Although the majority of this chapter is focused on foreign bodies located within the upper gastrointestinal tract and subsequent removal from this area, it is important to note that foreign bodies may also become lodged within the rectum. Recognizing the presence of rectal objects is key due risks of rectal perforation and peritonitis. Unlike objects lodged within the esophagus, rectal foreign bodies are most often associated with adults as opposed to children. In adults, objects lodged in the rectum are often intentionally placed for purposes of sexual acts, drug smuggling, or attention-seeking behaviors. In the case of pediatric rectal foreign bodies, accidentally retained objects are most common. The most commonly described item impacted in rectum in children reported is the rectal thermometer. Most often, rectal thermometer retention occurs in infants and young children after obtaining a rectal temperature. This places the infant at high risk, especially if the thermometer contains mercury. Chiu et al. described the unusual case of a teenage male with an anally placed rectal thermometer that caused a rectal perforation and subsequently migrated to the pelvic cavity. Because the patient was asymptomatic and had no knowledge of the inciting event, it was thought that the thermometer has been retained since infancy.[62] The removal of rectal foreign bodies can be challenging based on the nature of the object. In a case series of 13 adults with various items lodged in the rectum, seven items were retrieved without surgical intervention.[63] Removal techniques include manual removal under anesthesia, removal via sigmoidoscopy, or surgical removal. The successful removal of a rectal foreign body using sigmoidoscopy with balloon extraction under fluoroscopy in a 50-day-old infant has been reported.[64]

ACUTE MANAGEMENT OF FOREIGN BODIES

Initial Assessment

The American Society for Gastrointestinal Endoscopy has published guidelines for the management of ingested foreign bodies in both adults and children.[65] Controlled trials are mostly absent, so the guidelines rely on the best evidence with careful review of the literature.

The acuity of management of ingested foreign bodies is dependent on the presenting signs and symptoms of the patient and the duration of time since ingestion, as well as the type of object ingested. A brief medical history should be performed immediately to determine any underlying medical problems, regular medications, recent drug or alcohol exposure, medication allergies, or previous reaction to anesthetic agents. Physical examination should be performed to further determine the patient's respiratory status and severity of abdominal symptoms. For patient with signs and symptoms of acute abdomen, surgical services should be notified. A patient with obvious respiratory symptoms, difficulty controlling secretions, or repeated episodes of emesis should be managed emergently. For a patient with signs of impending respiratory failure, otolaryngology should be consulted immediately. In a 2006 series of 555 children presenting to the emergency room setting with a foreign body lodged in the esophagus and clinical symptoms, the most common clinical symptoms included

dysphagia in 37% of patients, drooling in 31% of patients, and choking in 17% of patients.[66] Other common symptoms include cough, abdominal pain, fever, chest pain, wheezing, stridor, vomiting, and refusal to eat. In large pediatric series, cases of asymptomatic foreign body ingestion have been reported to range from approximately 10% to 50% of all cases.[66-68]

The type and location of the item ingested plays key role in determining the management of the child. A host of different items have been reported in the literature with a wide variety of sizes, shapes, and textures. In a review of 325 consecutive cases of pediatric foreign body ingestions, 64% of patients ingested a radiopaque object whereas 35% of patients ingested a radiolucent object.[67] If the item swallowed is known to be radiopaque, such as a coin or any other metallic item, a plain frontal chest x-ray should be performed immediately. This will help determine if the object is in the gastrointestinal tract versus the airway. For example, an 'en face' appearance of a coin suggests that it is located in the esophagus, as opposed to the "edge" appearance suggesting that it is located in the trachea. Lateral films may occasionally be helpful in the setting of a radiopaque foreign body that overlies the vertebral column. These may not be visualized in the AP view, but can be visualized on the lateral view.[49] In some centers, metal detectors have also been used to identify metallic foreign bodies successfully; however, this practice is not currently widespread.[69,70]

Radiolucent foreign bodies can be more difficult to diagnose, because they will not be apparent on a chest x-ray. Radiolucent foreign bodies include items that are made from plastic, glass, and wood as well as food items such as bones or fibrous vegetable matter. Lateral films, a CT scan, or less often a barium swallow may be helpful in the setting of radiolucent foreign body ingestions. Features that can be suggestive of a radiolucent foreign body on a lateral plain film include tracheal compression, tracheal deviation, or air trapped within the esophagus.[71] The use of CT scan in these patients has also been described. Applegate et al. reported successful use of rapid, low-dose spiral CT scanning of the neck and chest in the detection of plastic Lego toys.[72] Caution should be taken when performing a contrast study in these patients. In symptomatic patients a contrast study is absolutely contraindicated because of risk of aspiration or barium entering the mediastinum. If the patient is symptomatic but radiologic evidence of a foreign body and its location cannot be determined, it is recommended that the patient undergo diagnostic endoscopy. If the item is visualized in the upper gastrointestinal tract, it can be removed at that time. If no object is seen, parents should inspect the stool for passage of the foreign body.

Finally, the length of time that the object has been present in the gastrointestinal tract has a significant effect on management. No foreign body should be left in the esophagus for more than 24 hours under any circumstances. As previously mentioned, the act of swallowing a foreign body may be unwitnessed, which can make the determination of duration of impaction difficult. If the child does not or cannot, as in the case of infants, inform the care provider of the act right away and is relatively asymptomatic, weeks may pass before the diagnosis is made. It has been reported that relative risk for developing complications related to foreign body aspiration is 1.88 if the duration of impaction is more than 24 hours, and the relative risk increases to 6.83 if the duration of impaction exceeds 72 hours.[50]

A wide variety of complications have been reported in relation to gastrointestinal tract foreign bodies including gastrointestinal perforation, tracheoesophageal fistula, aspiration, mediastinitis, esophageal-aortic fistula, stricture formation, and excessive bleeding.[73] Intra-abdominal complications have also included intussusception and peritonitis. Deaths related to foreign body ingestion in the United States have been estimated to occur at a rate of approximately 1500 per year.[74] Pediatric retrospective studies have reported complication rates related to foreign body ingestion in the range of 13 to 20%.[48,50]

Nature of the Object

Coins

Coins are the most frequent foreign body to require attention. For standard American money, pennies are 18 mm in diameter, dimes are 17 mm in diameter, nickels are 21 mm in diameter, and quarters are 24 mm in diameter. Given this size differential, pennies and dimes are more likely to pass readily through the esophagus, whereas quarters and nickels are more likely to become lodged when swallowed. If a coin is retained in the esophagus, but the patient is asymptomatic, it is reasonable to wait 6 to 12 hours before removing the coin. Previous studies have reported that the spontaneous passage of esophageal coins takes place in approximately 25% of patients over a period of 16 hours, with coins located distally in the esophagus more likely to pass.[75,76] During this observation period, the patient should be kept in nothing by mouth (NPO) status to provide ample time to clear food and other gastric material for proper administration of anesthesia. After the observation period, a repeat chest x-ray should be performed to note the position of the coin. If the coin remains in the esophagus after the observation period or the patient is symptomatic on initial presentation, upper endoscopy in indicated. Once the coin passes into the stomach, it is likely that it will traverse the pylorus and be passed in the stool without intervention. On occasion, coins will remain in the stomach after passing through the esophagus. This occurs most often with larger coins that may have difficulty passing through the pylorus, in patients with underlying gastric disease, or if the coin becomes impacted in the fundus of the stomach. In this case, after an observation period of 4 to 6 weeks, during which time serial x-rays are performed, it is reasonable to remove the coin endoscopically because it is unlikely that the coin will pass on its own.[43]

Magnets

Ingestion of a singe magnet does not impose increased risk over the ingestion of other types of foreign bodies. When multiple magnets are swallowed, there is increased concern. When multiple magnets are ingested, there is potential for the magnets attract each other within the gastrointestinal tract. If attracted magnets are left in place, significant complications may arise including fistula formation and gastrointestinal perforation. Cauchi and Shawis reported the case of a 9-year-old girl who had swallowed 12 magnets, which adhered together, 1 week before presentation. The patient underwent laparotomy that revealed five ileal perforations with the magnet aggregate lying within the peritoneal cavity.[77] It is recommended that immediate endoscopy take place in the setting of known or suspected multiple magnet ingestions. If the magnets are located beyond the duodenum, serial x-rays should be performed. Surgical intervention is required for magnets located beyond the level of the duodenum.

Batteries

Similar to esophagitis caused by tablets, battery ingestions also bridge the gap between caustic ingestion and foreign body ingestions. Button batteries are the most common type of battery

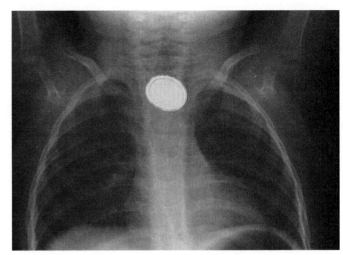

Figure 19-6. Disk battery impacted in the esophagus. Note the "double rim."

ingested by young children. Live disk button batteries used for electronic toys and watches discharge their current across tissue or liquid. Figure 19-6 shows a chest x-ray of a disk battery impacted in the esophagus, with the "double rim" sign that is useful in differentiating a disk battery from a coin. Children who ingest "live" disk batteries that impact in the esophagus invariably suffer deep electrical burns at the site if the batteries are left in place (Figure 19-7). This may result in perforation into the mediastinum (Figure 19-8). Several cases of severe battery-related injuries have recently been reported, including tracheo-esophageal and aortoesophageal fistulas and bilateral vocal cord paralysis.[73,78] Batteries should be removed urgently via endoscopy and the child observed in the hospital for at least 24 hours. Regular dry cell batteries may contain manganese dioxide, zinc, and potassium hydroxide. Rechargeable and disk batteries may contain lithium or cadmium.[79] Information from major battery manufacturers suggests that the risk of leakage is very small with modern cylindrical alkaline batteries; however, it is suggested that they be removed if still in the gastric lumen after 72 hours.[80,81]

Pins and Other Sharp Objects

Sharp objects, such as toys, hairclips, bones, and pins, should be removed urgently. Fish and chicken bones frequently impact in the hypopharynx. Usually, they can be removed easily with McGill forceps with anesthesia or by an ear, nose, and throat (ENT) surgeon under sedation. If sharp objects pass into the esophagus, there is a high risk of esophageal wall perforation. There is also an increased risk of gastric and intestinal perforation as the pin traverses the gastrointestinal tract.[82] Thus, any sharp objects within the duodenum or located proximally should be removed urgently.

Food Bolus

Food boluses usually impact in the mid-esophagus. Meat is the most common cause of food impaction, although candy, rice, and bread are also frequent causes. The "push technique" using a Hurst blunt-end dilator has been used in a large series of adult patients, but reported far less frequently in children. It has been advocated in the past to make an attempt to advance the food bolus from the esophagus to the stomach; however, given the increased recognition of potential underlying esophageal abnormalities, advancing the food bolus is no longer advised. Patients with underlying disorders, such as eosinophilic esophagitis, are

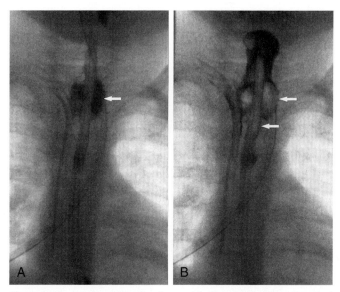

Figure 19-8. Esophageal perforation and leak on upper gastrointestinal radiograph due to disk battery impaction and secondary electrical burn. (**A**) Contrast media in the mediastinum. (**B**) Air in the mediastinum with air and contrast media leaking superiorly and inferiorly subsequent to "button battery" impaction and electrical burn.

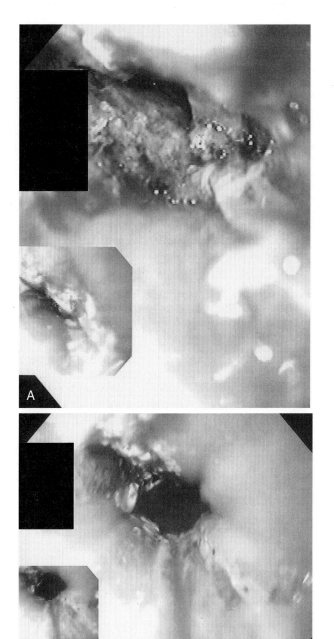

Figure 19-7. (**A**) Disk battery in the esophagus with necrotic debris at the burn site. (**B**) Typical bilateral esophageal burn after removal of a disk battery. *(See plate section for color.)*

at high risk of perforation during endoscopy and air insufflation, and esophageal manipulation should be minimized.[53]

Methods of Foreign Body Removal

Endoscopic Methods

Foreign bodies left in the esophagus may be removed a number of different ways. Objects have routinely been removed by gastroenterologists, otolaryngologists, or general pediatric surgeons using flexible endoscopy or rigid endoscopy. Endoscopic foreign body removal under amnesic sedation or propofol anesthesia has been the standard therapy in many centers. If there is a concern regarding aspiration of gastric contents or food material lodged

above a foreign body in the esophagus, orotracheal intubation is recommended. Endoscopic removal is absolutely required if there is a history of previous foreign body ingestion, esophageal surgery, or evidence of esophageal disease.

Under suitable sedation, the endoscope is passed to the level of the upper esophageal sphincter. A careful examination of these tissues ensures no damage from the ingestion and no foreign body impacted in this area. Most objects are identified immediately below the upper esophageal sphincter and can be grasped with a rat-tooth or similar forceps and removed. If the object is clearly sharp, impacted, and likely to perforate the esophagus, rigid endoscopy under general anesthesia with a wide-diameter tube may be required. An endoscope overtube can easily be used in adult-sized patients, but has not been proved useful in children because of the smaller size of the pharynx and upper esophageal sphincter, which are rarely of sufficient size to accept an overtube.

Objects that reach the stomach can usually be left to pass spontaneously down the bowel. The exception would be a large or long object that cannot negotiate the pylorus, duodenal C loop, or ileocecal valve. Nails and pins usually pass easily into the stomach and onward down the bowel with the blunt end forward. Objects longer than 2 inches (5 cm), such as nails, pencils, or pens, should be removed from the stomach or duodenum, if possible, because they will have a difficulty in passing the angulated portions of the bowel. Irregularly shaped objects that may stick to the cardia of the stomach during removal can be pulled up into a "hood," a device of thick latex that fits over the end of the endoscope (Figure 19-9). If unavailable, a hood can be made from a portion of thick latex surgical glove.[83] Table 19-3 lists some of the tools commonly used for foreign body removal during endoscopy. Figure 19-10 displays various devices that can be used to remove foreign bodies in the upper gastrointestinal tract. In case of doubt or difficulty with extraction, the endoscopist should consult a general surgeon with regard to gastrotomy to remove the object.

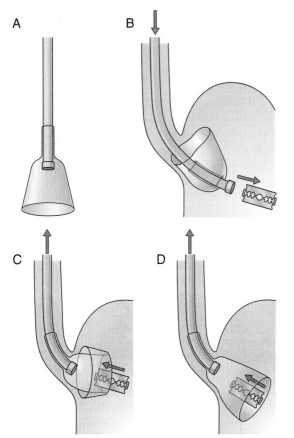

Figure 19-9. Latex hood fits over the endoscope tip. (**A**) Fitted. (**B**) Inverted before oral insertion and passed into the stomach. (**C**) Foreign body withdrawn into hood. (**D**) Hood flips over foreign body as endoscope is pulled back through lower esophageal sphincter.

TABLE 19-3. Foreign Body Removal Techniques

Object	Retrieval Tools
Coin and other blunt objects	Rat-tooth or alligator forceps, retrieval net
Food bolus	Retrieval net, tripod or pentapod forceps, friction fit adaptor
Sharp objects	Polypectomy snare, rat-tooth or alligator forceps
Smooth objects	Retrieval net or basket
Long objects	Polypectomy snare, double snare (consider rigid endoscopy)
Batteries	Retrieval net or basket
Safety pin	Combined forceps-snare technique
Objects with a hole	Suture technique

Reintroduction of the endoscope after the foreign body has been removed is key, because this may help identify any undiagnosed, underlying disease processes and to identify any other, unsuspected foreign bodies. Suitable biopsies can be taken to confirm a suspicion of inflammatory change.

Nonendoscopic Methods

Proteolytic enzymes such as papain have been used in the past in the case of a food impaction in the esophagus. In theory these enzymes aid in digestion of the food bolus and facilitate its

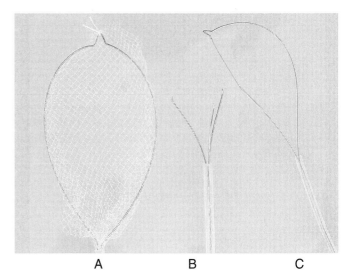

Figure 19-10. Various devices that can be used to remove foreign bodies. (**A**) Retrieval basket. (**B**) Three-pronged grasping forceps. (**C**) Polypectomy snare.

passage through the gastrointestinal tract. The use of proteolytic enzymes is now contraindicated because of possible side effects, including hypernatremia, erosion, and esophageal perforation, along with lack of efficacy.[65] The use of intravenous glucagon has also been attempted to aid in passage of esophageal foreign bodies, particularly coins, but does not appear to be efficacious.[84]

Balloon (Foley balloon catheter) removal of smooth objects is very successful in experienced hands.[66,85,86] The catheter, with the balloon deflated, is passed beyond the foreign body; the balloon is then inflated under fluoroscopic monitoring and the foreign body gradually withdrawn. Care must be taken to guard against aspiration of the foreign body into the airway as the object comes up into the hypopharynx, and to avoid vocal cord occlusion by a coin that "flips out." This method has a 94% efficacy rate with experienced personnel.[87]

Follow-up

Although discharge advice to observe for any evidence of dysphagia, odynophagia, or hematemesis is routine after foreign body removal, repeat endoscopy is required only if deep ulceration was found in the esophagus, or damage that might result in esophageal stricture. Management of concurrent disease discovered at endoscopy, such as eosinophilic esophagitis or peptic esophagitis, can be started immediately.

REFERENCES

12. Dogan Y, Erkan T, Cokugras FC, et al. Caustic gastroesophageal lesions in childhood: an analysis of 473 cases. Clin Pediatr 2006;45:435–438.
15. Kirkendall JM. Pill esophagitis. J Clin Gastroenterol 1999;28:298–305
23. Gupta SK, Croffie JM, Fitzgerald JF. Is esophagogastroduodenoscopy necessary in all caustic ingestions? J Pediatr Gastroenterol Nutr 2001;32:50–53.
43. Kay M, Wyllie R. Pediatric foreign bodies and their management. Curr Gastroenterol Rep 2005;7:212–218.
49. Smith MT, Wong RKH. Foreign bodies. Gastrointest Endosc Clin North Am 2007;17:361–382.
65. Eisen GM, Baron TH, Dominitz JA, et al. Guideline for the management of ingested foreign bodies. Gastrointest Endosc 2002;55:802–806.
See expertconsult.com for a complete list of references and the review questions for this chapter.

DEVELOPMENTAL ANATOMY AND PHYSIOLOGY OF THE ESOPHAGUS

20

Reema Gulati • Kadakkal Radhakrishnan • Mike A. Thomson

The pediatric esophagus has come of age. It is no longer regarded in gastrointestinal circles as just the tube that acts as a conduit from mouth to stomach, although this message still has some way to go in other medical spheres. Pathologic processes in the pediatric esophagus have received a disproportionately small amount of attention until recently, when appreciation of their pathophysiology and concordant clinical importance has been highlighted. This increase in interest and exposure is a phenomenon secondary to a number of important factors, including improved diagnostic yield from relatively recent technical advances in areas such as infant/pediatric endoscopy; advances in fields such as mucosal immunology, allowing for the realization that etiopathologic mechanisms for esophagitis are more complex than simple luminal chemical damage; and a shift in clinical opinion recognizing esophageal pathology as a major cause of ubiquitous nonspecific symptoms such as infant colic, feeding disorders, and recurrent abdominal pain. A state of knowledge such as this has made pediatric esophageal pathology, until recently, a relatively underdeveloped area of research and clinical understanding, but this is changing rapidly.

It is now clear, for example, that esophagitis in infants and children has many responsible etiologic pathways that may have complex interactions, and hence require equally complex diagnostic and therapeutic strategies. Such causative factors are now known to include cow's milk protein intolerance or allergy; pH-dependent and independent gastroesophageal reflux (GER); dysmotility of various causes; and infective, traumatic, and iatrogenic causes, among others.

This chapter paints the background in terms of the basic understanding of this structure's development, anatomy, and physiology to facilitate an understanding of the many clinical presentations of esophageal disease.

DEVELOPMENTAL ANATOMY

The primitive gut forms during the fourth fetal week as the head, tail, and lateral folds incorporate the dorsal part of the yolk sac into the embryo (Figure 20-1). The human esophagus develops from a fusiform swelling of the foregut at about 4 weeks' gestation. The endoderm of the primitive gut is responsible for the evolution of the epithelium and glands of the digestive tract (excepting the mouth and anus). The muscular and fibrous parts of the gastrointestinal tract, and the visceral peritoneum, come from the splanchnic mesenchyme surrounding the endodermal lining of the primitive gut. The foregut, midgut, and hindgut are terms used for descriptive purposes; the esophagus derives from the foregut, as do the pharynx, lower respiratory tract, stomach, duodenum, liver, biliary tree, and pancreas. The partitioning of the trachea from the esophagus by

the tracheoesophageal septum occurs (Figure 20-2). Thereafter the foregut is divided into a ventral portion, the laryngotracheal tube, and a dorsal portion, the esophagus.

Hence an abnormal communication, or fistula, connecting the trachea and esophagus can occur (once in every 2500 births) owing to incomplete division of the trachea and digestive portion of the foregut during the fourth and fifth weeks of fetal life. The four main variations are shown in Figure 20-3. Esophageal atresia probably develops from lack of deviation of the tracheoesophageal septum in a posterior direction, although isolated (very rare) esophageal atresia can develop from failure of recanalization of the esophagus in the embryonic period (see later discussion). This leads to polyhydramnios, because amniotic fluid cannot be swallowed. Congenital stenosis of the esophagus can occur in any area, but is usually present in the distal third as a web or band, or as a long segment of the esophagus with a very narrow lumen; again this is due to failure of recanalization of the esophagus in the embryonic period, by the eighth week of development. Occasionally a short esophagus may occur with a portion of the stomach displaced through the diaphragm as a hiatus hernia. Similarly, diverticuli, duplication cysts, and other anatomic abnormalities arise owing to failure of correct embryonic development, usually of the proximal esophagus.

Initially the esophagus is very short (see Figure 20-1), but it lengthens rapidly, reaching its final proportionate length by around 7 weeks of fetal life. This occurs as a result of cranial body growth – ascent of the pharynx rather than descent of the stomach.[1] The epithelium of the esophagus and the esophageal mucous glands are derived from the endoderm; although the squamous epithelium of the esophagus resembles the skin, the latter is derived from the ectoderm and is keratinized. Thence the epithelium of the esophagus proliferates and obliterates the lumen, with subsequent recanalization occurring before the end of the embryonic period. The striated muscle of the upper esophagus (muscularis externa) is derived from mesenchyme in the caudal branchial arches, and smooth muscle is derived from the surrounding splanchnic mesenchyme; both are supplied with innervation by the vagal nerve (Figure 20-4A-D).

Alternative Theories of Esophageal Development

Although separation of the foregut by a tracheoesophageal septum is the most commonly accepted theory of tracheoesophageal development, it is a matter of much controversy. This is because many studies of tracheoesophageal development have not been able to definitely identify the septum, creating uncertainty about its existence.[2-6] Conversely, there are other

207

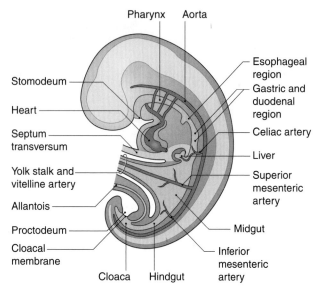

Figure 20-1. Median section of a 4-week-old embryo showing the early digestive system and its blood supply. The primitive gut is a tube extending the whole length of the embryo; it evolves from incorporation of the dorsal part of the yolk sac with its vascular supply into the embryo.

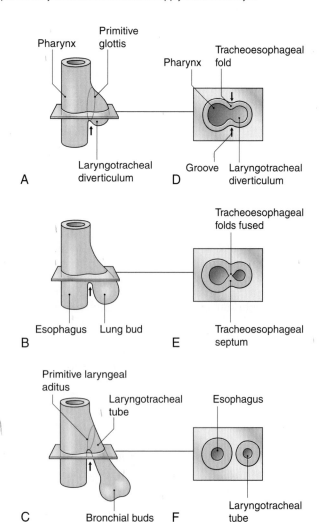

Figure 20-2. The tracheoesophageal septum evolves and separates the foregut into the laryngotracheal tube and the esophagus during the fourth week of embryonic development. (A-C) are longitudinal views, with corresponding cross-sectional views represented in (D-F).

morphogenetic mechanisms that have been suggested by various developmental biologists.

In the respiratory tap water theory, the respiratory diverticulum arises as a ventral outgrowth from the foregut and rapidly elongates to form the trachea, leading to the separation of the respiratory and gastrointestinal tracts. The mesenchyme that comes to lie between the two tracts is believed to constitute the septum.[2] It is also suggested that the point of bifurcation between the trachea and esophagus remains fixed at a constant somatic-vertebral level while the trachea descends.

Another theory suggests that separation of the foregut occurs due to fusion of the lateral walls of the foregut rather than due to an actual septum, and the fusion progresses in a caudorostral manner.[7]

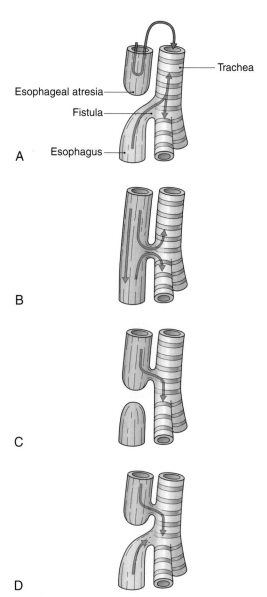

Figure 20-3. Tracheoesophageal fistulas. Ninety percent of cases are represented in (**A**) with esophageal atresia. Arrows indicate flow of luminal contents; it can be seen that in all but (**C**) the distal tracheoesophageal communication will lead to rapid intestinal accumulation of air. The "H" type represented in (**B**) will often not present in the neonatal period (with no oral intake possible and an attempt at nasogastric tube passage being unsuccessful, as in the other types), more usually presenting as a chronic aspiration syndrome.

In the foregut fold theory, yet another proposed mechanism, separation occurs as a result of development of three foregut folds: the laryngeal or anterocranial fold, the pharyngoesophageal or dorsal fold, and the tracheoesophageal or inferior fold. These folds approximate, leading to tracheoesophageal separation.[4,6]

GENETIC AND MOLECULAR ASPECTS OF TRACHEOESOPHAGEAL DEVELOPMENT

The characterization of human genetic disorders and development of teratogenic models with tracheoesophageal malformations[8] support the role of genetic and molecular mechanisms underlying these malformations. An ever increasing number of molecular pathways responsible for normal foregut patterning and differentiation are being elucidated.

The Sonic Hedgehog signaling pathway comprises the *Shh* glycoprotein and other downstream mediators that have multiple patterning roles in the developing embryo. Dorsoventral switch in *Shh* expression in the developing foregut has been found to be crucial for normal tracheoesophageal separation, and *Shh*–/– mice demonstrate a hypoplastic proximal esophagus that is not separated from the trachea.[9] Further, the Glioblastoma transcription factors (*Gli*), which are expressed in the mesoderm, also mediate hedgehog signaling in the gut. *Gli* mutant mice demonstrate hypoplastic foregut structures, further highlighting the importance of endo-mesodermal interaction during esophageal development.[10] Mutations in *Foxf1*[11] and *Hox C4*,[12] other transcriptional targets of *Shh*, are also associated with abnormal development of esophagus. *HoxD13* mutations have been recently described in a patient with VACTERL association.[12]

Although a detailed description of all the genes and molecular pathways known to be involved in development of the foregut is beyond the scope of the chapter, a brief description of genes/molecular pathways discovered by knockout studies in mice and chick embryos is presented in Table 20-1.

In humans, single-gene and chromosomal disorders that are associated with tracheoesophageal malformations are also

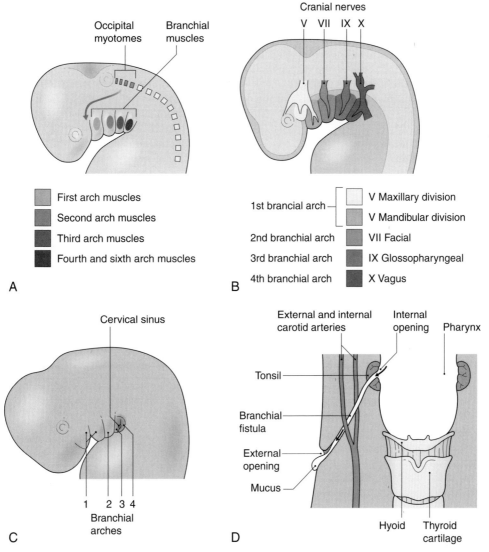

Figure 20-4. The branchial muscles, nervous supply and arches are represented in (**A**), (**B**), and (**C**), respectively, at 4 to 5 weeks' gestation. (**D**) shows the development of the pharynx, derived from pouches 2 and 3 with neuromuscular supply from branchial arches 2 and 3. The muscularis externa of the upper esophagus is derived from the distal branchial arches.

being increasingly described. A brief summary is presented in Table 20-2.[7]

ANATOMY

From this developmental discussion, it is understood that the esophagus becomes a structure that develops into a long muscular tube starting at the level of the lower cricoid cartilage border and sixth cervical vertebra, then descending mostly anterior to the vertebral column and through the superior and posterior mediastina. Given the juxtaposition of the esophagus to many mediastinal structures, including mediastinal and hilar lymph nodes, the possibility of linear endosonographic needle biopsies of these has been a breakthrough in the diagnosis of such pathologies as tuberculosis, sarcoid, and malignancy.[18] The esophagus then traverses the diaphragm at the level of the 10th thoracic vertebra and ends at the gastric cardia at the level of the 11th thoracic vertebra (Figure 20-5). The tube also bends in an anterior and posterior plane to follow the cervical and thoracic curvatures of the vertebral column (Figure 20-6). It has four narrow areas during its passage; these may be relevant to endoscopists, but are usually easily traversed: at its commencement at the oropharyngeal junction, where crossed by the aortic arch, where crossed by the left main bronchus, and, finally, where it traverses the diaphragm (see Figure 20-5). Other anatomic relationships can be seen in these figures. Emerging from the right crus of the diaphragm slightly left of the midline, in older children, as in adults, there is a short intra-abdominal portion (Figure 20-7). This portion

is absent in infants, and this is important in the pathogenesis of GER: the intra-abdominal portion, exposed to the relatively higher pressure of the abdominal cavity, compared with the lower (and during inspiration negative) pressure within the thoracic cavity, acts as an important "physiologic sphincter" or antireflux phenomenon (Figure 20-8). This is one part of the reason why infants have a much greater incidence of GER. It is also clear that the position of insertion of the esophagus into the stomach may be a contributory factor for GER in infants. In adults and older children, the insertion is much more oblique than the comparatively straight insertion in infants. Other anatomic factors invoked to explain the presence or absence of a sphincteric mechanism include reinforcement by the right crus of the circular muscle fibers at the junction of the esophagus and diaphragm (a factor not supported by one group)[19]; the phrenicoesophageal ligament, which is a layer of connective tissue extending from the inferior diaphragmatic surface and blending with the interfascicular septa and submucosa of the esophagus; the effects of spiral and longitudinal muscle; and various mucosal folds at the gastroesophageal junction. Hence some structures may exert a "physiologic sphincteric" control that may be compromised in the infant as anatomy matures; however, this remains poorly understood, and the main mechanism for infantile GER is thought more likely to be due to inappropriate relaxation of the gastroesophageal junction (see later discussion). It is therefore interesting to postulate how antireflux procedures such as open, laparoscopic, or even now endoscopic fundoplications work, given the lack of clear understanding of the reasons for GER.[20]

Vasculature supply is from the regional arteries such as the inferior thyroid branch of the thyrocervical trunk, descending aorta, bronchial arteries, left gastric branch of the celiac artery, and left phrenic artery. Veins drain in a similar longitudinal way to the inferior thyroid veins, the azygos vein, and left gastric vein. This left gastric vein is the most important of the portosystemic communications, and raised portal pressure will therefore lead to esophageal varices.

Nerve supply is considered further in the later section on physiology. In short, the parasympathetic is from the vagal and the sympathetic from the cervical and thoracic sympathetic trunks and greater splanchnic nerves. These form plexi between the two layers of the muscular coat and a second submucous plexus. This is shown in a cross-sectional diagram along with the layers of the esophagus that roughly translate to those in the rest of the gut (Figure 20-9)—except that the upper third of

TABLE 20-1. Mouse Genes Associated With Tracheoesophageal Malformations

Gene	Function	Foregut Phenotype
Nkx2.1[10]	Transcription factor	Undivided tracheoesophagus
Tbx4[15]	Affects Nkx 2.1 expression	Hypoplastic lungs; TEF
Sox2a[16]	HMG type transcriptional regulator	Anophthalmia-esophageal-genital syndrome
Nog[17]	BMP antagonist	TEF
RAR α/β₂[13]	Retinoic acid receptor	Undivided esophagotrachea

BMP, bone morphogenetic protein; HMG, high mobility group; TEF, tracheoesophageal fistula.

TABLE 20-2. Human Chromosomal and Single-Gene Disorders Associated With Esophageal Malformations

Name	Gene	Locus	Esophageal Defect
Anophthalmia- esophageal-genital	SOX2	3q26.3-g27	Laryngotracheoesophageal cleft
Feingold syndrome	MYCN	2p24.1	Esophageal atresia/TEF
CHARGE	CHD7	8q12	Esophageal atresia/TEF
Fanconi	FANCC	9p22.3	Esophageal atresia/TEF
Opitz	MID1	Xp22	Laryngotracheoesophageal cleft
Pallister-Hall	GLI3	7p13	Laryngotracheoesophageal cleft
Trisomies 21,13,18			Esophageal atresia/TEF
3p25 deletion			Esophageal atresia/TEF
5p15 deletion			Esophageal atresia/TEF
17q22q23.3 deletion			Esophageal atresia/TEF
13q34 deletion			Esophageal atresia/TEF
22q11.2 deletion			Esophageal atresia/TEF

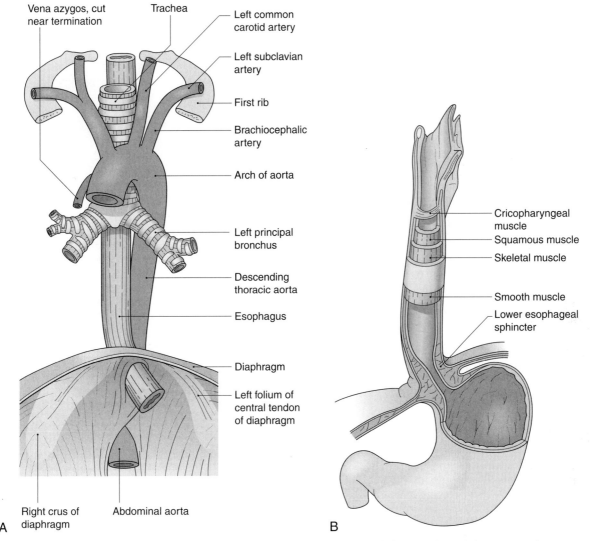

Figure 20-5. **(A,B)** Esophageal relationships in the posterior mediastinum and abdomen with muscle layers exposed.

the esophagus has a striated muscle layer, and the epithelium of the esophagus is nonkeratinized and stratified compared with that in other parts of the gut – leading to comparisons being drawn between cutaneous eczema and allergic esophagitis.[21] The recent development of endosonography has allowed differentiation of these seven layers at endoscopy (Figure 20-10), with identification of submucosal and muscle layer pathology in entities such as eosinophilic esophagitis.[22] At endoscopy, it is normally possible to biopsy only the mucosa and part of the submucosa, unless jumbo biopsy forceps are used, as is advocated in the Seattle protocol for the accurate detection of intestinal metaplasia signifying Barrett's esophagus.[23] Macroscopically the mucosa shows thickened folds that disappear on distention, except in the presence of edema, and this appearance may alert the endoscopist to the possibility of chronic esophagitis (Figure 20-11). If circumferential furrows on abnormally pale mucosa are detected, this may point to eosinophilic esophagitis (Figure 20-12). Histologic examination of the mucosal biopsy may allow conclusions to be drawn regarding the presence of GER and esophagitis. The site of biopsy should be above the distal 15% of the esophagus to avoid confusion with normal variation.[24] Biopsies should include epithelium, lamina propria,

and muscularis mucosae and should be oriented in a perpendicular plane to maximize diagnostic yield, such as evaluating properly the thickness of the basal zone, vascular ingrowth, and elongation of the stromal papillae. For definitive diagnosis, the presence of two of these three features is preferable; this will not be possible with poorly oriented tissue.[25,26] In an adult study, failure to use well-defined histologic criteria resulted in only 50% sensitivity for diagnosing esophagitis.[27] Elongation of stromal papillae is a useful indicator of reflux, and basal zone hyperplasia is defined when the papillae are more than 25% of the entire thickness of the epithelium; when more than 50%, the papillae are considered to be elongated[26,28,29] (Figure 20-13).

Anatomic variations from normal were partly dealt with in the earlier section on development of the esophagus. Tracheoesophageal fistulas, esophageal stenoses and atresia, and congenital webs were explained previously, but other abnormalities may occur, for instance rings. Two types of ring occur: the Schatzki ring, which is a submucosal fibrous thickening at the squamocolumnar junction and by far the more common, producing symptoms according to the degree of narrowness (Figure 20-14); and the muscular ring, accounting for 2 to 3% of all rings, which is a high-pressure zone of muscular

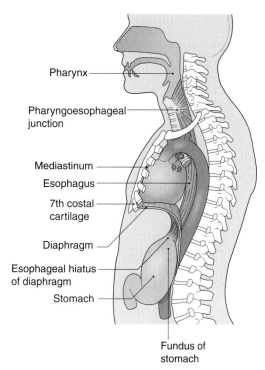

Figure 20-6. The esophagus descends posterior to the trachea and bends in a posterior and then anterior fashion to follow the contours of the cervical and thoracic vertebral columns.

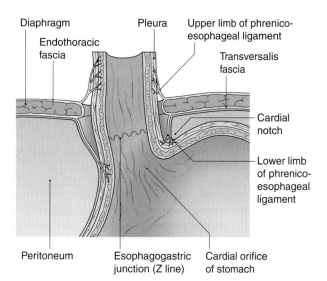

Figure 20-7. The upward movement of the esophagus is limited by the upper limb of the phrenicoesophageal ligament, which connects the esophagus flexibly to the diaphragm. The intra-abdominal portion of the esophagus is much shorter in the infant.

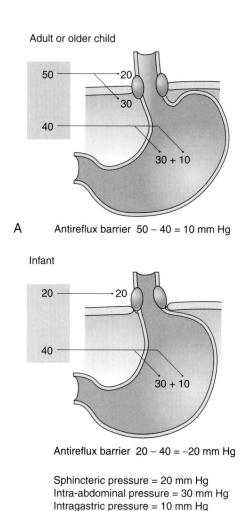

Adult or older child

A   Antireflux barrier 50 – 40 = 10 mm Hg

Infant

Antireflux barrier 20 – 40 = –20 mm Hg

Sphincteric pressure = 20 mm Hg
Intra-abdominal pressure = 30 mm Hg
Intragastric pressure = 10 mm Hg
B   (especially postprandial)

Figure 20-8. (**A**) Importance of the intra-abdominal portion of the esophagus in the maintenance of a pressure gradient to aid in the antireflux barrier. (**B**) The absence of this in an infant can be seen to predict the possibility of reflux.

hypertrophy, present at the junction of the uppermost portion of the lower esophageal sphincter with the distal esophagus. Webs are usually found in the upper third of the esophagus and may be due to iron deficiency (Plummer-Vinson), in which case they usually resolve with iron replenishment, although in practice most are ruptured at endoscopy performed for dysphagia. Diverticuli incorporate all layers of the esophagus and are of variable etiology. Pulsion (or epiphrenic) diverticuli occur in the distal third of the esophagus and are usually due to motor disorders such as diffuse esophageal spasm or achalasia; such

a diverticulum would be a contraindication to pneumatic dilation. Traction diverticuli, due to traction from a mediastinal lymph node usually in tuberculosis, occur in the middle third and are rare in childhood. Pseudodiverticuli occur rarely, as does Zenker's diverticulum, which is not a true diverticulum but a pressure-induced outpouching resulting from incoordination between pharyngeal contraction and relaxation of the upper esophageal sphincter as it passes through the cricopharyngeal muscle. The outpouching may become large enough extrinsically to compress the esophageal lumen, and it is important not to enter it by accident on endoscopic esophageal intubation as, unlike other diverticuli, it is made up only of mucosa and is therefore easily perforated. Occasionally esophageal polyps can occur and are either benign or inflammatory.

PHYSIOLOGY

Ontogeny of Esophageal Motor Function

The three components necessary to produce mature esophageal motor function are:
- An integrated enteric and autonomic neural system
- The inherent rhythmicity of smooth muscle
- Initial propagation of the peristaltic wave by the coordination of striated muscle

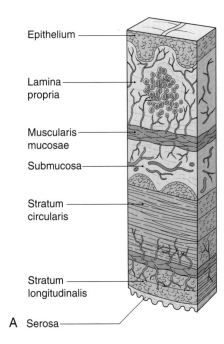

Epithelium

Lamina propria

Muscularis mucosae

Submucosa

Stratum circularis

Stratum longitudinalis

A Serosa

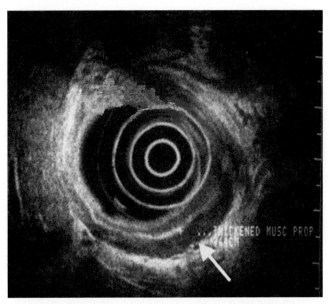

Figure 20-10. Endosonographic appearance of the esophagus showing the seven layers differentiated, corresponding to those seen in Figure 20-9. In this case, a thickened muscularis propria can be seen (arrow).

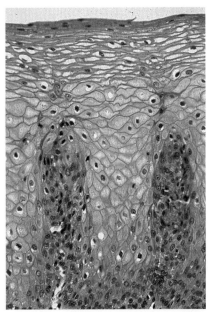

B

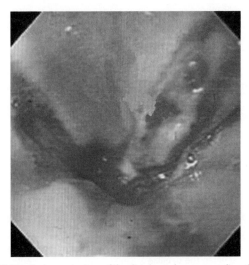

Figure 20-11. Endoscopic view of the distal esophagus revealing thickened folds resulting from edema, often a sign of chronic esophagitis. (*See plate section for color.*)

Figure 20-9. (A) Diagrammatic cross-section of the esophagus. **(B)** Histologic view of the normal esophagus (high-resolution image). Stratified squamous epithelium with mature squamous cells containing abundant clear (glycogen-rich) cytoplasm, and beneath, immature basal cells with little cytoplasm form a basophilic layer that is one to three cells in thickness. The invaginations of lamina propria form vascular papillae that extend into the epithelium for a distance equal to half of the epithelial thickness. Figure courtesy Ana Bennett, MD.

Like smooth muscle, the components of the enteric nervous system develop early in fetal life (Figure 20-15); in fact, as early as 12 weeks' gestation, however, it is much later that the integration with mature control of the smooth muscle by the enteric nervous system occurs.[30]

The previously simplistic understanding of the contradictory excitatory parasympathetic cholinergic pathways mediated by the vagal nerve, and the inhibitory sympathetic adrenergic control acting together to alter esophageal and intestinal smooth muscle activity via the submucosal and myenteric plexi

(Figure 20-16), has had to be adapted in the light of the recent, more in-depth, understanding of the complex processes at work in gut movement. These include the identification of a network of complex intrinsic innervation within the gut that begins and ends there. The intrinsic nerves of the submucosal and myenteric plexi are now known to be nonadrenergic noncholinergic (NANC) fibers, which contain a wide variety of neurotransmitters and are not involved solely with transmitting autonomic signals (see Figure 20-16).

Localized mechanical or chemical stimulation of the smooth muscle or stretch of the muscularis externa will elicit contraction above and relaxation below the point of stimulation. A stretch-sensitive neuron with connections in the myenteric plexus, and a chemosensitive or mechanosensitive neuron with connections in the submucosal plexus, may both be stimulated; this may result in ascending excitation (mediated by acetylcholine and substance P) and descending inhibition (mediated by

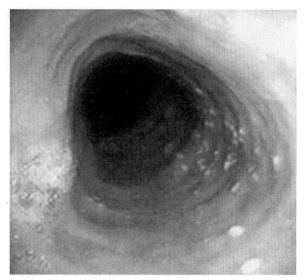

Figure 20-12. Endoscopic view of the distal esophagus revealing circumferential furrows, a sign of eosinophilic esophagitis. (*See plate section for color.*)

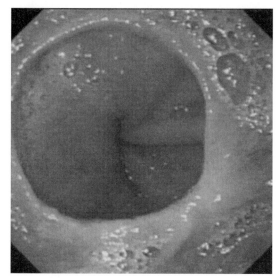

Figure 20-14. Endoscopic view of the distal esophagus revealing a Schatzki ring. (*See plate section for color.*)

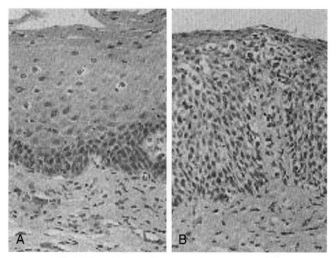

Figure 20-13. (A,B) Histologic cross-section of esophagus. Elongation of stromal papillae (P) is a useful indicator of reflux, and basal zone hyperplasia is defined when the papillae are more than 25% of the entire thickness of the epithelium; when more than 50%, the papillae are considered to be elongated.

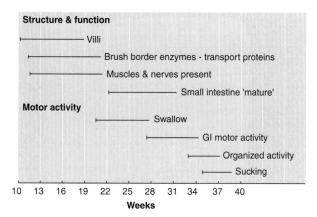

Figure 20-15. Ontogeny of intestinal function with gestational age.

vasoactive intestinal peptide [VIP] and nitric oxide) of contraction of the smooth muscle of the muscularis externa. Stimuli to the mucosa evoke release of serotonin (5-hydroxytryptamine; 5-HT) from enterochromaffin cells in the mucosa. Sensory neurons are simulated by 5-HT. The myenteric stretch receptors, however, respond directly to stretch. These sensory neurons then release intermediary substances, mainly calcitonin gene-related peptide, that act on the neurons within the myenteric and submucosal plexi, thus controlling motility of that portion of the gastrointestinal tract. This type of control is typical for each portion of the tract and is shown in Figure 20-16. The interaction of the local and central neural circuits involved in the control of esophageal motility is represented in Figure 20-17. The esophageal musculature, both striated and smooth, is innervated by branches of the vagal nerve.

The enteric neurons migrate from the neural crest. After a period of colonization, the first neurons to develop are serotonergic and cholinergic, then adrenergic and peptidinergic

(although the last not in the esophagus). Until quite late in fetal development, the neurons remain phenotypically undifferentiated, and it may be that external influences in fetal environment alter the developmental pathway (e.g., sympathomimetic use in preterm labor).

It should be mentioned that the central nervous system may play a part in overall esophageal motility, as evidenced by the derangement to normal esophageal peristalsis that occurs in neonates with peripartum cerebral insults leading to cerebral palsy.[31]

The neurohormonal influences on esophageal motility and lower esophageal sphincter (LES) pressure and function include substance P (increases LES pressure and motility), VIP (inhibits esophageal tone), and inducible nitric oxide synthase (iNOS; may decrease resting tone and allow LES relaxation) and may be altered by inflammation. Inhibitory neurotransmitter production is integral to LES relaxation, and the NANC neurotransmitter nitric oxide (NO) has received attention in animal[32] and human[33,34] studies. VIP is another candidate undergoing investigation, and the importance of the ontogeny of neuropeptides in the human fetus and infant is becoming increasingly apparent.[35] The complex interaction of the neural-enteric-hormonal axis has been the focus of recent work in such conditions as allergic and eosinophilic esophagitis, suggesting a role for other

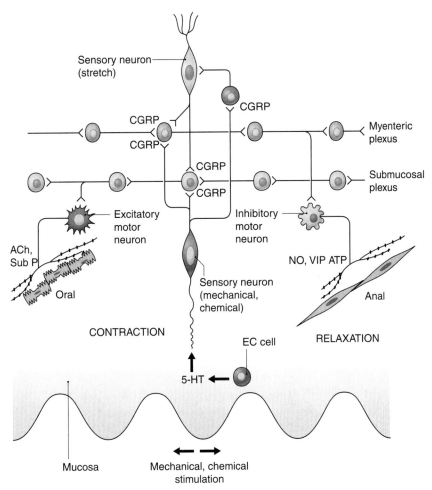

Figure 20-16. Mechanical or chemical stimulation of intestinal mucosa or stretch of the muscularis externa typically elicits contraction proximal to, and relaxation distal to, the point of stimulation or distention. Either of these stimuli leads to activation of ascending (oral) excitation or descending (anal) inhibition of contraction of the muscularis externa smooth muscle. Mucosal stimuli lead enterochromaffin cells (EC) to release 5-hydroxytryptamine (5-HT), which stimulates these sensory neurons, whereas myenteric stretch receptors respond directly to stretch. Having received one or other stimulus, the sensory neurons release predominantly calcitonin gene-related peptide (CGRP) on to interneurons in the enteric plexi. ACh, acetylcholinesterase; Sub P, substance P; VIP, vasoactive intestinal peptide; NO, nitric oxide.

inflammation-induced mediators in the pathogenesis of the associated LES dysfunction (e.g., interleukin [IL]-5, eotaxin, eosinophil-derived neurotoxin).[21,36,37] Of course, this is in the pathologic state, and this chapter is confined to discussion of the normal.

Fetal and Neonatal Motor Activity (Sucking and Swallowing)

The most self-evident function of the esophagus is that of transporting boluses from the mouth to the stomach by the process of voluntary and then involuntary propulsion. This has been observed as early as 16 weeks' gestation, and volumes swallows increase from around 2-7 mL/day at this age to 13-16 mL/day at 20 weeks and 450 mL/day at term.[38] Sucking, however, does not occur effectively until around 34 weeks' gestation, with implications for the institution of normal feeding in the preterm neonate. This is mainly due to the lack of maturation of the complex interactions required to produce coordinated oropharyngoesophageal phasic swallowing. Resultant failure of feeding with pooling in the pharynx and possible aspiration may then occur if feeding is attempted too early in life. Initially sucking is simply mouthing of the teat and is ineffective.

Subsequently bursts of 1-second interval sucking, four to seven at a time occur, associated with a swallow. Then, at around 34 weeks' gestation, 30-second bursts of sucking at 2-minute intervals develop, coordinated with swallowing.[39] At the same time esophageal contractions develop from disorganized tertiary contractions to coordinated propagating peristaltic waves initiated by swallowing.[40] All of these maturational changes are likely to be due to the alterations noted earlier in smooth muscle activity and enteric nerve fetal/neonatal development.[41] Nevertheless, the influence of nonnutritive sucking on esophageal and intestinal motor activity, and consequent enteral feeding tolerance, suggests that this can be manipulated, at least partially, by learned experience.[42]

Lower Esophageal Sphincter Development

Intraluminal pressure and postconceptional age are linked, and a number of perfused manometric systems have been used to produce data in support of this.[43] Effective sphincter pressure was shown to rise by a factor of 4 between 27 weeks' gestation and term. Interestingly, resting esophageal pressure does not change, but the effective sphincter pressure of the LES (difference between pressure in the fundus of the stomach and that

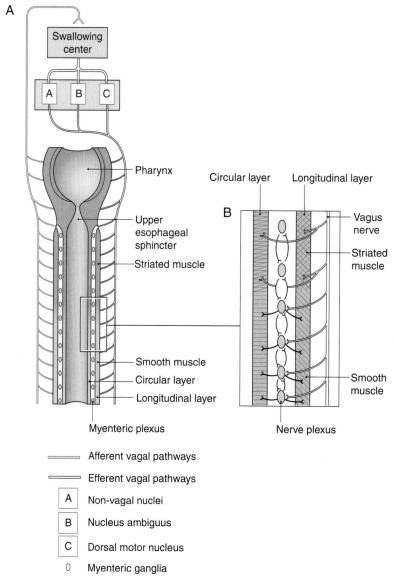

Figure 20-17. Local and central neural circuits controlling esophageal motility. (**A**) Vagal nerve branches provide motor neurons, and also sensory feedback to the swallowing center via vagal afferents. (**B**) Vagal visceral motor neurons innervate the lower esophageal smooth muscle, terminating mainly on the myenteric plexi neurons. These are both excitatory and inhibitory.

in the high-pressure area of the lower esophagus) rises significantly in line with postconceptional age: 3.8 mm Hg at 27 weeks' gestation, 8.5 mm Hg at 31 weeks, 12.2 mm Hg at 35 weeks, and 18.1 mm Hg at 37 weeks and above.[43] This suggests that the resting esophageal pressure itself is not the rate-limiting factor for the problem of GER. This study was undertaken with nasogastric tubes in situ; this may or may not have influenced the results. More recently, combined low-volume water perfusion manometric, pH, intraluminal esophageal impedance techniques have been employed in this population, and similar results have been obtained. This elegant experiment in a small number of preterm neonates (35 to 37 weeks postmenstruation), combined with assessment of gastric emptying by ^{13}C-Na octanoate breath test, showed unequivocally that transient lower esophageal relaxation episodes (TLESRs) are the factor that allows GER to occur; indeed, GER was also shown to be worse in the left lateral position than the right lateral position, in keeping with previous clinical studies. In addition, this work showed that gastric emptying was faster in the right lateral

position, leading to the conclusion that gastric emptying has little or no influence on GER in this population.[44] Development of effective gastric emptying, especially from the fundus, may have an influence on esophageal clearance.

Swallowing in the Normal Infant and Child

The process of swallowing consists of four phases for liquids and solids alike: oral preparatory, oral, pharyngeal and esophageal. Only the latter two are considered here (Figure 20-18).

Pharyngeal Phase

The pharyngeal phase begins with the production of a swallow and the elevation of the soft palate to close off the nasopharynx, and consists of peristaltic contraction of the pharyngeal constrictors to propel the bolus through the pharynx. Simultaneous closure of the larynx protects against airway penetration of the bolus. Simultaneously there is complete and automatic closure of the glottis, and the epiglottis is brought down over

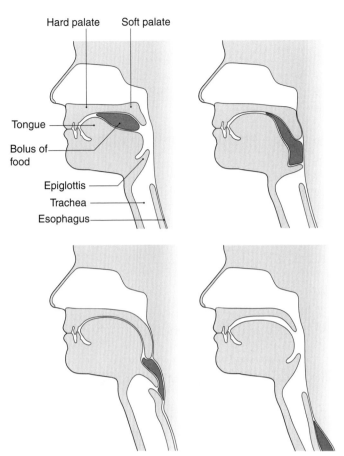

Figure 20-18. A bolus being transported through the four phases of swallowing.

the glottis, thereby deflecting the bolus laterally and posteriorly toward the upper esophageal sphincter (UES). With high-speed video fluoroscopy, four sequential events associated with laryngeal closure have been noted:

1. Adduction of the true vocal cords associated with the horizontal approximation of the arytenoids cartilages
2. Vertical approximation of the arytenoids to the base of the epiglottis
3. Laryngeal elevation
4. Epiglottic descent

The other major function of the laryngopharyngeal space is in eliciting a protective cough reflex, precipitated by a number of vagally mediated receptors (chemo-, thermo-, etc.) that detect the presence of potentially damaging noxious stimuli and cause laryngeal closure and a cough. This is becoming increasingly important to gastroenterologists as a phenomenon, with the recent appreciation of the pathologic importance of laryngopharyngeal reflux from the stomach in symptoms such as recurrent cough, hoarseness, and dysphonia. An increased resting pressure of the cricopharyngeal muscle is necessary to prevent pharyngeal penetration of the retrograde esophageal bolus.

The dynamics of UES function have been shown to be dependent on bolus size in adults, with increased opening size and prolongation of opening occurring with increase in bolus size.[45] Once complete bolus transfer through the UES, policed by coordinated cricopharyngeal relaxation and laryngeal closure, has occurred and the bolus has been transported into the esophagus by continuation of the peristaltic stripping

action of the pharyngeal muscles, the esophageal phase of swallowing begins.

Esophageal Phase

Swallow-induced automatic esophageal peristalsis usually propagates at 2 to 4 cm/s and will traverse the pediatric esophagus in around 6 to 10 seconds.[46,47] The peristalsis is more likely to traverse the entire esophageal length if the bolus is solid.[48] Peristalsis in the striated upper third of the esophageal muscular wall seems to be similar to that in the distal two thirds, which is smooth muscle, and the esophageal phase of swallowing is controlled by the swallowing center. Once the bolus has passed the UES, a reflex action causes the sphincter to constrict, then the primary peristaltic wave begins just below the UES. If this primary peristaltic wave does not clear the bolus completely, the continued distention of the esophagus initiates another peristaltic wave, termed secondary peristalsis (Figure 20-19). Real-time assessment of swallowed bolus transport is now possible with a new technique called intraluminal impedance; this can be combined with pH analysis and now even long-term manometry with low-flow water perfusion as part of the catheter.[49]

Lower Esophageal Sphincter Function

Differences in the function of the LES have been investigated.[50,51] This is an area that is tonically contracted at rest, at a pressure of about 20 mm Hg, and mediated mainly by vagal cholinergic fibers (see Figure 20-8) (although stimulation of the sympathetic nerves to the sphincter also causes contraction). Relaxation occurs consequent to an esophageal peristaltic wave. Hence the LES is innervated by both vagal excitatory fibers and vagal inhibitory fibers; increased activity of the inhibitory fibers and decreased activity of the excitatory fibers is associated with LES relaxation, and the opposite occurs as the LES regains its tone (Figure 20-20). Inhibitory neurotransmitter production is integral to LES relaxation, and the NANC neurotransmitter NO has received attention in animal[32] and human[33,34] studies. VIP is another candidate undergoing investigation, and the importance of the ontogeny of neuropeptides in the human fetus and infant is becoming increasingly apparent.[35] Rather than a "weak" LES in infants, it is more likely that a combination of anatomic relationships of the LES precluding effective pressure generation, and inappropriate LES relaxation, is responsible for infantile GER and its subsequent age-related improvement.[52,53] In adults, 90% of the refluxate is cleared in seconds and the remainder is neutralized by subsequent swallows.[54] Efficiency of esophageal clearance is therefore vitally important in the genesis of esophagitis. Propagation of a peristaltic wave in the esophagus with pressure generation and the contemporaneous LES relaxation is shown in Figure 20-19. The LES opens with the initiation of esophageal peristalsis.

Work exists suggesting that acid exposure of the distal esophagus induces dysmotility in pediatric patients,[55] allowing the potential for a "vicious cycle" of LES dysfunction to GER to LES dysmotility to further GER to esophagitis and back to LES dysmotility (Figure 20-21), but it is still not clear how an inflamed esophagus further impairs esophageal tone or motility. However, emerging work suggests a role for IL-5 and eotaxin in allergic neurohumoral modification and possible inappropriate relaxation of the gastroesophageal junction, with an interrelationship with mast cell degranulation and histamine release to

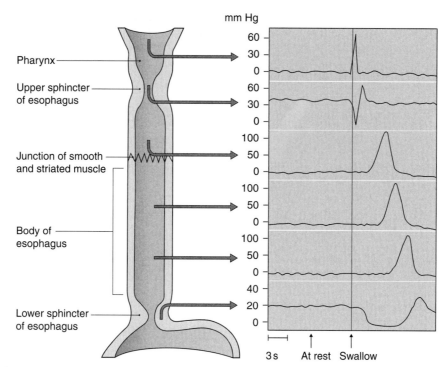

Figure 20-19. Swallowing pressures with timed relaxation of the upper and lower esophageal sphincters.

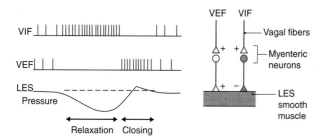

Figure 20-20. The lower esophageal sphincter (LES) is innervated by excitatory (VEF) and inhibitory (VIF) fibers from the vagus. Relaxation of the LES occurs with an increased activity of inhibitory fiber action potentials and a corresponding decrease in the action potential frequency from the excitatory fibers. The opposite occurs as the LES returns to resting tone.

afferent, then efferent, neurons that control TLESRs.[56] iNOS, which is markedly up-regulated in gastrointestinal inflammatory conditions such as Crohn's disease, is important in relaxation of the LES during TLESRs – which are the single most common mechanism underlying GER – but in one study was not up-regulated in the inflamed pediatric esophagus.[57] However, other workers have suggested an increased release of NO in the inflamed esophagus in children.[58] Other factors that affect clearance are posture-gravity interactions; volume, size, and content of a meal, for example breast milk[59,60]; defective peristalsis of the esophagus; gastric emptying; and increased noxiousness of refluxate.

PATHOPHYSIOLOGY

Mucosal Immunology and Inflammation

From the anatomic and physiologic discussion in this chapter it can be seen that the esophagus is relatively quiescent in the nonpathologic state from the immunologic standpoint, not having a major function as part of the largest immune organ in

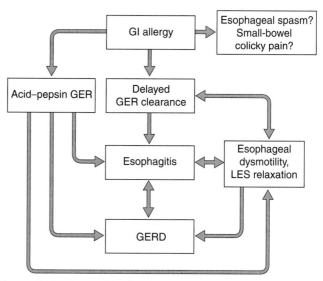

Figure 20-21. The relationships of gastroesophageal reflux (GER), physiology, allergy, and esophagitis in the child. GERD, gastroesophageal reflux disease; LES, lower esophageal sphincter.

the body – the gut. The esophagus has no Brunner's glands or Peyer's patches involved in antigen recognition and presentation, for instance, but if the epithelial barrier is breached, then immunologic functions can occur. Equally, in the pathologic state induced by T-cell-mediated allergy in the small bowel, homing of inflammatory cells to the esophagus can occur in the absence of luminal or epithelial damage.[21]

Acid, particularly when combined with pepsin, which, it is now realized, is still active up to around pH 5.5 or 6, is known to cause severe esophagitis in animals and humans.[54-57] Even an infant of 24 weeks' gestation in an intensive care setting has the ability to reduce intragastric pH to less than 2.[58] Pepsin plays a critical role in esophagitis as a result of acidic and possibly nonacidic refluxate. Animal work in dogs and rabbits has shown that the infusion of hydrochloric acid alone caused no damage, but that in combination with low concentrations of pepsin at pH below 2, severe esophagitis resulted.[59,60] Proteolysis may allow deeper penetration of harmful refluxate, and the simple notion that acid causes epithelial damage must therefore be questioned in favor of a more complex interplay of a number of noxious stimuli in the pathogenesis of reflux esophagitis in infants and children.

Furthermore, the role of duodenogastroesophageal reflux (DGER) remains controversial[61,62] and has not, to date, been studied adequately in the pediatric population. What is clear from adult studies is that alkaline reflux does not correlate well with bile reflux, the former being attributable to reasons other than DGER, such as saliva, food, oral infection, or an obstructed esophagus.[63] In fact, in one study, bile acid DGER correlated well with acid reflux, and those with more severe esophagitis had greater exposure to the simultaneously damaging effects of acid and bile acids.[61] Perfusion studies of the rabbit esophagus have shown that conjugated bile acids in an acidic environment produce mucosal injury, whereas unconjugated bile acids and trypsin are more harmful at more neutral pH values (pH 5 to 8).[59] It is further suggested by animal work that the hydrochloric acid–pepsin damage may actually be attenuated by the presence in the esophagus of conjugated bile acids, but that if damage is done to the squamous epithelium, the un-ionized forms of conjugated bile acids at low pH may be allowed access to mucosal cells and cause damage by the dissolution of cell membranes and mucosal tight junctions.

Recently, however, the place of intraluminal ambulant esophageal pH measurement as the "gold standard" for investigation of GER has been challenged. Mainly because pH-directed GER diagnosis is obscured by postprandial neutralization of gastric contents after milk ingestion and by drugs,[64-66] other tests have been developed to detect pH-independent GER (e.g., ultrasonography, barium radiography, scintigraphy, external electrical impedance tomography, and manometry).[67-72] However, disadvantages of these methods include short-term applicability, high incidence of artifact due to body movement, and the need for unphysiologic nonambulant body positioning. A new pH-independent intraluminal esophageal impedance technique, which relies on the higher conductivity of a liquid bolus compared with esophageal muscular wall or air, has been validated in adults.[73,74] When applied to GER in infants with simultaneous pH measurement over prolonged periods, this intraluminal impedance technique has shown that 73% of all GER occurs during or in the first 2 hours after feeding; furthermore, it is pH neutral and will therefore be missed by pHmetry. Even during so-called fasting, 34% of reflux events were missed by pHmetry. Some 75% of GER reached proximally as far as the pharyngeal space, and this has far-reaching implications for the study of GER-associated respiratory phenomena.[66] The intraluminal technique may also allow evaluation of GER in conditions associated with gastric hypoacidity or in infants receiving antacid therapy; at present, H_2 antagonists and proton pump inhibitors must be stopped for 2 and 5 days, respectively, before pHmetry can be performed reliably. The clinical importance of DGER may become evident with the recent advent of a spectrophotometric device that detects bilirubin in the esophageal refluxate.

Although it is now clear that multiple food antigens may induce esophagitis,[75] the most common precipitant is cow's-milk protein. Standard endoscopic biopsy and histology do not distinguish reliably between primary reflux esophagitis and the emerging clinical entity of cow's-milk-associated reflux esophagitis. This variant of cow's-milk allergy (CMA) appears to be a particularly common manifestation in infancy, with symptoms indistinguishable from those of primary GER, but settling on an exclusion diet.[76] In a recent study an association between GER and CMA was noted in 59% of the patients, and although simultaneous milk challenge and esophageal pH monitoring was not found to be diagnostically helpful, a significant decline in the reflux index was seen after elimination of milk in the GER-CMA group.[77] Some differentiation from primary reflux has been suggested on the basis of the esophageal pH testing pattern and β-lactoglobulin antibody response, although the former has not been substantiated by more than one center.[21,78,79]

Esophageal mucosal eosinophilia has been described in both suspected cow's-milk-associated[21,76] and primary[80] reflux esophagitis, as well as in other conditions such as primary eosinophilic esophagitis.[81,82] Primary eosinophilic esophagitis has a reported prevalence of up to 40 per 100,000 population in parts of the United States, with other countries reporting similar figures.[83] The clinical significance of eosinophils and their role in the pathogenesis of mucosal injury is poorly understood and the subject of recent debate.[80,84,85] Some have suggested an active role for eosinophils in the inflammatory process of esophagitis and have supported this with the observation of activation of the eosinophils by electron-microscopic criteria.[86] In addition to dietary exclusion of cow's milk,[61,76-79] oral steroids can induce remission of symptoms with decreased mucosal eosinophilia,[81,82] suggesting a pathoetiologic role for eosinophils. In addition, mepolizumab, a monoclonal anti-IL-5 antibody, has been used with success in a person with eosinophilic esophagitis, suggesting a pivotal role for IL-5 in recruitment, trafficking, and possible activation of eosinophils in mucosal eosinophilic conditions such as this.[87] As well as eosinophils, intraepithelial T lymphocytes, known as cells with irregular nuclear contours (CINCs), have been implicated as markers of reflux esophagitis.[88,89] In adults, such cells are of memory phenotype and display activation markers, although little is known of their pediatric equivalents. Mast cells may also serve as markers of allergic-type reflux.

A variety of immunohistochemical markers have been used to examine the esophageal mucosa, including eotaxin, a recently described eosinophil-specific chemokine,[84] and markers of T-cell lineage and activation. Despite the mild histologic abnormality in cow's-milk protein-associated esophagitis, an increased expression of eotaxin colocalized with activated T lymphocytes to the basal and papillary epithelium has been shown,[21] distinguishing this from primary reflux esophagitis. The molecular basis of the eotaxin upregulation in cow's-milk-sensitive enteropathy (CMSE) is unknown. However, there is evidence from murine models of asthma that antigen-specific up-regulation of eotaxin expression can be induced by T cells and blocked by anti-CD3 monoclonal antibodies. This suggests the possibility of a distinct mechanism in CMSE, in which mucosal homing to the esophagus occurs for lymphocytes activated within the small intestine.[89-91] This may explain the seemingly counterintuitive finding of basal, as opposed to superficial, chemokine expression and the common occurrence of mucosal eosinophilia in this condition.[21] The esophageal motility disturbance of CMSE-associated esophagitis is thus suggested to occur as a neurologic consequence of the inflammatory infiltration induced from lamina propria vessels into the epithelial compartment.[36,85] This proposed mechanism contrasts with the current concept of luminally induced inflammation found in primary reflux esophagitis and is consistent with the characteristically delayed onset and chronic nature of cow's-milk-associated reflux esophagitis.

SUMMARY

At first glance, this part of the gut is different in many respects from its cousins in the gastrointestinal tract and may be thought to be fairly uninspiring. However, if one takes the time to look more closely, the esophagus can clearly be seen as a more complex organ with many more responsibilities than simply acting as a conduit for bolus passage from pharynx to stomach. We are now in possession of a much greater understanding of many of the etiologic mechanisms that cause pathology in the esophagus, and with that acquisition of knowledge has come the realization that apparently simple pathologies such as esophagitis may have contributions from many different avenues: abnormal anatomy, disordered physiology, induction of newly identified neurohumoral pathways, presence of excess inflammatory cytokines such as IL-5 and excess chemoattractants such as eotaxin, and complex interactions of all of these and others. The conditions affecting the esophagus are increasingly common in children, and this is not merely acquisition bias: clearly, the

explosion in allergic conditions has had an impact on this, and indeed, other diseases of apparently idiopathic etiology, such as eosinophilic esophagitis, are rapidly rising in incidence and hence prevalence.

REFERENCES

2. Zaw-Tun HA. The tracheoesophageal septum – fact or fantasy? Origin and development of the respiratory primordium and esophagus. Acta Anat 1982;114:1–21.
4. Kluth D, Steding G, Siedl W. The embryology of foregut malformations. J Pediatr Surg 1987;22:389–393.
6. Kluth D, Fiegel H. The embryology of the foregut. Semin Ped Surg 2003;12:3–9.
7. Ioannides AS, Copp A. Embryology of oesophageal atresia. Semin Ped Surg 2009;18:2–11.
9. Ionnides AS, Henderson DJ, Spitz L, et al. Role of Sonic hedgehog in the development of the trachea and oesophagus. J Pediatr Surg 2003;38:29–36.
10. Van Den Brink GR. Hedgehog signaling in development and homeostasis of the gastrointestinal tract. Physiol Rev 2007;87:1343–1375.
16. Que J, Okubo T, Goldenring JR, et al. Multiple dose dependent roles for Sox2 in the patterning and differentiation of anterior foregut. Development 2007;134:2521–2531.

See expertconsult.com for a complete list of references and the review questions for this chapter.

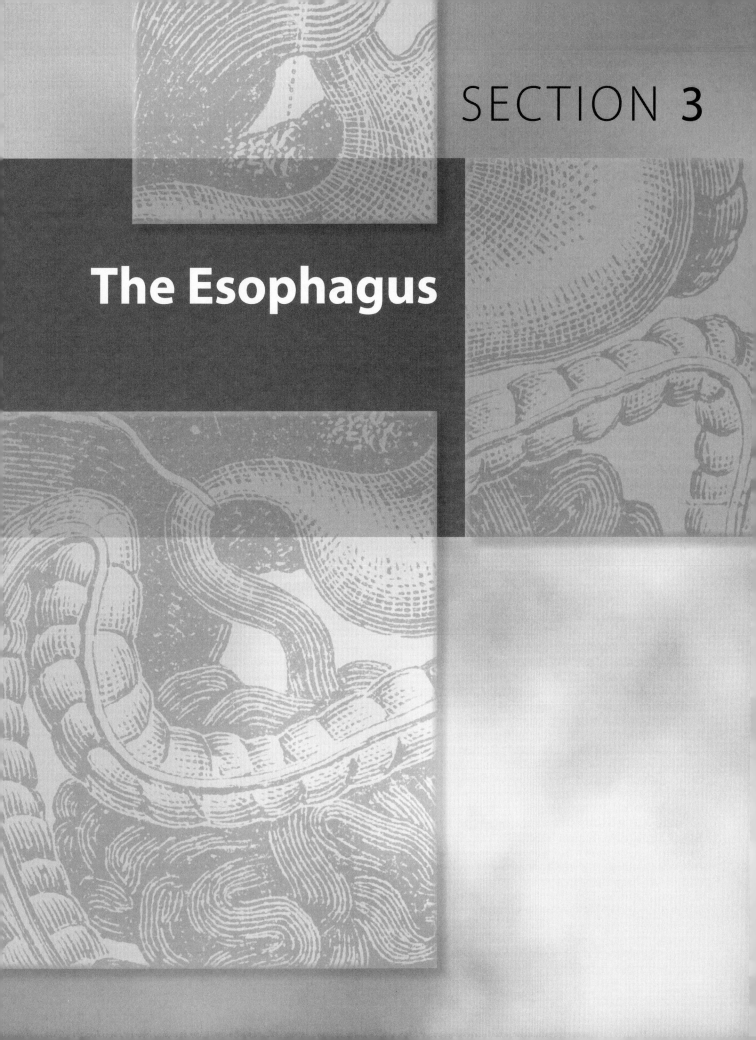

The Esophagus

SECTION 3

21 CONGENITAL MALFORMATIONS OF THE ESOPHAGUS

Steven W. Bruch • Arnold G. Coran

CONGENITAL LESIONS OF THE ESOPHAGUS

Congenital lesions of the esophagus fall into three categories: congenital esophageal stenosis, the variants of esophageal atresia and tracheoesophageal fistula, and laryngotracheoesophageal clefts.

CONGENITAL ESOPHAGEAL STENOSIS

Congenital esophageal stenosis presents in three variants; esophageal webs or diaphragms, fibromuscular stenosis, and stenosis due to cartilaginous tracheobronchial remnants. These lesions collectively are quite rare, occurring in 1 in 25,000 to 1 in 50,000 live births.[1] Most often, congenital esophageal stenosis presents as an isolated finding, but in 15 to 30% they are associated with other congenital anomalies.[2] Up to 8% of the babies with esophageal atresia and tracheoesophageal fistula have an associated distal congenital esophageal stenosis.[3] Other associated anomalies include cardiac defects, intestinal atresias, imperforate anus, and chromosomal abnormalities.

Clinical Manifestations and Diagnosis

Congenital esophageal stenosis may not manifest in the newborn period, because breast milk or formula passes through the stenotic area without difficulty. Symptoms often start at around 6 months of age when semisolid and solid foods are introduced into the diet. The babies then begin to regurgitate undigested foods and may develop recurrent respiratory infections due to aspiration. In unrecognized cases, the babies may present later with growth retardation. When these symptoms occur, babies are often studied with an esophagram that reveals the stenotic area and may show dilation of the esophagus proximal to the stenosis. The three variants give a different radiologic appearance. The esophageal diaphragms or webs are thin layers of tissue causing stenosis in the upper portion of the esophagus. The fibromuscular stenoses are thicker than the webs and tend to occur in the middle to lower esophagus. Cartilaginous remnants occur in the distal portion of the esophagus as shown in Figure 21-1. In a child with these radiologic findings and the appropriate clinical picture, the differential diagnosis would include achalasia and a stricture from gastroesophageal reflux disease. In order to make the distinction between these entities, additional work-up including endoscopy, manometrics, and 24-hour pH probe studies are useful. Recently, endoscopic ultrasound has been used to differentiate stenoses due to cartilaginous rests from those due to fibromuscular stenosis.[4]

Treatment

Therapy is dictated by the type of stenosis encountered. The thin proximal esophageal membrane or web can often be dilated at the time of endoscopy.[5] On occasion, these membranes require partial resection with electrocautery or laser through the endoscope followed by dilation.[6] The stenoses with cartilaginous remnants require resection and primary anastomosis, as dilation is not effective in this type of stenosis.[7] Fibromuscular stenosis can be dilated in most cases. A series from Japan used endoscopic ultrasound to differentiate fibromuscular stenosis from cartilaginous rests. Those with cartilaginous rests went on to surgery, and the children with fibromuscular stenosis were dilated. Ten of 13 children with fibromuscular stenoses were successfully dilated, and the remaining three required resection.[4] The exact location of the stenosis is often difficult to locate on the contrast studies. To find the stenotic area, it is helpful to place a Fogarty catheter past the stenosis, inflate the balloon, and pull back the catheter. Placing contrast in the esophagus will then verify the location of the stenosis. Intraoperatively, a lighted endoscope placed at the level of the stenosis aids in locating the stenosis, which is often impossible to accurately locate by palpation and inspection. The operative approach varies depending on the level of the stenosis. If the stenotic area is in the mid esophagus, the operative approach should be through a right thoracotomy, but if the stenosis is located in the distal esophagus, a left thoracotomy will provide the necessary exposure. The stenotic area of the esophagus is excised and a single-layer end-to-end anastomosis is performed. If the stenotic lesion is close to the gastroesophageal junction and resection may alter the antireflux mechanism, then a fundoplication should be added to the procedure.[1]

Outcome

Both dilation for webs and fibromuscular stenosis and resection for fibromuscular and cartilaginous remnant stenosis provide adequate relief of the stenosis. Compared to membranes or webs, fibromuscular stenosis required more frequent dilation over a longer period of time.[4] Postoperative dilations following resection of esophageal stenosis were required to prevent anastomotic strictures.[4,8]

ESOPHAGEAL ATRESIA AND TRACHEOESOPHAGEAL FISTULA

The treatment of esophageal atresia and tracheoesophageal fistula, which occurs in about 1 in 4000 live births, remains a challenge.[9] Since the first successful primary anastomosis by

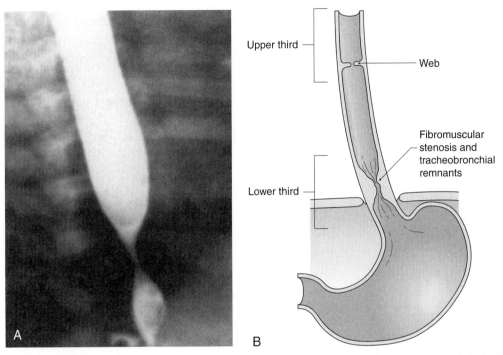

Figure 21-1. **(A)** Barium esophagram performed in a 1-month-old baby with dysphagia shows a congenital esophageal stenosis in the distal esophagus and proximal esophageal dilation. This is characteristic of a fibromuscular stenosis or a stenosis from a persistent cartilaginous remnant. **(B)** The usual location of the common forms of congenital esophageal stenosis: esophageal webs in the upper one third of the esophagus, and fibromuscular stenosis or persistent cartilaginous tracheobronchial remnants in the distal one third of the esophagus.

Haight in 1941,[10] improvements in surgical technique and neonatal care have increased the survival rate of babies born with esophageal atresia and tracheoesophageal fistula. Spitz et al. created a classification system in 1994 used to predict survival based on birth weight (greater or less than 1500 g) and the presence of associated complex anomalies, usually cardiac in nature.[11] In 2006, Spitz reexamined the survival data and found that the survival for babies with a birth weight greater than 1500 g and no cardiac abnormalities was similar in 1994 (97%) and 2006 (98.5%). However, the survival rates in babies who were small or had a major cardiac anomaly increased from 59% to 82%, and the survival rate in babies who were both small and had a major cardiac anomaly increased from 22% to 50% over the same time period.[12] In 2009, Okamoto refined the Spitz classification as depicted in Table 21-1.[13]

Anatomy

An understanding of the anatomy involved with each case of esophageal atresia and tracheoesophageal fistula is important when devising a treatment strategy. There have been several classification systems, but a description of each type is the easiest and most practical way to classify the five different types of esophageal atresia and tracheoesophageal fistula as shown in Figure 21-2. The most common configuration is esophageal atresia with a distal tracheoesophageal fistula. This configuration occurs in 86% of cases.[14] The proximal esophagus ends blindly in the upper mediastinum. The distal esophagus is connected to the tracheobronchial tree usually just above or at the carina. The second most common type is the isolated esophageal atresia without a tracheoesophageal fistula. This configuration occurs in 8% of cases.[14] The proximal esophagus ends blindly in the upper mediastinum, and the distal esophagus is

TABLE 21-1. Survival in Infants With Esophageal Atresia With or Without Tracheoesophageal Fistula Based on Birth Weight and Cardiac Anomalies

Class	Birth Weight	Major Cardiac Anomaly	Survival
I. Low risk	>2000 g	No	100%
II. Moderate risk	<2000 g	No	82%
III. Relatively high risk	>2000 g	Yes	72%
IV. High risk	<2000 g	Yes	27%

also blind ending and protrudes a varying distance above the diaphragm. The distance between the two ends is often too far to bring together shortly after birth. The third most common configuration, occurring in 4% of cases,[14] is a tracheoesophageal fistula without esophageal atresia. The esophagus extends in continuity to the stomach, but there is a fistula between the esophagus and the trachea. The fistula is usually located in the upper mediastinum running from a proximal orifice in the trachea to a more distal orifice in the esophagus. This is also known as an "H" type or "N" type tracheoesophageal fistula. Two more forms of esophageal atresia and tracheoesophageal fistula exist, both of which occur about 1% of cases.[14] These are esophageal atresia with both a proximal and distal tracheoesophageal fistula, and esophageal atresia with a proximal tracheoesophageal fistula. These two forms correspond to the first two forms described with the addition of a proximal fistula between the upper pouch and the trachea. A proximal fistula is often difficult to diagnose preoperatively even when bronchoscopy is performed, resulting[15] in the real incidence being higher than previously reported.[15] Again the esophageal atresia with proximal tracheoesophageal fistula, similar to its counterpart

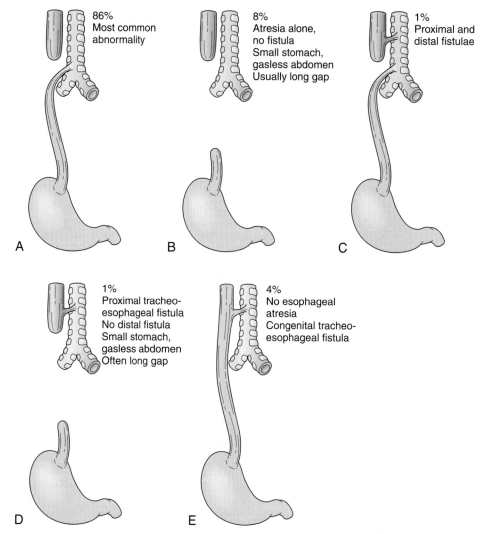

86%
Most common
abnormality

8%
Atresia alone,
no fistula
Small stomach,
gasless abdomen
Usually long gap

1%
Proximal and
distal fistulae

A   B   C

1%
Proximal tracheo-
esophageal fistula
No distal fistula
Small stomach,
gasless abdomen
Often long gap

4%
No esophageal
atresia
Congenital tracheo-
esophageal fistula

D   E

Figure 21-2. Types of esophageal atresia and tracheoesophageal fistula with rates of occurrence. (**A**) Esophageal atresia with distal tracheoesophageal fistula. (**B**) Isolated esophageal atresia. (**C**) Esophageal atresia with proximal and distal tracheoesophageal fistulas. (**D**) Esophageal atresia with proximal tracheoesophageal fistula. (**E**) H-type tracheoesophageal fistula.

without the proximal fistula, will have a long gap between the two ends of the esophagus, making it difficult to repair shortly after birth.

Associated Anomalies

As alluded to earlier, the main determinant of outcome in babies with esophageal atresia and tracheoesophageal fistula is degree of prematurity and the associated cardiac and chromosomal anomalies. Babies with esophageal atresia and tracheoesophageal fistula have a higher incidence of prematurity than the general population, most likely related to the polyhydramnios resulting from the fetal esophageal obstruction.[16] More than half of babies with esophageal atresia and tracheoesophageal fistula have one or more associated anomalies.[17] The majority of these associated anomalies are included in the VACTERL syndrome. This syndrome includes abnormalities in the following areas: vertebral, anorectal, cardiac, tracheal, esophageal, renal, and limb. A breakdown of the individual incidences of the anomalies in babies with esophageal atresia and tracheoesophageal fistula is presented in Table 21-2.[18] The presence of three or more of these anomalies constitutes

TABLE 21-2. Incidence of Associated Anomalies With Esophageal Atresia and Tracheoesophageal Fistula

Associated Anomalies	Occurrence (%)
Vertebral	24.1%
Atresia, anorectal and duodenal	14.3%
Cardiac	32.1%
Urinary	17%
Skeletal	16.1%
Other	10.8%

the VACTERL syndrome, which occurs in 19% of babies with esophageal atresia and tracheoesophageal fistula.[19] Of these children, 5% have chromosomal abnormalities including trisomy 13, 18, and 21.[19] Other syndromes associated with esophageal atresia and tracheoesophageal fistula are the CHARGE syndrome,[20] Potter's syndrome,[21] and the SCHISIS syndrome.[11] Infants with esophageal atresia and tracheoesophageal fistula also have a higher incidence of pyloric stenosis than expected in the normal population.[22]

Clinical Presentation and Diagnosis

Esophageal atresia can be suspected on prenatal ultrasound when the constellation of polyhydramnios, an absent or small fetal stomach bubble, and an upper pouch sign are present. These are nonspecific findings and when present have a positive predictive value for esophageal atresia of only 56%.[23] Babies with esophageal atresia and tracheoesophageal fistula present postnatally with inability to handle their saliva and will often cough, choke, and possibly develop cyanosis, especially with the first attempt to feed. The baby will spit up undigested formula after the feeding attempt. This usually leads to the placement of a tube in the esophagus, which does not go in as far as expected and meets resistance. Plain films of the chest and abdomen will show the tube coiled in the proximal mediastinum. This confirms the presence of esophageal atresia. The bowel gas pattern, or lack of bowel gas in the abdomen, determines if there is a distal tracheoesophageal fistula present (gas throughout the intestines), or if there is a pure esophageal atresia without a distal fistula (gasless abdomen). The remainder of the preoperative evaluation targets the associated anomalies and looks to determine the presence of a proximal fistula between the trachea and the esophagus. The associated anomalies of the VACTERL syndrome can be identified with four quick, simple evaluations. A physical exam evaluates limb and anorectal abnormalities. The plain film that demonstrated the esophageal and tracheal abnormalities is used to look for the vertebral and limb abnormalities. An ultrasound of the abdomen will delineate renal abnormalities. And an echocardiogram is required to evaluate for cardiac anomalies and to determine the position of the aortic arch, which helps in planning the surgical approach. If a right-sided aortic arch is encountered, further evaluation with a CT angiogram or MRI angiography to look for a vascular ring should be carried out, as a complete ring is found 37% of the time.[24] If suspicious, a chromosome analysis can be sent. The presence of a proximal fistula may be evaluated in one of three ways. A contrast evaluation of the esophageal pouch will often show a proximal fistula if it is present. An experienced radiologist should do this exam to decrease the risk of aspiration. Bronchoscopy just before the surgical repair to look for a proximal fistula may be useful. The last strategy is to look for a fistula during the proximal pouch dissection. A clue that a proximal fistula is present is that the proximal pouch will not be as dilated as usual since the fistula relieves the distending pressure in the proximal pouch both pre- and postnatally. Tracheoesophageal fistula without esophageal atresia (H-type fistula) may not present in the initial neonatal period and is more difficult to diagnose. The tube will go into the stomach when originally passed, but persistent coughing and choking with feeds by mouth should prompt a search for an isolated fistula. A prone pull-back esophagram or bronchoscopy with esophagoscopy are used to find the isolated fistula.

Treatment

After the diagnosis is confirmed, plans for operative repair should be made. In healthy newborns, the operation can take place within the first 24 hours of life to minimize the risk of aspiration and resulting pneumonitis. Before the operation, the baby should be kept supine with the head elevated 30° to 45°. A tube should be in the proximal pouch to constantly suction saliva and prevent aspiration. Intravenous access should

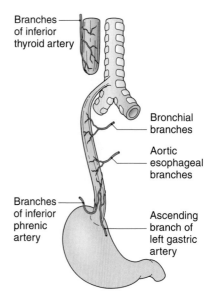

Figure 21-3. The vascular supply of the esophagus in esophageal atresia and tracheoesophageal fistula.

be established and fluids instilled along with broad-spectrum antibiotics and vitamin K.

The goal of operative therapy for esophageal atresia and tracheoesophageal fistula is to establish continuity of the native esophagus and repair the fistula in one setting. Most of the time primary repair can be achieved. There are special situations where this may not be possible or advisable. These situations will be described later. In the usual situation, the baby is stable both hemodynamically and from a pulmonary standpoint, is brought to the operating room, and is placed under a general anesthetic. Rigid bronchoscopy may be performed to locate the distal fistula, usually at or near the carina, and to look for a proximal fistula. The baby is then placed in the left lateral decubitus position in preparation for a right posterolateral thoracotomy. If the preoperative echocardiogram reveals a right-sided aortic arch, which occurs in 2% of cases, the repair should be approached from the left chest.[25] With a right-sided aortic arch, the two ends of the esophagus will need to be brought together over the arch, resulting in increased tension on the anastomosis and a high anastomotic leak rate in the range of 40%.[26] A right-sided aortic arch may be discovered intraoperatively, as the preoperative echocardiogram picks up only 20 to 62% of the right-sided arches correctly.[24,26] In that situation the repair is attempted through the right chest, and if it cannot be completed, the tracheoesophageal fistula is divided, the right chest is closed, and a left thoracotomy is used to complete the anastomosis. In the typical case, a right-sided posterolateral thoracotomy using a muscle-splitting, retropleural approach gives access to the mediastinal structures. The azygos vein is divided, revealing the tracheoesophageal connection. The distal esophagus is divided, and the tracheal connection is closed with 5-0 polypropylene monofilament suture. Manipulation of the distal esophagus is minimized to protect the segmental blood supply to this portion of the esophagus. The proximal esophagus has a rich blood supply coming from the thyrocervical trunk and may be extensively dissected as depicted in Figure 21-3. The dissection of the proximal esophageal pouch proceeds on the thickened wall of the proximal esophagus to prevent tracheal injury. Dissection

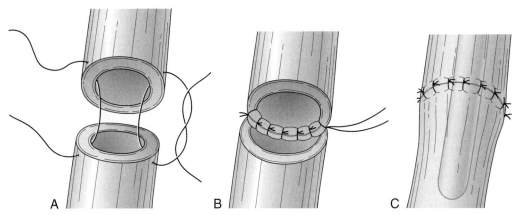

Figure 21-4. Single-layer end-to-end esophageal anastomosis. (**A**) Corner sutures are placed. (**B**) Posterior row sutures are placed. A tube is then passed through the anastomosis into the stomach. (**C**) Anterior row sutures complete the anastomosis.

is carried as high as possible to gain length for a tension-free anastomosis and to look for a proximal fistula, which occurs rarely. A single-layered end-to-end anastomosis is performed as depicted in Figure 21-4. A tube placed through the anastomosis into the stomach allows decompression of the stomach and eventual enteral feeding. A chest tube placed in the retropleural space next to the anastomosis controls any subsequent leak. Some surgeons prefer not to use a chest tube if the pleura remains intact. The advantage of a retropleural approach is that if the anastomosis leaks, the baby will not soil the entire hemithorax and develop an empyema. A leak into the retropleural space will result in a controlled esophagocutaneous fistula that will almost always close spontaneously. In 1999, Lobe performed the first thoracoscopic repair of esophageal atresia in a 2-month-old baby with pure esophageal atresia.[27] The next year, the first thoracoscopic repair of an esophageal atresia was performed in a newborn, and since then more than 210 thoracoscopic repairs have been reported in the literature, and many more unreported repairs have been done.[28-33] Thoracoscopic repair requires advanced laparoscopic skills to perform the intracorporeal anastomosis and requires a transpleural approach. Advantages include smaller, less traumatic incisions and better visualization. The results of thoracoscopic repairs compare well to historical reports of open repairs.[28]

Postoperatively, the baby is returned to the intensive care unit and continued on intravenous nutrition and antibiotics. Special care should is directed toward preventing aspiration with frequent oropharyngeal suctioning and elevation of the head of the bed 30° to 45°. Feedings may be started through the transanastomotic tube into the stomach 2 to 3 days after the operation. Acid suppressive therapy should be instituted to prevent acid irritation of the anastomosis and subsequent stricture. On postoperative day 5 to 7 an esophagram is obtained to check the integrity of the anastomosis. If there is no leak, the chest tube is removed and feeding is started orally. If a leak is present, it is treated conservatively with intravenous antibiotics and nutrition and chest tube drainage. Another esophagram is ordered in a week. These leaks will invariably close without further operative intervention.[34] Only a complete disruption of the anastomosis requires further operative procedures. In that case the proximal esophagus should be brought out of the left neck as a cervical esophagostomy, the distal esophagus should be tied off, and the mediastinum and chest should be adequately drained.

Special Situations

The majority of cases of esophageal atresia and tracheoesophageal fistula can be handled as just described. There are three variations that require further discussion. These three situations are babies with esophageal atresia and tracheoesophageal fistula who have severe respiratory disease where the fistula is contributing to the ventilatory insufficiency; babies with long-gap esophageal atresia; and babies with the H-type tracheoesophageal fistula. Babies with significant respiratory insufficiency and a tracheoesophageal fistula are usually premature neonates with lung immaturity requiring significant ventilatory support. The connection between the trachea and the distal esophagus may be the preferred path for air provided by the ventilator. The stiff lungs have a higher resistance than the fistulous tract, allowing a significant portion of each ventilation to go into the esophagus and then into the abdomen, resulting in abdominal distention and elevation of the hemidiaphragms, further impeding ventilation. Various strategies have been developed to deal with this situation. A change to high-frequency ventilation decreases the portion of tidal volume lost to the fistula. Advancing the endotracheal tube past the fistula opening prevents further loss of ventilation into the fistula, but is not always possible.[35] Bronchoscopically placed Fogarty catheters positioned in the fistula and inflated temporarily occlude the fistula, but have a tendency to become dislodged.[36] If a gastrostomy tube is present, the tube can be placed to underwater seal to increase the resistance of the tract and reduce airflow through the fistula.[14] However, to prevent further respiratory decompensation, and to ameliorate the risk of gastric perforation, these babies often require an urgent thoracotomy and control of the tracheoesophageal fistula. If the baby stabilizes, the remainder of the repair can proceed at that time, which is the usual case.[37] However, if the baby remains unstable, the esophagus is secured to the prevertebral fascia, the chest is closed, a gastrostomy tube is placed, and the definitive repair is completed when the baby is stabilized.

The second special situation occurs when there is a long gap between the two ends of the esophagus. This often occurs with pure esophageal atresia, or esophageal atresia with a proximal tracheoesophageal fistula. Both of these situations present with an x-ray picture of a gasless abdomen. On occasion, a baby with esophageal atresia and distal tracheoesophageal fistula may have a long gap between the two ends of the esophagus and fit into this special group. If the baby presents with a gasless abdomen, a long gap should be suspected. The baby is brought to the operating room for a gastrostomy tube placement to allow enteral feedings while waiting for the two ends of the esophagus to grow adequately so a primary anastomosis can be attempted. The stomach is quite small in these babies because it was unused during fetal life and has not yet stretched to its full capacity. Care must be taken to avoid injury to the small stomach and its blood supply while placing the gastrostomy tube. Careful placement will not compromise use of the stomach for an esophageal replacement if necessary. During gastrostomy tube placement, an estimate of the distance between the two ends of the esophagus is made using metal sounds and fluoroscopy. If the two ends of the esophagus are more than 3 vertebral bodies apart, they will not be easily connected. The baby is then nursed with a tube in the proximal pouch to remove the saliva and is fed via the gastrostomy tube. During the first several months of life, the gap between the two ends of the esophagus shortens because of spontaneous growth of the atretic esophagus.[38] The upper pouch may or may not undergo serial dilation to try to stretch the pouch depending on the surgeon's discretion.[39] The distance between the proximal and distal ends of the esophagus is measured every 2 to 4 weeks and, if the two ends are within 2 to 3 vertebral bodies, a thoracotomy and attempt at anastomosis is performed. If the gap remains greater than 3 vertebral bodies and the two ends of the esophagus are no longer approaching each other, the baby may require a cervical esophagostomy and esophageal replacement. Another option is to place traction sutures on both ends of the esophagus and either attach them under tension to the prevertebral fascia if the gap is moderate length, or bring them out through the back and increase the tension on

them sequentially over the ensuing 2 weeks. A repeat thoracotomy is then performed and a primary anastomosis is carried out after the two ends of esophagus are in close proximity.[40] Waiting longer than 4 months rarely provides extra growth of the esophageal ends resulting in primary anastomosis. The esophagostomy will allow the baby to take sham feeds to prevent oral aversion and subsequent feeding problems without the risk of aspiration while awaiting esophageal replacement. The replacement operation takes place between 9 and 12 months of age and consists of a gastric transposition, creation of a gastric tube, or a colonic interposition to replace the esophagus. If the gap reduces to 2 or 3 vertebral bodies, which occurs in close to 70% of the babies,[41] there are several techniques that can be used to gain length on the esophageal ends during the operation. These include complete dissection of the upper pouch to the thoracic inlet. A circular myotomy of Livaditis performed on the upper pouch produces about 1 cm of length for each myotomy.[42] Use of a circular myotomy is shown in Figure 21-5. A tubularization graft of the upper pouch can be created and connected to the distal esophagus.[43] If these techniques do not allow an adequate anastomosis, the distal esophagus is mobilized, despite its segmental blood supply, to gain length.[14] If these maneuvers do not allow an adequate anastomosis, then one of two options must be chosen. The first option is to create a cervical esophagostomy in the left neck and plan an esophageal substitution at a later time. The second option is to perform the esophageal substitution at the time using a gastric transposition, a gastric tube, or a colon interposition to replace the native esophagus. Currently, the second option using a gastric transposition is our preferred approach.

The third special situation that demands discussion is the H-type tracheoesophageal fistula without esophageal atresia.

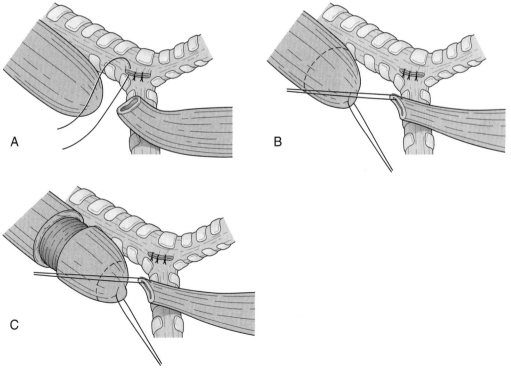

Figure 21-5. Repair of esophageal atresia and distal tracheoesophageal fistula using a circular myotomy to provide adequate length. (**A**) The tracheoesophageal fistula is closed with 5-0 Prolene. (**B**) The feasibility of primary anastomosis between the two esophageal segments is assessed. (**C**) A proximal esophagomyotomy provides extra length to allow for a primary anastomosis.

An H-type fistula will often escape discovery in the neonatal period, but will be found later during evaluation of coughing and choking episodes with feeds. Often the fistula is identified by contrast studies, usually a prone pull-back esophagram as shown in Figure 21-6. However, it is not unusual to require bronchoscopy and esophagoscopy to make the diagnosis. To repair this fistula, rigid bronchoscopy and esophagoscopy are used to find the fistula and place a Fogarty catheter through the fistula to aid in its identification during the exploration. The right neck is then explored through an incision just above the clavicle. The fistula is identified and divided. If possible, muscle or other available vascularized tissue is placed between the two suture lines to help prevent a recurrent fistula.

Postoperative Complications

Complications following repair of esophageal atresia and tracheoesophageal fistula relate to the anastomosis and to the underlying disease. The anastomotic problems include anastomotic leaks, anastomotic strictures, and recurrent tracheoesophageal fistulas. The issues related to the underlying disease include gastroesophageal reflux and tracheomalacia.

The number of anastomotic problems that occur after repair varies directly with the amount of tension that is used to create the anastomosis. The incidence of leak at the anastomosis varies from 5 to 20%.[44] The majority of these leaks seal within 1 to 2 weeks with conservative management including withholding oral feeds, intravenous antibiotics, parenteral nutrition, and chest tube drainage. Complete disruption of the anastomosis, a rare complication occurring in less than 2% of cases, presents with a tension pneumothorax and significant salivary drainage from the chest tube. This scenario may require early thoracotomy and revision of the anastomosis, or a cervical esophagostomy and gastrostomy for feeding with subsequent esophageal replacement.

Anastomotic strictures occur in one third to one half of repairs.[45] All repairs will show some degree of narrowing at the anastomosis, but dilations are not instituted unless the stricture is symptomatic, causing dysphagia, associated respiratory difficulties, or foreign body obstruction. Most strictures respond to repeated dilations. These are carried out every 3 to 6 weeks over a 3- to 6-month period. Strictures that are recalcitrant to dilations are often related to gastroesophageal reflux disease and will not resolve until the reflux is controlled.

The incidence of recurrent tracheoesophageal fistula formation ranges from less than 1% to 12% in various series.[44,46-48] These children present with coughing, choking, and occasional cyanotic episodes with feeding, and with recurrent pulmonary infections. Recurrent fistulas are often associated with anastomotic leaks, but the possibility of a missed proximal fistula must also be entertained. A prone, pull-back esophagram and bronchoscopy with esophagoscopy are useful to diagnose recurrent fistulas. A repeat right thoracotomy with closure of the fistula is a difficult operation. Identification of the fistula tract is improved with placement of a ureteral catheter in the fistula at bronchoscopy just before opening the chest. After the fistula is identified and divided, a viable piece of tissue, usually a vascularized muscle flap or a portion of pleura or pericardium, should be placed between the suture lines to prevent recurrence of the fistula, which occurs in up to 20% of these repairs.[49] Other means to close these fistulas have been attempted including endoscopic diathermy[50] and Nd:YAG laser obliteration of the fistula,[51] injection of sclerosing agents,[52] and injection of fibrin glue,[53] but surgical closure remains the treatment of choice.

Gastroesophageal reflux is commonly associated with esophageal atresia and tracheoesophageal fistula. This stems from the abnormal clearance of the distal esophagus due to poor motility, and the altered angle of His that occurs as a result of tension on the distal esophagus and proximal stomach to allow for an adequate anastomosis. Using videomanometry with topographic analysis, Kawahara et al. showed that there were two subgroups of patients with repaired esophageal atresia and tracheoesophageal fistula. Neither group had esophageal contractions at the anastomosis. One group had distal esophageal contractions and did not develop reflux, whereas the other group did not have distal contractions and 15 of 17 developed symptomatic gastroesophageal reflux.[54] Significant gastroesophageal reflux occurs in 30 to 60% of children following repair of esophageal atresia and tracheoesophageal fistula.[44,46,55] The reflux is treated medically with prokinetic and acid-reducing medication. Often a fundoplication will be required to control the reflux, especially if a stricture develops at the anastomosis that is resistant to dilation, or if repeated pulmonary aspiration associated with reflux complicates the postoperative course. Careful consideration should be given to a partial fundoplication in these children because of their abnormal distal esophageal motility. The choice of complete versus partial fundoplication is left to the surgeon, with proponents of both in the literature.[48,56,57] A comparison of fundoplications done in babies with and without esophageal

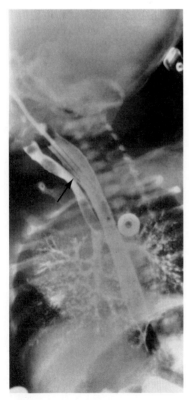

Figure 21-6. An H-type tracheoesophageal fistula is demonstrated as contrast is injected through a nasoesophageal tube. Contrast is noted passing from the esophagus, through the fistula, and filling the upper trachea and larynx.

atresia and tracheoesophageal fistula revealed that those with esophageal atresia had more intra- and postoperative complications and more problems with recurrent reflux, dysphagia, and dumping after the fundoplication.[58]

Symptomatic tracheomalacia occurs in 10 to 20% children after repair of esophageal atresia and tracheoesophageal fistula.[44,59] Tracheomalacia refers to collapse of the trachea on expiration leading to expiratory stridor and episodes of desaturations, apnea, cyanosis, and bradycardia that are often associated with feeds. This is thought to originate from weakening of the upper tracheal cartilage due to pressure exerted during fetal life from the fluid-filled dilated upper esophageal pouch. The tracheomalacia is sometimes severe enough to prevent extubation after the original repair of the esophageal atresia and tracheoesophageal fistula. Determining the etiology of this symptom complex can sometimes be difficult, because tracheomalacia and gastroesophageal reflux both occur frequently in this population and result in similar symptoms. Tracheomalacia is diagnosed with rigid bronchoscopy in the spontaneously breathing patient. The trachea will flatten anteroposteriorly, or "fishmouth" on expiration, as depicted in Figure 21-7. Tracheomalacia is often a self-limiting entity but may require intervention in children with severe life-threatening symptoms. If treatment with continuous positive airway pressure is not effective, then aortopexy[60] or tracheal stenting may be required.[61] Intervention for tracheomalacia is required in up to 5% of children with esophageal atresia.[62]

Outcome

The outcome for babies with esophageal atresia and tracheoesophageal fistula has improved over time to the point where now, unless the baby has major cardiac anomalies, significant chromosomal abnormalities, severe pulmonary complications, or birth weight less than 1500 g, almost all of these babies will survive. The long-term problems in children after repair of their esophageal atresia and tracheoesophageal fistula include pulmonary issues, especially reactive airway disease, bronchitis, and pneumonias, and upper gastrointestinal complaints of dysphagia and gastroesophageal reflux. Pulmonary symptoms severe enough to require hospitalization occur in close to half of children after repair of their esophageal atresia and tracheoesophageal fistulas.[63] Although the pulmonary symptoms tend to persist into adulthood, they tend to be mild and not affect activities of daily living.[19] The dysphagia and gastroesophageal reflux commonly seen in these children stem from the altered intrinsic innervation of the distal portion of the esophagus leading to the dysmotility that contributes to the dysphagia and reflux. This dysmotility continues into adulthood. In manometric studies of adults with repaired esophageal atresia, the main long-term motility deficits are uncoordinated peristaltic activity and low-amplitude contraction of the distal esophagus. Interestingly, the swallow-induced relaxation of the lower esophageal sphincter occurs normally. This abnormal esophageal motility results in dysphagia symptoms in up to 60% of adults and in gastroesophageal reflux. Using 24-hour pH probe and esophageal biopsy data, the incidence of gastroesophageal reflux has been documented in infants, in children up to the age of 10, and in adults after esophageal atresia repair. The incidence of reflux was similar in the three age groups: 41% in infants, 45 to 50% in children up to age 10, and 40% in adults. In the group of children up to age 10, no new cases of histologic esophagitis or abnormal pH probes occurred in children after age 5. The gastroesophageal reflux appears to develop early and persist in patients after esophageal atresia repair.[64] Esophageal strictures are uncommon as a late complication. If a stricture occurs late in the course, it is usually associated with gastroesophageal reflux. Barrett's esophagus occurs in up to 8% of these patients; how many of these progress on to esophageal adenocarcinoma remains uncertain.[65] Presently, there are six reported cases of esophageal cancer in patients who had their esophageal atresia repaired at birth. Three of these were squamous cell carcinomas, and three were adenocarcinoma. These cases developed early between the ages of 20 and 46.[64] However, a population-based, long-term follow-up study of 502 patients with repaired esophageal atresia over 50 years in Finland revealed three cases of cancer, none being esophageal or gastric.[66] Several quality-of-life measures have been used to assess the long-term outcomes of adults after repair as an infant. A Dutch study of quality of life in adults following repair of esophageal atresia and tracheoesophageal fistula compared to healthy subjects found no difference in overall physical and mental health between the two groups. However, former esophageal atresia patients reported worse "general health" and less "vitality" than the healthy subjects because of continued gastrointestinal difficulties reported in up to a quarter of the esophageal atresia group. Marital and family status did not differ from that of the general Dutch population.[67] The quality of life of adults after a colonic interposition as an infant is not as good as it is for adults who had a primary repair. In addition, children with esophageal atresia and tracheoesophageal fistula have more learning, emotional, and behavioral problems than the normal population of children, in part because of their associated anomalies including their varying degrees of prematurity, and their initial intensive care unit course often requiring mechanical ventilation for a period of time.[68]

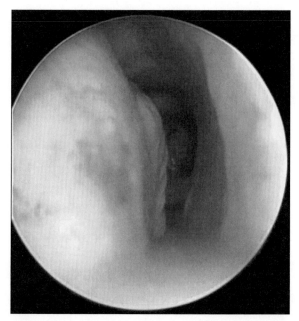

Figure 21-7. Tracheomalacia after repair of esophageal atresia and tracheoesophageal fistula. Bronchoscopic view of the tracheal lumen during spontaneous respirations shows almost complete collapse or the trachea during expiration.

LARYNGOTRACHEOESOPHAGEAL CLEFTS

Laryngotracheoesophageal cleft is a rare congenital anomaly consisting of a midline defect along the posterior portion of the larynx and trachea and the anterior portion of the esophagus leaving a communication between the these structures for varying lengths. Benjamin and Inglis classified laryngotracheoesophageal clefts into four types. Type I is a supraglottic interarytenoid cleft, type II extends into but not through the posterior cricoid lamina, type III extends through the cricoid and can involve the cervical trachea, and type IV extends below the thoracic inlet.[69]

Clinical Presentation and Diagnosis

Presentation of symptoms generally occurs shortly after birth and varies in severity depending on the extent of the cleft. Some of the type I clefts have minimal symptoms, but most babies will present with respiratory distress worsened by feedings, an absent or weak cry, hoarseness, stridor, and aspiration pneumonia. Evaluation of these symptoms involves contrast studies and bronchoscopy. Laryngotracheoesophageal clefts are often picked up on esophagram; however, it is sometimes difficult to differentiate a proximal cleft from spillover of contrast material from the pharynx and esophagus into the airway. Rigid bronchoscopy usually defines the defect, but a high index of suspicion must be maintained or the small proximal cleft may be overlooked. Careful examination of the posterior wall of the larynx is required because the mucosal folds in that area may obscure the cleft.

Treatment

Preoperatively, care should be taken to avoid aspiration episodes and to stabilize the airway. Depending on the severity of the cleft, some babies require intubation and gastrostomy tube placement before definitive repair. The type of repair is based on the level of the cleft. Often type I clefts require no surgical treatment or may be repaired with endoscopic techniques.[70] For type II and III clefts, an anterior approach to the larynx and upper trachea is used. Another option is a lateral approach that puts the recurrent laryngeal nerve at risk but leaves less laryngeal instability and may avoid prolonged postoperative intubation. The lower clefts, type IV, are best approached through a right thoracotomy or a median sternotomy. The esophagus and trachea are divided along the length of the cleft. A small strip of esophagus is left on the trachea to aid in closure and mimics the membranous portion of the trachea. Use of a special bifurcated endotracheal tube allows ventilation to continue during repair of the complete clefts as shown in Figure 21-8.[71] Cardiopulmonary bypass and extracorporeal membrane oxygenation may also be required for successful repair.

Outcome

Results continue to be rather poor. The postoperative survival rate is 75%, with anastomotic leaks occurring in up to 50% of the repairs.[70] A review of the experience at Great Ormond Street Hospital for Children showed that the longer the cleft, the worse the prognosis. All four of their patients with clefts that ended above the carina survived, whereas all five of the patients

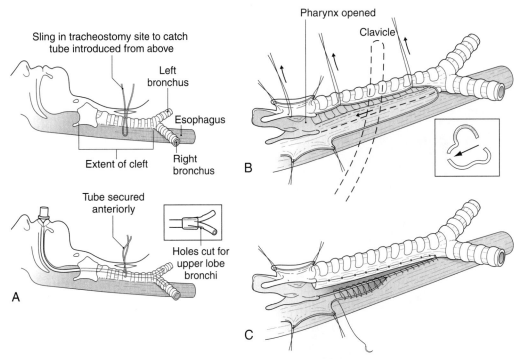

Figure 21-8. Repair of type III laryngotracheoesophageal cleft. **(A)** Stabilization of a bifurcated endotracheal tube at bronchoscopy using a loop passed through a tracheotomy that draws the endotracheal tube forward. **(B)** A cervical and thoracic approach allows retropleural exposure of the cleft. A longitudinal incision is made in the right tracheoesophageal grove below the tracheal rings. The incision is extended inferiorly, across the esophagus, and up the left side, leaving approximately 1 cm of esophageal wall attached to the trachea to allow adequate tissue to close the trachea. **(C)** The trachea has been closed with interrupted suture, and the esophagus is closed in a running fashion up to the thoracic inlet. Closure of the laryngeal portion of the cleft and the lateral pharyngeal wall is not yet accomplished.

with clefts extending all the way to the carina died.[72] Other common complications include pharyngoesophageal dysfunction, gastroesophageal reflux, and inability to wean from the ventilator. Early recognition, and, therefore, earlier treatment may prevent some of the secondary complications.

REFERENCES

4. Takamizawa S, Tsugawa C, Mouri N, et al. Congenital esophageal stenosis: therapeutic strategy based on etiology. J Pediatr Surg 2002;37:197–201.

10. Haight C, Towsley H. Congenital atresia of the esophagus with tracheoesophageal fistula: extrapleural ligation of the fistula and end-to-end anastomosis of esophageal segments. Surg Gynecol Obstet 1943;76:672.

12. Spitz L. Oesophageal atresia. Orphanet J Rare Dis 2007;2:24.

14. Harmon CM, Coran AG. Congenital anomalies of the esophagus. In: O'Neill Jr JA, Rowe MI, Grosfeld JL, editors. Pediatric Surgery. 6th ed St Louis, MO: Mosby; 2006:1051–1081.

72. Mathur NN, Peek GJ, Bailey CM, et al. Strategies for managing Type IV laryngotracheoesophageal clefts at Great Ormond Street Hospital for Children. Int J Pediatr Otorhinolaryngol 2006;70:1901–1910.

See expertconsult.com for a complete list of references and the review questions for this chapter.

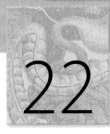

22 GASTROESOPHAGEAL REFLUX

Yvan Vandenplas

DEFINITIONS

Gastroesophageal reflux (GER) is the involuntary passage of gastric contents into the esophagus and is a normal physiological process occurring several times per day in every human, particularly after meals.[1,2] Most reflux episodes are of short duration, asymptomatic, and limited to the distal esophagus. Typically, a reflux episode is the consequence of a transient relaxation of the lower esophageal sphincter, unaccompanied by swallowing. A minority of reflux episodes occur as a consequence of increased abdominal pressure not accompanied by an increase of the LES pressure or when the LES pressure is chronically reduced. Physiologic GER is GER associated with absence of symptoms, or during the first months of life accompanied with regurgitation, and occasionally with vomiting. GER disease (GERD) is present when reflux of gastric contents is the cause of troublesome symptoms and/or complications.[2] Symptoms due to GER, esophageal and extraesophageal, are troublesome when they have an adverse effect on the well-being of the pediatric patient. To be defined as GERD, reflux symptoms must be troublesome to the infant, child, or adolescent and not simply troublesome for the caregiver.[2] GERD is reflux associated with mucosal damage or symptoms severe enough to impair quality of life. It is difficult to define when symptoms become troublesome in young children, because young children cannot adequately report symptoms.[3,4] Healthy and sick individuals do not differ in the presence or absence of GER, but in the frequency, duration, and intensity of GER and in its association with symptoms or complications. Physiologic reflux becomes pathologic if esophageal clearance is insufficient, if acid buffering is insufficient, if gastric emptying is delayed, if abnormalities in epithelial restitution or repair occur, if there are anatomical abnormalities such as hiatal hernia, and so forth.

Regurgitation, *spitting up*, *posseting*, and *spilling* are synonyms and are defined as the passage of refluxed gastric contents into the pharynx or mouth, sometimes being expelled out of the mouth.[1] Although regurgitation is mainly effortless, it may sometimes be forceful. Only a minority of physiologic reflux episodes are accompanied by regurgitation. Regurgitation is a characteristic symptom of reflux in infants, but is neither necessary nor sufficient for a diagnosis of GERD, because it is not sensitive or specific.[2] Because up to 50% of all infants under the age of 4 months present at least one to several episodes of spilling per day, this manifestation of reflux receives a lot of attention.[5] Regurgitation is distinguished from vomiting by the absence of a central nervous system emetic reflex, retrograde upper intestinal contractions, nausea, and retching. *Vomiting* is defined as expulsion with force of the refluxed gastric contents from the mouth.[3,4] Vomiting is a coordinated autonomic and voluntary motor response, causing forceful expulsion of gastric contents.[1] Vomiting associated with reflux is likely the result of the stimulation of pharyngeal sensory afferents by refluxed gastric contents. Bilious vomiting should not be diagnosed as GERD. Otherwise healthy infants and children with reflux symptoms that are not troublesome and are without complications should not be diagnosed with GERD.[2]

Rumination is characterized by a voluntary contraction of the abdominal muscles resulting in the habitual regurgitation of recently ingested food that is subsequently spitted up or reswallowed. Gagging, regurgitation, mouthing, and swallowing of refluxed material is identified as rumination.

ENVIRONMENTAL AND GENETIC FACTORS

In adults, the impact of lifestyle was suggested by showing that esophagitis and hiatus hernia were more common in a population with dyspeptic symptoms with the same genetic background living in England or in Singapore.[6] In adults, GERD affects whites more often than African Americans or Native Americans.[7] Because the lifestyle of women has become more similar to that of men, the difference in incidence in GERD between both sexes is disappearing. Alcohol, smoking, drugs, food components, intake, and weight are among many factors influencing the incidence of GER. Still in adults, over-the-counter use of low-dose aspirin and nonsteroidal anti-inflammatory drugs has a major impact on the incidence of severe GERD.[8] In children, erosive esophagitis was recently reported to be slightly more prevalent in boys.[9] Using pH monitoring, we could not demonstrate a male predominance of acid GER in children. Barrett's esophagus is partially genetically determined.[10]

In adults, race, sex, body mass index, and age are independently associated with hiatus hernia and esophagitis, race being the most important risk factor.[6] Carre et al. described autosomal dominant inheritance of hiatal hernia by discovering familial hiatal hernia in five generations of a large family, but without demonstrating the link to GERD.[11] The genetic influence on GERD is supported by increased GER-symptoms in relatives of GERD patients.[12] Moreover, the concordance for GER is higher in monozygotic than dizygotic twins.[13] Genes in question have been localized to chromosomes 9 and 13. A locus on chromosome 13q, between microsatellite D13S171 and D13S263, has been linked with severe GERD in five multiply affected families.[14] This could not be confirmed in another five families, probably because of the genetic heterogeneity of GERD and different clinical presentation of patients.[15] The relevance of these findings for the general population remains unclear.

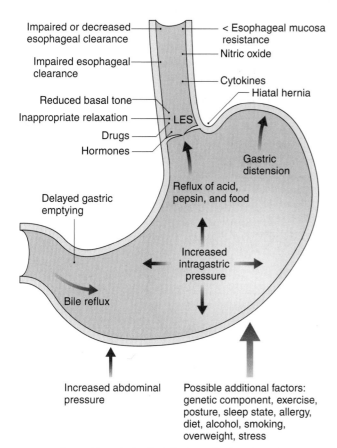

Figure 22-1. Pathophysiologic mechanisms for GER.

Labels on figure:
- Impaired or decreased esophageal clearance
- Impaired esophageal clearance
- Reduced basal tone
- Inappropriate relaxation
- Drugs
- Hormones
- Delayed gastric emptying
- Bile reflux
- < Esophageal mucosa resistance
- Nitric oxide
- Cytokines
- Hiatal hernia
- LES
- Gastric distension
- Reflux of acid, pepsin, and food
- Increased intragastric pressure
- Increased abdominal pressure
- Possible additional factors: genetic component, exercise, posture, sleep state, allergy, diet, alcohol, smoking, overweight, stress

PATHOPHYSIOLOGY

Transient lower esophageal sphincter relaxations (TLESRs) are the most important pathophysiologic mechanism causing GER at any age, from prematurity into adulthood.[16,17] TLESRs are a neural reflex, triggered mainly by the distention of the proximal stomach and organized in the brainstem, with efferent and afferent pathways traveling in the vagal nerve, activating an intramural inhibitory neuron that releases nitric oxide to relax the LES.

GER is influenced by genetic, environmental (e.g., diet, smoking), anatomic, hormonal, and neurogenic factors (Figure 22-1).[16] Three major tiers of defense serve to limit the degree of GER and to minimize the risk of reflux-induced injury to the esophagus. The first line of defense is the "antireflux barrier," consisting of the LES and the diaphragmatic pinchcock and angle of His. When this line of defense fails, the second, esophageal clearance, assumes greater importance and limits the duration of contact between luminal contents and the esophageal epithelium. Gravity and esophageal peristalsis serve to remove volume from the esophageal lumen, while salivary and esophageal secretions from esophageal submucosal glands serve to neutralize acid. The third line of defense, tissue or esophageal mucosal resistance, becomes relevant when (acid) contact time is prolonged.[16] Esophageal mucosal defense can be divided into preepithelial (protective factors in saliva and esophageal secretions containing bicarbonate, mucin, prostaglandin E2, epidermal growth factor, transforming growth factor), epithelial (tight junctions, intercellular glycoprotein material), and postepithelial factors.[16] There is a very important interindividual variation

of reflux perception suggesting different esophageal sensitivity thresholds. Capsaicin levels and the transient receptor potential vanilloid receptor-1 play a role in the sensation of heartburn.[18] The esophageal mucosa contains acid-, temperature-, and volume-sensitive receptors. A widening of the intercellular spaces is reported in patients with esophagitis and in patients with endoscopy-negative disease. Esophageal sensitivity to acid decreases when the esophagitis has healed. The presence of fat in the duodenum increases the sensitivity to reflux. Hyposensitivity as occurs in patients with Barrett's esophagus is a secondary phenomenon.

GER occurs during episodes of TLESR or inadequate adaptation of the sphincter tone to changes in abdominal pressure. Not all the factors responsible for maintaining LES tone have yet been determined, but nitric oxide likely plays an important role. Infants have a short intra-abdominal esophagus.

Infants ingest more than twice the volume than adults per kilogram body weight (100 to 150 mL/kg/day compared to 30 to 50 mL/kg/day), causing more gastric distention, and as a consequence more TLESRs. Feeding frequency is higher in infants than in adults, resulting in more postprandial periods during which TLESRs are more common. When investigated in supine position, the frequency of TLESRs in healthy adults and these with acid GERD does not differ. In healthy adults, only 30% of the TLESRs are accompanied by acid reflux, but in patients with GERD, reflux occurs in 65% of the TLESRs. Thus, in adults, controls and GERD patients have the same number of TLESRs, but in patients with GERD, these TLESRs are more than twice as frequently accompanied by acid GER.[19] Older studies performed in adults in the recumbent position may be more relevant to understanding the pathophysiologic mechanisms of acid reflux in infants. Normal individuals rarely experience TLESRs during sleep. Supine position removes all the beneficial gravitational effects of the erect position. Noxious materials, rather than air, are positioned at the cardia, available to move into the esophagus during TLESRs. A reflux is more likely to reach the pharynx in the recumbent than in the upright position. Both salivation and swallowing are markedly reduced during sleep, further impairing clearance. The upper esophageal sphincter is atonic during sleep, allowing reflux almost free access to the airways.

Delayed gastric emptying may increase postprandial reflux, possibly by increasing the rate of TLESRs and the likelihood of reflux during the TLESRs. Delayed gastric emptying has been documented in infants and children with symptomatic GER, particularly those with neurologic disorders.[20] Abnormal gastric accommodation to a meal and prolonged postprandial fundic relaxation have been described in patients with GERD.[21] Esophageal acid exposure in patients with GERD is directly correlated with the emptying time of the proximal stomach.[22] GERD was classically considered to be an acid peptic disease. But as a group, the majority of patients with reflux disease do not have a significant increase in gastric acid secretion. Recent analysis of postprandial acidity in the area of the gastroesophageal junction suggests that local acid distribution rather than total gastric secretion might be more relevant to the pathogenesis of GERD. Differences may exist in the degree of mixing of fundic contents leading to different distributions of acid in the stomach. Studies using pH monitoring, scintigraphy, and gastric magnetic resonance suggest that gastric mixing can be incomplete. Different layers of viscosity within the stomach might therefore influence the distribution of the gastric contents. A collection of acid in

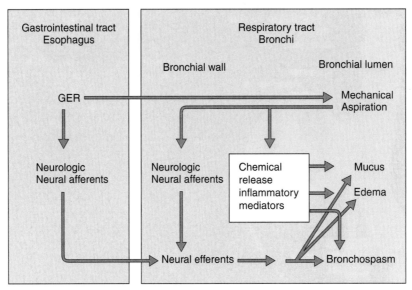

Figure 22-2. Pathophysiologic mechanisms of GER causing respiratory disease.

the gastric part of the esophageal junction was shown in adults in supine position, even in the postprandial period when stomach content was neutralized by the meal.[21]

Hiatal hernia increases the number of reflux episodes and delays esophageal clearance by promoting retrograde flow across the esophagogastric junction when the LES relaxes after a swallow. This mechanism underlies the so-called re-reflux phenomenon (acid reflux when the pH is still below 4).

The majority of the studies on pathophysiologic mechanisms have been performed in adults and did not consider weakly acid and nonacid reflux. The refluxed material can be acid, weakly acid, or nonacid. Reflux may be a mix of gas and liquid or pure liquid and may or may not contain bile. More than half of the acid and weakly acid reflux episodes are associated with reflux of gas.[19] Weakly acid reflux also occurs predominantly during TLESRs. With liquid meals, patients with GERD had a similar total rate of reflux episodes but a higher proportion of acid reflux events than controls.[23] Weakly acid reflux may be responsible for remaining symptoms in patients under antisecretory treatment. Components contributing to the noxiousness of refluxate are pepsin, bile acids and salts, and trypsin. The latter two depend on duodenogastric reflux preceding GER and are implicated in the genesis of strictures and Barrett's esophagus. Acid is emptied from the esophagus with one or two sequences of primary peristalsis, then the residual acidity is neutralized by swallowed saliva. Secondary peristalsis is the response to esophageal distention with air or water and is more important during sleep when peristalsis is reduced. Patients may have normal primary peristalsis but abnormal secondary peristalsis. Thus, nonacid reflux, as occurs in the postprandial period, may be inefficiently cleared and cause prolonged esophageal distention, and thus cause symptoms of discomfort. Esophageal clearance modulates the duration of reflux episodes, whereas mucosal resistance modulates the noxiousness of the components of refluxate.

Reflux may be causing respiratory symptoms through different pathways, such as (micro)aspiration or vagally mediated inflammation (Figure 22-2).

The relation between *Helicobacter pylori* infection and GER seems multifactorial and is still open for debate. But, because of the sharp fall in *H. pylori* infection, this issue has become less relevant. Eradication of *H. pylori* is not associated with increased symptoms of GER in children and adolescents.[24] Improvement in epigastric pain is significantly correlated with the improvement in GER symptoms but not with eradication of *H. pylori*.[24]

The role of the upper esophageal sphincter (and its role in GERD and chronic respiratory disease, laryngitis, hoarseness, coughing, etc.) has been insufficiently studied. Symptom presentation has not been linked to different pathophysiologic mechanisms. Children presenting with upper airway disease or ear, nose, and throat (ENT) manifestations may rather suffer from an insufficient upper esophageal sphincter, whereas patients with esophagitis may have more noxious reflux, insufficient clearing mechanisms, or a poor esophageal mucosal resistance.

SYMPTOMS AND SIGNS

Determination of the exact prevalence of GER and GERD at any age is virtually impossible for many reasons: most reflux episodes are asymptomatic, symptoms and signs are nonspecific, and self-treatment is common. Many factors influence the number of reflux episodes. In normal 3- to 4-month-old infants, three to four episodes of GER are detectable during 5 minutes of intermittent fluoroscopic evaluation.[25] Normal ranges of esophageal pH monitoring report up to 31 ± 21 acid reflux episodes recorded within a 24-hour period (but the frequency of sample frequency, data handling by the recording device, and program will determine this incidence).[26] There are no normal impedance data on the prevalence of acid and weakly acid reflux in healthy children.

Although reflux does occur physiologically at all ages, there is at all ages also a continuum between physiologic GER and GERD leading to significant symptoms, signs, and complications (Tables 22-1 and 22-2). GERD is a spectrum of a disease that can best be defined as manifestations of esophageal or adjacent organ injury secondary to the reflux of gastric contents into the esophagus or, beyond, into the oral cavity or airways. The presenting symptoms of GERD differ according to age (Table 22-3).

Table 22-1. Symptoms and Signs That May Be Associated With Gastroesophageal Reflux

Symptoms
  Recurrent regurgitation with or without vomiting
  Weight loss or poor weight gain
  Irritability in infants
  Ruminative behavior
  Heartburn or chest pain
  Hematemesis
  Dysphagia, odynophagia
  Wheezing
  Stridor
  Cough
  Hoarseness
Signs
  Esophagitis
  Esophageal stricture
  Barrett's esophagus
  Laryngeal/pharyngeal inflammation
  Recurrent pneumonia
  Anemia
  Dental erosion
  Feeding refusal
  Dystonic neck posturing (Sandifer syndrome)
  Apnea spells
  Apparent life-threatening events (ALTEs)

Table 22-2. Warning Signals Requiring Investigation in Infants With Regurgitation or Vomiting

Bilious vomiting
GI bleeding
  Hematemesis
  Hematochezia
Consistently forceful vomiting
Onset of vomiting after 6 months of life
Failure to thrive
Diarrhea
Constipation
Fever
Lethargy
Hepatosplenomegaly
Bulging fontanelle
Macro/microcephaly
Seizures
Abdominal tenderness or distention
Documented or suspected genetic/metabolic syndrome

Table 22-3. Symptoms According to Age

Manifestations	Infants	Children	Adults
Impaired quality of life	+++	+++	+++
Regurgitation	++++	+	+
Excessive crying/irritability	+++	+	−
Vomiting	++	++	+
Food refusal/feeding disturbances/anorexia	++	+	+
Persisting hiccups	++	+	+
Failure to thrive	++	+	−
Abnormal posturing/Sandifer's syndrome	++	+	−
Esophagitis	+	++	+++
Persistent cough/aspiration pneumonia	+	++	+
Wheezing/laryngitis/ear problems	+	++	+
Laryngomalacia/stridor/croup	+	++	−
Sleeping disturbances	+	+	+
Anemia/melena/hematemesis	+	+	+
Apnea/ALTE/desaturation	+	−	−
Bradycardia	+	?	?
Heartburn/pyrosis	?	++	+++
Epigastric pain	?	+	++
Chest pain	?	+	++
Dysphagia	?	+	++
Dental erosions/water brush	?	+	+
Hoarseness/globus pharyngeus	?	+	+
Chronic asthma/sinusitis	−	++	+
Laryngostenosis/vocal nodule problems	−	+	+
Stenosis	−	(+)	+
Barrett's/esophageal adenocarcinoma	−	(+)	+

Legend: +++ very common; ++ common; + possible; (+) rare; − absent; ? unknown.

Belching or eructation occurs during transient relaxation of the LES and is an important method of venting air from the stomach. The upper esophageal sphincter relaxes in response to esophageal body distention by gas, in contract to its contractile response to esophageal body distention by fluid. Hiccups are involuntary reflex contractions of the diaphragm followed by laryngeal closure. In some cases, hiccups cause GER.

Atypical symptoms as epigastric pain, nausea, flatulence, hiccups, chronic cough, asthma, chest pain, and hoarseness account for 30 to 60% of presentations of GERD[27,28] (Figure 22-3). Possible associations exist between GERD and asthma, pneumonia, bronchiectasis, ALTE (apparent life-threatening event), laryngotracheitis, sinusitis, and dental erosion, but causality or temporal association were not established.[28] The paucity of studies, small sample sizes, and varying disease definitions did not allow firm conclusions to be drawn.[28] Less than 10% of infants and children have (acid and troublesome) GERD.[26]

The clinician needs to be aware that not all regurgitation and vomiting in infants and young children is GER (or GER disease). Bilious vomiting, gastrointestinal bleeding, consistently forceful vomiting, weight loss or failure to thrive, diarrhea, constipation, fever, lethargy, hepatosplenomegaly, or abdominal tenderness or distention should raise the possibility of an alternate diagnosis. Bulging fontanelle, macro- and/or microcephaly, and seizures raise the possibility of genetic and/or metabolic syndromes (see Table 22-2).

GER and Uncomplicated Regurgitation

Regurgitation is the most common presentation of infantile GER, with occasional projectile vomiting.

About 70% of healthy infants have regurgitation that is physiologic, resolving without intervention in 95% of individuals by 12 to 14 months of age[5,29] (Figure 22-4). Daily regurgitation occurs more frequently in infants during the first 6 months of life than in older infants and children.[5] Frequent regurgitation, defined as more than three times per day, occurs in about 25% of infants during the first months of life.

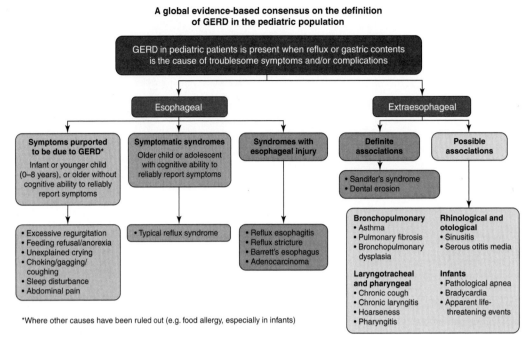

Figure 22-3. Symptoms and signs associated with GER.

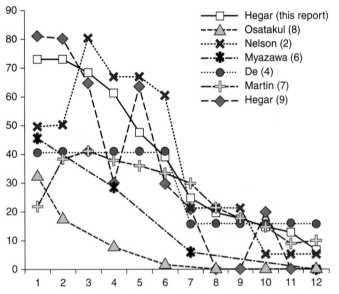

Figure 22-4. Natural evolution of physiologic regurgitation. Data from Hegar et al. (2009).[5]

A prospective follow-up reported disappearance of regurgitation in all subjects before 12 months, although an increased prevalence of feeding refusal, duration of meals, parental feeding-related distress, and impaired quality of life was observed, even after disappearance of symptoms.[30] Regurgitation occurs more frequently in infants than in adults because of the large liquid volume intake, the limited capacity of the esophagus (10 mL in newborn infants), the horizontal position of infants, and so on. "Excessive regurgitation" is one of the symptoms of GERD, but the terms *regurgitation* and *GERD* should not be used as synonyms.

Although most studies report a comparable incidence of regurgitation in unselected populations of formula versus breast-fed infants, Hegar et al. reported a higher incidence in formula-fed infants.[5] This observation fits with the knowledge that GER and symptoms of GERD may be indistinguishable from those of food allergy.[2] The incidence of cow's-milk protein allergy is 5 to 10 times higher in formula-fed than in breast-fed infants.[31] Despite the consensus that regurgitation is physiologic in the vast majority of infants, about 20 to 25% of parents seek medical advice because of infantile regurgitation.[29]

Regurgitation is a characteristic symptom of reflux in infants, but is neither necessary nor sufficient for a diagnosis of GERD, because regurgitation is not sensitive or specific. The physician's challenge is to separate regurgitation and vomiting caused by reflux from numerous other disorders provoking the same manifestations. Although the "happy spitter" certainly exists (and is not rare), many infants show some symptoms of distress and discomfort when regurgitating. Irritability may accompany regurgitation and vomiting; however, in the absence of other warning symptoms, it is not an indication for extensive testing.[1] But in fact, parental carrying capacity or anxiousness will determine whether a physician is contacted. Infant regurgitation is a benign condition with a good prognosis, needing no other intervention than parental education and anticipatory guidance, and intervention on feeding composition may contribute to parental reassurance. Overfeeding exacerbates recurrent regurgitation. Thickened or antiregurgitation (AR) formula decreases overt regurgitation.[1]

GER(D), Recurrent Regurgitation, and Poor Weight Gain

If poor weight gain is documented, it is obvious that the infant is not a happy spitter. Poor weight gain is a crucial warning sign that necessitates clinical management. These infants need a complete diagnostic work-up, starting with a dietary history to evaluate caloric intake. Hospitalization of these infants may be needed. Although usually regurgitation causes little more than a nuisance, important regurgitation also produces caloric insufficiency and malnutrition in a minority of infants. There may be abnormal sucking and swallowing, and weight gain may be poor. These infants have no apparent malformations and may be diagnosed as suffering "nonorganic failure to thrive" (NOFTT),[32] a "disorder" that sometimes is attributed to social/sensory deprivation or to socioeconomic or primary maternal-child problems. GERD is only one of the many etiologies of "feeding problems" in infancy. Poor weight gain, feeding refusal, back-arching, irritability, and sleep disturbances have been reported to be related as well as unrelated to GERD.[33,34]

GER(D) and Distressed Behavior

This group of patients is much more difficult to deal with than the infant with poor weight gain. A given amount of distress and crying may be evaluated by some parents as easily acceptable while the same amount of crying will be unbearable for other parents. Many factors, such as tobacco smoke, may cause infant irritability. Cow's-milk allergy is another well-identified cause of infant irritability. There is substantial individual variability, and some healthy infants may cry up to 6 hours a day.

The concept that infant irritability and sleep disturbances are manifestations of GER is largely derived from adult data.[1] Although this hypothesis seems an acceptable extrapolation, we should be aware that there are not many data on this topic. GERD affects quality of life significantly in adults, and probably also in children (and their parents); although quality of life is more difficult to evaluate in infants and young children. The developing nervous system of infants exposed to acid seems susceptible to pain hypersensitivity despite the absence of tissue damage. In adults, "nonerosive reflux disease" ("NERD") is a generally accepted entity. Again in adults, impaired quality of life, notably regarding pain, mental health, and social function, has been demonstrated in patients with GERD, regardless the presence of esophagitis.[35] In an unselected population, 28% of the adults report heartburn, almost half of them weekly, with a significant impact on the quality of life in 76%, especially if the symptoms are frequent and long lasting. Despite that, only half of the heartburn complainers seek medical help, although 60% takes medications. Thus, some adults "learn to live with their symptoms" and acquire tolerance to long-lasting symptoms, whereas others accept an impaired quality of life. In infants and young children, verbal expression of symptoms is often vague or impossible and persistent crying, irritability, back-arching, and feeding and sleeping difficulties have been proposed as possible equivalents of adult heartburn. Infants with GERD learn to associate eating with discomfort and thus subsequently tend to avoid eating and develop an aversive behavior around feeds, although behavioral feeding difficulties are also common in control toddlers.[30] Esophageal pain and behaviors perceived by the caregiver (usually the mother) to represent pain (e.g., crying and retching) potentially affect the response of the infant to visceral stimuli and the ability to cope with these sensations, both painful and nonpainful. Only one placebo-controlled study with proton pump inhibitors (PPIs) in distressed infants has been performed, showing an equal decrease in distressed behavior in the treatment and the placebo group.[1] To date,

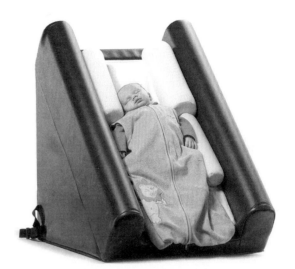

Figure 22-5. The Multicare-AR Bed.

there is no evidence that acid-suppressive therapy is effective in infants who present only with inconsolable crying. In infants and toddlers, there is no symptom or group of symptoms that can reliably diagnose GERD or predict treatment response. A pilot study suggested that a 40° supine position in a specially developed "Multicare-AR Bed" significantly decreased regurgitation and infant irritability (Figure 22-5).[36]

Cow's-milk protein allergy (CMPA) overlaps with many symptoms of GER disease and may coexist with or complicate GERD.[37] Treatment of CMPA implies the use of hydrolysates (or amino acid formula). Hydrolysates have a more rapid gastric emptying than intact protein. As a consequence, it can be speculated (the following is a hypothesis) that the number of TLESRs is decreased if an infant is fed an extensive hydrolysate. Moreover, improvement of GER (and GER-like) symptoms with hydrolysates is not proof of an underlying immunological mechanism such as allergy. In other words: infants who regurgitate and vomit may suffer CMPA, GER disease, both conditions, or neither.

GER(D) and Heartburn

Although the verbal child can communicate pain, descriptions of its intensity, location, and severity may be unreliable until the age of at least 8 years, and sometimes later.[2] In adults, adolescents, and older children, heartburn and regurgitation are the characteristic symptoms of GERD. In infants, the issue is more complicated; a symptom-based diagnosis of GERD in infants and young children remains difficult. Diagnosis and management of GERD in older children (more than 12 years of age) and adolescents follows the recommendations for adults.[1] According to parents, heartburn is present in 1.8% of 3- to 9-year-old healthy children and 3.5% of 10- to 17-year-old adolescents; regurgitation is said to occur in 2.3% and 1.4%, respectively, and 0.5% and 1.9% need antacid medication.[14] Heartburn is self-reported by 5.2% of adolescents, and regurgitation by up to 8.2%, whereas antacids are taken by 2.3% and histamine receptor antagonists (H$_2$RA) by 1.3%, suggesting that symptoms of GER are not rare during childhood and are underreported by parents or overestimated by adolescents.[38] GERD in adolescents is more adult-like. Heartburn is a symptom of GERD with or without esophagitis. Heartburn is the predominant

GER symptom in adults, occurring weekly in 15 to 20% and daily in 5 to 10% of subjects. The reason for the differences in presentation of GERD according to age remains unclear. The persistence of symptoms and progression to complications are unpredictable for a group of patients and for the individual patient. Overall, the correlation between symptoms, results of pH monitoring, acid perfusion test, and histology is poor.

GERD and Esophagitis

Esophagitis is defined as visible breaks of the esophageal mucosa.[1] Histology is recommended to rule out complications (Barrett's esophagus) or other causes of esophagitis (eosinophilic esophagitis). Reflux esophagitis is reported in 2 to 5% of the general population.[39] Reflux esophagitis is reported to occur in 2 to 5% of the population. Children with GER symptoms present esophagitis in 15 to 62%, Barrett's esophagus in 0.1 to 3%, and refractory GERD requiring surgery in 6 to 13%.[1,40] Erosive esophagitis in 0- to 17-year-old children with GERD symptoms was reported to be 12.4%, increasing with age.[9] The median age of the group with erosive esophagitis was 12.7 ± 4.9 years, versus 10.0 ± 5.1 years in those without erosive esophagitis.[9] The incidence of erosive esophagitis was only 5.5% in those younger than 1 year.[9] This finding is in sharp contrast with the extremely high incidence (24.8%) of antireflux medication prescribed in extremely low-birth-weight infants at the moment of discharge.[41] The huge differences in incidence of esophagitis are determined by patient recruitment, differences of definition of esophagitis, and availability of self-treatment. Hiatal hernia is more frequent in children with erosive esophagitis than in those without (7.7% versus 2.5%).[9]

The primary symptom of an esophageal stricture is dysphagia. Barrett's esophagus is not rare in adolescents with chronic GERD.[1] In adults, hospital discharges and mortality rates due to gastric cancer, gastric ulcer, and duodenal ulcer have declined during the past three decades, while those of esophageal adenocarcinoma and GERD have markedly risen.[42]

Esophagitis, identified by histology, occurs in 61 to 83% of infants with reflux symptoms severe enough to perform endoscopy. Although esophagitis may present with pain, it can also be asymptomatic. The group with asymptomatic esophagitis is in some ways the most problematic. Even severe esophagitis may remain asymptomatic, as demonstrated by children who present with peptic strictures without having experienced any discomfort attributable to esophagitis. Typical substernal burning pain ("heartburn," pyrosis) occurs in many children suffering from esophagitis. Odynophagia, which is pain on swallowing, usually represents esophageal inflammation. In nonverbal infants, behaviors suggesting esophagitis include crying, irritability, sleep disturbance, and "colic." Infants frequently also appear very hungry for the bottle until their first swallows and then become irritable and refuse to drink. Dysphagia ("typical" for eosinophilic esophagitis [EoE]), has also been linked to esophagitis.

The impressive rise in prevalence of EoE is still poorly understood,[43] and difficulty in distinguishing EoE from reflux esophagitis may be encountered.[44] In reflux esophagitis, the distal and lower eosinophilic infiltrate is limited to less than 5 eosinophils per high-power field (HPF) with 85% positive response to GER treatment, compared to primary eosinophilic esophagitis with more than 20 eosinophils per HPF. More recently, failure of PPI treatment as a condition to diagnose EoE

brought reflux esophagitis back in the picture of EoE.[45] EoE necessitates proper treatment (hypoallergenic feeding, corticoids, montelukast, etc.). Patients with allergic esophagitis are younger and have atopic features (allergic symptoms or positive allergic tests), but no specific symptoms. Atopic features are reported in more than 90% and peripheral eosinophilia in 50% of patients. At endoscopy, a pale, granular, furrowed, and occasional ringed esophageal mucosa may appear.[1]

GER(D) and Dysphagia, Odynophagia, and Food Refusal

Dysphagia is difficulty in swallowing; odynophagia is pain caused by swallowing. Although GERD is frequently mentioned as a cause of dysphagia or odynophagia, there are no pediatric data showing this relation. Dysphagia is a prominent symptom in patients with eosinophilic esophagitis. Feeding difficulty and/or refusal are often used to describe uncoordinated sucking and swallowing, gagging, vomiting, and irritability during feeding. A relation between GER, GERD, and feeding refusal has not been established. In case of feeding difficulties, achalasia and foreign body should be among the list of possible differential diagnoses.

GER(D) and Extraesophageal Manifestations

GER(D) and Reactive Airway Disease

An etiologic role for GER in reactive airway disease has not been demonstrated. Different pathophysiologic mechanisms are proposed: direct aspiration, vagally mediated bronchial and laryngeal spasm, neurally mediated inflammation. Old literature suggests that esophageal acidification in adults with asthma can produce airway hyperresponsiveness and airflow obstruction.[46] Few studies have been attempted to evaluate the opposite: the impact of asthma on the severity of GERD. Chronic hyperinflation as occurs in asthma favors many GER mechanisms. An association between asthma and reflux measured by pH or impedance probe has been reported in many studies.[28] Wheezing appears more related to GERD if it is nocturnal. A recent study reports a high prevalence of GER in children and adolescents with persistent asthma, equally distributed in the supine (nocturnal) and upright positions.[47] But, there was no correlation between the result of the pHmetry and pulmonary function tests.[47] There are no studies that help in selecting patients in whom reflux treatment may result in a reduction of asthma medication, if there are such patients at all.[1,28]

Very few prospective, randomized, and blinded treatment studies have been performed in children. In a series of 46 children with persistent moderate asthma despite bronchodilators, inhaled corticosteroids, and leukotriene antagonists, 59% (27/46) had an abnormal pHmetry.[48] Reflux treatment resulted in a significant reduction in asthma medication. Patients with a normal pHmetry were randomized to placebo or reflux treatment: 25% (2 of only 8 children) of the treated patients could reduce their asthma medication, whereas this was not possible in any patient on placebo.[48] Another study found omeprazole ineffective in improving asthma symptoms and parameters in children with asthma.[49] Overall, the literature on the causal role of GER in asthmatic adults is also not convincing.

If today there is no evidence for an etiologic role of GER in reactive airway disease in children, this is mainly due to lack of data. But this group of patients is particularly difficult to study.

Many possible diagnostic tools have been developed and are discussed elsewhere (see the following section on GER and recurrent pneumonia). But in the patient group with reactive airway disease, a "negative symptom association probability" does not exclude a causal role for GER because a certain "amount" of reflux may be necessary to start airway inflammation.

GER(D) and Recurrent Pneumonia

GER causing recurrent pneumonia has been reported in otherwise healthy infants and children, although with an incidence for reflux that was as low as 6%.[50] The reported mechanisms are similar to those for reactive airway disease. Direct aspiration during swallowing may be more relevant in this group.

No test can determine whether reflux is causing recurrent pneumonia. Upper esophageal and pharyngeal pH and impedance recordings provided contradictory information. Today, it is not yet clear if recording in the upper esophagus or pharynx will help in making therapeutic decisions.[51,52] A new technique to record pharyngeal reflux has been developed (Restech), with promising results needing confirmation.[52] Lipid-laden macrophages have been used as an indicator of aspiration, but this test's sensitivity and specificity for GER is poor. The measurement of pepsin seems to be more promising, although there is a substantial overlap between patients and controls.[53] One study evaluating nuclear scintigraphy with late imaging reported that 50% of patients with a variety of respiratory symptoms had pulmonary aspiration after 24 hours.[54] But aspiration also occurs in healthy subjects, especially during sleep.[1] Moreover, later studies failed to reproduce these findings.[55] Analysis of symptom association probability is also of questionable interest in this patient group.

Today, the clinician frequently has no other option than to make management decisions based on inconclusive diagnostic studies with no certainty regarding outcome. As in reactive airway disease, it is very likely (although not proven based on evidence) that (not all) reflux needs to be acid to cause airway manifestations. However, today, medical treatment options that are validated are limited to acid-reducing medication.

GER(D) and Cystic Fibrosis

The role of GER in adults and children with cystic fibrosis (CF) has been studied. Acid reflux exists in the majority of CF patients.[1] A high prevalence of acid GER was reported in very young infants with CF, even before respiratory symptoms developed. It is possible that the acid reflux is also a cause of aggravating respiratory symptoms, and that the respiratory symptoms aggravate the reflux. Aggressive medical and surgical reflux treatment in this patient group seems reasonable. In children with CF, a better weight gain was reported during PPI treatment (whether this is due to a reduction of acid reflux or better buffering of acid gastric content in the intestine is not clear).

GER(D) and ENT Manifestations

In some European countries, ENT doctors are prescribing more PPI medication than gastroenterologists. Many studies report a high incidence of reflux in patients with upper airway disease.[1]

In the future, more data on symptom-association probability between reflux measured with impedance and occurrence of symptoms such as coughing may provide helpful information. We demonstrated in a pilot study a positive symptom association in some children with recurrent coughing and normal "overall" parameters of GER investigations. Several studies revealed the presence of pepsin in the middle-ear fluid, but with a huge variation in incidence (14 to 73%).[1] Also, bile acids have been detected in middle-ear liquid, in higher concentrations than in serum.[56] However, several epidemiologic studies suggest a low incidence of reflux symptoms in patients with recurrent middle ear infections.

Data suggesting a causal relation between reflux and upper airway disease in children are limited. Data from several placebo-controlled studies and meta-analyses uniformly have shown no effect of antireflux therapy on upper airway symptoms or signs.[1] Well-designed, prospective, placebo-controlled, blinded studies are needed. Another bias might be selection of patients: these studies are frequently set up in tertiary care centers in highly selected patient populations. The question is how representative these patients are for the bulk of children with upper respiratory and/or ENT manifestations.

The presence of pepsin and bile in middle ear fluid might also be the consequence of reflux (and vomiting) at the moment of the acute middle ear infection, rather than an argument to hypothesize that chronic GER may be at the origin of the chronic middle-ear problem.

GER(D) and Dental Erosions

Young children and children with neurologic impairment appear to be at greatest risk of dental erosions caused by GER. Juice drinking, bulimia, and racial and genetic factors that affect dental enamel and saliva might be confounding variables that have been insufficiently considered.[1] There are no long-term (intervention) follow-up studies in high-risk populations.

GER(D) and Sandifer Syndrome

Sandifer syndrome (spasmodic torsional dystonia with arching of the back and opisthotonic posturing, mainly involving the neck and back) is an uncommon but specific manifestation of GERD.

GER(D) and Neurologic Impairment

The neurologically impaired child is a well-recognized group with increased GER and GERD. Diagnosis of reflux disease in these children is often difficult because of their underlying conditions. Whether this group of patients has more severe reflux disease, or has less effective defense mechanisms, or presents with more severe symptoms because of the inability to express and/or recognize symptoms remains open for debate. Response to treatment, both medical and surgical, is poor in the neurologically impaired child compared to the neurologically normal child.

GER(D) and Apnea and ALTE

Literature can best be summarized as follows: series fail most of the time to show a temporal association between GER and pathologic apnea, apparent life-threatening events (ALTE), and bradycardia.[1] However, a relation between GER and short, physiologic apnea has been shown.[57,58] There are well selected cases or small series that demonstrate that pathologic apnea can occur as a consequence of GER.

GER(D) and Other Risk Groups

Symptomatic GER is estimated to occur in 30 to 80% of children who have undergone repair of esophageal atresia.[20] Children with congenital abnormalities or after major thoracic or abdominal surgery are at risk for developing severe GERD. Children with neurologic impairment have more frequent, more severe, and more difficult-to-treat GERD than neurologically normal children. Neurologically impaired children accumulate many risk factors for severe GERD: spasticity or hypotonicity, supine position, constipation, etc. Children with anatomic abnormalities such as hiatal hernia, repaired esophageal atresia, and malrotation frequently have severe GERD. Although there is abundant literature on overweight and increased GER in adults, data in children are scarce. There are no data in literature that preterm babies have more (severe) reflux than full-term babies, although many premature babies are treated for reflux. The role of reflux in patients with bronchopulmonary dysplasia and other chronic respiratory disorders is not clear.

GERD and Complications

Barrett's esophagus, strictures, and esophageal adenocarcinoma are complications of chronic severe GERD. Barrett's esophagus is a premalignant condition in which metaplastic specialized columnar epithelium with goblet cells is present in the tubular esophagus. Differences in esophageal mucosal resistance and genetic factors may partially explain the diversity of lesions and symptoms.

More than 40 years ago, in the absence of reflux treatment, esophageal strictures were reported in about 5% of children with reflux symptoms.[59] Currently, esophageal stenosis and ulceration in children have become rare. In a series including 402 children with GERD without neurological or congenital anomalies, no case of Barrett's esophagus was detected.[40] In another series including 103 children with long-lasting GERD who were not previously treated with H_2RAs or a proton pump inhibitors (PPIs), Barrett's esophagus was detected in 13%. An esophageal stricture was present in 5 of the 13 patients with Barrett's (38%).[60] Reflux symptoms during childhood were not different in adults without than in adults with Barrett's.[61] Barrett's has a male predominance and increases with age. Patients with short segments of columnar-lined esophagus and intestinal metaplasia have similar esophageal acid exposure but significantly higher frequency of abnormal bilirubin exposure and longer median duration of reflux symptoms than patients without intestinal metaplasia.[62] There is a genetic predisposition in families in patients with Barrett's esophagus and esophageal carcinoma.[1]

Children with neurological impairment, chronic lung disease (especially cystic fibrosis), esophageal atresia, and chemotherapy have the most severe pathologic reflux and are at high risk for the development of complications of GERD.[1]

Peptic ulcer and esophageal and gastric neoplastic changes in children are extremely rare. In adults, over the past 30 years, a decreased prevalence of gastric cancer and peptic ulcer with an opposite increase of esophageal adenocarcinoma and GERD has been noted.[63] This has been attributed to independent factors, among which are changes in dietary habits such as a higher fat intake, an increased incidence of obesity, and a decreased incidence of *H. pylori* infection.[63] Frequency, severity, and duration of reflux symptoms are related to the risk of developing esophageal cancer. Among adults with long-standing and severe reflux, the odds ratios are 43.5 for esophageal adenocarcinoma and 4.4 for adenocarcinoma at the cardia.[64] It is unknown whether mild esophagitis or GER symptoms persisting from childhood are related to an increased risk for severe complications in adults.

DIAGNOSIS

Diagnostic procedures are not discussed in full detail. Detailed information regarding indications and pitfalls of radiologic contrast studies, nuclear reflux scintigraphy, ultrasound, pHmetry, intraluminal impedance, endoscopy, manometry, gastric emptying tests, and electrogastrography can be found in previous review papers and guidelines.[1]

In adults, diagnosis of GER disease is mainly based on clinical history.[65] However, history in children is difficult and considered poorly reliable up to the age of minimally 8 or even 12 years.[1] Therefore, questionnaires have been developed trying to improve history reliability. Orenstein developed the "infant GER-questionnaire."[66] The questionnaire results in an objective, validated, and repeatable quantification of symptoms suggesting GERD. The I-GER was revised (the "I-GERQ-R") in 185 patients and 93 controls, resulting in an internal consistency reliability from 0.86 to 0.87, and test-retest reliability was 0.85.[67] However, Aggarwal and coworkers showed that the I-GER-Q had a sensitivity of only 43% and a specificity of 79%.[68] Moreover, pHmetry results were not different according to a "positive" or "negative" score of the I-GER-Q.[68] Our group showed that not one question was significantly predictive for the presence of esophagitis. In our hands, the Orenstein I-GERQ cutoff score failed to identify 26% of infants with GERD (according to pHmetry results or presence of esophagitis), but was positive in 81% of infants with a normal histology of esophageal biopsies and normal pHmetry.[69] Deal et al. developed two different questionnaires, one for infants and one for older children, and showed that the score was higher in symptomatic than in asymptomatic children.[70] In other words: the correlation between the results of history obtained by questionnaires and of reflux investigations is poor.

Barium contrast radiography, nuclear scintiscanning, and ultrasound are techniques for evaluating postprandial reflux and provide limited information on gastric emptying. Normal ranges are not established for any of these procedures. Barium studies are not recommended as first-line investigation to diagnose GERD, but are of importance in diagnosing anatomic abnormalities such as malrotation, duodenal web, and stenosis and may suggest functional abnormalities such as achalasia. Nuclear scintigraphy may show pulmonary aspiration.[54] However, these data still need confirmation, because experience from many centers is that aspiration seldom occurs. Also, aspiration of saliva and gastric contents occurs during sleep in healthy adults.[71] Scintigraphy also can estimate gastric emptying. But the ^{13}C-octanoic acid (for solids) and ^{13}C-acetate (for liquids) breath tests are more appropriate to measure gastric emptying. The role of delayed gastric emptying in GER(D) remains controversial. The results of ultrasound are investigator dependent, and a relation between reflux seen on ultrasound and symptoms has not been established.[1] There is no indication for electrogastrography in the diagnostic work-up of a patient suspected of GERD.

Modern endoscopes are so miniaturized that endoscopy of preterm infants weighing less than 1000 g has become technically easy. Operator experience is an important component of interobserver reliability.[1] Endoscopy allows direct visual examination of the esophageal mucosa. Macroscopic lesions associated with GERD include esophagitis, erosions, exudate, ulcers, structures, and hiatal hernia. Redness of the distal esophagus in young infants is a normal observation because of the increased number of small blood vessels at the cardiac region. Endoscopy may also show a "sliding hernia," a stomach that is protruding into the esophagus during burping. Recent consensus guidelines define reflux esophagitis as the presence of endoscopically visible breaks in the esophageal mucosa at or immediately above the GE junction.[1,2] Endoscopy-negative reflux disease is common. There is a poor correlation between the severity of symptoms and presence and absence of esophagitis. There is insufficient evidence to support the use of histology to diagnose or exclude GERD. Biopsies of duodenal, gastric, and esophageal mucosa are mandatory to exclude other diseases.[1] More detailed information on the pros and cons of histology can be found in the recent consensus papers.[1,2]

Intraluminal esophageal acid perfusion provoking chest pain (Bernstein test) or using other end points has found expanded use in practice and research in the United States but was never popular in Europe. Ambulatory 24-hour esophageal pH monitoring measures the incidence and duration of acid reflux, whereas impedance measures all reflux episodes. Esophageal pHmetry is the best method to measure acid in the esophagus, but not all reflux that causes symptoms is acid, and not all acid reflux causes symptoms. Esophageal pHmetry is useful in evaluating the effect of a therapeutic intervention on reducing esophageal acid exposure. Medical treatment is currently focusing on the reduction of gastric acid secretion; the technique offers the possibility to measure intragastric and esophageal recording of pH simultaneously. Both hardware (electrodes, devices) and software influence the results.[1] Normal ranges have been established for pHmetry.[7] However, normal ranges also depend on the hard- and software used and are of limited value for reflux causing extraesophageal manifestations. It is becoming more and more obvious that the major indication for long-term recording of pH and/or impedance is the demonstration of an association between reflux and symptoms.

Manometry does not demonstrate reflux, but is of interest for analyzing pathophysiologic mechanisms causing the reflux, mainly by visualizing and measuring TLESRs, and is indicated in the diagnosis of specific conditions such as achalasia.[1] Ambulatory 24-hour esophageal manometry, in combination with pHmetry and/or impedance recording, is now technically feasible. This technique is mainly used in (clinical) research and allows the objective demonstration of reflux-symptom association (e.g., in patients presenting with chronic cough).

Intraluminal impedance measures electrical potential differences. As a consequence, the detection of reflux by impedance is not pH dependent, but in combination with pHmetry it allows detection of acid (pH below 4.0), weakly acid (pH 4.0 to 7.0) and alkaline reflux (pH above 7). Experience has shown that impedance needs to be performed in combination with pHmetry, because pH-only events occur (mainly during the night and mainly in young infants). Also, gas reflux can be measured, because liquid reflux causes a drop in impedance and gas reflux an increase. Interpretation of the recording is still laborious and necessitates sufficient experience, because the automatic analysis is not standardized and is not adequate in (young) children and infants. Impedance seems especially of interest in patients with symptoms suggesting reflux but not esophagitis. Obviously, "more" reflux episodes are detected with impedance-pHmetry than with pHmetry alone, but the question of whether "more is always necessary or better" remains unanswered at this time. The major clinical interest of impedance seems to be demonstration of symptom association, but normal data and validation of symptom association parameters in children are missing. Given the high cost of equipment and electrodes and the time needed for analysis and interpretation of impedance, the pros and cons in comparison to pHmetry are still debated. Impedance in combination with pHmetry definitively measures more reflux episodes than pHmetry alone. Interestingly, pH-only episodes, reflux episodes detected with pHmetry but not with impedance (drop in pH without bolus movement), occur in young children.[72]

Experience in children with spectrophotometric esophageal probes to detect bilirubin is still very limited. Orel and coworkers showed that some children with esophagitis suffer bile reflux.[73]

Indirect techniques have been developed, mainly to diagnose GER(D) in patients with extraesophageal manifestations. Accumulation of evidence regarding the determination of lipid-laden macrophages (LLMs) in bronchoalveolar liquid (BAL) resulted in the conclusion that this method lacks sensitivity and specificity.[1] More recent data show the presence of pepsin in BAL and middle-ear fluid.[1,55] Also, bile salts are detected in middle-ear fluid.[56] However, epidemiological data suggest a "protective" role of middle-ear infection for the prevalence of GERD.[1] There is no prospective, double-blind, placebo-controlled study treating reflux and evaluating the ENT outcome as primary endpoint.

All GER-investigation techniques test different aspects of reflux. Therefore, it is not unexpected that the correlation between the results of the different techniques is poor. There is no "always-best" investigation technique to diagnose GER(D) because the clinical situation of each individual patients differs. "Logic interpretation" (but not evidence-based medicine) suggests that if the question asked is, "Does this patient have esophagitis?" then endoscopy with biopsy is the best technique. If it is in the interest of the patient to measure acid GER episodes, 24-hour pHmetry is the preferred technique. But if quantification of all GER episodes is needed, impedance is likely to be the best. Impedance also measures weakly acid and alkaline reflux. However, postprandial reflux is mainly weakly acid or alkaline, and postprandial reflux was in general considered to be not really relevant, because the techniques measuring postprandial reflux (barium swallow, ultrasound, scintiscanning) are not recommended for this reason. Therapeutic options are mainly limited to acid-reducing medication. As a consequence, the real relevance of measuring weakly acid and alkaline reflux can be questioned.

TREATMENT OPTIONS

Because symptoms of GER and these suggesting GERD are frequent and nonspecific, especially during infancy, and because there is no "gold standard" diagnostic technique, many infants and children are exposed to antireflux treatment. Therapeutic options vary from reassurance, nutritional, and positional treatment and prokinetic and acid-reducing medication to surgery (Table 22-4). Physiologic GER does not need medical treatment. Attention in the paragraphs on therapeutic possibilities is focused on safety aspects. Therapeutic intervention should always be a balance between intended improvement of symptoms and risk for side effects.

Complications of Nonintervention

Although data on the natural evolution of regurgitation have been accumulated, there are only limited data on the natural history of GERD in infants and children because most patients

Table 22-4. Schematic Therapeutic Approach in 2010

Phase 1	Parental reassurance. Observation. Lifestyle changes. Exclude overfeeding.
Phase 2	Dietary treatment (decrease regurgitation)
	Thickened formula, thickening agents, extensive hydrolysates or amino acid based formula in cow's milk allergy
	Positional treatment (°)
Phase 3	For immediate symptom relief: alginates (some efficacy in moderate GERD); antacids only in older children
Phase 4	Proton pump inhibitors (drug of choice in severe GERD; more safety data needed)
	H_2 receptor antagonists less effective than PPIs
Phase 5	Prokinetics (but not one product available on the market in 2009 has been shown to be effective)
	Would treat pathophysiologic mechanism of GERD
Phase 6	Laparoscopic surgery

Efficacy and safety data in infants and children for most anti-GER medication are limited. (°): data on 40° supine sleeping position in infants are limited.

get treatment. Recent accumulation of data suggests a decreased quality of life in a number of frequently regurgitating infants and their parents, even if the regurgitation has disappeared.[30] Data suggest that pediatric GER is a heterogeneous disorder and that GERD occurring after infancy may be more predictive of the presence of GERD during adulthood.[74] Longitudinal follow-up of large numbers of children is still needed to answer the question of when classic adulthood GERD begins.[74] A 10-year follow-up of esophagitis (in adults) showed that more than 70% had persisting symptoms and 2% developed strictures.[75] Untreated GERD is associated with complications such as esophagitis, failure to thrive, esophageal stricture, and Barrett's esophagus.

It is not known whether mild esophagitis or GERD symptoms persisting from childhood into adulthood carry an increased risk for complications in adult life. Spontaneous improvement and healing of nonulcerated esophagitis may exist. But data suggest the opposite. Although symptoms improved in more than of the infants with reflux esophagitis followed longitudinally for 1 year without pharmacotherapy, histology remained abnormal in all.[76] There are also retrospective data suggesting that adults with reflux disease had more frequent reflux symptoms during infancy and childhood. However, there are no intervention data. In other words: we do not know if treatment of GER during infancy changes the outcome in adults. If treatment is prescribed, not only efficacy but also side effects of the treatment should be taken into account.

Nonpharmacological and Nonsurgical Therapies for GER

The first approach to (troublesome) infant regurgitation should be careful observation of feeding and handling of the child during and after feedings. Many infants are overfed or fed with an inappropriate technique.[1] Reassurance showing comprehension for the impaired quality of life is of importance.[1] Data from 10 randomized controlled trials of nonpharmacological and nonsurgical therapies for GER disease in healthy infants were reviewed[77]: such therapies may decrease regurgitation but have overall no proven efficacy on (acid) reflux.

Lifestyle Changes

Parental education, guidance, and support are required and often sufficient to manage infant regurgitation.[1] The impact of pacifier use on reflux frequency was equivocal and dependent on infant position. There are very limited data on lifestyle changes (dietary modification, alcohol avoidance, smoking cessation, etc.) in older children and adolescents. Most of these data are derived from adults. Expert opinion suggests that the older children with GERD should avoid caffeine, chocolate, alcohol, spicy foods, smoking, etc. Several studies have shown that chewing sugarless gum after a meal decreases reflux.

Dietary Treatment

Many infants presenting with frequent regurgitation also have distressed behavior and are irritable. Larger food volumes and higher osmolality increase the rate of TLESRs; a reduction of the food volume results in a decrease in the number of regurgitations but no change in acid reflux.[78] Dietary treatment requires control of appropriate formula preparation. A thickened or commercialized AR formula (not antireflux formula!) decreases visual regurgitation, but does not systematically decrease (acid) reflux.[79] However, data from three independent studies suggest that acid reflux is reduced with corn-starch-thickened formula.[80] Rice cereal may increase acid GER.[79] Commercialized thickened formula is preferred to thickening agents added to formula at home; the nutritional content of the thickening agent and its effect on osmolality have been considered in the commercial formula.[1] Corn-starch-thickened formula was shown to hasten gastric emptying.[81] Milk thickeners are often wrongly considered "inexpensive." Cow's-milk allergy may be a cause of reflux, regurgitation, and vomiting, often accompanied by distressed behavior. For a subgroup of infants presenting with recurrent regurgitation (with or without vomiting, with or without distress), cow's-milk protein allergy may be the culprit.[1,2] In these infants, extensive hydrolysates (or amino-acid-based formula, depending on local availability and cost) are recommended. However, improvement of symptoms with a hypoallergenic diet is not conclusive evidence for allergy (no proof of involvement of the immune system), because these formulas do have a more rapid gastric emptying than standard formulas. Ongoing pilot studies suggest promising results with thickened partial and extensive hydrolysates.

Conflicting results have been obtained with infants receiving milk thickeners or AR formula in whom cough was a manifestation of GER.[81,82] In vitro models testing the effect on one meal suggested that bean gum might be associated with malabsorption of minerals and micronutrients.[83] Studies of various thickening agents, including guar gum, carob bean gum, and soybean polysaccharides, indicate the potential for deceased intestinal absorption of carbohydrates, fats, calcium, iron, zinc, and copper.[84] Abdominal pain, colic, and diarrhea may ensue from fermentation of bean gum derivatives in the colon. In some, but not all, animal studies, adding carob bean gum to the diet decreased growth.[84] However, growth and nutritional parameters in infants receiving a casein-predominant formula thickened with bean gum were normal and were no different from those for a control group on standard infant formula.[85] Although rare, serious complications such as acute intestinal obstruction in newborns and preterm babies have been reported. Allergic reactions to carob bean gum have been reported in adults exposed to it at their workplaces and in infants after exposure to formula thickened with carob bean gum.[84]

In view of their safety and efficacy, milk thickeners and AR formula remain a valuable first-line measure in relieving overt regurgitation. In contrast, their efficacy in GER disease is questionable. Although the effect of thickened feeds is (mainly) cosmetic, it may help to bring reassurance to the parents and to improve the quality of life of infant and parents.[1] More data are needed on nutritional safety. Also, more epidemiological data are needed: how frequent is GERD unrecognized, and does the child suffer negative consequences because of the decrease of regurgitation with thickened feeds?

Positional Treatment

Despite gravity, the upright seated position leads to significantly more and longer reflux episodes than the simple prone and 30° elevated prone position, whether the infant is awake or asleep.[86] The supine (lying on back) and right lateral positions are associated with the highest incidence of GER; the prone position with the lowest, and the left lateral position with intermediate GER.[87] The prone anti-Trendelenburg position is the position with the lowest GER incidence. All studies have demonstrated significantly decreased acid reflux in the flat prone compared to flat supine position. Prone sleeping is considered an obsolete sleeping position in infants because of the increased risk for sudden death compared to supine sleeping. To date, the only other positional intervention proven to reduce reflux is the positioning of infants on their left sides after feeding.[87] Van Wijk et al.[88] concluded that optimal effect was achieved with a strategy of right lateral positioning for the first postprandial hour with a position change to the left thereafter to promote gastric emptying and reduces liquid GER in the late postprandial period. However, these position recommendations do not take the relation between side sleeping position and sudden death risk into account. At least two independent studies reported a significantly increased risk of sudden infant death syndrome (SIDS) in the side sleeping position compared to the supine sleeping position.[88] These data suggest that a further substantial decrease in the risk of SIDS could be expected if infants were placed to sleep on their backs.[88] The results of a pilot study with the "Multicare-AR Bed" suggest that a specially made bed that nurses the infant in a 40° supine body position reduces regurgitation, acid reflux (measured with pH monitoring), and reflux-associated symptoms (evaluated with the Infant-Gastro Esophageal Reflux Questionnaire) (see Figure 22-5).[36]

Prokinetics

From the pathophysiologic point of view, prokinetics seem a logical therapeutic approach to treat GERD in infants and children.

Metoclopramide

Data supporting the efficacy of metoclopramide are limited to observations with intravenous administration.[1] Application in infants is limited because of severe adverse events that occur in more than 20% of patients, including central nervous system effects and interactions with the endocrine system.[1] Irritability is the most frequently reported potential adverse effect of therapy. Other reported adverse effects included dystonic reactions, drowsiness, oculogyric crisis, emesis, and apnea.[1,89] Isolated cases of methemoglobinemia and sulfhemoglobinemia are reported. Neuroendocrine side effects such as galactorrhea and

gynecomastia occur.[90] Also metoclopramide has been reported to induce torsades de pointes.[91]

Domperidone

A recent systematic review of studies on domperidone identified only four randomized controlled trials in children, none providing "robust evidence" for efficacy of domperidone in pediatric GERD.[92] Most studies have been performed in older children or have investigated the effects of domperidone coadministered with other antireflux agents.[1] Somnolence was acknowledged by 49% of patients after 4 weeks of metoclopramide treatment compared with 29% of patients after 4 weeks of domperidone.[93] Prolactin plasma levels may increase because of pituitary gland stimulation.[94] Gynecomastia has been reported.[95] Domperidone occasionally causes extrapyramidal central nervous system and cardiac adverse effects.[96]

Erythromycin

Erythromycin, a dopamine-receptor antagonist, is sometimes used in patients with gastroparesis to hasten gastric emptying. Its role in therapy of GER and GERD has not been investigated. Systemic administration of erythromycin in young infants increases the risk for the infants to develop hypertrophic pyloric stenosis.[97] Intravenous (IV) erythromycin is reported to cause QT prolongation and ventricular fibrillation.[98] The use of erythromycin at doses far below the concentrations necessary for an inhibitory effect on susceptible bacteria provides close to ideal conditions for the induction of bacterial mutation and selection.[99] Azithromycin reduces GER in lung transplant recipients.[100] The effect of long-term administration of these antibiotics on gastrointestinal flora composition and resistance should be studied.

Cisapride

A Cochrane review on cisapride in children analyzed data from seven trials including 236 patients comparing cisapride to placebo on the effect on symptom presence and improvement and concluded that there was a statistical difference for the parameter "symptoms 'present/absent'" but not for "symptom change." The Cochrane review also concluded that cisapride compared to placebo significantly reduced the number and duration of acid reflux episodes, because there was a significant decrease in reflux index.[101] In other words, today cisapride is the only prokinetic with some evidence for efficacy, although this evidence is weak. Recently, in a small group of 20 patients, domperidone and cisapride were shown to have a similar decreasing effect on infant regurgitation, but acid reflux decreased more in the cisapride group.[102]

In general, cisapride is well tolerated. The most common adverse events are transient diarrhea and colic (in about 2%). There are isolated reports on more serious adverse events such as extrapyramidal reactions, seizures in epileptic patients, and cholestasis in very low-birth-weight infants. The effect of cisapride on cardiac events such as QT prolongation and arrhythmia is dose and risk-factor related. The relation between cisapride, the P450 cytochrome, and cardiac effect was for the first time considered in 1996.[103] Cisapride possesses Class III antiarrhythmic properties and prolongs the action potential duration delaying cardiac repolarization.[104] Torsades de pointes have been reported with cisapride.[105] Co-treatment with cisapride and macrolides such as clarithromycin and erythromycin prolongs the QT duration.[106] Underlying cardiac disease, drug interactions, and electrolyte imbalance are interfering factors.[94] Cytochrome P4503A4, which is involved in the metabolism of cisapride, is immature at birth and reaches adult activity by the age of 3 months.[107] A significant QTc prolongation occurs especially in infants younger than 3 months, but not in older infants.[108,109] This effect was related to higher plasma levels. A more frequent administration of lower doses (resulting in a recommended daily dose of 0.8 mg/kg/day) in premature infants results in lower peak levels.[109] Consumption of grapefruit juice also alters cisapride metabolism.[110] The use of cisapride is restricted to limited-access programs. In India, a copy of the original product is commercially available.

Other Molecules

Bethanechol, a direct cholinergic agonist studied in a few controlled trials, has uncertain efficacy and a high incidence of side effects in children with GERD. *Prucalopride*, a 5HT$_4$ agonist, is effective in adult constipation.[111] Prucalopride has received a positive opinion from the Committee for Medicinal Products for Human Use (CHMP) of the European Medicines Agency (EMEA) on the European Marketing Authorisation Application (MAA) for the treatment of chronic constipation in adults. *Mosapride* is a gastroprokinetic agent that acts as a selective 5HT$_4$ agonist that accelerates gastric emptying and is used for the treatment of acid reflux, irritable bowel syndrome, and functional dyspepsia. The data on reflux are very scarce and limited to adults. However, it has also cardiac side effects and was reported to induce torsades de pointes. *Clebopride* is a dopamine antagonist drug with antiemetic and prokinetic properties used to treat functional gastrointestinal disorders. Chemically, it is a substituted benzamide, closely related to metoclopramide. A small Spanish study found that more adverse reactions are reported with clebopride than with metoclopramide, particularly extrapyramidal symptoms. *Itopride* is a prokinetic benzamide derivative like metoclopramide or domperidone, but is not approved by FDA and EMEA. Itopride inhibits dopamine and have a gastrokinetic effect. Itopride is indicated for the treatment of functional dyspepsia and other gastrointestinal conditions. A limited number of data have been accumulated in small size Asian studies. The drug should not cause QT prolongation, because it does not involve the CYP3A4 system. *Ondansetron* is a 5HT$_3$ receptor antagonist that accelerates gastric emptying, inhibits chemotherapy-induced emesis, but prolongs colonic transit time.[112] There are no indications in GER disease. *Tegaserod*, a partial 5HT$_4$ agonist, was shown to accelerate small intestinal transit time and to increase proximal colonic emptying. Tegaserod also improves gastric emptying and decreases GER.[113] It was withdrawn from the market in 2007 because of the increased risks of heart attack or stroke.

Baclofen, 4-amino-3-(4-chlorophenyl)butanoic acid, is a γ-aminobutyric acid (GABA)-B receptor agonist, used to reduce spasticity in neurologically impaired patients. Given orally, it has been shown to decrease GER in healthy adults.[114] Baclofen was reported in a small series of eight neurologically impaired children to decrease significantly the number of acid reflux episodes, but did not change the reflux index (percent of esophageal acid exposure time).[115] In 2006, in a placebo-controlled study including 30 children, baclofen at 0.5 mg/kg/day was shown to reduce the number of TLESRs and acid GER during a 2-hour test period and to accelerate gastric emptying.[116] The data on baclofen are still very limited and do not support widespread use.

M0003 (from Movetis) is a "next generation gastrokinetic." M0003 is a specific and high-affinity 5-HT$_4$ agonist for the treatment of upper GI disorders, focusing initially on severe gastroparesis and pediatric reflux in children. Today, the drug is still in the phase of development and clinical trials in children have yet to start.

The NASPGHAN-ESPGHAN guidelines state that potential side effects of each currently available prokinetic agents outweigh the potential benefits.[1] There is insufficient evidence to justify the routine use of metoclopramide, erythromycin, bethanechol, or domperidone for GERD.[1]

(Alginate) Antacids

The key therapeutic advantage of antacids is their rapid onset of action, within minutes. Antacids include carbonate and bicarbonate salts (e.g., $NaHCO_3$ and Ca- or $MgCO_3$), alkali complexes of aluminum and/or magnesium (e.g., aluminum and magnesium hydroxides), aluminum and magnesium phosphates, magnesium trisilicate, and alginate-based raft-forming formulations. On-demand use of antacids may provide rapid symptom relief in some children and adolescents with nonerosive reflux disease. These products have mainly been validated in adults. Alginate-based raft-forming formulations have a quite different mode of action than antacids. In the presence of gastric acid, alginates precipitate, forming a gel. Alginate-based raft-forming formulations usually contain sodium or potassium bicarbonate; in the presence of gastric acid, the bicarbonate is converted to carbon dioxide which becomes entrapped within the gel precipitate, converting it into foam that floats on the surface of the gastric content, providing a relatively pH-neutral barrier.[117] Because alginate-based raft-forming formulations needs to float on the gastric contents for effectiveness, the time at which this medication is taken is of great importance. Optimal benefit is achieved when alginate-based raft-forming formulations are taken following a meal. Results showed a marginal but significant difference between Gaviscon Infant and placebo in average reflux height, and raises questions regarding any perceived clinical benefit of its use.[118] Data in infants and children remain limited.

Absorption from aluminum-containing antacids may cause serum aluminum concentrations to approach levels reported to cause osteopenia, rickets, microcytic anemia, and neurotoxicity with aluminum deposition in the brain tissue.[119] Side effects include diarrhea with magnesium-rich preparations. The presence of aluminum and magnesium in the majority of antacids means that such products have the potential to chelate drugs in the upper gastrointestinal tract. Important drug interactions with antacids include the prevention of the absorption of antibacterials such as tetracycline, azithromycin, and quinolones.[120] Antacid decreased the bioavailability of famotidine, ranitidine, and cimetidine by 20 to 25%, and the bioavailability of nizatidine by 12%.[121] Gaviscon contains a considerable amount of sodium carbonate, increasing the sodium content of feeding to an undesirable level, especially in preterm infants. Algicon, having a better taste than Gaviscon, has a lower sodium load but a higher aluminum content. Occasional formation of large bezoar-like masses of agglutinated intragastric material has been reported in association with Gaviscon. Data on compliance in infants and children (these products have an unpleasant taste) are missing.

Mucosal Protectors

The coating agent sucralfate is a basic aluminum salt of sucrose octasulfate. At an acid pH, it polymerizes to form a white paste-like substance that adheres selectively to ulcers or erosions via an electrostatic attraction between the negatively charged sucralfate polyanions and the positively charged protein moieties exposed by the inflamed mucosa. At these specific sites, sucralfate acts as a protective barrier by slowing back-diffusion of acid, pepsin, and bile salts. It also directly inhibits the binding of pepsin to ulcer protein. Other important effects of sucralfate include increased bicarbonate and mucus production, enhanced epithelial cell renewal, and restoration of a normal transmucosal potential difference.[122] The only randomized comparison study in children demonstrates that sucralfate was as effective as cimetidine for treatment of esophagitis.[123]

Besides constipation, sucralfate may cause bezoars, especially when given to patients in intensive care units. Patients with renal failure treated with sucralfate are exposed to aluminum toxicity. Aluminum accumulation has been observed in critically ill children with acute renal failure. The available data are inadequate to determine the safety or efficacy of sucralfate in the treatment of GERD in infants and children, particularly the risk of aluminum toxicity with long-term use. Extrapolation from adult data makes sucralfate unlikely to be effective in GERD.

H$_2$-Receptor Antagonists

Histamine-2 receptor antagonists (H$_2$RAs) decrease acid secretion by inhibiting histamine-2 receptors on gastric parietal cells. Historically, cimetidine was the first H$_2$RA available. Ranitidine, famotidine and nizatidine are the most popular, although very poorly studied in children. Pharmacokinetic studies in children suggest that peak plasma ranitidine concentration occurs 2.5 hours after dosing with a half-life of 2 hours. Gastric pH begins to increase within 30 minutes of administration, and the effect lasts for 6 hours.

Although no randomized controlled studies in children demonstrate the efficacy of ranitidine or famotidine for the treatment of esophagitis, expert opinion is that these agents are as effective as cimetidine and nizatidine. Extrapolation of the results of a large number of adult studies to older children and adolescents suggests that H$_2$RAs may be used in these patients for the treatment of GERD symptoms and for healing esophagitis, although H$_2$RAs are less effective than PPIs for both symptom relief and healing of esophagitis.[124,125]

Tachyphylaxis, or diminution of the response, to intravenous ranitidine and escape from its acid inhibitory effect have been observed after 6 weeks, and tolerance to oral H$_2$RA in adults and children is well recognized. In general, H$_2$RAs are considered safe. The endocrinologic side effects in adults associated with long-term administration of cimetidine preclude its long-term use in children.[126] Other side effects of acid-blocking medications are discussed in the following subsection.

Proton Pump Inhibitors

PPIs form a group of compounds called substituted benzimidazoles that concentrate within the parietal cells' intracellular canaliculi, irreversibly bind to the H$^+$,K$^+$-ATPase enzyme system, and strongly inhibit acid production. PPIs can be considered prodrugs, because protonation of the molecule in highly acidic environments results in a series of reactions that ultimately produce the active form of the PPI. Once covalently bound, the H$^+$,K$^+$-ATPase enzyme becomes nonfunctional, and activity only returns by parietal cell synthesis of new H$^+$,K$^+$-ATPase enzyme systems. In adults, the turnover of the H$^+$,K$^+$-ATPase is constant with a half-life about 48 hours. The maturation of this turnover is unknown in infants and children. The best access of the drug to the H$^+$,K$^+$-ATPase situated in the luminal side of the secretory membrane of the gastric parietal cells is provided by a meal, which is the stronger physiological event inducing the exteriorization of the H$^+$,K$^+$-ATPase. PPIs must be taken once a day, before breakfast, and must be protected from gastric acid by enteric coating. The achievement of "maximal acid-suppressant effect" can take up to 4 days. PPIs are almost completely absorbed in the small intestine. The granules and tablets should not be crushed, chewed, or dissolved, because gastric acid secretion may alter the drugs. If the microgranules are enteric coated, the capsules can be opened and administered orally or via a feeding tube, in suspension in an acidic medium such as fruit juice, yogurt, or applesauce. A "homemade" liquid formulation, produced by dissolving the granules, not the microgranules, in 8.4% bicarbonate solution, has been used in some reports.[1]

PPIs have been shown to be more effective than H$_2$RAs.[1] Omeprazole and esomeprazole are approved in the United States and Europe for pediatric use; in the United States, lansoprazole is approved as well. No PPI is approved for use in patients under the age of 1 year. In uncontrolled trials and case reports, omeprazole was used in dosages between 0.2 and 3.5 mg/kg/day for periods ranging from 14 days to 36 months. About 40% of children respond to a dosage of 0.73 mg/kg (equivalent to the adult dosage, i.e., 17 mg/m^2), 26% more respond to 1.44 mg/kg, and 35% failed to respond to this doubled dosage. The usual recommended starting dosage of omeprazole is 1 mg/kg once daily, i.e., with a maximum of 40 mg. IV omeprazole should be given once daily at 40 mg/1.73 m^2 (i.e., 1 mg/kg). As the benefit of a loading dose of IV omeprazole was demonstrated in adults, it is suggested to use a loading dose of 40 mg/1.73m^2, repeated after 12 hours in order to achieve a rapid antisecretory effect in similar critical situations in pediatric patients. The antisecretory effect of proton pump inhibitors is independent of plasma concentration but is correlated with the area under the plasma concentration-time curve. Most of the studies performed in children with GERD defined success of treatment by healing of esophagitis. Usual recommended starting dose for lansoprazole is less than 1 mg/kg once daily, i.e., 15 mg for children less than 30 kg in weight and 30 mg for those weighing more than 30 kg. At a rate similar to that observed with omeprazole, among the responders to lansoprazole, 80% of children had healing of esophagitis after 4 weeks of treatment. Overall, for both omeprazole and lansoprazole, the healing rate for peptic esophagitis is more than 75% after 4 to 8 weeks of treatment; the clinical symptoms improve in the same range. In adolescent patients with GERD, esomeprazole 20 or 40 mg daily for 8 weeks was well tolerated, and GERD-related symptoms were significantly reduced from baseline values in both groups.[127] Tolia showed that in 13 patients with esophagitis, esomeprazole 0.3 to 1.0 mg/kg/day for 8 weeks healed erosive esophagitis.[12] In children aged 1 to 11 years with endoscopically proven GERD, esomeprazole (at daily doses of 5, 10, or

20 mg) was generally well tolerated. The frequency and severity of GERD-related symptoms were significantly reduced during the active treatment period. Safety and tolerability of esomeprazole was also shown in 1- and 2-year-old children with GERD.[128] According to a recent systematic review, esomeprazole is the most effective PPI.[129]

Lansoprazole, omeprazole, and pantoprazole are metabolized by a genetically polymorphic enzyme, CYP2C19, absent in approximately 3% of whites and 20% of Asians. The potential for drug-drug interactions with omeprazole and esomeprazole is low. Salivary secretion is decreased with omeprazole.

PPIs are highly selective and effective in their action and have a few short- and long-term adverse effects. There is no relation between the dose and the side effects. PPIs are metabolized by the hepatocyte cytochrome P450 isoforms CYP2C19 and CYP3A4 to inactive metabolites (sulfide, sulfone, and hydroxy metabolites) that are excreted in urine.

There are four main categories of adverse effects related to PPI: idiosyncratic reactions, drug-drug interactions, drug-induced hypergastrinemia, and drug-induced hypochlorhydria.[1] Idiosyncratic reactions occur in up to 12 to 14% of children taking PPIs: headache, diarrhea, constipation, and nausea.[130,131] These may resolve with a lower dose or a switch to another PPI. Parietal cell hyperplasia and occasional fundic gland polyps are benign changes resulting from PPI-induced acid suppression and hypergastrinemia (occurring in up to 73% of the children, with no statistically significant differences in gastrin level by PPI type, dose, and dosing frequency or treatment duration). Long-term follow-up studies reported only mild grades of enterochromaffin-like cell hyperplasia. If more sensitive staining techniques are used, then up to 50% of the patient may have enterochromaffin-like cell hyperplasia.[130-132] Acid suppression, or hypochlorhydria, causes abnormal gastrointestinal flora and bacterial overgrowth.[133] As a consequence, the prevalence of infectious respiratory and gastrointestinal tract disease is increased.[134] The prevalence of bacterial gastroenteritis is increased.[135] *Clostridium difficile* is more prevalent.[136] In newborns in neonatal intensive care units, gastrointestinal colonization with *Candida* is increased.[137] Acid-blocking medication is associated with a higher incidence of necrotizing enterocolitis.[138] The prevalence of pneumonia is also increased.[139] Other adverse effects have been reported in elderly patients: deficiency of vitamin B_{12} and increased incidence of hip fractures. However, these findings have not been corroborated by more recent studies.[1] Interstitial nephritis (not in children) has as well been reported. This adverse effect is considered to be an idiosyncratic reaction, more frequent in the elderly. Animal studies suggest that acid suppression may predispose to the development of food allergy, but this needs confirmation in human studies.

The NASPGHAN-ESPGHAN guidelines state that for the treatment of chronic heartburn in older children or adolescents, lifestyle changes with a 4-week PPI trial are recommended.[1] If symptoms resolve, continue PPI for 3 months. If symptoms persist or recur after treatment, it is recommended that the patient be referred to a pediatric gastroenterologist.[1]

Therapeutic Endoscopic Procedures

In recent years, new endoscopic techniques intending to improve the function of the antireflux barrier have been developed. The first results of endoscopic gastroplasty (Endocinch

system), radiofrequency delivery at the cardia (Stretta system), and injection therapy (Enteryx procedure) in adults have been reported. The first series in adolescents have been reported.[140] Although experience is too limited to recommend broad use, the theoretical concept of these procedures is interesting. Further improvements to the techniques are still being introduced.

Peptic strictures are usually about one third of the esophageal length above the diaphragm. Strictures are best treated with balloon dilatation. Treatment of peptic strictures has two goals: dilating the stricture and arresting the reflux. Transendoscopic balloon dilators have the advantages of endoscopic visualization and safer radial forces, but, at a given diameter, mercury-weighted bougies may dilate more effectively. Occasionally, refractory strictures will benefit from injection of corticosteroids during endoscopic dilatation. Positive experience with mitomycin and biodegradable stents has been incidentally reported.

Surgery

Fundoplication decreases reflux by increasing the LES baseline pressure, decreasing the number of TLESRs and the nadir pressure during swallow-induced relaxation, increasing the length of the esophagus that is intra-abdominal, accentuating the angle of His, and reducing a hiatal hernia if present. The annual number of antireflux operations has been on the increase in the United States, especially in children under 2 years of age.[141] The prevalence of surgery is much higher in the United States than in Europe; reasons for this different approach are likely to be related to differences in health care organization and its cost and legal consequences. Most of the literature on surgical therapy in children with GERD consists of retrospective case series in which documentation of the diagnosis of GERD and details of previous medical therapy are deficient, making it difficult to assess the indications for and responses to surgery.[1] In general, outcomes of antireflux surgery have been more carefully evaluated in adults than in children. Adult series report that between 37% and 62% are taking PPI a few years after the intervention.[142,143] In adults, the mortality of the first operation is reported to be between 1 in 1000 and 1 in 330.[1] Although antireflux surgery in certain groups of children may be of considerable benefit, a failure rate of up to 22% has been reported.[144-150] Children with underlying conditions predisposing to the most severe GERD comprise a large percentage of many surgical series. In a study in adults, only 61% were satisfied with the outcome.[151] Laparoscopic Nissen fundoplication has largely replaced open Nissen fundoplication as the preferred antireflux surgery because of its decreased morbidity, shorter hospital stay, and fewer perioperative problems.

Total esophagogastric dissociation is an operative procedure that is useful in selected children with neurologic impairment or other conditions causing life-threatening aspiration during oral feedings.

CONCLUSION

GER and GERD are frequent conditions in infants, children, and adolescents. Symptoms differ with age, although the main pathophysiologic mechanism, transient relaxations of the lower esophageal sphincter associated with reflux, is identical at all ages. Although infant regurgitation is likely to disappear with age, little is known about the natural evolution of pediatric GER and GERD. The majority of reflux episodes are weakly acid, but the majority of symptomatic reflux is likely to be acid related. Symptoms are not specific and not sensitive. Esophageal and extraesophageal symptoms and signs caused by reflux do exist, although the evidence for causal relation between reflux and extraesophageal manifestations is at the most moderate. Complications of reflux disease may be severe and even life threatening, such as esophageal stenosis and Barrett's esophagus. There is no gold-standard diagnostic technique. The value of validated questionnaires for diagnosis and follow-up has been demonstrated. The best investigation to diagnose esophagitis is endoscopy with biopsies. In children with atypical reflux symptoms, pHmetry and impedance recording are the recommended techniques. Impedance in combination with pHmetry is likely to replace simple pHmetry. Treatment of regurgitation and moderate reflux disease should focus on reassurance with dietary and possibly also positional treatment. Dietary treatment for troublesome regurgitation and mild reflux disease should get more attention because there is growing evidence of efficacy. Alginates are useful when immediate symptom relief is required. Medical therapeutic options are mainly limited to acid-secretion-reducing medications, although not all reflux symptoms and disease are caused by acid reflux. Treatment possibilities struggle with the fact that there is no prokinetic drug with a convincing efficacy and safety profile. Laparoscopic surgery is the recommended surgical procedure.

REFERENCES

1. Vandenplas Y, Rudolph CD, Di Lorenzo C, et al. Pediatric Gastroesophageal Reflux Clinical Practice Guidelines: Joint Recommendations of the North American Society of Pediatric Gastroenterology, Hepatology, and Nutrition and the European Society of Pediatric Gastroenterology, Hepatology, and Nutrition. J Pediatr Gastroenterol Nutr 2009;49:498–547.
2. Sherman PM, Hassall E, Fagundes-Neto U, et al. A global, evidence-based consensus on the definition of gastroesophageal reflux disease in the pediatric population. Am J Gastroenterol 2009;104:1278–1295.
28. Tolia V, Vandenplas Y. Systematic review: the extra-oesophageal symptoms of gastro-oesophageal reflux disease in children. Aliment Pharmacol Ther 2009;29:258–272.
43. Spergel JM, Brown-Whitehorn TF, Beausoleil JL, et al. 14 years of eosinophilic esophagitis: clinical features and prognosis. J Pediatr Gastroenterol Nutr 2009;48:30–36.
79. Horvath A, Dziechciarz P, Szajewska H. The effect of thickened-feed interventions on gastroesophageal reflux in infants: systematic review and meta-analysis of randomized, controlled trials. Pediatrics 2008;122:e1268–e1277.
130. Edwards SJ, Lind T, Lundell L, Das R. Systematic review: standard- and double-dose proton pump inhibitors (PPIs) for the healing of severe erosive oesophagitis – a mixed treatment comparison of randomised controlled trials. Aliment Pharmacol Ther 2009;30:547–556.

See expertconsult.com for a complete list of references and the review questions for this chapter.

23 ACHALASIA AND OTHER MOTOR DISORDERS

Colin D. Rudolph • Manu R. Sood

The esophagus is a conduit that transports food, fluids and oropharyngeal secretions to the stomach. The lower esophageal sphincter (LES) prevents the reflux of gastric contents into the esophagus, and the upper esophageal sphincter (UES) into the hypopharynx. The term *esophageal motor disorder* is commonly used to describe abnormal motility patterns demonstrated during esophageal manometry studies. Some of these disorders, such as esophageal achalasia, have well-defined abnormalities of esophageal motility, which correlate with clinical symptoms. However, other esophageal motility disorders have a typical abnormal contraction pattern on manometry, but the clinical significance is not always clear. Thus, the classification of these disorders has been the subject of some controversy. Because of the differences in the neuromuscular anatomy of the proximal and the distal esophagus, the illnesses affecting these regions also differ. We have therefore separated the motor disorders affecting the proximal and distal esophagus into two sections (Table 23-1). In this chapter, we focus on specific esophageal motility disorders and discuss their clinical presentation, pathophysiology, and management.

DISORDERS OF THE PROXIMAL ESOPHAGUS

The upper esophageal sphincter (UES) is a manometrically defined high-pressure zone distal to the hypopharynx. It is formed primarily by the cricopharyngeal (CP) muscle with contribution from the lower fibers of the pharyngeal constrictor and the upper striated fibers lining the esophagus. The CP muscle is innervated by the vagus nerve, and sensory information is provided by the glossopharyngeal and sympathetic nervous systems. Pharyngeal, esophageal, and respiratory events can influence the UES pressure (Table 23-2). Relaxation of the UES with swallowing (Figure 23-1A) is initiated in the swallowing center located in the brainstem, and the programmed inhibition travels via the vagus nerve. Normal deglutition requires synchronized pharyngeal contraction, complete relaxation of the UES muscles, and traction by the neck muscles. This sequence of events pulls the larynx upward and forward, opening the sphincter as the pharyngeal contractions propel the bolus through the sphincter. When the sequence is uncoordinated or the UES sphincter fails to relax, the bolus is mishandled. Disorders affecting the UES are usually part of a generalized neurodevelopment problem, and oral and pharyngeal phases of swallowing may also be affected.

Upper Esophageal Sphincter Achalasia

Primary cricopharyngeal achalasia usually presents soon after birth with choking and coughing during feeds, nasal regurgitation of feeds, tracheal aspiration and dysphagia.[1,2] Diagnosis is often delayed because of the rarity of the disorder. A prominent posterior indentation (cricopharyngeal bar) is usually identified on a lateral radiograph in the pharyngoesophageal segment during a contrast swallow study, but this may be more difficult to identify in infants and children.[2] A dilated pharynx, lack of transit through the upper esophageal sphincter, a to-and-fro movement of contrast in the pharynx, aspiration, and nasal reflux are often observed during videofluoroscopic swallow studies. In older children, the administration of varying food bolus consistencies, rather than just liquid contrast, can help to evaluate the swallowing mechanism in detail. Similar findings can be observed in children with more generalized neuromuscular disorders, who do not initiate a coordinated pharyngeal swallow response on bolus entry into the pharynx. This can lead to the inappropriate diagnosis of CP achalasia by less experienced clinicians.

Manometric studies can confirm incomplete relaxation of the UES in some patients with radiographic abnormalities.[2-4] However, there is often a discrepancy between radiographic and manometric findings. This could be partly due to the inherent difficulty in performing manometric studies in this region, especially in an uncooperative infant. Maintaining the position of the transducers in the UES during swallowing can be difficult.[5] Use of a sleeve device or high-resolution manometry using manometry catheters with closely spaced circumferential pressure sensors can help overcome this problem.[6] It is imperative to recognize that a prominent cricopharyngeal muscle during radiographic studies can be seen in normal infants and has been observed in up to 5% of adults having barium swallow studies for various reasons, who did not have CP achalasia.

Several neuromuscular disorders have been associated with CP achalasia (Table 23-3). In Chiari malformation, swallowing difficulty usually predates other signs of brainstem compromise.[7-9] Associated esophageal motility abnormalities, such as spontaneous esophageal contractions and nonpropagation of swallows, are also present. In a vast majority of patients, normal swallowing is observed following craniocervical decompression surgery.[7] Severity of the preoperative brainstem dysfunction is a good predictor of outcome following surgery.

Symptoms of UES achalasia can spontaneously improve in some children; therefore, an initial conservative approach with aggressive pulmonary and nutritional support can be tried. However, one must be vigilant and aware of the risk of aspiration, which can be life threatening. When spontaneous recovery does not occur, dilatation[4] or cricopharyngeal myotomy[10] should be considered. In children, unlike adults, a single dilatation may be sufficient and is effective in babies as young as 5 months of age. An adult study of radiographic and

Table 23-1. **Classification of Esophageal Motor Disorders**

Disorders Affecting Proximal Esophagus

Primary
  Cricopharyngeal achalasia
  Cricopharyngeal incoordination
  Cricopharyngeal hypotension
Secondary
  Central nervous system
  Meningocele
  Arnold-Chiari malformation
  Cerebrovascular accidents
  Multiple sclerosis
  Autonomic nervous system
  Familial dysautonomia
  Motor neurons
  Bulbar poliomyelitis
  Neuromuscular junction
  Myasthenia gravis
  Botulism
  Striated muscle
  Polymyositis
  Dermatomyositis
  Muscular dystrophy

Diseases Affecting Distal Esophagus

Primary
  Achalasia
  Diffuse esophageal spasm
  Nutcracker esophagus
  Nonspecific esophageal motility disorder
Secondary esophageal motility disorders
  Gastroesophageal reflux
  Hirschsprung's disease
  Intestinal pseudo-obstruction
  Diabetes mellitus
  Scleroderma and CREST
  Inflammatory myopathies
  Esophageal scarring
  Tracheoesophageal fistula
  Esophageal atresia

Table 23-2. **Factors Influencing Upper Esophageal Sphincter Pressure**

Reduced Upper Esophageal Sphincter Pressure

Sleep
Belching
Expiration
Vomiting
Neuromuscular disorders:
  Myasthenia gravis
  Polymyositis
  Oculopharyngeal muscular dystrophy
  Amyotrophic lateral sclerosis

Increased Upper Esophageal Sphincter Pressure

Stress
Esophageal distension
Intra esophageal acid
Pharyngeal stimulation with air or water
Inspiration

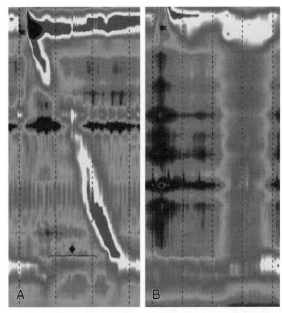

Figure 23-1. **(A)** High-resolution esophageal manometry showing a normal swallow. (Asterisk) Relaxation of the upper esophageal sphincter (UES). There is antegrade propagating contraction in the esophageal body with relaxation of the lower esophageal sphincter (LES) (diamond). **(B)** shows a typical swallow pattern in achalasia. There is relaxation of the UES during the swallow, but no propagating esophageal contractions and no LES relaxation, and a simultaneous increase in the intraluminal esophageal pressure. Image kindly provided by Dr. N. Tipnis, Medical College of Wisconsin, Milwaukee.

manometrically diagnosed patients with cricopharyngeal achalasia showed that cricopharyngeal myotomy was more beneficial when high pharyngeal pressures could be generated during swallows.[11] This suggests that when pharyngeal constrictors were able to generate contractions, the pharyngoesophageal bolus transit improved when the obstruction by the contracted UES was relieved.

Cricopharyngeal Incoordination

The pharynx receives frequent stimulation during breathing, bolus oral feeding, and gastroesophageal reflux. Depending on the type of stimulus, various reflex mechanisms help to adapt the anatomy and physiology of this region. This allows passage of the contents into the respiratory or the gastrointestinal tract. Cricopharyngeal incoordination is characterized by a delay in pharyngeal contraction in relation to cricopharyngeal relaxation during bolus oral feeding. It presents with swallowing difficulties, choking, and aspiration. Neonates with "transient cricopharyngeal incoordination" have a normal suck, but suffer from repeated choking and aspiration episodes. These symptoms can easily be confused with tracheoesophageal fistula or laryngotracheoesophageal cleft. Repeated choking and aspiration episodes can be life threatening, and early diagnosis is important. The clinical course is variable, and spontaneous improvement has been reported. Nutritional support and feeding advice are

essential. The aim should be to minimize the risk of aspiration, which can be life threatening.

Cricopharyngeal incoordination has also been reported in patients with central nervous system dysfunction such as Chiari malformation.[7] Cricopharyngeal incoordination may also result from cervical inflammation and constrictive processes, which restrict laryngeal and hyoid bone movement. In Pierre Robin sequence, sucking-swallowing electromyography and esophageal manometry reveal dysfunction in the motor organization of the tongue, the pharynx, and the esophagus.[12] Patients with familial dysautonomia (Riley-Day syndrome) have delayed, but complete, relaxation of UES and associated esophageal motility disorders.[13] Wyllie and colleagues reported two children with drooling following nitrazepam; both had delayed relaxation of

Table 23-3. **Conditions Associated With Cricopharyngeal Dysfunction**

Myoneural junction defect
  Myasthenia gravis
Muscular abnormality
  Dermato- and polymyositis
  Systemic lupus erythematosus
  Muscular dystrophy
  Acrosclerosis
  Thyrotoxic myopathy
  Paroxysmal hemoglobinuria
  Werdnig-Hoffman
  Tetanus
Neural defect
  Arnold-Chiari malformation
  Cerebral palsy
  Amyotrophic lateral sclerosis
  Syringobulbia
  Poliomyelitis
  Posterior inferior cerebellar artery syndrome
  Prematurity
  Meningomyelocele and hydrocephalus
Others
  Down syndrome

the UES in relation to pharyngeal contractions.[14] Cricopharyngeal incoordination with high-peaked esophageal peristalsis was reported in four patients with resistant myoclonic epilepsy being treated with nitrazepam. One patient required ventilation and improved following discontinuation of nitrazepam therapy.[15] UES dysfunction has also been reported in patients with Silver Russell syndrome, 5p⁻ (cri-du-chat) syndrome, and minimal change myopathy.[16]

Upper Esophageal Sphincter Hypotension

Reduced UES resting pressure is seen in a variety of neuromuscular disorders (see Table 23-2).[17] It is a manometric diagnosis, but the clinical significance is not clear because the UES is completely relaxed during sleep. It may predispose to regurgitation of esophageal contents into the oropharynx and risk of aspiration into the respiratory tract.

DISORDERS OF THE DISTAL ESOPHAGUS

Esophageal Achalasia
Incidence and Heredity

Achalasia is a motor disorder of the esophagus characterized by loss of esophageal peristalsis, increased LES pressure, and absent or incomplete relaxation of the LES with swallows. The incidence of achalasia has been estimated as 1 in 10,000.[18] Mayberry and Mayell, in a study of 129 children, determined an incidence rate of 0.1 to 0.3 cases per 100,000 children per year in the United Kingdom.[19] Patients with achalasia can present at any time from birth to the ninth decade of life. The majority of these are sporadic patients, and it is estimated that familial achalasia represents less than 1% of all achalasia cases. Most of these are horizontally transmitted and present in the first 5 years of life. Familial achalasia is more common in children born of consanguineous relationships, suggesting an autosomal recessive inheritance.[20,21] Concordance in monozygotic twins has also been reported.[22] Mayberry and Atkinson studied 167 families of patients with achalasia; 447 siblings were contacted and none had achalasia, suggesting that familial inheritance is rare.[23]

Pathogenesis

Autoimmune, infectious, and environmental causes have been implicated in studies of idiopathic achalasia. Neurons gradually disappear in the distal esophagus, and this is associated with localized infiltration of T lymphocytes, eosinophils, and mast cells. This would suggest a inflammatory neurodegeneration process. Identification of round cell infiltration of ganglion cells of the myenteric plexus and association with class II histocompatibility antigen, Dqw 1, favors an autoimmune hypothesis.[24] It has also been suggested that infectious or toxic inflammatory processes trigger interferon-γ release, thereby inducing the class II antigen expression on neural tissue. Neural tissue expressing class II antigen is recognized as a foreign by the T lymphocytes, which ultimately destroy the neural tissue. Serum antibodies to neurons of the myenteric plexus in patients with achalasia have been reported.[25,26] Measles and varicella zoster virus have been implicated in the pathogenesis of achalasia.[27,28] However, studies using polymerase chain reaction failed to identify herpes, measles, and human papillomavirus in esophageal specimens of achalasia patients.[29]

There may be minimal esophageal dilatation in early stages of the disease, and full-thickness esophageal biopsies show inflammation of the myenteric plexus, without a decrease in ganglion cells.[30] Later, there is a reduction in the ganglion cell number[31-33] and a decrease in varicose nerve fibers in the myenteric plexus.[34] Degenerative changes in the vagus nerve[31] have also been reported. However, it is not unusual for muscle biopsies obtained during surgery to be entirely normal with adequate numbers of ganglion cells. Quantitative and qualitative changes in the dorsal motor nucleus of the vagus, as well as a decrease in vasoactive intestinal peptide (VIP) and neuropeptide Y, have been reported in achalasia.[34,35] Vasoactive intestinal peptide is postulated as the major inhibitory transmitter released at the intramural postganglionic neurons of the LES, and low levels may be responsible for the lack of LES relaxation during swallowing. The intermediate mechanism by which VIP induces LES relaxation is not completely understood. In animal studies VIP and dopamine have been shown to activate adenylate cyclase and increase intracellular 3',5'-cyclic adenosine monophosphate concentration, which results in LES relaxation.[36,37] In guinea pig gastric fundic muscle cells, VIP released presynaptically stimulates intracellular nitric oxide synthase (NOS) and the production of nitric oxide (NO), resulting in muscle relaxation. Human studies have demonstrated the absence of NOS in the LES of patients with achalasia, and physiologic studies showed LES relaxation when NO was added to the muscle strips.[38,39] Similar pathologic findings are present in patients with triple A syndrome.[40]

Associations

Triple A Syndrome. Esophageal achalasia has been associated with adrenocorticotrophic hormone insensitivity and alacrima in triple A or Allgrove syndrome.[41] The gene for triple A syndrome has been localized to chromosome 12q13.[42,43] Alacrima is usually present from birth, and hypoglycemia due to adrenocortical deficiency develops within the first 5 years of life. However, symptoms can be subtle and may not be recognized well into adult life.[44]

Rozycki Syndrome. In this condition, achalasia is associated with autosomal recessive deafness, short stature, vitiligo, and muscle wasting.[45]

Other Associations. Achalasia is associated with Chagas' disease,[46] sarcoidoisis,[47] Hirschsprung's disease,[48] Down syndrome,[49] pyloric stenosis, paraneoplastic syndromes,[50] and Hodgkin's disease.[51] Achalasia has also been reported in association with neurodegenerative disorders such as hereditary cerebellar ataxia and myoneural disorders.[52]

Clinical Presentation

The clinical presentation depends on the duration of the disease and age of the child. The onset is usually gradual, and there can be a considerable delay from the time of onset of symptoms to diagnosis. In a review of 12 published studies, the mean duration of symptoms before the diagnosis was established was 23 months.[53] The mean age at diagnosis was 8.8 years.[53] In a worldwide survey of 175 children with achalasia, only 6% of the patients presented in infancy.[54] The youngest reported patient was a 900-g, 14-day-old premature baby.[55]

Infants and toddlers present with choking, cough, recurrent chest infections, feeding aversion, and failure to thrive. Older children usually present with vomiting, dysphagia, weight loss, respiratory symptoms, and slow eating (Table 23-4). Dysphagia may initially be confined to solids, but usually progresses to involve both liquids and solids. Stress is known to aggravate the symptoms. The child usually complains of food getting stuck in the chest, and repeated attempts at swallowing or washing the food down with liquid helps to relieve the symptom. Because of swallowing difficulty and discomfort the oral intake may be reduced, resulting in weight loss. Once the esophagus is dilated, the patient may regurgitate undigested, nonbilious, and generally nonacidic food eaten hours or days earlier. A large quantity of saliva can accumulate, especially at night, when the patient is lying flat. Early morning waking with choking episodes, bouts of coughing due to aspiration of esophageal contents, and vomiting whitish frothy saliva may be reported. Sudden death from aspiration is a serious risk. The patient may be aware of the gurgling sound from the fluid sloshing in the dilated esophagus.

Diagnosis

Radiography. In most instances, diagnosis of achalasia is considered following a barium swallow, which shows a variable degree of esophageal dilatation with tapering at the gastroesophageal junction[56,57] (Figure 23-2). One may also notice absent peristalsis or tertiary contractions. As the barium fills the dilated esophagus and the height of the barium column generates enough pressure to exceed the LES pressure, partial emptying of the barium column may be seen. Later in the disease process, the esophagus is grossly dilated and tortuous, with an S-shape described as the "sigmoid esophagus." Plain chest x-ray shows a widened mediastinum, an air fluid level, and an absent gastric air bubble. Radiography is also useful to evaluate the response to therapy. In adults, measurement of the height of the column of barium 5 minutes after barium ingestion in the upright position predicts a successful outcome following therapeutic interventions.[58]

Manometry. Manometry is the most sensitive and specific method for establishing the diagnosis of achalasia. The introduction of high-resolution manometry has enabled visualization of esophageal motility as a spatial continuum along the length of the esophagus with isobaric conditions represented as a color continuum (see Figure 23-1A). This, in conjunction with closely spaced manometry pressure sensors, has eliminated the problem of

Table 23-4. Symptoms of Achalasia in Children

Symptom	% of Children
Vomiting	80
Dysphagia	76
Weight loss	61
Respiratory symptoms	44
Chest pain/odynophagia	38
Failure to thrive	31
Nocturnal regurgitation	21

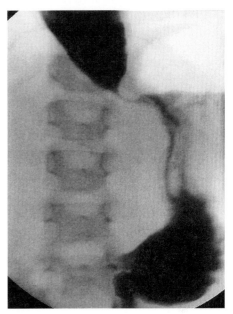

Figure 23-2. Barium swallow study in a child with achalasia showing esophageal dilatation and beaklike appearance.

movement-related artifact. The characteristic manometry findings in achalasia include absent esophageal peristalsis during dry and wet swallows, incomplete or absent LES relaxation, and elevated intraesophageal pressure (see Figure 23-1B). The LES pressure can be normal or elevated.[59] The lack of peristaltic contractions usually involves the entire length of the esophagus.[60] Abnormal or incomplete LES relaxation is seen in more than 70% of the patients. Because of obstruction at the distal end of the esophagus, the intraluminal pressure can be higher than the gastric fundal pressure.[61] Manometric abnormalities have been reported in babies as young as 2 weeks of age.[62] UES dysfunction including increased pressure, a short duration of relaxation with swallows, and a more rapid onset of pharyngeal contractions after UES relaxation has been reported.[63] The clinical significance of these findings is not clear.

Endoscopy. The esophagus appears patulous, and esophagitis secondary to food stasis and fermentation may be seen. The LES does not open during insufflations of air into the distal esophagus, and resistance may be noted with the passage of the endoscope through the gastroesophageal junction. Particular attention should be paid to the presence of a hiatal hernia, which can increase the risk of perforation during esophageal dilatation. Endoscopy also helps to exclude esophageal mucosal infection, carcinoma, and leiomyoma of the esophagus.

Table 23-5. Differential Diagnosis of Esophageal Achalasia

Esophageal stricture
Leiomyoma
Anorexia nervosa
Rumination
Chagas' disease
Candida esophagitis in chronic granulomatous disease
Adenocarcinoma of the stomach, oat cell carcinoma of the lung, and
    pancreatic carcinoma

Radionuclide Tests. A solid or liquid meal labeled with technetium-99m sulfur colloid can be used to measure esophageal emptying.[64] Patients with achalasia retain the tracer longer in the upright position.[65] The test may help to differentiate achalasia from other conditions such as scleroderma, because of the differing retention pattern. However, the usefulness of the test to assess patient response to therapy is debatable.

Differential Diagnosis

It is important to differentiate achalasia from other causes of esophageal obstruction (Table 23-5). Leiomyomas of the distal esophagus have been confused with achalasia in children.[66] Reluctance to eat because of difficulty in swallowing and associated weight loss may be confused with anorexia nervosa.[67] Regurgitating undigested food can mimic rumination symptoms in adolescents.[68] Esophageal motility abnormalities in Chagas' disease result from infection by *Trypanosoma cruzi*. The trypanosome causes destruction of the myenteric plexus, resulting in clinical and manometric findings similar to achalasia. This must be excluded in patients who have lived in or traveled to Latin America.[69] A transient achalasia-like motility disorder has been reported in a patient with underlying chronic granulomatous disease and *Candida* esophagitis.[70] In adults, gastric carcinoma involving the distal esophagus, oat cell carcinoma of the lung, and pancreatic carcinoma are associated with radiological and manometric findings similar to those in achalasia.

Treatment

Several treatment options are available for achalasia, including pneumatic dilatation, laparoscopic surgery, botulinum toxin injection into the lower esophageal sphincter, and pharmacologic therapies. In pediatric patients, pneumatic dilatation was previously considered as the best alternative because of its noninvasive nature and prolonged treatment response in many children. However, laparoscopic surgical approaches provide an alternative primary therapy. Regardless of treatment approach, several lifelong management considerations are recommended. First, patients remain at risk for recurrent aspiration due to residual food remaining in the esophagus following meals. This occurs particularly while recumbent and asleep. Therefore, patients should be encouraged to eat in an upright position, to clear solids by drinking fluids at the end of meals, and to minimize eating for several hours before bedtime. Second, all patients are at risk for chronic gastroesophageal reflux disease and resultant esophageal carcinoma, regardless of the approach to treatment. Thus, all patients require lifelong follow-up.

Pneumatic Dilatation. The objective of forceful esophageal dilatation is to stretch and rupture enough LES muscle to allow the passage of solids and liquids, without causing complete rupture of the esophagus or inducing gastroesophageal reflux. In a review of all published studies using dilatation therapy, 58% of patients had excellent or good outcome.[53] The rate of improvement varied from 35% to 100%. In the past two decades there has been a trend toward a general improvement in the number of patients with a "good" outcome with each subsequent study.[53]

Although the balloon dilatation techniques vary, several basic principles for successful dilatation have emerged over the years. The balloon must be positioned across the LES and the position confirmed radiographically, intermittently throughout the procedure. In patients with a dilated, tortuous esophagus, passing the balloon dilator over an endoscopically placed guidewire can reduce the risk of perforation. Using dilators with plastic balloons that are not elastic ensures a specific diameter and is safer.[71,72] Using a larger diameter balloon can increase the risk of perforation. The pressure applied during dilatation differs between published studies, but in general a minimum pressure of 300 mm Hg is used. The bag is inflated once or twice per session, and the inflation period can last from 15 to 20 seconds to several minutes. One study evaluated brief (6 seconds) with more prolonged (60 seconds) dilatation and found no difference.[73]

Successful dilatation allows the patient to eat regular meals without dysphagia. Very few studies have reported the long-term outcome following dilatation, and almost a quarter of adults require myotomy following unsuccessful dilatation.[74] If symptoms recur quickly or there is partial improvement, repeat dilation with a larger balloon or surgery is necessary. Some studies have suggested that children older than 9 years respond better to dilatation, and if symptoms reappear within 6 months, surgery is eventually required. With the introduction of minimally invasive surgical techniques, the role of dilatation therapy, with its inherent risk of perforation, as first-line treatment for achalasia has been challenged.

The main complications of pneumatic dilatation are esophageal perforation, fever, and pleural effusion.[75-77] Rare complications include persistent esophageal pain, aspiration pneumonia, and bleeding. Gastroesophageal reflux is a late complication in 5 to 12% of children.[53,78] The incidence of perforation in adults after pneumatic dilatation varies from 1 to 5%,[75,77] and estimated incidence in children is around 5.3%.[53] Most perforations occur at the distal left lateral aspect of the esophagus, usually 5 to 10 mm proximal to or 5 mm distal to the squamocolumnar junction,[79] suggesting that the LES muscle is fairly resistant to complete tearing. Esophageal perforation is accompanied with severe chest pain, fever, dysphagia, mediastinal and subcutaneous emphysema, or a pleural effusion. After dilatation, water-soluble contrast studies can identify perforation, and some units perform this routinely. In adults, the common postdilatation findings include linear mucosal tears; a contained perforation penetrating beyond the muscular wall; diverticular mucosal outpouching proximal to, within, or below the LES; and free perforation into the mediastinum, pleural space, or peritoneal cavity. Asymptomatic linear tears usually require no therapy; symptomatic tears and confined perforation beyond the muscular wall can be treated conservatively with intravenous antibiotics and nothing by mouth.[80] Immediate surgery and drainage is recommended for free perforation; however, medical treatment with intravenous antibiotics and parenteral nutrition has also been used successfully.

Surgery. Surgical treatment for achalasia in children previously was reserved for patients who developed perforation during dilatation, had residual dysphagia after multiple dilatations, or were poor candidates for dilatation because of associated comorbidities. The minimally invasive laparoscopic myotomy has outcomes comparable to open Heller myotomy and is now frequently offered as first-line treatment for achalasia. Most modern surgical procedures are variations of the Heller myotomy, and successful resolution of symptoms depends on the length of the myotomy. However, the adequate length of myotomy for children in different age groups is not known. It is argued that it must be long enough to relieve the obstruction, but not so long as to promote excessive gastroesophageal reflux. Intraoperative manometry has been used in adults to help guide the length of the myotomy.[81] The role of intraoperative manometry to document adequate reduction in lower esophageal sphincter pressure is not well studied in children. One small study has reported improved outcome following intraoperative manometry-guided myotomy in children.[82] The esophageal function is profoundly affected by general anesthesia and positive pressure ventilation, and the exact pressure and length of myotomy needed to be achieved is not known in children.

Good or excellent outcomes with symptom relief in 74 to 92% have been reported in children.[45,53,81,83-86,97-102] The best results are following a transabdominal myotomy with an antireflux procedure, resulting in long-term improvement in symptoms in more than 90% of patients. With the advent of laparoscopic techniques, the morbidity of achalasia surgery has been reduced significantly, and the majority of achalasia surgery in adults is now performed laparoscopically.[87] The surgical complications are comparable to those in open surgery, but laparoscopic myotomy is associated with a shorter hospital stay and quicker reintroduction of oral feeds.

The most common postoperative complications are residual dysphagia and gastroesophageal reflux. Postoperative gastroesophageal reflux is reported in 10 to 60%[53,88-90] of adult patients and 7 to 50% of pediatric patients.[53] Introducing an antireflux procedure at the time of a myotomy can reduce the risk of acid reflux, but increase the incidence of persistent dysphagia. Using a partial wrap and ensuring that it is not too tight can help reduce the risk of persistent dysphagia. Postsurgery dysphagia following open modified Heller myotomy was reported in 5% of patients. Dysphagia was more frequent when fundoplication was performed in association with Heller myotomy. Long-term follow-up and surveillance endoscopy, especially in adult life, is recommended because of an increased risk for developing esophageal carcinoma.[91]

Botulinum Toxin Injection. The botulinum toxin is a neurotoxin that binds to the presynaptic cholinergic terminals, thereby inhibiting the release of acetylcholine at the neuromuscular junction and producing chemical denervation. In achalasia, loss of inhibitory neurons in the myenteric plexus results in unopposed excitation of the smooth muscles of the lower esophageal sphincter. This excitatory effect is mediated through acetylcholine.[92] In adults, botulinum toxin has been used to treat achalasia and is a safe and simple therapeutic option. The toxin is injected endoscopically into the LES, and adult studies have reported a good initial response in 90% of patients. However, sustained response beyond 6 months was reported in a third of the patients.[93] Botulinum toxin treatment has been used successfully in children, but in a majority of children produces only short-term improvement, and most patients ultimately require dilatation or myotomy.[94-96] More

information is required before botulinum therapy can be recommended as first-line treatment for achalasia in children. The limited data indicate that like drug therapy, botulinum treatment may be a temporizing measure rather than a definitive treatment.

Drug Therapy. Isosorbide dinitrate, a smooth muscle relaxant, decreases LES pressure and improves esophageal emptying in achalasia.[97] However, headache and hypotension are common side effects, and drug resistance may develop with prolonged use. Nifedipine, a calcium channel blocker, also reduces LES pressure[98,99] and decreases the amplitude of esophageal contractions.[100] The pediatric experience is rather limited, but in one study of four adolescents with achalasia, LES pressure dropped by more than 50% after nifedipine therapy.[98] In one adult study, good long-term response was reported in two thirds of patients. It is generally accepted that drug treatment is a temporizing measure, and definitive therapy either by dilatation or surgical myotomy is generally required.

Nonachalasia Esophageal Motility Disorders

Diffuse Esophageal Spasm

Diffuse esophageal spasm (DES) is a clinical syndrome characterized by symptoms of sub-sternal distress, dysphagia, or both and an increased incidence of nonperistaltic esophageal contractions on manometry. Simultaneous contractions are rare in healthy individuals and usually seen with less than 10% of wet swallows. Manometry criteria for diagnosing DES include simultaneous esophageal contractions in 20% or greater of wet swallows intermixed with some normal peristalsis. If all contractions are simultaneous the diagnosis is achalasia. Very few studies have looked at DES as a possible cause of chest pain in children. Milov and colleagues reported DES in five adolescents with chest pain, and two had associated dysphagia.[101] Endoscopy was normal in all five. Three were successfully treated with sublingual isosorbide and one with diltiazem. Berezin and coworkers studied 27 children with chest pain; every child had an endoscopy, esophageal manometry, and the Bernstein test.[102] Esophageal manometry abnormalities were present in 4 patients: 3 had simultaneous esophageal contractions and associated esophagitis, and 1 patient had DES with normal endoscopy. Esophageal spasm has also been reported in a 22-month-old severely handicapped child who had significant acid reflux on pH study but no esophagitis on endoscopic examination.[103] Esophageal manometry, performed on three different occasions, showed DES that coincided with spells of crying and irritability and improved with verapamil, a calcium channel blocker. The etiology of DES is not known, but it has been suggested that it could be due to a defective deglutitive inhibitory reflex. Patients with DES show a hypersensitive response to cholinergic and hormonal stimulation, which may be related to a defect in neural inhibition due to decreased available nitric oxide.[104,36] Diffuse esophageal spasm is a dynamic disorder, and the manometric findings improve with time. The prognosis is generally good, and transition to achalasia occurs in only 3 to 5% of adults.[105]

Nutcracker Esophagus

The typical manometry finding of nutcracker esophagus (NE) is high-amplitude peristaltic contractions in a patient presenting with chest pain.[106] The amplitude of esophageal contraction should be at least two standard deviations above the normal. Prolonged duration contractions have also been described.[104] The manometric features may vary with time, and in one adult study only 54% of patients with an initial diagnosis of NE had the abnormality on subsequent study.[107] The psychological profile of patients with NE resembles that of irritable bowel syndrome[108] and can be associated with anxiety, depression, and somatization. Lower pain threshold to esophageal balloon distention, suggesting visceral hypersensitivity, has also been reported.[109] Barium studies are normal; tertiary waves or hiatal hernia are occasionally observed.[104] Some patients with NE may go on to develop achalasia.[106,110] The place of NE in the spectrum of esophageal motility disorders needs further clarification.

Nonspecific Esophageal Motility Disorder

Patients with abnormal esophageal motility, who do not fit any of the features described earlier in this chapter, are categorized as having a nonspecific esophageal motility disorder (NEMD). This includes patients who have low amplitude peristalsis (less than 12 mm Hg); nontransmitted contractions with more than 20% of wet swallow; and spontaneous, prolonged duration, retrograde, or triple-peaked esophageal contractions during manometric evaluation. Presenting symptoms include chest pain, dysphagia and gastroesophageal reflux. In one adult study 600 consecutive manometry recordings were reviewed and 61 patients were classified as NEMD.[111] The commonest abnormality recorded was nonpropagating esophageal contractions, observed in 40% of the wet swallows, followed by low-amplitude contractions in 22%, and 2% of wet swallows showed retrograde propagation or triple-peaked contractions.

NEMD is commonly seen in association with gastroesophageal reflux disease (GERD).[112] Absent esophageal contractions during swallowing are seen in infants with esophagitis.[113] Tertiary contraction, double-peaked peristaltic waves, and reduced amplitude of esophageal contractions have been reported in children with severe esophagitis.[114] These manometric abnormalities improved after effective treatment of esophagitis.

Treatment of Nonachalasia Esophageal Motility Disorders

There are very few published data in children regarding treatment of nonachalasia esophageal motor disorders. Reassurance and explanation of the underlying disorder responsible for the child's symptoms helps to relieve patient and parent anxiety. Advice regarding chewing food well, utilizing liquid chasers to ensure passage of solid food boluses, and avoiding food with extremes of temperature may be helpful. Nitrates and sublingual nifedipine reduce the amplitude of esophageal contraction and can improve dysphagia and chest pain. In adults, a placebo-controlled trial using trazodone[115] (an antidepressant) and imipramine[116] (a tricyclic antidepressant) reported improvement in chest pain. There are no similar trials in the pediatric age group.

Secondary Esophageal Motility Disorders

Intestinal Pseudo-obstruction

Low or absent LES pressure and low-amplitude tertiary esophageal contractions have been reported in children with intestinal pseudo-obstruction.[117]

Hirschsprung's Disease

Tertiary esophageal contractions, double- or multipeaked contractions, and nonpropagating contractions with more than 20% of swallows have been reported in children with Hirschsprung's disease.[118,119] Abnormal esophageal motility persists after surgical correction. Clinical significance of the manometry findings is unclear, because most of the patients have no symptoms due to this esophageal dysmotility.

Connective Tissue Disease

Scleroderma is a systemic disorder characterized by excessive connective tissue deposition in the skin and gastrointestinal tract. Esophageal motility disorders are common in adults and have also been reported in children.[120,121] These include low-amplitude contractions, tertiary contractions, and low LES resting pressure. Regurgitation, heartburn, and dysphagia are commonly reported,[122] and these symptoms are usually worse in patients with Raynaud's phenomenon. Abnormal esophageal motility is detected on barium swallow and manometry studies. Scintiscan studies demonstrate poor esophageal clearance.

Similar but less severe problems have also been reported in patients with polymyositis, dermatomyositis, systemic lupus erythematosus, the CREST syndrome, and mixed connective tissue disease. Corticosteroid treatment to control systemic symptoms may also improve esophageal symptoms. In Sjögren's syndrome, dysphagia due to lack of saliva is commonly noted. Decreased esophageal contraction time and an increased rate of propagation of esophageal contractions have been reported, but this is probably not clinically significant.

Esophageal Atresia and Tracheoesophageal Fistula

Abnormal esophageal motility is common and present from birth. Absent esophageal propagating contractions, tertiary contractions, low LES pressure, and GER with prolongation of acid clearance in the distal esophagus have been reported (see Chapter 21).

Dysmotility Due to Esophageal Scar Formation

Ingestion of corrosive poisons results in esophageal chemical burns that heal with scarring. Sclerotherapy for esophageal variceal bleeding may also lead to scarring and stricture formation. Dysphagia may result from stricture formation as well as a lack of esophageal propulsive activity in the area of the narrowed region.[123]

REFERENCES

3. Dinari G, Danziger Y, Mimouni M, et al. Cricopharyngeal dysfunction in childhood: treatment by dilatations. J Pediatr Gastroenterol Nutr 1987;6:212–216.
54. Myers NA, Jolley SG, Taylor R. Achalasia of the cardia in children: a worldwide survey. J Pediatr Surg 1994;29:1375–1379.
58. Vaezi MF, Baker ME, Achkar E, Richter JE. Timed barium oesophagram: better predictor of long term success after pneumatic dilation in achalasia than symptom assessment. Gut 2002;50:765–770.
81. Chapman JR, Joehl RJ, Murayama KM, et al. Achalasia treatment: improved outcome of laparoscopic myotomy with operative manometry. Arch Surg 2004;139:508–513; discussion 513.
114. Cucchiara S, Staiano A, Di Lorenzo C, et al. Esophageal motor abnormalities in children with gastroesophageal reflux and peptic esophagitis. J Pediatr 1986;108:907–910.

See expertconsult.com for a complete list of references and the review questions for this chapter.

OTHER DISEASES OF THE ESOPHAGUS

Shehzad A. Saeed • John T. Boyle

ESOPHAGEAL SYMPTOMS

Esophageal symptoms include heartburn, chest pain, dysphagia, and odynophagia, with or without associated vomiting or oral regurgitation. The differential diagnosis includes anatomical, infectious, and inflammatory disorders. Gastroesophageal reflux disease, eosinophilic esophagitis, structural abnormalities of the esophagus and chest, esophageal foreign body, caustic ingestion, and esophageal motility disorders are discussed in other chapters in this volume. This chapter addresses esophageal infections, chemotherapy/neutropenia-induced esophagitis, graft-versus-host disease, radiation esophagitis, medication-induced esophagitis, esophageal involvement by systemic immune-mediated disorders, and esophageal tumors.

ESOPHAGEAL INFECTIONS

Symptomatic esophageal infections are rare in healthy children. The most common infectious etiology in an immunocompetent host is herpes simplex.[1] Rarely, colonization and infection by *Candida* may be a complication of prolonged aggressive acid reduction therapy or chronic broad-spectrum antibiotic therapy. Colonization and infection by *Candida* may also complicate chronic disorders that alter esophageal anatomy, disorders that impair esophageal motility, or disorders that disrupt the esophageal mucosal barrier such as injury, radiation, or ulceration.

Most patients who develop infections of the esophagus have impaired immune function, particularly patients infected with human immunodeficiency virus (HIV), bone marrow or solid organ transplant recipients, patients with hematologic malignancies managed with cytotoxic drugs, and patients with immunodeficiency disorders that affect cellular immunity and/or granulocyte function.[2,3] At times patients with no obvious impaired immunity develop esophageal infection. Risk factors for esophageal infection also include conditions associated with alteration in cellular immunity including chronic corticosteroid usage (systemic or inhaled), radiation, severe burns, and generalized debilitation. Opportunistic esophageal infection by *Candida albicans*, herpes simplex virus, or cytomegalovirus (CMV) is most common, although a wide variety of other pathogens have been reported to cause esophageal infection in immunocompromised patients (Table 24-1).

Dysphagia, odynophagia, and chest pain are the most common symptoms of all causes of esophageal infection. Clinical presentation in immunocompromised patients may, however, be deceptive. Anorexia, nausea, heartburn, fever, or bleeding may be the predominant clinical presentation in immunocompromised children. Endoscopy with brushings and biopsy is the gold standard for diagnosis of esophageal infection.

Radiographic studies lack sensitivity to pick up early esophageal involvement and are of limited value in establishing an etiologic diagnosis of esophageal infection. An esophageal contrast study is most useful to exclude mechanical obstruction and to evaluate for the presence of perforation or fistula, which may complicate esophageal infection.

Candida Esophagitis

The most common infection of the esophagus is caused by *Candida albicans*, a yeast found in normal oral flora. Colonization entails superficial adherence and proliferation of *Candida* on the esophageal mucosa. Defenses against colonization include normal salivation, esophageal motility, a healthy esophageal epithelium, and a balance between oral bacterial and fungal flora. Infection results when *Candida* invades into esophageal epithelial cell layer, a process that usually requires defective mucosal immunity.[3,4] *Candida* esophagitis is an opportunistic infection that complicates disorders associated with granulocyte and/or lymphocyte numbers and dysfunction. Recent antibiotic exposure in such patients is a prominent risk factor. In a large pediatric study of HIV-positive patients, low CD4 counts (fewer than 50 cells per microliter) and antibiotic exposure were the most prominent risk factors for development of esophageal candidiasis.[5] Fungal virulence factors have also been implicated in the pathogenesis of infection, including ability of the specific species to colonize and adhere to esophageal mucosa by undergoing morphogenesis to the hyphal form or ability to express proteinases to lyse host cell membranes.

Oral thrush, a frequent finding among patients with esophageal infection, is often an indicator of an underlying pathologic esophageal process. In a large pediatric study of esophageal candidiasis, oral thrush was the single common presentation (94%), followed by odynophagia (80%), retrosternal chest pain (57%), fever (29%), nausea/vomiting (24%), dehydration (12%), and gastrointestinal (GI) bleeding (6%).[5] In adults, however, oral thrush was absent in 25% of *Candida* esophagitis cases.[6]

Endoscopy with brushings and biopsy is the gold standard for diagnosis and assessment of severity of *Candida* esophagitis.[7] Raised, white candidal plaques in the esophagus cannot be washed away with water. When plaques are brushed, there is usually bleeding at the site of attachment. The plaque represents desquamated epithelial cells with debris of fungal organisms, inflammatory cells, and bacteria. Esophagitis is assessed as grade 1 if the raised white plaques are 2 mm (tip of a biopsy forceps) or less in size, grade 2 if the raised white plaques are greater than 2 mm in size, grade 3 if mucosal ulceration is present or a confluent, thick plaquelike membrane coats the esophageal mucosa, and grade 4 if findings of grade 3 are

Table 24-1. Pathogens That Have Been Reported to Cause Esophageal Infection

Candida albicans
Mucormycosis
Herpes simplex virus
Varicella-zoster
Cytomegalovirus
Epstein-Barr virus
Miscellaneous *Candida* species
Papillomavirus
Tuberculosis
Cryptococcus
Miscellaneous bacterial species
Pneumocystis carinii
Aspergillosis
Leishmaniasis
Histoplasmosis
Bacillary angiomatosis
Blastomycosis
Cryptosporidiosis
Human herpes virus 6
Actinomycosis
Enterovirus
Mycobacterium avium

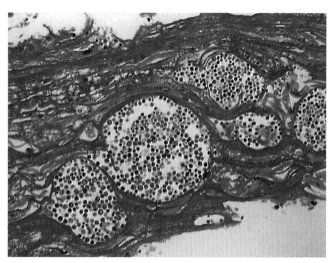

Figure 24-1. Invasive *Candida* esophagitis. The mucosa is necrotic, and the yeasts are within the mucosa (H&E, ×132). (*See plate section for color.*) Courtesy David R. Kelly, MD, Children's Hospital of Alabama and University of Alabama.

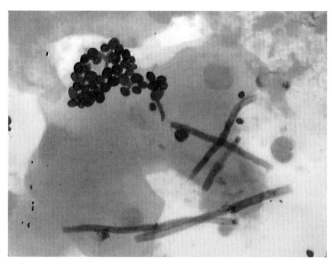

Figure 24-2. Yeasts, germ tubes (chlamydospores), and pseudohyphae of *Candida* in esophageal brushing specimen (GMS, ×330). (*See plate section for color.*) Courtesy David R. Kelly, MD, Children's Hospital of Alabama and University of Alabama,

associated with narrowing of the esophageal lumen.[6] Endoscopic appearance alone is insufficient for diagnosis of *Candida* esophagitis. Plaque-like material mimicking *Candida* may be found in severe reflux esophagitis, herpes simplex infection, CMV infection, pill esophagitis, eosinophilic esophagitis, and swallowed oropharyngeal debris. Cytologic examination of brushings is more sensitive than histologic examination of biopsy specimens to confirm diagnosis of esophagitis. Budding yeast cells, hyphae, and pseudohyphae are best seen by silver stain, periodic acid-Schiff (PAS) stain, or Gram stain. Brushings showing mycelial forms and budding yeast should be interpreted as confirming invasive *Candida* infection (Figures 24-1 and 24-2). Culture of the mucosa is usually not indicated, but should be sought if azole-resistant *Candida* species are suspected or if unusual pathogens (e.g., bacterial, *Mycobacterium tuberculosis*, or viral esophagitis) are being entertained in the differential diagnosis of the clinical presentation. Rarely, adherent plaques may not be present. An inflammatory stricture with no gross hint of a fungal cause may prove to have invasive fungal elements on biopsy.

In the past, treatment was usually dependent on the degree of immunosuppression and severity of mucosal involvement assessed at endoscopy. Patients with normal granulocytes, no or minimal lymphocyte defects and esophageal colonization, and grade 1 or 2 esophagitis were treated with topical antifungal agents including nystatin oral suspension or clotrimazole troches. Compliance was a factor in children because of the bitter taste of nystatin, the consistency of the troches, and the need for multiple daily doses. Topical agents are now reserved to treat candidal colonization in patients with normal immune function. Treatment of candidal infections was revolutionized in the 1990s by the availability of orally active triazole agents.[3] These agents inhibit the fungal cytochrome system required for fungal sterol synthesis to maintain cell wall integrity. The triazoles affect the fungal cell membrane permeability, leading to injury and cell death. They have excellent oral bioavailability, with levels after oral administration greater than 90% of the levels achieved with intravenous dosing. Intravenous therapy is only indicated in patients who are unable to swallow.

Absorption is facilitated by gastric acid; thus, it is important to avoid simultaneous acid reduction therapy if possible. Because triazole agents are much less potent inducers of the cytochrome P450 system in humans compared to earlier azole agents (ketoconazole), there is less potential for significant drug-drug interactions. Fluconazole is now the drug of choice for both treatment and prophylaxis of candidal esophagitis in patients with either granulocyte or lymphocyte dysfunction, with the exception described later (Table 24-2). Toxicities are uncommon and can include nausea, headache, and rash; significant hepatotoxicity is rare. The other oral triazole agent in clinical use, itraconazole, has a higher side effect potential, especially hepatotoxicity. It is reserved for patients who do not tolerate fluconazole or in fluconazole-resistant disease. Parenterally administered amphotericin B, complexed to a lipid or colloid carrier to reduce toxicity, remains the drug of choice for esophageal disease in the setting of disseminated candidal infection or in febrile neutropenic patients.

Table 24-2. **Treatment of *Candida* Esophagitis**

Suspected colonization or grade 1 infection in immunocompetent hosts
Nystatin, infants: 250,000 units qid; children: 500,000 units qid
Clotrimazole, 10-mg troche dissolved in mouth qid
Initial therapy of esophagitis
Fluconazole, 3 mg/kg per day, up to 200 mg PO daily for 3-4 weeks
Fluconazole-resistant disease
Fluconazole, 6-12 mg/kg per day, up to 400-600 mg PO daily for 3-4 weeks
Itraconazole oral solution, 3-5 mg/kg per day, up to 200 mg PO daily for 3-4 weeks
Amphotericin B, 0.3 mg/kg IV daily for 10-14 days
Patients with neutropenia and fever or documentation of disseminated *Candida* infection
Amphotericin B, 0.5-1.0 mg/kg IV daily for 3-4 weeks
Primary prophylaxis*
Fluconazole, 3 mg/kg per day, up to 100 mg PO daily
Secondary prophylaxis of HIV-infected patients
Fluconazole, 3 mg/kg per day, up to 100 mg PO daily, every third week

*Patients undergoing bone marrow or solid organ transplant, acute leukemia patients undergoing intensive cytotoxic chemotherapy, critically ill in intensive care units taking broad-spectrum antibiotics.

A predictable consequence of the increasing use of oral fluconazole therapy has been the emergence of resistant in vivo and in vitro strains. Risks for resistance include number of prior courses of fluconazole, cumulative exposure, and degree of immunosuppression. Another mechanism of clinically resistant disease is infection with more unusual species of *Candida*. Of potentially greater consequence are previously susceptible strains of *Candida albicans* that require progressively larger doses of fluconazole to achieve clinical response. Recent data suggest that in vitro susceptibility testing correlates well with clinical outcomes of treatment with fluconazole.[8] Many in vitro isolates intermediately or highly resistant to fluconazole remain susceptible to itraconazole. Although experience in pediatrics is limited, echinocandins including micafungin and anidulafungin have recently been shown to be effective following treatment failures with oral triazole agents.[9] Echinocandins are noncompetitive inhibitors of 1,3-beta-D-glucan synthase. Therapy results in reduced formation of 1,3-beta-D-glucan, an essential polysaccharide comprising 30% to 60% of *Candida* cell walls. Decreased glucan content leads to osmotic instability and cellular lysis. Also, low-dose, 10- to 14-day regimens of intravenous amphotericin B have been used effectively to treat local esophageal disease refractory to oral triazoles.

Several large adult studies have shown the benefit of oral fluconazole in the prevention of serious candidal infections in patients undergoing bone marrow or solid organ transplant, acute leukemia patients undergoing intensive cytotoxic chemotherapy, and critically ill patients in intensive care units who are taking broad-spectrum antibiotics.[10] Many treatment protocols now incorporate triazole agents as part of their standard prophylaxis regimen. The risk of emergence of acquired fluconazole resistance appears to be low in these settings. More controversial is the role of prophylaxis in HIV-infected patients. A large pediatric study of HIV-positive patients identified presence of oral candidiasis, low CD4+ counts (less than 200 CD4 cells/mm^3), and antibiotic exposure as the most prominent risk factors for development of esophageal candidiasis.[5] The main rationale for use of antifungal prophylaxis has been prevention of cryptococcal infections, which are associated with significant morbidity and mortality. Cyclical therapeutic protocols

have been reported in small populations. Because of concern of development of antifungal resistance, current U.S. Public Health Service/Infectious Disease Society of America guidelines do not recommend routine use of primary antifungal prophylaxis with triazole agents. Chronic secondary prophylaxis with fluconazole may be appropriate for patients with multiple or severe recurrences of *Candida* esophagitis.

Chronic mucocutaneous candidiasis is a rare clinical syndrome in which patients have persistent or recurrent candidal infections of the skin, nails, and mucous membranes. Invasive or disseminated infection is rare. A common immunologic abnormality is failure of the patient's T lymphocytes to produce cytokines that are essential for expression of cell-mediated immunity to *Candida*. Patients with chronic mucocutaneous candidiasis are at increased risk of developing autoimmune disorders (hemolytic anemia, idiopathic thrombocytopenic purpura, chronic active hepatitis, juvenile rheumatoid arthritis) and endocrinopathies (hypoparathyroidism, hypothyroidism, and Addison's disease). These patients require chronic prophylactic therapy and are at high risk to develop resistant strains.

Herpes Simplex Esophagitis

Most esophageal disease is caused by herpes simplex virus (HSV) type 1, which also causes the majority of oropharyngeal herpes infections.[1] Risk factors for esophageal disease include conditions that affect cellular immunity; unlike *Candida* esophagitis, granulocytopenia appears to be less important. There are numerous reports of cases in otherwise healthy children. Esophageal involvement can occur as a primary infection or as a manifestation of reactivated disease, because the virus may be latent in nerve ganglion cells. Unlike *Candida*, most esophageal infections occur in the absence of visible oral or nasolabial lesions. Fever is uncommon except during primary infection. Bleeding is more common in herpes infection, being reported in one-third of adult cases and ranging from heme-positive stool to massive hemorrhage.

The gold standard for diagnosis is upper endoscopy. The gross endoscopic appearance of HSV is nonspecific. Only a small percentage of patients have discrete 1- to 3-mm vesicles in the mid and distal esophagus. More common are sharply demarcated superficial ulcers with raised margins and yellow-gray bases, which form as vesicles slough. Plaque-like lesions with erythematous and friable mucosa that mimic *Candida* may also be present. Uninvolved mucosa appears normal. The diagnosis of HSV esophagitis is made by histopathology, viral culture, and polymerase chain reaction (PCR). Biopsies obtained from the margins of ulcers are more likely to show characteristic changes including multinucleated giant cells, cellular "ballooning," and the presence of eosinophilic intranuclear inclusions. Immunohistochemical stains for debris obtained from brushing ulcers may be useful in identifying sloughed infected HSV infected cells. Culture of HSV from esophageal biopsies is considered diagnostic and has been reported to have a higher yield than histologic techniques.

The decision to treat HSV esophagitis in immunocompetent patients is determined by the severity of the disease. HSV in healthy individuals tends to be self-limiting, and most require only supportive care. Resolution of symptoms may be gradual and take up to 2 weeks. The drug of choice for treatment in immunocompromised hosts is acyclovir[11] (oral, 80 mg/kg per day, up to 1000 mg/day in three to five doses for 7 to 14 days; IV, 15 to 30 mg/kg per day in three divided doses for 7 to 14 days). The decision to use parenteral therapy is based on the patient's ability to take oral medication and the severity of disease. Relapse may occur in immunocompromised patients, being reported in up to 15% of HIV-infected individuals. Such patients may require prolonged suppressive therapy. Acyclovir-resistant HSV infections have been described, especially in immunocompromised patients maintained on long-term therapy. Acyclovir-resistant mutant strains of HSV are usually susceptible to other systemic antivirals including foscarnet[12] (IV 80 to 120 mg/kg per day in two to three divided doses).

As with *Candida*, strategies for prevention of HSV infection have been incorporated into treatment protocols for patients with HSV-positive antibody status undergoing intensive immunosuppression regimens before bone marrow or solid organ transplant. Many of these regimens have started to use ganciclovir, which is effective against both HSV and CMV.

CMV Esophagitis

Unlike HSV esophagitis, which is found in a wide range of immunocompromised and healthy patients,[13] CMV esophagitis tends to be a complication of advanced HIV disease or iatrogenic immunosuppression in bone marrow and solid organ transplant recipients. HAART (highly active antiretroviral therapy) has significantly reduced the frequency of CMV infection in HIV disease. Esophageal disease can occur as a primary infection or from reactivation of latent infection. Esophageal infection also occurs in the setting of systemic viral dissemination. Thus, symptoms of fever, nausea, epigastric pain, diarrhea, and weight loss may be seen.

The gold standard for diagnosis is upper endoscopy. The gross endoscopic appearance of HSV is nonspecific. Shallow or deep ulcers against a background of normal mucosa are usually located in the mid-to-distal esophagus. Large ulcers greater than 1 cm in size suggest CMV. Because CMV-infected fibroblasts and endothelial cells are found in the base of esophageal ulcers and never in squamous epithelium, multiple biopsies should be taken from the center of the ulcer crater. Characteristic histologic features of CMV infection include large cells with amphiphilic intranuclear inclusions, halo surrounding the nucleus, and multiple small cytoplasmic inclusions (Figure 24-3). A biopsy of the ulcer base should also be obtained for culture and PCR.

Both intravenous ganciclovir and foscarnet appear to be very effective as initial therapy for CMV esophagitis. The dose of ganciclovir is 5 mg/kg per dose IV every 12 hours for 2 to 3 weeks with dosage adjustments for renal insufficiency. The primary toxicity of ganciclovir is marrow suppression, particularly neutropenia. This was an almost universal complication in HIV patients simultaneously receiving zidovudine, requiring the addition of granulocyte colony-stimulating factors. Recently, the wider choice of antiretroviral agents has reduced the need to maintain patients on zidovudine while being treated with ganciclovir. Other toxicities of ganciclovir include rash, nausea, vomiting, hepatotoxicity, and central nervous system toxicities. In patients who fail to respond to ganciclovir, the option is to switch to foscarnet (60 mg/kg per dose IV every 8 hours for 2 to 3 weeks), or to add foscarnet to ongoing ganciclovir therapy. The primary toxicity of foscarnet is nephrotoxicity. In several adult studies, only 50% of patients with gastrointestinal disease who respond to the initial course of therapy have relapse of symptoms.[13] All patients who do relapse should receive long-term maintenance therapy (ganciclovir, 5 mg/kg IV once daily) after acute treatment of their relapse.

All pediatric patients with HIV or candidates for bone marrow or solid organ transplant should be tested for prior

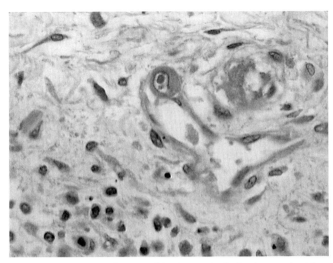

Figure 24-3. CMV esophagitis. This virus typically is characterized by a prominent eosinophilic intranuclear inclusion and displays vascular tropism (H&E, ×330). (*See plate section for color*) Courtesy David R. Kelly, MD, Children's Hospital of Alabama and University of Alabama.

exposure to CMV. In seronegative patients, every effort should be made to limit exposure to CMV-infected body fluids and blood products. A prophylaxis regimen, employing either acyclovir or ganciclovir, is now commonly used to treat transplant recipients who are CMV seropositive to prevent disease reactivation, or those are seronegative and receiving an organ from a CMV-seropositive donor. Routine primary prophylaxis is currently not recommended for HIV patients. Oral ganciclovir has been shown to be of benefit in decreasing the incidence of CMV infection in this population; however, the cost is high and no effect on overall mortality has been demonstrated.

Other Esophageal Pathogens

All additional esophageal pathogens listed in Table 24-1 are unusual and would need to be diagnosed specifically by culture, histopathological findings, or serology. Bacterial esophagitis is a possibility in severely immunocompromised neutropenic patients. Most reported infections are due to gram-positive pathogens. Endoscopic findings include diffuse esophageal inflammation, pseudomembranes, and ulcers. Histopathologic findings include evidence of deep bacterial invasion of mucosal layers without evidence of other pathogens. Culture of esophageal biopsies may or may not be specific, but at least guides therapy.

The esophagus is the gastrointestinal organ least likely to be infected by tuberculosis. Histoplasmosis and blastomycosis should be suspected in immunocompromised patients in areas where these organisms are endemic. Because itraconazole has increased activity against histoplasmosis and filamentous fungi including *Aspergillus*, this triazole should be considered for treatment of suspected superinfection with multiple opportunistic organisms.

Other Inflammatory Causes of "Esophageal Symptoms"

HIV-Associated Esophageal Ulcers

Patients with advanced HIV may develop single or multiple large ulcers in the mid to distal esophagus without evidence of specific infection. Onset is generally subacute. Patients may have coincident oropharyngeal aphthous ulceration. Patients generally have severe odynophagia and dysphagia. In the absence of a specific etiology, treatment is empiric. Some patients respond to high-dose systemic corticosteroids, sucralfate, and aggressive treatment of the underlying HIV infection.

Noninfectious Postchemotherapy Esophagitis

Leukopenic cancer patients or patients being conditioned for bone marrow transplant, especially those with hematologic malignancies, receiving intensive chemotherapy may develop fever, oropharyngeal mucositis or ulcers, odynophagia, dysphagia, and retrosternal chest pain. These symptoms often prevent adequate oral intake. The major differential diagnosis is *Candida* esophagitis versus chemotherapy-induced esophagitis.[14] The latter requires neutropenia and may represent a combination of immunosuppression and chemotherapy-induced cytotoxic mucosal injury or inhibition of mucosal cellular regeneration. Recovery from this severe complication is dependent on restoration of the leukocyte population. At endoscopy, the esophageal mucosa is friable, appears desquamated, or contains multiple mucosal ulcerations, raised white plaques, or thick confluent velvety whitish plaques. The appearance may be indistinguishable from that of *Candida* esophagitis. Because at least 50% of patients will have evidence of *Candida* in brushings or mucosal biopsies, strategies for the management of this clinical scenario have not been subjected to the same rigorous analysis as in patients with HIV disease. Fearing the high risk of systemic dissemination of mucosal infection, most pediatric oncologists will forgo endoscopic diagnosis and treat patients with this syndrome with broad-spectrum antibiotics and aggressive intravenous antifungal therapy.

Graft Versus Host Disease

The sudden onset of anorexia, dyspepsia, heartburn, nausea and vomiting may be the earliest manifestation of acute graft-versus-host disease (GVHD). Onset is usually 3 to 4 weeks after transplantation when the mucositis of conditioning chemotherapy have typically resolved. Gross esophageal involvement is rare, though biopsies of the esophageal mucosa may show characteristic intraepithelial cells with apoptotic keratinocytes diagnostic of GVHD. Diagnosis is more consistently achieved by biopsy of the gastric antrum, which is typically edematous and erythematous. Biopsy of this minimally abnormal mucosa may show the characteristic histologic findings of apoptosis of crypt epithelial cells, crypt dropout, and patchy lymphocytic infiltrates diagnostic of acute GVHD. Initial therapy for most patients consists of high-dose steroids with bowel rest.

A total of 25 to 40% of long-term survivors of bone marrow transplantation may develop chronic GVHD 3 to 12 months after engraftment.[15] Some 10% of these may manifest esophageal disease as dysphagia, odynophagia, and chest or retrosternal pain.[16] Radiology may reveal webs, ulcers, and strictures. Esophagogastroduodenoscopy reveals desquamation, vesicobullous lesions,[17] esophagitis, or normal-appearing mucosa. The procedure carries higher than normal risk of bleeding and perforation. The treatment of chronic GVHD is usually with prednisone and immunosuppression with imuran, cyclosporin, and tacrolimus.

Medication-Induced Esophagitis

Drug-induced esophagitis is an underdiagnosed entity. The drugs most commonly implicated in drug-induced esophagitis are doxycycline, tetracycline, slow-release potassium chloride, quinidine, alendronate, and nonsteroidal anti-inflammatory agents. Isolated reports have also implicated ferrous sulfate, clindamycin, rifampin, cromolyn sodium, oral theophylline, captopril, and ascorbic acid. Although patients with structural abnormalities and motility disorders of the esophagus are most at risk, drug-induced injury can develop in a normal esophagus. Symptoms are usually acute and follow immediately after ingestion of medication to several hours later. Most patients present with heartburn, odynophagia, and dysphagia, although hematemesis and melena have been reported from drug-induced esophageal damage. Single contrast x-rays will show changes only in severe cases where deep ulcers or stricture have occurred. Double-contrast studies may demonstrate discrete ovoid mucosal ulcerations. As with infectious esophagitis, endoscopy is far more sensitive than contrast x-ray for diagnosis of medication-induced esophagitis. The most common site of drug-induced esophagitis is the mid-esophagus at the level of the aortic arch. This area is characterized by external compression from the arch itself and by a physiologic reduction in amplitude of esophageal peristaltic waves. A common feature of most reported cases of esophageal ulceration due to slow-release potassium chloride is enlargement of the left atrium with compression of the esophagus. Antibiotics and anti-inflammatory drugs usually cause discrete ulcers, whereas injury due to potassium chloride is more likely to have smooth or ulcerated stricture. Esophageal biopsies show acute inflammation, ulceration, and edema.

The major differential diagnosis of acute dysphagia or odynophagia is GERD, infectious esophagitis, esophageal foreign body, medication-induced esophagitis, and caustic ingestion. In otherwise well patients taking doxycycline or tetracycline, it seems reasonable to stop the medication and treat with a time-limited 4-week course of acid reduction therapy with or without sucralfate. Rapid resolution of symptoms over a week would be expected. Although there may be a suspicion of medication-induced esophagitis, all other patients should undergo barium contrast x-ray to rule out esophageal stricture followed by upper endoscopy to establish a more objective diagnosis.

To reduce the risk of medication-induced esophageal injury, medications should be taken with adequate fluids and without immediately lying down for bed.

Radiation Esophagitis

Radiation injury to the esophagus usually affects the proximal esophagus and tends to be mild and self-limiting because the esophageal epithelium is relatively radiation resistant. Several predisposing factors have been implicated in radiation esophagitis, which include dose, schedule, and concomitant chemotherapy. The radiation damage usually begins within 2 weeks of initiation of radiation and resolves within a month or so after administration of the last dose.[18] Clinical symptoms include odynophagia, dysphagia, and chest pain. Rare complications include strictures, tracheoesophageal fistula, perforation, or gastrointestinal bleeding.[19] Treatment is empiric including acid reduction therapy, sucralfate, prokinetic drugs, and local anesthetics.[20] In some patients dilatation of strictures may be needed. There are no controlled studies assessing the efficacy of these modalities.

Esophageal Crohn's Disease and Behçet's Syndrome

Although Crohn's and Behçet's diseases need to be included in the differential diagnosis of patients presenting with dysphagia, odynophagia, or retrosternal pain, it is rare for esophageal symptoms to be the chief complaint in patients with these disorders. Ulcerating esophagitis with or without stricture formation has been described in case reports of both conditions. As more and more gastroenterologists have included upper endoscopy in the diagnostic evaluation of all patients with suspected inflammatory bowel disease, the incidence of nonspecific gross or histologic abnormalities in Crohn's disease has increased. Histology may vary from nonspecific chronic esophagitis suggesting GERD to characteristic noncaseating epithelial granuloma. Behçet's disease should be included in the differential of unexplained esophageal ulcers when there is a history of recurrent aphthous ulceration.

Epidermolysis Bullosa

Epidermolysis bullosa (EB) is a group of rare inherited disorders characterized by blister formation and scarring as a result of minor mechanical trauma. Major types of EB include epidermolysis bullosa simplex, hemidesmosomal epidermolysis bullosa, junctional epidermolysis bullosa, and recessive (dystrophic) epidermolysis bullosa (RDEB).[21] RDEB is most frequently associated with gastrointestinal lesions. Most of these types result from gene mutations encoding various types of collagen. Esophageal involvement can occur at any age, but usually occurs early in life. Mucosal bullae may occur spontaneously and may be precipitated by ingestion of food. This may lead to progressive dysphagia and near-total obstruction. Esophageal webs have also been reported, along with iron-deficiency anemia.[22] Most of these webs are in the cervical esophagus near the cricopharyngeal region. Strictures are also noted, most occurring in the proximal esophagus and one quarter in the lower esophagus. Radiological evaluation may help in assessing the location and severity of the anatomical lesions, but does not afford the potential for intervention. Management is symptomatic and geared toward minimizing blister formation and prevention of aspiration of food particles and secretions. Nutritional rehabilitation is the cornerstone of management and may require parenteral alimentation. Medical management has been tried with corticosteroids, phenytoin (doses adjusted for serum levels of 10 µg/L).[23] Recurrent strictures have been successfully treated with repeated balloon dilatations.[24,25] Colonic interposition is performed for nonresponding strictures or for perforation.[26,27]

ESOPHAGEAL TUMORS

Esophageal tumors are rare in children. Case series of esophageal lipomas,[28] fibromas,[29] leiomyomas,[30] granular cell tumors,[31] and adenocarcinomas (mostly in the setting of Barrett's esophagus)[32] have been reported in the literature. Clinical presentation may depend on the extension of the tumor mass into the lumen or surrounding organs. Patients may present with dysphagia, vomiting, anorexia, weight loss, or recurrent pulmonary symptoms and pneumonias. Endoscopic ultrasound may play a vital role in the diagnosis of these lesions, along with upper endoscopy. Treatment is tailored toward the specific lesion, and surgical resection remains the mainstay of treatment.

REFERENCES

1. Lavery EA, Coyle WJ. Herpes simplex virus and the alimentary tract. Curr Gastroenterol Rep 2008;10:417–423.
3. Pace F, Pallotta S, Antinori S. Nongastrointestinal reflux disease-related infectious, inflammatory and injurious disorders of the esophagus. Curr Opin Gastroenterol 2007;23:446–451.
4. Traeder C, Kowoll S, Arasteh K. *Candida* infection in HIV positive patients 1985-2007. Mycoses 2008;51(Suppl. 2):58–61.
9. de la Torre P, Meyer DK, Reboli AC. Anidulafungin: a novel echinocandin for candida infections. Future Microbiol 2008;3:593–601.
13. Baroco AL, Oldfield EC. Gastrointestinal cytomegalovirus disease in the immunocompromised patient. Curr Gastroenterol Rep 2008;10:409–416.

See expertconsult.com for a complete list of references and the review questions for this chapter.

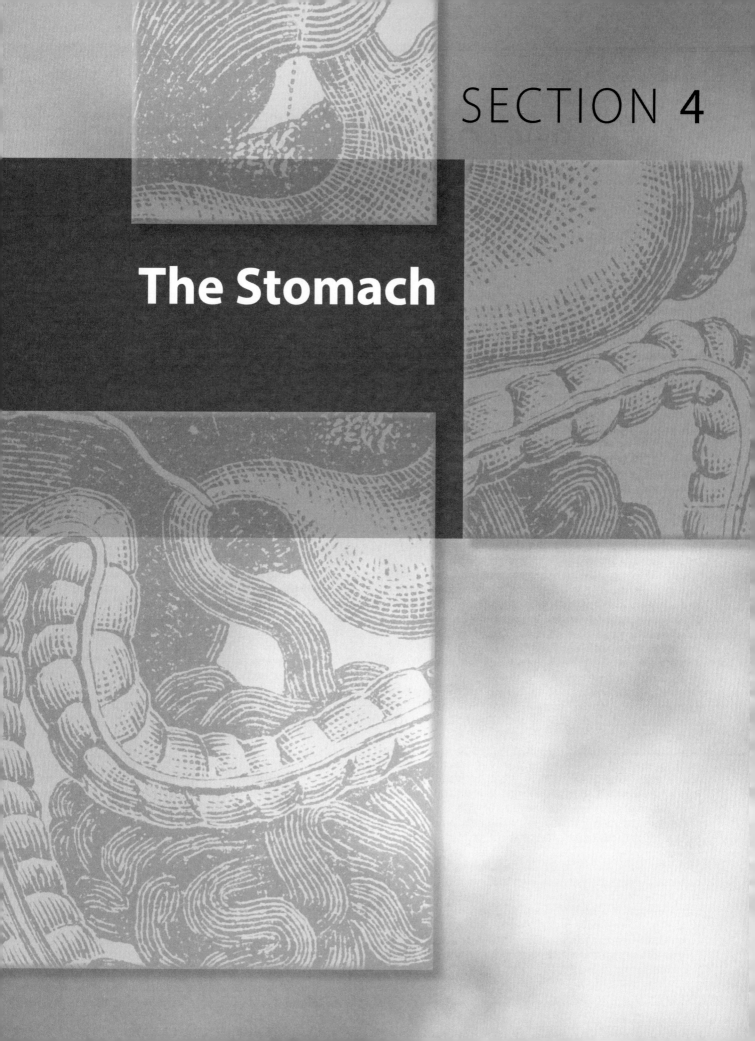

SECTION 4

The Stomach

25 DEVELOPMENTAL ANATOMY AND PHYSIOLOGY OF THE STOMACH

Steven J. Czinn • Samra S. Blanchard

The gastrointestinal tract begins as a primitive tubular system and is one of the first organs to polarize the embryo by forming an entry and exit with an anterior and posterior axis, also known as the craniocaudal axis, extending from the mouth to the cloaca (Figure 25-1). The nonneural elements of the gut are derived from endodermal and mesodermal cells. Bilateral folding of these layers forms the intestinal lumen, which is surrounded by concentric endodermal and splanchnic epithelia, creating a tubular gut. Cells from the outer epithelium migrate outward and form a loose mesenchyme, which later forms the muscle and connective tissue, while neural elements migrate from the neural crest at vagal and sacral levels to form the enteric nervous system.

The tubular gut has three distinct sections: the foregut, midgut, and hindgut. One of the first gross morphologic distinctions is the rotation and distention of the posterior foregut to begin differentiating the stomach just distal to esophagus. The stomach is also separated from the esophagus by the newly formed diaphragm from the developing abdominal cavity. At the end of the fourth and beginning of the fifth week, the stomach can be recognized as a fusiform dilation, which is initially oriented in the median plane. This primordial stomach soon enlarges and broadens ventrodorsally. During the next 2 weeks, the dorsal border of the primordial stomach grows faster than its ventral border (lesser curvature), demarcating the greater curvature of the stomach. As the stomach enlarges, it slowly rotates 90° in the clockwise direction around its longitudinal axis.[1] The ventral border moves to the right, and the dorsal border (greater curvature) moves to the left, changing the position of stomach. The original left side moves to the ventral surface, and the right side moves to the dorsal surface. During rotation and growth of the stomach, the cranial region moves to the left and slightly inferiorly, and its caudal region moves to the right and superiorly. After rotation, the stomach assumes its final position in the upper abdomen, with its long axis almost transverse to the long axis of the body. The rotation and growth of the stomach explains why the left vagus nerve supplies the anterior wall of the adult stomach and the right vagus nerve innervates the posterior wall of the stomach.[2]

Arterial blood supply to the distal esophagus, stomach, and proximal duodenum is derived from the branches of the celiac axis. The stomach is drained by the left gastric vein, right gastric vein, right and left gastroepiploic veins, and short gastric veins. These veins have no valves and can provide collateral blood flow when any portion of the portal system is obstructed. Esophageal and gastric varices usually involve the left gastric and short gastric veins.

The lymphatic drainage from the stomach enters the thoracic duct via the celiac nodes. Ultimately, the lymphatic drainage enters the venous system in the neck at the junction of the left internal jugular and left subclavian veins. Because of this anatomic relationship, gastric malignancies in adults may present with left supraclavicular lymph node metastasis.

Vagal and sympathetic fibers innervate the entire stomach by about 9 weeks of gestation.[3] Two major networks of nerve fibers are intrinsic to the gastrointestinal tract: the myenteric plexus (Auerbach's plexus), which can be found between the outer longitudinal and middle circular layers of muscle, and the submucosal plexus (Meissner's plexus), located between the middle circular muscular layer and the mucosa. Collectively, these neurons constitute the enteric nervous system. Catecholamines have been demonstrated in sympathetic fibers in Auerbach's plexus by week 10 and in Meissner's plexus by week 13.[4]

HISTOLOGY

Development of fetal human gastric mucosa occurs very early during fetal life. The first pit/gland structures are observed at 11 to 12 weeks of gestation. Between 11 and 17 weeks, the stratified surface epithelium is replaced by a simple mucous columnar epithelium, and gastric glands develop further. At this stage, the progenitor zone of the pit/gland structure is already localized in the isthmus,[5] as in adult mucosa.[1,6]

The gastric mucosa is organized in vertical tubular units consisting of an apical pit region, an isthmus, and the actual gland region that forms the lower part of the vertical unit. The progenitor cell of the gastric unit gives rise to all epithelial cells. The mucus-producing pit cells migrate up toward the gastric lumen, and acid-secreting parietal cells (oxyntic; *oxys* is Greek for acid) migrate downward to the middle and lower regions of the gland. Chief (zymogenic) cells secrete pepsinogen and predominate at the base of glands. Neuroendocrine cells, including enterochromaffin cells (serotonin), enterochromaffin-like (ECL) cells (histamine), and D cells (somatostatin), are also present at the base of the gland.

The glands of the different anatomic parts of stomach are lined with different types of cell (Figure 25-2). The cardiac glands are mostly populated by mucus-secreting or endocrine cells. The cardiac pits are irregular and shallow; the ratio of the lengths of pits:glands is approximately 1:1. In the body of the stomach, including the fundus, the glands are long and deep with straight pits. The ratio of the lengths of pits:glands is approximately 1:4. The gastric gland has parietal (oxyntic) cells that secrete hydrochloric acid and intrinsic factor, chief (zymogen, peptic) cells that secrete pepsinogens, endocrine cells, and mucous neck cells.

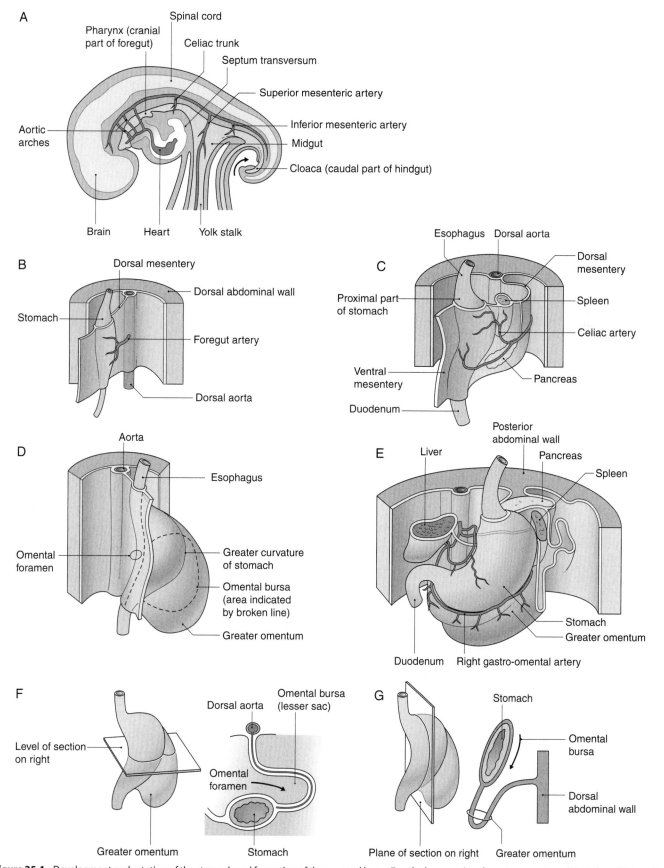

Figure 25-1. Development and rotation of the stomach and formation of the omental bursa (i.e., the lesser sac) and greater omentum. (**A**) 28 days. (**B**) Anterior lateral view at 28 days. (**C**) 35 days. (**D**) 40 days. (**E**) 48 days. (**F**) Lateral view at 52 days with a transverse section of the omental foramen and omental bursa. (**G**) Sagittal section of the omental bursa and greater omentum. Adapted from Moore and Persaud (1998), with permission.[47]

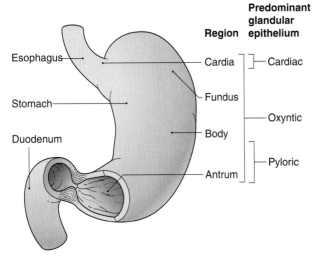

Figure 25-2. Anatomy of the stomach.

The antrum and pylorus contain the pyloric glands, composed of mainly mucous, endocrine, and G cells. There are very few parietal or chief cells. The glands here are characterized by deep pits but short glands, with a pit:gland ratio close to 1:1. Mucus is also secreted along with bicarbonate (HCO_3^-) by the surface mucous cells between glands. Surface mucous cells secrete neutral mucus, rather than the sulfated mucus secreted by mucous neck cells, which reside in close proximity to parietal cells. The surface mucous cells are cytoprotective, whereas the mucous neck cell functions as a stem cell precursor for surface mucous, parietal, chief, and endocrine cells.

NEUROMUSCULAR FUNCTIONS

Gastric motility is controlled centrally as well as by local neurohormonal control of the muscle layers, which include outer longitudinal, middle circular, and inner oblique fibers. Neuronal control involves the intrinsic myenteric plexus, the extrinsic postganglionic sympathetic fibers of the celiac plexus, and the preganglionic parasympathetic fibers of the vagus nerve. The vagal afferents are both relaxatory and excitatory.

Functionally, the stomach can be divided into two parts: the proximal stomach and the antrum. The proximal stomach, consisting of the cardia, fundus, and a portion of the body, is responsible for the storage of food and is capable of accommodating a large volume of nutrients with receptive relaxation and no dramatic rise in intragastric pressure.[5] Di Lorenzo et al.[7] demonstrated that the receptive relaxation of the proximal stomach is negligible in infants; this might explain in part the increased incidence of reflux in newborns.

The rate at which the stomach empties into the duodenum also depends on the type and components of food ingested. Liquids and solids have different mechanisms of emptying. An increased tonic intraluminal pressure in the fundus is necessary for the emptying of liquids. Liquid emptying has an exponential pattern of emptying that is dependent on the volume ingested as well as the osmolarity of the liquid. This is determined largely by the pressure differences between the stomach and duodenum and is modulated by receptors in the duodenum that slow gastric emptying when the caloric density or volume load reaching the duodenum is excessive.[8]

Solid food emptying has an initial lag phase followed by a linear phase. The distal stomach, which consists of the antrum and pylorus, is responsible for grinding and emptying solid food. Gastric peristaltic waves originating in the body of the stomach propagate toward the pylorus. The antral contractions allow only the small particles and liquids to pass into the duodenum and drive the larger particles (greater than 0.2 mm) back into the body of the stomach by retrograde propulsion. Food rich in carbohydrate leaves the stomach within a few hours. However, protein-rich food leaves more slowly, and emptying is slowest after a meal containing a significant amount of fat.[9] Finally, the rate of emptying also depends on antral distention (gastrogastric reflex), concentration of lipid, protein, and acid in the duodenum (duodenogastric reflex), and colonic distention (cologastric reflex).[10,11]

As a result of ingesting a meal, gastric distention stimulates "gastric mechanoreceptors" and hyperosmolality of the duodenal contents sensed by "duodenal osmoreceptors" initiate both enterogastric neural reflexes. Cholecystokinin (CCK) is released in response to this reflux and binds to CCK-1, previously termed CCK$_a$, receptors on gastric afferents, producing inhibition of the excitatory vagal efferents to the fundus. The primary inhibitory neurotransmitter is nitric oxide, which controls transpyloric flow, antral motility, and pyloric contraction. Serotonin is also involved in the inhibitory pathway. Appropriate propagation of gastric contractions or antroduodenal coordination is of great importance to the emptying of the stomach. Gastric motility is regulated by gastric myoelectric activity and consists of gastric slow waves and spike or second potentials. The gastric slow wave determines the propagation and maximum frequency of gastric contractions. It is generated in an area of the greater curvature that has the fastest rate of inherent rhythmicity and acts as a pacemaker controlling the rate and direction of propagation of gastric electrical activity. The normal frequency of gastric slow waves is 3 cycles per minute (cpm) in healthy humans. Abnormalities in the frequency of the gastric slow waves have been reported in a number of clinical settings, associated with gastric motor disorders and gastrointestinal symptoms. Gastric slow-wave activity can be measured noninvasively using the technique of electrogastrography (EGG).[12-14] Gastric motor activity initially appears between the gestational ages of 14 and 24 weeks.[15] EGG patterns at 35 weeks' gestation are similar to those of a full-term infant.[16] EGG patterns continue to mature over the first 6 to 24 months, reaching a stable pattern.[17]

A characteristic feature of fasting motor activity in the older child is the migrating motor complex (MMC), a highly organized propagated sequence of contractions that migrates from the stomach into the intestine and toward the ileum every 90 to 120 min. Three distinctive phases appear in sequence. Phase 1 is a pattern of quiescence that always follows phase 3. Phase 2 is a period of irregular contractions, varying in amplitude and periodicity. Because of this variation, some contractions are not propagated. Phase 3 is a distinctive pattern of regular high-amplitude contractions repeating at a maximal rate for 3 to 10 min and migrating from proximal to distal. The MMC begins anywhere from the esophagus to the ileum. About half of these contractions begin in the esophagus or the gastric body and migrate downward. Motilin is responsible for initiating phase 3 contractions that begin in the stomach. Gastric MMCs are present in newborns and preterm infants older than 32 weeks' gestational age. In younger preterm infants, only uncoordinated, nonmigrating contractions are present. The clinical implications of nonmigrating phase 3 contractions in very preterm infants are unknown. Theoretically, nonmigrating phase 3 contractions should not cause feeding intolerance, because liquid gastric emptying is related to the function of the fundus and not to antral peristalsis.

GASTRIC SECRETIONS

The stomach secretes water, electrolytes, hydrochloric acid, and glycoproteins, including mucin, intrinsic factor, and enzymes (Figure 25-3).

Gastric motility and secretion are regulated by neural and humoral mechanisms. For convenience, the physiologic regulation of gastric secretion is usually discussed as being either *cephalic* or *peripheral*, which includes both gastric and intestinal influences, although these overlap. The cephalic influences are vagally mediated responses induced by activity in the central nervous system. The vagus nerve contains afferent fibers that transmit sensory information from the gut to the brainstem, and efferent fibers that form the motor limb of the vasovagal reflexes. The cephalic phase of acid secretion is induced by sensory inputs of the thought, smell, sight, and taste of the food. The efferent fibers for this reflex are in the vagus nerves. Cephalic influences are responsible for one third to one half of the acid secreted in response to a normal meal and are abolished by vagotomy. Vagal stimulation increases gastrin secretion by release of gastrin-releasing peptide (GRP), or bombesin. Other vagal fibers release acetylcholine, which acts directly on the cells in the glands in the body and the fundus of the stomach. Acetylcholine binds to M_3 muscarinic receptors on the parietal cell and stimulates gastric acid secretion via calcium and phosphoinositol pathways.[18]

The peripheral mechanisms include gastric influences, consisting of local reflex responses to gastrin, and intestinal influences, reflex and hormonal feedback effects on gastric secretion initiated from the mucosa of the small intestine. Finally, the stomach also contains exocrine epithelial cells and endocrine-like neural regulatory cells.

GASTRIC ACID SECRETION

Hydrochloric Acid Secretion

Golgi first proposed that the parietal cell was the source of gastric acid and that it was formed within the surface invaginations, which he termed secretory canaliculi.[19] The ultrastructure of the parietal cell has numerous large mitochondria to provide adenosine triphosphate (ATP) for acid secretion. The H^+,K^+-ATPase (gastric acid pump, or proton pump) is a membrane-embedded protein identified and isolated in the 1970s. Parietal cells express receptors for acetylcholine, gastrin and histamine (Figure 25-4). The binding of these ligands to receptors on the surface of the parietal cell starts changes in second messengers that regulate the movement and location of the gastric proton pump. The H^+,K^+-ATPase exchanges protons for potassium and is responsible for gastric luminal acidification. In the resting state, the enzyme is stored in the cytoplasmic tubulovesicles. When the parietal cells are stimulated, the tubulovesicular structures fuse with the apical membrane to form secretory canaliculus, and the proton pumps start actively pumping H^+ ions in exchange for K^+. Pumping H^+ out of the parietal cells in exchange for K^+ requires appreciable energy, and this is provided by hydrolysis of ATP. Cl^- is also extruded

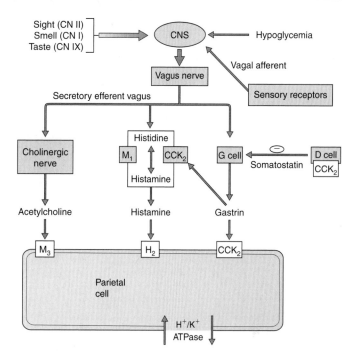

Figure 25-3. Secretory influences and hormones involved in the synthesis and secretion of hydrochloric acid by parietal cells. CCK, cholecystokinin; CNS, central nervous system.

down its electrochemical gradient through channels that are activated by cyclic adenosine monophosphate (cAMP) in the apical membrane. Ultimately, acid is generated from the dissociation of two molecules of water to form H_3O^+ and OH^-. The H_3O^+ is secreted via the proton pump in exchange for K^+, while the corresponding OH^- combines in the cell with carbon dioxide to form HCO_3^-. This reaction is catalyzed by carbonic anhydrase, and the parietal cells are particularly rich in this enzyme. The formed HCO_3^- is extruded by a conductance pathway on the basolateral membrane in exchange for Cl^- ions.

The H^+,K^+-ATPase is a heterodimer composed of two noncovalently linked subunits, α and β. The α subunit contains the catalytic site of the enzyme, which is important for functioning of the H^+,K^+-ATPase. It contains the cysteine residues where proton pump inhibitors bind. The β subunit appears to play a role in formation of tubulovesicle membranes and the transfer of enzyme to the apical membrane, and it may protect the enzyme from degradation.

In newborns, gastric pH ranges from 6.0 to 8.0. This is followed by a burst of acid secretion 24 to 48 hours after birth to adult levels (pH 1.0 to 3.0). Acid secretion then returns to low levels during the next few months of life, and adult pH levels are not reached again until 2 years of age.[20]

Stimulants of Gastric Acid Secretion

A variety of biological agents are present in the gastric mucosa including gastrin, histamine, GRP, ghrelin, and orexin, which stimulate the acid secretion, whereas leptin and glucagon-like peptide 1 released from the small intestine inhibit acid secretion.

Gastrin

Gastrin, produced by the antral G cell, is the most potent endogenous stimulant of gastric acid secretion during ingestion of a meal. The major stimulant of G cells in pyloric and

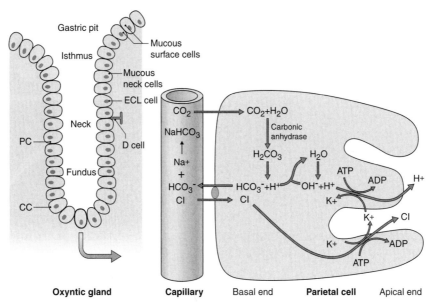

Figure 25-4. Steps involved in the secretion of hydrochloric acid into the gastric lumen. CC, chief cells; D cell, somatostatin-containing D cells; ECL, enterochromaffin-like cells; PC, parietal cell.

duodenal glands are luminal amino acids derived from peptic hydrolysis of dietary proteins. Gastrin stimulates the parietal cells directly, acting via CCK-2 receptor, a G protein-coupled receptor previously termed the CCK_b, and indirectly by stimulating enterochromaffin-like cells to secrete histamine. Histamine induces acid secretion by activating parietal cell H_2 receptors. The action of gastrin is mediated by an increase in intracellular calcium concentration compared with that of histamine, which is mediated by an increase in both calcium and cAMP levels.

As well as stimulating gastric acid secretion, gastrin has trophic effects on gastric oxyntic mucosa. Gastrin stimulates the migration of gastric epithelial cells directly and indirectly via multiple pathways that include the release of fibroblast growth factor, activation of the epidermal growth factor receptor, and activation of the mitogen-activated protein kinase pathway.[21]

Gastrin is also found in the pancreatic islets in fetal life. This may explain why gastrin-secreting tumors, called gastrinomas, occur in the pancreas. It is uncertain whether any gastrin is present in the pancreas of normal adults.

Chronic hypergastrinemia, whether induced by antisecretory medications, Zollinger-Ellison syndrome, or chronic atrophic gastritis, induces proliferation of gastric ECL cells.

Histamine

Histamine is stored primarily in the ECL cells that reside in the basal half of the oxyntic gland.[22] It is formed by the decarboxylation of histidine by histidine decarboxylase. Histamine receptors have been classified into four major subclasses: H_1, H_2, H_3, and, most recently, H_4.[23] Histamine, released from ECL cells, stimulates acid secretion primarily by interacting with H_2 receptors on parietal cells. H_3 receptor agonists have been reported to stimulate acid secretion in vitro and to inhibit acid secretion in vivo. The former is caused by inhibition of gastric somatostatin secretion, whereas the latter is more than likely caused by the central effects of these agents.[23-25] Gastrin, vasoactive intestinal peptide (VIP), and pituitary adenylate cyclase-activating peptide (PACAP)

directly stimulate histamine release from ECL cells, whereas somatostatin, peptide YY, and dopamine directly inhibit histamine release from ECL cells. Because VIP and PACAP also stimulate somatostatin secretion, the net effect depends on the relative contributions of the direct stimulatory and indirect inhibitory pathways.

Acetylcholine

Acetylcholine is released from postganglionic nerves in Meissner's plexus, stimulating the parietal cell directly via the muscarinic M_3-type receptors. Activation of M_3 receptors on the parietal cell leads to an increase in intracellular calcium. Calcium and cAMP then activate a set of protein kinases, resulting in the activation of the proton pump.

Other Stimulating Factors

Hypoglycemia acting via the brain and vagal efferents can also stimulate acid and pepsin secretion. Other stimulants include alcohol and caffeine, both of which act directly on the mucosa. Finally, glucocorticoids, acting via phosphoinositide 3 kinase and serum-inducible kinase and glucocorticoid-inducible kinase, stimulate acid secretion. This is one of the mechanisms whereby glucocorticoids promote the development of peptic ulcer disease.[18]

Inhibitors of Gastric Acid Secretion

Gastric acid secretion is also regulated by inhibitory mechanisms that are triggered by the stimulation of certain peptides as a result of the presence of nutrients in the intestine.

Somatostatin

In the stomach, somatostatin, which is present in D cells, inhibits acid secretion directly by acting on parietal cells and indirectly by inhibiting histamine secretion from ECL cells and gastrin secretion from G cells. Most of the somatostatin in the stomach is S14 and acts via a paracrine mechanism, whereas the somatostatin entering the circulation after a meal is mostly the S28 peptide derived from the small intestine.

Cholecystokinin

CCK inhibits acid secretion by binding to CCK-1 receptors on the gastric mucosal somatostatin cells, while stimulating acid secretion by binding to CCK-2 receptors on both parietal and ECL cells. Inhibitory function is more dominant.

Prostaglandins

Prostaglandin E_2 protects the gastric mucosa and inhibits acid secretion. The physiologic effects of prostaglandin E_2 on the gut are mediated by activation of four receptor subtypes that are expressed in parietal cells and one receptor on gastric mucous cells.

Secretin

Secretin-containing cells are located mainly in the upper small intestine. Secretin is released into the circulation from duodenal cells in response to gastric acid delivered into the lumen of the duodenum. In addition, bile salts and digested products of fat and protein can stimulate secretin release. Physiologic actions of secretin include stimulation of pancreatic exocrine secretion of water and bicarbonate, and inhibition of gastric acid secretion.

Structurally, secretin has sequence homology with other regulatory peptides that inhibit gastric acid, such as gastric inhibitory peptide (GIP), VIP, PACAP, and glucagon-like peptide (GLP) 1 and 2.

OTHER HORMONES AND PEPTIDES

Leptin

Leptin is a hormone produced mainly by the adipose tissue and plays a role in regulation of energy balance. Leptin has been detected in the fundic glands, both in the pepsinogen granules of chief cells and in the inhibitory peptide granules of endocrine-type cells. It is sensitive to the nutritional state and is rapidly mobilized in response to food ingestion following a fast, and may play a role in the regulation of short-term satiety.[26,27]

Ghrelin

Ghrelin, the natural ligand for the orphan growth hormone secretagogue receptor type I, was discovered in gastric extracts, localized to A-like (also termed Gr) cells in the basal part of oxyntic mucosa.

Plasma ghrelin concentrations increase before meals and decrease postprandially. Ghrelin has been shown to stimulate growth hormone, insulin secretion, gastric motility, and gastric acid secretion.[28-31] In conscious rats, ghrelin accelerates gastric emptying and small-bowel transit and reverses laparotomy-induced postoperative ileus. Thus, ghrelin holds promise as a treatment for postoperative ileus.

Orexin

Orexins (or hypocretins) are novel neuropeptides synthesized mainly in the lateral hypothalamic area (LHA) and are implicated in the regulation of food intake and arousal. Orexin-A colocalizes with gastrin in the antrum. Intracisternal and peripheral administration of orexin-A stimulates acid secretion.[32]

Adrenomedullin

Adrenomedullin, a novel peptide originally identified from pheochromocytoma tissue, has recently been localized to enterochromaffin-like cells in the gastric fundus. Hirsch et al. demonstrated that adrenomedullin stimulates fundic somatostatin via neural pathways and, as a consequence, inhibits histamine and gastric acid secretion.[33,34] Expression of adrenomedullin has also been reported as increased after mucosal injury, suggesting that it can promote epithelial restitution and support mucosal defense.[35,36]

PEPSINOGEN

Pepsinogen is a powerful and abundant protein digestive enzyme secreted by the gastric chief cells as a proenzyme and then converted by gastric acid in the gastric lumen to the active enzyme pepsin. The role of pepsin and its precursor in protein digestion was first described in the 19th century. Pepsinogens consist of a single polypeptide chain with a molecular weight of approximately 42,000 Da. Pepsinogens are synthesized and secreted primarily by the gastric chief cells of the human stomach before being converted into the proteolytic enzyme pepsin, which is crucial for digestive processes in the stomach. Furthermore, pepsin can activate additional pepsinogen autocatalytically. Pepsinogens belong to the endopeptidase family of aspartic proteinases. The aspartic proteinases are also called acid proteinases because they act between pH 1.5 and 5.0. The mucosal lining of human gastric mucosa produces four types of pepsinogen: pepsinogen I (PGA or PGI), pepsinogen II (PGC or PGII), cathepsin E, and cathepsin D. It has been reported that the moment of the first appearance of measurable pepsinogen in the fetal stomach varies considerably between species. In the human fetus, granules appear in the peptic cells at weeks 32 to 36. Cephalic vagal stimulation strongly stimulates pepsinogen secretion. Acetylcholine, cholecystokinin, gastrin, secretin, VIP, epidermal growth factor, and nitric oxide can stimulate pepsinogen.[21]

Anticholinergics, histamine H_2-receptor antagonists, and vagotomy decrease pepsinogen secretion. Raised serum levels of type 1 pepsinogen have been associated with duodenal ulcer and gastrinoma, whereas atrophic gastritis (with or without pernicious anemia) has been associated with low levels of type 1 pepsinogen.

MUCUS AND BICARBONATE SECRETION

Mucus is a highly hydrated gel that consists of 95% water, 5% mucin glycoprotein, and minor components such as electrolytes. Mucins are high-molecular-weight glycoproteins with 80% carbohydrate content; the remaining 20% is constituted by protein core. Mucin is the most important structural component of the mucus gel layer.

The integrity of gastric mucosa is maintained by multiple mechanisms. The mucus barrier forms a continuous gel into which a bicarbonate-rich fluid is secreted, forming a protective pH gradient. Gastric acid is secreted in a pulsatile manner through the mucus gel, allowing the formation of short-lived channels within the mucus gel that rapidly close to prevent the back-diffusion of luminal acid. This mechanism maintains the pH at the mucosa near neutrality, despite the low luminal pH.[37] The hydrophobicity of mucus is important for protection of gastric mucosa by preventing back-diffusion of hydrogen ions. Phospholipids secreted into mucus by gastric mucous cells also contribute to the hydrophobic effect. Dipalmitoylphosphatidylcholine, the predominant surface-active phospholipid found in pulmonary surfactant, is also found in high levels in the stomach and has been proposed to play a major role in mucosal defense.[38]

To date, nine human epithelial mucin genes have been identified and designated MUC1-4, MUC5B, MUC5AC, and MUC6-8. The secretory mucins MUC5AC and MUC6 are expressed in the gastric epithelium. The superficial epithelium and the cells in the upper part of gastric pits produce MUC5AC. MUC6 expression is confined to the lower mucous neck cells of the antral glands.[39]

A group of small cysteine-rich peptides, trefoil factor (TFF) peptides, also have an important role in the mucus layer. TFF1 is found in the foveolar cells of the stomach, and TFF2 in the distal stomach and lower portion of Brunner's glands of the duodenum.[40,41] Trefoils seem to play a role in gastric epithelial protection and mucosal healing, and they may play a part in mucus stabilization by crosslinking with mucins to aid the formation of the gel layer. When mucosal injury occurs, trefoils can stimulate repair by a process known as epithelial restitution.[42]

In the adult stomach, the gastric epithelium displays two well-characterized populations of mucus-secreting cells. Superficial epithelium synthesizes MUC5AC, and cells in the deep glands produce MUC6.[43]

GASTRIC LIPASE

The human stomach is also involved in the digestion of fat. Gastric lipase initiates the digestion of dietary fat and hydrolyzes about 20% of the triglycerides in a meal. It is resistant to the acidic environment of the stomach and does not require bile salts or cofactors for triglyceride hydrolysis. Gastric lipase has an important role in lipolysis in the perinatal period and in conditions where there is decreased pancreatic lipase activity. It is secreted by the chief cells located in the fundus. Gastric lipase activity is detectable at 10 weeks' gestation in gastric tissues and steadily increases until 20 weeks, correlating with gastric gland development.

INTRINSIC FACTOR

In addition to hydrochloric acid, the parietal cells in the gastric mucosa secrete intrinsic factor, a 49-kDa glycoprotein that binds to vitamin B_{12} (cyanocobalamin) and is necessary for its absorption from the small intestine. Intrinsic factor is a glycoprotein that contains 15% carbohydrate and is secreted by the parietal cells of the body and fundus of the stomach. The average daily diet in Western countries contains 5 to 30 μg vitamin B_{12}, of which 1 to 5 μg is absorbed. The total body stores of

the vitamin in adults range from 2 to 5 mg, of which approximately 1 mg is found in the liver. Human foods that contain the vitamin are of animal origin (meat, liver, fish, eggs, and milk). Dietary vitamin B_{12} is released from protein and peptide complexes in the stomach as a result of pepsin and an acidic environment; it attaches to both intrinsic factor and a second vitamin B_{12}-binding protein called R-binder.

As well as intrinsic factor, another vitamin B_{12}-binding protein is secreted into the stomach: R-binder. R-binder is degraded by pancreatic trypsin, and the released vitamin B_{12} released further binds to the intrinsic factor. This step is impaired in patients with pancreatic insufficiency, leading to reduced vitamin B_{12} absorption. The intrinsic factor–vitamin B_{12} complex then binds to a specific receptor, cubilin, in the ileal mucosa and is absorbed by endocytosis. An autosomal recessive mutation of the cubilin receptor can cause intrinsic factor–vitamin B_{12} malabsorption and megaloblastic anemia, also known as Imerslund-Graesbeck syndrome.[44] In enterocytes, cyanocobalamin is transferred from intrinsic factor to transcobalamin II, another cyanocobalamin-binding protein that transports cyanocobalamin in plasma. Cells then convert cobalamin to its active forms, methylcobalamin and 5-deoxyadenosyl cobalamin. Even small amounts of intrinsic factor secretion are sufficient for vitamin B_{12} absorption, preventing pernicious anemia in patients with hypochlorhydria due to acid blocker therapy.[45] Intrinsic factor deficiency, bacterial overgrowth, pancreatic insufficiency, ileal resection, or disease can cause vitamin B_{12} malabsorption with megaloblastic anemia.[46]

REFERENCES

1. Grand RJ, Watkins JB, Torti FM. Development of the human gastrointestinal tract. A review. Gastroenterology 1976;70:790–810.
2. Moore KL. The Developing Human. 6th ed. Philadelphia: Elsevier Science; 1998 p. 271-278.
11. Quigley E. Gastric motor and sensory function, and motor disorders of the stomach. In: Feldman M, Friedman LS, Sleisenger MH, editors. Gastrointestinal and Liver Disease. 7th ed. Philadelphia: Elsevier Science; 2002 p. 691–713.
18. Schubert ML. Gastric secretion. Curr Opin Gastroenterol 2008;24:659–664.
20. Schubert ML. Gastric exocrine and endocrine secretion. Curr Opin Gastroenterol 2009;25:529–536.
47. Moore KL, Persaud TVN. The Developing Human. 6th ed. Philadelphia: WB Saunders; 1998.

See expertconsult.com for a complete list of references and the review questions for this chapter.

CONGENITAL ANOMALIES AND SURGICAL DISORDERS OF THE STOMACH

Louisa W. Chiu • Oliver S. Soldes

EMBRYOLOGY

A general understanding of the embryologic development of the stomach is essential to the management of congenital and acquired surgical disorders of the stomach. The primordial stomach is a foregut organ that begins as a pharyngeal structure and then dilates and elongates to form the esophagus and stomach.[1] The dorsal border of the primordial stomach grows faster than the ventral border, resulting in the greater and lesser curvature, respectively. By the end of the seventh week of gestation, the stomach has undergone rotation around both the vertical and anteroposterior axes to come to rest in its normal anatomic position. See also Chapter 25 – Developmental Anatomy and Physiology of the Stomach.

HYPERTROPHIC PYLORIC STENOSIS

History, Incidence, and Etiology

Hypertrophic pyloric stenosis (HPS) is the most common gastric surgical disorder in neonates. It was first described clinically by Hildanus in 1627, with subsequent accounts given by Blair in 1717, Beardsley in 1788, and others.[2] Not until 1888 was the disease generally appreciated following Harald Hirschsprung's description with postmortem clinicopathologic correlation and introduction of the term *congenital pyloric stenosis*.[3] The first surgical treatment performed by Löbker in 1898 was a gastroenterostomy bypass of the pyloric obstruction.[4] Extramucosal pyloroplasty was demonstrated by Dufour and Fredet in 1908, and then modified to solely a muscle-splitting procedure by Ramstedt in 1911. Ramstedt's pyloromyotomy became the procedure of choice in the early 20th century.[5,6]

The incidence of HPS varies with geographical region,[7] but in general is about 2 to 5 per 1000 live births. It is more common in white populations. Some studies have shown a rise in incidence in the 1970s and 1980s,[8,9] other studies show a decline in incidence,[10] and still others show no significant change in trend.[11] The ratio of males to females remains constant at approximately 4:1. The prevalence of a positive family history demonstrates the polygenic mode of inheritance; the children of mothers who had pyloric stenosis are more likely to have the anomaly than children of fathers who had the disease.[12]

Hypertrophic pyloric stenosis is a result of progressive hypertrophy of the circular muscle, leading to a high-grade or complete gastric outlet obstruction. The exact etiology is unknown. Theories revolve around hyperacidity leading to spasms and edema, abnormal innervation, reduction of neuropeptides, deficiency of nitric oxide, and abnormal motility.[5,6]

Clinical Presentation

The typical infant presents between 3 and 6 weeks of age. Premature infants may present at an older age. Parents give a history of prolonged emesis that has progressively become more forceful and "projectile." The emesis is nonbilious, but may become brown-colored or have blood streaks due to minor mucosal hemorrhage from gastritis. Emesis occurs soon after feeds, and the infant will typically appear hungry following emesis. Often several formula changes have been made by the parent or pediatrician. A prolonged period of vomiting may lead to dehydration, lethargy, weight loss, and failure to thrive. Decreased urine output and hypochloremic, hypokalemic metabolic alkalosis develop in tandem. In response to hypovolemia, serum aldosterone levels rise, increasing renal absorption of sodium ions and water. A paradoxical aciduria and potassium diuresis may occur due to the aldosterone-mediated renal tubular excretion of hydrogen and potassium. Jaundice due to unconjugated hyperbilirubinemia occurs in 1 to 2% of infants and may be due to the effects of acute starvation on the immature liver and decreased levels of glucuronyltransferase activity.[13] The jaundice usually resolves following surgery. The differential diagnosis of nonbilious vomiting at this age includes overfeeding, gastroesophageal reflux, pylorospasm, increased intracranial pressure, infectious gastroenteritis, metabolic disorders, and other uncommon causes of gastric outlet obstruction.

Diagnostic Evaluation

The diagnosis of hypertrophic pyloric stenosis can be made by physical examination in the setting of an appropriate history. If a palpable olive-shaped mass is felt in the epigastric region under the liver edge, no further workup is necessary. Palpation may be assisted by placing a nasogastric (NG) tube briefly to decompress the distended stomach and then feeding the infant a small amount of dextrose water. The NG tube is removed when the examination is complete. With the ready availability of ultrasound, the patient will often have undergone sonographic investigation. The characteristic appearance of pyloric stenosis on ultrasound is a target sign consisting of an outer ring of low-echo-density musculature and an inner ring of high-echo-density mucosa. Measurements will typically reveal a pyloric channel length of greater than 16 mm and a pyloric muscle thickness of greater than 4 mm (Figure 26-1). The dimensions may be smaller in former premature infants with HPS or in cases of early presentation with HPS in evolution. Often the sonographer will also be able to comment on

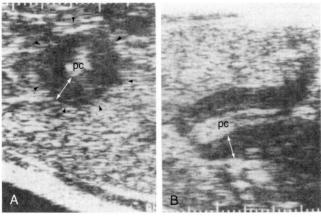

Figure 26-1. Pyloric ultrasound demonstrating (**A**) transverse and (**B**) longitudinal views of hypertrophic pyloric stenosis with increased muscle thickness and length. Black arrows outline the wall of the pylorus; the white line demonstrates the thickness of the pylorus in (**A**) and (**B**). pc, pyloric channel.

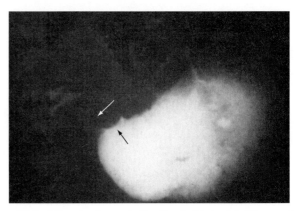

Figure 26-2. UGI series demonstrating the double tract (white arrow) and shoulder signs (black arrow) seen in HPS.

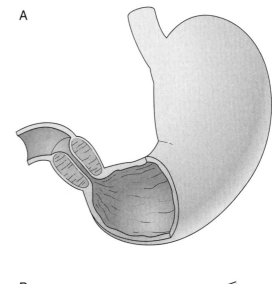

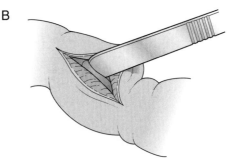

Figure 26-3. (**A**) Muscle hypertrophy in HPS produces a narrowed and elongated pyloric channel. (**B**) Extramucosal muscle-splitting pyloromyotomy relieves the obstruction of HPS.

whether there is passage of any gastric contents during the period of examination. Given that sonography is accurate, noninvasive, cost-effective, and without risk of contrast aspiration, it has replaced upper gastrointestinal (UGI) series as the gold standard for the imaging diagnosis of pyloric stenosis. Several studies have shown sensitivity and specificity of ultrasound to approach 100%.[14] Should there be any question about the diagnosis on ultrasound, an UGI series may be able to differentiate between pyloric stenosis and other possible causes of nonbilious emesis, such as gastroesophageal reflux, and antral or pyloric webs. On UGI, the narrowed pyloric channel of HPS produces a "string sign" of contrast, a "double track" sign illuminates the infolding mucosa, and a "shoulder sign" is caused by the muscle bulging into the distal antrum (Figure 26-2).[5]

Treatment

Treatment of hypertrophic pyloric stenosis is never a surgical emergency, but it may present as a medical emergency due to hypovolemia and electrolyte disturbances. The goal of initial therapy is to correct the dehydration and metabolic alkalosis before surgery. This requires rapid analysis of electrolytes and establishment of intravenous access. Fluids will normally be initiated with boluses of 10 to 20 mL/kg of normal saline to correct hypovolemia. Thereafter, an intravenous (IV) infusion of 5% dextrose in 0.45% saline is begun at 1.5 times the maintenance rate. Once urine output is established, 10 to 20 mEq/L of potassium chloride can be added to the infusion.[6] Electrolyte levels should be checked every 12 hours until they are normalized. The infant should be kept nothing by mouth (NPO), and NG tube suction should be avoided, because it will only further contribute to electrolyte disturbances.

Preoperative preparation may take 24 to 48 hours to correct electrolyte abnormalities in order to prevent postanesthetic apnea. Many pediatric anesthesiologists will require a chloride greater than 100 mmol/L and serum CO_2 less than 28 mmol/L before general anesthesia.[6] The stomach should be aspirated with an orogastric tube in the operating room immediately before induction, especially if the infant previously underwent a UGI contrast study.

Standard surgical correction of HPS is a muscle-splitting longitudinal extramucosal pyloromyotomy (Figure 26-3). The

means by which the surgeon accesses the abdominal cavity varies. An open pyloromyotomy may be performed through a traditional 2- to 3-cm right upper quadrant incision or the circumumbilical incision introduced by Tan and Bianchi in 1986.[15] Many surgeons today prefer to perform the pyloromyotomy laparoscopically, as first described by Alain et al. in 1991, with an umbilical incision and two stab incisions.[16] Regardless of the means of access, the elements of the procedure are the same. The serosa and outer muscle fibers are incised sharply from just proximal to the pyloroduodenal junction to just proximal to the antropyloric junction on the antrum. The deeper muscle fibers are bluntly split with the handle of the scalpel (open) or the retracted arthrotomy blade (laparoscopic). A Benson or laparoscopic pyloromyotomy spreader is used to complete the muscle-splitting down to submucosa. The adequacy of the pyloromyotomy is ensured when the two halves can move independently. The distal end, near the pyloroduodenal junction, is at the greatest risk for a mucosal tear and full-thickness myotomy into the lumen. The stomach can be insufflated with 45 to 60 mL of air via an oro-gastric tube to check for air bubbles or bilious fluid that would be indicative of a full-thickness enterotomy. A full-thickness myotomy can be repaired primarily with suture of the mucosa and submucosa with an omental patch, or closure of the initial myotomy and a new pyloromyotomy on the posterior or inferior side.[6]

Modifications to Alain's laparoscopic pyloromyotomy have been described, including Castañón's traumamyoplasty[17] and Rothenberg's slice and pull technique.[18] A nonlaparoscopic, transumbilical, intracavitary pyloromyotomy variation combining the advantages of open and laparoscopic techniques has been described by Gauderer.[19]

Postoperatively, many surgeons will initiate feeds within 4 to 8 hours. Protocols will vary depending on the surgeon's preference, but may start with ½ ounce of electrolyte solution and progress every 2 to 3 hours to 2 ounces of formula or breast milk. Many feeding protocols include nursing instructions to hold feeds for 1 to 2 hours for any emesis. Most infants can be discharged home within 24 to 48 hours without any antacids or prokinetic medications.

Surgical correction is the standard of care throughout the world. Under extenuating circumstances when surgical treatment is risky, unavailable, or undesirable, HPS may be medically treated with a prolonged course of intravenous and subsequent oral atropine (mean 51 days, range 29 to 137 days). Atropine suppresses muscular contractions and decreases gastrointestinal peristalsis. Kawahara et al. found a 87% success rate with atropine, but with a median 13-day hospital stay (range 6 to 36 days).[20] Medical treatment requires both prolonged hospitalization and oral atropine administration at home.[6]

Outcomes

Hypertrophic pyloric stenosis can be surgically corrected with minimal risk of mortality and morbidity. Transient small-volume postoperative emesis is common and generally thought to be caused by persistent edema, gastritis, and gastric atony, rather than a postoperative complication. Possible complications include a mucosal tear, incomplete pyloromyotomy, wound infection, and wound dehiscence. Significant complications are rare. Persistent vomiting may be a sign of an incomplete myotomy. Unexpected abdominal tenderness, abdominal distention, and clinical deterioration may be signs of an unrecognized full-thickness perforation. Postoperative sonography and water-soluble contrast studies are sometimes helpful, but edema and the radiological appearance of muscular hypertrophy are slow to resolve.

Studies have been performed comparing the right upper quadrant (RUQ) approach to the circumumbilical approach, and comparing open to laparoscopic repair. In 1999, Leinwand et al. retrospectively analyzed the RUQ approach compared to the circumumbilical approach and found the circumumbilical approach to be cosmetically superior but with an increased rate of mucosal perforation, serosal tears, and wound infections.[21]

Kim et al. performed a retrospective review in 2005 comparing laparoscopic, circumumbilical, and RUQ techniques and found that the laparoscopic approach resulted in a shorter operative time without higher complication or costs.[22] Recent prospective randomized studies by St. Peter et al., Fujimoto et al., Hall et al., Greason et al., and Leclair et al. have demonstrated that laparoscopic repair is as safe and effective as open repair, with the benefits of less pain and earlier return to feeding.[23-27] The latest meta-analysis in 2009 by Sola and Neville confirms that laparoscopic pyloromyotomy has a reduced rate of total complications and shorter postoperative time to feeding and length of stay.[28]

FOVEOLAR HYPERPLASIA

Focal foveolar hyperplasia (FFH) is a rare cause of gastric outlet obstruction and is characterized by mucosal hyperplasia and mucosal polyps. It is sometimes considered a localized Menetrier's disease (diffuse foveolar hyperplasia). Only a handful of cases have been reported, but histopathology reveals elongated, tortuous, polypoid gastric pits.[29] Its etiology is a mystery, but FFH has been reported to be associated with prostaglandin therapy for congenital cardiac disease[30,31] and cow's milk hypersensitivity.[32] Ultrasonography reveals a hyperechoic mucosa with polypoid mucosal thickening of the gastric antrum without extension into the lamina propria. The addition of Doppler sonography reveals an intense hyperemia of the antral wall deeper than the superficial mucosa.[33] Lesions are found in the antrum, are often multiple, and measure up to 5 mm. If the polyp is obstructive, then excision is indicated, whether endoscopically with snare polypectomy and electrocautery or surgically. In a retrospective review of ultrasound images of patients with hypertrophic pyloric stenosis managed by pyloromyotomy, 12% of patients were found to have coexisting foveolar cell hyperplasia, suggesting that perhaps foveolar hyperplasia is an unrecognized clinical entity that may lead to persistent postoperative emesis following myotomy. Tan et al. suggested that FFH occurring concurrently with HPS is adequately treated by routine extended pyloromyotomy.[34]

GASTRIC OUTLET OBSTRUCTION

Congenital gastric outlet obstruction (GOO) not due to HPS is very rare. These causes of GOO are primarily secondary to distal gastric webs or atresias or gastroduodenal duplications. Gerber classified distal gastric webs or atresia as pyloric or antral (1 cm or more proximal to pylorus) types.[35] Atresia may be subclassified as segmental gap atresia or pyloric aplasia (solid fibrous cord). Among these rare lesions, the frequencies are pyloric webs > pyloric atresia > antral webs > antral atresia (Figure 26-4).

Webs are obstructing membranes of mucosa and submucosa. Prepyloric webs may be windsock-like lesions with the redundant tissue prolapsing into the duodenum (Figure 26-5). Gastric web in the body of the stomach has also been reported.[36]

Pyloric atresia has an incidence of about 1 in 100,000 live births. Pyloric atresia is estimated to cause only 1% of intestinal atresias.[37] Associated anomalies are common and occur in 54% of children and include epidermolysis bullosa, other intestinal atresias, and gallbladder agenesis.[38,39] It may result from developmental arrest between the 5th and 12th gestational weeks. Because of the frequency of other anomalies, all patients with

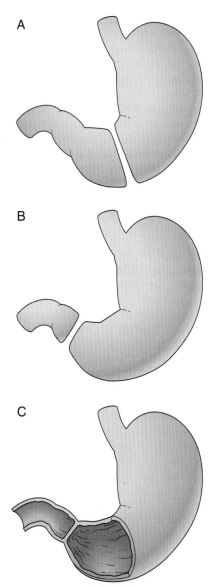

Figure 26-4. Congenital gastric outlet obstruction due to (**A**) antral segmental atresia, (**B**) pyloric segmental atresia, (**C**) pyloric web.

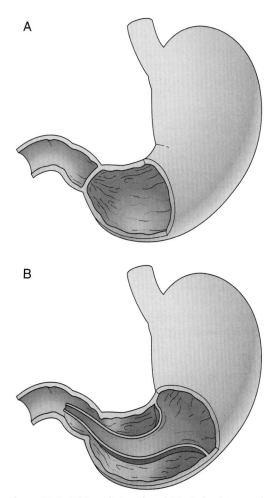

Figure 26-5. (**A**) Prepyloric web and (**B**) windsock type web.

pyloric atresia should be screened for other anomalies. Epidermolysis bullosa is most frequently associated with pyloric atresia and may involve the mucosa of the urinary tract, necessitating renal ultrasound to assess for vesicoureteric obstruction and hydronephrosis.[39]

Clinical Presentation

The presentation of antral or pyloric webs will depend on the degree of obstruction. Atresias may be suspected with antenatal polyhydramnios, gastric dilation, and narrowed gastric outlet. Neonates with high-grade or total obstruction present soon after birth with nonbilious vomiting, feeding intolerance, and gastric distention. Delayed diagnosis can lead to aspiration, dehydration, hypochloremic, hypokalemic metabolic alkalosis, and gastric perforation. Older children or adults with fenestrated webs are more likely to present with intermittent epigastric distention, nausea, vomiting, early satiety, and weight loss.

Diagnostic Evaluation

The diagnosis of gastric outlet obstruction will be suggested by gastric distention with minimal or no air distally on a plain abdominal film (solitary gastric bubble). Neonates and infants with nonbilious emesis will frequently undergo sonographic evaluation. Ultrasound of an antral web may demonstrate a persistent echogenic diaphragm-like structure in the antral region, gastric dilation, delay in gastric emptying, and a normal pylorus.[40] UGI contrast studies may reveal a stretched-out peak at the pylorus (complete obstruction) or a thin septum projecting into the antral lumen perpendicular to the longitudinal axis of the stomach (Figure 26-6). A pyloric dimple sign may be formed by the shallow pyloric cavity at the proximal end on UGI. A prolapsed prepyloric web may produce a double-bubble sign.[37,41] If the UGI series is inconclusive, upper endoscopy may be performed for direct visualization. The web is usually 1 to 4 mm thick and located 1 to 2 cm proximal to the pylorus with an aperture of varying size.[42]

Treatment

As in hypertrophic pyloric stenosis, correction of dehydration and electrolyte disturbances must be addressed first. Immediate NG decompression may be necessary in cases of complete obstruction. Webs may be treated by surgical excision via an incision over and across the web with transverse closure to widen the lumen (Heineke-Mikulicz type pyloroplasty) or by

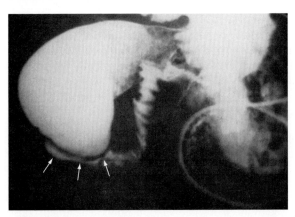

Figure 26-6. UGI series demonstrating an antral web. White arrows outline the obstructing web.

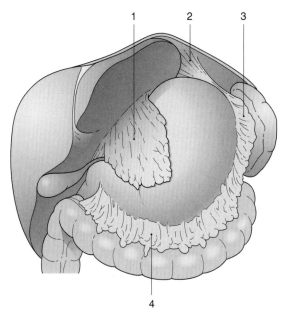

Figure 26-7. The peritoneal ligamentous attachments of the stomach are (1) gastrohepatic, (2) gastrophrenic, (3) gastrosplenic, and (4) gastrocolic ligaments. The stomach is also tethered by the duodenum and esophagus.

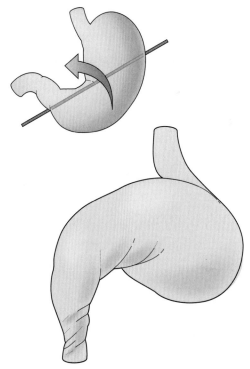

Figure 26-8. Organoaxial volvulus around the longitudinal axis of the stomach.

endoscopic incision or dilation. Gastrotomy with dilation without pyloroplasty has also been described.[43] Incidentally found or mildly symptomatic antral webs may be treated solely with small, thickened feeds and antispasmodics.[44]

For atresias, a short segment may be bypassed with a Finney or Heineke-Mikulicz pyloroplasty. For longer atresias or a segmental gap, a gastroduodenostomy is preferable to a gastrojejunostomy. A catheter must be passed distally to eliminate the possibility of any other atresias. Prokinetics may be useful for postoperative delayed gastric emptying. The overall mortality of pyloric atresia is greater than 50%, with the main cause of death related to associated anomalies or septicemia.[45] In the past, the association of pyloric atresia with epidermolysis bullosa translated to certain mortality, but this is no longer true. Hayashi et al. have reported long-term survival with aggressive treatment.[46]

GASTRIC VOLVULUS

Etiology and Pathophysiology

Gastric volvulus is an axial twisting of the stomach that causes foregut obstruction, and ischemia and necrosis of the stomach. It is a rare, potentially life-threatening cause of emesis, most often nonbilious, in children. Cribbs et al. reviewed 581 cases of gastric volvulus in children between 1929 and 2007, describing the disorder comprehensively.[47] Volvulus may occur due to absent or stretched gastric ligaments (primary volvulus) or due to abnormalities of the spleen or diaphragm (secondary volvulus), such as diaphragmatic hernia or eventration. Secondary volvulus may also be due to gastric dilation. The stomach is tethered by the four gastrohepatic, gastrosplenic, gastrocolic, and gastrophrenic ligaments and the duodenum and esophagus (Figure 26-7). Rotation can occur around the longitudinal axis of the stomach, producing an organoaxial volvulus (Figure 26-8), or around the transverse axis of the stomach, producing a mesenteroaxial volvulus (Figures 26-9 and 26-10). The majority of cases are of the organoaxial type, although mixed biplanar types can also occur. Acute volvulus is more likely to be associated with anomalies, whereas chronic volvulus more commonly has a primary etiology.[47,48]

Clinical Presentation

Gastric volvulus in adults was first described with the classic triad of sudden onset of epigastric pain, intractable retching without vomiting, and inability to pass a nasogastric tube.[49] Gastric volvulus may be described as acute, chronic, intermittent, recurrent, or acute-on-chronic in its presentation. The acute presentation in children includes nonbilious vomiting (75%), rather than intractable nonproductive retching, epigastric distention, and severe abdominal pain. Acute volvulus is more likely to occur in infants. The acute presentation also more often includes respiratory distress and cyanosis. Chronic volvulus is more common and more difficult to diagnose. Chronic or recurrent volvulus presents with signs of recurrent

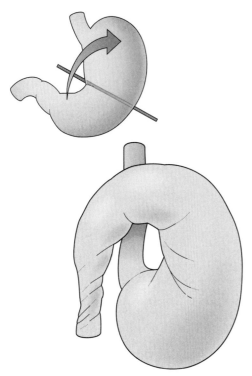

Figure 26-9. Mesenteroaxial volvulus around the transverse axis of the stomach.

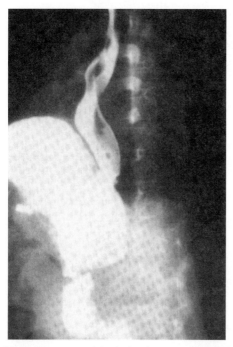

Figure 26-10. Mesenteroaxial volvulus demonstrated by UGI series.

emesis and respiratory infections, abdominal distention, feeding difficulties, and failure to thrive.[47,48,50]

Diagnostic Evaluation

Plain films and UGI contrast studies are the imaging modalities of choice. Plain abdominal film may demonstrate gastric distention in the epigastric region or left upper quadrant. UGI

series demonstrates esophageal obstruction and malposition of the stomach with a misplaced gastroesophageal junction or pylorus. An elevated hemidiaphragm on plain radiography is a sign of an underlying diaphragmatic abnormality precipitating a secondary volvulus.[48]

Treatment

Acute volvulus is a surgical emergency, and complete obstruction and strangulation can lead to perforation and necrosis of the stomach. Mortality remains high because of delayed diagnosis as well as strangulation and necrosis. Resuscitation and decompression with a nasogastric tube should be performed immediately, followed by an emergent operation. Surgical treatment consists of detorsion of the stomach, resection or repair of areas of perforation or necrosis, and gastric fixation. Gastric fixation may be performed by placement of a gastrostomy tube, fundic gastropexy,[51] or anterior gastropexy,[52,53] which can also be performed laparoscopically.[54] Any associated diaphragmatic abnormalities (hernia or eventration) should be repaired, and some surgeons perform a fundoplication in those infants with preexisting gastroesophageal reflux.[55] For chronic volvulus, reduction of the volvulus can sometimes be performed endoscopically or laparoscopically with gastropexy or gastrostomy tube placement. Nonoperative treatment involving positioning on the right side or prone with the head elevated following feeds has been more popular for mildly symptomatic chronic volvulus outside of North America.[47,50]

CONGENITAL MICROGASTRIA

Congenital microgastria is a rare anomaly of impaired foregut development, characterized by a hypoplastic tubular stomach with abnormal function and megaesophagus. There is subsequent gastroesophageal reflux, vomiting, and failure to thrive. The first case was described in 1894, and recent reviews have found approximately 60 reported cases.[56] Associated gastroesophageal reflux can lead to aspiration pneumonia and esophageal ulceration. Diarrhea may result from rapid gastric transit and dumping. Microgastria has been associated with numerous other malformations including malrotation, esophageal atresia, duodenal atresia, imperforate anus, situs inversus, asplenia, and renal, cardiac, and skeletal anomalies.[56-59] Microgastria is usually discovered on a UGI contrast study performed for the evaluation of reflux symptoms. A dilated esophagus and massive gastroesophageal reflux are also typically seen (Figure 26-11).

Medical treatment relies on continuous nasoenteral or nasogastric feeds, small frequent meals, prokinetic medications, and positioning precautions. Gastrostomy and jejunostomy tubes may assist in the feedings. Although the small stomach may adapt to the feeding regimen, long-term studies have demonstrated consistent growth retardation. The best outcomes are reported with gastric augmentation to create a larger gastric reservoir via a double lumen Roux-en-Y jejunal (Hunt-Lawrence) pouch.[56,58,59] The pouch also lessens the need for frequent feedings, facilitates oral intake, and reduces alkaline reflux esophagitis, all of which allows for improved nutrition and somatic development.[59]

GASTRIC PERFORATION

Gastric perforation is an acute abdominal surgical condition that can present with significant abdominal distention, peritoneal signs, vomiting, bloody gastric aspirates or hematemesis,

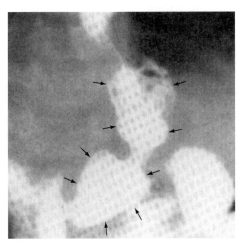

Figure 26-11. UGI series demonstrating congenital microgastria. Black arrows outline the stomach.

and sepsis. The diagnosis is suspected based on physical exam and confirmed by the presence of large amounts of free air on an abdominal x-ray. Occasionally, abdominal distention may compromise respiration. Massive amounts of free air in the presence of peritoneal signs (tenderness, rigidity) mandates surgical exploration without the need for additional imaging.

In the discussion of the etiology of gastric perforations, neonatal cases are a distinct entity from perforation in older infants and children. Neonatal perforation is generally thought to be spontaneous, ischemic, or due to iatrogenic trauma.[5,60,61] Spontaneous neonatal perforations occur in about 1 in 2900 live births. One hypothesis of the etiology is a defect of normal musculature in the stomach resulting in a focal weakness, prone to rupture.[62] Kawase et al. found an association of antenatal nonsteroidal anti-inflammatory drugs in very low birth weight infants with spontaneous isolated gastrointestinal perforation.[63] Ischemic perforations may be due to severe sepsis, necrotizing enterocolitis, volvulus, or stress ulcers. These lesions often have a surrounding zone of necrosis or devitalized tissue. Iatrogenic perforations occur secondary to the placement of a nasogastric or orogastric tube[61] or with aggressive positive pressure ventilation. These perforations tend to be puncture wounds or short lacerations along the greater curvature.[5,62] Gastric perforation may be a complication of mechanical ventilation in neonates with distal tracheoesophageal fistula.[64]

The leading cause of gastric perforation in children is trauma, whether it is accidental, nonaccidental, or iatrogenic. The incidence of gastric injury in blunt abdominal trauma is around 1%.[65] A full stomach followed by blunt trauma may be a predisposing factor.[65,66] It is essential to remember child abuse as a cause of gastric perforation.[66]

Surgical treatment consists of minor debridement and primary closure of small, clean perforations, or may require extensive debridement, resection, and temporary gastrostomy in the case of significant necrosis of tissue. Mortality is generally high, from 12.5 to 60%, especially in premature neonates, in whom 100% mortality has been reported.[60-62,64]

GASTRIC AND DUODENAL DUPLICATIONS

In 1951 Gross popularized the use of the term *duplication* to describe any anomaly along the gastrointestinal tract that had a contiguous wall with the alimentary tract, had a

developed smooth muscle layer, and was lined with alimentary epithelium.[67] Duplications can occur anywhere from the mouth to the anus. The incidence of gastrointestinal duplications is about 1 in 4500.[68] Accumulation of mucosal secretions within the duplications produces a progressive mass effect on the lumen of the adjacent segment of the gastrointestinal tract. They may be lined with gastric mucosa or ectopic pancreatic tissue and may lead to ulceration, hemorrhage, and pancreatitis. Proposed theories of their etiology include the split notochord syndrome, defects in recanalization, and remnants of embryonic diverticula.[69]

Gastric duplication represent about 7% of gastrointestinal duplications.[70] They typically lie along the greater curvature, are more likely cystic than tubular, and usually do not communicate with the stomach, but may communicate with aberrant pancreatic ducts. Ectopic pancreatic tissue is found in about a third of gastric duplications.[71] Associated anomalies include esophageal or duodenal duplications and vertebral or pancreatic anomalies. The clinical presentation of a gastric duplication is typically vomiting, feeding intolerance, and sometimes a palpable abdominal mass. There may be weight loss or abdominal pain. The presentation may be similar to that of gastritis or peptic ulcer disease, with signs of hematemesis, melena, or even perforation.

Duodenal duplications make up 5 to 7% of alimentary tract duplications and most commonly occur in the first or second portion of the duodenum.[72] Extrinsic compression may lead to duodenal obstruction, biliary obstruction, or pancreatitis. Endoscopic retrograde cholangiopancreatography (ERCP) or magnetic resonance cholangiopancreatography (MRCP) assist in delineating pancreatic and duodenal involvement.

Duplications are more frequently being diagnosed on antenatal ultrasound as an inner echoic mucosa surrounded by hypoechoic muscular layers and the presence of debris within the lesion.[70] Postnatal ultrasound and computed tomography (CT) are useful for defining the lesion's location. A UGI series may demonstrate an extrinsic defect, and technetium-99m scanning can demonstrate the presence of ectopic gastric mucosa.

The treatment of duplications largely depends on their location and involvement of critical structures. Broadly, the treatment of a gastrointestinal duplication is complete excision when possible, and laparoscopic-assisted success has been reported.[73] If this is not possible because of hazards related to the anatomic location, other techniques, such as partial excision and mucosal stripping or fenestration and internal drainage into the intestinal lumen or a Roux-en-Y loop of jejunum, provide another option.

POLYPS

Gastric polyps are uncommonly encountered in children during diagnostic esophagogastroduodenoscopy. Gastric polyps may rarely cause obstructive or bleeding symptoms. Most are asymptomatic, and solitary polyps are relatively rare. Hyperplastic inflammatory type polyps are the most common gastric polyps encountered.[74] Gastric polyps more often occur in association with polyposis syndromes such as familial adenomatous polyposis (FAP), Peutz-Jeghers syndrome, or juvenile polyposis. They are frequently encountered in these patients during surveillance endoscopy. All three syndromes are autosomal dominant and associated with an increase risk of malignancy. They require lifelong surveillance of both the upper and lower

GI tract. The risk of malignancy is greatest in patients with FAP and adenomatous and fundic gland polyps. The hamartomatous polyps of juvenile polyposis and Peutz-Jeghers syndrome have lesser malignant potential.[74,75] Gastric polyps are typically removed endoscopically. Those polyps that cannot be removed endoscopically may be removed via gastrotomy or partial gastrectomy when necessary. See also Chapter 43.

TUMORS

Gastric tumors of all types are rare and include lymphomas, leiomyomas, leiomyosarcomas, teratomas, carcinomas, gastrointestinal stromal tumors (GISTs), carcinoid tumors, and inflammatory pseudotumors. See also Chapter 49 – Neoplasms of the Gastrointestinal Tract and Liver. Masses may be found incidentally or due to abdominal pain and/or distention, a palpable mass, gastrointestinal hemorrhage, obstruction, or perforation.

Non-Hodgkin's lymphoma is the most common GI malignancy in children and in the stomach.[76] Gastric lymphomas may be primary or secondary following treatment for leukemia. For isolated gastrointestinal lymphoma, the primary treatment is complete surgical resection, including regional lymph nodes. Patients with metastatic disease are treated with surgery and adjuvant chemotherapy and radiotherapy.[75,76]

Leiomyomas and leiomyosarcomas are soft-tissue tumors of smooth muscle origin that involve the gastric wall. The most common presentation is gastrointestinal hemorrhage, obstruction, and perforation. Wide surgical excision with resection of the lymph node basin is the primary treatment.[75]

Gastric teratomas comprise only 1% of all pediatric teratomas, which are more often found in the ovaries, testes, sacrococcygeal region, retroperitoneum, and mediastinum. In a 2000 review, only 102 cases were identified, with less than 10% of cases in girls. Although the germ cell tumors are mostly benign, there are case reports of malignant gastric teratomas.[75,77] Diagnosis by plain x-ray, ultrasound, or CT may be made based on the findings of an irregular soft tissue mass with both solid and cystic components and the presence of calcifications. Complete resection is required because of the malignant potential, and prognosis is excellent whether or not malignant elements are found.[77]

Gastric adenocarcinomas account for significantly fewer than 1% of pediatric malignancies, and fewer than 25 cases have been documented. The median age of presentation is 15 years, although the youngest reported was a 2.5-year-old.[75,78,79] Presenting symptoms include pain, anorexia, vomiting, gastrointestinal bleeding, upper abdominal mass, and weight loss. Delay in diagnosis is not uncommon.[79,80] Given the frequency of delayed diagnosis and the poor prognosis, any child with the symptoms just listed should be considered for upper endoscopy.[81] Surgical and adjuvant treatment is based on adult protocols, and the outcome is poor.[75] Median survival is only about 5 months following diagnosis.[80]

Gastrointestinal stromal tumors are mesenchymal tumors that have characteristics of interstitial cells of Cajal, and only 16 cases have been reported in children. For unknown reasons they occur predominantly in girls, and the presence of metastasis at diagnosis is more common in the pediatric population.[75,82] In a review of five patients treated at Memorial Sloan-Kettering between 1982 and 2003, all pediatric patients were female with multiple tumor nodules in the stomach.[82] Treatment is en bloc resection. Adjuvant therapy with the tyrosine kinase inhibitor imatinib mesylate is under study in pediatrics.

Although carcinoid tumors are most likely to be found in the appendix, cases have been reported along the whole gastrointestinal tract. The majority of GI carcinoid tumors in children are benign and rarely metastasize. The treatment of tumors without metastases consists primarily of complete resection alone. Tumors that penetrate the serosa or mesentery require mesenteric resection and surveillance. Patients with tumors over 2 cm in size should undergo screening for metastases with 5-hydroxyindoleacetic acid (5-HIAA) levels and CT or MR imaging.[75]

Inflammatory pseudotumors (IPTs) are composed of spindle cells, myofibroblasts, plasma cells, and histiocytes. They are also known as inflammatory myofibroblastic tumors or plasma cell granulomas and are thought to be a result of aberrant response to tissue injury. Although IPT occurs most commonly in the lung, gastrointestinal occurrences are reported. The stomach is the most common of gastrointestinal sites. Surgical resection of primary tumors is recommended, and recurrence and metastases are common.[83]

REFERENCES

6. Aspelund G, Langer JC. Current management of hypertrophic pyloric stenosis. Semin Pediatr Surg 2007;16:27–33.
28. Sola JE, Neville HL. Laparoscopic vs open pyloromyotomy: a systematic review and meta-analysis. J Pediatr Surg 2009;44:1631–1637.
47. Cribbs RK, Gow KW, Wulkan ML. Gastric volvulus in infants and children. Pediatrics 2008;122:e752–e762.
59. Velasco AL, Holcomb 3rd GW, Templeton Jr JM, Ziegler MM. Management of congenital microgastria. J Pediatr Surg 1990;25:192–197.
71. Holcomb 3rd GW, Gheissari A, O'Neill Jr JA, et al. Surgical management of alimentary tract duplications. Ann Surg 1989;209:167–174.
75. Ladd AP, Grosfeld JL. Gastrointestinal tumors in children and adolescents. Semin Pediatr Surg 2006;15:37–47.

See expertconsult.com for a complete list of references and the review questions for this chapter.

GASTRITIS, GASTROPATHY, AND ULCER DISEASE

Ranjan Dohil • Eric Hassall

The terms *acid peptic diseases*, *peptic diseases*, and *acid-related disorders* are used synonymously to describe conditions that involve gastric acid and pepsin in their pathogenesis; they refer to a number of disorders including esophagitis, gastritis, gastropathy, peptic ulcer disease, and duodenitis. This chapter addresses acid peptic disorders other than esophagitis.

Gastritis and peptic ulcer disease are important for several reasons. They have significant associated morbidity and are usually amenable to treatment; in addition, some forms of chronic, severe gastritis may destroy mucosal elements, resulting in atrophic gastritis and intestinal metaplasia, which may be preneoplastic. Thus, as with many conditions that develop in childhood, there may be lifelong implications. Although gastritis and ulcer disease are both clinically important stand-alone entities, they often are part of a continuum of disease, from mild gastritis or gastropathy through to severe forms in which ulceration of the gastric mucosa is present.[1-3] Conversely, when primary duodenal ulcer disease is present, gastritis is usually present – in the case of *Helicobacter pylori*–related disease. *Helicobacter pylori* is the most important cause of gastritis and of peptic ulcer disease, and it is a classic illustration of the continuum principle. Aspects of *H. pylori* infection other than gastritis and associated ulcer disease are addressed elsewhere in this book.

Gastritis is characterized by the presence of inflammatory cells. Thus the diagnosis is purely histologic, made only by evaluation of biopsies (random or targeted) of the stomach, and not by endoscopic findings, which may be variable. Often gastritis is found to be present in biopsies taken from gastric mucosa that appears normal at endoscopy. In contrast, *gastropathy* refers to those entities in which inflammation is not a prominent feature, although there is often epithelial damage and regeneration, and perhaps vascular abnormalities. Gastropathies often have a typical endoscopic appearance (e.g., portal hypertensive gastropathy, prolapse gastropathy) but are not usually associated with biopsy evidence of inflammatory infiltrate. Gastritis and gastropathy are not diagnosed clinically or on radiologic studies – they are diagnosed by upper gastrointestinal (GI) endoscopy with biopsy.[1-5] Patients with these conditions may or may not have symptoms; symptoms that do occur are those of upper GI disorders and are often not specific.

Gastric Mucosal Anatomy ("Endoscopic Anatomy")

The gastric body or corpus is characterized at endoscopy by thick mucosal folds or rugae; it extends distally to the incisura on the lesser curvature (Figure 27-1). The fundus is the dome-shaped area immediately above the gastric body and, like the corpus, is lined with oxyntic mucosa. The foveolae or gastric pits occupy the upper 20 to 25% of the mucosa, the tightly packed oxyntic glands occupying the rest. The lower half of the gland is lined by pepsinogen-secreting chief cells, and the upper half by parietal cells that secrete acid and intrinsic factor. Endocrine cells, found between the basement membrane of the gland and the parietal and chief cells, are primarily enterochromaffin-like (ECL) cells, which secrete histamine; some are D cells that secrete somatostatin, and some are enterochromaffin (EC) cells, which secrete serotonin. The gastric antrum extends from where the gastric folds of the body end to the pylorus and consists of clear-staining mucous glands and endocrine cells. Of the latter, gastrin-producing G cells are predominant, with some D and EC cells. Although different histologic zones of the stomach correspond generally to the different gross anatomic zones, there is always some overlap and interdigitation of histologic zones at areas of transition – hence the term *transitional mucosa* for these. Examples of transitional zones are the antrum-body interface, especially the region of the incisura, and also the gastric cardia.

Gastric Secretions

The stomach secretes water, acid, bicarbonate, other electrolytes (K^+, Cl^-, Na^+), enzymes that are active at low pH (pepsin from chief cells and lipase from gastric body epithelium), intrinsic factor from parietal cells, and mucins.[6,7] Hydrochloric acid is secreted by the parietal cells of the gastric body and fundus via an energy-requiring process. See Chapter 25.

CLINICAL PRESENTATION

The spectrum of symptoms caused by upper GI disorders is limited, but there are a number of entities in the differential diagnosis. For example, it may be difficult to clinically distinguish upper abdominal pain due to peptic disease, hepatobiliary disease, pancreatitis, and esophagitis (reflux, eosinophilic or other) from functional disorders such as nonulcer dyspepsia or functional heartburn, unless a specific esophageal symptom, such as dysphagia, is present. Nevertheless, as a start, with a thorough history and physical examination, the physician can often determine whether the child's presenting symptoms are likely of upper or lower GI origin. A detailed approach to history taking and differential diagnosis in childhood abdominal pain and upper GI disorders is given elsewhere.[8]

Peptic disorders are far less prevalent in children than adults, accounting for probably no more than 10 to 20% of children with abdominal pain in an outpatient GI subspecialty clinic setting. Esophagitis due to reflux and other causes is included in this estimate, as it may present with upper abdominal pain.[8] The commonest causes of abdominal pain in children are constipation and irritable bowel syndrome, and although these conditions usually present with pain that is not epigastric, difficulties may arise when the child is unclear about the nature and location of the pain.[8,9] Children under the age of about 8 to 10 years are often unable to reliably localize pain.[10] Nocturnal wakening should be clearly differentiated from difficulty falling asleep, which is more likely to be caused by a functional disorder.[9,11,12]

The symptoms caused by gastritis are highly variable, depending on the etiology, severity, and extent of disease. In the absence of ulceration, the chronic gastritis associated with *H. pylori* infection is unlikely to be a cause of recurrent abdominal pain in childhood or nonulcer dyspepsia in adults[13-17]; however, more recent (although small) studies have suggested an association with chronic pain symptoms and *H. pylori* gastritis.[18-20] (Regardless of this, consensus recommendations are to treat if *H. pylori* infection is found – see the later section on Management.) Younger children with peptic disorders often have irritability, vomiting, poor appetite, and occasionally weight loss. Older children, aged 10 years and above, may present with more adult-typical symptoms such as epigastric pain, nausea, early satiety, vomiting, anemia, and weight loss. Symptoms of frank gastric outlet obstruction are uncommon in children.

The combination of abdominal pain, vomiting, and nocturnal wakening is suggestive of peptic ulcer disease, but a temporal relationship with meals occurs in only about half of children with diagnosed peptic ulcer disease.[21-23] GI bleeding may occur with long-standing antecedent epigastric pain or other symptoms, but painless bleeding may be the only manifestation of ulcer disease. Up to 25% of children with duodenal ulcer have this "silent" presentation; about 25% present with bleeding and antecedent pain, and the rest present only with abdominal pain or recurrent vomiting.[24,25] Pain that is truly epigastric is relatively uncommon in children and, when present, always requires investigation, as does upper GI bleeding

with or without pain; peptic ulcer disease is but one cause of these presentations. On physical examination, epigastric tenderness does not correlate with the presence or absence of peptic ulcer disease. Iron deficiency anemia may be a consequence of *H. pylori* gastritis, even in the absence of ulcer disease.[26] The diagnosis of nonulcer dyspepsia is made by ruling out other conditions at endoscopy. Many patients will have been treated empirically with antacids, histamine (H) 2 blockers, or proton pump inhibitors (PPIs) before seeing a pediatric gastroenterologist. Those who have a significant and repeated response to this therapy most likely have some form of acid peptic disease. For symptoms that are chronic or relapsing, an upper GI endoscopy with biopsy is required to help differentiate among the varying causes of symptoms, preferably while off acid-suppressing therapy for at least 1 to 2 weeks. In deciding which patients require endoscopy, the acuity, frequency, and severity of the symptoms should be taken into account as well as the degree to which symptoms are disruptive to the child's normal daily activities. Patients may needlessly come to endoscopy in order to exclude acid peptic disease, when a thorough history and examination would indicate that constipation or irritable bowel syndrome is a more likely diagnosis. Others may have only mild upper GI symptoms, and a short trial with antacids or acid-suppressing therapy may be more appropriate.

DIAGNOSTIC METHODS

Upper Gastrointestinal Contrast Radiography ("Upper GI Series")

Upper gastrointestinal radiologic contrast studies can define only gross mucosal changes in the stomach. These studies are frequently falsely positive or negative for gastric mucosal disorders, including ulcers, and therefore often are misleading. For these reasons, barium studies have little or no role in the diagnosis of gastritis or uncomplicated peptic ulcer disease. Thus "gastritis" is not a radiologic or clinical diagnosis. In the relatively uncommon circumstance where gastric outlet obstruction is suspected, either by symptoms or endoscopy, this test is useful.

Upper Gastrointestinal Endoscopy and Biopsy

Once the decision to undertake endoscopy has been made, it is important that the endoscopist make every reasonable effort to maximize the diagnostic potential of the procedure. Endoscopic and biopsy findings can often be interpreted only in combination with the patient's history, physical examination findings, and sometimes other tests. Close collaboration with an experienced pathologist who is knowledgeable about gastrointestinal disorders is central to the process.[27] In pediatrics, there is often a tendency to overcall the diagnosis of gastritis, based on cellular infiltrates that are marginally increased and that may often be explained by a recent viral infection. As always, it is for the endoscopist/gastroenterologist to review the histology and the case with the pathologist, and to determine the clinical significance, if any, of histopathology in the context of the patient's symptoms. "Chronic nonspecific inflammation" is a "finding" that is often of little help in managing patients, though the exclusion of other entities sometimes is of help.

There are some "normal" parameters for cellular infiltrates in the gastric mucosa in children, based on biopsies called

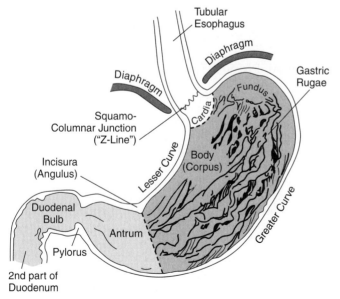

Figure 27-1. Gastric mucosal anatomy. Adapted from Rudolph CD, Rudolph AM, Hostetter MK, Lister G, Siegel NJ, eds. Rudolph's Pediatrics, 21st ed. Stamford, CT: McGraw-Hill; 2002.

"normal" retrospectively.[5] Drugs that may significantly change endoscopic or histologic findings include bismuth compounds (Pepto-Bismol, DeNol), antibiotics, acid-suppressing drugs, nonsteroidal anti-inflammatory drugs (NSAIDs), oral iron, systemic/inhaled corticosteroids, and chemotherapeutic agents. Ideally drugs would be discontinued for at least 2 weeks before endoscopy so that endoscopic findings are not masked, for example by acid-suppressing agents. Some drugs are better not used at all, especially where there is an adequate substitute for symptomatic relief. Specific foods may play an active role in the disease process, and patients suspected of having celiac disease or allergic or eosinophilic gastroenteropathy should remain on a regular diet until the endoscopy has been performed, if at all possible, so that the suspected offending agent is active at the time of the investigation.

Reporting of Endoscopic Findings

The endoscopist should report only what is *seen*, using terminology that is standard, factual, and unambiguous – the report should be descriptive rather than interpretive. Jargon or "-itis" terms should be avoided in the objective part of the endoscopy report. For example, use of the term *gastritis* could mean anything from erythema to distinct erosions; if the mucosa is red, it should be documented as *red* or *erythematous* (mild, moderate, intense, or hemorrhagic) and not as *antritis* or *gastritis*, because inflammation may not be present.[3,28] Another endoscopic finding, antral nodularity, may indicate *H. pylori* gastritis, past or present; the nodules may persist for months or years after eradication of *H. pylori* and resolution of gastritis, and inflammation may not be present on biopsy.[24,29] See Figure 27-2.

An *erosion* is a mucosal break that does not penetrate the muscularis mucosae, whereas an *ulcer* extends through the muscularis into the submucosa. However, this histologic definition does not have much practical application for endoscopists, who are seldom able to obtain (nor do they need to obtain) histologic evidence of the depth of the mucosal defect. Lesions may be described generally as superficial or deep, using some clues: erosions are often multiple and usually have white bases, and each is surrounded by a ring of erythema. When an erosion

has recently bled, its base may be black. Ulcers are deeper, more punched-out, and, when they are chronic, often have raised, rolled edges. For the purposes of clinical trials, lesions greater than 5 mm in diameter are termed ulcers, and smaller lesions are called erosions. This definition does not take into account the actual definition of erosion versus ulcer. *Hemorrhage* refers to a bright, shiny red appearance of the mucosa in patches, streaks, or discrete petechiae, not associated with a visible mucosal break. Although the term *submucosal hemorrhage* sometimes is used, endoscopists cannot see through the muscularis mucosae; therefore the term *subepithelial hemorrhage* is more accurate, to allow for varying depths of hemorrhage. Other confusing terms used for subepithelial hemorrhage (and best avoided) are *acute gastritis*, *hemorrhagic gastritis* (inflammation is usually absent from hemorrhagic lesions), and *hemorrhagic erosion* (usually no erosion is present) (see Figure 27-1). If gastric rugae are large, accurate descriptive terms are *thick folds* or *swollen folds*, not *edematous folds* or *hypertrophic folds*, because *edema* and *hypertrophy* are histologic, not endoscopic, findings; the swelling might be due to infiltrative disease, edema, or hypertrophy.[2,5] In those conditions the folds remain thick in appearance despite adequate insufflation of air at endoscopy. Causes of swollen gastric folds are shown in Table 27-1.

When erosions or ulcers are seen, important descriptors should include specific anatomic location in the stomach or duodenum, size, shape, number, depth (superficial or deep), nature of the edge (raised, rolled, in the case of ulcers/deep

TABLE 27-1. Causes of Swollen or Thick Folds

Ménétrier's disease
Chronic varioliform gastritis
H. pylori infection
Chronic granulomatous disease
Eosinophilic gastritis
Adenocarcinoma
Lymphoma (mucosa-associated lymphoid tumor)
Plasmacytoma
Zollinger-Ellison syndrome

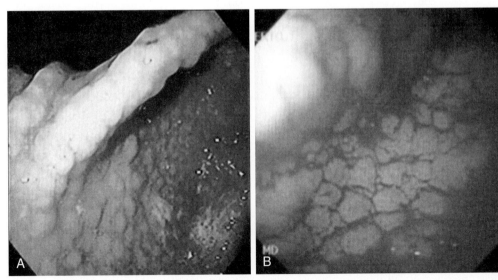

Figure 27-2. (A) Diffuse antral nodularity seen on endoscopy in a teenager with epigastric pain. **(B)** Following biopsy, blood acts as a "vital" stain to highlight the nodules. This is particularly useful when nodules are not so apparent. Histologic examination demonstrated *H. pylori* infection with chronic active pangastritis. The patient responded well to anti–*H. pylori* therapy. (*See plate section for color.*)

lesions), and the base – exudate, red-based, black (sign of recent bleeding), presence of a visible vessel or clot, active bleeding. Ulcers in the duodenal bulb may be missed if they are active or have recently bled, because part of the bulb may be in spasm, and the ulcer(s) can be hidden between folds.

It is also important to describe *nodules* in the stomach carefully. On close examination of the mucosa, a patch of nodules is often seen at the antral-body junction; these usually represent a prominent areae gastricae,[30] which is a normal finding, more evident in some patients than others. Nodules or mucosal "bumps" or pseudopolyps may also occur in disorders such as chronic varioliform gastritis, Crohn's disease, eosinophilic gastritis, cytomegalovirus (CMV) gastritis, Henoch-Schönlein disease, and cystinosis, entities described later, and with different zonal distributions in the stomach.

Biopsy Sampling

Different disorders often have a predilection for one topographic zone or another of the stomach. However, the same agent may cause different patterns of injury in different populations (e.g., *H. pylori*). Sometimes there may be disease in more than one zone of the stomach (e.g., *H. pylori*, Crohn's disease, eosinophilic gastritis, atrophic gastritis, CMV gastritis), as indicated later. In addition, the distribution of disease may be influenced by treatment. Thus, the topography of endoscopic or histologic findings may give important clues to the etiology. Although the antrum is the major repository of histologic abnormalities for many pathologies that occur in children, biopsies should be taken from different topographic zones of the stomach.[4,31-36] When *H. pylori* chronic gastritis is suspected, biopsies should be taken from the greater and lesser curves of the antrum and body, from the incisura, and from the gastric cardia.[31,36,37]

The number and locations of biopsies depends on the disease suspected and the endoscopic findings. Even when mucosa is normal, biopsies should be taken.[2,32-34,36] Biopsies should be taken from the gastric cardia when *H. pylori* infection, gastroesophageal reflux disease (GERD), or mucosa-associated lymphoid tissue (MALT) tumor[38] may be present.[31,35,38-40]

The size of biopsies is also important. In most children over 2 or 3 months of age, an endoscope with a 2.8-mm biopsy channel can usually be used, and biopsies with these forceps are often adequate, if several are taken. Biopsies taken with "jumbo" or large-cup forceps offer about two or three times the amount of mucosa for diagnosis; these can often be obtained in children older than 5 or 6 years. The enhanced tissue yield with jumbo biopsy forceps must be weighed against the risk of complications when large forceps are used. However, when careful technique is used, the risk is tiny. On occasion, endoscopic mucosal resection or full-thickness surgical biopsies are required. This may be the case in the infiltrative disorders, which can present with "thick folds," mass, or ulceration, such as cancer, lymphoma, plasmacytoma,[41] or leiomyoma/leiomyosarcoma, or with certain gastric polyposes.[42]

APPROACH TO GASTRITIS

Histologic

There are many ways to approach the histologic description or classification of gastritis. The diversity of approaches reflects the fact that no single one can meet all the descriptive needs of pathologists, and the diagnostic or "action plan" goals of endoscopists/clinicians.

The Sydney "classification" or system of gastritis has been widely accepted in adults. The current Sydney system incorporates topographic, morphologic, and etiologic information,[32,43] that is, location (antrum or body) and histologic parameters – inflammation, activity, atrophy, intestinal metaplasia, and *H. pylori* infection. Each of these is graded semiquantitatively as mild, moderate, or marked. It is based on the findings in endoscopic biopsies taken on protocol from specified areas of the stomach – two biopsies from the antrum within 2 to 3 cm of the pylorus, two from the gastric body, and one from the incisura.

The Sydney system has little broad application to children. Pediatric gastroenterologists should focus on getting good tissue in individual patients and analyzing the findings with an experienced GI pathologist

Inflammation

It is typical to describe the types of cell present and their distribution in the mucosa. "Acute" or "active" refers to the presence of neutrophils, "chronic" refers to the presence of round cells (lymphocytes, monocytes, plasma cells), and "chronic active" refers to a combination of a chronic process with some neutrophils present. There are no precise definitions for chronic gastric inflammation because the "normal" number of mononuclear "allowable" is unknown.[32,43,44] Although adult "normal" or asymptomatic volunteers sometimes undergo endoscopy and biopsy as a baseline for studies, their histology even in "health" may reflect many variables, such as normal aging, smoking, intake of alcohol, or NSAIDs.

A working definition of chronic inflammation in adults that is widely accepted is the presence of more than a few lymphocytes, plasma cells, and/or macrophages per high-power field,[32] but this definition cannot be extrapolated to children. In childhood, some acceptable numbers are available from "retrospective normals." The information is summarized elsewhere,[5] but in cells per millimeter.[21] Unlike the presence of round cells in the mucosa, the presence of any number of neutrophils is regarded as abnormal, indicating acute or active inflammation. The presence of lymphoid follicles is strongly suggestive of active *H. pylori* infection in children[16,24,45] and adults,[29,43] and although initially considered to be a feature of *H. pylori* only in children, if specifically sought, they are said to be present in 100% of adult patients with *H. pylori*.[43] If lymphoid follicles and inflammation are present in the absence of *H. pylori*, it is likely that the organism has been missed. In *H. pylori* infection, lymphoid follicles may be absent if biopsies of sufficient size and number are not taken. The distinction between a lymphoid follicle (active germinal center) and a lymphoid aggregate (no active germinal center) is important – the former are generally found only in active gastritis due to *H. pylori* or other causes, whereas the latter may be found in noninflamed, noninfected gastric mucosa.[24,29,45]

In addition to the types of cells and lymphoid collections, descriptive terminology also includes the extent or depth of inflammation in the mucosa. This may be described as "superficial," "deep" or "pan-mucosal," and as "diffuse" or "focal." These terms can be combined, to provide an overall description, for instance "chronic active, pan-mucosal." The severity of gastritis can be quantitated by a scoring system[55] for comparison of effect of treatment.

Atrophy and Intestinal Metaplasia

Gastric atrophy (also known as "atrophic gastritis") is an important consequence of gastritis. It is considered to be a preneoplastic lesion when a certain type of intestinal metaplasia develops in the atrophic mucosa.[46-54] Although *H. pylori* infection is far and away the most important cause of atrophic gastritis worldwide, it may result from any severe, chronic mucosal injury to the gastric mucosa. In children, the authors have seen it occur with intestinal metaplasia in severe chronic varioliform gastritis and in autoimmune disease (scleroderma) with GI tract involvement. Severity of inflammation appears to be a factor in addition to chronicity.

True atrophy is present when there is gland loss, no regeneration, and fibrosis is present, with or without metaplasia. In advanced atrophy there may be relatively little inflammation, as the acute and chronic injury may have passed and left a "quiescent" damaged mucosa. It is widely accepted that intestinal metaplasia per se constitutes a form of atrophic gastritis, even if gland loss is not striking.[51,52] More recently, some have expanded the definition to include the presence of pseudopyloric metaplasia of the corpus, which is identified by the presence of pepsinogen I in mucosa that is topographically corpus but phenotypically antrum.[52] Atrophy may be missed if pseudopyloric mucosa is not sought and recognized to be metaplastic.

Atrophic gastritis is a patchy lesion and may be missed by sampling error, if sufficient tissue is not obtained from multiple sites.[47,50,53] This is a particularly important issue in populations with high rates of *H. pylori* infection and of gastric cancer.

Caution should be exercised in interpreting or acting on reports of "atrophic gastritis" and "intestinal metaplasia." There is some subjectivity in calling gland loss, even among experts. In addition, when active inflammation is present, inflammatory cells and edema may push glands apart and give an appearance of atrophy that is reversible by treatment of the underlying *H. pylori* infection, so-called "pseudo-atrophy."[53] Thus, atrophy can be easily overcalled. For all of these reasons, interobserver reliability in calling atrophy is less than ideal.[52-54]

Recently, multiple biopsy regimens in such children have been reported, with studies in Japan[46] and Colombia[52] showing atrophy in up to 10% of *H. pylori*–infected patients coming to endoscopy. Focal intestinal metaplasia may be found very rarely as a congenital occurrence, as has been observed in an autopsy study of neonatal stomachs.[55] If a single focus of a few intestinalized cells is found on random biopsy (usually antrum), this may be congenital or could represent evidence of healing of some previous focal injury. However, if more than a few cells are metaplastic, or more than one focus is found, this may represent a more widespread mucosal disorder. Such findings cannot be interpreted in the absence of detailed mucosal mapping. Patterns of chronic atrophic gastritis are discussed further under *H. pylori* gastritis.

Endoscopic/Clinical

Categorization into gastritides and gastropathies can be helpful in narrowing the diagnostic possibilities in a given case. Further classification of gastritides and peptic ulcer disease according to underlying cause may help to understand the natural history of a lesion. In the past, we proposed an arbitrary classification into erosive and nonerosive types, but we now rather term them simply by etiology. *Of central importance is that even when endoscopic findings are minimal or absent, histology is necessary to diagnose or rule out a gastritis or gastropathy.* Next and in Table 27-2, we list the types and causes of gastritis and gastropathy, approximately in sequence of perceived importance or frequency in children – this will differ between centers, and between countries.

TABLE 27-2. Causes of Gastritis and Gastropathy

Helicobacter pylori
"Stress" gastropathy
Neonatal gastropathies
Traumatic gastropathy
Inflammatory bowel disease
Eosinophilic (allergic) gastritis
Aspirin and other NSAIDs
Other drugs
Nonspecific gastritis
Portal hypertensive gastropathy
Proton pump inhibitor gastropathy and polyps
Celiac gastritis
Lymphocytic gastritis
Graft versus host disease
Cytomegalovirus gastritis
Chronic granulomatous disease
Other granulomatous gastritides
Uremic gastropathy
Bile gastropathy
Henoch-Schönlein gastritis
Corrosive gastropathy
Exercise-induced gastropathy/gastritis
Collagenous gastritis
Gastritis with autoimmune diseases
Pernicious anemia
Ménétrier's disease
Chronic varioliform gastritis
Radiation gastropathy
Cystinosis
Phlegmonous and emphysematous gastritis
Other infectious gastritides
Plasmacytoma, cancer, gastric (MALT) lymphoma

GASTRITIS

Helicobacter pylori Gastritis

H. pylori is the most common cause of gastritis in the world. In addition, given its association with peptic ulcer disease, atrophic gastritis, and adenocarcinoma and with the rare entity of gastric lymphoma, it is the most important.[24,25,56-58] The majority of individuals with *H. pylori* gastritis are asymptomatic, unless they develop ulcer disease, adenocarcinoma, or lymphoma.[14-16] The prevalence of *H. pylori* varies widely between socioeconomic classes and countries. This and other aspects pertinent to the infection itself are addressed in Chapter 28.

Acute Infection

In infected adults and children *H. pylori* induces an acute neutrophilic infiltrate, followed by a chronic gastritis,[24,56,57] which remains present for the duration of the infection. Acute infection has been studied in a number of individuals,[59-62] some of whom infected themselves for study purposes. The acute infection may cause epigastric pain, nausea, vomiting, halitosis, and headache.[59-62] An early consequence of acute infection appears to be increased gastric acid secretion followed by achlorhydria within a week or so, lasting for 6 weeks or more. The decrease in acid secretion seems to correlate with the timing and degree of inflammation of the gastric oxyntic mucosa.

Chronic Infection

Some studies have suggested that acute infection with *H. pylori* quite often clears spontaneously in children,[63] although this does not appear to be the case in adults, in whom infection likely is lifelong if untreated. Most infected individuals develop a chronic, active, nonatrophic gastritis, which is typically asymptomatic. There is focal epithelial cell damage and an inflammatory infiltrate in the lamina propria, consisting of neutrophils, eosinophils, and monocytes, largely B and T lymphocytes. There is also development of lymphoid follicles and a plasma cell infiltrate.[29] In children and adults, the gastric antrum appears to be the commonest site of bacterial colonization and active gastritis.[24,25,37,51,64-66] In the only pediatric study to compare the yield of *H. pylori*–positive biopsies from different zones of the stomach, the gastric cardia had a higher yield than the antrum and body;[31] In children, the antral-predominant chronic active gastritis is usually superficial, although panmucosal involvement does occur.[24] The cellular infiltrate is predominantly lymphocytic with neutrophils, although the latter may not be as abundant as seen in adults.[24,56,67,68] The intensity of inflammation present may vary between different countries, possibly related to the strain of *H. pylori* involved. Regional differences in patterns or severity of inflammation may also be due to socioeconomic status, age at time of infection, and exposure to other organisms. In some individuals, chronic *H. pylori* gastritis progresses with time to atrophic gastritis, with an annual increase in prevalence among otherwise normal subjects of 1 to 3%.[69] This progression leads to three patterns of atrophic gastritis: body predominant, antral predominant, and multifocal.[39,40,56] As the degree of atrophy progresses, the presence of active *H. pylori* infection decreases, owing to the loss of *H. pylori*–friendly acid-secreting superficial gastric mucosa to intestinal metaplasia, which does not harbor *H. pylori*. The supervention of hypochlorhydria is also somewhat hostile to *H. pylori* colonization, because in the absence of acid, other organisms can proliferate and offer competition for *H. pylori*. The acid–*H. pylori* relationship, and mechanisms of development of atrophy, have been well described elsewhere.[69] An uncommon manifestation of *H. pylori* infection is granulomatous gastritis, with superficial epithelioid granulomas.[70,71]

Different patterns of inflammation are associated with different "disease states" that *H. pylori* may cause.[72] Duodenal ulcer disease is usually accompanied by an antral-predominant gastritis and very little involvement of the corpus; thus, a high acid-output state is maintained. In contrast, gastric ulcer, atrophic gastritis, and cancer risk are associated with a panmucosal or body-predominant gastritis; this gives rise to a low acid-output state. The two patterns appear to be largely mutually exclusive: the duodenal ulcer disease state appears to "protect" against atrophic gastritis and cancer or, perhaps more accurately, is simply unassociated with these conditions.[69,72] The chronic atrophic gastritis that may result from chronic *H. pylori* infection can give rise to "pernicious anemia," a hypochlorhydric state with megaloblastic anemia but without the autoantibodies associated with the "classic" condition of pernicious anemia (see the later section on pernicious anemia).

Endoscopy and Biopsy

This is the most reliable way to diagnose *H. pylori* infection in children.[14-16] A striking, diffuse, and continuous nodularity of the antrum is the hallmark endoscopic feature of *H. pylori* infection.[24,65,73] When *H. pylori* gastritis is associated with duodenal ulcer in children, the nodularity is always present; however, when *H. pylori* causes gastritis alone ("primary gastritis"), the nodularity is seen in only some 50 to 60% of cases.[24] Eradication of the infection results in healing of the gastritis in children, but the mucosal nodularity and histologic lymphoid hyperplasia may persist for months or years,[24,56,74,75] so the presence

of nodules at endoscopy does not mean that *H. pylori* or active gastritis is present. Use of acid-suppressing therapy may change the pattern of inflammation, causing a preferential colonization and inflammation in the body, fundus, and cardia.

"Stress" Gastropathy

The term refers to physiological stress – shock, hypoxemia, acidosis, sepsis, burns, major surgery, multiple organ system failure, or head injury. Stress erosions are typically asymptomatic, multiple, and superficial and do not perforate; however, when they do present, they do so with overt upper GI hemorrhage. They usually involve the oxyntic mucosa, with early lesions predominantly in the fundus and proximal body, later spreading to the antrum to produce a diffuse erosive and hemorrhagic appearance; antral involvement alone is uncommon. They are not usually associated with significant underlying mucosal inflammation. Lesions usually occur within 24 hours of the onset of physiologic stress. Risk factors for hemorrhage include gastric hypersecretion, mechanical ventilation, and use of corticosteroids. Newborns and infants appear to be more prone to perforation.

Neonatal Gastropathies

Most neonatal gastropathies are stress gastropathies (see preceding paragraph), including prematurity, hypoxemia, prolonged ventilatory support, sepsis, and acid-base imbalance. Although hemorrhagic gastropathy has been reported in otherwise healthy full-term infants presenting with severe upper GI hemorrhage,[76] and also as antenatal hemorrhage,[77] most cases of hemorrhagic gastropathy are reported in sick neonates in the intensive care unit.

Upper GI endoscopy is unlikely to reveal specific lesions that alter the infant's supportive management, and in sick small infants, the procedure is not without risk. More often than not, a conservative approach will better serve the patient. An unusual gastropathy may occur in infants with congenital heart disease receiving prolonged infusions of prostaglandin E to maintain patency of the ductus arteriosus. This consists of antral mucosal thickening or a focal mass due to foveolar cell hyperplasia, presenting as gastric outlet obstruction.[78]

Traumatic Gastropathy

Forceful retching or vomiting produces typical subepithelial hemorrhages in the fundus and proximal body of the stomach. This is due to "knuckling" or trapping of the proximal stomach into the distal esophagus, resulting in vascular congestion, and is also known as *prolapse gastropathy*. Mallory-Weiss tears immediately above or below the gastroesophageal junction also may occur. Although both prolapse gastropathy and tears tend to resolve quickly, they can result in significant blood loss. By a similar mechanism of trauma, linear erosions may occur in the herniated gastric mucosa of patients with a large hiatal hernia, resulting in chronic blood loss anemia.[79] Gastric erosions may result from trauma secondary to long-term nasogastric tube placement. Aggressive continuous suction through nasogastric tubes, especially in children who are receiving anticoagulants, can cause severe subepithelial hemorrhage and bleeding. Ingestion of foreign bodies, gastrostomy feeding devices, and endoscopic procedures such as diathermy[80-82] are also common causes of subepithelial hemorrhage, erosion, and ulcer. Gastric prolapse through the gastrostomy tract may occur, particularly after laparoscopic G-tube placement, especially in those with developmental delay, poor nutritional status, and ventilator dependence. This condition usually requires surgical intervention.[83]

Inflammatory Bowel Disease

Crohn's disease is the commonest cause of granulomatous disease of the stomach.[5] Although gastroduodenal involvement is relatively common, Crohn's disease is rarely isolated to the stomach and usually also involves more distal intestinal disease.[84]

Macroscopic and/or histologic abnormalities are present in the esophagus, stomach, or duodenum in up to 80% of children with Crohn's disease.[1,5]

Eosinophilic (Allergic) Gastritis

The terms *eosinophilic gastritis* and *allergic gastritis* are often used interchangeably, though in the past, eosinophilic gastritis was more commonly applied to a more intractable form of disease that occurred in older children or adults.

Eosinophilic gastritis (EG) is one of the EGIDs – eosinophilic gastrointestinal disorders, including eosinophilic esophagitis, gastritis, gastroenteritis, and colitis. These are characterized by the presence of symptoms, a prominent eosinophilic infiltrate, and exclusion of other causes of this infiltrate. Disorders such as Crohn's disease, collagen vascular disease (e.g., scleroderma), parasite infection and also with acute/chronic infections (e.g., *H. pylori*, anisakis) may be accompanied by mucosal eosinophilia,[114] but in general, the eosinophilia is much more marked in allergic disease.

Some patients with EG have a history of seasonal allergies, food sensitivities, eczema, asthma, and atopy. The EGIDs in general are typically secondary to mixed IgE and non-IgE allergic reactions resulting in increased levels of interleukin-3, interleukin-5, and granulocyte/monocyte-colony stimulating factor – all strongly proinflammatory cytokines.[114,116]

The eosinophilia may be mucosal (the most common subtype), muscular, or serosal. These may also occur in combination. Symptoms depend on the severity and extent of involvement. The mucosa form typically presents with symptoms similar to other forms of gastritis, sometimes including symptoms of gastric outlet obstruction. In infants or younger children, failure to thrive or food refusal occur. Anemia due to occult blood loss and hypoalbuminemia occur commonly.[85] If muscular and/or serosal involvement occur, abdominal pain and ascites may be present. Eosinophilic gastritis more commonly presents as part of an eosinophilic gastroenteritis than as an isolated entity.

Eosinophilic gastritis is usually associated with a specific allergen, and in infants and children, cow's or soy milk protein, egg, and wheat are the most frequently identified antigens.[86-88] A temporal relationship between characteristic symptoms and the ingestion of certain foods is particularly helpful in establishing the diagnosis, with symptoms such as growth failure in infants, irritability, abdominal pain and vomiting occurring within 1 to 2 hours of ingestion.[85-87] In most infants and young children, reintroduction of the antigen is almost always possible by 24 months of age or earlier,

although some allergies such as those to peanuts, tree nuts, and seafood may persist.[85] An allergen is not always identified, but food allergen is often assumed because in more severe cases, replacement of all whole protein in the diet with hydrolyzed protein or elemental diet results in symptomatic and endoscopic resolution, as well as resolution of anemia and hypoalbuminemia.

When present, gastroscopic features are nonspecific and include friability and erythema, erosions, swollen mucosal folds, and scattered mucosal nodular lesions or pseudopolyps, particularly in the gastric antrum, sometimes with ulceration.[89,90] The mucosa in milder cases may be macroscopically normal. The histologic features include an eosinophilic infiltrate in the lamina propria and the surface and foveolar epithelium; occasionally lymphocytes, plasma cells, and neutrophils are present.

If deeper layers are involved, endoscopy may not be diagnostic, and endoscopic ultrasound or MRI may demonstrate gastric wall thickening; full-thickness surgical biopsy may be required for diagnosis. Only about half the patients with EGIDs have a peripheral eosinophilia, which may be due to coexisting atopy. Raised serum IgE levels and positive radioallergosorbent testing for specific allergens are often present.

Treatments include removal of the presumed allergen, the leukotriene receptor antagonist montelukast, the mast cell stabilizer ketotifen, systemic corticosteroids, azathioprine, and elemental diet. It is difficult to deliver topic steroids to the gastric mucosa. Cromoglycate preparations are hardly ever effective.[91-94]

Aspirin and Other NSAIDs

NSAIDs are the most commonly prescribed drugs in the world.[95] Although invaluable for the treatment of many disorders, the usefulness of NSAIDs is limited largely by their adverse effects on the GI tract. NSAIDs can result in mucosal damage, ranging from histologic changes alone to frank ulceration; patients may be asymptomatic or suffer life-threatening ulcer bleeding or perforation. Less frequent but well-recognized effects occur in the small and large bowel and esophagus.[96]

It is the topical action of NSAIDs on gastric mucosa that most likely causes acute hemorrhage and erosions within 15 to 30 minutes of ingestion, primarily in the antrum, even with low doses of NSAID.[96] These early lesions are often asymptomatic and are not predictive of clinically significant ulcer formation per se. Aside from the topical effects, the systemic presence alone of an NSAID compromises mucosal integrity and may produce severe ulceration of the mucosa. The beneficial and deleterious effects of NSAIDs arise primarily through their ability to inhibit the cyclooxygenase (COX)-catalyzed conversion of arachidonic acid to prostaglandins.[97]

In young children, ulceration of the incisura presenting with upper GI bleeding is a typical NSAID lesion, and bleeding may occur after just one or two doses of drug, or with more chronic use. The characteristic histologic NSAID lesion in adults and children is a reactive gastropathy, that is, epithelial hyperplasia, mucin depletion, enlarged (reactive) nuclei, fibromuscular (smooth muscle) hyperplasia, vascular ectasia, and edema.[98] Less often, NSAIDs may cause a reactive gastritis.

The main area of concern is long-term use of NSAIDs. Upper GI bleeding following NSAID ingestion in children has been well documented.[99-103] Naproxen is the most commonly used

NSAID in pediatric rheumatologic practice.[104] In one study, 75% of children with juvenile rheumatoid arthritis who had taken one or more NSAIDs for over 2 months had endoscopic evidence of gastropathy, antral erosions, or ulcers[101]; of these, 64% had anemia and abdominal pain. Another study in children with rheumatoid disease showed a relative risk for gastroduodenal injury of 4.8 in those taking NSAIDs versus those not taking these drugs.[102] In that study, abdominal pain was present in 28% of patients taking NSAIDs compared with 15% in those not. Because NSAIDs are protein-bound, and hypoalbuminemia may occur in systemic juvenile rheumatoid arthritis (JRA) there is theoretical potential for greater NSAID toxicity due to higher levels of free drug.[104] A recent large pediatric study[105] comparing naproxen with two different doses of celecoxib for JRA showed rates of gastrointestinal side effects in 24 to 36% of patients, and higher, but not significantly, in the naproxen-treated group.

Factors that place patients at higher risk for severe gastroduodenal ulceration and complications of NSAIDs include a history of ulcer (complicated or uncomplicated), drug dose, concomitant use of aspirin and another NSAID, comorbidities, concomitant use of a corticosteroid, age over 65 years, use of an anticoagulant, and *H. pylori* infection.[72,95,106]

Other Drugs

Although many drugs can cause nonulcer dyspepsia, erosive or hemorrhagic gastropathies have been described with valproic acid, dexamethasone, chemotherapeutic agents, alcohol, potassium chloride, iron, and long-term fluoride ingestion.[107,108-117]

Nonspecific Gastritis

In the authors' experience, a significant number of children have chronic gastritis for which no cause can be identified.[5] In these cases, the inflammation is chronic, lymphoplasma cellular, more focal than diffuse within the biopsy, and usually superficial. Although it appears to be more prevalent in the antrum than the corpus, this may reflect sampling bias.

IBD Gastritis

Gastritis can be associated with either Crohn's disease or colitis. Treatment of upper GI Crohn's disease is often challenging, but it may be responsive to therapy with corticosteroids, 6-mercaptopurine, and infliximab.[118,119] Diagnosis and management of Crohn's disease is discussed further in Chapter 44.

Portal Hypertensive Gastropathy

This congestive gastropathy is common in children with both cirrhotic and noncirrhotic portal hypertension, but is not related to the severity of underlying liver disease, the size of esophageal varices, the presence of hypersplenism, or a previous history of bleeding and variceal sclerotherapy.[120-122] The endoscopic findings of postal hypertensive gastropathy (PHG) vary from a mild gastropathy with a mosaic pattern of 2- to 5-mm erythematous patches separated by a fine white lattice, to a severe gastropathy typified by the presence of cherry-red spots or even a confluent hemorrhagic appearance (Figure 27-3). Although hemorrhage from PHG is not usually catastrophic, bleeding may occur and result in severe blood-loss anemia. The histologic findings

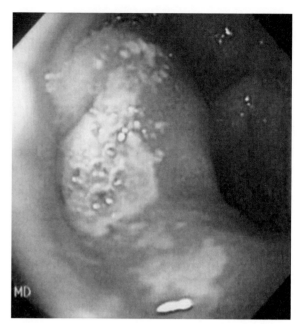

Figure 27-3. A chronic punched-out duodenal ulcer with overlying exudate, surrounded by swollen erythematous mucosa. This picture was from a 14-year-old boy with epigastric pain and nausea. He was positive for *H. pylori* infection. (*See plate section for color.*)

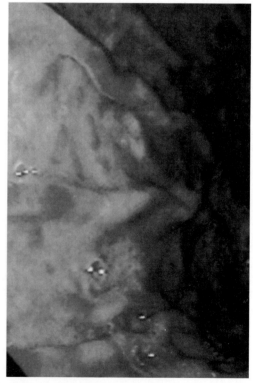

Figure 27-4. Endoscopic view of the stomach demonstrates cherry-red spots overlying a mildly swollen erythematous gastric body mucosa in a patient with portal hypertensive gastropathy and esophageal varices secondary to biliary atresia. (*See plate section for color.*)

in PHG are ectasia of mucosal capillaries and venules, and submucosal venous dilation, without any significant inflammatory infiltrate.[123,124] However, PHG is an endoscopic diagnosis; biopsy is not required and is potentially dangerous. See Figure 27-4.

Proton Pump Inhibitor Gastropathy and Gastric Polyps

Long-term or high-dose PPI therapy often causes a characteristic hyperplasia of parietal cells, with a thickened parietal cell zone, and lingular pseudohypertrophy of individual parietal cells. Endoscopic evidence of polyps and/or nodules has been reported in children within 10 to 48 months of starting PPI therapy.[125] Whereas some of the nodules were reported to have disappeared spontaneously, all polyps persisted during the 31-month follow-up.[125] No evidence of dysplasia has been reported, even after 10 years of therapy.[126] In children on long-term PPIs up to 11 years' duration, 61% developed ECL hyperplasia, of only the lowest grades.[127]

In a national study of more than 120,000 adult EGDs,[128] more than 6% included the finding of gastric polyps, of which 77% were fundic gland polyps. Most were in stomachs of patients not infected with *H. pylori*, receiving chronic PPI therapy. Fundic gland polyps and other PPI related gastric changes are thought to be reversible and have no significant risk for cancer.[129-131]

Gastric polyps unrelated to PPI therapy, "nodules," and pseudopolyps (due to any inflammatory process, such as Crohn's disease, allergic gastritis) should be considered in the differential diagnosis of PPI polyps.[128] These include other hyperplastic polyps such as occur in familial adenomatous polyposis, which may be premalignant, or due to inflammation; or the hamartomatous polyps of Peutz-Jeghers syndrome, which are not premalignant.

Celiac Gastritis

Celiac disease exists when an immune reaction to gluten occurs. More than 95% of patients are HLA DQ2 positive and, although symptoms may appear during infancy, more typical features will occur afterwards. Although gastroscopy is usually normal, if looked for, a lymphocytic gastritis is often detected[132-135]; this is characterized by the intraepithelial location of the lymphocytic infiltrate.

A recent study in children reported intraepithelial lymphocytic gastritis (antrum > body) in 29 of 33 children with untreated celiac disease; 15 of these also had evidence of focal or diffuse chronic gastritis within the lamina propria.[135] Mucin depletion was often seen when increased intraepithelial lymphocytes were associated with chronic gastritis. The number of intraepithelial lymphocytes returned to normal with a gluten-free diet.[135]

Lymphocytic Gastritis

Although lymphocytic gastritis is a pattern of gastritis, rather than a cause (unless it is idiopathic), it is a common histologic finding deserving special mention. It may be seen in disorders as diverse as celiac disease, CMV gastritis, Ménétrier's disease, *H. pylori* infection, and chronic varioliform gastritis (Table 27-3). It is also mentioned under each of those disease entities.

Graft Versus Host Disease

Acute graft versus host disease (GVHD) occurs between 21 and 100 days after transplantation, with varying degrees of mucositis, dermatitis, enteritis, and hepatic dysfunction.[136] GVHD

TABLE 27-3. Lymphocytic Gastritis

Celiac disease
Ménétrier's disease in adults
Cytomegalovirus infection
Chronic varioliform gastritis
Helicobacter pylori infection
Crohn's disease
Idiopathic

occurs most often after allogeneic bone marrow transplantation and only occasionally after solid organ transplantation. Although acute GVHD more often involves the small and large intestine, when the stomach and/or esophagus are involved, symptoms such as nausea, vomiting, and upper abdominal pain are commonly reported. The stomach is an important area for the histologic diagnosis of gastrointestinal GVHD, even when diarrhea is the main symptom.[137,138] The gastric endoscopic and histologic findings, however, may also underestimate the severity of GVHD elsewhere in the gut. Endoscopy with biopsies is not routinely required for the diagnosis of GVHD, but when performed for investigation of upper GI symptoms or bleeding, or to exclude opportunistic infection, the findings vary considerably. They range from normal, or subtle changes, even when most or all of the epithelium is lost, to patchy erythema with erosions, to extensive mucosal sloughing. The early biopsy findings are unique to GVHD, consisting of crypt epithelial cell apoptosis and drop-out. In more severe cases, whole crypts may drop out. There is variable lymphocytic infiltration of the epithelium and lamina propria. In advanced cases, there may be ulceration, edema, fibrosis, and perforation. When acute GVHD is suspected, the duodenum and esophagus should be biopsied, in addition to the proximal and distal stomach, but with recognition that duodenal biopsy carries higher risk in these patients.[137,138] Histologic distinction among GVHD, CMV infection, human immunodeficiency virus, and other immunodeficiencies may be difficult.[137] Chronic GVHD (more than 100 days posttransplant) rarely involves the stomach. Endoscopy and biopsy is safe if patient is not coagulopathic and has a platelet count above 50,000.[175] PPI therapy may be associated with increased apoptosis in the antral biopsies; therefore it is important to also biopsy from the gastric body.[139]

Cytomegalovirus Gastritis

CMV infection occurs most often in immunosuppressed children and adults, such as those with acquired immunodeficiency syndrome (AIDS) or following solid organ or bone marrow transplant.[140] In the immunocompetent child, CMV infection is usually associated with Ménétrier's disease. CMV infection is so uncommon in apparently immunocompetent adults[141] that its finding suggests an occult malignancy or early immune deficiency.[142] In such patients, this compounds the diagnostic difficulty in distinguishing between gross or histologic lesions caused by infection, GVHD, and physiologic stress, or that due to chemotherapy. However, if the highly distinctive pattern of injury is present, it is more likely that CMV is the cause. The infection tends to occur in the gastric fundus and body and may cause wall thickening, ulceration, hemorrhage, and perforation.[143,144] Histologic findings include acute and chronic inflammation with edema, necrosis, and cytomegalic inclusion bodies in epithelial and endothelial cells, as well as in ulcer bases and mucosa adjacent to ulcers. In contrast to herpes virus infection, which tends to be superficial, CMV usually affects deeper portions of the mucosa, and the active inflammation may be focal or panmucosal. The diagnostic yield is increased by viral culture of mucosal biopsies and immunohistochemical detection of CMV early antigen. Treatment with ganciclovir may be beneficial in immunosuppressed patients, but otherwise spontaneous recovery usually occurs within 1 to 2 months.[145]

Chronic Granulomatous Disease

Chronic granulomatous disease (CGD) is a rare inherited immune deficiency disorder, occurring more frequently in boys, in which granulomatous gastric wall involvement is common. CGD may present with upper GI symptoms. Severe gastroenteritis and oral aphthous ulceration may occur in some patients.[146] This disease should be differentiated from Crohn's disease. When present, symptoms of delayed gastric emptying occur, with a narrowed, poorly mobile antrum on contrast radiography.[140,147,148] There are no specific endoscopic findings, but often the antral mucosa is pale, lusterless, and swollen. Histologic findings include focal, chronic active inflammation in the antrum, with granulomata or multinuclear giant cells. In the authors' experience of six cases, the diagnostic lipochrome-pigmented histiocytes were absent in gastric biopsies, but were found in the lower gastrointestinal tract.[5]

Other Granulomatous Gastritides

Granulomatous gastritis is only sometimes the primary process; often, it is a reaction to other disorders, listed in Table 27-4, such as infection, foreign body, immune-mediated etiologies, carcinomas, lymphomas,[149] and *H. pylori* infection.[70,71] Burkitt's lymphoma is the most prevalent type of lymphoma in children, and it may occur as a primary tumor of the stomach.

In most cases, the morphologic appearance of granulomas does not provide useful clues as to the cause. Rarely, necrotizing granulomatous inflammation that occurs in association with lymphoma may be the predominant component causing diagnostic error.[149]

In the developed world, granulomatous gastritis other than that due to Crohn's disease is rare. The differential diagnosis includes foreign body reaction, tuberculosis, histoplasmosis, and Wegener's disease, among other disorders.[150-153] Idiopathic isolated granulomatous gastritis is a rare condition of a chronic granulomatous reaction limited to the stomach, and a diagnosis of exclusion. Langerhans cell histiocytosis (histiocytosis X), a rare condition in which organs are infiltrated by proliferating histiocytes, can cause granulomatous gastritis[154] and gastric polyps.[155] Sarcoidosis of the stomach is rare but does occur in children[156,157] and adults.[158-160] In areas where tuberculosis is endemic, care is required in diagnosing and treating isolated gastric Crohn's disease, especially with steroids or immunosuppressives.[150]

Uremic Gastropathy

In acute renal failure, gastropathy may be due to physiologic stress rather than renal failure itself. When GI bleeding occurs in acute renal failure, it is associated with erosions and/or ulcers. Gastric pH may be less acid than expected; this may reflect neutralization of gastric acid with ammonia, a breakdown product

TABLE 27-4. Causes of Gastric Granulomas

Noninfectious Causes
Crohn's disease
Chronic granulomatous disease
Vasculitis associated
Sarcoidosis
Lymphoma
Idiopathic
Infectious Causes
Tuberculosis
Syphilis
Histoplasmosis
Parasites
Foreign body granulomas

of urea that is very high in the gastric juice of patients with chronic renal failure.[161,162]

Bile Gastropathy

Bile reflux or duodenogastroesophageal reflux (DGER) is well documented following gastric surgery such as Billroth I and II, and after selective vagotomy with pyloroplasty.[163] Reports of DGER in the intact stomach, however, are confined mainly to the adult literature.[164,165] The mere finding of bile in the stomach at endoscopy is common and unlikely to be of any significance. Typical endoscopic features of DGER include "beefy" redness or erythema, bile staining of the gastric mucosa, and occasionally erosions. Despite this, there is little or no increased cellular infiltrate in the lamina propria, the main histologic features of this condition being epithelial-foveolar hyperplasia (occasionally with a corkscrew appearance), lamina propria edema, and venous congestion. These changes constitute the entity of a so-called reactive gastropathy.[2,166] After surgery they are found more commonly in the stomach than at the anastomosis. Other features include anastomotic erosions, lipid islands, and mucosal cysts

Henoch-Schönlein Gastritis

Henoch-Schönlein purpura (HSP) is a frequently recognized multisystem disorder due to an immune complex–mediated vasculitis involving small and medium-sized vessels. Although it can present in all age groups, the peak incidence occurs in 4- to 6-year-olds.[167,168] It can present in children and adults of all ages with involvement of skin, GI tract, kidneys, and joints. GI symptoms and signs include colicky periumbilical or epigastric pain, nausea and vomiting, and gastrointestinal bleeding.[168,169] Less common serious abdominal complications include intramural hematoma, intussusception, bowel infarction, bowel perforation, pancreatitis, appendicitis, and cholecystitis. Endoscopic findings in the stomach include erythematous or hemorrhagic mucosa and mucosal edema, with erosions or ulcers.[170-172] Similar lesions are often present in the duodenum and jejunum. Although gastric mucosal biopsies are usually too superficial to show typical histologic changes, they may show a leukoclastic vasculitis similar to that seen in the skin.[170] Endoscopy is seldom required for the diagnosis of this condition, although it may be helpful in children with persistent abdominal pain or vomiting who have not yet demonstrated the typical nonthrombocytopenic rash of HSP. A few may never develop the rash.[173-175]

Corrosive Gastropathy

The ingestion of strong acids and alkalis usually results in damage to the esophagus, but may involve the stomach. When gastric injury does occur, the pre-pyloric area is particularly vulnerable,[176,177] probably because of pylorospasm and pooling of secretions.

Exercise-Induced Gastropathy or Gastritis

This condition is well recognized in long-distance runners, usually presenting with blood loss anemia, with or without upper GI symptoms. Symptoms often occur postexercise and include abdominal cramps or epigastric pain, nausea, gastroesophageal reflux, and vomiting.[233] These symptoms may arise following altered blood circulation and also altered motility occurring in marathon runners.[178] Both erosive gastropathy and nonerosive gastritis have been described with mucosal lesions, occurring almost equally in the gastric antrum, body, and fundus.[179,180]

Collagenous Gastritis

This rare entity, characterized by subepithelial collagen deposition and an associated gastritis, may not itself comprise a distinct disorder, but rather a consequence of inflammation or a local immune response in the stomach, or as one histologic feature of a more diffuse disease process.[181]

Gastritis Associated With Autoimmune Diseases

In autoimmune pernicious anemia, the stomach is the primary affected organ.[182] In addition, gastritis with and without atrophy has been seen in children with autoimmune thyroiditis and nongoitrous juvenile hypothyroidism, some with achlorhydria and gastric parietal cell antibodies.[183] Autoimmune atrophic gastritis has also been described in 15% of adults with vitiligo.[184]

Conversely, hypertrophic gastropathy has been associated with systemic lupus erythematosus.[185] In children and adults with connective tissue diseases, a mast cell gastritis and a combination mast cell and eosinophilic gastritis have been described.[186]

Pernicious Anemia

The term *pernicious anemia* is applied to the anemia and condition that results from a deficiency of intrinsic factor, although megaloblastic anemia may arise from poor dietary intake or malabsorption of vitamin B_{12}.[187] The result is absolute achlorhydria, with megaloblastic anemia due to vitamin B_{12} deficiency. Pernicious anemia is thus the manifestation of the most severe, end-stage form of diffuse atrophic body gastritis. It is associated with endocrinopathies such as autoimmune thyroid disease and diabetes mellitus, vitiligo, selective IgA deficiency, abnormal cellular immunity, chronic candidiasis, and collagen vascular disease.[188,189] Untreated pernicious anemia may result in neurologic deficits such as seizures in infants of vitamin B_{12}–deficient mothers[190] and reversible ataxia in older children.[191] The typical finding at endoscopy is absent or thin rugae of the gastric body, sometimes with blood vessels visible through the mucosa. Histologic examination shows severe atrophic fundic gland gastritis with absence of parietal cells. Adenocarcinoma of the stomach occurs as a complication.

Although gastric adenocarcinoma is rare in children, it does occur,[192-194] and endoscopic surveillance of pernicious anemia is indicated. Atrophic gastritis has long been considered to be of "autoimmune" origin, because of the presence of antibodies to secretory elements and the association with other autoimmune conditions. Nevertheless, the condition can occur as a result of chronic *H. pylori* infection, typically associated with multifocal atrophic gastritis, and thus differing from typical autoimmune pernicious anemia in which the antral mucosa is normal.[195]

A separate condition and category entirely is so-called childhood or juvenile pernicious anemia. This is a heterogeneous group of conditions that can be considered as "metabolic" rather than autoimmune. There is no gastric gastropathy and ulcer disease atrophy, but megaloblastic anemia and hypochlorhydria or achlorhydria are present.[196]

Ménétrier's Disease

This rare condition is characterized by giant gastric folds, excess mucus secretion, decreased acid secretion, and protein-losing gastropathy. Although this condition is reported from the neonatal period onwards, the mean age of onset in children is 4.7 years.[197] In children, it is generally a benign disorder, self-resolving within weeks or months, considered due to CMV infection.[198-200] In contrast, in adults, Ménétrier's disease is an acquired premalignant disorder that may even present with malignancy. It is rare for an immunocompetent adult to have CMV-induced transient protein-losing hypertrophic gastropathy. In making a diagnosis of Ménétrier's disease, other more common causes of large gastric folds should be considered, for example lymphoma; infections such as *H. pylori*, CMV, and anisakiasis; granulomatous gastritides; eosinophilic and allergic gastritis; and other rare causes such as plasmocytoma and systemic lupus erythematosus.[185]

The combination of endoscopic and histologic findings is diagnostic. Endoscopy shows swollen, convoluted rugae, sometimes with polypoid or nodular configuration. The histologic appearance is typically of elongated, tortuous foveolae, with reduction of chief and parietal cell glands, and often with cystic dilations that may extend into muscularis mucosae and submucosa. The lamina propria is edematous with increased eosinophils, lymphocytes, and round cells, and the muscularis mucosa may be hyperplastic with extensions into the mucosa. Ménétrier's disease has been strongly associated with CMV infection in immune-competent children, and raised CMV IgM levels, positive CMV testing by polymerase chain reaction (PCR), or positive culture of gastric tissue may be helpful in confirming the diagnosis.[198,200]

Chronic Varioliform Gastritis

Also known as chronic erosive gastritis, CVG is a rare disorder of unknown etiology that is associated with a dense lymphocytic infiltrate. Although occurring largely in middle-aged and elderly men of European descent,[201,202] CVG has also been reported in a few children[203-206] who present with varying combinations of upper GI symptoms, anemia, protein-losing enteropathy, peripheral eosinophilia, and raised serum IgE levels. Endoscopically, the gastric folds appear thickened, but the most striking features are the innumerable prominent nodules in the fundus and proximal body of the stomach. Other causes of lymphocytic gastritis are shown in Table 27-3.

Radiation Gastropathy

This uncommon condition, described primarily in adults, is associated with abdominal irradiation of patients with malignancy and causes erosions or ulcers particularly in the gastric antrum and pre-pyloric regions,[136] as well as severe diffuse hemorrhagic gastritis or gastropathy.[207,208]

Cystinosis

This rare autosomal recessive lysosomal storage disorder is characterized by the deposition of cystine within macrophages of most body organs. Cysteamine is found to be an acid stimulant, but only some patients will suffer regular upper GI symptoms.[209] At endoscopy, 2 of 11 poorly controlled children with cystinosis had a distinctive diffuse fine nodular appearance throughout the stomach.[210]

Phlegmonous Gastritis and Emphysematous Gastritis

Phlegmonous gastritis is a rare life-threatening condition in which a rapidly progressive bacterial inflammation of the gastric submucosa results in necrosis and gangrene.[211] Although some adult reports associate this condition with excessive alcohol ingestion, upper respiratory infections and AIDS, most cases are associated with β-hemolytic streptococci, *Staphylococcus aureus*, *Escherichia coli*, and *Clostridium welchii*, but other organisms such as *Candida albicans* and *Mucor* spp. may be involved.[212] Patients may have infections elsewhere in the body or be immunocompromised. Some patients may present with severe peritonitis with gastric perforation.[213] Acute emphysematous gastritis is a complication of phlegmonous gastritis in which gastric wall infection is due to gas-forming bacteria such as *C. perfringens*.[214-217] This often fatal condition is characterized by severe abdominal pain and systemic toxicity, with radiologic evidence of gas bubbles and thickening of the gastric wall. Predisposing factors include ingestion of caustic agents and abdominal surgery. It has also been reported in a leukemic child,[300] in a child with a phytobezoar,[214] in a patient who ingested large volumes of a carbonated beverage,[217] and in hepatic cirrhosis.[218]

Other Infectious Gastritides

Giardia lamblia is said to be the commonest of all gastrointestinal parasites and occurs worldwide.[219] It is characteristically a small-bowel parasite. Gastric colonization with *Giardia* was reported in 41 (0.4%) of 11,000 patients who underwent gastroscopy and biopsies over a 5-year period at one institution.[220] The patients had presented with symptoms including dyspepsia, epigastric pain, and abdominal distention. Hypochlorhydria was a likely prerequisite for the organisms to infect the stomach. Given the evidence, *Giardia* may be a pathogen in the stomach in some patients, and may be a regurgitant contaminant from the duodenum in others. *Helicobacter heilmannii* (previously *Gastrospirillum hominis*) is probably transmitted from cats and dogs[221,222] and may cause chronic active gastritis similar to that of *H. pylori*, but with less severe inflammation, which is focal and usually restricted to the antrum.[222-225] However, as yet, a definite association between *H. heilmannii* infection and ulcer disease

has not been established.[225] Herpes simplex virus is a rare cause of gastritis and erosions in immunosuppressed patients, with biopsy showing the characteristic intranuclear inclusion bodies.[226,227] Evidence of herpes simplex virus type 1 was identified in 4 of 22 gastric or duodenal ulcers by means of immunohistochemistry and molecular probes.[228] The herpes zostervaricella virus is a very rare cause of gastritis in adults and possibly in children.[229,230]

Influenza A is a rare cause of bleeding from hemorrhagic gastropathy in children and is sometimes fatal. Bleeding may have been due to a stress gastropathy resulting from a severe systemic illness, rather than directly due to virus. A gastropathy with hypertrophic gastric folds and protein-losing enteropathy has been described in a 3-year-old with a rising titer of IgM to *Mycoplasma pneumoniae* and no evidence of recent CMV infection.[231] Epstein-Barr virus has been associated with gastritis and diffuse lymphoid hyperplasia within the gastric mucosa.[232] *Mycobacterium tuberculosis* involvement of the stomach is very rare and usually associated with tuberculosis elsewhere or with immune deficiency.[233-235] Syphilis involving the stomach is very rare.[236] Fungal infections of the stomach, such as candidiasis, histoplasmosis, and mucormycosis, may occur, especially in sick neonates, malnourished children. and those with burns or immune deficiency.[237-242] If gastric ulceration is seen in immunodeficient patients, fungal infection should be sought and, if present, treated, along with peptic ulcer therapy. Infection with fungi of the Mucoraceae family (*Rhizopus*, *Mucor*, and *Absidia*) can cause the systemic disease mucormycosis, which is fatal in malnourished or immunosuppressed children and in preterm neonates. Fungal infection of the stomach with *Histoplasma* and *Aspergillus* or the parasite *Strongyloides stercoralis* occurs rarely.[243] *Ascaris lumbricoides* was reported to cause bleeding duodenal ulcer with perforation in an infant.[244] Early endoscopy is diagnostic and therapeutic, allowing for removal of worms and relief of symptoms.[245-248]

PEPTIC ULCER DISEASE

Peptic ulcers can be classified as primary, secondary, or due to hypersecretory states (Table 27-5). Secondary ulcers are those occurring in the presence of systemic underlying disease, whereas in primary ulcer disease this is usually not present, and the cause is either *H. pylori* or idiopathic (true *Hp*-negative disease). Primary peptic ulcers are more often duodenal, whereas secondary ulcers are more often gastric, or may be both. In children, primary ulcers may be single, with a punched-out appearance and raised rolled edges, sometimes with satellite erosions; or they may be multiple and shallower. Most primary peptic ulcers in children occur between the ages of 8 and 17 (mean 11.5) years,[21,24,25] whereas secondary ulcer disease occurs at all ages, depending on the cause of the underlying gastritis. Ulcer disease due to hypersecretory states is more commonly duodenal.

Historical Perspective

Until the late twentieth century, peptic ulcer disease was regarded as a chronic relapsing, largely incurable disorder. By the mid to late 1980s, it came to be recognized that most primary duodenal ulcers were associated with gastric infection by a bacterium, *Helicobacter pylori*, the eradication of which resulted in cure of ulcer disease in most cases. In 2005, Warren and Marshall[57] received the Nobel Prize in Physiology or Medicine

TABLE 27-5. **Classification of Peptic Ulcer Disease in Children**

Primary Peptic Ulcer Disease
H pylori associated
H pylori negative or idiopathic
Secondary Peptic Ulcer Disease
Most causes of gastritis and gastropathy, as listed in Table 27-2
Ulcer Disease Due to Hypersecretory States
Zollinger-Ellison syndrome
G-cell hyperplasia or hyperfunction
Systemic mastocytosis
Cystic fibrosis
Short bowel syndrome
Hyperparathyroidism

for their discovery of "the bacterium *Helicobacter pylori* and its role in gastritis and peptic ulcer disease."

Approximately 20 to 40% of chronic duodenal ulcers are not related to *H. pylori*, or to NSAIDs or other identifiable causes. Given the success of medical treatment of peptic ulcer disease with either *H. pylori* eradication and/or PPIs, acid-reducing operations are now hardly ever performed for peptic ulcer disease.

Epidemiology

The prevalence of peptic ulcer disease is so low in children that it is not possible to comment on time trends in the frequency of this disorder in the pediatric age group. A number of factors are alleged to cause or predispose to peptic ulcer disease. Current evidence is discussed and referenced in an excellent review.[6]

Diet. Although spicy foods may cause dyspepsia in some individuals, there is no evidence that they cause peptic ulceration. There is no evidence that any dietary factors contribute to peptic ulcer disease. Coffee, tea, and cola are potent acid secretagogues, but no link to peptic ulceration has been established. Decaffeinated coffee is as potent a secretagogue as caffeinated coffee. Bland diets have not been shown to be of benefit in treatment.

Genetics. Some familial clustering of peptic ulcer disease may be due to *H. pylori* infection, but there appears to be a genetic predisposition independent of this, for example among concordant twins, HLA subtypes, and in carriers of blood group antigens. These factors may be important in non–*H. pylori* peptic ulcer disease.[72]

Emotional Stress. Emotional stress alone, without the contribution of *H. pylori* and NSAIDs, is unlikely to cause ulceration. However, even modern studies have suggested that emotional distress may be a contributing factor to the occurrence of peptic ulcer complications; for example, after an earthquake in Kobe, Japan, in the 1990s, the incidence of gastric ulcers and bleeding from these increased.[249] Emotional stress may well play a role in genetically susceptible individuals. The term *stress ulcer* is reserved for organic stress: burns, sepsis, hypoxemia, etc.

Smoking. Cigarette smoking predisposes to ulcer formation and complications, probably by inhibiting prostaglandin synthesis and thereby compromising preepithelial or mucosal integrity. In addition, tobacco is a gastric acid secretagogue and inhibitor of duodenal bicarbonate secretion.

Alcohol. There is little evidence that alcohol in the concentration found in commercially available alcoholic beverages causes peptic ulceration, although it may cause petechiae of uncertain significance. There is no increased incidence of peptic ulceration in noncirrhotic humans. Modest alcohol ingestion may be protective of gastric mucosa, via stimulation of prostaglandin synthesis.

Associated Diseases. A strong association exists between chronic pulmonary disease in adults and peptic ulceration. This is poorly understood, but may be related to cigarette smoking. Peptic ulcer disease is associated with hepatic cirrhosis and chronic renal disease, although studies on the latter are contradictory.

Primary Peptic Ulcer Disease

Helicobacter pylori Associated

Although *H. pylori* infection is the commonest cause of peptic ulcer disease in children, these ulcers are rare in children under 8 years of age.[14-16,24,25] Peptic ulcers that are *H. pylori* related cannot be distinguished by their endoscopic appearance from *H. pylori*–negative ulcers – it is the presence of *H. pylori* gastritis that makes the distinction. Exactly how many patients with chronic gastritis actually go on to develop ulcer disease is not known in children, but the lifetime risk of an infected patient developing peptic ulcer disease is estimated as 15 to 20% in adults.[250] The mechanism by which *H. pylori*–associated gastritis causes ulceration in the duodenum appears to involve a complex interplay among infection, acid production, gastric metaplasia, proinflammatory cytokine production and bacterial virulence factors.[72] The pathogenesis of *H. pylori* ulcer disease is summarized in Figure 27-5.

Helicobacter pylori–Negative Disease

"True" *H. pylori*–negative ulcer disease can be diagnosed only when *H. pylori* infection has been reliably excluded. Other conditions must also be excluded,[251] i.e., secondary causes of ulcer disease, such as Crohn's disease, Zollinger-Ellison syndrome, G-cell hyperplasia, CMV infection, allergic disease, and even sarcoidosis.

Reports of prevalence vary widely in both the adult and the pediatric populations. Adult studies report prevalences in North America of *H. pylori*–negative duodenal and gastric ulceration of 11 to 48%.[72,252,253] The few data in children indicate a prevalence of up to 29 to 44%.[254-256] The prevalence of *H. pylori*–negative patients with duodenal ulcers appears to be increasing, possibly due to the relative decrease *H. pylori*–associated ulcer disease.

Though *H. pylori*–related and *H. pylori*–negative ulcer disease (duodenal and gastric) are endoscopically indistinguishable, that is, an ulcer looks like an ulcer, they behave differently. Studies have shown consistently that gastric or duodenal ulcer patients who have bled and subsequently healed have significantly higher rates of rebleeding and mortality.[252,257] Some of the latter is due to more comorbidities in *H. pylori*–negative patients, e.g., cancers and renal failure, which themselves may be associated with peptic ulcer disease, so it is not necessarily primary ulcer disease under study.[252] Possible explanations for the differences in rebleeding are that a subset of the *H. pylori*–negative patients have

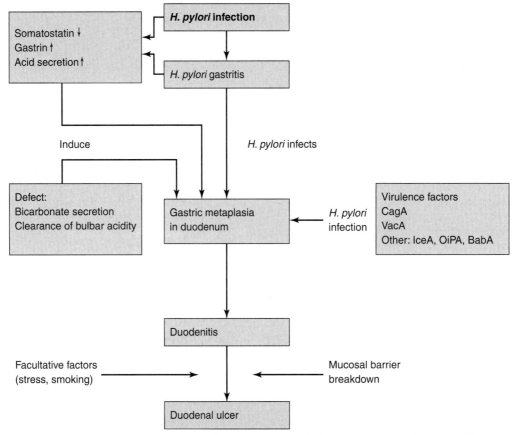

Figure 27-5. Pathogenesis of *H. pylori* ulcer disease. From Malfertheiner et al. (2009), with permission.[72]

acid hypersecretion[258] or that *H. pylori*–positive patients respond better to acid suppression therapy[251] or that they are different types of ulcer genetically.

A recent study[259] showed that some duodenal ulcer patients with negative antral biopsies and even negative urea breath tests had colonization of metaplastic gastric epithelium in the duodenal bulb, and that some ulcers healed with *H. pylori* eradication therapy. Thus, the widely differing prevalences of *H. pylori*–negative ulcer disease may reflect different degrees of thoroughness of exclusion of *H. pylori* infection, as well as truly changing prevalences of *H. pylori* infection within communities as eradication treatments are used. (See Figure 27-6.)

Secondary Peptic Ulcer Disease

All the causes of gastritis and gastropathy may be considered as causes of secondary peptic ulcer disease, except for *H. pylori*.

Ulcer Disease due to Hypersecretory States

Zollinger-Ellison (ZE) syndrome is caused by gastrinomas – i.e., gastrin-secreting tumors.[260] ZE syndrome and G-cell hyperplasia do occur in children, but are extremely rare.[261-263] Although elevated plasma gastrin levels are commonly present in patients receiving PPIs, they are seldom in the ZE range. An elevated plasma gastrin together with gastric pH below 2 is strongly suggestive of ZE syndrome. However, a false-positive secretin test can occur during PPI therapy; hence the importance of discontinuing this at least 2 weeks before testing.[264] The syndrome may occur in association with multiple endocrine neoplasia type 1 (MEN1) or as a sporadic form. Patients with MEN1

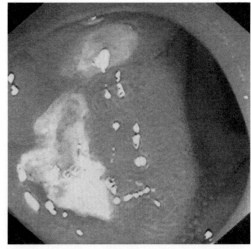

Figure 27-6. Ulcer in the duodenal bulb in a 12-year-old patient who presented with abdominal pain and loss of appetite with early satiety. His gastric biopsies were normal, and no *H. pylori* was present. He had no history of use of NSAIDs, and no antibiotics in the prior 6 months. He had true *H. pylori*-negative duodenal ulcer disease. (*See plate section for color.*)

and ZE syndrome may present earlier in childhood than those with sporadic ZE syndrome.[265] In addition to the pancreatic gastrinomas, ZE syndrome can be associated with extrapancreatic gastrinomas in the stomach, duodenum, liver, kidney, and lymph nodes.[260]

Typically, patients with sporadic ZE syndrome present with multiple ulcerations that are refractory to standard doses of acid-suppressing therapy and may occur in atypical sites such as the jejunum. Symptoms include abdominal pain, persistent diarrhea, heartburn, weight loss, and GI bleeding. Endoscopy reveals prominent gastric folds in most, and esophageal, pyloric, or duodenal stricturing in up to 10% of cases. Acid-reducing surgery may be unnecessary in most cases, as acid hypersecretion can usually be controlled with high-dose PPIs.

Systemic mastocytosis is a condition in which mast cells accumulate in skin, bone, bone marrow, liver, spleen, and GI tract.[266] Mast cell products such as histamine and cytokines produce a variety of effects, including gastric hypersecretion, so, as in ZE syndrome, nausea, vomiting, abdominal pain, peptic ulceration, diarrhea, and malabsorption may occur. Musculoskeletal pain and hypotension or shock may also occur. The commonest form of mastocytosis is cutaneous alone, i.e., with no systemic involvement, most commonly as "urticaria pigmentosa." The cutaneous form commonly presents in the first few months of life and is a benign disorder. In the systemic form, serum gastrin levels typically are normal. Gastric and duodenal mucosa may have ulcers and urticaria-like papules (the latter also in colon), but anesthesia poses particular risks to these patients, and special precautions must be taken if a procedure really is required. Management with H_1 and H_2 antagonists and acid suppression is usually effective.

Other conditions associated with gastric acid hypersecretion include short bowel syndrome, hyperparathyroidism, and cystic fibrosis. Peptic ulcer disease is reported in children and adults with short bowel syndrome, but the exact mechanism remains unclear.[360,361] Peptic ulceration, usually duodenal, can occur in patients with primary hyperparathyroidism as a result of hypercalcemia-induced gastric acid hypersecretion.[267] The incidence of peptic ulcer disease in patients with cystic fibrosis is not known, but they do occur.[268,269]

DIAGNOSIS

The definitive diagnosis of gastritis and peptic ulcer disease is by upper GI endoscopy and biopsies (Figure 27-7). Visceral penetration, a rare complication in children, may be diagnosed or confirmed by CT or MRI. In patients who present with significant vomiting, an upper GI contrast study is necessary to rule out malrotation. Specific recommendations for the diagnostic approach to suspected ulcer disease and possible *H. pylori* infection are given in published Consensus Guidelines[14-16] and discussed in detail in Chapter 28.

MANAGEMENT

Regardless of the cause of ulcer disease, gastric acid and pepsin are major factors in the final pathway leading to deeper mucosal damage. Therefore, acid-suppressing or buffering therapy is often important in the management of gastritis, gastropathy, and peptic ulcer disease. In addition, where applicable, treatment specific to the underlying cause of the mucosal injury should be administered. For example, in NSAID-associated mucosal injury, allergic or eosinophilic gastritis, or celiac disease, specific strategies of drug discontinuation or antigen removal should ideally be undertaken. When it is of advantage or necessity to the patient to continue the offending drug, co-treatment with acid suppression may prevent mucosal damage and heal that already present. The use of

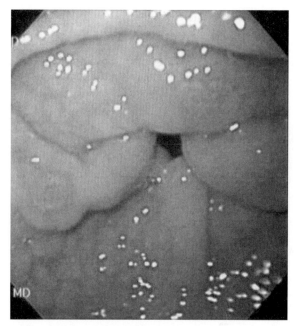

Figure 27-7. Endoscopic appearance of the gastric antrum in a 14-year-old Vietnamese boy with chronic abdominal pain. Multiple gastric antral erosions with surrounding erythema and nodularity are seen. *H. pylori* infection was confirmed on biopsy. There was no history of NSAID use. (*See plate section for color.*)

acid-suppressing drugs may not always be helpful in upper GI tract mucosal injury; for example, in allergic or eosinophilic gastritis, the pathogenic process is immune in nature, and removal of the offending allergen, or treatment with corticosteroids, may be required. Upper GI tract Crohn's disease is best managed with immune modulation directed at Crohn's disease. Stress-induced gastritis is treated through the management of underlying acidosis, hypoxemia, or sepsis. Traumatic gastropathy requires supportive therapy as well as attention to the underlying cause of forceful emesis. Acid suppression is best accomplished with PPIs; their use in children is detailed elsewhere.[270-272] Most PPI data in children pertain to treatment of GERD, as that is the most common indication for their use, but in practice the drugs are used for other acid peptic disorders. Their use as one component of eradication therapy in *H. pylori*–related disease is addressed in Chapter 28. H_2-receptor antagonists (e.g., ranitidine, cimetidine, famotidine) are also commonly used in children. They are of lower efficacy than PPIs but less expensive, and their safety and dosing is established in children. A major drawback of H_2-receptor antagonists is the tachyphylaxis that develops with chronic use.[370,371] Over-the-counter antacids are frequently employed and remain useful for the treatment of relatively minor symptoms on an as-needed basis. Antacids remain valuable when used in intensive regimens in severely ill patients in intensive care units, usually in combination with a parenterally administered H_2-receptor antagonist or PPI. Sucralfate is a complex aluminum of sulfated sucrose, with little acid-neutralizing ability. When exposed to an acid pH, the molecule dissociates and binds to damaged tissue.[273,274] The drug is generally well tolerated. In children with renal failure, aluminum may be inadequately excreted; hence, caution is advised.[275]

The greater efficacy and generally more easily tolerated formulations of PPIs and H_2-receptor antagonists have rendered the use of sucralfate quite uncommon in children. It may be useful in management of duodenogastric reflux[273] and was used in children with peptic ulcer disease in the pre-PPI era.[276] Diet plays little role in the prevention or treatment of acid peptic disease. For ulcer disease recalcitrant to therapy, it may be useful to exclude from the diet beverages causing increased acid secretion, such as tea, coffee, and cola.[277] Bland diets are not of any proven benefit in the treatment of peptic ulcers and serve only to diminish quality of life. There is no need specifically to exclude spicy food from the diet, unless the patient complains that these cause symptoms; the same principle applies to other foods. Complications of peptic ulcers, such as perforation, bleeding refractory to endoscopic hemostasis, and gastric outlet obstruction, are rare in children. The last complication may occur as a result of primary peptic ulcer disease, Crohn's disease, chronic granulomatous disease, or ingestion of iron or NSAIDs.[278-282] Use of PPIs and eradication of *H. pylori* infection have made acid-reducing operations for peptic ulcer disease all but obsolete in children. Such surgery as might be required is discussed elsewhere.[6,283]

REFERENCES

3. Carpenter HA, Talley NJ. Gastroscopy is incomplete without biopsy: clinical relevance of distinguishing gastropathy from gastritis. Gastroenterology 1995;108:917–924.

6. Spechler SJ. Peptic ulcer disease and its complications. In: Feldman M, Friedman LS, Sleisenger MH, editors. Gastrointestinal and Liver Disease: Pathophysiology, Diagnosis, Management, 7th ed. Philadelphia: Saunders; 2002 p. 747–781.

15. Gold BD, Colletti RB, Abbott M, et al. *Helicobacter pylori* infection in children: recommendations for diagnosis and treatment. J Pediatr Gastroenterol Nutr 2000;31:490–497.

36. Yantiss RK, Odze RD. Optimal approach to obtaining mucosal biopsies for assessment of inflammatory disorders of the gastrointestinal tract. Am J Gastroenterol 2009;104:774–783.

72. Malfertheiner P, Chan FK, McColl KE. Peptic ulcer disease. Lancet 2009;374:1449–1461.

251. McColl KE. *Helicobacter pylori*-negative nonsteroidal anti-inflammatory drug-negative ulcer. Gastroenterol Clin North Am 2009;38:353–361.

See expertconsult.com for a complete list of references and the review questions for this chapter.

HELICOBACTER PYLORI IN CHILDHOOD

28

Séamus Hussey • Nicola L. Jones

Three decades ago, pediatric gastritis and peptic ulcer disease lacked a putative microbial causative agent. Pediatric flexible upper endoscopy was becoming more available. Speculation regarding pathogenesis of gastroduodenal ulceration and inflammation included immune-mediated duodenal ulcer disease, postprandial hyperacidity, primary defective mucosal healing and inherited gastric hypersecretion; investigation still included barium radiography, and treatments included antacids, carbenoxolone sodium, and cimetidine at bedtime.[1-4] In 1983 Warren and Marshall proposed that colonization of the human stomach with an organism, now known as *Helicobacter pylori* (*H. pylori*), was associated with human disease, specifically peptic ulcer disease.[5] Earliest reports of this bacterium in children noted its coincidence with gastritis and ulcer disease.[6,7] In February 1994, the National Institutes of Health Consensus Development Conference concluded that *H. pylori* represented the major cause of peptic ulcer disease.[8] Later that year the International Agency for Research on Cancer Working Group of the World Health Organization classified *H. pylori* as a group I (definite) human carcinogen.

H. pylori is a slow-growing gram-negative, curved or S-shaped rod with a single tuft of polar flagella.[9] Large-scale analysis of *H. pylori* protein expression has been used to identify possible disease markers associated with the wide spectrum of putative *Helicobacter*-associated diseases, as well as being utilized in selecting potential vaccine candidates.[10-12]

Although *H. pylori* infects both children and adults worldwide, its role in certain pediatric diseases is a matter of some contention.[13] Pediatricians and pediatric gastroenterologists must therefore avoid inappropriate investigation and potentially toxic therapies, while ensuring appropriate utilization of preventive medicine in minimizing future ill health.

EPIDEMIOLOGY

The interface between *Homo sapiens* and *H. pylori* has been ongoing for many millennia. *H. pylori* haplotype analysis has recently been used as a tool to trace historic human migration patterns.[14-16] Although it is possible that other primates could act as a reservoir of infection, to date humans are the only established natural reservoir of *H. pylori* in the animal kingdom. At least five different gastric non-*H. pylori Helicobacter* species have been isolated from patients at endoscopy.[17] Pigs, dogs, and cats constitute reservoir hosts for gastric *Helicobacter* species with zoonotic potential.[18] Nonhuman primates rapidly acquire *H. pylori* and can been used as animal models of disease.[19-21]

Socioeconomic Risk Factors

Within populations where socioeconomic disparity exists, indices of lower socioeconomic status – including low household income, lower parental educational level, higher housing density, and poor sanitary conditions – continue to influence a higher *H. pylori* prevalence among children, in comparison with their noninfected peers.[22-29] In a 21-year longitudinal study, Malaty et al. observed a marked difference between African American children (increasing from an initial prevalence of 13% to 43%) and white children (increasing from 4% to 8%) by 21 to 23 years of age.[30] Co-infection among parents (especially mothers), siblings, and nonsibling household contacts are established risk factors for childhood *H. pylori* acquisition.[31-35] Child-rearing practices may also influence transmission of infection.[31]

Transmission of Infection

Direct person-to-person contact has been long thought of as a major mode of transmission. Rowland et al. showed that maternal infection was an independent risk factor for childhood *H. pylori* infection.[31] Data from studies of a German birth cohort suggested an odds ratio (OR) of 13 for the effect on the index child of the mother being infected.[35] Biofilm formation by *H. pylori* strains is a possible mechanism of survival outside the body.[36] A strain found in marine zooplankton was able to form biofilms in a more structured way than clinical strains. *H. pylori* has been identified in water systems, by polymerase chain reaction (PCR) rather than culture, and whether these strains are subsequently infectious remains uncertain.[37] As there is no valid assessment of the physiologic status of *H. pylori* found in external environments, it is not possible to clarify the role of particular external reservoirs in *H. pylori* transmission.

Prevalence

H. pylori is rapidly acquired early in our life cycle, generally during early childhood years.[31,38] Cross-sectional prevalence studies outnumber longitudinal studies examining *H. pylori* infection acquisition and loss. Many published studies have been of heterogeneous design and population base and used diverse methods of *H. pylori* detection, not all of which have been validated for use in pediatric populations.

Higher rates of childhood *H. pylori* infection earlier in the 20th century likely account for the persisting higher disease prevalence with advancing age in developed countries. This "birth cohort effect" has been unmasked by cross-sectional seroprevalence studies from around the world.[39-41] Historically, it was held that disease prevalence and burden was much less in Africa. Recent publications in which objective data were available (e.g., obtained by endoscopy) have also confirmed original observations that the prevalence of peptic ulcer disease in Africa is not unusually or unexpectedly low, discounting the "African enigma."[42,43]

Limitations aside, epidemiological studies have contributed greatly to our understanding of the prevalence of *H. pylori* disease. As an example, recent studies from China, Tunisia, Turkey, the Netherlands, rural Alaska, and Israel have reported childhood *H. pylori* prevalence rates of 13.1, 51.4, 30.9, 1.2, 86, and 32.5%, respectively.[25,26,44-46] A Canadian study from three tertiary centers reported a 5.8% prevalence of infection in 204 symptomatic children undergoing endoscopic evaluation as outpatients.[47] A Turkish study found that 26.3% of children younger than 2 years of age undergoing endoscopy were *H. pylori* positive, many with histopathologic abnormalities.[48]

Data from both developed and developing regions of the world suggest that the prevalence of *H. pylori* infection in children is continuing to decline. Notwithstanding the higher prevalence of infection among populations of lower socioeconomic class, seroprevalence studies still show an overall downward trend in infection over the past decade across age groups.[49,50] *H. pylori* is sensitive to improved housing and sanitary conditions in countries experiencing improvements in general economic and social conditions and provides an interesting example of the birth cohort effect. Tkachenko et al. described a dramatic example in their study of seroprevalence changes in St. Petersburg, Russia.[51] Using two cross-sectional studies in children from 1995 and 2005 (and using the same enzyme-linked immunosorbent assay (ELISA) method for anti-*H. pylori* IgG), they showed that the overall prevalence of *H. pylori* infection had decreased from 44 to 13% 10 years later. Among children under 5 years, the prevalence decreased from 30 to 2%. This trend is mirrored in similar reports from Europe, Asia, and the Americas.[49,50,52] A study of Korean children demonstrated a fall in seroprevalence among 6- to 8-year-olds from 8.1% in 1993 to 1.6% in 2002.[53] In a retrospective longitudinal observational study of 1743 symptomatic U.S. children, Elitsur et al. reported an overall *H. pylori* prevalence of 12.1% but interestingly also observed a significant decrease in the mean annual infection rate in patients, from 18.3% before 2000 to 7.3% by 2005.[54]

Incidence

Beyond our first decade of life, annual incidence of newly acquired infection is remarkably low.[13] Accurate studies of the incidence of *H. pylori* infection in childhood are few in number. In the first prospective study of age-specific incidence of *H. pylori* infection, Rowland et al. described the incidence of infection in 327 Irish children enrolled between 2 and 4 years of age using the validated ^{13}C-urea breath test (UBT).[31] Adopting strict criteria, they showed that acquisition of *H. pylori* infection occurred in early childhood years and that co-infection of household contacts and prolonged use of feeding bottles, but not pacifiers, beyond the age of 2 years were risk factors for infection. Over 4 years of follow-up, 279 index children not infected at baseline contributed 970 person-years of follow-up to the study. During this time, 20 children became infected with *H. pylori*. The age-specific rate of infection per 100 person years was 5.05, 4.2, and 2.07 for children aged 2-3, 3-4, and 4-5 years, respectively. Only 1 of 48 children was infected

after the age of 5 years during 416 person-years of follow-up. The authors did not find evidence of spontaneous infection clearance in their study children. The use of serological, stool, and urine tests to detect *H. pylori* in other studies of infection incidence may potentially weaken the data, but the majority conclude that the incidence of *H. pylori* infection is highest in children under 5 years of age.[55]

Many confounding factors that influence the epidemiology of *H. pylori* infection are difficult to control and must be borne in mind when interpreting published data. Given that *H. pylori* is acquired in childhood, environmental factors that influence infection most likely exert their greatest influence during childhood. These are among the most difficult factors to control in cross-sectional or retrospective studies. As an example, lower standards of housing, water quality, and sanitary conditions have historically been associated with increased risk of infection, and yet not all studies have corroborated these findings.

Spontaneous Bacterial Clearance

Spontaneous clearance of *H. pylori* infection in early childhood has been reported. Clearance of IgG seen in very young infants is more likely to represent the detection and then clearance of maternal antibodies.[56,57] However, more recent investigative data suggest that spontaneous elimination of *H. pylori* in childhood may be influenced by antibiotic use for systemic childhood infections, albeit an incomplete explanation.

Reinfection and Recrudescence

The risk of reinfection in the pediatric setting following successful eradication is low in developed countries. Generally, recolonization of the same strain within 12 months of eradication (recrudescence) rather than reinfection (colonization with a new strain, more than 12 months after eradication) is considered to be responsible for most documented "cases." A prospective study by Rowland et al. followed 52 children for a mean of 2 years following successful eradication therapy.[58] Reinfection was identified by UBT; age below 5 years was the only risk factor for reinfection identified by logistic regression. Neither socioeconomic status nor number of infected family members influenced reinfection rates. The estimated reinfection rate for children older than 5 years was 2.0% per person per year. Other studies have estimated reinfection rates in children of between 2 and 13% per patient per year.[59-61] Reported results may be overrepresentative, given that strains are often not isolated and positive tests could represent recrudescence (i.e., possible treatment failure) rather than de novo reinfection. The risk of reinfection in developing countries is less clear. A recent meta-analysis of studies involving predominantly adult subjects suggested that reinfection rates may be higher in developing than developed countries.[62] Continuing poor sanitary and water standards and household density may account in part for the differential reinfection rates between countries at economic extremes.

HOST FACTORS AND RESPONSES

H. pylori is a formidable pathogen. Its natural reservoir is the human population, and it is carried and transmitted asymptomatically by the majority of infected hosts. Following infection, *H. pylori* activates signal transduction pathways that culminate in a rapid host response, both locally and systemically. However, the variable nature and outcome of this response in individuals has generated considerable interest in host and bacterial determinants of infection and disease outcomes. Gastric cancer and duodenal ulceration are mutually exclusive outcomes of *H. pylori* infection.[63] However, various *H. pylori* strains are equally associated with both diseases, suggesting that host factors are also important.

Host Genotype

Cytokine gene polymorphisms are important host factors that can alter *H. pylori* disease outcomes. Proinflammatory polymorphisms of the IL-1β gene have been associated with the development of gastritis predominantly involving the body of the stomach (corpus gastritis), hypochlorhydria, gastric atrophy, and gastric adenocarcinoma, but a reduced risk of duodenal ulceration.[64-68] In the absence of these polymorphisms, *H. pylori* gastritis predominantly involves the antrum and is associated with normal to high acid secretion. Polymorphisms of the TNFα and IL-10 genes demonstrate a similar but less pronounced association with the development of gastric cancer.[69]

Host innate and adaptive immune responses are ordinarily under genetic influence. Scientific advances in the past decade have underscored the importance of host genetic polymorphisms on functional immune responses and disease susceptibility.[70,71] Harboring genetic polymorphisms in key immunity-related genes offers an attractive explanation in part for diverse host phenotypic responses to this bacterium within given ethnic populations.

Polymorphisms in IL-1β and its receptor have been linked to gastric cancer susceptibility. Individuals with the *IL-1Bβ31*C* or _511*T and *IL-1RN*2/*2* genotypes were shown to be at increased risk of developing hypochlorhydria and gastric atrophy in response to *H. pylori* infection.[66,68,72-78] In children, polymorphisms in the IL-1 receptor antagonist gene, *IL1RN*, but not the IL1B gene cluster were associated with susceptibility to duodenal ulcer.[79] This polymorphism, along with cagA+ *H. pylori* strain infection, is independently associated with duodenal ulcer. Complementary transgenic animal model studies have underscored the additive risk of combined host and bacterial disease risk factors leading to *H. pylori* disease and ultimately gastric cancer.[73,80] Polymorphisms in cytokine genes including TNFα, IL-8, and IL-10, which result in a proinflammatory phenotype in the host, have been linked to increased severity of *H. pylori* disease in children and cancer susceptibility in adulthood.[65,81]

Pattern recognition receptors are germline-encoded proteins which detect conserved microbial molecular motifs and danger signals. They include the membrane associated Toll-like receptor family (TLR) and cytosolic nod-like receptor family (NLR). Polymorphisms in TLRs and NLRs have been associated with a variety of gastrointestinal diseases. Polymorphisms in TLR4, which senses bacterial lipopolysaccharide (LPS), have been linked with susceptibility to *H. pylori*–induced gastritis and gastric cancer.[82,83] However, these findings have not been consistently replicated, albeit in populations of different ethnicity.[84-86] A study of 486 Brazilian children undergoing gastroscopy for abdominal pain failed to show an association between polymorphisms in *TLR2*, *TLR4*, and *TLR5* and *H. pylori* infection or duodenal ulceration.[87] However, children with *TLR4* polymorphisms were more likely to have infection with cagA+ *H. pylori*

strains and enhanced mucosal IL-8 and IL-10 levels as measured by ELISA. Interestingly, HLA class I and II allele studies have not shown a predisposition to *H. pylori* infection, although they may affect susceptibility to gastric cancer.[88-90]

These limited data suggest that in the genetically susceptible host, failure to attenuate the inflammatory response to *H. pylori* infection locally leads to chronic inflammation and reduced acidity. This milieu may favor subsequent colonization with non–*H. pylori* species and/or production of genotoxic effects. It is likely that in this era of genome-wide association studies, more elaborate research methodologies may uncover more clues to the influence of host genotype on *H. pylori* infection and disease.

Host Immune Response

The seemingly robust, complex acute host immune response to *H. pylori* infection is surprisingly ineffective at clearing this bacterium and preventing *H. pylori* from establishing a bacterial niche that often lasts several decades.[91] Host and bacterial factors are clearly at play in moderating infection and disease spectrum and severity.

Antral gastritis is associated with increased stimulated acid production and predisposes to duodenal ulceration, whereas corpus-predominant or pangastritis is associated with reduced acid production and predisposes to gastric ulcer and gastric adenocarcinoma.[92] The degree of gastric infiltration by neutrophils also correlates with the development of gastroduodenal ulcerations, and this is in part dependent on the release of damaging inflammatory mediators such as reactive oxygen species.[93]

Innate Immune Receptors

H. pylori is a predominantly extracellular organism that generally adheres to the gastric mucosal surface. Gastric epithelial cells and to a lesser extent intraepithelial myeloid cells effect the first host responses to infection. Innate immune sensing of microbial associated molecular patterns such as lipopolysaccharide, peptidoglycan, and flagellin by their specific pattern-recognition receptors is responsible for the earliest detection of and response to infection. TLRs and NLRs constitute the majority of our innate receptor arsenal. Cell-surface TLRs, including TLR2, TLR4, and TLR5, do not seem to mediate significant initial immune responses to *H. pylori*.[94-97] Indeed, *H. pylori* LPS is less potent than that of *Salmonella* spp. or *Escherichia coli*, and modification of *H. pylori* LPS facilitates immune evasion.[98,99]

Given that *H. pylori* is primarily an extracellular pathogen, it may seem intriguing that it engages NLRs at all. This interaction is in part mediated by its gene-encoded type IV secretion system (TFSS), a molecular syringe that facilitates translocation of bacterial effector proteins and products into cells.[100,101] *H. pylori* peptidoglycan is translocated into host cells where it engages with its receptor, Nod1.[102] Downstream effects of Nod1 activation include instigation of NFκB-mediated inflammatory cascades and subsequent IL-8 production.

Autophagy

Autophagy is a process in eukaryotic cells whereby cytosolic elements and organisms are enclosed in multilamellar vacuoles and transferred to the lysosome for degradation and processing.[103] Its role in processing intracellular bacteria has become apparent over the past decade. Recently, an interaction between autophagy and *H. pylori,* and its role in disease pathogenesis, has been uncovered. VacA toxin induces autophagy in gastric epithelial cells in vitro and also facilitates bacterial replication and survival (Figure 28-1).[104,105] *H. pylori* multiplies within autophagosomes in macrophages in vitro, suggesting that it may be subverting autophagy for its own benefit.[106,107] Further studies in this field are awaited.

Myeloid Cells – Macrophages

H. pylori induces chronic gastritis in almost all hosts.[108] Initial neutrophil recruitment gives way to mononuclear cell infiltrates with lymphocytes and macrophages and the attendant epithelial cell damage.[109] Following *H. pylori* infection, enhanced levels of IL-1β, IL-2, IL-6, IL-8, and tumor necrosis factor α (TNF-α) are detected in the gastric epithelium.[110] Phagocytosis of *H. pylori* by macrophages results in marked IL-6 production.[101] The precise role of TLRs in macrophage chemokine and cytokine responses to *H. pylori* remains unclear, although recent reports suggest that mouse macrophages deficient in MyD88, a downstream adaptor of certain TLRs, have diminished cytokine responses to *H. pylori* infection.[99,111] As effector cells, macrophages generate nitric oxide (NO), catalyzed by the enzyme inducible NO synthase (iNOS), which is up-regulated in macrophages following *H. pylori* infection in vitro.[112] Through its arginase enzyme, encoded by the gene *rocF, H. pylori* competes with the eukaryotic macrophage for the iNOS substrate L-arginine (L-Arg) to enhance its survival.[113] The enzyme generates urea from L-Arg, which is then utilized by urease to synthesize ammonia and neutralize the gastric luminal HCl. Reduced macrophage NO generation therefore confers an immune evasion advantage.

Myeloid Cells – Dendritic Cells

Mucosal dendritic cells (DCs) are an important component of our antigen presenting cell repertoire. They express an array of innate immune receptors and their cytokine responses influence the differentiation of T helper cells.[114,115] Transepithelial and lamina propria DCs identified in patients with chronic gastritis respond to both live bacteria and *H. pylori* antigens, releasing varying quantities of IL-6, IL-8, IL-10, and IL-12.[116-119] In contrast to macrophages, TLR and Myd88 expression in DCs is not dispensable for complete *H. pylori* recognition and DC activation.[120] Endosomal TLRs recognizing microbial nucleic acids were recently identified as important components of DC responses to *H. pylori*. C-type lectin receptors (CLRs) expressed by DCs are crucial for directing immune responses to pathogens.[121] DC-specific ICAM3-grabbing nonintegrin (DC-SIGN) recognizes *H. pylori* fructose residues and, following pathogen binding, triggers the expression of specific cytokines that influence T cell differentiation.[122] DC-SIGN binding of *H. pylori* was recently shown to result in enhanced IL-10 and reduced IL-12 and IL-6 expression that could subsequently favor Th-2 polarization.[123]

Myeloid Cells – B Lymphocytes

H. pylori also induces a vigorous mucosal humoral response that does not lead to eradication but does contribute to tissue damage. Infiltrating B lymphocytes and plasma cells give rise to *H. pylori*–specific IgA and IgG antibodies. CD4+ T cells help B lymphocytes to produce antibodies, and also contribute to inflammation in the gastric mucosa by producing high amount of interferon-γ (IFN-γ).[92] *H. pylori*–specific IgG or IgA antibodies can be detected in peripheral blood from early stages of infection. Some have reported that peripheral blood lymphocytes from patients with duodenal ulcer and chronic antral gastritis show no significant alteration in systemic immune responses to *H. pylori*, whereas others report proliferation and activation of CD4+ and CD8+ T lymphocytes.[124-128] B cell deficient mice infected with *H. pylori* have reduced colonization at 8 and 16 weeks postinoculation, compared with wild-type mice, which is associated with increased gastric inflammation and infiltration of CD4+ T cells.[129] The IgG and IgA responses to *H. pylori*

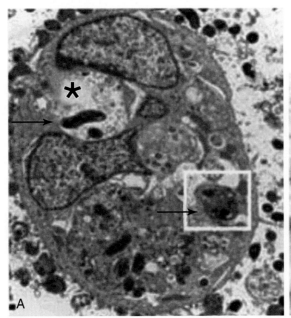
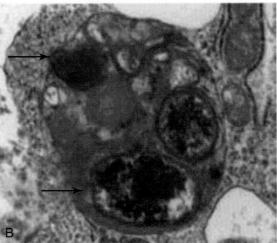

Figure 28-1. *H. pylori* induces autophagy. Transmission electron micrographs depicting a gastric epithelial cell infected with *H. pylori* (**A**). The asterisk denotes intracellular *H. pylori* inside a VacA-induced large vacuole (arrow). **B** is an enlargement of the framed area in A, showing details of the autophagic compartment and bacteria within the autophagosome (arrows). Adapted from Terebiznik et al. (2009),[105] with permission.

in the serum and gastric mucosa have been well described and may be involved in protective immunity, but these B cell-mediated antibody responses could also be counterproductive. The development of gastric mucosa-associated lymphoid tissue lymphoma stems from activated B cells. Recently it has been reported that chronic gastric infection with *H. pylori* protected splenic B cells from apoptosis, indicating a B cell activation/survival phenotype that may have implications for mucosa-associated lymphoid tissue lymphoma.[130] In addition to producing antigen-specific antibodies, B cells can also produce potentially harmful autoantibodies.[131] The implications of T-cell–B-cell interactions in the pathology of the immune response remain to be fully explained.

Myeloid Cells – T Lymphocytes

A variety of T cell responses, both in the gastric mucosa and in the periphery, have been characterized.[132-135] Immature T helper (Th) cells can differentiate into Th1, Th2, and Th17 functional subtypes. Th1 cells secrete IL-2 and interferon gamma (IFN-γ) and induce cell-mediated immune responses that regulate the response to infection with intracellular pathogens. Th2 cells produce IL-4, IL-5, IL-6, and IL-10 and are generally traditionally induced in response to extracellular pathogens. The data on *H. pylori*–induced effects on T cell differentiation, both locally and systemically, have been difficult to reconcile. In the human gastric mucosa, *H. pylori* induces recruitment of CD4+ and CD8+ T cells and murine studies have shown that the gastric inflammation is T cell-dependent, as, experimentally *H. pylori* does not induce gastritis in T cell-deficient mice.[136,137] *H. pylori*–specific T cells with a Th1 phenotype (i.e., secreting IFN-γ) have been cloned from *H. pylori*–infected gastric mucosa and, through the production of IFN-γ, were cytotoxic to gastric epithelial cells.[138] Conversely, it has been suggested that activation of a Th2 cell response, and production of Th2 cell cytokines such as IL-4, is protective against severe pathology and curbs potentially detrimental effects of Th1-related cytokines.[139]

Recently, a significant expansion of granulocytes and γδ-TCR+ T lymphocytes and high concentrations of IL-10 were observed in the peripheral blood of *H. pylori*–infected subjects in comparison to healthy controls.[140] No differences were detected between infected and noninfected subjects in regard to the frequencies of CD3,+ CD19,+ CD4,+ and CD8+ T cells and their subsets. A mixed T cell response, though favoring a Th2 profile, was reported in a study of gastric T cells from subjects with and without *H. pylori* infection.[141] Using flow cytometry and RT-PCR, mixed *H. pylori*–specific T regulatory and T helper subsets with a predominant CD4+ IL10+ response were found in the gastric antrum. This more "tolerant" response could in part explain incomplete clearance of *H. pylori* and chronicity of infection. Previous investigations had reported predominant Th1 responses to *H. pylori*, which could be partly explained by methodological differences.[134,142-145] Interestingly, patients in this study with ulceration had reduced T regulatory and increased Th1 and Th2 response profiles compared to those without ulceration.

A specific subset of CD4+ T cells termed T helper-17 (Th17) cells, which are distinct from and antagonized by the classical Th1 or Th2 cells, has been described recently.[146] Th17 cells produce IL-17 and play a prominent role in the development of chronic inflammation associated with inflammatory and autoimmune disorders.[147] T cell production of IL-17 stimulates the production of IL-1, IL-6, TNF-α, and matrix metalloproteinases

by fibroblasts, endothelial cells, epithelial cells, and macrophages. IL-17 up-regulation occurs at both RNA and protein levels in *H. pylori* infection.[148] IL-17 activates ERK1/2 MAP kinases in gastric epithelial cells, and IL-17 expression levels correlate with the IL-8 content and number of infiltrating neutrophils in *H. pylori*–infected mucosa.[149] Furthermore, IL-23 is overexpressed in *H. pylori*–infected gastric mucosa, which could contribute to sustaining IL-17 production.[150] The exact molecular mechanism by which IL-23 regulates IL-17 in *H. pylori*–infected mucosa remains to be ascertained, but the signal transducer and activator of transcription 3 (STAT3) likely plays a key role in IL-23-driven IL-17 production during *H. pylori* infection.

Apoptosis and Neoplasia

H. pylori induces apoptosis both in vitro and in vivo by several mechanisms.[151] *H. pylori* or its products can induce apoptosis directly. For example, VacA induces the release of cytochrome *c* from mitochondria.[152,153] Alternatively, the bacterium induces host immune responses which then mediate apoptosis. For instance, Th1 cell cytokines (TNF-α and IFN-γ) markedly potentiate *H. pylori*–induced epithelial cell apoptosis.[154,155] *H. pylori* also up-regulates expression of the Fas death receptor.[156,157] The absence of Fas signaling has been associated with less apoptosis and enhanced premalignant gastric mucosal changes.[158,159]

The mechanisms of *H. pylori*–related carcinogenesis are unclear and are likely the result of both bacterial and host factors, and environmental factors such as smoking, high-salt diet, and antioxidant ingestion.[63] *H. pylori* disrupts the DNA mismatch repair system.[152,160,161] By leading to gastric atrophy, *H. pylori* may be permitting its own replacement by more genotoxic bacteria.[69]

Carcinomas occur with pangastritis. The more common type occurs following progressive atrophy, hypochlorhydria, intestinal metaplasia, and dysplasia.[162,163] Disturbance of the balance between epithelial cell proliferation and apoptosis is considered a risk factor for gastric atrophy and, later, neoplastic transformation. Studies in humans demonstrate that, in the absence of premalignant lesions or gastric cancer, *H. pylori*–induced apoptosis is associated with increased epithelial proliferation. However, in the presence of metaplasia and *H. pylori* infection, apoptosis returns to normal levels, whereas proliferation remains increased.

Acid Homeostasis

H. pylori infection can cause hypergastrinemia by both reducing D-cell somatostatin production and increasing G-cell gastrin production. Removal of *H. pylori* reverses these effects.[69] However, the ultimate effect of infection on acid homeostasis depends on the topographic distribution of *H. pylori*–induced inflammation within the stomach. In antral-predominant gastritis, gastrin release leads to higher acid levels, and persistently high gastrin levels increase the parietal cell mass.[164,165] This in turn results in increased acid delivery to the duodenum, inducing gastric metaplasia. *H. pylori* can colonize gastric metaplasia, resulting in inflammation and, possibly, ulceration.[165-168]

With pangastritis or corpus-predominant gastritis, *H. pylori* infection suppresses acid production both directly and indirectly. Inflammatory mediators inhibit parietal cell acid secretion and enterochromaffin-like cell histamine production.[169,170] Reduced acid secretion further increases gastrin levels, promoting gastric epithelial cell proliferation. Epithelial cell characteristics become altered, leading to progressive gastric gland loss, and thus gastric atrophy. Gastric atrophy increases the risk of gastric ulceration and noncardia gastric adenocarcinoma.[171]

Putative Hormonal Effects

H. pylori infection can affect the expression of the appetite- and satiety-controlling hormones leptin and ghrelin.[172-176] In children, an inverse relationship between serum ghrelin concentration and the severity of *H. pylori*–induced gastritis has been demonstrated.[177] *H. pylori* infection leads to a reduction of the density of gastric ghrelin-positive cells. The decrease in ghrelin is associated with neutrophil activity, chronic inflammation, glandular atrophy, and low serum pepsinogen. *H. pylori* infection decreases gastric D cells that produce somatostatin, and the subsequent loss of gastric G cells' inhibition is a mechanism for hypergastrinemia in *H. pylori*–infected individuals.[178] The decrease of somatostatin-mediated inhibition on leptin-producing cells in the gastric mucosa may be responsible for an increase of gastric leptin but cannot explain the decrease in G cells.

H. pylori eradication has been shown to lead to an increase of body weight.[179] The underlying mechanism has been suggested to be of gastric hormonal origin, with both ghrelin and leptin contributing to this effect. Although the prevalence of *H. pylori* infection was previously shown to be significantly higher in lean rather than obese patients, there is neither a sound scientific basis nor robust data to support the hypothesis that *H. pylori* is a protective factor against obesity.[180,181]

BACTERIAL FACTORS AND ADAPTATIONS

Genetic Diversity

The *H. pylori* genome (1.65 million base pairs) codes for more than 1500 proteins including enzymes that modify the antigenic structure of surface molecules, control the entry of foreign DNA into the bacterium, and influence bacterial motility.[182,183] These factors are essential for *H. pylori* to effectively colonize humans. More than 100 bacterial genes are required for gastric colonization, and their expression can be up-regulated within the stomach.[184,185] *H. pylori* lacks a genetic mismatch-repair system to control the confidentiality of replication, which results in a high mutation rate.[186] Genetic diversity of *H. pylori* has likely resulted from endogenous mutations and recombination.[187,188] Many *H. pylori* isolates have a hyper-mutator phenotype, which favors the emergence of variants after selective pressure; the rapid development of high-level resistance to commonly used antibiotics such as clarithromycin is one such example.[188] *H. pylori* are also highly competent to uptake DNA; thus, the *H. pylori* genome continuously changes during chronic colonization by acquiring fragments of DNA from other *H. pylori* strains.[189] In essence, each host is colonized not by a single clone, but by a variety of usually closely related organisms.

Colonization and Environmental Adaptation

After ingestion, *H. pylori* colonizes the gastric mucus layer and can adhere to and invade gastric epithelial cells. Gastric acidity, motility, nutrient availability, and host immune responses are but some of the barriers to colonization. *H. pylori* has adapted remarkably to many of these barriers. *H. pylori* can hydrolyze urea to generate ammonia and modify the local pH.[190-193] Its urease activity is governed by a unique pH-gated urea channel, UreI, encoded by the *ureI* gene. UreI opens at low pH and closes at neutral pH conditions.[194,195] *H. pylori*'s urease binds substrate with a much higher affinity than that of other bacterial species. *H. pylori* also depends on strong motility to persist in the viscous mucous layer of the human stomach. Polar flagella confer motility, and nonmotile mutants are unable to establish persistent infection in experimental animals.[196] Bacterial nutrients are derived locally, and *H. pylori* has numerous mechanisms to counteract the actions of reactive oxygen and nitrogen species and reduce competition from other microbes.[197,198]

Mucosal Adherence

The adherence of *H. pylori* to the gastric mucosa is important for initial colonization and subsequent persistence in the human gastric mucosa. The *H. pylori* genome encodes five major outer membrane protein (OMP) families that can bind to antigens (receptors) on gastric epithelial cells, anchoring bacteria to counteract mechanical clearance.[199,200] The Hop (*Helicobacter* outer membrane protein) family can act as adhesion molecules and include the blood group antigen binding adhesin (BabA), sialic acid binding adhesin (SabA), adherence-associated lipoprotein (AlpA and AlpB), outer membrane inflammatory protein (OipA), and HopZ.[201] Lewis b and related blood group antigens are recognized by BabA, whereas sialyl-Lewis x and sialyl-Lewis a antigens are recognized by SabA. The corresponding receptors for AlpAB, OipA, and HopZ remain unknown. *H. pylori* binds tightly and specifically to gastric epithelial cells using these adhesins.[202] The adhesin BabA2 is associated with higher levels of bacterial colonization, neutrophil infiltration, and IL-8 secretion in the gastric mucosa, suggesting that BabA2 facilitates colonization and augments host immune responses.[200] Infections with *babA2*-positive strains are associated with peptic ulcer disease and preneoplastic gastric lesions.[203,204] Sialyl-Lewis x expression on the gastric epithelium is promoted by both gastric inflammation and malignant transformation.[199,205] A suggested model proposes that in chronic *H. pylori* infection, the bacteria initially utilize BabA2 to recognize and bind to the gastric epithelium; the resulting inflammation up-regulates the expression of sialyl-Lewis x antigens, which the bacteria then in turn exploit for increased adherence by utilizing SabA.

The dimeric form of trefoil factor 1 (TFF1) can interact with *H. pylori*.[206] This small protein is coexpressed with the gastric mucin, MUC5AC. TFF-1 acts as a linker molecule, binding to both MUC5AC and *H. pylori* LPS in a pH-dependent manner, and may be a factor in determining the tropism of this organism for gastric tissue.[207]

cag Pathogenicity Island

Type IV secretion systems (T4SS) are biological "molecular syringes" produced by many gram-negative bacteria that transport proteins or DNA-protein complexes into other cells.[208] T4SS typically consist of core, metabolic, and pilus-associated components. The *H. pylori* T4SS is a filamentous sheathed organelle with a rigid, needle-like pilus protruding from the bacterial surface.[209-211] These pili are often located at one bacterial pole and are induced on cell contact. CagF is a chaperone-like protein which is crucial for the translocation of CagA.[212,213]

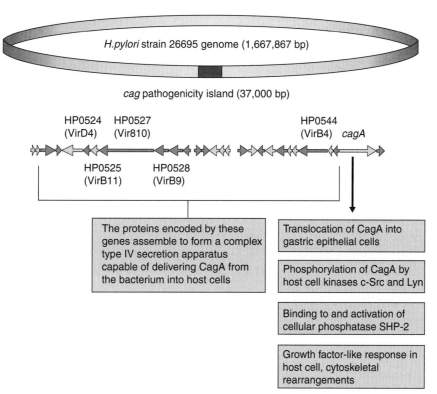

Figure 28-2. The *cag* pathogenicity island. Most *H. pylori* strains that cause disease (so-called type I strains) contain the *cag* pathogenicity island, a chromosomal region with about 37,000 base pairs and 29 genes, whose location is indicated by the arrows. The figure shows the arrangement of genes in strain 26695, whose genome sequence was the first to be published. The island is split into two parts in some strains. Most of the *cag* genes are probably involved in the assembly of secretory machinery that translocates the protein CagA into the cytoplasm of gastric epithelial cells. Five genes (denoted by Vir) are similar to components of the type IV secretion system of the plant pathogen *Agrobacterium tumefaciens* (Vir proteins). Proteins encoded by the island are involved in two major processes, the induction of IL-8 production by gastric epithelial cells and the translocation of CagA from the bacterium into the host cell. From Suerbaum and Michetti (2002).[218]

CagL is a pilus-covering protein which anchors and targets the T4SS to the host transmembrane cell adhesion molecule, integrin $\alpha_5\beta_1$, where CagA is then injected.[210]

One distinguishing feature of *H. pylori* strains is the presence or absence of the cag pathogenicity island (PAI). The cytotoxin-associated gene (*cagA*) encodes for a 120- to 140-kDa immune-dominant protein, CagA, a marker for the cag pathogenicity island (PAI). This 37-kb fragment of chromosomal DNA is acquired by horizontal transfer and encodes for components of the T4SS that transports CagA and peptidoglycan into host cells.[102,214] CagA can modulate cell growth and motility, alter tight junctions, disturb cell polarity, and activate STAT3 in vitro and in vivo.[215,216] Translocated CagA can also induce IL-8 release in infected cells and activate NF-κB in a strain- and time-dependent manner.[217]

As shown in Figure 28-2, CagA modulates several signal transduction cascades in host cells.[218] Following translocation, CagA becomes phosphorylated at conserved EPIYA motifs located near the C terminus by the host-cell Src kinase.[219] Phosphorylated CagA interacts with SHP-2, a tyrosine phosphatase, resulting in a conformational change in SHP-2 and inhibition of its phosphatase activity.[220] The increased Erk/MAP kinase activation can lead to a deregulation of cell growth.[221] Phosphorylated CagA can also interact with the C-terminal Src kinase, Csk, which results in inhibition of Src kinase activity.[222] The role of cagA in disease pathogenesis is not completely understood. Numerous studies, particularly in Western countries, have shown that *cag* PAI-positive *H. pylori* strains confer an increased risk for peptic ulcer disease and gastric cancer over strains that lack the *cag* PAI.[223-226] In children, infection with a CagA+ strain has been associated with peptic ulcer disease in some populations but not others.[227-230]

A second T4SS expressed by *H. pylori* involves ComB proteins, encoded by *comB* genes.[231] These proteins have all the characteristics of a pore-forming transmembrane complex suitable for DNA translocation through the cellular envelope. ComB is functionally unrelated to the *cag* PAI system, such that mutations within *comB* do not affect the function of *cag* PAI, and vice versa.

Plasticity Region

A comparison of two fully sequenced genomes of *H. pylori* identified a large single hypervariable region that contained almost half of the strain-specific genes.[232] This region, called the plasticity region, has an altered G and C content and contains several insertion sequences, suggesting that it may be acquired from horizontal transfer. Because of these features, investigators have begun to search for putative virulence factors in this region. A study of *H. pylori* strains isolated from 200 Brazilian patients identified an association between the presence of a gene located in the plasticity region, *JHP947*, and the presence of duodenal ulcer and gastric carcinoma.[233] A further study also indicated that *JHP947* was associated with secretion of IL-12 and duodenal ulcer disease.[234] In addition, a cluster of genes with homology to genes of the T4SS has been located in the plasticity region.[235]

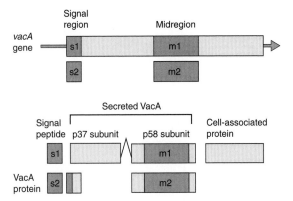

Figure 28-3. *vacA* polymorphism and function. The gene *vacA* is a polymorphic mosaic with two possible signal regions, s1 and s2, and two possible mid-regions, m1 and m2. The transplanted protein is an autotransporter with N- and C-terminal processing during bacterial secretion. The s1 signal region is fully active, but the s2 region encodes a protein with a different signal-peptide cleavage cite, resulting in a short N-terminal extension to the mature toxin that blocks vacuolating activity and attenuates pore-forming activity. The mid-region encodes a cell-binding site, but the m2 type binds to and vacuolates fewer cell lines in vitro. From Blaser and Atherton (2004),[69] with permission.

Vacuolating Cytotoxin, VacA

Vacuolating cytotoxin (VacA) is an 88-kDa pore-forming protein produced by approximately 50% of *H. pylori* strains. VacA was originally named for its ability to induce massive vacuolation in epithelial tissue culture cells.[69] *vacA* is a polymorphic gene that appears to be conserved among all *H. pylori* strains.[236] As shown in Figure 28-3, the *vacA* gene possesses variable signal (s1 or s2) and mid-regions (m1 or m2). Strains of *H. pylori* that express active forms of the toxin are associated with more severe cases of disease.[236] The toxin inserts into lipid membranes to form a hexameric anion-selective, voltage-dependent channel through which bicarbonate, urea, and organic anions can be released, providing substrate for urea hydrolysis and hence protection from gastric acidity.[237] A wide range of cellular effects have been attributed to VacA as illustrated in Figure 28-4, including induction of apoptosis, alteration of the process of antigen presentation, disruption of macrophage phagosome maturation, inhibition of T cell activation and proliferation, and autophagy induction.[104,105,238-241] The role of VacA in mediating disease in humans is unclear. In certain populations, specific *vacA* alleles are associated with the presence of disease such as gastric adenocarcinoma.[242] Association between *vacA* alleles and disease presentation and outcome in children has been variably reported.[228,243,244]

Host Immune Evasion and Manipulation

Despite the presence of a vigorous immune response, *H. pylori* eradication is not usually observed unless specific antibiotic therapy is provided. This demonstrates the effectiveness of *H. pylori*'s strategies in evading host immunity. Although not completely resistant to host immune activation, *H. pylori* has evolved a variety of mechanisms to reduce recognition by immune sensors, down-regulate activation of immune cells, and escape immune effectors.

Many bacteria have unmethylated cytosine-guanine-rich DNA (CpG DNA) that is recognized by TLR9.[245] However, *H. pylori* DNA is highly methylated, which likely minimizes detection by TLR9, at least in certain cell types.[69] Bacterial flagella are usually recognized by TLR5, but *H. pylori* flagellin does not strongly activate the TLR5 signaling pathway.[96] TLR4 recognizes bacterial LPS.[246] Owing to modifications within the lipid A core, *H. pylori* LPS is relatively anergic, stimulating TLR4 on macrophages but not on gastric epithelial cells.[95] *H. pylori* counteracts macrophage function by inhibiting phagocytosis, disrupting phagosome maturation, and promoting apoptosis.[247-249] *H. pylori* VacA interferes with both the uptake and processing of antigens, suppresses T-cell proliferation and activation, and induces selective T-cell apoptosis.[250-252] *H. pylori* is also able to disrupt cytokine signaling pathways in vitro.[253] In addition, by mimicking gastric epithelial Lewis antigens and by antigenic variation of surface proteins, the bacterium evades host adaptive responses.[254] The relative importance of each of these strategies is not yet established and may well vary from host to host.

Antibiotic Resistance–the Bacterial Perspective

Antimicrobial drug resistance is a major cause of treatment failure and has led to declining eradication rates. *H. pylori* antibiotic resistance mechanisms are mainly based on point mutations located on the bacterial chromosome. Given its lack of DNA repair-mismatch mechanisms, it is not surprising that antibiotic resistance easily develops de novo, although horizontal gene transfer is another possible resistance mechanism.[255] Resistance of *H. pylori* to commonly used antibiotic groups including nitroimidazoles, macrolides, penicillins, tetracyclines, and fluoroquinolones has been characterized and provides the basis for designing current and future treatment regimens.

Metronidazole and tinidazole are bactericidal antibiotics administered in prodrug form that need to be activated within the target cell by electron transfer processes. This leads to the formation of nitro-anion radicals and imidazole intermediates that cause lethal damage to subcellular structures and DNA.[256] In *H. pylori*, resistance is mediated by reduced or abolished activity of any of several putative electron acceptors, including ferredoxin (FdxA), flavodoxin (FldA), ferredoxin-like protein (FdxB), NAD(P)H flavin nitroreductase (FrxA), 2-oxoglutarate oxidoreductase (OorD), pyruvate:ferredoxin oxidoreductase (PorD), and oxygen-insensitive NAD(P)H nitroreductase (RdxA).[182,257] Regardless of whether mutations in these factors alter the expression of the corresponding protein, or result in a truncated protein or changed amino acid sequence, the finding that mutations in multiple proteins all result in an increased minimum inhibitory concentration of antibiotic might explain the wide range in levels of resistance.

Clarithromycin is a bacteriostatic antibiotic that binds reversibly to 23S ribosomal RNA (rRNA) to interfere with protein synthesis. In *H. pylori*, resistance to clarithromycin and other related macrolides is mostly because of point mutations in one of two adjacent 23S rRNA nucleotides.[258] These substitutions decrease ribosomal affinity for macrolides, resulting in increased resistance.

Amoxicillin binds to penicillin-binding proteins (PBPs) and interferes with bacterial cell wall synthesis, resulting in lysis of replicating bacteria. Resistance to penicillins generally results from beta-lactamase activity or mutational changes in one or more PBPs. In *H. pylori*, resistance is primarily mediated by alterations to PBPs.[259] Many *H. pylori* isolates described as being amoxicillin resistant are often just tolerant of penicillins – i.e., their resistance is transient and not stable. Stable amoxicillin resistance in *H. pylori* is rare and is mediated by mutational

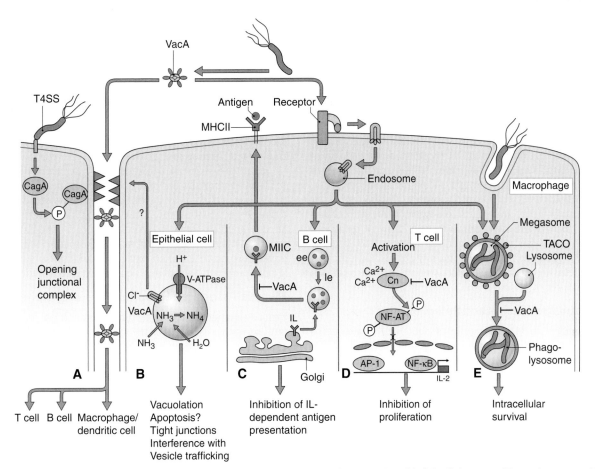

Figure 28-4. Multiple functions of VacA in different cell types. CagA protein is injected into gastric epithelial cells by a type IV secretion system (T4SS) and tyrosine-phosphorylated. CagA opens tight junctions between epithelial cells (**A**). VacA is secreted by *H. pylori* and comes first into contact with epithelial cells, where it is internalized and subsequently induces vacuoles, possibly by constituting anion-selective membrane channels (**B**). VacA may also interact with cells of the immune system after passing opened tight junctions. VacA inhibits antigen presentation in B cells, possibly by blocking the maturation of endosomes to major histocompatibility complex (MHC) class II compartments, where antigen loading takes place (**C**); the inhibition of interleukin (IL)-2 secretion in T cells and thus of T-cell activation and proliferation by blocking the transcription factor, nuclear factor (NF)-AT (**D**); and the inhibition of phagosome-lysosome fusion in macrophages by recruiting the coat protein, tryptophan aspartate-containing coat protein (TACO) (**E**). ee, early endosome; le, late endosome; li, invariant chain; MIIC, MHC class II compartment; Cn, calcineurin; V-ATPase, vacuolar-ATPase. From Fischer W, Gebert B, Haas R. Novel activities of the *Helicobacter pylori* vacuolating cytotoxin: from epithelial cells towards the immune system. Int J Med Microbiol 2004; 293:539-547.

changes in PBP1A. Amoxicillin resistance in *H. pylori* also ensues from alterations in outer membrane protein composition, resulting in an increased diffusion barrier effect.[260,261]

Tetracycline is a bacteriostatic antibiotic that binds to the 16S rRNA, resulting in inhibition of protein synthesis and bacterial growth.[262] The main mechanism of tetracycline resistance in *H. pylori* arises from base-pair substitutions in the 16S rRNA primary binding site of tetracycline, although reduced membrane permeability could contribute to tetracycline resistance.[263,264]

Fluoroquinolones are bactericidal antibiotics that inhibit DNA gyrase, an enzyme that catalyses the negative supercoiling of DNA. In *H. pylori*, resistance to fluoroquinolones is caused by point mutations in the DNA gyrase-encoding gene *gyrA*.[265]

DISEASE ASSOCIATIONS

Various diseases are suspected as being associated with *H. pylori* infection. The evidence for some is compelling if not conclusive. For others it is highly suggestive. For many, conclusive evidence of association is notably sparse. The spectrum of *H. pylori*–related disease encountered in childhood varies somewhat from that recognized in the adult population.

Gastrointestinal Manifestations

Gastritis

Infection with *H. pylori* is associated with chronic gastritis in both children and adults. The first reports of this came from Warren and Marshall, who ingested the organism and subsequently developed gastritis. Eradication of *H. pylori* results in the healing of gastritis. Whether gastritis, in the absence of ulcer disease, has any manifest symptoms, including recurrent abdominal pain or nonulcer dyspepsia, has been a source of controversy.[266-268] Best available evidence from multiple geographic areas of the world suggests that *H. pylori* gastritis remains largely asymptomatic in children and is not a causal factor in recurrent abdominal pain.[269-277]

Ulcer Disease

H. pylori infection plays a causal role in the development of duodenal and gastric ulcers and should be eradicated when detected in such settings.[268] The lifetime risk of peptic ulcer disease in the setting of *H. pylori*–positive gastritis in adults varies geographically. In the United States it is reported to be as low as 3%, whereas in Japan the rate is 25%.[278] Reinfection with *H. pylori* and the recurrence rate of *H. pylori*–associated peptic ulcers after successful eradication therapy in adults is very low. This applies even in geographic regions where *H. pylori* is highly prevalent.[279]

In children, ulcer disease is thought to be less common than adults, with reported rates in symptomatic children of 2 to 22.5%.[227,280-284] The recent pediatric European treatment registry report noted gastritis in 87% of 518 children, with the remainder having duodenal or gastric ulceration. The pattern of *H. pylori* gastritis and the age of *H. pylori* acquisition both appear to be important determinants of future sequelae. Antral-predominant gastritis has a higher risk of duodenal ulcer, whereas subjects with corpus-predominant gastritis are more prone to gastric ulcers and gastric malignancy. A combination of bacterial factors and host genotype and immune responses also likely determine whether children proceed to develop ulceration.[230] A duodenal ulcer promoting gene (*dupA*), located in the plasticity region of the *H. pylori* genome, may be one such virulence marker.[285]

Gastroesophageal Reflux and Reflux Disease

Currently there is no convincing clinical data that *H. pylori* status or eradication affects gastroesophageal reflux disease (GERD) in children. Various epidemiologic studies have demonstrated an inverse relationship between rates of *H. pylori* infection and the prevalence of GERD and/or the aggravation of esophagitis with *H. pylori* eradication.[286,287] Conversely, many studies have found no relationship between reflux symptoms and *H. pylori* eradication.[288-290] The first prospective evaluations of the effect of *H. pylori* eradication on GER symptoms in pediatric patients were published in 2004.[291,292] Both symptoms of GER and epigastric pain were unrelated to *H. pylori* status and eradication outcome. Similar results have been found in adult and pediatric studies.[293-297]

Gastric Carcinoma

Gastric cancer is the second most frequent cause of cancer-related death in the world and the fourth most common cause of cancer-related death in Europe.[298,299] *H. pylori* infection is mostly associated with noncardia adenocarcinomas.[300] The initial sero-epidemiologic evidence for this association came from three nested case-control studies that all showed that patients with cancer had a higher *H. pylori* seroprevalence compared with controls. The attributable risk with positive serology ranged from 2.1 to 8.7.[162,301] Several subsequent studies have placed the relative risk of gastric cancer in infected individuals between two- and sixfold.[302,303] One study that subsequently controlled for bias even suggested that the risk is much higher.[304] A meta-analysis of *H. pylori* association with early gastric cancer suggested an OR of 3 compared with noncancer controls.[305] Several studies have examined the role of *H. pylori* eradication in cancer prevention. A recent meta-analysis suggests a beneficial role in Asian countries with a high prevalence of gastric cancer, whereas benefits in the West were less clear.[306] A prospective study of 1526 Japanese subjects conducted over an 8-year period reported that, during follow-up, gastric cancer developed in infected patients only; no cases were detected in eradicated or uninfected patients.[303] Interestingly, in the West, around 60% *of H. pylori* isolates possess CagA compared with virtually all isolates in Japan.[307] A randomized primary prevention trial from China appeared to show no effect of *H. pylori* treatment on gastric cancer, but on subgroup analysis, subjects without endoscopic precancerous lesions at baseline had significantly less gastric cancer.[308] Perhaps there is an optimal time to adopt such a treatment-prevention strategy, beyond which *H. pylori* eradication is ineffective at preventing the progression to carcinoma.

As mentioned previously, bacterial, host, and environmental factors modulate the sequelae of infection. Gastric cancer has been more strongly linked to *cagA*+ strains and host gene polymorphisms including *IL-1, TNFα*, and *IL-10*.[309] Environmental factors such as smoking and dietary intake play an important role in determining disease risk.[310-312]

Acquiring *H. pylori* infection at a very early age has been related to a much higher gastric cancer risk, especially in the setting of a positive family history of gastric cancer.[313] The familial aggregation of stomach cancer may, in part, be explained by familial aggregation of *H. pylori* infection.[314] The implications of this on diagnosis and treatment in the broader pediatric setting have yet to be determined, but physicians must be cognizant of a close family history of gastric cancer in their patients.[268]

Mucosa-Associated Lymphoid Tissue Lymphoma

Primary malignant tumors of the stomach are uncommon in children and usually consist of lymphoma and sarcoma.[315] Primary gastric lymphoma can be divided histologically into mucosa-associated lymphoid tissue (MALT) lymphoma and non-MALT lymphoma. Primary gastric lymphoma is a very rare malignancy in children.[316] The risk of gastric MALT lymphoma is significantly increased with *H. pylori* infection.[317] Some 72 to 98% of patients with gastric MALT lymphoma are infected with *H. pylori*. The eradication of *H. pylori* alone induces regression (and remission) of gastric MALT lymphoma in 70 to 80% of cases.[318] Failure of the lymphoma to respond to eradication therapy has been associated with certain genetic abnormalities within the host, including the presence of the specific genetic translocations t(11;18)(q21;q21). Such cases usually progress to high-grade tumors.[319] Most subjects who respond to eradication therapy remain in remission for many years.

Extraintestinal Manifestations

Iron Deficiency Anemia

Most of the published studies describing anemia in the setting of *H. pylori* infection have been in pediatric populations.[320] In general, within developed countries, iron deficiency anemia (IDA) is seen more frequently in children and adolescents than adults.[321] Thus, if *H. pylori* infection does lead to IDA, then children are more likely to be affected than adults.

Epidemiologic studies have indicated an association between *H. pylori* seropositivity and low serum ferritin and hemoglobin levels.[322] A seroepidemiologic study of 937 children found iron deficiency to be twice as common in *H. pylori*-positive children compared with uninfected children.[323] A number of case reports have demonstrated IDA, previously resistant to iron replacement therapy, responding to the eradication of *H. pylori*, with a few reports of *H. pylori* eradication resulting in improvement of anemia even without iron supplementation.[324-326] Recent studies have reported conflicting evidence regarding the influence of *H. pylori* status and eradication on iron deficiency and on iron treatment failure.[327-332] Whether iron deficiency, like *H. pylori*, is an index of dietary or socioeconomic status rather than a cause of anemia per se remains to be fully elucidated.

Several mechanisms responsible for *H. pylori*–mediated iron-deficiency anemia have been postulated. Chronic gastrointestinal bleeding due to gastritis, erosions, or ulceration may be to blame, although most studies have not detected occult gastrointestinal blood loss in infected patients with anemia. The levels of gastric acidity and gastric ascorbic acid are important for the absorption of dietary iron, and hypochlorhydria could affect iron bioavailability.[333] Acid production and its regulation during bacterial colonization are not well understood in children; however, it is doubtful whether children with mild pangastritis have functional changes identical to those seen in adults. In most children, the mucosal and glandular structure within the gastric body remains completely normal during chronic *H. pylori* infection, with atrophy being an unusual, later phenomenon.[334] Another suggested mechanism is related to the sequestration of iron by antral *H. pylori* infection. *H. pylori* is known to possess genes with an iron-scavenging function, thus enabling the bacterium to extract iron from its host.[335] Children with low iron intake or increased iron requirements form an obvious risk group for IDA. In this vulnerable group, it is possible that even minor disturbances in the iron absorption mechanisms that may occur due to *H. pylori* infection might quickly lead to a deficiency state.[336] Guidelines for *H. pylori* infection in children suggest that children presenting with unexplained iron deficiency anemia that is refractory to therapy may warrant investigation for *H. pylori* infection.[268]

Short Stature

A number of studies have suggested that *H. pylori* infection may have a negative effect on growth, although reports are conflicting.[337-344] Most studies are longitudinal in design, utilizing either serology or UBT for diagnosis, and include children over a fairly wide age range. In 2001, Richter et al. conducted a cross-sectional population-based study in Germany involving 3315 children aged 5 to 7 years.[345] This group represented 88% of all preschool and school-aged children born in the area over a 12-month period. The overall prevalence of *H. pylori* infection was about 7%. A small, but statistically significant, difference in height (before and after age and sex adjustment) was detected between *H. pylori*–positive and -negative children and was more pronounced in males. In contrast to other studies, no significant difference in socioeconomic status was found between the two groups. It has been suggested that growth retardation could be a result of either gastritis or comorbidity, such as anemia.[346,347] Alternatively, *H. pylori* infection and growth retardation may be caused coincidentally by the same confounding factors, such as socioeconomic factors.[348] Notwithstanding the considerable literature on an association between *H. pylori* and short stature, no study to date has demonstrated a causal relationship between *H. pylori* and short stature by showing increase in growth velocity in children following eradication of *H. pylori*. Furthermore, the lack of standardization of *H. pylori* testing, anthropometric measurements, documentation of height velocity, mid-parental height recording, and other potential confounding factors within the available literature means that any inference must be regarded with caution.

Other Suggested Associations

A wide variety of extraintestinal manifestations have been suggested to have an association with *H. pylori* infection. These range in diversity from dermatologic and autoimmune problems such as chronic urticaria and atopy to idiopathic

thrombocytopenia (ITP). Current data suggests that a role for *H. pylori* in adult ITP is plausible and that treatment is justifiable and beneficial.[349-351] This has now been reflected in the latest European and Asian treatment guidelines.[352,353] Data from pediatric studies to date are less convincing, however.[354-356]

A critical assessment of the evidence on a relationship with sudden infant death syndrome (SIDS) has concluded that a causal association is very unlikely.[357] A recent analysis of data from NHANES suggested an inverse correlation with asthma.[358] Current evidence for other putative associations in children is not compelling.

Benefits of Disease

It is postulated that there may be potential benefits to *H. pylori* infection. *H. pylori* may stimulate specific local and systemic immunoglobulin secretion and thus participate in host defense against exogenous pathogens. *H. pylori* may synthesize antibacterial peptides that would prevent other faster-growing bacteria from colonizing the gastric mucosa and gastrointestinal tract.[198] Some, but not all, studies suggest that *H. pylori* may be associated with protection from diarrheal diseases in both children and adults in developed countries.[359] Given that only a small proportion of *H. pylori* carriers develop clinically related disease, it may well be that there are benefits to colonization. However, the potential positive final consequences of *H. pylori* elimination for human health should not be overlooked.

DIAGNOSIS

The ideal test for *H. pylori* would be noninvasive, highly accurate, inexpensive, and readily available. The test would differentiate between active and past infection and discriminate between *H. pylori* infection and *H. pylori*–associated disease. No such test currently exists. Thus it is important to appraise the advantages and disadvantages of the tests that are available and assess their suitability for use in children.[268]

Among all the diagnostic tests currently available, there is no single "reference standard" for the diagnosis of *H. pylori* infection. A variety of studies have now been completed confirming the accuracy of the various diagnostic methods in children. There are only a few data, however, validating these methods in diverse populations.

Two categories of test are available to diagnose *H. pylori* infection: invasive (requiring endoscopy) and noninvasive (or nonendoscopic). Within each broad category there are a variety of different options.

Invasive Tests

Endoscopy and Biopsy

Upper gastrointestinal endoscopy and biopsy remains the current reference standard in the diagnosis and identification of *H. pylori* infection and its consequences in childhood.[267,268] It allows visualization of the upper gastrointestinal tract and also facilitates the diagnosis of diseases other than those related to *H. pylori* infection. Gastric inflammation caused by *H. pylori* is not always observed macroscopically.[360] Nodularity within the stomach is seen more frequently in children than in adults. It was described by Hassall and Dimmick in 1991.[361] The mucosa is irregular in appearance, resembling a cobblestone pavement.

Nodules measure 1 to 4 mm in diameter, have a smooth surface, and are the same color as the surrounding mucosa. Seen most often within the gastric antrum, it is frequently referred to as antral nodular gastritis. Antral nodularity correlates with the severity of histologic gastritis.[360] Nodules are often best appreciated following biopsy, when blood from the biopsy site surrounds and highlights them. Endoscopy facilitates the collection of mucosal biopsies, on which a variety of direct tests can then be performed. Procedural risk, anesthetic/sedation requirements, relative expense, and limited access to appropriate pediatric expertise all remain disadvantages.

Culture

Culture is a potential reference standard for the diagnosis of suspected *H. pylori* infection. However, the bacterium has fastidious growth requirements, and under adverse conditions its morphology transforms.[362] Cultivation requires a microaerophilic environment and complex media and, although specific, its sensitivity can vary greatly between laboratories.[363] Even experienced laboratories recover the organism from only 50 to 70% of infected biopsies.[364] Diagnostic yield is improved when multiple biopsies are collected.[365] It is important that specimens for culture are processed within 2 to 3 hours of collection, because *H. pylori* lacks regulatory genes, rendering its survival for long periods outside the gastric environment poor.[182]

In summary, culture of *H. pylori* is a tedious but reliable procedure with a high degree of sensitivity if performed carefully. Its major advantage is in the ability to perform antibiotic sensitivity testing on the isolates, which can influence the outcome of therapy. Both phenotypic and genotypic methods are available for antimicrobial susceptibility testing.

Rapid Urease Test

The urease activity of *H. pylori* enabled the development of a variety of diagnostic tests, including the rapid urease test (RUT). Urease catalyzes the hydrolysis of urea into ammonia and carbon dioxide. The production of ammonia leads to an increase in the local pH. Samples are placed within a gel containing urea and a pH indicator. A color change occurs as urea is broken down by the bacteria.[267] The use of RUTs in pediatrics is limited by a significantly lower sensitivity compared with that of histology; this is possibly related to a lower mucosal bacterial load.[6] A variety of studies have validated this method in children. Elitsur and Neace examined a group of 94 children in West Virginia. Using histology as the reference standard, 19% of their study population was *H. pylori* positive.[366] When utilizing a combination rather than a single investigation as the comparative standard, the sensitivity of the RUT in childhood is significantly improved.[367] In a study of 59 Mexican children with a disease prevalence of 37%, of the three invasive techniques (culture, histologic examination of antrum and corpus biopsies with hematoxylin and eosin [H&E] and Giemsa staining, and RUT), RUT was the most sensitive and had the best negative predictive value (NPV) (100%).[368]

Histopathology

On H&E staining of gastric mucosal biopsies obtained from *H. pylori*–infected patients, a superficial infiltrate is usually seen with substantial numbers of plasma cells and lymphocytes within the mucosa.[369] Biopsies obtained from children infected with *H. pylori* generally have less neutrophil infiltration compared with tissue obtained from infected adults.

Methods of *H. pylori* detection include routinely stained H&E slides, modified Romanovsky methods (Giemsa, Diff-3), Sayeed stains, or silver stains (Dieterle, Warthin-Starry, Steiner, Genta).[370] Silver stains are very sensitive, but also stain a wide variety of bacteria and rely on demonstrating the typical morphology of the bacterium.[371] They have shown 82% concordance with immunohistochemistry. Immunohistochemical techniques utilizing anti–*H. pylori* antibodies are quite effective.[372] In children, H&E and Giemsa stains have shown a sensitivity of 82% and specificity of 95%.[368]

Although *H. pylori* colonization results in chronic gastritis, not all chronic gastritis is due to *H. pylori*.[373] Eshun et al. retrospectively reviewed 37 patients and 12 controls and found that higher grades of gastritis were associated with greater numbers of organisms.[371] When biopsies in children display chronic inflammation and a negative urease test result, immunohistochemical stains should be utilized to further investigate for *H. pylori* infection.

The site from which the biopsy is taken can affect the accuracy of diagnosis. Elitsur et al. studied 206 children to determine the optimal biopsy location.[374] After sampling six different sites, they concluded the mid-antrum at the lesser curvature was the best location for detecting *H. pylori* histologically in children. More recently, of biopsies from 89 consecutive children undergoing upper gastrointestinal endoscopy for symptoms suggestive of acid peptic disease, 25% were *H. pylori* positive.[373] All *H. pylori* cases had a positive RUT and positive histology (*H. pylori* demonstrated with Giemsa staining) on biopsies from the cardia, but not the antrum. Adult studies have demonstrated the cardia to be second only to the antrum in yield of *H. pylori* on biopsy.[375]

Recently, techniques such as fluorescent in situ hybridization (FISH) and PCR analysis have been used to detect *H. pylori* in biopsy specimens and even identify those with particular antibiotic resistance properties. However, these are neither routinely used nor available widely.[376-379]

Noninvasive Tests

Urea Breath Test

The urea breath test (UBT) is still considered to be the most accurate noninvasive method to detect *H. pylori* infection. Urea is labeled with the ^{13}C isotope and then ingested. ^{13}C is a naturally occurring nonradioactive isotope. It can be safely used in even very young infants and can be repeated without risk to the child.[380] Urea hydrolysis by *H. pylori* produces ammonia and labeled carbon dioxide. Urea rapidly passes down its concentration gradient into the epithelial blood supply, and within minutes appears in the breath (Figure 28-5). Labeled urea (50 to 100 mg) is usually given with a test meal to delay gastric emptying. Breath samples are collected at variable times postingestion.[381] For optimal results, the gastric environment should be acidic.[382] Detection requires a mass spectrometer and results are reported as delta over baseline (DOB) values for the measured ratio $^{13}CO_2/^{12}CO_2$. DOB values exceeding a fixed cutoff value are considered indicative of *H. pylori* infection.[383]

Validation of this technique in childhood is ongoing.[384-386] However, comparative evaluations of different protocols are scarce. A multicenter trial in 2000 demonstrated that the DOB cutoff value varied with changes in ^{13}C-urea dose, type of test meal, and time of breath collection. Test meals that contain citric acid result in higher DOB values in *H. pylori*–positive patients and thus may improve the sensitivity of the test in children.[387] A study by

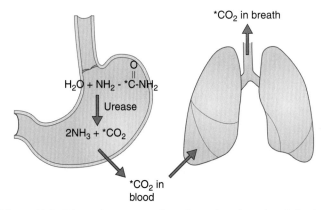

Figure 28-5. Schematic representation of urea breath testing. Following ingestion, labeled urea comes into contact with the mucosa and diffuses through the mucus. It is hydrolyzed by *H. pylori* urease, producing ammonia and labeled carbon dioxide, which passes rapidly into the blood supply and into the breath, within minutes. The expired concentration of labeled carbon dioxide is then measured. For optimal results, the gastric environment should be acidic. From Fischer W, Gebert B, Haas R. Novel activities of the *Helicobacter pylori* vacuolating cytotoxin: from epithelial cells towards the immune system. Int J Med Microbiol 2004; 293:539-547.

Kindermann et al. of 1499 German children confirmed UBT utility in children over 6 years of age, with 149 cases being validated histologically.[388] The positive predictive value (PPV) and NPV for children over 6 years of age were 98% and 100%, but for children under the age of 6 years, they were 69% and 100%, respectively. Koletzko and Feydt-Schmidt have demonstrated a significant inverse relationship between DOB values and age in both infected and noninfected children.[383] Kindermann's analysis demonstrates a false-positive rate of about 8%.[388] These findings support the concept that the DOB cutoff value needs to be calculated by the ROC curve for each protocol in each patient population.

The accuracy of noninvasive tests remains questionable in young toddlers and infants. One difficulty posed by this patient group is the lack of sufficient numbers of study patients.[283] In 2005, the Canadian Consensus group concluded that UBT is the best available and most reliable noninvasive test in children, but it is far less accurate in younger children.[268] Recent attempts to address this by modifying the analysis protocol suggest improvements in the false positive rate in children under the age of 6 years.[389,390] The optimal cutoff for a positive test in children younger than 5 years is higher than in adults.[391] Increasing the cutoff from a DOB of 5 to 8 improved UBT specificity from 95.5 to 98.1%. Another study reported a sensitivity and specificity of the UBT of just 83% and 91% respectively, in comparison to histology and rapid urease test in 40 children.[392] In Brazilian children, histologic grades for mononuclear infiltrate, neutrophilic infiltrate, and bacterial density did not correlate with the UBT results.[393] Such heterogeneous results suggest that UBT in children should be interpreted qualitatively and cautiously and underscores the importance of consistency in UBT protocol and analysis.

Serologic Tests

H. pylori infection induces both cellular and humoral immune responses, resulting in an early increase in specific IgM, and a later and persistent increase in specific IgA and IgG.[394] In general, serologic assays cannot be used on their own in children for diagnosis or monitoring of *H. pylori* infection because of widely variable sensitivity and specificity for detection of antibodies (IgG or IgA) against *H. pylori* in children. IgA-based tests

detect only 20 to 50% of *H. pylori*–infected patients.[395] Tests based on the detection of specific anti-*H. pylori* IgG antibodies in the serum offer a better sensitivity than IgA-based tests but cannot distinguish active from past infection. A number of different techniques are available, including enzyme immunoassay (IgG or IgA), agglutination tests, and Western blotting. The duration of infection and the ability of the host to mount an immune response influence the results of this test. In some children, the duration and degree of infection may not have been present long enough to generate an immune response in all cases.[368] The inaccuracy of these tests means they cannot be justified for clinical use, on either clinical or economic grounds, and they should be restricted to large epidemiology studies. Given the low test sensitivities in infants and toddlers, epidemiologic studies based on antibody testing may underestimate the prevalence and transmission of *H. pylori* infection in the very young.[383,396] Office-based serology tests, although technically simple to perform and attractively convenient, are not recommended for diagnosis. Their inaccuracy was such that 33% of positive tests in dyspeptic patients in a primary care setting were false positives.[397]

The identification and validation of a panel of biomarkers of *H. pylori* infection in children including pepsinogen I and II and gastrin 17 is awaited. Although the data are promising, adult studies have failed to produce convincing results to advocate its routine use to date.[398,399]

Results with salivary antibody tests have been disappointing.[400-403] Urine antibody results have been variable. A pilot study of 132 adult patients demonstrated a sensitivity of 86% and a specificity of 91%. A follow-up European multicenter trial using the same assay had a sensitivity and specificity of 89% and 69%.[381,404] Validation of these alternative noninvasive methods in children is hampered by inconsistent use of an acceptable reference standard, and so they are not currently recommended for clinical use.[405-407]

Stool Antigen Test

Stool testing for *H. pylori* antigen is an inexpensive, noninvasive method of determining *H. pylori* infection. When comparing the cost-effectiveness of this method against UBT, the stool test requires an optical spectrophotometer, usually present in any laboratory; has negligible maintenance costs; and does not require dedicated personnel.[381]

Both polyclonal and monoclonal assays have been developed and tested in children. A large review of studies from 1999 to 2001, evaluating 3419 patients, suggested that the polyclonal test is not as reliable as the UBT.[408] Kato et al. studied 264 children aged 2 to 17 years and demonstrated an overall sensitivity of 96%, specificity of 96.8%, PPV of 93.2%, and NPV of 98.4%.[409] Results were independent of age.

In contrast, monoclonal antibody testing has shown greater promise. A multicenter study evaluated the test in 302 symptomatic children and compared it with UBT, RUT, histologic examination, and biopsy.[410] The sensitivity, specificity, PPV, and NPV were 98%, 99%, 98%, and 99%, respectively. Similar findings were demonstrated previously in a pediatric group.[411] A more recent meta-analysis of monoclonal stool antigen detection reported a pooled sensitivity of 94% and specificity of 97%.[412] Validation in children under 5 years, those with gastrointestinal bleeding, and those taking acid suppressive therapy is awaited. It is likely that in the near future, monoclonal stool antigen testing will be sanctioned as an alternative to the currently recommended UBT in the posttherapy setting.

Commercially available stool immune-chromatography kits are also available, but interobserver variability and equivocal results are problematic. Two studies found high sensitivities (94.6 and 100%) and specificities (98.4 and 100%) for this test, whereas another reported far less accurate results (pre- and posttreatment: specificity 92.3 and 100%, respectively; sensitivity 65 and 60%, respectively).[413-417]

Sophisticated molecular technologies have recently become more widely available and have been used to detect *H. pylori* in stool. Whereas bi-probe real-time PCR assays in adults have shown excellent results, testing in children has been somewhat disappointing to date. Reports by Falsafi and Lottspeich and their coworkers found a reasonable specificity but a poor sensitivity in children.[418,419] An association between higher scores of *H. pylori* in histology and more severe gastritis with positivity of stool PCR was also observed and may explain the insufficient sensitivity in children who, for the most part, have less severe gastritis.

Summary

Noninvasive methods are particularly promising for the accurate diagnosis of *H. pylori* infection. Currently there is insufficient evidence to recommend them over invasive tests in symptomatic children, because they cannot be used reliably to diagnose or distinguish *H. pylori*-associated diseases in children from conditions that are not *H. pylori* related. Current guidelines recommend treatment only in children with confirmed *H. pylori*–related diseases.[266-268] However, with further knowledge of the measurable health risks for *H. pylori*–infected children, or with the availability of vaccination and other treatment options, the risk-benefit relationship and recommendations regarding noninvasive testing may change.

When Is Testing Indicated?

At present, the primary goal of testing is to diagnose the cause of clinical symptoms and not simply to detect the presence of *H. pylori*. As in many clinical scenarios, testing is not helpful unless it will alter the management of the disease. As knowledge of the intestinal and extraintestinal manifestations of *H. pylori* expands, so too will the appropriate indications for *H. pylori* testing in children. Table 28-1 summarizes the current indications for testing developed by the 2004 Canadian *Helicobacter pylori* Paediatric Consensus Conference.[268] A summary of recommendations generated from this conference is given in Table 28-2. Revised guidelines are anticipated in the near future, arising from the recent joint NASPGHAN/ESPGHAN consensus conference.

TREATMENT

Children with peptic ulcer disease and *H. pylori* infection should receive treatment; the treatment endpoint should be the eradication of infection. However, as previously discussed, the majority of children infected with *H. pylori* do not have peptic ulcer disease. For many, the diagnosis of *H. pylori* infection is incidental and their management is controversial.

Conventional Regimens

Clinically relevant *H. pylori* eradication regimens should have cure rates of at least 80% (according to intention-to-treat analysis), be without major side effects, and induce minimal bacterial

TABLE 28-1. When Is Testing for *H. pylori* Indicated in Children?

Endoscopically diagnosed peptic ulcer disease	Yes
There is a family history of gastric cancer	Yes
Documented MALT lymphoma	Yes
Refractory iron deficient anemia without other cause	Yes
Recurrent abdominal pain or nonulcer dyspepsia	No
Newly diagnosed gastroesophageal reflux disease	No
Before long-term PPI therapy is commenced	Perhaps
Asymptomatic children	No

MALT, mucosa-associated lymphoid tissue; PPI, proton pump inhibitor.

TABLE 28-2. Recommendations

Investigation and Testing
Population screening for *H. pylori* in asymptomatic children to prevent gastric cancer is not warranted
Testing for *H. pylori* in children should be considered if there is a family history of gastric cancer
The goal of diagnostic interventions should be to determine the cause of presenting symptoms, not the presence of *H. pylori* infection
Recurrent abdominal pain is not an indication to test for *H. pylori* infection
H. pylori testing is not required in patients with newly diagnosed gastroesophageal reflux disease
H. pylori testing may be considered before long-term PPI therapy
Testing for *H. pylori* infection should be considered in children with refractory iron deficient anemia when no other cause has been found
When investigation of children with persistent or severe upper abdominal symptoms is indicated, GI endoscopy with biopsy is the investigation of choice
The urea breath test is the best noninvasive diagnostic test for *H. pylori* infection in children
Serological antibody tests are not recommended as a diagnostic tool for *H. pylori* in children

How to Treat
First-line therapy for *H. pylori* infection is a twice daily, triple-drug regimen comprising a PPI plus two antibiotics (clarithromycin plus amoxicillin or metronidazole)
Optimal treatment duration is 14 days
H. pylori culture and antibiotic sensitivity testing should be available to monitor population antibiotic resistance and to manage treatment failures

Adapted from the Canadian Helicobacter Study Group Consensus Conference. Jones NL et al. Can J Gastroenterol 2005; 19:399-408.
PPI, proton pump inhibitor.

resistance.[218] Antibiotics alone have not achieved this. Luminal acidity influences both the effectiveness of some antimicrobial agents and the survival of the bacterium; thus antibiotics have been combined with acid suppression such as proton pump inhibitors (PPIs), bismuth, or H_2 antagonists. So-called "triple" (TT) and "quadruple" (QT) therapies are a combination of an antisecretory agent with two or three antimicrobial agents for 7 to 14 days. These regimens have been investigated extensively and approved in adult populations. The "classic" regimen is treatment twice daily for 7 days with a PPI and clarithromycin plus either amoxicillin or metronidazole.[420] A meta-analysis in 1999 of 666 studies in 53,228 adult subjects demonstrated parity between all regimens that included a PPI plus any two of three antibiotics (clarithromycin, amoxicillin, and a nitroimidazole), with cure rates ranging from 79 to 83%.[421]

Bismuth has been used in the treatment of peptic ulcer disease for many years. The exact mechanism of action in *H. pylori* eradication is not known. A variety of regimens involving bismuth have been described in both the pediatric and adult literature. Concern has been expressed about the potential toxic effects of bismuth salts in children, because chronic ingestion of high-dose bismuth associated with encephalopathy and/or acute renal impairment has been reported, but not in children being treated for *H. pylori* disease.[422] It has also been suggested that the strong taste of ammonia associated with liquid bismuth may reduce compliance.[423] Treatment regimens utilizing PPIs are often felt to be more attractive in the pediatric setting.

Many early treatment studies in children were open trials with small numbers of participants. In 2000, Oderda et al. performed a systematic review of all published eradication treatment schedules in children, but given the limited number of adequate studies and the marked heterogeneity, it was difficult to make any definitive statements from the data.[424] Recommendations for eradication therapy outlined in the various pediatric consensus statements are based on the extrapolation from adult data. The first pediatric randomized controlled double-blind trial compared 1week of triple therapy with omeprazole, amoxicillin, and clarithromycin (OAC) to dual antibiotic therapy with amoxicillin and clarithromycin (AC).[425] Eradication was 75% versus 9.4%, respectively: a finding in keeping with adult data. A Brazilian study of 25 children demonstrated eradication rates of only 50% after 7 days' therapy, improving to 73% after 10 days.[426] open randomized study of 106 Russian children demonstrated eradication rates of 80 to 89% after 7 days' therapy with omeprazole, amoxicillin, and metronidazole (OAM).[427] A prospective study of QT for 1 week, utilizing omeprazole, amoxicillin, clarithromycin, and metronidazole (OACM), demonstrated an eradication rate of 94%.[428] Recent trials in different geographic areas and ethnic backgrounds have not achieved eradication rates above 75%.[327,429-431] Furthermore, the spectrum of clinical practice was highlighted in the report of the European pediatric treatment registry, which reported use of 27 different regimens in 518 children with *H. pylori*.[283] Overall eradication rate was 65.6% but was significantly higher in children with ulcer (79.7%) than without (63.9%). Bismuth-containing triple therapies were more efficacious than PPI-containing ones (77% versus 64%) when used as first-line treatment. There was no difference between treatments given for 1 or 2 weeks, or whether given as first or second therapies.

Sequential Regimens

Declining eradication rates with established regimens have led researchers to explore alternative treatment options. Sequential therapy involves dual therapy with a PPI and amoxicillin for 5 days followed sequentially by 5 days of triple therapy (a PPI with two alternative antibiotics). Amoxicillin is speculated to reduce bacterial load and possibly confer protection against clarithromycin resistance. The regimen was first proposed over a decade ago in a small adult trial with excellent results (98% eradication).[432] Since then, several trials have been published and subsequent meta-analyses show a 90 to 94% eradication rate with sequential therapy by intention to treat analysis compared with 75 to 80% for 7 to 10 days' TT.[433-435] The data from these analyses are interesting and promising, although certain caveats must be borne in mind. Only one study was double-blinded, most patients lived in Italy, methods of detection were not comparable across all studies, and publication bias

was evident. Meanwhile, sequential therapy does not address the problem of increasing clarithromycin resistance; comparison between sequential therapy and combined first-line and second-line therapy might be more appropriate, given that it involves the deployment of four pharmacological agents.

In 2005, 74 children were randomized to receive either sequential treatment (omeprazole plus amoxicillin for 5 days, followed by omeprazole plus clarithromycin plus tinidazole for another 5 days) or triple therapy (OAM) for 1 week.[436] Eradication was assessed by UBT 8 weeks after therapy. Sequential therapy achieved eradication in 97.3% of children compared with 75.7% on standard triple therapy. This remains the only published randomized trial in children to date that shows a benefit of sequential therapy over standard regimens. In a later study of probiotic supplementation, 82.5% overall eradication was obtained from a group of 40 children, each receiving sequential therapy.[437] The authors have subsequently communicated an eradication success rate of 85% in 108 clinic patients, albeit an uncontrolled patient group.[438]

Table 28-3 summarizes the existing *H. pylori* treatment guidelines recommended by the North American Society of Pediatric Gastroenterology and Nutrition and indicates particular guidelines likely to undergo modification in forthcoming revisions.

Treatment Failure

A variety of host and bacterial factors contribute to treatment failure including antibiotic resistance, virulence factors, bacterial load, patient adherence to therapy, adequacy of drug delivery, and possibly host *CYP2C19* genotype (either extensive or poor PPI metabolizers).[439,440]

Antibiotic Resistance – a Clinical Perspective

The most commonly prescribed antimicrobial agents to eradicate *H. pylori* are amoxicillin, clarithromycin, metronidazole, and tetracycline. *H. pylori* resistance to these is an important variable in successful eradication. In general, rates of resistance are increasing with time.[441] Antibiotic resistance may be primary (present before therapy) or secondary (developing during therapy). Antimicrobial resistance from a prospective 4-year European study of 1233 patients reported 24% resistance to clarithromycin (higher in children under 6 years and those living in southern Europe); 25% resistance to metronidazole (higher in children born outside Europe); and dual resistance in 6.9%, whereas resistance to amoxicillin was rare (0.6%).[442] The use of antibiotics for other indications was suggested as the major risk factor for developing primary resistance. Tailoring first-line regimens following antibiotic sensitivity testing of cultured bacteria has been shown to enhance eradication in children, and some centers may consider this in the setting of increasing antibiotic resistance.[443]

Adjunctive Therapies

A number of studies have explored the potential benefits of probiotic therapy in *H. pylori* treatment regimens. Studies using fermented milk products have shown up to 10% improved eradication rates when they were used in addition to standard regimens.[444] In pediatric populations, there have been few randomized controlled trials evaluating whether consumption of lactic acid bacteria increases *H. pylori* eradication and reduces the

TABLE 28-3. 2000 NASGHAN Recommendations

2000 NASGHAN Recommendations	Change Likely in Pending Revision
Testing Recommendations	
The diagnosis of *H. pylori* can only be made reliably through the use of endoscopy with biopsy	✓
Commercial serologic tests are frequently unreliable for screening children for the presence of *H. pylori* infection	
Urea breath testing has not been studied sufficiently in children	✓
Testing should be performed in children with endoscopically diagnosed or radiologically definitive duodenal or gastric ulcers	
Children with recurrent abdominal pain without documented ulcer disease should not be tested for *H. pylori*	
Testing in asymptomatic children is not recommended	
Routine screening of children with a family history of gastric cancer or recurrent peptic ulcer disease is not recommended	
Testing following treatment of documented *H. pylori* is recommended, especially with complicated peptic ulcer disease	
Where pathological evidence of MALT lymphoma is documented, testing for *H. pylori* is recommended	
Treatment Indications	
Eradication is recommended for children who have a duodenal or gastric ulcer identified at endoscopy and *H. pylori* detected on histology	
Eradication is recommended if active *H. pylori* infection is documented in children with a prior history of documented duodenal or gastric ulcer disease	
There is no compelling evidence for treating children with *H. pylori* and nonulcer dyspepsia or functional abdominal pain	
Treatment is not recommended for *H. pylori* infected children residing in chronic care facilities; children with unexplained short stature; children at risk of acquisition of infection, including asymptomatic children who have a family member with either peptic ulcer disease or gastric cancer	
Treatment Recommendations	
Treatment is recommended to consist of 3 or 4 medications, given once or twice daily, for 1 to 2 weeks	✓

Adapted from Gold BD et al. J Pediatr Gastroenterol Nutr 2000; 31:490–497.

side effects of treatment, but the results are conflicting.[437,445,446] A recent randomized double-blind placebo controlled trial in children undergoing 7-day triple therapy with or without *Lactobacillus GG* failed to show a benefit in either eradication or reported side effects.[429] A previous study had reported a beneficial effect of *Lactobacillus reuteri* on the side effect profile of children taking sequential therapy for eradication.[437] *Saccharomyces boulardii* has shown a negligible effect on *H. pylori* eradication in children, either alone or as an adjunct, but is associated with a reduction in side effects of treatment regimens.[447,448] Taken together, the trend of results from trials in children to date suggests that probiotic therapy alone is inadequate, but

as an adjunct to established therapies, it may slightly improve eradication and possibly ameliorate treatment side effects.

Vaccination

Vaccination against *H. pylori* should be feasible. It offers an attractive, cost-effective approach to preventing infectious disease.[449,450] Given the evolving problems with antimicrobial resistance, vaccination is enticing. Several key proteins involved in *H. pylori* pathogenesis, such as urease, VacA, and cagA, have been shown to confer protection against infectious challenge with *H. pylori* in experimental animal models.[450-452] The effector mechanisms of this protection are unknown. Nevertheless, urease or mixtures of *H. pylori* antigens were immunogenic in *H. pylori*–negative volunteers in a number of clinical trials, using aluminum hydroxide as an adjuvant.[453,454] Results of ongoing trials are eagerly awaited.

CONCLUSION

Our understanding of the pathogenesis of infectious disease, cancer, inflammatory diseases, and of course peptic ulcer disease has been revolutionized over the past quarter century since the identification of *H. pylori*. Our medical management of children with suspected gastroduodenal ulceration differs radically from that of our peers 30 years ago and has achieved marked improvements in clinical outcomes. The *H. pylori* literature encompasses the very best in cutting-edge hypotheses and methodologies in clinical, epidemiologic, and basic science research. However, it also provides a salutary lesson to the reader on the need for standardization and validation of our investigative methodologies and for rigorous interpretation of the resulting data. The next quarter century of research will no doubt be just as exciting. Meanwhile, revised clinical guidelines from the major pediatric gastroenterology bodies are keenly awaited.

REFERENCES

31. Rowland M, Daly L, Vaughan M, et al. Age-specific incidence of *Helicobacter pylori*. Gastroenterology 2006;130:65–72.
69. Blaser MJ, Atherton JC. *Helicobacter pylori* persistence: biology and disease. J Clin Invest 2004;113:321–333.
115. Medzhitov R. Recognition of microorganisms and activation of the immune response. Nature 2007;449:819–826.
146. Steinman L. A brief history of T(H)17, the first major revision in the T(H)1/T(H)2 hypothesis of T cell-mediated tissue damage. Nat Med 2007;13:139–145.
186. Dong QJ, Wang Q, Xin YN, et al. Comparative genomics of *Helicobacter pylori*. World J Gastroenterol 2009;15:3984–3991.
267. Gold BD, Colletti RB, Abbott M, et al. *Helicobacter pylori* infection in children: recommendations for diagnosis and treatment. J Pediatr Gastroenterol Nutr 2000;31:490–497.
268. Bourke B, Ceponis P, Chiba N, et al. Canadian Helicobacter Study Group Consensus Conference: Update on the approach to *Helicobacter pylori* infection in children and adolescents – an evidence-based evaluation. Can J Gastroenterol 2005;19:399–408.
412. Gisbert JP, de la Morena F, Abraira V. Accuracy of monoclonal stool antigen test for the diagnosis of *H. pylori* infection: a systematic review and meta-analysis. Am J Gastroenterol 2006;101:1921–1930.

See expertconsult.com for a complete list of references and the review questions for this chapter

GASTRIC MOTILITY DISORDERS

29

Miguel Saps • Carlo Di Lorenzo

GASTRIC MOTOR PHYSIOLOGY AND GASTRIC EMPTYING

The stomach is a hollow organ with distinct anatomical areas: cardias, fundus, body or corpus, antrum, and pylorus. Functionally, the stomach is formed by a proximal portion (fundus and proximal corpus) and a distal portion (distal corpus and antrum). Gastric emptying results from the coordinated motor activity of the proximal and distal parts of the stomach. Gastric contractions are regulated by slow waves generated in an electric pacemaker located near the proximal one third of the corpus along the greater curvature. The gastric pacemaker generates continuous rhythmic changes in membrane potential (slow waves) of 3 cycles per minute (cpm) that propagate toward the antrum and regulate the frequency and timing of the smooth muscle contractions. When an additional wave of depolarization (spike potential) is superimposed on the slow waves, a critical threshold is reached and a contraction occurs. The origin of the depolarization of the slow waves is thought to be in the interstitial cells of Cajal.[1] The gastrointestinal motor function is characterized by two distinct periods: postprandial or digestive and fasting or interdigestive period.

Postprandial Motility

Proper digestion and absorption of nutrients requires optimal interaction among gastrointestinal transit, endocrine and exocrine secretion, and gut-brain responses involved in the induction of satiety. During the consumption of a meal, the proximal stomach relaxes, allowing ingestion of considerable amounts of food with a limited increase in intraluminal pressure. Gastric relaxation is accomplished through two vagally mediated phases. The initial phase is initiated by deglutition and leads to the relaxation of the lower esophageal sphincter and the rapid relaxation of the proximal stomach. This is called "receptive relaxation" and is mediated by a vagovagal reflex. Once the bolus reaches the stomach it stimulates mechanoreceptors in the gastric wall that maintain the gastric relaxation (long-lasting relaxation) through intramural and vagal reflex pathways. This mechanism is called "adaptive relaxation" or "gastric accommodation."[2] This sustained relaxation delays gastric emptying, providing sufficient time for contact with gastric enzymes, and is recognized as a "lag phase" during gastric emptying studies. The proximal part of the stomach regulates the intragastric pressure through slow, tonic fundic contractions, producing a pressure gradient between the stomach and duodenum that enables liquid emptying.[3] Fundic contractions also contribute to the transfer of solid contents from the proximal stomach to the antrum for grinding. The mechanisms for

the functional coordination between the proximal and distal stomach remain largely unknown, although the presence of fundo-antral reflexes[3,4] suggests the existence of a neural connection between the two regions. During the postprandial state, waves of circular propagated contractions originating in the corpus move the solid bolus toward the pylorus. Intermittent, isolated, powerful antral peristaltic waves acting against a closed pylorus mix and grind the solid particles. A contracted pylorus does not allow the passage of the chyme promoting the retropulsion and further trituration of the bolus in the antrum. Once the bolus has been triturated to small particles suitable for intestinal absorption, the pyloric sphincter relaxes to permit the passage of the chyme into the duodenum. Peristaltic antral activity moves the gastric content into the duodenum until complete emptying is achieved. Antral and duodenal motility are coordinated via neurotransmitters and hormones. The distention of the antrum leads to relaxation of the pylorus through the antrosphincteric reflex and duodenum through the antroduodenal reflex. The distention of the duodenum causes antral relaxation through the duodenoantral reflex, and the relaxation of the pylorus causes antral contraction through the sphincteroantral reflex.[5,6] During the fed state, the duodenal bulb contracts and cease contracting intermittently to allow gastric emptying.[5] The presence of nutrients in the duodenum activates intestinal receptors triggering a neurohumoral enterogastric feedback mechanism that regulates both proximal and distal motility. The activation of this mechanism leads to a reduction in antegrade propagating pressure waves and antral activity and an increase in pyloric tone,[7,8] resulting in a decrease in transpyloric flow.[6] Retrograde duodenal peristalsis occurs frequently in the proximal duodenum, leading to the movement of the chyme back into the distal antrum, slowing gastric emptying.[7]

Gastric emptying rate varies according to the volume, consistency, caloric content, osmolality, temperature, chemical properties of the ingested fluid, metabolic state, diurnal variation, and ambient temperature[8] (Table 29-1). Although the temperature of the meal is known to influence gastric emptying,[9] data from studies on the effects of various temperatures in gastric emptying are conflicting, and the mechanisms as to how meal temperature influences gastric emptying have not been completely elucidated. It has been proposed that thermoreceptors are involved in the mechanisms that affect gastric motility.[10] A human study investigating the effect of temperature on gastric emptying found that hot meals accelerated gastric emptying compared to warm (body temperature) and cold meals.[11] A study on the manometric effects of temperature found that warm and cold drinks suppressed antral pressure waves and stimulated isolated pyloric pressure waves.[10] Temperature of the meal does not have a similar effect on

TABLE 29-1. Factors Affecting Gastric Emptying

	Slows	Accelerates
Intraluminal Content		
Lipids	Slows	
High osmolar load	Slows	
High caloric density	Slows	
Solids	Slows	
Hot meals		Accelerates
High gastric pH	Slows	
Other Factors		
GLP-1	Slows	
Leptin	Slows	
Cholecystokinin	Slows	
Hyperglycemia	Slows	
Hypoglycemia		Accelerates
PYY	Slows	
Ghrelin		Accelerates
Motilin		Accelerates
Melatonin	Slows	
Stress	Slows	
Intense exercise	Slows	
Rectal/colonic distention	Slows	

intestinal transit, as it takes between 5 and 30 minutes for the meal to reach body temperature in the stomach.[11] The understanding of the effect of meal temperature may be relevant in the management of patients with gastroparesis and functional dyspepsia, in whom delayed gastric emptying of both liquid and solid meals is frequently found.[12] The caloric content is the most important variable affecting the gastric emptying of liquids.[8] Plain water empties the stomach at rates faster than solutions containing calories, whereas a higher caloric content decreases the gastric emptying rate. Water and isotonic saline follow an exponential pattern in which the volume of liquid leaving the stomach is a constant fraction of the remaining volume in the stomach.[13] Gastric emptying occurs at a similar rate during rest or moderate exercise, whereas intense exercise inhibits gastric emptying.[14] Gastric emptying is an important factor in the digestion and absorption of fat. Oil empties more slowly than low-nutrient aqueous liquids.[15] Nuclear medicine studies show that oil is retained in the proximal stomach and there is retrograde movement of oil but not of low-nutrient liquids from the distal to the proximal stomach.[15] Because of the exclusive secretion of gastric lipase by the fundic mucosa in humans,[16] the retention of fat in the proximal stomach may facilitate gastric digestion of lipids. The consistency of the meal also affects gastric emptying. Homogenized fat and aqueous liquids empty from the stomach at similar rates.[17] The gastric emptying of fat and other nutrients is regulated by the effect of their digestion products with receptors in the small intestinal wall. Because of a comparable effect on small intestinal receptors, the gastric emptying rate of protein, fat, and carbohydrate meals of similar caloric content is approximately 2.5 kcal/min.[18] The effect of nutrients in the small intestine is important in the regulation of gastrointestinal motility, appetite, energy intake, and glucose homeostasis. Small-intestinal fat infusion results in greater suppression of energy intake than does an equivalent intravenous fat load.[19] The presence of lipolytic products in the small intestine diminishes antral[6] and duodenal pressures and increases basal pyloric pressure modulating gastric emptying. Intraduodenal fat stimulates the secretion

of intestinal hormones such as cholecystokinin (CCK) and peptide YY and suppresses appetite and energy intake.[20] CCK has a powerful inhibitory effect on appetite and gastric emptying. Fat is the most potent stimulator of intestinal chemosensors, but protein and carbohydrate also trigger the "ileal brake." This mechanism activates a distal-to-proximal intestinointestinal and intestinogastric feedback loop that result in the inhibition of gastric emptying and small bowel transit.[21] The presence of carbohydrates and lipids at the luminal level triggers the postprandial release of incretin hormones such as gastric inhibitory peptide (GIP) and glucagon-like peptide-1 (GLP-1) into the circulation.[22] GIP and GLP-1 are critical in glucose homeostasis in both health and diabetes. Both hormones are part of the enteropancreatic axis that stimulates insulin release while inhibiting glucagon release following a meal when blood glucose levels are elevated. GLP-1 relaxes the gastric fundus, inhibits antropyloroduodenal propagated waves, and stimulates both the tonic and phasic motility of the pylorus, serving as a brake to gastric emptying.[23] GLP-1 effect in decreasing glucagon production while stimulating insulin levels and delaying the delivery of nutrients from the stomach, minimizing the postprandial glycemic increase, provides the rationale for the use of GLP-1 analogues in the treatment of diabetes mellitus.[24] GLP-1 and possibly neural factors may play a role as a mediator of the ileal brake. In addition, GLP-1 seems to enhance unpleasant visceral perception during the postprandial state, reducing food intake.[25]

Gastric emptying plays a considerable role in regulating food intake. Rapid gastric motility is associated with overeating and obesity.[26] Ghrelin is a brain-gut peptide hormone predominantly secreted by the stomach with endocrine, orexigenic, and gastrointestinal effects.[27] Ghrelin increases proximal gastric tone, accelerates gastric emptying, and increases the activity of migrating motor complexes (MMCs) in the stomach and small bowel.[28] Ghrelin administration also affects plasma levels of gastrointestinal hormones involved in the control of interdigestive motility such as pancreatic polypeptide (PP), somatostatin, and glucagon.[29] Ghrelin's potent prokinetic effects are being investigated in the treatment of postoperative ileus and gastroparesis.[29] Similarities in structure and function have been found between ghrelin and motilin.

Motilin, a 22-amino-acid residue polypeptide hormone secreted by the enterochromaffin cells of the gut, is a potent stimulant of gastrointestinal motility. Similarly to ghrelin, motilin also induces antral phase III activity of the MMC in the stomach. Whereas GIP and GLP-1 are released in response to ingestion of nutrients, ghrelin and motilin release is inhibited by ingestion of nutrients. The mechanisms inducing the release of motilin are unclear, but absence of nutrients in the proximal small intestine is an important requirement for its release. Plasma motilin concentration remains low as long as the gastric motor activity remains in the digestive pattern.[30] Once the stomach and small intestine are emptied, motilin is intermittently released at 100-minute intervals during the interdigestive period.[30] Smooth muscle and neural subtype motilin receptors have been demonstrated in the antrum of various species. Motilin regulates fasting antral motility via a predominantly cholinergic mechanism.[31] It has been proposed that the neural receptors may play a role in the initiation of MMC cycling, whereas the smooth muscle receptors may only enhance the contractile activity without resulting in phase III.[32] In the duodenum, motilin receptors are of the smooth muscle subtype and less numerous, indicating that motilin has a less important motility effect more distally in the gastrointestinal tract.[33] Motilin infusion induces gallbladder emptying in the fasting state shortly after its administration and preceding an antral phase III cluster.[34] The effect is similar to the physiologic situation in which the gallbladder contracts preceding the initiation of antral phase III activity.[35] Motilin stimulates both the exocrine and endocrine pancreas via cholinergic pathways.[36]

Leptin is a protein produced by adipocytes that affects neural and endocrine systems and regulates appetite, body weight, and energy expenditure. Increase in plasma levels of leptin leads to satiety related to delay in gastric emptying, whereas leptin deficiency accelerates gastric emptying.[37]

Stress response affects gastrointestinal motility in a differential manner in the proximal (stomach) and distal (colon) portions of the gastrointestinal tract. In the stomach, stress leads to antral hypomotility, reduced propagated antral waves, and increased retrograde contractions, resulting in delayed gastric emptying.[38] Corticotropin-releasing factor (CRF, also known as corticotropin-releasing hormone) and other CRF-related molecules such as urocortins[39] seem to mediate the gastrointestinal response to stress. These neuropeptides elicit their action on a series of widely distributed protein-coupled receptors. Animal studies have shown that intracisternal administration of CRF and urocortin decreases appetite and delays solid gastric transit[40,41] via stimulation of central CRF type 2 receptors.[42]

The appropriate response to food is one of the most helpful indicators to determine the normalcy of gastric function. The postprandial period can be calculated in manometric studies as the period of time from the onset of the meal to the time of return of the interdigestive period characterized by the return of MMC. A normal postprandial motility indicates vagal integrity and normal enteroenteric reflexes.[43]

Interdigestive or Fasting Motility

The MMC constitutes a cyclic "program" involving the stomach, intestine, pancreas, and gallbladder that integrates mechanical, physical, biologic, chemical, and immunologic components.[19] The secretory components of the MMC include duodenal release of bile and pancreatic juices and increased secretion of gastric and duodenal bicarbonate, gastric acid, and intestinal chloride.[44,45] The motility component of the MMC is responsible for sweeping secretions and undigested food through the small intestine (the "gastrointestinal housekeeper") during the fasting state, avoiding the development of bacterial overgrowth. The rhythm of the MMC seems to be regulated by the cholinergic neurons of the enteric nervous system,[46] but the secretory coordination depends on the presence of an intact extrinsic innervation.[47] The MMC is composed of four phases that together last 90 to 180 minutes. The total cycle length between MMC periods shows no age-dependent variation in children and is similar in adults and children without upper gastrointestinal symptoms.[48] Phase I is a period of motor quiescence, and it occupies less than 10% of the fasting time in the small bowel.[48] Phase II contractions follow phase I and are characterized by intermittent and irregular amplitude and frequency.[48] Phase III activity is the most characteristic feature of fasting motility and is known as the "activity front" (Figure 29-1). The presence of normal phase III contractions indicates the presence of an intact gut neuromuscular function.[49] During phase III, repetitive contractions occur at 3 to 4 per minute in the antrum, 10

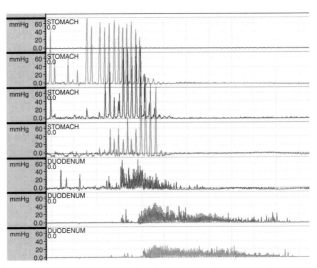

Figure 29-1. Normal antroduodenal manometry. The tracing shows a normally propagated phase III of the motor migrating complex.

to 13 per minute in the duodenum, and 7 to 8 per minute in the ileum, migrate aborally, and last longer than 2 minutes.[50] Phase III contractions propagate for longer distances but more slowly than phase II contractions and are associated with shortening of the small intestine. The average duration of phase III is approximately 7 minutes in both genders.[50] Phase IIIs are considered nonmigrating or stationary when the propagation velocity is greater than 25 cm/min. Phase III should be followed by a transition period of irregular contractions (phase IV) that leads to phase I. The fact that a different rate of contractions is present in the stomach and duodenum reflects the presence of separate but coordinated gastric and intestinal pacemakers. Most of the phase III activity is generated in the stomach and duodenum with a minority being generated more distally. The longer the fasting, the more proximally the MMC is initiated. During sleep the motility cycle tends to be shorter and is characterized by longer phase I and shorter phase II components as compared to daytime.

DISORDERS OF GASTRIC FUNCTION

Gastroparesis

Gastroparesis is a disorder of gastric motility in which the ability of the stomach to contract and empty is impaired. Gastroparesis is characterized by the presence of symptoms such as bloating, early satiety, nausea, vomiting of "old" undigested food, and abdominal discomfort in the absence of a mechanical obstruction. In pediatrics, gastroparesis is mostly seen in preterm infants, with allergy to cow's-milk protein[51] or immaturity of the gastrointestinal tract, and is less common during childhood. Acquired cases most commonly occur following infections or surgery. Viral infections have been associated with gastroparesis, but reports of gastric dysfunction following *Mycoplasma* infections have also been published.[52] Postviral cases usually present with persistent vomiting for days or months after an intercurrent illness. By the time the physician becomes involved, the acute illness has often resolved and the etiologic agent cannot be isolated. Multiple viruses have been associated with postviral gastroparesis, including rotavirus,[53] Epstein-Barr virus, and cytomegalovirus,[54] but other viruses can also result in alterations of motility. Diagnosis is based on the clinical presentation, the exclusion of other causes of persistent vomiting, and the demonstration of delayed gastric emptying. A pediatric study showed that gastroparesis that developed after an acute viral illness resolved in 6 months to 2 years in all cases.[53]

Patients with alterations of the central nervous system frequently have gastric dysrhythmias that lead to persistent vomiting.[55] A study of 18 neurologically impaired children showed abnormal antroduodenal motility in all cases.[56] Possible mechanisms involved in foregut dysmotility in this group of children include abnormal modulation of the enteric nervous system by the central nervous system or involvement of the enteric nervous system in the same process affecting the central nervous system. Gastroparesis may occur as a consequence of vagal nerve injury following upper abdominal surgery, in particular after fundoplication or bariatric surgery. Gastroparesis has also been reported after lung and heart transplantation,[57] possibly due to a combination of factors that include motor inhibitory effects of immunosuppressive drugs, opportunistic viral infections, and vagal nerve injury. Symptoms of postsurgical gastroparesis frequently improve with time, possibly because of vagal reinnervation and the ability of the enteric nervous system to adapt to the loss of vagal input.[58] Other causes of gastroparesis described in children include cystic fibrosis, juvenile diabetes, chronic intestinal pseudo-obstruction, muscular dystrophy, and systemic autoimmune conditions such as scleroderma and Crohn's disease. Gastric motor and electrical abnormalities are frequent in adult patients with diabetes, and delayed gastric emptying is found in 30 to 50% of patients with long-standing diabetes mellitus. Visceral autonomic neuropathy is an important underlying factor in the gastroparesis associated with diabetes.[59] Hyperglycemia delays gastric emptying of liquid and solid meals. Alterations in gastric emptying do not occur in patients with euglycemic hyperinsulinemia. Thus, the effects of alterations in emptying are not likely to be attributable to the effect of hyperinsulinemia.[60] Conversely, gastric emptying of solids and liquids is faster in healthy and diabetic patients during acute episodes of hypoglycemia. This is probably due to cholinergic stimulation[60]; however, both sympathetic and parasympathetic mechanisms may be involved in this response.[61] Thus, it is possible that anticholinergic drugs could be beneficial in the stomach response to hypoglycemia. Gastric dysmotility may also contribute to the poor metabolic control of diabetes secondary to a mismatch between the delivery of the nutrient load to the duodenum and the onset of insulin action. Several reports have been published on gastric dysfunction in children with diabetes mellitus,[62-64] and postprandial antral hypomotility seems to be the most common motor abnormality in this scenario.[65]

Patients with Hirschsprung's disease may also have alterations in gastric emptying. Abnormal motility of the upper gastrointestinal tract and autonomic nervous system (sympathetic and parasympathetic) dysfunction has been reported in some of these patients.[66,67] A controlled study on adolescent and adult patients who had surgery for Hirschsprung's disease in early childhood showed an abnormal pattern of gastric emptying for solids and caloric liquids. Most patients had delayed gastric emptying, whereas some patients had a prolonged period in which no emptying occurred followed by a period of rapid gastric emptying. An abnormal glucose and insulin homeostasis was also found in a subset of these patients.

Multiple drugs may cause alterations in gastric emptying. Anticholinergics, opioids, tricyclic antidepressants, diphenhydramine,

proton-pump inhibitors,[68] H$_2$ receptor antagonists, antacids, sucralfate,[69] octreotide,[70] beta-adrenergic receptor agonists, calcium channel blockers, interferon alfa, and levodopa among others may delay gastric emptying. Gastroparesis enhances the absorption of drugs such as hydrochlorothiazide, nitrofurantoin, phenytoin, and spirolactone.[57] Caustic ingestion was also shown to lead to delayed liquid gastric emptying even in the absence of symptoms.[71]

Dyspepsia

Functional dyspepsia is defined by the pediatric Rome III criteria as a clinical syndrome characterized by at least 2 months of persistent or recurrent pain or discomfort centered in the upper abdomen, not relieved by defecation or associated with changes in stool frequency or stool form and in the absence of an underlying disease that is likely to explain the symptoms.[72] The symptom complex frequently includes other symptoms such as early satiety, postprandial fullness, nausea, vomiting, belching, bloating, and anorexia. Symptoms are usually associated with the ingestion of a meal. The pathophysiology underlying functional dyspepsia is still to be elucidated. Studies conducted in adult patients with functional dyspepsia have uncovered abnormalities of gastric sensory and motor function. Several putative mechanisms including delayed gastric emptying, impaired gastric accommodation in response to a meal, and hypersensitivity to gastric distention have been proposed. Several studies have shown a significant association between delayed gastric emptying of solids and symptoms of nausea, vomiting, and meal-related fullness.[73-75] However, the correlation between symptoms and results from gastric emptying studies is generally poor, and some studies seem to indicate that delayed gastric emptying does not play an important role in the pathogenesis of meal-related symptoms.[76] In fact, the main motility abnormality in patients with dyspepsia and autonomic dysfunction may even be rapid gastric emptying.[77] A possible explanation is that an accelerated early phase of emptying may lead to feedback inhibition by the duodeno-antral reflex that may result in delayed late emptying phase.[5] Impaired gastric accommodation is common in patients with functional dyspepsia, and it may result in rapid initial gastric emptying.[78] However, similarly to the abnormalities in emptying, disturbances in accommodation alone cannot reliably predict the presence of symptoms in patients with dyspepsia.[79] Thus, dyspepsia may be better conceptualized as the end result of a multifactorial dysfunction of the enteric nervous system. There is a paucity of studies investigating the pathophysiology of dyspepsia in children. A study of 57 children with functional dyspepsia showed that fast gastric emptying at 4 hours was associated with bloating.[80] A study in adolescents with functional dyspepsia using the satiation nutrient drink test, breath test for gastric emptying of solids, and single photon emission computed tomography (SPECT) demonstrated increased postprandial symptoms after meal challenge, delayed gastric emptying, and a reduced gastric volume response to feeding.[80]

Rumination

Rumination syndrome is a functional gastrointestinal disorder that has been recently defined by the infant and adolescent versions of the Rome III criteria.[81] It is characterized by the repetitive effortless regurgitation of recently swallowed food from the stomach into the mouth within 30 minutes from the ingestion of a meal. Occasionally, the regurgitation may even begin during the meal. Once the stomach content reaches the mouth, the partially digested food is reswallowed or expelled. The characteristics of rumination change in the different age groups. In infants and young children, rumination mainly occurs in developmentally delayed or neurologically impaired children. In adolescents, rumination generally occurs in otherwise healthy children. Rumination is frequently denied by the parents and unrecognized by medical providers. A study of adolescents with rumination showed that the average duration of symptoms at diagnosis was 17 months.[82] In children and adolescents, rumination is frequently confused with other conditions that cause vomiting, such as gastroesophageal reflux disease, gastroparesis, eating disorders, and cyclic vomiting.

Children with rumination frequently present with other symptoms including weight loss and abdominal pain.[82] Characteristically, retching and heartburn are absent. The diagnosis is clinical, and diagnostic tests should be kept to a minimum as they generally are negative.[82,83] Gastric emptying studies may demonstrate a delay in emptying due to the constant regurgitation and reswallowing, which keeps the radiolabeled meal from emptying the stomach normally. Antroduodenal manometry shows a characteristic pattern in many of these patients (Figure 29-2), with brief, simultaneous increases in abdominal pressure recorded in the stomach and in the small intestine that manifest clinically by regurgitation ("r" waves).[82,84] It remains unclear whether these increases in pressure are elicited by diaphragmatic descent or by abdominal wall contraction or both.[85] In children and adolescents, rumination has been associated with significant functional disability with weight loss, hospitalization, and school and work absenteeism.[84] A history of trauma, surgery, or infection preceding the onset of symptoms is frequently elicited.[83] A history of psychiatric illnesses including anxiety and depression is frequently associated with rumination.[83] Barostat studies showed that patients with rumination have higher gastric sensitivity and experience more nausea and bloating than healthy controls during balloon distention. There seems to be also a greater lower esophageal sphincter pressure reduction in response to gastric distention than in healthy controls. Data are conflicting regarding gastric accommodation function in patients with rumination.[85,86]

It has been hypothesized that rumination constitutes an abnormal belch reflex that eventually overcomes the resistance provided by the lower esophageal sphincter. A multidisciplinary approach is recommended for the treatment of children with rumination.[87] The modalities of this approach should be individualized in each case, especially when associated psychiatric conditions are present. Education of patients and families, psychotherapy, and behavioral interventions such as biofeedback, hypnosis, and diaphragmatic breathing are the mainstays of treatment.[88] There is no evidence to support the use of antireflux medications or antireflux surgery in patients with rumination. The prognosis of rumination in children and adolescents is benign, although symptoms may persist for years.[82]

Dumping Syndrome

Dumping syndrome is caused by the rapid passage of partially digested contents from the stomach to the small intestine. It is characterized by an early phase that occurs 10 to 30 minutes

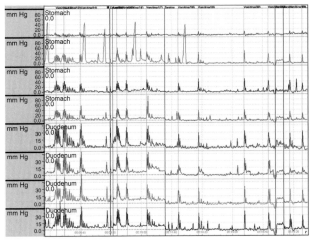

Figure 29-2. Antroduodenal manometry in a patient with rumination. The tracing shows simultaneous contractions in the stomach and in the small bowel ("r" waves), associated with the act of regurgitation.

after the meal and a late phase that occurs approximately 1 to 3 hours after eating. Clinical manifestations of one or both of these phases may be present in each patient. It is estimated that manifestations of early phases of dumping occur in 75% of all affected patients.[89] In the early phase, the rapid arrival of a hyperosmolar chyme into the duodenum leads to a large shift of fluids from the intravascular space to the intestinal lumen, resulting in hypovolemia, duodenal distention, and high-amplitude intestinal contractions. Clinical manifestations of early dumping comprise both vasomotor and gastrointestinal complaints including nausea, diaphoresis, weakness, dizziness, palpitations, cramping, and diarrhea.[90] It remains unclear how critical the fluid shift is in generating symptoms because the administration of intravenous fluids does not prevent clinical manifestations of early dumping syndrome.[91] Late dumping results from reactive hypoglycemia that is attributed to the rapid delivery of carbohydrates to the small intestine, leading to exaggerated insulin release. Symptoms of late dumping include hypoglycemia, tremors, sweating, weakness, and dizziness.

Dumping syndrome may be seen after surgical procedures such as esophagectomy, gastrectomy, vagotomy with pyloroplasty, bariatric surgery, and fundoplication. It has been reported to occur in up to 30% of children undergoing antireflux surgery.[92] In patients with symptoms suggestive of dumping syndrome, a modified oral glucose tolerance test may help to establish the diagnosis.[93] Gastric emptying studies typically demonstrate rapid stomach emptying. Initial treatment includes lifestyle modifications and dietary measures. Patients are advised to lie down for at least 30 minutes after meals to decrease gastric emptying and prevent symptoms of hypovolemia. Dietary recommendations include eating smaller portions; increasing the viscosity of food by adding uncooked cornstarch, guar gum, or pectin to the meals[94]; and delaying liquid intake up to 30 minutes after the meal. Readily absorbable carbohydrates should be minimized in the diet to prevent late dumping. Use of acarbose is recommended in patients with manifestations of late dumping, because it interferes with carbohydrate absorption in the small intestine and has been shown to improve glucose tolerance and reduce hypoglycemia.[95] However, treatment with acarbose may result in bloating, flatulence, and diarrhea because of its bacterial fermentation. Octreotide has been reported to be beneficial in patients with dumping syndrome who fail to respond to dietary measures. Octreotide delays gastric emptying and small bowel transit, inhibits the release of gastrointestinal hormones, delays monosaccharide absorption, decreases insulin secretion and prevents hemodynamic changes.[94,95] Surgical reintervention or continuous enteral feeding may be considered in refractory cases.

ASSESSMENT OF GASTRIC MOTOR AND SENSORY FUNCTION

Scintigraphy

Scintigraphy provides a cost-effective physiologic, noninvasive, and quantitative measurement of gastric emptying with limited radiation exposure. Following the ingestion of a radiolabeled meal, the proportion of radioactivity retained in the stomach is measured at various times. The result of a scintigraphic gastric emptying is influenced by the phase of the meal evaluated (solid or liquid), its caloric content, and the duration of the scanning. A consensus document from the American Neurogastroenterology and Motility Society and the Society of Nuclear Medicine[96] has established standardized methodology and reference values for performing gastric emptying studies in adults. The report provides recommendations on meals to be used, patient positioning, and frequency and duration of measurements. The statement on solid-meal gastric emptying recommends the use of a low-fat, egg-white meal labeled with technetium-99m sulfur colloid. This meal consists of the equivalent of two large eggs, plus two slices of bread and jam with water. Delayed emptying is considered to be gastric retention of more than 90% at 1 hour, more than 60% at 2 hours, and more than 10% at 4 hours. The composition of the meal may be altered in patients who report severe symptoms after eating foods rich in fat, who have specific allergies to some of the components of the standardized meal, or in whom the ingestion of gluten is contraindicated. However, no normal values are provided for these exceptional situations.

Because the symptoms of rapid emptying may sometimes be similar to those of delayed emptying[97] and the treatment is different, it is important to determine values for accelerated transit time. The consensus document recommended less than 30% of gastric retention at 1 hour as indicative of rapid gastric emptying. It is suggested to acquire images at 0, 1, 2, and 4 hours after meal ingestion (the document does not provide normal values for imaging at 3 hours). The report advocates extending the test up to 4 hours based on data from adult studies that indicate that longer testing increases the detection rate of clinically significant delayed emptying.[98] There are patients with delayed emptying at certain time points who later normalize their emptying, and some individuals with early normal emptying and delayed later emptying.[98] Although the experts recognized this possibility, they did not provide recommendations for the interpretation of this situation, because the clinical importance of an isolated delay in emptying at only certain time points remains unknown. It is recommended to stop drugs that may affect motility such as metoclopramide, erythromycin, domperidone, opiate analgesics, and anticholinergic agents 2 days before the test. The study ought to be performed in the morning after an overnight fast or after at least 6 hours of fasting. Although the

report was based mostly on a large adult multicenter study[99] and has not established normal values for pediatric patients, the use of these reference values provides an opportunity to standardize the interpretation of gastric emptying testing in children as well.

Scintigraphic gastric emptying is commonly indicated to diagnose gastric stasis or dumping syndrome. Solid-phase gastric emptying testing is the preferred test to document gastroparesis because gastric emptying of liquids is frequently maintained even in the setting of severe gastroparesis.[100] Regurgitation or vomiting of a portion of the ingested meal after the initial baseline measurement requires adjusting count values because it may lead to lower estimated gastric retention. Critics of gastric scintigraphy have argued that the projection method on which this technique is based leads to important pitfalls. Scintigraphy may not accurately distinguish between the stomach and superimposed areas of intestine containing radiolabeled chyme, possibly resulting in an overestimation of the amount of retained gastric contents.[101]

Ultrasonography

Ultrasonography is a noninvasive and validated technique[102] that can be used to estimate whole stomach and antropyloric volume, antral area, and transpyloric flow during fasting and feeding states. Functional three-dimensional ultrasonography allows the simultaneous determination of gastric emptying and gastric accommodation. However, the disadvantages of ultrasonographic techniques – that it is operator dependent and technically demanding, and the fact that it only measures liquid emptying – has limited its use in clinical practice. Additional limitations of ultrasonography include difficulties in measuring proximal and distal gastric regions simultaneously and the fact that gastric secretions cannot be accounted for.

Magnetic Resonance Imaging

Magnetic resonance imaging (MRI) assessment of gastric emptying has been validated as a diagnostic and research tool.[101] MRI allows the assessment of gastric emptying of any type of meal with excellent correlation with scintigraphic techniques. MRI is a sensitive technique that can detect differences in gastric emptying between meals of different consistency and energy content and is an ideal test to assess the effects of pharmacologic manipulation without radiation exposure. It allows the simultaneous assessment of gastric contractile activity, emptying, and accommodation. Despite the proven benefits of this technique, the limited availability of MRI and the high cost of the test have restricted its use in clinical practice.

Breath Testing

Breath testing is a noninvasive technique that assesses gastric emptying of solids or liquids using stable isotope substrates and the sequential measurement of breath $^{13}CO_2$ by isotope ratio mass spectrometry.[103] Gastric emptying is the rate-limiting step in the final delivery of $^{13}CO_2$ to the breath. Several pitfalls of this technique may confound its interpretation. Breath testing excretion of ^{13}C-octanoic acid or ^{13}C-acetate is based on the assumption of normal small bowel, pulmonary, pancreatic, and liver function and the absence of visceral hemodynamic changes. Therefore, the results may not be easily interpreted in patients with various illnesses.[104]

Acetaminophen Absorption Test

Acetaminophen absorption test is a sensitive method for detecting delayed and accelerated gastric emptying.[105] Some of the drawbacks of this test are that it only measures liquid gastric emptying and it requires repeated blood sampling and normal small bowel absorption.[106] A study comparing acetaminophen absorption and ^{13}C-acetate breath test to scintigraphic gastric emptying assessment in healthy subjects found good agreement between the acetaminophen absorption test and the liquid scintigraphic gastric emptying, but poor agreement between the ^{13}C-acetate breath test and the scintigraphic test.[107]

Single Photon Emission Computed Tomography

SPECT is a reliable scintigraphic technique that allows the assessment of gastric volume and the relation between different gastric functions such as accommodation and emptying by radioisotope imaging of the gastric wall. SPECT is based on the intravenous injection of ^{99m}Tc pertechnetate that selectively accumulates in the gastric mucosa.[108] SPECT imaging has been validated for the measurement of gastric volumes in comparison with the barostat as the gold standard.[109] SPECT has been used in the investigation of adolescents with functional dyspepsia.[80]

Barostat

The barostat is a computerized air pump device that can be used to measure visceral tone, compliance, and sensation of hollow organs. The barostat is the gold standard test for the assessment of fundic relaxation in response to a meal. It measures fundic tone by monitoring the volume of air within an intragastric bag that is clamped at a constant, preset pressure level.[110] The technique involves the intubation of the esophagus to advance an infinitely compliant polyethylene balloon (similar to a sandwich bag) (Figure 29-3) into the fundus. The system maintains a constant intrabag pressure by inflating or withdrawing air when the pressure falls or exceeds a selected level. As the intraballoon pressure is fixed, changes in intraballoon volume reflect changes in tone due to gastric relaxation or contraction. Accommodation is assessed by measuring and comparing intragastric volumes in the fasting and postprandial periods.[4] Postprandial accommodation usually reaches a peak approximately 10 minutes after completion of meal ingestion and lasts for a minimum of 30 minutes. A major methodologic drawback that limits a more widespread use of barostat testing is the need for orogastric intubation and the inability of many patients to ingest a meal with the tube and the balloon in place. It has been argued that the barostat balloon could potentially induce artifacts secondary to the positive intraluminal balloon pressure. This technique has been shown to cause dilatation of the antrum due to meal displacement by the balloon in the gastric fundus, leading to an exaggerated proximal gastric relaxation.[111] In addition, the orogastric balloon may stimulate the swallowing reflex and induce

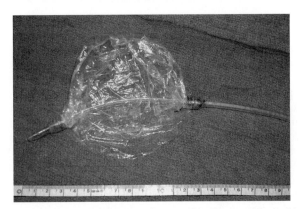

Figure 29-3. Picture of a barostat balloon used to assess gastric sensitivity, compliance, and accommodation.

receptive relaxation. The barostat technique has been used in children with chronic abdominal pain to assess visceral hypersensitivity and gastric compliance.[112] Currently, its use in pediatrics is limited to research settings.[113]

Drinking Tests

Noninvasive methods of assessing gastric accommodation include the satiety drinking test and water load test. These techniques assume that the volume of water or liquid meal that the patient drinks reflects the volume of the stomach. The nutrient drink test uses a liquid meal of known caloric content to measure the maximum tolerated volume. The amount of calories ingested at maximum satiety after an overnight fast is considered a surrogate of gastric accommodation. Studies comparing gastric accommodation values by nutrient drink test and gastric volume measurements by SPECT have shown poor agreement.[114] The water load test has been used in adult and pediatric investigations to study sensation in patients with functional dyspepsia. In the water load test, subjects are requested to drink room-temperature water from an unmarked flask over a certain period of time until reaching satiety. Different protocols have been used in adults including ad libitum ingestion of water over 3 to 5 minutes (rapid water load) or at a fixed rate at 100 mL/min until the patient reaches satiety. Results have varied, and the agreement among different satiety tests remains controversial.[115,116] Similarly to other gastric function tests, drink tests are prone to intrasubject variation,[115] and it is unclear whether the conditions under which these tests are conducted accurately reflect what occurs under physiologic conditions and how much personality characteristics and quality of life influence the results.[114,116] Sood et al. have established water normal load values in 176 healthy school children who were asked to drink as much water as possible over 3 minutes until the feeling of fullness was achieved.[117] Diagnostic value of the water load test in children with abdominal pain remains controversial, with studies using the rapid load test indicating that although the test has an acceptable specificity for the diagnosis of functional dyspepsia, it has poor sensitivity.[118] Conversely, another study comparing 110 children with functional abdominal pain and 120 healthy controls using a 15-minute water load test concluded that the test is useful because of its good convergent and discriminant validity. In this study and in a similar investigation the test reproduced naturally occurring abdominal pain episodes.[119,120]

Antroduodenal Manometry

Antroduodenal manometry measures intraluminal pressures in the distal stomach and duodenum. The test is performed by introducing a motility catheter transnasally or through an existing gastrostomy site. The catheter should have at least two pressure sensors in the antrum. The distance between sensors varies from 1 cm in the antrum to 3-5 cm in the duodenum and jejunum depending on the child's size. Studies should measure at least 3 hours of fasting motility (or the recording of two MMCs) and 1 hour of postprandial motility after ingestion of a mixed solid-liquid meal of at least 10 kcal/kg or 400 kcal.

Alterations of the normal pattern of interdigestive motility may be seen in several clinical conditions including scleroderma, diabetes, intestinal pseudo-obstruction, dumping syndrome, surgical damage to the vagal nerve, and functional bowel disorders.[121] In children, several abnormal manometric patterns have been described in association with specific clinical entities. Intestinal myopathy is identified by the presence of coordinated contractions that do not exceed 10 to 20 mm Hg in the absence of a dilated bowel. Intestinal neuropathy is characterized by the presence of normal amplitude but uncoordinated contractions.

Wireless Motility Capsule

The SmartPill GI Monitoring System is a novel device currently used in adults to evaluate motility in patients with suspected gastroparesis. It consists of a capsule that is ingested by the patient and transmits wireless data on intraluminal pH, pressure, and temperature to a receiver as it moves throughout the gastrointestinal tract. The information is stored and later downloaded to a computer that displays the data graphically. The gastric emptying time measured by the wireless motility capsule correlates well with the emptying measured by scintigraphy and discriminates between healthy and gastroparetic subjects.[122] This technique offers a nonradioactive, ambulatory alternative to scintigraphy. The device has not yet been approved for use in children, and it remains to be demonstrated whether the information it provides can obviate the need for manometry testing in children with symptoms suggestive of gastric dysfunction.

Electrogastrogram

The electrogastrogram (EGG) is a noninvasive method that allows recording of myoelectric activity of the stomach through cutaneous electrodes positioned on the skin in the upper abdomen. Although EGG provides an attractive means of detecting abnormalities in electric rhythm that are associated with disturbed gastric function,[123,124] the interpretation, clinical significance, and usefulness of this technique remain controversial. EGG is sometimes not interpretable or may show results that overlap between children with normal and abnormal manometry. It is unclear whether postprandial EGG changes in amplitude reflect increased gastric contractility or mere distention of the stomach that brings the organ closer to the cutaneous electrodes.[125] A recent study using EGG, ultrasonographic assessment of gastric emptying rate, and antral motility testing showed impaired gastric emptying and antral motility as well as changes in the EGG in patients with childhood functional recurrent abdominal pain.[126]

TREATMENT

Management of gastroparesis is based on dietary and lifestyle measures (small-volume and frequent meals low in fat and fiber content), correction of existing fluid and electrolyte deficiencies, nutritional optimization, and improvement in gastric motility. A detailed dietary history should be obtained to investigate the composition, size, and time of meal intake and tolerance of solids, semisolids, and liquids. Fluids should be ingested throughout the meal. Patients are instructed to avoid carbonated beverages in attempt to limit gastric distention and to sit or walk for 1 to 2 hours following meals. In cases of unremitting symptoms, most calories should be provided in a liquid form, because liquid emptying is often preserved. A thorough history should uncover use of drugs potentially causing gastric dysfunction. Gastric emptying delay may result from the combination of several motor defects, including exaggerated fundic relaxation, impaired antral contractility, abnormal antroduodenal coordination, and pylorospasm. Motor disturbances frequently coexist with visceral hyperalgesia. Thus, pharmacologic therapy should try to target the different pathophysiologic mechanisms with the use of prokinetics in combination with symptomatic agents including antiemetics and visceral analgesics and fundic relaxants. Visceral analgesics are used when pain is a significant component of the symptom complex and include psychoactive medications such as low-dose tricyclic antidepressants, selective serotonin reuptake inhibitors, selective noradrenaline reuptake inhibitors, and combined serotonin/noradrenaline reuptake inhibitors. An in-depth discussion of antiemetic and pain medications is beyond the scope of this chapter. Patients should be informed that multiple drug trials may be attempted before finding the optimal therapeutic regimen and that improvement of symptoms and not necessarily resolving the underlying abnormality is the goal of treatment.

Prokinetics

Prokinetics are a group of drugs that stimulate gastric smooth muscle contractions and enhance gastric emptying. There are few available prokinetics in the United States, and there has been no placebo-controlled randomized intervention study in children with gastroparesis.

Dopamine receptors are widely distributed throughout the gastrointestinal wall. Selective stimulation of dopamine receptors inhibits proximal gastrointestinal motility. Metoclopramide elicits its prokinetic effect as a dopamine D2 receptor antagonist, serotonin (5HT) receptor type-4 agonist, and direct stimulant of stomach and small intestine smooth muscle. Metoclopramide has been shown in some but not all studies to increase the duration and frequency of antral and duodenal contractions,[127] increase lower esophageal sphincter pressure,[128] and relax the pyloric sphincter.[129] In addition, metoclopramide has a centrally mediated effect, suppressing nausea and vomiting in the area postrema. It can be administered by the oral, subcutaneous, or intravenous route. Side effects common to all dopamine receptor antagonists include neuroendocrine actions, including a rise in prolactin levels resulting in galactorrhea[130,131] and central nervous system effects such as extrapyramidal dyskinetic reactions. Long-term use of metoclopramide at high doses puts children at risk for persistence of tardive dyskinesia.[132] These potentially severe adverse effects have led to a "black box" warning by the U.S.

Food and Drug Administration, advising against the use of metoclopramide for more than 3 months.

Domperidone has a mechanism of action similar to metoclopramide with the benefit of not crossing the brain-blood barrier, minimizing side effects.[63,65] Among the mechanisms of action of domperidone are the enhancement of acetylcholine release, inhibition of cholinesterase activity, and antagonism of adrenergic alpha-1 receptors.[65] Although domperidone is considered a safe drug,[133] there have been reports of cardiac arrhythmias, cardiac arrest, and even sudden death associated with its use.[134] A pediatric study found oral domperidone effective in improving gastric motility and metabolic control in children with gastroparesis and insulin dependent diabetes.[65] It can be used in the United States by an investigational new drug (IND) application for conditions causing chronic nausea and vomiting and for treatment of gastroparesis.[135]

Erythromycin is a macrolide antibiotic with agonistic effects on motilin receptors of the smooth muscle cells of the gastrointestinal tract. Erythromycin administration induces phase III of the MMC in the antrum and duodenum. Erythromycin effect is limited to the stomach and small bowel because it lacks colonic activity.[136] Erythromycin used at subtherapeutic doses (3 to 5 mg/kg/dose every 6 hours) is a powerful prokinetic. It has been shown to be safe and effective in improving feeding intolerance in preterm infants and children in several studies.[137,138] On the other hand, multiple reports have shown that early exposure to erythromycin in the neonatal period is associated with a significant risk for the development of pyloric stenosis in infants.[139] A common theme of multiple studies on prokinetics is the poor correlation between the reduction of symptoms and improvement in gastric emptying.[140-143]

Botulinum Toxin

Botulinum toxin is currently been used in the treatment of different disorders of smooth muscle hypertonicity in the gastrointestinal tract.[144] Intrapyloric injection of botulinum toxin type A has been used in severe refractory cases of gastroparesis in adults and children. The toxin is injected endoscopically using a sclerotherapy needle in each quadrant of the pylorus, usually at a dose of 25 units per site (Figure 29-4). By blocking the release of acetylcholine from cholinergic nerve endings, botulinum toxin can potentially inhibit the barrier function at the level of the pylorus, enhancing emptying and providing symptomatic relief. Several case series[145,146] and nonrandomized clinical trials support the use of botulinum toxin in the treatment of gastroparesis.[147,148] The largest published study showed an overall symptomatic improvement in 43% of 63 patients with gastroparesis with a median duration of response of approximately 5 months.[149] However, the largest controlled clinical trial in adults with gastroparesis who were randomized to 200 units of botulinum toxin or placebo showed essentially negative results. Symptomatic improvement was achieved in 37% of patients who received the active drug; however, 56% of the patients in the placebo group also improved.[147] The improvement in gastric emptying was not significantly different between the two groups. Similar results were found in a crossover trial that showed that the toxin was not superior to placebo in improving symptoms or gastric emptying.[150] Although botulinum toxin is occasionally used in children with refractory gastroparesis, no study has been published evaluating the efficacy of this intervention in children.

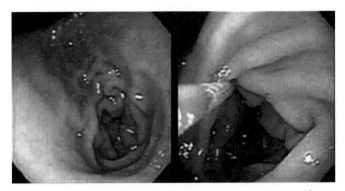

Figure 29-4. Intrapyloric injection of botulinum toxin in a patient with gastroparesis. A sclerotherapy needle is inserted through the biopsy channel of the endoscope to inject the toxin in the four pyloric quadrants.

Medications That Promote Fundic Relaxation

These include nitrates, buspirone, sumatriptan, and selective serotonin reuptake inhibitors. In patients with functional dyspepsia, early satiety has been associated with defects in fundic accommodation. Although the use of fundic relaxants for the treatment of gastroparesis has not been investigated, these drugs may be empirically tried in the management of early satiety associated with gastroparesis.

Buspirone is a serotonin 1A (5-HT$_{1A}$) receptor agonist that is used in the treatment of anxiety and depression. It has been shown to reduce symptoms and enhance gastric accommodation in adults with functional dyspepsia.[151] Studies on healthy volunteers who received paroxetine showed conflicting results. Whereas one study showed a beneficial effect on accommodation,[152] another study showed no effect on accommodation or gastric emptying.[153] Sumatriptan, a 5-HT$_{1B/1D}$ receptor agonist used to abort symptoms in migraines and cyclic vomiting syndrome, has been shown to relax the stomach in patients with dyspepsia and healthy subjects.[154,155] Clonidine, an α_2-agonist that is used to reduce intestinal fluid losses,[156,157] has been shown to enhance gastric accommodation.[158]

Gastric Electrical Stimulation

Patients who fail standard medical and dietary therapy may benefit from gastric electrical stimulation. The technique consists of implanting two electrodes connected to a pacemaker into the seromuscular layer of the stomach. The electrodes are placed by laparoscopy, and the position is confirmed by upper endoscopy before the electrodes are secured with sutures and clips. The electrodes are then connected to a pulse generator placed in an anterior abdominal pocket and programmed through a radiofrequency wand. There are several variations of the technique, with some centers endoscopically placing an initial testing probe that remains in place for a few days in order to assess success and tolerance before the definitive implantation, whereas others do not use a testing phase. Stimulation protocols vary in amplitude, pulse width, frequency, and interval of cycling. The largest prospective adult study published on patients with gastroparesis showed improvement in frequency and severity of nausea and vomiting. There was normalization of gastric emptying time in 11 of 27 patients. The study also showed reduction of gastric emptying time at 2 hours but not at 4 hours.[159] Epigastric pain was unchanged at 12 months, indicating that gastric electrical stimulation may not be useful in patients with predominant pain symptoms. Other adult studies using gastric electrical stimulation have shown improvement in quality of life and nutritional status.[160] A pediatric study described nine children with chronic nausea and vomiting with a mean age of 14 years who underwent temporary gastric electrical stimulation followed by placement of the permanent device. There was a sustained benefit in seven patients in symptom scores and quality of life.[161] There were no significant changes in gastric emptying and electrogastrogram values. The mechanism by which gastric electrical stimulation leads to symptomatic improvement remains unclear. Although it was initially thought that gastric electrical stimulation altered gastric dysrhythmias and improved gastric emptying,[160] it has become evident that the high-frequency, short-duration pulses used by the currently commercially available gastric stimulators do not regulate gastric slow waves.[162] Studies on gastric emptying have shown conflicting results, with some studies showing improvement whereas others do not.[159,163,164] Similarly, these stimulation parameters do not modify efferent vagal activity.[165] Tack et al. found that pacing decreased the sensitivity to gastric distention and improved gastric accommodation in response to meals.[166] Animal studies have also shown that gastric electrical stimulation enhances fundic relaxation. The results of those studies may explain the beneficial symptomatic effect of gastric electrical stimulation in the absence of a consistent effect on gastric emptying.

REFERENCES

28. Tack J, Depoortere I, Bisschops R, et al. Influence of ghrelin on interdigestive gastrointestinal motility in humans. Gut 2006;55:327–333.

34. Luiking YC, Akkermans LM, Peeters TL, et al. Effects of motilin on human interdigestive gastrointestinal and gallbladder motility, and involvement of 5HT3 receptors. Neurogastroenterol Motil 2002;14:151–159.

49. Tomomasa T, DiLorenzo C, Morikawa A, et al. Analysis of fasting antroduodenal manometry in children. Dig Dis Sci 1996;41:2195–2203.

51. Vandenplas Y, Hauser B, Salvatore S. Current pharmacological treatment of gastroparesis. Expert Opin Pharmacother 2004;5:2251–2254.

66. Miele E, Tozzi A, Staiano A, et al. Persistence of abnormal gastrointestinal motility after operation for Hirschsprung's disease. Am J Gastroenterol 2000;95:1226–1230.

79. Tack J, Caenepeel P, Corsetti M, et al. Role of tension receptors in dyspeptic patients with hypersensitivity to gastric distention. Gastroenterology 2004;127:1058–1066.

84. Chial HJ, Camilleri M, Williams DE, et al. Rumination syndrome in children and adolescents: diagnosis, treatment, and prognosis. Pediatrics 2003;111:158–162.

90. Tack J, Arts J, Caenepeel P, et al. Pathophysiology, diagnosis and management of postoperative dumping syndrome. Nat Rev Gastroenterol Hepatol 2009;6:583–590.

97. Delgado-Aros S, Camilleri M, Cremonini F, et al. Contributions of gastric volumes and gastric emptying to meal size and postmeal symptoms in functional dyspepsia. Gastroenterology 2004;127:1685–1694.

See expertconsult.com for a complete list of references and the review questions for this chapter.

BEZOARS 30

Benjamin R. Kuhn • Adam G. Mezoff

The term *bezoar* comes from the Persian word *badzehr*, which refers to the material found in sacrificed animals such as goats. In ancient times, this material was thought to have magical or medicinal powers and was used as an antidote to poisons from snake bites, infections, diverse diseases, and even as a means of combating aging.[1,2] The Indian physician Charak reported the presence of bezoars in his work in the second and third centuries BC.[3] Baudamant was the first to describe bezoars in the Western world, in an autopsy performed in 1779.[4] Matas performed the first extensive review in 1915; subsequently Debakey and Oschner published their landmark review in 1938.[1,2] Schonbon first published a description of the surgical removal of bezoars in the 19th century.[3]

DEFINITIONS

Bezoars are defined as aggregates of undigested or inedible material found anywhere in the gastrointestinal tract, although most commonly found in the stomach. Plant fiber, hair. and medication bezoars have all been well described.

EPIDEMIOLOGY

Predisposing factors are indicated in Table 30-1. Case reports of bezoars secondary to gastric surgery are now increasing, even in children.[5,6] This category is anticipated to expand with the increasing frequency of adolescents receiving Roux-en-Y gastric bypass for obesity. Common pediatric gastric surgeries include fundoplication, gastrostomy, pyloroplasty, and now the Roux-en Y gastric bypass. The adult literature commonly includes vagotomy for peptic ulcer disease as a predisposing factor to bezoar formation, and potentially any gastric surgery may alter vagus nerve function, leading to dysmotility.[7] An esophageal tricho-bezoar is reported in a pediatric patient postfundoplication as well.[8]

ETIOLOGY AND PATHOGENESIS

Phytobezoars

Phytobezoars are the most frequently observed type and account for approximately 40% of the total number of reported bezoars. They are composed of indigestible vegetable fibers, most commonly from pulpy fruits, orange pits, seeds, roots or leaves. Predisposing factors are indicated in Table 30-1. A case of a "cotton" bezoar was reported in a heroin addict who swallowed the cotton ball used to filter a water-methadone pill preparation for intravenous infusion.[9] These bezoars are usually found in the stomach (78%), although up to 17% may occur in the small intestine.[10] Sunflower seed concretions have been described in the colons of children.[11]

Diospyrobezoars (Persimmon Bezoars)

Although made of vegetable matter, persimmon bezoars represent a class by themselves and account for up to 29% of all bezoars in some series.[1] Persimmon bezoars are named for a Native American tree that also is present in Iran and the Middle East, *Diospyros virginiana*. Its fruit, a berry, contains a material called shiboul or phobatanin. This substance is present in the unripened fruit and under the skin of the ripe fruit.[12]

Trichobezoars

Trichobezoars occur predominantly (up to 90%) in females under the age of 20, and often in children.[1] They have been described in children as young as 1 year old. They consist of an aggregation of hair and foodstuff and are black regardless of the patient's hair color, because of the chemical reaction of hair with gastric acid (Figure 30-1). The hair in the trichobezoar is usually from the patient, although hair from animals, carpet, or toys is occasionally recovered.[13] Trichobezoars are usually the site for intense food putrefaction and can generate a very foul-smelling odor and halitosis. The act of hair swallowing is thought to be akin to pica or nail biting. Only about 9% of patients with trichobezoars have proven psychiatric problems.[14] Trichobezoars usually are present in the stomach but may have very long tails. These tails can invade the esophagus proximally and extend to the small intestine. Involvement from the stomach extending to the entire length of the small intestine is referred to as Rapunzel syndrome.[3] Trichobezoars may weigh up to 6.5 pounds.

Lactobezoars

Lactobezoars are gastric masses made of milk protein. They occur primarily in premature, low-birth-weight infants. Although the exact cause remains unclear, formation is thought to be related to formula composition, protein flocculation, thickening agents, immature gastric motility, and rapidity of feeding.[15] Most reported cases have occurred in infants fed high-calorie formula for premature babies.[16] However, human milk bezoars have also been described.[17] The formation of lactobezoars may be precipitated by the addition of thickening agents, such as gel of pectin, to the infant's formula.[18] Lactobezoars have also been reported in adults fed Osmolite (Ross Nutritionals, Columbus, OH).[19]

Paper Bezoars

At least two case reports of paper bezoars, one in a child and one in an adult, have been described. The undigested material was toilet paper, ingested over several days.[20]

TABLE 30-1. Factors Predisposing to the Formation of Phytobezoars

Factor	Prevalence in Patients (%)
Poor mastication	80
Gastric surgery with vagotomy	56
Gastroparesis	20
Histamine H$_2$ receptor antagonists	12
Diabetes mellitus	6
Excessive intake of fibers	44

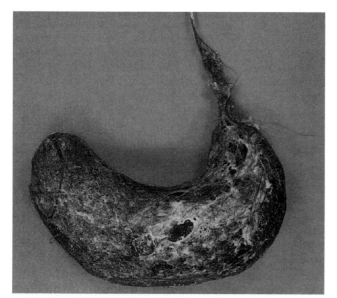

Figure 30-1. Hair cast of the stomach. Courtesy D. Mirkin, MD, Children's Medical Center, Dayton, OH.

Medication Bezoars (Pharmacobezoars)

A large number of case reports have documented the formation of concretions from various medications, leading to gastric bezoars. The medications implicated include nifedipine XL,[21] sucralfate,[22] bromide,[23] enteric-coated aspirin,[24] iron,[25] meprobamate,[26] slow-release theophylline,[27] and antacids.[28] Along with the typical obstructive symptoms of bezoars, these foreign bodies may also induce symptoms based on their intrinsic pharmacologic effects. Bezoar formation is probably related to the composition of the inert compound in the medication (e.g., cellulose). This has been a particular problem with medications packaged in insoluble material for long, continuous delivery of the active drug.[21]

Cement Bezoars

Cement contains oxides of silica, aluminum, iron, and calcium, sulfuric anhydroxide, magnesium hydroxide, and calcium carbonate. It is easily accessible to children. Several cases of cement bezoars have been reported in young children, with the formation of solidified concretions. Different types of cement require various lengths of time to "set." After this time has elapsed, attempts at gastric lavage are futile and surgery is required.

TABLE 30-2. Clinical Manifestation of Bezoars

Characteristic	Incidence in Patients (%)
Halitosis	20-40
Abdominal/epigastric pain	40-70
Fullness after meal	20-60
Nausea/vomiting	10-50
Abdominal mass	10-88
Perforation/pneumatosis/acute abdomen	7-10
Dysphagia	5
Intestinal obstruction, partial or complete	≤75
Weakness/weight loss	6-30
Peptic ulcer disease	10-24
Hematemesis	≤71

Yeast Bezoars

Yeast bezoars have been reported primarily in patients undergoing gastric surgery, particularly vagotomy, although one was described in a newborn and was composed of *Candida albicans* and polystyrene resin.[29] Of the 43 patients with yeast bezoars reported in a Finnish study in 1974, 48% had undergone a Billroth I procedure and vagotomy. The most common species of fungus noted were *C. albicans* and *C. glabrata*.[30] Yeast bezoars are usually asymptomatic and are discovered incidentally. They have a tendency to recur.

Shellac Bezoars

Although glue bezoars have been described in experimenting adolescents, most shellac bezoars occur in adult alcoholics who drink shellac to intensify the effect of their alcohol. Shellac can be found in furniture polish and is readily available to children.[1]

Polybezoars

The term *polybezoars* refers to bezoars composed of multiple objects (metallic, plastic, or even wood) encased in trichobezoars. These usually are found in children or in neurologically impaired adults. Polybezoars often contain a large number of metal pins or clips[31] (Table 30-2).

Chewing Gum Bezoars

Although rare, three cases are reported in the literature of chewing gum bezoars. Two of these were chewing gum fecomas removed by manual disimpaction under anesthesia. The characteristic "taffy-pull" appearance of colorful material was diagnostic.[32]

CLINICAL PRESENTATION

A summary of the clinical manifestations of bezoars is shown in Table 30-2.[1,33-37] The initial presentation of many bezoars depends on their type. In premature infants and newborns, the most common bezoar is the lactobezoar. The most common symptom is feeding intolerance.[15] With time, symptoms may include abdominal distention, irritability, and vomiting. Physical examination often discloses a palpable midabdominal mass.

Trichobezoars and phytobezoars are more common in older children and adults. Trichobezoars form over long periods (several years), and early in their course, their signs and symptoms can be subtle, such as early satiety or nausea.[1] These bezoars can grow to a substantial size and mass, causing pressure necrosis of the gastric mucosa, ulceration, gastrointestinal bleeding, and even gastric perforation.[36] Most trichobezoars have "tails," either up into the esophagus, or distally into the small intestine, which can lead to partial or complete obstruction. Trichobezoars can often be identified by abdominal palpation. Crepitus, caused by putrefaction and bacterial growth, may be elicited. Phytobezoars are formed much more rapidly than trichobezoars. Symptoms include nausea, vomiting, and signs of gastric outlet obstruction, which may persist even after the bezoar has been removed. Serious complications such as gastric perforation are rare but have been the subject of case reports in both adult and pediatric patients.[36] Not only may pharmacobezoars induce symptoms as a result of their gastric mass, but they also carry the potential for drug intoxication.[21-27,38] Concretion of foreign objects in the duodenum and in the biliary tract can cause pancreatitis (toxic "sock" syndrome).[39] Symptoms such as malabsorption and protein-losing enteropathy can also arise from bezoars in these locations.[1]

DIAGNOSIS

The diagnosis of bezoars in adult patients can often be made by history and physical examination. Knowledge of predisposing factors may heighten clinical suspicion. Laboratory studies are of limited value, although occasionally a mild microcytic anemia or leukocytosis may develop. Imaging studies such as plain abdominal radiographs are the initial diagnostic modality identifying most bezoars. Barium studies may be useful to identify the bezoar and to determine the extent of the mass (Figure 30-2). However, upper gastrointestinal series may fail to diagnose bezoars in 36 to 50% of patients.[28,39] Moreover, in a reported case of enteric-coated aspirin bezoar, the use of barium changed the acid environment, leading to its distribution and a subsequent increase in the salicylate level.[24] Other methods, such as ultrasound or computed tomography, have also been used to document gastric bezoars.[40,41] These studies do not add to the diagnostic accuracy. Endoscopy remains the diagnostic modality of choice for identifying the type of gastric bezoar. Endoscopy also allows further therapeutic interventions.[27]

TREATMENT

Various methods have been used to both dissolve and/or retrieve the bezoar mass. Often they are used in concert depending on the type of bezoar and its location in the gastrointestinal (GI) tract. They can be divided into categories based on an attempt at (1) lavaging or dissolving the bezoar, (2) retrieval, or (3) fragmentation.

Lavage/Dissolution

Instillation of various pharmacologic agents have been attempted to chemically dissolve bezoars. This may require direct access to the GI tract via nasogastric tube, endoscope, or even laparotomy. Various solutions have been attempted:

1. *Acetylcysteine*. Schlang described lavaging with 15 mL of an acetylcysteine solution diluted in normal saline. This was instilled per nasogastric tube, and the bezoar was successfully dissolved.[42]

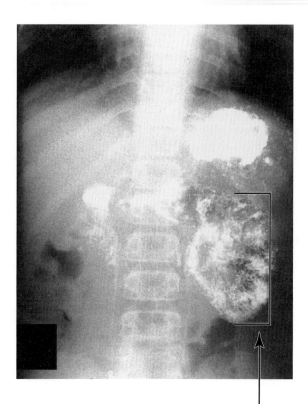

Figure 30-2. Barium swallow, showing a mass effect in the body of the stomach. This mass was a trichobezoar that had to be removed surgically. Courtesy F. Unger, MD, Children's Medical Center, Dayton, OH.

2. *Papain*. This enzyme, although no longer available in tablet form, is found in high concentrations in commercial meat tenderizers, along with high concentrations of sodium (1880 mg/5 mL).[43] It has been used successfully to enzymatically break protein bonds in phytobezoars and can be administered in a lavage solution.[44] Care must by used with this modality, because complications such as hypernatremia and perforation of the esophagus or stomach have been reported.[45,46]
3. *Cellulose*. It is believed that this enzyme cleaves the bond between leukoanthocyanidine-hemicellulose-cellulose. Several cases of successful dissolution of a bezoar with the use of a 3 to 5 g cellulose solution diluted with up to 500 mL water administered orally for 2 to 5 days have been reported.[44,47]
4. *Coca-Cola*. Phytobezoars have been successfully dissolved using nasogastric installation of 3 liters of Coca-Cola over a 12-hour period.[48]
5. *Polyethylene-glycol*. This is often reported as an adjunct in the removal of colonic bezoars, along with colonoscopy and attempts at retrieval.[49]
6. *Enemas*. Various enema preparations have been utilized to help soften and dissolve colonic bezoars. Koneru et al. describe the use of serial water-soluble contrast enemas to dissolve a colonic bezoar found in a 532-g premature infant.[50]
7. Steinberg et al. described a method whereby they laparoscopically discovered a large bezoar, then performed an appendectomy in order to insert a catheter through the appendiceal stump in order to lavage the hard mass without further surgical intervention.[51]

Retrieval

Various retrieval methods have been utilized to remove bezoars *en bloc*. Endoscopic retrieval has been the first choice for treatment in this category; however, surgical enterotomy is often necessary to remove large or difficult-to-dissolve bezoars such as shellac or cement bezoars. The facilitation of esophageal bezoar and food impaction removal by a Saeed Banding Device is well described in unique cases.[52-54]

Kanetaka et al. reported on a dual technique whereby a trichobezoar was fragmented by accessing the stomach with a laparoscope and utilizing laparoscopic scissors to fragment the bezoar so it could be retrieved endoscopically.[55]

Fragmentation

Fragmentation can be accomplished endoscopically or by extracorporeal means.

1. *Endoscopically*. This is the procedure of choice, often utilizing a snare to help break the large, hard bezoar into smaller pieces, which can pass through the intestinal tract. Lavage solutions or metoclopramide have been utilized to augment the passage of gastric bezoars that have been fragmented endoscopically.[56] Gaya et al. described the successful removal of persimmon bezoars with a combination of snare fragmentation and administration of cellulase, cysteine, and metaclopramide.[57] The authors cautioned that large fragments may not pass the pylorus and may lead to obstruction.

2. *Electrohydraulic lithotripsy*. Kuo et al. reported on 11 patients successfully undergoing lithotripsy to fragment gastric phytobezoars.[58]

PREVENTION

Gastric motility disorders, previous gastric surgery, poor mastication, and hypochlorhydria are major risk factors for the development and recurrence of many forms of gastric phytobezoars. Dietary counseling to avoid pulpy and fiber-rich foods should be provided to patients with these problems. Prokinetic agents such as metoclopramide or cisapride may be useful in preventing recurrences in certain patient populations. Identification of pica-like behavior in children should initiate counseling to prevent the ingestion of foreign substances. A history of significant trichotillomania may prompt psychological evaluation.

REFERENCES

1. Debakey M, Ochsner A. Bezoars and concretions. Surgery 1938;4: 934–963.
2. Debakey M, Ochsner A. Bezoars and concretions. Part 2. Surgery 1939;5:132–160.
6. Zamir D, Goldblum C, Linova L, et al. Phytobezoars and trichobezoars: a 10-year experience. J Clin Gastroenterol 2004;38:873–876.
28. Lee J. Bezoars and foreign bodies of the stomach. Gastrintest Endosc Clin North Am 1966;6:605–619.
36. Robles R, Parrilla P, Escamilla C, et al. Gastrointestinal bezoars. Br J Surg 1994;81:1000–1001.
44. Walker-Renard P. Update on the medical management of phytobezoar. Am J Gastroenterol 1993;10:1663–1666.

See expertconsult.com for a complete list of references and the review questions for this chapter.

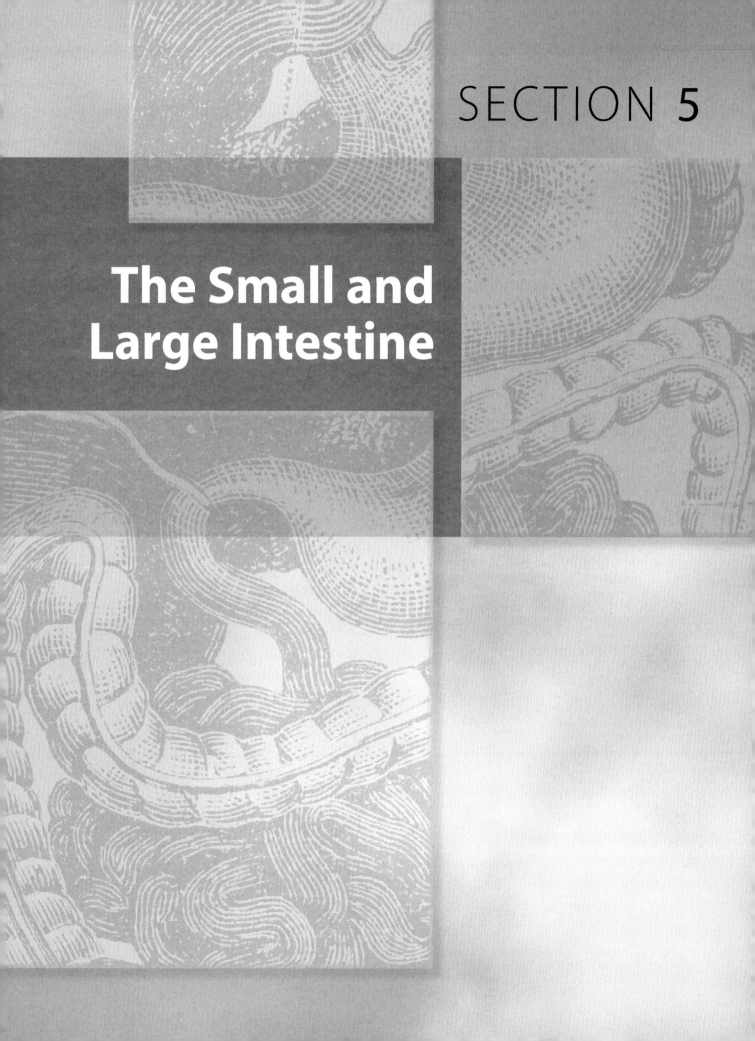

SECTION **5**

The Small and Large Intestine

31

ANATOMY AND PHYSIOLOGY OF THE SMALL AND LARGE INTESTINES

Noah F. Shroyer • Samuel A. Kocoshis

The small and large intestines are contiguous and occupy most of the abdominal cavity. Working in concert, and with remarkable efficiency, they are responsible for several complex functions including digestion and the absorption of nutrients, among them vitamins and trace elements. Other functions include fluid and electrolyte transport, excretion, and physical and immunologic defense mechanisms.

The intestines are morphologically adapted to serve these functions, with distinct regional and anatomic variations. The digestion and absorption of nutrients is almost solely restricted to the small intestine. Fluid and electrolyte transport occur along the entire length of small and large intestines, with most of it taking place in the small intestine.

The mucosal surface of the small intestine is covered by finger-like lumenal projections, called villi, which provide extensive surface area for nutrient absorption. However, this remarkable adaptation unfortunately serves as a double-edged sword, providing a massive interface for possible antigenic interaction with the environment. This interface is modulated via the activity of the immunoendocrine system and the integrative functions of the enteric nervous system. The enteric nervous system is an independent nervous system within the wall of the digestive tract, now often referred to as the second brain, because of its ability to generate and modulate essential gastrointestinal tract functions without input from the autonomic or central nervous system.

There is a growing understanding of the complex processes of nutrient digestion and absorption and the roles of hormones and neurotransmitters in intestinal motility regulation, as well as the vast field of enteric neuroimmunophysiology; these are all beyond the scope of this chapter. This chapter focuses on the morphology of the small and large intestines along with the physiologic roles of fluid and electrolyte transport.

INTESTINAL ANATOMY

Development of the Intestines

The mature intestine develops during embryogenesis from all three germ layers: endoderm, mesoderm, and ectoderm. The endoderm gives rise to the simple columnar epithelial cell lining of the surface of the small and large intestines. Cells of the lamina propria and muscularis layers derive from the embryonic mesoderm. The enteric neurons derive from embryonic ectoderm, specifically from migrating neural crest cells. This schema is true for the esophagus, stomach, pancreas, and liver; organs

of the digestive system are therefore ontogenically and functionally related. Development of the intestine is covered in detail in Chapter 1.

Anatomy of the Small Intestine

The small intestine is a convoluted tubular organ, extending from the pylorus to the ileocecal valve, occupying the central and lower parts of the abdominal cavity. Mostly circumscribed by the large intestines, it is divided into three segments: duodenum, jejunum, and ileum. The average length of the small intestine is between 250 and 300 cm in the newborn,[1,2] increasing to as much as 600 to 800 cm in the adult. The caliber of the small intestine gradually diminishes from its origin to its termination. The duodenum constitutes approximately the first 25 cm of the small intestine in adults; the remaining length is arbitrarily divided into the proximal two fifths, designated as the jejunum, and the distal three fifths, designated as the ileum. The transition from jejunum to ileum is arbitrary, because there are no histologic or gross anatomic demarcations between these segments. The duodenum is derived from the distal foregut during embryologic development. It is partly retroperitoneal. The proximal 2 to 5 cm of the duodenum are occasionally supported on a short mesentery, and the remainder lies firmly fixed in a retroperitoneal position, forming an incomplete circle around the head of the pancreas, where it is devoid of mesenteric cover. The duodenum emerges from this retroperitoneal position at the ligament of Treitz in the left upper quadrant. The duodenum is arbitrarily divided into four segments:

- The first portion of the duodenum, which begins at the pylorus and ends at the neck of the gallbladder, is the most mobile segment.
- The second portion, often referred to as the descending portion, descends from the neck of the gallbladder along the right side of the vertebral column to the level of the third lumbar vertebra.
- The third portion, or the horizontal part, courses over the lower boarder to the third lumbar vertebra, passing from right to left, with a slight inclination upward, lying just inferior to the origin of the superior mesenteric artery in front of the aorta.
- The fourth portion, or ascending part, usually ascends immediately to the left of the aorta, up to the level of the second lumbar vertebra, where it makes a ventral turn to unite with jejunum (duodenojejunal flexure or ligament of Treitz).

The biliary and pancreatic ducts drain into the second portion of the duodenum. In most children, both ducts join together approximately 1 to 2 cm from the outer margins of the duodenal wall, and thereafter traverse the posteromedial aspect of the duodenal wall, through the sphincter of Oddi, to empty into the lumen of the second part of the duodenum at the ampulla of Vater. In 5 to 10% of individuals, an accessory pancreatic duct also enters 1 to 2 cm proximal to the ampulla of Vater, as the duct of Santorini. [3]

The jejunum and ileum are derived from the endodermal midgut. There is no distinct demarcation between them, but progressive structural differences are present from the proximal jejunum to the distal ileum. The jejunum is thicker and more vascular than the ileum, diminishing in size with distal progression. The intestinal luminal diameter is also greatest in the jejunum, shrinking in diameter as it progresses distally.

The jejunum and ileum, attached to and loosely suspended from the posterior abdominal wall by the mesentery, are freely mobile, enabling each coil to accommodate easily to changes in form and position with propulsive peristaltic contractions.

The mesentery begins as an anterior reflection of the posterior peritoneum, attached to the posterior abdominal wall along a line extending from the left side of the body of the lumbar vertebra to the right sacroiliac joint, where it crosses over the duodenum along with other retroperitoneal structures, enveloping the jejunum, ileum, the jejunal and ileal branches of the superior mesenteric blood vessels, nerves, lacteals, lymph nodes, and a variable amount of fat.[3] The mesentery is fan-shaped, with the breadth greater in the middle than at its upper and lower ends. The entire length of the jejunum and the ileum is suspended in the mesentery, with the exception of the very distal ileum, which is retroperitoneal along with the cecum.

The duodenum derives its arterial supply from the right gastric, supraduodenal, right gastroepiploic, and superior and inferior pancreaticoduodenal arteries, whereas the venous drainage is via the superior mesenteric, splenic, and portal veins. The jejunal and ileal branches of the superior mesenteric artery form the arterial arcade that courses through the mesentery to supply the jejunum and ileum. The main venous drainage of the jejunum and ileum is through the portal and superior mesenteric veins.

Lymphatic drainage, coursing through the mesentery from the villous lacteals and the lymph follicles, converges to the preaortic lymph nodes around the superior mesenteric and celiac arteries. Approximately 70% of the lymph passes via the intestinal trunk and about 25% via the thoracic duct to the main subclavian vein.[4] The intestines are overall quite rich in lymphoid tissue; the Peyer's patches are small aggregates of lymphoid tissue located along the antimesenteric border of the small intestine. They are most abundant in the region of the midileum to the ileocecal valve. The Peyer's patches are more prominent during childhood and regress in size and number with advancing age.

The plicae circulares, which are crescentic luminal protrusions of the submucosa covered by mucosa, running almost circumferentially in a circular fashion along the inside diameter of the intestinal wall, are most prominent in the distal duodenum and proximal jejunum, decreasing in number and size with progression through the ileum. They are permanent structures and do not smooth out when the intestine is distended.[3] Together with the continuous reduction in caliber and villus height, these anatomical differences amount to a fourfold reduction in the surface area, occurring over the course of the small intestine from distal duodenum and jejunum to the ileum.

The junction of the small intestines with the large intestines is referred to as the ileocecal valve, partly because of its structural appearance in most individuals and partly because the end of the terminal ileum (being wedged into the wall of the cecum) functions like a flutter valve. The ileocecal valve (sphincter) opens when a peristaltic wave strong enough to overcome the resistance of the valve arrives at the terminal ileum. The cecum, in concert, will manifest reflexive relaxation. Overdistention or peristaltic contraction of the cecum causes a reflexive contraction of the sphincter. This protective mechanism prevents overfilling of the cecum or cecoileal reflux. This is an important factor to be remembered by endoscopists when attempting to intubate the terminal ileum during colonoscopy. Reflexive contraction of the sphincter due to overdistention with air will often thwart successful intubation of the ileum.

Anatomy of the Large Intestine

The large intestine commences at the cecum as a blind pouch below the termination of the small intestine. It curves around, usually encircling the convolutions of the small intestine, and terminates at the rectum. From cephalad to caudad, the large intestine consists of the following segments:
- Cecum and vermiform appendix
- Colon, which in turn is composed of four sections – ascending, transverse, descending, and sigmoid colon
- Rectum
- Anal canal

The colon is approximately 60 cm long in the newborn, increasing to approximately 150 cm in the adult. The caliber of the large intestine is greatest at the cecum and gradually diminishes as it approaches the rectum, where it balloons out considerably in size just above the anal canal.[3] The colonic wall remains fairly constant in thickness throughout its entire length and lacks the villi that are a hallmark of the small intestine. The colon functions as a receptacle and reservoir for fecal matter; periodic high-amplitude contractions propel the contents caudally. Absorption of fluids and electrolytes, which is its main function, takes place along the entire length. The colon is easily distinguished from the small intestine by several distinctive characteristic features:
- It lacks villi.
- It is larger in caliber.
- It is mostly fixed in position.
- Its outer longitudinal muscular layer is congregated into three distinct longitudinal bands, or teniae coli, extending from the cecum to the rectum.
- It has a characteristic sacculated and puckered appearance due to outpouchings (termed haustra) of its walls. The luminal surface is interrupted by intermittent creases (called plicae semilunares) that can be visualized as irregular folds in the luminal surface.
- Fatty projections of the mesentery and the serosa (termed appendices epiploicae) are found scattered over the free surface of the entire large intestine, with the exception of the cecum, vermiform appendix, and rectum.

Extending as a reflection of the peritoneal lining, the mesentery envelops the colon just as it does the small intestine. However, most of the large intestine is fixed in a retroperitoneal manner with only a small portion suspended by the mesentery.

The transverse colon and sigmoid colon are fully suspended by the mesentery, whereas only a portion of the cecum is fully suspended. The prominent mesentery of the transverse colon is termed the transverse mesocolon, and the appendix is anchored by a short and well-defined mesentery referred to as the mesoappendix. The proximal cecum, ascending colon, descending colon, and rectum have only partial mesenteric covering on their anterior surfaces.

Originating from the midgut, the proximal colon, cecum, ascending colon, and proximal two thirds of the transverse colon all derive their blood supply from the superior mesenteric artery. The inferior mesenteric artery supplies the remaining one third of the transverse colon, descending colon, sigmoid colon, and rectum. In addition to the blood supply from the inferior mesenteric artery, the rectum and anal canal also receive blood from the internal iliac and median sacral arteries. The superior and inferior mesenteric veins drain the same regions of the large intestine supplied by the corresponding arteries.[3] With the exception of the lower half of the anal canal, the large intestine derives its nerve supply from the parasympathetic and sympathetic systems. The nerve distribution pattern closely mimics the arterial supply. The proximal colon receives its sympathetic neuronal innervation from the celiac and superior mesenteric ganglia, whereas the parasympathetic supply is from the vagus nerve. In each case the nerves are distributed to the proximal colon in plexuses around the branches of the superior mesenteric artery.[3] The distal colon receives its sympathetic nerve supply via branches from the lumbar segments of the sympathetic trunk, and the parasympathetic nerves originate from the pelvic splanchnic nerves.[5] The lymphatic drainage of the large intestine courses through the mesentery in close proximity to the arterial and venous supplies. First draining through groups of small pericolic nodes along the right and middle colic arteries and their branches, lymph flow from the colon drains into intermediate nodes located within the mesentery. The lymph ultimately terminates in the large colic preaortic nodes surrounding the superior and inferior mesenteric arteries. The rectum and anal canal drain into inferior mesenteric and iliac nodes via perirectal nodes, which lie in close apposition to the rectal walls.

As stated previously, the primary function of the large intestine is water and electrolyte absorption; however, the large intestine is capable of absorbing small quantities of short-chain fatty acids (SCFAs), which are by-products of the anaerobic bacterial fermentation of polysaccharides. The SCFAs absorbed by the colon contribute only about 7% of overall total body energy requirements,[6] with slightly higher amounts being contributed during infancy.[6,7] More importantly, the colonic epithelium depends on the luminal SCFAs for their energy supply,[8] as evidenced by the development of diversion colitis after surgical diversion of the fecal stream and resolution of the colitis with colonic instillation of *n*-butyric acid.[9]

Cecum

The cecum commences as a large pouchlike cul-de-sac in the right iliac fossa and continues superiorly with the ascending colon. Its diameter is greater than its length; the adult cecum measures approximately 6 cm in length and 7.5 cm in width.[3] The ileocecal valve, opening into the posteromedial wall of the cecum at its defined proximal end, passes through the wall in a perpendicular manner pointing slightly

downward. The superior and inferior folds of the ileocecal valve formed by the protrusion of the ileum are arranged in an elliptical manner, forming the orifice of the ileocecal valve. This arrangement allows the valve to function as a sphincter. The appendiceal orifice lies about 2.5 cm inferior to the ileocecal valve. Being supported by a distinct mesentery, the cecum, appendix, and last segment of the ileum are mobile. This mobility accounts for the observed positional variability of these structures within the right lower abdominal quadrant[3] and the rare predisposition for developing a cecal volvulus.[10,11]

Vermiform Appendix

The adjective *vermiform* literally means "worm-like" and describes the narrow, elongated shape of the appendix. The appendix descends inferiorly as a small finger-sized tubular appendage of the cecum. It is typically anywhere between 2 and 20 cm long,[5] being longest in childhood. It generally shrinks during development and throughout adult life. The appendiceal wall is composed of all layers typical of the intestine. Its outer layer and that of the cecum are circumferential, and the teniae coli are not apparent until the level of the ileocecal valve. The appendix, once regarded as a vestigial organ, is now recognized as an important component of the mammalian mucosal immune system, particularly B lymphocyte-mediated immune responses and extrathymically derived T lymphocytes.[12] It shares functional similarities with the pharyngeal tonsils and Peyer's patches. The vermiform appendix may vary greatly in location and be situated either dependently below the distal cecal pouch or behind the cecum, anteriorly or posteriorly to the ileum in a retroperitoneal manner.

Ascending Colon

Originating at the level of the ileocecal valve, the ascending colon is narrower than the cecum.[3] It ascends in a cephalad manner to the inferior surface of the posterior lobe of the liver, where it angulates sharply to the left and slightly forward, forming the hepatic flexure. It measures about 20 cm in length in the adult[13] and is situated retroperitoneally in about 75% of individuals.[5]

Transverse Colon

The ascending colon emerges from its retroperitoneal position, coursing anteriorly and medially to become the transverse colon. It becomes fully enveloped in mesentery (transverse mesocolon) and dips down to a variable extent toward the pelvis as it crosses the abdomen medially to the left upper abdominal quadrant. Here it curves acutely on itself, downward and then upward, forming the splenic flexure.[3] A thickened reflection of the peritoneum, termed the phrenicocolic ligament, anchors the splenic flexure, suspending it higher than the hepatic flexure. The transverse colon lies anterior to the stomach and the small intestine throughout its course and measures approximately 40 to 50 cm in length.[5]

Descending Colon

The descending colon emerges from the splenic flexure, continuing downward and posteriorly to take up a retroperitoneal position with only a partial peritoneal cover on its anterior surface in about 65% of individuals.[5] It measures approximately 25 to 45 cm in length, extending from the splenic flexure to the level of the left iliac crest.[3,5]

Sigmoid Colon

The sigmoid colon begins at the pelvic brim, where it is continuous with the descending colon as it emerges from a retroperitoneal position. The sigmoid colon forms a loop that varies greatly in length, averaging about 40 cm in an adult.[3] It is surrounded and supported by a mesentery termed the sigmoid mesocolon, longest at the center of the loop, then shortening and disappearing as it approaches the rectum. Thus, the sigmoid colon is somewhat fixed at its junctions with descending colon and rectum, respectively. Enjoying a great range of mobility in its central region,[3] it is predisposed to volvulus depending on the length of its mesocolon and/or the degree of distention. The sharpest angulations of the loop occur as the sigmoid turns downward to join the rectum.

Rectum

The rectum extends from the sigmoid colon at the level of the third sacral vertebra following the sacral curvature to the anal canal distally. It initially passes downward and posteriorly, and then directly downward before finally passing downward and anteriorly to join the anus.[3] It measures approximately 12 to 15 cm in length in the adult.[5] The peritoneum is reflected anteriorly at the rectosigmoid junction in most individuals; hence, the entire rectum lies below the peritoneum in close relationship to structures within the pelvis. The anorectal junction usually lies 2 to 3 cm in front of and just below the tip of the coccyx.[3] The rectum is narrowest at its junction with the sigmoid, expanding out into the rectal ampulla at its lower end just before joining the anus. Unlike the sigmoid, the rectum lacks sacculations, appendices epiploicae, and mesentery. The teniae coli converge and blend with the outer muscular layer about 5 to 6 cm above the rectosigmoid junction. The outer rectal wall becomes progressively thickened, forming prominent anterior and posterior muscular bands as it descends toward the anus. The luminal surface of the rectum has two longitudinal and transverse folds; the longitudinal folds are more apparent in the empty state, being easily effaced by rectal distention. The transverse folds or shelves are permanent and more prominent; commonly three folds are present, but this number may vary.[3]

Anorectal Margin

The proximal portion of the anorectal margin is located at the most proximal portion of the anal columns, a grouping of 6 to 10 folds that surround the anorectal canal and project from a cephalad to caudad direction. These columns are more prominent in children than among adults.[3] The depressions between the columns are called the anal folds. These columns converge distally to form small crescentic folds of tissue termed the anal valves. The level at which the anal columns converge to form the anal valves is termed the pectinate line, which is thought to represent the junction between the endodermal and ectodermal portions of the anal canal. Beyond the pectinate line, the epithelial cell layer of the anal canal transitions abruptly from columnar to stratified squamous epithelium, which in turn continues and terminates in an irregular line or "white" zone at the anal opening, termed the zona alba. Differing from the external skin, the zona alba is composed of *nonkeratinized* stratified squamous epithelium, whereas beyond the zona alba, the epithelial layer changes to the typical *keratinized* squamous epithelium of the skin, with the full complement of sweat glands, sebaceous glands, and hair follicles.[3]

Anal Canal

The anal canal begins where the distal end of the rectal ampulla sharply narrows and passes inferiorly and outward to the anal opening. The anal canal is about 2 cm long in the infant, increasing to about 4.5 cm in the adult.[69] The canal occupies the ischiorectal fossa, where it is supported by a number of ligaments and muscular attachments as it pierces the pelvic diaphragm. The physiologic anorectal junction is situated within the pelvic diaphragm, which is made up of the levator ani and coccygeus muscles. The segment of the levator ani sling that encircles the anorectal junction is termed the puborectalis muscle. The contraction of this muscle pulls the rectum forward to retain stool, and the relaxation straightens the anal canal, allowing defecation. The walls of the anal canal are surrounded by a complex of muscular fibers, arranged as the internal and external anal sphincters.[3] Commencing at the anorectal junction, the circular muscle layer of the large intestine thickens to become the internal anal sphincter. This sphincter, composed of smooth muscle fibers, surrounds the upper three quarters of the anal canal.[3] The external sphincter is made up of striated muscle. Surrounding the entire length of the anal canal, the external anal sphincter consists of three parts, namely the subcutaneous, superficial, and deep parts.

Intestinal Histology and Cellular Morphology

The intestinal wall is made up of four layers. From outside inwardly, these consist of the serosa or adventitia, the muscularis propria, the submucosa, and the mucosa. The mucosa is further subdivided into distinct layers, again starting from the outside inwardly: the muscularis mucosa, lamina propria, and epithelial cell layer (Figure 31-1).

The serosa, or the outermost layer, is a simple extension of the visceral peritoneum and mesentery as it envelops the tubular

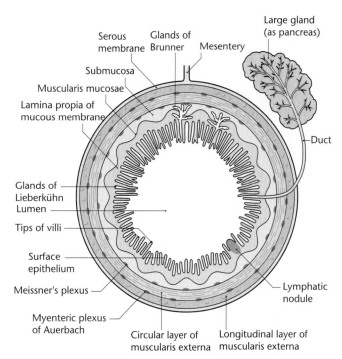

Figure 31-1. Schematic diagram of a cross-section of intestinal mucosa. Adapted from Bloom and Fawcett, 1968.[86]

intestines. It consists of a single layer of flattened mesothelial cells supported by a small amount of connective tissue, the adventitia. All segments of the small intestine are fully invested in the serosal coat with the exception of the retroperitoneal portions (the duodenum and the very terminal portion of the ileum), which have serosal covering only on their anterior or anterolateral surfaces. The large intestine is surrounded by a loose layer of connective tissue termed the adventitia, called the serosa when covered by the peritoneal reflection containing squamous mesothelial cells. Scattered macrophages, eosinophils, mast cells, and fibroblasts are occasionally encountered within the serosa.

The muscularis propria is made up of two distinct layers of smooth muscle: the thinner outer longitudinal layer and the thicker inner circular layer. In the large intestine, the outer longitudinal muscle layer is thickened to form three prominent muscular bands, the teniae coli, which run in parallel to the long axis of colon throughout its entire length. The width of the teniae ranges from 6 to 12 mm in different individuals,[3] and their thickness increases caudally from the cecum to the sigmoid colon. The inner circular muscle layer is thin over the cecum and colon, running circumferentially, but maintaining a slightly oblique orientation to the long axis of the large intestine.[5] Its fibers are especially thickened in the rectum, and in the anal canal they become numerous, forming the internal anal sphincter.

There are two major ganglionated enteric nervous system plexi embedded within the wall of the intestines, the submucosal (Meissner's) plexus and the myenteric (Auerbach's) plexus. Meissner's plexus is found within the submucosa, and the myenteric plexus is located in the plane between the longitudinal and circular layers of the muscularis. The numerous ganglia and localized collection of nerve cell bodies that make up the submucosal and myenteric plexi are extensively interconnected by nerve bundles, giving the appearance of a flat meshwork. Some of the nerve bundles do not connect to ganglia; they ramify over the smooth muscles within the plane of the myenteric plexus to contact individual smooth muscle cells.[4]

The plexi extend without discontinuity within the circumference of the intestinal wall throughout the gastrointestinal tract. The ganglia of the myenteric plexus are more prominent and contain more nerve cell bodies than those of the submucosal plexus.

Interstitial cells of Cajal, present within the myenteric plexus at the interface between the circular muscle and the submucosa, are now recognized as pacemakers of intestinal contractile activity, regulating intestinal tone.[14,15] Abnormalities of the interstitial cells of Cajal have been demonstrated in several intestinal motility disorders.[16,17]

The submucosa consists of a band of loose connective tissue with a scattering of cellular elements, which include lymphocytes, macrophages, mast cells, plasma cells, eosinophils, and fibroblasts. It is bounded below by the muscularis and above by the outermost layer of the mucosa, the muscularis mucosa. The submucosa, lying next to the mucosa, supports it in its specialized function of nutrient, fluid, and electrolyte absorption by carrying a rich network of blood vessels, lymphatics, and nerves. The rich vascular supply and lymphatic drainage ensures efficient handling of absorbed nutrients and fluids following a meal. The extensive nerve network, working via the enteric nervous system, ensures adequate agitation and propulsion of the ingesta, and hormonal secretion and control necessary for efficient digestion and absorption.

Brunner's glands are located almost exclusively in the submucosa of the duodenum; they begin at the pylorus, where they are most numerous, and extend for a variable length within the walls of the proximal jejunum (Figure 31-2). They form

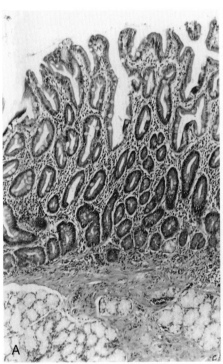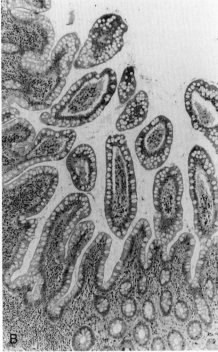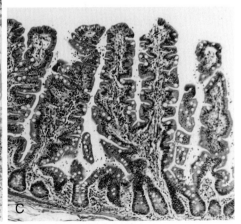

Figure 31-2. Light micrographs of normal human mucosa of the intestine. (**A**) Duodenal mucosa. Brunner's glands are readily identifiable within the submucosa. (**B**) Jejunal mucosa. Villi are tall, thin, and most prominently developed within the jejunum. (**C**) Ileal mucosa. Villi are broader and shorter, goblet cells are prominent, and the lamina propria contains more lymph follicles and lymphoid cells. Hematoxylin and eosin stain, ×100. Courtesy of R. S. Markin, MD.

an array of extensively branched epithelial tubules that contain mainly mucus and serous secretions. Brunner's glands secrete a layer of mucus, forming a slippery viscoelastic gel that lubricates the mucosal lining of the proximal intestinal tract.[5] The mucous layer also possesses the capacity to protect the delicate epithelia surface from peptic digestion. This unique property is due primarily to the gel-forming properties of the glycoprotein molecules (Pb1), class III mucin glycoproteins, and is thought to be the product of mucin gene *MUC6*, assigned to chromosome 11.[18]

Brunner's glands interconnect and drain into the base of the duodenal crypts, where they secrete mucin and bicarbonate to a limited extent, along with a host of additional factors including epidermal growth factor, trefoil peptides, bactericidal factors, proteinase inhibitor, and surface-active lipids.[5] These factors are said to guard against the degradation of the mucin-protective barrier coat and the underlying mucosa by digestive enzymes and other surface-active agents produced in this region. Some of these factors also play important roles in passive and active immunologic defense mechanisms. Brunner's gland secretion, along with bicarbonate, contributes to the increased luminal pH of the region by promoting pancreatic secretion and gallbladder contraction.

The muscularis mucosae is the deepest layer of mucosa, lying next to the submucosa. It consists of an outer longitudinal and inner circular layer of smooth muscle cells. It is a fairly thin layer, being only 3 to 10 cells thick, extending into the circular folds (plicae circularis). The colonic muscularis mucosae is thicker, and the thickness increases progressively from the cecum to the anal canal.[5]

Lying above the muscularis mucosae, the lamina propria provides structural support for the basement membrane of the epithelium. It is composed of a thin layer of connective tissue that embraces the crypts and extends into the villous protrusions. The lamina propria is rich in arterioles, veins, lacteals, nerve fibrils and fibroblasts, as well as various cell types, including lymphocytes, macrophages, eosinophils, mast cells, and neutrophils.

The mucosa is thick and highly vascularized in the proximal portion of the small intestine, but thinner and less vascular in the distal small intestine. The mucosa is thrown into crescentic folds, the plicae circulares (also termed the valves of Kerckring). The small intestinal surface is studded with finger-like or leaflike protrusions, the intestinal villi. These two striking morphologic and physiologic features, along with the formation of microvilli on the epithelial surface, combine to produce a 400- to 500-fold increase in the surface area of the mucosa.[19] The mucosa of the colon is devoid of villi that characterize the small intestine, but contains crypts of Lieberkühn (which are larger than those found in the ileum) and crescentic folds (plicae circulares) that correspond to the external sacculations termed haustra.

The luminal surface of small intestine is covered by millions of tiny hairlike, highly vascularized structures called villi (Figure 31-3). The villi project for about 0.5 to 1.5 mm into the lumen, giving it a velvety appearance and feel. The height of the villi decreases progressively from the duodenum to the ileum. Villi are larger and denser in the duodenum and jejunum, and smaller and fewer in the ileum. [5] They are wider and ridge-shaped in the proximal duodenum, whereas in the distal duodenum and proximal jejunum they are predominantly leaf-shaped and only occasionally finger-shaped. Finger-shaped villi predominate in the distal jejunum and ileum. Villi are covered primarily with mature absorptive enterocytes, interspersed with a few mucus-secreting goblet cells and rare enteroendocrine cells. Each villus contains a central artery, a vein, and a central lacteal. A cascading capillary bed is formed at the tips of the villi in close proximity to the basal surfaces of the epithelium, allowing for rapid clearance of absorbed nutrients, fluids, and electrolytes into the systemic circulation. The capillary walls are fenestrated with diaphragmatic covers, greatly facilitating the absorptive process.[20] The core of the villus also contains some small nerve fibers, plasma cells, macrophages,

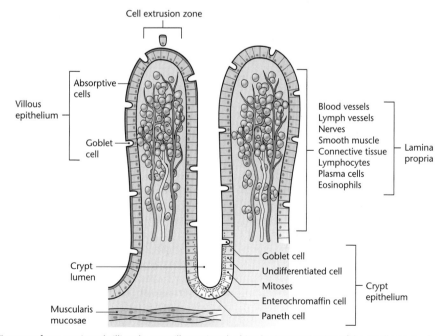

Figure 31-3. Schematic diagram of two sectioned villi and a crypt illustrating the histologic organization of the small intestinal mucosa. Adapted from Sleisenger and Fordtran, 1989.[13]

mast cells, lymphocytes, eosinophils, and fibroblasts. The bases of the villi are surrounded by several pitlike crypts, the crypts of Lieberkühn, extending down through the lamina propria to the muscularis mucosa.

The epithelial cell lining of the small intestine is continuous, but the cell population differs between the villi, the crypts, and the epithelium overlying the Peyer's patches. The crypts are populated primarily by undifferentiated columnar epithelial cells, with a minor scattering of goblet cells, Paneth cells, tuft cells, cuplike cells, and enteroendocrine cells. The villous epithelium contains the same array of cells, with the exception of Paneth cells. The undifferentiated cells are replaced with mature enterocytes. The epithelial cells overlying the Peyer's patches contain all of the aforementioned cells plus functionally and structurally distinct membranous cells (M cells), which are thought to be key sites of antigen and luminal bacteria sampling for the mucosa-associated lymphoid system.[21] M cells are responsible for transepithelial transport, delivering foreign antigens and microorganisms to the mucosal lymphoid tissue for recognition and handling, an attribute currently being exploited in vaccine production.[22] Structurally distinct, the M cells usually assume an oval or globular configuration, but with a widened base and narrowed apex. Some enteroinvasive pathogens are known to exploit these features of M cells to bridge the intestinal epithelial barrier.[23] The M cells are also found in other parts of the body, especially where there is an interface between the mucosal and the external environment; these sites include, but are not limited to, the tonsils, adenoids, airways, and ocular mucosa.[24] The apical microvilli overlying Peyer's patches are randomly shortened and occasionally fused into folds or ridges.

The mucosal epithelial cells are turned over every 5 to 7 days; hence, intense mitotic activity occurs within the intestinal crypts. All intestinal epithelial cells derive from long-lived, resident progenitors or "stem cells." These intestinal stem cells are located near the base of the crypts, where they divide to produce additional stem cells (to maintain their numbers) as well as rapidly dividing progenitors, termed "transit amplifying" cells, that will differentiate into the various epithelial cell types. The transit amplifying cells undergo several additional cell divisions as they migrate upward along the intestinal crypt wall. Cell cycle arrest and differentiation as a distinct cell type (terminal differentiation) occurs near the top of the crypt. In the small intestine, most terminally differentiated cells migrate out of the crypt and onto the villi and are fully mature by the time they reach the upper third of the villus; Paneth cells migrate to the base of the crypt where they reside in close proximity to the stem cells. In the large intestine, terminal differentiation occurs in the upper one third of the crypt, and most cells migrate onto the mucosal surface; in some regions of the large intestine, terminally differentiated cells also migrate to the crypt base, displacing the proliferating cells upward. Old and spent cells are extruded into the intestinal lumen in a process termed anoikis, usually at the tip of the villi or the surface of the colon, to face the same fate of digestion and absorption along with the ingesta. Overlying the Peyer's patches, epithelial cell differentiation includes the production of M cells from nearby stem cells.

Differentiation and homeostasis of the intestinal epithelium is regulated by several key developmental pathways including the WNT (Wingless), NOTCH, BMP (Bone Morphogenetic Protein), and HEDGEHOG pathways.[25,26] These pathways involve signaling between epithelial cells as well as between the epithelium and the underlying lamina propria, particularly the

myofibroblasts.[27] In addition, the growth and integrity of the intestinal mucosa are maintained under the influence of the ingesta and several luminal factors as well as autocrine, endocrine, and paracrine secretion from the surrounding cells. Thus, enteral, humoral, and tissue factors are all essential for the well-being of intestinal mucosa.

It is now clear that therapeutic drugs can be developed to target these developmental pathways. Keratinocyte growth factor (KGF, also termed fibroblast growth factor 7, or palifermin) has been approved for the treatment of radiation- or chemotherapy-induced alimentary canal mucositis.[28] Other peptides secreted from enteroendocrine cells play a major cytoprotective and reparative role in the survival and proliferation of the intestinal mucosa, such as the glucagon-like peptides.[29-32] Glucagon-like peptide (GLP) 1 and GLP-2 are released from enteroendocrine cells in response to nutrient ingestion. GLP-1 enhances glucose-stimulated insulin secretion and inhibits glucagon secretion, gastric emptying and feeding. It also has proliferative and antiapoptotic effects on pancreatic β cells. GLP-2 is a 33-amino-acid peptide, encoded carboxy-terminal to the sequence of GLP-1 in the proglucagon gene. It is an intestinal trophic peptide that stimulates cell proliferation and inhibits apoptosis in the intestinal crypts. Recent clinical trials using GLP-2 suggest that it may have utility in treating patients with short bowel syndrome and Crohn's disease.[33-35]

Absorptive Cells

Lining both the villi and crypts is a layer of cells referred to as the enterocytes, or absorptive cells. These are tall columnar cells, each possessing a basally located, clear, oval nucleus and several nucleoli. The cells are tightly cemented to the basal lamina and are joined to the adjacent enterocytes at the apical pole by intercellular tight junctions. The luminal surface is studded with densely packed (1000 to 2000 per cell) finger-like, cylindrical projections termed microvilli. Each microvillus is about 1 µm long and 0.1 µm wide.[3] The microvilli are constantly bathed by luminal contents and contain the membrane-bound digestive proteins, transport proteins, and other cellular elements necessary for nutrient absorption.

The intestinal microvillus is supported by a central core of cytoskeleton, which consists of highly concentrated microfilaments made up of five major proteins: actin, villin, fimbrin, brush border myosin I, and spectrin.[36] Villin and fimbrin are bundling proteins that crosslink to support a central core of about 20 to 30 actin filaments (Figure 31-4). The microfilaments are continuous and linked at the apical bases of the microvillus, forming a plexiform band called the terminal web, which consists mainly of spectrin. The terminal webs are also interconnected with the junctional complexes or tight junctions. The microvillus is rich in glycoprotein, cholesterol, and glycolipids.

The apical surfaces of the intestinal epithelial cells carry multiple brush-border transporters that couple ion influxes to organic solute influxes, or exchange one ion for another. Three Na/H exchangers (NHEs) have been localized to intestinal brush-border membranes. NHE2 and NHE3 are found in both small intestine and colon.[37] NHE1 is present only in the basolateral membrane of enterocytes and is thought to be involved with HCO_3 secretion. Two anion exchangers have also been localized to small-intestinal and colonic brush-border membranes and cloned. They are named "down-regulated in adenoma" (DRA) and putative anion transporter 1 (PAT1).

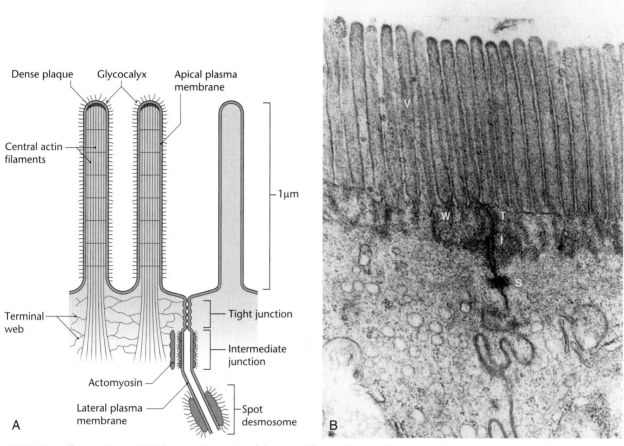

Figure 31-4. Microvillus membrane. (**A**) Schematic illustration of the microvillus membrane and specialized supporting structures of the apical cytoplasm of adjacent intestinal absorptive cells. (**B**) Electron micrograph of adjacent villous absorptive cells. The adjacent cells are tightly adherent through the formation of a junctional complex, containing a tight junction (T), intermediate junction (I), and spot desmosome (S). Thin supporting central filaments of actin are present within the microvillus (V) and terminate by embedding with filaments in the terminal web (W). Magnification ×15,000.

Contiguous enterocytes are tightly apposed at their apicolateral poles by the formation of junctional complexes. These consist of adherence membranes in three areas:

• The most proximal tight junction, or zonula occludens
• An intermediate junction, or zonula adherens
• A deeper junction, the spot desmosome or macular adherence zone

Movements of fluid and ions through this intercellular space from the apical to the basolateral compartment is termed *paracellular transport* and is the dominant pathway for passive fluid and ion flow across the intestinal epithelial barrier into the endothelial cells. Permeability depends on the regulation of the tight junctions.[38]

The tight junction, or zonula occludens, measures approximately 100 to 600 nm in depth,[39] serving as a regulatable, semipermeable diffusion barrier and permitting the passage of ions while restricting the movement of large molecules. The tight junction is leakier and has a lower resistance in the proximal intestine, where absorption is most efficient, and tighter with a higher resistance in the ileum and large intestine. There is also strong evidence suggesting variations in the functional states of the junctional complexes, maintaining a relatively high resistance in the fasting state and a low resistance in the fed state.[19]

Tight junctions contain of a family of transmembrane proteins—claudins, occludins, and junctional adhesion molecules—which are anchored to the membranes of two adjacent cells and interact with one another to bind the cells together and prevent the passage of molecules between them. These membrane proteins are connected with the various signal transduction and transcriptional pathways involved in the regulation of tight junction function via interaction with scaffold proteins.[40,41]

Knowledge about the tight junction has evolved from a relatively simplistic view of it being a physical and permeability barrier in the paracellular space to one of a multicomponent, multifunctional complex that is involved in regulating numerous and diverse cell functions. The tight junction membrane proteins interact with an increasingly complex array of tight junction plaque proteins to regulate paracellular solute and water flux and to integrate diverse processes such as gene transcription, tumor suppression, cell proliferation, and cell polarity.

The zonula adherens, also called the adherens or intermediate junction, is located just below the zonula occludens on the lateral aspect of contiguous cells and is less adherent, with cells being separated by a 15- to 20-nm gap. Forming a beltlike region of cell-to-cell adhesion, the zonula adherens represents the intercellular linkage of transmembrane cadherins to the actin cytoskeleton via the catenins. The zonula adherens component β-catenin plays a dual role as a structural component of those junctions and as a key molecule in the WNT signaling pathway, where it functions as a transcriptional activator.[42]

The most distal portion of the junctional complex is a small circular junction located just below the zonula adherens, often referred to as the macula adherens or spot desmosome. The adjacent lateral membranes here are separated by a gap of about 30 to 50 nm.[5] Unlike the zonula occludens, spot desmosomes are not continuous around the circumference of the cell, but are rather scattered around the cell perimeter in an uneven row. Three calcium-dependent adhesion molecules belonging to the cadherin family – desmoglein I and desmocollins I and II – mediate intercellular attachment. These proteins bind to keratin intermediate filaments via desmoplakins. The overall function of desmosomes appears to be primarily to support cell-cell adhesion and to provide mechanical stability to the epithelium.

The remainder of the lateral wall of the enterocyte below the macula adherens is termed the basolateral membrane. This membrane has unique structural and biologic characteristics that differentiate it from the apical membrane. The basolateral membrane is often plicated and interdigitates with the adjacent lateral cellular membranes. Lacking the brush-border transporters, Na/H exchangers, and digestive enzymes present on the apical membrane, it is embedded with basolateral membrane carriers that facilitate diffusion of organic solutes and are not coupled to ion movements. The basolateral membrane K^+ channels are responsible for K^+ extrusion from the cell and NaK_2Cl co-transporter, which determines the maximal rate of chloride entry into the cell. Na,K-ATPase in the basolateral membrane uses energy from ATP hydrolysis to drive Na^+ extrusion and K^+ uptake.[37]

Gap junctions are communication junctions, consisting of small, circular structures between contiguous cell membranes with a narrow gap in between. The gaps are connected by tiny tubular channels called connexons, composed of connexin proteins, which allow the intercellular passage of ions and low-molecular-weight nutrients and intracellular messengers such as cyclic adenosine monophosphate (cAMP).

In addition to the basally located nuclei, other cellular organelles are present within the enterocyte in anticipated polarity. The Golgi apparatus, responsible for terminal glycosylation of synthesized proteins, lies in a supranuclear position, and just below the terminal web at the apical portion are numerous membrane-bound lysosomes.[3] Also scattered throughout the cytoplasm are free ribosomes, mitochondria, lysosomes, microtubules, and smooth and rough endoplasmic reticulum. The cellular structure and organelles are efficiently arranged and coordinated to work in concert for the absorption, packaging, and subsequent extrusion of absorbed lipids, carbohydrate, and peptides.

Surface Epithelial Cell

Corresponding to the absorptive cells of the small intestine, surface epithelial cells (also termed principal cells[5]) line the large intestinal epithelial surface and the upper one third of the crypts. The luminal surfaces of these columnar cells are capped by apical membranes containing numerous microvilli supported by well-developed terminal webs. The lateral borders of the luminal surfaces are bound by junctional complexes similar to those found in the small intestine. Their cytoplasm contains the usual cytoplasmic organelles. The nucleus is centrally located with a scattering of endoplasmic reticulum located both above and below it. The apical cytoplasm is particularly rich in secretory granules along with scant amounts of Golgi apparatus.

Goblet Cells

Goblet cells are mucin-producing cells found scattered among other cells of the intestinal villi and crypts in lesser numbers than the absorptive cells. Overall, they are found in greater numbers in the large intestine and distal ileum than in the rest of the intestine. The term *goblet cell* derives from the characteristic wineglass shape of these cells in conventionally fixed tissue: a narrow base and an oval apical portion (expanded with mucin-secreting granules) that sometimes extends into the intestinal lumen. If special precautions are taken during tissue fixation, goblet cells can be seen as cylindrically shaped.

Goblet cells usually assume a distinctly polarized morphology, with the nucleus and Golgi apparatus basally situated. The remaining cellular organelles are aligned along the lateral margins of the cell, compressed to these regions by the abundant, membrane-bound mucus-secreting granules within the cell interior.[43-45] Mucin secreted from the goblet cells is largely composed of highly glycosylated proteins suspended in an electrolyte solution. The mucin is secreted via two pathways: (1) a low-level, unregulated, and essentially continuous secretion dependent on cytoskeletal movement of secretory granules; and (2) stimulated secretion via regulated exocytosis of granules in response to irritating extracellular stimuli. This second pathway ensures that mucin production and secretion can rapidly be increased. The goblet cell mucin provides a protective lubricant barrier against shear stress and shields the intestinal mucosa from peptic digestion and chemical damage. It is also thought to bind surface antigens and inhibit their attachment to the epithelial surfaces. The copious amounts of mucin produced by goblet cells is crucial in providing lubrication for the passage of feces.[3]

Gut Endocrine Cells

Enteroendocrine cells, or gut endocrine cells, are a highly specialized mucosal cell subpopulation, sparsely distributed throughout the entire length of the small intestine. The enteroendocrine lineage consists of at least 15 different cell types that are categorized based on their morphology, specific regional distribution, and peptide hormone expression.[46,47] These cells are typically tall and columnar in appearance, and the apical surface is studded with microvilli. They are present in both crypts and villi. Their large nucleus is usually basally located, with the Golgi apparatus situated above the nucleus. The most distinct feature of gut endocrine cells is the prominent cytoplasmic secretory granules, distributed mainly in the basal region of the cell. The secretory granules of the individual gut endocrine cell appear relatively uniform in size, shape, and density, suggesting that the granules may be specific for a single active amine or peptide hormone.

The hormone products are discharged into the extracellular space on the basal and basolateral side of the cell. The hormone diffuses a short distance and passes into the capillary bed underneath, exerting paracrine effects locally within the gastrointestinal tract and endocrine effects regionally or at distal target-organ sites. Some of the specific products of the different cells are shown in Table 31-1. Two pathways of secretion are recognized in gut endocrine cells: one regulating secretion of large, dense-core vesicles (LDCVs), and a second regulating secretion of synaptic-like microvesicles (SLMVs).

TABLE 31-1. **Enteroendocrine Cell Products and Functions**

Secreted Product	Cell Type	Stimuli	Effect
Cholecystokinin (CCK)	I/CCK	Fat and protein	Increases gallbladder contraction and pancreatic secretion; decreases gastric emptying; anorectic
Gastrin	G	Food/nutrient/protein	Increases gastric acid secretion via ECL cells
Ghrelin	P/D1 (gastric), M	Fasting	Increases gastric emptying; orectic
Glucagon-like peptide 1 (GLP-1)	L	Fat	Decreases gastric emptying; incretin effect; anorectic
Glucagon-like peptide 2 (GLP-2)	L	Fat	Intestinal trophic factor; enhances digestive enzyme activity; decreases gastric emptying
Glucose-dependent insulinotropic polypeptide (GIP)	GIP	Fat	Incretin effect
Histamine	ECL	Gastrin	Increases acid secretion
Melatonin		Food/nutrient	Circadian entrainment; increases pancreatic secretion
Motilin	M	Fasting	Cyclic increase regulates migrating motor complex
Neurotensin	N	Fat	Increases pancreatic and biliary secretion and colonic motility; decreases gastric and small intestinal motility; anorectic
Oxyntomodulin (OXM)	L	Nutrients	Anorectic; incretin effect
Pancreatic polypeptide	PP	Food/nutrient	Decreases gastric emptying; anorectic
Peptide YY (PYY)	L	Fat	Decreases gastric emptying and small intestinal motility; anorectic
Secretin	S	Acid	Increases pancreatic secretion
Serotonin (5-HT)	Enterochromaffin, S	Luminal distention	Multiple effects on gastrointestinal motility
Somatostatin (SST)	D	Multiple, complex	Inhibits hormone and exocrine secretion
Uroguanylin		Salt	Regulates sodium homeostasis; mucosal protection

Paneth Cells

Paneth cells are sparse in number and located exclusively at the base of the crypts of Lieberkühn. Their primary function is to secrete antimicrobial products, and they are thought to protect the nearby intestinal stem cells from colonization by potentially pathogenic microbes, thereby conferring protection from enteric infection and contributing to maintenance of the gastrointestinal antimicrobial barrier. They are often pyramidal in shape, with the widest portion at the base. The nucleus is basally located, and the cytoplasm is rich in eosinophilic granules. Paneth cells secrete α-defensins and adenosine monophosphates in response to cholinergic stimulation. When exposed to bacteria or bacterial antigens, they also secrete lysozyme and phospholipase A$_2$, both of which have antimicrobial activity.[48-51]

Animal studies indicate that Paneth cell numbers, location, and granule morphology are altered by infection and zinc status. To date, the most compelling evidence in support of the role of Paneth cells in providing protection against enteric infection is from studies of mice transgenic to overproduce a human Paneth cell α-defensin, HD-5. These mice are completely immune to infection and systemic disease from orally administered *Salmonella typhimurium*.[52]

α-Defensins are the principal antimicrobial molecules secreted by Paneth cells.[53] They are peptides with hydrophobic and positively charged domains that can interact with phospholipids in cell membranes. This structure enables defensins to bind and insert into membranes, where they interlink to form pores that disrupt membrane integrity, leading to cell killing. Owing to the higher density of negatively charged phospholipids in bacterial membranes compared with vertebrate membranes, defensins preferentially bind to and disrupt bacterial cell walls, sparing the cells they are destined to protect.[54,55]

Cup Cells

Constituting 1 to 6% of cells in the crypts and on the villi of the small intestine are intestinal cup cells.[56-58] These are largely limited to the ileum, suggesting a specific but undetermined function. The cells, being narrower than surrounding enterocytes, are tall and columnar with a characteristic cuplike depression of the apical surface. A distinctive feature of the cup cell is the shorter microvilli and the presence of a thickened and extensive glycocalyx coat. Cup cells also have higher cholesterol levels on their microvillus membranes than other enterocytes. The significance of these unique features is yet to be elaborated, and the exact function of the cups remains unknown at present.

Tuft Cells

Tuft cells (also called brush or caveolated cells) are present in the intestinal epithelium in very sparse numbers.[59-62] Their distinctive morphologic features include a wide base, a narrow apex, and a tuft of long microvilli projecting from the apical surface into the gastrointestinal lumen. The microvilli are attached via a core of long microfilaments passing deep into the apical cytoplasm. Between the microvilli are parallel arrays of vesicles (caveoli) containing flocculent material. Tuft cells express chemosensory proteins similar to taste receptor cells of the taste bud and therefore may regulate physiologic responses to nutrients.[63-65]

PHYSIOLOGY OF WATER AND ION TRANSPORT

The epithelial lining of all segments of the intestines from the duodenum to the distal colon is equipped with mechanisms for both absorption and secretion of water and electrolytes[66,67] (Figure 31-5). Water and ions can move in a bidirectional manner across the intestinal mucosa (i.e., from the luminal side

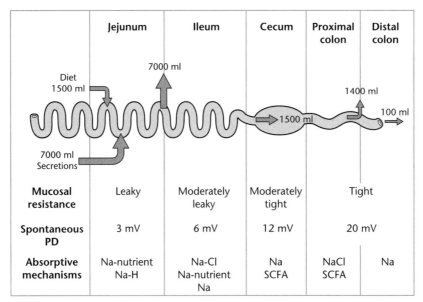

	Jejunum	Ileum	Cecum	Proximal colon	Distal colon
Mucosal resistance	Leaky	Moderately leaky	Moderately tight	Tight	
Spontaneous PD	3 mV	6 mV	12 mV	20 mV	
Absorptive mechanisms	Na-nutrient Na-H	Na-Cl Na-nutrient Na	Na SCFA	NaCl SCFA	Na

Figure 31-5. Overview of intestinal fluid balance. Some 8 to 9 L of fluid flow into the intestine; salivary, gastric, biliary, pancreatic and intestinal secretions make up the bulk of this amount. Most intestinal fluid is absorbed in the small bowel, with approximately 1500 mL of fluid crossing the ileocecal valve. The colon extracts most of this fluid, leaving 100-200 mL of water daily. On progression down the intestine, it becomes increasingly "tight"; potential difference (PD) measurements demonstrate a corresponding rise. Absorptive mechanisms in each segment of the gut differ, but chloride secretion is found throughout the gut. SCFA, short-chain fatty acids. Adapted from Sleisenger and Fordtran, 1989.[13]

into the blood and lymphatics, or from the serosal side into the intestinal lumen). In the physiologic state, the two opposing processes (absorption and secretion) result in a net absorption of fluid and electrolytes, maintaining normal homeostasis. The difference between the two unidirectional fluxes, or the "net" ion flux, determines the direction of net transport.

Absorption

Water, ion, and solute absorption across the intestinal mucosa occurs via three distinct routes and mechanisms.

The first is via active ion-coupled solute transport. A Na^+ gradient is the driving force of solute absorption via this route. Organic solutes such as glucose, galactose, amino acids, and oligopeptides are absorbed across the small intestinal apical mucosa via carriers whose movement is coupled to that of Na^+. Na^+ coupling provides the electrical and chemical forces that drive organic solutes uphill against a concentration gradient (i.e., from a low intraluminal concentration to a higher concentration in the intracellular environment) – a gradient opposing that of sodium. The organic solute is then transported by basolateral membrane carriers independent of ion movement, downhill from the enterocyte via the basolateral membrane into the intestinal capillaries. Some oligopeptides are absorbed unhydrolyzed and intact across the intestinal apical membrane via a proton-coupled mechanism. The oligopeptide uptake is indirectly coupled to Na^+ transport, and the proton needed for this is provided by Na^+/H^+ exchange, a process that acidifies the unstirred layer just above the enterocyte apical membrane.[37]

Salt is absorbed along with these organic solutes, creating an osmotic gradient for water to follow. It is thought that about 80% of water absorption takes places via the paracellular pathways under the influence of local osmotic gradient within these paracellular channels.[68-70]

The second absorptive mechanism involves absorption of electrolytes in the absence of nutrients via activity of intestinal brush-border proteins now known as Na^+/H^+ exchangers (NHEs). Available data suggest different transport mechanisms in the jejunum and ileum. In the jejunum, sodium bicarbonate ($NaHCO_3$) is absorbed via an exchange of an equivalent amount of luminal HCO_3 because secreted H^+ and Cl^- movement is purely passive, whereas in the ileum NaCl is absorbed via equal rates of Na^+/H^+ and Cl^-/HCO_3^- exchanges.

Three NHEs have been identified, localized to intestinal apical membranes and cloned. NHE1 was the first to be identified and is present only in the basolateral membrane of enterocytes. It is involved in HCO_3 secretion. NHE2 and NHE3 are found in both the small and the large intestine. NHE activity and expression are stimulated by nutrients and regulated by pathological processes such as inflammation.[71] NHE3 appears to play a more important role in intestinal absorption, as NHE2 knockout mice have normal intestines but develop gastric dysfunction, whereas NHE3 knockout mice are plagued by chronic diarrhea.[37,72,73] A family of anion exchangers, namely "down-regulated in adenoma" (DRA or SLC26A3), pendrin (PDS or SLC26A4), and putative anion transporter 1 (PAT1 or SLC26A6), have been localized to small intestinal and colonic apical membranes and cloned.[74,75] DRA and pendrin are thought to mediate Cl^-/base exchange.[76] DRA was identified and first cloned from the colonic mucosa. Subsequently, it was found to be down-regulated in villous adenomas and carcinomas. The *DRA* gene encodes a chloride transporter defective in the rare congenital chloride diarrhea, and mutations in *DRA* result in a recessively inherited disorder characterized by massive loss of chloride in stool.[77] The functional identity and distribution of PAT1 (SLC26A6) was initially not clear. However, recent functional studies demonstrated that PAT1 plays a central role in Cl^-/HCO_3^- exchange in the small intestine, mediating absorption of chloride and secretion of bicarbonate. It may also be involved in the absorption of anionic organic weak acids in the small intestine.[78,79] PAT1 expression is limited predominantly to the small intestine and stomach, with minimal expression in the large intestine. This pattern of expression is essentially opposite that of *DRA*, which is predominantly expressed in colon but scantily expressed in small intestine, with the duodenum being the site of greatest small intestinal expression.

The upper gastrointestinal tract, particularly the duodenum, is constantly exposed to an acidic chyme delivered from stomach, with a pH that is sometimes as low as 1.5.[80,81] Mucin production from the goblet cells (as previously discussed) and secretion of bicarbonate to buffer the acid are the main defense mechanisms for protecting the duodenal mucosa against acid injury. DRA and PAT1 are abundant in the duodenum and present at higher density there than NHE2 and NHE3, suggesting a role in duodenal alkalinization.

To engage efficiently in the transcellular transport of ions, the enterocyte requires the simultaneous function and operation of more than two ion exchangers. In addition to the increased turnover of the Na^+/K^+ pump, the opening of basolateral membrane Cl^- and K^+ channels is essential to prevent swelling of the enterocyte by allowing serosal exit of the Cl^- taken up from the lumen and extrusion of the K^+ taken up by the Na^+/K^+ pump.

The third and final route of solute absorption is via the paracellular pathway. This is the dominant route for passive solute transport across the intestinal epithelial membrane.[82] The permeability of this pathway is modulated via the regulation of the intracellular tight junctions or zonula occludens, which function as a barrier between apical and basolateral compartments, restricting the flow of luminal contents into the blood and lymphatics, and vice versa. The tight junctions counterregulate the gradient generated by the transcellular pathways by selectively allowing passive diffusion of small hydrophilic molecules and ions from the intestinal lumen into the bloodstream and the lymphatics. Tight junctions are dynamic structures constantly subjected to changes that dictate their functional status under a variety of physiologic and pathologic conditions.

The electrical resistance and permeability of these tight junctions are thought to be dependent on a complex interaction of transmembrane protein microfilaments and discrete extracellular proteins, as described previously.

Secretion

Chloride secretion occurs in the intestinal crypt cells throughout the small intestine, whereas chloride is generally absorbed in the large intestine.[83] Four separate transmembrane transporters are now recognized to regulate intestinal chloride secretion. These are the apical chloride channel (the cystic fibrosis transmembrane conductance regulator, CFTR), basolateral membrane K^+ channel, basolateral membrane Na^+,K^+,Cl^- co-transporter, and basolateral membrane Na^+,K^+ ATPase. Chloride secretion is activated by phosphorylation and opening of the CFTR chloride channel by protein kinases, which are in turn activated by various stimuli including pathogenic enterotoxins, endogenous secretagogues, and enteric neurotransmitters. Additional members of the chloride channel family (ClC family) can also contribute to chloride secretion. Chloride secretion into the lumen is driven by the electronegative intracellular environment relative to the electroneutral lumen. Sodium and water are drawn to the luminal chloride via the paracellular pathway, resulting in net fluid and ion secretion. The Na^+,K^+ ATPase maintains the high extracellular Na^+ required for this effect. The basolateral membrane K^+ channels, including the IK1 and KvLQT1 proteins, then open to repolarize the cell, counteracting the

TABLE 31-2. Daily Average Influx of Fluid Into the Gastrointestinal Tract (Volume, Liters)

Ingestion	1-1.5
Saliva production	0.25-0.5
Gastric secretions	0.5-1
Bile production	0.5-1
Pancreatic secretion	0.5-5
Small bowel secretion	2-3

depolarizing effect of the Cl^- channel. This sequence ensures the sustenance of the electrical driving force, namely chloride secretion into the intestinal lumen. Once the apical channels and the basolateral K^+ channels have been mobilized and activated, the basolateral membrane Na^+,K^+,Cl^- co-transporter is the rate-limiting factor for chloride entry into the cell from the serosa through the basolateral membrane.

In the ileum and colon, NHEs and Cl^-/HCO_3^- exchangers in the apical membranes produce net electroneutral absorption of NaCl and secretion of H^+ HCO_3^-. The dual action of the DRA (SLC26A3) and PAT1 (SLC26A6) proteins produces an electroneutral secretion of HCO_3^- and absorption of Cl^-. Chloride-independent mechanisms of bicarbonate secretion include cAMP-dependent secretion and HCO_3^- secretion associated with absorption of short-chain fatty acids.[84]

Daily Gastrointestinal Tract Fluid Fluxes

On average, an adult secretes or ingests 7 to 8 liters of fluid into the gastrointestinal tract daily (Table 31-2). Saliva and oral intake accounts for about 1.5 liters per day; 1.5 liters of gastric acid and digestive enzymes is sequestered daily, whereas bile and pancreatic secretion respectively contribute 1 liter each.

During the initial phase of intestinal digestion, a net flux of about 3 liters of fluid is secreted into the lumen following the osmotic gradient across the relatively loose "tight" junction of the jejunal mucosa. However, about 6 liters of secreted fluid and electrolytes is reabsorbed back within the jejunum and ileum, and only about 1.2 liters of fluid is released into the colon daily. The colon absorbs about 1 liter of fluid, releasing about 0.2 liters in the feces.

Endogenous Neuroendocrine and Paracrine Regulation of Absorption and Secretion

Two distinct groups of regulatory compounds are known to mediate the intestinal epithelial function. One group inhibits active electrolyte absorption and stimulates active secretion (Table 31-3). The other group has the opposite effect, stimulating active absorption and inhibiting secretion (Table 31-4).[85]

The first group (prosecretory and antiabsorptive) includes four classes of agents:
- Neurotransmitters, including acetylcholine, substance P, vasoactive intestinal peptide (VIP), and nucleotides (ATP and UDP)
- Paracrine agents, including serotonin and neurotensin
- Proinflammatory agents, including but not limited to histamine, serotonin, prostaglandins, leukotrienes, and platelet-activating factor
- Guanylin

TABLE 31-3. Endogenous Control of Ion and Water Transport: Secretory Agents

Agent	Source	Target	Intracellular mediator(s)
Prostaglandin	Mesenchymal cells	Epithelial and neural cells	cAMP, Ca^{2+}, and protein kinase C
Neurotensin	Epithelial endocrine cells	Enteric neurons	Protein kinase C and Ca^{2+}
Guanylin	Goblet cells	Epithelial cells	cGMP
Serotonin (5-hydroxytryptamine; 5-HT)	Mast and epithelial endocrine cells	Epithelial and neural cells	Protein kinase C and Ca^{2+}
Vasoactive intestinal peptide (VIP)	Enteric neural cells	Epithelial cells	Protein kinase C and Ca^{2+}
Acetylcholine (Ach)	Enteric neural cells	Epithelial, mesenchymal, and neural cells	Ca^{2+} and protein kinase C
Substance P	Enteric neural cells	Mast, epithelial, and neural cells	Ca^{2+} and protein kinase C
Histamine	Mast cells	Mesenchymal and neural cells	Ca^{2+}, cAMP, and protein kinase C
Platelet-activating factors	Ca^{2+}, cAMP, and protein kinase C	Mesenchymal cells	Ca^{2+}, cAMP, and protein kinase C
Adenosine	Epithelial cells	Epithelial and mesenchymal cells	Ca^{2+}, cAMP, and protein kinase C
Leukotrienes	Mesenchymal cells	Epithelial and neural cells	Ca^{2+}, cAMP, and protein kinase C
Bradykinin	Vascular	Mesenchymal cells	Ca^{2+}, cAMP, and protein kinase C
ATP/ADP	Enteric neurons	Epithelial and mesenchymal cells	Protein kinase C and Ca^{2+}

TABLE 31-4. Endogenous Control of Ion and Water Transport: Antisecretory Agents

Agent	Source	Target Cell	Intracellular Mediator(s)
12-Hydroxyeicosatetraenoic acid (12-HETE)	Mesenchymal cells	Epithelial and neural cells	Blockage of basolateral K^+ channel
Neuropeptide Y	Enteric neural and epithelial endocrine cells	Epithelial and neural cells	Unknown
Norepinephrine	Neural cells	Epithelial and neural cells	Activation of inhibitory G protein
Somatostatin	Enteric neural and epithelial endocrine cells	Epithelial and neural cells	Activation of somatostatin receptors

The second group consists of compounds that promote active ion absorption and inhibit active bicarbonate and chloride secretion. These compounds include neuropeptide Y, norepinephrine, somatostatin, and most neurotransmitters.

Mast cells are the major effector cells for immediate hypersensitivity and chronic allergic reactions. Acting on the extensive interface between intestinal surface epithelium and the external environment, they elaborate a variety of autocrine/paracrine secretions including adenosine, leukotriene B_4, substance P, acetylcholine, histamine, serotonin, and several chemokines. The presence of antigenic threats is detected by receptor-bound antigen-specific immunoglobulin E (IgE), priming the mast cells to recognize the sensitizing antigens and regulate the response to these threats. During subsequent encounters, the mast cells signal the presence of the inciting antigen to the enteric nervous system. The signal is interpreted as a threat, and the enteric nervous system initiates a programmed secretory and propulsive motor behavior organized to eliminate the threat rapidly and effectively. This programmed alarm system protects the individual, but at the expense of often uncomfortable symptoms that include cramping abdominal pain, fecal urgency, and diarrhea.

REFERENCES

25. Scoville DH, Sato T, He XC, Li L. Current view: intestinal stem cells and signaling. Gastroenterology 2008;134:849–864.
35. Yazbeck R, Howarth GS, Abbott CA. Growth factor based therapies and intestinal disease: is glucagon-like peptide-2 the new way forward?. Cytokine Growth Factor Rev 2009;20:175–184.
42. Brembeck FH, Rosario M, Birchmeier W. Balancing cell adhesion and Wnt signaling, the key role of beta-catenin. Curr Opin Genet Dev 2006; 16:51–59.
47. Rindi G, Leiter AB, Kopin AS, et al. The "normal" endocrine cell of the gut: changing concepts and new evidences. Ann N Y Acad Sci 2004;1014: 1–12.
63. Bezencon C, le Coutre J, Damak S. Taste-signaling proteins are coexpressed in solitary intestinal epithelial cells. Chem Senses 2007;32:41–49.
71. Kiela PR, Xu H, Ghishan FK. Apical NA^+/H^+ exchangers in the mammalian gastrointestinal tract. J Physiol Pharmacol 2006;57(Suppl 7):51–79.

See expertconsult.com for a complete list of references and the review questions for this chapter.

MALDIGESTION AND MALABSORPTION

32

Reinaldo Garcia-Naveiro • John N. Udall, Jr.

Food assimilation is the major function of the gastrointestinal tract. Most nutrients cannot be absorbed in their natural form, and for this reason they need to be digested. Food is chemically reduced to digestive end products, small enough to participate in the absorption process across the intestinal epithelium. An understanding of the pathophysiology of maldigestion and malabsorption should be based on a knowledge of the normal steps of digestion and absorption. Normal intestinal assimilation can be divided into sequential physiologic stages: (1) hydrolysis and solubilization in the lumen and at the enterocyte membrane and (2) absorption across the intestinal mucosa and into systemic body fluids.

Hydrolysis is the basic process of digestion. Carbohydrates, fats, and proteins undergo digestion by hydrolysis. The difference in the process for each nutrient lies in the enzymes required to promote the digestive reaction. Different physiologic processes, such as solubilization, intestinal motility, and hormone secretion, are also involved in normal digestion and absorption. Following digestion in the intestinal lumen and at the brush border, monosaccharides, monoglycerides, fatty acids, small peptides, and amino acids are then absorbed and processed by the enterocyte. Vitamins, minerals, and water also participate in the process. A nutrient must be transported into blood and lymph in order to be stored or metabolized in distant organs. Any disease that interrupts the delicate sequence of reactions important in digestion and absorption may lead to maldigestion and malabsorption and end in malassimilation.

These physiologic stages may be altered in intestinal disease (Table 32-1). For clinical purposes, maldigestion and malabsorption are discussed by nutrient group, starting with carbohydrates, then lipids, proteins, vitamins, minerals, and water.

CLASSES OF NUTRIENTS

Carbohydrates

The type of carbohydrates ingested varies with age. During infancy, lactose accounts for most of the dietary carbohydrate.[1] However, in older children and adults, starch makes up much of the ingested carbohydrates, with smaller amounts of lactose and sucrose.[2] Even when considered on a worldwide basis, carbohydrates constitute the major source of calories in the human diet. They are divided into four major groups: (1) monosaccharides or simple sugars, which cannot be hydrolyzed into a simpler form; (2) disaccharides, which yield two molecules when hydrolyzed; (3) oligosaccharides, which yield 2 to 10 monosaccharides when hydrolyzed; and (4) polysaccharides, which yield more than 10 molecules on hydrolysis. A schematic representation of digestion and absorption of dietary carbohydrates is shown in Figure 32-1.

People in the Western world consume about 400 g of carbohydrates daily. Starches (glucose polymers), as noted previously, represent the largest portion of ingested carbohydrates. Much of the starch in the diet is present in wheat, rice, and corn as polysaccharides whose molecular weight ranges from 100,000 to greater than 1,000,000. The two chief constituents of starch are amylose, which is nonbranching in structure, and amylopectin, which consists of highly branched chains.[2] Each is composed of a number of α-glucosidic chains having 24 to 30 glucose molecules apiece. The glucose residues are united by 1:4 or 1:6 linkages (branch point). Dietary fiber, which is nonstarch polysaccharides and lignin from plants, is not subject to digestion in the intestine of humans but is an important source of "bulk" in the diet.

Digestion of carbohydrates starts in the mouth. The carbohydrate comes in contact with saliva, produced by three pairs of salivary glands: the parotid, submandibular, and sublingual. These three pairs of glands contribute 20, 60, and 20%, respectively, to the total amount of saliva.[3] Numerous smaller glands are located in the lips, palate, tongue, and cheeks; these glands also contribute to the exocrine fluid. Saliva contains mucin, a "slimy" glycoprotein important for lubrication and a serous secretion rich in ptyalin, an α-amylase, which participates in the hydrolysis of starch.

Salivary and pancreatic α-amylases act on interior α1,4 glucose-glucose links of starch but cannot attack α1,4 linkages close to α1,6 branch points or the α1,6 branch point. Pancreatic α-amylase is normally secreted in excess. For this reason, carbohydrate hydrolysis is impaired only in severe forms of pancreatic insufficiency. Because α-amylase cannot hydrolyze the 1,6 branching links and has relatively little specificity for 1,4 links adjacent to these branch points, large oligosaccharides containing five to nine glucose units and consisting of one or more 1,6 branching links are produced by α-amylase action. The products of this digestion are the disaccharide maltose, the trisaccharide Maltotriose. and α-limit dextrins, branched polymers containing an average of about eight glucose molecules.[2]

The final stages of carbohydrate digestion occur by enterocyte membrane-associated enzymes. Disaccharides are hydrolyzed to monosaccharides by specific enzymes located in the brush border of intestinal epithelial cells (see Figure 32-1). The disaccharidases are, in fact, mostly oligosaccharidases, which hydrolyze sugars containing three or more hexose units. They are present in highest concentration at the villous tips in the jejunum and persist throughout most of the ileum, but not in the colon.

TABLE 32-1. **Gastrointestinal Diseases Associated With Maldigestion and Malabsorption**

Disease/Condition	Pathophysiology	Disease/Condition	Pathophysiology
Intraluminal Digestion		Lowe's syndrome	X-linked trait with defect in transport of lysine and arginine
Stomach		Glucose-galactose malabsorption	Selective defect in glucose and galactose sodium co-transport system
Protein-calorie malnutrition	Decreased acid production, hypochlorhydria	Congenital chloride diarrhea	Selective defect in chloride transport by the intestine
Zollinger-Ellison syndrome	Inactivation of pancreatic enzymes at a low duodenal pH, and decreased ionization of conjugated bile salts	A-β-lipoproteinemia	Absent production of apolipoprotein B, lipoproteins, and chylomicrons
Pernicious anemia	Decreased intrinsic factor secretion, vitamin B_{12} malabsorption	Hypobetalipoproteinemia	Impaired production of apolipoprotein B
Dumping syndrome	Rapid emptying of stomach contents into the small intestine, dilution of enzymes	Celiac disease	Damage to absorptive/digestive surface
		Short bowel syndrome	Loss of absorptive/digestive surface, abnormal transit
Pancreas		Mucosal injury syndromes	Damage to digestive/absorptive surface
Cystic fibrosis	Impaired secretion of enzymes and bicarbonate	Milk/soy protein intolerance	
Shwachman-Diamond syndrome	Impaired secretion of enzymes	Postenteritis syndrome	
Acute/chronic pancreatitis	Impaired secretion of enzymes and bicarbonate	Tropical sprue	Damage to digestive/absorptive surface
Protein-caloric malnutrition	Impaired secretion of enzymes	Bacterial infection/ inflammation	
Trypsinogen deficiency	Impaired secretion of enzymes	*Shigella*	Damage to digestive/absorptive surface, abnormal motility
Lipase deficiency	Impaired secretion of enzymes	*Salmonella*	Damage to digestive/absorptive surface, abnormal motility
Amylase deficiency	Impaired secretion of enzymes	*Campylobacter*	Damage to digestive/absorptive surface, abnormal motility
Liver		Cholera	Secretory water and electrolyte loss
Cholestasis syndromes	Impaired secretion of bile salts with deficient micelle formation	Giardiasis	Disruption of epithelial function secondary to adhesion or toxin (?)
Surgery	Intestinal malabsorption of bile salts, deficient bile salt pool	Crohn's disease	Damage to digestive/absorptive surface, chronic gastrointestinal blood loss
Intestine		Whipple's disease	Lymphatic obstruction, impaired lipid transport (?), patchy enteropathy
Enterokinase deficiency	Impaired activation of luminal pancreatic enzymes	Viral infection	
Protein-caloric malnutrition	Bacterial overgrowth with consumption of nutrients, toxin production, and deconjugation of bile acids	Rotavirus	Damage to digestive/absorptive area
		Human immunodeficiency virus	Damage to digestive/absorptive area, bacterial overgrowth, exocrine pancreatic and hepatic insufficiency
Anatomic duplication	Bacterial overgrowth with consumption of nutrients	Acrodermatitis enteropathica	Impaired absorption of zinc
Blind loop syndrome	Bacterial overgrowth with consumption of nutrients	*Uptake Into Blood and Lymph*	
Short bowel syndrome	Bacterial overgrowth with consumption of nutrients	Congestive heart failure	Venous distention, bowel wall edema
Pseudo-obstruction	Bacterial overgrowth with consumption of nutrients	Intestinal lymphangiectasia	Obstructed lymphatic transport of lipid and fat-soluble vitamins, intestinal protein loss
Digestion at the Enterocyte Membrane		*Miscellaneous Disorders*	
Congenital disaccharidase deficiency	Impaired digestion of a specific disaccharide leading to bacterial fermentation in the colon	Immune deficiency syndromes	Altered bacterial flora
Lactase		Allergic gastroenteropathy	Unknown immune mechanism
Sucrase-isomaltase		Eosinophilic gastroenteropathy	Unknown immune mechanism
Trehalase		Drugs	
Acquired/late-onset disaccharidase deficiency	Loss of enzyme activity due to mucosal injury or loss of activity with age	Methotrexate	Damage to mucosal surface by interference with enterocyte replication
Lactase		Cholestyramine	Blocked reabsorption of bile salts in the ileum by drug; malabsorption of calcium, fat, bile acids, and fat-soluble vitamins
Sucrase-isomaltase			
Glucoamylase			
Enterocyte Absorption		Phenytoin	Calcium, folic acid malabsorption
Protein-calorie malnutrition	"Damage" vs. "adaptive regulation," altered mucosal architecture	Sulfasalazine	Folic acid malabsorption
Hartnup's disease	Transport defect of neutral amino acids	Histamine H_2 receptor antagonists	Impaired acid/proteolytic liberation of vitamin B_{12}
Lysinuric protein intolerance	Transport defect of dibasic amino acids in intestine and kidney		
Blue diaper syndrome	Transport defect of tryptophan		
Oasthouse syndrome	Transport defect of methionine in intestine and kidney		

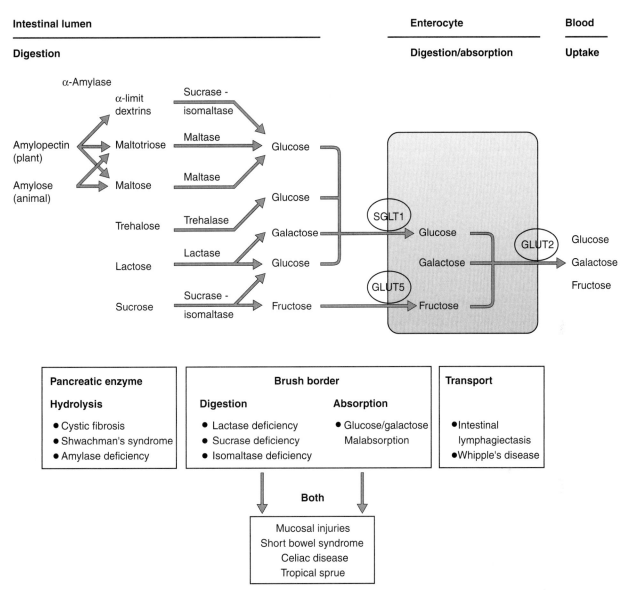

Figure 32-1. Digestion of carbohydrates is initiated by salivary and pancreatic α-amylase (endoenzymes). They digest the linear "internal" α-1,4 linkages between glucose residues, but cannot break "terminal" α-1,4 linkages. They also cannot split the α-1,6 linkages at the branch points of amylopectin or the adjacent α-1,6 linkages. The products of α-amylase action are linear glucose oligomers, maltotriose, maltose, trehalose, lactose, and sucrose. Brush border oligosaccharidases, intrinsic membrane proteins with their catalytic domains facing the lumen, hydrolyze the products of α-amylase digestion. Absorption occurs by way of SGLT1, which is the sodium-coupled transporter that mediates the uptake of glucose and galactose from the lumen into the enterocyte, and GLUT5, which mediates the facilitated diffusion of fructose into the enterocyte. Uptake of monosaccharides across the basolateral membrane and into the interstitial space occurs by GLUT2. GLUT, glucose transporter; SGLT, sodium/glucose co-transporter.

Digestion and absorption of carbohydrates from the diet leads to the entry of three monosaccharides into the circulation: glucose, fructose, and galactose. In normal subjects, the capacity of the small intestine is such that virtually all the free mono- and disaccharides present in the normal diet are completely absorbed. However, when there is malabsorption of disaccharides, monosaccharides, or other carbohydrates, such as sorbitol or xylitol, these sugars are emptied into the colon. The unabsorbed carbohydrates may then be fermented by colonic bacteria, which leads to the production of carbon dioxide, hydrogen, and methane. Propionic and butyric acids, both short-chain fatty acids, are also produced. Butyric acid can be utilized by colonic mucosal cells as an energy source, and the bulk of the absorbed propionate is cleared by the liver.[4]

The most common type of carbohydrate maldigestion and malabsorption is caused by intestinal lactase deficiency. There are several types of lactase deficiency: congenital, adult-onset, and secondary lactase deficiency. Congenital lactase deficiency is rare and is associated with symptoms occurring a short time after birth when lactose is present in the diet.[5] The largest group of patients with this disorder is from Finland, where at least 16 cases have been described.[6] Adult-onset lactase deficiency is extremely common and "normal" for most humans, beginning as early as 2 years of age in some racial groups and as late as adolescence in others. Individuals with adult-onset lactase deficiency comprise the majority of the world's population. Individuals of northern European ancestry and certain groups in Africa and India, however, maintain lactase activity throughout adulthood. This ethnically related lactase deficiency is the most common cause of lactose intolerance. On a global scale, it is obvious that persistence of the ability to digest lactose is the exception rather than the rule. Mutation of a regulatory gene for lactase has been postulated to explain the delayed onset of hypolactasia. There may be a genetically controlled "switching off" of the lactase gene in susceptible individuals.[7-9] Continuing milk intake in populations known to become lactase deficient beyond the childhood years can affect the age of onset. Lactase does not behave as an inducible enzyme, but continued exposure to milk products can, to a certain degree, affect the regulatory gene.[10,11]

The prevalence of lactose intolerance in the white population of the United States is about 20%, whereas in American Indians, Eskimos, Japanese and Chinese, the prevalence is 80 to 100%. In the Scandinavian countries, lactose intolerance occurs in 2 to 15% of the population. As noted earlier, the age of onset of this ethnically associated lactase deficiency varies from early childhood to late teenage years. In African Americans, symptomatic lactose intolerance increases after 10 years of age.

Secondary lactase deficiency occurs following infectious gastroenteritis or injury to the small intestinal mucosa caused by gluten or other sensitizing substances. Recovery of full function of this disaccharidase might take months, because lactase is the last disaccharidase to return to normal following injury. This secondary lactose intolerance has popularized the use of formulas containing sucrose or glucose polymers for children recovering from gastroenteritis. In addition, damage to the intestinal mucosa may increase the likelihood not only of lactose malabsorption, but also of a cow's-milk protein sensitivity. This has also encouraged the use of soy protein, protein hydrolysates, and amino acid–based formulas. There is evidence that implicates protein hypersensitivity in prolonged diarrhea seen in some children, with progression to a more chronic form of diarrhea. The damaged mucosa is thought to have decreased levels of disaccharidases. Continued ingestion of disaccharide when the enzyme important in hydrolysis is deficient may perpetuate the diarrhea.

The presence of malabsorbed substrate in the intestinal lumen is responsible for the fluid shifts that occur in osmotic diarrhea. Fermentation by colonic bacteria contributes to cramps and bloating. It seems prudent to withhold lactose, or at least to decrease its total intake, in children with severe gastroenteritis for a period of 1 to 3 weeks if there is evidence of lactose intolerance. An exception to this guideline is the recommended practice of continuing breast feedings during acute gastroenteritis.[12,13]

Sucrase is a hybrid molecule consisting of two enzymes – one hydrolyzing sucrose into glucose and fructose and the other enzyme hydrolyzing the $\alpha1,6$ branch points of α-limit dextrins. Therefore, sucrase-isomaltase and not "sucrase" is the preferred term for this disaccharidase. The molecular relation and sharing of active sites between sucrase and isomaltase is still of great interest to geneticists and biochemists, because deficiency of one enzyme is accompanied by abnormal activity of the second. Congenital sucrase-isomaltase deficiency was first described in 1961 by Weijers and co-workers.[14] Although it is generally considered to be a rare condition, the heterozygote frequency in white subjects is 2%. The homozygote condition, rare in whites, is as high as 5% in Greenlanders.[15] Symptoms vary from severe diarrhea in infancy to intermittent diarrhea, cramps, and gas in the older child. The correct diagnosis may be missed for years, with symptoms being attributed to "toddler's diarrhea" or "maternal anxiety." When the diagnosis is suspected on clinical grounds, a breath hydrogen test after an oral sucrose load

or an abnormal sucrose tolerance test will help identify sucrose as the offending carbohydrate. The diagnosis is established by the demonstration of deficient sucrase-isomaltase activity in a morphologically normal jejunal biopsy. Treatment of sucrase-isomaltase deficiency consists of strict avoidance of sucrose. A commercial preparation of sucrase is available and efficacious.[16] Starch can still be consumed in sucrase-isomaltase deficiency because most of its chemical makeup consists of amylose, which is digested by pancreatic α-amylase or by brush border glucoamylase.

Several maltases (glucoamylases) have been identified. Maltases are responsible for the digestion of maltotriose. The enzyme differs from pancreatic α-amylase because maltase sequentially removes a single glucose from the nonreducing end of a linear $\alpha1,4$ glucose chain, breaking down maltose into glucose. Theoretically, maltase deficiency may lead to carbohydrate maldigestion, although its clinical significance appears to be minimal.

Trehalose (α-D-glucopyranoside) is a nonreducing disaccharide that occurs in mushrooms, in some microorganisms, and in many insects. Trehalase deficiency can cause symptoms similar to those of lactase malabsorption.[17] An autosomal dominant type of inheritance has been suggested.

Brush border enzyme deficiencies are frequently acquired. The most common disaccharide deficiencies occur following infectious gastroenteritis or other damaging insults to the intestine, including gluten-induced enteropathy, cow's-milk protein sensitivity, giardiasis, and rotavirus infection. A congenital defect involving the transport of glucose and galactose is extremely rare.

Once monosaccharides have been produced on the brush border, absorption depends on mechanisms coupled to energy-dependent, active sodium transport, requiring specific carrier proteins known as SGTL1. Glucose and galactose are two monosaccharides known to be absorbed through this pathway, whereas fructose and xylose appear to be absorbed by a process of facilitated diffusion where GLUT5 is the specific carrier for fructose.[18] Not all carbohydrate hydrolyzed at one site is absorbed at that site; rather, the sugar may be carried in intestinal juice to be absorbed further downstream. Glucose-galactose malabsorption was first described in 1962 by Lindquist and Meeuwisse.[19] In vivo and in vitro studies have shown markedly impaired or absent sodium-coupled mucosal uptake of glucose in this disease.[20] In many patients, clinical tolerance to the offending carbohydrates improves with age, despite the fact that the enzyme deficiency and transport defect persist.

Maldigestion and malabsorption can accompany severe disease of the pancreas. In addition, pancreatic amylase deficiency has been described. Lowe and May reported a 13-year-old boy whose duodenal juice showed a persistent absence of amylase with decreased levels of trypsin but a normal amount of lipase.[21] Another case of amylase deficiency was reported by Lilibridge and Townes.[22] They described a 2-year-old child who showed poor weight gain on a diet containing starch, despite a more than adequate caloric intake. Weight gain and growth improved when starch was eliminated from the diet and replaced by disaccharides.

Lipids

Greater than 90% of ingested lipid in the diet is in the form of neutral fats or triglycerides. The diet also contains small amounts of phospholipids, cholesterol, and cholesterol esters.

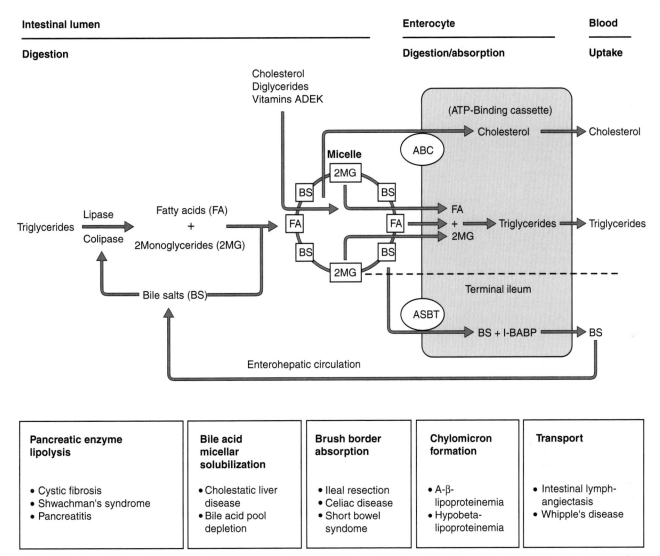

Figure 32-2. Digestion of triglycerides in the intestinal lumen occurs initially by lipase and colipase. Bile salts combine with the digestive products (fatty acids and monoglycerides). Mixed micelles of bile acids and lipid digestion products diffuse through the unstirred layer. Transport proteins such as ABC mediate the transport of cholesterol across the brush border membrane. Fatty acids and monoglycerides diffuse across the membrane. In the cytosol, fatty acids are bound to fatty acid–binding protein and cholesterol is bound to sterol carrier proteins. Uptake of cholesterol and triglycerides into the systemic circulation occurs at the basolateral membrane. In the terminal ileum, the uptake of bile salts occurs via ASBT. Intracellular I-BABP bind bile salts and transport them to the basolateral membrane where uptake occurs. ABC, ATP-binding cassette; BS, bile salts; FA, fatty acids; 2MG, 2-monoglyceride; ASBT, apical sodium-dependent bile transporter; I-BABP, ileal bile-acid binding protein.

A schematic representation of the digestion and absorption of dietary lipids is shown in Figure 32-2.

Many of the steps in fat digestion, absorption, and metabolism are not well developed in the newborn human and even less so in the preterm infant.[23] The full-term infant, if fed with mother's milk, receives nutrients that are well adapted to the needs of the rapidly growing newborn. The fat in human milk is ideally suited to the requirements of full-term infants; however, in infants born extremely premature, the gastrointestinal tract is not always able to digest and absorb nutrients.[23]

As noted previously, triglycerides are the main dietary fat throughout life, and this applies to the infant as well. However, phospholipids and cholesterol also have important nutritional functions. It is open to question whether formulas that contain only trace amounts of cholesterol, compared with the cholesterol content of human milk (10 to 15 mg/dL) provide an adequate amount of this lipid. Cholesterol not only is a precursor

for steroid hormones and bile acids, but also is an essential component of cell membranes. At an average milk consumption of 750 to 850 mL/day, the rapidly growing infant absorbs 75 to 125 mg of cholesterol a day.

The newborn and especially the premature infant are deficient in pancreatic lipase and bile salts that are needed for digestion and solubilization of dietary fat. Pancreatic enzyme activity measured in the duodenum of full-term and preterm newborn infants under basal conditions shows considerable protease (trypsin and chymotrypsin) activity, but only trace amounts of lipase and no amylase.[23] During the first month of life, pancreatic lipase remains very low or absent not only under basal conditions, but also after cholecystokinin-pancreozymin stimulation.[23,24] At 2 years of age, basal activity and secretory response of pancreatic lipase are well developed.[23,24]

Fat digestion in the newborn depends on the activities of the infant's lingual lipase, gastric lipase, and the activity of a specific digestive lipase present in human milk. Gastric lipase is stable at a pH of 1.5 to 2.0 and has optimum activity at a pH of 3.0 to 6.5. This is different from pancreatic lipase, which requires a higher pH. Gastric lipase is also resistant to pepsin present in the stomach. In formula-fed premature infants, 30% of the fat is digested in the stomach. This compares with 40% of the ingested fat hydrolyzed in the stomach of the breast-fed infant. Overall fat absorption attributable to lipolysis by nonpancreatic digestive lipase amounts to about 50 to 70% of ingested fat, suggesting that the excellent absorption of milk fat in the newborn depends on additional digestive enzymes, such as milk lipase.[23]

Little is known concerning the postnatal changes in pancreatic lipase activity from birth until adult levels are achieved.[23] However, with age, pancreatic lipase and colipase become more important in fat digestion. The products of pancreatic lipolysis, fatty acids and monoglycerides, must be solubilized. The mechanism to do this develops during maturation as bile salt production by the liver increases. The fatty acids and monoglycerides are solubilized in the intestinal lumen by bile salts to form micelles with the polar end facing the aqueous phase of intestinal fluid and the nonpolar hydrocarbon end inserted into the interior of the micelle. Bile salt micelles increase the capacity of water to carry fatty acids and allow for more efficient absorption.

In contrast to the immaturity of digestive function, fat uptake by the enterocyte from the intestine seems to be well developed at birth. However, most of the studies on the mechanism of fat absorption have been carried out in suckling animals with only occasional observations in humans. Once inside the enterocyte, long-chain fatty acids are transported to the reesterification site, the endoplasmic reticulum, by means of a cytosolic fatty-acid-binding protein.[25] Fatty-acid binding proteins (FABPs) are a family of cytosolic proteins that bind hydrophobic ligands and are thought to be important in the uptake and intracellular transport of fatty acids in the enterocyte. Much knowledge concerning these carrier proteins has accumulated since their initial description.[26-29] The fatty acids are activated to acyl CoA and their reesterification to triglyceride then occurs. The newly synthesized triglyceride, together with phospholipids, cholesterol, and protein, is assembled into lipoproteins (chylomicrons and low-density lipoproteins [LDLs]). These large particles are released in the intercellular space by reverse pinocytosis and move across the basement membrane into lymphatics.[23,30] This complex sequence of events is necessary for the absorption of long-chain triglycerides. Short-chain and medium-chain triglycerides, because they are more water soluble, may be absorbed directly into the portal blood system.

Failure to digest or absorb fats results in a variety of clinical symptoms and laboratory abnormalities. These manifestations are the result of both fat malassimilation per se and a deficiency of the fat-soluble vitamins. In general, malabsorption of fat deprives the body of calories and contributes to weight loss and malnutrition. Unabsorbed long-chain fatty acids interact with colonic mucosa to cause diarrhea by an irritant effect on the colon.[30] In addition, unabsorbed fatty acids bind calcium, a mineral normally present in the intestinal lumen. The calcium is then not available to bind oxalate. In fat malabsorption, oxalate not bound to calcium remains free and the oxalate is readily absorbed. This results in oxaluria and calcium oxalate kidney stones, which may occur in Crohn's disease.[31,32]

Recognition of fat malabsorption or steatorrhea is usually not difficult. The stools tend to be large and bulky. Because of their increased gas content, they tend to float in toilet water. In the infant, a film of oil can be seen or oiliness noticed when changing diapers. The smell is typically foul.

Fat malabsorption may occur in diseases that impair bile production or excretion, or it may occur in pancreatic insufficiency. In certain conditions, bile acid excretion is impaired, but serum bilirubin concentration may be normal or near normal. This is seen in children with a paucity of intrahepatic bile ducts. They may not be jaundiced, but have other biochemical signs of cholestasis such as pruritus or increased serum cholesterol, alkaline phosphatase, or gamma glutamyl transpeptidase. Steatorrhea may be mild to severe in these children.

The most common cause of pancreatic insufficiency is cystic fibrosis. This disease affects not only enzymes important in fat digestion, but also those important in carbohydrate and protein digestion. Cystic fibrosis is a multiorgan disease that is characterized by the triad of malabsorption, failure to thrive, and chronic sinopulmonary infections. The many potential features of cystic fibrosis include pancreatic insufficiency (approximately 85%), liver dysfunction (15 to 30%), and raised concentrations of sodium and chloride in the sweat, as well as obstructive azoospermia in postpubertal males.[33]

Some 15% of the patients have growth percentiles for height and weight exceeding the 75th percentile. Therefore, good stature does not exclude the diagnosis. The expression of the gene is highly variable, with hundreds of mutations: some patients are seriously handicapped physically, whereas others, who are experiencing minimal symptoms, are not identified until later in adulthood. Dr. Harry Shwachman in Boston reported 70 patients who were not diagnosed until they were over 25 years of age.[34] Moreover, there are patients in whom a single clinical feature is the dominant finding, such as electrolyte abnormalities, pancreatitis, liver disease, sinusitis, or obstructive azoospermia and infertility.

Nutritional problems in cystic fibrosis are multifactorial, including not only maldigestion and malabsorption, but also increased energy expenditure, increased intestinal losses, and increased caloric requirements.[35]

Pancreatic insufficiency is also part of Shwachman's syndrome, an inherited disease with abnormal bone marrow function, metaphyseal dysostosis, neutropenia, thrombocytopenia, anemia, and eczema. Shwachman's syndrome may result in severe failure to thrive, and the neutropenia is responsible for frequent and generalized infections, including chronic purulent otitis, mastoiditis, and meningitis. The primary defect in this syndrome remains unknown.[36]

A-β-lipoproteinemia must be considered in the differential diagnosis of a child with steatorrhea, failure to thrive, and anemia. A biochemical clue is the presence of very low serum cholesterol concentration, generally less than 50 mg/dL. The presence of acanthocytes or spiculated red blood cells in a peripheral blood smear is also suggestive. The serum is not turbid after a fatty meal because of the basic inability to form chylomicrons and transport lipid from the enterocyte. The diagnosis is confirmed by serum lipoprotein electrophoresis along with a jejunal biopsy that shows fat-laden villi.[37,38] The progressive neurological deterioration, including retinitis pigmentosa, ataxia, and ophthalmoplegia, was until recently considered an inseparable part of the disease; it has now been correlated with chronic vitamin E deficiency.[39] Early diagnosis and institution of adequate vitamin E replacement will prevent or modify the neurological deterioration.[40]

In congenital lipase deficiency, steatorrhea is present from birth.[41] Although pancreatic lipase, but not colipase, is deficient, a functioning gastric source of this lipolytic enzyme is present. There is also evidence of lingual/pharyngeal lipase activity. The diagnosis is confirmed by a secretin-pancreozymin test, which demonstrates normal proteolytic and amylolytic enzymes, but absent lipase activity in duodenal fluid.

Proteins

Infants fed 750 to 850 mL formula a day ingest approximately 12 g protein. Digestion of this protein begins in the stomach under the influence of pepsin. Although gastric proteolysis is extremely limited, intestinal protein digestion in the infant is probably adequate.[42] The efficiency with which proteins are digested and absorbed in the newborn relates more to the highly glycosylated form of some of the proteins in human milk than to the immaturity of neonatal digestive enzymes.

In the adult, the average protein intake varies considerably. The usual diet in a developed country provides 70 to 100 g protein/day.[43] Endogenous protein from secretions along the oro-gastro-intestinal tract contributes an additional 50 to 60 g/day. The bulk of dietary protein is hydrolyzed by pancreatic proteases secreted into the proximal duodenum in inactive form. Activation is catalyzed by the duodenal surface enzyme enterokinase, which converts trypsinogen to activated trypsin. Activation is virtually instantaneous. Intraluminal digestion of dietary protein occurs by sequential action of pancreatic endopeptidases and exopeptidases. The endopeptidases trypsin, chymotrypsin, elastase, DNase, and RNase act on the peptide at the interior of the molecule. The peptides are then hydrolyzed by the exopeptidases carboxypeptidase A and B, which remove a single amino acid from the carboxy-terminal end of the peptide, yielding basic and neutral amino acids (AAs) as well as small peptides.[43] As shown in Figure 32-3, peptidases in the brush border then hydrolyze the residual di-, tri-, and tetrapeptides.

The brush border proteases generate a large quantity and variety of short- and medium-sized peptides, as well as free amino

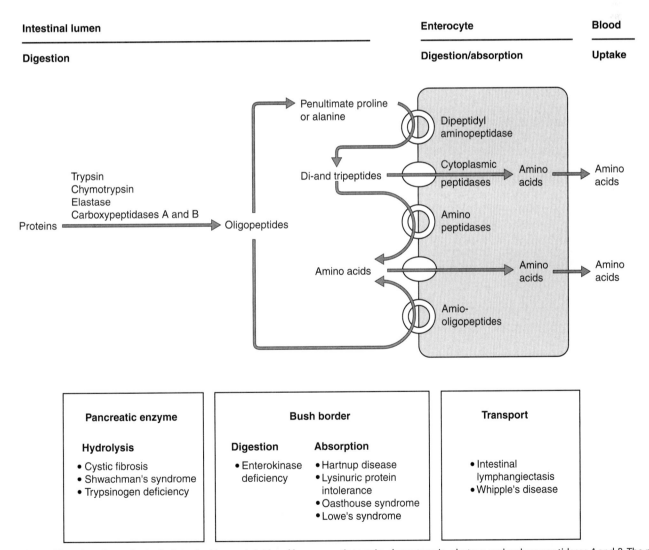

Figure 32-3. Digestion of proteins in the intestinal lumen is initiated by pancreatic trypsin, chymotrypsin, elastase, and carboxypeptidases *A* and *B*. The pancreatic proteases convert dietary proteins to oligopeptides. Brush border peptidases (open circles) then hydrolyze the oligopeptides to amino acids, dipeptides, tripeptides, and larger peptides. The amino acids are absorbed across the brush border membrane by amino acid transporters (closed circles) and the small peptides by a peptide transporter (closed circles). In the cytosol of the enterocyte, dipeptides, tripeptides, and larger peptides are cleaved to single amino acids. Uptake of the single amino acids occurs across the basolateral membrane of the enterocyte.

acids. Most proteins and oligopeptides are rapidly degraded. However, some structures are fairly resistant to hydrolysis, and the rapidity of the digestive process is dependent on the protein's amino acid sequence and on posttranslation modifications, such as glycosylation, that render peptides more resistant to hydrolysis.[42,43] Although oligopeptides of medium chain length are the primary products of the luminal phase of protein digestion, they are further cleaved by a spectra of membrane anchored peptidases at the brush border of intestinal epithelial cells. In vitro models used to study this have shown that when dipeptides are used as substrates, almost 90% of total mucosal hydrolysis is attributed to cytosolic enzymes, whereas with tripeptides, only around 50% of the hydrolytic activity originates from the soluble cytosolic fraction. In the case of tripeptides and those peptides with more than four amino residues, essentially all hydrolytic activity is brush border membrane bound.[43] Luminal hydrolysis of normal di- and tripeptides occurs rapidly when the enzymes are not overloaded with substrates. When overloading does occur, some peptides then bypass hydrolysis and are taken up intact into the cell.

Multiple peptide transporters for the different substrate groups were initially postulated. Indeed, findings from experiments with intact tissue preparations have suggested, on the basis of cross-inhibition studies, that there could be more than one type of peptide carrier. However, cloning of the cDNA of the intestinal di-tripeptide carrier now designated as PEPT1, extensive analysis of mammalian genome databases, screening of intestinal tissue banks, and immunohistology have not yet provided evidence for more than one peptide carrier in the brush border membrane of small intestinal epithelial cells.[43]

From these physiological considerations, protein malabsorption would be expected in diseases causing (1) pancreatic insufficiency; (2) loss of mucosal surface such as occurs in short bowel syndrome and celiac disease; (3) generalized impaired enterocyte function accompanying celiac disease; and (4) impaired dipeptide or amino acid transport by the enterocyte. The last possibility, impaired dipeptide or amino acid transport at the enterocyte membrane is extremely rare. Several of these diseases are noted in Table 32-1.

Severe loss of body protein may occur in protein maldigestion or malabsorption before there is evidence of laboratory abnormalities. This loss is more likely to occur when there is insufficient protein intake. Impaired protein synthesis from liver diseases and excessive protein loss in renal disease can further aggravate protein deficiencies. Clinically, protein deficiency results in edema and diminished muscle mass. Because the immune system is dependent on adequate protein, protein deficiency can manifest as recurrent or severe infections. Alternatively, there may be growth retardation, mental apathy, and irritability. Other features of protein deficiency include weakness, muscle atrophy, edema, hair loss, deformity of skeletal bone, anorexia, vomiting, and diarrhea.

Vitamins

Fat-Soluble Vitamins

Diseases causing malabsorption of dietary fat commonly cause malabsorption of fat-soluble vitamins. This is especially important in diseases that also result in impaired micelle formation due to bile salt deficiency, such as biliary atresia. Failure to absorb the fat-soluble vitamins A, D, E, and K results in a variety of symptoms. Vitamin A deficiency is associated with follicular hyperkeratosis. Vitamin E deficiency leads to a progressive demyelination of the central nervous system. Malabsorption of vitamin D causes osteopenia and rickets. Vitamin K deficiency may be associated with easy bruisability and/or bleeding into the nose, bladder, vagina, or gastrointestinal tract.

Water-Soluble Vitamins

Folic Acid. The principal source of folic acid comes from dietary folates (folacins) that are widely distributed in foods: liver, yeast, leafy vegetables, legumes, and some fruits. All folacins are hydrolyzed to folic acid, or pteroylglutamic acid, during digestion absorption. Pteroylglutamic acid is absorbed at a faster rate than larger polymers. Only 25 to 50% of dietary folacin is nutritionally available. Boiling destroys folate activity. The daily requirement for folate is approximately 100 μg. On the basis of a 50% food folate absorption, the recommended dietary allowance is 200 μg. Tissue stores of folate are only about 3 mg; therefore, malabsorption can deplete the body of folate within 1 month.

Polyglutamate forms of folate are hydrolyzed to the monoglutamate form. This hydrolysis takes place at the brush border by the enzyme folate conjugase. Folic acid is absorbed from the intestinal lumen by a sodium-dependent carrier. Once in the intestinal epithelial cell, folic acid is methylated and reduced to the tetrahydric form.

Interference with folic acid absorption at the brush-border carrier site occurs with drugs such as phenytoin and sulfasalazine. In addition, folic acid deficiency itself can impair folic acid absorption by producing "megaloblastic" changes in columnar epithelial cells of the intestine, creating an abnormal epithelium. Congenital isolated folate in malabsorption is rare, but has been described.[44]

Vitamin B$_{12}$. Vitamin B$_{12}$ is the generic term for compounds with bioactivity. Cobalamin refers to cobalt-containing compounds with a corrin ring. Cobalamin is the preferred term to distinguish those compounds that are active in humans from the many analogs produced by bacteria. Microorganisms in the human colon synthesize cobalamin, which is absorbed in small amounts. However, strict vegetarians who do not eat cobalamin-containing meats may develop cobalamin deficiency. The average Western diet contains 10-20 μg/day. The daily requirement for cobalamin is 0.3 μg for infants and 2.0 μg for adult males. The human liver is the repository of approximately 5 mg of cobalamin. The large hepatic stores account for the delay of several years in the clinical appearance of vitamin B$_{12}$ deficiency once cobalamin malabsorption begins.

When cobalamin is liberated from food, it is bound at acid pH to haptocorrin (R binder).[45] R binders or proteins are glycoproteins present in many body secretions, including serum, bile, saliva, and gastric and pancreatic juices. Most of the gastric R protein is from swallowed saliva. The haptocorrin cannot mediate the absorption of cobalamin alone, and its physiologic function is incompletely understood.

The cobalamin/haptocorrin complex, bound in the upper intestinal tract, leaves the stomach along with free intrinsic factor. In the duodenum, pancreatic proteases in the presence of bicarbonate hydrolyze the haptocorrin, thereby liberating free cobalamin. The cobalamin now combines with gastric intrinsic factor. A conformational change takes place, allowing the cobalamin–intrinsic factor complex to be resistant to proteolytic digestion. This resistance allows the complex to safely traverse the small intestine and reach the ileum, its site of active absorption. In the ileum, the cobalamin–intrinsic factor complex binds to a specific receptor located on the brush border. Free cobalamin without intrinsic factor does not bind to the ileal receptor. After passage across the enterocytes, cobalamin is transported in blood bound to circulating proteins known as transcobalamins.

Pancreatic insufficiency may lead to cobalamin deficiency, but lack of intrinsic factor or pernicious anemia is the most common cause of cobalamin deficiency. Bacterial overgrowth of the small intestine disrupts the cobalamin-intrinsic factor complex, decreasing cobalamin absorption. *Giardia lamblia* infestation is also associated with cobalamin malabsorption. Cobalamin absorption may be impaired after ileal resection or by diseases affecting more than 50 cm of the terminal ileum, such as Crohn's disease, celiac disease, tuberculosis, and lymphoma. Finally, bariatric surgery is being performed on a limited number of morbidly obese teenagers. Vitamin B_{12} absorption has been shown to be compromised following gastric bypass surgery.[46] Clearly there is a wide diversity in the etiology of cobalamin deficiency, and this requires a versatile diagnostic approach.

Other Water-Soluble Vitamins. Most of the water-soluble vitamins, such as the B vitamins and vitamin C (ascorbic acid), are absorbed in the small intestine either by carrier-mediated transport or by passive diffusion. Generalized malabsorption syndromes, such as occurs in Crohn's disease, impair the absorption of these vitamins and can lead to a deficiency state. However, water-soluble vitamin malabsorption and deficiency is less frequent in the pediatric population than are malabsorption and deficiencies of fat-soluble vitamins.

Minerals

Iron

Iron is available for absorption from vegetables (nonheme iron) and from meats (heme iron). Heme iron is better absorbed (10 to 20%) than nonheme iron (1 to 6%). It is also less affected by intraluminal factors or dietary composition. The average dietary intake of iron is 10 to 20 mg/day. Men absorb 1 to 2 mg/day, whereas menstruating women and iron-deficient patients absorb 3 to 4 mg/day. In acute blood loss, increased absorption of iron does not occur for 3 days. Nonheme iron, in the ferric iron (Fe^{3+}) state, when ingested into a stomach unable to produce acid, forms insoluble iron complexes, which are not available for absorption. In the presence of gastric acid and ascorbic acid, ferrous iron (Fe^{2+}) forms. The ferrous iron complexes to a mucopolysaccharide of about 200,000 MW and is transported as a complex into the duodenum and proximal jejunum. There, in the presence of ascorbic acid, glucose and cysteine, the iron is absorbed. Dietary factors such as phosphate, phytate, and phosphoproteins can render the iron insoluble and inhibit iron absorption.

Both heme and nonheme iron are absorbed most rapidly in the duodenum. Some of the iron absorbed is deposited as ferritin within the enterocyte, and the remainder is transferred to plasma-bound transferrin. When the enterocyte defoliates, iron deposited as ferritin is lost into the intestinal lumen. This mechanism for loss is probably overwhelmed by the large amount of iron ingested. The amount of iron absorbed from the intestine depends largely on two factors: (1) total body iron content and (2) rate of erythropoiesis.

Any disease that is associated with mucosal atrophy of the small intestine may be associated with iron malabsorption. Drugs that suppress gastric acid secretion can also contribute to the malabsorption of this mineral. Recent studies of *Helicobacter pylori* gastritis have shown that this infection raises gastric pH, depresses levels of gastric ascorbic acid, and may contribute to the development of iron deficiency anemia.[47,48]

Calcium

Calcium absorption occurs in the proximal small intestine and is dependent on vitamin D intake. Calcium needs are greater during puberty than at any other time in life.[49] The efficiency of calcium absorption is increased during puberty as bone formation is optimized. Balance studies have indicated that for most healthy subjects, the maximal net calcium balance during puberty is achieved with intakes between 1200 and 1500 mg calcium/day. During puberty, the efficiency of conversion of 25-hydroxy-vitamin D to $1,25(OH)_2$ vitamin D increases.

Calcium malabsorption is most frequently related to the direct damage of small intestine mucosa as occurs in celiac disease, with a significant reduction of the intestinal surface area. It also accompanies diseases causing fatty acid malabsorption. The malabsorbed fats complex with calcium, forming insoluble calcium soaps. Deficiency of vitamin D and renal disease will contribute to calcium malabsorption, as will hypoparathyroidism and inborn defects either in $1,25(OH)_2$ vitamin D formation or in the intestinal vitamin D receptor.

Magnesium

In small intestine disorders, such as Crohn's disease, celiac disease, and autoimmune enteropathies, magnesium absorption may be affected by direct damage to the small intestine surface. In addition, the absorption of magnesium may be compromised by the luminal binding of the magnesium to the malabsorbed fat that occurs in these diseases. A congenital form of selective intestinal magnesium malabsorption has been reported.[50]

Zinc

Like other minerals, zinc is malabsorbed in mucosal disease of the small intestine. There is also zinc malabsorption in acrodermatitis enteropathica. Differentiating acrodermatitis from acquired zinc deficiencies can be difficult because both conditions present in the same manner. Some studies have shown that low zinc levels in the mother's milk may produce an acquired zinc deficiency in full-term, breast-fed infants. Acrodermatitis enteropathica tends to occur in the first few months of life shortly after discontinuation of breast feeding. Two new proteins that are absent in the fibroblasts of patients with acrodermatitis enteropathica have recently been discovered.[51] These proteins may be responsible for the decreased zinc absorption and abnormal zinc metabolism that occurs in dermatitis enteropathica.

Water

Malabsorption of water can occur in diseases affecting the intestine. The epithelium of the small intestine exhibits passive permeability to salt and water. Osmotic equilibration between plasma and the intestinal lumen is fairly rapid; therefore, large differences in ion concentration do not develop. Intercellular junctions are more permeable to cations (positively charged ions) than anions (negatively charged ions). Therefore, intestinal lumen-to-blood concentration differences for Na^+ and K^+ are generally smaller than those for Cl^- and HCO_3^-. The colonic epithelium displays lower passive permeability to salt and water than the epithelium of the small intestine. One consequence of this lower passive ionic permeability (higher electrical resistance) is that electric potential differences across the colonic epithelium are an order of magnitude greater than those in the small intestine. Active Na^+ absorption, which is the main transport activity of the distal colon, generates a serosa-positive charge or potential difference (PD). Under the influence of aldosterone, this PD can be 60 mV or even higher. A 60-mV PD will sustain a 10-fold concentration difference for a monovalent ion such as K^+. Most of the high K^+ concentration in the rectum is accounted for by the PD. Despite the high fecal K^+ level, little K^+ is lost in the stool, because stool volume (about 200 to 300 mL/day) is normally so low. In contrast, during high-volume (more than 1000 mL/day) diarrhea of small bowel origin (rotavirus, cholera), the stool K^+ concentration is considerably lower, but stool K^+ loss is nonetheless great because of the large fluid volume that is malabsorbed. In such states, the stool K^+ concentration is low and the Na^+ concentration relatively high because diarrheal fluid passes through the colon too rapidly to equilibrate across the colonic epithelium.

In the small intestine, active electrolyte and fluid absorption can be conceived of as either nutrient-dependent or nutrient-independent. The absorptive processes for glucose and neutral amino acids are Na^+ dependent so that one Na^+ molecule is translocated across the brush border with each glucose or amino acid molecule. The sodium pump (Na^+,K^+-ATPase), which is located exclusively in the basolateral membrane of the enterocyte of the small intestine, extrudes Na^+ that has entered the cell from the lumen, thereby maintaining a low intracellular Na^+, a high intracellular K^+, and a negative intracellular to extracellular electric potential. This Na^+,K^+ pump provides the potential energy for uphill sugar and amino acid absorption. Glucose is co-transported with sodium. Patients in intestinal secretory states such as cholera can absorb glucose normally. Sodium and water are also absorbed, accompanying the transport of glucose. As a consequence, the fluid losses of these patients can be replaced by oral glucose-electrolyte solutions.[52] These individuals generally do not require intravenous fluids unless they are comatose or too nauseated to drink the necessary large volumes of fluid to correct the dehydration. Application of this knowledge has had a major impact on the health of children worldwide. The oral rehydration therapy can be life-saving for children and adults with cholera-like diarrheas, which are so prevalent in developing countries, and state-of-the-art facilities and hospitals are not required for this simple therapy.

In the distal colon, the luminal membrane contains Na^+ channels, which can be blocked by low concentrations of the diuretic amiloride. The Na^+ entering through these channels is then extruded across the basolateral membrane by the Na^+,K^+-ATPase pump discussed previously. Aldosterone increases the number of these channels and also increases the number of Na^+,K^+-ATPase pumps. Aldosterone therefore enhances active Na^+ absorption in the distal colon. Chloride is absorbed along with Na^+ and traverses the epithelium by both cellular and paracellular routes. The transcellular route involves a Cl^-/HCO_3^- exchanger in the luminal membrane and Cl^- channels in the basolateral membrane. Intracellular mediators such as cyclic AMP (cAMP) do not appear to affect these Na^+ channels. Thus, patients with secretory diarrheas, especially those who are salt-depleted and therefore have elevated blood levels of aldosterone, are able to reabsorb some of the secreted fluid in their distal colon. Spironolactone, which inhibits the action of aldosterone, can increase the severity of diarrhea in such patients.

Water and electrolyte absorption and secretion in the small and large intestine can be adversely affected by a variety of hormones, bile salts, endotoxins, fatty acids, and pathologic conditions. When this occurs and this finely tuned system of absorption and secretion is disrupted, water and electrolyte flux may be altered with significant or even massive losses of intestinal water and electrolytes.

DIAGNOSTIC APPROACH

History

A good history, a physical examination, and judicious use of laboratory studies usually provide the information necessary to diagnose a maldigestion or malabsorption disorder.

The symptoms of diarrhea, weight loss, and poor growth are not unique to malabsorption. Many disorders that do not directly affect the gastrointestinal tract may produce similar symptoms. Urinary tract infections and certain diseases of the central nervous system may cause diarrhea and other signs or symptoms suggestive of malabsorption. However, with other clues from a complete and accurate clinical history, a cause can often be postulated. Important aspects of the history include the following:

1. A chronologic description of all symptoms (e.g., fever, diarrhea, abdominal pain), the relation of symptoms to changes in lifestyle or stress, and information concerning the introduction of antibiotics or other medications should be obtained. Exacerbation of chronic medical problems should also be considered.

2. Assessment of appetite, activity, and sleeping habits before the onset of the symptoms is important.

3. A dietary history is necessary to assess intake in terms of nutritional type and quantity. Note should be made of the dietary manipulations employed in an attempt to resolve symptoms. The physician should ascertain whether there has been prolonged dietary restriction initiated to control diarrhea. Dietary restrictions can result in malnutrition.

4. A perinatal history should be obtained. Signs and symptoms present from birth suggest a congenital disorder but do not rule out acquired causes of malabsorption. A history of prior abdominal surgery can suggest an anatomic cause for malabsorption, such as an intestinal stricture or partial small bowel obstruction.

5. A history of serial infections can implicate cystic fibrosis or an immune deficiency syndrome as a possible cause of maldigestion or malabsorption.

6. Inquire about recent travel on the part of the patient or immediate family members to tropical or underdeveloped areas. If a child is cared for in a day-care nursery, infections such as giardiasis may be implicated as a cause of malabsorption.

7. Many maldigestive and malabsorptive disorders affect organ systems other than the intestinal tract. Systemic complaints not directly related to the digestive tract (e.g., malaise, edema, fever, delayed onset of menses, secondary amenorrhea, weight loss) may suggest inflammatory bowel disease or early liver disease. Evidence of bleeding, bruising, or rashes may be secondary to a deficiency state that accompanies malabsorption.

8. A family history should be obtained because other family members may have similar signs and symptoms. This can suggest a genetically determined or infectious disorder.

Physical Examination

The number and prominence of physical findings may parallel the severity and chronicity of the malabsorptive disorder. The physical examination may be unremarkable or show subtle abnormalities known to be associated with mild malabsorption. During the examination, it may be noticed that the child is depressed and passive in response. This is common in moderate to severe malnutrition. Many chronically malnourished children also show evidence of developmental delay. Accurate measurement of height, weight, and head circumference; calculation of weight for length; and construction of a growth curve are fundamental parts of the physical examination. The plotted growth curves for weight and length can provide valuable information in the assessment of growth problems secondary to the nutritional inadequacies of chronic maldigestive and malabsorptive disorders.[53] Examination of the head, face, and neck may reveal evidence of fat-soluble or water-soluble vitamin deficiencies (e.g., xerophthalmia in vitamin A deficiency, cheilitis and smooth tongue in vitamin B complex deficiencies). Examination of the trunk, buttocks, and extremities can give a subjective impression of muscle wasting or decreased fat stores. A more accurate measurement of muscle mass and fat stores can be provided by skinfold thickness measurements.

The cardiac examination may reveal a rapid heart rate from anemia, or bradycardia secondary to protein-calorie malnutrition. Abdominal distention may be detected, reflecting fatty infiltration of the liver, laxity of abdominal musculature, or both. This can be associated with protein-calorie malnutrition. Tenderness of the liver may be present secondary to fatty infiltration or congestive heart failure. A prominent abdominal venous pattern, a palpable spleen, or a noticeable fluid wave on abdominal examination may herald chronic liver disease with portal hypertension and ascites. A delay in the appearance of secondary sex characteristics is common with chronic malabsorption in older children. Nail-bed pallor from decreased blood hemoglobin and clubbing of the nail beds can occur in both celiac disease and inflammatory bowel disease.[54-56] Joint pain, swelling, and erythema can be extraintestinal manifestations of inflammatory bowel disease. Abnormalities of color and texture of the skin and hair can be seen in fat-soluble vitamin and trace element deficiency states. The neurologic examination may reveal the abnormal reflexes of Chvostek's or Trousseau's sign from hypocalcemia. There may also be abnormal cerebellar signs from a vitamin E- or vitamin B-complex deficiency.

Laboratory Testing

Laboratory studies can help confirm the presence of maldigestion and malabsorption and, more importantly, help identify the cause. They can elucidate specific vitamin or trace element deficiency states as well as document adequate serum levels during supplemental vitamin therapy. Studies can be divided into several categories based on availability, expense, and invasiveness (Table 32-2).

Initial Phase Testing

Stool Examination. Fecal testing is a lost art. A comprehensive evaluation of feces is a most beautiful and gracious examination and can be helpful in interpreting a disease process. For example, the identification of occult blood, fecal leukocytes, or fecal calprotectin in a stool specimen suggests an inflammatory

TABLE 32-2. Diagnostic Studies in the Evaluation of Maldigestion and Malabsorption

Initial studies
  Stool examination for blood, leukocytes, reducing substances and *Clostridium difficile* toxin; stool examination for ova and parasites and cultures for infectious bacterial pathogens
  Complete blood count
  Serum electrolytes, blood urea nitrogen, creatinine, calcium, phosphorus, albumin, total protein
  Urinalysis and culture
Second-phase studies
  Sweat chloride test
  Breath analysis
  D-Xylose test
  Serum carotene, folate, B_{12}, and iron levels
  Fecal α1-antitrypsin level
  Fecal fat studies or coefficient of fat absorption studies
  Fatty test meal, Lundh test meal
  Serum vitamin levels
Third-phase studies
  25-Hydroxy-D, and
  Contrast radiographic studies: upper gastrointestinal series, barium enema
  Small intestinal biopsy for histology and mucosal enzyme determination
  Bentiromide excretion test
Specialized studies
  Schilling test
  Serum/urine bile acid determination
  Endoscopic retrograde pancreatography
  Provocative pancreatic secretion testing

condition. Decreased stool pH and positive reducing substances may reflect carbohydrate maldigestion and malabsorption in the small intestine and subsequent fermentation by colonic bacteria. Qualitative fecal fat excretion or stain for fat globules (Sudan stain) can be a quick and simple way to screen for fat malabsorption.[57] If properly performed, a Sudan stain on a spot sample of stool can detect more than 90% of patients with clinically significant steatorrhea.[58] Additionally, and more importantly, the method can differentiate between neutral and split fat. By definition, a neutral fat is a triglyceride that contains three fatty acids and glycerol. Split fats are simple fatty acids that are reduced by the action of lipase. In patients with pancreatic insufficiency, the predominant stool fat stained by the Sudan agent will be the neutral fat (intact triglyceride). This is different in patients with normal pancreatic function and abnormal small intestinal mucosa, where the simple fatty acids are present in large amounts in stool.

Fecal enzymes such as stool trypsin or chymotrypsin may be helpful in obtaining a diagnosis in patients with fat malabsorption. The fecal elastase-1 test has been used to evaluate pancreatic insufficiency in both diabetes and cystic fibrosis and is especially useful in patients with abnormally high neutral fat on Sudan staining.[59,60]

If there is suspicion of a gastrointestinal pathogen, stool samples should be obtained for bacterial culture, ova and parasites, and virology examination. For some enteric pathogens, the diagnostic value of fecal testing is lost if the stool is not taken to the laboratory quickly and tested immediately. Collection of a stool sample can be a challenge for the mother of a child with liquid stools. Rectal aspiration using an 8- to 10F feeding tube and a 20-mL syringe may be tried.[57] Other techniques include lining a disposable diaper with plastic wrap to prevent absorption and using a urine collection bag that has been placed over the anus. Stool samples that cannot be processed immediately and examined for bacterial pathogens, ova, and parasites can be placed in an appropriate preservative or transport medium for later analysis.

Complete Blood Count. Anemia is common in malabsorption syndromes, including celiac disease, cystic fibrosis, and inflammatory bowel disease. The microcytic, hypochromic anemia of iron deficiency is prevalent and may be caused by chronic blood loss through the gastrointestinal tract or by iron malabsorption. Less commonly, megaloblastic anemia can occur. In untreated celiac disease, this can result from reduced serum and red blood cell folate levels.[61] The chronic malabsorption of folate and vitamin B_{12} may also produce megaloblastic anemia. In cystic fibrosis, iron deficiency anemia with low serum ferritin is seen frequently, even in stable patients.[62] In cystic fibrosis patients with advanced pulmonary disease, polycythemia is seen less frequently than with other pulmonary disorders of comparable severity. The anemia associated with inflammatory bowel disease can present as an iron deficiency anemia, megaloblastic anemia, or the anemia of chronic disease.

Additional Blood Tests. In patients with malabsorption, the chronic loss of electrolytes and base can be reflected by low serum levels of sodium, potassium, chloride, and bicarbonate. Depending on the degree of malnutrition, total serum proteins, including albumin, can be depressed. Because of its relatively long half-life, serum albumin may not reflect current nutritional status. Serum proteins with a relatively shorter half-life may be used as nutritional markers. These include prealbumin (transthyretin), somatomedin C, retinol-binding protein, and transferrin.

Second Phase Testing

Serum concentrations of carotene, folate, and vitamins B_{12}, A, and E are also used to assess maldigestive and malabsorptive states. Monitoring of absorbed lipids after a standardized meal may be helpful in assessing maldigestion and malabsorption.[63,64] Healthy adults generally consume 70 to 120 grams of fat per day; the fecal fat excretion is less than 6 g/day. A quantification of the daily fecal fat output should be a reasonable test to evaluate for fat malabsorption. Ideally, an adequate quantitative fecal fat test needs a 3- to 5-day stool collection, to reduce errors and variability that may occur if a shorter collection period is used. More than 6 grams of fat in stool per 24 hours is pathologic, although adult patients with steatorrhea may have more than 20 g/day. Sometimes fecal fat excretion can be moderately increased in diarrheal diseases even without fat malabsorption; for example, values of up to 14 g/day have been reported in volunteers in whom diarrhea was intentionally induced and in patients with a stool weight of greater than 1000 g/day.[65,66]

Keeping a good record of all dietary intake beginning the day before, and extending for the remainder of the stool collection, improves the interpretation of the test. Knowing the daily fat intake (FI) and the fat output (FO) can allow for calculation of fractional fat absorption (FFA) or coefficient of fat absorption. Usually, a value above 94% is normal.

$$FFA = FI - FO/FI \times 100 = normal\ greater\ than\ 94\%$$

The fractional fat absorption may be more useful than a simple fecal fat output in pediatric patients. But importantly,

quantitative fecal fat determination does not discriminate between causes of steatorrhea. Additionally, a 72-hour stool collection is difficult to obtain from a small child. For these reasons, quantitative fecal fat excretion studies are not commonly used. Instead, other tests such as the acid steatocrit for detecting steatorrhea on a spot stool specimen may be used.[67] The steatocrit (a gravimetric assay performed on a spot stool sample) may provide an accurate and simplified method to assess fat malabsorption. It is based on the principle that when a stool sample is homogenized and centrifuged at 15,000 rpm for 15 min, the lipid portion rises to the top and the solid aqueous portion gravitates to the bottom. If this is done in a hematocrit tube, the amount of fat in a given stool sample can be estimated. This provides a crude estimate of fat malabsorption. A study evaluating this technique found a sensitivity of 100%, a specificity of 95%, and a positive predictive value of 90% compared to a 72-hour fecal fat collection that was used as the gold standard.[68] However, the value of the steatocrit in assessing fat malabsorption has been challenged.[69]

Breath Tests. Breath hydrogen testing is performed principally for the investigation of lactose malabsorption or bacterial overgrowth of the small intestine, although other applications show promise. Similarly, malabsorption of sucrose, fructose, and other sugars can be diagnosed by breath hydrogen testing. A test for fat malabsorption is the ^{14}C-triolein breath test. The test involves measurement of breath CO_2 after ingestion of the radiolabeled triglyceride triolein and provides a measure of fat absorption. However, interpretation of results may be difficult because several disease states can lead to erroneous values and normal values are affected by aging. As a result, the test is not commonly used. Stable isotope breath testing for fat malabsorption is primarily used as a research tool.

D-Xylose. The absorption of D-xylose is thought to be a passive process that reflects the functional surface area of the proximal small intestine. The test is not dependent on bile salts, pancreatic exocrine secretion, or intestinal brush border enzymes. A standard dose is given by mouth. It is based on body surface area ($14.5\ g/m^2$ up to a maximum dose of 25 g as a 10% aqueous solution). Approximately 50% of the absorbed dose is metabolized in the liver and the remainder is excreted in the urine. The serum D-xylose concentration at 1 hour can be used to assess D-xylose absorption after a standard dose. The serum level should exceed 25 mg/dL. A timed urine collection after the standard oral dose can also be used to approximate D-xylose absorption. The sensitivity and specificity of this test is somewhat controversial.[70,71] However, it does remain a relatively noninvasive screen for adequate proximal small intestinal surface area.

Third Phase Testing

Wireless Capsule Endoscopy. Recently, Fritscher-Ravens et al. reported the use of wireless capsule endoscopy in detecting small intestinal pathology.[72] In their study of children under 8 years of age ($n = 83$), their primary endpoint was gastrointestinal (GI) pathology. They found that GI bleeding was the leading cause; however, excessive protein loss occurred in 9 patients and malabsorption in 12. They confirmed that wireless capsule endoscopy was safe down to 1.5 years of age and could be helpful in establishing small intestinal pathology.

Intestinal Biopsy. The diagnostic value of a small intestinal biopsy varies with the disease process. Capsule biopsy specimens are obtained from the area of the duodenojejunal junction, and endoscopic biopsies are usually obtained from the proximal to middle duodenum. Serial biopsy specimens from other areas of the proximal small bowel can be considered when intermittent or patchy disease distribution is suspected. The careful mounting of the biopsy sample before fixation allows for proper orientation.

Disaccharidase Activities. The relationship between symptoms, intestinal mucosal histology, and disaccharidase activities is not well defined. Gupta et al. analyzed a total of 246 endoscopically obtained duodenal biopsies in 232 patients.[73] They found that the geometric means (95% confidence interval) in children aged less than 24 months (in units) are lactase, 36.7 (13.4 to 100.4); maltase, 178.5 (88.9 to 356.3); palatinase, 12.7 (3.8 to 41.5); and sucrase 60.0 (24.0 to 148.1). In children 24 months of age or older, the values were similar except for lactase at 23.2 (3.9 to 108.1). Only lactase activity decreased with age ($p < 0.05$). Additionally, no differences in disaccharidase activities were noted in patients with and without diarrhea if the mucosal histology was normal.

Pancreatic Testing. Finally, there are a variety of specific tests for assessment of pancreatic secretory function. These include provocative pancreatic secretion testing. The bentiromide excretion test and, more recently, a noninvasive stable-isotope method to assess pancreatic exocrine function have also been used.[74]

MANAGEMENT

Only selected management principles are outlined here, because treatment principles have been noted elsewhere in this volume.

Therapy for malabsorptive disorders is based on first identifying the disease process and then applying specific treatment principles for the disease. Second, if protein-calorie malnutrition and/or any vitamin or trace mineral deficiency is present, it should be vigorously treated enterally, parenterally, or using both approaches. The goal of nutritional support in pediatric practice is to provide adequate calories, lipids, protein, vitamins, and trace minerals for catch-up growth and maintenance of normal growth.

Maldigestion

For altered luminal digestion, specific therapies can be initiated, depending on the cause of the maldigestion. Supplemental enzymes may be provided to augment depressed enzyme secretion by the pancreas, as in cystic fibrosis and Shwachman-Diamond syndrome. The enzymes can be given along with a histamine receptor antagonist or proton pump inhibitor to minimize acid-mediated degradation of the enzymes. However, with the high-potency pancreatic enzyme supplements used

today, colonic strictures (fibrosing colonopathy) have been described, and there are now specific recommendations for the use of these replacement enzymes.[75,76] Fat-soluble vitamin supplements can be provided in an attempt to overcome disorders of absorption. New pharmacologic strategies have been developed to enhance the absorption of vitamin E with the use of polyethylene glycol.[77,78] Dietary medium-chain triglycerides can improve fat absorption in patients with impaired triglyceride digestion and absorption. Liver disease and cholestasis can occur with cystic fibrosis. Some disorders of cholestasis can be improved by the use of ursodeoxycholic acid, which stimulates bile flow, resulting in improvement in fat digestion. Cotting and colleagues demonstrated improved liver function and nutritional status in eight cystic fibrosis patients treated with ursodeoxycholic acid.[79]

Dumping syndrome has been shown to be a complication of the Nissen fundoplication. Symptoms associated with dumping syndrome can be alleviated with the use of uncooked starch.[80]

Malabsorption

In patients with mild to moderate malabsorption, a slow continuous infusion of nutrients by way of a nasogastric tube or through a gastrostomy may increase absorption. The slow rate increases the contact time between nutrients and the absorptive surface. This form of therapy is ideal for nocturnal feedings, but an enteral infusion pump is necessary. Other methods, such as the use of taurine, may improve fat absorption in patients with cystic fibrosis.[81]

Patients with severe malabsorption that has resulted in significant protein-calorie malnutrition may require parenteral nutritional support, which can provide the necessary nutrients, including minerals, vitamins, and iron.

In the future, new drugs as well as designer formulas and nutrients may allow health care professionals to optimize intestinal digestion and absorption in patients with diseases of the intestinal tract.

REFERENCES

1. Ushijima K, Riby JE, Kretchmer N. Carbohydrate malabsorption. Pediatr Clin North Am 1995;42(4):899–915.
20. Wright EM. Genetic disorders of membrane transport. I. Glucose galactose malabsorption. Am J Physiol 1998;275(38):G879–G882.
23. Hamosh M. Lipid metabolism in pediatric nutrition. Pediatr Clin North Am 1995;42(4):839–862.
24. Lebenthal E, Lee PC. Development of functional response in human exocrine pancreas. Pediatrics 1980;66:556–660.
26. Pelsers MM, Namiot Z, Kisielewski W, et al. Intestinal-type and liver-type fatty acid-binding protein in the intestine. Tissue distribution and clinical utility. Clin Biochem 2003;36(7):529–535.
43. Hannelore D. Molecular and integrative physiology of intestinal peptide transport. Annu Rev Physiol 2004;66:361–384.

See expertconsult.com for a complete list of references and the review questions for this chapter.

PROTRACTED DIARRHEA

Jonathan Evans

Protracted diarrheal disease is a major cause of global child-hood morbidity and mortality. Despite the ongoing individual and population-based burdens of protracted diarrhea, there has been a significant reduction in the number of related publications devoted to this topic. This most likely reflects decreases in resource allocation to this problem and not the advances in care achieved over the past three decades. Many issues remain unresolved, and protracted diarrhea continues to pose definitional, epidemiologic, diagnostic, and risk-factor challenges.[1] The greatest advances have been made in developed countries, and the causal profile of chronic diarrheal disease is now generally distinct from that found in developing nations.

In developing countries, infection remains the primary cause of most protracted diarrheal diseases. Persistent or repeated infections may lead to a postenteritis enteropathy, contributing further to malnutrition and a downward spiral toward debilitation and death.

In developed nations, death from infectious diarrhea is now uncommon. Specific preventive measures have contributed to the decrease in mortality and morbidity from chronic diarrheal disease in developed nations. These include improved sanitation and access to medical care at a societal level, renewed emphasis on breast-feeding, reduction in the use of partial starvation regimens during diarrheal episodes, and increased availability of nutritious, age-appropriate foods for the most vulnerable populations (e.g., the WIC program in the United States). As morbidity from infectious etiologies has declined in developed countries, a concomitant increase in autoimmune and inflammatory-based diseases has been documented.

This chapter defines protracted diarrhea, describes global epidemiologic differences and risk factors, and reviews the pathophysiology and most important etiologies. It should be emphasized that although rare causes of intractable diarrhea contribute little to the global burden of disease, they provide unique insight into our understanding of human physiology and are deserving of detailed descriptions. General principles of management are covered in a separate chapter.

DEFINITIONS, EPIDEMIOLOGY, AND RISK FACTORS

Diarrhea can be defined by measured stool volume of greater than 10 mL/kg/day.[2] Practical definitions of diarrhea can vary. The World Health Organization (WHO), for example, defines diarrhea as the "the passage of loose or watery stools at least 3 times in a 24 hour period." It emphasizes however the change in consistency over frequency and the caregiver's insight into whether the child has diarrhea or not.[3] An arbitrary limit has been set at 14 days to delineate acute from chronic diarrheal episodes,[3,4] although it is recognized that even episodes of 7 to 14 days can carry a nutritional penalty.[1] The terms *chronic*,

persistent or *protracted* diarrhea can be used interchangeably. The term *intractable diarrhea of infancy* was first used by Avery et al. in 1968[5] and thought to describe a single, but unexplained, clinical entity. It is now used to describe a symptom complex comprising multiple etiologies but for the most part postenteritis enteropathy.

Mortality from diarrheal diseases has decreased from 4.6 million deaths per year in the early 1980s to the most recent estimates in 1999 of 2.5 million per year for both children and adults.[2,3] More than 70% of these deaths occur in children.[1] This decrease in mortality is mainly due to improved sanitation practices but also the introduction of oral rehydration therapy in 1979. The major burden of diarrheal disease continues to be carried by developing countries with an excess of infectious etiologies. Reducing the rates of malnutrition and provision of safe water, better sanitation, and better hygiene is expected to reduce the inequalities between developing and developed countries.[3]

As infectious etiologies have significantly decreased in developed countries, there has been an upsurge in atopic and other immune-mediated disorders, including inflammatory bowel disease and celiac disease. This has been attributed to the "hygiene hypothesis" whereby decreased exposure to pathogens in early life has led to immunodysregulatory responses, notably in the fine balance, between T-helper cells (Th1 and Th2) and T-regulatory cells.[6-8]

Malnutrition can both predispose and follow chronic diarrhea. It is considered the most important epidemiologic risk factor for developing protracted diarrhea and is predominant in developing areas of the world.[4,9] It can be found in up to 40% of deaths associated with prolonged diarrhea.[10] Malnutrition can lead to protracted diarrhea by several mechanisms including achlorhydria predisposing to small bowel contamination, systemic immune deficiencies, and altered repair mechanisms. Zinc deficiency, lack of breast-feeding, male sex, enteric infection with *Escherichia coli* or *Cryptosporidium*, systemic infections, intrauterine growth retardation, and immune status are other important risk factors.[4,11]

PATHOPHSYSIOLOGY OF PROTRACTED DIARRHEA

The pathophysiology of protracted diarrhea is complex and still incompletely understood. Two core processes are classically described: secretory and osmotic. Each can occur separately or together, as is the case in severe enteropathies. It should be emphasized that additional factors and mechanisms may play a role in increasing stool fluid output, such as increased intestinal motility (e.g., diarrhea predominant irritable bowel syndrome), pancreatic insufficiency (e.g., cystic fibrosis), or excessive fluid intake (e.g., chronic nonspecific diarrhea of childhood) amongst others. A simplified schematic of the interplay between the two core processes and other factors is shown in Figure 33-1.

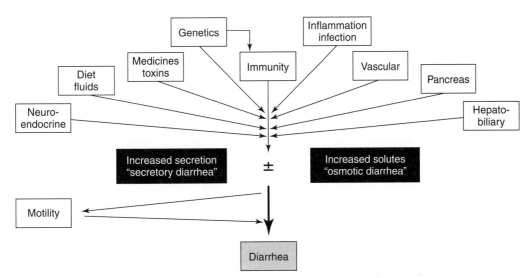

Figure 33-1. The pathophysiology of protracted diarrhea.

Secretory diarrhea occurs when there is excess fluid secretion compared to absorption, most often the result of impaired electrolyte transport. The activation of chloride channels (e.g., the cystic fibrosis transmembrane regulator or CFTR) is the common final pathway resulting in increased electrolyte and water secretion. Phosphorylation-induced activation of these channels may be mediated by increased intracellular concentrations of cAMP, cGMP, or calcium.[12] This cascade of intracellular processes may be triggered by either exogenous or endogenous substances. Exogenous mediators classically include bacterial toxins such as *Vibrio cholerae* toxin or heat-stable *E. coli* toxin, but may also involve viruses (e.g., rotavirus, human immunodeficiency virus [HIV]) or parasites (e.g., *Cryptosporidium parvum, Giardia lamblia*).[13-16] Endogenous mediators may be endocrine, such as vasoactive intestinal peptide or serotonin, or released by the immune system, such as histamine, serotonin, prostaglandins, or interleukin-1. Finally, loss of tight junction integrity with increased intestinal permeability can also contribute to increased intestinal fluid secretion. Mediators of this mechanism may be again exogenous (e.g., zonula occludens toxin of *Vibrio cholerae, Salmonella, Shigella*) or endogenous (e.g., epidermal growth factor).[12]

Osmotic diarrhea is the second core process resulting in diarrhea. Homeostasis dictates that fluid shifts will neutralize osmotic gradients between the intraluminal and extraluminal spaces of the intestinal tract. The osmolality of the succus entericus is determined by the quantity of solutes it contains. These solutes are composed of carbohydrates, proteins, lipids, minerals, and electrolytes from ingested nutrients and endogenous secretions from the hepatobiliary tree, pancreas, and intestinal epithelial cells. In the proximal small bowel, where the intraluminal osmolality is high from recently ingested meals, water is secreted into the lumen and an isotonic balance can be achieved as early as the proximal jejunum.[17] In adults approximately 120 mL/kg/day of fluid (±8 L in a 65-kg adult) can pass through the duodenum and 285 mL/kg/day in an infant. As nutrients are absorbed along the length of the small bowel, the osmolality decreases and water is reabsorbed such that in the adult only 25 mL/kg/day enters the cecum and 61 mL/kg/day in the infant. The colon, through several efficient Na transport mechanisms

operating within the apical membranes of colonocytes, both on the colonic surface and within the crypts, can extract daily an additional 20 to 30 mL/kg of water in the adult and 50 mL/kg in the infant.[3,18,19] Osmotic diarrhea occurs when intraluminal solutes are not sufficiently absorbed because of maldigestion and or malabsorption, creating an osmotic gradient that can only be neutralized by maintaining excessive amounts of water within the intestine.

Carbohydrate malabsorption is the most common cause of osmotic diarrhea in childhood. Lactose intolerance, the prototype for carbohydrate-induced diarrhea, is the result of maldigestion of this disaccharide due to decreased levels of the enzyme lactase contained on the brush border membrane of the enterocyte. The unabsorbed carbohydrate, along with its obligate excess fluid, enters the colon, where it is digested by colonic bacteria, producing short-chain fatty acids (acetate, butyrate, and propionate organic anions). This further increases the osmotic load, resulting in more fluid fluxes into the colon. Taking advantage of this process, for example, lactulose, a fructose-galactose disaccharide that cannot be digested by humans, has been used in medical therapeutics as a laxative for children and adults with constipation.

Less common causes of osmotic diarrhea may be due to malabsorption of peptides, amino acids, and fats such as in Hartnup disease (malabsorption of neutral amino acids), cystic fibrosis (pancreatic insufficiency), and ileal resection in short bowel syndrome (bile salt depletion with fat malabsorption). Enteric loss of larger proteins may occur as a result of increased gut permeability (e.g., Crohn's disease) or obstruction to lymphatic outflow (e.g., intestinal lymphangiectasia).

Decreased absorptive area either through decreased intestinal length (e.g., short bowel syndrome) or inflammation (e.g., celiac disease) can also lead to malabsorption and osmotic diarrhea. Increased motor activity of the gut can lead to malabsorption by functionally decreasing the absorptive surface through decreased contact time between chyme and the intestinal epithelial lining. Diarrhea caused primarily by abnormal motor activity (*diarrhee motrice*) is rare but may contribute to the diarrhea seen in diseases of autonomic dysfunction[20] and diarrhea predominant irritable bowel syndrome. Allergic dysmotility due to non-IGE-mediated food allergy has been described

TABLE 33-1. Causes of Protracted Diarrhea

Infection	***Specific Absorption Defects***
Bacterial: *Vibrio cholerae*, *Escherichia coli* (e.g., enteropathogenic, enteroaggregative), *Salmonella*, *Campylobacter*	Carbohydrates
	Sucrase-isomaltase deficiency
Viral: HIV, rotavirus	Lactase deficiency: developmental, congenital, primary, secondary
Parasite: *Cryptosporidium parvum*, *Giardia lamblia*	Glucose-galactose malabsorption
Others	Proteins/amino acids
Small bowel bacterial overgrowth syndrome	Hartnup disease
Postenteritis enteropathy	Cystinuria
Tropical sprue	Lipids
	Abetalipoproteinemia
Food-Sensitive Diseases	Hypobetalipoproteinemia
Celiac disease	Electrolytes
Allergic and eosinophilic enteropathies	Congenital chloridorrhea
Postenteritis enteropathy	Congenital sodium diarrhea
Chronic nonspecific diarrhea of childhood ("toddler's diarrhea")	Minerals
	Acrodermatitis enteropathica
Immune-Mediated Diseases	Other
Primary immune deficiencies: SCID, thymic hypoplasia, CD40 ligand deficiency, IgA deficiency	Ileal bile acid receptor defect
Secondary immune deficiencies: AIDS	***Syndromes of Intractable Diarrhea of Infancy***
Autoimmune enteropathy/IPEX/APCED syndromes	Microvillous inclusion disease
Intestinal graft vs. host disease	Intestinal epithelial dysplasia (tufting enteropathy)
Celiac disease	Autoimmune enteropathy/IPEX/APCED
	Enterocyte heparan sulfate deficiency (CDG-1c)
Inflammatory Enteropathies	Enterokinase deficiency
Inflammatory bowel disease: Crohn's disease, ulcerative colitis	Syndromatic diarrhea
Behçet's disease	
Intractable ulcerating enterocolitis of infancy	***Pancreatic Insufficiency***
	Cystic fibrosis
Anatomic Abnormalities	Schwachman's syndrome
Malrotation	
Short gut syndrome	***Other***
Intestinal lymphangiectasia	Factitious diarrhea or Munchausen's syndrome by proxy
Congenital	Anorexia nervosa ("purging")
Constrictive pericarditis	Dietary
Fontan procedure	Chronic nonspecific diarrhea of childhood ("toddler's diarrhea")
	Mismanagement: formula mixing
Intestinal Motility-Mediated Diseases	Additives: sorbitol, Olestra (nonabsorbable fat substitute)
Allergic dysmotility	Iatrogenic/medicines/toxins:
Chronic nonspecific diarrhea of childhood ("toddler's diarrhea")	Laxatives
Chronic intestinal pseudo-obstruction	Orlistat (lipase inhibitor)
Irritable bowel syndrome	Radiation enteritis
	Heavy metals: arsenic
Primary Metabolic Diseases	Organophosphates
Mitochondrial cytopathies	Polyposis syndromes
Mucopolysaccharidosis syndromes	Hirschsprung's enterocolitis
Congenital disorders of glycosylation	Constipation with overflow incontinence
	Hyperthyroidism
Malignancy	
VIPoma	
Carcinoid syndrome	
Small bowel lymphoma	
Medullary carcinoma of the thyroid	

AIDS, acquired immunodeficiency syndrome; HIV, human immunodeficiency virus; SCID, severe combined immunodeficiency.
Some etiologies may be found under several headings, either because they involve different mechanisms of disease or because their disease causation is still incompletely understood.

and involves antigen-induced degranulation of mast cells and eosinophils leading to abnormal gut motility.[21,22] In most cases, however, abnormal motor activity is secondary, aggravating existing diarrhea that is the result of increased fluid secretion and inflammation.

Causes of Protracted Diarrhea

The causes of protracted diarrhea are numerous. Reviewed herein are those that are most important from an epidemiologic standpoint, are frequently encountered in pediatric gastroenterology practice, or, even though rarely encountered, provide valuable insight into the pathophysiology of diarrheal syndromes. A nonexhaustive listing is provided in Table 33-1.

Infection-Induced Enteropathies

Many organisms are capable of causing chronic diarrheal disease, particularly when host immunity is impaired. Some organisms are however notable causes of chronic diarrhea on a global scale. Enteropathogenic *E. coli* (EPEC) and enteroaggregative *E. coli* (EAEC) are the most commonly implicated bacterial causes of persistent diarrhea among children in developing countries.[16] Small intestinal biopsy in these children shows marked enteropathy, and there may be direct signs of bacterial overgrowth. The exact mechanism by which EAEC leads to diarrhea is not known. In EPEC, the characteristic finding is revealed by electron microscopy as the "attaching-effacing lesion," due to induced cytoskeletal rearrangement within infected enterocytes. This provides a form of pedestal on which adherent bacteria may be seen and disrupts the brush border, leading to loss of absorptive area.[16,23] In developed countries, *Clostridium difficile* is increasingly considered a cause of chronic diarrhea as it becomes more prevalent in the community and more difficult to treat. Interestingly, and because they are most commonly thought of as causing only acute disease, *Campylobacter*, *Shigella*, and *Salmonella* can be responsible for chronic diarrheal states.[11]

Viral agents are also usually associated with acute, short-duration infections. However, it has been shown that some viruses, such as rotavirus, can cause protracted diarrhea in immunodeficient and immunocompetent children alike.[24] Children with acquired immunodeficiency syndrome (AIDS) can have persistent diarrhea, and although the most commonly accepted mechanism is due to opportunistic infections from chronic immunodeficiency, a direct effect of HIV on the enterocyte has been postulated.[14] In immunocompromised children, cytomegalovirus and other enteric viruses (e.g., adenovirus) may also cause chronic diarrhea.

Many parasites cause protracted diarrhea including *Microsporidium*, *Isospora belli*, *Entamoeba histolytica*, *Strongyloides stercoralis*, *Cyclospora cayetanensis*, *Giardia lamblia*, and *Cryptosporidium parvum*.[11]

Giardia lamblia trophozoites may be found in the duodenum and jejunum, particularly in children with IgA deficiency,[25] and may cause acute or chronic diarrhea. Histologic examination may show increased numbers of intraepithelial lymphocytes and sometimes partial villous atrophy, although findings are patchy.[26]

Cryptosporidium parvum has become accepted as an important human pathogen since the recognition of AIDS. However, it is now known that immunocompetent hosts may also be at risk. A study in West African children has shown that *Cryptosporidium* was the most significant risk factor in the development of chronic diarrhea after an acute enteritis episode.[27] Small bowel histology may sometimes demonstrate schizonts, in association with a mild or moderate enteropathy in children with no known immunodeficiency.[28]

Strongyloides stercoralis infestation is a major cause of chronic diarrhea, protein-losing enteropathy, and malnutrition in tropical, developing countries. Sporadic cases may be seen in developed countries brought back by travelers or immigrants. Diagnosis may be suggested by peripheral eosinophilia but is established by examination of histologic specimens or duodenal aspirates for the parasite.[29]

Postenteritis syndrome, also called intractable diarrhea of infancy, postenteritis enteropathy, or "slick gut" syndrome, is a chronic small intestinal condition with a worldwide distribution. It remains an important clinical problem in developing countries where access to medical care and adequate nutrition and hygiene is limited. Its clinical and histologic features can overlap with those of tropical sprue, which is perhaps its adult equivalent. The downward spiral of postenteritis syndrome may begin with a persistent infection or a sequence of infections, following one after the other, and providing an apparent clinical picture of a single continuing illness. The sequential nature of these infections can be determined only by repeated testing for

infective agents.[30,31] Enteric infection with inflammation and resulting loss of intake can lead to disaccharidase deficiency (so-called postinfectious or secondary lactase deficiency) in its mildest form and profound, generalized malabsorption in its most severe forms. In this latter instance malnutrition can ensue with death in up to 50%.[32,33] Although this most severe form is common in developing countries, it can also be seen in developed-world infants with immunodeficiencies or other debilitating diseases.

Food-Sensitive Enteropathies

Diarrhea caused by food can occur under different guises: antigen sensitivities, carbohydrate intolerance, or feeding mismanagement due to issues of either excess or composition.

It has been recognized for many years that food antigens may induce chronic small intestinal enteropathy presenting as persistent diarrhea. The most important specific enteropathy in this category is celiac disease. This immune-mediated disease is covered in depth in its own chapter of this book. Certain misconceptions surrounding celiac disease persist, such as that there is only one pediatric presentation: diarrhea with explosive floating stools, bloating, malnutrition, and failure to thrive. It is now recognized that this classic clinical presentation is only the tip of the celiac disease iceberg and that many other presentations exist. Another misconception is that celiac disease occurs only in developed countries; it has now been found to be an important cause of chronic diarrhea in the developing countries of the Saharan regions and Indian subcontinent.[34,35]

There is additional evidence that some cases of postenteritis enteropathy show a food-sensitive component, thought to be due to lost oral tolerance for food antigens after breach of the intestinal barrier.[36,37] Cow's-milk enteropathy is the most frequent overlap condition, in which mucosal damage may be initiated by infection and perpetuated by continued antigen ingestion. Treatment with a lactose-free milk-derived formula may improve symptoms but leaves the underlying pathology untreated.

True food allergies and eosinophilic gastroenteritis should be part of the differential diagnosis of children with chronic diarrhea and are covered in another chapter of this book.

Cow's-milk protein intolerance of infancy is a well-documented cause of enterocolitis in children. It typically presents with diarrhea and hematochezia within days to months after exposure to cow's-milk protein in neonates and young infants. Up to 50% of infants may cross-react with soy protein, and rarely this entity may be seen in exclusively breast-fed babies. Treatment includes exclusion of the offending proteins in the diet of the formula-fed infant and in the maternal diet of the breast-fed infant. This may involve changing to a protein-hydrolysate formula, or rarely to an amino acid–based formula. In the great majority of cases, soy and cow's-milk protein can be reintroduced into the diet after 1 year of age without recurrence.[38-40]

Chronic nonspecific diarrhea of childhood is a common cause of protracted diarrhea in affluent societies.[18,41] For the lay person it is also known as toddler's diarrhea, peas and carrots diarrhea, or sloppy stool syndrome. It typically presents in otherwise healthy children between the ages of 1 and 5 years. It can be continuous or episodic with usually variable stool consistencies from watery to soft. Parents can be particularly frustrated because of their (or their family's) expectations of what normal stools should be, or because of the inability to keep the children at day care. Although there is evidence supporting abnormal gut motility,[42] the history often identifies an "unbalanced" diet. This may be the result of parental manipulation of the diet in an attempt to control the output of what may have started as a self-limited acute infectious enteritis (e.g., dairy restriction, "BRAT" diet) or manipulation of the diet by a child in the midst of their "terrible twos" and facilitated by the parents' misperception of poor appetite. In many instances, the consumption of excessive quantities of hypertonic fluids such as fruit juices is identified. Certain juices such as apple, grape, or peach contain large amounts of poorly absorbable fructose and sorbitol. In some children, the juice intake can be so excessive that failure to thrive can ensue.[43] Another subset of children, however, may be exquisitely sensitive to juices such that a single 240-mL serving causes carbohydrate malabsorption as evidenced by diarrhea and abnormal breath hydrogen testing.[44] Diagnosis is often suspected by a careful history and a physical exam supporting good health. It is confirmed by an empiric trial of therapy without any need for further testing. Treatment involves parental reassurance, removing or severely limiting hypertonic juices from the diet, decreasing excessive volume intakes to reasonable amounts, and removing any unfounded food restrictions. A balanced diet is recommended. This should include encouraging the consumption of fiber-rich and fatty foods (e.g., cheeses, whole milk). Fat is known to slow gastric emptying and to increase small-intestinal transit time by activating the "ileal brake" and decreasing colonic motility.[41]

Rarely, infants may present with chronic diarrhea due to errors in milk formula mixing as inexperienced parents reconstitute formula from powder, creating a concentrated, hypertonic feeding. The diagnosis is again made by taking a careful history.

Immune-Mediated Enteropathies

It is well recognized that infants and children with severe immunodeficiency syndromes have chronic diarrhea and failure to thrive. There is still only imperfect knowledge about specific patterns of injury in different syndromes.[45,46] Primary immunodeficiency syndromes are thought to cause persistent diarrhea either by enteropathy or chronic infection. These syndromes include severe combined immunodeficiency syndrome (SCID), thymic hypoplasia, class II major histocompatibility class defect, and CD40 ligand deficiency.[46] The early presentation is usually diagnosed as the first major pathogen identified in the stool, and immunodeficiency is suspected subsequently when the illness becomes persistent and difficult to treat with accompanying failing health, or when there are unexplained repeated infections with different organisms. The histology of the intestinal mucosa may be normal or show variable abnormalities (e.g., villous blunting, absent plasma cells).

It is not just major immunodeficiency that may be associated with gastrointestinal diseases causing chronic diarrhea. The association of minor immunodeficiency with dietary sensitization has been noted for many years, following the finding in 1973 of low IgA in children with milk allergy.[47] This condition, transient IgA deficiency of infancy, occurs as a result of a developmental delay in maturation of IgA responses, possibly reflecting a relative lack of infectious exposures in early life, as it is not seen in developing-world infants. Transient IgA deficiency of infancy may be part of a broader pattern of delayed immune maturation that includes low circulating CD8 and natural killer cells, and IgG subclass deficiency.[48,49] In addition

to chronic loose stools, children may present in early life with variable combinations of eczema and immediate hypersensitivity responses.

Secondary immunodeficiencies can also lead to protracted or relapsing diarrhea, as is the case for AIDS as described previously.

Autoimmune enteropathy (AIE) is a rare disorder recognized since the early 1980s and characterized by severe and unrelenting diarrhea, failure to thrive, and immune-mediated intestinal injury.[50,51] It occurs in infants and young children for the most part, although adult-onset cases have recently been described.[52] Recent and significant understanding of its pathophysiology, including disease-causing gene mutations, allows us to recognize at least four types:

1. Isolated AIE with typical anti-enterocyte antibodies occurring in both sexes
2. IPEX occurring only in males
3. IPEX-like syndrome occurring in both sexes
4. APECED syndrome (APS-1)

The pathogenesis of AIE continues to be elucidated, but it appears that a common pathway is the disruption of normal regulatory T cell homeostasis. In IPEX syndrome, for example, abnormal expression of the FOXP3 gene results in defective regulatory function of T cells. The now 30 recognized mutations of the FOXP3 gene can lead to a multisystemic, autoaggressive T cell-mediated disorder.[53] The well documented anti-enterocyte antibodies of AIE are now thought to be an epiphenomenon of intestinal inflammation, rather than its cause. They are also no longer thought to be pathognomonic of AIE because they can be also seen in low titers in other intestinal diseases such as Crohn's disease or cow's-milk allergy.[54,55]

Clinical features are characterized by severe and protracted secretory diarrhea starting for most in the first few weeks of life and leading to frequent episodes of dehydration, electrolyte imbalances, and malnutrition requiring parenteral nutritional support.[52,53] Complications such as septicemia, rashes, and impaired development, the result of chronic malnutrition and hospitalizations, are not unexpected. Prognosis, before the advent of immunomodulator therapy and transplantation, was poor but even today remains dependent on the extent and severity of the intestinal injury and the presence of extraintestinal manifestations.

IPEX syndrome (immune dysregulation *p*olyendocrinopathy *e*nteropathy *X*-linked) is a form of AIE associated at the onset with insulin-dependent diabetes mellitus, hematologic abnormalities (e.g., Coombs-positive anemia), and eczema. Other endocrinopathies (e.g., thyroid disease) or renal disease may develop later.[53] The variable expressions of IPEX syndrome may be related to poorly defined genotype-phenotype relations. An IPEX-like syndrome that is unrelated to FOXP3 gene mutations and can occur in boys and girls alike has been described but is poorly understood.[53]

In the APECED syndrome (also called autoimmune polyglandular syndrome 1 or APS-1), AIE is associated with *auto*immune phenomena, *p*olyendocrinopathy, *m*ucocutaneous *candidiasis*, and *ectodermal dysplasia.*[52] The gene associated with the disease, AIRE (autoimmune regulator), has been mapped to the chromosome 21q22.3. The disease is described most frequently in certain populations such as Finns, Iranian Jews, and Sardinians.[56] The clinical manifestations may be milder because the immune target is within the enteroendocrine cells rather than the absorptive cells.[57]

TABLE 33-2. Diagnostic Criteria for Autoimmune Enteropathy[57,58]

Protracted diarrhea with severe enteropathy and villous atrophy
No response to exclusion diets
Presence of circulating anti-enterocyte antibodies, anti-goblet cell
 antibodies, or evidence of other autoimmune disease
No severe immunodeficiency
Abnormal T-cell activation studies
Genotyping of suspected mutations based on clinical presentation

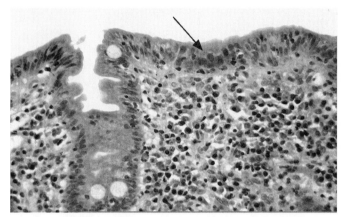

Figure 33-2. Villous atrophy in a patient with autoimmune enteropathy due to IPEX syndrome. Despite the dense increase in T cells within the lamina propria, there is minimal increase in intracellular lymphocyte numbers (arrow). This finding provides contrast to the high density of intraepithelial lymphocytes in celiac disease. (*See plate section for color.*)

Diagnosis of AIE should be considered in any infant with severe, unexplained diarrhea requiring parenteral nutritional support. The diagnostic criteria first described by Walker-Smith et al.[58] still apply and with recent updates[57] are shown in Table 33-2.

The histopathology of AIE, central to the diagnosis, can be confused with celiac disease demonstrating villous atrophy but with a paucity of intraepithelial lymphocytes. Also described is a dense lymphoplasmacytic infiltration of the lamina propria, and crypt abscesses can be demonstrated in the most severe cases (Figure 33-2).

A rational basis for treatment is guided by our recent understanding of T cell dysregulation in AIE and involves immunosuppression that targets T cell function, including steroids, tacrolimus, rapamycin, and others.[52,53] IPEX syndrome is generally considered more difficult to treat with poorer outcomes. Those children in whom AIE cannot be stabilized with immunosuppressives have been referred for bone marrow transplantation with variable but improving results.[59-61]

Inflammatory Enteropathies

True inflammatory bowel disease, usually considered uncommon in young children, is now being described increasingly in this age group. The differential diagnosis should include chronic granulomatous disease, Behçet's disease, or intractable ulcerating enterocolitis of infancy.[62,63] A full diagnostic assessment may be needed to differentiate between these diseases and early-onset Crohn's disease and ulcerative colitis. Intractable ulcerating enterocolitis of infancy is a rare autosomal recessive condition. It runs a severe course, often requiring early colectomy, and children are at risk for Epstein-Barr virus

(EBV)-associated lymphomatous proliferations including non-Hodgkin's lymphoma. Immunosuppressive agents and bone marrow transplantation have been used to control the disease.[64]

Specific Absorption Defects

Specific nutrient absorption defects are important causes of protracted diarrhea, due either to their common occurrence (e.g., primary lactase deficiency) or to their rare appearance with early onset and daunting diagnostic challenges such as normal histologic features (e.g., congenital chloridorrhea). They may cover the gamut of all nutrients including carbohydrates, proteins, lipids, electrolytes, and minerals.

Primary lactase deficiency is the most frequently encountered carbohydrate deficiency in daily clinical practice. It is also referred to as adult-onset hypolactasia, or hereditary lactase deficiency. It develops in childhood at various ages and has a worldwide distribution in a variety of racial groups. It can be found in up to 70% of the world's population.[65,66] Diagnosis is suspected by the clinical history and confirmed by brush border hydrolase assay. Less invasive breath hydrogen testing may also confirm the diagnosis if other mucosal diseases such as celiac or Crohn's disease are not suspected. Diagnosis by empiric trial alone of a lactose-restricted diet may also be used in the otherwise healthy child. Treatment includes avoidance of lactose-containing foods or addition of oral lactase replacement capsules to the diet.[66] Secondary lactase deficiency may be seen after an acute infectious illness, and rarely congenital lactase deficiency has been described in a few isolated populations.[67,68] In the neonatal intensive care nursery, developmental lactase deficiency may be seen in infants below 34 weeks gestational age at birth.[65]

Congenital glucose-galactose malabsorption is a rare disorder presenting in infants receiving a glucose or lactose-based milk. When recognized early, it is treated with a fructose-based formula; otherwise it can lead to neurologic complications and death. Mutations in the sodium-glucose luminal co-transporter (SGTL-1) have been described, leading to early-onset diarrhea.[69]

Congenital sucrase-isomaltase deficiency presents with an osmotic diarrhea when sucrose is introduced into the diet. Typically, a breast-fed infant will develop diarrhea when juices, solid foods, or sucrose-sweetened medicines are introduced. Measurement of intestinal disaccharidases remains the gold standard for diagnosis.[70]

Two rare conditions caused by defective electrolyte exchange mechanisms cause early-onset secretory diarrhea. Congenital chloridorrhea, the more common of the two, is an autosomal recessive disorder of intestinal $Cl^--HCO_3^-$ exchange caused by a mutation in the SLC26A3 gene.[71] More than 30 mutations have been described, occurring mainly in Finnish, Polish, and Arab populations. Diarrhea begins in utero with polyhydramnios and prematurity. Affected infants present with metabolic acidosis, hypochloremia, and a stool Cl^- concentration greater than 90 mmol/L, usually greater than the sum of Na^+ and K^+ concentrations. When diagnosed early and treated with replacement of ongoing electrolyte losses, the prognosis is good. Congenital sodium diarrhea due to defective Na^+H^+ coupled transport in the brush border membrane is even less common. Stool sodium levels are high, less than for chloride. Stool pH is alkaline as opposed to the other congenital diarrheas.[72]

Acrodermatitis enteropathica is an inherited disorder, the result of a mutation in the Zip-4 transporter, leading to severe

TABLE 33-3. Causes of Intractable Diarrhea of Infancy

Normal Villous-Crypt Architecture
Transport defects
    Congenital chloridorrhea
    Congenital sodium diarrhea
    Glucose-galactose malabsorption
    Sucrase-isomaltase deficiency
    Ileal bile salt receptor defect
    Acrodermatitis enteropathica
Enterokinase deficiency
Congenital enterocyte heparan sulfate deficiency
Congenital short bowel syndrome

Villous Atrophy
Microvillous inclusion disease
Intestinal epithelial dysplasia (tufting enteropathy)
Autoimmune enteropathy/IPEX/APCED
Infectious and postinfectious enteropathies
Allergic enteropathy
Syndromatic diarrhea
Idiopathic

Adapted from Sherman et al.[78]

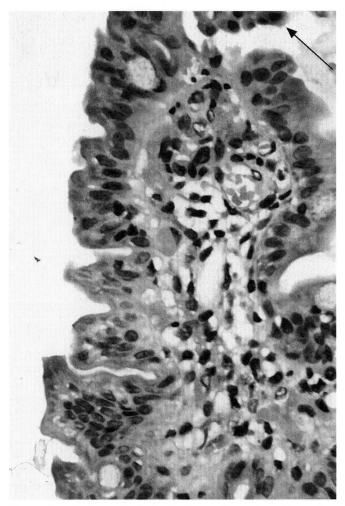

Figure 33-3. Shedding of surface epithelium at villus tip (arrow) in a patient with tufting enteropathy. (*See plate section for color.*)

zinc deficiency. Symptoms develop after weaning and begin with chronic diarrhea and skin rash, mainly periorally and perianally. It may progress to a bullous pustular dermatitis of the hands and feet, alopecia and nail dystrophy, developmental delay, failure to thrive, and infections secondary to dysregulation of cell-mediated immunity. The disease is fatal if left untreated. Plasma zinc levels are usually low and response to zinc supplementation effective.[45,73]

Abetalipoproteinemia is a rare defect in chylomicron formation due to absent beta lipoprotein. This causes postmucosal transport of fat with accumulation in the enterocyte, resulting in steatorrhea. Early clinical findings may be similar to celiac disease. It is one of the few diseases in the category of specific absorptive defects where histologic abnormalities can be seen: the intracellular accumulation of fats on Sudan red stains of frozen biopsy specimens. The diagnosis is confirmed by assay of absent plasma beta lipoprotein. Hypobetalipoproteinemia also involves defective chylomicron formation with intracellular fat accumulation but without the other characteristic features.[45]

Syndromes of Intractable Diarrhea of Infancy

Protracted diarrhea occurring during the first 6 months of life can be a challenging diagnostic and management problem once common causes such as infection, celiac disease, or cystic fibrosis among others have been eliminated. They are commonly grouped under the descriptive title of intractable diarrhea syndromes of infancy. Some have been previously described (e.g., autoimmune enteropathy). A practical listing according to the presence or absence of histologic changes will help in the approach to these difficult patients (Table 33-3).

Enterocyte heparan sulfate deficiency, first described in 1996, is a congenital condition resulting in severe protein-losing enteropathy.[74,75] The pathogenesis is thought to be similar to congenital nephrotic syndrome. Heparan sulfate is a negatively charged sulfated glycosaminoglycan that prevents albumin leakage by electrostatic interaction.[76] Another form of enterocyte heparan sulfate dysregulation can occur as part of the congenital disorders of glycosylation (CDG-1). In this instance, the mislocalization of heparan sulfate within the enterocyte may explain the protein-losing enteropathy seen in this condition.[77]

Tufting enteropathy, now known as intestinal epithelial dysplasia (IED), is a severe, early-onset syndrome of secretory diarrhea that persists despite bowel rest and parenteral nutrition and can lead to intestinal failure.[78-80] Consanguineous parents or affected siblings suggests an autosomal recessive inheritance but the causative gene(s) have not been identified. Associated dysmorphic features, choanal, esophageal, or rectal atresia, have been described with this condition. Light microscopy of small bowel biopsies show variable villous atrophy, crypt hyperplasia, and normal or slightly increased inflammatory cells in the lamina propria. The characteristic finding, however, is the presence of focally crowded enterocytes forming a "tuft." The apical plasma membrane can be rounded, giving the enterocyte a tear-shaped appearance[78] (Figure 33-3). Small bowel transplantation is indicated in those affected infants with intestinal failure and complications from parenteral nutrition.[81]

Microvillous inclusion disease was one of the first recognized syndromes of intractable diarrhea. It is severe and life threatening with diarrhea beginning in the first days of life. Fluid losses can be as high as 300 mL/kg while nil per os, and stool sodium and chloride concentrations approach those of serum.[78,82] History of polyhydramnios is absent. Affected infants require massive fluid support and parenteral nutrition, which is often

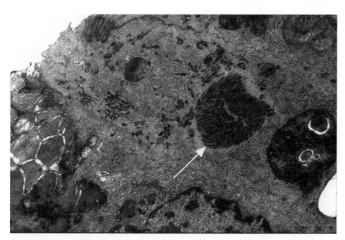

Figure 33-4. Intracellular inclusions (arrow) in microvillous inclusion disease. Electron micrograph courtesy of Dr. Alan Phillips.

complicated by early cholestasis and sepsis. Prognosis is generally poor without intestinal transplantation.[83] A genetic cause is suspected with clustering of cases in specific populations (e.g., Navajo Indians), but the target genes and the pathogenesis is still unknown. Light microscopy shows villous atrophy with little inflammatory infiltrate. On higher magnification, the surface enterocytes are focally piled up with vacuolization of the apical cytoplasm and loss of brush border definition. Immunostaining demonstrates alkaline phosphatase within cytoplasmic circular structures corresponding to the microvillous inclusions. Diagnostic features are also found on electron microscopy of the small intestine and include intracellular inclusions in the apical enterocytes and secretory granules within the crypts[78,82] (Figure 33-4).

Syndromic diarrhea, also referred to as phenotypic diarrhea or tricho-hepato-enteric syndrome, is another rare form of intractable diarrhea presenting within the first 6 months of life. The persistent diarrhea is associated with facial dysmorphism (hypertelorism, broad midface and nose) and hair that is wooly, underpigmented, and easily plucked. Half of patients develop hepatic fibrosis or cirrhosis. The enteropathy may be severe, requiring long-term parenteral nutrition. Histopathology shows nonspecific villous atrophy, and a functional T-cell immune deficiency has been reported. The etiology is unknown, but an autosomal recessive inheritance is suspected.[84,85]

Anatomic Abnormalities

Protracted diarrhea as the presenting symptom of intestinal malrotation may not occur until after infancy. Intestinal strictures or dysmotile loops of bowel may predispose to bacterial overgrowth syndrome and worsen malabsorption and diarrhea. Primary intestinal lymphangiectasia is an important anatomic abnormality that causes protein-losing enteropathy, often also causing a low circulating lymphocyte count and visibly dilated lymphatics at endoscopy. This may also occur secondary to cardiac conditions such as constrictive pericarditis or following a Fontan procedure for repair of congenital heart disease. The presentation may mimic celiac disease, with diarrhea and failure to thrive, and eventual hypoproteinemic edema. Small intestinal biopsy may show gross lymphatic dilation, but the lesion may be patchy and biopsies may be normal.

ASSESSMENT OF THE PATIENT WITH PROTRACTED DIARRHEA

The large number of diagnostic possibilities and available investigative studies mandates a rational approach to each child presenting with diarrhea. However, a single unifying diagnostic protocol cannot be recommended, because the physician's approach will need to vary dependent on the clinical circumstances. The evaluation of a malnourished child in a developing country where infection is most prevalent, for example, will be different from that of a same-age child who is healthy, thriving, and living in a developed urban environment. Other distinguishing variables may include the age of the patient, available medical resources, and finally the physician's own clinical acumen.

Clinical History and Physical Examination

A careful clinical history and physical exam is the single most important element in the evaluation of any patient with persistent diarrhea. It will decide the other elements of the diagnostic evaluation: whether to pursue invasive endoscopic testing or an empiric trial of dietary changes (e.g., suspicion of celiac disease versus toddler's diarrhea). The age of symptom onset may give an important clue to the diagnosis: primary epithelial disorders may present within the first days of life, immune-mediated disorders during the first weeks, and inflammatory bowel disease after early childhood. A detailed dietary history can often provide the diagnosis in cases of chronic nonspecific diarrhea of childhood, primary lactase deficiency, or errors in milk formula mixing. The relation between onset of symptoms and introduction to new foods may also be an important clue in food-sensitive enteropathies such as celiac disease or allergic enteropathy. The stooling pattern including size, consistency, and frequency should be recorded. Often it will steer the clinician toward the right diagnosis: small, frequent, painful, and mucoid stools with tenesmus may be suggestive of colitis, as opposed to large, watery, and relatively painless stools indicative of a small bowel origin.

Nutritional assessment as part of the physical exam is necessary and should include, height, weight, and global nutritional appearance. The numerical data should be plotted on normative, relevant percentile graphs including the body mass index for age (or weight for length index in infants). Past growth parameters are very helpful in constructing growth curves and estimating growth velocities: a body mass index for age that has fallen from the 75th percentile to the 15th percentile over 1 year is suspicious of organic disease and more worrisome than a child that has maintained that same low percentile over the same period.

Often neglected by physicians in training is an examination of the perianal area, which can provide important diagnostic clues. The presence of a significant diaper dermatitis in infants can be suggestive of a carbohydrate intolerance brought on by the acidic quality of their stools. In the older child, the presence of anal fissures, skin tags, or drainage, in the absence of constipation, should be suggestive of Crohn's disease. A digital rectal examination may be helpful when considering inflammatory bowel disease or to distinguish between the child with true diarrhea and overflow incontinence.

Diagnostic Stool Studies

Observation of the stool is an important part of the assessment: whether it is watery, or contains blood, mucus, or pus. Stool output, although equally important, may be difficult to quantitate, especially when dealing with highly absorbent diapers, reduced nursing care in hospitals, and the inability to accurately separate stool from urine in young children. This may be circumvented in difficult cases by use of a urinary catheter, reversal of the diaper (or alternatively lining the inside of the diaper with plastic wrap), and attentive care by parents or nursing staff. The change in output following a short period of nil per os may help differentiate osmotic from secretory causes of diarrhea. Routine laboratory examination of the stool may include fecal leukocytes ("the nongastroenterologist's colonoscopy") indicative of inflammation, and pH and reducing substances in the younger child looking for carbohydrate malabsorption. More specialized stool assays include quantitative α1-antitrypsin for protein-losing enteropathy, fecal elastase for pancreatic insufficiency, and lactoferrin or calprotectin for inflammatory conditions. Fecal calprotectin in particular has been reported as an accurate marker of inflammatory bowel conditions in both adults and children with a sensitivity and specificity of 70% and 96%, respectively, in this latter group.[86]

Measurement of stool electrolytes and osmolality gap may also be helpful to distinguish between secretory and osmotic conditions. Measurement of stool osmolality by the laboratory may be inaccurate because of bacterial degradation of carbohydrate, and consequently the osmolality gap should be calculated by subtracting the sum of stool Na^+ and K^+ multiplied by 2, from 290 (the osmolality of serum). Secretory diarrhea is suspected if the stool Na^+ is greater than 90 mM and the osmotic gap is less than 50.

In all cases of chronic diarrhea, it is important that stools be examined by culture for bacterial pathogens and by microscopy for ova, cysts, and parasites. It is imperative to communicate with the laboratory regarding availability of tests, proper handling of specimens, and any suspicions regarding possible nonroutine pathogens. When available, most laboratories have replaced culture and microscopy of fecal samples with enzyme-linked immunosorbent (ELISA) assays, which are more sensitive and specific but also less observer dependent. Examples include detection of *Giardia* and *Cryptosporidium*. *Giardia* may also be isolated from duodenal aspirates collected at the time of upper endoscopy.

Hematologic, Biochemical, and Immunologic Studies

These tests are important in the child with unexplained chronic diarrheal disease, not only to aid in diagnosing the underlying condition, but also to assess the degree of injury. A complete blood count may show anemia, and abnormal red blood cell indices may emphasize its chronicity. Inflammatory indices such as the erythrocyte sedimentation rate, C-reactive protein, or platelet count may indicate Crohn's disease, ulcerative colitis, or other inflammatory conditions if elevated. Serum assays are also helpful to assess the depth of nutritional deficits and general state of debilitation. These may include electrolyte, total protein, albumin, vitamin, and mineral levels. A prealbumin assay may be helpful in distinguishing malnutrition from protein-losing enteropathy in the hypoalbuminemic child, with the caveat that the two states may often coexist.

Chronic diarrhea may be an important manifestation of underlying immunodeficiency, especially if there is a history of recurrent infections or eczema. Baseline immunologic testing should include quantitative immunoglobulin, T-cell, and IgG subsets. Anti-endomysial antibodies or tissue transglutaminase antibodies should be collected if celiac disease is suspected.

Anti-enterocyte antibodies should be requested if autoimmune enteropathy is being considered, especially if there is evidence of other autoimmune disorders, an endocrinopathy, or a family history of autoimmunity. Commercially available serologic profiles can be useful in the evaluation of the child with possible inflammatory bowel disease. Genetic testing may be helpful in the diagnosis of some viral diseases (e.g., DNA polymerase chain reaction [PCR] for cytomegalovirus) or inherited disorders (e.g., cystic fibrosis).

Hydrogen Breath Tests

Hydrogen breath testing can be a valuable, noninvasive, office-based tool to diagnose carbohydrate malabsorption (e.g., lactose or fructose), small bowel bacterial overgrowth syndrome, or orocecal transit times. Its main indication is in the cooperative child in whom no other disease other than a carbohydrate-sensitive enteropathy is suspected. Up to 25% of patients may have a non-hydrogen-producing fecal flora and be responsible for false negatives. Positive results may be misleading if there is another diffuse mucosal disease such as Crohn's or celiac disease. In these instances the carbohydrate malabsorption is secondary to the mucosal inflammation and villous blunting and not a primary deficiency as may be thought.[87-89]

Sweat Test

It is important to exclude cystic fibrosis in any child with persistent diarrhea and failure to thrive. Sweat chloride testing remains the gold standard for diagnosis. In young infants, the inability to collect sufficient volumes of sweat for analysis may be circumvented by serum assays for immunoreactive trypsinogen or DNA mutational analysis. Elevated serum trypsinogen levels, a sign of pancreatic inflammation and impending exocrine failure, are now part of many newborn screening programs in Western developed countries. In white populations the ΔF508 mutation of the CFTR gene is most commonly encountered (70% of patients); however, a negative result does not exclude the carriage of a rare mutation. In particular, children carrying a single ΔF508 mutation may still have the disease if they have a rare mutation, inherited from the other parent, that was not screened by the assay used.

Endoscopy and Histologic Sampling

Endoscopy with biopsy is the most accurate tool to diagnose most chronic enteropathies when routine stool and hematologic studies have failed or are inconclusive. It remains the cornerstone of diagnosis for diseases such as Crohn's disease, ulcerative colitis, graft-versus-host disease, celiac disease, and primary specific absorption defects.[65,90,91] Esophagogastroduodenoscopy and ileocolonoscopy have been part of the pediatric gastroenterologist's diagnostic armamentarium for decades, allowing detailed examinations of the upper and lower intestinal tracts. The recent additions of wireless capsule endoscopy and balloon-assisted enteroscopy now allow examination of the entire small bowel with improved diagnostic yields. Wireless capsule endoscopy, despite its inability to obtain histologic samples, can be an important diagnostic tool in the evaluation of children with suspected or established inflammatory bowel disease.[92,93] It may confirm the disease in children with suspected Crohn's disease, or it may help to differentiate ulcerative colitis from Crohn's disease in patients with indeterminate colitis when standard techniques have failed. It has limited applications to the diagnosis of celiac disease (e.g., disease unresponsive to therapy) and may provide benefit in evaluating children with graft-versus-host disease or polyposis syndromes.[94-96] When histologic sampling of the small bowel is required, push enteroscopy for the proximal jejunum and balloon-assisted enteroscopy for the remainder of the small bowel may be considered.[97] This latter technique is now being used on a limited basis in some pediatric centers.

Regardless of the technique, multiple and adequate-size biopsy samples should be obtained when possible. In addition to routine histology, frozen samples can be sent for disaccharidase assay and snap-frozen specimens for immunohistochemical analysis. In cases of intractable diarrhea of infancy, additional biopsies should be processed for electron microscopy.

Intestinal Imaging

Standard contrast follow-through studies continue to provide valuable information in the diagnosis and evaluation of inflammatory bowel diseases,[98] short bowel syndrome, and other anatomic abnormalities. Increasingly, ultrasonography with Doppler flow analysis[99] and labeled white blood cell scans have been used to detect intestinal inflammation. Recent developments in computed tomographic (CT) enterography, using special contrast media to highlight the mucosa, and magnetic resonance (MR) enterography are expected to replace standard imaging modalities, allowing visualization of both the intraluminal and extraintestinal spaces.[100-102] This latter technique eliminates the ionizing radiation exposure brought about by CT scans, a significant benefit in children with Crohn's disease who will require multiple scans over their lifetime.

ACKNOWLEDGMENTS

I would like to acknowledge Dr. Simon Murch for his exceptional contribution to the previous edition of this manuscript, and for his advice and help in the preparation of the current version of this chapter.

REFERENCES

3. Thapar N, Sanderson IR. Diarrhoea in children: an interface between developing and developed countries. Lancet 2004;363:641–653.
12. Fasano A. Cellular microbiology: How enteric pathogens socialize with their intestinal host. J Pediatr Gastroenterol Nutr 1998;26:520–532.
18. Treem WR. Chronic nonspecific diarrhea of childhood. Clin Pediatr 1992;3:413–420.
53. Ruemmele FM, Moes N, Patey-Mariaud de Serre N, et al. Clinical and molecular aspects of autoimmune enteropathy and immune dysregulation polyendocrinopathy autoimmune enteropathy X-linked syndrome. Curr Opin Gastroenterol 2008;24:742–748.

See expertconsult.com for a complete list of references and the review questions for this chapter.

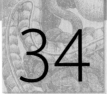

34 PROTEIN-LOSING ENTEROPATHY

Francisco A. Sylvester

Protein-losing enteropathy (PLE) is defined as abnormal protein loss from the digestive tract, often resulting in decreased concentration of serum proteins. PLE is not a discrete clinical entity, but rather a manifestation of a wide variety of gastrointestinal and extraintestinal diseases. PLE can result from abnormal protein leakage across the gut or diminished uptake by intestinal lymphatics. PLE can be secondary to altered mucosal permeability at any level of the digestive tract due to active inflammation. PLE can also occur when intestinal lymphatics are obstructed, such as in intestinal lymphangiectasia (Table 34-1). Finally, some congenital disorders of glycosylation can also present with PLE. Intestinal protein loss may be intermittent, may go into remission, and can be exacerbated by intercurrent infection.

PATHOPHYSIOLOGY

Murch has proposed a unifying mechanism to explain PLE caused by a variety of disorders.[1] Normally the presence of sulfated glycosaminoglycan in the epithelium confines albumin to the intravascular compartment by strong electrostatic interactions between anionic sites in the glycosaminoglycan carbohydrate chains and arginyl residues within protein molecules.[2] In pathological states, in a manner similar to the nephrotic syndrome, loss of normal intestinal epithelial heparan sulfate proteoglycan (HSPG) expression allows the diffusion of albumin and other proteins from the bloodstream into the lumen of the digestive tract. More specifically, syndecan-1 (Sdc1), the predominant HSPG on intestinal epithelial cells, is absent from the basolateral surface of intestinal epithelial cells during PLE exacerbations.[2] The return of Sdc1 and other HSPG is associated with remission of PLE, suggesting a role for these sulfated glycosaminoglycans in its pathogenesis. The critical role for these molecules was recently confirmed in vivo in two mouse models of PLE.[3]

One can propose three mechanisms that affect normal intestinal epithelial expression of HSPG and produce the development of PLE (Figure 34-1): (1) focal degradation in the inflamed digestive tract, (2) failed synthesis in rare genetic defects (enterocyte heparan sulfate deficiency), and (3) mislocalization in congenital disorders of glycosylation, where the HSPG does not reach the cell surface. Many digestive diseases can present with associated with PLE (see Table 34-1). The presence of PLE does not localize the pathological process to any specific portion of the gastrointestinal tract. These entities are discussed in detail elsewhere in this text, including esophagitis, gastritis, enteritis, and colitis due to different etiologies. In this chapter we focus our discussion on clinical entities associated with PLE that are not addressed in detail in other chapters.

CAUSES OF PLE

Abnormal Enterocyte Expression of HPSG
Focal Degradation of Glycosaminoglycan During Intestinal Inflammation

Inflammation in any portion of the digestive tract can lead to PLE. Intestinal inflammation is characterized by complex events that give rise to the release of mediators capable of degrading and modifying bowel wall structure. One family of these mediators is matrix metalloproteinases (MMPs). These are enzymes that are capable of degrading extracellular matrix components and have been implicated in tissue remodeling and ulceration in inflammatory bowel disease (IBD), celiac disease, and *Helicobacter pylori* infection.[4-7] The intestinal expression of inhibitors of MMPs is decreased during active intestinal inflammation.[4] Therefore, epithelial proteoglycans may be degraded, with consequent protein leakage. In addition, increased epithelial permeability, local hyperemia, and disruption of the integrity of the epithelial barrier (ulceration) can also contribute to the loss of intestinal protein (see Figure 34-1). Local production of interferon (IFN)-γ[8] and tumor necrosis factor (TNF)-α, cytokines that are commonly implicated in acute and chronic gastrointestinal inflammation, can disrupt the integrity of the epithelial cell barrier[9,10] and increase its permeability to proteins.[11,12] Moreover, TNF-α can decrease the synthesis of HSPG[13] and promote its shedding.[14] In an in vitro model of PLE, the combination of these cytokines, reduced HSPG, and increased hydrostatic pressure (mimicking venous or lymphatic congestion) causes maximum protein leakage.[12] Therefore, factors present in seemingly disparate diseases can result in PLE.

Failed Synthesis of Enterocyte Glycosaminoglycans

Murch et al. described three young male infants who presented within the first weeks of life with massive enteric protein loss, secretory diarrhea, and intolerance of enteral feeds in spite of normal intestinal biopsies.[15] All required total parenteral nutrition and repeated albumin infusions. By specific histochemistry, Murch and coworkers detected a gross abnormality in the distribution of small intestinal glycosaminoglycans in all three infants, with complete absence of enterocyte heparan sulfate (HS). The distribution of vascular and lamina propria glycosaminoglycans was, however, normal. They suggested that these children had a congenital defect in the synthesis of enterocyte proteoglycans, and that these were important in normal intestinal function.

In protein-calorie malnutrition (kwashiorkor), the expression of HSPG and sulfated glycosaminoglycan is lower in the epithelium and lamina propria compared to well-nourished children or children with marasmus.[16] This may contribute to intestinal protein loss and edema in children with kwashiorkor.

TABLE 34-1. **Causes of Protein-Losing Enteropathy in Children**

Metabolic

Enterocyte heparin sulfate deficiency (lack of synthesis)
Congenital disorders of glycosylation (mislocalization)

Mucosal Erosion or Ulceration

Infectious causes
  Acute infectious diarrhea[90,99,104,105,107,108]
  Clostridium difficile[109-111]
  Clostridium perfringens[112]
  Cytomegalovirus[113]
  Giardiasis[117-121]
  Helicobacter pylori[122,123]
  Hypertrophic gastropathy (Ménétrier disease)[83,124-127]
  Measles[128]
  Strongyloides stercoralis[121,129]
Noninfectious causes
  Allergic gastroenteropathy[130-137]
  Anastomotic ulceration/ischemia[138]
  Celiac disease
  Gastrointestinal tumors
  Graft-versus-host disease
  Henoch-Schönlein purpura[139]
  Inflammatory bowel disease
  Multiple polyposis
  Portal hypertension[140]
  Neonatal necrotizing enterocolitis
  Systemic lupus erythematosus

Lymphatic Obstruction (Intestinal Lymphangiectasia)

Primary
Secondary
  Arsenic poisoning[141]
  Congestive heart failure
  Constrictive pericarditis[38,39,142-145]
  Damage to the thoracic duct
  Familial[32,146]
  Inflammatory
  Noonan syndrome[147]
  Retroperitoneal tumors
  Vascular thrombosis after liver transplantation[148]

Includes selected references for causes not discussed in the text.

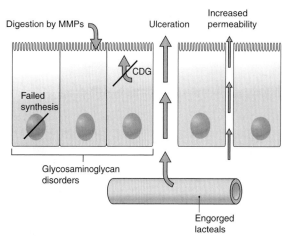

Figure 34-1. Mechanisms of protein-losing enteropathy. Protein can be lost through several mechanisms in the digestive tract, including increased permeability and discontinuity of the epithelial barrier (ulceration) due to inflammation, primary or secondary lymphangiectasia (due to engorged lacteals), or disorders of epithelial glycosaminoglycans (most importantly syndecan-1). These can be mislocalized (as in the case of congenital glycosylation disorders), not synthesized (as in enterocyte heparin sulfate deficiency), or digested at the surface of the enterocyte by matrix metalloproteases (MMPs). Any of these mechanisms will result in leakage of vascular proteins into the gut lumen.

Because many of these children also suffer from intestinal infection, it is likely that inflammation also plays a role.

Congenital Disorders of Glycosylation

Congenital disorders of glycosylation (CDGs) are multisystemic disorders characterized by defects in N-glycosylation of proteins.[17] CDGs can present with multisystemic involvement, including liver disease, protein-losing enteropathy, cyclic vomiting, and diarrhea.[2,18,19]

The pathophysiology of CDGs involves abnormalities in intracellular processing of proteins. Most secreted, cell surface, and extracellular proteins are glycosylated. During normal N-glycosylation there are two distinct steps. In the first phase there is assembly and transfer of a 14-sugar unit precursor from a lipid carrier to protein in the endoplasmic reticulum. This precursor is called the lipid-linked oligosaccharide. In the second step there is subsequent modification of the protein-bound sugar chains in the endoplasmic reticulum and Golgi apparatus to produce a properly folded protein. These proteins can then be directed to the cell membrane or exported by the cell.[19] When protein glycosylation is defective because of congenital causes, it can lead to disease in humans, the so-called CDGs. Defects in the steps up to and including the synthesis and transfer of the lipid-linked oligosaccharide to protein are

called group I CDGs. Group II consists of defects in subsequent oligosaccharide processing.

Perhaps the most interesting form of CDG for the pediatric gastroenterologist is CDGIb (OMIM 602579, 154550).[20] This disorder is caused by phosphomannose isomerase (PMI) deficiency. Loss of PMI decreases the GDP-mannose pools and limits the amount of available lipid-linked oligosaccharide that can bind to proteins. Although other forms of CDG are characterized by a wide variety of neurological manifestations, patients with CDGIb have normal motor and mental development, and their clinical presentation is dominated by symptoms of gastrointestinal and liver disease.[18,19] These children may present with chronic diarrhea, cyclic vomiting, protein-losing enteropathy, coagulopathy, hypoglycemia, and hepatomegaly. Hypoalbuminemia, elevated aminotransferases, and low antithrombin-III are characteristic. Partial villous atrophy from intestinal biopsies can falsely suggest celiac disease. Liver biopsy can reveal hepatic fibrosis with ductal plate malformations. Children with evidence of hepatomegaly, portal hypertension, hepatic fibrosis and/or steatosis, hypoglycemia, failure to thrive, coagulopathy, or hypoglycemia should be tested for CDG-Ib by transferrin isoelectric focusing. This is based on the observation that underglycosylation of glycoproteins in CDG-Ib produces transferrin with incomplete glycosylation that has a lower molecular mass than normal. Other diagnostic modalities include enzymatic analysis, plasma aspartylglucosaminidase activity,[21] transferrin mass spectrometry, and molecular analysis of PMI mutations.[19,22]

PLE Caused by Lymphangiectasia

Intestinal lymphangiectasia is characterized histologically by dilatation of the lacteals in the small intestine that distorts the villous architecture (Figures 34-2 through 34-4). Classically, there is absence of inflammation. Poor lymphatic drainage

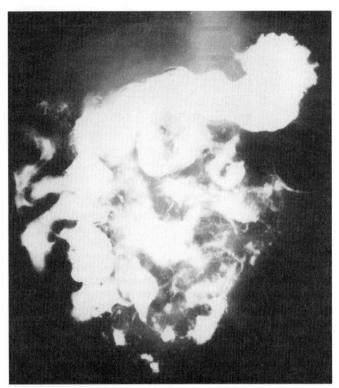

Figure 34-2. Intestinal lymphangiectasia. Prominent valvulae conniventes are present throughout the small bowel.

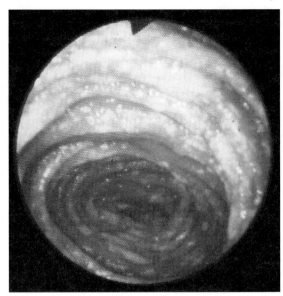

Figure 34-3. Endoscopic view of the duodenum showing snowflake-like lesions; histologically these represent dilated lacteals.

causes elevated intestinal lymphatic pressure and leakage of lymph into the intestinal lumen, with consequent loss of protein and lymphocytes.[23] Intestinal lymphangiectasia can be congenital or secondary to a disease that interferes with intestinal lymphatic drainage.

Primary Intestinal Lymphangiectasia (OMIM 152800)

Waldmann and Schwab reported that patients with edema of the legs and low serum protein had intestinal protein loss, presumably due to lymphangiectasia.[24] Subsequently, Murphy observed that these patients were lymphopenic and had double vortex pilorum ("hair whorl") and prominent "floating ribs" (ribs 11 and 12). Strober then reported the presence of hypogammaglobulinemia, skin anergy, and impaired allograft rejection in these patients.[23] Later it was suggested that increased fibrinolysis in the gastrointestinal mucosa may play an important role in enhancing mucosal permeability to plasma proteins in intestinal lymphangiectasia.[25]

Patients with intestinal lymphangiectasia can present at any age during childhood, from premature infants[26] to adolescents.[27] Children typically complain of diarrhea as their first symptom, often before 3 years of age. Vomiting, growth retardation, and peripheral lymphedema are also common. Children can present with seizures due to hypocalcemia. In some cases there is a family history of lymphedema. Lymphopenia can be present initially, but may appear years after the protein loss begins. Spontaneous remissions can occur.[28]

A number of distinct syndromes characterized by intestinal lymphangiectasia and a variety of congenital malformations have been described, including Hennekam lymphangiectasia-lymphedema syndrome (OMIM 235510), Urioste syndrome (OMIM 235255), and a variant of macrocephaly-cutis marmorata

telangiectatica congenita (OMIM 602501).[29] Intestinal lymphangiectasia has also been reported in some patients with autoimmune polyglandular disease type 1 (OMIM 240300),[30] aplasia cutis congenita,[31] and Noonan syndrome (OMIM 163950). Other organ systems can be affected in patients with intestinal lymphangiectasia, including the lung, uterus, and conjunctiva.[32] Enamel changes and other dental problems have been described.[33] Rarely, some patients can present with gastrointestinal blood loss.[27,34,35]

Secondary Lymphangiectasia

Cardiovascular Causes. Although structural heart defects,[36] constrictive pericarditis,[37-39] and obstruction of the venous drainage can all engorge intestinal lymphatics and lead to PLE, the largest cardiac group with PLE is children with the cavopulmonary anastomosis for palliation of the univentricular heart, the so-called Fontan procedure. The Fontan operation has been revised over the years. However, the surgical principle remains the same, to separate the systemic and pulmonary venous return by excluding the systemic venous return from the systemic single ventricle, with or without a residual atrial communication or baffle fenestration. Therefore, blood flow is provided in series to the pulmonary and systemic circulation without the requirement for a right ventricular pumping chamber.[40] For reasons that are not well understood, PLE develops in 4% to 11% of patients after Fontan palliation.[41] Chronically elevated systemic venous pressure and increased thoracic duct pressure are thought to be responsible for the development of PLE in these patients, with immunologic or inflammatory factors perhaps superimposed.[41] Raised pulmonary resistance or obstruction to pulmonary blood flow can cause elevated systemic venous pressure. However, it remains unclear what finally triggers the development of PLE and why it sometimes develops many years after surgery in children who are doing well from the hemodynamic point of view. Patient risk factors for the development of PLE post-Fontan include heterotaxia, polysplenia, anomalies of systemic venous return, ventricular anatomic variants (other than dominant left ventricle), increased pulmonary arteriolar resistance, and increased left

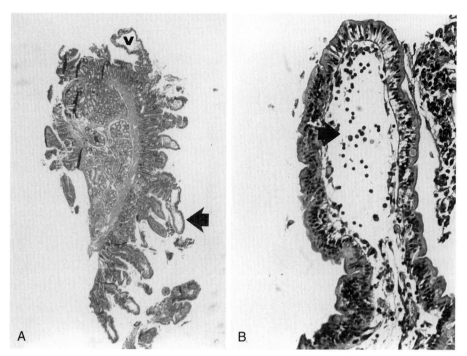

Figure 34-4. Lymphangiectasia. (**A**) Low-power magnification of expanded villi (V) with dilated lymphatic channels (arrow) (hematoxylin and eosin stain, ×50). (**B**) Higher-power magnification of a villus with dilated lacteal (arrow) (hematoxylin and eosin stain, ×200).

ventricular pressure. Interestingly, patients with tricuspid atresia are less likely to develop PLE than other groups.[41] Perioperative risk factors include longer cardiopulmonary bypass time, increased left atrial pressure after the operation, longer length hospital stay, and presence of postoperative renal failure.[42] Some laboratory findings have suggested an immune-mediated or autoimmune disorder with immune complex formation, complement activation, and endothelial damage.[43] Coagulation disorders with low protein C levels correlate with the very early stage of PLE without clinical signs. PLE can start, as judged by increased fecal α1-antitrypsin concentration, before symptoms of diarrhea or hypoproteinemia appear.[44-46] A study of 44 consecutive Fontan patients with PLE, short deceleration time, poor New York Heart Association (NYHA) class, and low serum albumin identified a group of patients at the greatest risk for death.[47] Once the symptoms of PLE are established, there seems to be an ongoing progression, with intestinal lymphatic dysfunction and poor prognosis. In a recent large retrospective review of outcomes of the Fontan procedure in 261 patients 3 decades after their surgery, the mortality hazard ratio of patients who developed PLE was 2.2- to 2.5-fold higher.[47]

Systemic Lupus Erythematosus. Hypoalbuminemia in systemic lupus erythematosus (SLE) is usually secondary to protein renal loss. The most common immune-mediated pathological conditions involving the gastrointestinal tract during the course of SLE are represented by arterial vasculitis and abdominal vessel thrombosis. PLE is an uncommon cause of hypoalbuminemia in SLE, and may or may not be associated with lymphangiectasia.[48-59] Rarely can it present in association with chylothorax and chylous ascites.[60] PLE has been reported to respond to oral corticosteroids in adult patients, although in some patients more aggressive immunosuppression is needed to alleviate symptoms.[61] In addition, diet and octreotide have also been used in patients with SLE with reported benefit.[61]

Tumors. The presence of a retroperitoneal tumor can compress the lymphatic drainage from the splanchnic bed, causing obstruction, increased pressure in the system, and leakage of protein from intestinal lymphatics into the gut lumen. This phenomenon has been reported as a complication of several tumors, including neuroblastoma,[62-64] metastatic melanoma,[65,66] and others. Rarely, intestinal tumors, both benign and malignant, can present with PLE, including lymphoma,[67-70] leukemic infiltration,[71] lymphangioma,[72] hemangioma,[73,74] Kaposi sarcoma,[75,76] melanoma,[77] polyps,[78-80] and posttransplant lymphoproliferative disease.[81] The diagnosis of these tumors may require a high index of suspicion, because their manifestation may be primarily gastrointestinal. PLE secondary to lymphangiectasia induced by chemotherapy has also been reported.[82]

Other Causes. Transient secondary intestinal lymphangiectasia of the terminal ileum was reported in an 8-year old immunocompetent child with primary cytomegalovirus (CMV) infection, in the absence of Ménétrier disease.[83] Lymphangiectasia can accompany autoimmune polyglandular syndrome,[84] familial pachydermoperiostosis,[85] and the yellow nail syndrome (slow-growing, thickened, excessively curved nails of yellowish-grey hue with absent cuticle and lunula and onycholysis).[86] Junctional epidermolysis bullosa, which is caused by mutations in α6 or β4 integrins, can present with failure to thrive, PLE, and pyloric atresia.[87] Recently, a mutation in β4 integrin was also associated with desquamative enteropathy, pyloric atresia, and severe PLE, without significant skin disease in two Kuwaiti children.[88] In addition, infantile systemic hyalinosis, a rare, progressive, and often fatal autosomal recessive disease characterized by joint contractures, perianal nodules, failure to thrive, gingival hypertrophy, diarrhea, and frequent infections, is associated with PLE.[89]

TABLE 34-2.   Manifestations of Protein-Losing Enteropathy

Clinical Symptoms and Signs

Diarrhea
    Fat malabsorption
    Carbohydrate malabsorption
Edema
    Dependent
    Extremity (may be unilateral)
    Facial
Pleural effusion
Pericardial effusion

Laboratory Findings

Decreased serum proteins
    Albumin
    α1-Antitrypsin
    Ceruloplasmin
    Fibrinogen
    Hormone binding proteins
    Transferrin
Malabsorption of fat-soluble vitamins (A, D, E, K)
Hypogammaglobulinemia (IgA, IgG, IgM)
Lymphocytopenia – altered cellular immunity

DIAGNOSIS

The clinical manifestations of PLE are highly variable and are determined by the degree of enteral protein loss and the nature of the underlying disease (Table 34-2). The most common symptom is diarrhea. The main serological findings include reduced levels of albumin, transferrin, gamma globulins (including IgA, IgG, and IgM), ceruloplasmin, and fibrinogen. Peripheral edema or ascites can appear in severe cases secondary to decreased plasma oncotic pressure. Pleural effusions and pericardial effusions may also develop, particularly if the thoracic duct is obstructed. Associated fat and carbohydrate malabsorption may occur as a result of small bowel involvement in the primary disease process, and fat-soluble vitamin deficiency may develop. Changes in clotting factors may develop, but rarely produce clinical findings, and the hypogammaglobulinemia is not typically associated with infections. Lymphopenia can be present in patients with lymphangiectasia and may result in alterations in cellular immunity.

Urinary protein loss and hypoalbuminemia secondary to decreased protein synthesis (liver disease) and malnutrition should be excluded. Often an underlying inflammatory enteropathy such as eosinophilic gastroenteritis, inflammatory bowel disease, or celiac disease can be identified by history, laboratory and imaging studies, and endoscopic examination with biopsies.

The diagnosis of PLE can be established noninvasively by measuring the fecal concentration of α1 antitrypsin[90] or fecal calprotectin.[91] α1-Antitrypsin is a serum protein and is not ingested in the diet. Its molecular weight is similar to that of albumin. It is a protease inhibitor, so it is relatively resistant to digestion and is stable for 72 hours in stool samples. Its excretion is fairly constant in the same individual over several days. These characteristics make it a suitable marker for intestinal protein loss. However, α1 antitrypsin can be degraded by acid digestion in the stomach, and therefore its fecal concentration may be normal in spite of the presence of inflammation in the esophageal or gastric mucosa. A fecal α1-antitrypsin concentration of less than 54 mg/dL is considered normal in most laboratories. The protein concentration can be measured in a random stool sample, although clearance studies can also be performed.[90] This assay is widely available in the United States. Calprotectin constitutes about 60% of the soluble cytosol proteins in neutrophil granulocytes and plays a central role in neutrophil defense. Calprotectin is resistant to protein digestion in the intestinal tract and can be measured in feces as a marker of inflammation and protein loss.[92] It is stable at room temperature for up to 5 days. In the United States, the assay for fecal calprotectin is still not widely available commercially. It is measured by an enzyme-linked immunoassay, and a concentration of less than 50 µg/g stool is considered normal. Higher concentrations can be present normally in infants before 10 weeks of age.[93] Other leukocyte proteins, including lactoferrin, S100A12, and pyruvate kinase, are also used clinically or in the research setting to screen for intestinal inflammation[94-98] Increased fecal concentration of these proteins is not specific to any particular disease associated with PLE.

Small bowel contrast studies typically demonstrate thickened or edematous folds in patients with hypoalbuminemia. The radiologic appearance has been described as stacked coins. Radiologic evaluation may also identify a variety of mucosal abnormalities. Endoscopy may demonstrate white specks giving the mucosa a "snowflake" pattern. Some lesions, such as lymphangiectasia, can be patchy, so multiple biopsies at different locations are helpful in establishing a diagnosis. Random capsule biopsies may miss the lesions and are generally not recommended. Endoscopy is particularly useful in patients where noninvasive testing for leakage of protein into the gastrointestinal tract is normal but PLE is suspected, such as inflammatory processes limited to the esophagus and stomach. Endoscopy is routinely used to identify the presence of mucosal inflammation or polyps that may involve the small bowel or colon. Characteristic histological findings include dilated lacteals that are most prominent at the tips of the villi. There may be other mucosal changes dependent on the nature of the underlying condition. In lymphangiectasia or lymphatic duct obstruction, the mucosa will be normal without evidence of inflammation or villous atrophy. The sensitivity of endoscopy to detect lymphangiectasia may be enhanced by the ingestion of a fatty meal before the procedure.[99]

Wireless capsule endoscopy may also be helpful to detect discrete or patchy small bowel lesions that are beyond the reach of conventional endoscopes.[100,101] Additional diagnostic modalities include double-balloon enteroscopy,[102,103] radionuclide scans,[104,105] magnetic resonance enterography, and computed tomography with intravenous and oral contrast.

TREATMENT

PLE associated with many forms of gastrointestinal inflammation improves with treatment of the underlying disease. The specific therapies for these disorders are reviewed elsewhere in this text.

CDGIb is a treatable disorder. Mannose supplementation circumvents the enzymatic defect and can correct defective glycosylation in patients. Doses of 0.1 to 0.15 g/kg four times daily are effective without apparent side effects. Free mannose does not occur in foods, and therefore it needs to be supplemented in these patients. Unfractionated heparin has been used anecdotally.[106]

Intestinal lymphangiectasia can be treated with a high-protein, low-fat diet that is supplemented with medium-chain triglycerides (MCTs), which will be absorbed directly into the portal circulation. Octreotide has been helpful,[107-110] but it probably should be reserved for those patients who fail dietary therapy with MCT oil because of its cost and inconvenience. Antiplasmin therapy (*trans*-4-aminomethylcyclohexane carboxylic acid) may have some role, based on the hypothesis that mucosal fibrinolysis increases mucosal permeability in patients with lymphangiectasia.[25,111] Surgery is reserved for palliation of large chylous ascites[112] or resection of isolated lesions.[113]

In PLE secondary to the Fontan procedure, the success rate of medical and surgical treatments aimed at treating PLE by reducing systemic venous pressure is very limited and ranges only from 19 to 40%. Medical treatments seem more promising than surgical revision. Some experts believe that therapeutic intervention may be most beneficial if started before the manifestation of symptoms of PLE and advocate following serum albumin levels and serial fecal α1antitrypsin after surgery. Surgical management options include the correction of small hemodynamic lesions and alteration of the primary hemodynamic derangement via fenestration of the systemic venous baffle. In refractory cases, resolution of PLE has been reported after heart transplant. Medical modalities include anticoagulation, improving hemodynamics, and intestinal cell membrane stabilization with high-dose steroids or subcutaneous high-molecular-weight heparin. It is not clear how parenteral heparin stops intestinal protein leakage. One possibility is that it binds and sequesters cytokines such as IFN-γ and TNF-α,[114,115] or that it restores HS

on the basolateral surface of epithelial cells.[11,12] However, the efficacy of heparin in this context has recently been put into question. In a retrospective review of 17 patients post-Fontan procedure who developed PLE and treated with heparin, 13 patients reported subjective symptom improvement (decreased abdominal pain, diarrhea, and edema with improved sense of well-being), but only 3 patients went into complete remission. For all patients, there was no significant difference between the number of hospital admissions or albumin infusions before starting heparin and during the first year of heparin therapy.[116] There is some evidence that performing the Fontan operation at an earlier age before ventricular dysfunction occurs may lead to improved long-term results.

REFERENCES

1. Murch SH. Toward a molecular understanding of complex childhood enteropathies. J Pediatr Gastroenterol Nutr 2002;34(Suppl 1):S4–S10.
3. Bode L, Salvestrini C, Park PW, et al. Heparan sulfate and syndecan-1 are essential in maintaining murine and human intestinal epithelial barrier function. J Clin Invest 2008;118:229–238.
20. Damen G, de Klerk H, Huijmans J, et al. Gastrointestinal and other clinical manifestations in 17 children with congenital disorders of glycosylation type Ia, Ib, and Ic. J Pediatr Gastroenterol Nutr 2004;38:282–287.
47. Silvilairat S, Cabalka AK, Cetta F, et al. Protein-losing enteropathy after the Fontan operation: associations and predictors of clinical outcome. Congenit Heart Dis 2008;3:262–268.

35

CELIAC DISEASE

Riccardo Troncone • Salvatore Auricchio

DEFINITION

Celiac disease (CD) is an immune-mediated systemic disorder elicited by the ingestion of wheat gliadin and related prolamins, affecting individuals HLA DQ2 and/or DQ8 positive, and characterized by the presence of anti-tissue transglutaminase antibodies and/or gluten-dependent manifestations including enteropathy.

HISTORICAL BACKGROUND

CD was first accurately described by Samuel Gee in 1888, but it was not until the early 1950s that Dicke in The Netherlands established the role of wheat and rye flour in the pathogenesis of the disease and identified the protein known as gluten as the harmful factor in those cereals.[1] A major contribution to the understanding of the disease came from the development of methods for peroral biopsy of the jejunal mucosa, which allowed definition of the mucosal lesion,[2] and from the definition of diagnostic criteria published in 1969 by the European Society of Pediatric Gastroenterology and Nutrition (ESPGAN).[3] In recent years substantial numbers of data have been produced that have profoundly changed our understanding of epidemiology, clinical aspects, and pathogenesis of CD, opening new perspectives for treatment.

CEREAL PROTEINS AND OTHER ENVIRONMENTAL FACTORS

Cereal Proteins

The cereals that are toxic for patients with CD are wheat, rye and barley; rice and maize are nontoxic and are usually used as wheat substitutes in the diet of patients with CD. The toxicity of oats has been reassessed in recent years. It has in fact been shown that the use of oats as part of a gluten-free diet has no unfavorable effects on adult patients in remission and does not prevent mucosal healing in patients with newly diagnosed disease.[4,5] Nonetheless, a few patients with CD seem not to tolerate oats[6]; furthermore, the fear that small amounts of gliadin could contaminate oats suggests caution before advocating the inclusion of oats in the diet of celiac patients. Cereal grains belong to the grass family (Gramineae); grains considered toxic for celiac patients (rye, barley, and, to a lesser extent, oats) bear a close taxonomic relationship to wheat, whereas nontoxic grains (rice and maize) are taxonomically dissimilar (Figure 35-1). Wheat seed endosperm contains heterogeneous protein classes differentiated, according to their extractability and solubility in different solvents, into albumins, globulins, gliadins, and glutenins. Gliadins are monomers, whereas glutenins form large polymeric structures. The gliadins (classified according to their N-terminal amino acid sequences into alpha, gamma, and omega types) and the glutenins (subdivided into high-molecular-weight glutenins and low-molecular-weight glutenins) are the typical gluten components and determine respectively the viscosity and elasticity (strength) of the dough.[7] The wheat toxicity results from the gliadin protein fraction, and the toxicity of cereals other than wheat is most likely associated with prolamin fractions equivalent to gliadins in the grain of these other species; on the other hand, glutenin peptides have been shown to be immunogenic for mucosal T cells from celiac patients.[8] The richness in proline and glutamine confers an unusual resistance to gastrointestinal enzymes[9] and renders them a good substrate for tissue transglutaminase,[10] both these phenomena favoring the reactivity with mucosal CD4 T cells. Several HLA-DQ2 restricted T-cell epitopes have in fact been found clustering in regions of gliadin rich in proline residues,[11] target of the tissue transglutaminase (TG2) deamidating activity (see Pathogenesis). Variations in immunogenicity exist among cultivars, and work is in progress to identify wheat varieties with a reduced amount of T epitopes to be used in breeding programs. However, toxicity seems not to be restricted to CD4 T cell epitopes, as in vitro[12,13] and in vivo[14,15] studies have shown that other peptides not reacting with CD4 T cells could also be involved in pathogenesis, being able to activate innate immunity mechanisms,[12] or interact with CD8+ cytotoxic T cells.[16]

Other Environmental Factors

The high concordance rate for monozygotic twins and the similar risk shown by dizygotic twins and other siblings suggest that a shared environment (gluten antigen aside) has little effect.[17] On the other hand, the relevance of environmental factors other than gluten in CD is suggested by the significant changes in the incidence of the disease by time and place. Feeding practices seem to be relevant. Recently, Sweden has experienced an epidemic of symptomatic celiac disease in children aged less than 2 years. The abrupt increase and decline in the incidence of the disease coincided with changes in the dietary pattern of infants.[18] The risk of celiac disease was found to be greater when gluten was introduced in the diet in large amounts[18]; in contrast, it was reduced if children were still breast-fed when dietary gluten was introduced.[19] This finding adds to previous case referent studies showing that breast-feeding is protective.[20] Still uncertain is the relevance of the age of introduction of gluten in an infant's diet.[21] An important question is whether favorable dietary habits simply postpone the onset of celiac disease, or reduce the overall lifetime risk of the disease; a challenging possibility that requires further studies is that celiac disease might be delayed, or even prevented, by intervening in the dietary patterns of genetically susceptible individuals during the first year of life. Among other environmental factors that

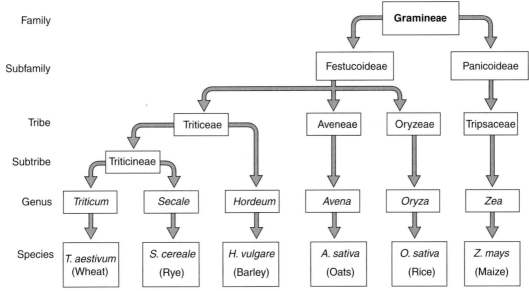

Figure 35-1. Taxonomic relationships of major cereal grains. From Kasarda DD, Qualset CO, Mecham DK, et al. A test of toxicity of bread made from wheat lacking alpha-gliadins coded for by the 6A chromosome. In: McNicholl B, McCarthy CF, Fottrell PF, eds. Perspectives in Celiac Disease. Lancaster, UK: MTP Press; 1978:55, with permission.

could play a possible role in CD, infective factors have also been considered. The possible role played in pathogenesis by alpha interferon,[22] and the epidemiological evidence of increased risk in relation to the month of birth,[23] have suggested the possible involvement of a viral infection. Infectious episodes could potentially contribute because they might increase gut permeability with increased antigen penetration and/or may drive the immune system toward a Th1 response. Rotavirus appears to be a good candidate. In fact, frequent rotavirus infection predicted a higher risk of CD autoimmunity[24]; moreover, homology between the rotavirus neutralizing protein VP7 and tissue transglutaminase has been reported.[25]

GENETICS OF CELIAC DISEASE

Family Studies

Susceptibility to CD is determined to a significant extent by genetic factors. That is suggested by the occurrence of multiple cases in families, the prevalence of CD found among first-degree relatives being approximately 10%.[26] Moreover, as many as 75% of monozygotic twins have been found to be concordant with the disease.[17] The concordance rate among HLA-identical siblings is about 30%, indicating that a significant part of the genetic susceptibility maps to the HLA region on chromosome 6.

Genetic Markers

The strongest association of CD is with the HLA class II D region markers, class I and class II region gene associations being secondary to linkage disequilibrium. It has been suggested that the primary association of CD is with the DQ αβ heterodimer encoded by the DQA1*05 and the DQB1*02 genes.[27] Such a DQ molecule has been found to be present in 95% or more of celiac patients compared with 20 to 30% of controls. The data available on DQ2-negative celiac patients indicate that they almost invariably are HLA DQ8 positive (DQA1*0301/DQB1*0302).[28] A gene dosage effect has been reported allowing classification of cases in classes of risk, and a molecular hypothesis for such

a phenomenon has been proposed based on the impact of the number and quality of the HLA DQ2 molecules on gluten peptide presentation to T cells.[29] The most likely mechanism to explain the association with HLA class II genes is, in fact, that the DQ molecule binds a peptide fragment of an antigen involved in the pathogenesis of CD to present it to T cells. Less clear is the gene dosage effect on the clinical presentation of the disease.[30]

HLA explains 40% of the disease heritability; the remaining 60% is shared by an unknown number of non-HLA genes whose contribution taken singularly is modest. Genetic linkage studies[31] have identified apart from the HLA region (CELIAC 1) several loci: CELIAC 2 on 5q 31-33 (cytokine cluster),[32] CELIAC 3 on 2q33[33] (CD28, CTLA4, ICOS), and CELIAC 4[34] on 19p13.1 (MYO9B). Recent genome-wide associated studies[35,36] have identified nine loci that contribute to CD risk; interestingly, some are shared with type 1 diabetes. The identification of non-HLA risk factors will improve the identification of high-risk individuals for a more precise diagnosis and implementation of possible prevention strategies.

EPIDEMIOLOGY

The reported prevalence of symptomatic CD is 1 in 1000 live births, with a range from 1 in 250 (observed in Sweden) to 1 in 4000 (observed in Denmark).[37] The prevalence in women appears to be greater than in men. Population-based screening studies have clearly shown that CD is underdiagnosed, clinical CD representing the top of the iceberg. A recent Finnish study has shown that the prevalence of biopsy proven CD is at least 1:99 children,[38] indicating CD as one of the most common genetically based diseases. Similar prevalence have been indicated in most European countries, in North Africa, in South America, and in the United States.[39] The highest rate has been reported in the Sarahawi population.[40] Increased awareness of the disease coupled with a low threshold for serological screening is uncovering a large number of undiagnosed cases who carry an increased mortality risk. It is still debated whether it is

TABLE 35-1. **Who Should Be Screened for Celiac Disease**

Extraintestinal Presentations	Associated Disease
Unexplained anemia	Insulin-dependent diabetes mellitus
Short stature	Autoimmune endocrinopathies
Aphthous stomatitis	IgA deficiency
Enamel hypoplasia	Connective tissue disorders
Infertility	Down syndrome
Intractable seizures	Turner's syndrome
Ataxy	
Polyneuropathy	
Hypertransaminasemia	First-degree relatives
Osteoporosis	
Alopecia	

more cost effective to focus attention on at-risk subjects such as family members and other at-risk groups (Table 35-1), or adopt mass screening of the general population.[41,42] Interestingly, in recent years there has been evidence for a further real increase of the prevalence of the disease that cannot be attributed to a better detection rate. The environmental factors responsible for this trend common to other immune-mediated disease remain to be identified.[43]

PATHOGENESIS

Celiac disease is a T-cell-mediated, chronic inflammatory disorder with an autoimmune component. The loss of tolerance observed in CD depends on the special physical and chemical properties of gliadin. Altered processing of gliadin by intraluminal enzymes, changes in intestinal permeability, and activation of the innate immune system precede the adaptive immune response observed in established CD. The inflammatory reaction occurs in the epithelial layer and deeper in the lamina propria as well (Figure 35-2).

Gliadin Resistance to Enzymes and Passage Through the Epithelium

Because of their high content of proline and glutamine, gliadins show an unusual resistance to gastrointestinal enzymes. It has been demonstrated that the lack of endoprolylpeptidase activity, in gastric and pancreatic enzymes and in the human brush border, prevents efficient enzymatic attack of proline-rich domains in gluten proteins.[9]

It is still unclear whether a primary defect of intestinal permeability exists in CD. An increased passage through a paracellular route has been postulated on the basis of the increased expression of zonulin,[44] and a transcellular protected transport pathway by retrotranscytosis of secretory IgA through the transferring receptor CD71 has been described.[45]

Activation of the Innate Immune System

Gliadin can activate both the innate immune and the adaptive immune system in patients with CD. The nonimmunodominant peptide fragment of gliadin (amino acids number 31-43) has been shown to rapidly induce the activation of the innate immune response in treated celiac disease mucosa cultured in vitro.[13,46] This results in the expression of epithelial stress molecules and production of interleukin-15, which among other effects inhibits the immunoregulatory signaling of transforming growth factor β (TGF-β).[47] The biological basis of the stress induced by 31-43 is still unclear. The peptide may induce tyrosine phosphorylation[48] and actin rearrangement[48] and potentiate EGF receptor stimulation.[49] In the context of the activated innate immunity, an important role is also played by interferon-α produced by plasmacytoid dendritic cells.[50]

CD4+ T-cell Activation in the Lamina Propria: the Adaptive Immune Response

One of the key events in the pathogenesis of CD is the activation of lamina propria T cells by gliadin peptides presented with MHC class II molecules HLA-DQ2 or HLA-DQ8. Gluten proteins contain a large number of peptides capable of stimulating T cells.[8] The interplay among gliadin, tissue transglutaminase 2 enzyme, and DQ2 or DQ8 is now better understood, and a model has been developed from studies by Sollid and Koning. It has been found that TG2 enzymatically converts particular glutamine residues in gliadin to glutamic acid. This greatly increases the affinity of these peptide fragments for HLA-DQ 2 or HLA-DQ 8, resulting in more effective antigen presentation to naïve T cells.[51] The alpha-2 gliadin 33mer fragment is the most immunogenic, as it contains six partly overlapping DQ2-restricted epitopes.[9] TG2 then enhances gliadin-specific T cell responses in celiac disease; interestingly, TG2 is inactive under normal physiological conditions,[52] and a key step in the pathogenesis of CD is its activation possibly by viral components or gluten itself.

Cytokine Production

The pattern of cytokines produced following activation of T cells by gliadin has been characterized and shown to be TH1 predominant, with interferon-γ present in the mucosa. Interestingly, IL-12, another TH1 cytokine, has not been detected. Both IL-18[53] and interferon-α[22] are potential candidates as the driving factors favoring TH-1 T-cell differentiation and IFN-γ production in CD. Other proinflammatory cytokines whose expression is enhanced in the CD mucosa include IL-6, IL-18, and IL-21.[54] The immunosuppressive and immunoregulatory cytokine IL-10 is also increased in CD mucosa, but is not sufficient to negate the proinflammatory actions of interferon-γ.[55,56] It is still unclear whether there is a problem of T cell regulation. Gliadin-specific T regulatory cells have been demonstrated in the CD mucosa[57] and increased number of FOXP3-positive T cells counted in the active phase of the disease.[58] Additional effector cells are recruited and activated, downstream of T cell signaling. Increased expression of metalloproteinases,[59] which degrade matrix structures, and of angiogenesis and other growth factors[60] contribute to the complex remodeling process that ultimately results in the classical flat mucosa of CD.

Intraepithelial Lymphocytes

Increased intraepithelial lymphocytes (IELs) are a hallmark of CD. Mechanisms in addition to activation of lamina propria T cells are involved in IEL recruitment. For example, marked alterations in the expression of MIC and HLA-E occur on the intestinal epithelium of untreated CD patients. MIC and HLA-E are induced as part of the stress response of intestinal epithelial

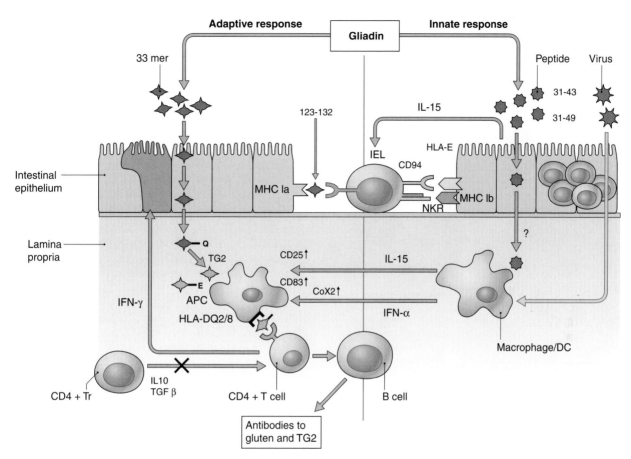

Figure 35-2. CD pathogenesis. The left part of the figure illustrates the contribution of the adaptive T-cell response orchestrated by lamina propria CD4+ T cells. Intraluminal and brush border proteolysis releases immunostimulatory peptides, likely within large peptides containing oligomerized epitopes. They are deamidated by tissue transglutaminase (TG2) and bind into the peptide pocket of HLA-DQ2/8 molecules of antigen-presenting cells (APC), allowing their presentation to CD4+ T cells in lamina propria. Activated T cells help the production of antibodies against gliadin and TG2 and release large amounts of interferon gamma (IFN-γ) and other proinflammatory molecules. Specific activation of CD8 TcRαβIEL by some gliadin peptides might also occur via MHC class I molecules. The mechanisms that favor the triggering of the adaptive response are not elucidated, but might implicate a primary regulatory defect or a permissive activation by innate immune mechanisms (e.g., IL15 or α-interferon) specifically triggered by gliadin.[9,18] The right part of the figure shows the possible role of innate immunity activated by specific A gliadin sequences (e.g., 31-43) and orchestrated around the production of IL-15. IL-15 produced by lamina propria macrophages promotes the antigen-presentation activity of dendritic cells and thereby the adaptive T-cell response. IL-15 produced by enterocytes enhances the recruitment of IEL, promotes their survival and expansion, and induces their cytotoxicity and IFN-γ production, as well as the expression of some innate receptors. The ligands for these receptors are atypical MHC class I molecules (MHC class Ib) induced by inflammation or stress on epithelial cells. From Cerf-Bensussan N, Cellier C, Heyman M, et al. J Pediatr Gastroenterol Nutr 2003; 37:412-421; modified, with permission.

cells, by interferon-γ and by gluten itself. MIC and HLA-E are ligands for receptors NKG2D and CD94, respectively, present on intraepithelial lymphocytes. IL-15 up-regulates NKG2D and CD94 expression by these immune cells.[61] Most recently, it has also been shown that CD8+ lymphocytes can directly recognize gliadin peptides.[62] Activation of intraepithelial lymphocytes, with increased FAS Ligand expression, results in epithelial cell apoptosis and villous atrophy via interactions with FAS on intestinal epithelial cells.[63] Increased perforin-granzyme production by activated IELs, which can form holes in target cell membranes, further contributes to GI mucosal epithelial cell destruction.[64] IL-15 may also promote the emergence of T cell clonal proliferation because of its antiapoptotic action on IELs.

Autoimmune Phenomena in CD

There is significant and increasing evidence to support the categorization of CD as an autoimmune disorder. CD associates with multiple other well-recognized autoimmune disorders, and there are multiple autoimmune phenomena observed in CD.

The most characteristic and widely evident expression of autoimmunity in CD is the presence of antibodies to tissue transglutaminase 2 in patient sera.[65] These antibodies have more recently been shown to contribute to CD pathogenesis. Antibodies to TG2 inhibit its enzymatic activity in a dose-dependent manner in vivo and in vitro, although only partially.[66] Further, in vitro these antibodies also interfere with epithelial cell differentiation, disturbing TGF-β-mediated crosstalk between epithelial cells and fibroblasts beneath[67]; finally, they induce proliferation of epithelial cells.[68] Recent data support that TG2 auto antibodies are primarily produced in the gut mucosa,[69] where they can be detected before appearing in the circulation. IgA against extracellular forms of TG2 present in the liver, muscle, and lymph nodes has been detected in CD patients, indicating that this TG2 is accessible to the gut-derived autoantibodies.[70] Several of the extraintestinal clinical manifestations of CD (fatty liver/hepatitis, neurological disturbances, and cardiac disease) may be related to the presence and action of these anti-TG2 antibodies in situ in these target organs.

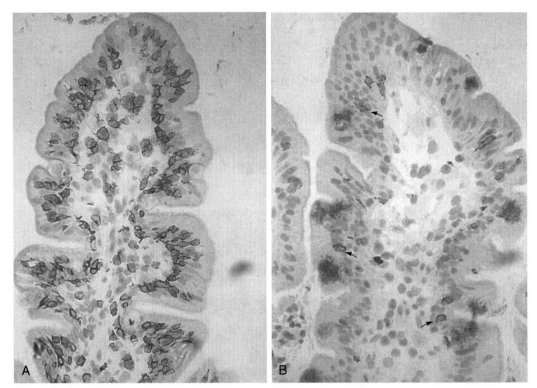

Figure 35-3. Increased density of (**A**) intraepithelial lymphocytes CD3+ and (**B**) intraepithelial lymphocytes expressing the gamma/delta T-cell receptor, in a celiac patient with serum positive antiendomysial antibodies, but normal jejunal architecture. (*See plate section for color.*)

The mechanisms leading to autoimmunity in CD are not completely known. The up-regulation of TG2 observed in inflamed sites may generate additional antigenic epitopes, by crosslinking or deamidating external or endogenous protein "epitope spreading." Unmasking of normally hidden epitopes in an inflamed environment, with more efficient antigen processing and presentation, has also been hypothesized as an important mechanism resulting in autoimmunity. T cell help from gliadin-specific T-cell cones, favoring the production of autoantibodies by B cells, has been suggested as an explanation for the observed dependence on the presence of dietary gluten for the production of anti-TG2 autoantibodies.[71] It is notable that TG2 are not the only autoantibodies present in CD patients. Antibodies to actin[72] and calreticulin[73] have been detected in the sera of celiac patients. New autoantigens (to enolase and to the beta chain of ATP synthase) have recently been identified by the mass fingerprinting approach (proteomics).[74] Their role in CD pathogenesis is not known.

PATHOLOGY

CD manifests itself pathologically as a disease of the small intestine. A distinct pattern of abnormalities has been observed; the features include (1) partial to total villous atrophy; (2) elongated crypts; (3) increased mitotic index in the crypts; (4) increased IELs; (5) infiltrations of plasma cells and lymphocytes as well as mast cells, eosinophils, and basophils in the lamina propria; and (6) absence of identifiable brush border and abnormalities in the epithelial cells, which become flattened, cuboidal, and pseudostratified (Figure 35-3A, B). However, these changes are not pathognomic of CD, and most of them may be seen in other entities, such as cow's-milk or soy-protein hypersensitivity,

intractable diarrhea of infancy, heavy infestation with *Giardia lamblia*, primary immunodeficiencies, tropical sprue, bacterial overgrowth, and intestinal lymphoma. Hence, it is crucial to establish the gluten dependence of the jejunal lesion.

It has now become clear that, from a pathological point of view, the small intestinal enteropathy in celiac disease may be of variable severity. A spectrum of histological signs could be present. According to the Marsh classification, they include infiltrative (IELs more than 25 per 100 epithelial cells), hyperplastic, and destructive patterns. This classification has been modified and validated by Oberhuber et al.[75] and later by Corazza et al.[76] The changes, even the most severe, are not pathognomonic and should always be interpreted in the context of the clinical and serological setting. The presence of only infiltrative changes (Marsh 1) is nonspecific (only 10% of subjects presenting this pattern have CD),[77] but positive serology increases the possibility of CD. Immunohistochemistry allows a more precise identification of IELs (CD3 staining). It also allows count of γδ cells: high count of γδ cells (or γδ/CD3 ratio) increases the specificity for CD in Marsh 1-2 mucosae,[78] but requires frozen, nonfixed biopsies. In paraffin-embedded biopsies, counting villous tip IELs also increases the specificity for CD. The presence of IgA anti-tissue transglutaminase deposits seems to be very specific to CD and to predict the evolution to more severe histological patterns.[79]

CLINICAL PRESENTATION

Clinical features of CD differ considerably. Intestinal symptoms are common in children diagnosed within the first 2 years of life; failure to thrive, chronic diarrhea, vomiting, abdominal distention, muscle wasting, anorexia, and irritability are present in most cases. With the shifting of the age at presentation of the

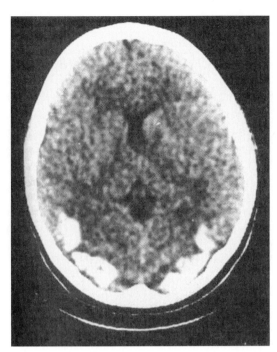

Figure 35-4. CT scan showing bilateral parieto-occipital calcifications in the cortico-subcortical layers in a patient with epilepsy and celiac disease.

disease later in childhood and with the wider and more liberal use of serological screening tests, extraintestinal manifestations, without any accompanying digestive symptom, have increasingly been recognized, affecting almost all organs.

Short stature has probably been the first isolated extraintestinal presentation of CD to be recognized; already in the early 1980s, approximately 10% of patients with isolated short stature undergoing jejunal biopsy were found to have a total villous atrophy.[80] Nonetheless, both in children and in adults, the most frequent extraintestinal manifestation of CD is iron deficiency anemia.[81] The prevalence of CD in adult patients with microcytic anemia unresponsive to iron therapy is as high as 8.5%.[82] As far as the locomotor apparatus is concerned, arthritis and arthralgia as presentation symptoms of CD were described by Maki et al.[83] The majority of adult celiac patients suffer from metabolic osteopathy; gluten-free diet normalizes bone mass only in a proportion of subjects. However, patients whose CD was diagnosed in childhood and who have since then been receiving a gluten-free diet have a bone mineral density similar to that of healthy controls.[84] The nervous system is also involved in CD. An Italian report has proposed an association between CD and epilepsy in patients with bilateral occipital calcifications[85] (Figure 35-4); in such patients gluten-free diet beneficially affects the course of epilepsy only when started soon after epilepsy onset. Moreover, gluten sensitivity is proposed to be common in patients with neurological diseases of unknown etiology, such as gluten ataxia.[86] Peripheral neuropathies of axonal and demyelinating types have also been reported and may respond to elimination of gluten from the diet. There is no doubt that the liver is a target of gluten toxicity in CD. Isolated hypertransaminasemia has been recognized as a possible presentation of CD; it may be expression of chronic "cryptogenic" hepatitis resolving on a gluten-free diet.[87] Serological screening for CD is mandatory in such patients.[88] Patients with severe liver disease have been described in whom gluten-free diet prevented progression to hepatic failure, even in cases in which liver transplantation was considered.[89] Patients having fertility problems may have subclinical CD: unexplained infertility may be the only sign of CD.[90] Similarly, unfavorable outcomes of pregnancy such as recurrent abortions, premature delivery, or low weight at birth are more often observed in undiagnosed or untreated CD patients.[91] Different degrees of dental abnormalities have been described in children with CD; severe enamel hypoplasia is present in up to 30% of untreated CD children.[92] Alopecia areata has been reported to be the only clinical manifestation of CD.[93]

A special place in this list is taken by dermatitis herpetiformis (DH), a gluten-dependent condition characterized by a symmetric pruritic skin rash with subepidermal blisters and granular subepidermal deposits of IgA in remote uninvolved skin. Most patients with DH have abnormal small intestinal biopsy pathology, histologically indistinguishable from that of CD, although usually less severe. Approximately 60% of children with DH have been reported to have subtotal villous atrophy and 30% have partial villous atrophy on jejunal biopsy.[94] The histologic changes return to normal after dietary exclusion of gluten. Therapy with dapsone usually leads to prompt clinical improvement; a strict gluten-free diet permits a reduction or discontinuation of dapsone over a period of months. Improvement of skin lesions on a gluten-free diet seems to occur also in patients with no evident mucosal abnormality; in the same patients the rash recurs with a gluten rechallenge.

Finally, there are patients clinically silent and identified during screening programs, for example in at-risk groups (first-degree relatives, patients with type 1 diabetes). Although they report no symptoms, more careful history, examination, or laboratory investigations may reveal subtle abnormalities (e.g., osteopenia).

There is no relation between severity of the clinical picture and severity or extension of the mucosal lesions. Conflicting results have been reported on the relation between HLA dose and clinical presentation.[30] The mechanisms operating in the different manifestations of the disease may be different. Extradigestive manifestations may more likely result from the intestinal damage and consequent nutritional deficiencies (e.g., anemia, osteopenia) and/or due to the deranged (auto)immune response (e.g., skin, liver, joints, central nervous system involvement).

Because of the raised attention for CD and the more diffused screening of "at risk" subjects, an increasingly frequent problem is posed by children with positive serology for CD, but with a normal intestinal mucosa; they are named "potential" celiac patients.[95] Unlike "latent" celiac patients, they have never experienced intestinal villous atrophy, and in fact we do not know how many and which of them will in the future develop damage of the jejunal mucosa. Anti-TG2 titers are usually lower than that showed by celiac patients with atrophy; in some of them titers become negative or fluctuate during follow-up. There is no agreement on how those subjects should be managed. In most cases they are left on a normal diet, particularly if they are clinically silent. In this case a careful surveillance of the nutritional status of those patients, including a thorough evaluation of the bone status, is mandatory.

ASSOCIATED DISEASES

Some diseases, many with an autoimmune pathogenesis, are found with a higher than normal frequency in celiac patients; among these are thyroid diseases,[96] Addison's disease,[97] pernicious anemia,[98] autoimmune thrombocytopenia,[99] sarcoidosis,[100] insulin-dependent diabetes mellitus,[101] alopecia,[102] and cardiomyopathies.[103] Such associations have been interpreted as a consequence of the sharing of identical HLA haplotypes (e.g., B8, DR3). Nevertheless, the relation between CD and autoimmunity is more complex. In CD patients there is evidence that the risk of developing autoimmune diseases seems to be directly correlated to the duration of gluten exposure.[104] However, studies in adults have challenged this concept.[105]

An increased incidence of CD has been found in Down syndrome patients compared with the general population.[106] Similarly, in Turner's syndrome and Williams syndrome a higher number of CD cases was also observed.[107,108] Selective IgA deficiency is also a condition associated with celiac disease.[109] Screening test alternatives to those based on the measurement of IgA isotype antibodies must be adopted in such patients.

LABORATORY FINDINGS

Serological Tests

Serological tests have acquired great importance in recent years. After the demonstration that tissue transglutaminase is the main autoantigen recognized by endomysial antibodies,[65] anti-tissue transglutaminase antibodies, whose measurement is now based on the use of recombinant human enzyme as coating antigen in enzyme-linked immunosorbent assay (ELISA), have shown a great sensitivity and specificity for the diagnosis of celiac disease[110] (Table 35-2). The specificity is almost absolute, considering that subjects with positive serum endomysial antibodies and normal histology have a high chance of developing enteropathy in subsequent years.[111] On the other hand, a note of caution comes from studies in adult patients indicating a lower sensitivity, particularly in subjects with a milder form of enteropathy.[112] Recent guidelines[113] suggest using IgA anti-tissue transglutaminase as the first-choice test and endomysial antibody testing if the results of IgA anti-tissue transglutaminase are equivocal. It is mandatory to check for IgA deficiency, particularly when the laboratory detects a low optical density on IgA anti-tissue transglutaminase test. In case of confirmed IgA deficiency, IgG anti-tissue transglutaminase and endomysium should be assessed.

Finally, although it has now been clearly shown that the site of production of endomysial and tissue transglutaminase antibodies is the gut mucosa[114] and that their presence in the serum is the result of their spillover, it is more than a working hypothesis that there are "seronegative" subjects with presence of such antibodies only in their intestinal secretions.[115]

HLA

As already mentioned, celiac disease is strongly associated with some HLA allele specificities, namely those serologically recognized as HLA DQ2 (90 to 95% of cases) and HLA DQ8 (approximately 5% of cases). Fewer than 2% of celiac patients lack both HLA specificities; at the same time approximately one third of our "normal" population has one or the other marker. This means that the demonstration of being DQ2 and/or DQ8 positive has a strong negative predictive value, but a very weak positive predictive value for the diagnosis of celiac disease. With these limitations, it may prove useful to exclude

TABLE 35-2. Serological Tests for Celiac Disease

Test	Sensitivity	Specificity	PPV	NPD
AGA IgG	57-100	42-98	20-95	41-88
AGA IgA	53-100	65-100	s28-100	65-100
AEA IgA	75-98	96-100	98-100	80-95
Guinea pig tTG	90.2	95		
Human tTg	98.5	98		

Reproduced from Fasano and Catassi (2001),[39] with permission from the American Gastroenterological Association.

celiac disease in subjects on a gluten-free diet, or in subjects belonging to at-risk groups (e.g., first-degree relatives, insulin-dependent diabetics, patients with Down syndrome), to avoid long-term follow-up.

Biopsy

Biopsy could be performed by a Crosby capsule or by upper endoscopy. Although jejunal biopsies obtained by means of a Crosby capsule are usually of a better quality, the general consensus is that biopsies should be taken during upper endoscopy. Such a policy has several advantages (shorter procedure time, absence of radiation, possibility of inspecting the mucosa, more fragments obtained to overcome the possibility of focal lesions). Biopsies (at least four) should be taken from the first (the bulb) and second or third portions of the duodenum.[113] Correct orientation of the biopsy is necessary. A spectrum of histological signs are considered to be consistent with CD.

DIAGNOSIS

According to the current ESPGHAN criteria,[116] the two requirements mandatory for the diagnosis of CD remain (1) the finding of villous atrophy with hyperplasia of the crypts and abnormal surface epithelium, while the patient is eating adequate amounts of gluten; and (2) a full clinical remission after withdrawal of gluten from the diet. The finding of circulating IgA antibodies to gliadin, reticulin, and endomysium at the time of diagnosis, and their disappearance on a gluten-free diet, adds weight to the diagnosis. A control biopsy to verify the consequences on the mucosal architecture of the gluten-free diet is considered mandatory only in patients with equivocal clinical response to the diet and in patients asymptomatic at first presentation (as is often the case in patients diagnosed during screening programs, such as first-degree relatives of celiac patients).

Gluten challenge is not considered mandatory, except under unusual circumstances. These include situations where there is doubt about the initial diagnosis, for example when no initial biopsy was done, or when the biopsy specimen was inadequate or not typical of CD. Gluten challenge should be discouraged before the age of 7 years and during the pubertal growth spurt. Once decided, gluten challenge should always be performed under strict medical supervision. It should be preceded by an assessment of mucosal histology and performed with a standard dose of at least 10 g gluten per day without disrupting established dietary habits. A further biopsy is taken when there is a noticeable clinical relapse or, in any event, after 3 to 6 months. Serological tests (IgA gliadin, reticulin, and endomysium antibodies, absorptive and permeability tests), more than clinical symptoms, can be of help in assessing the timing of the biopsy to shorten the duration of the challenge.[117]

A recent survey indicates that most pediatricians still follow these criteria.[118] However, the current guidelines for CD are almost 20 years old,[116] and since then significant changes have occurred. A wider spectrum of histological lesions (not only villous atrophy) have been associated to CD, HLA typing is increasingly used in some clinical situations, and, finally, evidence has accumulated for the diagnostic value of CD-related antibodies. It could then possible to switch from a situation where the biopsy was the only criterion to a new one where clinical presentation, serology, histology, and genetics all contribute to the diagnosis.

THERAPY

Gluten-Free Diet

Since the identification of gluten as the etiologic factor in CD, a strict gluten-free diet has become the cornerstone of the management of such patients. Their diet should exclude wheat, rye, and barley. Although oats seem to be tolerated by the great majority of CD patients, it seems wise to add oats to a gluten-free diet only when the latter is well established, so that possible adverse reactions can be readily identified. Rice and maize are nontoxic and are usually used as wheat substitutes.

The clinical response to withdrawal of gluten is often dramatic, but it must be stressed that the gluten-free diet is recommended for both symptomatic and asymptomatic patients with CD. A gluten-free diet is thought to be protective against the development of malignant disease. Patients with celiac disease have a risk of small bowel adenocarcinoma that is about 80-fold greater than that of the general population.[119] The predominant celiac-associated lymphoma is the enteropathy-associated T-cell lymphoma. Malignancies are not the main risk that celiac patients not compliant with gluten-free diet are exposed to; nutritional deficiencies,[120] in particular osteoporosis, are additional concerns. The most likely cause of lack of response is failure to adhere strictly to the diet. More studies are needed to establish the need of a gluten-free diet for those patients with immunological stigmata of CD and no or minimal enteropathy (latent and potential cases).

All the present evidence strongly supports the view that restriction of gliadin and related prolamines should be complete and for life for all patients. If analytical methods for gluten detection have already reached a satisfactory sensitivity, more information is needed on the daily gluten amount that is tolerated by CD patients. The data so far available seem to suggest that the threshold should be set below 50 mg/day.[121]

Therapeutic Strategies for the Future

Significant progress has been made in recent years in the understanding of the cellular and molecular basis of CD and in the consequent identification of possible targets for therapy. Recently it has been shown that, because of the high proline content, gliadin peptides are highly resistant to digestive processing by pancreatic and brush border proteases. Enzyme supplement therapy using bacterial endopeptidases has been proposed to promote complete digestion of cereal proteins and thus destroy T-cell multipotent epitopes. The identification of gliadin peptide sequences having biological effects, either through non-immune-mediated mechanisms or by activation of T cells, is important. Breeding programs and/or transgenic technology may lead to production of wheat that is devoid of biologically active peptide sequences. The identification of specific epitopes may also provide a target for immunomodulation of antigenic peptides. Engineered peptides may potentially bind to HLA molecules but not T-cell receptors (TCR), or bind TCRs but switch a proinflammatory Th1 to a Th2 or protective Th3 response. Other promising areas include inhibition of the innate immune response activated by gliadin peptides, preventing gliadin presentation to T cells by blocking HLA binding sites, use of TG2 inhibitors, and assessing IL-10 as a tool to promote tolerance. An immunomodulatory approach will need to have a safety profile equivalent to that of the gluten-free diet, but with the advantage of increased compliance.[122]

REFERENCES

36. Hunt KA, Zhernakova A, Turner G, et al. Newly identified genetic risk variants for celiac disease related to the immune response. Nat Genet 2008;40:395–402.
51. Sollid L. Coeliac disease dissecting a complex inflammatory disorder. Nat Rev Immunol 2002;9:647–655.
65. Dieterich W, Ehnis T, Bauer M, et al. Identification of tissue transglutaminase as the autoantigen of celiac disease. Nat Med 1997;3:797–801.
75. Oberhuber G, Granditsch G, Vogelsang H. The histopathology of coeliac disease: time for a standardized report scheme for pathologists. Eur J Gastroenterol Hepatol 1999;11:1185–1194.
113. Richey R, Howdle P, Shaw E, Stokes T. Guideline Development Group. Recognition and assessment of coeliac disease in children and adults: summary of NICE guidance. BMJ 2009;338:b1684.
122. Troncone R, Ivarsson A, Szajewska H, Mearin ML. Members of European Multistakeholder Platform on CD (CDEUSSA). Review article: future research on coeliac disease – a position report from the European multistakeholder platform on coeliac disease (CDEUSSA). Aliment Pharmacol Ther 2008;27:1030–1043.

See expertconsult.com for a complete list of references and the review questions for this chapter.

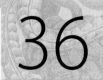

36 SHORT BOWEL SYNDROME

Stuart S. Kaufman

DEFINITION

Short bowel syndrome (SBS) refers to the sum of functional impairments that result from a critical reduction in intestinal length. In the absence of therapy, features of SBS include diarrhea and chronic dehydration, malnutrition with weight loss and growth failure, and numerous electrolyte and micronutrient deficiencies. Parenteral nutrition (PN) is the primary therapy that defines SBS. The term *intestinal failure* has been used recently in reference to severely compromised intestinal function of any etiology that requires PN irrespective of bowel length. Thus, mucosal disorders such as microvillus inclusion disease and tufting enteropathy, as well as severe intestinal pseudo-obstruction, are also forms of intestinal failure.[1] SBS is by far the most common cause of intestinal failure and continues to represent the model for management of these complex disorders.

ETIOLOGY

Frequency of pediatric SBS worldwide is unclear in the absence of a uniform reporting system. Sigalet has estimated an incidence in children of 4.8 per million, which is roughly twofold greater than incidence in adults.[1,2] SBS most often originates in infancy as a result of congenital malformation of the gastrointestinal tract (Table 36-1). Common causes include extensive small intestinal atresia, particularly when multiple or "apple-peel" in configuration, and gastroschisis.[3-7] The incidence of gastroschisis is increasing,[8] and the relative risk is sixfold higher in infants born to teenage compared to older mothers.[9] Small intestinal volvulus secondary to intestinal malrotation is another common cause of SBS, about one third of the total. These malformations are not mutually exclusive; malrotation occurs in about 10 to 15% of patients with intestinal atresia,[10] and malrotation and atresia may accompany severe gastroschisis. The other main etiology of pediatric SBS is necrotizing enterocolitis (NEC). Severity of NEC and resultant bowel loss is proportional to the degree of prematurity; most extensive gut necrosis occurs in infants under 32 weeks' gestation. However, NEC also occurs in full-term infants, often precipitated by preexisting disorders that include severe congenital heart disease.[11] Omphalocele and aganglionosis involving the small bowel as well as colon are much less common.

An amalgam of disorders that overlap the common etiologies in infancy and adulthood cause SBS beginning in later childhood and adolescence.[12] Volvulus resulting from previously asymptomatic intestinal malrotation is a relatively common cause in this age group. Massive abdominal trauma and intra-abdominal neoplasia that requires abdominal and pelvic exenteration to complete tumor resection, particularly desmoid tumors in patients with familial adenomatous polyposis, also contribute.

INTESTINAL FUNCTION AND THE IMPACT OF INTESTINAL LOSS

Absorption and secretion in the gastrointestinal tract occur in steady state when the gastrointestinal tract is anatomically intact and functionally normal. The upper digestive tract, including stomach, duodenum, and proximal jejunum, is principally secretory. In these regions, water flows into the lumen passively in response to ion gradients established by their active transport across the epithelial basolateral plasma membrane and ultimately into the bowel lumen. Approximately 8000 mL of fluid passes into the gut lumen daily in adults under the stimulus of food and dietary water.[13] Proximal gut secretion of water is essential, because dietary solids must first be liquefied before they can be absorbed. Net absorption occurs in all but the most proximal jejunoileum (6500 mL daily) and colon (1000 to 1500 mL daily) in adults, resulting in only about 200 mL of daily fecal water loss. Net water absorption in the distal bowel is also passive in response to movement of solutes from the lumen to the mucosal epithelium. Diarrhea in SBS results when aggregate fluid secretion exceeds maximal absorption by remnant distal bowel. Often, both electrolytes secreted by proximal bowel (secretory diarrhea) and unabsorbed dietary solutes, especially carbohydrates (osmotic diarrhea), contribute to total fluid losses.

Proximal Intestinal Loss

When mainly proximal intestine is lost, which is unusual in pediatric SBS, clinical impact on digestion is generally small. In some patients, increased gastric fluid output offsets the usual contribution of the small bowel to the total volume secreted.[14] Gastric acid secretion increases in proportion to the magnitude of the resection, possibly because of a parallel reduction in release of enteric hormones such as somatostatin that inhibit acid production. In some patients, gastric hyperacidity may cause transient malabsorption by inactivating pancreatic enzymes and precipitating bile acids. However, diarrhea is rarely substantial after proximal intestinal resection, because the more distal jejunum, ileum, and colon have sufficient functional reserve to increase fluid uptake three- to fivefold.[13] Similarly, protein and carbohydrate absorption are minimally affected, because their complete assimilation requires only about one third of normal small bowel length.[15] Only lipids require the entire small bowel for normal uptake, so intestinal resection from any region may produce nutritionally significant lipid malabsorption.

TABLE 36-1. Etiology of Short Bowel Syndrome in Children

Neonates

Congenital malformation – 60%
   Gastroschisis
   Volvulus (secondary to malrotation, mainly; also Meckel's
     diverticulum, persistent omphalomesenteric duct)
   Small intestinal atresia, especially multiple jejunal
   Omphalocele
   Congenital short bowel
Necrotizing enterocolitis – 40%

Older Children and Adolescents

Volvulus secondary to malrotation
Trauma
Intra-abdominal neoplasia
Rare: Radiation enteropathy (associated with infantile abdominal/pelvic
   malignancy)

Distal Intestinal Loss

Resection of more distal small intestine, particularly ileum, generally reduces nutrient, fluid, and electrolyte absorption more than resection of an equivalent length of proximal jejunum.[13,16] The concept that loss of ileum should significantly impair nutrient assimilation is counterintuitive, because most macronutrients are assimilated in the upper small bowel. However, loss of all or most of this region of the small intestine has two consequences in addition to loss of length per se.

First, in contrast with the duodenum and jejunum, only ileum actively reabsorbs bile acids. If around one third or more of the ileum is lost, about 100 cm in adults and 50 cm in children, the compensatory increase in hepatic bile acid synthesis will not keep pace with increased fecal bile acid loss.[1] In that case, the proximal intestinal lumen bile salt concentration will be inadequate for efficient lipid emulsification, contributing to fat malabsorption. Furthermore, fat malabsorption increases colon fluid loss, both because long-chain fatty acids hydroxylated by colonic bacteria stimulate colonocyte electrolyte (and thereby water) secretion, particularly potassium and bicarbonate, and because long-chain fatty acids are themselves impermeable to colon epithelium, further increasing the total solute concentration in the colon lumen. A lesser amount of ileal loss may produce bile acid malabsorption without causing total body bile acid depletion or fat malabsorption. However, diarrhea may still result, because bile acids as well as long-chain fatty acids may stimulate colonic water secretion.[17]

Second, loss of ileum and probably the ileocecal valve and colon adversely affect motility of more proximal gut. Ileal loss, that is, removal of the "ileal brake," accelerates gastric emptying of liquids and increases proximal small bowel motility directly, thereby shortening total intestinal transit time independent of that resulting from reduction in intestinal length per se.[18] The result is a further reduction in contact between luminal contents and the mucosal surface, adding to the aggregate reduction in nutrient, fluid, and electrolyte assimilation. Hormones normally secreted by the distal ileal and colonic mucosa, including peptide PYY and GLP-1, probably mediate the ileal brake.[19,20] The relative contributions of the distal ileum, ileocecal valve, and proximal colon in slowing proximal motility remain incompletely defined.

Colon Loss

The colon normally absorbs only a small fraction of water reclaimed during digestion, about 10 to 15% of the total. The colon also normally plays only a secondary role in digestion; at most, 20% of complex dietary starch and even less (less than 5%) of dietary nitrogen and lipid escape small intestinal absorption.[13] Starches that escape absorption in the small intestine and also soluble fibers are salvaged to a considerable degree in the colon via fermentation to bioavailable short-chain fatty acids, primarily acetic, propionic, and butyric acid, by resident anaerobic bacteria.[19,21] An increased load of carbohydrates (and proteins) enters the colon following massive small intestinal resection, thereby increasing substrate available for fermentation; up to 1100 calories may be recovered daily in this fashion.[22-25] Uptake of short-chain fatty acid molecules in the colon also creates an osmotic gradient that enhances water absorption, thereby limiting total fecal fluid loss.

When all or most of the colon is lost, outcome depends on the magnitude of concurrent small intestinal loss. Patients who have relatively preserved small bowel that ends in an ileostomy do not generally lose enough calories to affect nutrition, and it is possible to maintain positive fluid and electrolyte balance with increased enteral intake because of the absorptive reserve of distal small bowel. In contrast, loss of most of the ileum in addition to the colon, resulting in an end-jejunostomy, generally produces negative fluid balance that is driven by the secretory character of proximal small bowel.[16] Attempted compensation with increased enteral fluid intake disproportionately increases fluid loss from the stoma, and in this situation, only intravenous (IV) fluid therapy can maintain a positive fluid balance.

FACTORS THAT DETERMINE PROGNOSIS OF SBS

Small Intestinal Length and Absorptive Function

The intestinal tract approximately doubles in length during the last trimester of a normal pregnancy. By term, small intestinal length ranges between 200 and 250 cm. Postnatal growth, which occurs predominantly in the first few years after birth,[26] is highly variable. Usual small bowel length is about 550 to 600 cm by adulthood but may range from 400 to 700 cm; approximately one third or 200 to 300 cm is functional jejunum. Because of this variability, the amount of small intestine remaining after a resection, not the amount removed, is the single most import factor determining whether SBS will develop and if so, whether PN dependence will be permanent (Figure 36-1).[3,5,26] Children and adults who retain only about 30% of normal small intestinal length after resection, about 70 cm in infants and 150 to 200 cm in adults, are at risk to develop SBS.[27,28] In adults, PN is likely when total enteral macronutrient absorption by the remnant gastrointestinal tract is less than one third of that ingested, or about 84% of the basal metabolic rate.[29] Medical and nutritional interventions short of PN are typical when nutrient assimilation ranges between one third and two thirds of that ingested. Similarly, parenteral fluid therapy can be expected when net assimilation falls below 1.4 kg per day.[29] The implication is that adult patients with an extreme intestinal loss must become profoundly hyperphagic, increasing caloric intake up to threefold, in order to avoid PN. Comparable data

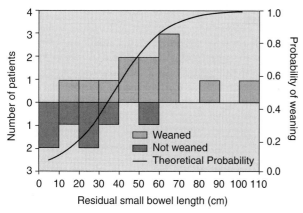

Figure 36-1. Theoretical relationship between probability of autonomy from PN and residual measured small bowel length. From Figure 2 in Andorsky et al. (2001).[5]

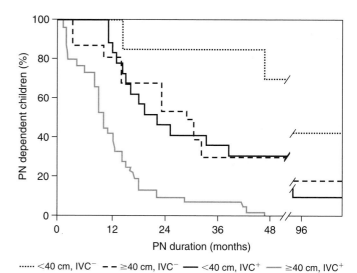

····· <40 cm, IVC⁻   – – ≥40 cm, IVC⁻   —— <40 cm, IVC⁺   —— ≥40 cm, IVC⁺

Figure 36-2. Interaction between remnant small bowel length and presence or absence of ICV on duration of PN. Data from Goulet et al. (2005).[35]

have not been definitively established in children. However, given the metabolic demands of growth and development, children probably need to tolerate an enteral intake twofold greater than normal, that is, to assimilate at least 50% of calories consumed, to avoid PN.

Impact of Colon Anatomy

Outcome of SBS is strongly influenced by coincident colon resection and, by implication, resection of the ileocecal valve (ICV). Because the ICV is rarely removed without some colon and ileum, prognostic significance of ICV loss by itself is difficult to judge.[30,31] In adult- and, by implication, child- and adolescent-onset SBS, a remnant small bowel that is less than 100 to 115 cm and ends as a stoma results in lifelong PN dependence in the overwhelming majority of affected patients.[12,28] In these older patients, preservation of at least 60 cm of proximal jejunum anastomosed to some length of colon (no ICV) yields an 85 to 90% probability of ending PN, whereas no more than half can end PN if remnant jejunal length is only 30 to 35 cm. In contrast, if the same length of remnant small bowel (30 to 35 cm) is in continuity with the ICV and entire colon, which implies at least some ileal preservation, then PN can usually be discontinued eventually. In infant-onset SBS, PN is usually permanent if remnant small bowel is less than 70 cm and ends with an abdominal wall stoma. Infants with as little as 20 to 25 cm of small bowel may end PN if the remnant small bowel retains continuity with an intact colon including the ICV,[32-34] and indefinite PN is rare when a remnant jejunoileum of at least 40 cm is in continuity with an ICV and intact colon.[31,35] In contrast, no more than half of infants with a partial colon, that is, no ICV, and 40 cm or less of small bowel are able to end PN.[4,36] The combined impact of remnant small bowel length and presence or absence of an ICV is depicted in Figure 36-2. A limitation of these prognostic criteria is the rapid intestinal growth that occurs in the third trimester, which may explain the greater probability of premature infants ending PN compared to full-term infants with equivalent lengths of remnant small bowel.[3] For that reason, remnant small bowel in premature patients is increasingly expressed as the percentage of bowel normally present at the given gestational age; most end PN if the amount remaining is greater than or equal to 10% of expected.[30]

Function of Remnant Gut

Lengths of small intestine and colon remaining after surgical resection are not the sole determinants of outcome in SBS, specifically whether or not PN will be permanent. In addition to gut anatomy, health of remaining bowel undoubtedly has an impact, because there are indications that nonnecrotic bowel retained after extensive resection may be sublethally but permanently damaged by the original event. This situation is most apparent in the 10 to 25% of infants with gastroschisis coassociated with intestinal atresia or stenosis. In this group, prolonged dysmotility often mandates PN despite seemingly adequate bowel length[37,38]; those with jejunoileal atresia alone do not appear to have this risk.[39] Overall, however, etiology of SBS is not an independent predictor of outcome.[3,30,40] Gut function after resection is difficult to quantify directly, particularly in infants, and early tolerance of enteral nutrition (EN) serves as a surrogate measure. Thus, in infants with 25 cm of small bowel remaining after neonatal resection, tolerance of 75% of calories via the gastrointestinal tract by age 3 months predicts a 90% probability of ending PN. Conversely, tolerance of only 25% of daily calories via the gastrointestinal tract with 25 cm of remnant small bowel at age 3 months predicts a 50% chance of ending PN (Figure 36-3).[26]

Intestinal Adaptation

Alimentary tract function gradually improves following massive intestinal resection, thereby diminishing impact of gut loss to a variable degree through compensatory events collectively referred to as "adaptation." Central to the concept of adaptation is that global absorptive function of a segment of adapted remnant bowel is greater than that of an equivalent length of bowel immediately after resection. Most information about adaptation is derived from adult laboratory animal models of massive intestinal resection.[18] Applicability of this information to humans in general and to small infants in particular is uncertain. Apart from species-specific differences in physiology, animal models usually do not account for congenital or acquired abnormalities of remnant bowel that might undermine subsequent reparative processes. Nonetheless, animal data are a useful framework on which SBS may be understood and physiologic patient care practices developed. Following massive intestinal loss, generalized *cellular hyperplasia*, most notably affecting myocytes and enterocytes, ensues under the stimulus of enteral nutrients.[41,42] Mucosal hypoplasia occurs in the absence of enteral feeding, although this phenomenon may not be nearly as pronounced in humans as in experimental animals.[43,44] Complex nutrients are most effective in stimulating cellular hyperplasia, intact proteins more than free amino acids or peptides, and long-chain triglycerides (LCTs) more than medium-chain triglycerides (MCTs). Increased numbers of enterocytes lengthen the villus-crypt unit, increase the total surface area available for absorption, and increase the total number of the various enzyme and transport molecules per crypt, although the absolute number of these molecules in individual enterocytes decreases. Expansion of enterocyte and myocyte mass presumably contributes to expected *dilatation of remnant bowel*, further increasing total absorptive surface area.

The time frame over which hyperplasia occurs following resection is not precisely established in humans.[43] One indication that enterocyte hyperplasia does continue for months after resection is the rise in plasma citrulline concentration that frequently accompanies successful withdrawal of PN.[45] Enterocytes are the sole source of plasma citrulline, concentration of which varies in proportion to the length of small intestine remaining after resection.[46] Either an initial postresection plasma citrulline concentration of at least roughly 12 μmol/L or a rise to this level or greater following initiation of EN appears to predict successful PN withdrawal. Clinical tolerance of enteral feeding improves for about 2 years after resection in adults[28] and for at least 3 to 4 years in children,[3,26,47] even though adaptation at the molecular and cellular levels may be restricted to a shorter period. Patients continuing to require PN after these intervals may need PN indefinitely. The obvious disparity in clinical adaptation between infants and adults is not surprising given the natural *linear growth of the intestinal tract* during early childhood; the degree to which adaptation to SBS increases linear intestinal growth in children has not been established.

In the clinical setting, apparent adaptation may continue over time without obvious change in small intestinal structure or function. Efficiency of bacterial fermentation in the colon may increase as additional carbohydrate and protein substrate becomes available. Increases in colonic bacterial fermentation may be gradual and clinically indistinguishable from more efficient nutrient assimilation by the small intestine. Evidence concerning systemic metabolic adjustments to massive intestinal resection is scant. Limited data in children suggest that there is no significant alteration in total energy expenditure in SBS.[48] In contrast, adults may discontinue PN despite aggregate nutrient absorption well below the predicted basal metabolic rate, suggesting that metabolic compensation following massive intestinal resection and severe malabsorption can, in fact, occur. In infancy and childhood, energy expenditures, expressed per kilogram of total bodyweight or lean body mass, fall with advancing chronologic age, which may also contribute to apparent adaptation, because the magnitude of increase in calories required to sustain growth gradually falls over time.

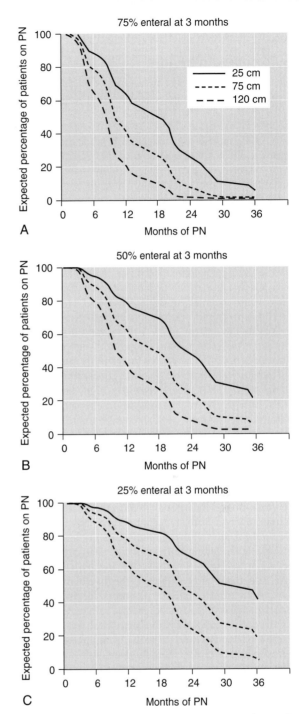

Figure 36-3. Three plots derived from the Cox Proportional Hazard equation for three groups of patients with short-bowel syndrome. Patients who receive (**A**) 75%, (**B**) 50%, and (**C**) 25% of their daily calories by the enteral route at 3 months' adjusted age. The vertical axis shows expected percentage of patients who depend on PN at any age (months). Patients with three different residual intestinal lengths after initial surgery are shown (25, 75, and 120 cm residual intestine, respectively). By using the Cox Proportional Hazard equations, survival curves such as these can be generated for any combination of the two variables. Care must be taken in applying these plots to patients whose medical management differs significantly from that described for subjects of this study. Variation of the model will require a prospective evaluation of its accuracy in more patients with neonatal intestinal resection. From Figure 2 of Sondheimer et al. (1998).[26]

CLINICAL MANAGEMENT OF SBS

Early Postoperative Phase

The period of postoperative ileus ordinarily lasts less than 1 week if ongoing abdominal sepsis or other complications do not occur. At this time, fecal output is low as upper gastrointestinal secretions are drained, usually via a nasogastric or concurrently placed gastrostomy tube. Recovery of motility permits discontinuation of upper gastrointestinal tract decompression, following which fecal output may variably increase. The clinical challenge is appropriate replacement of ongoing losses to maintain fluid and electrolyte balance. Proper water and electrolyte replacement is most difficult when the small bowel ends as a proximal jejunostomy. Given the fundamentally secretory character of proximal small bowel, a high enterostomy is associated with an output that approximates 30 to 50 mL/kg per day even while the patient remains nil per os, in effect, a secretory diarrhea. Gastric hypersecretion may contribute to early, high fluid loss from an enterostomy. Histamine-2 receptor antagonists and proton pump inhibitors delivered intravenously have been advocated to reduce gastric hypersecretion during the first months after massive intestinal resection, although evidence that supports the efficacy of this practice in infants and children is lacking. Sodium and chloride concentrations in proximal jejunostomy effluent are relatively high, both up to 120 mEq/L, and these electrolytes must also be replaced adequately in addition to fluid in order to prevent hyponatremia and hypochloremia. In contrast, potassium and bicarbonate losses are low. Progressively distal placement of an enterostomy reduces fluid loss as additional, predominantly absorptive small bowel modifies the fecal stream. Retention of a substantial length of colon generally precludes significant secretory fluid loss; however, potassium and bicarbonate requirements tend to climb as requirements for sodium and chloride generally fall.

PN should begin following establishment of stable fluid and electrolyte status. When remnant bowel anatomy predicts prolonged if not indefinite PN, a semipermanent, cuffed catheter (Broviac, Hickman) can be placed at the time of original surgery or soon thereafter. Alternatively, parenteral feeding may be initiated via a peripherally inserted central catheter ("PICC line"). During the early period of PN in the hospital, it is usually useful to deliver replacement fluids separate from PN, because volume and composition of replacement fluid are likely to change much more frequently than PN, especially after EN is initiated.

Initiation of Feeding

Criteria to start EN are resolution of postoperative ileus, cessation of upper gastrointestinal tract decompression, and achievement of stable metabolic, fluid, and electrolyte status with PN and ancillary fluid and electrolyte support. In all ages, proprietary liquid diets are usually used. Most attention concerning EN in pediatric SBS has focused on young infants, the most common time that SBS is diagnosed. Optimal formula composition for infant SBS remains controversial. Controversies include nitrogen source, free amino acid, a mixture of amino acids and short peptides (protein hydrolysates), or intact protein; and also quantity and type of lipid, medium-chain versus long-chain triglycerides. In the past, hydrolysate formulas were favored based on the assumption that assimilation of peptides by a short gut should be superior to that of intact proteins,

TABLE 36-2. Anatomic Considerations in Management

Terminal enterostomy (or very short colon remnant in continuity)
  No lipid restriction – use LCT
  High dose anti-motility agents
  Soluble fiber to increase viscosity/slow gastric emptying
  Oral hydration solution with high sodium (90-120 mEq/L)
Small bowel remnant in continuity with all or most of colon
  Lipid restriction – use LCT and MCT
  Low dose anti-motility agents
  Soluble fiber to increase viscosity and colon fermentation to short-chain fatty acids
  Oral hydration solution with low sodium (50 mEq/L) with potassium and bicarbonate/citrate

which, in fact, may not be the case.[49] Amino acid–based formulas were discouraged because of indications that enterocyte peptide uptake is superior to amino acid uptake. Recently, there have been indications that amino acid–based formulas are best tolerated, possibly because of a reduced tendency to precipitate hypersensitivity reactions.[5,50] Furthermore, including breast milk in the diet also appears to promote intestinal adaptation. In contrast, adult patients with SBS including those with terminal enterostomies do not benefit from peptide formulas in comparison with diets and formulas containing intact proteins,[51] and it is logical to infer the same in older children and adolescents. Continuous intragastric infusion is the usual mode of delivery in order to maximize nutrient and fluid absorption and to circumvent typically rapid gastric emptying that contributes to very short gastrointestinal transit times.[52] Occasionally, gastric feeding tolerance is poor following massive intestinal resection, usually in the setting of small bowel dilatation secondary to obstruction in utero and chronic lung disease. In these situations, infusion of feeding directly into the proximal small bowel, usually via transpyloric feeding tube, may produce superior tolerance.

Impact of Intestinal Anatomy

A temporary end-enterostomy is commonly placed at the time of initial resection. It is generally highly desirable to reestablish continuity of remnant small bowel and colon at the earliest practicable time, because total fluid and nutrient absorption usually improve afterward for the reasons noted previously. Gut anatomy also influences formula selection, particularly carbohydrate and lipid composition (Table 36-2). Extreme resections that require a permanent enterostomy are rare in infants and children, but patients who retain an enterostomy or whose remaining small bowel is in continuity with a short length of rectosigmoid colon do best with diets or formulas with a standard, relatively high, lipid content. The reason is that enterocyte lipid absorption, being nonsaturable, is a fixed fraction of the total ingested; the greater the amount ingested, the greater the amount absorbed. Because dietary lipids do not contribute substantially to osmolarity of enteric succus, lipid malabsorption, unlike carbohydrate malabsorption, does not markedly increase water loss in patients with an enterostomy.[15] In these patients, substitution of some dietary LCTs with MCTs offers no significant absorptive advantage and may actually be deleterious, because MCTs may stimulate adaptive enterocyte hyperplasia less than do LCTs.[53] Furthermore, MCTs are only useful as an energy source and are not incorporated into structural lipids essential for tissue growth.

Patients with substantial colon length in continuity with small bowel benefit from a diet that includes MCTs, because medium-chain fatty acids, which are more water soluble than long-chain fatty acids, can be assimilated by the colon if not absorbed by the small bowel.[21] Consequently, medium-chain fatty acids may be less prone to stimulate colonic salt and water secretion than malabsorbed long-chain fatty acids. Because bacterial production of short-chain fatty acids occurs predominantly in the colon, patients with enterocolonic continuity benefit more from diets enriched with complex carbohydrates, including both starches and soluble fibers, than do patients with enterostomies.

Advancement of EN and Reduction in PN

The primary objective in managing the patient with SBS is prevention of permanent intestinal failure, that is, elimination of PN and removal of the central venous catheter required to deliver it. In practice, PN is gradually curtailed as enteral feeding, initially consisting predominantly of a liquid formula delivered by tube, is increased. Enteral feeding is increased based on two interrelated criteria, the ability to increase body mass appropriately as parenteral calories are diminished and the ability to maintain hydration as PN volume is curtailed.

Enteral feeds are generally initially increased by 0.5 to 1.0 cal/kg every 1 to 3 days; continued and preferably accelerated weight gain justifies reductions in parenteral calories. Decreases in PN are usually quantitatively less than concomitant increases in EN in light of the malabsorption inherent to SBS. Aggregate enteral absorption of nitrogen, carbohydrate, and lipid calories is not routinely measured directly, but fractional intestinal absorption probably varies between 33 and 67% of the total ingested depending on the magnitude and region(s) of remnant bowel. Fractional enteric absorption can be estimated as the difference between estimated total energy expenditure and delivered PN calories divided by the quantity of calories actually infused into the gastrointestinal tract. Total energy expenditure is initially equivalent to parenteral caloric intake before initiation of EN under the key assumption that PN had established appropriate body growth. Continuing estimation of enteric absorption can guide future PN weaning, quantifies adaptation of remnant bowel, and helps to identify reductions in bowel function that suggest development of complications such as small intestinal bacterial overgrowth (see the later section "Complications of SBS and PN"). A constant or increasing percentage of enteral nutrient absorption over time is expected. Macronutrient absorption is often superior to that of fluid and electrolytes, so PN calories may be weaned by reducing the concentrations of macronutrients in PN rather than by reducing PN volume.

A reduction in PN volume as well as parenteral calories is indicated when stable hydration is maintained with increasing EN as demonstrated by physical examination, estimated stool output, and relevant laboratory data, including urea nitrogen, hematocrit, and albumin. Estimating hydration is often challenging, because subcutaneous fluid may be difficult to distinguish from body fat. Fecal volume may also be difficult to estimate, because liquid stools blend with urine in diapers of infants without stomas. Useful indicators of a moderate stool pattern include the finding of diapers that contain only urine several times daily, fewer than six to eight stools daily, absence of diaper rash attributable to liquid feces, and, in the case of infants with an enterostomy or colostomy, outputs less than

TABLE 36-3. Supplementation Following Discontinuation of PN

Vitamins
  Vitamin D (calciferol, calcitriol)
  Vitamin E (tocopheryl polyethylene glycol succinate, Aqua-E)
  Vitamin B$_{12}$ (oral, sublingual, subcutaneous)
  Vitamin A – rarely needed
  Vitamin K – very rarely needed
Electrolytes
  Sodium/potassium citrate (Bicitra, Polycitra, Polycitra-K, Polycitra-LC)
  Calcium (carbonate/citrate)
  Magnesium (oxide, gluconate [Magonate])
Elements
  Iron (ferrous sulfate – enteral, iron sucrose [Venofer], sodium ferric gluconate [Ferrlecit] -parenteral)
  Zinc (sulfate, gluconate)

50 mL/kg per day. It is important to resist the tendency to increase PN volume to prevent or reverse dehydration in response to increased enteral feeding unless the increased enteral feeding confers the benefit of a reduced need for PN calories.

As PN is curtailed, it becomes increasingly necessary to deliver electrolytes, trace elements, and vitamins via the gastrointestinal tract that were formerly delivered intravenously (Table 36-3). Patients who retain a substantial length of colon often need supplemental potassium and bicarbonate. Those with predominantly small bowel resection may need extra calcium, magnesium, and zinc. When intravenous vitamin therapy ends, patients lacking all or most of the ileum are particularly likely to develop deficiencies of vitamin D and vitamin E due to bile acid malabsorption. The amount of remnant terminal ileum necessary to permit adequate vitamin B$_{12}$ absorption may be as little as 15 cm.[54] Blood levels should be checked every 3 to 6 months; an elevated plasma methylmalonic acid concentration may be more sensitive than serum vitamin B$_{12}$ concentration in detecting early deficiency.[55] Hypophosphatemia is unusual and, when present, usually indicates vitamin D deficiency, possibly calcium deficiency, and secondary hyperparathyroidism. Because of the rarity of duodenal resection, pharmacologic iron supplementation is unusual in the absence of chronic gastrointestinal blood loss.

Because ending of PN is the first nutritional priority for patients with SBS, liquid diets are generally infused continuously and without interruption well beyond the initial feeding period, because this strategy is most likely to achieve maximal retention of calories and fluid delivered into the gastrointestinal tract.[56,57] The desirability of delivering EN continuously over the longest period possible must be weighed against the desirability of permitting some oral feeding for the purpose of preserving and promoting feeding skills. Maintaining feeding skills is especially important for those patients who have a high probability of ending PN, because eventual achievement of a normal to near-normal lifestyle includes eating by mouth, a skill that is quickly lost during infancy if all oral intake is forbidden. If fluid balance is tenuous, consumption of limited quantities of glucose-electrolyte solution in lieu of formula may minimize stool output while preserving the ability to swallow. When all or most of the colon is present, proprietary solutions containing 50 mEq/L of sodium (Pedialyte) are satisfactory, but when there is only a short segment of colon in continuity with proximal jejunum or there is no colon, customized solutions containing 90 to 120 mEq/L of sodium are needed for optimal water absorption.[58] Solids rich in complex carbohydrates, particularly those that are high in soluble fiber such as cereals and unsweetened fruits and lean meats, are best tolerated in those retaining a significant length of colon. Patients with little or no colon may experience few if any problems following ingestion of items with high fat content. Given the high degree of individual variation, some trial and error with feeding is often necessary. The combination of formula infusion and oral solids while awake may produce smaller and more formed stools than formula infusion alone, which may be a function of a net increase in viscosity of the diet.[59] Reducing the rate of infusion while asleep may be justified, because infrequent diaper changes during the night may promote skin breakdown.

An additional test of tolerance to EN is the ability to deliver PN intermittently, that is, to "cycle" PN. The two rationales for cycling are the potential reduction in hepatic stress of PN and the potential developmental benefit of improved mobility that results from being disconnected from an intravenous infusion pump.[60] As no prospective data establish optimal duration of the "off" period, this interval is based largely on the ability to maintain stable hydration and metabolic status, especially blood glucose level. Typical periods of interruption range from 4 hours in young infants to 12 hours in older children and adolescents. As increasingly larger quantities of enteral feeding are tolerated, duration of the "off" period can also be increased. Timing of the PN infusion is based largely on caretaker convenience. Adults with SBS customarily receive PN at night, because freedom from intravenous infusion during the daytime usually outweighs the inconvenience of frequent nocturnal urination. Nighttime infusion may be less advantageous to incontinent children, because associated increases in urine production may further increase the risk of local skin breakdown. The ultimate test of successful PN withdrawal is the ability to sustain the growth trajectory established during the period of PN therapy.[35] Patients are most likely to fail a trial of PN withdrawal when small intestinal anatomy is marginal, that is, the length is around 40 cm or less, with absent ICV and partial colon resection. Despite an initial failure, a later trial of PN cessation may be successful as metabolic requirements relative to body size decrease.

Home PN in SBS

Pediatric as well as adult patients with SBS fare better when receiving PN in the home than in the institutional setting.[61] The benefit to patient life quality and family social structure is obvious. PN at home is relatively safe[62] and cost may be reduced by as much as 25 to 50% compared to the expense of continued hospitalization.[63] Planning for discharge to home should begin soon after surgery, once patient survival appears to be a reasonable certainty. Teaching should emphasize the primary responsibility of parents and/or other family providers for all aspects of intravenous fluid delivery and routine central venous catheter care. After discharge, a multidisciplinary team that includes physician, nursing, dietary, social work, and pharmacy components directs care. Professional nursing care should be provided in the home only as necessary to facilitate a smooth transition from the hospital. Formal mechanisms for regular communication between family care providers and the team, delivery of fluids, drugs, and other supplies to the home, and ambulatory laboratory support are established. This organization permits weaning of PN and advancement of EN as rapidly as possible, as caregivers assess response to dietary interventions, evaluate

hydration, and obtain scheduled and unscheduled laboratory testing, all in telephone, e-mail, and office consultation with the team.

ADDITIONAL MEDICAL INTERVENTIONS

Antimotility agents such as loperamide (Imodium) and diphenoxylate/atropine (Lomotil) are not routinely used in pediatrics. An appropriate exception is the patient with SBS. These agents slow transit time with the intention of improving fluid absorption and reducing fecal fluid loss. Efficacy often requires relatively high doses, particularly in patients with an enterostomy.[64] Indications of overdose include abdominal distention, vomiting, and lethargy. Although reducing water losses incurred by enteral feeding, antimotility agents by themselves rarely permit complete withdrawal of intravenous fluid therapy.

As a *bile acid binding resin*, cholestyramine has a limited role in pediatric short bowel syndrome. A trial of cholestyramine therapy may be useful in pediatric patients with a limited ileal resection, probably 50 cm or less, that is sufficient to produce ileal bile acid malabsorption and spillover into the colon that results in secretory diarrhea. In this setting, accelerated hepatic bile acid synthesis should be adequate to maintain the body bile salt pool, leaving lipid absorption unaltered by cholestyramine treatment. With more extensive ileal resection, a high-lipid diet may provoke colonic secretory diarrhea directly, and bile acid sequestration is unlikely to be helpful. Octreotide also has a limited role in pediatric SBS. The primary rationale for octreotide is to reduce output from proximal enterostomies, which may amount to several liters per day, thereby complicating fluid and electrolyte management.[65] Octreotide does not eliminate the need for intravenous fluid entirely in this setting, nor does it improve macronutrient absorption.

Some experimental evidence supports therapy with enterocyte/colonocyte growth factors and hormones to promote adaptation to massive intestinal loss. Employment of *glutamine* in SBS is largely discredited irrespective of age.[66] Although *growth hormone* is approved in the United States in adults with short bowel syndrome, improvements in energy absorption are relatively small, appear limited to those with intact colon, and disappear following termination of therapy.[67] There are isolated reports suggesting improvement in macronutrient absorption in nonrandomized trials of epidermal growth factor (EGF) in pediatric patients with SBS, but no evidence has been presented to indicate that the effect is sufficiently potent to shorten duration of PN significantly.[68] *Glucagon-like peptide-2* (GLP-2) and its longer acting analogue, teduglutide, improve fluid absorption in adults following intestinal resection, thereby reducing IV fluid requirements, but sustained treatment does not appear to improve energy absorption significantly.[69] No controlled trials have been reported on human infants using any of these agents, alone or in combination, and confinement of their use to the research setting is the current care standard.[67]

COMPLICATIONS OF SBS AND PN

Hepatobiliary Disease

Patients with SBS who are receiving PN are more prone to develop *progressive liver disease* and liver failure than those receiving PN for other reasons. Histologic features include variable portal and lobular inflammation, cellular bilirubin and cholate stasis, macrophage hyperplasia, and interlobular bile duct proliferation with varying degrees of portal and lobular fibrosis that may progress to fully established cirrhosis.[70] Cholestasis of any severity is more common in premature as compared to full-term infants; however, progression of PN-associated liver disease to liver failure in infant SBS does not directly relate to degree of prematurity.[5,71] Evidence is equivocal as to whether infants with the most extreme small bowel loss are most vulnerable to develop liver failure,[30,31,72] whereas extreme small intestinal loss per se does appear to pose a risk for progression to liver failure in older children and adults.[73] Incidence of progressive liver disease in infants with SBS appears to be increased by sepsis developing within the first months following resection.[71] Potential causes of, or contributors to, PN-associated liver disease include lack of EN, loss of immunologic protection associated with deficiency of gut-associated lymphoid tissue, lack of certain conditionally essential nutrients in PN such as choline, and hepatotoxicity of some PN components including intravenous lipid emulsion, copper, and manganese.[74,75] There is currently no proven therapy for PN-associated liver disease other than reduction in PN that presumably must occur over a finite interval as tolerance of EN by remnant bowel increases.[71,76] The absolute quantity or proportion of enteral calories that prevents or reverses PN-associated liver disease may vary based in part on the function as well as length of remnant bowel.[77] The most promising investigational therapy for PN-associated liver disease is intravenous lipid emulsion derived from fish oil (Omegaven, Fresenius Kabi AG, Bad Homburg, Germany).[78,79] Complete or partial substitution of standard preparations derived from vegetable oil with Omegaven may reverse or ameliorate apparently advanced and irreversible liver disease. Postulated mechanisms include reduced exposure to potentially hepatotoxic constituents of vegetable oils, particularly phytosterols, the ability of very long-chain fatty acids in fish oil to counteract the purported proinflammatory state inherent to SBS, or both.[80]

Chronic *cholecystitis* with pigmented (calcium bilirubinate) stones is part of the spectrum of PN-associated liver disease in patients with SBS.[81] Loss of the ileum and enterohepatic circulation of bile acids and a lack of EN contribute. Also important in the development of gallstones is absolute duration of PN, which is about 30 months in affected patients.[82] The extent to which established parenchymal liver disease also contributes to formation of stones is unclear. Evidence of biliary tract obstruction and symptoms and signs of gallbladder inflammation indicate cholecystectomy.[83]

Small Intestinal Bacterial Overgrowth

Small intestinal bacterial overgrowth (SIBO), defined as more than 10^5 fecal bacteria per milliliter in duodenal-jejunal fluid,[3] can develop in dysmotile or partially obstructed bowel segments if sufficient luminal nutrients are available to support bacterial proliferation. An ICV reduces occurrence of SIBO but does not completely prevent it. SIBO may undermine tolerance of EN and thereby delay the ending of PN in patients with SBS by mechanisms that include direct enterocyte injury and inactivation of bile acids via deconjugation. Symptoms of SIBO are similar to those of partial bowel obstruction and include abdominal distention, nausea and vomiting, and increased stools with flatulence. Affected patients may have elevated concentrations of breath hydrogen when fasting or following oral glucose challenge.[84] Acquisition of fat-soluble vitamin deficiencies caused by bile acid depletion and vitamin B_{12} deficiency produced by bacterial

competition for vitamin B_{12} uptake provides additional evidence that may warrant confirmation by proximal small intestinal fluid culture.[54] In contrast with other vitamins, serum folate may be high owing to bacterial production.[55] Studies in adults demonstrate efficacy of amoxicillin-clavulanic acid and norfloxacin.[85] No comparable controlled studies have been performed in children, but trimethoprim-sulfamethoxazole and gentamicin (given by mouth) are often used for SIBO attributed to coliforms. The dose of gentamicin employed is usually about 10 mg/kg per day, although markedly higher doses have been tested clinically.[86] Verifying the absence of gentamicin absorption with blood levels is often recommended. Agents with efficacy against strict anaerobes such as metronidazole should be used with more caution, because they have the potential to suppress organisms largely responsible for converting complex carbohydrates to short-chain fatty acids. Recently, there have been anecdotal reports of therapy with rifaximin, which is approved for treatment of traveler's diarrhea, for SIBO due to SBS. The purported advantages of rifaximin include a lack of absorption and broad efficacy against gram-positive and gram-negative aerobic and anaerobic bacteria[87]; formal trials are lacking. Use of antibiotics to treat bacterial overgrowth in SBS requires caution even when the diagnosis is clear, because antibiotics may promote bowel colonization with resistant organisms that may be the source of catheter-related bloodstream infections and related infective complications. Because acid-suppressing agents promote SIBO,[88] their administration should be based on specific indications rather than empiric prophylaxis beyond the initial postoperative period. Disadvantages of conventional antibiotic therapy of SIBO have led to therapy with probiotic bacteria, nonpathogenic organisms including *Lactobacillus* and *Bifidobacterium* species that colonize the gastrointestinal tract and displace potentially pathogenic organisms.[89] Although isolated case reports suggest a benefit of probiotics in SBS,[90] these organisms may themselves pose a systemic infectious risk[91]; confirmation of benefit in controlled trials is lacking, and current indications for probiotic therapy do not include SBS.[92]

A special form of SIBO in patients with colon in continuity with the small bowel is overgrowth of lactobacilli strains that produce large quantities of d-lactic acid rather than hydrogen or other short-chain fatty acids.[93,94] *D-Lactic acidosis* may be especially prone to develop when a high rate of gut lactic acid production and absorption is associated with impaired clearance, leading to encephalopathy characterized by lethargy and ataxia reminiscent of alcohol intoxication in association with metabolic acidosis and increased ion gap. Nystagmus may be present.[93] Large numbers of gram-positive rods in stools may suggest the diagnosis that is confirmed by an elevated plasma concentration of d-lactic acid. Effective treatment of d-lactic acidosis includes suppressing production by reducing intake of mono- and disaccharides that are primary food substrates and by treatment with antibiotics; oral gentamicin appears to be particularly effective,[86,95] whereas response to vancomycin is inconsistent.[96] Probiotic therapy has also been successfully employed in isolated cases[97] but should be used with caution based on the considerations noted earlier.

Enterocolitis

The prevalence of enterocolitis in pediatric patients with SBS has not been precisely established but is probably more common than the few published reports suggest (Figure 36-4).[3,98]

Aphthous ulceration is occasionally present that is distinct from perianastomotic ulceration that can complicate ileocolonic resection.[99,100] Eosinophils are often a prominent component of the inflammatory infiltrate. Symptoms include increased, bloody stools and secondary iron deficiency; abdominal pain may not be apparent. Enterocolitis associated with SBS may occur in infants early after resection, even when EN consists of an amino acid–based formula. Enterocolitis also develops in older children who are approaching complete adaptation to a broad enteral diet, implying that both SIBO and food allergy may contribute to pathophysiology in this group. Treatment is largely empiric and includes mesalamine, corticosteroids, and oral antibiotics in addition to iron replacement. Therapy

is important, because inflammation may be severe enough to delay ending of PN.[3] Testing for food allergies may also be appropriate.

Anatomic and Functional Bowel Obstruction

Marked dilatation of small bowel that remains after resection is common in disorders associated with obstruction in utero, especially jejunal atresia and gastroschisis; the result is often inefficient peristalsis that directly contributes to SIBO, malabsorption, and feeding intolerance. Compounding the deleterious effects of *dysmotility*, strictures may evolve in persistently ischemic regions, particularly at anastomoses, leading to chronic partial or progressive mechanical obstruction. Development of recurrent vomiting, abdominal distention, and/or abdominal pain suggest that either mechanical obstruction or dysmotility is the culprit, often in conjunction with SIBO, and should be evaluated with radiologic imaging, endoscopy, and biopsy (Figure 36-5). Diagnosis and management may be difficult, because de facto pseudo-obstruction may be hard to discriminate from mechanical obstruction in the setting of previous intestinal surgery. Medical therapy for symptomatic dysmotility may include antibiotics, anti-inflammatory drugs, and prokinetic agents. These treatments may have limited efficacy, and when symptoms are severe or interfere with advancement of EN, surgical intervention may be desirable.

Numerous operations correct bowel dysmotility that may be present with or without concurrent mechanical obstruction. Simple antimesenteric longitudinal tapering efficiently reduces intestinal caliber, reduces stools, and improves feeding tolerance in the short term.[101] Because longitudinal tapering further reduces already diminished intestinal absorptive surface area, Bianchi devised the longitudinal intestinal lengthening operation in order to preserve surface area while improving motility.[74]

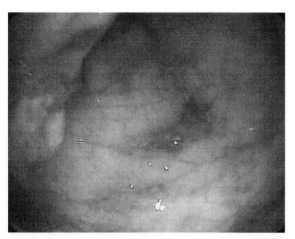

Figure 36-4. Short gut enterocolitis. Endoscopic view of sigmoid colon demonstrating intense, focal erythema. Microscopy demonstrated eosinophilia in lamina propria and eosinophilic cryptitis with lymphoid hyperplasia.

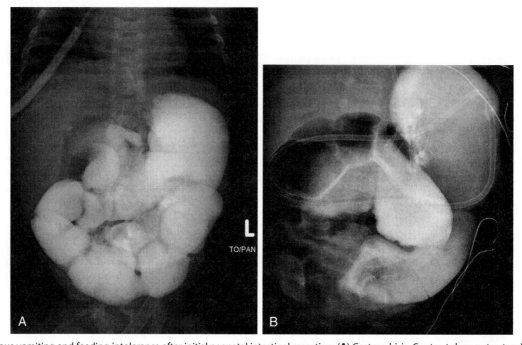

Figure 36-5. Bilious vomiting and feeding intolerance after initial neonatal intestinal resection. (**A**) Gastroschisis. Contrast does not extend beyond a dilated loop to the right of the midline. Complete obstruction at jejunocolonic anastomosis found at surgery. (**B**) Jejunal atresia. Dilatation of the duodenum and proximal jejunum beyond which caliber is markedly reduced without complete obstruction. Patent jejunojejunal anastomosis with proximal blind loop found at surgery.

In this operation, a dilated bowel segment is divided into two tubes in the mesenteric-anti-mesenteric plane with a stapler followed by anastomosis of the two narrowed segments end to end. Thus, the Bianchi procedure doubles the length of the affected segment while reducing its diameter by one half. Longitudinal intestinal lengthening has largely been replaced by a technically simpler but apparently equally effective procedure developed by Kim et al., serial transverse enteroplasty, more popularly referred to as the "STEP" procedure.[102,103] In this operation, a series of staple lines, all perpendicular to the long axis of the dilated bowel, are placed, each staple line originating alternately from either side to create a maze-like tunnel within the dilated segment. Like longitudinal intestinal lengthening, the STEP procedure roughly doubles the length of the dilated segment (Figure 36-6).[104,105] The STEP procedure improves carbohydrate assimilation, but a beneficial effect on lipid absorption is less clear. Reductions in PN dependence with preserved or improved growth appear to persist for several years.[106] Intestinal lengthening operations are most beneficial to patients who meet the following criteria: EN at maximal tolerance; significant small bowel dilatation, that is, greater than twice-normal diameter; and absence of liver disease complicated by portal hypertension or marked hepatocellular synthetic dysfunction. Hyperbilirubinemia alone is not a contraindication.[103]

Pancreatitis

Recurrent acute and chronic pancreatitis that may progress to pancreatic insufficiency occurs in some patients with SBS, the cause of which is often unknown.[107,108] The presence of gallstones is an obvious risk factor, but pancreatitis may occur in the absence of overt hepatobiliary tract disease. Other potential but unproven causes include organ ischemia resulting from chronic underhydration, vasculitis associated with the systemic inflammatory response inherent to SBS, hypertriglyceridemia secondary to intolerance of intravenous lipid emulsion, and ampullary spasm.[109] Exocrine pancreatic insufficiency may worsen fat malabsorption in SBS, but the number of patients benefiting from replacement therapy in addition to usual dietary intervention is conjectural. Cystic fibrosis, present in about 10% of patients with intestinal atresia, may contribute to steatorrhea, and routine testing of these patients has been advocated.[10]

Renal Disease

Prolonged PN for SBS and SBS itself may produce renal complications, of which the best characterized is nephrolithiasis associated with oxaluria. Oxalic acid stones develop as a result of lipid malabsorption; calcium binds preferentially to lumen fatty acids compared to oxalate, leaving free oxalate available for uptake by the colon if in continuity with remnant small bowel.[81] Patients with a terminal enterostomy are also susceptible to this complication if inadequate replacement of high stoma output leads to chronic dehydration. Consumption of solid foods with low oxalate content and maintenance of high urine output are the best ways to prevent this problem. Hyperuricemia with tubulointerstitial disease and nephrolithiasis have also been reported in SBS.[110] Although dietary factors and arginine depletion may contribute to development of these complications,[111] chronic dehydration is the easiest factor to correct.

Chronic underhydration and sodium depletion due to high fecal or stoma losses and excessive PN cycling are probably more frequent in SBS than commonly realized.[69] Along with repeated exposure to numerous nephrotoxic drugs, chronic underhydration and sodium depletion almost certainly contribute to the tendency of the glomerular filtration rate to fall over time in proportion to duration of PN.[112] Chronic dehydration and sodium depletion produce extended activation of the renin-angiotensin system, and in recognition of that principle, some advocate periodic measurement of urine electrolytes. Verification that the absolute urine sodium concentration is greater than 20 mmol/L or that the urine sodium/potassium ratio is greater than 1 supports a clinical impression of a quiescent renin-angiotensin system and appropriate fluid and electrolyte balance.[67,112]

Complications Associated With Central Venous Catheters

Patients with PN-dependent SBS may experience the same catheter-related complications as patients who receive PN for other reasons. These include recurring bloodstream infections and mechanical problems related to catheter insertion and long duration of placement, including pleural effusion, pericardial tamponade, thromboembolism, and lumen occlusion with fibrin, lipid, or calcium phosphate precipitates. Therapy

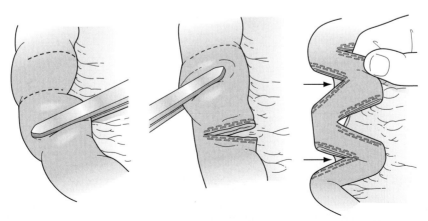

Figure 36-6. Serial transverse enteroplasty procedure. The small arrows show the direction of insertion of the GIA stapler and the sites of the mesenteric defects. The staplers are placed in the 90° and 270° orientations using the mesentery as the 0° reference point. From Figure 1 of Kim et al. (2003).[104]

with warfarin is appropriate to preserve central vein access in pediatric patients with SBS in the event of recurrent thrombosis.[113] Presence of vitamin K in standard parenteral vitamin formulations does not undermine efficacy. Although catheter-related infections are less frequent in patients at home than in the hospital, infection remains the most common reason for rehospitalization.[61] In pediatric patients with SBS, rates of infection have ranged between about one and six per 1000 days of PN.[3,4,34,114,115] The ultimate catheter-related complication is loss of central venous access due to thrombotic occlusion of all available sites. When there is no reasonable chance to end PN, the only remedy for loss of central venous access is a successful intestinal transplant (see the later section "Referral for Intestinal Transplantation").

SURVIVAL AND ITS COSTS IN PEDIATRIC SBS

About 60 to 70% of infants with SBS of neonatal onset eventually end PN and subsist purely on EN with varying degrees of ongoing disability related to the complications discussed earlier.[30,116] There is promise that outcomes in pediatric SBS will improve in the future with wider application of newer medical and surgical therapies including enteroplasty and PN incorporating fish oil–based lipid.[8] Even without the benefit of newer therapies, complete adaptation to EN occurs more frequently in infants than in older patients for two reasons. First, the inherent growth potential of infant bowel probably provides a very favorable climate for adaptation if EN is aggressively administered. Second, most infants with SBS do not have life-threatening comorbidities such as malignancy and atherosclerotic disease that are commonly present in adults with SBS.

Reported death rates of patients remaining dependent on PN range from 24 to 92%.[3,5,26,31] The wide variation probably reflects disparate enrollment criteria and follow-up among the case series reported.[116] An initial peak in mortality occurs in the early perioperative period, and a second peak occurs around 1 to 1.5 years of age, usually of complications directly related to SBS and PN, particularly PN-associated liver failure and sepsis.[8,30,72,117] The distinction between death from liver failure and death from sepsis is artificial, because bacterial and fungal infection in infants with SBS is most likely to be fatal when advanced liver disease is present. Fatal SBS is most frequent in the setting of *extreme short bowel*, that is, preservation of only some duodenum or at most, duodenum and a few centimeters of jejunum, usually terminating as an end-duodenostomy or jejunostomy. This anatomy is equivalent to 95% or greater small intestine resection and may be encountered following necrotizing enterocolitis, small intestinal volvulus, multiple intestinal atresia, and total intestinal aganglionosis.[118] Before the advent of intestinal transplantation, therapy was commonly withheld from infants with extreme short bowel, as survival on PN was extremely poor; most succumbed within 6 to 12 months after diagnosis. The increasing availability of intestinal transplant has required modification of this practice. Diagnosis of extreme SBS clearly incompatible with survival on PN requires a joint yet rapid decision by the surgical-neonatal team and the child's parents or guardians whether to proceed with or to withhold surgical therapy. A decision in favor of early surgery to remove nonviable gut and to initiate PN indicates the intention to list for and perform intestinal transplantation as soon as practicable, preferably before advanced liver disease supervenes if possible.[34]

Whereas the overall cost of care during the first year after diagnosis of SBS averages US$500,000, cost of care thereafter is more strongly influenced by prognosis.[47] Patients who survive, the majority of whom eventually end PN, incur an average annual cost while receiving PN of about US$200,000 per year after the first year, which is only about one half the cost of care for those who ultimately die from their disease.

Referral for Intestinal Transplantation

Intestinal transplantation is appropriate when indications are that PN will be permanent and that the probability of fatality is high. Perception of threatened or actual liver failure in the setting of little or no prospect of ending PN is the most common indication for transplant.[119] Progressive liver disease may be present when hyperbilirubinemia fails to remit following several months of enteral feeding, particularly when greater than 6 mg/dL, in conjunction with indications of evolving portal hypertension, especially progressive splenomegaly with thrombocytopenia, and falling serum albumin concentration.[72] Patients with progressively worsening liver disease *without* severe portal hypertension who have failed all previous medical and surgical efforts at ending PN may be candidates for isolated intestinal transplantation, because less advanced liver disease may resolve following a successful operation that allows withdrawal of PN.[120] Historically, a liver biopsy that demonstrates stage 1 or 2 fibrosis has been thought to support a diagnosis of reversible liver disease and feasibility of isolated intestinal transplant; however, the prognostic value of liver biopsy for this purpose is questionable.[76] Conversely, PN-associated liver disease occasionally progresses to end-stage, that is, *with* portal hypertension, in patients who have the potential for complete intestinal adaptation, often because other medical problems interfered with early, postnatal delivery of EN. Transplantation of the liver alone in infants and children with SBS is indicated when approximately 50% of caloric requirements are delivered by EN and intestinal anatomy predicts complete intestinal adaptation.[76,121,122]

The other major indication for intestinal transplantation is the threatened inability to continue PN because of impending loss of adequate venous access. Successful intestinal transplantation depends in part on the ability to maintain stable central venous access through the perioperative period. For that reason, consensus of the intestinal transplant community is that loss of half or more of all standard access sites justifies transplantation when the need for PN appears indefinite.[119] In infants, standard sites include the two internal jugular and two subclavian veins. In older children, the femoral veins are included. Although recurring, life-threatening sepsis is an indication for transplant, transplantation solely because of recurring, life-threatening sepsis is infrequent in practice.

SUMMARY

SBS is an important chronic gastrointestinal disorder of infancy and childhood. Type and magnitude of intestinal loss influence pathophysiology, clinical management, and prognosis. Appropriate management requires an understanding of normal intestinal growth and regional intestinal function as well as PN, fluid and electrolyte physiology and intestinal microbiology. Optimal care of the patient with SBS occurs in the home setting with family members operating as an integral part of the multidisciplinary health care team. Continuous reevaluation of the prognosis is essential, particularly during the phase of PN dependence. Nontransplant surgical and transplant options should be pursued when a relatively benign, self-limited outcome appears unlikely without them.

REFERENCES

15. Jeppesen PB, Mortensen PB. Colonic digestion and absorption of energy from carbohydrates and medium-chain fat in small bowel failure. J Parenter Enteral Nutr 1999;23:S101–S105.

35. Goulet O, Baglin-Gobet S, Talbotec C, et al. Outcome and long-term growth after extensive small bowel resection in the neonatal period: a survey of 87 children. Eur J Pediatr Surg 2005;15:95–101.

47. Spencer AU, Kovacevich D, McKinney-Barnett M, et al. Pediatric short-bowel syndrome: the cost of comprehensive care. Am J Clin Nutr 2008;88:1552–1559.

50. Bines J, Francis D, Hill D. Reducing parenteral requirement in children with short bowel syndrome: impact of an amino acid–based complete infant formula. J Pediatr Gastroenterol Nutr 1998;26:123–128.

106. Ching YA, Fitzgibbons S, Valim C, et al. Long-term nutritional and clinical outcomes after serial transverse enteroplasty at a single institution. J Pediatr Surg 2009;44:939–943.

116. Wales PW, de Silva N, Kim JH, et al. Neonatal short bowel syndrome: a cohort study. J Pediatr Surg 2005;40:755–762

See expertconsult.com for a complete list of references and the review questions for this chapter.

SMALL BOWEL TRANSPLANT

Hiroshi Sogawa • Kishore R. Iyer

Outcomes of intestinal transplant (Tx) have dramatically improved over the past decade. In experienced centers, patient survival exceeds 90% 1 year after intestinal Tx.[1,2] The improved outcome may be in equal parts because of technical advances, improved monitoring for opportunistic viral infections with measurement of levels of viral replication by polymerase chain reaction (PCR), and improvements in immunosuppression regimens, as well as a better understanding of histopathology. Thus, although data are lacking to make robust claims, we believe that current low rates of rejection may relate to dramatic improvements in immunosuppressive strategies with widespread adoption of antibody induction, but may also in part be due to greater reluctance to treat nonspecific histological abnormalities as rejection.

Parenteral nutrition (PN) remains a life-saving therapeutic option for patients with short bowel syndrome and in those with intestinal failure due to a variety of causes. Although PN prolongs life in patients with these conditions, it is sometimes complicated by life-threatening central venous catheter-related infections, loss of venous access sites, and liver disease that may progress to cirrhosis. For the subset of patients who have failed PN and are at an increased mortality risk from the frequency or severity of PN-related complications, intestinal Tx provides an alternative approach that is rapidly emerging as the standard of care.

HISTORY

Carrell[3] established the vascular basis for intestinal Tx more than 100 years ago. Lillehei et al.[4] carried out intestinal Tx studies in dogs, but success from an intestinal graft was not achieved until Starzl et al.,[5] in 1989, reported survival for 192 days in 1 of 2 children who received a multivisceral graft. Williams et al.[6] reported a similar outcome in the same year in 1 of 2 children; immunosuppression was based on cyclosporine and corticosteroids with low-dose irradiation of the graft in an attempt to induce graft lymphoid depletion. Death in both instances occurred from consequences of over-immunosuppression in the form of lymphoproliferative disease and sepsis. In 1988, Grant et al.[7] reported the first successful liver–small bowel Tx in a 41-year-old patient, who was discharged from the hospital 8 months after Tx on an unrestricted oral diet; the patient continued to do well for about 4 years. Immunosuppression was achieved using cyclosporine, prednisone, and azathioprine with antibody induction using OKT3. Between 1987 and 1995, Goulet et al.[8] reported on 9 intestinal transplants carried out in 7 children, with cyclosporine-based immunosuppression; 1 patient remains alive more than 16 years after her original Tx. These seminal cases paved the way for reports of improved results in multiple centers.[1,2,9-13]

INDICATIONS AND REFERRAL

Quigley[14] observed in 1996 that for the well-adapted patient who is stable on home PN, small intestinal Tx could not rival the established role of PN. The home PN registry data maintained by Howard and Malone[15] suggests that for long-term adult patients on home PN, 1- and 4-year survival rates are in the order of 94% and 80%, respectively. Spencer et al. reported 10-year survival on PN of 94.6% in a pediatric population with bilirubin less than 2.5 mg/dL.[16] Therefore, for the majority of patients with intestinal failure, an effective therapy in the form of PN is readily available. For intestinal Tx to become the first-line therapy for the patient with refractory intestinal failure, the results of Tx have to be better than those of long-term PN. Thus, the indications for intestinal Tx are simply stated as follows:
1. Presence of irreversible and permanent intestinal failure *and*
2. Presence or onset of life-threatening complications of PN.

The latter are mainly in the form of the onset of liver disease or central venous catheter-related complications such as recurrent or life-threatening sepsis and loss of venous access sites. Although there is general agreement that liver disease in the setting of intestinal failure and proven refractory PN dependence is a clear indication for intestinal Tx, indications related to venous access are more contentious. Development of metastatic infectious foci, such as infective endocarditis or recurring severe septic episodes resulting in multiple organ-system failure, in the individual patient constitute clear indications for intestinal Tx. The American Society of Transplantation, in a position paper, suggested that in infancy, referral for intestinal transplant is appropriate when two of the four available standard access sites, the right and left subclavian veins and right and left internal jugular veins, have been lost to thrombosis.[17] In the older child (and the adult patient), referral for intestinal Tx would probably be appropriate when three of the six available standard access sites – the right and left internal jugular, right and left subclavian, and right and left femoral veins – have been lost to thrombosis. Consideration must also be given to the inevitable wait for an appropriate donor organ, which, depending on size and blood type, can sometimes be many months, and across the United States carries a mortality risk on the order of 28%. It is true to state that "on the intestinal transplant waiting list" may be one of the riskiest places for a patient with intestinal failure to be.

Contraindications to Intestinal Transplant

The fundamental goal in intestinal transplantation must be the hope of a good quality of life in the long term. Contraindications to Tx of the intestine are similar to those for other solid organs (malignancy, severe systemic disease, etc.), but they may be even more absolute because of the considerable morbidity and mortality following this procedure. Thus, patients with multiple severe congenital anomalies, recent malignancy, or severe neurologic disability are not appropriate candidates for Tx. Multisystem autoimmune diseases and severe immune deficiencies also represent relative contraindications to intestinal Tx.

Recipient Evaluation and Selection

Recipient evaluation must be carried out by a multidisciplinary team, paying special attention to the following:
1. Irreversibility of intestinal failure and potential for intestinal salvage
2. Presence of liver disease and potential for reversibility
3. State of vascular access and remaining available sites
4. Psychosocial issues
5. Potential contraindications to Tx

The importance of a careful evaluation cannot be overemphasized. At Mount Sinai Medical Center in New York, this has led to alternative therapies (intestinal rehabilitation) in the majority of patients and in some cases has even allowed patients to be weaned off PN. In carefully selected patients, we have attempted intestinal salvage even in the face of advanced liver disease, using conservative, nontransplant surgical procedures such as longitudinal intestinal lengthening and tapering (Bianchi procedure), STEP (serial transverse enteroplasty), or other tapering procedures and aggressive repair of fistulas with attempts at recruitment of distal unused bowel. The encouraging results with multidisciplinary evaluation and management of these patients has led to establishment of Intestinal Rehabilitation Programs at our center and others, with the focus being on management of the disease state rather than viewing intestinal transplantation as an end in itself.[18] Unfortunately, for many patients, late referral, often with advanced liver disease or precarious venous access, is the most common reason for lack of alternatives to transplant, or the obligatory requirement for a combined liver-intestinal graft when an isolated intestinal graft may have sufficed if only the patient had been referred just a few months prior.

PRETRANSPLANT NUTRITIONAL MANAGEMENT

A thorough nutritional assessment is completed when patients are evaluated for transplantation. This includes current height, weight, head circumference, triceps skinfold thickness (TSF), and mid-arm circumference (MAC). Growth is evaluated, and a history of enteral feeding tolerance and oral intake is also assessed. In infants, it is important to try to provide oral intake of formula, infant foods, or other age-appropriate foods to allow normal feeding and swallowing development. At this time, if there are no contraindications such as gastrointestinal bleeding or excessive stool output, attempts are made to maximize enteral feedings and oral intake, especially in the face of minimal or no liver disease. The current PN prescription is assessed for appropriate calories, protein, lipid, vitamins, and minerals. Calorie and protein needs in the PN-dependent pediatric patient are normally less than the recommended daily allowance (RDA). Our experience has shown that these children may need as little as 70% of the RDA for calories to maintain weight. In contrast, during the adaptation phase, caloric provision to maintain growth has to take into account a potential malabsorption factor of 30 to 50%, due to rapid transit and diarrhea. Growth

may be difficult to accomplish in the sick child awaiting intestinal transplant; overfeeding through PN may contribute to the advancement of liver disease. Other factors that may contribute to PN-related cholestasis include the influence of lipid emulsions,[19,20] recurrent catheter sepsis, and bacterial overgrowth.[21] Steps to minimize the risk of liver disease include cycling PN, monitoring for cholelithiasis, and most importantly, maximizing enteral feedings while providing adequate nutrition for growth without overfeeding.[21] Blood levels of vitamins A, D, and E, zinc, carnitine, selenium, copper, and manganese are also measured at evaluation. Manganese and copper are excreted primarily by the liver. Therefore, patients with cholestatic liver disease may have a decreased need for these minerals.[20] Vitamin and mineral supplementation in total PN (TPN) is adjusted based on blood levels. Copper deficiency can result in pancytopenia. For this reason, copper is supplemented in the TPN according to blood levels and not routinely eliminated in patients with significant liver disease. The recent dramatic reports of the reversal of parenteral nutrition-associated cholestasis produced by substitution of soy-based lipid emulsions with fish-oil based emulsions (Omegaven, Fresenius, Germany) in growing numbers of children may be the basis for a paradigm shift in approach to the patient with parenteral nutrition-associated cholestasis.[22,23] If vitamin and mineral levels are within normal limits at evaluation, levels do not need to be checked again for 6 months. However, if levels are decreased or elevated and changes are made in the TPN, levels should be monitored in 1 to 2 months to ensure that the changes were appropriate. When the transplant evaluation is complete, nutritional recommendations are forwarded to the referring physicians. Patients are normally not seen by the nutritionist again until transplantation unless the patient's medical status changes and reevaluation is necessary. Variceal bleeding is not usually a feature of end-stage PN-associated liver disease in the setting of short bowel syndrome. Significant gastrointestinal bleeding particularly from mucocutaneous junctions at gastrostomies or jejunostomies can be a serious and sometimes life-threatening complication that is precipitated or worsened by attempts to push enteral feeding beyond tolerance in the face of significant portal hypertension. We have successfully used the transjugular intrahepatic portosystemic shunting (TIPS) procedure in a small number of children with refractory gastrointestinal bleeding to successfully bridge them to combined liver–small bowel Tx.

CHOICE OF ALLOGRAFT

Once a decision is made to list a patient for Tx, a careful evaluation allows for a rational choice of allograft. The results of isolated intestinal Tx seem to be superior to those obtained from Tx with the larger composite grafts.[24-28] These improved results may be even better when viewed on an "intent-to-transplant" basis, because of the significantly higher mortality on the waiting list for patients awaiting combined liver–small bowel or multivisceral grafts. Our own recent experience suggests that patients awaiting isolated intestinal grafts appear to have a much greater chance of receiving intestinal grafts even outside their own United Network for Organ Sharing (UNOS) region. This is likely because the liver from any potential deceased donor is allocated first to local recipients awaiting isolated liver transplantation and only subsequently to regional or national intestinal recipients, only when there are no potential local recipients. Because of the much greater numbers of liver recipients awaiting transplant, if the liver is allocated locally, then the intestine can no longer be allocated to patients requiring combined liver-intestine grafts and is allocated in sequence to the first isolated intestine candidate awaiting transplant.

In our experience, mild to moderate degrees of liver dysfunction with portal and even bridging fibrosis on a liver biopsy are not contraindications to Tx with an isolated small bowel graft, as opposed to a combined liver intestine allograft.[27,29] We have recently reported regression of liver fibrosis after successful isolated intestinal Tx.[30,31] More advanced degrees of liver dysfunction and the presence of cirrhosis or clinical stigmata of significant portal hypertension mandate a combined liver–small bowel allograft. In carefully selected patients with PN-associated end-stage liver disease, occasionally an isolated liver transplant may allow for intestinal adaptation to occur with eventual nutritional autonomy from PN.[32] It must be recognized that for this high-risk subset of patients undergoing isolated liver transplantation, a team experienced in transplantation and in the management of the short bowel syndrome is required.

From an immunologic standpoint, multivisceral or combined liver-intestine transplant may have an advantage over isolated intestinal transplantation. The Pittsburgh group has recently reported their observations that allografts that include the liver (liver-intestine or multivisceral) had a better chronic rejection-free graft survival compared to isolated intestinal transplant.[1] Additional long-term follow-up in larger numbers of patients is required before these conflicting observations can be fully understood and reconciled into meaningful clinical practice.

DONOR AND RECIPIENT OPERATIONS

Donor and recipient operations have been described in considerable detail elsewhere; highlights of the different procedures are described later[33-35] (Figures 37-1 and 37-2). Cadaveric

donors should be 50% to 60% of recipient weight, ABO blood group compatible, and hemodynamically stable. Thymoglobulin 1.5 mg/kg is given to the donor at the time of surgery to deplete the donor-derived lymphocytes as prophylaxis against the risk of graft-versus-host disease (GVHD).

In isolated intestinal transplants, the intestinal graft is separated from the donor pancreas just below the lower edge of the pancreas while preserving the first jejunal branch of the SMA. The graft receives arterial inflow through an anastomosis between the donor SMA and the infrarenal aorta. Venous drainage of the graft is accomplished by an anastomosis between the donor portal vein and the recipient's SMV at the inferior border of the pancreas or between the donor portal vein and the inferior vena cava. The latter is favored in the presence of liver dysfunction. The proximal donor jejunum is anastomosed to the recipient jejunum or duodenum. The donor distal ileum is connected to the recipient's colon with a loop ileostomy to provide access for endoscopic monitoring of the graft.

In principle, the composite multivisceral graft in the donor is conceptualized as a grape cluster, with a double stem consisting of the celiac axis and the SMA, from which individual grafts can be removed on their vascular pedicles as appropriate.[36,37] The technique of liver–small bowel transplantation developed by Langnas et al. avoids all hilar dissection.[34] The stomach and colon are excluded from the standard isolated intestinal grafts; inclusion of the stomach, in cases of gastric dysmotility, appears to be on an institutional basis. The duodenum just beyond the pylorus and the terminal ileum is transected between double rows of staples. A long segment of thoracic aorta is procured in continuity with the SMA and celiac trunk in cases of combined liver–small bowel grafts. On the back table, the celiac axis is dissected to the level of the splenic artery, which is ligated and divided. The donor aorta inferior to the origin of the SMA is oversewn. The pancreas is transected just to the right of the

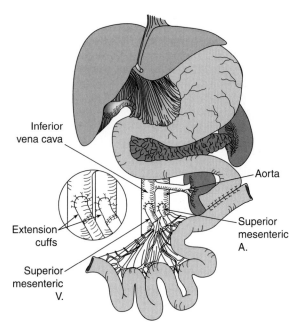

Figure 37-1. Isolated intestinal transplant: The donor SMA (superior mesenteric artery) is anastomosed to the recipient aorta. The donor SMV (superior mesenteric vein) is anastomosed to the recipient inferior vena cava. From Iyer K: Small bowel transplantation. In: Spitz L, Coran A, editors. Operative Pediatric Surgery, 6th ed. London: Hodder-Arnold; 2006 p. 1015–1023. Reproduced with permission.

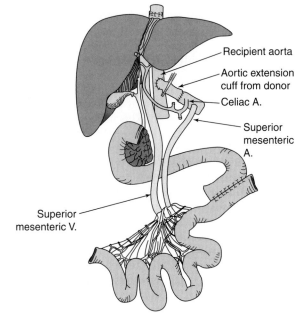

Figure 37-2. Combined liver and intestinal transplant: The donor aortic conduit was anastomosed to the recipient aorta. Only two vascular anastomosis (aortic and vena cava) are needed. Adapted from Iyer K: Small bowel transplantation. In: Spitz L, Coran A, editors. Operative Pediatric Surgery, 6th ed. London: Hodder-Arnold; 2006 p. 1015–1023. Reproduced with permission.

portal vein and its cut edge oversewn, allowing the bile duct to be preserved intact, though transection of the graft pancreas may be avoided in very small donors. Arterial inflow to the combined liver–small bowel graft is accomplished through anastomosis between the donor thoracic aorta and the recipient supraceliac aorta, and venous outflow is through a standard caval anastomosis, with a piggyback technique if size disparity between the donor and recipient cava requires it. A recipient portacaval or portoportal shunt allows for decompression of native remnant viscera, such as stomach and pancreas. Intestinal continuity is restored in nearly all cases with a loop ileostomy to allow access for endoscopy and graft biopsy.

POSTOPERATIVE MANAGEMENT

Intestinal transplant recipients need high levels of immunosuppression to prevent rejection. Tacrolimus (Prograf, FK 506, Astellas Pharma US, Inc, Deerfield, IL), in addition to corticosteroids, is one of the primary immunosuppressants used by most transplant centers. Tacrolimus is a macrolide antibiotic derived from the fungus *Streptomyces tsukubaensis* and acts by inhibiting calcineurin through an FK-binding protein (FKBP-12)-FK506 complex. This calcineurin inhibition indirectly blocks the cytokine driven proliferation of cytotoxic T-cells and interleukin (IL)-2 synthesis. In vitro, it is approximately 100-fold more potent than cyclosporine.[31] Corticosteroids inhibit the expression of IL-1, IL-2, IL-3, IL-6, interferon, and tumor necrosis factor (TNF). Through this inhibition, all stages of T-cell activation are suppressed. Sirolimus (Rapamune, Wyeth-Ayerst Laboratories, Philadelphia, PA), from the fungus *Streptomyces hygroscopicus*, is a target of rapamycin (TOR) inhibitor, that is used in some centers as maintenance therapy in addition to corticosteroids and allows use of a reduced dose of tacrolimus, particularly in patients with renal dysfunction. Sirolimus binds to FKBP-12, and the sirolimus-FKBP-12-complex does not inhibit calcineurin, but rather inhibits TOR, leading to a reduction in cytokine-dependent cellular proliferation.[38] Basiliximab (Simulect; Novartis Pharmaceutical, Eastover, NJ) and daclizumab (Zenapax; Roche U.S. Pharmaceuticals, Nutley, NJ) are both monoclonal antibody IL-2 receptor antagonists that inhibit proliferation of activated T cells.[38] These agents are being used more frequently in immunosuppressive protocols to offer increased immunosuppression without the adverse effects of the high-dose standard therapy. At our institution, tacrolimus, corticosteroids, and basiliximab are used for primary immunosuppression. Tacrolimus is started orally within 12 to 24 hours after surgery. Intravenous tacrolimus is avoided unless therapeutic trough concentrations cannot be maintained with oral therapy. In our practice, this has never been required, though some centers favor use of intravenous tacrolimus in the early postoperative period. Trough concentrations are maintained between 20 and 30 ng/mL for the first month, followed by 15 to 20 ng/mL for months 1 to 3, 12 to 18 ng/mL for months 3 to 6, 10 to 15 ng/mL for months 6 to 12, and 8 to 10 ng/mL thereafter. These concentrations are modified based on patient-specific criteria such as rejection episodes, infections, or other adverse effects the patient may be experiencing. Most patients will achieve these concentrations while being dosed twice daily; however, in some patients, three times a day dosing may be necessary because of increased metabolism or decreased absorption. When enteral feedings are started, tacrolimus doses will often need to be increased. Although Murray et al.[39] demonstrated

no difference in absorption when tacrolimus was administered with Osmolite (Ross Products Division, Abbott Laboratories, Columbus, OH) nutritional feedings, we have frequently observed decreased levels of tacrolimus in our patients when enteral feedings are started.[39] This observation has been regardless of the type of feedings used. Corticosteroids are quickly tapered over 7 days to 1 mg/kg/day, then tapered further to 0.25 mg/kg/day by 3 months. Basiliximab is administered as an intravenous (IV) infusion of 10 mg for patients weighing less than 35 kg or 20 mg for patients above 35 kg, twice (pre-reperfusion and post-reperfusion if blood loss is significant) on the day of surgery (day 0) and again on postoperative day 4. One of the major side effects of tacrolimus is nephrotoxicity, and it is common to see some degree of this in all patients after intestinal transplant. Tacrolimus causes vasoconstriction in the afferent arterioles of the glomeruli.[38] This decreased blood flow is dose dependent and, initially, reversible. Dose reduction and addition of other immunosuppressants, such as sirolimus, may help decrease nephrotoxicity while maintaining adequate immunosuppression. When possible, concurrent use of other nephrotoxic agents should be avoided. Electrolyte abnormalities may be caused by absorption problems or nephrotoxicity, or may be drug induced. Tacrolimus has been shown to cause hyperkalemia and hypomagnesemia.[40] Potassium intake must be monitored closely, and excess potassium in parenteral and enteral nutrition should be avoided. Potassium-sparing diuretics, and other medications causing hyperkalemia, including angiotensin-converting enzyme (ACE) inhibitors, should be used with caution. Tacrolimus also leads to magnesium loss, which frequently needs correction with supplemental magnesium therapy.[41] Oral magnesium may lead to increased ostomy output; therefore, magnesium replacement in the PN or through intravenous boluses should be tried first.

Although hypertension in transplant recipients may be multifactorial, immunosuppression may be the major offender. Tacrolimus causes renal vasoconstriction, and corticosteroid administration may lead to fluid retention, both of which can cause high blood pressure. If fluid retention is the cause, diuretics are the first line of therapy. If a patient is not fluid overloaded, a dihydropyridine calcium channel blocker, such as amlodipine, is started. Calcium channel blockers decrease the arterial vasoconstriction caused by tacrolimus. Amlodipine has less effect on tacrolimus concentrations than nondihydropyridine calcium channel blockers, such as verapamil. Other medications that may be added include beta-blockers, clonidine, and ACE inhibitors. Tacrolimus, cyclosporine, and corticosteroids can cause hyperglycemia, and it is not uncommon for intestinal transplant recipients to receive insulin during the initial postoperative period. As corticosteroids are tapered to maintenance doses, most patients will not need further treatment. If hyperglycemia persists, dietary and lifestyle modifications, exercise, and insulin or oral hypoglycemic medications may need to be added. Corticosteroids, cyclosporine, and sirolimus are immunosuppressants that have profound effects on serum lipid levels. Patients who are receiving lipid emulsion with their PN or other medications, such as propofol, diuretics, or beta-blockers, are also at risk for hyperlipidemia. If patient serum triglyceride levels are between 250 and 350 mg/dL, lipids in their PN are decreased. At levels above 350 mg/dL, Intralipid (Clinter, Deerfield, IL) is discontinued. When levels fall below 200 mg/dL, lipids are restarted at a lower rate. If a patient does have increased serum lipid levels, lipids should be discontinued, and the patient's medication profile should be reexamined. Offending agents should be reduced or discontinued if possible.

Even with higher levels of immunosuppression, rejection is still common in intestinal transplant recipients. Historically, 70% to 90% of recipients experienced at least one rejection episode.[42,43] With the use of various forms of antibody induction, the incidence of rejection has decreased to less than 25 to 30%.[1,44,45] Rejection episodes are initially treated with a 2- to 3-day intravenous methylprednisolone bolus of 10 to 20 mg/kg per day. If a rejection episode does not respond to corticosteroids, antibody therapy consisting of anti-thymocyte globulin (Thymoglobulin; Sangstat Medical Corp, Fremont, CA) is initiated.

The quest for noninvasive tests such as blood citrulline, granzyme B, and perforin to diagnose acute rejection in intestinal transplant recipients remains in preclinical trials.[46] At the present time, it is our practice to carry out protocol surveillance intestinal biopsies at day 5 to 7, followed by weekly biopsies until week 6, and then as indicated. Indications for biopsies are often nonspecific and include unexplained fever, change in stoma output or appearance, and gastrointestinal bleeding. It seems that the gross appearance of the mucosa does not correlate with histologic appearances.[47] Although there is a lack of clear endoscopic criteria for diagnosis of rejection, endoscopy (Figure 37-3A) with biopsy remains the gold standard for diagnosis of rejection in intestinal allografts. Acute rejection of an intestinal allograft is characterized by a varying combination of findings and an increase in crypt cell apoptosis on biopsy[48] (Figure 37-3B). Although crypt cell apoptosis is not a specific or absolute finding, it represents a distinctive feature of acute cellular rejection even when other changes are minimal. Chronic rejection is characterized by vasculopathy (Figure 37-3C), with intimal thickening affecting the medium-sized vessels; unfortunately, mucosal changes in the presence of chronic rejection are nonspecific or may even be absent, making the diagnosis very difficult.

Infectious complications are very common after intestinal transplantation. There is a high incidence of bacterial, viral, and fungal infections because of high levels of immunosuppression, multiple invasive procedures, and perhaps bacterial translocation. The most common pathogens include enterococci, enteric gram-negative rods, *Pseudomonas* spp., staphylococci, *Candida albicans*, Epstein-Barr virus (EBV), and cytomegalovirus (CMV).[49]

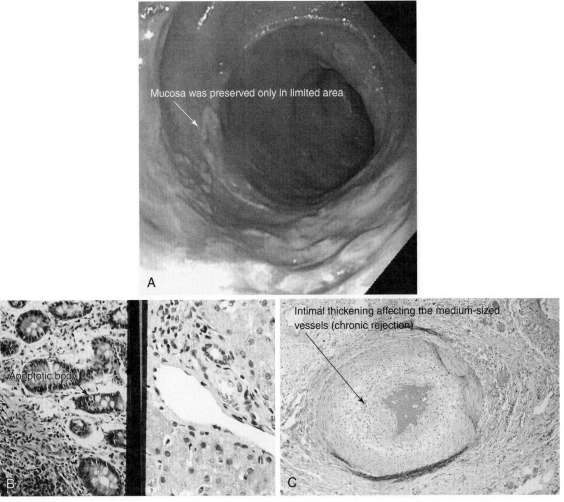

Figure 37-3. (**A**) Endoscopic picture of severe acute rejection of the intestinal allograft with extensive loss of intestinal mucosa. (**B**) Photomicrograph of an H&E-stained section of a mucosal biopsy from an intestinal allograft. Acute cellular rejection is objectively defined as more than six apoptotic cells per 10 consecutive crypts with accompanying enterocyte injury, characterized by mucin depletion, cytoplasmic basophilia, and nuclear hyperchromasia. (**C**) Although not as well defined as acute cellular rejection, this photomicrograph of an H&E-stained section demonstrates obliterative arteriopathy that is characteristic of chronic allograft rejection. These vascular changes are usually only encountered at the time of explant. *(See plate section for color.)*

Prophylactic broad-spectrum antibiotics with gram-negative and anaerobic coverage are administered for the first week after Tx. Ganciclovir, followed by valganciclovir, is administered to prevent viral infections, specifically cytomegalovirus, herpes simplex virus, and EBV. Prophylactic antifungal therapy is also routinely used at our center for 2 weeks postoperatively. In addition, trimethoprim/sulfamethoxazole is given three times weekly for *Pneumocystis jirovecii*, formerly known as *Pneumocystis carinii*, pneumonia prophylaxis for the life of the allograft.

POSTTRANSPLANT NUTRITIONAL MANAGEMENT

Short- and long-term nutritional goals for the pediatric patient after intestinal transplant are as follows:

1. Autonomy from parenteral nutrition
2. Discontinuation of intravenous replacement fluids
3. Eventual removal of the central venous catheter
4. Transition to oral feedings and discontinuation of tube feedings
5. Appropriate long-term growth

Patients are given intravenous fluids for the first 24 hours after intestinal transplant because of fluid shifts and electrolyte imbalances. Pediatric intestinal transplant patients, especially those with respiratory or renal impairment before or after transplant, are very sensitive to fluid status changes. Adequate fluid intake is important to maintain satisfactory perfusion of the new graft and to replace gastric and ileostomy losses. For these reasons, daily monitoring of weights, intake and output, and electrolytes is crucial. Ventilated patients must be monitored closely for the effects of fluid on respiratory status.

Once fluid and electrolyte status have stabilized, PN is initiated 24 to 48 hours after transplant and adjusted according to electrolytes and fluid status. Calorie and protein requirements vary depending on ventilation status, sepsis, wound healing, fevers, and nutritional status. Requirements are calculated using actual body weight unless the patient is severely under- or overweight at transplant. Ventilated, sedated patients who are well nourished before transplant may need only 70% to 80% of the RDA for calories if there are no complications such as fever or open abdominal wounds. However, patients who are septic or malnourished before transplant or after extubation may need up to 120% of RDA for calories. Protein is normally provided at 2 to 2.5 g/kg per day. Patients with renal disease may be restricted to 1 g/kg per day. Elevated tacrolimus levels may affect kidney function, as discussed earlier, resulting in fluid and electrolyte imbalances. Hyperglycemia, hypertriglyceridemia, or fluid restriction can contribute to the inadequate provision of calories and protein during the immediate postoperative period.

Continuous tube feedings are initiated when there is evidence of bowel function with ileostomy output, usually 5 to 7 days after transplant. We use a low-fat, low-osmolarity, elemental formula for the first 4 to 6 weeks after transplant. Other centers have reported acceptable stool outputs with high medium-chain triglyceride (MCT), peptide-based formulas.[50] Tube feedings are initiated at 5 mL/h and increased by 5 or 10 mL/h daily based on ileostomy output, electrolytes, and clinical status. Fat malabsorption is common after intestinal transplant. The use of pancreatic enzymes has been reported to decrease stomal outputs and increase weight gain in the posttransplant period. It is not uncommon for Tx patients to have poor gastric motility in the months after transplant. Prokinetic agents can be used to assist gastric emptying. Jejunal tube feedings are often required for a few weeks or months, with transition to gastric feedings when gastric motility improves. Percutaneously placed gastric or gastrojejunal feeding tubes are appropriate for this patient population because of the long duration of tube feedings after transplant. Ideally, stool output should be <30 mL/kg/day after transplant. Stomal outputs >50 mL/kg/day are considered excessive, and antidiarrheal agents or dietary fiber may be initiated to increase intestinal transit time. Depending on fluid status, stool output in excess of 30 to 50 mL/kg/day is replaced with an IV solution such as 0.45% saline, to maintain hydration. Bicarbonate and other electrolytes such as magnesium are often added based on serum electrolyte values.

Most often, patients are placed on a dilute enteral formula to provide adequate enteral hydration because of high fluid losses from the ileostomy. Formulas are normally diluted to between one-half and three-fourths strength with free water, depending on fluid requirements. Patients may need up to 150 mL/kg/day of enteral fluid to maintain hydration and discontinue intravenous replacement fluids. A small number of patients will continue to have large fluid losses from their ostomy in the absence of viral infection or rejection. For these patients, recruitment of the colon with stoma closure may be required before replacement fluids can be discontinued.

Discontinuation of fluid replacement and removal of the central venous catheter is an important milestone after intestinal transplantation, because of the morbidity and mortality associated with central line infections. Patients are transitioned to an age-appropriate, fiber-containing, intact protein formula approximately 4 to 6 weeks after transplant. However, if there is a history of milk or soy protein intolerance, or stool output increases with the transition, an elemental formula with appropriate fat content will be used for an extended period of time. Parenteral nutrition is discontinued when 100% of nutritional needs are met enterally. A multivitamin appropriate for age is started when TPN is discontinued. Oral intake is initiated when tube feedings are well established, 10 to 14 days after transplant. Infants and children who have been PN dependent since infancy present a unique challenge for therapists when attempting to introduce oral intake because of severe oral aversions the child may have acquired from past experiences. In view of this, no dietary restrictions (other than avoiding foods and beverages high in simple sugars and caffeine) are recommended to encourage oral intake. For patients who have the desire to eat a significant amount of food after transplant, a low-lactose and low-fat diet is followed for the first 4 to 6 weeks after transplant. A diet low in concentrated sweets is continued indefinitely to avoid osmotic diarrhea. During times of increased stool output caused by viral infection or rejection, patients may need to avoid lactose and milk protein because in our experience these foods can increase stool output. Food allergies, especially to milk protein, are not uncommon. Once patients have been stable without TPN for a period of a few weeks, transition to bolus feedings or nocturnal drip can begin with an increased focus on oral intake.

NURSING IMPLICATIONS

Children transplanted for short gut syndrome provide some of the most complex and challenging situations for the nursing staff in the postoperative period. Not only are nurses expected to monitor issues surrounding routine postoperative care, but issues such as immunosuppression, rejection, increased risk of infection, nutrition and dehydration, family education, and social issues must also be addressed. Immediately after transplantation, organ system assessments must be made quickly and accurately. Assessments include respiratory status, oxygenation and ventilation, cardiovascular status, renal function, fluid and electrolyte balance, surgical dressings and drains, bleeding, pain management, and medication administration. Many short gut patients have low albumin levels before transplantation because of related liver dysfunction and increased enteral losses. Large volumes of fluids are often administered intraoperatively to maintain stability of blood pressure. This, in combination with the high prevalence of hypoalbuminemia, leads to fluid shifts from intravascular spaces to interstitial spaces, which may involve the lungs. A delicate balance between fluids is needed to maintain blood pressure, and administration of diuretics to reduce fluid overload may be required. Blood pressure, weight, intake and outputs (urinary, nasogastric, ostomy, dressings, and drains), and laboratory values should be monitored closely.[51]

Cardiac complications may include hypovolemia and hypertension. Postoperative bleeding may cause hypovolemia. Immunosuppressive medications may produce a drug-induced hypertension. This is usually dose-related. Oral antihypertensive agents are most commonly used to control hypertension, but occasionally short-acting intravenous medications may be needed. Urine output in the pediatric population should be maintained at or above 1 mL/kg/hr. Decreased output may be caused by decreased intravascular volume or an alteration in kidney function. Renal laboratory values and medication levels should be routinely monitored. Surgical wounds that require attention include the transplant incision, the ileostomy site, central line sites, surgical drains, and arterial lines. The surgical incision may be stapled closed or, more often, left open for secondary closure. Accurate marking and monitoring of surgical dressings for bleeding is important with changes reported immediately to the surgeon. Surgical drains should be monitored for changes in color or amount of drainage. Drainage should usually be serosanguineous; changes to frank blood or bilious drainage should be reported to the surgeon immediately. Intravenous analgesic medications are generally discontinued around the second or third postoperative day, and the use of acetaminophen suspension usually provides adequate control of incision discomfort.[52] Infectious complications pose a significant problem postoperatively for any solid organ transplant recipient because of the use of immunosuppressive medications to control rejection. Any fever above 38° C needs to be brought to the attention of the physician. Blood cultures, wound cultures, urine cultures, chest x-ray, and stool cultures may be done as indicated by each episode of fever. As enteral feedings are slowly advanced and parenteral nutrition is weaned, monitoring of fluid status and electrolyte balance becomes even more challenging. Working closely with the dietitian and physician, the nurse must be vigilant for early signs of dehydration. Maintenance of hydration is paramount because an episode of severe dehydration can lead to loss of the graft, perhaps because of an as-yet-unexplained loss of autoregulation of splanchnic blood flow. The nurse caring for the transplant patient must be familiar with the side effects of the various immunosuppressive agents and report adverse events to the physician. Organ rejection is a frightening experience for patients and families. Careful explanation of the immune system and how immunosuppressive medications work is needed for families.

Clinical Transplant Nurse Coordinator

Although the clinical transplant nurse coordinator is not directly at the bedside, it is that person's responsibility to educate the patient and family about the transplant process from evaluation through transplantation and on through the period of outpatient care. The nurse coordinator focuses heavily on reinforcement of information given by other members of the transplant team. Answering any questions that arise from the family and assisting in finding practicable solutions to ongoing concerns are major priorities of the coordinator. Continued follow-up of transplant patients in the long term is also monitored by the nurse coordinator through routine laboratory testing and frequent telephone conversations with families. The nurse coordinator also works closely with social services to assess psychosocial issues that arise and to coordinate appropriate referrals to address any areas of concern. Major issues that repeatedly arise with these patients are emotional support, spiritual support, financial issues, and role changes. Many families face the reality of death of their child before and after transplant, and emotional support through family, friends, religious organization, and medical staff is vital. Families are often separated by long distances from their support systems. Families may be separated with one parent present with the child and the other parent at home working. Siblings may be present or may remain at home with other family members. Loss of income because of one parent continually being with the patient can cause great financial burdens on the families. Many families feel isolated, scared, and totally out of control of their lives as they work through the transplant process. It is the responsibility of the nurse coordinator to ensure that these concerns are addressed early before reaching crisis levels and that the transplant team is aware of and sensitive to these peripheral, nevertheless important issues.

OUTCOMES

According to U.S. Organ Procurement and Transplantation Network (OPTN) Scientific Registry of Transplant Recipients (SRTR) data in 2005, the 1-year patient- and graft-survival figures are 81% and 73%, respectively, for intestine alone; 76% and 75%, respectively, for small bowel–liver grafts.[11] Five-year survival was 54% for intestine alone. Those survival figures have improved remarkably between 1997 and 2005.[11] Despite the apparent immunologic advantage conferred by simultaneous liver grafting at the time of small bowel transplantation, isolated intestinal Tx seems to provide better patient survival and graft function at all follow-up,[25,28,53,54] although the Pittsburgh group reported a better chronic rejection-free graft survival in multivisceral or combined liver-intestinal transplant.[1] An important observation was the finding that programs that had performed at least 10 intestinal Tx had better patient and graft survival than programs that had performed fewer than 10 procedures.[42] In experienced centers, 1-year patient survival appears to exceed 90% from various reports.[1,2,45,54]

Retransplantation had been considered to have poor results until recently. Recent reports suggest that retransplantation can be achieved with reasonably good 5-year survival (47%) in multivisceral or combined liver-intestinal transplantation.[1] Our own experience suggests good outcomes with intestinal retransplantation, admittedly with a clear trend, predictably, toward increased length of stay following transplant.

Figures from the Intestinal Transplant Registry suggest that of 126 survivors of intestinal Tx, 95 (77%) were weaned from PN, 17 (14%) required partial PN, 4 (3%) were receiving PN with their graft intact, and 8 (6%) were receiving PN after removal of their graft.[42] In our experience, the median time to weaning PN was just over 1 month. Oral zinc supplementation is often required until ostomy takedown. Normally 10 to 20 mg/d of oral zinc is provided in addition to the oral multivitamin. Levels are monitored quarterly and doses adjusted accordingly.

Children may not grow well in the first 2 years after intestinal transplant.[55] This may be because of multiple factors including high doses of corticosteroids used to prevent or treat rejection. Also, acute complications such as viral infections and sepsis requiring recurrent hospitalization are more common in the first 2 years after transplant. This may have a deleterious effect on growth. In the absence of growth hormone deficiency or chronic rejection, patients seem to experience some degree of catch-up growth by about 5 years after transplantation.[55,56] Of pediatric patients 5 years posttransplant, 85% meet all of their nutritional needs orally. The remaining patients need supplemental tube feedings. Seventy-eight percent of patients have albumin levels above 3.6 g/dL. All patients 5 years posttransplant have discontinued PN and replacement fluids. Quality of life after intestinal Tx has been examined.[57-59] The data suggest a quality of life very similar to that of patients receiving long-term home PN and a trend toward improvement in this parameter over time as anxiety over allograft function decreases. The group from Nebraska showed that pediatric intestinal transplant recipients report a quality of life that was similar to normal school children and one that was overall better than children with other chronic diseases. Interestingly, the parents of intestinal transplant recipients report significant limitations, primarily in the domain of physical well-being of their children, compared with normal school children. The reasons for this apparent discrepancy between the children's perceptions and that of their parents acting as proxy is unclear and merits further study.[59]

Complications

Registry figures for the incidence of acute rejection after intestinal Tx remain high: 57% for intestine transplant alone, 39% for liver and intestine, and 48% for multivisceral transplants.[42,60] Immunosuppression was based on tacrolimus in 90% of these cases.[12] Registry data support other observations that simultaneous liver grafting may reduce the risk of intestinal graft rejection.[7,42,61] Despite this apparent immunological advantage, isolated intestinal grafts perform better at all follow-up times.[53] With the use of various induction agents such as basiliximab (an anti-IL-2 antibody), alemtuzumab (an anti-CD52 antibody), or anti-thymocyte globulin, a marked reduction in the incidence of acute rejection and in the severity of the rejection episodes was observed.[2,44,62,63]

There has been a predictable decrease in the incidence of infectious complications, particularly fungal and viral infections paralleling the use of antibody induction regimens, because of the reduced need to treat episodes of rejection with augmented immunosuppression. Infectious complications are frequent after Tx and are the major source of morbidity and

mortality after the procedure. Bacterial infections are almost ubiquitous, occurring in more than 90% of cases after Tx. Bacteremia is frequently related to intraperitoneal infection, central venous catheter, or pulmonary sepsis. Fungal infections occur in about 25% of cases. Registry data for CMV disease indicates **infection in 24% of patients** for isolated intestinal grafts, 18% for liver-intestinal grafts, and 40% for multivisceral grafts.[7] Risk factors for CMV infections include transplantation from CMV-positive donors to CMV-negative recipients, increased tacrolimus levels, and increased numbers of corticosteroid boluses to treat acute rejection episodes.[64,65] Adenovirus was isolated in 44 of 117 patients after Tx at Nebraska; the exact significance remains unclear because of the natural prevalence of the virus in the pediatric population. The bowel was the primary site of isolation in the majority of patients; isolation of the virus was occasionally associated with nonspecific enteritis that was usually self-limiting and did not seem to need specific treatment. Adenovirus and calicivirus[66] might cause severe infection in the transplanted bowel. Three of four patients in whom the virus was isolated from bronchoalveolar lavage died from a severe pneumonitis, which in the absence of other isolates was deemed to be adenoviral in etiology. All four were treated with reduced immunosuppression, and one patient, who eventually died, additionally received IV ribavirin.[5] We have recently experienced a case of severe adenoviral enteritis that caused recurrent intestinal perforations and refractory enterocutaneous fistulas. The patient was successfully treated with intravenous cidofovir and withdrawal of immunosuppression. This patient is alive over a year after transplant with full graft function.

The incidence of GVHD would be expected to be high in an allograft with a large lymphocyte mass such as the gut. Our own experience indicates that the complication is rare; Reyes et al.[53] reported an incidence of 7%. Histopathological criteria for diagnosis include keratinocyte necrosis in biopsies of skin lesions, epithelial apoptosis of native gastrointestinal tract, or necrosis of oral mucosa. Immunohistochemical demonstration of donor cell infiltration into the lesions is required for confirmation.

Figures from the International Intestinal Transplant Registry for the incidence of posttransplantation lymphoproliferative disease (PTLD) are 7% for intestinal grafts, 11% for liver–small bowel grafts, and 13% for multivisceral grafts. The Pittsburgh group reported PTLD in 13% (52/395) of patients recently.[67] Risk factors for the development of PTLD include the number of rejection episodes, use of the monoclonal antibody OKT3, splenectomy, and younger age.[53] Use of a low-dose chemotherapy regimen may be sufficient to control disseminated PTLD without excessive side effects. Rebound rejection remains a significant contributor to morbidity and even mortality.[68,69] The exact implications of early detection of EBV infection by quantitative PCR remain to be defined. Surgical complications in the form of anastomotic leaks and intestinal perforations occur frequently; the latter are sometimes precipitated by endoscopic biopsies. Chylous ascites may be seen occasionally and treated with low-fat formula and PN. Another significant source of morbidity and even mortality seems to be sudden ischemic necrosis of the graft in the setting of a nonspecific diarrheal illness with attendant dehydration and hypovolemia. This catastrophic complication is frequently heralded by the appearance of pneumatosis intestinalis and sepsis. It is unclear if the process represents "necrotizing enterocolitis" in the graft as has been described[70] or, in late cases, may simply be a consequence of failed autoregulation of splanchnic blood flow in a vulnerable graft that is undergoing hitherto-unrecognized chronic rejection.

Chronic rejection was reported in 15% of intestinal transplant patients in Pittsburgh.[1] Most patients with chronic rejection present with diarrhea or chronic abdominal cramps, but the symptoms of rejection can be subtle. A high index of suspicion is needed to diagnose chronic rejection, but very frequently histology obtained from an endoscopic biopsy may fail to reveal chronic rejection, and a full-thickness intestinal biopsy obtained in the operating room is required. If suspicion for chronic rejection is high and the patient is a potential retransplant candidate, exploratory laparotomy with possible graft enterectomy can be justified after detailed discussion of risks and benefits with the patient and family. No effective treatment for chronic rejection has been reported except for retransplantation.

FUTURE PROSPECTS

Because patient survival has improved at 1 and 5 years,[1,2,71] long-term management and chronic allograft enteropathy are the biggest challenges to solve.[72] With the increased frequency of retransplantation, at least in the larger centers, attention needs to be focused on improving outcomes in these very challenging patients. Concern has been expressed that isolated small bowel transplants as opposed to the liver–small bowel transplants would carry a much higher rate of graft loss from chronic rejection.[1,73] In any event, it is clear that late graft loss caused by chronic rejection is a frustrating issue that needs to be addressed with newer immunosuppressive strategies or immune-tolerance induction protocols.[74,75] The choice of appropriate allograft will continue to have an important bearing on outcome while remaining an issue for debate.[28] We believe that "less is better" in the context of transplantation for intestinal failure. We have shown that improved results are obtainable with isolated intestinal transplantation even in the face of moderate degrees of liver dysfunction.[27] It would seem that a functioning intestinal allograft is capable of reversing mild to moderate degrees of PN-associated liver dysfunction.[30,31] Likewise, in select patients who have a history of some enteral tolerance with loss of enteral tolerance coinciding with development of liver disease, an isolated liver allograft may be capable of salvaging the short bowel from permanent "failure."[32] We continue to have philosophical concerns regarding living-related intestinal Tx. The technical feasibility of the procedure has been clearly established. We believe that recipient outcomes will need to improve considerably before the procedure can be applied more liberally.[76,77] With the advent of emerging immunosuppressive strategies, results of intestinal Tx may continue to improve. Intestinal Tx is here to stay, and the day may not be far when Tx may replace PN as the standard of care for the patient with intestinal failure – the day may indeed not be far.

REFERENCES

1. Abu-Elmagd KM, Costa G, Bond GJ, et al. Five Hundred Intestinal and Multivisceral Transplantations at a Single Center: major Advances With New Challenges. Ann Surg 2009;250:567–581.
12. Grant D, Abu-Elmagd K, Reyes J, et al. 2003 report of the Intestine Transplant Registry: a new era has dawned. Ann Surg 2005;241:607–613.
23. Puder M, Valim C, Meisel JA, et al. Parenteral fish oil improves outcomes in patients with parenteral nutrition-associated liver injury. Ann Surg 2009;250:395–402.
30. Fiel MI, Wu HS, Iyer K, et al. Rapid reversal of parenteral-nutrition-associated cirrhosis following isolated intestinal transplantation. J Gastrointest Surg 2009;13:1717–1723.
44. Abu-Elmagd KM, Costa G, Bond GJ, et al. Evolution of the immunosuppressive strategies for the intestinal and multivisceral recipients with special reference to allograft immunity and achievement of partial tolerance. Transpl Int 2009;22:96–109.
45. Mazariegos GV, Soltys K, Bond G, et al. Pediatric intestinal retransplantation: techniques, management, and outcomes. Transplantation 2008;86:1777–1782.
54. Fishbein TM, Kaufman SS, Florman SS, et al. Isolated intestinal transplantation: proof of clinical efficacy. Transplantation 2003;76:636–640.

See expertconsult.com for a complete list of references and the review questions for this chapter.

ALLERGIC AND EOSINOPHILIC GASTROINTESTINAL DISEASE

38

Jonathan E. Markowitz • Chris A. Liacouras

Gastrointestinal disorders involving an accumulation of eosinophils include a variety of conditions including classic IgE-mediated food allergy, inflammatory bowel disease, gastroesophageal reflux, and the primary eosinophilic gastrointestinal disorders (eosinophilic esophagitis, eosinophilic gastroenteritis, and eosinophilic colitis). The goal of this chapter is to provide an overview of those conditions that are characterized by an eosinophilic infiltration in the gastrointestinal (GI) tract and are largely driven by food-specific antigens. Food hypersensitivity is briefly reviewed; the majority of the discussion focuses on the primary eosinophilic GI disorders.

FOOD ALLERGY OR HYPERSENSITIVITY

Type I (IgE-mediated) immediate hypersensitivity reactions to foods are most common in young children, with 50% of these reactions occurring in the first year of life. The majority are reactions to cow's milk or to soy protein from infant formulas.[1] Other food allergies begin to predominate in older children, including egg, fish, peanut, and wheat. Together with milk and soy, these account for more than 90% of food allergy in children.[2]

Blinded food challenges have shown that symptoms referable to the GI tract in IgE-mediated allergy typically begin within minutes of the ingestion, although occasionally may be delayed for up to 2 hours. They tend to be short-lived, lasting 1 to 2 hours.[3,4] Symptoms include nausea, vomiting, abdominal pain, and diarrhea; they may also include oral symptoms, skin manifestations, wheezing, or airway edema.

Anaphylactic reactions to food ingestion are life-threatening. For the purpose of this discussion, the term *anaphylaxis* is limited to those IgE-mediated reactions causing upper airway obstruction, hypotension, and circulatory collapse. Although any protein may be implicated, certain foods have a propensity to cause severe reactions in susceptible persons: cow's milk, egg, peanut, and shellfish. The altering of food protein antigens through cooking or prior hydrolysis does not preclude a type I allergic reaction because some proteins are relatively resistant to denaturation.

Meanwhile, the oral allergy syndrome (OAS) is another IgE-mediated allergy, where the reaction is typically oral itching or tingling. Occasionally, facial or throat swelling may occur as well; it is unclear whether OAS causes other GI symptoms such as pain and diarrhea. With IgE-mediated food allergy, the rapid onset of GI symptoms after food ingestion correlates highly with positive IgE-RAST or skin prick tests to the offending antigen, demonstrating that these reactions are related to typical type-I hypersensitivity.[4] On the other hand, in patients with OAS, symptoms relate to cross reaction between similar epitopes on certain pollens and certain fruits and vegetables.[5]

Patients with a history of a significant reaction to one or more foods should be tested by skin prick against those foods and against a limited battery of common food allergens (milk, soy, egg, peanut, fish, wheat). Skin testing has a sensitivity of 90% to 100% depending on the antigen, so patients with negative skin testing are very unlikely to have IgE-mediated disease and should be challenged openly with the food in question. Non-IgE-mediated hypersensitivity may still cause symptoms on challenge, but these may be delayed for hours or days. IgE-RAST testing for specific foods does not have greater positive or negative predictive value than skin prick testing, and combining the two does not improve the diagnostic yield.[6] The specificity of skin prick testing for food allergies ranges from 40 to 80%, which implies that the possibility of a false positive skin test is not inconsequential.[7] Therefore, the use of skin testing in the evaluation of food allergy should be limited to cases where there is a high clinical suspicion of allergies as the etiology of symptoms, which increases the positive predictive value of the test.

If IgE-RAST or skin prick tests are positive, the food should be avoided for at least 3 weeks; if symptoms improve, the elimination diet should be continued. If there is no improvement, then open or single-blind challenges with the food can be given to try to elicit a response. These challenges should be performed in a setting in which access to emergency treatment of allergic reactions is available, and this is generally best handled by an allergist.

Positive challenges should lead to consultation with a dietitian to educate the patient and family concerning avoidance of the food and to ensure that adequate nutrition is maintained. Groups such as the Food Allergy and Anaphylaxis Network and the American Partnership for Eosinophilic Disorders provide support and educational materials for families. Patients with a history of serious reactions to foods should be provided with an epinephrine kit for home use, proper instruction on how the device is used, and a medical alert bracelet.

EOSINOPHILIC GASTROENTEROPATHIES

The eosinophilic gastroenteropathies are an interesting yet somewhat poorly defined set of disorders that must include the infiltration of at least one layer of the GI tract with eosinophils, in the absence of other known causes for eosinophilia (e.g., parasitic infections or drug reactions).[8,9] Peripheral eosinophilia is not required for diagnosis, although it is a frequent finding.

395

TABLE 38-1. Typical Number of Gastrointestinal Mucosal Eosinophils per Microscopic High-Powered Field in Normal Individuals

Gastric antrum	<10
Duodenum	<20
Colon	10-20
In infants	<10
Esophagus	0

First reported more than 50 years ago, the clinical spectrum of these disorders was defined solely by various case reports. As these reports became more frequent, various aspects of the disease became better described and stratified. Additional insight into the role of the eosinophil in health and disease has allowed further description of these disorders with respect to the underlying defect that drives the inflammatory response in those afflicted. Perhaps most important to the definition of these disorders has been the understanding of the heterogeneity of the sites affected within the GI tract (Table 38-1).

Eosinophilic gastroenteropathies are thought to arise from the interaction of genetic and environmental factors. Of note, approximately 10% of individuals with one of these disorders has a family history in an immediate family member.[10] In addition there is evidence for the role of allergy in the etiology of these conditions, including the observations that up to 75% of patients are atopic[11,12] and that an allergen-free diet can sometimes reverse disease activity.[11-14] Interestingly, only a minority of individuals with eosinophilic gastroenteropathies have food-induced anaphylaxis,[15] and therefore these disorders exhibit properties that are intermediate between pure IgE-mediated allergy and cellular mediated hypersensitivity disorders.

EOSINOPHILIC ESOPHAGITIS

Eosinophilic esophagitis (EoE) is characterized by an isolated, severe eosinophilic infiltration of the esophagus manifested by gastroesophageal reflux-like symptoms, but refractory to typical reflux therapies. This disorder has been given several names including eosinophilic esophagitis, allergic esophagitis, primary eosinophilic esophagitis, and idiopathic eosinophilic esophagitis.

Etiology

EoE is caused by an abnormal immunologic response to specific antigens. In the vast majority of cases the antigens responsible are food antigens, although there appears to be a contribution from other environmental antigens in certain individuals.[16] Although several studies have documented resolution of EoE with the strict avoidance of food antigens, in 1995 Kelly et al. published the seminal paper on EoE.[17] Because the suspected etiology was an abnormal immunologic response to specific unidentifiable food antigens, each patient was treated with a strict elimination diet that included an amino acid–based formula. Patients were also allowed clear liquids, corn, and apples. Seventeen patients were initially offered a dietary elimination trial with 10 patients adhering to the protocol. The initial trial was determined by a history of anaphylaxis to specific foods and abnormal skin testing. These patients were subsequently placed on a strict diet consisting of an amino acid–based formula for a median of 17 weeks. Symptomatic improvement

was seen within an average of 3 weeks after the introduction of the elemental diet (resolution in eight patients, improvement in two). In addition, all 10 patients demonstrated a significant improvement in esophageal eosinophilia. All patients reverted to previous symptoms on reintroduction of foods.

Although an exact explanation for this type of response was not determined, Kelly et al. suggested an immunologic basis, secondary to a delayed hypersensitivity or a cell-mediated hypersensitivity response, as the cause for EoE. More recently, Spergel et al. demonstrated that foods that cause EoE do not do so through immediate hypersensitivity reactions.[12] By using a combination of traditional skin prick testing and a less-used technique of atopy patch testing, they established that a delayed cellular mediated allergic response may be responsible for many cases of EoE. Further supporting a delayed type response, CD8+ lymphocytes have been identified as the predominant T cell within the squamous epithelium of patients diagnosed with EoE.[18]

A link between eosinophilic esophagitis and atopy has been established.[14,19] It is these links between atopy and EoE that originally suggested that food allergies play a role in the pathogenesis of this disease. The role of food allergy was confirmed as patients improved on elemental diets. Elimination of the responsible food usually does not lead to rapid resolution of the symptoms. Rather, improvement of symptoms occurs approximately 1 to 2 weeks after the removal of the causative antigen. Also, in patients with EoE, symptoms do not always occur immediately after reintroduction to the foods. It may take several days for symptoms to develop, suggesting either a mixed IgE and T-cell mediated allergic response or strictly a T-cell delayed mechanism in the pathogenesis of this disease. Although both IgE and T-cell mediated reactions have been identified as possible causative factors, T-cell mediated reactions seem to be the predominant mechanism of disease.

Several authors have suggested that aeroallergens may contribute to the development of EoE. Mishra et al. used a mouse model to show that the inhalation of *Aspergillus* caused EoE.[20] They found that the allergen-challenged mice developed elevated levels of esophageal eosinophils and features of epithelial cell hyperplasia that mimic EoE. In addition, Spergel and coworkers reported a case of a 21-year-old female with asthma and allergic rhinoconjunctivitis who also had EoE.[21] The patient's EoE became symptomatic with exacerbations during pollen seasons, followed by resolution during winter months.

Clinical Manifestations

Eosinophilic esophagitis can occur in all ages, but traditionally presents in younger patients with a male-to-female ratio of about 3:1. However, with increased awareness of the disorder among internist-gastroenterologists, there has also been increased recognition of the disorder in adults. Patients typically present with one or more of the following symptoms: vomiting, regurgitation, nausea, epigastric or chest pain, water brash, globus, and decreased appetite (Table 38-2).[14,22] Less common symptoms include growth failure and hematemesis. Esophageal dysmotility and dysphagia are less common in younger children, but become increasingly prevalent in adolescents and adults. Symptoms can be frequent and severe in some patients but extremely intermittent and mild in others. The majority of patients may experience daily dysphagia or chronic nausea or regurgitation, whereas others may have infrequent

TABLE 38-2.   Characteristics of Eosinophilic Esophagitis

Clinical Symptoms
Similar to symptoms of GERD
  Vomiting, regurgitation
  Heartburn
  Epigastric pain
  Dysphagia
Symptoms different in infants and adolescents
Often intermittent symptoms
Male > female

Associated Signs and Symptoms (>50% of patients)
Bronchospasm
Eczema
Allergic rhinitis

Family History (35-45% of patients)
Food allergy
Asthma

TABLE 38-3.   Contrasting Characteristics of Eosinophilic Esophagitis and Gastroesophageal Reflux

Eosinophilic Esophagitis
Intermittent symptoms
pH probe
  Normal
Acid blockade
  Unresponsive
Number of esophageal eosinophils
  >20 eosinophils/high-power field (HPF)

Gastroesophageal Reflux
Persistent symptoms
pH probe
  Abnormal
Acid blockade
  Responsive
Number of esophageal eosinophils
  1-5 eosinophils/HPF

or rare episodes of dysphagia. Up to 50% of patients manifest additional allergy-related symptoms such as asthma, eczema, or rhinitis. Furthermore, more than 50% of patients have one or more parents with history of allergy.

Children with EoE have been studied in comparison to those with gastroesophageal reflux.[11,12] Although the symptoms of vomiting and abdominal pain occurred similarly in both groups, dysphagia, diarrhea, and growth failure are predominant in those with EoE. In addition, patients with EoE are more likely to have had allergic symptoms, another family member with an allergic history, and peripheral eosinophilia. Patients with EoE have higher numbers of eosinophils in their esophagus and also tend to have relatively normal pH-metry when compared to those with gastroesophageal reflux (GER) (Table 38-3).

Evaluation and Diagnosis

Children with chronic refractory symptoms of gastroesophageal reflux disease or dysphagia should undergo evaluation for EoE. Although laboratory and radiologic assessment may be appropriate, the majority of these patients should undergo an upper endoscopy with biopsy. The diagnosis of EoE is often made when an isolated severe histologic esophagitis is seen that is unresponsive to aggressive acid blockade and associated with symptoms similar to those seen in gastroesophageal reflux disease.[23] The diagnosis is further supported if the patient responds both clinically and histologically to the elimination of a specific food(s). In the past, a 24-hour pH probe was required to demonstrate that the esophageal disease was not acid induced; however, more recent guidelines allow for diagnosis in the setting of appropriate clinical and histologic findings. As a general guideline, patients with EoE tend to have 20 or more eosinophils per high-power field (HPF) on biopsies, while those with GER tend to have 5 or less. However, very high levels of esophageal eosinophilia have been demonstrated with GER alone,[24] emphasizing that failure of appropriate medical therapy is an important feature of the diagnosis. Currently, upper endoscopy with biopsy is the only diagnostic test that can accurately determine if the esophageal inflammation of EoE is present.

Once EoE is suspected, patients should be encouraged to seek an allergy consultation. Skin prick testing and serum RAST tests may provide some clues to possible food allergens. Unfortunately, these tests are most useful in determining IgE-based allergic disorders. Because EoE is considered to be either a T-cell mediated disease or a mixed IgE and T-cell mediated disorder, the sensitivity and specificity of skin prick tests alone are low. Atopy patch testing (the placement of an antigen on the skin for several days followed by assessment for localized skin reaction) may be more useful in determining the antigens responsible for causing esophageal eosinophilia[12] and should be utilized if available. If no specific antigen(s) are found through allergy testing, a trial of an elimination diet, consisting of removal of the antigens that most commonly cause EoE, can be attempted.[25] The most common foods identified as causing EoE are milk, soy, egg, wheat, nuts, fish, and shellfish. If all of these measures fail, an elemental diet utilizing an amino acid–based formula should be considered. The assessment of success should be based on both the improvement of clinical symptoms and histologic improvement.

Once EoE has resolved, foods should be reintroduced individually no more frequently than one every 5 to 6 days. This time period is usually sufficient to see a recurrence of symptoms; if symptoms develop, the food should be discontinued. However, in some cases symptoms do not occur despite recurrence of eosinophilic infiltration. A repeat endoscopy with biopsy is required in order to evaluate for the presence of esophageal mucosal injury. Because clinical symptoms often occur sporadically, biopsy remains the most important way to accurately determine the presence or resolution of EoE.

Although upper endoscopy with biopsy can precisely determine the diagnosis, noninvasive diagnostic tests have proven to be less useful. These include the evaluation of serum IgE levels and quantitative peripheral eosinophils, radiographic upper gastrointestinal (UGI) series, pH probe and manometry, RAST testing, and skin prick and patch testing. When used alone, serum IgE levels and serum eosinophils have been found to be unreliable, as these tests usually respond to environmental allergens as well as ingested or inhaled allergens. Although radiographs determine anatomic abnormalities, these tests cannot identify tissue eosinophilia. Patients with EoE usually have normal or borderline pH-metry. These patients may have mild GERD secondary to abnormalities in esophageal motility due to tissue eosinophilic infiltration.

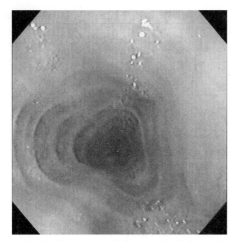

Figure 38-1. "Trachealization" or "felinization" of the midesophagus in a patient with eosinophilic esophagitis. The terms arise from the ringed appearance of the esophagus that cause it to resemble a human trachea or a cat esophagus (which has rings of cartilage).

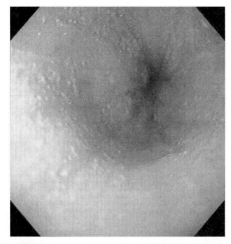

Figure 38-2. White plaques seen in the midesophagus in a patient with eosinophilic esophagitis.

EoE should be considered only when the eosinophilia is isolated strictly to the esophageal mucosa. In the past, early reports suggested that eosinophilia in EoE was more characteristic in the midesophagus than the distal (which is more likely to have eosinophils relating to acid reflux); however, recent information demonstrates that a severe mucosal eosinophilia can occur in either the distal or proximal esophagus.[26-28] To make an accurate diagnosis, the remainder of the GI tract must be normal. When EoE is suspected, the sensitivity for detecting the disease is increased when more biopsies are obtained from the esophagus. Sensitivity seems to be highest when at least five biopsies are obtained.[29]

EoE has been associated with visual findings on endoscopy: concentric ring formation called "trachealization" or a "feline esophagus," longitudinal linear furrows, and patches of small, white papules on the esophageal surface (Figures 38-1 and 38-2).[30] Most investigators believe that the esophageal rings and furrows are a response to full-thickness esophageal tissue

inflammation. The white papules appear to represent the formation of eosinophilic microabscesses.

In 1999, Ruchelli et al. evaluated 102 patients presenting with GER disease (GERD) symptoms who also were found to have at least 1 esophageal eosinophil per HPF without any other GI abnormalities.[31] Patients were subsequently treated with aggressive acid blockade. It was demonstrated that the treatment response could be classified into three categories. Patients who improved had on average 1.1 eosinophils per HPF, patients who relapsed on completion of therapy had 6.4 eosinophils per HPF, and patients who remained symptomatic had on average 24.5 eosinophils per HPF.

In 2000, Fox et al. utilized high-resolution probe endosonography in patients with EoE in order to determine the extent of tissue involvement.[32] They compared eight patients identified with EoE to four control patients without esophagitis. They discovered that the layers of the esophageal wall were thicker in EoE patients than in control group (2.8 to 2.2 mm). Additionally, the mucosa-to-submucosa ratio was greater in EoE patients (1.6 to 1.1 mm) and the muscularis propria thickness was greater in EoE pts (1.3 to 1.0 mm). These findings suggested that EoE patients had more than just surface involvement of eosinophils.

Management

The identification and removal of allergic dietary antigens is the mainstay of treatment for EoE. Although removal of the offending food(s) reverses the disease process in patients with EoE, in many cases the isolation of these foods is difficult. Often, patients with EoE cannot correlate their GI symptoms with the ingestion of a specific food. This occurs because of the delayed hypersensitivity response. Several reports have demonstrated several days for symptoms to recur on ingestion of antigens that cause EoE.[17,22] Even when a particular food causing EoE has been isolated, it may take days or weeks for the symptoms to resolve. In addition, although one food may be identified, there may be several other foods (not identified) that could also be contributing.

Although attempts should be made to identify and eliminate potential food allergens through a careful history and the use of allergy testing, it may be difficult to determine the responsible allergic foods; the administration of a strict diet, utilizing an amino acid–based formula, is often necessary to do so. As established previously, the use of an elemental diet rapidly improves both clinical symptoms and histology in patients with EoE.[13,14,17] Because of poor palatability, the elemental formula is commonly administered by continuous nasogastric feeding, although there are some more palatable options that have emerged in the past few years. The diet may be supplemented with water, and some have also approved the use of a protein-free single-antigen juice such as white grape or apple. Many patients also tolerate foods made solely of highly refined carbohydrates, such as certain lollipops; however, it is usually better to introduce these other foods somewhat later in the elemental diet.

Reversal of symptoms typically occurs within 10 days with histologic improvement within 4 weeks. Although the strict use of an amino acid–based formula may initially be difficult for patients (and parents) to accept, its benefits outweigh the risks of other treatments and the rapid improvement in symptoms proves very reinforcing to families. The use of other medications, such as corticosteroids, may temporarily improve the disease and its symptoms; however, on their discontinuation the disease recurs. In contrast, when foods that cause EoE are identified through a combination of allergy testing, endoscopy, elimination, and selective reintroduction, a lifelong remission without medication can be attained.

Treatment of true EoE with aggressive acid blockade, including medical and surgical therapy, has not been proven effective. Several published reports have demonstrated the failure of H_2 blocker and proton pump therapy in patients with EoE.[18,31,33] Although acid blockade may improve clinical symptoms by improving acid reflux that occurs secondary to the underlying inflamed esophageal mucosa, it does not reverse the esophageal histologic abnormality. Although some case reports suggested that fundoplication was beneficial for patients with EoE, in 1997, Liacouras reported on two cases of failed Nissen fundoplication in patients who were diagnosed with severe eosinophilic esophagitis.[34] Both patients underwent fundoplication for presumed acid reflux esophagitis unresponsive to medical therapy. However, postsurgical evaluation of both patients revealed ongoing clinical symptoms. Repeat esophagogastroduodenoscopy (EGD) demonstrated persistent esophageal eosinophilia. Subsequently, both patients responded to oral corticosteroids with resolution of symptoms and histologic improvement.

Before 1997, reports suggested that systemic corticosteroids improved the symptoms of EoE in adults identified with a severe eosinophilic esophagitis.[35,36] In 1998, Liacouras et al. were the first to publish the use of oral corticosteroids in 20 children diagnosed with EoE.[33] These patients were treated with oral methylprednisolone (average dose 1.5 mg/kg/day; maximum dose 48 mg/day) for 1 month. Symptoms were significantly improved in 19 of 20 patients by an average of 8 days. A repeat endoscopy with biopsy, 4 weeks after the initiation of therapy, demonstrated a significant reduction of esophageal eosinophils, from 34 to 1.5 eosinophils per HPF. However, on discontinuation of corticosteroids, 90% had recurrence of symptoms.

In 1998, Faubion reported that swallowing a metered dose of aerosolized corticosteroids was also effective in treating the symptoms of EoE in children.[37] Four patients diagnosed with EoE manifested by epigastric pain, dysphagia, and a severe esophageal eosinophilia unresponsive to aggressive acid blockade were given fluticasone, four puffs twice a day. Patients were instructed to use an inhaler but to immediately swallow after inhalation in order to deliver the medication to the esophagus. Histologic improvement was not determined. Within 2 months, all four patients responded with an improvement in symptoms. Two patients required repeat use of inhalation therapy. Success with this therapy was recently confirmed.[18]

Later, Konikoff et al. performed a randomized double-blind placebo-controlled trial utilizing swallowed fluticasone in patients with EoE.[38] The study revealed symptom improvement and decreased esophageal eosinophils in those who received study drug compared to those who received placebo. In addition to swallowed fluticasone, Aceves et al. reported an effective alternative by using liquid budesonide mixed with a sucralose suspension.[39]

Although topical therapy such as these can improve symptoms of EoE, to date there is no evidence that topical steroids result in histologic remission (as opposed to histologic improvement). Additionally, the side effects can include esophageal candidiasis and growth failure.[40,41] As with all therapies that do not involve removal of antigens, symptoms often recur in patients on discontinuation of the therapy.[18]

TABLE 38-4. **Characteristics of Eosinophilic Gastroenteritis**

Clinical characteristics
Nausea, vomiting, regurgitation
Severe abdominal pain
Diarrhea, protein-losing enteropathy
Gastrointestinal bleeding
Ascites
Intestinal obstruction
>95%, gastric antrum involved
Peripheral eosinophilia (>50%)
Associated allergies, eczema, asthma, rhinitis, atopy

Other forms of medical therapy that have been evaluated previously include the mast-cell-stabilizing agent cromolyn sodium and the leukotriene antagonist montelukast.[42-46] Although each of these medications represents an appealing option from a pathophysiologic standpoint, the available data do not support their use, based on either lack of clinical improvement or minimal to no histologic resolution.

The latest innovation in therapy includes the use of biologic agents directed at the cytokine interleukin-5 (IL-5). IL-5 plays in important role in eosinophil recruitment, activation, and proliferation. In the past, two small studies demonstrated the effectiveness of anti-IL-5 in improving both symptoms and esophageal histology.[47,48] In 2009, the first large-scale pediatric trials utilizing an anti-IL-5 monoclonal antibody were underway, although to date the results are still pending. If effective, this therapy may represent an additional option to a subset of patients with EoE.

EOSINOPHILIC GASTROENTERITIS

Eosinophilic gastroenteritis (EoG) is a general term that describes a constellation of symptoms attributable to the GI tract, in combination with pathologic infiltration by eosinophils (Table 38-4). This group includes eosinophilic gastritis, gastroenteritis, and enterocolitis. There are no strict diagnostic criteria for this disorder, and it has been largely shaped by multiple case reports and series. A combination of GI complaints with supportive histologic findings is sufficient to make the diagnosis. These conditions are grouped together under the term EoG for the discussion here, though it is likely that they are distinct entities in most patients.

EoG was originally described by Kaijser in 1937.[49] It is a disorder characterized by tissue eosinophilia that can affect different layers of the bowel wall, anywhere from mouth to anus. The gastric antrum and small bowel are most frequently affected. In 1970, Klein et al. classified EoG into three categories: mucosal, muscular, and serosal forms.[50]

Etiology

EoG affects patients of all ages, with a slight male predominance. Most commonly, eosinophils infiltrate only the mucosa, leading to symptoms associated with malabsorption, such as growth failure, weight loss, diarrhea, and hypoalbuminemia. Mucosal EoG may affect any portion of the GI tract. A review of the biopsy findings in 38 children with EoG revealed that all patients examined had mucosal eosinophilia of the gastric antrum.[51] Seventy-nine percent of the patients also demonstrated eosinophilia of the proximal small intestine, with 60%

having esophageal involvement and 52% having involvement of the gastric corpus. Those with colonic involvement tended to be under 6 months of age and were ultimately classified as having allergic colitis.

The exact etiology of EoG remains unknown, although it is now recognized as a result of both IgE- and non-IgE-mediated sensitivity.[12] The association between IgE-mediated inflammatory response (typical allergy) and EoG is supported by the increased likelihood of other allergic disorders such as atopic disease, food allergies, and seasonal allergies.[52,53] Specific foods have been implicated in the cause of EoG in some patients.[54,55] In contrast, the role of non-IgE-mediated immune dysfunction, in particular the interplay between lymphocyte-produced cytokines and eosinophils, has also received attention. IL-5 is a chemoattractant responsible for tissue eosinophilia.[56] Desreumaux et al. found that among patients with EoG, the levels of IL-3, IL-5, and granulocyte-macrophage colony-stimulating factor (GM-CSF) were significantly increased as compared to control patients.[57] Once recruited to the tissue, eosinophils may further recruit similar cells through their own production of IL-3 and IL-5, as well as production of leukotrienes.[58] This mixed type of immune dysregulation in EoG has implications in the way this disorder is diagnosed, as well as the way it is treated.

Clinical Manifestations

The most common symptoms of EoG include colicky abdominal pain, bloating, diarrhea, weight loss, dysphagia. and vomiting.[43,59] In addition, up to 50% have a past or family history of atopy.[51] Other features of severe disease include GI bleeding, iron deficiency anemia, protein-losing enteropathy (hypoalbuminemia), and growth failure.[59] Approximately 75% of affected patients have an elevated blood eosinophilia.[60] Males are more commonly affected than females. Rarely, ascites can occur.[60,61]

In an infant, EoG may present in a manner similar to hypertrophic pyloric stenosis, with progressive vomiting, dehydration, electrolyte abnormalities, and thickening of the gastric outlet.[62,63] When an infant presents with this constellation of symptoms, in addition to atopic symptoms such as eczema and reactive airway disease, an elevated eosinophil count, or a strong family history of atopic disease, then EoG should be considered in the diagnosis before surgical intervention if possible.

Uncommon presentations of EoG include acute abdomen (even mimicking acute appendicitis)[64] or colonic obstruction.[65] There have also been reports of serosal infiltration with eosinophils, with associated complaints of abdominal distention, eosinophilic ascites, and bowel perforation.[61,66-70]

Evaluation and Diagnosis

EoG should be considered in any patient with a history of chronic symptoms including vomiting, abdominal pain, diarrhea, anemia, hypoalbuminemia, or poor weight gain in combination with the presence of eosinophils in the GI tract. Other causes of eosinophilic infiltration of the GI tract include the other disorders of the eosinophilic gastroenteropathy spectrum, as well as parasitic infection, inflammatory bowel disease, neoplasm, chronic granulomatous disease, collagen vascular disease, and the hypereosinophilic syndrome.[71-75]

A number of tests may aid in the diagnosis of EoG; however, no single test is pathognomonic, and there are no standards for diagnosis. Eosinophils in the GI tract must be documented before EoG can be truly entertained as a diagnosis. This is most readily done with biopsies of either the upper GI tract through esophagogastroduodenoscopy or the lower tract through flexible sigmoidoscopy or colonoscopy. A history of atopy supports the diagnosis, but is not a necessary feature. Peripheral eosinophilia or an elevated IgE level occurs in approximately 70% of affected individuals.[76] Measures of absorptive activity such as the D-xylose absorption test and lactose hydrogen breath testing may reveal evidence of malabsorption, reflecting small intestinal damage. Radiographic contrast studies may demonstrate mucosal irregularities or edema, wall thickening, ulceration, or luminal narrowing. A lacy mucosal pattern of the gastric antrum known as *areae gastricae* is a unique finding that may be present in patients with EoG.[77]

Evaluation of other causes of eosinophilia should be undertaken, including stool analysis for ova and parasites and serologic tests for specific parasites in endemic areas. Signs of intestinal obstruction warrant abdominal imaging. RAST testing, as well as skin testing for environmental antigens, is rarely useful. Skin testing using both traditional prick tests and patch tests may increase the sensitivity for identifying foods responsible for EoG by evaluating both IgE-mediated and T-cell mediated sensitivities.[12]

Management

There is as much ambiguity in the treatment of EoG as there is in its diagnosis. This is in large part because the entity of EoG was defined mainly by case series, each of which employed its own mode of treatment. Because EoG is a difficult disease to diagnose and relatively rare in prevalence, randomized trials for its treatment are uncommon, leading to considerable debate as to which treatment is best.

Food allergy is considered one of the potential underlying causes of EoG. The elimination of pathogenic foods, as identified by any form of allergy testing, or by random removal of the most likely antigens, should be a first-line consideration. Unfortunately, this approach results in improvement in a limited number of patients. In severe cases, or when other treatment options have failed, the administration of a strict diet, utilizing an elemental formula, has been shown to be successful.[53,78] In these cases, elemental formula provided as the sole source of nutrition has been reported to be effective in the resolution of clinical symptoms and tissue eosinophilia.

When the use of a restricted or elemental diet fails, corticosteroids are often employed because of their high likelihood of success in attaining remission.[43] However, when the patient is weaned from the drug, the duration of remission is variable and can be short-lived, leading to the need for repeated courses or continuous low doses of steroids. In addition, the chronic use of corticosteroids carries an increased likelihood of undesirable side effects, including cosmetic problems (cushingoid facies, hirsutism, acne), decreased bone density, impaired growth, and personality changes. A response to these side effects has been to look for substitutes that may act as steroid-sparing agents, while still allowing for control of symptoms. Anecdotally, immunomodulators more commonly used as steroid-sparing agents in inflammatory bowel disease, such as mercaptopurine or azathioprine, have been used with some success.

Orally administered cromolyn sodium also has been effective in some patients,[43,79-81] and recent reports have detailed the efficacy of other oral anti-inflammatory medications.

Montelukast, a selective leukotriene receptor antagonist used to treat asthma, has been reported to successfully treat two patients with EoG.[45,82] Treatment of EoG with inhibition of leukotriene D4, a potent chemotactic factor for eosinophils, relies on the theory that the inflammatory response in EoG is perpetuated by the presence of the eosinophils already present in the mucosa causing an interruption in the chemotactic cascade breaking the inflammatory cycle. Suplatast tosilate, another suppressor of cytokine production, has also been reported as a treatment for EoG.[83]

Given the possibilities for treatment of EoG, the combination of therapies incorporating the best chance of success with the smallest likelihood of side effects should be employed. When particular food antigens that may be causing disease can be identified, elimination of those antigens should be employed as a first-line therapy. When testing fails to identify potentially pathogenic foods, a systematic elimination of the most commonly involved foods[84] can be employed. If this approach fails, total elimination diet with an amino acid-based formula should be considered. Trials of nonsteroidal anti-inflammatory medications such as cromolyn, montelukast, and suplatast are a reasonable option, although some might prefer to wait for more detailed studies. Monoclonal antibodies against interleukin-5 may also hold some promise in the future, although current studies are limited to those with EoE; further research will be necessary in the EoG population.

When other treatments fail, corticosteroids remain a reliable treatment for EoG, with attempts at limiting the total dose or the number of treatment courses where possible. Because of the diffuse and inconsistent nature of symptoms in this disease, serial endoscopy with biopsy is a useful and important modality for monitoring disease progression.

EOSINOPHILIC PROCTOCOLITIS

Eosinophilic proctocolitis (EoP), also known as allergic proctocolitis (AP) or milk-protein proctocolitis, has been recognized as one of the most common etiologies of rectal bleeding in infants.[51,85] This disorder is characterized by the onset of rectal bleeding, generally in children less than 2 months of age.

Etiology

The gastrointestinal tract plays a major role in the development of oral tolerance to foods. Through the process of endocytosis by the enterocyte, food antigens are generally degraded into nonantigenic proteins.[86,87] Although the GI tract serves as an efficient barrier to ingested food antigens, this barrier may not be mature for the first few months of life.[88] As a result, ingested antigens may have an increased propensity for being presented intact to the immune system. These intact antigens have the potential for stimulating the immune system and driving an inappropriate response directed at the GI tract. Because the major component of the young infant's diet is milk or formula, it stands to reason that the inciting antigens in EoP are derived from the proteins found in them. Cow's milk and soy proteins are the foods most frequently implicated in EoP.

Commercially available infant formulas most commonly utilize cow's milk as the protein source. There are at least 25 known immunogenic proteins within cow's milk, with β-lactoglobulin and casein serving as the most antigenic.[89] It is felt that up to 7.5% of the population in developed countries exhibit cow's-milk allergy, although there is wide variation in the reported data.[90-92] Soy protein allergy is felt to be less common than cow's-milk allergy, with reported prevalence of approximately 0.5%.[89] However, soy protein intolerance becomes more prominent in individuals who have developed milk protein allergy, as there is significant cross-reactivity between these proteins, with prevalence from 15 to 50% or more in milk-protein sensitized individuals.[93] For this reason, substitution of a soy protein-based formula for a milk protein-based formula in patients with suspected milk-protein proctocolitis is often unsuccessful.

Maternal breast milk represents a different challenge to the immune system. Up to 50% of the cases of EoP occur in breast-fed infants; but, rather than developing an allergy to human milk protein, it is felt that the infants are manifesting allergy to antigens ingested by the mother and transferred via the breast milk. The transfer of maternal dietary protein via breast milk was first demonstrated in 1921.[94] More recently, the presence of cow's-milk antigens in breast milk has been established.[95-97]

When a problem with antigen handling occurs, whether secondary to increased absorption through an immature GI tract or though a damaged epithelium secondary to gastroenteritis, sensitization of the immune system results. Once sensitized, the inflammatory response is perpetuated with continued exposure to the inciting antigen. This may explain the reported relationship between early exposures to cow's-milk protein or viral gastroenteritis and the development of allergy.[98-100]

Clinical Manifestations

Diarrhea, rectal bleeding, and increased mucus production are the typical symptoms seen in patients who present with EoP.[51,101] There is a bimodal age distribution with the majority of patients presenting in infancy (mean age at diagnosis of 60 days[102]) and the other group presenting in adolescence and early adulthood.

The typical infant with EoP is well-appearing with no constitutional symptoms. Rectal bleeding begins gradually, initially appearing as small flecks of blood. Usually, increased stool frequency occurs accompanied by water loss or mucus streaks. The development of irritability or straining with stools is also common and can falsely lead to the initial assumption of anal fissuring. Atopic symptoms, such as eczema and reactive airway disease, may be associated. Continued exposure to the inciting antigen causes increased bleeding and may, on rare occasions, cause anemia and poor weight gain. Despite the progression of symptoms, the infants are generally well appearing and rarely appear ill. Other manifestations of GI tract inflammation, such as vomiting, abdominal distention, or weight loss, almost never occur (Table 38-5).

Evaluation and Diagnosis

EoP is primarily a clinical diagnosis, although several laboratory parameters and diagnostic procedures may be useful. Initial assessment should be directed at the overall health of the child. A toxic-appearing infant is not consistent with the diagnosis of EoP and should prompt evaluation for other causes of GI bleeding. A complete blood count is useful, as the majority of infants with EoP have a normal or borderline low hemoglobin. An elevated serum eosinophil count may be present. Stool studies for bacterial pathogens, such as *Salmonella* and *Shigella*,

TABLE 38-5.   Characteristics of Eosinophilic Proctocolitis

Clinical Symptoms
Blood-streaked stools
Diarrhea
Mild abdominal pain
<3 months of age
Usually normal weight gain
Well-appearing
Eczema, atopy – rare

Laboratory Features
Fecal leukocytes
Mild peripheral eosinophilia
Rarely
  Hypoalbuminemia
  Anemia
Pin prick, RAST testing negative

should be considered in the setting of rectal bleeding. An assay for *Clostridium difficile* toxins A and B should also be considered, although infants may be asymptomatically colonized with this organism.[103,104] A stool specimen may be analyzed for the presence of white blood cells, and specifically for eosinophils. The sensitivity of these tests is not well documented, and the absence of a positive finding on these tests does not exclude the diagnosis.[105] Eosinophils can also accumulate in the colon in other conditions such as pinworm and hookworm infections, drug reactions, vasculitis, and inflammatory bowel disease, and it may be important to exclude these, especially in older children.

Although not always necessary, flexible sigmoidoscopy may be useful to demonstrate the presence of colitis. Visually, one may find erythema, friability, or frank ulceration of the colonic mucosa. Alternatively, the mucosa may appear normal or show evidence of lymphoid hyperplasia.[106,107] Histologic findings typically include increased eosinophils in focal aggregates within the lamina propria, with generally preserved crypt architecture. Findings may be patchy, so that care should be taken to examine many levels of each specimen if necessary.[108,109]

Management

In a well-appearing patient with a history consistent with EoP, it is acceptable to make an empiric change in the protein source of the formula. Because of the high degree of cross-reactivity between milk and soy protein in sensitized individuals, a protein-hydrolysate formula is often the best choice.[99] Resolution of symptoms begins almost immediately after the elimination of the problematic food. Although symptoms may linger for several days to weeks, continued improvement is the rule. If symptoms do not quickly improve, or persist beyond 4 to 6 weeks, other antigens should be considered, as well as other potential causes of rectal bleeding. In breast-fed infants, dietary restriction of milk- and soy-containing products for the mother may result in improvement; however, care should be taken to ensure that the mother maintains adequate protein and calcium intake from other sources.

EoP in infancy is generally benign, and withdrawing the milk protein trigger resolves the condition. Though gross blood in the stool usually disappears within 72 hours, occult blood loss may persist for longer.[102] The prognosis is excellent, and the majority of patients are able to tolerate the culprit milk protein

by 1 to 3 years of age. In older individuals, it is more difficult to identify the food triggers, and therefore patients usually require medical management. Though there is a paucity of clinical data regarding therapy for this condition, it appears that glucocorticoids and aminosalicylates are efficacious.[9] The prognosis for older-onset EoP is less favorable than the infant presentation and is typically chronic and relapsing.

OTHER MANIFESTATIONS OF GASTROINTESTINAL ALLERGY

Although we have described several specific manifestations of allergic bowel disease in the preceding sections, there remain numerous nonspecific complaints that may occur in the infant that have also been linked to food allergy. These nonspecific complaints create an especially difficult situation for the practitioner, because only a proportion of infants with these complaints will have them as a result of allergy. Further, there are no specific findings that independently can confirm or exclude the diagnosis. Among these potential nonspecific manifestations are gastroesophageal reflux, colic, constipation, and diarrhea.

Gastroesophageal Reflux

GER is a common complaint among infants, children, and adults. Up to two thirds of 4-month-old infants experience regurgitation on a daily basis,[110] with other complaints such as forceful vomiting, arching, irritability, and feeding refusal occurring to varying degrees. Furthermore, many infants and children may experience GER without the presence of any overt signs or symptoms. Most cases of GER are not attributable to a specific underlying cause; however, one of the leading identifiable causes of GER in this population is food allergy.[111,112]

Relatively recently, the association between GER and cow's-milk allergy (CMA) was prospectively investigated.[112] In a 3-year prospective study, infants with symptoms compatible with GER underwent pH monitoring and endoscopy to confirm the presence of GER. Patients with a reflux index (percentage of time with acid reflux) of greater than 5% and the presence of esophagitis were considered to have GER. The presence of CMA in these patients was assessed using skin prick tests, by the presence of eosinophils in fecal mucus, nasal mucus, or peripheral blood, and by circulating levels of anti-β-lactoglobulin IgG. Patients who had positive assays for CMA and GER were placed on a cow's-milk restricted diet with a protein hydrolysate formula. After 3 months, a double-blind cow's milk challenge was performed to confirm the diagnosis of CMA.

This stringent method of diagnosing both GER and CMA revealed a surprisingly high prevalence (42%) of patients with GER who also had CMA. Further, this author group went on to show that 14 of 47 patients (30%) had GER that was attributable to the CMA itself, based on resolution of symptoms on restricted diet followed by return of symptoms when rechallenged. Whether cow's milk or other food allergies are responsible for such a high proportion of GER in all populations remains to be seen; however, these results imply that refractory cases of GER warrant consideration of food allergy as a contributing factor.

Infantile Colic

Infantile colic is a term that is generally used to describe acute self-limited episodes of irritability (presumably due to abdominal pain) that occur in otherwise healthy infants in the first several months of life.[113] Although labeling an infant as having "colic" implies that there is no organic disease responsible, a subset of infants diagnosed with colic will have an underlying organic cause. Food allergies, and specifically CMA, have been highly implicated in the organic etiologies of infantile colic.

In a trial of 70 formula-fed infants, 50 (71%) had resolution of colic symptoms when cow's-milk protein was removed from the diet, with 100% relapse rate after two successive reintroductions of the protein.[114] Similarly, in a double-blind crossover study, cow's-milk allergy was implicated in 24 of 27 infants with colic, with significant reductions in daily crying when cow's-milk protein was removed from the diet,[115] and worsening of symptoms when whey was reintroduced into the diet in a blinded fashion.

Traditionally, changing the infant's formula is a common way of dealing with colic; often several formula changes are made (e.g., from cow's-milk based to soy based to hydrolyzed protein). It is often unclear, however, whether the formula change is responsible for the eventual resolution of symptoms, as colic by definition begins to resolve by 4 to 5 months of age.

Diarrhea

The presence of diarrhea in the context of food allergies can be multifactorial. As discussed in previous sections, EoG and AP may both lead to intestinal mucosal damage and subsequent diarrhea. However, food allergy may also result in diarrhea in the absence of mucosal damage or eosinophilic infiltration.

Gastrointestinal symptoms, in particular diarrhea, are commonly seen among children with atopic eczema[116,117]; avoidance of particular foods in these patients will alleviate the symptoms.[117] In patients with GI symptoms related to milk ingestion (confirmed by double-blind challenge), the instillation of milk into the intestinal lumen resulted in increased production of histamine and eosinophil cationic protein within 20 minutes.[118] Albumin concentration in the intestine also increased, suggesting increased gut permeability and leakage; none of these findings were seen in normal controls.

Animal models suggest that food allergy may also increase intestinal motility, which in turn may lead to diarrhea.[119] Increased intestinal mast cell counts have been seen in subjects with increased intestinal motility.[120] However, diarrhea in relation to food allergy is almost certainly a multifactorial event that may involve other processes such as secondary carbohydrate malabsorption or overingestion of nonabsorbable sugars.

Constipation

Constipation is a common problem among infants and children, and although often short-lived or self-limited, a substantial proportion may have symptoms that persist for 6 months or more.[121] It has long been suggested that cow's milk plays a role in the development of chronic constipation,[122] and there is evidence that CMA is a causative factor. One of the most compelling studies involved a blinded cross-over study of cow's milk restriction in children with chronic constipation.[123] In this trial, 65 children with chronic constipation (all of whom received cow's milk in their regular diet) were randomized to receive either cow's milk or soy milk for 15 days, followed by a washout period and reversal of the previous diet. Sixty-eight percent of the children had improvement in their constipation while taking soy milk, whereas none had improvement on cow's milk. Rechallenging the responders with cow's milk resulted in return of constipation. Evidence of CMA was based

on higher frequencies of coexistent rhinitis, dermatitis, and bronchospasm in responders, as well as increased likelihood of elevated IgE to cow's-milk antigens and inflammatory cells on rectal biopsy. A subsequent study revealed further evidence of the causative nature of CMA in constipation.[124]

Approach to the Potentially Allergic Infant With Nonspecific GI Symptoms

Because GI complaints such as those listed previously are quite common in the infant population, the practitioner who cares for infants will commonly be faced with the issue of when to implicate food allergy. Further complicating the issue is that general allergic complaints such as atopic eczema and rhinitis are also quite common in this population. Optimally, the allergic contribution to any GI complaint would be investigated through double-blind food challenges. However, this is not practical for most practitioners.

Any infant with GI symptoms refractory to standard treatment may be manifesting signs of food allergy. Because CMA is implicated most commonly in this population, removal of this antigen from the diet is a reasonable approach. However, this change should be made in concert with appropriate investigations for other etiological factors (e.g., anatomic studies such as upper GI series in chronic reflux, stool cultures in chronic diarrhea). Soy formula may be substituted for cow's milk formula, with the understanding that there is a high cross-reactivity between cow's milk and soy protein in sensitized individuals. Protein-hydrolysate formulas represent a good option, more likely to result in improvement in a truly allergic infant. Breast-feeding mothers may need to restrict their intake of milk and soy for several weeks before the antigens no longer appear in breast milk. The use of amino acid–based elemental formulas should be reserved for those who have failed hydrolyzed protein formulas, and preferably in those who have some other objective positive findings of allergy. It should be remembered that the natural history of allergy in the infant is often self-limited, and thus improvement with dietary elimination does not independently confirm food allergy. Formally rechallenging the infant with the suspected food antigen is a better way to confirm that allergy existed and was responsible for the symptoms in question. Formal consultation with an allergist in this context is highly advisable.

CONCLUSION

Eosinophilic disorders of the GI tract are becoming increasingly recognized as distinct clinical entities with specific management strategies. Whereas EoG is rare and difficult to diagnose, EoP and EoE are much more common and easily diagnosed by endoscopic biopsy. Although EoP is a well-accepted entity, the diagnosis of EoE has recently been receiving a great deal of attention. Recent literature suggests a miniepidemic of EoE in the pediatric population, though controversy still exists regarding the etiology and treatment.

Future research should focus on clarifying the prevalence and natural history (e.g., the potential development of strictures) and optimizing the diagnostic approach and treatment options of all gastrointestinal eosinophilic disorders. The particular management challenges posed by these conditions warrants close liaison between gastroenterologists, allergists, and dietitians. In addition, patients and families require particular support, especially when trying to adopt restricted diets. Patient-founded support advocacy groups have been established for this purpose (e.g., the American Partnership for Eosinophilic Disorders, www.APFED.org).

Awareness of food-induced allergic and eosinophilic disease of the GI tract has increased, but many unanswered questions remain. The variation in geographical distribution of EoG and EoE has yet to be explained. The pathogenesis of these conditions has to be fully elucidated, in particular the role of environmental and infectious agents. Advances need to be made in diagnosing these conditions, especially with the use of less invasive techniques than endoscopy with biopsy and also in better identifying offending food antigens and allergens. In addition, biochemical studies need to be pursued so that we can determine a cause of these disorders. Is the eosinophil dysregulation due to an immunologic defect or an allergy? These and other research questions reinforce the limitations of our current understanding of GI eosinophilic disease.

REFERENCES

9. Rothenberg ME. Eosinophilic gastrointestinal disorders (EGID). J Allergy Clin Immunol 2004;113:11–28; quiz 9.

12. Spergel JM, Beausoleil JL, Mascarenhas M, Liacouras CA. The use of skin prick tests and patch tests to identify causative foods in eosinophilic esophagitis. J Allergy Clin Immunol 2002;109:363–368.

13. Markowitz JE, Spergel JM, Ruchelli E, Liacouras CA. Elemental diet is an effective treatment for eosinophilic esophagitis in children and adolescents. Am J Gastroenterol 2003;98:777–782.

14. Liacouras CA, Spergel JM, Ruchelli E, et al. Eosinophilic esophagitis: a 10-year experience in 381 children. Clin Gastroenterol Hepatol 2005;3:1198–1206.

23. Furuta GT, Liacouras CA, Collins MH, et al. Eosinophilic esophagitis in children and adults: a systematic review and consensus recommendations for diagnosis and treatment. Gastroenterology 2007;133:1342–1363.

27. Straumann A, Spichtin HP, Grize L, et al. Natural history of primary eosinophilic esophagitis: a follow-up of 30 adult patients for up to 11.5 years. Gastroenterology 2003;125:1660–1669.

91. Høst A, Jacobsen HP, Halken S, Holmenlund D. The natural history of cow's milk protein allergy/intolerance. Eur J Clin Nutr 1995;49(Suppl 1):S13–S18.

See expertconsult.com for a complete list of references and the review questions for this chapter.

INFECTIOUS DIARRHEA

39

José M. Garza • Mitchell B. Cohen

In the United States, an estimated 21 to 37 million episodes of diarrhea occur annually in children younger than 5 years of age.[1] Ten percent of these children are seen by a physician, more than 200,000 are hospitalized, and between 300 and 400 die from the illness. Worldwide, the number of childhood deaths from diarrhea is higher than 4 million per year.

Knowledge of diarrheal disease has increased remarkably during the past few decades.[2] This increased understanding of pathogenic mechanisms has led to improvements in therapy. This chapter discusses the major viral and bacterial agents of infectious diarrhea, including their epidemiology, pathogenesis, clinical manifestations, diagnosis, and therapy.

VIRAL GASTROENTERITIS

Diarrheal disease caused by viral agents occurs far more frequently than does similar disease of bacterial origin. In fact, viral gastroenteritis is the second most common illness in the United States, after the common cold.[3] Despite the frequent occurrence of viral enteritides, the identification of a specific virus as causative agent is a relatively recent development. Rotavirus and a number of other small round structured viruses have been identified as a major cause of nonbacterial gastroenteritis in children and adults. This discussion focuses on these established pathogens, then continues with a brief summary of several newer viral enteropathogens and the current status of several candidate pathogens.

Rotavirus

Rotavirus was first identified as a specific viral pathogen in duodenal cells of children with diarrhea by Bishop and associates in 1973. Subsequent studies indicated that rotavirus is responsible not only for more cases of diarrheal disease in infants and children than any other single cause but also for a significant portion of deaths caused by diarrhea in both developed and developing countries throughout the world.[4] Rotavirus is responsible for 20 to 70% of hospitalizations for diarrhea among children worldwide.[5] Compared with other causes of gastroenteritis, rotavirus is more frequently associated with severe symptoms.[6] Before the initiation of the rotavirus vaccination program in 2006, nearly every child in the United States was infected with rotavirus by age 5 years.[7]

Virology

The genus *Rotavirus* is classified as a member of the family Reoviridae of the RNA viruses. Rotaviruses are round particles 68 nm in diameter and are composed of two separate shells (capsids). The capsids surround a 38-nm icosahedral core structure, which in turn encloses the 11 double strands of RNA in the core. This structure gives the virus its characteristic appearance of a wide-rimmed wheel with spokes radiating from the hub, from which its name was derived (*rota* is Latin for "wheel").[8]

Rotaviruses are classified based on antigenic properties of various proteins found in the capsid structure. The VP6 protein on the inner capsid of the virus determines the rotavirus group.[9] Most viruses infecting humans are classified as group A, although rotaviruses from groups B and C have occasionally been associated with human diarrheal disease as well. The next level of classification is the subgroup, which is determined by other antigenic differences among the VP6 proteins. At least two subgroups are known to exist.[9] Subgroup typing has proved important in the study of patients who experience more than one episode of rotaviral infection. In these patients, recurrent infections usually but not necessarily involve agents of different subgroups, which suggests that subgroup antigens are not sufficient for inducing the production of protective antibodies.[10] Finally, the rotaviruses are classified into a variety of serotypes based on the antigenic differences of VP7 glycoprotein or the VP4 protease-sensitive hemagglutinin proteins that are found in the outer capsid.[11] VP4 is designated as the P antigenic protein because it is cleaved by the protease trypsin at the intestinal level, and VP7 is designated as the G antigenic protein because it is a glycosylated structure. There are at least 42 different G/P strains with different serotype combinations. However, five serotypes, G1P8, G2P4, GP8, G4P8, and G9P8, are the predominant circulation rotavirus G/P serotypes.[12] The prevalence of serotypes can fluctuate from year to year,[13] and although the five most common serotypes are responsible for approximately 95% of infections worldwide, there are substantial geographical differences. For example, in a recent global study, G1P8 was responsible for more than 70% of infections in North America, Australia, and Europe but less than 30% in South America, Asia, and Africa.[14]

Epidemiology

Rotavirus infection appears to occur throughout the world. In temperate climates, a sharp increase in incidence of cases occurs during the winter months.[4] In the United States, the peak rotavirus season begins in November in the Southwest and ends in the Northeast in April.[4] In the tropics, year-round transmission occurs, with seasonal variation in some areas.[15] Transmission is primarily from person to person, through contact with feces or contaminated fomites. Respiratory transmission has been suggested but not proved.[16] Rotavirus is highly contagious because very few infectious virions are needed to cause disease in susceptible hosts.[17]

Although the virus may affect all age groups, it most commonly produces disease in children between 6 and 24 months of age. Before vaccination, most children developed rotavirus antibodies by the age of 2 years, which helps to explain the observed decreased incidence of rotaviral infection in later childhood. Rotavirus infection also occurs in adult populations with approximately half the frequency seen in children. Those adults whose children had rotavirus were more likely to be infected than were adults without infected children.[18] Most adults found to have rotavirus infection were asymptomatic; if symptoms were present, they were generally mild. This would seem to indicate that the antibody acquired earlier in life provides protective benefit.

The other age group that appears to have relative protection from rotavirus infection is the neonate. The virus can be found in stool samples from asymptomatic neonates. Neonatal epidemics of rotavirus excretion have been described in which approximately half of the nursery patients examined were found to have rotavirus. Many of these infants were asymptomatic, and those with disease had only mild symptoms.[19,20] Breast-fed infants are less likely to be infected, and, when infected, these infants are apparently less likely than their bottle-fed counterparts to suffer symptoms of disease. This may reflect the protective effect of maternal antibodies in colostrum and breast milk.[21] Nosocomial spread of rotaviral illness among hospitalized infants has also been documented.[22]

Factors associated with increased risk for hospitalization for rotavirus gastroenteritis among U.S. children include lack of breast-feeding, low birth weight, day-care attendance, the presence of another child younger than 24 months in the household, and having Medicaid or no medical insurance.[23]

Clinical Manifestations

Once a susceptible patient has come in contact with rotavirus, a 48- to 72-hour incubation period occurs before the onset of symptoms.[16] Illness typically begins with the sudden onset of diarrhea and vomiting, and fever is present in most patients.[16] The diarrhea is usually watery and rarely may be associated with gross or occult blood in the stool.[24] The fluid loss from diarrhea and vomiting may be severe enough to cause dehydration. Diarrhea caused by rotavirus usually lasts from 2 to 8 days.[25] Shedding of virus into the intestinal lumen begins about 3 days after infection and may persist for as long as 3 weeks.[26] A comparison of the characteristics of rotaviral infections with those of other enteric viruses is presented in Table 39-1. In addition to gastrointestinal symptoms, patients with rotavirus often have respiratory tract symptoms.[16] Unlike fever and vomiting, none of the respiratory manifestations associated with rotavirus infection are helpful in the recognition of rotaviral disease.[27] The clinical symptoms of rotavirus infection are more severe in patients with underlying malnutrition. In the malnourished murine rotavirus model, a smaller inoculum is required for infection, less time is required for incubation, and the symptoms are more severe.[28] In addition, rotavirus replication can occur in the liver and kidney, at least in immunocompromised hosts.[29] Children and adults who are immunocompromised because of congenital immunodeficiency or because of bone marrow or solid organ transplantation sometimes experience

severe or prolonged rotavirus gastroenteritis.[7] The severity of rotavirus disease among children infected with human immunodeficiency virus (HIV) is thought to be similar to that among children without HIV infection.[7]

Pathophysiology

Rotavirus invades the villus intestinal epithelial cells and replicates, causing cell death and sloughing. Histologically, this is manifest as blunting of the intestinal villi, and in response to the loss of villus cells, there is crypt hypertrophy. The lytic infection of highly differentiated absorptive enterocytes and the sparing of undifferentiated crypt cells results in both a loss of absorptive capacity with "unopposed" crypt cell secretion (causing secretory diarrhea) and loss of brush border hydrolase activity (causing osmotic diarrhea).

Another possible mechanism for rotaviral diarrhea also has been demonstrated. The rotavirus nonstructural glycoprotein NSP4 has been shown to mediate age-dependent intestinal secretion in mice.[30] The relevance of this novel viral enterotoxin to human rotaviral infection is uncertain. Other models, including vasoactive inflammatory agents, have also been proposed; consistent with this, in rotavirus infection there may be an increase in the number of inflammatory cells in the lamina propria. Disease effects are apparently limited to the duodenum and the proximal jejunum,[16] because studies in patients with known rotavirus disease have yielded normal gastric and rectal biopsies.[31]

Diagnosis

Rotavirus was initially linked to acute gastroenteritis through electron-microscopic evidence of viral particles in biopsy specimens of affected patients. This technique continues to be used in rotavirus detection, especially in conjunction with monoclonal or polyclonal antibodies (immunoelectron microscopy).[25] The obvious drawback of this approach is the need for specialized personnel and equipment. Consequently, a variety of immunoassays have been developed for detecting group A rotavirus antigen in stool[31]; most immunoassays have sensitivities and specificities in the range of 90%.

Treatment

Currently, supportive care with oral or intravenous rehydration is the mainstay of therapy.[32] Although novel antisecretory therapies have been reported,[33] no antiviral agents effective against rotavirus have yet been developed. However, probiotic therapy has been shown to be effective in preventing and treating rotaviral infection. Treatment with *Lactobacillus* GG has been shown to shorten the course of rotaviral diarrhea by at least 1 day.[34-36] In addition, other probiotic agents (*Bifidobacterium bifidum* and *Streptococcus thermophilus*) have been shown to prevent diarrheal disease and shedding of rotavirus in a chronic hospital setting when given to formula-fed infants.[36] Oral administration of immunoglobulin has been shown to promote faster recovery

TABLE 39-1. **Viral Enteric Pathogens**

Virus	Predominant Age Group Affected	Seasonality	Duration of Symptoms
Rotavirus	6-24 months	↑ in winter months	2-8 days
Norovirus/caliciviruses	Older children, adults, infants	Winter and summer	12-48 hours
Enteric adenovirus	<2 years	↑ in summer months	Up to 14 days
Astrovirus	1-3 years	Unknown	1-4 days

from rotaviral infection[37]; this therapy should be reserved for severely affected hospitalized infants.

Prevention

In infants, natural rotavirus infection confers protection against subsequent infection. This protection increases with each new infection and reduces the severity of diarrhea.[38] A rotavirus vaccine (Rotashield J, Wyeth-Ayerst, St. David's, PA) was approved for use in the United States and was placed on the American Academy of Pediatrics' recommended vaccination schedule. Although the vaccine was efficacious, an increased incidence of intussusception within 2 weeks of receiving the vaccine was identified by the Vaccine Adverse Event Reporting System (VAERS), leading to voluntary withdrawal by the manufacturer.[39]

Two different rotavirus vaccine products are licensed and widely used in infants in the United States; they differ in composition and schedule administration. Safety and efficacy has been demonstrated for both vaccines; there is 85 to 98% protection against severe rotavirus disease and 74 to 87% protection against rotavirus disease of any severity through at least the first rotavirus season.[7] Neither vaccine was associated with intussusception, and the Advisory Committee on Immunization Practices (ACIP) does not express a preference for either one.[7]

Pentavalent Human-Bovine Reassortant Rotavirus Vaccine (RotaTeq [RV5]). Licensed in the United States in 2006, RotaTeq is a live, oral vaccine that contains five reassortant rotaviruses developed from human and bovine parent rotavirus strains (G1,G2,G3,G4, and P1A). The efficacy has been evaluated in two phase III trials among healthy infants.[40,41] The vaccine is to be administered orally in a three-dose series at ages 2, 4, and 6 months with a minimum age for first dose at 6 weeks and maximum at 14 weeks and 6 days. The minimal interval between doses is 4 weeks and maximum age for last dose 8 months.[7]

Monovalent Human Rotavirus Vaccine (Rotarix [RV1]). Licensed in the United States in 2008, Rotarix is a live, oral vaccine that contains a human rotavirus strain (G1P1A). The efficacy has been evaluated in two phase III trials.[42,43] The vaccine is to be administered orally in a two-dose series at ages 2 and 4 months with the same minimum and maximum age ranges and intervals as RotaTeq.[7]

Early success from the vaccines has been documented; the National Respiratory and Enteric Virus Surveillance System (NREVSS) and the New Vaccine Surveillance Network (NVSN) indicated that the onset and peak of the 2008 rotavirus season were delayed by 15 and 8 weeks, respectively. as compared with the six previous consecutive seasons.[44] Further data indicate that the number of tests positive for rotavirus during the 2008 season decreased by more than two thirds as compared with the seven preceding rotavirus seasons.[7]

Small Round Structured Viruses

Caliciviruses

"Winter vomiting disease" was thought to be caused by nonbacterial gastroenteritis for decades before an etiologic agent was identified from an outbreak, in 1968, in Norwalk, Ohio. In this outbreak, only some of the patients had diarrhea; the predominant clinical manifestation was vomiting and nausea. Virus particles were visualized by immune electron microscopy on fecal material derived from the Norwalk outbreak. This represented the first definitive association between a specific virus (Norwalk virus) and acute gastroenteritis. Subsequently a number of similar etiologic agents were identified; before the cloning of the prototype Norwalk virus genome,[45] these viruses, which were a group of morphologically diverse, positive-stranded RNA viruses that caused acute gastroenteritis, were identified as Norwalk-like agents. These organisms were also named for the communities in which they were first isolated (e.g., Montgomery County, Hawaii, Snow Mountain, Taunton, Otofuke, and Sapporo viruses). Based on reverse transcription–polymerase chain reaction (RT-PCR), the sequence structure of these viruses has enabled their classification as human caliciviruses (HuCV). Human caliciviruses are now recognized as a leading cause of diarrhea worldwide among persons of all ages.[46]

With the use of molecular tools, HuCV have now been preliminarily classified into four genotypes, represented by Norwalk virus, Snow Mountain agent, Sapporo virus, and hepatitis E virus.[47,48] Recently the nomenclature of two genotypes has changed, renaming Norwalk virus as norovirus and Sapporo virus as sapovirus.[49] This HuCV classification system may allow the development of assays based on recombinant HuCV antigens or PCR products rather than the current cumbersome classification schemes that rely on human reagents (convalescent outbreak sera) of varying sensitivity and specificity. Molecular tools have already allowed the identification of HuCV as agents of both pediatric and adult viral gastroenteritis in foodborne outbreaks as well as outbreaks in nursing homes, hospitals, and a university setting. Despite the potential for future understanding of the contribution of individual HuCV to outbreaks of nonbacterial gastroenteritis, Norwalk virus still remains the prototypic agent of HuCV, and it is described in greater detail in the following section.

Norovirus

Epidemiology. Norovirus is worldwide in distribution. Of patients exposed to norovirus either naturally or experimentally, 50% develop clinical symptoms.[50] Studies evaluating the prevalence of anti-norovirus antibody among populations of various age groups initially demonstrated that the group from 3 months to 12 years of age had only a 5% antibody-positive rate. More recent epidemiologic studies, using baculovirus-expressed recombinant norovirus antigen in an enzyme-linked immunosorbent assay (ELISA), have demonstrated a serologic response in 49% of Finnish infants between 3 and 24 months of age.[51] These data contradict previous beliefs that norovirus most often caused disease in older children and adults.

Transmission of norovirus is most often fecal-oral. Unlike rotavirus, this usually involves the spread of infection to a large population through a common source rather than from direct, person-to-person contact. In one outbreak, an infected bakery employee transmitted the virus through food products to approximately 3000 people.[52] Outbreaks have also been related to ingestion of raw oysters and clams and to contaminated water supplies. Spread of this disease has been documented in closed-in populations such as those in long-term care facilities and cruise ships.[53] In addition to its fecal-oral spread, there is some evidence that norovirus is transmitted through a respiratory route in the form of aerosolized particles from vomitus. Contamination of environmental surfaces with norovirus has been documented during outbreaks.[54] Although previously referred to as "winter vomiting disease," norovirus produces outbreaks of disease that can occur throughout the year.[55] Several characteristics of norovirus facilitate their spread in epidemics: (1) low infectious dose (fewer than 10 viral particles), (2) prolonged viral shedding, (3) stability of the virus in relatively high concentrations of chlorine and a wide range of temperatures, and (4) the fact that repeated infections can occur with reexposure.[46]

Pathophysiology. The histologic changes induced by norovirus in an infected host have been studied in small bowel biopsies from infected volunteers. Those volunteers who remained free of clinical symptoms had normal biopsy specimens, whereas those with symptoms exhibited marked, but not specific, changes, including focal areas of villous flattening and disorganization of epithelial cells. On electron microscopy, microvilli were shortened, and there was dilatation of the endoplasmic reticulum. These volunteers had repeat biopsies 2 weeks after the illness, and normal histology was again present. Other investigators have demonstrated the presence of normal gastric and rectal histology in patients affected by norovirus as is typical of viral gastroenteritis. Using norovirus virus-like particles (derived from capsid proteins) researchers have recently demonstrated that human histo-blood group antigens may act as receptors for norovirus infection[56,57] and may explain the varying host susceptibility observed in outbreaks and volunteer studies.[58]

Clinical Manifestations. The clinical manifestations of disease produced by the norovirus include nausea, vomiting, and cramping abdominal pain (see Table 39-1). Diarrhea is said to be a less consistent feature of this illness. In the original outbreak, only 44% of patients experienced diarrhea, whereas 84% had vomiting. Other studies, however, have found that diarrhea occurs in most children and experimentally infected adult volunteers who become ill from this virus. Fever occurs in approximately one third of affected patients, but respiratory symptoms are not typically a part of this illness. An incubation period of approximately 24 to 48 hours has been noted before the onset of symptoms,[50] and symptoms persist for 12 to 48 hours. The typical symptoms of infection are in part also seen in premature infants but with a huge variety of clinical courses including abdominal distention, apnea, and sepsis-like appearance.[59]

Diagnosis and Treatment. Norwalk virus could be detected in fecal samples for a median of 4 weeks and for up to 8 weeks after virus inoculation; peak virus titers are most commonly found in fecal samples collected after resolution of symptoms, and presymptomatic shedding was more common in persons who did not meet the definition of clinical gastroenteritis.[60] RT-PCR assays have been developed for detection of noroviruses in clinical and environmental specimens, such as water and food.[61,62] RT-PCR followed by nucleotide sequencing has been useful in epidemiologic studies, and also various commercial stool enzyme immunoassay (EIA) detection methods have been developed[46]; the sensitivity is genotype dependent.[63] A rapid and accurate diagnostic assay is not widely available, but the presence of four epidemiologic features of norovirus disease can be useful in confirming norovirus as a cause of outbreaks: (1) vomiting in more than half of affected persons, (2) mean incubation period of 24 to 48 hours, (3) mean duration of illness of

12 to 60 hours, and (4) absence of bacterial pathogen in stool culture.[64]

The treatment for norovirus is supportive; oral rehydration solutions are used if necessary. Significant dehydration is uncommon, and the need for hospitalization is rare. A number of candidate vaccines are currently being evaluated.

Enteric Adenovirus

The enteric adenoviruses are among the more recently recognized viral pathogens that cause acute gastroenteritis. Adenoviruses are a large group of viruses long recognized for their role in the pathogenesis of respiratory infections and keratoconjunctivitis. Most of the 47 serotypes are known to be shed in the feces of infected patients. In patients with predominantly gastrointestinal symptoms, the organisms are detectable by electron microscopy of stool samples; however, they fail to grow in standard tissue culture conditions. Their unique cell culture requirements allow for the differentiation of nonenteric adenoviruses from the enteric serotypes (Ad40 and Ad41), which are recognized to be among the common causes of viral childhood gastroenteritis.[65]

Infection with enteric adenoviruses apparently occurs throughout the year, with only slight seasonal variation.[66] This disease tends to affect predominantly younger children, with most patients being younger than 2 years of age.[66,67] Enteric adenovirus is spread by the fecal-oral route. Transmission of the disease to family contacts is unusual.

Diarrhea is the most commonly reported symptom of enteric adenoviral infection. In contrast with diarrhea from other viral enteritides, diarrhea from enteric adenovirus typically persists for a prolonged period, sometimes as long as 14 days. Viruses may be excreted in the feces of infected patients for 1 to 2 weeks. Vomiting frequently occurs but is usually mild and of a much shorter duration than is the diarrhea. Dehydration has been seen in approximately half of affected patients, and hospitalization is sometimes necessary. The frequency of association of respiratory symptoms with enteric adenovirus infection is unclear.[67]

The diagnosis of enteric adenovirus is best made by electron microscopy or immunoelectron microscopy of stool samples or from intestinal biopsy specimens. ELISA and PCR techniques have also been used successfully in enteric adenovirus diagnosis. Treatment is mainly supportive, and oral rehydration solutions are useful in cases of dehydration.

Astrovirus

Astrovirus, similar to HuCV, is a single-stranded RNA virus grouped with the small round structured viruses. However, the recently derived sequence of the astrovirus RNA genome reveals that this agent is sufficiently different to be classified in its own family as Astroviridae.[68] Astrovirus is worldwide in distribution and tends to infect mainly children in the 1- to 3-year age group. In controlled studies in Thailand, astrovirus infection was the second most common cause of enteritis, after rotavirus infection, in symptomatic children.[69] Astrovirus infection occurred in 9% of children with diarrhea, compared with 2% of controls. Comparable findings have been reported in day-care centers in North America and Japan. Most children infected with astrovirus develop symptoms. Vomiting, diarrhea, abdominal pain, and fever all are commonly seen with infection by this agent, and symptoms typically last 1 to 4 days. Spread of the virus may occur via the fecal-oral route from person-to-person contact or through contaminated food or water. Asymptomatic shedding of astrovirus has also been reported.

Other Viruses

A variety of other viruses are being studied to determine what role, if any, they may play in the pathogenesis of human enteric infections. With the exception of those viruses previously discussed in detail, insufficient data are available to ascertain clinical and epidemiologic differences, if any, among the various small round viruses.

Pestivirus, a single-stranded RNA virus of the togavirus family, has been found in the feces of 24% of children living on an American Indian reservation who had diarrhea attributable to no other infectious agent.[70] These children experienced only mild diarrhea but had more severe respiratory complaints.

Coronavirus is known to cause an upper respiratory illness in humans and has been shown to cause diarrhea in some animals.[71] The role of this agent in human diarrheal disease is unclear, and at least one study found coronavirus more commonly in children without diarrhea than in those who were ill.[72] Coronavirus was implicated in an outbreak of necrotizing enterocolitis.[73]

Toroviruses are pleomorphic viruses recognized to cause enteric illness in a variety of animals. Members of this group, originally described in Berne, Switzerland, and Breda, Iowa, and named for those cities, have been seen in the feces of humans with diarrheal disease.[74] Because of the pleomorphic structure of toroviruses, electron microscopy was inadequate to prove an etiopathogenic role of these viruses in diarrheal disease. The more recent findings of torovirus-like particles by immunoassay, using validated anti-Breda virus antiserum, lends additional weight to the hypothesis that these are agents of human gastroenteritis.[75] Their causative role in human disease, however, remains unproved. Similarly, picobirnavirus is known to cause disease in animals and has been isolated from stools of humans with diarrheal illness.[76]

Cytomegalovirus has been associated with enteritis and colitis. Except for Ménétrier's disease, caused by gastric cytomegalovirus infection, enteritis and colitis seem to occur almost exclusively among immunocompromised patients. In this population, cytomegalovirus causes viremia and is carried by the blood stream to a variety of sites, including organs of the gastrointestinal tract. Diagnosis may be made by virus detection in feces, by demonstration of typical cytomegalic inclusion cells, or by in situ hybridization.[66]

BACTERIAL GASTROENTERITIS

Host-Defense Factors

For an infecting bacterial agent to cause diarrhea, it must first overcome the following gastrointestinal tract defenses: (1) gastric acidity, (2) intestinal motility, (3) mucus secretion, (4) normal intestinal microflora, and (5) specific mucosal and systemic immune mechanisms. Gastric acidity is the first barrier encountered by infecting organisms. Many studies have demonstrated the bactericidal properties of gastric juice at pH less than 4. In patients with achlorhydria or decreased gastric acid secretion, the gastric pH is higher, and this bactericidal effect is diminished. Gastric acidity serves to decrease the number of viable bacteria that proceed to the small intestine.

Organisms surviving the gastric acidity barrier are trapped within the mucous layer of the small intestine, facilitating their movement through the intestine by peristalsis. If motility in the intestine is abnormal or absent, organisms are more readily able to initiate the infectious process. Some organisms can elaborate toxic substances that impair intestinal motility. Increased intestinal peristalsis, which occurs during some enteric infections, may be an attempt by the host to rid itself of infective organisms.

In addition to its role in conjunction with intestinal motility, mucus also serves to provide a nonspecific barrier to bacterial proliferation and mucosal colonization. This barrier has been shown to be effective in preventing toxins from exerting their effects. Exfoliated mucosal cells trapped in the mucous layer may trap invading microorganisms. Mucus also contains carbohydrate analogues of surface receptors, which may prevent invading organisms from binding to actual receptors.

The normal endogenous microflora of the gut serves as its next line of defense. Anaerobes, which are a large component of the normal flora, elaborate short-chain fatty acids and lactic acid, which are toxic to many potential pathogens. In breastfed infants, this line of defense is enhanced by the presence of anaerobic lactobacilli, which produce fermentative products that act as toxins to foreign bacteria. Further evidence in support of the importance of endogenous microflora is the increase in susceptibility to infection after one's normal flora has been reduced by antibiotic administration, as is seen with *Clostridium difficile* infection.

The most complex element in the host-defense armamentarium involves the mucosal and systemic immune systems. Both serum and secretory antibodies may exert their protective effects at the intestinal level, even though the serum components are produced outside the gut. An immune response may be *specific* to a particular infective agent or *generalized* to a common group of bacterial antigens.

Mechanisms of Bacterial Disease Production

Bacteria have developed a variety of virulence factors (Table 39-2) to overcome host defense mechanisms: (1) *invasion* of the mucosa, followed by intraepithelial cell multiplication or invasion of the lamina propria; (2) production of *cytotoxins*, which disrupt cell function via direct alteration of the mucosal surface; (3) production of *enterotoxins*, polypeptides that alter cellular salt and water balance yet leave cell morphology undisturbed; and (4) *adherence* to the mucosal surface with resultant flattening of the microvilli and disruption of normal cell functioning. Each of the bacterial virulence mechanisms acts on specific regions of the intestine. Enterotoxins are primarily effective in the small bowel but can affect the colon; the effects of cytotoxins and direct epithelial cell invasion occur predominantly in the colon. Enteroadhesive mechanisms appear to function in both the small intestine and colon.

Salmonella

Members of the species *Salmonella* are currently recognized as the most common cause of bacterial diarrhea among children in the United States. Surveillance data from the Centers for Disease Control and Prevention show that in 2008 the incidence of *Salmonella* was 16.2 per 100,000, and although there was an apparent increase in *Salmonella* infections, this rate has not changed significantly over the past 3 years.[77] Infection caused by *Salmonella* may result in several different clinical syndromes, including

TABLE 39-2. Bacterial Pathogens Grouped by Pathogenic Mechanism

Invasive	Cytotoxic	Toxigenic	Adherent
Shigella	*Shigella*	*Shigella*	Enteropathogenic *E. coli*
Salmonella	Enteropathogenic *Escherichia coli*	Enterotoxigenic *E. coli*	Shiga toxin-producing *E. coli*
Yersinia enterocolitica	Shiga toxin-producing *E. coli*	*Yersinia enterocolitica*	Enteroaggregative *E. coli*
Campylobacter jejuni	*Clostridium difficile*	*Aeromonas*	Diffusely adherent *E. coli*
Vibrio parahaemolyticus		*V. cholerae* and non-O1 vibrios	

Modified from Cohen MB. Etiology and mechanisms of acute infectious diarrhea in infants in the United States. J Pediatr 1991; 118:S34-S43,[92] with permission.

(1) acute gastroenteritis; (2) focal, nonintestinal infections; (3) bacteremia; (4) asymptomatic carrier state; and (5) enteric fever (including typhoid fever). Each of these entities may be caused by any of the commonly recognized species of *Salmonella*.

Microbiology

Salmonella is a motile, gram-negative bacillus of the family Enterobacteriaceae. It can be identified on selective media because it does not ferment lactose. Three distinct species of *Salmonella* are recognized: *Salmonella enteritidis*, *Salmonella choleraesuis*, and *Salmonella typhi*. *S. enteritidis* is further subdivided into approximately 1700 serotypes. Each serotype is referred to by its genus and serotype names (e.g., *Salmonella typhimurium*) rather than the formally correct *S. enteritidis*, serotype *typhimurium*. *S. choleraesuis* and *S. typhi* are known to have only one serotype each. The most common serotypes in infants are Typhimurium, Newport, Javiana, Enteritidis, and Heidelberg.[78]

Epidemiology

Salmonella is estimated to cause 1 to 2 million gastrointestinal infections each year in the United States.[79] At Cincinnati Children's Hospital Medical Center, salmonellae are the most commonly isolated bacterial enteropathogens (Figure 39-1). The highest attack rate for salmonellosis is in infancy, with a lower incidence of symptomatic infection in patients older than 6 years of age.[79] Nontyphoidal *Salmonella* is usually spread via contaminated water supplies or foods, with meat, fresh produce, fowl, eggs, and raw milk frequently implicated.

A wide variety of foods have caused outbreaks of salmonella; a large outbreak involved contaminated alfalfa sprouts that were shipped worldwide.[80] Most of the egg-associated outbreaks have involved products such as mayonnaise, ice cream,[81] and cold desserts, in which salmonella can multiply profusely and which are eaten without cooking after the addition of, or contamination by, raw egg. Although "shell" eggs are frequently contaminated, the number of bacteria in infected eggs is often near or below the human infective dose. In contrast, with a generation time of 80 minutes at 20° C, one bacterium can become a billion in 40 hours, and with a generation time of 40 minutes at 25° C, it can do so in 20 hours.

Although any of these food sources may become contaminated through contact with an infected food handler, the farm animals themselves are often infected. Pets, notably cats, turtles, lizards, snakes, and chicks, may also harbor *Salmonella*. Person-to-person spread of infection also occurs and is especially common in cases involving infants. A population-based case-control study was done in infants less than 1 year of age and identified the following risk factors: (1) travel outside the United States, (2) attending day care with a child with diarrhea, (3) riding in a shopping cart next to meat or poultry; and (4) exposure to reptiles. Breast-feeding was found to be protective.[82]

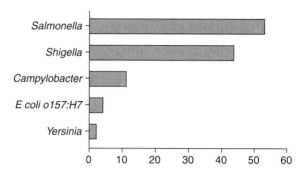

Figure 39-1. Bacterial enteropathogens isolated at Cincinnati Children's Hospital Medical Center (CCHMC) in the year 2008. In addition to stool cultures above, 256 specimens tested positive for *C. difficile* by toxin assay in the year 2008. A total of 4601 stool cultures and 2950 tests for *C. difficile* were sent in 2008. Data from Infection Control Office, CCHMC.

Pathogenesis

Inocula of fewer than 10^3 salmonellae are probably sufficient to cause disease.[83] Patients in whom host defenses are diminished are more likely to develop clinical manifestations of the disease. This has been demonstrated in patients who have reduced levels of gastric acid. Patients with lymphoproliferative diseases and hemolytic diseases, especially sickle cell anemia, are more likely to experience severe disease and develop complications from *Salmonella* infection. The mechanisms for this increased susceptibility may involve altered macrophage function, defective complement activation, or damage to the bones from thromboses.

Having overcome host defenses, *Salmonella* produces disease through a process that begins with colonization of the ileum and the colon. The organisms next invade enterocytes and colonocytes and proliferate within epithelial cells and in the lamina propria (Figure 39-2). From the lamina propria, *Salmonella* may then move to the mesenteric lymph nodes and eventually to the systemic circulation, causing bacteremia. Because these organisms invade enterocytes and colonocytes, both enteritis, with watery diarrhea, and colitis, with bloody diarrhea, may result. This multistage infection of the host is directed by *Salmonella*-mediated delivery of an array of specialized effector proteins into the eukaryotic host cells via two distinct secretion systems. Additional secretion systems appear to be functional and contribute toward virulence but are not currently well characterized.[84]

Clinical Manifestations

After an incubation period of 12 to 72 hours, *Salmonella* usually produces a mild, self-limited illness characterized by fever and watery diarrhea. Blood, mucus, or both are commonly present in the stool. Bacteremia occurs in approximately 6%

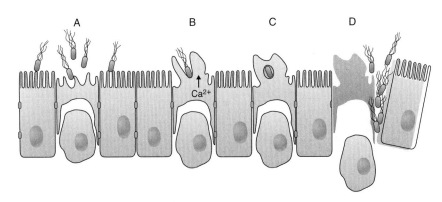

Figure 39-2. Interaction of enteropathogenic *Salmonella* species with the intestinal epithelium. Diagrammed are the interaction and invasion of salmonellae with an M cell and an absorptive epithelial cell overlying the Peyer's patch follicle. *Salmonella* invasion is shown for an M cell. Adherence of salmonellae to an M cell (**A**) is followed by *Salmonella* invasion-induced membrane ruffle (**B**). (**C**), Bacterium localized within an intracellular vacuole. (**D**), Destruction of the invaded M cell followed by an influx of bacteria into the epithelial cell breach and entry into Peyer's patch. From Hromockyj A, Falkow S. Interactions of bacteria with the gut epithelium. In: Blaser MJ, Smith PD, Ravdin JI, et al., eds. Infections of the Gastrointestinal Tract. New York: Raven Press; 1995.[97] Courtesy Brad Jones, PhD.

of *Salmonella* infections in children but much less frequently in adults. Patients may develop nonintestinal sequelae after *Salmonella* infection, including pneumonia, meningitis, and osteomyelitis.

Even in those patients in whom no sequelae occur, excretion of the organisms may persist for several weeks. In patients younger than 5 years of age, the median time of excretion is 7 weeks, with 2.6% of patients continuing to shed organisms for 1 year or longer.[85] Studies have also shown a higher incidence of the carrier state among children with salmonellosis than is seen in adults.[85] Localization of *Salmonella* organisms in chronic carriers is often in the biliary tract and is frequently associated with cholelithiasis.

Diagnosis and Treatment

Diagnosis of *Salmonella* infection can be made through stool or blood culture. Use of enriched media and culture of material from freshly passed stools, rather than from rectal swab, increase the likelihood of recovering the organism.[85] Owing to the increased risk of developing the carrier state, antimicrobial treatment of uncomplicated cases of *Salmonella* gastroenteritis is not recommended. Treatment is recommended in patients at high risk for the development of disseminated disease, including those who are immunocompromised, those with hematologic disease, patients with artificial implants, those with severe colitis, and pregnant women. Treatment is also recommended for patients at any age who appear toxic.

Treatment of all children younger than 1 year of age with salmonellosis remains controversial because of the risk of bacteremia and secondary infections. Antimicrobial therapy is recommended for infants with *Salmonella* bacteremia. Parenteral antibiotics are recommended for any infant (younger than 3 months of age) with a stool culture that is positive for *Salmonella*.[86]

Most *Salmonella* are sensitive to a wide variety of antibiotics, including ampicillin (35 mg/kg [maximum 1 g] per dose, given every 4 hours, intravenously, for 14 days), chloramphenicol (20 mg/kg [maximum 1 g] per dose, given every 6 hours, intravenously or orally, for 14 days), trimethoprim-sulfamethoxazole (trimethoprim, 5 mg/kg [maximum 160 mg], plus sulfamethoxazole, 25 mg/kg [maximum 800 mg] per dose, given every 12 hours, orally, for 14 days), and the third-generation cephalosporins. Resistance to ampicillin is increasing.[87] Ceftriaxone, cefotaxime, or a fluoroquinolone (not approved for use in children younger than 18 years of age) are often effective when resistance to other agents is demonstrated.

A follow-up stool culture usually is not warranted unless the patient is employed in the preparation of food. If evidence of a "cure" is necessary, two to three consecutive negative stool cultures, obtained 1 to 3 days apart, are sufficient.

Typhoid Fever

Although uncommon in the United States, typhoid fever, caused by *S. typhi*, commonly affects children in developing countries. *S. typhi* differs from other salmonellae in that it requires a human host. The disease it causes also differs in severity from the typically mild gastroenteritis caused by other members of the genus; *S. typhi* infection also has a higher case-fatality rate.

Typhoid fever typically begins with a period of fever lasting approximately 1 week. Patients then complain of headache and abdominal pain. Diarrhea is not usually a manifestation of typhoid fever, and many patients experience constipation. Hepatomegaly and splenomegaly have also been frequently noted. The characteristic "rose spots" (palpable, erythematous lesions), typical in adult cases of typhoid fever, occur with far less frequency in pediatric patients. Patients may become chronic carriers.

Diagnosis of typhoid fever is made on the basis of positive blood cultures. *S. typhi* is usually sensitive to several antimicrobial agents, including ampicillin, chloramphenicol, trimethoprim-sulfamethoxazole, cefotaxime, and ceftriaxone. Drug choice is based on site of infection and susceptibility of the organism. A recent Cochrane review[88] showed that azithromycin appears to be better than fluoroquinolones in populations with drug-resistant strains and that it may also perform better than ceftriaxone.

Two typhoid vaccines are commercially available; a live, oral Ty21a and injectable Vi polysaccharide. They have been shown to be safe and efficacious and are licensed for people aged more than 2 years.[89,90] Immunization of school-age or preschool-age children is recommended in areas where typhoid fever is shown to be a significant public health problem, particularly where antibiotic-resistant *S. typhi* is prevalent. Vaccination may be offered to travelers to destinations where the risk of typhoid fever is high, especially to those staying in endemic areas for longer than 1 month.[89]

Other vaccines, such as a new modified, conjugated Vi vaccine called Vi-rEPA, are in development and may confer longer immunity.[90]

Shigella

Bacillary dysentery, an illness caused by *Shigella*, was described in ancient Greece. Osler, in 1892, referred to the disease as "one of the four great epidemic diseases of the world." He further stated: "In the tropics it destroys more lives than cholera, and it has been more fatal to armies than powder and shot." Despite our increased knowledge of the pathogenesis and treatment of shigellosis, this organism continues to be a significant cause of diarrheal disease.

Microbiology

Shigella is a gram-negative, nonmotile, non-lactose-fermenting aerobic bacillus, closely related to members of the genus *Escherichia*. The organisms are classified into four species or groups known as *Shigella dysenteriae*, *Shigella flexneri*, *Shigella boydii*, and *Shigella sonnei* (groups A, B, C, and D, respectively). Members of groups A, B, and C exist in numerous serotypes, but only one serotype of group D is known. *S. sonnei* is the most commonly recovered *Shigella* species in the developed world, accounting for 70% of isolates in the United States. *S. dysenteriae* and *S. flexneri* are the most commonly recovered species of *Shigella* in the developing world.[91]

Epidemiology

Shigella is worldwide in its distribution, and the incidence and severity of shigellosis span an equally broad range. In 2008, FoodNet calculated the incidence of *Shigella* infection in the United States to be 6.59 per 100,000.[77] Although *Shigella* occurs much less frequently in the developed world, in some studies it is the second most common pathogen identified in cases of bacterial diarrhea in children aged 6 months to 10 years.[92] It may also be the most common bacterial cause of outbreaks of diarrhea in day-care settings. Outbreaks of shigellosis have also been described in residential institutions and on cruise ships. This disease is endemic on American Indian reservations in the Southwest.

Shigella is predominantly spread via the fecal-oral route, with person-to-person contact the most likely method. Secondary spread to household contacts may occur. The infection may be spread through contamination of food and water, as often occurs in areas of poor sanitation and inadequate personal hygiene.

Risk exposures for cases include international travel in the week before symptom onset, attending or working in day care, contact with a child or household member with diarrheal illness, using untreated drinking water or recreational water, and sexual contact with someone with diarrhea.[78] It is important to know that shigellosis should still be considered in patients with watery diarrhea even without a contact history.[93]

Clinical Manifestations

Patients infected with *Shigella* may experience a mild, self-limited, watery diarrhea that is clinically indistinguishable from gastroenteritis caused by a variety of other agents. The more classic form of shigellosis, however, is bacillary dysentery. This illness usually begins with fever and malaise, followed by watery diarrhea and cramping abdominal pain. By the second day of illness, blood and mucus are usually present in the stools, and tenesmus has become a prominent symptom. At this point, in approximately 50% of affected patients, the stool volume decreases, with only scant amounts of blood and mucus being passed.[91] This pattern of bloody, mucus-containing stools is referred to as *dysentery*. Bacteremia is an uncommon feature of this illness, but several other complications have been reported, including seizures (in children),

arthritis, purulent keratitis, and the hemolytic-uremic syndrome (HUS). Nonsuppurative arthritis is the most commonly occurring extraintestinal complication of shigellosis. Patients who carry the histocompatibility locus antigen HLA-B27 may be predisposed to the development of this complication as well as to the development of Reiter's syndrome. The association of seizures with shigellosis was earlier attributed to the neurotoxic effect of the *Shigella* toxin (Shiga toxin). It now seems likely, however, that the seizures may simply represent a subgroup of common febrile seizures and have no direct relation to the effects of Shiga toxin.

Pathogenesis

Shigella has been found to cause disease only in humans and in the higher apes.[91] The organisms are potent, with as few as 10 organisms being able to cause disease in a healthy adult.[91] Patients infected with *Shigella* may excrete 10^5 to 10^8 organisms per gram of feces. This high rate of excretion and the relatively low number of organisms required to produce disease make possible the widespread distribution of disease.

For *Shigella* to exert its pathologic effect on a host, the bacteria must first come into contact with the surface of an intestinal epithelial cell and induce cytoskeletal rearrangements resulting in phagocytosis.[94,95] The bacteria then secrete enzymes that degrade the phagosomal membrane, releasing the bacteria into the host cytoplasm. Intracytoplasmic bacteria move rapidly, in association with a comet tail made up of host-cell actin filaments. When moving bacteria reach the cell margin, they push out long protrusions with the bacteria at the tips that are then taken up by neighboring cells, allowing the infection to spread from cell to cell (Figure 39-3).

Shiga toxin is elaborated by all species, although in greater amounts by *S. dysenteriae* than by other species,[91] and may play a role in the pathogenesis of *Shigella* infection. The toxin has neurotoxic, enterotoxic, and cytotoxic effects.[91] Structurally, it is composed of an active, or A, subunit (molecular weight 32 kDa) surrounded by five binding, or B, subunits (77 kDa).[91] The B subunits bind to cell-specific receptors and are taken up by endocytosis. Within the cells, the B subunits are cleaved away, and the remaining A subunit is shortened by proteolysis. This molecule is thought then to bind to the 60S ribosome and inhibit protein synthesis, leading to cell death and sloughing.[96] This is the presumed mechanism for the cytotoxic effect. An enterotoxic effect of Shiga toxin in the ileum may account for the early watery diarrhea.

Diagnosis and Treatment

In patients with signs and symptoms of colitis, the diagnosis of shigellosis should be considered. Stool culture provides the only definitive means to differentiate this organism from other invasive pathogens. *Shigella* may be cultured from stool specimens or rectal swabs, especially if mucus is present, but there may be a delay of several days from the onset of symptoms to the recovery of organisms. Sigmoidoscopy or colonoscopy typically reveals a friable mucosa, possibly with discrete ulcers. Rectal biopsy may be useful to differentiate shigellosis from ulcerative colitis.

In addition to rehydration, antimicrobial therapy has been recommended for *Shigella* (1) to shorten the course of the disease, (2) to decrease the period of excretion of the organisms, and (3) to decrease the secondary attack rate, because humans provide the only reservoir for the organism. However,

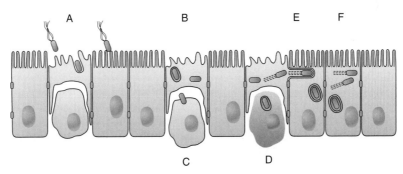

Figure 39-3. Interaction of *Shigella* species with the gut epithelium. Diagrammed is the putative interaction of shigellae with M cells overlying Peyer's patch follicles as well as absorptive epithelial cells. Invasion is diagrammed for an M cell. (**A, B**) Adherence to and intimate association of shigellae with an M cell followed by localization of the invading organism with an intracellular cytoplasmic vacuole. (**C-E**) Bacteria, having transcytosed the M cell, may interact with Peyer's patch macrophages and induce macrophage apoptosis. Bacteria free within the target cell cytoplasm also move within the host cell via an actin-associated tail. (**F**) *Shigella* intercellular invasion through a host cell membrane protrusion, followed by residence of the invading organism within a double-membraned intracellular cytoplasmic vacuole and escape from that vacuole. From Hromockyj A, Falkow S. Interactions of bacteria with the gut epithelium. In: Blaser MJ, Smith PD, Ravdin JI, et al., eds. Infections of the Gastrointestinal Tract. New York: Raven Press; 1995,[97] with permission.

handwashing, rather than use of antimicrobials, is the most effective method to prevent person-to-person spread. Those clinicians who advise against the routine treatment of shigellosis with antibiotics argue that (1) the disease is most often self-limited and (2) the use of antibiotics may facilitate the development of resistant strains and may increase the likelihood of developing HUS.

We recommend antibiotic therapy only for patients who are severely ill at the time of diagnosis or who remain ill at the time of identification of *Shigella* in a stool culture. A wide range of antibiotics has been used to treat *Shigella*, necessitated by the development of resistant strains. Currently, the agent of choice is trimethoprim-sulfamethoxazole (trimethoprim, 5 mg/kg [maximum 160 mg], plus sulfamethoxazole, 25 mg/kg [maximum 800 mg] per dose, given every 12 hours, orally or intravenously, for 5 days). Ampicillin (25 mg/kg [maximum 500 mg] per dose, given every 6 hours, orally or intravenously, for 5 days) may be used if local strains are typically susceptible.[97] Amoxicillin is ineffective against *Shigella*. Nalidixic acid (55 mg/kg per day given every 6 hours for 5 days) has proved effective. Cefixime and ceftriaxone are alternative agents for resistant organisms.[91] Tetracycline, ciprofloxacin, and norfloxacin have been used successfully for the treatment of *Shigella*, but these agents are approved for use only in adult patients. Multidrug-resistant strains have occurred in Latin America, central Africa, and Southeast Asia.[98]

Development of a vaccine for shigellosis continues to be a challenge. These efforts include vaccines using a modified *Escherichia coli* strain; one using a mutant strain of *S. flexneri*, which lacks the ability to proliferate intracellularly; and one based on a strain with mutations in its virulence genes. Vaccine development continues to be limited by the lack of a suitable animal model.[99]

Campylobacter

Campylobacter is a gram-negative, motile, curved or spiral-shaped rod, exhibiting a "seagull" appearance when identified in stained stool smears. Multiple species of *Campylobacter* have been recognized, including *Campylobacter jejuni*, *Campylobacter fetus*, *Campylobacter coli*, and *Campylobacter laridis*, with *C. jejuni* being the one most commonly associated with disease in humans. *Campylobacter upsaliensis* has been reported

as another member of this group that causes diarrhea,[100] and it seems probable that still others may be identified.

Epidemiology

Campylobacter is recognized to be worldwide in distribution. In developing countries, *Campylobacter* is a significant bacterial cause of diarrhea in children younger than 2 years of age, yet it rarely occurs in developing nations in older children and adults. When infection does occur in the population older than 2 years of age, it tends to be asymptomatic.[101] It is likely that patients in these countries are infected with *Campylobacter* early in life and then develop immunity, thus making asymptomatic infection more typical in older children and adults.

In the industrialized world, most patients infected with *Campylobacter* develop symptoms.[101] The number of *Campylobacter* infections in these countries is now recognized to be quite high, with some studies finding this organism to be the most common cause of bacterial diarrhea. *Campylobacter* tends to infect people in two distinct age groups: children in the first year of life and young adults. *Campylobacter* spp. is the most common cause of bacterial enteric infections in the United States, causing an estimated 2 million infections annually.[102]

Campylobacter may be spread by direct contact or through contaminated sources of food and water. Milk, meat, and eggs, especially if undercooked, have been implicated in outbreaks. These sources may be contaminated from human fecal shedding, or the organisms may be harbored in the asymptomatic farm animals. *Campylobacter* is commonly spread among populations of children in day-care centers. A population-based case-control study showed that risk factors for campylobacteriosis were drinking well water, eating fruits and vegetables prepared in the home, having a pet in the home with diarrhea, visiting or living on a farm, riding in a shopping cart next to meat or poultry, and traveling outside of the United States. Infants with campylobacteriosis were less likely to be breast-fed or to be in a household where hamburger was prepared.[103]

Pathogenesis

The mechanisms through which *Campylobacter* produces disease are not fully understood but likely involve three potential mechanisms[104]: (1) adherence to the intestinal mucosa followed by the elaboration of toxin; (2) invasion of the mucosa in the terminal ileum and colon; and (3) "translocation," in which the organisms penetrate the mucosa and replicate in the lamina propria and mesenteric lymph nodes. The variety of pathogenic mechanisms may account for the spectrum of disease caused by *Campylobacter*. It is also conceivable that different strains or serotypes of *Campylobacter* may demonstrate different pathogenic mechanisms, as is seen with diarrheagenic *E. coli*.

Clinical Manifestations

Campylobacter may cause disease ranging from mild diarrhea to frank dysentery. Typically, patients experience fever and malaise followed by diarrhea, nausea, and abdominal pain that may mimic appendicitis or inflammatory bowel disease. The symptoms usually resolve in less than 1 week. Bacteremia may rarely occur, with some species implicated more often than are others. *Campylobacter* is also known to cause meningitis, abscesses, septic abortions, pancreatitis, and pneumonia. Guillain-Barré syndrome and Reiter's syndrome are documented to occur as sequelae of *Campylobacter* infection. Increasing evidence has implicated *C. jejuni* as the most common antecedent of Guillain-Barré syndrome and the variant form, Miller-Fisher syndrome, a neuropathy associated with ataxia, areflexia, and ophthalmoplegia.[105,106] Although evidence for molecular mimicry is still preliminary, it is likely that peripheral nerves share epitopes with *C. jejuni*; therefore, the immune response initially mounted to attack *C. jejuni* is misdirected to peripheral nerves.[106] After the resolution of symptoms, patients may continue to shed organisms for as long as 7 weeks.

Diagnosis and Treatment

Culture of the organisms, the gold standard for diagnosis, is routinely accomplished in most laboratories if selective media are used and cultures are incubated at 42° C. Because disease caused by *Campylobacter* is usually mild and self-limited, supportive treatment alone should suffice. In cases of severe disease, erythromycin (10 mg/kg [maximum 500 mg] per dose, given every 6 hours for 5 to 7 days) has been recommended.[97] The need for antibiotic therapy has been questioned, based in part on several studies demonstrating a decrease in the duration of excretion of *Campylobacter* after antibiotic treatment but no decrease in the duration of symptoms. In general, in these studies, antimicrobial therapy was begun late in the course of the illness. In a placebo-controlled, double-blind trial, Salazar-Lindo and colleagues[107] demonstrated a shortened duration of illness, from 4.2 to 2.5 days, in patients who received erythromycin by day 4 of their illness. For cases of *Campylobacter* septicemia, gentamicin (1.5 to 2.5 mg/kg per dose, intramuscularly or intravenously, given every 8 hours) is recommended, with chloramphenicol and erythromycin acceptable as alternatives. Tetracycline (250 to 500 mg per dose, intravenously, given every 6 to 12 hours) may be used in patients older than 8 years of age.[97] Ciprofloxacin is an effective alternative agent but is not approved for use in children younger than 18 years of age. Antibiotic treatment is recommended for outbreaks of *Campylobacter* in day-care settings, because treatment has been shown to eliminate fecal shedding of organisms within 48 hours.[104]

Yersinia

Microbiology

The genus *Yersinia* includes the species *Yersinia pestis*, which causes plague; *Yersinia pseudotuberculosis*, known to cause pseudoappendicitis, mesenteric adenitis, and gastroenteritis; and *Yersinia enterocolitica*, recognized with increasing frequency as a cause of bacterial diarrhea. *Yersinia* is a gram-negative, coccoid bacillus that is facultatively anaerobic. It is non-lactose-fermenting and is observed to be motile at temperatures of 25° C but nonmotile at 37° C.

Epidemiology

Yersinia was initially thought to occur with greater frequency in countries with cooler climates but is now recognized to be worldwide in distribution. Although the true incidence and prevalence of this organism are not known, in some areas yersiniosis occurs more frequently than does shigellosis.[108] Outbreaks due to *Yersinia* have been associated with spread through contaminated water and foods, including bean sprouts, tofu, and chocolate milk.[108] Pork has also been implicated as a source, as in the Fulton County, Georgia, outbreak in 1990, in which chitterlings were found to be the vehicle of infection.[109,110] The organism tends to cause disease more frequently in young children, with 24 months the median age in one study.[111] *Yersinia* may also be spread among household contacts. In addition, there may be an increased incidence in the summer months.[111,108] A case control study from Sweden reported that risk factors for acquiring *Y. enterocolitica* in children less than 6 years of age were foods prepared from unprocessed raw pork products and treated sausages. Other factors were the use of pacifiers and contact with domestic animals.[112]

Pathogenesis

Y. enterocolitica constitutes a heterogeneous group of serotypes with many identified virulence factors.[113] *Y. enterocolitica* produces disease in the intestine through an invasive route. After penetrating the mucosal epithelium, primarily in the ileum, organisms replicate in Peyer's patches and accumulate in the mesenteric lymph nodes.[108] Most serotypes produce an enterotoxin similar to the *E. coli* heat-stable toxin but only at temperatures lower than 30° C; therefore, this toxin may *not* have an important role in disease production by *Yersinia* in the human intestine. There is speculation on the role of preformed toxin in causing disease, because toxin may be produced when the organisms are present in refrigerated foods.[108]

The virulence of *Y. enterocolitica* has been shown to be plasmid related. Different serotypes exhibit different degrees of virulence. Serotypes O:3, and O:9 are the ones most frequently associated with diarrheal disease in Europe and Japan, whereas a larger number of serotypes are seen in North America.[113]

Clinical Manifestations

The most frequent clinical syndrome caused by *Y. enterocolitica* is gastroenteritis, which typically affects young children. After an incubation period of 1 to 11 days, patients develop diarrhea, fever, and abdominal pain.[108] A marked increase in the leukocyte count is common. The symptoms usually resolve in 5 to 14 days but have been known to persist for several months. Excretion of organisms occurs for about 6 weeks.[111] Several complications, including appendicitis, have been documented after *Y. enterocolitica* infection. However, in older children and young adults, *Yersinia* is more likely to produce the pseudoappendicular syndrome, in which the signs and symptoms mimic appendicitis.[108] In this same age group, there has also been an association of *Y. enterocolitica* with nonspecific abdominal pain. Radiographic changes in the terminal ileum more often associated with Crohn's disease, namely mucosal thickening and aphthous ulcers, have been seen with yersiniosis in young adults.

Yersinia bacteremia occurs and, despite therapy with appropriate antibiotics, has a case-fatality rate of 34 to 50%. The finding of *Yersinia* in blood from asymptomatic donors, however, makes the possibility of transient bacteremia seem likely as well.[108]

Sequelae of *Yersinia* infection include erythema nodosum and reactive arthropathy; however, these are more commonly seen in adults.[113] This arthropathy tends to involve the weight-bearing joints of the lower extremities and has been noted to occur most often in *Yersinia* patients who carry the histocompatibility antigen HLA-B27.

Diagnosis and Treatment

Yersinia may be cultured with the use of selective media, preferably with "cold enrichment." Despite the best of methods, culture of *Yersinia* may require as long as 4 weeks. In addition to diagnosis by culture, *Yersinia* may also be detected serologically, through the use of agglutinin titers. These measurements appear to be useful only in conjunction with cultures, because agglutinin titers may be affected by a number of factors, including the patient's age, the underlying disease, and previous use of antibiotics and immunosuppressive agents. These titers may also be more useful in Europe and Japan, where infection is caused by a restricted number of serotypes.

Antibiotics have not been proved effective in alleviating symptoms of *Yersinia* or in shortening the period of its excretion.[108] Pai and associates[114] compared the efficacy of trimethoprim-sulfamethoxazole versus placebo in the treatment of *Yersinia* gastroenteritis and found no significant difference. It should be noted, however, that therapy was not begun until near the end of the course of the illness. In cases of severe disease and in patients with underlying illness, treatment is recommended. Trimethoprim-sulfamethoxazole, aminoglycosides, chloramphenicol, and third-generation cephalosporins are generally recommended. Tetracycline and quinolones are alternative choices for adult patients.[97] Gentamicin or chloramphenicol is recommended for treatment of septicemia. Because septicemia may be associated with an iron overload state,[115] cessation of iron therapy is also recommended during infection.

Cholera

Although cholera is a disease rarely encountered in developed countries, it remains an important entity.[116,117] Investigation of the pathogenesis of cholera led to the recognition and understanding of the mechanism of action of cholera toxin, which remains the prototype for bacterial enterotoxins. Cholera is also important, from a therapeutic perspective, in that initial efforts in the use of oral rehydration solutions were carried out in patients with cholera. However, most importantly, on a worldwide basis, cholera continues to be a major public health problem in almost all developing countries.[118] Cholera afflicts both children and adults, and cholera exists as an endemic disease in more than 100 countries. The death rate is highly dependent on the treatment facilities; the highest mortality rates are in Africa, where case-fatality rates have approximated 10%, especially during epidemic attacks. It is likely that cholera as an endemic infection causes 100,000 to 150,000 deaths annually.

Microbiology

Vibrio cholerae is a gram-negative, motile, curved bacillus that is free-living in bodies of salt water. *V. cholerae* is classified on the basis of lipopolysaccharide antigens. Until recently, all epidemic strains of *V. cholerae* were of the O1 serotype. Group O1 is further subdivided into two biotypes: classic and El Tor. Other serotypes were thought to cause sporadic cases of diarrhea but not epidemic disease. This dictum was discarded after the development of an ongoing epidemic in Asia and South America caused by a new serotype, O139, synonym Bengal.[119] Although the pathogenesis and clinical features of O139 cholera are identical to those of O1 cholera, persons having immunity to serotype O1 are not immune to the Bengal serotype. This lack of immunity is primarily a result of the unique O139 cell surface antigen.

Epidemiology

V. cholerae is spread via contamination of food and water supplies. There is no evidence of an animal reservoir, but humans may serve as transient carriers. On rare occasions, humans may chronically carry the organism. Owing to the nature of its spread, persons living in areas with adequate sanitation are at minimal, if any, risk for encountering cholera. Cholera does occur in the United States, but usually as a result of imported food brought back by returning international travelers. Travelers from the United States to endemic areas are at low risk (incidence of 1 per 30,000 travelers).[120] Cholera has also been isolated from oysters in the Gulf Coast.[121] However, owing to the frequency of international travel, it is important for the clinician who encounters a patient with severe cholera symptoms (dehydration and rice-water stools) to suspect this infection even in nonendemic areas.

Pathogenesis

V. cholerae enters its potential host through the oral route, usually in contaminated food or water. Volunteer studies have shown that a relatively large number of organisms (approximately 10^{11}) must be ingested to produce symptoms. Similar to other ingested organisms, *V. cholerae* must survive the acidic gastric environment. The importance of gastric acidity as a host-protective factor is borne out by the increased occurrence of cholera in patients with absent or reduced gastric acidity.

The organisms travel to the small intestine, where they adhere to the epithelium. This process may be aided by production of mucinase. The intestinal epithelium remains intact with normal morphology. *Vibrio* species produce a toxin that is composed of a central subunit (A) surrounded by five B subunits; the latter bind to a ganglioside, GM_1, which serves as the toxin receptor. This binding facilitates the transfer of the A subunit across the cell membrane, where it is cleaved into two components, denoted A_1 and A_2. The disulfide linkage between A_1 and A_2 is reduced to liberate an active A_1 peptide, which acts as a catalyst to facilitate the transfer of adenosine diphosphate-ribose from nicotinamide adenine dinucleotide to a guanyl nucleotide-binding regulatory protein (G_s). G_s then stimulates adenylate cyclase, located on the basolateral membrane, thereby increasing cyclic adenosine monophosphate. This result in turn leads to chloride secretion and a net flux of fluid into the intestinal lumen.

Although this mechanism of toxin action adequately explains the clinical symptoms of cholera, similar symptoms have been noted in patients infected with strains that do *not* produce the classic cholera toxin. This has led to the recognition that *V. cholerae* harbors additional virulence factors in the bacterial genome that may contribute to diarrheal disease and must be considered in the design of a nonreactigenic vaccine.

Newly recognized toxins produced by *V. cholerae* include zonula occludens toxin and the accessory cholera toxin.[122,123]

Clinical Manifestations

After an incubation period, commonly 1 to 3 days, the symptoms of cholera usually begin abruptly with profuse, watery diarrhea and sometimes with vomiting. The stool soon becomes clear, with bits of mucus giving it the so-called rice-water appearance. Patients do not experience tenesmus but rather a sense of relief with defecation. Typically there is no fever. The rate of fluid loss with cholera can be remarkable in severe disease, with purging rates in excess of 1 L/hour reported in adult patients. Despite the dramatic presentation and health risk of "*cholera gravis*," most patients with cholera infection are asymptomatic or experience mild symptoms. In addition to people with reduced gastric acidity, people with blood group O are at increased risk for more severe disease. Other host factors that predispose to increased purging are less clear, but there is great variability in clinical symptoms after infection.

Diagnosis and Treatment

V. cholerae is identified by colonial morphology and pigmentation on selective agar (e.g., thiosulfate citrate bile salt-sucrose agar). Further identification depends on biochemical markers (e.g., positive oxidase reaction) and motility of the organism. Specific serotyping is used to confirm the identification.

The mainstay of cholera treatment is rehydration. In cases in which the disease is less severe and is recognized early, oral rehydration solutions are appropriate and effective. When purging is excessive (more than 10 mL/kg per hour), intravenous rehydration is required.

Antibiotics have been shown to cause a decrease in duration of the diarrhea, total amount of fluid lost, and length of time organisms are excreted. Tetracycline (250 to 500 mg per dose, given every 6 hours for 3 to 5 days) has been recommended as an appropriate antibiotic for adults, and furazolidone (1.25 mg/kg [maximum 100 mg] per dose, given every 6 hours for 10 days) has been suggested for children and pregnant patients. Ampicillin, chloramphenicol, trimethoprim-sulfamethoxazole, and doxycycline may also be used. Single-dose ciprofloxacin has also been shown to be effective in the treatment of *V. cholerae* O1 or O139,[124] although this drug is not approved for use in children. A recent randomized controlled trial showed that a single dose of azithromycin 20 mg/kg was superior to ciprofloxacin for treating cholera in children.[125]

Despite much progress, an ideal cholera vaccine is not yet available. An ideal vaccine would provide a high level of long-term protection even to those at high risk for severe illness (e.g., people with blood group type O), and this protection would commence shortly after administration of a single oral dose. New oral vaccines have been developed for cholera, including both killed vaccines and live attenuated strains.[126,127] CVD 103-HgR, a vaccine strain with a 94% deletion of the *ctxA*, proved efficacious against experimental challenge with *V. cholerae* El Tor Inaba 3 months after inoculation, suggesting it may be useful for travelers to endemic areas.[128] Unfortunately CVD 103-HgR was not effective in a field trial.[129] Peru-15, a nonmotile strain that colonizes better than CVD 103-HgR, has been shown to be highly effective in volunteer studies.[130] A reformulated bivalent (*V. cholerae* O1 and O139) killed whole cell oral vaccine was also found to be safe and immunogenic in a cholera-endemic area in India.[131] Other live attenuated O1 oral cholera vaccines are in earlier stages of development including VA1.3 vaccine from India, IEM 108 from China,[132] and an intranasal vaccine.[133]

Other Vibrios

The noncholera vibrios, *V. parahaemolyticus*, *V. pluvialis*, *V. mimicus*, *V. hollisae*, *V. furnissii*, and *V. vulnificans*, have been shown to cause gastrointestinal illness, wound infections, and septicemia.[134] Although each organism has its own characteristics, most noncholera vibrios produce a protein toxin identical to the classic cholera toxin. Some species also produce a heat-stable toxin similar to *E. coli* heat-stable toxin.[135] Although these organisms produce a cholera-like illness, the stool may sometimes contain blood and leukocytes, and sepsis can occur. This has led to speculation that some members of this group, namely *V. parahaemolyticus*, may be capable of invasiveness as well as toxin production.[134] In the United States, gastroenteritis caused by these vibrios is most often associated with the ingestion of raw oysters.[136]

Gastroenteritis caused by non-O1 vibrios tends to be far milder than that caused by *V. cholerae*. In severe cases of diarrhea or septicemia, antibiotics may be helpful, with the agents used for *V. cholerae* recommended.

Escherichia coli

E. coli constitutes a diverse group of organisms, including both nonpathogenic strains, which are among the most common bacteria in the normal flora of the human intestine, and pathogenic strains. Pathogenic *E. coli* strains that cause diarrheal illness have been recognized since the 1940s.[137]

These diarrheagenic *E. coli* have been studied extensively and are currently classified, on the basis of serogrouping or pathogenic mechanisms, into six major groups: (1) enteropathogenic *E. coli* (EPEC), an important cause of diarrhea in infants in developing countries; (2) enterotoxigenic *E. coli* (ETEC), a cause of diarrhea in infants in developing areas of the world and a cause of traveler's diarrhea in adults; (3) enteroinvasive *E. coli* (EIEC), which cause either a watery ETEC-like illness or, less commonly, a dysentery-like illness; (4) Shiga toxin-producing *E. coli* (Stx-producing; formerly known as enterohemorrhagic *E. coli*), which cause hemorrhagic colitis and HUS; (5) enteroaggregative *E. coli* (EAggEC); and (6) diffusely adherent *E. coli* (DAEC), which along with EPEC have been implicated as causes of acute and persistent diarrhea. Each of these groups of *E. coli* has unique properties (Table 39-3).

Enteropathogenic *Escherichia coli*

EPEC is a major cause of diarrhea in developing countries. As much as 30% to 40% of infant diarrhea, particularly in those less than 6 months of age, may be caused by EPEC, and in some studies EPEC infection exceeds that of rotavirus.[138-141] In North America and the United Kingdom, EPEC infections were common during the 1940s through the 1960s; now they are most commonly associated with sporadic cases and nosocomial or day-care outbreaks.[142,143] However, because of the general unavailability of serotyping, the true incidence of EPEC-associated diarrhea may be underestimated. A 1997 study in Seattle children with diarrhea, and a 2005 study in Cincinnati in which DNA probes were used to screen *E. coli* present in stool, found a high incidence of EPEC-like organisms (atypical EPEC) in this population.[144,145]

TABLE 39-3. **Diarrheagenic** *Escherichia coli*

Name	Abbreviation	Pathogenic Mechanisms	Illness
Enteropathogenic *E. coli*	EPEC	Adherence to enterocytes	Infantile diarrhea in developing countries
Enterotoxigenic *E. coli*	ETEC	Enterotoxin elaboration	Infantile diarrhea in developing countries; traveler's diarrhea
Enteroinvasive *E. coli*	EIEC	Invasion of epithelial cells; toxin elaboration	Watery diarrhea/dysentery
Stx-producing *E. coli**	Stx	Cytotoxin elaboration Adherence	Hemorrhagic colitis; hemolytic-uremic syndrome
Enteroaggregative *E. coli*	EAggEC	Adherence Enterotoxin elaboration	Persistent diarrhea in developing countries
Diffusely adherent *E. coli*	DAEC	Adherence	Diarrhea

*Formerly enterohemorrhagic *E. coli* (EHEC).

The hallmark of EPEC infection is the "attaching and effacing" lesion seen in the intestine. This lesion is characterized by destruction of microvilli and intimate adherence between the bacterium and the epithelial cell membrane. Directly beneath the surface of the adherent organism, there are marked cytoskeletal changes in the enterocyte, including accumulation of actin polymers. Often, the bacteria are raised on a pedestal-like structure as a result of this actin accumulation. A number of steps are probably responsible for the development of this attaching and effacing lesion. As proposed by Donnenberg and Kaper,[146] EPEC pathogenesis consists of three phases: (1) localized adherence, which brings the bacteria in close contact with the enterocyte (e.g., docking); (2) signal transduction, including increases in intracellular calcium and protein phosphorylation; and (3) intimate adherence, a multigene process encoded in the bacterium by a locus of enterocyte effacement.[147,148] The dramatic loss of absorptive microvilli in the intestine presumably leads to diarrhea via malabsorption. Although this is probably the predominant mechanism, some evidence suggests that a separate secretory mechanism is also involved.

Patients with symptomatic EPEC infection typically experience diarrhea, vomiting, malaise, and fever. The stool may contain mucus but does not usually contain blood. Symptoms with EPEC infection are more severe than with some other enteric infections and may persist for 2 weeks or longer.[137] In some patients, EPEC has caused protracted diarrhea with dehydration, malnutrition, and zinc deficiency as complications; treatment with parenteral hyperalimentation has been required.[143] EPEC can be detected by serotyping of isolated *E. coli*,[142] by demonstration of the presence of the enterocyte adherence factor or other virulence genes using molecular probes,[149] or by identification of the attaching and effacing phenotype using tissue culture cells.[150] These assays are not commonly used in the clinical microbiology laboratory. Diagnosis of EPEC may be made by demonstrating the presence of adherent organisms on small intestinal or rectal biopsy.[142,143]

Although controlled studies of antibiotic therapy for EPEC have been few, the significant morbidity associated with this agent argues for treatment with antibiotics in most cases. Trimethoprim-sulfamethoxazole (trimethoprim, 5 mg/kg [maximum 160 mg], plus sulfamethoxazole, 25 mg/kg [maximum 800 mg] per dose, given every 12 hours) has been used with some success, as have oral neomycin and gentamicin.

Enterotoxigenic *Escherichia coli*

ETEC are recognized as an important cause of diarrhea in infants in developing areas of the world. In endemic areas, children in the first few years of life may be infected several times each year. It is an important cause of diarrhea in infants and in travelers from developed to undeveloped countries, especially in regions of poor sanitation.[151] In the United States, cases of ETEC among children are uncommon. ETEC is also a major cause of traveler's diarrhea in adults. Fecal-oral transmission and consumption of heavily contaminated food or water are the most common vehicles for ETEC infection. The prevention of the spread of ETEC depends on ensuring appropriate sanitary measures: handwashing and proper preparation of food, chlorination of water supplies, and appropriate sewage treatment and disposal.[151]

The production of disease by ETEC begins with colonization of the small intestine. There the bacteria depend on fimbriae (also called *pili*) to facilitate attachment to the mucosal surface and overcome the forward motion of peristalsis. This attachment process causes no detectable structural changes in the architecture of the brush border membrane but does allow the bacteria to release their enterotoxins, heat-labile toxin (LT) and heat-stable toxin (ST), in close proximity to the enterocyte brush border membrane where toxin receptors are present.[152] These toxins in turn stimulate adenylate cyclase (in the case of LT) or guanylate cyclase (in the case of ST), and both ultimately result in a net fluid secretion from the intestine (see the reviews by Cohen and Giannella[153] and by Sears and Kaper[154]). Two endogenous ligands for the ST receptor, guanylin and uroguanylin, have been identified.[155,156] This discovery is consistent with the hypothesis that ST is a superagonist and exerts its diarrheal action by means of usurping a normal secretory mechanisms in the intestine (e.g., by molecular mimicry of these less potent endogenous ligands). Uroguanylin may also act as a hormone regulating salt and water excretion in the kidney in response to an oral salt load.[157]

Clinically, ETEC infection causes nausea, abdominal pain, and watery diarrhea. Stools typically contain neither mucus nor leukocytes. ETEC can be diagnosed with the use of bioassays such as the suckling mouse assay, immunoassays, or gene probes specific for either ST or LT. PCR assays are also available. However, none of these assays is commonly used in the clinical microbiology laboratory. Supportive measures are sufficient therapy for most cases of ETEC diarrhea, with oral rehydration a mainstay of therapy. Antibiotics, including trimethoprim-sulfamethoxazole, have been shown to decrease the duration of fecal excretion of the organisms. Quinolone antibiotics may be more effective,[158] but they are not recommended for use in children. Rifaximin was also shown to provide protection against and treatment for travelers' diarrhea.[159-161]

Cholera toxin (CT) is more than 80% homologous to LT, and vaccination with CT-B subunit (CT-B) based vaccines elicits a protective immune response against LT-producing ETEC strains. Peru-15 (an oral live attenuated candidate cholera vaccine) has been engineered to express and secrete high levels of CT-B; this candidate vaccine Peru-15pCTB has promising characteristics of an oral, single-dose, bivalent cholera/ETEC vaccine[162] and is currently undergoing Phase 1 clinical trial.

Enteroinvasive *Escherichia coli*

EIEC share many common features, including virulence mechanisms, with *Shigella*. These organisms preferentially colonize the colon and invade and replicate within epithelial cells, where they cause cell death.[137] In addition, both organisms elaborate one or more secretory enterotoxins. Clinically, both *Shigella* and EIEC infections are characterized by a period of watery diarrhea that precedes the onset of dysentery (scanty stools containing mucus, pus, and blood). More commonly, in contrast to *Shigella*, only this first phase of watery diarrhea is seen in EIEC infection. This illness is clinically indistinguishable from other causes of bacterial diarrhea (e.g., ETEC) or nonbacterial infectious diarrhea. In a minority of patients with EIEC infections, the dysentery syndrome of characteristic stools, tenesmus, and fever is also seen. Bacteremia is not reported.

Infection due to EIEC is uncommon, but foodborne outbreaks of disease have occurred in the United States and aboard cruise ships. Diagnosis is dependent on bioassay (the Sereny test), serotyping, ELISA, or DNA probe techniques. None of these tests is commonly available in the clinical laboratory. Treatment is currently limited to supportive measures, although ampicillin given intramuscularly has been associated with bacteriologic cure and clinical improvement.

Shiga Toxin-Producing *Escherichia coli*

Stx-producing *E. coli* are a distinct class of organisms that have been identified since 1983 as the cause of two recognizable syndromes: hemorrhagic colitis and HUS.[163,164] Hemorrhagic colitis is an illness characterized by crampy abdominal pain, initial watery diarrhea, and subsequent development of grossly bloody diarrhea with little or no fever. Although there may be more than 100 serotypes in this class of diarrheagenic *E. coli*, in North America the *E. coli* serotype O157:H7 is the prototypic member of this family of organisms. *E. coli* O157:H7 is the most common cause of infectious bloody diarrhea in the United States.[165] Similarly, HUS, which is defined as the triad of acute renal failure, thrombocytopenia, and microangiopathic hemolytic anemia, is also highly associated with antecedent *E. coli* O157:H7 infection.

Stx-producing *E. coli* infections may occur in sporadic cases, but they have also been associated with outbreaks of disease in nursing homes, day-care centers, and other institutions; several reviews have been published.[166-169] It is estimated that *E. coli* O157:H7 causes approximately 10,000 to 20,000 infections per year in the United States alone and may be responsible for 250 deaths annually.[170] Inadequately cooked hamburgers were most likely the source of the first outbreak and remain the most common vehicle of transmission. In 1993 there was a large epidemic in the western United States; inadequately cooked hamburgers were again implicated as the cause. Aside from ground beef, many other food vectors have been implicated. Epidemics have been attributed to apple juice or cider, and large-scale outbreaks in Japan have been associated with bean sprouts. Contaminated water has also been a source of infection.[171,172] Common to all of these outbreaks is a reservoir of Stx-producing *E. coli* in the intestines of cattle and other animals that are asymptomatic. Infection is spread either by direct contact with intestinal contents or through droppings or water runoff from contaminated pastures. A low infectious dose for Stx-producing *E. coli* and the resistance of these organisms to gastric acid and to the food preserving process (high salt and drying) contribute to the high attack rate. The low infectious dose also contributes to frequent person-to-person transmission.[166-169] Nonfoodborne outbreaks have been associated with attending child day care,[173] drinking contaminated water,[174] and swimming in unchlorinated water.[175]

Both the very old and the very young appear to be at increased risk for Stx-producing *E. coli* infection and its complications.[166-169] Clinical features and complications of *E. coli* O157:H7 infection include bloody diarrhea, nonbloody diarrhea, HUS, thrombotic thrombocytopenic purpura, and, uncommonly, asymptomatic infection.[166] Symptoms may persist for several days or, less commonly, for several weeks. Early reports suggested that carriage of the organism was brief and that prompt culture was necessary to recover these organisms.[176,177] More recently, prolonged shedding has been observed.[173,178] This has led to the recommendation that two negative stool cultures be obtained before a child is allowed to return to day care.[173]

The identification of Stx-producing *E. coli* is made difficult because it is not possible to differentiate disease-producing *E. coli* from normal enteric flora on the basis of standard microbiologic techniques. There are currently six techniques for identification of Stx-producing *E. coli*: biochemical markers with serotyping (most commonly used), serum antibody tests, cytotoxin bioassays, DNA hybridization, PCR-based tests, and cytotoxin detection (including ELISAs). Some of these methods (e.g., toxin-based assays) detect the presence of cytotoxin-producing organisms, including non-O157 serotypes. It may be important to use both biochemical markers and toxin-based assays in clinical practice to identify organisms that are truly pathogenic.[179] The increased use of non-culture-based methods, such as Shiga toxin enzyme immunoassays, has resulted in a dramatic increase in reports of non-O157 Stx-producing *E. coli*.

Prevention of disease transmission is made difficult by the fact that these organisms colonize the intestine of healthy cattle and other food animals, including beef, pork, lamb, and poultry. Therefore, they can survive and multiply in the food chain. Proper cooking destroys these organisms; in hamburgers, an internal cooking temperature of 70° C (157° F) renders the meat safe. Practically, safe cooking most commonly results in a gray hamburger (not pink), with clear juices. Risk can be lowered by educating consumers about cross-contamination, use of warning labels now affixed to meat in the United States, and improvements in meat processing and microbial contamination detection.

At present there is no effective therapy to treat Stx-producing *E. coli* disease, so prevention is the most important strategy. Hemorrhagic colitis has been confused with a number of other conditions, including ischemic colitis, appendicitis, Crohn's disease, ulcerative colitis, cecal polyp, pseudomembranous colitis, and an acute abdomen (ileitis). Therefore, an important aspect of treatment of Stx-associated hemorrhagic colitis is making the correct diagnosis and avoiding unnecessary diagnostic studies such as angiography and laparotomy. The mainstay of therapy for hemorrhagic colitis is the management of dehydration, electrolyte abnormalities, and gastrointestinal blood loss. Antimicrobial agents may help by killing the bacterial pathogens, but they may also cause harm by increasing the release and subsequent absorption of Stx.[180] Trials of antibiotic treatment of Stx-producing *E. coli* infection are inconclusive. Although these organisms are uniformly sensitive to antimicrobials in vitro, at present there is no evidence that antimicrobial therapy is helpful in diminishing the severity of illness, shortening the duration of fecal excretion, or preventing HUS.[181] Of greater concern is a study suggesting an increased incidence of HUS in those treated with antimicrobials.[182] An attempt to assimilate findings of published series on the subject via a meta-analysis failed to identify an increased risk of HUS in those treated with antimicrobials.[183] Regardless, until more data are available on this topic, most experts would agree that treatment of Stx-producing *E. coli* with antimicrobials is not advisable.[184] Rifaximin does not cause replication of phage or strain lysis and therefore might not increase the risk of HUS, but it has not been studied in humans with O157 infection.[185,186] A multicenter trial failed to demonstrate an improved clinical course in pediatric patients treated with Stx-binding resin.[223] Other toxin neutralizing therapies are currently under investigation, including the use of G3 receptor analogues and monoclonal antibodies.[186,187]

Enteroaggregative and Diffusely Adherent *Escherichia coli*

EAggEc and DAEC were initially categorized as part of a larger group of enteroadherent *E. coli*. These strains differed from classical EPEC strains in that they did not show localized adherence in the Hep-2 cell assay.[188] The aggregative or "stacked brick" appearance of EAggEC in this bioassay permitted epidemiologic investigation, and EAggEc were found to be associated with persistent diarrhea in developing counties. There was uncertainty about EAggEc pathogenicity because these organisms are found in apparently healthy individuals and because some epidemiologic studies failed to show an association with disease.[189,190] However, evidence from volunteer studies[191,192] and outbreaks[193] has confirmed the pathogenicity of some EAggEC strains. Studies at Cincinnati Children's Hospital Medical Center have shown that EAggEC are an important unrecognized cause of acute infant diarrhea.[145] The mechanisms by which these organisms cause disease is thought to involve adherence to the intestinal mucosa including dispersin protein, a newly identified EAggEC virulence factor, followed by secretion of one or more enterotoxins and/or stimulation of IL-8 release by a flagellar protein.[194-196] DAEC are less well characterized but have also been associated with diarrheal disease. Both the HEp-2 cell assay and DNA probes have been used to identify these organisms, but these are not routinely available in the clinical microbiology laboratory.

Clostridium difficile

C. difficile is a spore forming gram-positive anaerobic bacillus. Disease caused by this organism can manifest in a variety of ways, ranging from asymptomatic carriage to potentially life-threatening pseudomembranous colitis. It is a frequent cause of antibiotic-associated diarrhea and a common nosocomial pathogen.

Epidemiology

Of great interest in the study of *C. difficile* is the difference in the incidence of isolation of the organism and its toxin in various age groups. *C. difficile* toxin has been found in the feces of

10% of normal-term neonates and 55% of those in a neonatal intensive care unit.[197] Most infants found to have toxin in their stools are asymptomatic. A small group of toxin-positive infants have signs and symptoms of necrotizing enterocolitis, but no clear relation to *C. difficile* or its toxin has been demonstrated. The presence of *C. difficile* toxin in these asymptomatic infants may indicate the coexistence of some protective antitoxic substance[198] or may reflect a lack of appropriate toxin receptors in patients in this age group.[199]

The incidence of *C. difficile* toxin positivity decreases beyond the neonatal period. The incidence of asymptomatic carriage in children older than 2 years of age approaches that in healthy adults (about 3%). Furthermore, not all of these organisms are toxin producers. Adults who develop disease from *C. difficile* infection are also more likely than children to experience severe colitis symptoms, although there are some reports of severe infection in infants, especially those with underlying intestinal pathology such as patients with Hirschsprung's disease or necrotizing enterocolitis.[200]

Beginning in December 2002, outbreaks of an unexpectedly large number of *C. difficile* cases were reported in Quebec, Canada.[201] These outbreaks were characterized by a 4.5-fold increased prevalence over historical incidence rates, a 5-fold increase in mortality, and a 2.5-fold increase in the proportion of complicated cases. During the outbreaks in Canada, a new hypervirulent strain, identified as BI/NAP1/027, was found to be responsible for the increased prevalence and severity.[201] All pathogenic strains of *C. difficile* produce toxin A or B or both. This BI/NAP1/027 hypervirulent strain produces 16 times more toxin A and 23 times more toxin B than other strains and has now been found throughout the United States and in many parts of the world. Although rates of *C. difficile* infection are increasing coincidentally with this new strain, it does not appear that the increased prevalence is predominantly due to the emergence of the BI/NAP1/027 strain. Non-BI/NAP1/027 community-acquired strains appear to be more important to the overall increased disease burden. During 2005, nonhypervirulent strains caused severe disease in generally healthy persons in the community at a rate of 7.6 cases per 100,000 population without the usual risk factors of older age, exposure to health care facilities, or antimicrobial use.[202] A 5-year retrospective study revealed an increase in the number of patients seen in the emergency department with community-acquired *C. difficile* infection.[203] A recent prospective cohort study found *C. difficile* toxin in 6.7% of stool samples tested in children seen for diarrhea in a children's hospital emergency department in Seattle; this rate is may be an underestimate because in this study only toxin B positive strains were identified.[204] A similar incidence of community-acquired *C. difficile* associated diarrhea was found in Connecticut.[205]

Pathogenesis

C. difficile elaborates two important toxins responsible for the inflammation, fluid, and mucus secretion as well as damage to the intestinal mucosa. Toxin A, which is responsible for the activation and recruitment of inflammatory mediators, is a large protein (308 kDa) that binds to an enterocyte surface receptor and activates an intracellular G protein-dependent signal transduction mechanism.[206] Bound toxin results in altered permeability, inhibition of protein synthesis, and direct cytotoxicity. Toxin B demonstrates cytotoxic effects. Most strains produce both toxins, but there are some that elaborate only one or none.[207] A third "binary toxin" or cytodistending toxin (CDT) (actin-specific ADP-ribosyltransferase) is found in 1 to 16% of infected patients and may be associated with more severe diarrhea. Binary toxin has enterotoxic activity in vitro, but its role, if any, in the pathogenesis of C. difficile infection is not yet clear. It may act synergistically with toxins A and B in causing severe colitis.[208]

The ability to form spores is thought to be a key feature in enabling the bacteria to persist in patients and the physical environment for long periods, thereby facilitating its transmission. C. difficile is transmitted through the fecal-oral route. Postulated risk factors include contact with a contaminated health care environment, contact with persons who are infected with and shedding C. difficile, and ingestion of contaminated food.[205] Some studies reveal increase risk in patients on gastric acid-suppressing medication.[207]

Clinical Manifestations

Most patients experience mild, watery diarrhea; abdominal pain and/or tenderness may be present. Although symptoms often last only a few days and spontaneously resolve, in some patients, symptoms persist for weeks to months. There is a broad range of symptoms ranging from asymptomatic carrier, mild to moderate diarrhea with or without blood, colitis with mucopus, and, less frequently, pseudomembranous enterocolitis, where patients are often extremely ill, with high fever, leukocytosis, and hypoalbuminemia. Any mucosal disease, including inflammatory bowel disease, is thought to be a risk factor. In children, inflammatory bowel disease is associated with increased prevalence of C. difficile infection.[209] C. difficile–related diarrhea frequently occurs in the setting of antimicrobial administration, and hospitalization is another major risk factor for the acquisition of infection.

Diagnosis and Treatment

C. difficile should be suspected in cases of colitis or mild diarrhea in which blood and leukocytes are noted in the stools. Concurrent or recent exposure (within several weeks) to antibiotics should increase the suspicion for C. difficile as the causative agent. The use of virtually any antibiotic may predispose to C. difficile disease.

The "gold standard" for diagnosis of C. difficile is the detection of toxin from fecal samples, using a cell cytotoxicity neutralization assay, and it is based on identifying C. difficile toxin B in cell culture. This assay has a high sensitivity and specificity, but it can take up to 48 hours. Stool culture requires specialized laboratory technique, and it will identify organisms that are not toxin producers, making interpreting a stool culture a challenge. Enzyme immunoassays can detect toxins A and/or B, are rapid, and are less expensive, with a turnaround time of a few hours. They have high specificity, but sensitivity is between 65 to 85% because of the high level of toxin that needs to be present.[207] Sigmoidoscopy in cases of pseudomembranous colitis typically reveals friable white exudate overlying multiple ulcerated areas. The histologic findings of such lesions are depicted in Figure 39-4. Less commonly, pseudomembranes may not be present in the rectosigmoid but may be present in the more proximal colon.

Pending additional data, for now it seems prudent to restrict routine testing for C. difficile in children with appropriate symptoms who are younger than 12 months to those with unusual risk factors and to test children between 1 and 2 years of age with appropriate symptoms and antimicrobial exposure. Children older than 2 years of age should be evaluated in the same manner as older children and adults, and infection should be considered even in the absence of prior antimicrobial exposure.[200]

In cases of mild diarrheal illness caused by C. difficile, discontinuation of any antibiotics the patient is receiving may be sufficient therapy. Although vancomycin is the only U.S. FDA-approved drug for treatment of C. difficile infection, oral metronidazole remains the first-line therapy for mild infection. Compared with vancomycin, metronidazole is much less expensive and has similar efficacy, but in severe infection vancomycin is more effective.[208] In cases of severe illness and especially in cases of pseudomembranous colitis, treatment should include oral vancomycin.

There is a fairly high rate of relapse of illness, generally 15 to 20%, after treatment of C. difficile. These relapses usually occur within 1 month of completion of therapy and sometimes but not always result from the activation of C. difficile spores remaining from the primary infection.[206] Most of these cases of

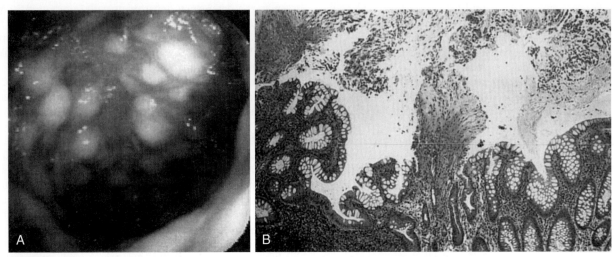

Figure 39-4. (**A**) The endoscopic appearance of the sigmoid colon with multiple densely adherent plaques (pseudomembranes). (**B**) Mucosal biopsy shows a focus of necrotizing enterocolitis with a typical volcano lesion (accumulated fibropurulent exudate intermixed with mucus). *From Bates M, Bove K, Cohen MB. Pseudomembranous colitis caused by C. difficile. J Pediatr 1997;130:146, with permission.*

relapse are responsive to a second course of metronidazole or vancomycin. The first relapse episode can be treated with the same agent that was used for the initial episode. For the second recurrence, vancomycin or a vancomycin taper or pulse therapy has been recommended. Recurrences can be multiple, and recurrent *C. difficile* treatment is a challenge. Other treatment options include alternative antibiotics such as rifaximin in conjunction with vancomycin[210] or nitazoxanide.[211] *Lactobacillus GG* and *Saccharomyces boulardii* have been beneficial for the prevention of antibiotic-associated diarrhea.[212] For treatment of *C. difficile* diarrhea recurrence, *S. boulardii* was found to be effective in adults but has not been well studied in children. Other therapies for recurrent infection include fecal transplantation[213] and intravenous immunoglobulin.[214] None of the toxin binding agents are currently proven to be effective.[215]

Aeromonas and Plesiomonas

Several organisms not previously recognized as enteric pathogens have been linked to diarrheal disease. This includes organisms of the genus *Aeromonas* and the closely related bacterium *Plesiomonas shigelloides* (previously classified as *Aeromonas shigelloides*). These organisms are gram-negative, facultatively anaerobic bacilli classified in the family Vibrionaceae. They are oxidase-positive, differentiating them from members of the Enterobacteriaceae.[216]

Aeromonas

Several members of the genus *Aeromonas*, including *Aeromonas hydrophila,* are common inhabitants of fresh and brackish water in the United States. These organisms were initially recognized as opportunistic pathogens in immunocompromised hosts, especially those with malignant hematologic diseases. The organisms also have been known to cause disease in patients with underlying hepatobiliary disease.[216] *Aeromonas* has been isolated from healthy persons as well and has therefore been thought to be part of the normal flora. Despite initial studies that yielded conflicting results,[217] it is now generally accepted that *A. hydrophila* is an enteric pathogen.

Studies in Australian children with diarrhea have found *Aeromonas* species present in 10% of patients.[218] Infection appears to occur most frequently in children younger than 2 years of age.[219] Of patients with *Aeromonas* isolated from stool cultures at Cincinnati Children's Hospital Medical Center, approximately 50% were younger than 3 months. *Aeromonas* infection is also seasonal, occurring more often in the summer months.[216]

Not all *Aeromonas* species are pathogenic. In a prospective control study of children with diarrhea, *Aeromonas* was isolated only from control subjects.[145] The method of pathogenesis remains unclear. Both cytotoxic[219] and enterotoxic[216] properties have been observed, but neither these nor other pathogenic mechanisms are found consistently in strains isolated from patients with *Aeromonas*-associated disease.[217] *Aeromonas caviae*, a commonly isolated species, demonstrates both adherence and cytotoxin production.[220]

Clinical symptoms attributed to *Aeromonas* can be grouped into three categories: (1) acute watery diarrhea, the most common syndrome; (2) dysentery, which usually is self-limited; and (3) persistent watery diarrhea. Cramping abdominal pain and vomiting may also occur.[219] Symptoms may occasionally be severe and, especially when dysentery is present, have been incorrectly diagnosed as ulcerative colitis.[218]

In mild cases of *Aeromonas* infection, supportive treatment should suffice. In patients who are immunocompromised, are otherwise acutely ill, or have persistent illness, treatment with antibiotics is recommended. Trimethoprim-sulfamethoxazole is usually effective (trimethoprim, 5 mg/kg [maximum 160 mg], plus sulfamethoxazole, 25 mg/kg [maximum 800 mg] per dose, given every 12 hours for 14 days), as are tetracycline, chloramphenicol, and the aminoglycosides.[216] Most strains of *Aeromonas* are resistant to the penicillins, including ampicillin.[216]

Plesiomonas

P. shigelloides, like *Aeromonas*, is commonly found in the environment,[221] especially in bodies of water, including water from a home aquarium.[222] Unlike *Aeromonas*, however, *Plesiomonas* has been reported to occur in epidemics, with contaminated water often found to be the cause.[221] *Plesiomonas* is also known to be spread through improperly cooked seafood.[223]

The pathogenesis of disease caused by *P. shigelloides* is not well understood. A cytotoxin has been found in some strains[221] but not in others. An invasive mechanism is also suspected, because of the colitis symptoms.[223] In addition to small-volume stools with leukocytes and possible blood, patients may also experience severe abdominal pain. Fever has been seen in approximately one third of patients.[223] In one group of adult patients, symptoms persisted longer than 2 weeks in 75% and longer than 4 weeks in 32%.[223]

Diagnosis of *P. shigelloides* is made by stool culture. Although this illness is usually self-limited, treatment with antimicrobial agents has been shown to decrease the duration of symptoms,[223] with trimethoprim-sulfamethoxazole or aminoglycosides suggested as appropriate choices. There are no controlled trials of antimicrobial treatment of gastroenteritis caused by this organism.

Mycobacterium avium-intracellulare

Mycobacterium avium and *Mycobacterium intracellulare*, known collectively as *Mycobacterium avium-intracellulare* or *Mycobacterium avium* complex (MAC), are acid-fast bacilli that have been recognized primarily for their role in cases of atypical tuberculosis. These organisms are now recognized as causative agents of diarrheal symptoms as well. In a review of pediatric cases of atypical mycobacterial infections, Lincoln and Gilbert[224] described two immunocompetent patients whose clinical findings included diarrhea and colonic ulceration.

Of even greater significance than these sporadic cases of MAC infection in immunocompetent hosts is its occurrence among immunocompromised patients. In patients with the acquired immunodeficiency syndrome, MAC is among the most commonly isolated agents causing systemic bacterial infections.[225] These patients may also have chronic diarrhea and abdominal pain.[226,227] MAC has also been noted to cause diarrhea in patients undergoing bone marrow transplantation[228] and in a patient with cystic fibrosis.[229]

The MAC organisms may be cultured from gastric and duodenal aspirates obtained endoscopically and from the stool, the bone marrow, and the blood.[225] Endoscopic examination in patients with MAC may reveal findings similar to those seen in Whipple's disease, with minute superficial ulcerations in the small bowel.[227] Treatment of MAC infections with conventional antituberculosis agents usually is unsuccessful in eradicating the organisms or alleviating symptoms.[225]

POTENTIAL DIARRHEAGENIC ORGANISMS

Enterotoxigenic Bacteroides fragilis

Bacteroides fragilis is an anaerobic organism that is commonly isolated from normal stool flora. However, some investigators have identified a toxin-producing variant that is enteropathogenic. Enterotoxigenic *Bacteroides fragilis* (ETBF) organisms have been isolated from both healthy persons and those with diarrhea.[230] The only known virulence factor of ETBF is the *B. fragilis* toxin that stimulates secretion of the proinflammatory cytokine, IL-8.[231] Epidemiologic associations with diarrhea in children have been shown for ETBF in several studies[232-235] but not others.[236]

A recent observational study in Bangladesh followed children more than 1 year of age and adults to identify individuals infected with *B. fragilis*.[231] A total of 1209 patients with diarrhea were screened, and 417 (34.5%) yielded *B. fragilis*, of which 86 (7%) were ETBF. The clinical presentation of infection included abdominal pain, tenesmus, and nocturnal diarrhea that lasted a median of 3 days and resulted in dehydration in 14% of individuals. Fecal leukocytes, lactoferrin, and proinflammatory cytokines increased in the ETBF-infected patients.

Brachyspira aalborgi

Intestinal spirochetosis, or the colonization of the large bowel by *Brachyspira aalborgi* and related spirochetes, has been implicated as a cause of diarrhea,[237] but its clinical relevance is still controversial.[238,239] Some studies have shown an association between this organism and bloody diarrhea,[240] although asymptomatic colonization have also been reported.[241] A recent study assessed adult patients with chronic watery diarrhea; of 1174 patients, only 8 were positive for intestinal spirochetosis, it was not diagnosed in the controls (n = 104), and histological resolution of the infection with metronidazole paralleled clinical recovery in 6 patients.[242] The potential of this organism to cause diarrhea requires further evaluation.

Hafnia alvei

This organism has been associated with diarrhea in sporadic cases and in at least one hospital outbreak. Although a causal relation between *Hafnia alvei* and diarrhea has not been clearly established, a subset of this organism may be enteropathogenic. Organisms isolated from patients with diarrhea typically demonstrate the attaching and effacing lesion seen with EPEC, whereas nonpathogenic isolates do not show this characteristic.[243]

Listeria monocytogenes

Invasive illness caused by *Listeria* is well known, but it was only recently that convincing evidence was obtained that *Listeria* can cause acute, self-limited, febrile gastroenteritis in healthy persons. At least seven outbreaks of foodborne gastroenteritis for which *L. monocytogenes* was the most likely etiology have been described.[244] Convincing evidence came from an outbreak of febrile gastroenteritis associated with the consumption of contaminated chocolate milk.[245]

Commonly reported symptoms from outbreaks are fever, diarrhea, arthromyalgia, and headache. Diarrhea is typically nonbloody and watery. Fatigue and sleepiness is frequently reported after an incubation period of 24 hours or less. This gastrointestinal infection is typically self-limited without serious complications in healthy individuals with symptoms lasting 1 to 3 days. A wide variety of foods have been implicated including rice salad, corn-and-tuna salad, chocolate milk, cold smoked rainbow trout, corned beef, cheese, and cold cuts.[244] No data exist regarding the efficacy of treatment with antimicrobials in this illness, and it is not warranted in most instances.

CONCLUSION

Despite this chapter's extensive catalog of both bacterial and viral infectious agents, from 40 to 60% of cases of diarrhea are currently not attributable to any known cause. Undoubtedly, as techniques for identification and culture become more sophisticated, other causative agents will be identified and the percentage of diarrheal illnesses described as idiopathic or nonspecific will continue to decline. Advances in the widespread use of improved oral rehydration solutions have led to a decline in the morbidity and mortality associated with diarrhea. Future advances in preventive measures, including vaccines, may lead to a reduction of the incidence of diarrheal disease.

REFERENCES

36. Guandalini S, Pensabene L, Zikri MA, et al. *Lactobacillus* GG administered in oral rehydration solution to children with acute diarrhea: a multicenter European trial. J Pediatr Gastroenterol Nutr 2000;30:54–60.
41. Vesikari T, Matson DO, Dennehy P, et al. Safety and efficacy of a pentavalent human-bovine (WC3) reassortant rotavirus vaccine. N Engl J Med 2006;354:23–33.
42. Ruiz-Palacios GM, Perez-Schael I, Velazquez FR, et al. Safety and efficacy of an attenuated vaccine against severe rotavirus gastroenteritis. N Engl J Med 2006;354:11–22.
145. Cohen MB, Nataro JP, Bernstein DI, et al. Prevalence of diarrheagenic *Escherichia coli* in acute childhood enteritis: a prospective controlled study. J Pediatr 2005;146:54–61.
208. Kelly CP, LaMont JT. *Clostridium difficile* – more difficult than ever. N Engl J Med 2008;359:1932–1940.

See expertconsult.com for a complete list of references and the review questions for this chapter.

ENTERIC PARASITES 40

Judy Fuentebella · Jacqueline L. Fridge · Dorsey M. Bass

Enteric parasites are important agents of disease throughout the world. Although the frequency and severity of parasitic diseases are most extreme in the developing world, changes in worldwide travel, immigration, commerce, and day care for young children and increasing numbers of patients with immune compromise have led to increased incidences of parasitic diseases in the developed world. Parasitic disease may mimic other gastrointestinal disorders, such as inflammatory bowel disease, hepatitis, sclerosing cholangitis, peptic ulcer disease, and celiac disease. Parasitic infection can also trigger overt manifestations of quiescent chronic intestinal disorders.

EPIDEMIOLOGY

A variety of epidemiologic factors predispose patients to parasitic infestation worldwide, but the single most important factor is socioeconomic status. It has been shown repeatedly, in both the developed and developing world, that children of lower socioeconomic status have higher parasite loads and a greater prevalence of multiple infestations.[1,2] Travel to developing countries can expose an individual to parasites that may not cause symptoms until weeks, months, or years later. Immigrants from developing countries often harbor pathogens that are unfamiliar to physicians in their new homelands and may pass them on to their new countrymen. Less obvious sources of parasites include foodstuffs increasingly imported from all areas of the world. The United States has experienced outbreaks of intestinal cyclosporiasis from imported raspberries.[3]

Protozoan infections endemic to the developed world, such as giardiasis, are transmitted with great efficiency in day-care centers, where fecal-oral contamination is quite common. Institutions for the mentally retarded are also common reservoirs for *Giardia*, *Entamoeba histolytica*, and other protozoans. Pets and livestock are potential sources of *Cryptosporidium*, *Giardia*, and *Toxocara* species, canine hookworm, *Balantidium coli*, and other organisms.

Dietary habits can also be risk factors. Consumption of raw or undercooked fish can lead to *Diphyllobothrium latum*, *Capillaria philippinensis*, or *Anisakis* infection. Inadequate cooking of pork predisposes to *Taenia solium* and *Trichinella* infections. Beefsteak tartare and other raw or rare bovine delicacies can harbor *Taenia saginata*. Furthermore, a variety of protozoan organisms can be transmitted via produce that has been exposed to human or animal waste. Unpasteurized apple juice has been reported as a cause of *Cryptosporidium* outbreaks.[4]

HOST FACTORS

Children, particularly toddlers, are more susceptible to these infestations, owing to their habits of "mouthing" all sorts of environmental objects, their propensity to go barefoot, and their immunologic "naiveté." Patients with compromised immune systems, whether due to congenital defects, infections such as human immunodeficiency virus (HIV), or medical ministrations (transplant and oncology patients), may have severe, protracted, or unusual manifestations of parasitic disease. Patients with hypogammaglobulinemia and immunoglobulin A (IgA) deficiency may suffer severe protozoan infections such as giardiasis. Patients with acquired immunodeficiency syndrome (AIDS) infected with *Cryptosporidium* organisms may have severe, prolonged diarrhea as well as unusual manifestations in the biliary tree and lungs, despite high levels of luminal IgA antibody directed against *Cryptosporidium*.[5] Sexual practices, particularly those that involve anal penetration, are also associated with transmission of parasitic diseases.[6,7]

CLINICAL PRESENTATIONS

Enteric parasites most often produce gastrointestinal symptoms—abdominal pain, diarrhea, flatulence, and distention.[8] In a children's hospital laboratory survey of stool ova and parasite tests, it was found that stools sent from the gastroenterology clinic were most likely to be positive, as compared with stools submitted from other outpatient clinics, the emergency room, or inpatient settings.[9] Heavy infestations of large worms such as *Ascaris* can lead to intestinal obstruction or, if they migrate into the biliary system, biliary obstruction with cholangitis or pancreatitis. *Amoeba* and *Trichuris* organisms can cause enterocolitis with tenesmus and mucoid, bloody stool.

Liver disease from enteric parasites can be due to bile duct obstruction by organisms such as *Ascaris* worms or liver flukes or from portal hypertension due to inflammatory reactions to ova, as in schistosomiasis. Some protozoans such as *Cryptosporidium* can infect biliary epithelium and produce syndromes such as cholangitis and cholecystitis. Other protozoans such as *E. histolytica* can cause hepatic parenchymal necrosis resulting in liver abscesses.

Systemic manifestations of parasitic infestation are also common. Intestinal luminal blood and protein loss can lead to anemia and edema. Fever is often the most prominent feature of amebic liver abscess. Malabsorption is common in giardiasis and cryptosporidiosis and can lead to wasting, fat soluble-vitamin deficiency, and failure to thrive. Onset of nephrotic syndrome has been associated with *Giardia lamblia*, *Strongyloides stercoralis*, and possibly hookworm species.[10]

DIAGNOSIS

Stool Examination

The mainstay of diagnosing enteric parasites is a skilled microscopist in the parasitology laboratory. At least 35 species of enteric parasites may be identified by stool examination.[11]

Furthermore, the observation of fecal leukocytes, eosinophils, and macrophages in preserved specimens may provide clues to parasitic gastrointestinal diseases. Because microscopists' skills vary, clinicians are advised to select reference laboratories with care. Careful attention to the appropriate collection, preservation, and examination of samples is critical to successful diagnosis of enteric parasites.

Appropriate sample collection begins with ascertaining that no interfering substances are present in the stool that will invalidate the results. Common interfering substances include barium (from contrast radiography), bismuth preparations, antacids, and mineral oil. Antibiotics can also make detection of protozoans difficult. It is preferable to wait 2 weeks after the ingestion of any of these substances before obtaining a specimen. Clinicians evaluating gastrointestinal symptoms should obtain stool specimens before initiating gastrointestinal radiology studies and certain forms of empiric therapy. Water and urine contamination of stool lead to rapid lysis of trophozoites and should be avoided.

Although examination of a fresh stool specimen is useful for identification of motile trophozoites, it is rarely performed in laboratories in the United States. Most stools are collected in preservatives, which allows for convenience in both collection and examination. The commonly used preservatives, such as formalin and poly(vinyl alcohol), are quite toxic if ingested.

The appropriate number and frequency of stool examinations are matters of some controversy. It is clear that repeated samples obtained on separate days enhance sensitivity by at least 20%, owing to variable shedding of eggs, cysts, and trophozoites.[12] For patients with very low clinical-epidemiologic risk factors, one sample may be adequate, but for those with a high index of suspicion, more than three samples may be needed, particularly for *E. histolytica* and *Dientamoeba fragilis*.

Some enteric parasites, most notably *Cryptosporidium* and *Cyclospora* species, are not detected on routine ova and parasite examinations. These organisms require either acid-fast staining or special immunofluorescence techniques.

Immunoassay

Enzyme-linked immunosorbent assay (ELISA) tests for antigen in stool samples are widely available for *Giardia* and *Cryptosporidium* species. These sensitive and specific assays can be useful adjuncts to standard stool examinations. Because several common organisms can cause the clinical picture of giardiasis, ELISA is not recommended as the sole means of evaluating patients, except in the context of a known outbreak. Centers for Disease Control and Prevention (CDC) ELISA has a sensitivity of up to 95% and specificity of 90% for strongyloidiasis.[13]

Macroscopic Examination

Ascaris lumbricoides worms can be passed intact in the stool or vomited, particularly during febrile illness. They are easily recognized because of their size (15 to 40 cm) and resemblance to earthworms. Cestodes, or more commonly, segments of cestodes, can also be passed per rectum. Species identification is possible by microscopic examination. *Enterobius* organisms venture nocturnally onto the perianal area to lay eggs. The small threadlike worms may be visualized, or the "Scotch tape" test may be employed to identify the eggs of this common parasite.

Serology

Serologic detection of antibodies to *E. histolytica* is possible in 85% of patients with dysentery and 95% of infected patients who have liver abscesses in nonendemic areas. Specific IgM serology for *Giardia* and *Strongyloides* may be useful in obscure cases.

Eosinophilia

Eosinophils are granulocytes with cytoplasm that stains strongly with acid dyes such as eosin. They normally make up less than 5% of circulating granulocytes, or an absolute count of fewer than 500/mm^3. Elevation of eosinophils in the peripheral blood is associated with allergy, connective tissue disease, infections, and malignancy.[14] Only invasive parasitic infections are associated with a peripheral eosinophilia, and the degree of elevation is proportional to the degree of invasion.[15] Protozoal infections rarely cause eosinophilia. Circulating eosinophils are a marker of much higher tissue aggregations of eosinophils, usually in the skin and epithelial tissues. Eosinophil production is stimulated by cytokines released by Th2 cells. The Th2 immune response is triggered by allergens and helminths and differs from the Th1 response involved in bacterial and viral infections. Eosinophilia is not a sensitive screening tool for parasitic infection. However, if eosinophilia is present, infection with *Ascaris*, hookworm, visceral or cutaneous larva migrans, *Strongyloides*, *Trichinella*, *Trichuris*, or tapeworm must be considered.

Intestinal Fluid and Biopsy

Duodenal fluid may be useful in diagnosis of giardiasis or strongyloidiasis when stool specimens are negative. Fluid may be obtained by duodenal intubation or during endoscopy. It should be examined immediately. The Entero-Test is a gelatin capsule that contains a string that adsorbs duodenal fluid. It is swallowed and then retrieved by a string taped to the patient's cheek. This technique may be difficult to perform in young children.

In selected patients, duodenal biopsy may reveal *Giardia*, *Cryptosporidium*, microsporidia, or *Strongyloides* organisms. Biopsy of the edges of colon ulcers may reveal trophozoites of *E. histolytica*. The sensitivity of intestinal biopsy for diagnosis of parasitic disease depends to a large degree on the interest and experience of the pathologist.

BENEFITS OF PARASITES

Interest is growing in a hypothesized link between lack of exposure to helminth infection and the development of allergy. Several studies have shown that children with chronic parasitic infections have reduced skin reactivity to common environmental allergens such as the house dust mite, as compared to noninfected children with otherwise similar exposures.[16] There seems to be benefit both from current parasite infection and from repetitive infection in infancy.[17] Inflammation triggers CD4+ T cell production of either a Th1 or Th2 predominant response. Th1 cytokines stimulated by bacterial and viral infections are the cytokines that mediate a normal inflammatory response. Th2 cytokines are stimulated by parasites and allergens and cause an allergic response, but in the case of parasitic infections the response is modified and IgE degranulation is inhibited. Recurrent exposure to parasites in infancy is thought to down-regulate the Th2 response and lessens the likelihood of induction of allergy. Current parasite infection also down-regulates the inflammatory response, possibly to allow the parasite to mature and reproduce. The role of the anti-inflammatory cytokines such as interleukin 10 (IL-10) is important, because repetitive parasitic and other infections up-regulate IL-10 and ensure a normal termination of inflammation.[18]

As with allergy, the incidence of inflammatory bowel disease is said to be inversely related to the prevalence of parasitic infection. Immune tolerance and autoimmunity, mediated by Th3/Tr1 cells, also depends on the balance of anti-inflammatory cytokines IL-10 and transforming growth factor β (TGF-β) with pro-inflammatory cytokines from the Th1 pathway. Parasitic infections down-regulate Th1 responses that are implicated in the mucosal inflammation seen in inflammatory bowel disease.[19] After promising experiments on mice, humans with inflammatory bowel disease have been dosed with *Trichuris suis* (pig whipworm). The results suggest efficacy, but repeated dosing is needed to sustain remission.[20]

PATHOGENIC ORGANISMS

Protozoa

Giardia lamblia

Giardiasis is the most common pathogenic intestinal protozoan infection in the world. It has been estimated that some 2 to 5% of the population of the industrialized world and up to 30% of those in the developing world are infected at any time.[21-26] It is increasingly recognized in day-care center outbreaks and in food- and waterborne outbreaks in industrialized countries. The majority of these infections are asymptomatic. Prevalence of infection increases through infancy and early childhood, not decreasing until early adolescence. A major pediatric health concern is that this protozoan may be contributing to failure of growth and cognitive development in the developing world.[27] However, *Giardia* was only recognized as a major pathogen in the 1970s and was listed as a parasitic pathogen by the World Health Organization in 1981.[28] *Giardia* was also the first described human protozoan agent of intestinal disease. Von Leeuwenhoek observed them in 1681 in his own diarrheal stool and described them as "animalcules." *Giardia* is an ancient organism and was recently demonstrated in the stools of prehistoric Peruvian human populations.[29] It is a primitive eukaryocyte and relies on anaerobic metabolism as it lacks mitochondria. These organisms share many properties with bacteria and hence are susceptible to antibiotics. *Giardia* are also of interest because of their relationship to archaebacteria by comparison of ribosomal RNA sequence.[30] This relationship suggests that organisms such as *Giardia* may have been among the first eukaryotic life forms. The *Giardia* Genome Project has successfully sequenced 90% the genetic material of *Giardia* and is a valuable resource for further study of this organism (www.mbl.edu/Giardia).[31]

G. lamblia exists in two forms: the encysted, environmentally stable form that is responsible for transmission and the small intestine-dwelling trophozoite, which is the motile form observed by von Leeuwenhoek. The process of excystation is thought to be pH dependent and follows the transition of the cyst from acid stomach to alkaline duodenum, causing the characteristic heavy infestation in the proximal small bowel.[32]

In the small intestine, the trophozoites adhere to enterocytes by a ventral disk, causing local effacement of the microvilli. *Giardia* is a waterborne pathogen that can be transmitted via the fecal-oral route. The study of *Giardia* species has been hampered by multiple naming systems. The *Giardia* pathogenic to mammals is known as *Giardia lamblia* and also as *G. intestinalis* and *G. duodenalis*.[33] Several different assemblage types identified within *G. lamblia* have relevance for host specificity, but evidence is lacking for effect on clinical disease severity.[34] A variety of domestic mammals including dogs and cats, wild mammals such as beavers, raccoons, and rodents, and domestic livestock such as cattle and sheep can harbor the organism.[35-38] The role of animals in the transmission of *Giardia* to humans remains controversial, partly because of emerging data about the relevance of assemblage types within the *G. lamblia* species that may determine host specificity.[39]

The pathophysiology of giardiasis is unclear. Pathologic changes in the small intestine are quite variable. Although most symptomatic patients have normal or nearly normal villi,[40] 5 to 10% or more have subtotal villus atrophy. Patients with immunoglobulin deficiency are particularly prone to histological abnormality, but AIDS patients do not seem to be at increased risk of severe or persistent giardiasis.[27] There are no reported cases of giardiasis associated with commonly used immunosuppressive agents such as steroids or cyclosporine. Secretory IgA is thought to have an important role in host defenses to *Giardia*, but the deficiency must be severe to be clinically relevant.[41,42] Invasive disease may rarely occur with spread to the gallbladder and urinary system. Most symptomatic patients have lactose intolerance, both clinically and as measured by the hydrogen breath test.

Symptoms of giardiasis can include diarrhea, flatulence, malabsorption with weight loss, constipation, and abdominal pain. The 2- to 3-week incubation period may be followed by a phase of acute illness, but more than half of infected children will be asymptomatic. Symptoms can be intermittent or continuous. Stools may be watery, malabsorptive, or formed, but are not bloody and do not contain leukocytes. Urticaria may occur and may be prolonged.[43]

Laboratory findings are generally nonspecific. Fat may be found in the stool. Rarely, serum albumin is decreased and fecal α_1-antitrypsin is increased. Eosinophilia does not occur. Radiological findings are generally nonspecific. Giardiasis localized to the terminal ileum may radiologically mimic Crohn's disease.[44] Ophthalmoscopy may demonstrate salt-and-pepper retinal degeneration in preschool children, but progressive retinal disease does not occur.[45]

Diagnosis is based on demonstration of *Giardia* trophozoites, cysts, or antigen in stool, duodenal fluid, or intestinal biopsy specimens (Figure 40-1). Microscopic examination of a single stool specimen is approximately 70% sensitive for detection. Sensitivity increases to approximately 85% with three samples. Examination of duodenal fluid has been reported to be 40 to 90% sensitive. Antigen detection assays by direct fluorescence antibody (DFA) or enzyme immunoassay (EIA) on stool offer 89 to 100% sensitivity and 99.3 to 100% specificity on a single specimen, but do not identify other protozoans that can cause similar symptoms.[46-48]

Treatment options for giardiasis include metronidazole (and its derivatives), nitazoxanide, paromomycin, quinacrine, and furazolidone (Table 40-1). Immunocompromised patients may require prolonged therapy to clear the organism. Some apparent

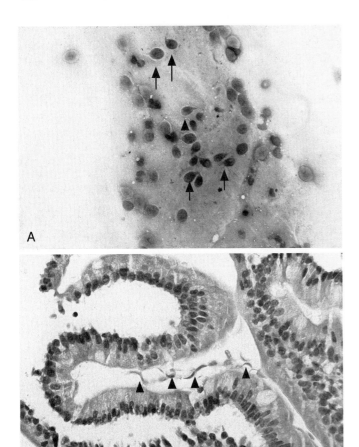

Figure 40-1. Trophozoites (arrows) of *Giardia lamblia* from small bowel biopsy. (**A**) Giemsa stain of touch prep. (**B**) Routine section (hematoxylin and eosin). (*See plate section for color.*) Courtesy Drs. Gerald Berry and Terry Longacre.

clinical treatment failures are due to lactose intolerance, which can persist for weeks after successful treatment. There is no clear role for the use of probiotics in the treatment or prevention of *Giardia* infection.[49] No treatment is recommended for asymptomatic children carrying cysts. However, treatment may be considered in outbreak control and in patients with cystic fibrosis, celiac disease, or hypogammaglobinemia.[26]

Prevention of infection is a major public health concern. An inoculum of only 10 to 100 cysts can cause infection in humans. *Giardia* is more resistant than bacteria and the cyst can survive 3 months in water at 4° C. Waterborne infections account for 60% of cases in the United States.[50] Standard iodine water purification tablets will not reliably kill *Giardia* in infected water, and it is relatively resistant to chlorination and ozonolysis.[34,51] Swimming pools and even tap water are common sources of infection. Filtration of water and ultraviolet light treatment are most effective at eradicating *Giardia* from the water supply.[52] Foodborne infection outbreaks are usually secondary to infected or excreting food handlers, but viable *Giardia* have been found on fruits and vegetables such as lettuce and strawberries.[50] Outbreaks in day-care centers are also common. Thorough handwashing is essential to disease prevention. Antigenic variation in the *Giardia* surface antigens has slowed development of a vaccine for humans, but a veterinary vaccine for cats and dogs is commercially available.[53] Breast-feeding is protective for preventing infection and symptomatic infection.[54]

Entamoeba histolytica

Although a variety of species of amebae inhabit the human intestine, only *E. histolytica* is clearly pathogenic. Although identical on light microscopy, newer biochemical, immunologic, and DNA analyses exist that distinguish between pathogenic and nonpathogenic strains.[59-62] Nonpathogenic strains are named *Entamoeba dispar*.[63,64] Even in patients with symptomatic AIDS, *E. dispar* is not pathogenic. In addition, only certain strains of *E. histolytica* are capable of invading the mucosa and causing disease. Even within an endemic area, there are genetically distinct strains of *E. histolytica* that cause intestinal versus hepatic disease.[65] Virulence factors are related to a number of proteins produced by the parasite, including a lectin that mediates adherence to epithelial cells, a peptide that lyses cells by creating a pore, and matrix-digesting proteases.[66] Indeed, the name *histolytica* refers to the ameba's ability to break down extracellular matrix proteins and cause necrosis of host cells.[67]

The life cycle of these unicellular eukaryocytes is quite similar to that of *Giardia*. Ingested cysts are stimulated by gastric acid to excystate in the small intestine. The resulting trophozoites colonize the large intestine, where they multiply in the mucin layer. The trophozoites then either invade the mucosa or encystate, depending on local conditions and the nature of the particular strain. The interaction of the genetic capabilities of the strain and host factors such as the bacterial flora of the gut determine virulence.[68] Invading trophozoites destroy epithelial target cells by releasing substances such as hemolysins, which disrupt cell membranes by creating an amoebapore. A variety of excreted cysteine proteases disrupt the extracellular matrix. Injury to epithelial cells triggers release of cytokines leading to chemotaxis of leukocytes, which also contribute to the local inflammatory response. Eventually, ulceration of the mucosa occurs and invading amebae may enter the portal circulation and eventually the liver. In vitro, the trophozoites have a powerful ability to kill T lymphocytes, neutrophils, and macrophages. Virulence may also be related to the trophozoites' ability to cause apoptosis in these inflammatory cells and then phagocytose them, thus limiting further inflammatory response.[66] Unlike intestinal lesions, hepatic abscesses contain few inflammatory cells, consisting almost entirely of necrotic liver cells. In patients treated with large doses of steroids, amebae may spread to a variety of organs, including the lungs, brain, and eyes. For unknown reasons, such systemic dissemination is not common in AIDS patients, who are often infected with *Entamoeba* species.[69]

The WHO estimates there are 100,000 deaths per year due to *E. histolytica*, second only to malaria for parasite-related death.[64] Risk factors for amebiasis include poverty, crowding, poor hygiene, travel in endemic areas, and male homosexual promiscuity. Risk factors for severe disease include young age (particularly infants), malnutrition, and corticosteroid use. Although physicians in the United States think of amebic disease as exotic, prevalence of infection here has been estimated as high as 5% among the general population and 30% among homosexual men. However, most prevalence data predate the ability to distinguish *histolytica* from *dispar*.[7,70] Recent prevalence data show varying distribution of the two species throughout the world.[71] *E. histolytica* accounts for about 10 to 20% of diarrheal illnesses in children in endemic areas.[72] The rate of infection in travelers returning from endemic areas is 2.7%. Asymptomatic infections commonly last more than a year, and latency periods as long as several years are possible.[73] Clinicians

TABLE 40-1. **Treatment of Enteric Parasites**[55-58]

Disease	Drug	Dosage	Comments
Amebiasis (*E. histolytica*)			
Asymptomatic and luminal clearance	Iodoquinol or	30-40 mg/kg per day in 3 doses × 20 days (max. 2 g/day)	Currently suggested that asymptomatic cyst passers in nonendemic areas be treated
	Paromomycin or	25-35 mg/kg per day in 3 doses × 7 days (max. 1.5 g/day)	
	Diloxanide furoate or	20 mg/kg per day in 3 doses × 10 days (max. 1.5 g/day)	Not commercially available in United States
Colitis, liver abscess	Metronidazole or	35-50 mg/kg per day in 3 doses × 7-10 days (max. 2.25 g/day)	Metronidazole absorbed very well orally. Follow with luminal clearance
	Tinidazole or	50 mg/kg per day in 1 dose × 3 days (max. 2 g/day)	May be less effective but better tolerated. Follow with luminal clearance as above
	Ornidazole	25 mg/kg per day × 5-10 days	Alternates include dehydroemetine or combination therapy with chloroquine phosphate
Ancylostoma caninum (dog hookworm, eosinophilic enterocolitis)	Albendazole or	400 mg once (may repeat in 3 weeks)	Serologic/clinical diagnosis; no ova or parasites are found in stool
	Pyrantel pamoate or	11 mg/kg per day × 3 days (max. 1 g/day)	
	Mebendazole or Endoscopic removal	100 mg bid × 3 days	
Anisakiasis (fish worm)	Surgical or endoscopic removal		For symptoms of obstruction, use nasogastric infusion of piperazine citrate 75 mg/kg per day (max. 3.5 g)
Ascariasis	Albendazole or	400 mg once	
	Mebendazole or	100 mg bid × 3 days or 500 mg once	
	Pyrantel pamoate or	11 mg/kg once (max. 1 g)	
	Ivermectin	150-200 μg/kg once	
Balantidium coli	Tetracycline or	40 mg/kg per day in 4 doses × 10 days (max. 2 g/day)	Contraindicated in pregnant women and children less than 8 years old. Paromomycin is alternate for pregnant women
	Iodoquinol or	30-40 mg/kg per day in 3 doses × 20 days (max. 2 g/day)	
	Metronidazole	35-50 mg/kg per day in 3 doses × 5 days (max. 2.25 g/day)	
Blastocystis hominis	Metronidazole or	35-50 mg/kg per day in 3 doses × 5-10 days (max. 2.25 g/day)	Clinical importance of infection is debatable.
	Iodoquinol	40 mg/kg per day in 3 doses × 20 days (max. 2 g/day)	Alternate trimethoprim-sulfamethoxazole and nitazoxanide
Capillaria philippinensis	Mebendazole or	200 mg bid × 20 days	Noncompliance with prolonged course leads to frequent relapse
	Albendazole or	400 mg daily × 10 days	
	Thiabendazole	25 mg/kg per day in 2 doses × 30 days	
Cryptosporidiosis	Nitazoxanide or	100 mg bid × 3 days (children 1-3 years old), 200 mg bid × 3 days (children 4-11 years old), 500mg bid × 3 days (≥12 years old)	Consider oral human immune globulin or bovine colostrum in immunocompromised patients. Improved immune function is best prognosis[53]
	Azithromycin dihydrate alone or with paromomycin (minimally effective)	25 mg/kg per day bid × 14 days 30 mg/kg per day in 3 doses (max. 4 g/day)	
Cyclospora	Trimethoprim-sulfamethoxazole (TMP-SMZ)	TMP 10 mg/kg per day, SMZ 50 mg/kg per day bid × 7-10 days (max. 1 DS tablet bid)	HIV-infected patients may need higher dose and longer treatment. Ciprofloxacin is an alternate for sulfa-allergic patients
Dientamoeba fragilis	Iodoquinol or	30-40 mg/kg per day in 3 doses × 20 days (max. 2 g/day)	Contraindicated in pregnant women and children less than 8 years old
	Tetracycline or	40 mg/kg per day in 4 doses × 10 days (max. 2 g/day)	
	Metronidazole or	35-50 mg/kg per day in 3 doses × 10 days (max. 2.25 g/day)	
	Paromomycin	25-35 mg/kg per day in 3 doses × 7 days	
Enterobius vermicularis (pinworm)	Pyrantel pamoate or	11 mg/kg (max. 1 g) once; repeat in 2 weeks	Treatment of household contacts is often advised
	Mebendazole or	100 mg once; repeat in 2 weeks	
	Albendazole	400 mg × once; repeat in 2 weeks	

Continued

TABLE 40-1. Treatment of Enteric Parasites—cont'd

Disease	Drug	Dosage	Comments
Giardiasis	Metronidazole or	15 mg/kg per day in 3 doses × 5-7 days (max. 750 mg/dose)	Other alternates include bacitracin.
	Tinidazole or Ornidazole or Nitroimidazole	50 mg/kg once (max. 2 g)	
	Furazolidone or	6 mg/kg per day in 4 doses × 7-10 days (max. 400 mg/day)	For resistant Giardia[55]
	Albendazole or	400 mg once × 5 days	
	Nitazoxanide or	100 mg bid × 3 days (children 1-3 years old), 200 mg bid × 3 days (children 4-11 years old), 500mg bid × 3 days (≥12 years old)	With metronidazole for resistant strains.[56]
	Paromomycin or	25-35 mg/kg per day in 3 doses × 5-10 days (max. 1.5 g/day)	Least efficacious, but recommended for pregnant women
	Quinacrine	6 mg/kg tid × 5 days (max. 300 mg/day)	Colors skin yellow
Hookworm (*Ancylostoma duodenale, Necator americanus*)	Albendazole or Pyrantel pamoate or Mebendazole	400 mg once 11 mg/kg per day × 3 days (max. 1 g) 100 mg bid × 3 days or 500 mg once	
Isospora belli	TMP-SMZ	TMP 10 mg/kg per day, SMZ 50 mg/kg per day bid × 10 days (max. 1 DS tab bid)	Pyrimethamine and ciprofloxacin are alternates for sulfa allergic patients
Microsporidiosis (intestinal) (*Enterocytozoon bieneusi, Ecephalitozoon [Septata] intestinalis*)	Fumagillin or Albendazole	60 mg/d × 14 days (adult dose) 400 mg bid × 21 days (adult dose)	*E. intestinalis* responds much better to treatment Alternatives include metronidazole, atovaquone, and nitazoxanide
Schistosomiasis S. *japonicum*	Praziquantel	60 mg/kg in 3 doses × 1 day	Treatment does not reverse established portal hypertension
S. *mansoni*	Praziquantel or Oxamniquine	40 mg/kg in 2 doses × 1 day 20 mg/kg in 2 doses × 1 day	Contraindicated in pregnancy
S. *haematobium*	Praziquantel	40 mg/kg in 2 doses × 1 day	
S. *mekongi*	Praziquantel	60 mg/kg in 3 doses × 1 day	
Strongyloidiasis (*Strongyloides stercoralis*)	Ivermectin or	200 µg/kg per day × 2 days	Discontinuing large doses of steroids is important in fulminant, disseminated disease
	Thiabendazole or	50 mg/kg per day in 2 doses × 2 days (max. 3 g/day)	
	Albendazole	400 mg bid × 7 days	
Tapeworm (adult worm) (*D. latum, T. solium, T. saginata, D. canium*)	Praziquantel or Niclosamide	5-10 mg/kg once 50 mg/kg once	
Tapeworm (*Hymenolepis nana*)	Praziquantel or Nitazoxanide	25 mg/kg once 200 mg bid × 3 days (children 4-11 years old), 100 mg bid × 3 days (children 1-3 years old)	
Trichuris trichiura (whipworm)	Mebendazole or Albendazole or Ivermectin	100 mg bid × 3 days or 500 mg once 400 mg × 3 days 200 µg/kg per day × 3 days	

need to take a detailed and distant travel history and maintain a high index of suspicion for late development of liver abscesses.

Symptoms of intestinal amebiasis vary with the location and extent of the infection. *E. histolytica* may invade any portion of the colon, though the cecum and ascending colon are most commonly affected. Patients often complain of abdominal pain, anorexia, malaise, and intermittent diarrhea. Patients with rectosigmoid involvement suffer from tenesmus and more frequent diarrhea. Patients with extensive involvement have symptoms similar to those of ulcerative colitis, with frequent mucous, bloody stools. In nonfulminant cases, fever is uncommon, but with fulminant colitis or hepatic abscess, fever can be prominent. Toxic megacolon or perforation can occur and are

leading causes of mortality in untreated patients. In some cases, a localized granulomatous reaction to *E. histolytica* known as an *ameboma* occurs. Amebomas are difficult to distinguish from colon carcinoma. Amebic dysentery may mimic inflammatory bowel disease, leading to institution of high-dose steroid therapy, which can be lethal in persons with amebiasis. Painful cutaneous ulcers may complicate colitis. Salpingitis and lymphadenitis due to *E. histolytica* have also been reported.[74,75]

Amebic liver abscess is manifested by right upper quadrant pain, leukocytosis, fever, and hepatomegaly. Liver abscess usually occurs in the absence of current or recent overt intestinal disease. Liver function tests, including bilirubin and transaminases, are often normal. Ultrasonography shows one or more cystic masses in the hepatic parenchyma. Complications of abscesses include rupture, with possible pericardial or pleural spread. Cases of postinfectious glomerulonephritis have been reported following amebic liver abscess.[76]

Diagnosis of colonic amebiasis is best made by microscopic examination of fresh stool. Three to six samples should be adequate to identify 90% of cases. Biopsies taken from the edge of colon ulcers may also be useful in identifying trophozoites, particularly with periodic acid-Schiff (PAS) stain (Figure 40-2). Indications for biopsy include negative stool exams and negative serum antibodies, chronic syndrome or mass lesions noted in a highly suspicious setting for amebiasis.[77] Stool EIA panels are available to detect E. histolytica/E. dispar with 96% sensitivity and 99% specificity.[78,79] ELISA tests are available to distinguish histolytica from dispar. Polymerase chain reaction (PCR) tests are slightly more reliable, although costly, time consuming, and not yet commercially available.[80] PCR and ELISA cannot be performed on fixed stool; the stool must be fresh or frozen.[81]

Serologic EIA detects the IgG specific for E. histolytica in 95% of patients with extraintestinal amebiasis, 70% of patients with luminal infection, and 10% of asymptomatic cyst passers.[82] Most patients with amebic liver abscess have neither overt intestinal symptoms nor detectable cysts or trophozoites in their stool. Thus, EIA is particularly useful for suspected amebic liver abscess. Unfortunately, standard serology is difficult to interpret in endemic areas. Newer serum antigen tests are available that can distinguish E. histolytica from dispar and become negative with successful treatment. If the EIA is negative during the acute presentation, a repeat serology testing is recommended in 1 week. If the second serology remains negative, other etiologies should be considered. EIA serology usually revert to negative 6 to 12 months after infection is cleared. In an aspirated abscess, the parasite is identified 15% of the time, antigen detection via ELISA has 20% sensitivity, and PCR has a sensitivity of 83% and specificity of 100%. However, PCR assays are not widely available.[82,83] In nonendemic areas, suspected liver abscesses may require aspiration to exclude bacterial causes.

Treatment of amebiasis is highly effective. The importance of correct diagnosis must again be emphasized, as only about 10% of people with stools testing positive for Entamoeba will have the pathogenic histolytica strain.[81] The drug of choice for invasive colon or liver disease is metronidazole (or the related drugs, tinidazole and ornidazole). The recommended dosage (30 to 50 mg/kg/day tid to a maximum of 750 mg/dose) is three times that employed for giardiasis. The drug is absorbed extremely well from the gut, and oral therapy is usually quite effective. Indications for drainage of liver abscesses include diagnosis, imminent rupture (cavity greater than 10 cm in adults), or failure to respond to 72 hours of metronidazole. All symptomatic patients as well as asymptomatic cyst passers require a luminal agent to prevent disease spread. Iodoquinol or paromomycin is administered for this purpose (see Table 40-1). Organisms resistant to metronidazole can be treated with nitazoxanide or tizoxanide.[84,85]

Outbreaks of infection can be prevented by attention to water supplies, good handwashing, and general hygiene. As with Giardia, a very low inoculum is needed, perhaps only a single cyst. Humans and primates are thought to be the only reservoirs of E. histolytica, but insect vectors such as cockroaches may contribute to spread.[86] Because immunity to E. histolytica is related to mucosal IgA, oral vaccines are under development.[87-89]

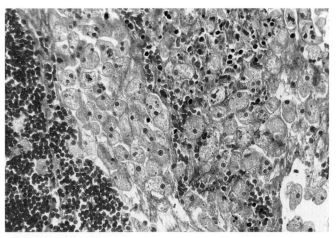

Figure 40-2. *Entamoeba histolytica* trophozoites in a colonic biopsy. (*See plate section for color.*) Courtesy Drs. Gerald Berry and Terry Longacre.

Dientamoeba fragilis

D. fragilis is a binucleate flagellate related to Trichomonas. It is 5 to 12 μm in diameter and inhabits the large intestine. It has worldwide distribution; infection is found most often in children, day-care center attendees, and persons with poor hygiene.[90] It is also associated with traveler's diarrhea. Seroprevalence studies suggest that 90% of children have experienced infection by age 5 years.[91] The vast majority of infections are asymptomatic. There is an association with pinworm infestation: patients with D. fragilis are 8 to 20 times more likely than uninfected persons to have pinworms.[92] Experimental ingestion of pinworm ova has led to D. fragilis infection. Coinfection with Blastocystis hominis has also been described. D. fragilis alone has not been shown to infect volunteers, and the organism is unstable in water and gastric juice.

Symptoms of D. fragilis infestation include diarrhea (predominantly during the first or second week), abdominal pain, flatulence, and weight loss.[93,94] Occasionally, mild colitis has been described that mimics allergic colitis.[95] But D. fragilis is not known to cause invasive disease, even in the immunocompromised. Unlike most protozoan infections, eosinophilia is reported to be associated with D. fragilis, although this may be due to associated pinworm infestation. Diagnosis is made by stool examination. The stool must be placed in preservative immediately to fix the trophozoite, because there is no cyst form of Dientamoeba. Invasive organisms have not been reported in biopsy specimens. A Scotch tape test for pinworm should be performed to look for concurrent Enterobius infestation. Treatment is usually metronidazole, although iodoquinol, tetracycline, paromomycin, and secnidazole have also been effective.[96] Because Dientamoeba has no cyst form, it exists poorly outside of hosts. The fragilis name refers to this fragile nature noted by early researchers.[97] The transmission is person-to-person rather than through contaminated foods or water. Prevention is therefore achieved by good handwashing.

Blastocystis hominis

B. hominis is a strict anaerobic protozoan that is a common inhabitant of the human cecum and colon. Its pathogenic role is controversial, because some studies have failed to note different prevalences of infection in symptomatic and asymptomatic persons.[98,99] One study that has shown such a difference was in children in Malaysia and another in German tourists.[100,101]

Infection causes chronic diarrhea in AIDS patients and may be a significant pathogen in other immunocompromised groups.[102-104] Zoonotic spread from cattle, horses, and pigs may occur.[105] Some studies suggest that the number of organisms observed in fecal smears correlates with symptoms. Symptoms are similar to those with *D. fragilis* and may be chronic.[106] A possible link between *B. hominis* and irritable bowel syndrome has been proposed.[107] Diagnosis is by stool examination, but culture is more sensitive.[108] As the pathogenic role of *B. hominis* remains questionable, treatment is not recommended by some, unless there is no other identifiable agent.[26] Treatment is usually metronidazole; furazolidone, emetine, co-trimazole, and iodoquinol are alternatives.[107]

Balantidium coli

B. coli are very large (50 to 200 μm) ciliate protozoa that may invade the colonic mucosa to induce abdominal pain, diarrhea, and frank dysentery. Fulminant colitis has also been reported. Distribution is worldwide, although most infections occur in the tropics, in association with poor hygiene and intimate contact with livestock. Swine are a major reservoir of *B. coli*, and farmers and slaughterhouse workers are at increased risk. Immunocompromised patients are at risk of severe or even fatal infection.[110,111] Diagnosis is made by finding the characteristic large trophozoites in fresh stool. Tetracycline, metronidazole, paromomycin, and iodoquinol are used to treat this infection.

Cryptosporidium

Cryptosporidium organisms were described early in this century as a veterinary pathogen, but it was not until 1976 that human disease was recognized.[112] These small protozoans are classified in the order Eucoccidiida, along with *Plasmodium* (malaria), *Isospora*, and *Toxoplasma gondii*. Cryptosporidia infect a wide variety of mammals and may complete their complex life cycle, which involves both asexual and sexual multiplication, in the intestinal epithelia of one host. They are intracellular but do not enter the cytoplasm of host cells. The final product of the life cycle is the oocyst, which measures 4 to 6 μm in diameter and contains four infectious sporozoites.

With the advent of improved diagnostic testing and increased physician awareness, a great deal has been learned about the epidemiology of *Cryptosporidium* infection. *Cryptosporidium parvum* is quite prevalent among livestock such as cattle, pigs, and sheep and domestic pets such as kittens and puppies.[113,114] More recently the presence of *C. parvum* in wildlife such as rodents, geese, flies, and shellfish has been demonstrated.[115-118] The contamination of wildlife leads to the continual reinfecting of water sources. Genotype analysis has shown that, as with *Giardia* and *Entamoeba*, there are different subgroups of *C. parvum*. Genotype 1 (or H) is thought to only infect humans and is called *C. hominis*, whereas genotype 2 (or C) infects both humans and animals.[119,120] The discovery of these genotypes add weight to the theory that human-to-human as well as zoonotic spread occurs.[39,121] Occasionally, other *Cryptosporidium* species such as those unique to cats, dogs, or deer can infect humans. *Cryptosporidium* is a relatively common cause of human diarrhea, accounting for as many as 6% of cases in the developing world and 1.5% in the developed world.[122-126] Infection may contribute to failure of height growth in endemic areas.[127] However, measurement of *C. parvum* IgG and IgA antibodies suggests that the majority of children have been exposed to the parasite.[128] This protozoan is transmitted primarily via the fecal-oral route. The respiratory route has also been reported.[26] Aside from contact with animals, other known risk factors include day-care center attendance, drinking untreated and recreational waters, employment in hospitals, and immunosuppression.[129] Prior infection offers some protection against reinfection.[130]

Parasite replication occurs mainly in the apical border of jejunal, ileal, and colonic enterocytes (Figure 40-3). Pathologic examination shows variable villus atrophy with crypt hyperplasia, usually with a mild mixed inflammatory infiltrate.

The associated clinical illness begins after approximately a week's incubation and consists of voluminous watery stools, flatulence, malaise, and abdominal pain lasting from 3 to 30 days in a normal host. Fever is not a major feature. Considerable weight loss can occur, and the disease can be devastating to previously malnourished hosts. In immunocompromised hosts, such as patients with AIDS, the diarrhea can be severe, "cholera-like," and fatal. Immunocompromised patients may develop symptomatic *Cryptosporidium* infection of pancreatic ducts, the biliary tree and gallbladder, lungs, and sinuses.[131-133] Diagnosis usually requires special stains of stool samples. In many laboratories these special stains must be specifically requested. Commercial DFA and EIA kits, as well as PCR assays with good sensitivity and specificity, are available.[134] Cryptosporidia can also be found in bronchial wash material and in biopsies of affected organs.

Treatment remains problematic. Normal hosts recover spontaneously in 1 to 3 weeks, but the immunocompromised host may suffer unremitting severe disease. Such patients may require meticulous supportive care, including intravenous fluids and nutritional support. A variety of drugs have been used with limited efficacy in patients with AIDS, including metronidazole, sulfonamides, rifaximin, and spiromycin.[135,136] A short course of nitazoxanide has shown good efficacy in clinical trials, but is not effective in children with HIV.[26,57] The luminal amebicide paromomycin has been helpful in reducing oocyst shedding and improving symptoms in some patients, but it does not clear the organism from extraluminal sites such as the biliary system. Azithromycin has shown promise in recent studies but has not yet been formally evaluated with placebo controls.[137,138] Enteric immunoglobulins from either human serum or bovine colostrum have also been administered, with varying results.[139,140] Reversal of immunosuppression by

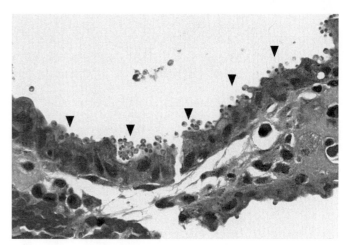

Figure 40-3. Cryptosporidia on the surface of a small intestinal biopsy. (*See plate section for color.*) Courtesy Drs. Gerald Berry and Terry Longacre.

effective antiretroviral therapy usually leads to improvement in diarrhea.[141] The probiotics *Lactobacillus reuteri* and *L. acidophilus* have reduced oocyst shedding in immunosuppressed mice.[142]

Because the oocysts are chlorine resistant and small enough to pass through conventional water purification filtration devices, huge waterborne outbreaks affecting hundreds of thousands of people are possible.[143,144] These characteristics have led the WHO to classify cryptosporidia as a "reference pathogen" for water quality.[145] Foodborne outbreaks have occurred and have been linked to soft fruit, salad vegetables, and unpasteurized apple juice. Vaccines for humans and animals are not yet available.[26]

Other Coccidia

Sarcocystis, *Cyclospora*, and *Isospora belli* are obligate intracellular protozoans that may produce intestinal coccidian infestations. *Sarcocystis* organisms produce a zoonosis in carnivores and can also cause human disease after consumption of undercooked beef or pork.[146] Infection seems to be most prevalent in Southeast Asia. *Sarcocystis hominis* and *S. suihominis* complete their life cycles in the intestines of humans. Other species of *Sarcocystis* can cause an invasive disease such as myositis.[147] Intestinal symptoms range from mild abdominal pain to acute obstruction requiring resection of heavily infested small bowel. Other than surgical resection, optimal therapy is not known.

Cyclospora species are coccidia that produce a spectrum of infection quite similar to that of *Cryptosporidium*.[148] Oocysts of *Cyclospora* are larger than those of *Cryptosporidium*, measuring 8 to 10 µm in diameter and are best seen with acid-fast stains.[149,150] These tests are not routine and must be specifically requested when infection is suspected. *Cyclospora* is a known cause of traveler's diarrhea, but prolonged illness has been reported in patients with AIDS. Invasive disease of the biliary tree has been reported in several cases.[151] Most reported cases to date have originated in developing countries where asymptomatic carriage may be relatively common among local children and may increase in the rainy season.[152] There is no clear animal host. Infection is waterborne and not person-to-person because oocysts excreted in stool are not immediately infectious. Several large foodborne outbreaks have been documented. For example, in the United States, a multistate outbreak due to *C. cayetanensis* was traced to raspberries imported from Guatemala.[153] Treatment is trimethoprim-sulfamethoxazole; ciprofloxacin is a less effective alternate for sulfa-allergic patients.[154] Prophylaxis against relapses may be needed for immunocompromised patients.

Isospora belli is a cause of traveler's diarrhea in normal hosts and of protracted diarrhea in immunocompromised hosts.[155] Although infection is much more common in the tropics, daycare outbreaks have been reported in the United States. Unlike *Cryptosporidium*, scant numbers of the large 30-µm oocysts are excreted in the stool, making diagnosis difficult. However, excreted oocysts may be infectious, and person-to-person transmission is possible.[150] Small intestine biopsy may be helpful in establishing the diagnosis. Accurate diagnosis is important because the organism is usually sensitive to trimethoprim-sulfamethoxazole. As with *Cyclospora*, ciprofloxacin is a less effective alternate. Maintenance therapy to prevent relapses may be necessary for immunocompromised patients.

Microsporidia comprise a unique group of unicellular protozoa of the Microspora phylum with 1000 separate species.[150]

Human pathogens include *Enterocytozoon bieneusi*, *Encephalitozoon* (*Septata*) *intestinalis*, *Trachipleistophora hominis*, and *Vittaforma corneae*. They are all intracellular parasites that have been reported principally in patients with AIDS and more recently in recipients of solid organ transplants.[155-159] However, cases in apparently normal patients have been described, especially in those with a travel history to the tropics. Animal reservoirs such as pigs, domestic pets, and rodents exist, and zoonotic infection is possible, but waterborne or sexual spread is probably the more common mode of infection.[160,161] The illness is similar to that found with *Cryptosporidium* infection: prolonged watery diarrhea with weight loss. Microsporidia can also cause cholangiopathy, keratoconjunctivitis, and respiratory tract infections in patients with AIDS.[131,162-165] Although special techniques for visualizing spores are reported, diagnosis often requires intestinal biopsy, preferably jejunal.[166] Experienced or reference laboratories should be used when possible.[167] The more common *E. bieneusi* is difficult to recognize in standard paraffin hematoxylin and eosin sections and may require embedding in plastic resin, special stains, or electron microscopy. *E. intestinalis* is larger and more easily seen on routine sections. Albendazole has been reported helpful for these infections, particularly for *E. intestinalis*. It has been noted that albendazole improves clinical status in *E. bieneusi* infections but does not clear the organism from the stool. PCR may be useful in differentiating between *E. intestinalis* and *E. bieneusi*, in light of the drug's efficacy.[168] Fumagillin and nitazoxanide can be used as alternatives.[169,170] The combination of albendazole and furazolidone has been proposed for *E. bieneusi* infections in AIDS patients.[171] The organisms are very resistant to environmental conditions, and immunocompromised patients may reduce risk of infection by avoidance of swimming, drinking unfiltered tap water, and contact with pets such as rabbits, birds, and dogs.[172]

Nematodes (Roundworms)

Ascaris lumbricoides

A. lumbricoides is the largest and most common helminthic infection worldwide.[173] Adult worms live in the jejunum, where the 20- to 49-cm-long females may produce 200,000 eggs per day. The fertilized eggs are excreted in the feces and must mature in the soil for 10 to 14 days before the first-stage larvae, which are infectious, develop. When such embryonated eggs are ingested and reach the intestine, second-stage larvae develop that penetrate the intestinal mucosa to migrate via the liver to the lungs. The tiny larvae then pass through the alveolar wall to the respiratory tract and back to the gut after being swallowed. Then mature worms develop that may live 12 to 18 months. The respiratory phase may induce an eosinophilic pneumonitis, Loeffler's syndrome, which may clinically resemble seasonal asthma.

Under normal circumstances, the intestinal phase of infection is asymptomatic. Serious complications arise either during heavy infestations, which may produce intestinal obstruction, or during migration of worms, which is frequently precipitated by an unrelated febrile illness. Infected patients may vomit or cough up the large earthworm-like ascarids during such illnesses. Alternatively, the worms can obstruct the biliary or pancreatic ducts, producing cholangitis or pancreatitis.[174-176] *Ascaris* obstruction of the bowel lumen may lead to volvulus or perforation.[177]

The role of *Ascaris* worms in chronic malnutrition of children in the tropics is unclear. Heavy infestation is probably one of many factors affecting such children. Some studies have shown improvement in nutritional status after *Ascaris* eradication.[178]

Diagnosis of ascariasis can be made by finding the eggs in stools. Adult worms may be expelled from the mouth or anus, observed during endoscopy, or outlined by barium during radiologic studies. Eosinophilia is prominent only during larval migrations through tissues.

Treatments include pyrantel pamoate, which paralyzes *Ascaris* worms and can be given by nasogastric tube for cases of intestinal obstruction. Mebendazole and albendazole are also effective in uncomplicated cases. Endoscopic or surgical therapy is necessary for some complications, although most cases of biliary ascariasis and intestinal obstruction respond to conservative medical management. Indications for surgical intervention include lack of response to medical treatment within 24 to 48 hours, complete obstruction, intussusception, volvulus, or perforation.[179] Mass treatment programs are useful in communities with high prevalences of infection.

Trichuris trichiura

T. trichiura (whipworm) is named for the morphology of adult worms. *Trichuris* worms differ from other human nematodes in two ways. First, there is no tissue migration during its life cycle. Second, adult *Trichuris* worms reside in the colon rather than the small intestine (Figure 40-4). Like *Ascaris* eggs, those of *Trichuris* must mature in the soil before being ingested, making direct person-to-person transmission impossible. The larvae hatch and mature in the distal small bowel before migrating to the cecum, where they attach to the bowel wall via their narrow anterior ("whip") end. They may reside in the colon for as long as 8 years.

Trichuris has a worldwide distribution similar to that of *Ascaris*. The infection is most common in the tropics, especially Asia, but an estimated 2 million people are infected in the United States. Toddlers and young children tend to have the heaviest worm burdens.

Most light infections are asymptomatic. Moderate infections produce a picture of chronic colitis with diarrhea, abdominal pain, and weight loss.[180] Heavy infections can produce a dysentery-like picture that may feature rectal prolapse.[181] Chronic infections in children are associated with stunted growth, anemia, and delayed cognitive development.[182] Treatment is with albendazole or mebendazole (see Table 40-1).

Necator americanus and *Ancylostoma duodenale* (hookworms)

Hookworm infestation affects approximately 1 billion people.[181,183] There are two species of human hookworms, *N. americanus* and *A. duodenale*. Transmission of hookworm requires contamination of soil with human fecal material and an unshod population (usually young children). Filiform infective larvae in the contaminated soil invade the host via the skin (usually the bare foot) and are carried by the circulation to the lungs, where they penetrate the alveoli. They then proceed up the airway until they are swallowed into the gut. Hookworms reside in the small intestine, where they attach to the mucosa with their specialized mouthparts. Each worm is capable of ingesting up to 250 μL of blood per day. Symptoms of hookworm are the sequelae of this blood loss—mainly anemia and hypoproteinemia.[184] Patients may also report intense pruritic rashes on the feet during the initial larval penetration, known as "ground itch." Some patients with heavy worm burdens also

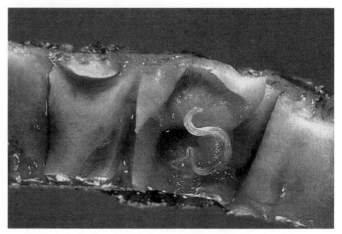

Figure 40-4. *Trichuris trichiura* in a resected colon. (*See plate section for color.*) Courtesy of Drs. Gerald Berry and Terry Longacre.

report epigastric distress. Diagnosis of significant hookworm infection is made by finding the characteristic ova in fresh or preserved stool specimens. Treatment of choice is mebendazole or albendazole (see Table 40-1).

Strongyloides stercoralis

Strongyloides is a small (1 to 10 mm long) nematode that is capable of replicating completely within the host.[185] Because of this capability, patients with suppressed immune systems can acquire an enormous worm burden, with potentially fatal dissemination. Infection begins when filiform larvae in contaminated soil penetrate the skin. The larvae then migrate via blood or lymph to the lungs, where they penetrate the alveoli and proceed up the airway to the pharynx and are swallowed. The larvae mature in the proximal small intestine, and females burrow into the lamina propria to lay eggs (Figure 40-5). The eggs hatch locally, and the resulting rhabditiform larvae migrate into the intestinal lumen. Most of the rhabditiform larvae are passed with stool into the environment, where they mature into infectious filiform larvae. A variable number are able to differentiate into filiform larvae in the host colon. These infectious progeny are capable of reinfecting the host and maintaining a state of chronic infection.

In most hosts, an equilibrium state seems to be reached in which a small number of adult worms are maintained. In severely malnourished or steroid-treated hosts, the equilibrium becomes impaired and huge worm burdens can develop. In such circumstances larvae may disseminate to all organs, carrying with them associated enteric bacteria. This syndrome, known as disseminated strongyloidiasis or hyperinfection syndrome, is usually fatal.[186] *Strongyloides* organisms are present in virtually all tropical and subtropical regions. They are also found in the southern United States and in small pockets of industrialized nations. Institutionalized patients are often infected.

Whereas most normal patients with chronic low-grade infections are asymptomatic, *Strongyloides* can cause significant gastrointestinal illness. Most common is a syndrome similar to giardiasis, with bloating, heartburn, and malabsorptive stools. Intractable diarrhea has been described in infants. Rarely, an ulcerative colitis-like picture may be seen with prominent pseudopolyp formation.[187] Some patients develop recurrent urticarial or maculopapular rash, and migrating larvae may produce a serpiginous rash known as larva currens, which is pathognomonic.[179]

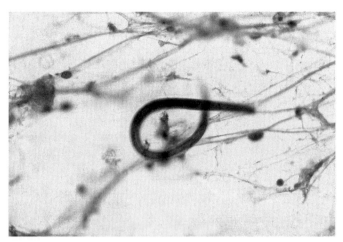

Figure 40-5. *Strongyloides stercoralis* (adult form). (*See plate section for color.*) Courtesy Drs. Gerald Berry and Terry Longacre.

The disseminated strongyloidiasis syndrome most often follows high-dose corticosteroid therapy.[188] Interestingly, the hyperinfection syndrome does not appear to be very common in patients with AIDS, even in tropical areas.[189] The hyperinfection syndrome usually results in a severe mucoid, bloody diarrhea, as a result of millions of adult worms and larvae migrating through the mucosa of the intestine. Prostration, shock, perforation, and associated gram-negative sepsis are common. Larvae can carry gram-negative organisms to every organ, including those of the central nervous system. Even with treatment, mortality can be more than 25% in this syndrome.[179]

Diagnosis of *S. stercoralis* infection is principally by identification of larvae in the stool. Repeat stool studies may be needed, because the sensitivity of a single stool exam can be as low as 30%, especially in chronic infections that have a low worm output.[179] Eggs and adult worms are seldom identified. Duodenal fluid or biopsy may also be helpful in the diagnosis. Eosinophilia is common but often not impressive and is not a feature of the disseminated disease. CDC immunoassay has sensitivity up to 95% and specificity up to 90%.

Treatment of choice is ivermectin.[190] Albendazole and mebendazole have some efficacy as well. For disseminated strongyloidiasis, treatment is daily until symptoms resolve and larvae are no longer detected for at least 2 weeks, which is the length of the autoinfection cycle. For follow-up after treatment, serology and eosinophilia may be better monitoring tools than stool studies.[179]

Capillaria philippinensis

C. philippinensis normally parasitizes freshwater fish and birds, but it can be acquired by humans who consume raw or undercooked fish. As with *S. stercoralis*, a complete cycle of reproduction can occur within the human host, allowing for great amplification of the worm burden. The worms primarily colonize the upper small intestine. The human disease has been mainly reported in Southeast Asia, Thailand, and the Philippines. Symptoms are chronic abdominal pain, diarrhea, severe wasting, and edema.[191] The disease is often fatal when untreated. Eggs, larvae, and adult worms may be found in the stool or in duodenal aspirates. Treatment is a prolonged (20-day) course of mebendazole or albendazole.

Enterobius vermicularis (pinworm)

These small nematodes are a common infection of children throughout the world and are the most common helminth infection in the United States.[179] They inhabit the cecum, appendix, and adjacent bowel and cause anal pruritus when the females emerge from the rectum to lay eggs in the perianal skin. The migrating females can also cause urinary tract infections, vaginitis, and salpingitis in girls. The eggs are best found by placing a piece of clear adhesive tape sticky side down over the perianal area during the night or early morning and then examining it under the microscope. The sensitivity for a single tape test is 50% and is 99% for five tape tests. Obtaining three consecutive specimens is recommended. Treatment is with mebendazole. Because of frequent environmental contamination, most clinicians treat the household. Reinfection is common, and repeated treatment courses may be needed.[58]

Cestodes (Tapeworms)

The most important tapeworms of humans are *D. latum*, *T. saginata*, *T. solium*, and *Hymenolepis nana*. The first three are spread by the ingestion of undercooked fish or meat, whereas *H. nana* has a classic fecal-oral route of contagion. All of the adult worms consist of a scolex, or head, which attaches to the host intestine, and numerous proglottids, the egg-producing segments.

D. latum is a fish tapeworm that can measure 3 to 10 m in length. Most infections are asymptomatic, although vitamin B_{12} deficiency may occur because of competition with the host. Diagnosis is made by finding eggs or proglottids in the stool. Treatment is praziquantel.

Taenia solium

T. solium is the pork tapeworm. Humans acquire the intestinal infection by eating undercooked pork containing the infectious cysticerci. Intestinal infection is largely asymptomatic, but a potentially serious condition can be transmitted by eggs passed in the stools of humans infected with the pork tapeworm. Cysticercosis results from ingestion of eggs from *T. solium*–infected humans. The ingested eggs hatch into oncospheres, which penetrate the mucosa and are carried by the blood to a variety of tissues, including muscle and brain. Seizures and other neurologic problems may follow.

Taenia saginata

T. saginata, the beef tapeworm, is acquired by eating undercooked beef. This largest human parasite may be 25 m long. Nevertheless, infection is usually asymptomatic except for the passage of proglottids in the feces or the occasional crawling out of the anus of active proglottids. The eggs of *T. saginata* are not infectious in humans, so there is no equivalent of cysticercosis from the beef tapeworm.

Hymenolepis nana

H. nana does not require an intermediate host and spreads easily via the fecal-oral route. Furthermore, autoinfection may allow the worm burden to increase without additional exposure. Symptoms of heavy worm burden may include diarrhea, cramping, and anorexia. The diagnosis is made by finding ova in the stool. Niclosamide and praziquantel are the drugs of choice.

Flukes

Schistosomiasis

Schistosoma mansoni, *S. japonicum*, and *S. haematobium* are trematodes whose complex life cycles require an intermediate snail host.[192-194] *S. mansoni* is found in the Caribbean, South America, the Middle East, and Africa. *S. japonicum* is found in the Far East: Japan, China, and the Philippines. *S. haematobium* is found mainly in the Nile valley and elsewhere in Africa. Humans are infected when skin is exposed to contaminated water containing cercariae, which penetrate the skin and are carried to the lungs. They eventually reach the systemic circulation and the intrahepatic portal circulation, where they mature into adult forms. As the male and female worms couple, they migrate upstream to the terminal mesenteric venules, where the female lays 300 to 3000 eggs per day for several years. Some eggs erode into the gut lumen and are excreted with feces, to continue their life cycle in snails; other eggs remain trapped in tissues or are swept upstream into the liver. As the eggs erode into the bowel lumen, they evoke an inflammatory response that may produce a dysentery-like picture with bleeding, ulceration, and pseudopolyp formation. With severe chronic infection, eggs that have been carried to the liver cause fibrosis and severe portal hypertension. Diagnosis can be made by stool examination in the more acute phases. Rectal biopsy and liver biopsy can also be diagnostic. Serologic testing is also available (but not helpful) for persons in endemic regions, where light exposure is common. Treatment with praziquantel is effective but does not reverse the severe chronic portal hypertension seen in long-standing cases.

Liver Flukes

Clonorchis sinensis, *Opisthorchis viverrini*, and *O. felineus* are trematode liver flukes. The first two are common in southern Asia, and *O. felineus* is found in eastern Europe. After ingestion of undercooked fish or crab, the metacercariae excyst in the small intestine and migrate to the small intestine. Most mild infections are asymptomatic, although heavier infections may manifest as recurrent cholangitis or biliary obstruction. Radiographically, the infection may mimic sclerosing cholangitis.[195] Long-term infection may lead to cholangiocarcinoma. Diagnosis is made by finding eggs in the stool. Treatment is praziquantel.[196]

Zoonotic Infections

For most of the parasitic infections described previously, humans are primary, or at least intermediate, hosts (i.e., the infecting parasites can complete or partially complete their reproductive cycle in humans). Infection with parasites from other native hosts can lead to unusual manifestations, as these "strangers in a strange land" often migrate aimlessly away from the intestine.

Cutaneous Larva Migrans

Nematode larvae from a variety of species can wander in the skin, producing severe pruritus. "Swimmer's itch" is usually due to cercariae from bird schistosomes, whereas "ground itch" syndromes may be due to a variety of nematodes.

Anisakiasis

Anisakis larvae (from raw or undercooked fish) can produce intense abdominal distress as they flee the gastric or intestinal lumen across the epithelium. These parasites are quite common in a variety of popular food fish, such as salmon, mackerel, rockfish, and cod.[197] Symptoms usually begin within 12 hours of eating the fish. The worms have a propensity for the greater curve of the stomach and can produce an impressive local inflammatory response as well as systemic leukocytosis.[198] Some data suggest that symptoms result from hypersensitivity to the worms. Diagnosis is based on history, radiology, and endoscopy. Treatment consists of physically removing the worms by endoscopy or surgery.

Ancylostoma caninum

Canine hookworms can cause eosinophilic ileocolitis during their abortive infection of humans.[197,199] Although most cases have been reported from western Australia, at least one case has been described in the southern United States.[200] *A. caninum* is common in dogs worldwide, and further reports are anticipated. Because the canine hookworm does not produce eggs in human hosts, diagnosis has depended on finding the usually solitary worm during colonoscopy or by serology. Mebendazole and albendazole are said to be helpful.

Visceral Larva Migrans

The larvae of ascarids of cats and dogs (*Toxocara cati* and *T. canis*) disseminate in the viscera and eyes of the child host who ingests the ova, which are common in sandboxes and playground soil.[201,202] Typical clinical manifestations include fever, hepatomegaly, lymphadenopathy, cough, and wheezing. Serious sequelae, including blindness, can result from ocular involvement. Diagnosis is based on the clinical picture and serology. Although most cases resolve spontaneously, severe pulmonary disease responds to steroids. Larvicidal drugs such as diethylcarbamazine and albendazole are also used.

REFERENCES

26. Escobedo AA, Almirall P, Alfonson M, et al. Treatment of intestinal protozoan infections in children. Arch Dis Child 2009;94:478–482.

57. The Medical Letter. Drugs for parasitic infections. July 2007; 5(Suppl): 1–15. Last modified July 2009. Available at http://www.medletter.com/.

58. American Academy of Pediatrics. Red Book: 2006 Report of the Committee on Infectious Diseases. Elk Grove Village: IL: American Academy of Pediatrics; 2006.

77. Ravdin J, Stauffer W. *Entamoeba histolytica* (amebiasis). In: Mandell GL, Bennett JE, Dolin R, eds. Mandell, Douglas and Bennett's Principles and Practice of Infectious Diseases. 6th ed. Philadelphia: Elsevier; 2005 p. 3097–3111.

82. Centers for Disease Control and Prevention. 2009 Parasite and Health, amebiasis. Available at http://www.dpd.cdc.gov. Accessed September 7, 2009.

179. Maguire J. Introduction to helminth infections. In: Mandell GL, Bennett JE, Dolin R, eds. Mandell, Douglas and Bennett's Principles and Practice of Infectious Diseases. 6th ed. Philadelphia: Elsevier; 2005 p. 3258–3267.

See expertconsult.com for a complete list of references and the review questions for this chapter.

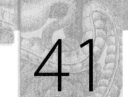

GASTROINTESTINAL MANIFESTATIONS OF PRIMARY IMMUNODEFICIENCY

41

Cary Qualia • Athos Bousvaros

Since the last edition of this book, advances in the understanding of the adaptive and innate immune systems have led to the characterization of a number of novel primary immune deficiencies, including IPEX syndrome and NEMO mutations. In addition, it is now recognized that "idiopathic inflammatory bowel disease" (aka IBD, Crohn's disease, and ulcerative colitis) may also be in part caused by genetic mutations in the innate and adaptive immune system. An expert panel of the World Health Organization has identified more than 80 primary and secondary immunodeficiency syndromes.[1] The most common of these primary immune deficiencies is selective IgA deficiency, which is very often asymptomatic. However, other primary immune deficiency syndromes have more severe complications, and frequently affect the intestine and liver. This chapter first gives an overview of the immunologic pathways that can be affected in primary immune deficiency and then reviews the gastrointestinal manifestations and complications of the more common primary immunodeficiency syndromes (Table 41-1). A more detailed discussion of the systemic complications of each specific syndrome can be found elsewhere.[2,3]

INNATE VERSUS ADAPTIVE IMMUNITY

The immune response is a complex process that can be divided into innate and adaptive responses. This distinction is somewhat arbitrary, as the innate immune response can initiate the adaptive immune response. The differences between these two arms of the immune system are summarized in Table 41-2. The *innate immune system* is the first line of defense against invading microorganisms and involves a response to a limited number of microbial products, including lipopolysaccharides, peptidoglycans, and flagellins. The microbial products that activate the innate immune system are called *pathogen-associated molecular patterns* (PAMPs), and the cellular receptors that bind these products are called *pattern-recognition receptors* (PRRs). The innate system serves a prominent protective function in all tissues and organs, especially the intestinal tract, genitourinary tract, respiratory tract, and skin, where there is greater exposure to the external environment and foreign antigens. Components of the innate immune system include epithelial surfaces that form physical barriers (e.g., the skin, lung, or gut epithelia), antimicrobial peptides (defensins, cathelicidins), complement, intraepithelial lymphocytes, dendritic cells, macrophages, and neutrophils.[4,5]

The initial interaction involved in the initiation of an innate immune response involves the interaction of a PAMP microbial substance (protein, lipopeptide, or lipopolysaccharide) with a pattern recognition receptor on a cell (e.g., a dendritic cells or a macrophage). The PRR may be either on the surface of a cell (e.g., a Toll-like receptor (TLR)) or an intracellular molecule (e.g., an intracellular NOD protein). The interaction of an organism's PAMP product with a cell's PRR triggers a signaling cascade involving MAP kinases and IkB kinases, ultimately resulting in transcription of NF-κB responsive cytokine producing genes. The end result is cytokine (e.g., interleukin-6, tumor necrosis factor) production. The cytokines can in turn produce a rapid but limited immune response. The initial immune response generated by the innate immune system may include the production of additional cytokines by dendritic cells, the phagocytosis of a microbe by a macrophage or neutrophil, or the killing of bacteria and infected cells by natural killer (NK) cells[5,6] (Figure 41-1).

The innate immune system is limited in its repertoire. It can only respond to a small number of bacterial molecules, and bacteria have evolved proteins (e.g., virulence factors) that are not recognized by innate immune receptors. In contrast, the adaptive immune system has the ability to generate receptors and antibodies that recognize a much wider array of microbial pathogens. The principal effector cell components of the adaptive immune system are antibody-producing B cells, phagocytes, and cytotoxic T cells. To activate the adaptive immune system, macrophages and dendritic cells take up and digest antigens, then process and present the antigen to T cells. Activated helper T cells in turn stimulate the production of antibody-producing B cells and cytotoxic cells.[4]

Thus, the human immune system can generate new antibodies and new cellular receptors to allow it to recognize pathogens and fight infections more efficiently. However, these responses often take days to weeks to achieve maximal activity and require a somatic gene rearrangement, which results in immunologic memory. The majority of immunodeficiency syndromes described in this chapter represent defects in adaptive immunity.

COMPONENTS OF THE ADAPTIVE IMMUNE RESPONSE

To trigger the cascade of immunologic events summarized in Table 41-3, an exogenous antigen must penetrate the physical barriers at epithelial surfaces. In certain specialized regions of gut epithelium termed *follicle-associated epithelium* (dome epithelium), modified epithelial cells (M cells) preferentially bind bacteria and viruses. These M cells are located over lymphoid nodules and Peyer's patches in the gut. They provide a portal of

435

TABLE 41-1. **Common Primary Immunodeficiency Syndromes**[164-167]

Immunodeficiency	Mechanism	Laboratory Findings	Gastrointestinal Manifestations	Extraintestinal Manifestations
Humoral				
Selective IgA deficiency	Inability of B cells to differentiate into IgA-secreting plasma cells	Low or absent IgA with normal IgM and IgG levels	Diarrhea, celiac sprue, nodular lymphoid hyperplasia, cholelithiasis, primary biliary cirrhosis	Recurrent sinusitis and other respiratory tract infections, atopy, anaphylaxis to blood products and IVIg, achlorhydria, Henoch-Schönlein purpura
X-linked agammaglobulinemia	Arrest of cell maturation in pre-B lymphocyte stage	Decreased levels of all serum immunoglobulins, reduced number of B cells with normal precursor levels	Diarrhea, malabsorption, sclerosing cholangitis	Recurrent sinusitis and other respiratory tract infections, arthritis, enteroviral encephalitis, dermatomyositis
Hyper-IgM syndrome	Defective expression of CD154 on T cells, impaired B-cell isotype switching	Normal/elevated IgM with low IgA and IgG levels	Diarrhea, sclerosing cholangitis, abnormal aminotransaminases, hepatosplenomegaly, recurrent oral ulcers, severe hepatitis B infections	Chronic encephalitis and meningitis, lymphoid hyperplasia, autoimmune diseases (diabetes mellitus, rheumatoid arthritis, uveitis)
Transient hypogammaglobulinemia of infancy	Accentuation and prolongation of "physiologic" hypogammaglobulinemia of infancy as IgG derived from mother declines and infant production is not fully developed	Low serum IgG levels, IgA and IgM levels may be low	Chronic diarrhea, lactose intolerance	Recurrent respiratory tract infections
Cellular				
DiGeorge syndrome	Thymic aplasia with impaired T lymphocyte maturation	Decreased levels of T lymphocytes with normal B and natural killer (NK) cells, normal immunoglobulin levels	Mucocutaneous candidiasis	Cardiac defects (e.g., truncus arteriosus), hypocalcemia, tetany, seizures, facial abnormalities
Chronic mucocutaneous candidiasis	Failure of T cells to proliferate or stimulate cytokines in response to *Candida albicans*	Mucosal swabs, scrapings, and biopsy specimens positive for *Candida*	Candidal thrush and esophagitis	Skin lesions, autoimmune endocrinopathies (e.g., thyroiditis, adrenal insufficiency), dental enamel dysplasia, vitiligo
Combined Cellular-Humoral				
Common variable immunodeficiency	Normal levels of B cells that are unable to differentiate into plasma cells	Reduced levels of IgG accompanied by low IgA and/or low IgM levels, normal or reduced B cell numbers	Diarrhea, IBD-like disease, pernicious anemia, nodular lymphoid hyperplasia, malabsorption, MALT lymphoma	Chronic respiratory tract infections
Severe combined immunodeficiency	Failure of maturation of lymphoid stem cells	Reduced T cells with normal B and NK cells	Diarrhea, oral candidiasis, esophageal candidiasis	Pneumonia, bronchitis, failure to thrive, illnesses following vaccinations
Disorders of Phagocyte Function				
Chronic granulomatous disease	Defects in NADPH oxidase activity, impairing oxidative burst and killing activity	Dihydrorhodamine reductase (DHR) or nitroblue tetrazolium (NBT) tests show diminished neutrophil respiratory burst activity	Colitis, hepatic abscess, gastric outlet obstruction, small bowel obstruction, granulomatous stomatitis, oral ulcers, esophageal dysmotility	Recurrent skin infections and abscesses, lymphadenitis

TABLE 41-1. **Common Primary Immunodeficiency Syndromes[164-167]—cont'd**

Immunodeficiency	Mechanism	Laboratory Findings	Gastrointestinal Manifestations	Extraintestinal Manifestations
Leukocyte adhesion deficiency	Defects in adhesion to endothelium and migration into tissue	Increased neutrophils	Mucositis, necrotizing enterocolitis, perirectal abscesses	Delayed separation of umbilical cord, periodontitis, absent pus formation, impaired wound healing
Other				
Wiskott-Aldrich syndrome	Disruption of membrane receptors, interrupting integrity of cytoskeletal elements	Thrombocytopenia with small platelets	Colitis, bloody diarrhea, malabsorption	Eczema, recurrent upper respiratory tract infections, bleeding
NF-κB essential modifier (NEMO) mutations	Impaired B cell switching and APC activation	Increased IgA and IgE levels, decreased IgM and normal IgG levels	Vomiting, diarrhea, CMV colitis, Giardiasis	Features of hypohidrotic ectodermal dysplasia, growth delay
IPEX	FOX P3 mutation leads to impaired T cell development	Eosinophilia; may have increased IgE and IgA levels	Severe enteropathy with watery/bloody diarrhea	Eczema, atopy, lymphadenopathy, diabetes mellitus

APC, antigen-presenting cell; CMV, cytomegalovirus; IBD, inflammatory bowel disease; IPEX, immune dysfunction, polyendocrinopathy, enteropathy, X-linked; IVIg, intravenous immunoglobulin; MALT, mucosa-associated lymphoid tissue; NF-κB, nuclear transcription factor-κB.

TABLE 41-2. **Innate Versus Adaptive Immunity**

	Innate Immunity	Adaptive Immunity
Response	Immediate	Delayed (days to weeks)
Stimuli	Limited (bacterial LPS, HSP, etc.)	Variable
Receptors	Toll-like receptors	MHC–TCR
Cells	Dendritic cells, macrophages, NK cells, intraepithelial	T and B lymphocytes, lymphocytes of the gut
Mechanisms	Variety	Cellular and humoral immune responses
	Mechanical barriers – epithelial cells, cytotoxic (defensins and other secretory enzymes), gastric acid, mucins, commensal intestinal flora, intestinal motility	

HSP, heat shock protein; LPS, lipopolysaccharide; MHC, major histocompatibility complex; NK, natural killer T cells; TCR, T-cell receptor.

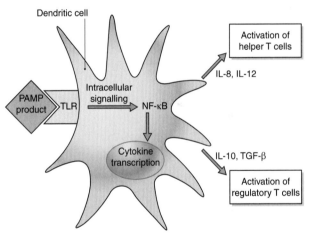

Figure 41-1. Mechanisms of innate immune response. Binding of bacterial proteins with pathogen-associated molecular patterns (PAMP products, e.g., lipopolysaccharide) to Toll-like receptors (TLR) on dendritic cells results in signal transduction. The signal generated at the cell membrane results in the activation of a complex signaling pathway involving the proteins MyD88, TNF receptor-associated factor 6 (TRAF-6), NIK, and IKK. As a result, the protein NF-κB enters the nucleus and stimulates cytokine transcription. Depending on the cytokines released, different T-cell populations may be activated.

entry that directly exposes potential pathogens to the systemic and mucosal components of the adaptive immune systems.[7]

The adaptive immune system has different methods of responding to microbial proteins. The "classical pathway" of antigen presentation involves endocytosis of a microbial protein or peptide by antigen-presenting cells (APCs, including macrophages and dendritic cells). APCs are characterized by their ability to phagocytose proteins or peptides, degrade them intracellularly, complex these peptides with proteins of the major histocompatibility complex (MHC), and transport the peptide-MHC protein to the APC surface.[8,9] Antigen presentation to a CD4 (helper) T lymphocyte occurs when a peptide complexed to an MHC class II protein on the surface of an APC comes in contact with the T-cell receptor complex on the surface of the lymphocyte. Binding to the T-cell receptor alone is not

sufficient to promote T-lymphocyte activation, however. The CD4 molecule on the surface of the T lymphocyte stabilizes the T cell–APC interaction. In addition, to propagate the signaling pathway that leads to T-cell activation, a second co-stimulatory signal must be delivered to another molecule on the surface of the T cell. The co-stimulatory signal can be delivered in a number of ways (e.g., macrophage CD80 binding to T cell CD28, or macrophageLFA-3 binding to T cell CD2). Failure to deliver the second signal may result in a clone of T cells that do not respond to antigen and may be a mechanism by which the host develops tolerance to certain antigens.[8,10]

If antigenic stimulation and co-stimulation occur, a signal is transduced through the CD3 complex, characterized by phosphorylation of tyrosine molecules in the CD3 and zeta chains (Figure 41-2). Subsequently, tyrosine kinases, including Lck and zeta-associated protein 70 (ZAP-70), are activated and induce phosphorylation of phospholipase Cγ1, which in turn converts inositol 4,5-biphosphate to inositol 1,4,5-triphosphate (IP_3). IP_3 formation results in increased cytosolic free calcium from intracellular stores, and activation of the molecule calcineurin. A second intracellular signal transduction pathway initiated by phospholipase Cγ1 involves the molecules diacylglycerol and protein kinase C (see Figure 41-2). These pathways are separate but synergistic, and inhibition of one or the other may abrogate T-cell activation.[11,12]

Calcineurin and protein kinase C enzymes in turn promote increased transcription of cytokine gene products mediated by nuclear binding factors, including the nuclear factor of activated

TABLE 41-3. Components of the Adaptive Immune Response

Antigen uptake by antigen-presenting cells (dendritic cells, macrophages)
Antigen processing
Antigen presentation to T cells
T-lymphocyte activation
B-cell activation, switching, and immunoglobulin production
Leukocyte homing and adhesion to tissues
Effector cell recruitment
Release of inflammatory mediators (e.g., prostaglandin, leukotriene, complement)

Adapted from Rhee and Bousvaros, 2004, with permission.[168]

T cells (NF-AT) and NF-κB. NF-κB essential modifier (NEMO), also known as inhibitor of NF-κB kinase γ (IKK-γ), is required for the activation and subsequent translocation to the nucleus of the transcription factor NF-κB, where NF-κB activates multiple target genes.[13,14] A third T-cell activation pathway triggered by antigen recognition involves a group of kinases termed mitogen-activated protein (MAP) kinases, which in turn activate the transcription factor AP-1.[15,16]

Based on studies performed with murine T-lymphocyte clones, helper (CD4) T lymphocytes have been categorized into two broad types, Th1 and Th2. Both of these functional T cell subtypes mature from naïve CD4 helper T cells. Cytokines secreted by dendritic cells and other antigen-presenting cells are essential in determining whether Th1 or Th2 cells are generated; release of interferon-gamma and IL-12 preferentially promotes differentiation of Th1 cells, whereas release of IL-4 promotes Th2 cell formation. Type 1 helper T cells (Th1) promote cellular immune responses and delayed-type hypersensitivity by secreting interleukin (IL) 2, interferon γ (IFN-γ) and tumor necrosis factor β (TNF-β). In contrast, type 2 helper T cells (Th2) promote B lymphocyte differentiation into plasma cells and antibody formation by secreting IL-4, IL-5, IL-10, and IL-13.[17,18] Thus, a Th1 cytokine pattern promotes macrophage activation with the aim of eliminating intracellular microbes, whereas a Th2 response results in mast cell activation, clearing of parasites and allergic reactions. A third type of CD4 cell, called Th17, has recently been identified and assists in recruitment of leukocytes to areas of inflammation by producing IL-17.[19] Th1 cells have been implicated in the pathogenesis of

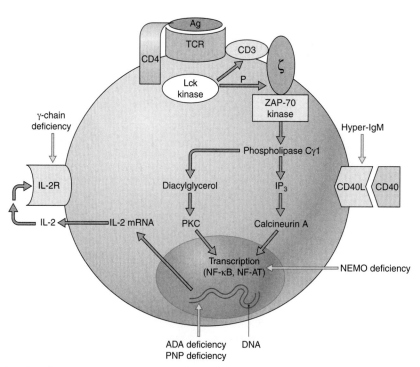

Figure 41-2. Signaling effects in T-lymphocyte activation and sites of effects of immunodeficiency syndromes. Binding of antigen (Ag), in association with MHC proteins, to the T-cell receptor (TCR)-CD3 complex activates two intracellular pathways of signaling. The first pathway involves diacylglycerol (DAG) and protein kinase C (PKC); the second involves inositol triphosphate (IP_3) and calcineurin. The end-result of this intracellular signaling is increased DNA synthesis by T cells and increased synthesis of cytokine (e.g., IL-2) messenger RNA as mediated by the nuclear factor of activated T cells (NF-AT). The activated T-cell expresses CD40 ligand (CD40L). Patients with adenosine deaminase (ADA) deficiency and purine nucleotidyl phosphorylase (PNP) deficiency have impaired synthesis of DNA; patients with X-linked severe combined immunodeficiency have defective IL-2 receptor (-chain expression. Patients with hyper-IgM syndrome have defective expression of CD40L. Adapted from Rhee SJ, Bousvaros A. Immunosuppressive therapies. In: Walker WA, Goulet O, Kleinman RE, et al., eds. Pediatric Gastrointestinal Disease, 4th ed. Lewiston, NY: BC Decker; 2004.

Crohn's disease, whereas Th2 cells have been implicated in the pathogenesis of ulcerative colitis and allergic disorders.

Another group of T cells termed regulatory T cells serves to down-regulate the immune response and promote immunologic tolerance. The best characterized regulatory T cell subset is the CD4+CD25+ T cell, which secretes anti-inflammatory cytokines, such as IL-10 and transforming growth factor β (TGF-β). The IL-10 inhibits macrophage activation and antagonizes the pro-inflammatory cytokine IFN-γ, whereas TGF-β inhibits B- and T-cell proliferation.[20] These regulatory T cells are characterized by a transcription factor called FoxP3, and mutations in this gene in humans result in IPEX, a rare cause of infantile autoimmunity (discussed later in this chapter).

Humoral immunity is generated by B lymphocytes, which, on exposure to antigen, proliferate and differentiate into plasma cells.[21] All B cells are initially programmed to synthesize IgM (Figure 41-3). For a B cell to switch its class of antibody produced to IgG or IgA (isotype switching), several other molecular stimuli need to occur. The CD40 ligand (gp39, CD154) is a molecule on the surface of the T cell that binds to CD40 on B cells. This interaction promotes B-cell activation and differentiation, as well as isotype switching from IgM to IgG, IgA, or IgE. Conversely, the CD40-CD154 interaction also promotes activation of CD4+ T cells. Deficiency of this molecule results in an unusual form of immunodeficiency termed the hyper-IgM syndrome.[22] Another T-cell protein termed ICOS is also important in B-cell differentiation, and ICOS mutations have been associated with common variable immune deficiencies.[23] Subsequent differentiation to immunoglobulin-producing plasma cells depends on a number of B-cell genes, including the transmembrane activator and CAML interactor (TACI) gene. Cytokines, such as IL-4, are responsible in switching B cells from IgM to IgE production, and TGF-β has been shown to play a

role in B-cell switching to IgA production.[24] Thus, humoral immunodeficiencies may arise either from direct mutations in B cell genes (e.g., TACI, which results in selective IgA or common variable immune deficiency), or by mutations in T cell genes (e.g., CD 40 ligand) that are essential for B-cell differentiation.[25]

The end result of the immune response is the recruitment of activated effector cells (cytotoxic lymphocytes, macrophages, neutrophils, eosinophils, and mast cells) to an infected or inflamed tissue. In bacterial infections, neutrophils can phagocytose and degrade microorganisms; this process is facilitated by opsonization of bacteria by immunoglobulin and complement.[4] In viral infections, infected cells are typically lysed by CD8 (cytotoxic) T cells, which have two distinct mechanisms of cytotoxicity: perforin and Fas ligand.[26] Perforin is a membrane pore-forming molecule, which allows release of granular enzymes (e.g., granzymes) directly into the cytosol of the target cells. Granzyme B induces rapid apoptosis of the target cell in caspase-dependent and caspase-independent manners.

Derangements at any point in this complex pathway may result in three principal types of clinical disorder in immunodeficient patients:

- Susceptibility to infection may be increased.
- Autoimmune disease, including enteropathy, colitis, and hepatitis, may occur because dysfunctional mononuclear cells may be unable to suppress unwanted immune responses properly.
- Risk of malignancy may increase.

HUMORAL IMMUNODEFICIENCIES

Selective IgA Deficiency

Selective IgA deficiency is the most common primary immunodeficiency, with a prevalence of approximately 1 in 500. It has a male predominance, and in patients with IgA deficiency the serum IgA

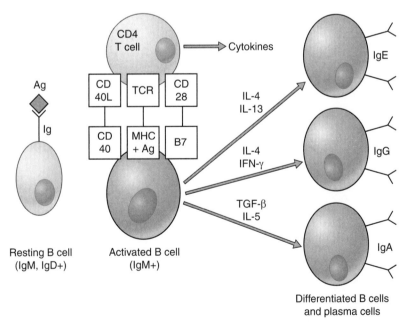

Figure 41-3. B-cell differentiation and the role of helper T cells. For a resting B cell to differentiate into an antibody-producing plasma cell, three steps are necessary. The first step involves binding of antigen (Ag) on to immunoglobulin molecules (Ig) on the surface of the B cell, which provides an initial signal for B-cell activation. The second step involves physical contact with a helper T lymphocyte, which further activates both the B cell and the T cell. The three major molecular interactions mediating the B- and T-cell contact involve CD40-CD40 ligand, MHC+ antigen with the T-cell receptor (TCR), and B7-CD28. This physical contact promotes B-cell proliferation and differentiation. The third step in B-cell differentiation involves cytokine stimulation. The activated T cell may produce different cytokines that promote immunoglobulin class switching (isotype switching). Differentiation into IgE-producing B cells and plasma cells is promoted by IL-4 and IL-5; IgG-producing B cells are promoted by IL-4 and IFN-γ; and IgA-producing B cells are promoted by TGF-β and IL-5.

levels are significantly higher in winter than in other seasons.[27] The decreased IgA production may result from a wide variety of potential immunologic derangements including alterations in B-cell switching. Individuals with this disorder have extremely low levels (less than 5 mg/dL) of serum and mucosal IgA; in addition, 15 to 20% of patients with selective IgA deficiency also have low levels of IgG subclasses IgG$_2$ and IgG$_4$. A compensatory increase in biologically active secretory IgM frequently protects against infection.[28] The pathogenesis of IgA deficiency is not known, though mutations in the TACI gene have been identified in a small number of patients.[25] In addition, certain human leukocyte antigen (HLA) haplotypes, including B8 and DR-3, are associated with selective IgA deficiency.[29] Studies of T-cell function have been normal in most patients with selective IgA deficiency.

Most persons with selective IgA deficiency are asymptomatic. The precise mechanism of this lack of disease in IgA deficiency is unclear and is thought in part to be due to a compensatory increase in secretory IgM, and possibly in IgG as well.[30] However, patients with IgA deficiency are at increased risk for infections, gastrointestinal disease and autoimmune disease[30] (Table 41-4). Children with selective IgA deficiency have been show to be at an increased risk of developing dental caries.[31] Recurrent giardiasis refractory to antibiotic therapy may result in partial villus atrophy and secondary malabsorption.[32] Chronic *Strongyloides* infection, poorly responsive to anthelmintic therapy, has also been reported.[33] Interestingly, individuals with selective IgA deficiency are able to resolve rotavirus disease and actually show higher total IgG and IgG1 subclass antibody titers to rotavirus than people with normal IgA levels. This suggests that IgA is not needed to clear rotavirus in humans.[34]

The most common noninfectious complication of selective IgA deficiency is celiac disease, which is estimated to occur in approximately 5 to 15% of patients with selective IgA deficiency.[35] Antigliadin IgA, antiendomysial IgA, and anti-tissue transglutaminase IgA antibodies commonly yield false-negative results and are unreliable screening tools in this population; the tissue transglutaminase IgG antibody may be a better screening test, but has not been well validataed.[36,37] Heneghan et al. found that, of 604 subjects with celiac sprue, 14 (2.3%) had IgA deficiency.[38] In a prospective study in which jejunal biopsy was performed in 65 consecutive children with selective IgA

TABLE 41-4. Disorders Associated With Selective Immunoglobulin A Deficiency

Upper respiratory infections
Otitis media
Sinusitis
Bronchiectasis
Allergic disorders (including food allergies, asthma, eczema)
Anaphylaxis to intravenous immunoglobulin
Giardiasis
Strongyloidiasis
Nodular lymphoid hyperplasia
Celiac disease (with false-negative antiendomysial antibody)
Achlorhydria
Malabsorption villus atrophy
Cholelithiasis
Inflammatory bowel disease
Primary biliary cirrhosis
Gastrointestinal carcinoma and lymphoma
Henoch-Schönlein purpura
Hepatitis C

Data from Cunningham-Rundles,[30] Leung et al.[33] and Meini et al.[39]

deficiency, 7.7% showed diagnostic features of celiac disease.[39] Additional gastrointestinal (GI) complications reported in selective IgA deficiency have included ulcerative colitis, Crohn's disease, and nodular lymphoid hyperplasia.[30,40,41,46,48] However, it is unclear whether these are true associations, or simply represent two conditions that occur coincidentally.

Antibiotic therapy with metronidazole or nitazoxanide should be administered to patients with selective IgA deficiency and giardiasis.[42] If diarrhea persists and biopsy demonstrates villous atrophy, a gluten-free diet may be therapeutic. Intravenous immunoglobulin (IVIg) should be avoided in patients with selective IgA deficiency, because it does not cross mucosal surfaces and may result in systemic anaphylaxis.[43] Finally, a small number of patients with selective IgA deficiency may develop common variable immunodeficiency (CVID), which has a much higher prevalence of gastrointestinal complications.[44]

X-Linked Agammaglobulinemia

X-linked (Bruton's) agammaglobulinemia (XLA) manifests with recurrent infections after 9 months of age. In a study by Conley and Howard, the mean age at diagnosis in the 60 patients with sporadic XLA was 35 (median 26, range 2 to 11) months.[45] Affected boys have a paucity of peripheral lymphoid tissue and low serum levels of all classes of immunoglobulin. Humoral responses to specific antigens are markedly depressed or absent. The gene for XLA has been localized to chromosome Xq21.3-q22. B cells from affected persons have different mutations affecting the function of a B cell-specific tyrosine kinase gene (*BtK*).[46] Defects in the *Btk* gene affect the early stages of B-cell differentiation.[47]

The onset of recurrent bacterial infections is typically during the latter part of the first year of life, when the levels of maternal antibodies acquired passively through the placenta are no longer protective. Recurrent sinusitis, otitis media, pneumonia, and bronchitis are the most common reported illnesses in persons with XLA. Autoimmune disease (including arthritis and dermatomyosis) may also develop.[48] Chronic enteritis develops in 10%; identifiable causes of the enteritis include *Giardia*, *Salmonella*, *Campylobacter*, *Cryptosporidium*, rotavirus, coxsackievirus, and poliovirus. In a multicenter survey, gastrointestinal infections with recurrent diarrhea were seen in 13% of patients with XLA.[49] Associations with sclerosing cholangitis and a sprue-like illness have also been noted.[50,51] Patients with XLA, small bowel strictures, and transmural intestinal fissures resembling Crohn's disease have been seen. In contrast to Crohn's disease, however, no granulomas or plasma cells are identified when strictures are resected.[52] In a reported case, the regional enteritis of the terminal ileum in a patient with XLA was thought to be due to enterovirus infection.[53] Patients with XLA may also be at increased risk for small and large bowel cancers.[51,54]

Treatment of XLA is aimed at replacing IgG either intravenously or subcutaneously. Neither IgA nor IgM can be replaced. Antibiotic treatment of recurrent infections is necessary. Vaccinations containing live viruses are contraindicated.[55,56] A recent study suggests that children with X-linked agammaglobulinemia have a quality of life that is superior to children with rheumatic disease.[57]

Hyper-IgM Syndrome

This syndrome is a rare humoral immune disorder that affects mainly boys (55 to 65%) and is characterized by severe recurrent bacterial infections with decreased serum levels of IgG,

IgA, and IgE but raised IgM levels. The molecular basis for the X-linked form of immunodeficiency with hyper-IgM (HIGM) has been identified as a T-cell defect, in which mutations in the gene that encodes the CD40 ligand molecule are present. The T cell's CD40 ligand cannot interact with the CD40 molecule on the B-cell surface, resulting in impaired isotype switching from IgM to IgG or IgA, and reduced functional antibody.[58,59] In a recently published study of 23 patients with HIGM, six different CD40L mutations were identified. An underlying genetic defect was not identified in 6 of 14 patients analyzed.[60] An autosomal recessive form of hyper-IgM syndrome has also been reported, which involves is a mutation in the gene that encodes activation-induced cytidine deaminase (AICD).[61]

Boys with hyper-IgM syndrome present at between 1 month and 10 years of life with opportunistic infections. Chronic encephalitis and idiopathic neurologic deterioration may occur. Gastrointestinal complications reported include histoplasmosis of the esophagus, cryptosporidiosis, giardiasis, hepatosplenomegaly, intestinal lymphoid hyperplasia, and recurrent large painful oral ulcerations (Figures 41-4 and 41-5).[56,61-64] Protracted or recurrent diarrhea is common, occurring in about one third of the patients, and *Cryptosporidium* is the most frequently isolated pathogen.[65] Patients with hyper-IgM syndrome are also at increased risk for intestinal lymphoma.

Liver disease and other autoimmune disorders are frequently seen in hyper IgM syndrome.[22,66] Abnormal transaminase and alkaline phosphatase levels are seen in 50% of patients. Two separate series have suggested that sclerosing cholangitis and cirrhosis occur in up to 35% of patients older than 10 years of age.[62,67] Pancreatic and hepatobiliary malignancies have been reported in patients as young as 7 years of age.[67]

Therapy of hyper-IgM involves gamma globulin replacement therapy and treatment of specific infectious complications. Gamma globulin administration may reduce the frequency of bacterial infections and the incidence of lymphoid hyperplasia associated with HIGM. Treatment of the autoimmune conditions may include corticosteroids, immune-modulating agents, or biologic therapies.[22,56,66]

Transient Hypogammaglobulinemia of Infancy

Transient hypogammaglobulinemia of infancy (THI) is a poorly defined condition characterized by low serum immunoglobulin levels in infancy, with attainment of normal levels at a later time. Serum IgG is typically low, without any subclass specificity; IgA or IgM levels may also be decreased. The prevalence of this condition in infants with recurrent infections ranges from 0.1% to 5% in different studies.[68-70] Children with THI typically present with recurrent respiratory infections at 6 to 12 months of age. In a multicenter survey of 77 children with this disorder, 91% of patients presented with recurrent infections, 47% had environmental allergies, and 4% had autoimmune disease. The immunoglobulin deficiency and clinical symptoms usually resolve within 24 months.[70] However, a small subset of children initially diagnosed with THI may ultimately be diagnosed with other immune deficiencies, such as common variable immune deficiency.[3]

Chronic diarrhea is the second most common complication in these patients after respiratory illness. Lactose intolerance, *Giardia lamblia* infestation, or *Clostridium difficile* infection were found in one third of 55 children with low serum immunoglobulin levels and chronic diarrhea. Small bowel histology demonstrated enteritis or villus atrophy in up to 50% of these patients. It is unclear whether these patients had THI or enteric protein loss from the intestinal illness.[71] In children with recurrent *C. difficile* infection unresponsive to antibiotics and low antibody titers to *C. difficile*, IVIg has resulted in clearance of the infection.[72]

CELLULAR IMMUNODEFICIENCIES

DiGeorge Syndrome

DiGeorge syndrome arises from a defect in the differentiation of the third and fourth pharyngeal pouches during embryologic development, usually due to a chromosome 22q11 deletion.

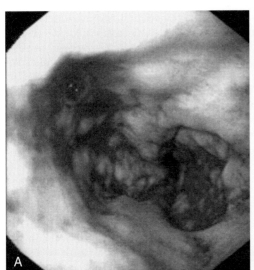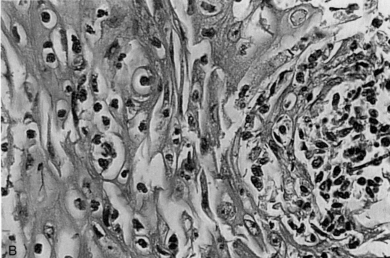

Figure 41-4. Esophageal candidiasis in a patient with the hyper-IgM syndrome. (**A**) Endoscopic view of the esophagus demonstrates near-complete coating of the esophageal mucosa with a creamy white exudate. (**B**) Esophageal histology demonstrates inflammatory cells and pseudohyphae. **A**, Courtesy Drs. Carine Lenders and Samuel Nurko; **B**, courtesy of Dr. Kameran Badizadegan, Children's Hospital, Boston.

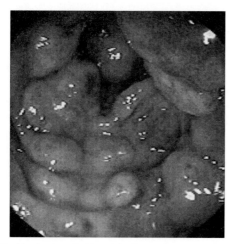

Figure 41-5. Massive lymphoid nodular hyperplasia seen in the colon of a patient with hyper-IgM syndrome. Courtesy Dr. Victor Fox, Children's Hospital, Boston.

The syndrome consists of conotruncal cardiac anomalies, hypoparathyroidism, velopharyngeal insufficiency, craniofacial dysmorphism, and thymic hypoplasia. Patients may have absent T- cells or normal T-cell numbers. In addition to immunologic dysfunction, anatomic abnormalities such as bronchomalacia and aspiration can lead to recurrent respiratory tract infections.[73]

Most infants with DiGeorge syndrome experience developmental delay, facial dysmorphia, and palatal dysfunction. Feeding difficulties arise from poor coordination of the tongue, pharyngeal, and esophageal muscles. Infants with cleft palates can have difficulty breast-feeding, and patients with cardiac anomalies can fatigue easily while trying to feed. Two to 5 percent of affected children have delayed eruption of teeth and enamel hypoplasia. Many children experience constipation and gastroesophageal reflux, which may be partially due hypotonia. Malrotation of the intestines can occur. Treatment involves transplantation of either mature T cells, or thymus tissue for patients with absent T cells.[74]

Chronic Mucocutaneous Candidiasis and APECED Syndrome

Chronic mucocutaneous candidiasis is characterized by a diminished T-cell response to candidal antigens. Infants with this disorder present with persistent thrush or candidal dermatitis, failure to thrive, and dystrophic nails. Candidal esophagitis may result in feeding refusal. A subset of children with chronic candidiasis have the APECED syndrome (autoimmune polyendocrinopathy, candidiasis, and ectodermal dysplasia). The molecular basis of APECED involves mutations in the AIRE (autoimmune regulator) gene, and perhaps defective regulatory T cells. The clinical features of APECED in addition to the candidiasis include hypoparathyroidism, adrenal insufficiency, pernicious anemia, type 1 diabetes, and gonadal failure.[75,76] Malabsorption secondary to pancreatic insufficiency contributes to poor weight gain in 10% of patients. Therapy includes eradication of *Candida* with topical antibiotics plus ketoconazole or fluconazole, as well as hormone or pancreatic enzyme replacement when appropriate.[77]

COMBINED CELLULAR-HUMORAL IMMUNODEFICIENCIES

Common Variable Immunodeficiency

CVID, also called acquired hypogammaglobulinemia, adult-onset hypogammaglobulinemia, or dysgammaglobulinemia, is a rare heterogeneous group of disorders affecting between 1 in 50,000 and 1 in 200,000 persons. It is characterized by hypogammaglobulinemia, recurrent infections, enteropathy, autoimmune disease, and malignancy. Up to 45% of cases are diagnosed in childhood.[86] The cause of CVID is unknown, but B-lymphocyte differentiation into plasma cells is impaired, and mutation in the TACI gene has been identified in a subset of patients.[25,78] The different abnormalities reflect the variability of CVID and support the concept that more than one gene is probably responsible for the immune abnormalities in CVID.

Patients typically present in late childhood and young adulthood with recurrent sinusitis, bronchitis, and pneumonia. Common causes of the respiratory illness include *Streptococcus pneumoniae*, *Haemophilus influenzae*, and *Mycoplasma pneumoniae*; mycobacteria, *Pneumocystis*, and fungi are less frequent pathogens. Diagnosis of CVID is established by demonstration of persistently low antibody levels over time and impaired responses to standard pediatric immunizations. In a male, XLA must be excluded.[79,80]

Gastrointestinal disease occurs in up to 70% of patients and accounts for much of the morbidity (Table 41-5).[81] Infectious diarrhea caused by a wide variety of pathogens may occur. Nodular lymphoid hyperplasia is detected radiographically or endoscopically in up to 20% of patients and may predispose to either malabsorption or gastrointestinal bleeding.[82,83] In one case report, a 40-year-old patient with CVID developed cytomegalovirus infection of the stomach and small bowel with multiple ulcers and strictures, resulting in intestinal obstruction.[84]

Between 10% and 20% of patients with CVID have an enteropathy characterized by weight loss, abdominal pain, and severe diarrhea in the absence of enteric infection. Small bowel biopsy in these patients demonstrates partial or subtotal villus atrophy, hyperplastic crypts, and apoptotic bodies.[52,85-87] Although the diagnosis of CVID is suspected when plasma cells are absent in a gastrointestinal biopsy, this finding is only present in about two thirds of patients with this disease.[85] Gluten- or lactose-free diets may help a subset of patients, but most improve when treated with an elemental diet, although parenteral nutrition may also be required.[88] The severe malabsorption may result in vitamin B_{12} deficiency and/or zinc deficiency.[89] An IBD-like syndrome, characterized by small intestinal strictures and microscopic colitis, may also occur.[81,87]

Patients with CVID are at a 30-fold increased risk for the development of gastric carcinoma or malignant lymphoma. The lymphomas in CVID are extranodal and usually B cell in type. Cunningham-Rundles et al. studied 22 B-cell lymphomas in patients with CVID over a period of 25 years and found that five lymphomas arose in mucosal sites—mucosa-associated lymphoid tissue (MALT) lymphomas.[90] These MALT lymphomas are low-grade B-cell lymphomas and tend to occur in organs that have acquired lymphoid tissue as a result of long-term infectious or autoimmune stimulation (e.g., chronic gastric *Helicobacter pylori* infection and chronic hepatitis C infection of the liver).[90] *H. pylori* infection and *p53* gene mutation may play a role in the gastric carcinogenesis.[91] The small bowel

TABLE 41-5. Gastrointestinal Complications of Common Variable Immunodeficiency

Enteric infections (including *Shigella*, *Salmonella*, and dysgonic fermenter 3)
Giardiasis
Cryptosporidiosis
Nodular lymphoid hyperplasia
Enterocolitis
Enteropathy, malabsorption, wasting syndrome
Perirectal abscess
Short stature
Zinc deficiency
Inflammatory bowel disease
Ménétrier's disease
Atrophic gastritis or pernicious anemia
Gastric adenocarcinoma
Intestinal lymphoma
Cecal carcinoma (undifferentiated)
Hepatitis C with cirrhosis

Data from Sneller et al.,[169] Cunningham-Rundles,[79] Sperber and Mayer,[170] de Bruin et al.,[92] Quinti et al.,[171] Eisenstein and Sneller,[172] and Cunningham-Rundles and Bodian.[173]

lymphomas reported may manifest with intestinal malabsorption. In addition, a cecal carcinoma of neuroendocrine origin has been reported in a 16-year-old patient with CVID.[92]

Some 20% of patients with CVID have a persistent mild increase in transaminase levels. The cause is unknown, with liver biopsies demonstrating mild periportal changes or granulomas.[48] Hepatitis C is can occur as a complication of IVIg infusion in patients with CVID and may have an aggressive course.[93] Treatment includes interferon and liver transplantation.[94,95]

Therapy for CVID consists of monthly IVIg infusions and symptomatic treatment of infections and malabsorption.[96] Epstein-Barr virus infections in patients with CVID may respond to IFN-α.[97]

Severe Combined Immunodeficiency

The term *severe combined immunodeficiency* (SCID) refers to a group of diseases characterized by molecular defects interfering with T- and/or B-cell differentiation and resulting in an infant with failure to thrive and extreme susceptibility to infections.[97-99] Approximately 20 defective genes have been associated with SCID; patients are classified according to the specific mutation present, the associated lymphocyte phenotype, and mode of inheritance[97-102] (see Table 41-1). Presenting features include growth impairment, chronic diarrhea, persistent thrush or candidiasis, and overwhelming sepsis. Graft-versus-host disease from transfusions of unirradiated blood, or disseminated illness from live vaccines, may occur if the diagnosis is delayed. Diagnosis is established by the demonstration of low or absent T-lymphocyte numbers in peripheral blood; B-cell and neutrophil counts may also be depressed, depending on the variant of SCID.[100]

Gastrointestinal illness occurs in up to 90% of patients. Organisms frequently associated with illness include rotavirus, *Candida*, cytomegalovirus, Epstein-Barr virus, and *Escherichia coli*. Although candidiasis rarely involves the intestine, candidal esophagitis should be suspected in infants with SCID and decreased oral intake.[103] Chronic viral infection is the most frequent cause of enteritis and may be responsible for death in

80% of cases.[104] Chronic rotavirus infection has been reported after administration of the live attenuated rotavirus vaccine.[105] Other less common causes of enteropathy include *Salmonella*, *Shigella*, and *Cryptosporidium* infections.

Autoimmune manifestations of SCID may include enteropathy, hemolytic anemia, and glomerulonephritis.[103] Boeck et al. found clinically significant gastroesophageal reflux in 20.5% of patients with SCID, much higher than that reported for the normal population (0.1 to 0.3%), but the mechanism is unknown.[106]

Hepatic abnormalities are also common in patients with SCID and include graft-versus-host disease of the liver, adenovirus and cytomegalovirus hepatitis, rotavirus hepatitis, parenteral nutrition-associated liver disease, and lymphoproliferative disorder.[107,108] Pancreatic infection by viruses has also been described.[109]

One variant of SCID that seems to render a patient particularly prone to gastrointestinal complications is *bare lymphocyte syndrome*. Gastrointestinal candidiasis is common in addition to giardiasis, cryptosporidiosis, and other bacterial enteritides. A high incidence of hepatobiliary abnormalities is noted, including sclerosing cholangitis associated with biliary cryptosporidiosis. Bacterial cholangitis secondary to *Pseudomonas*, *Enterococcus*, and *Streptococcus* infections has been described.[110]

The principal therapy for patients with SCID is bone marrow transplantation, ideally from a matched sibling.[111] In patients with SCID with adenosine deaminase deficiency, infusions of a long-acting form of adenosine deaminase correct metabolic abnormalities and provide some restoration of immune function.[112] In addition, gene replacement therapy is also being studied.[111,113]

NF-κB Essential Modifier Mutations

NEMO mutations have been identified in patients with X-linked hyper-IgM and hypohidrotic ectodermal dysplasia (HED).[114] B-cell switching and antigen-presenting cell activation are impaired with NEMO mutations. Certain mutations of NEMO are associated with deficient NK cell cytotoxicity[115] and dysgammaglobulinemia with very poor specific antibody production.[116] Patients display features of HED with conical teeth and absence (or hypoplasia) of hair, teeth, and sweat glands. Recurrent bacterial and viral infections often occur in infancy.

Gastrointestinal symptoms include persistent vomiting, chronic diarrhea, recurrent cytomegalovirus colitis, and giardiasis.[180-182] Growth delay is common as a result of infection and poor nutrition due to gastrointestinal symptoms. Parenteral nutrition is often used to provide adequate nutritional support. Patients with NEMO mutations may also develop enterocolitis.[117] The clinical presentation and endoscopic appearance of enterocolitis in patients with NEMO may be similar to that of patients with idiopathic IBD (e.g., Crohn's disease) (Figure 41-6). Whereas IBD causes signs of chronic active enterocolitis (granulomas, deep cryptitis, and lymphocyte-predominant inflammation), a relative paucity of lymphocytes and an absence of granulomas is seen in mucosal biopsies taken from patients with NEMO. Although the neutrophil-predominant inflammation seen in NEMO is suggestive of acute inflammation, clinical improvement usually requires glucocorticoid therapy.[117] For patients with complications of NEMO, stem cell transplant has been utilized and may alleviate the intestinal symptoms.[118]

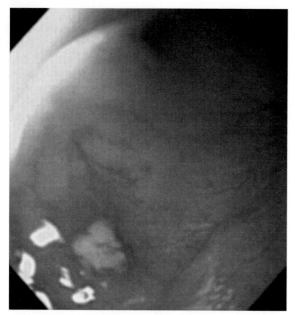

Figure 41-6. Endoscopic photo of colonic inflammation in patient with ectodermal dysplasia and NEMO mutation. The patient's colitis resolved after bone marrow transplantation. *Courtesy Dr. Samuel Nurko.*

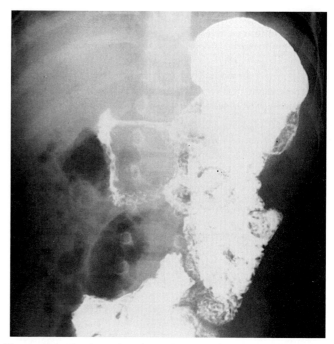

Figure 41-7. Gastric outlet obstruction secondary to antral narrowing in a patient with chronic granulomatous disease. The patient underwent partial gastrectomy, with inflammatory cells and granulomas identified in the hypertrophied antral tissue. *Courtesy Dr. Thorne Griscom and Children's Hospital, Boston, Radiology Teaching File.*

DISORDERS OF PHAGOCYTE FUNCTION

Chronic Granulomatous Disease

Chronic granulomatous disease (CGD) refers to a group of immunodeficiencies characterized by the inability of an affected patient's neutrophils to generate superoxide and hydrogen peroxide, leaving the patient susceptible to infections with catalase-positive organisms.[119] The disease has an estimated incidence of 1 in 250,000 persons, with an X-linked inheritance pattern seen in two thirds of patients and autosomal recessive inheritance in the remainder.[138,139] The diagnosis is currently established by demonstrating defective uptake of dihydrorhodamine by neutrophils using flow cytometry.[120] The X-linked form is due to a mutation in the gene for the phagocytic oxidase cytochrome glycoprotein of 91 kDa (gp91phox), and the autosomal recessive form is due to a mutation in the gene for a cytosolic component of 47-kDa (p47phox) protein.[121] The most common presenting features involve suppurative infections by catalase-positive organisms, such as *Staphylococcus aureus*, *Serratia*, *Aspergillus*, *Candida*, and *Nocardia*.[122,123]

Gastrointestinal involvement occurs in approximately 50% of patients.[124] Many patients with CGD present with gastric outlet obstruction secondary to pronounced antral narrowing[125] (Figure 41-7). The antral narrowing is usually caused by a combination of infection and granulomatous inflammation. It may resolve with a combination of antibiotics and corticosteroid therapy, but may also require surgical intervention.[126] Small bowel involvement may mimic Crohn's disease, with multifocal abscesses, fistulas, and granulomatous colitis. The presence of lipid-containing histiocytes in the mucosa and submucosa of colonic biopsies strongly suggests CGD colitis (Figure 41-8).[127,128] Such colitis may respond to therapy with corticosteroids, IFN-γ, or cyclosporin, but surgical resection may be necessary for intractable colitis or acute obstruction.[122,129] Pyogenic or fungal liver abscess is also a common complication of CGD; it is treated with appropriate antimicrobial agents,

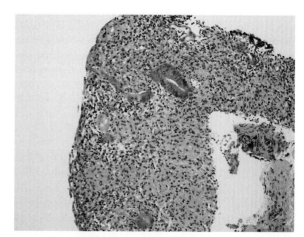

Figure 41-8. Crohn's-like colitis in a 2-year-old with chronic granulomatous disease. The colitis responded to therapy with IFN-γ.

surgical drainage, and possibly IFN-γ.[130-133] Prophylactic IFN-γ may reduce the frequency of opportunistic infections.[131] Antibiotic prophylaxis with trimethoprim-sulfamethoxazole and itraconazole is also used. Linezolid and antifungal medications (e.g., voriconazole) will allow most patients to survive into adulthood. Hematopoietic stem cell transplantation from an HLA-identical donor is the only proven curative treatment for CGD.[132] Gene transfer into hematopoietic stem cells with retroviral vectors and low-intensity chemotherapy conditioning has led to partial correction of granulocyte function and symptom improvement in patients.[133] This treatment approach is considered experimental and may be tried for patients who do not have a suitable stem-cell donor.[132]

Leukocyte-Adhesion Deficiency

Leukocyte-adhesion deficiency type I is characterized by impaired phagocytic function secondary to deficiencies of adhesion molecules (CD18/β2 integrin) necessary for cell migration and interactions and is an autosomal recessive disorder.[3] Leukocyte-adhesion deficiency type II is a defect of carbohydrate fucosylation and is associated with growth retardation, dysmorphic features, and neurologic deficits.[3,134-136] Necrotic infections of the skin (including pyoderma gangrenosum) and mucous membranes, otitis media, and episodes of microbial sepsis are the principal features.[137,138] Gastrointestinal complications include intraoral infections and periodontitis, candidal esophagitis, gastritis, appendicitis, necrotizing enterocolitis, and perirectal abscess.[139,140] Fatal enterocolitis similar to that of necrotizing enterocolitis or Hirschsprung's disease has been described in an infant with leukocyte adhesion deficiency.[141] A syndrome of leukocyte adhesion deficiency combined with a severe bleeding disorder has been recognized as LAD-1/variant syndrome. Children affected with this disease develop nonpurulent bacterial and fungal infections and a severe bleeding tendency.[142]

Hematopoietic stem cell transplantation from an HLA-matched donor can be curative for patients with LAD.[135] A recently published study of 36 children with leukocyte adhesion deficiency who had undergone stem cell transplantation showed an overall survival rate of 75% at a median follow-up of 62 months. All of the patients who received myeloablative or reduced-intensity conditioning regimens survived.[143] Antibiotic therapy is required for recurrent infections. Prophylactic antibiotics are sometimes necessary. Meticulous dental care and oral hygiene are recommended. Patients with type II disease may benefit from oral fructose supplementation before neurological manifestations occur.[144]

OTHER PRIMARY IMMUNODEFICIENCIES

Wiskott-Aldrich Syndrome

Wiskott-Aldrich syndrome (WAS) is an X-linked immunodeficiency. There is a wide spectrum of clinical manifestations, with some patients only developing mild X-linked thrombocytopenia, whereas others develop a severe phenotype defined by thrombocytopenia, immunodeficiency, eczema, and a high susceptibility to tumors and autoimmune manifestations.[145] The gene for this syndrome has been identified on the short arm of the X chromosome at Xp11.22-p11.23.[146] The gene product, WAS protein (WASP), is expressed only in hematopoietic cells and belongs to a unique family of proteins that are responsible for transduction of signals from the cell membrane to the actin cytoskeleton. The interaction between WASP, the Rho family GTPase CDC42, and the cytoskeletal organizing complex Arp2/3 is critical to many of these functions, which, when disturbed as a result of WASP mutations, translate into measurable defects of cell signaling, polarization, motility, and phagocytosis.[147,148] The WAS protein is also important in the function of regulatory T cells.[149] Children are usually diagnosed before 2 years of age, after presenting with epistaxis, purpura, recurrent otitis, sinusitis, pneumonia, opportunistic infections, or diarrhea.[150]

Gastrointestinal complications occur in 10 to 30% of patients. Gastrointestinal bleeding from thrombocytopenia can antedate the diagnosis. Infectious diarrhea occurs in up to 25% of cases, although opportunistic pathogens are unusual. WAS is one of the rare conditions that can trigger inflammatory bowel disease in early infancy. A steroid-responsive inflammatory bowel disease characterized by bloody diarrhea and colonic pseudopolyps has been seen.[151] Finally, patients with Wiskott-Aldrich syndrome are at a 100-fold increased risk of developing lymphoma, which may originate in the gut.[150]

The only curative option for patients with Wiskott-Aldrich syndrome is hematopoietic stem cell transplantation.[145] Using an HLA-matched sibling as the donor is preferred. The procedure is most likely to be successful when performed on patients younger than 5 years. Supportive care with IVIg and prophylactic antibiotics (especially against pneumococcal infections) can be helpful. Performing a splenectomy can increase platelet number and size and decrease the number of required platelet transfusions.

X-Linked Lymphoproliferative Disease

X-linked lymphoproliferative disease (XLP) is characterized by three major clinical phenotypes: fulminant infectious mononucleosis (50%), B-cell lymphomas (20%), and dysgammaglobulinemia (20%).[152,153] An XLP registry was established in 1978 and has approximately 300 patients registered from more than 80 families.[153] The mutated gene in XLP has been identified on the long arm of the X chromosome at Xq24-25, encoding for the protein SH2D1A, also known as SAP for SLAM (signaling lymphocytic activation molecule)-associated protein.[154-156] This protein plays an important role in intracellular signaling by associating with the surface activating receptors SLAM (CD105) and 2B4 (CD244) that are present on T and NK cells.[157]

Hepatosplenomegaly, fulminant hepatitis, and hepatic necrosis are the common gastrointestinal manifestations in patients with XLP with fulminant infectious mononucleosis. Uncontrolled lymphocyte proliferation, organ infiltration, and T-cell cytotoxic activity lead to multiorgan failure; hepatic necrosis and bone marrow failure constitute the most common events that determine death in these patients.[158] Intestinal lymphoma involving the ileum and cecum is well described, and the malignant lymphomas are usually non-Hodgkin's lymphoma of the Burkitt type.[159] Chemotherapy is often used for treatment, but outcome is generally poor. The mortality rate of XLP is 100% by the age of 40 years, and XLP is generally fatal in the first decade of life in patients with XLP with either fulminant infectious mononucleosis or B-cell lymphoma.

IPEX

IPEX (immune dysfunction, polyendocrinopathy, enteropathy, X-linked) typically presents during the first few months of life with diabetes mellitus, intractable diarrhea, failure to thrive, eczema, and hemolytic anemia. Affected males may also develop thrombocytopenia, autoimmune hypothyroidism, and lymphadenopathy associated with splenomegaly. Mutations in the FOXP3 gene mapped to chromosome Xp11.23-q13.3 lead to IPEX. Interestingly, there is genetic overlap of this gene interval with that of WAS. The human FOXP3 protein is a transcriptional regulator required for normal T-cell function.[160] Characteristic histopathologic findings include severe villus atrophy and mucosal erosion with lymphocytic infiltrates of the submucosa or lamina propria. Lymphocytic infiltrates can also be seen in the pancreas and thyroid.[160] A graft-versus-host disease–like pattern associated with anti-enterocyte antibodies has been shown to be the most frequent intestinal presentation of IPEX syndrome.[161]

The diagnosis of IPEX is often made by genetic analysis. As this testing may take weeks to complete and thereby delay initiation of treatment, at least one attempt has been made to develop a screening tool for this disease. Heltzer et al. found markedly decreased immunocytochemical staining of FOXP3+ T cells in bowel biopsies of two patients with classic IPEX syndrome. Another patient with a mild form of the disease had intact staining.[162]

Symptomatic treatment involves total parenteral nutrition, red blood cell transfusions, platelet transfusions, and insulin injections. Cyclosporin A or tacrolimus, with or without corticosteroids, may be effective for limited periods of time. Sirolimus is less nephrotoxic and has also been utilized.[163] Stem cell transplantation is the only effective cure. Endocrinopathies often persist as a result of permanent cell damage (e.g., diabetes mellitus due to destruction of insulin-producing B cells). If untreated, most affected boys die at an early age.[163]

REFERENCES

8. Abbas A, Lichtman A, Pillai S. Antigen processing and presentation to T lymphocytes. In: Abbas AK, editor. Cellular and Molecular Immunology. 6th ed. Philadelphia: Saunders; 2010. p. 113–136.
28. Ballow M. Primary immunodeficiency disorders: antibody deficiency. J Allergy Clin Immunol 2002;109:581–591.
49. Plebani A, Soresina A, Rondelli R, et al. Clinical, immunological, and molecular analysis in a large cohort of patients with X-linked agammaglobulinemia: an Italian multicenter study. Clin Immunol 2002;104:221–230.
67. Hayward AR, Levy J, Facchetti F, et al. Cholangiopathy and tumors of the pancreas, liver, and biliary tree in boys with X-linked immunodeficiency with hyper-IgM. J Immunol 1997;158:977–983.
121. Winkelstein JA, Marino MC, Johnston Jr RB, et al. Chronic granulomatous disease. Report on a national registry of 368 patients. Medicine (Baltimore) 2000;79:155–169.
137. Bonilla FA, Geha RS. 12. Primary immunodeficiency diseases. J Allergy Clin Immunol 2003;111:S571–S581.

See expertconsult.com for a complete list of references and the review questions for this chapter.

42

GASTROINTESTINAL COMPLICATIONS OF SECONDARY IMMUNODEFICIENCY SYNDROMES

Tracie L. Miller • Laura L. Cushman

Secondary immunodeficiency syndromes constitute a spectrum of disorders. Infections of the gastrointestinal tract pose the greatest risk for children with secondary immunodeficiencies. Cellular changes in the gastrointestinal tract (the largest immune organ in the body) that lead to diarrhea and malabsorption, peptic disease, dysmotility, and liver disease are among some of the other disorders of the gastrointestinal tract faced by these children. Worldwide, human immunodeficiency virus (HIV-1) infection and malnutrition are by far the most common secondary immunodeficiency states. However, in the United States and other developed countries, severe malnutrition and new cases of perinatal HIV-1 disease are rare because of relatively high standards of living and effective highly active antiretroviral therapies (HAART) given to pregnant HIV-infected women that prevent transmission of HIV to the infants.[1] Between 2004 and 2005, there were 67 reported cases of perinatally acquired HIV and 4883 new diagnoses of unspecified origin in adolescents 13 to 24 years of age.[2] HIV-infected children and adolescents are now surviving because of effective antiretroviral strategies, yet there is increased horizontal acquisition of HIV in adolescents owing to risky social behaviors. Furthermore, children with chronic illness are among the highest population at risk for malnutrition and its sequelae.[3] Thus these two disorders serve as models for complications of other secondary immunodeficiency states.

PEDIATRIC HIV INFECTION

The first cases of the acquired immunodeficiency syndrome (AIDS) were described in the early 1980s. Later, in 1984,[4] HIV-1 was determined to be the causative agent, and HIV-1 infection was recognized as a spectrum of disease, ranging from asymptomatic infection to full-blown AIDS. The AIDS epidemic claimed an estimated 2 million lives in 2007, and an estimated 2.7 million people acquired HIV-1 in 2007. An estimated 33 million people globally are living with the virus.[5] With the successful preventive strategies of elective cesarean section delivery and chemoprophylaxis of pregnant HIV-1-infected women, the transmission rates plummeted from 15 to 30% to less than 1 to 2% of all HIV-1-infected women delivering infants.[6] The advent of HAART in 1996 changed the natural history of HIV-1 in children in many countries.[7] However, the successes of prevention and prophylaxis have not been realized as much in developing countries, where HIV infection continues to increase. For this reason, there are disparate accounts of opportunistic infections and other diseases in regions with high HAART accessibility and those with limited HAART accessibility.[8]

HIV-1 is an RNA virus that belongs to the lentivirus family. It has a particular tropism for the CD4 surface antigen of cells, and the binding of HIV-1 to the CD4 receptor initiates the viral cycle. The virus may subsequently replicate within the host cell or, alternatively, the proviral DNA within the host cells may remain latent until cellular activation occurs. Human T lymphocytes and monocytes-macrophages are the primary cells that are infected with HIV-1, although other cell lines may be infected as well. The net effect is suppression of the immune system and a progressive decline in CD4+ T lymphocytes, which leaves patients susceptible to opportunistic and recurrent bacterial infections.

HIV AND THE CELLULAR COMPONENTS OF THE GASTROINTESTINAL TRACT

The gastrointestinal tract is the main source of HIV-1 infection when parenteral transmission is excluded. In vertical transmission, HIV-1 is found in the gastrointestinal tract after the fetus swallows infected amniotic fluid, blood, cervical secretions, or breast milk. The virus, inoculated in the gastrointestinal tract, infects the fetus as it enters into the gut-associated lymphoid tissue (GALT) through the tonsil or upper intestinal tract. Examination of both acute simian immunodeficiency virus (SIV) and HIV infection have documented reduced CD4 cell levels in GALT prior to a detectable reduction in T cells of the peripheral blood, highlighting the gastrointestinal tract's role and susceptibility.[9-12] The rates of acquisition of HIV-1 through the gastrointestinal tract are likely related to the quantity of virus in the person transmitting it[13-15] and the immunologic function and maturity of the patient being infected. Mucosal infections with opportunistic infections may increase HIV-1 transmission. Mycobacterial infections up-regulate CC chemokine receptor 5 (CCR5) expression in monocytes, which facilitates the entry of CCR5-tropic HIV-1. Other factors, such as tumor necrosis factor-α (TNF-α), which is induced by nuclear factor (NF)-κB (which itself is pathogen induced), are potent inducers of HIV-1.[16,17]

Cellular routes that potentially can transmit HIV-1 across the gastrointestinal tract include M cells, dendritic cells, and epithelial cells. M cells are specialized epithelial cells that overlie the Peyer's patches and transport large macromolecules and microorganisms from the apical surface to the basolateral surface. Human transport of HIV-1 by M cells in vivo has not been reported. Dendritic cells bind HIV-1 through a dendritic cell-specific adhesion molecule. In vitro studies support the role of dendritic cells in transmitting HIV-1[18-21]; however, the role of the dendritic cell in in vivo transmission of HIV-1 has yet to be determined. Epithelial cells express CCR5 and can selectively transfer CCR5-tropic HIV-1. The epithelial cell can transport HIV-1 in vitro from the apical to the basolateral surface.[22,23] The R5-tropic viruses are transferred in vitro through epithelial cell lines.[24]

Once transmitted, the lamina propria lymphocytes express CCR5 and CXC4 chemokine receptor 4 (CXCR4), which support HIV-1 replication.[25,26] Early after infection, there is a greater proportion of infected lymphocytes in the lamina propria than in peripheral blood.[27,28] For the patients actively receiving HAART, Poles et al.[29] described "cryptic replication" occurring in GALT reservoirs in which viral replication is actively taking place at slower rates but HIV-1 RNA levels remain undetected in peripheral blood. Further, GALT contained more than twice as many lymphoid cells (160,000) than peripheral blood mononuclear cells (70,000) possessing HIV-1 DNA with viral replication capacity. There was no significant reduction in these values when the analysis was repeated after 12 months. Lymphocytes are able to disseminate the virus to distant sites, with depletion of CD4 cells in the lamina propria[27,30] and then in the blood. Even with aggressive suppression of HIV-1 during the primary stages by highly active antiretroviral agents, CD4 cell depletion is observed in the effector subcompartment gut mucosa when CD4 levels in the peripheral blood have stabilized.[10] As mucosal and peripheral T cells are depleted, monocytes and macrophages become important reservoirs for the virus. The intestinal macrophages do not promote inflammation and do not carry the receptor for CCR5 or CXCR4; however, the blood monocytes are different in their profile and are infected by HIV-1. They are found infected in the blood and thereafter take up residence in the gut.[31] They are stimulated by opportunistic agents and proinflammatory cytokines.[32] Recent in vitro studies have implicated the integrin receptor α4β7 on which the HIV-1 envelope binds and transmits signals mediated by an epitope in the V2loop of gp120. This in turn activates LFA-1 and is pivotal in virological synapse formation, allowing rapid cellular dissemination of HIV-1.[33]

Villous atrophy and gastrointestinal tract dysfunction are coincident with high levels of HIV-1 viral load in the gut.[34] Altered epithelial permeability may permit microbial translocation and generalized immune activation leading to localized cytokine production and further replication of HIV.[35] A dysfunctional gastrointestinal tract can produce clinical symptoms that contribute to both morbidity and mortality in children with HIV-1 infection. These symptoms include weight loss, vomiting, diarrhea, and malabsorption (Table 42-1). The advent of antiretroviral treatment induces debilitating effects on mechanisms within the gut that promote chronic HIV infection. Mainly, high levels of lipopolysaccharides (LPS) are associated with marked systemic immune activation sustaining this infection; antiretroviral therapy decreases levels of LPS, promotes CD4+ T cell reconstitution, and may subsequently decrease the systemic immune activation.[36] Additional studies examining this relationship stand to offer greater insight into HIV pathogenesis.

TABLE 42-1. Gastrointestinal Symptoms and Causes in HIV-1-Infected Childre

Anorexia, Nausea, Weight Loss, Vomiting	
Peptic disease	Idiopathic, gastroesophageal reflux, medications, *H. pylori*
Opportunistic infections of upper gastrointestinal tract	*Candida*, CMV, HSV
Pancreatic or hepatobiliary disease	Pancreatitis, cholangitis, infectious
Encephalopathy/CNS disorders	HIV
Idiopathic aphthous ulcers	HIV
Primary anorexia	HIV
Gastrointestinal dysmotility	HIV, autonomic, infectious, inflammatory
Medication toxicity	Specified in Table 3
Gastrointestinal Malabsorption, Diarrhea, Mucosal Disease	
Infectious	Bacterial, parasitic, viral
Inflammatory	HIV enteropathy, IBD
Disaccharidase deficiency	Infectious, inflammatory
Protein-losing enteropathy	Infectious, inflammatory
Fat malabsorption	Infectious, inflammatory
Hepatobiliary Disease	
Sclerosing cholangitis	Infectious
Chronic pancreatitis	Infectious, drug-induced
Cirrhosis	Hepatitis B and C co-infection

CMV, cytomegalovirus; CNS, central nervous system; HSV, herpes simplex virus; IBD, inflammatory bowel disease

STRUCTURE AND FUNCTION OF THE INTESTINAL TRACT IN HIV INFECTION

As mentioned, there are distinct changes in the cellular milieu of the gastrointestinal tract in HIV-1-infected patients. Previous studies have shown that activated mucosal T cells play a role in the pathogenesis of enteropathy in the human small intestine[37] and can affect the morphology of the villi and crypts in a manner similar to that seen in patients with HIV-1 infection. The magnitude of viral burden in the gastrointestinal tract is associated with villous blunting and other abnormal morphology.[34] A number of studies in the 1980s associated a distinct enteropathy with HIV-1.[38] Diarrhea, weight loss, an abnormally low D-xylose absorption, and steatorrhea, without evidence of intestinal infection, were common findings. Jejunal biopsies showed partial villous atrophy with crypt hyperplasia and increased numbers of intraepithelial lymphocytes. This was the first histologic description of a specific pathologic process that occurred in the lamina propria of the small intestine in some patients with HIV-1. Others[39] found low-grade small bowel atrophy and maturational defects of enterocytes, supporting an HIV-1 enteropathy characterized by mucosal atrophy with hyporegeneration. However, some investigators have challenged this concept, suggesting that the findings could be attributed to an undiagnosed enteric infection. Recently, genotype profiling for genes responsible for endothelial barrier maintenance and metabolic functioning has shown a decreased expression in the presence of increased viral replication in the GALT and reduced CD4+ T cell levels.[40] These findings are significant, because they offer an additional modality for evaluating microenvironmental alterations within the gastrointestinal tract of the patient. Additional studies will help to determine the efficacy of gene expression profiling in HIV-infected individuals.

Miller et al.[41] published histologic findings in 43 children with HIV-1 infection. The majority of patients had normal villous architecture, and many of the children with villous blunting had an associated intercurrent enteric infection. Distinct features of hyperplasia of the lamina propria and increased intraepithelial lymphocytes were not apparent.

Bjarnason et al.[42] studied intestinal inflammation and ileal structure and function in patients with a wide spectrum of HIV-1 disease states. HIV-1-infected patients who were minimally symptomatic had normal intestinal absorption and permeability, yet had greater gastrointestinal dysfunction as they progressed to AIDS. Malabsorption of bile acids and vitamin B_{12} did not correlate with morphometric analysis of ileal biopsies and was unremarkable in these patients. Thus, there was significant mucosal dysfunction with only minor ileal morphologic changes. Malabsorption of bile acids may play a pathologic role in patients with AIDS diarrhea. The absorptive defect of AIDS enteropathy using a D-xylose kinetic model of proximal absorption was studied[43] and correlated with the results of a Schilling test for cobalamin absorption, which measures distal intestinal function. There were minimal histologic abnormalities in both the proximal and distal biopsy sites in patients with diarrhea and no enteric infection. D-Xylose absorption was low, and the absorptive defect was more severe and greater than would be expected from the histologic abnormalities found. Thus, these findings support the theory that there is little association between histologic characteristics of the small bowel and its absorptive function in patients with HIV-1 infection.

Most studies do not support a direct role for gastrointestinal malabsorption on growth failure or weight loss. Ullrich et al.[39] described gastrointestinal malabsorption in HIV-1-infected patients who had low levels of lactase enzyme in the brush border, crypt death, decreased villous surface area, and decreased mitotic figures per crypt when compared with control patients. In addition, Keating et al.[44] described absorptive capacity and intestinal permeability in HIV-1-infected patients. Malabsorption was prevalent in all groups of patients with AIDS, but was not as common in the asymptomatic HIV-1-infected patients. Malabsorption correlated with the degree of immune suppression and with body mass index. There were mild decreases in the ratio of jejunal villous height to crypt depth, yet not as severe as the subtotal villous atrophy found in celiac disease. Lim et al.[45] found disaccharidase activity decreased proportionately with greater HIV-1 disease severity, although there was no association between disaccharidase levels and weight loss. In addition, Mosavi et al.[46] found no correlation between diarrhea and weight loss in HIV-1-positive patients. Taylor et al.[47] found mild histologic changes accompanied by severe disaccharidase abnormalities; however, symptoms were severe enough to withdraw lactose in only 25% of the patients. Collectively these studies suggest that gastrointestinal malabsorption may be present, but is not always associated with weight loss and diarrhea.

Formal studies of intestinal absorption in children with HIV-1 are more limited. Malabsorption occurs frequently in HIV-1-infected children and may progress with the disease. In one study, 40% of children had nonphysiologic lactose malabsorption and 61% had generalized carbohydrate malabsorption

that was not associated with gastrointestinal symptoms or nutritional status.[48] These findings have been confirmed by others.[49] Another study in children revealed an association between diarrhea and nutrition.[50] Abnormal D-xylose absorption has also been associated with enteric infections in children.[48] Fat and protein loss or malabsorption have also been described. Sentongo et al.[51] evaluated fat malabsorption and pancreatic exocrine insufficiency using fecal elastase-1 enzyme assay in 44 HIV-1-infected children. Hormone-stimulated pancreatic function testing and 72-hour stool and dietary fat sample collection were performed in children with abnormal fecal elastase levels. The prevalence of steatorrhea was 39% and that of pancreatic insufficiency was 0% (95% confidence interval 0 to 9%). There were no associations between steatorrhea and pancreatic insufficiency, growth, HIV-1 RNA viral load, CD4 status, or type of antiretroviral therapy. Other studies support the absence of association.[52] Thus, the clinical significance of steatorrhea in pediatric HIV-1, similar to absorption of other nutrients, is unclear.

The etiology of malabsorption in HIV-1 infection is probably multifactorial. The cellular milieu of the lamina propria is altered significantly with HIV-1 infection.[34,53] The depletion of the CD4 T lymphocytes in the intestinal tract may cause change in the cytokine environment and alter intestinal function. Viral load in the intestinal tract may be considerably higher than that measured peripherally, and this can also affect mucosal gastrointestinal structure and function. Recently, the HIV-1 Tat protein was found to decrease glucose absorption through decreasing the activity of the sodium D-glucose symporter.[54] Studies suggesting these hypotheses include that of Kotler et al.,[55] which looked at intestinal mucosal inflammation in 74 HIV-1-infected individuals. These authors found abnormal histopathology in 69% of the patients, and this finding was associated with altered bowel habits. High tissue P24 antigen levels were observed, and these correlated with more advanced HIV-1 disease. Tissue P24 detection was associated with both abnormal bowel habits and mucosal histology. The tissue content of cytokines, including TNF, α-interferon, and interleukin-1β, was higher in HIV-1-infected individuals than in controls, and these increases were independent of intestinal infection. Thus, HIV-1 reactivation in the intestinal mucosa could be associated with an inflammatory bowel-like syndrome in the absence of other enteric pathogens.

Small bowel bacterial overgrowth can be another source of gastrointestinal dysfunction leading to malabsorption. Bacterial overgrowth may be due to AIDS gastropathy,[56,57] in which the stomach produces only small amounts of hydrogen chloride, allowing bacterial pathogens to escape the acid barrier of the stomach and colonize the duodenum. Additionally, iatrogenic hypochlorhydria may be due to the use of acid-blocking agents as treatment for peptic disease. Interestingly, some authors have found no relationship between gastric pH and small bowel bacterial colonization and diarrhea in HIV-1-infected patients.[58] Enteric pathogens[59] have been associated with enteric dysfunction, as discussed later.

With the advent of HAART, gastrointestinal symptoms, especially those associated with opportunistic infections, are less common.[60] As viral burden decreases, immunosuppression has less effect on gastrointestinal function. Compared to untreated patients, HAART-treated patients had greater integrity of intestinal mucosal barrier and decreased villous atrophy.[61] Ritonavir, a protease inhibitor, in combination therapy resulted in restoration of gastrointestinal function in 10 children with carbohydrate malabsorption, steatorrhea, protein loss, and iron deficiency.[62] However, one study in adults found similar rates of fat malabsorption in patients taking HAART and in those not taking HAART.[63]

INFECTIONS OF THE GASTROINTESTINAL TRACT

The gastrointestinal tract is a major target for opportunistic infections in HIV-1-infected children. The spectrum of these infections is dependent on HIV-1 disease progression. In developed countries, with improved HIV-1 viral suppression associated with HAART, opportunistic infections of the gut and elsewhere are less common.[64] However, immunocompromised children are still at risk for infections with cytomegalovirus (CMV), herpes simplex virus (HSV), *Cryptosporidium*, and microsporidia. Previous dogma that much of the diarrhea found in children with HIV-1 infection is not associated with enteric pathogens has been challenged. Unusual viral and parasitic infections can be diagnosed as a result of better diagnostic techniques. However, the cause of diarrhea in a significant number of patients with HIV-1 remains undiagnosed.[65]

Occurrence of opportunistic disease and infection of the gastrointestinal tract in immunocompromised patients relies heavily on the accessibility of HAART. As a result, there is great disparity of documented incidence of gastrointestinal infections dependent on access to HAART in particular regions. For this reason, we have divided this section into two subsections: gastrointestinal infections in regions with low HAART accessibility or in patients with CD4 T-lymphocyte counts less than 200 cells/mm³, and gastrointestinal infections in regions with high HAART accessibility and successful viral suppression. This does not imply that any of the infections discussed here occur in isolation contingent on HAART accessibility, because all HIV-1 patients regardless of HAART may encounter these complications. In the post-HAART era, it is helpful for a physician to know which backdrop lends itself to specific vulnerabilities.

INFECTIONS OF THE GASTROINTESTINAL TRACT IN REGIONS WITH LOW HAART ACCESSIBILITY OR IN PATIENTS WITH CD4 COUNTS BELOW 200 CELLS/mm³

Viral Infections

The detection of viral gastrointestinal infections in HIV-1-infected children can sometimes be difficult owing to the limitations of diagnostic techniques. The most common gastrointestinal viral pathogen in HIV-1-infected children is CMV. Other pathogens, such as HSV, adenovirus, Epstein-Barr virus, and a variety of other unusual viruses, can also contribute to intestinal dysfunction and diarrhea.

Herpes Simplex Virus

HSV infection in an immunocompromised child usually represents reactivation of a latent virus that had been acquired earlier in life. Gastrointestinal infection with HSV most commonly involves the esophagus and causes multiple small, discrete ulcers. HSV can also involve other areas of the intestinal tract, including the colon and small bowel. The diagnosis of HSV relies on recognizing the multinucleated intranuclear inclusion bodies (Cowdry type A) with a ground-glass appearance and molding of the nuclei. The squamous epithelium is usually infected, although there may also be involvement of intestinal glandular epithelium in the mesenchymal cells. HSV monoclonal antibody staining is confirmatory for the diagnosis. In extensive involvement, there may be transmural necrosis and development of tracheoesophageal fistulas. Treatment of HSV and other common gastrointestinal pathogens and their primary sites of involvement are outlined in Table 42-2.

Other herpes viruses have also been detected in the gut of HIV-1-infected individuals. A case report of one 34-year-old HIV-1-infected man with intestinal pseudo-obstruction and disseminated cutaneous herpes zoster revealed positive immunohistochemistry against herpes zoster in a resected portion of the terminal ileum. This area had focal ulceration. The virus was localized to the muscularis propria and myenteric plexi throughout the entire length of the specimen. The authors postulated that the location of the virus in the gut may have been the etiologic factor for the pseudo-obstruction.[66]

Cytomegalovirus

CMV in the immunocompromised child, like HSV, represents reactivation of a latent virus that was acquired in earlier life. CMV is one of the more common viral pathogens of HIV-1-infected children. The reported incidence of gastrointestinal involvement in the pre-HAART era varied from 4.4% to 52% of patients studied. The incidence rates may have varied based on the techniques of diagnosis.[57] CMV infection is rare in patients with CD4 T-lymphocyte counts greater than 50 cells/mm³.[67] CMV may involve any part of the gastrointestinal tract, with an increased incidence in the esophagus or colon. CMV infection usually results in one or two discrete single and large ulcers of the esophagus and colon. Lesions may lead to severe gastrointestinal bleeding and hemodynamic instability. CMV inclusion bodies can be discovered incidentally in an asymptomatic patient, and this does not necessarily reflect disease.

In patients with upper intestinal CMV disease, there can be dysphagia and upper abdominal symptoms, whereas diarrhea is more common with colitis. The diarrhea can be watery or bloody. Children may be systemically ill.[68] The colitis from CMV infection is patchy and can be associated with severe necrotizing colitis and hemorrhage.[69] CMV usually affects the cecum and the right colon. Diagnosis is confirmed by endoscopy and biopsy. The histologic appearance of CMV-infected cells is unique (Figure 42-1). These cells are enlarged and contain intranuclear and cytoplasmic inclusion bodies. The nuclear inclusion bodies are acidophilic and are often surrounded by a halo. Cytoplasm inclusion bodies are multiple, granular, and often basophilic. Cells that are dying may appear smaller and smudged, with poorly defined inclusion bodies. Staining for CMV antigen shows that many of the infected cells are endothelial cells with others being perivascular mesenchymal cells. CMV can cause vasculitis because of its target cell population. Thus, the spread of CMV occurs with circulating infected endothelial cells. Treatment options are outlined in Table 42-2. Once HAART is established, with decreased viral burden (both HIV-1 and CMV) and improved CD4 counts, CMV treatment may be discontinued without concern for reactivation.[70]

TABLE 42-2. Primary Location and Drug Therapy for Common Enteric Pathogens Infecting Immunocompromised Children

Pathogen	Drug Treatment
Bacteria	
Salmonella (SI, C)	Ampicillin; TMP-SMZ; cefotaxime sodium, ceftriaxone sodium; fluoroquinolones (>18 years)
Shigella (SI, C)	Ampicillin, TMP-SMZ; ceftriaxone sodium; azithromycin; fluoroquinolones (>18 years)
Campylobacter (SI)	Erythromycin; azithromycin dihydrate; doxycycline (>8 years); fluoroquinolones (>18 years)
Yersinia (SI, C)	TMP-SMZ; tetracycline (>8 years); cefotaxime sodium; chloramphenicol; fluoroquinolones (>18 years)
Clostridium difficile (C)	Discontinue antibiotics, if possible; metronidazole; vancomycin; bacitracin; cholestyramine (may bind toxin and relieve symptoms); Lactobacillus GG
Mycobacteria	
Mycobacterium tuberculosis (SI)	Isoniazid; rifampin; pyrazinamide; ethambutol; aminoglycoside
MAC (SI)	(1) Clarithromycin or azithromycin combined with (2) ethambutol with adding (3) rifabutin (not in combination with PIs) or rifampin, plus (4) amikacin or streptomycin
Viruses	
Cytomegalovirus (SI, C)	Ganciclovir; foscarnet; CMV-IVIG; valganciclovir hydrochloride
Herpes simplex virus (O/P, E)	Aciclovir; foscarnet; famciclovir; penciclovir
Fungi	
Candida albicans (O/P, E)	Fluconazole, itraconazole, ketoconazole, amphotericin B
Histoplasma (SI)	Amphotericin B; fluconazole; itraconazole
Cryptococcus (SI)	Amphotericin B with oral flucytosine (serious systemic infections); fluconazole; itraconazole
Pneumocystis jiroveci (SI)	TMP-SMZ; pentamidine; atovaquone; dapsone
Parasites	
Cryptosporidia (SI)	Nitazoxanide; azithromycin; paromomycin, octreotide; human immune globulin; bovine hyperimmune colostrum
Microsporidia (SI)	Albendazole; metronidazole; atovaquone; nitazoxanide; fumagillin
Isospora belli (SI)	TMP-SMZ; pyrimethamine; fluoroquinolones (> 18 years)
Giardia lamblia (SI)	Metronidazole; furazolidone; nitazoxanide

C, colon; E, esophagus; MAC, *Mycobacterium avium-intracellulare* complex; O/P, oropharynx; PI, protease inhibitor; S, stomach; SI, small intestine; TMP-SMZ, trimethoprim-sulfamethoxazole.

Other Viral Infections

Infections with other unusual viral pathogens have been described. These include the human papilloma virus and Epstein-Barr virus, which have been identified in esophageal ulcers of patients with HIV-1. Adenovirus of the stomach and

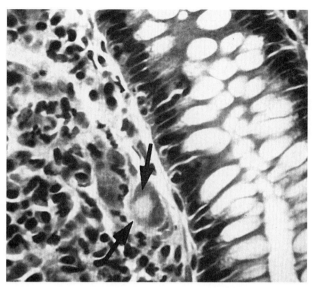

Figure 42-1. Small bowel biopsy showing cytomegalovirus inclusion (arrows) within the lamina propria.

colon have also been reported and are often difficult to identify.[71] In the pre-HAART era, patients who excreted adenovirus from their gastrointestinal tract had a shorter survival.[72] There are unusual enteric viruses that have been associated with diarrhea in HIV-1-infected children.[73] These viruses, among others, include astrovirus and picobirnavirus.[74] Cegielski et al.[75] studied 59 children with HIV-1 infection in Tanzania. They looked for enteric viruses identified by electron microscopy of fecal specimens. Small round structured viruses (SRSVs) were found more frequently in HIV-1-infected children than in uninfected children with chronic diarrhea. Rotavirus and coronavirus-like particles were not associated with HIV-1 infection. These authors considered that these SRSVs may be associated with HIV-1 infection and could lead to chronic diarrhea in Tanzanian children.

Bacterial Infections

Bacterial infections that involve the gastrointestinal tract of children with HIV-1 infection may be divided into three groups: bacterial overgrowth of normal gut flora; pathogens that can affect immunocompromised children as well as immunocompetent children (*Salmonella, Shigella, Campylobacter, Clostridium difficile*, and *Aeromonas*); and bacterial infections that are more common in immunocompromised children (*Mycobacterium avium-intracellulare* complex; MAC).

Few studies have evaluated bacterial overgrowth in HIV-1-infected children, although gastric hypoacidity has been associated with opportunistic enteric infections and bacterial overgrowth in adult patients with HIV-1.[76] Other studies have not found this association. Small bowel bacterial overgrowth was not a common finding in a group of 32 HIV-1-infected patients, regardless of the presence of diarrhea, and it was not associated with hypochlorhydria.[58] Lactose hydrogen breath testing has shown high baseline readings in children that may indirectly suggest bacterial overgrowth of the small intestinal tract.[48] Detection of bacterial overgrowth in the small bowel is usually performed by quantitative duodenal aspirate for bacterial culture, with therapy directed at treating the organisms, which are often anaerobic.

Common Bacterial Infections

Common bacterial pathogens include *Salmonella*, *Shigella*, *Campylobacter*, *Clostridium difficile*, and *Aeromonas*. Infection with these organisms occurs more frequently in immunocompromised patients. Combined morbidity and mortality rates associated with HIV-1 and these bacterial pathogens in developing countries approach 50% in some studies.[77] HIV-1-infected patients with *Campylobacter* infection have higher rates of bacteremia than the general population. Deaths from sepsis due to this organism have been reported in severely immunodeficient patients with AIDS, despite HAART.[78]

Escherichia coli

Other entities, such as bacterial enteritis, have been described in adults with HIV-1. A study by Orenstein and Kotler[79] evaluated ileal and colonic biopsies in patients with AIDS and diarrhea and found bacteria similar to adherent *E. coli* along the intestinal epithelial border. Similar findings were documented by Kotler et al.,[80] who showed adherent bacteria in 17% of all adult patients with AIDS. The infection was localized primarily to the cecum and right colon, and three distinct histopathologic patterns of adherence were observed: attachment on effacing lesions, bacteria intercalated between microvilli, and aggregates of bacteria more loosely attached to the damaged epithelium. The bacterial cultures of frozen rectal biopsies yielded *E. coli* in 12 of the 18 patients. These findings suggest that chronic infection with adherent bacteria can also produce the syndrome of AIDS-associated diarrhea. In a "look back" evaluation, Orenstein and Dieterich[71] found that enteropathogenic bacterial infections were overlooked on initial examination and concluded that, for accurate diagnoses, specimens should be evaluated by laboratories with expertise in HIV.

Mycobacteria

Intestinal infections with mycobacteria, including *Mycobacterium tuberculosis*, MAC, and other atypical mycobacteria, were the most frequently encountered bacterial infections in HIV-1-infected patients in the pre-HAART era[81] and became more prevalent in the pre-HAART era as patients were living longer with CD4 counts below 200 cells/mm³.[82,83] In the HAART era, disseminated MAC in colonized patients can be successfully prevented; however, the effects of HAART on restoration of CD4 counts do not prevent MAC colonization.[84]

Infection with MAC usually occurs in the very late stages of AIDS in children, when CD4 counts are lower than 200 cells/mm³. The most common clinical manifestations of gastrointestinal infections with MAC include fever, weight loss, malabsorption, and diarrhea. Intestinal obstruction, resulting from lymph node involvement and intussusception; terminal ileitis, which resembles Crohn's disease; and refractory gastric ulcers are often found. Severe gastrointestinal hemorrhage has also been described.[85] Endoscopically, fine white nodules may be seen in the duodenum, or the duodenal mucosa may look velvety and grayish in appearance. Segments of the gastrointestinal tract can become infected with MAC. Histologically, there is a diffuse histiocytic infiltrate in the lamina propria with blunting of the small intestinal villi. These histiocytic infiltrates can be recognized on hematoxylin and eosin staining and on acid-fast stains and are pathognomonic for infection (Figure 42-2). With the advent of HAART, immune reconstitution disease has been described.[86,87] This is likely an immune reaction in which previously quiescent organisms become active because of the improved immune

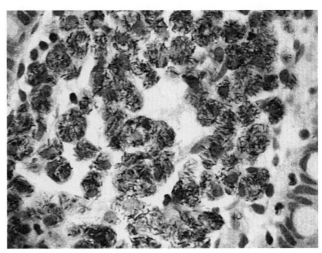

Figure 42-2. Small bowel biopsy showing histiocytes infiltrated with *Mycobacterium avium-intracellulare* within the lamina propria.

function associated with HAART. This can occur in as many as 25% of patients who respond to HAART.[88] Lymphadenitis is the most common condition, although abscesses can appear anywhere. Severe abdominal complaints may result.

Appropriate therapies are outlined in Table 42-2, yet this organism is often frustrating to treat. Azithromycin 600 mg, when given in combination with ethambutol, is an effective agent for the treatment of disseminated *M. avium* disease in patients infected with HIV-1.[89] Caution must be exercised in administering these multidrug regimens for MAC in patients receiving concurrent HAART. Rifamycins induce cytochrome P450 enzymes and accelerate the metabolism of clarithromycin and HIV-1 protease inhibitors. Conversely, clarithromycin inhibits these enzymes, resulting in increased rifabutin toxicity. The net result is treatment regimens that can be extremely difficult to tolerate and manage, especially for sicker patients. Clarithromycin and azithromycin must be administered in combination with other agents, such as ethambutol, to prevent the emergence of macrolide resistance.[90]

Parasitic infections

Cryptosporidium parvum

In the early 1980s, cryptosporidiosis was regarded as an AIDS-defining disease and an opportunistic intestinal pathogen. It became an important cause of chronic diarrhea, leading to high morbidity and mortality rates in immunocompromised patients. To date, no effective chemotherapy is available. With the introduction of protease inhibitors in HAART regimens, the incidence of cryptosporidiosis in patients with AIDS has declined substantially in developed countries.[91] However, in developing nations, gastrointestinal infection with *C. parvum* is prevalent and carries high morbidity and mortality rates.[92,93]

Although *Cryptosporidium* was initially described in animals, it was first noted to cause an enterocolitis in both immunocompromised and immunocompetent humans in 1976.[94,95] An intact T-cell response is the primary mechanism that confers protection against this organism; thus, patients with abnormal T-cell function or number are at risk. The spectrum and severity of disease in immunocompromised individuals with cryptosporidiosis correlates with most severe disease found in individuals with defects in the T-cell response.[91] The overall frequency of infection seems to be related to the severity of immunodeficiency and not the specific disorder.[96]

Cryptosporidium usually affects the gastrointestinal tract, although it has been found in other organs including the biliary tract,[97] pancreas,[98] and respiratory tract.[99] In immunocompetent individuals, the diarrhea is self-limiting, whereas in immunocompromised patients, it may be protracted and associated with significant malabsorption and nutritional compromise. The small intestine is the primary target, although it can occur in any part of the intestinal tract. Esophageal cryptosporidiosis has also been described in one child[100] and in adults. Clayton et al.[101] described two patterns of enteric cryptosporidiosis. One was accompanied by severe clinical disease with significant malabsorption, with the majority of the organisms found in the proximal small bowel, whereas less severe clinical disease was seen in patients with colonic disease or with infection noted only in the stool. Patients with proximal small bowel infection with *Cryptosporidium* showed crypt hyperplasia, villous atrophy, lamina propria inflammatory infiltrates, abnormal D-xylose absorption, greater weight loss, and shorter survival, with greater need for intravenous hydration and hyperalimentation than patients with colonic disease. In other studies, absorption of nutrients showed an inverse correlation with active infection,[102] as shown by altered vitamin B_{12} and D-xylose absorption and lactulose and mannitol urinary excretion ratios. Intestinal function improved in patients whose oocyte counts were reduced by treatment with paromomycin.

Symptomatic cryptosporidiosis has been documented in as many as 6.4% of immunocompetent children and 22% of immunodeficient children, whereas in an asymptomatic population, *Cryptosporidium* was found in 4.4% of immunocompetent and 4.8% of immunodeficient children.[103] Spiramycin at 100 mg per kg daily for 14 days caused a significant reduction in the shedding of infectious oocysts, and no gastrointestinal symptoms developed in children treated for asymptomatic infection, whereas children who were not treated developed gastrointestinal symptoms.[103]

The diagnosis of cryptosporidiosis is made by identifying the organisms in a duodenal aspirate, stool, or tissue sample (biopsies). On hematoxylin and eosin-stained sections, these organisms can be found as rows or clusters of basophilic spherical structures 2 to 4 μm in diameter, attached to the microvillous border of the epithelial cells (Figure 42-3). The tips in the lateral aspect of the villi show the greatest number of organisms in the small intestine. In the colonic epithelium, the crypt and surface epithelial involvement appears equal. *Cryptosporidium* also stain positively with Giemsa and negatively with mucous stains. The acid-fast stain on a stool sample is one of the most widely used methods of determining whether a patient has cryptosporidiosis. More recent sensitive and specific methods for diagnosing cryptosporidiosis include fluorescein-labeled IgG monoclonal antibodies.[104,105]

Treatment of cryptosporidiosis in children with HIV-1 infection is often difficult. The disease can be chronic and protracted with diffuse watery diarrhea and dehydration. Several different agents are used to eradicate the organism, with varying success rates. The most effective treatment is to improve immunologic function and nutritional status. With the advent of HAART, many children's immune function has been restored with a lower incidence and prevalence of *Cryptosporidium* infection.[106] The introduction of HAART in a patient with severe debilitating *Cryptosporidium* infection not only

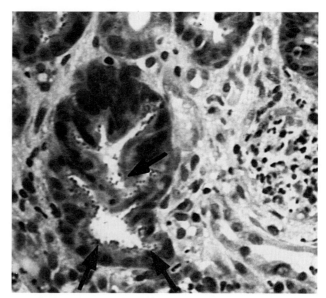

Figure 42-3. Small bowel biopsy showing *Cryptosporidium* attached to the villus (arrows).

resulted in an increased CD4 count in the peripheral blood and clearance of the organism, but also produced a marked increase in CD4 count in the rectal mucosa on biopsy, suggesting this may have been the main mechanism of clearing the parasite.[107] Octreotide therapy of acute and chronic diarrhea, with coincident improvement in nutritional status, eradicated *Cryptosporidium* in one patient.[105,108] Other investigators have used bovine hyperimmune colostrum with benefit.[109,110] The macrolides, such as azithromycin, have shown some promise in the treatment of *Cryptosporidium* infection.[111,112] The effect of protease inhibitors as therapy against *Cryptosporidium* has been tested in a cell culture system.[113] Nelfinavir moderately inhibited the host cell invasion over a period of 2 hours. Indinavir, nelfinavir, and ritonavir inhibited parasite development significantly. The inhibitory effect was increased when the aminoglycoside paromomycin was combined with the protease inhibitors indinavir, ritonavir and, to a lesser extent, saquinavir, compared with the protease inhibitor alone. Thus, protease inhibitor therapy may directly (rather than indirectly, through its effects on the immune system) inhibit growth of *Cryptosporidium*. Amadi et al.[92] found that a 3-day course of nitazoxanide improved diarrhea, helped eradicate the parasite, and improved mortality in HIV-1-seronegative, but not HIV-1-seropositive, children in Zambia. Treatment with nitazoxanide on immunocompetent patients demonstrated parasitic load reduction, but its effects on immunocompromised patients are not yet palpable.[114]

Microsporidia

Microsporidia are obligate intracellular protozoal parasites that infect a variety of cell types in many different species of animals. These organisms were first described in 1857, when recognized as a cause of disease in nonhuman hosts.[115] The first description of microsporidia (*Enterocytozoon bieneusi*) as a human pathogen was in 1985, and microsporidia have since been described as more common human pathogens.[116] Infection with microsporidia typically occurs in patients with severely depressed CD4 T-lymphocyte counts. One of the largest case studies of intestinal microsporidiosis in patients with HIV-1 infection was described by Orenstein et al.[117] in 67 adult patients with AIDS and AIDS-related complex and chronic nonpathogenic diarrhea. *E. bieneusi* was diagnosed by electron microscopy in 20 of the patients. Jejunal biopsies were more positive than duodenal biopsies. The parasites and spores were clearly visible by light microscopy in 17 of the 21 biopsies. Infection was confined to enterocytes located at the tip of the intestinal villus, and the histologic findings included villous atrophy, cell degeneration, necrosis, and sloughing. Other investigators[118-120] found microsporidia in as many as 50% of HIV-1-infected patients with chronic and unexplained diarrhea evaluated in the pre-HAART era. *E. bieneusi* has been documented in 15 to 25% of children with[121] or without[122] diarrhea in developing countries, making it fairly ubiquitous in these regions of the world. Other species of microsporidia, including *Encephalitozoon (Septata) intestinalis*, can cause significant enteric disease with diarrhea, wasting and malabsorption. *Encephalitozoon intestinalis* differs from *Enterocytozoon bieneusi* in its tendency to disseminate, and it can infect enterocytes as well as macrophages, fibroblasts, and endothelial cells.

Microsporidia are found with increasing frequency in HIV-1-negative patients.[123] Infection has been documented in almost every tissue and organ in the body, and in epithelial, mesenchymal, and neural cells. Microsporidia can cause inflammation and cell death and a variety of symptoms including shortness of breath, sinusitis, and diarrhea with wasting. If left untreated, microsporidiosis can be a significant cause of mortality.

Treatments for microsporidia include albendazole, which can relieve clinical symptoms and eliminate microsporidial spores in the feces, especially of the less common pathogen, *E. intestinalis*. *E. bieneusi* is more challenging to treat, although therapy with fumagillin or its analogue, TNP-470 (antiangiogenesis agents), has shown promising results.[124-126] Other studies show atovaquone as an effective treatment as well.[127] Indirect treatment by improving the immune system with HAART has also effectively cleared these organisms.[106,128,129]

Isospora belli

Isospora belli is recognized as an opportunistic small bowel pathogen in patients with HIV-1 infection. This organism is most common in tropical and subtropical climates. Isosporiasis can be diagnosed by identification of the oocyte in the stool or by biopsy. The diagnosis is critical because, in contrast to cryptosporidiosis or microsporidiosis, the therapy is very effective. *I. belli* is found within the enterocyte and within the cytoplasm. The organism stains poorly, although the central nucleus, large nucleolus, and perinuclear halo give it a characteristic appearance. The infection produces mucosal atrophy and tissue eosinophilia. A 10-day course of trimethoprim-sulfamethoxazole is effective therapy, and recurrent disease can be prevented by ongoing prophylaxis with this combination drug.[130] Ciprofloxacin, although not as effective, is an acceptable alternative for those with sulfa allergies.[130] Other therapies for *Isospora* include pyrimethamine, also indicated for patients with sulfa allergies.[131]

Other Parasites

Blastocystis hominis is usually considered a nonpathologic parasite, but it has been described in patients with chronic diarrhea and HIV-1 infection.[132] This organism is more pathogenic in immunocompromised patients and can cause mild, prolonged, or recurrent diarrhea. Effective therapy includes diiodohydroxyquinoline 650 mg orally three times daily for 21 days. Other protozoan infections that can be found in HIV-1-infected patients are *Entamoeba histolytica*, *Entamoeba coli*, *Entamoeba hartmanni*, *Endolimax nana*, and *Giardia lamblia* in 4% of cases.

Fungal Infections

Candida albicans

Candidiasis of the gastrointestinal tract is the most common fungal infection in HIV-1-infected children. The esophagus is the primary target of *Candida*, and this infection occurred in the majority of patients during the course of their illness in the pre-HAART era. It was also the second most frequent AIDS-defining disease, second in prevalence only to *Pneumocystis jirovecii*. Patients with *Candida* esophagitis complain of odynophagia or dysphagia and may often have vomiting and recurrent abdominal pain. Children often have oral thrush, coincident with more disseminated and invasive *Candida* esophagitis, although the absence of oral thrush does not preclude the diagnosis of *Candida* esophagitis.[41] In one study, oral candidiasis preceded the diagnosis of *Candida* esophagitis in 94% of children.[133] Other risk factors include low CD4 count and prior antibiotic use.[133] Histopathologically, yeast forms within an intact mucosa confirm invasive disease. This is in contrast to colonization, where the yeast is found overlying intact mucosal surfaces or necrotic tissue. These organisms are best seen with Grocott's methenamine silver method or periodic acid-Schiff stain. Upper gastrointestinal studies are suggestive of *Candida* esophagitis with diffuse mucosal irregularities (Figure 42-4). Upper gastrointestinal endoscopy with biopsy and appropriate staining is the most sensitive test for determining invasive candidiasis of the esophagus. Candidiasis can also occur in the stomach, as well as the small bowel if the acid barrier has been suppressed either through an intrinsic decrease in gastric acid production or iatrogenically with the use of potent acid blockers. Numerous effective therapies have been described to treat *Candida* of the upper gastrointestinal tract, including fluconazole, ketoconazole, and itraconazole.[134,135] Ketoconazole has more hepatic side effects than fluconazole. Itraconazole is usually well tolerated and is effective. In severe and invasive disease, either topical or intravenous amphotericin can be used. Agents such as oral miconazole and nystatin are not indicated for invasive *Candida*.

Other Fungal Infections

Disseminated histoplasmosis develops in 5% of adult patients with AIDS in the Midwestern region of the United States, and elsewhere. The clinical signs and symptoms related to this infection may be indolent, but left untreated can carry significant morbidity and mortality.[136] The likelihood of disease is higher in patients with CD4 counts under 200 cells/mm^3.[137] There is enterocolitis associated with infection, and at colonoscopy, plaques, ulcers, pseudopolyps, and skip areas are frequently seen. Cryptococcal gastrointestinal disease has been identified in patients with disseminated *Cryptococcus* infection. The esophagus and colon are involved most frequently. *P. jirovecii* infection of the gastrointestinal tract has also been described.[59] Gastrointestinal pneumocystosis develops after hematogenous or lymphatic dissemination from the lungs, or reactivation of latent gastrointestinal infection. The administration of aerosolized pentamidine has increased the risk of

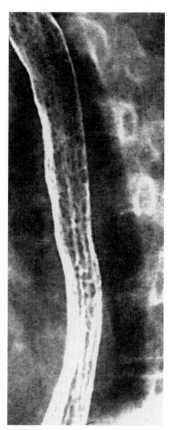

Figure 42-4. Radiographic contrast study showing mucosal irregularities seen with *Candida* esophagitis.

developing extrapulmonary spread of *P. jirovecii* pneumonia. *P. jirovecii* pneumonia infection can occur throughout the gastrointestinal tract. In the lamina propria there are foamy exudates with *P. jirovecii* organisms found within them. Although more rare, infection of the colon can also cause diarrhea.

INFECTIONS OF THE GASTROINTESTINAL TRACT IN REGIONS WITH HIGH HAART ACCESSIBILITY AND SUCCESSFUL HIV VIRAL SUPPRESSION

The effect of HAART on rates of infection of the gastrointestinal tract are twofold. First, on a macro level, the advent of HAART has led to a dramatic decrease in perinatal transmission of HIV, and therefore the rates of newly infected children have plummeted,[138] with reports of vertical transmission falling between 1 and 2%.[139] Second, HAART has been successful in immune reconstitution, and therefore in regions with high HAART accessibility, there has been a marked decrease in the number of HIV patients presenting with opportunistic infections. These infections have not been eradicated, but the majority of patients adhering to HAART are able to achieve CD4+ cell reconstitution and therefore stave these off. Patients who sustain chronically low CD4+ T lymphocyte levels in spite of HAART accessibility and usage continue to be at risk for the opportunistic infections[140] described in the previous section. When comparing incidence rates of opportunistic infection in the pre- (before January 1, 1997) and post-HAART era, there was an overall decrease.[8,141] Specifically: incidence rates of

CMV decreased from 1.4 to 0.1; esophageal candidiasis from 0.9 to 0.4; herpes simplex virus from 0.2 to 0; and chronic intestinal and cryptosporidiosis from 1.3 to 0 per 100 persons per year.[141] Additionally, Nachman et al.[142] reported successful withdrawal of opportunistic infection prophylaxis for a period of 132 weeks in pediatric HIV-positive patients more than 2 years old who had achieved CD4 reconstitution without significant incidence when compared to demographically matched HIV-negative patients. In light of this progress, we have integrated additional immunocompromised patient populations into our discussion of gastrointestinal vulnerabilities.

Bacterial Infections

Clostridium difficile

Colitis from *C. difficile* is also more common in the immunosuppressed population owing to chronic antibiotic use and impaired immune system.[143] Pulvirenti et al.[144] studied 161 HIV-1-infected patients with *C. difficile* and found that they had longer hospital stays and more admissions than patients without *C. difficile* infection, as well as other opportunistic infections such as herpes virus. They found *C. difficile*–associated diarrhea in 32% of all study patients with diarrhea. However, infection with *C. difficile* appeared to have little impact on morbidity or mortality. In a 1998, New York state screening study[145] of hospitalized HIV-1-infected patients in the HAART era, 2.8% were admitted with a diarrheal diagnosis, with 51.3% of these having a *C. difficile* infection. Thus, even with HAART, diarrhea is prevalent and is often associated with identifiable pathogens. *C. difficile* infection has been reported to be one of the most common bacterial diarrheal pathogens among HIV-infected patients although its rates have decreased with HAART.[146] Because of the serious complications that are associated with active bacterial enteric infections in immunodeficient children, treatment options are outlined in Table 42-2.

Helicobacter pylori

H. pylori prevalence is not significantly different between HIV-1-infected patients and HIV-1-negative patients.[147,148] Some investigators have found the seroprevalence of *H. pylori* to be lower in HIV-1-infected patients,[149] especially as CD4 counts decline with advancing disease.[147] The protection from *H. pylori* may be a result of frequent antibiotic use or correlated with a more advanced, dysfunctional immune state that results in a decreased inflammatory response to the organism.[150] Remission of a high-grade gastric mucosa-associated lymphoid tissue (MALT) lymphoma followed *H. pylori* eradication and HAART in a patient with AIDS.[151] However, a recent study of HIV-infected adults showed that 32% of patients with peptic symptoms had *H. pylori* on biopsy, with those having CD4 counts above 200 cells/mm^3 at a higher risk.[152] Treatment of *H. pylori* in HIV-1-infected children is similar to that in noninfected children, with special attention to drug interactions.

MOTILITY OF THE GASTROINTESTINAL TRACT IN HIV INFECTION

In up to 15 to 25% of HIV-1-infected children, the etiology of the diarrhea is unclear. Autonomic dysfunction is another potential mechanism of noninfectious diarrhea not previously described. Clinically, children with autonomic neuropathy have sweating, urinary retention, and abnormal cardiovascular hemodynamics. It is possible that this autonomic denervation contributes to diarrhea in patients with HIV-1 infection, as suggested by Griffin et al.[153] When neuron-specific polyclonal antibodies were applied to jejunal biopsies, there was a significant reduction in axonal density in both villi and pericryptal lamina propria in patients with HIV-1 infection compared with controls, with the greatest reduction in patients with diarrhea. Octreotide therapy has shown promising results in some patients.[154] Finally, drug side effects should be considered, with many of the antiretroviral therapies causing chronic diarrhea and other gastrointestinal toxicities (Table 42-3).

Motility problems of the esophagus and stomach have been reported[155-157] and can be a source of upper gastrointestinal complaints including vomiting, dysphagia, nausea, and dyspepsia. The motility abnormalities may be primary, or they may be secondary to infectious or inflammatory disease of the respective organ. Hypertension of the lower esophageal sphincter with incomplete relaxation, esophageal hypocontraction, and nonspecific motility disorders have been described in patients with normal intact esophageal mucosa.[156] Gastric emptying, especially in patients with infections or advanced disease, may be delayed, as documented by gastric scintigraphy.[155] However, delayed gastric emptying does not always correlate with upper gastrointestinal symptoms or small bowel motility studies. In adults with HIV-1 infection and minimally advanced disease, gastric emptying of solids was delayed and emptying of liquids accelerated compared with that in controls. No abnormal esophageal motility patterns were found. All patients had

TABLE 42-3. HIV-Related Medications and Common Gastrointestinal Side Effects

Medication	Action	Side Effects
Abacavir	NRTI	Nausea, vomiting, abdominal pain, pancreatitis, abnormal liver function
Aciclovir	Antiviral	Nausea, abdominal pain, diarrhea, abnormal liver function
Amprenavir	PI	Abdominal pain, diarrhea
Atazanavir	PI	Nausea, diarrhea, abdominal pain, hyperbilirubinemia
Atripla (tenofovir, emtricitabine, efavirenz)	Combination	Nausea, vomiting, diarrhea, abdominal pain, hepatitis, bone loss, pancreatitis, lactic acidosis
Azithromycin	Antibacterial	Nausea, vomiting, melena, jaundice
Ciprofloxacin	Antibacterial	Ileus, jaundice, bleeding, diarrhea, anorexia, oral ulcers, hepatitis, pancreatitis, vomiting, abdominal pain
Clarithromycin	Antibacterial	Nausea, diarrhea, abdominal pain, abnormal taste
Combivir (zidovudine-lamivudine)	Combination	Nausea, vomiting, abdominal pain, abnormal liver function, pancreatitis, lactic acidosis
Darunavir	PI	Nausea, vomiting, diarrhea, abdominal pain, pancreatitis, hepatitis, constipation
Didanosine (ddl)	NRTI	Nausea, vomiting, abdominal pain, pancreatitis, abnormal liver function
Efavirenz	NNRTI	Nausea, vomiting, abnormal liver function
Emtricitabine	NRTI	Lactic acidosis, hepatomegaly
Epzicom (zidovudine, abacavir)	Combination	Nausea, vomiting, abdominal pain, abnormal liver function, lactic acidosis, pancreatitis
Erythromycin	Antibacterial	Nausea, vomiting, abdominal pain
Etravirine	NNRTI	Nausea, vomiting, diarrhea, abdominal pain, hepatitis
Fosamprenavir	PI	Nausea, diarrhea, vomiting, abdominal pain
Enfuvirtide (Fuzeon)	FI	Nausea, diarrhea, abdominal pain, hepatitis, pancreatitis, dry mouth, anorexia
Ganciclovir	Antiviral	Nausea, vomiting, diarrhea, anorexia, abnormal liver function
Indinavir	PI	Nausea, vomiting, abdominal pain, diarrhea, changes in taste, jaundice, abnormal liver function
Ketoconazole	Antifungal	Hepatotoxicity
Lamivudine (3TC)	NRTI	Nausea, diarrhea, vomiting, abdominal pain, pancreatitis, abnormal liver function
Lopinavir/ritonavir	PI	Diarrhea, nausea, abdominal pain
Maraviroc	FI	Nausea, constipation, diarrhea, flatulence, abdominal pain, hepatitis, dysgeusia, stomatitis
Nelfinavir	PI	Nausea, diarrhea, fatigue, abnormal liver function
Nevirapine	NNRTI	Stomatitis, nausea, abdominal pain, raised gamma-glutamyl transpeptidase level, hepatotoxicity
Pentamidine	Antiparasitic	Abdominal pain, bleeding, hepatitis, pancreatitis, nausea, vomiting
Raltegravir	II	Gastritis, hepatitis, nausea, hyperbilirubinemia
Rifampin	Antibacterial	Abdominal pain, nausea, vomiting, diarrhea, jaundice
Ritonavir	PI	Nausea, vomiting, diarrhea, abdominal pain, pancreatitis, abnormal liver function
Saquinavir	PI	Mouth ulcers, nausea, abdominal pain, diarrhea, pancreatitis, abnormal liver function
Stavudine (d4T)	NRTI	Nausea, vomiting, abdominal pain, diarrhea, pancreatitis, abnormal liver function, hepatic failure
Sulfonamides	Antibacterial	Hepatitis, pancreatitis, stomatitis, nausea, vomiting, abdominal pain
Tenofovir	NRTI	Nausea, vomiting, diarrhea, abdominal pain, hepatitis, bone loss, pancreatitis
Tipranavir	PI	Hyperlipidemia, nausea, vomiting, diarrhea, abdominal pain, pancreatitis, hepatitis
Trizivir (abacavir-lamivudine-zidovudine)	Combination	Nausea, vomiting, abdominal pain, pancreatitis, abnormal liver function
Truvada (emtricitabine, tenofovir)	Combination	Lactic acidosis, nausea, vomiting, diarrhea, abdominal pain, hepatitis, bone loss, pancreatitis
Zalcitabine	NRTI	Pancreatitis, hepatic failure (with HBV), steatosis, lactic acidosis
Zidovudine (ZDV)	NRTI	Nausea, vomiting, abdominal pain, abnormal liver function

FI, fusion inhibitor; HBV, hepatitis B virus; II, integrase inhibitor; NNRTI, nonnucleoside–reverse transcriptase inhibitor; NRTI, nucleoside analogue–reverse transcriptase inhibitor; PI, protease inhibitor.

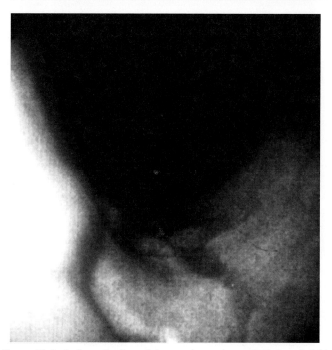

Figure 42-5. Endoscopic view of the esophagus in an HIV-infected child with a large idiopathic esophageal ulcer.

TABLE 42-4. **Approach to Diagnosis of Gastrointestinal Tract Disease in the Immunocompromised Child**

Preliminary Evaluation
1. Complete history and physical examination
    Caloric intake, anthropometrics, gastrointestinal symptoms
    Drug interactions
    Oropharyngeal, abdominal, and rectal examinations
2. Laboratory
    Complete blood count, viral load (if chronic viral infection), immune function, chemistries (liver function studies, lactate dehydrogenase, pancreatic studies)
3. Evaluation for enteric pathogens
    Bacterial, viral, parasite cultures, examination of stool

Secondary Evaluation (if enteric pathogens are not present)
1. Malabsorption studies
    Hydrogen breath test analysis
    Fecal fat determination
    Fecal elastase
    D-Xylose absorption
    Stool α1-antitrypsin
2. Radiographic studies (contrast, computed tomography, ultrasonography)

Tertiary Evaluation
1. Diagnostic endoscopy
    Biopsies, routine stains
    Brushings, cytology
    Duodenal aspirate (quantitative bacterial culture, ova and parasite)
    MAC culture, AFB stains (if HIV, CD4 count < 200 cells/mm³)
    Electron microscopy
2. Motility studies (in the appropriate clinical setting)

AFB, acid-fast bacilli; MAC, *Mycobacterium avium-intracellulare* complex.

a normal endoscopy prior to the motility studies.[157] Thus, in the absence of infectious and inflammatory disease in patients with appropriate symptoms, motility studies or empiric trials of prokinetic agents should be considered, with careful consideration of drug interactions.

IDIOPATHIC ESOPHAGEAL ULCERATION

Esophageal ulceration can be a result of an intercurrent opportunistic infection. Idiopathic oral and esophageal ulcers have been described in both children and adults with HIV-1.[158] These ulcers are characteristically large and may be single or multiple (Figure 42-5). The ulcers are located in the mid to distal esophagus. Controversy exists regarding the pathogenesis of these ulcers; some investigators have identified HIV-1 at the ulcer base,[159] whereas others have not.[160] Treatment options for these ulcers are limited, but include steroid therapy, with encouraging results,[159] and thalidomide.[161,162] However, chronic low-dose thalidomide does not prevent recurrence of the oral or esophageal aphthous ulcers.[163] In addition to the potentially teratogenic effects, a significant portion of children receiving thalidomide develop a rash, which precludes use of the drug. Significant caution should be exercised when using thalidomide. Overall, HAART has had a positive impact on esophageal disease occurrence and relapse.[164]

CLINICAL MANAGEMENT OF GASTROINTESTINAL DISORDERS IN HIV INFECTION AND OTHER IMMUNODEFICIENCIES

The diagnostic approach to the child with HIV-1 or other immunodeficiencies and gastrointestinal symptoms is outlined in Table 42-4. A comprehensive clinical history should be taken with a focus on estimating caloric intake and evaluating abdominal symptoms, such as diarrhea, vomiting, and abdominal pain. Growth history should also be reviewed. The physical examination should focus on an assessment of nutritional state and the possibility of intestinal or hepatobiliary disease. With diarrheal symptoms, every HIV-1-infected child should have a complete evaluation for bowel pathogens. This should precede all other diagnostic studies, as treatment of the pathogen may result in resolution of the symptoms. Investigation for enteric infections should include studies for the organisms outlined in the preceding section on infectious diarrhea. The child's antiretroviral regimen and initiation of new medications should be noted as many of these medications produce significant gastrointestinal side effects (see Table 42-2). Every effort should be made to correlate timing of the initiation of a drug with onset of symptoms. The clinician should keep in mind that children with active enteric infections may also have secondary problems with malabsorption.

If the clinical history and physical examination are suspicious for malabsorption without enteric infection, the next step should include an evaluation of specific nutrient absorption. Carbohydrate malabsorption can be detected through lactose breath hydrogen testing, which measures hydrogen production as a response to an oral lactose load. A raised baseline breath hydrogen or early peak of hydrogen production suggests bacterial overgrowth, and appropriate treatment can be initiated. Lactose malabsorption results in a level of hydrogen production more than 10 to 15 parts per million over baseline, 60 minutes after ingestion. Dietary changes can then be made.

D-Xylose absorption testing also helps to determine the absorptive capacity of the gastrointestinal tract. D-Xylose is an absorbable sugar that does not require active transport for uptake by enterocytes. Thus, the D-xylose serum level, after administration of a test dose, reflects the absorptive ability of the gastrointestinal tract and the integrity of the mucosal surface. In younger children, the administered dose is 0.5 g per kg bodyweight, given orally after an overnight fast. In older children and adolescents, the maximum dose is 25 g. A serum level is obtained 1 hour after ingestion. Urine samples may be obtained for 5 hours after ingestion as well. Plasma citrulline levels correlate with enterocyte mass and function and may be used to indicate gastrointestinal function.[165]

Fat malabsorption is determined by a 72-hour fecal fat collection. A high-fat diet is administered several days before the collection is initiated and throughout the collection period. An alternative method is to keep a dietary fat intake record during the period of fecal fat collection. The stool is analyzed for total fat content, and the fecal fat is compared with the amount ingested; a coefficient of fat absorption is then calculated. Ten percent or more of ingested fat in the stool is considered abnormal. Alternatively, a Sudan stain may be performed on a random stool sample. This may be helpful as a quick test for fat malabsorption, although it is not so reliable. Quantification of fecal elastase may help to determine whether the fat malabsorption is pancreatic in origin. Lastly, raised fecal α_1-antitrypsin levels suggest protein loss from the gut.

If noninvasive studies, such as those described above, are not helpful in documenting and determining the etiology of the malabsorption, diarrhea, or vomiting, endoscopy (either upper or lower) with biopsy and appropriate culture of fluid may be useful. Miller et al.[41] confirmed histologic abnormalities in 72% of children undergoing upper endoscopy. In 70% of patients in this series, the clinical management of the child was changed because of the endoscopic evaluation. A high diagnostic yield has been supported by other investigators.[166] Specific gastrointestinal symptoms are not predictive of abnormal findings at endoscopy; advanced HIV-1 disease stage and an increased number of symptoms seem to be more predictive.[41] Histologic studies of the small bowel may aid in determining the degree of the villous blunting, and electron microscopy and special staining for opportunistic pathogens can be performed. Quantitative bacterial cultures and parasite evaluation of the duodenal fluid should be obtained when an endoscopy is performed. Characteristically, the detection of more than 10^5 organisms per milliliter of duodenal fluid confirms bacterial overgrowth. It is important to obtain both anaerobic and quantitative cultures. However, other studies have shown that endoscopy does not improve the diagnostic yield compared with stool examination in patients with intestinal infection. The only exception is the diagnosis of CMV.[167] An additional study found that flexible sigmoidoscopy was as useful as a full colonoscopy for diagnosing infection.[168] Special histologic stains for fungal, mycobacterial, or viral infections did not increase the diagnostic yield over routine hematoxylin and eosin staining.[169]

Treatment for intestinal infections has been outlined in Table 42-2 and previous sections. Therapy for gastrointestinal malabsorption should be directed toward the underlying diagnosis. If clinically symptomatic lactose malabsorption is found, a lactose-free diet should be initiated. Compliance may be difficult, because many foods contain lactose. Children can limit the effects of dietary lactose by taking exogenous lactase or using lactase-treated milk. There should be careful consideration of calcium and vitamin D intake, because children with HIV-1

infection are susceptible to low bone mineral density.[170-172] If there is malabsorption of protein and fat, a protein hydrolysate diet should be tried. Many of these supplements are poorly tolerated because they are unpalatable. In some circumstances, specialized supplements may need to be administered through a supplemental feeding tube.[173,174] Peptic and motility disorders can be treated as in other, non-HIV-1-infected children, paying careful attention to potential drug interactions with antiretroviral regimens.

OTHER SECONDARY IMMUNODEFICIENCIES

A variety of other disorders (Table 42-5) can cause secondary immunodeficiencies with effects on the gastrointestinal tract. Overall, these disorders are more prevalent than either primary or HIV-1-associated immunodeficiencies. Premature infants, children with cancer and associated exposure to immunosuppressant and cytotoxic medications (including children with graft-versus-host disease), and children with protein-losing enteropathy with associated loss of immunoglobulins from the gastrointestinal tract can all be immunodeficient because of the underlying disorder. In general, children with these immunodeficiencies are at risk for many of the same complications that are experienced by children with HIV-1 infection. Gastrointestinal tract infections are among the most common problems facing children with other secondary immunodeficiencies.

Malnutrition and Micronutrient Deficiencies

Malnutrition is the most common cause of immunodeficiency worldwide. Nutritional status and immunity have long been linked in many disease states. Before HIV-1 was described, *P. carinii* (now *jirovecii*) pneumonia and Kaposi's sarcoma,

TABLE 42-5. Causes of Secondary Immunodeficiencies

Prematurity
Metabolic disorders
  Down syndrome
  Malnutrition
  Micronutrient deficiency
  Uremia, nephrotic syndrome
  Sickle cell disease
  Diabetes mellitus
  Protein-losing enteropathy
Immunosuppression
  Drug
  Radiation
Infectious diseases
  HIV
  Congenital rubella
  Cytomegalovirus
  Epstein-Barr virus
  Acute bacterial disease
  Disseminated fungal disease
Hematologic or malignancy
  Leukemia, lymphoma, other malignancies
  Graft-versus-host disease
  Aplastic anemia, agranulocytosis
Surgery or trauma
  Splenectomy
  Burns
Inflammatory bowel disease
Systemic lupus erythematosus, other autoimmune diseases
Cirrhosis
Morbid obesity
Other chronic diseases of childhood

known opportunistic diseases, were first described in otherwise healthy, but malnourished, children and adults in developing nations.[175,176] This association led investigators to conclude that nutrition alone can affect the immunologic response of an individual. In malnourished children there is a profound involution of lymphoid tissues, including thymic atrophy and diminished paracortical regions of lymph nodes.[177] In young infants and children, protein-calorie malnutrition increases the risk of death by severalfold by increasing the susceptibility to infection.[178] In many countries, the mortality rate increases from 0.5% in children whose weight-for-height percentage of standard is greater than 80%, to 18% in children whose weight-for-height percentage of standard is less than 60%.[179] In other diseases such as cystic fibrosis and cancer, nutritional status has been linked closely to survival and morbidity. Malnourished children with leukemia and lymphoma have a higher risk of *P. jirovecii* pneumonia than children who have normal nutrition.[175]

Biochemically, protein-calorie malnutrition leads to changes in several aspects of the immune system. Cell-mediated immunity, microbial function of phagocytes, complement systems, secretory antibodies, and antibody affinity are consistently impaired in patients with significant malnutrition. Additionally, deficiencies of micronutrients, especially zinc and iron, as well as many others, may also have deleterious effects on the immune system. Other aspects of immunity that are altered by protein-calorie malnutrition include impaired chemotaxis of neutrophils, decreased lysozyme levels in serum and secretions, and interferon production in antibody response to T-cell-dependent antigens. A child with protein-calorie malnutrition may also have impaired mucosal immunity with lowered concentrations of secretory IgA in saliva, nasopharynx, tears, and the gastrointestinal tract compared with well-nourished control children.

Similar to children and adults with HIV-1 infection, patients with malnutrition have depressed T-cell function not only in the peripheral circulation but also in the intestinal tract. Subsequently, plasma cell function and macrophage activity may be impaired, leading to more frequent intestinal infections in children with severe protein-calorie malnutrition. Not only does nutrition improve the immunologic functioning of the intestinal tract, but nutrients themselves are trophic and essential for the maintenance of the absorptive capacity of the intestines. In some studies, weight loss greater than 30%, due to other disorders, is associated with a reduction in pancreatic enzyme secretion of over 80%, villous atrophy, and impaired carbohydrate and fat absorption.[180] These disorders are promptly reversed with appropriate nutritional rehabilitation. With villous blunting, antigen uptake can increase, leaving the child at higher risk of enteric infection. The pathogenesis of villous blunting is unclear but may be due to crypt hyperplasia as the primary event with premature sloughing at the villus tip[181] versus loss of enterocytes at the villus tip with resultant proliferation at the crypts.[182]

Malnutrition and its associated immunodeficiency are of global concern, and researchers have experimented with both dietary regimens and micronutrient supplementation to improve, and perhaps ultimately restore, adequate immunological function.[183,184] Because of the low cost of many micronutrients when compared to pharmacological agents, success in such experimentation could have profound implications for those suffering from malnutrition, as well as other immunocompromised patients.

Zinc is accepted as a promoter of immune function and consequently has been evaluated in HIV-1 immunocompromised patients. In a South African study that treated patients with 10 mg of zinc (elemental) daily for 6 months and compared them to a control group receiving a placebo, there was a significant difference in patient presentation of diarrhea favoring zinc supplementation.[185] Further demonstrating its potential alleviatory effects, Canani et al.[186] observed that the transactivating peptide's (Tat) secretory mechanism was inhibited by zinc and subsequently prevented diarrhea in pediatric HIV-1 patients. Both of these positive outcomes, although documented in HIV-1 patients, present zinc as an additional treatment option for symptoms of malnutrition-related immunodeficiency.

Some studies have administered multivitamins to HIV-1 patients including adults and children and evaluated effects of specific micronutrients. Adequate levels of vitamin A, when bolstered by supplementation in HIV-1 positive and HIV-1 negative children older than 6 months, correlated with reduced mortality and morbidity.[187] Although not yet well-documented in children, multivitamin intake of HIV-1 positive adults demonstrated retarded progression of the virus.[187] Improved hematologic status, mainly decreased rates of anemia, was observed in women and their children in Tanzania who were treated with iron supplements during and after pregnancy. This was marked by an average hemoglobin count that was 0.33 g/dL greater than that of the patient group who did not receive multivitamin treatment.[188] These findings underscore the need for additional randomized control trials in pediatric populations to further understand the role of micronutrient supplementation as a complimentary treatment component.

Immunosuppressive Therapy

Immunosuppressant medications are the mainstay of therapy for many diseases in children with autoimmune disorders, inflammatory bowel disease, chronic pulmonary disease, cancer, and organ transplantation. The best known immunosuppressants include corticosteroids, azathioprine, cyclosporin, tacrolimus, and anti-thymocyte globulin. Unfortunately, the effects of these medications are not targeted toward specific organs, but rather indiscriminately suppress immune function throughout the child. Thus, several immunologic functions including a decrease in monocyte adherence, neutrophil chemotaxis, and overall suppression of the inflammatory response are present. Children are at risk of enteric infections, similar to those described in children with HIV-1 infection. Pediatric patients undergoing transplant procedures, specifically solid organ transplant, are at increased risk of acquiring gastrointestinal infections when compared to their healthy counterparts. Acutely, these complications present with vomiting, diarrhea, and cramping. The most frequently diagnosed posttransplant infection is CMV,[189-191] but its onset has been reduced significantly with the administration of prophylactic drugs such as ganciclovir.[189-192]

LIVER COMPLICATIONS IN SECONDARY IMMUNODEFICIENCY

Another aspect of the gastrointestinal tract that renders importance in secondary immunodeficiency is the liver. Although data regarding liver complications in pediatric HIV-1 patients are lacking, there are considerable reports on HIV-1 infected adults. Hepatitis coinfection, biliary tract disease, and drug-derived illness are some of the major complications we discuss in this section. Liver complications in secondary immunodeficiency, in their own right, deserve extensive coverage beyond the scope of this chapter, and so this section offers only a snapshot of this complex topic.

Hepatitis A, B, C Coinfection

Both hepatitis and HIV infections share similar transmission pathways, and for this reason, it is not surprising that rates of viral coinfections are considerable. Hepatitis A is often thought of as the less serious of the hepatitis viruses when treated promptly, and coinfection with HIV does not seem to predispose an individual to adverse outcomes. In 2006, coinfection rates of hepatitis B were reported to be between 5 and 10% in the global HIV population. Prolonged hepatitis B infection is one of the greatest concerns of for coinfected patients.[193] Hepatitis B virus e antigen (HBeAg) is the protein associated with active hepatitis B in patients and is used by clinicians to determine efficacy of medications. For monoinfected hepatitis B patients, proper treatment can result in significant reduction of HBeAg in 90 to 95% of patients; however, this success is not mirrored in HIV-coinfected populations.[194] There is also evidence for greater reactivation and replication in hepatitis B-HIV coinfected patients.[193,195-197] Explanation for this focuses on HIV patients' increased proinflammatory cytokine production and their inability to eliminate hepatocytes infected with hepatitis B.[196,198] Balancing dual treatment for both hepatitis B and HIV viruses presents a unique challenge for clinicians. Acquired mutations of hepatitis B render additional treatment considerations, deepening the challenge. Resistant hepatitis B strains have been identified, many of them falling under the tyrosine-methionine-aspartate-aspartate category, YMDD. Iacomi et al.[199] determined that 28 of 29 hepatitis B–HIV coinfected patients exhibited this specified resistance. Lamivudine, once commonly prescribed, has become less effective because of developed resistance. Of the various treatment options, only tenofovir is used in HIV treatment and is effective in both the wild-type hepatitis B virus and the resistant YMDD strain, and it is often concomitantly administered with emtricitabine.[200,201]

Mothers coinfected with hepatitis C and HIV are more likely to transmit HIV to their children, indicating greater risk of perinatal transmission in coinfected patients.[202,203] Liver disease in coinfected patients may be accelerated when compared to their monoinfected counterparts. Pathways that have been proposed to accelerate fibrosis in coinfected patients include direct viral effects, dysregulation of the immune system toward a profibrotic state, and other metabolic pathways that lead to liver toxicity and processes such as steatosis and insulin resistance.[204] Giovaninni et al.[203] studied 49 HIV-infected children, 11 of whom were coinfected with hepatitis C. Six of the coinfected patients had abnormal alanine aminotransferase (ALT) levels. Three of the six children had AIDS, and three had AIDS-related complex. Five children with normal aminotransferase had no detectable viral progression. Following acute hepatitis C infection, hepatitis C–HIV coinfected patients are over 20% more likely than monoinfected patients to develop chronic hepatitis C infection.[205-207] Interferon with ribavirin therapy is widespread in chronic hepatitis-C monoinfected patients, and its efficacy in hepatitis C–HIV coinfected patients is yet to be fully realized.[208,209] When compared to conventional interferon therapy

(IFNα-2a), 180 μg/week pegylated interferon (pegIFNα-2a) plus 800 mg/day ribavirin demonstrated enhanced histological effects that were also associated with improved virological response in hepatitis C–HIV coinfected patients.[210] End-stage liver failure, cirrhosis, and hepatocellular carcinoma have been observed with greater frequency in hepatitis C–HIV coinfected patients.[205] These findings reflect adult populations and may or may not be indicative of outcomes in pediatric patients.

Biliary Tract Complications

Children with acute biliary tract disease may present with right-sided abdominal pain, vomiting, and jaundice. Also, elevated serum bile levels may induce pruritus. Despite a disproportionate increase in alkaline phosphatase levels, ALT levels may or may not be elevated. An ultrasound of the biliary system may be needed when serum sampling is equivocal. Biliary tract disease is often obstructive; thus, use of endoscopic retrograde cholangiopancreatography (ERCP) will help to identify the obstruction, perhaps provide bile sampling, and even mitigate the obstruction via sphincterotomy. Bile sampling may indicate the presence of CMV, *Cryptosporidium*, *Mycobacterium*, or microsporidia, which were all discussed in previous sections. In one study employing sonography, 26 of 41 HIV-infected children displayed hepatobiliary abnormalities, yet there was no evidence of infection.[211] AIDS cholangiopathy is defined by intra- and extrahepatic sclerosing cholangitis and is commonly linked to CMV and *Cryptosporidium* infections. Incidence in pediatric HIV populations remains to be thoroughly evaluated.

Treatment-Derived Complications

The advent of HAART, as discussed previously, has had profound effects on reducing many infections within the gastrointestinal tract. In the liver, however, there has been a negative association between receipt of antiretroviral therapy and development of liver complications, defined as *immune restoration hepatitis*.[193] Serum ALT elevation is associated with liver tissue damage and therefore is used to detect liver disease. Hepatitis-HIV patients on HAART present with elevated ALT levels in the blood principally derived from HAART-induced hepatotoxicity, resistance to antiretrovirals, and HAART noncompliancy.[212] Specifically, mitochondrial damage has been implicated as a contributor to liver death, which stems from coinfection and drug treatments.[213,214] Current research aims to determine effective methodology for detecting hepatic mitochondrial toxicity as a means to identify patients at risk of developing liver complications due to treatment.[213]

SUMMARY

Gastrointestinal disorders in children with secondary immunodeficiencies cause considerable comorbidity. Infection of the gastrointestinal tract is one the most common complications associated with secondary immunodeficiencies. However, malabsorption, peptic disease, and liver and biliary tract disease are also prevalent. These gastrointestinal complications contribute negatively to the overall clinical outcomes of children who have other chronic medical conditions, and they can often become life-threatening. Thus, clinicians should be vigilant and aggressive in the evaluation and treatment of gastrointestinal tract dysfunction in children with secondary immunodeficiencies.

REFERENCES

8. Gona P, Van Dyke RB, Williams PL, et al. Incidence of opportunistic and other infections in HIV-infected children in the HAART era. JAMA 2006;296:292–300.

35. Brenchley JM, Price DA, Schacker TW, et al. Microbial translocation is a cause of systemic immune activation in chronic HIV infection. Nat Med 2006;12:1365–1371.

62. Canani RB, Spagnuolo MI, Cirillo P, Guarino A. Ritonavir combination therapy restores intestinal function in children with advanced HIV disease. J Acquir Immune Defic Syndr 1999;21:307–312.

165. Crenn P, De Truchis P, Neveux N, et al. Plasma citrulline is a biomarker of enterocyte mass and an indicator of parenteral nutrition in HIV-infected patients. Am J Clin Nutr 2009;90:587–594.

178. Scrimshaw NS, Taylor CE, Gordon JE. Interactions of nutrition and infection. WHO Monograph Series World Health Organ 1968:57.

204. Kim AY, Chung RT. Coinfection with HIV-1 and HCV – a one-two punch. Gastroenterology 2009;137:795–814.

See expertconsult.com for a complete list of references and the review questions for this chapter.

PEDIATRIC POLYPOSIS SYNDROMES

Warren Hyer

Gastrointestinal polyps in children commonly present with rectal bleeding, abdominal pain, or intussusception. Other children are asymptomatic, and their polyps may be detected only as part of a screening program for an inheritable polyposis syndrome. In the case of the latter, or if the patient presents with multiple polyps, there is a risk of malignant change.

HISTOPATHOLOGIC CLASSIFICATION

Gastrointestinal polyps in children fall into two major categories: hamartomas and adenomas (Table 43-1). Solitary polyps in children are most commonly hamartomas, predominantly of the juvenile type, and such polyps are benign. Of the familial syndromes, familial adenomatous polyposis is more common than juvenile polyposis or Peutz-Jeghers polyposis. Table 43-2 outlines the different histologic features.

CLINICAL MANAGEMENT

The most common manifestation of a large bowel polyp is painless rectal bleeding. Other symptoms attributed to polyps include abdominal pain, altered bowel habit, or prolapse of polyp or rectum. Diagnosis will be made at full colonoscopy and polypectomy, which serves to remove the symptomatic polyp, that is, the source of bleeding or intussusception (Table 43-3). The clinical presentation, pathologic findings, and the histologic description of the polyp are all necessary to establish the correct diagnosis. Once a polyp has been identified at endoscopy, a carefully targeted family history must be taken asking about family members with cancer, the site of the cancers, age of onset (particularly asking whether cancer or polyps have occurred in first or second degree relatives before the age of 50 years) (Table 43-4). Such a history may require the expertise of a multidisciplinary familial cancer clinic or polyposis registry to develop a detailed family cancer pedigree.[1] Genetic studies can further assist determining the type and prognosis of the polyposis syndrome.

FAMILIAL ADENOMATOUS POLYPOSIS

In children, gastrointestinal (GI) adenomas are almost always associated with hereditary adenomatous polyposis syndromes. Familial adenomatous polyposis (FAP) is characterized by the development of hundreds and thousands of adenomas in the colon and rectum as well as several extracolonic manifestations. Almost all affected patients will develop a colorectal cancer if FAP is not detected and treated at an early stage.

Clinical Features

Patients with FAP typically develop multiple adenomas throughout the large bowel: usually more than 100 and sometimes more than 1000 polyps (Figure 43-1) begin to appear in childhood or adolescence and increase in number with age. The standard clinical diagnosis of typical or classical FAP is based on the identification of more than 100 colorectal adenomatous polyps. By the fifth decade, colorectal cancer (CRC) is almost inevitable if colectomy is not performed. A milder form of disease is observed in 8% of cases: attenuated FAP (AFAP), characterized by fewer adenomas and later presentation. These cases are less likely to present in childhood.[2]

Gastric fundic gland polyps in the antrum and small-bowel adenomas occur, yet neither require intervention in the pediatric age group. Dysplastic changes can occur but very rarely lead to cancers. Gastric cancers are reported in the Asian population. Children under 5 years of age may develop hepatoblastoma, with an increased risk in boys.[3] Adult patients with FAP are also at increased risk of malignancies of the duodenum and ampulla of Vater. Duodenal adenomas will progress to malignancy if untreated in 5% of adults. In addition, FAP is associated with an increased risk of cancers of the thyroid, brain, and pancreas, whereas papillary carcinoma of the thyroid has been reported in adolescence.

Extraintestinal manifestations are common (Table 43-5). The presence of these manifestations was previously described as "Gardner's syndrome"; however, because these lesions are commonly found in many patients affected by FAP, this term is no longer used. Pigmented ocular lesions (previously termed congenital hypertrophy of the retinal epithelium, or CHRPE) are found in some but not all cases. The presence on indirect ophthalmoscopy of more than four pigmented ocular fundus lesions carries a 100% positive predictive value for FAP in at-risk families, particularly if the lesions are large. The absence of pigmentation, however, is of no predictive value.

Genetics of FAP

FAP is an autosomal dominant inherited condition caused by a mutation in the APC gene occurring in 1:10,000 births. In 20 to 30% of cases, the condition is caused by a spontaneous mutation with no clinical or genetic evidence of FAP in the parents or family.[4]

The gene responsible for FAP, APC (adenomatous polyposis coli), is located on chromosome 5q21 and appears to be a tumor suppressor gene.[5] Most mutations are small deletions or insertions that result in the production of a truncated APC protein. In FAP, a germline mutation inactivates one of the two APC

TABLE 43-1. Polyps and Polyposis Syndromes Seen in Childhood

Adenomatous Polyposis Syndromes
Familial adenomatous polyposis
Turcot's syndrome

Hamartomatous Polyps
Solitary juvenile polyp
Juvenile polyposis syndrome
PTEN – hamartoma tumor syndrome, such as:
  Bannayan-Riley-Ruvalcaba syndrome
  Gorlin's syndrome
  Cowden's syndrome
Peutz-Jeghers syndrome

Inflammatory Polyps

Mixed polyposis Syndrome

TABLE 43-2. Pathologic Features of Polyps Seen in Children

Polyp Type	Macroscopic Appearance
Juvenile polyp	Pedunculated 1-3 cm in size, rarely larger, with smooth red surface. At microscopy, dilated cysts filed with mucin, abundant lamina propria with prominent inflammatory infiltrate, haphazardly arranged
Peutz-Jeghers	Sessile or pedunculated with lobulated surface 0.5-5 cm in size. At microscopy, frondlike structure, elongated branching arborizing strands of smooth muscle
Tubular and villous adenoma	Pedunculated smooth, red lobulated surface, 0.5-5 cm in size. At microscopy, glands and tubules with or without inflammatory infiltrate. Villous adenomas are sessile and broad based. Dysplasia is always present

TABLE 43-3. Endoscopic Polypectomy in Children

1. Only skilled endoscopists should be performing colonoscopic polypectomy in children – if experienced, the risk of perforation and significant bleeding should be <1%.
2. Tiny adenomas, <1 mm in size, confirm the diagnosis of familial adenomatous polyposis (FAP) and can be seen more easily by spraying 0.2% indigo carmine dye onto the colonic surface either via specially designed spray catheters or directly down the biopsy channel.
3. Position change and endoscopic rotation are also important to place the polyp in the convenient 5 o'clock position before attempting polypectomy.
4. Polyps > 5 mm should be removed by snare polypectomy.
5. Pedunculated polyps, in which larger vessels may be present within the stalk, are best removed using coagulating diathermy. Newer noncontact techniques such as argon plasma coagulation offer safe and rapid destruction of multiple polyps but do not provide histology.
6. The risk of removing larger (>1 cm) sessile polyps is considerable, particularly in the right colon, and requires more advanced polypectomy techniques such as submucosal injection of 1:10,000 adrenaline or hypertonic saline to lift the mucosa away from the underlying muscle layer.

TABLE 43-4. History and Examination in a Child With Possible Gastrointestinal Polyps

History
Nature of bleeding and frequency
Painful or painless rectal bleeding
History of GI obstructive symptoms
Detailed family history exploring early deaths or diagnosis of GI cancer
Weight loss, anorexia (tumor)
Learning difficulties (JPS or PTEN hamartoma)

Examination
Mucosal pigmentation (PJS)
Dysmorphic features (JPS)
Edema (hypoalbuminemia in infantile JPS)
Extraintestinal manifestations of FAP – see Table 43-5, e.g., subcutaneous cysts, exostosis, congenital hypertrophy of the retinal pigment epithelium
Hepatic mass (FAP)
Thyroid mass (FAP or Cowden's)

GI, gastrointestinal; JPS, juvenile polyposis syndrome; PJS, Peutz-Jeghers syndrome.

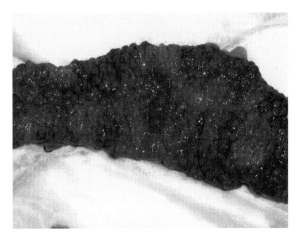

Figure 43-1. Colectomy specimen from a child with dense adenomatous polyposis.

codon 1309, are associated with a severe form of FAP, whereas mutations localized at the extreme ends of the gene and in the alternatively spliced part of exon 9 are associated with a mild form of FAP, and an intermediate expression of disease is found in patients with mutations in the remaining parts of the gene. Other phenotype-genotype correlations have been observed.[6] These correlations are not absolute, and there may be considerable intrafamilial variation, suggesting that there are other factors involved in the pathogenesis of the disease. Some of the phenotypic variability seen in patients cannot be explained by the location of their *APC* mutation. Environmental factors and other genes – often termed *modifier genes* – may have critical effects on *APC* function and disease expression.[7] More than 300 different germline mutations have been described, and finding the mutation may be a formidable task. Families need to be aware that the mutation may only be detected in 70 to 90% of cases.

In addition, another polyposis gene has been identified – the MUTYH gene (mutY human homologue). Mutations in this gene cause an autosomal recessive form of adenomatous polyposis (also called MYH-associated polyposis), but this does not present in childhood.

alleles, which underlies the predisposition to adenoma formation. Many mutations have been identified on this large gene, and there is a correlation between the genetic site and severity of clinical manifestation. Mutations between codons 1250 and 1464 (Figure 43-2), especially those with a mutation at

Diagnosis: Interpretation of the Genetic Test and Clinical Screening in FAP

In order to determine the appropriate screening protocol for a given family, the first step would be to seek which mutation is present in the FAP affected index case. The mutation will only be found in 70 to 90% of the patients who are affected. If a mutation cannot be found, the genetic testing is noninformative, and it will not be possible to offer predictive testing to asymptomatic at-risk relatives (Figure 43-3).

TABLE 43-5. **Extracolonic Manifestations of FAP in Children and Young Adults**

Site	Examples
Bone	Osteomas, mandibular and maxillary Exostosis Sclerosis
Dental abnormalities	Impacted or supernumerary teeth Unerupted teeth
Connective tissue	Desmoid tumors Excessive intra-abdominal adhesions Fibroma Subcutaneous cysts
Eyes	Congenital hypertrophy of the retinal pigment epithelium
CNS	Glioblastomas, e.g., Turcot's syndrome
Adenomas	Stomach Duodenum Small intestine Adrenal cortex Thyroid gland
Carcinomas	Thyroid gland Adrenal gland
Liver	Hepatoblastoma

CNS, central nervous system.

Once the family-specific mutation has been identified, directed DNA diagnostic techniques can be readily used to predict FAP in other family members. The absence of the gene mutation in other family members is considered accurate in excluding FAP, and the subject should be considered to hold an average population risk for the subsequent development of adenomas and cancer. Such genotype-negative individuals can be discharged from follow-up.

The presence of the family-specific gene mutation confirms the diagnosis of FAP, and such patients should undergo endoscopic assessment. The diagnosis is confirmed by finding polyps at flexible sigmoidoscopy or colonoscopy, histologically confirmed as adenomas (Figure 43-4). Affected individuals should undergo annual flexible sigmoidoscopy beginning at the age of 10 to 14 years and continuing until adenomas are found.[8] Gene positive children will require a full colonoscopy by the age of 14 to 16 years to determine polyp density and location and degree of dysplasia. Dye spraying the rectal mucosa with indigo carmine or methylene blue increases the sensitivity of the examination. Endoscopy in asymptomatic adolescents must be performed in a sensitive and nontraumatic fashion to ensure compliance and cooperation for future examinations.

For families in which the genotype is not known, protocols vary. It is necessary to perform annual sigmoidoscopy on all first-degree relatives until adenomas are found. In addition, from the age of 20 years, colonoscopy with dye spray is performed at 5-year intervals.

No patient should undergo screening for FAP without detailed counseling. The individual being screened must understand the nature of the test and its possible outcomes. Many authorities feel that the child should be involved in the decision-making process, and the diagnosis should be delayed until the child is old enough to contribute to the screening program, for example, from the age of 11 years onward.[9,10] Some children understand the genetic screening and its consequences at a younger age, such as 8 years. Each family situation should

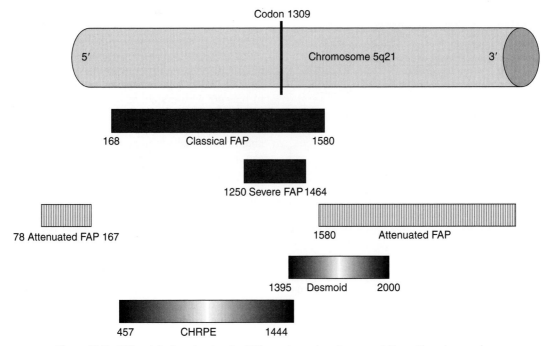

Figure 43-2. APC protein domains showing FAP genotype-phenotype correlation with codon number.

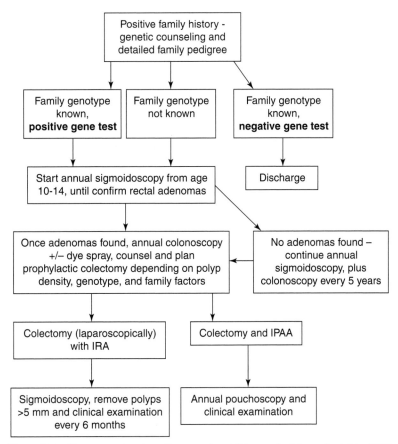

Figure 43-3. Management protocol for screening children and adolescents at risk of FAP.

be considered individually. Well-informed consent, as a mature minor, before predictive testing is the most desirable outcome. There are psychologic issues as well as family, insurance, and employment implications that may arise in the case of a positive result. These should be discussed before testing, and there should be a clear protocol for posttest management.[11]

The current advice is to commence endoscopic surveillance from the early teens. Because some patients, especially those with a mutation located at codon 1309 in the APC gene, may develop severe polyposis of the colorectum before the age of 10, attention must be paid to FAP-related symptoms. These symptoms may include increasing bowel movements, looser stools, mucous discharge, rectal bleeding, and abdominal or back pain. In symptomatic patients, endoscopic investigation may be indicated at any age. Severe dysplasia and even malignancy have been documented in children with FAP under the age of 12 years. Consequently, those children from families in which severe dysplasia or carcinomas have been found at a young age should undergo screening at an earlier age.[12]

Management of FAP

If adenomas are detected, colonoscopic investigations should be performed annually until colectomy is planned.[13] Colectomy is the only effective therapy that eliminates the inevitable risk of colorectal cancer. In the absence of severe dysplasia, colectomy is usually performed in the mid to late teens or early 20s to accommodate work and school schedules. Almost all screen-detected adolescents are asymptomatic and may not contemplate interruptions in their schooling or effects on

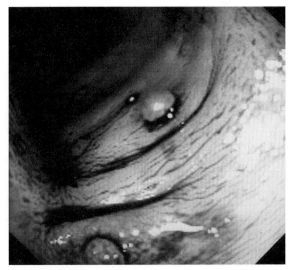

Figure 43-4. Adenomas found at colonoscopy with dye spray. (*See plate section for color.*)

relationships. The surgical option, therefore, must not only be carefully timed but also have low morbidity and excellent functional result.

Colectomy is indicated as soon as there are large numbers of adenomas (measuring up to 5 mm), or adenomas showing a high degree of dysplasia. The timing of primary preventative surgery may be influenced by knowledge of the mutation site and the likely severity of the polyposis. For example, patients with a deletion at codon 1309 should be offered earlier surgery, because this phenotype is characterized by a large numbers of polyps and a higher risk of cancer.[14] Even though a low polyp density suggests a lower risk of developing malignancy,[15] it is unsafe to delay surgery on the grounds of polyp density alone.[16]

Surgical options include subtotal colectomy with ileorectal anastomosis (IRA), or restorative proctocolectomy with ileo pouch anal anastomosis (IPAA or pouch procedure).

The IRA is a low-risk operation with good functional results and can be performed laparoscopically. There is no pelvic dissection with its attendant risks of hemorrhage, loss of fertility in women, or damage to adjacent organs such as ureters. Complication rates after IRA are low, and postoperative bowel function is almost always good, averaging four semiformed stools daily. After the IRA, the rectum remains at risk of cancer. Although initially there may be regression of rectal polyposis, the adenomas may recur and progress leading to cancer; hence 6-monthly surveillance of the rectum is needed postoperatively, and despite this, inexperience can result in early cancers being missed.

An IPAA procedure removes the colorectal cancer risk almost completely, but is more complicated than an IRA, carrying a higher morbidity, and often requires a temporary ileostomy. The pouch procedure may carry a higher risk of complications, need for a loop ileostomy, reoperations, longer hospital stays, night evacuation, and decreased fertility in women.[17] Bowel frequency is generally higher than that for an IRA. The risk of cancer still exists after IPAA, because tumors may develop at the anastomosis or below. Adenomas can develop in the ileal pouch. Pouch creation is associated with an as yet unknown risk of pouch neoplasia, and the pouch should be examined regularly.[18]

The advantages of an IPAA with a lower risk of cancer must be compared against the higher operative morbidity – the patients and parents must be carefully counseled. Conversion to an ileo-anal pouch can be carried out when the patient is much older.[19] An IPAA is the treatment of choice if the patient has a large number of rectal adenomas (for example, more than 15 to 20 adenomas); in the presence of adenoma with severe dysplasia; if the colon has more than 1000 adenomas; or in those with high-risk genotypes (e.g., codon 1309).[20,21] In patients with only a few rectal adenomas or with a polyp-free rectum, both options are possible. An IRA may be preferable, and the decision can be made on an individual basis, considering preoperative sphincter function, patient compliance, and risk of desmoid. In patients with desmoids, it has been reported that conversion of IRA to IPAA might be difficult because of (asymptomatic) mesenteric desmoid tumors and shortening of the mesentery. For this reason, a primary IPAA might be the best option in patients with an increased risk of desmoid development.[7]

Prognosis

Genetic investigations, colonic surveillance, and prophylactic colectomy have had a favorable impact on mortality in affected patients. Studies that evaluated the mortality of patients with FAP reported that surveillance policies and prophylactic colectomy have resulted in a reduction in the number of FAP patients who died from CRC. Currently, a greater proportion of deaths are attributable to extracolonic manifestations of the disease (desmoid tumors, duodenal cancer). Upper endoscopic surveillance of the stomach, duodenum, and periampullary region with a side-viewing endoscope is recommended after the age 20 years, unless the patient has symptoms such as upper abdominal pain that warrant earlier investigation. Central registration in a family cancer registry and prophylactic examination lead to a reduction of CRC-associated mortality and ensure appropriate follow-up and patient support.

Desmoid Disease

Desmoids are locally aggressive but nonmetastasizing myofibroblastic lesions that occur with disproportionate high frequency in patients with FAP. Possible risk factors include abdominal surgery, positive family history for desmoids, and site of the mutation (mutations beyond codon 1444). In contrast to sporadic desmoid tumors, the majority of the tumors associated with FAP are located in the abdominal wall or intra-abdominally. The tumors can be diagnosed by computed tomographic (CT) scanning or magnetic resonance imaging (MRI). The latter procedure may also provide information on the activity of the tumor. Associated etiologic factors include the germline mutation, estrogens, and surgical trauma.[22] Desmoids occur most commonly in the peritoneal cavity (Figure 43-5) and may infiltrate locally, leading to small bowel, ureteric, or vascular obstruction. Desmoid tumors are frequently encountered incidentally in patients requiring further surgery. These lesions may progress rapidly or may resolve spontaneously, their unpredictable nature making them difficult to treat.[23] Attempted surgical resection carries a high morbidity and mortality (10 to 60%) and usually stimulates further growth. The options for treatment are pharmacologic treatment (nonsteroidal anti-inflammatory drugs and/or anti-estrogens), chemotherapy, surgical excision, or radiotherapy. Evidence for the efficacy of these treatments is poor and is based on small, noncontrolled studies. Evaluating efficacy of different treatments is complicated by a variable natural history in desmoid disease, with some tumors showing spontaneous regression in the absence of treatment. Pediatricians treating children with extraintestinal desmoid tumors should consider the possibility of FAP in the family.

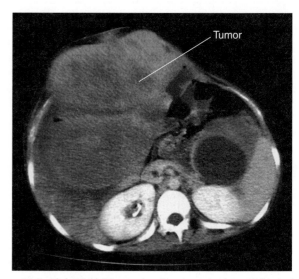

Figure 43-5. Abdominal CT scan showing a massive intra-abdominal desmoid tumor in a 14-year-old with FAP.

Future Chemoprevention

Nonsteroidal anti-inflammatory drugs (NSAIDs) may be protective against colon cancer by inhibiting prostaglandin synthesis via their effects on cyclooxygenase (COX). Since the initial studies in 1983 using the NSAID sulindac,[24] subsequent publications have shown a significant reduction in the number of rectal polyps in patients taking sulindac after colectomy; however, not all polyps regressed. Despite protracted drug use, the adenomas still progressed with case reports of rectal cancer.[25] Sulindac administered before the development of polyps in genotype-positive adolescents did not prevent the development of adenomas.[26]

COX-2 (cyclooxygenase-2) enzyme is induced in inflammatory and neoplastic tissue. NSAIDs inhibit COX enzyme, which is integral in the production of prostaglandin. Selective COX-2 inhibitors generate fewer GI-related side effects compared to the classical nonselective NSAIDs. One of these drugs (celecoxib) was found to reduce the number of colorectal adenomas by 28%.[27] Unlike sulindac, this drug also reduced the number of duodenal adenomas.[28] Celecoxib was well tolerated with fewer side effects than sulindac caused. Unfortunately, cardiovascular side effects have recently been reported in patients using another selective COX-2 inhibitor, rofecoxib. In a trial involving 2600 patients with colon polyps, 3.5% of the patients assigned to rofecoxib had a myocardial infarction or stroke, as compared with 1.9% of the patients assigned to placebo: this necessitated premature cessation of the trial.[29] Meta-analysis of different NSAIDs confirmed the increased risk of cardiovascular diseases with rofecoxib[30]: however, a dose of around 200 mg per day of celecoxib did not lead to this increased risk. These data did not exclude a potential increased risk when used at the typical higher doses administered to patients with FAP. As a result, some specialists dealing with FAP patients are reluctant to prescribe these drugs, especially because most patients have to use the drug in high doses on a long-term basis.

Although NSAIDs do not replace surgical treatment for colonic FAP, they may yet play a role in postponing surgery in patients with mild colonic polyposis, or patients with rectal polyposis after prior colectomy. They may also be used in patients who refuse surgical treatment, or in patients for whom operation is not an option due to extensive desmoid disease.

Although NSAIDs have been shown to reduce the number of adenomas, it has not been proven that these drugs prevent the development of CRC. Patients treated with NSAIDs, despite manifesting a reduction of the size and number of rectal adenomas, have still developed cancer.

Diet plays an important role in protecting against the development of sporadic cancer, and studies exploring whether dietary manipulation can modify disease are in progress. Other agents investigated but so far with inconclusive effect on polyp burden include vitamin C, oral calcium, and the ornithine decarboxylase inhibitor difluoromethylornithine (DFMO).[31]

JUVENILE POLYP (SOLITARY AT DIAGNOSIS)

Children with a solitary juvenile polyp present at a mean age of 4 years with painless rectal bleeding or perianal polyp protrusion. Up to 40% of children with a juvenile polyp have multiple polyps – and 60% are proximal to the rectosigmoid, confirming the need for full colonoscopy even if a polyp is found in the rectum. Polyps should be removed even when discovered incidentally. If a polyp is found to be solitary after full colonoscopy,

and there is no relevant family history, endoscopic polypectomy is sufficient treatment. There appears to be no increased risk of colorectal cancer as a result of the polyp in patients with a solitary juvenile polyp. After polypectomy, parents must be aware that juvenile polyps may be the first feature of a hamartomatous polyposis syndrome; if fresh symptoms arise, the child should be reinvestigated. If multiple juvenile polyps are found or there is a positive family history (e.g., colonic polyps or early-onset CRC), juvenile polyposis syndrome (JPS) should be considered and an alternative approach taken.

JUVENILE POLYPOSIS SYNDROME

JPS is a rare polyposis syndrome with an estimated prevalence of 1 in 100,000 individuals presenting with multiple hamartomatous polyps and an increased risk of gastrointestinal malignancies. The condition should be considered in patients with more than five juvenile polyps in the colon, or juvenile polyps found in other parts of the gastrointestinal tract, or any juvenile polyps in a child with a positive family history.

There are three forms:
1. Juvenile polyposis of infancy
2. Juvenile polyposis coli (colonic involvement only)
3. Generalized juvenile polyposis

Juvenile polyposis of infancy has an onset in infancy presenting with anemia and hemorrhage, diarrhea, protein-losing enteropathy, intussusception, and rectal bleeding. The course in such infants is fulminant, and death frequently occurs before the age of 2 years in severe cases despite colectomy.

Patients with juvenile polyposis coli and generalized juvenile polyposis develop 50 to 200 polyps in their lifetime. The total number of polyps needed to make the diagnosis remains controversial (between three and five).[32] Patients present with chronic and acute gastrointestinal bleeding, anemia, prolapsed rectal polyps, abdominal pain, and diarrhea. These hamartomatous polyps occur throughout the gastrointestinal tract including the colon, rectum, stomach, and small bowel. A significant proportion of patients with juvenile polyposis have been reported to have other morphologic abnormalities including digital clubbing, macrocephaly, alopecia, cleft lip or palate, congenital heart disease, genitourinary abnormalities, and mental retardation.

Complications

There is little doubt that juvenile polyposis is a premalignant condition. There is a 15% incidence of colorectal carcinoma occurring in patients under the age of 35 years, leading to a cumulative risk of colorectal cancer of 68% by age 60 years with a mean age of onset of colonic neoplasia of 38 years (range of 6 to 58 years). Neoplastic changes have been documented both in the polyps and in flat, apparently normal colonic mucosa.

The risk of neoplastic change is more likely to occur in patients with the generalized form of polyposis compared with those with colorectal polyposis alone. The youngest patient reported with a cancer to date is a 15-year-old.

Genetics of Juvenile Polyposis

JPS is a fully penetrant condition with variable expression – 60% of cases are familial, and the others occur sporadically. Germline mutations in *SMAD4, BMPR1A,* and *ENG1* cause JPS.

Approximately 54% of cases will have a detectable mutation. *SMAD4* on chromosome 18q21.2 is a tumor suppressor gene in the transforming growth factor β (TGF-β) signal transduction pathway and will be found in about 20% of JPS patients.[33] *SMAD4* mutations predispose to hamartomas and cancer through disruption of the TGF-β signaling pathway. Patients with the *SMAD4* mutation appear to have a higher risk of gastric polyps and hereditary hemorrhagic telangiectasia (HHT) – the latter condition is characterized by cutaneous telangiectasia and risk of arteriovenous malformations.

BMPR1A is located on chromosome 10q22.3 and accounts for another 20% of JPS patients. *ENG1* mutation on gene 9q has recently been described in two patients without HHT.

Treatment and Follow-Up

Once the gene mutation has been identified in the index patient, other at-risk family members should be tested – approximately 75% of patients will have an affected parent. All children in that proband will have a 50% chance of inheriting the mutation if a parent is found to carry the mutation and, after counseling in the teenage years, should undergo testing.

Affected children should undergo colonoscopic surveillance every 2 years, or earlier if symptoms arise. In those families where the gene mutation is not known, first-degree relatives of patients with JPS should be screened by colonoscopy starting at age 12 years, even when the subject is asymptomatic (Figure 43-6).

Full colonoscopy is necessary as right-sided polyps are common in this condition as compared with their frequency in FAP or solitary juvenile polyps, and all polyps should be resected. Annual colonoscopy is performed until all polyps have been resected and then the screening interval is stretched to every 2 to 3 years. Gastroscopy is commenced from the mid teens. Colectomy is warranted for patients with cancer, dysplasia, or high polyp burden with symptoms who cannot be controlled endoscopically, or those patients who may fail to turn up for screening. Colectomy with IRA would be unusual in the pediatric or adolescent group.

PTEN – HAMARTOMA TUMOR SYNDROME

This group comprises of rare genetic syndromes of Bannayan-Riley-Ruvalcaba syndrome (BRRS), Cowden's syndrome, and Proteus syndrome – all three affiliated with a mutation in the tumor suppressor gene PTEN located at 10q23.3.[34] Cowden's syndrome rarely presents in childhood and manifests with macrocephaly, papillomatous papules, and acral keratosis. It carries a 50% risk of breast cancer in adult women and a 10% lifetime risk of epithelial thyroid cancer. Up to 90% of patients have small hamartomatous colonic polyps distal to the hepatic flexure.

BRRS presents in childhood with gastrointestinal hamartomas, particularly in the ileum and colon, causing intussusception, rectal bleeding, and hypoalbuminemia. There are additional characteristics including macrocephaly, developmental delay, lipomatosis, and hemangiomatosis.

Proteus syndrome is characterized by hemihypertrophy and congenital malformations but has few gastrointestinal implications – it is included in the PTEN group because it shares the PTEN gene mutation.

The PTEN mutation can be detected in 80% of patients with Cowden's, 60% with BRRS, and 50% with Proteus syndrome. All offspring of an affected individual have a 50% chance of inheriting the mutation. BRRS presents before adolescence, and there is value in genetic testing in early childhood in a family where the mutation has been identified.

Patients with BRRS need regular colonoscopy and small bowel surveillance and are at risk of anemia, intussusception, and hypoalbuminemia from the polyps. They carry a lifetime increased risk of cancer, and surveillance is recommended from age 18 years focusing on renal, thyroid, and breast cancer.

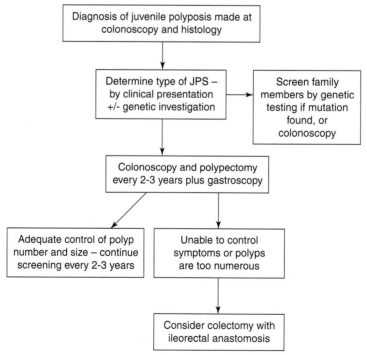

Figure 43-6. Management of juvenile polyposis in childhood.

PEUTZ-JEGHERS SYNDROME (PJS)
Clinical Features and Diagnosis

PJS is a rare (prevalence 1 in 50,000 to 1 in 200,000 live births) autosomal dominant condition characterized by mucocutaneous pigmentation and the presence of hamartomatous polyps throughout the gastrointestinal tract. Polyps arise primarily in the small bowel, and to a lesser extent in the stomach and colon. Polyps are most commonly found in the jejunum and cause bleeding and anemia or intussusception and obstruction from an early age. Presumptive diagnosis can be made in those with a positive family history and typical PJS freckling.[35] Rarely, polyps have been described in the renal pelvis and bladder, lungs, or nares.

Pigmentation tend to arise in infancy, occurring around the mouth, nostrils, perianal area, fingers and toes, and the dorsal and volar aspects of hands and feet (Figure 43-7). They may fade after puberty but tend to persist in the buccal mucosa. Lip freckling is not unique to PJS. The primary concern to the pediatrician is the risk of small bowel intussusception causing intestinal obstruction, vomiting, and pain. In addition, intestinal bleeding leading to anemia can occur. In a child/adolescent, the clinical diagnosis of PJS may be made when any one of the following is present:

1. Two or more histologically confirmed PJ polyps
2. Any number of PJ polyps detected in one individual who has a family history of PJS in close relative(s)
3. Characteristic mucocutaneous pigmentation in an individual who has a family history of PJS in close relative(s)
4. Any number of PJ polyps in an individual who also has characteristic mucocutaneous pigmentation

Genetics of Peutz-Jeghers Syndrome

The mutated gene *STK11(LKB1)* located on chromosome 19p 13.3 is associated with PJS and encodes a serine/threonine kinase.[36] It appears that *STK11* is a tumor suppressor gene that might act as a gatekeeper regulating the development of hamartomas and adenocarcinomas in PJS.[37] The gene mutation can be identified in up to 90% of patients. Once the mutation has been identified, at-risk family members can be tested for the family-specific mutation. Parents of apparently isolated PJS cases should be carefully assessed, and all siblings should be tested if a parent is found to be affected. After appropriate genetic counseling and informed consent, testing at-risk family members may be performed early in childhood so that gastrointestinal surveillance can start early.

There is marked inter- and intrafamilial phenotypic variability in PJS. Therefore, the availability of predictive genetic testing may have some value but cannot determine the likely severity of phenotype.[38] In studies of larger PJS cohorts, no difference was seen between individuals with missense and truncating mutations, or between familial and sporadic cases, although it was suggested that there was a higher risk of cancer in individuals with mutations in exon 3 of the gene. Of 419 PJS patients, 297 with documented mutations, the type and site of mutation did not influence cancer risk.[39]

If the gene mutation is known in previous affected cases in the family, there is value in presymptomatic testing in those patients with no pigmentation (or even potential prenatal diagnosis).

Management and Complications

The management of a young child with midgut PJS polyps is controversial. In a retrospective review, 68% of children had undergone a laparotomy for bowel obstruction by the age of 18 years, and many of these proceeded to a second laparotomy within 5 years.[40] There is a high reoperation rate after initial laparotomy for small bowel obstruction.

Children who present with midgut complications need polypectomy either by double-balloon enteroscopy (DBE), or by laparotomy and intraoperative enteroscopy (IOE) (Figure 43-8). The latter is recommended in any patient with PJS undergoing laparotomy, because careful endoscopy via an enterotomy in the small bowel allows identification and removal of polyps, thus avoiding multiple enterotomies and the risk of short bowel syndrome associated with resection. This technique is superior to palpation and transillumination in identifying polyps, and removal of all detected polyps ("clean sweep") reduces relaparotomy rate significantly.[41,42]

Endoscopic evaluation of the upper and lower gastrointestinal tract and imaging of the small bowel should be performed from the age of 8 years. If symptoms are present before this, screening should start earlier. The development of video capsule endoscopy (VCE) has replaced the barium enterography as the preferred technique for assessing the small bowel.[43] VCE is more sensitive, preferred by patients, and reduces the lifetime risk from cumulative radiation exposure. Children younger

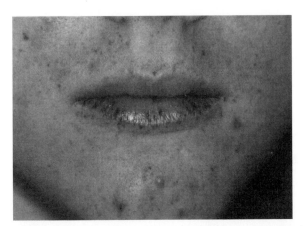

Figure 43-7. Typical mucocutaneous pigmentation seen in PJS. (*See plate section for color.*)

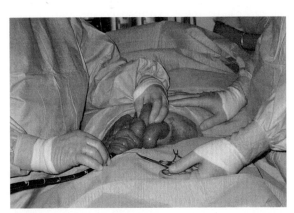

Figure 43-8. Intraoperative enteroscopy performed at laparotomy for intussusception in a patient with PJS.

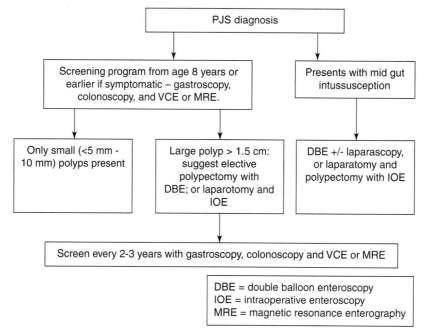

Figure 43-9. Management protocol for screening children and adolescents at risk of PJS.

than 6 years may require the VCE to be placed endoscopically, and the risk of capsule retention is less than 1%. Careful selection of patients for VCE will help reduce the risk of retention, and in those where a concern remains, a patency capsule can be used before VCE. An acceptable alternative to VCE is MRI enterography with a close correlation between the two modalities, especially with polyps larger than 15 mm.

The advantages and disadvantages of prophylactic polypectomy for asymptomatic patients should be discussed with the family. Management is influenced by the size of the polyps and their location (Figure 43-9). Prophylactic polypectomy of larger small-bowel polyps (more than 1.5 cm) by IOE or DBE should be performed to reduce the incidence of subsequent complications and the requirement for emergency laparotomy. For children who are asymptomatic with small polyps (less than 1.0 cm), the parents should be counseled about the risk of intussusception.

Symptomatic children with sizable midgut polyps (larger than 1.5 cm in size) should be referred for DBE or laparotomy and IOE. DBE with polypectomy of PJS polyps in the small bowel carries a significant risk of perforation and should be performed only by those expert in polypectomy. Muscularis mucosa commonly invaginates into the large pedunculated stalk, increasing the risk of perforation at electrocautery (Figure 43-10). DBE can be combined with laparoscopy to assess perforations that may arise at polypectomy.

No single pharmacologic agent has been shown to affect the clinical course of PJS, but animal studies have suggested that rapamycin, celecoxib, and metformin may reduce polyp burden; none of these are in routine clinical use.[44]

Malignancy Risk

The risk of neoplasia is well documented in young adults and includes development of unusual tumors such as Sertoli cell tumor of the ovary and testicular tumors in prepubescent boys. A meta-analysis to assess the risk of cancer in PJS identified a

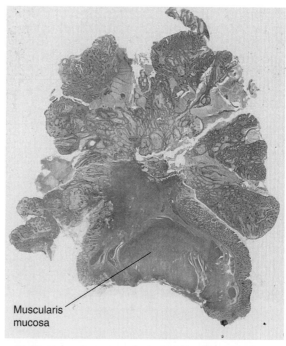

Figure 43-10. Light microscopy of a large PJS polyp showing muscularis mucosa invaginating into the polyp, increasing the likelihood of perforation at snare polypectomy.

relative risk for all cancers in PJS patients (aged 15 to 64) of 15.2 compared to the normal population, with tumors reported throughout the GI tract including colon (39%), pancreas (36%), stomach (29%), and extraintestinal tumors of the lung, testes, breast (54%), uterus, ovary, and cervix.[45]

Clinicians caring for adolescents with PJS should be aware of unusual symptoms, such as those due to a feminizing testicular tumor, and have a low threshold for investigating potential malignancies. A recommended screening program for PJS

TABLE 43-6. Suggested Program for Screening for Malignancies in Peutz-Jeghers Syndrome After Adolescence

General
Annual hemoglobin and liver function tests
Annual clinical examination

Genital Tract
Annual examination and consider testicular ultrasound biennially from birth until 12 years
Cervical smear with liquid-based cytology every 3 years from age 25 years

Gastrointestinal
Baseline EGD/colonoscopy, age 8
  If polyps detected, continue every 3 years until age 50 years
  If no polyps detected, repeat at age 18 years, then every 3 years until age 50 years
VCE every 3 years from age 8 years

Breast
Monthly self-examination from age 18 years
Annual breast MRI from age 25 to age 50, thereafter annual mammography

EGD, esophagogastroduodenoscopy.

patients after adolescence is shown in Table 43-6, but it is not proven that such a program will reduce morbidity or mortality.

OTHER POLYPOSIS SYNDROMES

Gorlin's syndrome is an autosomal dominant condition comprising upper gastrointestinal hamartomas and pink or brown macules in exposed areas such as the face and hands. In addition, patients may have frontal and parietal bossing, hypertelorism and variable skeletal abnormalities, or intracranial calcification and are at risk of medulloblastoma.

Turcot's syndrome is characterized by concurrence of a primary brain tumor (most often glioblastoma multiforme) and multiple colorectal adenomas. The number of adenomas is often not high, but many of the reported patients have been adolescents. Patients with a polyposis syndrome and neurologic symptoms should undergo thorough neurologic examination and investigation for possible brain tumor. The management of the colonic polyps in Turcot's syndrome is the same as for FAP.

In patients with long-standing inflammatory colitis, inflammatory polyps (pseudopolyps) may develop. They are usually found in the colon and rarely in the rectum. Inflammatory polyps are of no significance and have no malignant potential. As the colitis heals, they may regress.

In the vast majority of patients with polyposis, a clear-cut diagnosis can be made, such as FAP or PJS. However, there are

some rare cases where distinctions cannot be made on histology – the mixed polyposis syndromes (HMPS).[46] This condition is a dominant genetic disorder localized to a mutation in the area of 15q13-14 (CRAC1) or in the BMPR1A gene and characterized by the occurrence of colorectal polyps of mixed histology, namely hyperplastic, atypical juvenile, serrated adenomas, and eventually colorectal cancer. HMPS families have been identified in many countries where Jewish migration occurred from Europe. Affected patients require systematic and frequent colonoscopic examinations, polypectomies, and decisions on elective prophylactic colectomy.

SUMMARY

Colonic polyps in children are often solitary and carry no long-term implications; however, a detailed cancer family history is required when a child presents with multiple gastrointestinal polyps. Those patients should be classified by clinical presentation, endoscopic appearance, polyp histology, and family history. The identification of the gene mutations responsible for most of the polyposis syndromes has enabled genetic screening for other family members, affected the choice of therapies and surgery, and assisted in classifying patients and determining their prognosis. Gastrointestinal polyposis is associated with an increased lifetime risk of cancer necessitating colectomy in FAP, or surveillance in PJS and JPS. Multidisciplinary care managed by polyposis registries ensures timely genetic counseling, endoscopic surveillance, and surgery. Future chemopreventative strategies may also affect the clinical course and timing of surgery.

The management of polyposis syndromes exemplifies the practice of combining clinicopathologic findings with genetic investigations, enabling appropriate patient care to prevent CRC in at-risk children.

REFERENCES

1. Rozen P, Macrae F. Familial adenomatous polyposis: the practical applications of clinical and molecular screening. Familial Cancer 2006;5:227–235.
13. Vasen HFA, Möslein G, Alonso A. Guidelines for the clinical management of FAP. Gut 2008;57:704–713.
27. Steinbach GD, Lynch PM, Phillips RKS, et al. The effect of celecoxib, a specific cyclo-oxygenase inhibitor in familial adenomatous polyposis. N Engl J Med 2000;342:1946–1952.
40. Hinds R, Philp C, Hyer W, et al. Complications of childhood Peutz Jeghers syndrome: implications for pediatric screening. J Pediatr Gastroenterol Nutr 2004;39:219–220.

See expertconsult.com for a complete list of references and the review questions for this chapter.

44

CROHN'S DISEASE

Shervin Rabizadeh • Jeffrey S. Hyams • Marla Dubinsky

Crohn's disease, a condition of chronic intestinal inflammation, continues to impair the quality of life for hundreds of thousands of children and adults. Although a considerable amount of research has been put forth, the exact etiology of Crohn's disease remains unclear. There is limited understanding of the initiation and propagation of the pathophysiology that leads to this heterogeneous inflammatory process. This makes Crohn's disease a challenging disorder for both basic scientists and clinicians, currently limiting our therapies to those that mitigate inflammation rather than prevent it. Nonetheless, significant strides have been made in management of Crohn's disease patients and individualizing treatment according to the patient's genotype-phenotype interactions.

EPIDEMIOLOGY

Defining the exact epidemiology of Crohn's disease has been made difficult by the insidious onset of disease, frequent marked delay in diagnosis, occasional presentation with extraintestinal manifestations, and occasional misclassification of patients. Despite these limitations, recent data suggest that the incidence of Crohn's disease has increased dramatically.[1] In Sweden, the incidence is 4.9 per 100,000 children, more than twice that of ulcerative colitis, with a marked increase noted between 1990 and 2001.[2] A more recent study from Norway evaluating a cohort of children observed between 2005 and 2007 demonstrated an incidence of 10.9 per 100,000 children.[3] A statewide population-based study of children in Wisconsin revealed an overall inflammatory bowel disease (IBD) incidence of 7.05 per 100,000, with that for Crohn's disease of 4.56 – more than twice that of ulcerative colitis.[4] There is generally a slight female preponderance and a bimodal distribution of age at diagnosis, with a peak in the second to third decades of life, followed by a smaller peak in the sixth and seventh decades. Although Crohn's disease can be found in infancy, most pediatric cases occur in the early adolescent years, with a peak incidence at 11 to 12 years of age.

Recent observations have challenged many of the old tenets of IBD epidemiology. The emerging pattern suggests similar patterns of disease incidence in whites and nonwhites, those who live in urban and those who live in rural areas, and those in more northern and southern latitudes.[4,5] The large discrepancy between disease incidence in Jews and non-Jews has greatly decreased.[6] Interestingly, there appears to be a difference in geographical location and disease incidence. Incidence rates differ between studies from different countries and within regions in countries. In the United States, there is a lower prevalence of Crohn's disease in the South compared to the Northeast, Midwest, and West regions of the country.[7]

The most important risk factor for developing Crohn's disease is a family history of IBD (see later discussion), but several other risk factors have emerged. Improved living conditions early in life increase the likelihood of developing the condition.[8,9] Other factors that appear to increase risk include previous appendectomy,[10] older maternal age during pregnancy for females developing Crohn's disease,[11] and possibly maternal smoking. Data concerning the permissive or protective role of breast-feeding and the development of IBD are conflicting.[12] There are conflicting reports as to whether measles vaccination or exposure in early life is associated with a greater risk of Crohn's disease, but the bulk of evidence argues against an association.[13] Conditions associated with a higher frequency of Crohn's disease include Turner's syndrome,[14] Hermansky-Pudlak syndrome,[15] and glycogen storage disease type Ib.[16]

ETIOLOGY

Though the etiology is unclear, Crohn's disease is thought to result from a complex interaction of genetic, host immune, and environmental factors. Animal models have provided important insight into this relationship.[17]

Genetics

The single greatest risk factor for the development of IBD is having a first-degree relative with the condition, with the estimated risk 30 to 100 times greater than in the general population.[18] The age-adjusted risk for a first-degree relative of a proband with Crohn's disease developing the condition during their lifetime is about 4%, with a slightly greater risk for females than for males.[19] Daughters of an individual with Crohn's disease have a 12.6% lifetime risk of developing IBD, compared with a 7.9% risk for male offspring.[19] If both parents have Crohn's disease, offspring have a 33% risk of developing the condition by the age of 28 years.[20] At the time of diagnosis of Crohn's disease, the likelihood of finding IBD in a first-degree relative of the proband is 10 to 25%.[19,21] Concordance in monozygotic twins is greater for Crohn's disease (50%)[22] than for insulin-dependent diabetes, asthma, or schizophrenia. Although early observations of families with multiple affected members suggested genetic anticipation (earlier onset of disease, increased severity, or both, in succeeding generations of affected families), more recent evidence has not supported this finding.[23] Subclinical intestinal inflammation has been demonstrated in healthy relatives of patients with Crohn's disease, suggesting a possible inherited defect with less destructive expression in some individuals than in others.[24] This subclinical inflammation may also be associated with increased gut permeability,[25] another phenomenon demonstrated in the relatives of patients with Crohn's disease.[26] A similar phenomenon with subclinical intestinal inflammation has been described in the relatives of patients with ankylosing spondylitis, a condition that shares many similarities with Crohn's disease.[27]

The number of susceptibility loci associated with Crohn's disease as identified by genetic linkage analyses, through genome-wide screens, has grown exponentially. Original studies identified a number of susceptibility loci, designated *IBD1* through *IBD6* on chromosomes 16, 12, 6, 14, 5, and 19 respectively.[28] The *IBD1* locus in the pericentromeric region of chromosome 16 is the best replicated region, showing strong evidence for linkage in Crohn's disease in both Jewish and non-Jewish cohorts.[29] Three main polymorphisms of this gene, known as *NOD2/CARD15* (caspase activation recruitment domain), increase susceptibility to Crohn's disease (R702W, G908R, 1007fs). Having one copy of the risk allele confers a small increased risk (two- to fourfold), whereas having two copies increases the risk of developing Crohn's disease 20- to 40-fold.[28]

More recently, a meta-analysis of three genome-wide association studies (GWAS) identified over 30 independent gene loci associated with Crohn's disease.[30] These genes highlight, in particular, the key importance of autophagy and adaptive and innate immunity. The GWAS supported the previously identified association between NOD2/CARD15 and Crohn's. Further, other genes that have strongly been associated with Crohn's disease include an autophagy gene, ATG16L1, the gene encoding the interleukin-23 (IL-23) receptor subunit, and IL12B, IL10, and STAT3 genes.[30,31] ATG16L1, similar to *NOD2/CARD15*, affects the intracellular processing of bacterial components. The IL-23 and STAT3 genes are part of the T helper 17 (Th17) cell pathway, which appears to play a role in other dysregulated immune disorders. A separate GWAS in children and young adults reproduced 23 of the 32 loci implicated in the large meta-analysis GWAS of adult-onset Crohn's disease.[32] Furthermore, this study also identified crossover of genes between Crohn's and ulcerative colitis, revealing some commonality in the disease mechanism of these two conditions.[31,32]

Microbial Factors

A complex interaction of gut mucosal immune mechanisms with intestinal flora is thought to be critical in the development of Crohn's disease.[33] This interaction could include:

- An appropriate response to a persistent pathogenic infection
- An inappropriate response to normal luminal flora because of a defective epithelial barrier or disordered immune response
- Alterations in bacterial function and composition

However, no pathogen has reproducibly been identified as a potential cause of Crohn's disease. Persistent infection with measles virus is not supported by current data.[34] Conflicting data have associated Crohn's disease with *Mycobacterium avium pseudotuberculosis*, which causes granulomatous enteritis in ruminants,[35] as well as *Listeria monocytogenes* and *Helicobacter hepaticus*.[33] Compared with healthy persons or those with nonspecific colitis, individuals with Crohn's disease have much higher concentrations of adherent colonic bacteria,[36] with noninflamed mucosal surfaces having more bacteria than inflamed surfaces. The significance of this finding is unclear.

Epidemiologic data suggest the onset of IBD in a small proportion of patients following well-defined enteric infection with common pathogens such as *Salmonella*, *Shigella*, *Campylobacter*, or *Yersinia*.[37] A recent large population-based cohort study identified an increased risk of IBD in individuals with previous *Salmonella* or *Campylobacter* gastroenteritis.[38] Exacerbation of known Crohn's disease can follow intercurrent bacterial

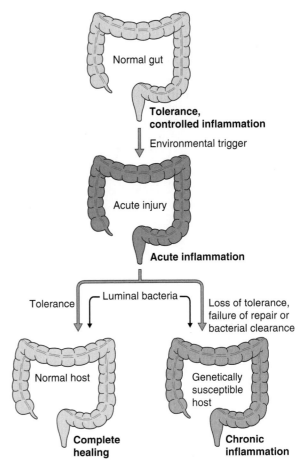

Figure 44-1. Variable responses to environmental triggers (e.g., viral infection, nonsteroidal anti-inflammatory drugs) in genetically susceptible and normal hosts. In the normal host, injury leads to self-limited acute inflammation. In genetically predisposed hosts, the inflammatory response continues, leading to chronic inflammation and tissue damage. Adapted from Sartor (2004).[43]

or viral infection,[37] and recent data have highlighted the role of cytomegalovirus and *Clostridium difficile* in some of these patients.[39-41]

Immune Mechanisms

Intestinal epithelium and the enteric immune system represent the primary mechanical and immunologic forces mediating the interaction between the gut and enteric bacteria and other antigenic and noxious compounds that traverse it. In normal gut mucosa there is a dynamic interplay between appropriate response to mucosal immune stimulation and down-regulatory forces mitigating accompanying tissue injury. This balanced relationship results in "physiologic" inflammation (Figure 44-1). Defective barrier function (genetically induced or secondary to mucosal injury) may allow increased permeability to bacterial or other antigens, leading to unchecked stimulation of local immune cells.[42] Defective down-regulation of an appropriate response to luminal stimulation may also result in more exuberant inflammation, resulting in the tissue injury characteristic of Crohn's disease.[43]

The inflammatory response in the gut has been characterized by the designation of T helper cell (Th) 1, Th2, Th17, and T regulatory (Tr) pathways. It has been suggested that the Th1

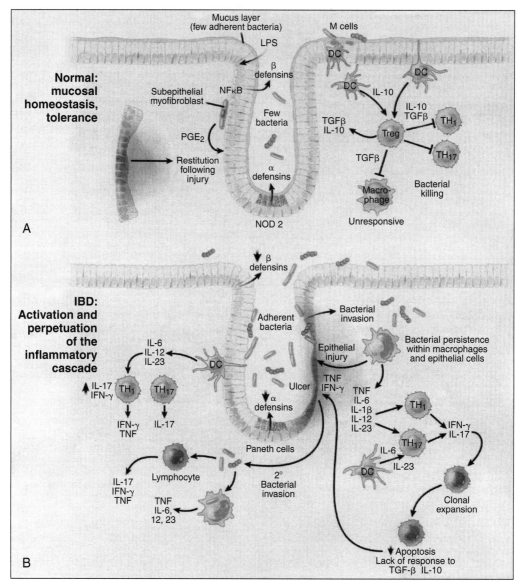

Figure 44-2. Mucosal immunity and cytokine profile in normal mucosa and in patients with IBD with predominance of Th1 and Th17 mediated response. Adapted from Sartor (2008).[261]

pathway is important in the pathogenesis of Crohn's disease (Figure 44-2).[44] Th1 polarizing cytokines (tumor necrosis factor (TNF), IL-12, IL-18) are proinflammatory cytokines that induce differentiation of CD4+ T cells to the Th1 phenotype. TNF, in particular, appears to have great importance as it promotes chemokine secretion from intestinal epithelial cells, disrupts the epithelial barrier, and promotes apoptosis of intestinal epithelial cells.[45] Th2-derived cytokines, IL-4, IL-5, and IL-13, are produced by Th2 CD4+ T cells and mediate intestinal inflammation. Although abnormalities in tissue and circulating mononuclear cell activity have been demonstrated in Crohn's disease,[46] their role in perpetuating chronic inflammation is unclear. It has been proposed that Th2 pathways may play a role in early, acute inflammation.[47]

Th17 cells have derived the name by their ability to produce IL-17, also termed IL-17A. Additionally, the Th17 pathway involves cytokines IL-17F, IL-21, IL-22, IL-23, TNF-α, and IL-6.[48] Th17 pathway cytokines are postulated to play a role in the protection of the host against microorganisms.[49] The Th17

pathway has recently been associated with Crohn's disease (see Figure 44-2). IL-23R gene polymorphisms that influence IBD susceptibility have been identified in Crohn's disease patients and validated in multiple different populations.[50] Several further studies have identified changes in cytokine levels of the Th17 pathway in Crohn's disease patients. An example of this is the demonstration of increased number of IL-17 producing cells in the inflamed gut of patients with Crohn's disease.[51] The importance of the Th17 pathway in Crohn's disease is an active focus of both basic and translational research, because it appears to be an important mediator in the abnormal immune response to the environment promoting intestinal tissue damage.

Multiple other cytokines (IL-1, IL-6, IL-7, IL-11, IL-15) have been implicated as possible participants in the mediation of chronic inflammation in Crohn's disease. Recently, a novel paradigm has been suggested for the pathogenesis of Crohn's disease in which an "immunodeficiency" exists.[52] This hypothesis has been supported by the observation of Crohn's-like disease in immunodeficiency states such as chronic granulomatous disease, glycogen storage disease type Ib, leukocyte adhesion deficiency, Chediak-Higashi syndrome, and a variety of neutropenias. Further, granulocyte-macrophage colony-stimulating factor (GM-CSF) has been useful in some patients with Crohn's disease.[53]

Neuroendocrine

Inflammatory mediators may alter the structure and function of enteric nerves, and enteric neurotransmitters (e.g., substance P) may have a proinflammatory effect.[54] Calcitonin gene-related peptide (CGRP)-containing nerves are prominent in Crohn's disease tissue;[55] in experimental models of colitis, CGRP appears to have an anti-inflammatory effect.[56]

Pathway for Tissue Injury

The signature feature of Crohn's disease is the intense bowel infiltration with inflammatory cells. Levels of vascular adhesion molecules are greatly increased, resulting in exaggerated migration of circulating inflammatory cells into the mucosa.[57] Tissue concentrations of prostaglandins, leukotrienes, free radicals, nitric oxide, proinflammatory cytokines and various chemokines are increased. These substances induce various proteases that result in degradation of extracellular matrix and ulceration. The matrix metalloproteinases (MMPs) are divided into four groups (collagenases, gelatinases, stromelysins, and membrane type) and are produced by mesenchymal cells, mononuclear inflammatory cells, and neutrophils. MMPs are overexpressed in IBD tissue.[58] They are inhibited by several molecules, the most important of which is α_2-microglobulin.[59] In addition, lipoxins, lipoxygenase-derived eicosanoids produced during cell-cell interactions, serve to mitigate inflammation by inhibiting neutrophil chemotaxis and adhesion to epithelium, epithelial chemokine release, TNF-α-stimulated inflammatory responses, cyclooxygenase product generation, and epithelial cell apoptosis.[60]

Bowel wall thickening and fibrosis is common in Crohn's disease. Mucosal thickening comes from both the epithelium and the lamina propria. Keratinocyte growth factors are overexpressed in the mucosa in IBD.[61] Lamina propria expansion appears to be mediated by multiple cytokines including TNF-α and IL-1β, which are mitogens for subepithelial colonic myofibroblasts,[62] and connective tissue growth factor (CTGF), which promotes extracellular matrix formation and proliferation.[63]

The balance between ongoing inflammatory tissue injury, healing, and remodeling appears to dictate the degree to which there is growth of the intestinal muscularis and eventually fibrosis and stenosis. Microvessels from chronically inflamed Crohn's disease tissue demonstrate microvascular endothelial cell dysfunction, characterized by loss of nitric oxide–mediated vasodilation that may lead to reduced perfusion, impaired healing, and maintenance of inflammation.[64] Fibrosis results from the deposition of excessive fibrillar collagen and other extracellular matrix materials, and by the overgrowth of smooth muscle. Up-regulation of fibrogenic activity by subepithelial myofibroblasts,[65] increased type III collagen production by fibroblasts in response to transforming growth factor β (TGF-β),[66] and possible mediation of fibrogenic activity by mast cells[67] occurs.

A schematic representation of the theoretical pathogenesis of Crohn's disease is shown in Figure 44-3.

PATHOLOGY

Macroscopic Pathology

Gross inspection of the bowel in well-established Crohn's disease reveals marked wall thickening as a result of transmural edema and chronic inflammation. Mural thickening is accompanied by narrowing of the bowel lumen and may be severe enough to cause clinical obstruction. The mesentery is thickened with edematous, indurated fat that migrates over the serosal surface of the bowel (Figure 44-4). Mesenteric lymph nodes are frequently enlarged. The bowel mucosa may reveal small aphthous lesions, which may coalesce into larger irregular and deeper ulcers (Figure 44-5). Bowel inflammation and ulceration may be confluent, but more characteristically is punctuated by "skip areas" of grossly and even microscopically normal mucosa. Cobblestoning of the surface lining may occur as a result of extensive linear and serpiginous mucosal ulceration with associated regeneration and hyperplasia, in addition to marked submucosal thickening (Figure 44-6). Stricture formation may occur in the setting of chronic inflammation as a result of fibrous tissue proliferation involving first the submucosa and then the deeper layers of the bowel wall.

Loops of adjacent bowel may become matted together because of serosal and mesenteric inflammation. Fistulas are thought to arise when transmural bowel inflammation extends through the serosa into adjacent structures, such as bowel, abdominal wall, bladder, vagina, or perineum. Frequently, a fistulous tract may end blindly in an inflammatory mass (phlegmon) adjacent to the bowel and involves the bowel itself as well as the mesentery, lymph nodes, and, occasionally, a chronic active abscess cavity.

Microscopic Appearance

The findings on histologic examination of the bowel in Crohn's disease are highly dependent on the duration of disease involvement. Early disease may manifest as superficial aphthoid lesions of the mucosa, usually overlying a lymphoid follicle (Figure 44-7). Mucosal ulcers may become confluent, producing broad, depressed ulcer beds. There is sequential progression from mucosal disease to profound transmural infiltration of the bowel with lymphocytes, histiocytes, and plasma cells. The inflammation is characteristically extensive in the submucosa and is characterized by edema, lymphatic dilation, and collagen deposition. The last is responsible for obliteration of the submucosa, resulting in stricture, obstruction, or both. Deep fissuring ulceration into the muscularis propria frequently occurs and, when prominent, is highly characteristic of Crohn's disease even in the absence of granulomas. Crypt abscesses and goblet cell depletion are common but may not be as marked as in ulcerative colitis (Figure 44-8). Mucosa that is thought to be normal grossly often reveals abnormalities such as edema and an increase in mononuclear cell density in the lamina propria.

Granulomas are not always found in pathologic specimens from individuals with Crohn's disease, being absent in up to 40% of surgically resected specimens and 60 to 80% of mucosal biopsies.[68] Granulomas may be found in any layer of the bowel wall, although most commonly in the superficial submucosa (Figure 44-9). Biopsies from ulcers or the edge of aphthoid lesions may have the highest yield of granuloma. Granulomas may also be present in extraintestinal structures such as lymph nodes, mesentery, and peritoneum.

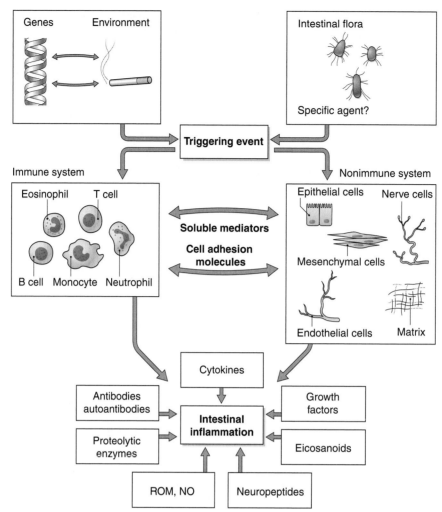

Figure 44-3. Schematic representation of possible contributing factors to the development of Crohn's disease. NO, nitric oxide; ROM, reactive oxygen metabolites. Courtesy Claudio Fiocchi, MD.

PATHOPHYSIOLOGY OF GASTROINTESTINAL SYMPTOMS

The presence of inflammation in the small and large intestine, bowel wall thickening, or both leads to a number of derangements that culminate in symptoms consistent with Crohn's disease, such as abdominal pain, diarrhea, and gastrointestinal bleeding. Inflammatory mediators released by activated immune cells lead to increased mucosal electrolyte secretion. Extensive jejunal and ileal disease may result in malabsorption. Malabsorbed fatty acids entering the colon impair electrolyte and water absorption. Abnormal terminal ileal function may result in bile acid loss, with an eventual decrease in the luminal bile acid concentration, worsening steatorrhea. Bile salts may significantly impair colonic absorption of electrolytes. Bacterial overgrowth in the small intestine associated with obstruction, stasis, or enteroenteric fistula may lead to mucosal damage and bile salt deconjugation, further worsening symptoms. Diffuse mucosal disease leads to exudation of serum proteins and bleeding. Cramping abdominal pain may result from gut distention, usually associated with obstruction or abnormalities in intestinal motility. The pain of Crohn's disease may also result from the inflammation-mediated recruitment of silent nociceptors in the ileocecal region.

CLASSIFICATION OF SUBGROUPS IN CROHN'S DISEASE

The complex interaction of an individual's genetic composition, immunologic status, and environment lead to the heterogeneous manifestations of Crohn's disease. Attempts to categorize patients with Crohn's disease by their variable clinical and laboratory manifestations is called *phenomics* (Table 44-1).

The Montreal classification was published by an international panel of experts to define subgroups of patients with Crohn's disease.[69] Age at diagnosis, disease location, and disease behavior were identified as the most important factors for subclassification. Disease location was classified as ileal, colonic, ileocolonic, or isolated upper gastrointestinal, which reflected any involvement proximal to the terminal ileum. Biologic behavior was classified as nonstricturing nonperforating (inflammatory), stricturing (persistent luminal narrowing with proximal dilatation without evidence of penetrating disease), penetrating (intra-abdominal fistula, inflammatory masses, and/or abscesses), or perianal.

Longitudinal observation of patients shows considerable evolution of biologic behavior, with many patients presenting with inflammatory disease and then manifesting stricturing or penetrating disease over time. A high degree of concordance for

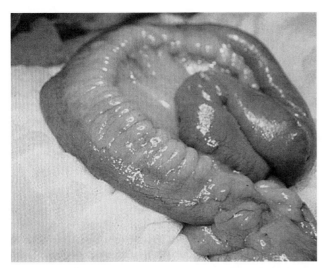

Figure 44-4. Mesenteric fat creeping over inflamed bowel.

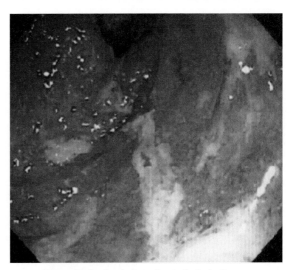

Figure 44-5. Cecal ulceration in Crohn's disease.

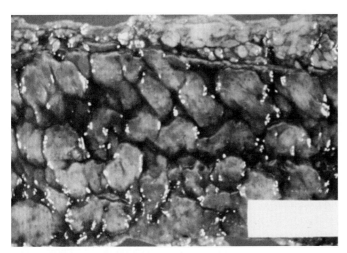

Figure 44-6. Colonic resection specimen showing marked bowel wall thickening with cobblestoning.

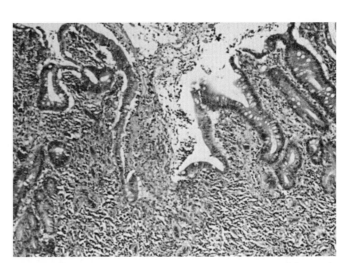

Figure 44-7. Solitary aphthoid lesion overlying a lymphoid nodule in early Crohn's disease.

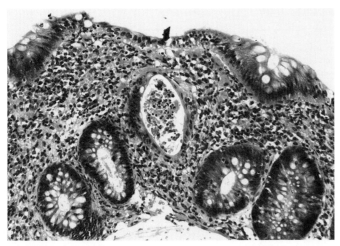

Figure 44-8. Neutrophilic crypt abscess and crypt architectural distortion. (*See plate section for color.*)

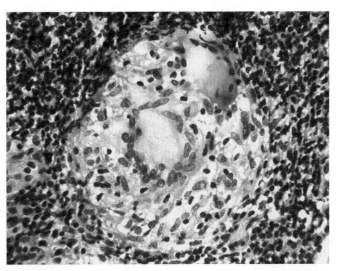

Figure 44-9. Epithelioid granuloma with multinucleated giant cells. (*See plate section for color.*)

anatomic site and biologic behavior is often noted in families with more than one affected member.

The presence or absence of immunologic markers has been used to categorize patients with IBD. Anti-neutrophil cytoplasmic antibody (ANCA), anti-*Saccharomyces cerevisiae* antibody (ASCA), an antibody to the *Escherichia coli*-related outer membrane porin C (anti-OmpC), and anti-Cbir1 antibody (antibody against flagellin) have been examined most closely. Perinuclear (p)ANCA associated with IBD is produced by mucosal B cells responding to various antigens.[70] Although present in the serum of 60 to 70% of patients with ulcerative colitis, pANCA is also detected in 15 to 25% of patients with Crohn's disease.[71,72] Patients with Crohn's disease who are pANCA positive exhibit an ulcerative colitis-like picture with left-sided colonic disease and histopathologic expression similar to that of ulcerative colitis.[73] Also, Crohn's patients with pANCA were more reactive to Cbir1 than were pANCA-positive ulcerative colitis patients.[74] Levels of ASCA (IgG or IgA) are detected in about 50 to 60% of patients with Crohn's disease.[72] The presence of high-titer ASCA in the absence of ANCA is highly predictive of Crohn's disease.[72,75] Higher levels of IgG and IgA ASCA correlate with the presence of small bowel involvement, as well as with fibrostenosing or perforating disease.[76] Antibodies to I2 (Crohn's disease-associated bacterial sequence) and OmpC are associated with a greater number of strictures and internal perforations.[77] Anti-Cbir1 is associated with Crohn's disease, especially patients with internal penetrating disease, fibrostenotic disease, and small bowel disease.[78] pANCA-positive patients with Crohn's disease are less likely to respond to infliximab than those who are ASCA positive or totally seronegative for these markers.[79] Antibodies to OmpC are present in 38% of patients with Crohn's disease, particularly in those who are ASCA negative.[80] Antibody profiles also appear to be different based on the age of presentation, with younger patients (less than 7 years of age) more likely to express anti-Cbir1 while older children have higher rates of ASCA positivity.[81] Also, the total number of antibodies seems important clinically. Complicated Crohn's disease increases in children in relation to escalating number and magnitude of these immune reactivity antibodies.[82]

TABLE 44-1. Clinical and Laboratory Subgroups of Patients With Crohn's Disease

Anatomic Location
Gastroduodenal (30-40% of subjects)
Jejunoileal (15-20%)
Ileal (30-35%)
Ileocolonic (50-60%)
Colonic (15-20%)
Perirectal (20-30%)

Biologic Behavior
Inflammatory
Stricturing (fibrostenosing)
Penetrating

Laboratory Markers
ANCA
ASCA
Anti-OmpC
Anti I2
Anti-Cbir1
Genetic markers
NOD2/CARD15 (multiple polymorphisms)

CLINICAL FEATURES

The presenting clinical features of Crohn's disease are depicted in Table 44-2. Minor discrepancies are seen in different case series, but the most common geographic distribution of disease is ileocolitis (40 to 60%), followed by small bowel alone (20 to 30%) and colon alone (20%). Children under 5 years of age have a higher likelihood of colonic involvement.[83] Gastroduodenal involvement is found in up to 30% of children with Crohn's disease.[84]

Terminal ileal and cecal disease is associated with right lower quadrant discomfort; examination often reveals tenderness on palpation and a fullness or distinct mass in this area. Periumbilical pain is common with colonic disease or more diffuse small bowel disease. Gastroduodenal inflammation is common and may be associated with epigastric pain. Odynophagia and dysphagia are observed in most patients with Crohn's disease of the esophagus. The abdominal pain associated with Crohn's disease tends to be persistent and severe and frequently awakens the child from sleep. At times the acute development of right lower quadrant pain without a well-established previous history of illness suggests a diagnosis of appendicitis, but laparotomy findings are consistent with Crohn's disease.

Diarrhea is seen in two thirds of children and may be severe and nocturnal. Gross blood in the stool is unusual with isolated small bowel disease, and more common when the colon is involved. Severe hemorrhage, however, may be seen in the setting of small bowel disease when bowel ulceration extends deeply into the bowel wall and involves a larger blood vessel.

Fever can be low-grade or spiking and may persist for extended periods before a diagnosis is made. Nausea and vomiting are frequent and may be seen with involvement of any part of the bowel; they are particularly common in the setting of severe colitis. Fatigue is a common complaint. Anorexia, weight loss, and diminution in growth velocity may be seen in 20 to 60% of children.

About 20 to 30% of affected children develop perirectal inflammation with fissures, fistulas, or tags and may be misdiagnosed as having hemorrhoids or perianal condyloma. The perirectal disease may prompt a suspicion of abuse. Drainage from these fistulas may be impressive, but perirectal pain is unusual unless there is actual abscess formation.

Gastrointestinal Complications

Hemorrhage

Massive acute gastrointestinal hemorrhage is seen in less than 1% of patients with Crohn's disease, but may be severe enough to cause exsanguination. Mesenteric angiography is used to guide surgical resection.

TABLE 44-2. Clinical Features of Crohn's Disease

Feature	Proportion Affected (%)
Abdominal pain	75
Diarrhea	65
Weight loss	65
Growth retardation	25
Nausea/vomiting	25
Perirectal disease	25
Rectal bleeding	20
Extraintestinal manifestations	25

Obstruction

Intestinal obstruction may occur secondary to severe bowel wall inflammation with or without localized phlegmon or abscess formation, stricture formation associated with chronic inflammation, undigested food occluding the lumen of a strictured bowel, carcinoma, or adhesions associated with previous surgery. Chronic low-grade obstruction may lead to proximal small bowel bacterial overgrowth.

Perforation

Free perforation (i.e., that not accompanying an abscess or chronic fistula) is unusual in Crohn's disease. It is most common in the ileum. Rarely it can be the initial presentation of the disease. No relationship to perforation has been established between corticosteroid therapy, duration of disease, toxic dilation, or obstruction.[85] Classic signs of peritonitis may be masked in the presence of corticosteroid therapy.

Abscess

Transmural bowel inflammation with fistulization and perforation may lead to the formation of abscesses. Fever and abdominal pain are usually present, although it may be difficult to differentiate clinically between an abscess and an exacerbation of the underlying disease with phlegmon formation. Fecal flora is found when these abscesses are cultured. Hip pain may indicate the presence of an iliopsoas abscess.

Fistula Formation

Although perianal and perirectal fistulization are most common, other types of fistula include enteroenteric, enterovesical, enterovaginal, and enterocutaneous. A small proportion of children have highly destructive perianal disease, which often does not respond well to medical therapy. The most common enteroenteric fistula is between the ileum and the sigmoid colon. Enterocolic fistulas may lead to bacterial overgrowth of the proximal bowel.

Toxic Megacolon

Toxic megacolon is rare in Crohn's disease.

Carcinoma

Subjects with Crohn's colitis may be at similar risk of developing carcinoma of the colon as those with ulcerative colitis related to chronic inflammation.[86] Carcinoma of the small bowel and lymphoma, independent of immunosuppressive medication exposure, have also been described.[86]

Extraintestinal Manifestations

Extraintestinal manifestations are seen in 25 to 35% of patients with IBD. In on large cohort of pediatric IBD patients, 6% had at least one extraintestinal manifestation before disease diagnosis, and at least one extraintestinal manifestation developed in 29% of the children within 15 years of diagnosis.[87] Extraintestinal manifestations can be classified in four groups[88]:

- Those related directly to intestinal disease activity; these usually respond to therapy directed against bowel disease
- Those whose course appears to be unrelated to bowel disease activity
- Those that are a direct result of the presence of disease bowel, such as ureteral obstruction or nephrolithiasis
- Complications arising from therapy

Joints

Arthralgia (30 to 40% of patients) and frank arthritis (10%) may be seen.[89] Either the axial skeleton or peripheral joints may be involved. A schema has recently been proposed to classify peripheral joint problems in patients with Crohn's disease.[90] Type 1 arthropathy involves fewer than five joints (pauciarticular), usually involves large joints, is brief in duration, and temporally is related to flares of intestinal inflammation. It is clinically and genetically similar to the reactive arthritis that is associated with human leukocyte antigen (HLA) class I genes. Type 2 arthritis involves multiple small joints and has a course independent of intestinal inflammation; it is not associated with HLA class I genes. In children, arthritis may precede clinical evidence of gastrointestinal inflammation, and occasionally children are diagnosed as having juvenile rheumatoid arthritis only to have the diagnosis change once diarrhea and rectal bleeding have begun.

Ankylosing spondylitis is a seronegative arthropathy affecting the vertebral column and is characterized by sacroiliitis and progressive ankylosis or fusion of the vertebral column. It is strongly associated with HLA-B27: up to 50% of patients with IBD who are positive for HLA-B27 develop ankylosing spondylitis. Ileocolonoscopy in individuals with idiopathic ankylosing spondylitis demonstrates gut inflammation resembling early IBD.[91]

Musculoskeletal

Muscle diseases described include vasculitic myositis, granulomatous myositis, pyomyositis, and dermatomyositis. Proximal muscle weakness is rarely associated with high-dose daily corticosteroid therapy.

Cutaneous

The most common cutaneous manifestation is perianal disease. Erythema nodosum occurs in up to 10% of patients with Crohn's disease, usually during a period of increased intestinal inflammatory activity; recurrence is common. Pyoderma gangrenosum is reported in up to 1 to 2% of patients with Crohn's disease; its course is not necessarily related to bowel disease activity. Metastatic Crohn's disease is characterized by granulomatous skin lesions distant from the perineum (often the lower extremities), and its course is independent of bowel activity.[92] Epidermolysis bullosa acquisita, a blistering condition of the skin and mucous membranes, is rarely seen. Trace metal deficiency (zinc) and vitamin deficiency (pyridoxine) may be complicated by rashes. Acne is often worsened by corticosteroid therapy, which can also produce striae.

Oral

Oral ulceration (canker sores) ranges in severity from painless to severe. Biopsy may contain granuloma. Orofacial granulomatosis is a rare condition associated with inflammation and cobblestone ulceration of the oral cavity and may precede overt intestinal inflammation. Pyostomatitis vegetans is characterized by friable erythematous plaques and is considered the mucosal equivalent of pyoderma gangrenosum.

Ocular

Ocular problems such as uveitis, episcleritis, and iritis are often seen in the setting of other extraintestinal manifestations, such as arthritis and erythema nodosum.[93] Slitlamp examination reveals uveitis in about 6% of children with Crohn's disease; most are asymptomatic.[94] Increased intraocular pressure and posterior subcapsular cataracts may be seen with prolonged corticosteroid therapy.

Vascular

Hypercoagulability from thrombocytosis, hyperfibrinogenemia, raised levels of factor V, and factor VIII, and depression in free protein S concentration is seen in some patients with IBD.[95] Vascular complications have included deep vein thrombosis, pulmonary emboli, and neurovascular disease. Vasculitis is a rare complication of Crohn's disease.

Renal

Urinary tract abnormalities may include ureteral obstruction and hydronephrosis secondary to an ileocecal phlegmon encasing the right ureter, enterovesical fistula, perinephric abscess, and nephrolithiasis. Oxalate, urate, and phosphate stones may be found. The development of proteinuria or raised creatinine levels in a patient with long-standing Crohn's disease suggests amyloidosis. Drug related interstitial nephritis has been described following 5-aminosalicylic acid (5-ASA) therapy[96]; however, some patients develop chronic interstitial nephritis before taking any medication.[97]

Hepatobiliary

Abnormal serum levels of aminotransferases are seen during the course of disease in approximately 14% of children with IBD.[98] When increased enzyme levels are prolonged (for more than 6 months), the patient usually has either sclerosing cholangitis or autoimmune hepatitis.[98] A brief increase in serum aminotransferase levels may be associated with increased bowel disease activity, medications (e.g., 6-mercaptopurine, methotrexate), parenteral nutrition, and massive weight gain. Other hepatobiliary disorders include hepatic granuloma, hepatic abscess, cholelithiasis, and acalculous cholecystitis. Terminal ileal resection or significant ileal disease is associated with increased enteric bile acid loss and an interruption of the enterohepatic circulation of bile acids. Bile may then become supersaturated with cholesterol, leading to gallstone formation.

Autoimmune hepatitis or primary sclerosing cholangitis (PSC) occurs in less than 1% of children with Crohn's disease. Of children with IBD who develop sclerosing cholangitis, about 10% have Crohn's disease.[99] In contrast to adults, there may be significant overlap in the clinical and histologic expression of autoimmune hepatitis and PSC in children with IBD.[100] Serum γ-glutamyl transpeptidase (GGT) appears to be a better screen for PSC than serum alkaline phosphatase.[100]

Pancreas

Pancreatitis may develop as a reaction to drug therapy (6-mercaptopurine, sulfasalazine), from periampullary duodenal disease, associated with sclerosing cholangitis, and in an idiopathic form.[101,102]

Bone

Osteopenia may result from malnutrition, inadequate calcium intake or malabsorption, vitamin D deficiency, excessive proinflammatory cytokine production by diseased bowel, prolonged inactivity, and corticosteroid therapy.[103] Reduced bone mineral density can occur before diagnosis or during the course of illness.[104,105] It has been proposed that bone formation may be inhibited in the presence of bowel inflammation.[106] Both cortical and trabecular bone loss may occur, with resultant fractures, loss of height, severe pain, and disability. Although the absolute risk of fracture development in children and adolescents is unknown, data in adults suggest an increase compared with a control population.[107] Risk likely relates to disease severity and duration and the total amount of corticosteroids taken.

Hematologic

Anemia may be secondary to iron deficiency, folic acid deficiency, vitamin B_{12} deficiency, hemolysis (drug-induced or autoimmune), and bone marrow suppression (drug-induced). Immune activation with the elaboration of proinflammatory cytokines may suppress erythrocyte production. It may also be the operative mechanism for thrombocytosis seen in many patients. Neutropenia is a rare accompanying condition.

Malnutrition

Weight loss is seen in most children with Crohn's disease at the time of presentation, and anthropometric observations during the course of disease commonly show abnormalities compared with age-matched control children.[108] Causes of malnutrition in these patients include suboptimal dietary intake, increased gastrointestinal losses, malabsorption, and possibly increased requirements associated with marked inflammatory activity (Figure 44-10). Anorexia may be severe enough to mimic anorexia nervosa. Children who fear exacerbation of gastrointestinal symptoms as a result of eating decrease their intake. Delayed gastric emptying may be associated with early satiety. Marked mucosal inflammation leads to the loss of cellular constituents and hematochezia, with the development of protein-losing enteropathy and iron deficiency anemia. Fecal calcium and magnesium losses may be increased.[109] Deficiency states for iron, folic acid, vitamin B_{12}, nicotinic acid, vitamin D, vitamin K, calcium, magnesium, and zinc have been noted.[110] Vitamin D deficiency is highly prevalent in pediatric patients with IBD as up to 35% demonstrated low mean serum 25-hydroxyvitamin D concentration.[111] Abnormalities in lipoprotein composition and oxidant antioxidant status have been demonstrated, along with essential fatty acid deficiency.[112]

Limited studies have suggested increased resting energy expenditure,[113,114] together with decreased diet-induced thermogenesis.

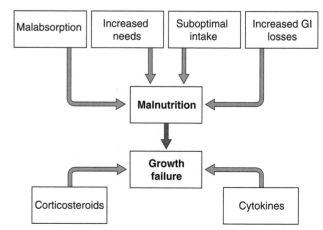

Figure 44-10. Factors contributing to the development of malnutrition and growth failure in children and adolescents with Crohn's disease.

Corticosteroid therapy affects both energy expenditure and lipid oxidation.[115]

Growth Failure

A decrease in growth velocity may precede overt gastrointestinal symptoms in up to 40% of children with Crohn's disease,[116] and evidence of impaired linear growth at the time of diagnosis may be present in 30%.[116,117] There is evidence that some patients with disease onset early in life fail to reach predicted adult height.[118]

There are likely several pathogenetic mechanisms that lead to growth failure (see Figure 44-10), including chronic undernutrition secondary to inadequate intake, excessive losses, and increased energy requirement, as well as the effect of bowel inflammation on the growth process.[119,120] The anorexia present in some patients with Crohn's disease is striking and out of proportion to the severity of abdominal pain or diarrhea. In most patients, both basal and stimulated growth hormone levels are normal, but the concentration of insulinlike growth factor (IGF) 1 is reduced, suggesting a degree of hepatic growth hormone insensitivity. In an animal model of colitis, data suggest that part of the diminution in IGF-1 levels is from malnutrition and the remainder secondary to the effects of inflammation.[121] In this same animal model, appetite suppression appeared to be linked to increased serotonin release from the paraventricular nucleus of the hypothalamus, possibly induced by circulating proinflammatory cytokines.[122]

Chronic administration of high-dose daily corticosteroid therapy may be an iatrogenic cause of growth failure. Daily corticosteroid therapy for a period as short as 7 to 14 days is associated with decreased type I collagen production, a prerequisite for linear growth.[123] Alternate-day therapy appears to have little impact on growth velocity[123] or on type I or III collagen production.[124] It is often difficult to separate the growth-retarding effects of increased disease severity from those of the concomitant use of high doses of corticosteroids.

Psychologic Disturbances

In the 1950s, IBD was thought to be a psychosomatic disorder.[125] As knowledge regarding the pathology of Crohn's has grown, less research has focused on the interplay of psychologic disturbances and disease activity. However, recently there has been a resurgence of in evaluating the role of various psychologic stress factors on Crohn's disease. Depression and anxiety have been most extensively evaluated. Patients with inactive disease had a significantly higher relapse rate if they had a raised depression score.[125] Multiple studies have shown conflicting results regarding the benefit in disease activity with treatment of psychologic stress. The majority of these have shown some benefit including decrease in health care utilization; however, further studies are still needed.[125,126]

DIAGNOSIS

A combination of clinical and laboratory observations suggests a diagnosis of Crohn's disease, which is then confirmed with radiologic, endoscopic, and histologic findings (Table 44-3). Delayed diagnosis is common because the clinical findings may involve systems outside the gastrointestinal tract.

TABLE 44-3. Clinical and Laboratory Findings Used to Establish a Diagnosis of Crohn's Disease

History
Abdominal pain
Diarrhea
Rectal bleeding
Fever
Arthritis
Rash
Family history of IBD

Physical Examination
Abdominal tenderness
Abdominal mass
Perirectal disease
Clubbing
Stomatitis
Erythema nodosum
Pyoderma gangrenosum

Growth Data
Height and weight velocity
Decreased for age
Delayed puberty

Laboratory Tests
Anemia
Increased erythrocyte sedimentation rate
Increased C-reactive protein level
Hypoalbuminemia
Thrombocytosis
Positive stool occult blood
Serology (ANCA, ASCA, anti-Cbir1, anti-OmpC)

Imaging Including Ultrasound, Fluoroscopy, CT, MRI
Nodularity
Luminal narrowing, strictures
Bowel wall thickening
Abscess, phlegmon
Fistula

Endoscopy Including Wireless Capsule Endoscopy
Ulcers
Inflammation
Cobblestoning
Rectal sparing

CT, computed tomography; MRI, magnetic resonance imaging.

History and Physical Examination

A complete clinical history is mandatory and will elicit both gastrointestinal and extraintestinal manifestations detailed previously. Physical examination should include careful abdominal palpation with particular attention to tenderness, fullness, or mass. Careful inspection of the perirectal area and perineum is mandatory. One should consider rectal examination and stool guaiac as part of the routine physical examination in a child suspected of having IBD. The presence of stomatitis, clubbing, arthritis, erythema nodosum, or pyoderma gangrenosum is suggestive of IBD. Height and weight should be measured and compared with previous values to calculate the rate of change and to compare with expected values from standard growth curves.

Laboratory Evaluation

Appropriate stool cultures and examination should be made to exclude enteric bacterial pathogens and parasites including *Salmonella, Shigella, Campylobacter, E. coli* 0157:H7, *Yersinia,*

Aeromonas, Clostridium difficile, Cryptosporidium, and *Giardia.* Acute onset of bloody diarrhea with fever and vomiting is more suggestive of a bacterial pathogen than Crohn's disease.

Laboratory abnormalities frequently found include anemia (70% of patients), raised erythrocyte sedimentation rate (ESR) (80%) and/or C-reactive protein (CRP) (70%), hypoalbuminemia (60%) and guaiac-positive stools (35%).[127,128] Although thrombocytosis is common (60%), total leukocyte count is often normal. However, 21% of children with mild Crohn's disease had normal ESR, hemoglobin, platelet count, and albumin, though this was in contrast to patients with moderate to severe disease, who had normal parameters in only 3.8% of the cohort.[129] There may be bandemia. In the nutritionally depleted patient, serum zinc, magnesium, calcium, and phosphorus levels may be low. Serum aminotransferase levels are raised at the time of diagnosis in approximately 10% of patients.[98] Testing for ASCA, ANCA, anti-Cbir1, and anti-OmpC may be performed as described previously and usually serves as adjunctive evidence in the diagnosis.

Breath hydrogen testing for lactose malabsorption may be helpful in subsequent dietary management. Urinalysis should be performed to explore pyuria or infection associated with enterovesical fistula. Though not performed at all centers, fecal calprotectin can be complementary to other testing for diagnosis of Crohn's disease.[130]

Radiographic Evaluation

Small bowel imaging is strongly recommended and considered gold standard in all children suspected with Crohn's disease. Historically, the small bowel follow-through (SBFT) examination has been the radiological technique of choice in Crohn's disease. With the advancement in other modalities such as ultrasound, computed tomography (CT), and magnetic resonance imaging (MRI), more options are now available to assist in disease characterization.

Contrast Fluoroscopy

SBFT contrast imaging is used to identify irregular, nodular (cobblestoned), and thickened bowel loops, as well as stenotic areas (string sign), ulcers, and fistulas (Figure 44-11). Pathologic terminal ileal nodularity is common in Crohn's disease and must be distinguished from nonpathologic nodular lymphoid hyperplasia. In the latter the nodules are usually 3 mm or less in diameter.

Ultrasonography

Ultrasound is a noninvasive and radiation-free technique that permits better access than other radiologic techniques. Its role in Crohn's disease has been growing as it has a high negative-predictive value for disease diagnosis if bowel wall thickening is absent.[131] In a meta-analysis, ultrasound evidence of bowel wall thickness had a sensitivity of 75 to 95% with specificity of 67 to 100% for the diagnosis of Crohn's disease.[132] Similar values have been demonstrated in smaller pediatric studies, with the highest sensitivity in patients having terminal ileal involvement.[130] However, ultrasound can be limited by technical difficulties (obese patients) as well as its ability to evaluate for superficial lesions.[131] Ultrasound may also play a role in monitoring response to treatment (extent of disease, bowel-wall thickening, hyperemia on Doppler studies) as well as disease complications such as abscess formation or stenosis of bowel.

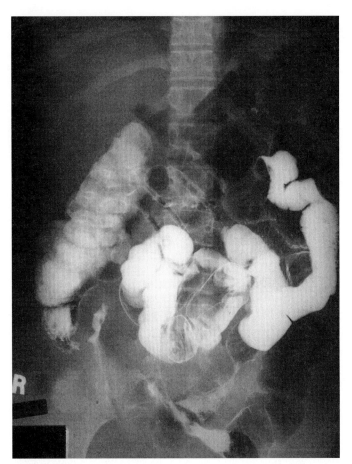

Figure 44-11. Distal ileal narrowing and distortion in an adolescent with newly diagnosed Crohn's disease.

This technique is very operator dependent and has not been adopted routinely in North America.

Computed Tomography

CT has become an important tool in the diagnosis and follow-up of patients with Crohn's disease. It may be useful in delineating bowel-wall inflammation and extramural extension of inflammation by fistulization to adjacent structures and in diagnosing abscesses (Figure 44-12). The use of negative luminal contrast (either orally or via a nasojejunal tube) in CT enterography or CT enteroclysis studies has improved mucosal detailing and luminal visualization and hence the diagnostic capabilities of the technique, as mural attenuation and wall thickness correlate highly with endoscopic and histologic findings.[133,134] This is different from the positive contrast use for standard CT scanning, and it is helpful to detect extraintestinal abnormalities not detected on SBFT. However, the clinician must be aware of the significant radiation exposure associated with abdominal CT, especially in the situation of repeated imaging in a child with Crohn's disease.

Magnetic Resonance Imaging

Although more costly than CT, MRI involves no radiation exposure and appears to have similar sensitivity to other imaging techniques.[135,136] MRI also has the advantage of revealing extraintestinal pathology. Intraluminal contrast is necessary for bowel loop separation and good contrast resolution between lumen, wall, and extraluminal structures. Further, the addition

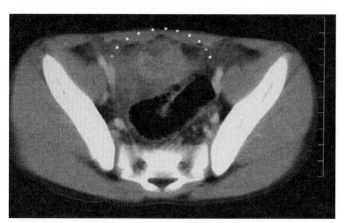

Figure 44-12. Marked distal small bowel wall thickening in an 8-year-old with Crohn's disease.

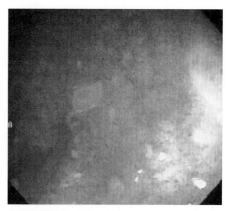

Figure 44-13. Colonic aphthous lesions in an adolescent with newly diagnosed Crohn's disease.

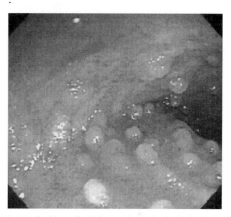

Figure 44-14. Marked lymphoid hyperplasia in Crohn's disease. (*See plate section for color.*)

of gadolinium has improved identification of small bowel abnormalities.[132] Similar to CT studies, luminal contrast can be given orally or via a nasojejunal tube. The latter technique may improve bowel distention of the small intestine; however, many practitioners prefer the oral enterographic approach because of its less invasive nature.[132,137] A recent study showed that MR enterography was diagnostically as effective as CT enterography and superior to SBFT for detection of ileitis and extraenteric complications of Crohn's disease, with the added benefit of being radiation free.[138] Pelvic MRI has also established itself as a reliable technique for assessment of perianal disease activity and fistulization.[139,140]

Endoscopic and Histologic Evaluation

Examination of the colon is often performed early in the evaluation of a child with chronic diarrhea, hematochezia, and abdominal pain with the aim of diagnosing IBD and helping to distinguish ulcerative colitis from Crohn's disease. The finding of aphthous lesions (small ulcers on an erythematous base) in the setting of an otherwise normal-looking colon is highly suggestive of Crohn's disease (Figure 44-13). Rectal sparing is unusual in ulcerative colitis and common in Crohn's disease. Patchiness of inflammation with abnormal areas interspersed with grossly normal-appearing areas is characteristic of Crohn's disease. Deep fissuring ulcers and heaped-up edematous mucosa (pseudopolyps) may be present. The ileocecal valve may appear granular, friable, and edematous. Intubation of the terminal ileum is critical in the diagnosis of Crohn's disease, often revealing marked nodularity, ulceration, and inflammation (Figure 44-14).

Mucosal biopsies should be taken from normal- and abnormal-appearing areas. Biopsies of normal-appearing areas may reveal inflammation and, rarely, granuloma, diagnostic of Crohn's disease. Although focally enhanced gastritis is common in Crohn's disease, it can also be present in patients with ulcerative colitis, and so its presence does not reliably differentiate between the two disorders.[141]

Wireless capsule endoscopy has become an adjunct diagnostic technique and is being used with increasing frequency in both children and adults in whom conventional evaluative techniques have been unrevealing, but in whom a high suspicion for Crohn's disease of the small bowel still exists.[142] Before capsule endoscopy, it is important that any bowel stenosis or stricture that might impair passage of the capsule has been evaluated by small bowel imaging.[143] Also, in an effort to avoid retention of the capsule, a dissolving test capsule or patency capsule has been developed. This capsule is constructed with dissolvable material and has a radiotag allowing for identification of the location of stenosis or stricture.[143]

DIFFERENTIAL DIAGNOSIS

The protean manifestations of Crohn's disease create a long differential diagnosis. Disease entities to be considered are reviewed in Table 44-4.

THERAPY

There is no cure for Crohn's disease, but emerging therapies have improved the therapeutic goal of bowel healing and long-lasting remission. Care must also be taken to use common sense, and treatment should be directed toward symptoms and quality of life, not just abnormal laboratory tests, biopsies, or radiographs. Management can be complex and must focus on the individual patient. Inflammation may be present without symptoms,[144] and symptoms may be present without inflammation (e.g., stricture, irritable bowel syndrome). There may be a considerable dissociation between abnormal test results and clinical activity.[144,145] The clinician must decide whether the target of therapy is to reduce inflammation, alleviate a surgical

TABLE 44-4. Differential Diagnosis of Presenting Symptoms of Crohn's Disease

Primary Presenting Symptom	Diagnostic Considerations
Right lower quadrant abdominal pain, with or without mass	Appendicitis, infection (e.g., *Campylobacter, Yersinia*), lymphoma, intussusception, mesenteric adenitis, Meckel's diverticulum, ovarian cyst
Chronic periumbilical or epigastric abdominal pain	Irritable bowel, constipation, lactose intolerance, peptic disease, celiac disease
Rectal bleeding, no diarrhea	Fissure, polyp, Meckel's diverticulum, rectal ulcer syndrome
Bloody diarrhea	Infection, hemolytic-uremic syndrome, Henoch-Schönlein purpura
Watery diarrhea	Irritable bowel, lactose intolerance, giardiasis, *Cryptosporidium*, sorbitol, laxatives
Perirectal disease	Fissure, hemorrhoid (rare), streptococcal infection, condyloma (rare)
Growth delay	Celiac disease, endocrinopathy
Anorexia, weight loss	Anorexia nervosa
Arthritis	Collagen vascular disease, infection
Liver abnormalities	Chronic hepatitis

condition, promote growth, improve quality of life, or a combination of these.

Pharmacologic Therapy

Multiple medications have proven efficacy in reducing symptoms, inducing remission, and maintaining remission. Traditionally, Crohn's disease was treated by a stepwise approach with less "powerful" and presumably safer agents tried first, and more "powerful" agents used subsequently as goals of treatment were not met. Individualization of treatment regimens and increasing experience with immunomodulators and biologic therapy has challenged this approach. Pharmacologic agents used to treat Crohn's disease can be divided into the following categories: aminosalicylates, corticosteroids, immunomodulators, antibiotics, and biologics[146,147] (Table 44-5).

Aminosalicylates

Aminosalicylates act at multiple levels in the inflammatory response. Actions include inhibition of leukotriene and thromboxane synthesis, scavenging of reactive oxygen metabolites, inhibition of platelet-activating factor synthesis and formation of nitric oxide, and alteration of mucosal prostaglandin profiles.[148]

Sulfasalazine (Azulfidine) and mesalamine (Asacol, Pentasa, Lialda, Apriso, Rowasa, Canasa) are used to treat mild to moderate Crohn's disease. Vehicles differ between the various forms of mesalamine medication, allowing for differences in dispersion in the intestinal tract.

Induction. Sulfasalazine is usually effective for mild to moderate Crohn's colitis but has no documented efficacy in small bowel disease.[149] The efficacy of mesalamine in the treatment of active Crohn's disease is more questionable.[150] Several studies have shown improvement in symptoms with mesalamine products as compared to placebo, especially with increasing doses.[151,152]

However, more recent studies have not replicated these results, and though meta-analysis showed an improvement in the Crohn's disease activity index (CDAI) in patients treated with drug compared to placebo, the observed numeric difference did not appear clinically significant.[153] Mesalamine enemas or suppositories may be used for distal colonic disease, especially when patients have significant symptoms of tenesmus. All of these studies are done in adult IBD patients, and thus the true efficacy in children remains unknown.

Maintenance and Postoperative Therapy. Similar to induction therapy, there is considerable controversy as to the role of 5-ASA in maintaining remission.[154] A large meta-analysis of 2097 adult patients showed that mesalamine significantly reduced the relapse rate following surgical induction of remission, but not medically induced remission.[155] Another study failed to show postsurgical benefit.[156]

Toxicity. 5-ASA is usually well tolerated, but dose-related and idiosyncratic reactions can occur. Worsening disease can be seen with any of these agents. Nausea and vomiting are more common with sulfasalazine. Less common but important complications include pancreatitis, blood dyscrasias, hair loss, hepatitis, nephritis, and pericarditis.[157,158]

Corticosteroids

The effects of corticosteroids in mitigating the inflammation have been reviewed in detail elsewhere.[159] Corticosteroids bind to corticosteroid receptors on target cells, regulating the expression of certain genes. An interaction between NF-κB and activated corticosteroid receptors may be crucial in the downregulation of proinflammatory mediators[160,161] such as IL-1, IL-6, IL-8, IFN-γ, TNF-α, adhesion molecules, and leukotrienes. The two corticosteroids used in clinical practice are prednisone (and its equivalents) and budesonide.

Induction. Systemic corticosteroids are very effective in the treatment of active disease in virtually all distributions of Crohn's disease.[149,162] Response rates of up to 90% have been demonstrated.[144,162] Oral therapy is usually initiated with prednisone at a dose of 1 mg/kg daily with a maximum of 40 to 60 mg/day. Intravenous therapy is occasionally used for particularly severe disease. The dose is tapered over several weeks to months and then discontinued depending on the patient's response. Corticosteroid dependence demonstrated by recurrent symptoms on tapering or shortly after withdrawal is common[163] and often necessitates the use of additional therapy. Resistance to corticosteroids can develop over time and appears to result from several mechanisms, including decreased cytoplasmic glucocorticoid concentration associated with overexpression of the multidrug resistance gene (*MDR1*), impaired glucocorticoid signaling because of dysfunction at the level of the glucocorticoid receptor, and proinflammatory mediator-induced inhibition of glucocorticoid receptor transcriptional activity.[164]

Budesonide, a synthetic steroid with high affinity for the glucocorticoid receptor (15 times that of prednisone), with potent anti-inflammatory activity and low systemic bioavailability (85% first-pass metabolism), is being used in the treatment of Crohn's disease.[159] Studies have shown that budesonide is superior to placebo[165] and mesalamine[166] in the treatment of ileal or ileocolonic disease, and similar to but not quite as good as prednisolone.[167,168] Efficacy in adults is greatest at a

TABLE 44-5. **Pharmacologic Therapy for Pediatric Crohn's Disease**

Drug Category	Indications	Daily Dose (mg/kg)	Maximum Dose
Aminosalicylates			
Sulfasalazine	Mild colonic disease	50-75	3-4 g
Mesalamine			
Pentasa	Mild small bowel or colonic disease	50-100	4 g
Asacol	Mild distal small bowel or colonic disease	50-100	4.8 g
Corticosteroids			
Prednisone	Moderate to severe small bowel or colonic disease	1	40-60 mg
Budesonide	Distal small bowel or ascending colon disease	n/a	6-9 mg
Immunomodulators			
Azathioprine	Steroid-dependent or refractory disease; minimize	2.5-3	250 mg*
6-Mercaptopurine	steroid use prospectively; perirectal disease	1-1.5	175 mg
Methotrexate	Steroid dependent or refractory disease	10-15 mg/m² (weekly, SQ)	25 mg (weekly, SQ)
Antibiotics			
Metronidazole	Perirectal disease; colonic disease	20-30	1.0 g
Ciprofloxacin	Perirectal disease	20 mg/kg	1 g
Anti-TNF			
Infliximab	Steroid-dependent or refractory disease; steroid sparing; perirectal disease; maintenance of remission; refractory extraintestinal disease	5-10 mg/kg[†] (IV)	n/a
Adalimumab[‡]	Steroid-dependent or refractory disease	160 mg, 80 mg, 40 mg at 0, 2, and 4 weeks, then 40 mg every other week	n/a
Certolizumab[‡]	Steroid-dependent or refractory disease	400 mg at 0, 2 and 4 weeks then every 4 weeks	n/a
Anti-adhesion Therapy			
Natalizumab	Previous treatment with anti-TNF therapy and continued active symptoms	300 mg IV every 4 weeks	n/a

*Maximum doses of azathioprine or 6-mercaptopurine are relative values and will be determined by clinical response, laboratory tolerance as reflected by complete blood count and serum aminotransferase levels, and 6-thioguanine levels.
†Infliximab is generally initially administered as a three-infusion series at 0, 2, and 6 weeks. Maintenance therapy is initially given every 8 weeks, and then every 6 to 12 weeks as determined by clinical course.
‡Currently adalimumab, certolizumab, and natalizumab are only approved for Crohn's patients over 18 years of age. Pediatric trials of adalimumab and certolizumab are ongoing.

dose of 9 mg/day. A nonblinded pediatric report showed similar findings.[169] Compared with prednisone, budesonide generally has fewer corticosteroid side effects and a diminished effect on the pituitary-adrenal axis, but these problems may still be found.[167,168,170] Some data suggest a switch from prednisone to budesonide in patients with prednisone-dependent remission to decrease corticosteroid-associated side effects.[171] Corticosteroid enemas may be used for relief of symptoms caused by inflammation of the sigmoid and rectum.

Maintenance and Postoperative Therapy. Prednisone does not decrease the risk of relapse in patients with medically induced remission.[162] In comparison with placebo, budesonide has no beneficial effect in decreasing relapse rates at 1 year following medically or surgically induced remission.[172-174] This was confirmed in a recent Cochrane Database systemic review.[175] However, in a small study of corticosteroid-dependent patients in remission, those switched to budesonide had a lower relapse rate at 1 year than patients tapered off prednisone and switched to mesalamine (55% versus 82%).[176]

Toxicity. The toxicity of corticosteroid therapy relates to the size and duration of the dose administered and causes significant morbidity, especially in pediatric patients. Growth inhibition is a major problem with daily therapy, but normal growth rates may be preserved with alternate-day therapy.[123] In one small study, budesonide did not appear to improve growth in children who had decreased gastrointestinal symptoms.[177] Compliance with corticosteroid therapy may be problematic in children and adolescents, who suffer mood swings and develop cosmetic problems such as acne and cushingoid facies. Adequate calcium intake and maintaining physical activity are important in preventing corticosteroid-induced bone disease. Avascular necrosis has been noted in 0.3 to 0.5% of patients with Crohn's disease.[178,179] Though some of the patients with this complication had not been exposed to steroids, Crohn's disease appears to predispose patients to chronic steroid usage-induced osteonecrosis.[180]

Immunomodulators

Immunomodulator therapy is commonly used in the treatment of Crohn's disease refractory to corticosteroids or when patients cannot be weaned from corticosteroids, and increasingly as primary therapy. The potential mechanisms of action and pharmacology of these medications have been reviewed previously.[181] Azathioprine and 6-mercaptopurine (6-MP) remain the most commonly used immunomodulators. The metabolism of 6-MP and its prodrug azathioprine are shown in Figure 44-15. Deficiency of the enzyme thiopurine methyltransferase (TPMT) (severe in 0.3% of the population and moderate in 11%) can lead to high 6-thioguanine levels, which may exert severe bone marrow toxicity. Patients should have quantitative measurement

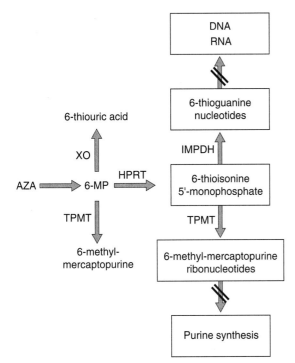

Figure 44-15. Metabolism of azathioprine (AZA) and 6-mercaptopurine (6-MP). HPRT, hypoxanthine phosphoribosyl transferase; IMPDH, inosine 5'-monophosphate dehydrogenase; TPMT, thiopurine methyltranferase; XO, xanthine oxidase.

of TPMT before starting therapy to assist in choosing the appropriate starting dose for a patient.[182] Methotrexate has also been used in the treatment of Crohn's disease, given its success in other immune-related disorders such as rheumatoid arthritis and psoriasis.[183]

Induction. 6-MP (1 to 1.5 mg/kg daily) and azathioprine (2.5 to 3 mg/kg daily) are effective in patients with active disease when added to corticosteroid therapy. They facilitate the development of remission and promote tapering of corticosteroids.[184,185] Either medication usually requires 2 to 4 months to show efficacy, and neither is very effective as primary induction therapy as a single agent. A double-blind placebo-controlled trial showed that the addition of 6-MP to corticosteroids at initiation of therapy in children was associated with lower cumulative corticosteroid requirements and prolonged remission.[184] Therapeutic effect and toxicity correlate with 6-MP metabolite levels, and these can be utilized to assist in dose adjustment.[186-188] TPMT enzyme activity level can be measured before initiating therapy, and if it is normal, full-dose therapy can be started. If TPMT is not measured, it is preferable to start at a lower dose and to monitor blood counts frequently (at 1 to 2 weeks × 1 month, then every 2 to 4 weeks × 2 months, followed by monthly × 3 months, and then every 2 to 3 months). 6-Thioguanine therapy should not be used because of the risk of serious liver injury.[187]

Methotrexate (25 mg subcutaneously, once weekly) was more effective than placebo in facilitating remission in adult patients receiving prednisone for chronically active disease.[189] Published data in children are limited, but several small nonblinded studies suggest efficacy in children refractory to or intolerant of 6-MP.[190,191] The mandatory coadministration of folic acid may minimize side effects such as nausea and hair loss.

The utility of cyclosporin to treat active inflammatory disease is uncertain, with conflicting studies on efficacy.[192,193] It may be helpful in the treatment of severe perirectal fistula.[194] Oral tacrolimus is associated with fistula improvement but not resolution.[195]

Maintenance Therapy. 6-MP and azathioprine have been shown to decrease significantly the likelihood of recurrent disease in patients in remission.[196,197] Methotrexate has also shown ability to maintain remission when compared to placebo.[191] Maintenance is hard to achieve with cyclosporin. Immunomodulator therapy was shown to lessen intra-abdominal septic complications in adults with Crohn's disease undergoing bowel reanastomosis or strictureplasty.[198]

Toxicity. All immunomodulators predispose patients to an increased risk of infection. Myelosuppression is a potentially serious side effect of azathioprine/6-MP, particularly in those with TPMT deficiency; however, leukopenia can be seen with 6-MP therapy in the absence of TPMT deficiency at any time during administration, and blood counts should be monitored periodically (every 2 to 3 months).[199] TPMT activity may be inhibited by aminosalicylates, and leukopenia may be more common with the coadministration of mesalamine and has also been reported with infliximab.[200,201] Other side effects associated with azathioprine/6-MP include pancreatitis, hepatitis, fever, rash, and arthralgia. A theoretical risk for the development of malignancy has been suggested for long-term therapy, but is thought to be quite low.[202] Methotrexate therapy has been associated with hepatitis, hypersensitivity pneumonitis (1 in every 300 patients), nausea, and rash. The risk of hepatic fibrosis is thought to be low in patients with IBD treated with methotrexate.

Biologic Therapy

Antibodies that neutralize tumor necrosis factor-α (TNF-α) are the biologic therapy most commonly used in Crohn's disease. The most experience in children exists with the anti-TNF-α antibody infliximab. Infliximab is a chimeric (70% human, 30% mouse) IgG$_1$ monoclonal antibody that binds TNF-α. Infliximab has been used for moderate to severe luminal disease, corticosteroid-dependent or -refractory disease, and fistulous disease and to address a variety of extraintestinal manifestations. Adalimumab, a fully human monoclonal antibody, and certolizumab, a recombinant humanized antibody, are newer to the market and approved for use in adult patients with Crohn's disease. Pediatric trials with these medications are ongoing.

Natalizumab, an IgG4 monoclonal antibody that blocks adhesion and migration of leukocytes into the gut by binding the α$_4$-integrin, is approved for adults only with Crohn's disease. Natalizumab has been shown to be efficacious in inducing remission in Crohn's patients, especially those with an elevated C-reactive protein and active disease.[203] Published experience in children has demonstrated efficacy equal to adult studies but limited to 38 children and adolescents treated with low-dose therapy.[204] Monotherapy with this agent is mandatory, because concerns for progressive multifocal leukoencephalopathy (PML) have been raised.[205]

Induction. Controlled data in adults have shown efficacy of infliximab, adalimumab, and certolizumab in inducing response in patients with moderate to severe disease.[206-208] These results have been replicated in pediatric studies for infliximab and adalimumab.[209,210] Infliximab has also been shown effective for treatment of fistulous[211] disease. The ability of anti-TNF therapy to allow a decrease in dosage or elimination of corticosteroid therapy in some patients has proven very beneficial.[212] In luminal inflammatory disease, short-term response rates range from 50% to 80%, and endoscopic healing of diseased bowel has been demonstrated in some patients. Healing of perirectal fistula occurs in some patients. Extraintestinal complications of Crohn's disease such as pyoderma gangrenosum have been treated successfully with infliximab.[213] Infliximab is given initially as three infusions of 5 mg per kg per dose at 0, 2, and 6 weeks. Higher dosing (up to 10 mg per kg per dose) can be given if necessary. Episodic dosing appears to be associated with a higher risk of subsequent allergic reactions. Adalimumab induction dosing for individuals weighing more than 40 kg is 160 mg, then 80 mg, followed by 40 mg; certolizumab induction dosing is 400 mg at 0, 2, and 4 weeks.

Maintenance Therapy. Infliximab (every 8 to 12 weeks), adalimumab (every 2 weeks), and certolizumab (every 4 weeks) are more effective than placebo in maintaining remission in adults with luminal Crohn's disease.[214-216] Furthermore, regularly scheduled maintenance treatment regimens of infliximab improve outcomes compared with those in patients receiving maintenance therapy in an episodic fashion.[217] Remission of active fistula is also improved with maintenance infliximab, but recurrence is common once therapy is stopped.[218] Maintenance of remission has been demonstrated in pediatric studies with infliximab at least 3 years after initiation of therapy,[209,219] as well as adalimumab 1 year after initiation of therapy.[210] Studies are ongoing with certolizumab.

Special Issues. One of the challenges that emerged with the introduction of biologic therapy in Crohn's disease relates to the role of monotherapy (i.e., biologic therapy only) versus concomitant therapy (i.e., biologic plus immunomodulator). The controversy over concomitant therapies centers around balancing potential increased efficacy with possible increased risk of malignancy, specifically hepatosplenic T-cell lymphoma (HSTCL). This is a rare and often fatal subtype of peripheral T-cell non-Hodgkin's lymphoma.[220] HSTCL has been reported in a handful of IBD patients (primarily males and less than age of 21) treated with 6-MP/azathioprine alone, or with these thiopurines combined with infliximab or adalimumab.[220,221] Signs and symptoms associated with HSTCL can include fever, fatigue, elevation in liver enzymes, anemia, leukopenia, splenomegaly, and hepatomegaly. In the randomized control trials performed on biologics, response rate was not significantly different between patients who were on immunomodulators and those who were not at the time of starting the biologic.[207,222] Further, withdrawal of immunomodulators 6 months after starting infliximab did not result in a difference in treatment outcomes or mucosal healing compared to those who were continued on concomitant therapy.[223] Recent data, however, have shown improved response rates in adults naïve to immunomodulators on concomitant therapy versus monotherapy.[224] In this study, 508 adult Crohn's disease patients who were naïve to both biologics and immunomodulators were randomized to receive azathioprine plus placebo, infliximab plus placebo, or azathioprine and infliximab. At 50 weeks post initiation of treatment, steroid-free remission was significantly higher in the

concomitant treatment group (46%) versus 35% and 24% in the infliximab monotherapy and azathioprine monotherapy groups, respectively.[224] There was no increased risk of adverse events including malignancies in the dual therapy group, but the follow-up is too short to support any conclusions about lymphoma risk.

Toxicity. Numerous minor and significant acute and late complications have been seen with infliximab therapy. Infusion reactions are most common (5 to 10% of patients) and are generally associated with the presence of higher-titer antibody to infliximab (ATI).[225-227] High-titer ATI may also be associated with shorter duration of action of the drug.[225,228] Concomitant immunomodulator therapy as well as regular dosing of infliximab (every 8 weeks) reduces ATI formation.[225,229] Intravenous hydrocortisone premedication before infliximab infusion reduces ATI levels but does not eliminate formation or infusion reactions.[229] Maintenance scheduled infusions also appear to be associated with a lower likelihood of antibody development.[229] A delayed serum sickness-like reaction has been described in 1 to 3% of patients.[226,230] A high percentage of treated adult patients develop antinuclear antibodies (more than 50%), but clinical autoimmunity is rare.[231] Fatal tuberculosis as well as other opportunistic infections such as cytomegalovirus, histoplasmosis, aspergillosis, *Listeria*, *Pneumocystis*, and varicella infection among others have been seen. Purified protein derivative (PPD) testing should always precede infliximab therapy. Intra-abdominal infection is an absolute contraindication to infliximab therapy, and any abscess should be drained and treated before therapy. Lymphoproliferative disease has been described in adults[232] and pediatric patients[220,221] in the setting of infliximab therapy as well as hepatosplenic T-cell lymphoma as discussed previously. Cause and effect of this serious latter problem is not established, but great care is required in selecting patients for this therapy and in monitoring their course. Any patient with a previous history of lymphoma should not receive infliximab. Further contraindications to infliximab therapy include multiple sclerosis or optic neuritis, and congestive heart failure.

Antibiotics and Probiotics

These medications have long been used as both primary treatment and to address the complications of Crohn's disease.

Antibiotics

ACTIVE DISEASE. Metronidazole has similar efficacy to sulfasalazine in the treatment of Crohn's disease of the colon.[233] It has been used as the drug of choice for perirectal fistula, although the problem usually flares on discontinuation of therapy. Metronidazole plus ciprofloxacin had a similar efficacy to methylprednisolone in a small group of adults with active disease.[234] Ciprofloxacin is commonly used to treat perirectal disease, although controlled data are lacking.

MAINTENANCE THERAPY. Metronidazole (20 mg/kg daily) decreases the likelihood of endoscopic recurrence at 3 months and clinical recurrence by 1 year following ileal resection.[235]

TOXICITY. Peripheral neuropathy is the most serious side effect of metronidazole therapy. Rarely, paresthesias may persist despite discontinuing the medication. Nausea and a metallic taste are common. *Candida* esophagitis has been seen in adolescents treated with broad-spectrum antibiotics who are also receiving immunosuppressive therapy (personal observation).

Probiotics. Though widely used by patients because of anecdotal and word-of-mouth evidence of benefit, at present there are no controlled data suggesting efficacy of prebiotics or probiotics in the acute or chronic management of Crohn's disease.[236] A study in adults showed no efficacy of *Lactobacillus* GG in preventing recurrent disease after definitive resection.[237]

Adjunctive Therapy

Enteric-coated fish oil preparation has been used to maintain remission in Crohn's patients.[238] Other treatments have focused on symptom control. Loperamide may help control diarrhea. Anticholinergics such as dicycloverine may be helpful in subjects with Crohn's disease who also have irritable bowel syndrome-like symptoms. Low-dose tricyclic antidepressant therapy (e.g., amitriptyline 10 to 20 mg/day) may also be helpful in this situation. Cholestyramine, a bile acid-binding resin, may decrease diarrhea in patients who have had terminal ileal resection or extensive ileal disease with the attendant loss of bile acids into the colon stimulating colonic secretion. Individuals with extensive resection of the terminal ileum are at risk for developing vitamin B_{12} deficiency and should receive parenteral supplementation. Calcium supplementation should be provided to at least meet the recommended daily requirement if not met by dietary intake. Nonsteroidal anti-inflammatory drugs (NSAIDs) may exacerbate Crohn's disease and should be avoided if possible.

Nutritional Therapy

Nutritional therapy can be used as primary therapy without accompanying pharmacologic intervention or as adjunctive therapy with medications. It should always be used in patients suffering malnutrition.

Active Disease. Total parenteral nutrition and bowel rest may be effective in inducing remission in up to 60 to 80% of subjects.[239] A large meta-analysis of exclusive enteral nutrition therapy, with either elemental or polymeric diets, showed a large range (20 to 80%) of remission.[240] In general, enteral therapy was less effective than corticosteroids in effecting remission in studies where a comparison was made. No differences have been demonstrated between elemental and nonelemental diets. Relapse rate after enteral nutrition-induced remission is greater than that following remission achieved with prednisolone.[241] In selected children with growth failure, particularly those with predominantly small bowel disease, enteral nutritional therapy may be preferable to corticosteroids as initial therapy. Most children require nasogastric tube administration of these formulas, as oral acceptance is low. It has been suggested and disputed that the fat content of these enteral formulas might affect the success rate, with fat blends that promote proinflammatory mediator production (n6 polyunsaturated fatty acids) being inferior to those containing monounsaturated fatty acids.[242,243] Glutamine supplementation of the enteral formula appears to offer no advantage.

Maintenance Therapy. Data are limited. One study showed that after successful treatment of active Crohn's disease in children and adolescents by exclusive enteral nutritional therapy, supplementary enteral nutrition prolonged remission and was associated with improved growth.[244] Gastrostomy placement is safe and well tolerated in children being treated with long-term enteral therapy who do not want to use a nasogastric tube.

Other Indications. Intensive nutritional support, primarily through enteral supplementation via tube feedings, has been shown to be effective in reversing growth retardation in most patients.[116] It is *imperative* that nutritional support be started well before physiologic bone maturation and fusion of epiphyses if catch-up growth is to be expected, and that noncorticosteroid regimens be used to suppress bowel inflammation.

Surgery

Following terminal ileal resection, endoscopic evidence of recurrent disease is present at the neoterminal ileum in more than 70% of adults at 1 year after surgery, although only 35% are symptomatic.[245] In one pediatric series, clinical recurrence rates were 17%, 38%, and 60% at 1, 3, and 5 years, respectively.[246] In patients with higher pediatric Crohn's disease activity index (PCDAI) scores, the preoperative use of 6-MP and colonic disease were associated with higher recurrence rates, perhaps reflecting more aggressive disease at the time of surgery. Segmental colonic resection with reanastomosis is associated with a higher risk of recurrence than ileal or ileocecal resection.[246,247] The recurrence rate at the neoterminal ileum 5 to 10 years after panproctocolectomy and ileostomy is 70% when ileal disease was present at the time of surgery versus only 10% when disease was limited to the colon.[248] Postsurgical therapy with immunomodulators or biologics should be considered in patients at increased risk for recurrence.

Strictureplasty is a well-accepted method in the surgical management of adult and pediatric patients with Crohn's disease.[249,250] In this procedure, a longitudinal incision is made through the stenotic bowel and the opening is then closed transversely. The risk of reoperation following strictureplasty is no greater than when resection is performed. Strictureplasty is generally performed on small intestinal strictures or at an ileocolonic anastomosis in the presence of mostly fibrotic disease. Mild inflammation does not preclude strictureplasty.

Unless perianal hygiene is severely compromised, perianal skin tags are generally not excised. A variety of surgical techniques has been developed to help address severe perirectal disease refractory to medical management. Anal fissures generally heal and should not be treated surgically. Superficial perianal abscesses can be treated with incision and drainage. Deep abscesses are frequently associated with high perianal fistula and are treated with incision and drainage followed by placement of a noncutting seton. While the seton facilitates drainage of the abscess, it also perpetuates the fistula. Complex fistulas may require long-term drainage and staged fistulotomy. Control of symptoms is the realistic goal of such therapy. Proctectomy and diversion of the fecal stream may be required for particularly severe perirectal disease. Marked rectal disease, with or without complex fistula formation, may eventually lead to rectal stenosis requiring dilation.

Despite intensive medical and nutritional therapy, growth failure still persists in some children with Crohn's disease. Provided the subject is prepubertal or in early puberty, surgery may significantly improve growth in most of these children if good nutrition can be maintained, and corticosteroid therapy can be discontinued or weaned to an alternate-day schedule.[251]

Homeopathy

Homeopathic remedies are frequently used by patients and families in the management of Crohn's disease. To date, no controlled data have shown efficacy. These remedies are often used without the knowledge of the attending physician, because families may want to avoid confrontation.

Psychologic Therapy

Education of both patient and family is essential in the management of Crohn's disease. Demystification of the disease course and thorough explanation of the rationale for and complications of therapy often relieve unjustified fears. Counseling and attendance at age- and sex-matched peer groups may be helpful. Antidepressant and antianxiety therapy can be offered and are quite helpful when indicated.

NATURAL HISTORY

Disease Course

Crohn's disease is marked by periods of exacerbation and remission. Historically, only 1% of adult patients with well-documented Crohn's disease do not suffer at least one relapse following diagnosis and initial therapy[252]; of a cohort of 480 adults, only 10% maintained long-term remission free of corticosteroids following their initial presentation.[253] Children with ileocolitis generally have a poorer response to medications and a greater need for surgery than those with small bowel disease alone. Yet to be determined in either of these populations is whether current immunomodulatory therapy and emerging biologic therapy will affect the likelihood of disease exacerbation and need for surgery. Data have suggested that markers of inflammation such as C-reactive protein, orosomucoid, and erythrocyte sedimentation rate identify patients at higher risk for recurrence.[254] Younger age (less than 25 years) appears to be associated with a greater risk of relapse. A history of multiple previous relapses is probably the greatest predictor of subsequent relapses. Smoking is a significant risk factor for recurrence.

Malignancy

There have been concerns raised regarding three types of malignancy and Crohn's disease: colorectal cancer, small bowel cancer, and lymphoma.

The risk of colorectal cancer appears to be similar in ulcerative colitis and Crohn's colitis and is affected by disease duration and severity,[255] occurring a median of 18 years after the onset of Crohn's disease.[256] Chronic 5-ASA administration may decrease the risk.[255] Yearly screening colonoscopy for patients with colonic inflammation of greater than 8 to 10 years' duration appears warranted. Adenocarcinoma of the small bowel is rare, but occurs more frequently than in the general population; the rare affected patients often have disease for more than

20 years at the time of cancer development, tend to be male, have fistulizing disease, and often have surgically excluded loops.[255,257]

It is controversial whether there is a primary relationship between Crohn's disease and an increased risk of non-Hodgkin's lymphoma.[221,258,259] A slightly increased risk may be observed with the administration of azathioprine or 6-MP,[258,259] but improved quality-adjusted life expectancy because of therapeutic effect on the disease course may outweigh this incremental risk. Lymphoproliferative disease has been described in recipients of anti-TNF-α therapy[232]; after discontinuation of this therapy, outcome has ranged from lymphoma regression to death. Hepatosplenic T cell lymphoma in patients on concomitant treatment of infliximab or adalimumab with azathioprine or 6-MP in mostly teenage males, though very rare, is certainly concerning and needs to be discussed with families on initiation of various treatment regimens.[221]

Mortality

Death from Crohn's disease in the pediatric population is extremely rare. Adults with Crohn's disease appear to have a slight increased mortality risk compared with age-matched controls.[260]

ACKNOWLEDGMENT

The author is indebted to Andrew Ricci, Jr, MD, and Fabiola Balerezo, MD, for their contribution to the pathology section of this chapter.

REFERENCES

30. Barret JC, Hansoul S, Nicolae DL, et al. Genome-wide association defines more than thirty distinct susceptibility loci for Crohn's disease. Nat Genet 2008;40:955–962.
184. Markowitz J, Grancher K, Kohn N, et al. A multicenter trial of 6-mercaptopurine and prednisone in children with newly diagnosed Crohn's disease. Gastroenterology 2000;119:895–902.
202. Siegel CA, Marden SM, Persing SM, et al. Risk of lymphoma associated with combination anti-tumor necrosis factor and immunomodulator therapy for the treatment of Crohn's disease: a meta-analysis. Clin Gastroenterol Hepatol 2009;7:874–881.
209. Hyams J, Crandall W, Kugathasan S, et al. Induction and maintenance infliximab therapy for the treatment of moderate-to-severe Crohn's disease in children. Gastroenterology 2007;132:863–873.
210. Rosh J, Lerer T, Markowitz J, et al. Retrospective evaluation of the safety and effect of adalimumab therapy (RESEAT) in pediatric Crohn's disease. Am J Gastroenterol 2009;104:3042–3049.
220. Rosh JR, Gross T, Mamula P, et al. Hepatosplenic T-cell lymphoma in adolescents and young adults with Crohn's disease: a cautionary tale? Inflamm Bowel Dis 2007;13:1024–1030.
261. Sartor RB. Microbial influences in inflammatory bowel diseases. Gastroenterology 2008;134:577–594.

See expertconsult.com for a complete list of references and the review questions for this chapter.

45 ULCERATIVE COLITIS IN CHILDREN AND ADOLESCENTS

James F. Markowitz

Ulcerative colitis (UC) is an important pediatric gastrointestinal disease, given its potential for significant morbidity and even mortality during childhood, its chronicity, and its premalignant nature. Although significant advances in our understanding of its immunologic basis have led to novel approaches to its therapy, UC remains medically incurable. Nevertheless, current medical and surgical therapeutic options have improved the overall outlook for children with this condition.

EPIDEMIOLOGY

As opposed to the documented rise in incidence of pediatric Crohn's disease over the past few decades, incidence rates of UC in children appear to have remained fairly stable in some parts of the world while rising in other areas. Population-based studies from Wisconsin[1] and northern Stockholm[2] describe incidence rates of 2.1 and 2.2 per 100,000 population per year, respectively, rates that fall in the middle of the range of estimates of 0.5 to 4.3 per 100,000 population per year reported in earlier studies.[3] By contrast, incidence rates in eastern Europe are at the lower end of those reported. For instance, in central and western Slovenia the incidence of UC in children was 0.77 per 100,000 per year in the late 1990s, increasing to 1.57 per 100,000 per year in data collected between 2000 and 2005.[4] Although the incidence rates for UC appear to be about half of that seen for Crohn's disease in the same population,[1,2,4] anomalies exist, such as recent studies from Poland and Italy that report incidence rates of UC in children to be greater than that of CD.[5,6] Estimated prevalence rates in children are 18 to 30 per 100,000.

Males and females are equally affected. Although the majority of pediatric patients with UC present as adolescents (87% of subjects in a review from the Cleveland Clinic),[7] very young children with UC are not unusual[8,9] and about 40% of children with UC present by the age of 10 years.[10] Care must be exercised in diagnosing the youngest children, however, given the predilection for children under age 10 years with Crohn's disease to present with isolated colitis.[11] When followed over time, a significant number of these children with apparent UC will demonstrate features consistent with Crohn's.[9]

Overall, 10 to 15% of children with UC have first-degree relatives with inflammatory bowel disease (IBD).[10,12] However, 22.6% of Jewish children with UC have affected relatives, compared with only 13.7% of non-Jewish children.[12] Children with UC are more likely than their unaffected siblings to have had diarrhea during infancy.[13] However, children who received formula feedings as infants appear to be at no greater risk of developing UC than those who were breast-fed.[14]

Appendectomy for acute appendicitis before 20 years of age clearly protects against the development of UC in adults.[15] Interestingly, it appears that protection against UC is not conferred by the appendectomy itself, but rather by the acute appendicitis or mesenteric lymphadenitis prompting appendectomy. This has recently been demonstrated convincingly using population based data from 709,353 people from Denmark and Sweden with a total duration of follow-up of 11.1 million years.[16] Whereas appendectomy before age 20 years in patients with documented appendicitis or mesenteric lymphadenitis reduced the risk of subsequent UC by about half, appendectomy performed in patients without these underlying inflammatory disorders has no effect on the subsequent rate of developing UC. It is not clear, however, to what degree this factor protects against the development of UC during childhood.

The effect of either active or passive cigarette smoking on the risk of developing UC during childhood is also not clear. Epidemiologic studies have documented that passive smoking during childhood protects against developing UC as an adult.[17] However, although passive smoking may increase the risk of developing Crohn's disease as a child, a protective effect against the development of UC during childhood has not been clearly demonstrated.[13,18] In fact, one study has suggested that becoming a smoker before the age of 10 years is associated with an earlier age of developing UC compared to patients who never smoked.[19] In addition, a case-control study questions whether cigarette smoking is protective against UC in adults at all, as adults who had never smoked could not be shown to have an increased risk of UC compared with active smokers.[20] In this study, the risk of UC appeared to be increased only in smokers who had stopped smoking, suggesting the possibility that the disease was either triggered or unmasked by the removal of an immunosuppressive effect exerted by cigarette smoke.

GENETICS

Genetic factors are important in UC, although to a lesser degree than in Crohn's disease. Studies consistently demonstrate a lower rate of IBD in relatives of probands with UC than in those with Crohn's disease.[12,21,22] Similarly, the rate of concordant disease is much less for monozygotic twin pairs with UC than it is for those with Crohn's disease.[23]

Despite this, a number of genetic breakthroughs in UC have been made. Among the first was the recognition of an association between HLA class II alleles and UC. HLA-DR2 has been found in 40% of a U.S. population with UC, confirming previous studies in which 70% of a Japanese population with UC was found to have the same association.[24,25] Further work has demonstrated additional UC-associated histocompatibility gene loci in the Japanese population, including HLA-B and HLA-DRB1.[25] A specific allele of another HLA-associated gene, major histocompatibility complex (MHC) class I chain-related gene A, has been shown to be associated with UC in a Japanese population, and homozygosity for the allele is associated with earlier age of disease onset.[27]

Another gene of interest is the multidrug resistance 1 (MDR1) gene, located on chromosome 7 in a region identified by genome-wide scans as a potential site of an IBD susceptibility gene. Abnormal gene expression is characterized by decreased production of P-glycoprotein, an important barrier to microbial invasion of the intestine. Studies have identified genetic polymorphisms in the MDR1 gene more frequently in white patients with UC than in normal controls or those with Crohn's disease.[28] Similar abnormalities have been replicated in a genetically heterogeneous population from northern India.[29] This abnormality potentially impairs colonic defenses against luminal bacteria or toxins, a defect that could result in a chronic immune response. This observation is of particular importance, as an MDR1 knockout mouse has been shown to develop a form of colitis similar to UC that can be prevented by antibiotics.[30]

A number of other genes or gene loci have been identified as potentially important in the susceptibility to or development of UC (Table 45-1). Many have been identified as the result of genome-wide association studies. Variants associated with either increased or decreased odds ratios for association with UC have been identified. In most cases, the specific genes involved and the role that the gene products play in the development of UC have not been clarified.

ETIOLOGY

Despite significant advances in unraveling the pathophysiology of UC, its etiology remains unknown. Numerous theories have been proposed over the years.

Immunity

Current opinion appears to favor a defect in immune regulation as the primary cause of UC. As opposed to the predominantly cell-mediated response seen in Crohn's disease, the immunologic profile of patients with UC is characterized by a predominantly humoral response.[39] In UC, there is marked overproduction of IgG_1 by both intestinal lymphocytes and those in the peripheral circulation.[40] Autoantibodies have been identified that are directed against colonic epithelial proteins such as the cytoskeletal protein tropomyosin.[41] In addition, these autoantibodies cross-react with antigens in tissues commonly affected by the extraintestinal manifestations of UC, including the biliary epithelium, skin, chondrocyte, and ciliary body of the eye.[42] Which factor or factors initiate this autoimmune process remains to be elucidated.

The genetic discoveries of the past few years, however, appear to confirm the hypothesis that UC is caused by a defect in immune regulation. The genes that have been shown to be associated with UC potentially play important roles in preventing enteric organisms from accessing the lamina propria (e.g., decreased production of P-glycoprotein due to defective MDR1 gene expression) or in immune response (e.g., HLA genes, interleukin (IL) 11, TNF-α).[24-38] These functions suggest that the driving force for the unremitting inflammation characterizing

TABLE 45-1. **Putative UC-Associated Genes and Gene Loci**

UC-Associated Genes
HLA genes
HLA-DR2[24,225]
HLA-B[26]
HLA-DRB1[26]
MHC class 1 chain relayed gene A[27]
MDR-1[28,29]
TNF-α receptor 1B[31]
ICAM-1[32]
IL-11[33]
IL-1 receptor antagonist[34]
IL-10 gene promoter[35]
IL-10[36]
ARPC2[36]
UC-Associated Gene Loci
4q27 (IL2, IL21)[37]
1p36[38]
12q15[38]
6p21[38]
1p31 (IL23R)[38]

UC appears to be the normal enteric flora rather than an enteric pathogen. How these genes promote the chronic inflammation of UC, and whether they predispose to the development of autoantibodies, remains to be determined.

Infectious Agents

Although there is great clinical similarity between UC and infectious colitides, no solid evidence supports the theory that an infectious agent is the primary cause of colonic inflammation in UC. Children can initially present with documented enteric infection such as *Salmonella* or *Clostridium difficile*, only to be found after clearance of the pathogen to have persistent, chronic inflammation. In fact, compared to controls who never had a documented infection with either *Salmonella* or *Campylobacter*, a population-based study from Denmark identified a nearly threefold increase in IBD (both UC and Crohn's disease) in subjects in the 15-year period following one of these infections.[43] Despite this, the majority of patients lack such a history. Although cytomegalovirus is probably not an etiologic agent in the development of UC, it does appear to be associated with up to 25% of cases of steroid-resistant fulminant disease.[44]

Food Allergy

Allergic reactions, especially to dietary antigens such as milk, have been investigated extensively, but data supporting an allergic etiology for UC are lacking. High titers of antibodies to dietary antigens such as milk are not specific to UC.[45] Patients with UC at times respond to elemental or elimination diets, but when the particular food that appeared to induce symptoms is reintroduced, symptoms are only rarely reproduced consistently.[46]

Psychologic Factors

In the past, UC has been considered to be a psychosomatic disorder. However, although children with UC often demonstrate psychologic profiles that distinguish them from healthy children and other chronic disease controls,[47-51] these traits do not appear to be the cause of the illness. An analysis of the literature on the psychosomatic etiology of UC demonstrates many methodologic deficiencies, including lack of controls, lack of diagnostic criteria, and nonblinded collection of data.[52] None of the well-designed studies in the literature shows an association between UC and psychiatric disturbance.

Metabolic Deficiencies – Short-Chain Fatty Acids

Short-chain fatty acids extracted from the luminal contents are a major source of energy for the colonocyte. The observation that fecal butyrate is increased in UC has suggested the possibility that UC might represent a form of colonic mucosal "malnutrition."[53,54] It is not clear, however, that the observed increase in fecal butyrate in UC is due to the colonocyte's inability to utilize short-chain fatty acids as metabolic fuel.

Diet

Little is known about the effect of diet on the development of UC in children. However, a recent prospective study in adults has demonstrated that subjects with the highest intake of n-6 polyunsaturated fatty acids (PUFAs) (as linoleic acid) were more than twice as likely (OR = 2.49, 95% CI 1.23 to 5.07, p = .01) as those with the lowest intake to develop UC.[55] Thirty percent of the identified UC cases could be attributed to the highest consumption of linoleic acid. By contrast, those with the highest intake of the n-3 PUFA, docosahexaenoic acid, had a significantly reduced odds ratio (0.23, 95% CI 0.06 to 0.97) for the development of UC. As n-6 PUFAs are converted into proinflammatory molecules including arachidonic acid, prostaglandin E2, leukotriene B4, and thromboxane A2, there is biologic plausibility for the hypothesis that high consumption of linoleic acid (found in red meats and cooking oils) might contribute to the development of UC. Similarly, n-3 PUFA promote the production of antiinflammatory molecules, such that a diet high in these fatty acids might plausibly protect against the development of UC.

PATHOLOGY

Anatomic Distribution

The extent of UC at the time of diagnosis appears to have varied over the years, possibly as a function of the area of the world being described. Before the mid-1970s, the extent of disease in UC determined by barium enema and sigmoidoscopy estimated that 60% of children had pancolitis, 22% left-sided colitis, and 17% proctitis or proctosigmoiditis.[56,57] A study from the northeastern United States in the 1980s and early 1990s, however, found that at diagnosis only 41% of children have pancolitis, whereas 34% have left-sided disease and 26% proctitis or proctosigmoiditis.[10] A similar distribution of disease (37% extensive colitis, 35% left-sided colitis, 28% proctitis) has been described at diagnosis in a French pediatric UC population.[58] However, 49% of this French population demonstrated more extensive colonic involvement over time. By contrast, 75% of a Scottish pediatric population had extensive colitis at diagnosis, and 46% of the remaining children demonstrated extensive disease at the end of follow-up.[59] The most recent data available, drawn from the Pediatric IBD Collaborative Research Group's prospective multicenter North American registry of children less than 16 years of age diagnosed between 2002 and 2009 reveals that 267 of 332 (80%) have extensive colitis at diagnosis. There has

been a suggestion that pancolitis is more common in younger children, with one report from the United States identifying pancolitis in 71% of children under 10 years of age presenting with UC.[8] However, a Danish study identified pancolitis in only 13% of children aged less than 10 years,[60] and a U.S. study of children under the age of 5 years at diagnosis identified pancolitis in only 40%.[9] However, when follow-up studies are reported, it is estimated that there is proximal extension of disease within 3 years of initial UC diagnosis in up to 25% of children initially presenting with proctosigmoiditis and 29 to 70% over the course of follow-up.[60-62]

Although UC has classically been described as a diffuse inflammation confined to the rectum and colon, careful endoscopic and pathologic studies demonstrate that this is not entirely true. Upper gastrointestinal involvement has been found, with esophageal disease in 15 to 50% of cases and gastroduodenal inflammation in 25 to 69%.[63,64] Gastric biopsies examined by immunostaining reveal lymphocytes expressing markers characteristic of a T helper cell type 2 (Th2) immune response, similar to that found in the rectums of children with UC.[65] Descriptions of distal colonic UC associated with periappendiceal or appendiceal inflammation have also been published.[66] Therefore, in a patient with colitis, inflammation in the proximal gastrointestinal tract or partial colonic involvement with associated "skip" lesions is not necessarily evidence of Crohn's disease.[67]

Macroscopic Findings

The inflammatory changes characteristic of UC are confined to the mucosal surface. Therefore, to the surgeon or pathologist, the external surface of the colon appears normal. On the other hand, macroscopic changes are immediately apparent to the endoscopist. Classically, mucosal abnormalities begin at the anal verge and extend proximally to a variable extent. In the untreated patient, rectal sparing should suggest Crohn's disease, although a few children with well-documented UC have been described to have rectal sparing at initial presentation.[68-70] Because treatment (both systemic and rectal) can significantly change the appearance of the mucosa, particular care must be taken in interpreting the finding of rectal sparing in the child undergoing endoscopy once therapy has been initiated.

The gross appearance of the mucosa in UC depends on the severity of inflammation (Figure 45-1). Mild disease is characterized by diffuse erythema and loss of the normal mucosal vascular pattern. A fine granularity can also be present. Moderate inflammation results in numerous small surface ulcerations, scattered flecks of exudate, and spontaneous or contact bleeding from the mucosal surface. With more active disease, larger, deep ulcerations covered with shaggy exudate become widespread. As these ulcers surround less involved areas of mucosa, single or multiple pseudopolyps form (Figure 45-2). All of these changes are present diffusely in involved areas of the large bowel, but the severity of the inflammatory process can vary from location to location.

Microscopic Findings

Neutrophilic infiltration of crypts (cryptitis) often accompanied by crypt abscesses, depletion of goblet cell mucin, and chronic inflammatory cells in the lamina propria constitute the primary histologic findings in UC (Figure 45-3). In addition, signs of chronicity include evidence of crypt damage such as crypt

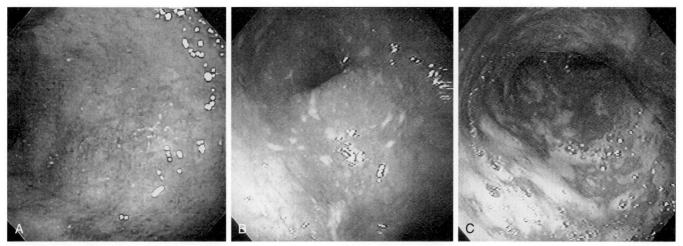

Figure 45-1. Endoscopic appearance of the colon in ulcerative colitis. (**A**) Mild inflammation. (**B**) Moderate inflammation. (**C**) Severe inflammation. (*See plate section for color.*)

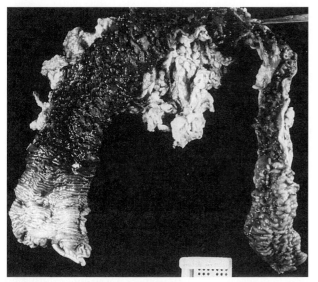

Figure 45-2. Macroscopic appearance of the colon of a 16-year-old patient with ulcerative colitis at the time of subtotal colectomy. Note the mucosa characterized by diffuse ulceration and multiple pseudopolyps. Courtesy Ellen Kahn, MD.

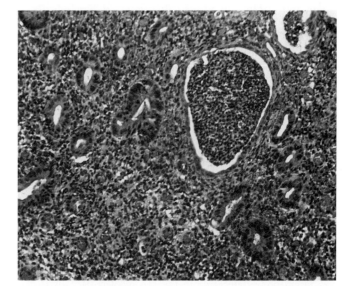

Figure 45-3. Colonic biopsy. Active ulcerative colitis, characterized by neutrophilic infiltration of the crypts, crypt abscesses and crypt distortion. Hematoxylin-eosin stain, ×125. Courtesy Ellen Kahn, MD.

distortion, a papillary configuration to the surface epithelium, and Paneth cell metaplasia. None of these findings is pathognomonic for UC, as similar changes can be seen in severe Crohn's colitis. Infectious colitis may also have a similar appearance, although histologic differentiation of UC from acute self-limiting colitis is generally possible.[71] Although diffuse histologic involvement of the affected bowel is typical in the untreated patient, a few children have manifested patchy inflammation and rectal sparing.[68-70] In surgical specimens obtained from patients with severe or fulminant disease, ulceration can, at times, extend into the submucosa or rarely the deeper layers of the bowel wall.

CLINICAL FEATURES

Symptoms and Signs

Children with UC most commonly present with diarrhea, rectal bleeding, and abdominal pain (Table 45-2). Frequent watery stools can contain either streaks of blood or clots, and are most common on arising in the morning, after eating and during the night. Children often describe both tenesmus and urgency, although the former symptom is at times misinterpreted as constipation by the child or parent. Acute weight loss is common, but abnormalities of linear growth are unusual (see later discussion).

The severity of symptoms at presentation is variable. Some 40-50% of children and adolescents present with mild symptoms, characterized by fewer than four stools per day, only intermittent hematochezia, and minimal (if any) systemic symptoms or weight loss.[10] These children generally have normal findings on physical examination, or only minimal tenderness on palpation of the lower abdomen. Stools may have streaks of blood or may be positive only for occult blood. Laboratory studies can reveal mild anemia and raised acute-phase reactants such as the erythrocyte sedimentation rate. However, some children have entirely normal laboratory findings.

Another third of children are moderately ill, often displaying weight loss, more frequent diarrhea, and systemic symptoms. Physical examination demonstrates abdominal tenderness,

TABLE 45-2. Symptoms at Diagnosis of Ulcerative Colitis

	Toronto* (Diagnosed 1970-1978)		Cleveland† (Diagnosed before 1967)	
	No. of Patients (n = 87)	**% of Population**	**No. of Patients (n = 125)**	**% of Population**
Hematochezia	84	96	107	86
Diarrhea	82	94	116	93
Abdominal pain	77	88	107	86
Anorexia	44	50	–	–
Nocturnal diarrhea	43	49	–	–
Weight loss	37	42	64	51
Fever	12	13	46	37
Vomiting	10	11	53	42

*Data from Hamilton et al.[57]
†Data from Michener.[259]

whereas laboratory studies often are characterized by moderate leukocytosis, mild anemia, and raised acute-phase reactants.

The final 10 to 15% of the pediatric UC population has an acute fulminant disease presentation. These patients appear moderately to severely toxic and have severe crampy abdominal pain, fever, more than six diarrheal stools per day, and, at times, copious rectal bleeding. They frequently manifest tachycardia, orthostatic hypotension, diffuse abdominal tenderness without peritoneal signs, and distention. Laboratory studies reveal leukocytosis, often with numerous band forms, anemia, thrombocytosis, and hypoproteinemia. Toxic megacolon represents the most dangerous extreme of acute fulminant colitis and is quite rare in the pediatric age group.

EXTRAINTESTINAL MANIFESTATIONS

Extraintestinal manifestations are common in children with UC and can affect almost every organ system of the body. The more common sites of involvement are the skin, eye, biliary tree, and joints. Although the etiology for these extraintestinal manifestations remains unknown, it has been shown that an anti-colonocyte antibody detectable in the serum of patients with UC cross-reacts with antigens present in the skin, ciliary body of the eye, bile duct, and joints.[41,42,72] Many of the extraintestinal manifestations tend to occur at times of increased colitis activity. It is therefore tempting to speculate that extraintestinal symptoms develop when autoantibodies capable of recognizing these nonintestinal tissues are produced as part of the humoral response characteristic of UC.

Hepatobiliary

The most serious hepatobiliary diseases associated with UC are primary sclerosing cholangitis (PSC) and autoimmune hepatitis. The presentation and severity of these manifestations are generally independent of the activity of colitis and often do not appear to be affected by medical management of UC or by colectomy. PSC occurs in 3.5% of children and adolescents with UC,[73] although with long-term follow-up into adulthood rates as high as 9.8% have been described.[74] Autoimmune hepatitis is seen in less than 1%.[73] Either may be present at the time of, or even precede, the initial diagnosis of UC, or may develop during the course of the illness.

Both illnesses cause variable degrees of chronic liver disease, ranging from mild to end-stage liver disease requiring transplantation, or death.[73,75,76] PSC also is a risk factor for the development of cholangiocarcinoma.

Compared to patients with UC alone, adults with PSC and UC tend to present at a younger age and have a greater likelihood of having more extensive, but less severe, colitis.[77] It has also been shown that the presence of PSC enhances the risk of colorectal aneuploidy, dysplasia, and cancer in patients with UC.[78] The absolute cumulative risk for colorectal cancer in patients with UC and PSC is 9%, 31%, and 50% after 10, 20, and 25 years of disease, respectively, compared with 2%, 5%, and 10% in patients with UC without PSC.[79] In patients with UC and PSC who have a colectomy and ileal pouch, the risk of severe mucosal atrophy, aneuploidy, and dysplasia in the pouch also appears to be increased.[80] In addition, those with PSC and UC complicated by colorectal cancer are at increased risk of cholangiocarcinoma, compared with patients with PSC and UC but no colorectal malignancy.[79] Although treatment with ursodeoxycholic acid has shown some potential benefit in decreasing the risk of colonic cancer in adult patients with UC and PSC,[81] earlier initiation and increased frequency of colonic surveillance is indicated.

In addition, liver function abnormalities can be seen in a variety of other clinical circumstances, for instance during periods of increased colitis activity, as well as in association with specific therapies used for colitis including corticosteroids, sulfasalazine, parenteral hyperalimentation, azathioprine, and 6-mercaptopurine (6-MP), or with fatty changes associated with massive acute weight gain.[73]

Joints

Arthralgia has been described in up to 32% of children with UC at some time during their course.[82] Arthritis, either a peripheral migratory type affecting the large joints or a monoarticular nondeforming arthritis primarily affecting the knees or ankles, has been reported in 10 to 20% of children.[82,83] The presence and activity of arthritis and arthralgia generally, but not invariably, correlate with the activity of the bowel disease. Ankylosing spondylitis occurs in up to 6% of adults with UC, but is rare during childhood.

Skin

Cutaneous manifestations occur during periods of enhanced colitis activity, with erythema nodosum occurring more commonly than pyoderma gangrenosum.[84] Erythema nodosum lesions appear as raised, erythematous, painful circular nodules

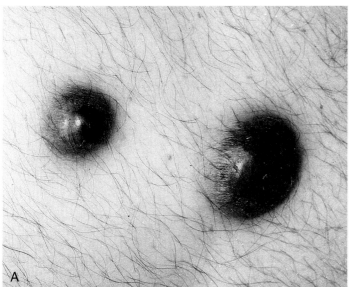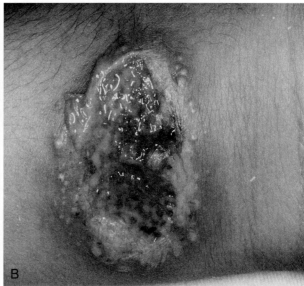

Figure 45-4. **(A)** Pustular phase of pyoderma gangrenosum in a 15-year-old boy with ulcerative colitis. Cutaneous lesions began to appear 2 weeks after initial gastrointestinal symptoms. **(B)** Typical chronic ulcer of pyoderma gangrenosum from the same patient, located on the dorsal surface of the forearm.

that usually occur over the tibia, but may also be present on the lower leg, ankle, or extensor surface of the arm. Lesions persist for several days to a few weeks and generally remit with treatments directed at the enhanced colitis activity.[84] Pyoderma gangrenosum usually appears as small, painful, sterile pustules that coalesce into a larger sterile abscess (Figure 45-4). This ultimately drains, forming a deep, necrotic ulcer. Lesions usually occur on the lower extremities, although the upper extremities, trunk, and head are not spared. A variety of possibly beneficial therapies have been reported, although at present systemic or local ciclosporin, tacrolimus, and intravenous infliximab appear to be the treatments of choice.[85-89]

Thromboembolic Disorders

Case reports document the occurrence of thromboembolic complications in children with UC. Sites of venous or arterial thrombosis include the extremities, portal or hepatic vein, lung, and central nervous system. Although thromobophilia,[90] hyperhomocysteinemia possibly due to folate deficiency[91] or vitamin B_6 deficiency,[92] and specific mutations of coagulation factors such as factor V Leiden[93] have been described in individual patients with UC and a history of thrombosis, no consistent abnormality has been identified to explain why only a subset of patients develops thrombotic complications.

Ocular Disorders

Eye involvement in UC is rare in children, although episcleritis and asymptomatic uveitis have been described.[94] Other ocular disorders such as posterior subcapsular cataracts or increased ocular pressure may be the result of corticosteroid therapy.[95,96]

COMPLICATIONS

Bleeding

Hematochezia is nearly universal in UC, but severe hemorrhage requiring urgent or multiple transfusions occurs in less than 5% of cases. When present, severe hemorrhage is usually the result of diffuse, active, mucosal ulceration. Children who continue to require blood transfusions after 7 to 14 days of intensive medical therapy have been shown to be at risk for significant complications and colectomy.[97]

Perforation

Free perforation of the colon is an emergent complication of UC that occurs rarely. Circumstances that predispose to perforation include acute fulminant colitis, toxic megacolon and diagnostic interventions such as barium enema or colonoscopy. In these settings, gaseous distention or direct pressure from an endoscope can generate sufficient force to perforate the inflamed colon. Peritonitis and septic shock can result. These potentially life-threatening complications require appropriate fluid resuscitation, broad-spectrum antibiotics, and emergent surgery. Plain radiographs of the abdomen may be required to identify a possible free perforation in children with UC who develop worsening symptoms or shoulder pain, as concomitant corticosteroid therapy may mask physical findings such as boardlike rigidity or diffuse rebound tenderness.

Toxic Megacolon

This complication represents a medical and potentially surgical emergency.[56,97] It has been described in up to 5% of children and adolescents with UC, although data gathered in the 1980s and 1990s described only one patient with toxic megacolon in 171 children followed for a total of 823 patient-years.[10] At the time of diagnosis of toxic megacolon, altered levels of consciousness and hypotension appear to be rare in children, whereas fever, tachycardia, electrolyte disturbance, and dehydration are more common.[98] Radiographic signs suggestive of toxic megacolon include intestinal thickening, abnormal colonic haustra, and a transverse colon diameter of 56 mm or greater.[98] Improper diagnosis or treatment can lead to a rapidly progressive deterioration complicated by severe electrolyte disturbances, hypoalbuminemia, hemorrhage, perforation, sepsis, and/or shock. Precipitating factors include the use of antidiarrheal agents such as anticholinergics or opiates, and excessive colonic distention during barium enema or colonoscopy.

Carcinoma

The colorectal tumors that develop in the setting of chronic ulcerative colitis are adenocarcinomas. In contrast to sporadic adenocarcinomas, tumors that arise in UC do not begin as adenomatous polyps, but rather as flat lesions characterized by the presence of dysplasia.[99] The genetic alterations that precede the development of dysplasia occur multifocally in the colon, so that the resulting adenocarcinomas are evenly distributed about the colon.[100] Multifocal or synchronous tumors are present in 10 to 20% of patients.[101]

Individuals who develop UC during childhood have a particularly high lifetime risk of colorectal cancer because duration (greater than 10 years) and extent (pancolitis > left-sided colitis > proctitis) of colitis are the two most critical risk factors for cancer in this condition.[102-104] Other less well characterized risk factors include concomitant sclerosing cholangitis[78,79]; an excluded, defunctionalized, or bypassed segment[89,105]; depressed red blood cell folate levels[106]; and having a family history for non-colitis-associated colon cancer.[100] Patients as young as 16 years of age have been demonstrated to have colonic aneuploidy, dysplasia, or cancer, although, as in adults, the risk for these changes does not appear to be significant in the first decade of illness.[56,102,108]

Population-based studies support the observation that children with UC have an increased lifetime risk of colorectal cancer.[109-112] A large Swedish study revealed that children with onset of UC before the age of 15 years have a standardized incidence ratio (SIR, the ratio of observed to expected cases) of colorectal cancer of 118 (162 for those with pancolitis), compared with a SIR ranging from 2.2 to 16.5 in individuals older than 15 years at diagnosis.[109] These values translate into cumulative colorectal cancer incidence rates of 5% at 20 years and 40% at 35 years for patients with colitis onset at ages 0 to 14 years, and 5% and 30%, respectively, for those whose colitis began between the ages of 15 and 39 years.[109] These values are strikingly similar to those originally reported by Devroede from the Mayo Clinic in children with onset of colitis at less than 14 years of age (3% in the first 10 years, 43% at 35 years).[102] In addition, 52 to 68% of patients with colitis-associated cancers detected because of symptoms have regional node involvement or distant metastasis, resulting in an overall 5-year survival rate of 31 to 55%.[113-115] Therefore, it is estimated that there is an 8% risk of dying from colonic cancer 10 to 25 years after diagnosis of colitis if colectomy is not performed for control of disease symptoms.[116]

Given the high risk of colorectal cancer, surveillance colonoscopy has been advocated as an approach that might lessen the need for prophylactic proctocolectomy. Surveillance programs as currently practiced suffer from lack of objective premalignant markers and the problems associated with invasive testing. A standardized definition of dysplasia (negative, indefinite, low grade, high grade)[99] is in widespread use, but interobserver variability using these definitions results in major discrepancy rates of 4 to 7.5% between expert pathologists reviewing the same slides.[117,118] In addition, evaluations must be made, but have not always been reported, based on an "intent to treat" model, because noncompliance with the surveillance protocol (refusal to enroll or maintain a regular examination schedule)

and inability to evaluate the entire colon adequately because of stricture, poor bowel preparation, or active disease constitute realities of surveillance that have a direct bearing on the efficacy of the surveillance strategy.

The literature generally reflects the practice of performing colectomy only when high-grade dysplasia or cancer is detected. With this approach, a review of prospective cohort studies has revealed that surveillance detects cancer at an early and potentially curable stage 65% of the time, thereby reducing the frequency of detecting advanced lesions from 60% to 35%.[116] However, the data suggest that 33 patients would have to be under regular surveillance for 15 years to prevent one incurable cancer. With biannual examinations resulting in seven to eight colonoscopies per patient, a total of about 250 procedures would be performed to prevent one incurable cancer.[116] Analyses such as these have led to a vigorous discussion regarding the cost-effectiveness of surveillance as currently practiced.[119,120]

These data have led to a search for better markers to enhance the predictive accuracy of surveillance. Meta-analysis supports the inclusion of low-grade dysplasia as an indication for colectomy, as identification of low-grade dysplasia during surveillance colonoscopy is associated with a ninefold increased risk of developing colorectal cancer and a 12-fold risk of any advanced lesion.[121] Other markers, including aneuploidy,[108,122-124] loss of tumor suppressor gene (e.g., *p53*)[125] function, expression of proto-oncogenes (e.g., K-*ras*),[126] and expression of abnormal mucin-associated antigens (e.g., sialosyl-Tn),[127] have also been investigated as adjuncts to surveillance for dysplasia.

No prospective studies have assessed the optimal schedule of surveillance, although a cost-benefit analysis has suggested colonoscopies every 3 years for the first 10 years of surveillance, with more frequent investigations as the duration of colitis increases.[128] Current practice generally begins with biyearly colonoscopies 7 to 10 years after diagnosis. Although many advocate initiating surveillance only after 15 to 20 years of disease in adults with left-sided colitis or proctosigmoiditis, the frequent proximal extension of these disease distributions in patients with onset of disease during childhood suggests that all patients with childhood-onset UC of any extent be enrolled in a surveillance program within 10 years of initial diagnosis. Procedures require panendoscopy to the cecum, with two to four biopsies every 10 cm from the cecum to the sigmoid, and every 5 cm in the sigmoid and rectum. Additional biopsies must be performed if a mass or other suspicious lesion is identified. Newer endoscopic modalities including chromoendoscopy, narrow-band imaging, and the use of magnifying colonoscopes allow better visualization of dysplastic changes and potentially more accurate, directed biopsy sampling.[129] Current recommendations for colectomy include any identification of dysplasia (low or high grade) confirmed by two independent experienced pathologists. Repeat colonoscopy for confirmation of dysplasia on new biopsies is not recommended, because there is no way to guarantee that the identical site can be biopsied on a subsequent procedure. If indefinite dysplasia is identified, aggressive medical management to reduce active inflammation followed by repeat surveillance colonoscopy within 3 to 6 months is indicated.

Growth and Development

It is common for children to demonstrate acute weight loss at the time of diagnosis or during periods of increased disease activity. However, children who develop UC are not immune to obesity, and studies from two independent North American populations have identified that 20% to 30% of children with UC have elevated BMI at diagnosis consistent with overweight or risk for overweight.[130] However, as opposed to Crohn's disease, only about 10% of children with UC demonstrate significantly impaired linear growth.[122] Why linear growth impairment is so unusual in UC, compared with Crohn's disease, remains to be fully explained, although the different cytokine profiles seen in the two diseases may be important. Although serum from children with Crohn's disease produced marked impairment in bone growth in an in vitro animal model, serum from children with UC and from normal controls does not.[132] Further study is necessary before it can be determined whether this effect is mediated by circulating proinflammatory cytokines or some other serum factor.

DIAGNOSIS

History

Many children present with obvious symptoms of diarrhea and rectal bleeding. However, in others, symptoms are less obvious and more difficult to elicit, especially in children or adolescents who are unwilling or too embarrassed to discuss the frequency and consistency of their bowel movements. Awakening with pain or the need to defecate is an especially important symptom to elicit, as it often helps to differentiate the child with organic illness from one with a functional condition. The history should seek to identify evidence of recent weight loss, poor growth, arrested sexual development, or, in the postmenarchal adolescent, secondary amenorrhea. When family history reveals other relatives with IBD, the possibility that UC is present is increased.

Physical Examination

A careful physical examination may demonstrate a number of findings that help suggest the appropriate diagnosis. Children with active colitis often have mild to moderate abdominal tenderness, especially in the left lower quadrant or midepigastric area. Tender bowel loops may be palpable, although inflammatory masses are lacking. With fulminant disease, marked tenderness can be present. Perianal inspection is generally normal, and the presence of perianal tags or fistulas suggests Crohn's disease. The presence of skin lesions, such as erythema nodosum, pyoderma gangrenosum, or cutaneous vasculitis, or of arthritis is an important clue to the autoimmune nature of the child's illness.

Laboratory Studies

Once UC is suspected, the laboratory studies outlined in Table 45-3 help to exclude other illnesses and provide evidence to support proceeding to more invasive radiologic and endoscopic diagnostic procedures. Microcytic anemia, mild to moderate thrombocytosis, raised erythrocyte sedimentation rate, C-reactive protein, and hypoalbuminemia are present in 40 to 80% of patients. Total white blood cell count is normal to only mildly increased, unless the illness is complicated by acute fulminant colitis. Abnormal liver function is found in 3% of children at the time of initial diagnosis and reflects signs of potentially serious concomitant liver disease (chronic active hepatitis or sclerosing cholangitis) in about half of them.[73] In a number of children, however, all laboratory studies can be normal.[133] Fecal levels of calprotectin, a neutrophil-associated protein present in the stools in conditions associated with intestinal inflammation, are higher in patients with active UC than in healthy controls and correlate well with the severity of endoscopically determined mucosal inflammation.[134,135] Although calprotectin levels can also be raised in patients with enteric infection or Crohn's disease, an increased fecal calprotectin assay can help determine which children with abdominal pain or diarrhea should undergo more invasive testing for UC or Crohn's disease.[134,136] An elevated fecal calprotectin level has also been shown to predict relapse in patients with apparent quiescent UC.[137]

Enteric pathogens must be excluded in all patients, both at the time of diagnosis and during acute flares of active disease after diagnosis. Particular attention should be given to the possibility of *Clostridium difficile*–mediated colitis. If a pathogen is identified, it must be treated and the patient followed, as it is not unusual for children with UC to present initially with superimposed infection. If symptoms persist despite eradication of the identified pathogen, work-up should continue.

Serologic tests for the detection of circulating perinuclear antineutrophil cytoplasmic antibody (pANCA) can be useful in differentiating UC from other colitides, including Crohn's disease.[138,139] pANCA can be detected in about 70% of patients with UC, but is present in only 6% of Crohn's patients and 3% of controls. However, pANCA-positive Crohn's patients tend to have "UC-like" disease, making reliance on this serologic marker as a means of differentiating UC from CD problematic. Although the other serologic markers commonly identified in patients with IBD (anti-*Saccharomyces cerevisiae* antibody [ASCA] and anti-outer membrane porin of *Escherichia coli* [anti-ompC]) are found only rarely, the anti-flagellin antibody (anti-CBir1) can be found in up to 30% of children with UC. The use of these antibodies for differentiating inflammatory bowel disease from functional disorders has also been made more problematic by the recognition that anti-flagellin antibodies can also be identified in adults with irritable bowel syndrome.[140] Despite this, a positive pANCA coupled with a negative ASCA titer has a sensitivity of 69.2%, specificity of 95.1%, positive predictive value of 90.0%, and negative predictive value of 87.1% for the diagnosis of UC in children.[141] Although children with indeterminate colitis may be negative for all serologic markers, at times the markers can be helpful in determining whether the child actually has Crohn's disease or UC. In adults with indeterminate colitis, a finding of pANCA+/ASCA– predicts UC in 64%, whereas pANCA–/ASCA+ findings predict Crohn's disease in 80%.[142]

TABLE 45-3. Laboratory Studies in Suspected Ulcerative Colitis

Complete blood count, differential, reticulocyte count
Erythrocyte sedimentation rate, C-reactive protein
Electrolytes, serum chemistries (including total protein, albumin, liver function)
Serum iron, total iron binding capacity, ferritin
Stools for enteric pathogens (including *Salmonella, Shigella, Campylobacter, Yersinia, Aeromonas, Escherichia coli*)
Stool for *Clostridium difficile* toxins
Direct microscopic examination of the stool for ova and parasites, Charcot-Leyden crystals, leukocytes
Perinuclear anti-neutrophilic cytoplasmic antibody, anti-*Saccharomyces cerevisiae* antibody, anti-ompC (anti-outer membrane porin of *E. coli*) antibody
Fecal calprotectin

Radiography

Traditionally, when UC was suspected, a barium enema was performed to identify radiographic signs of inflammation. Barium enema can, at times, differentiate between Crohn's and UC, but the classic radiographic findings attributed to one form of colitis can be mimicked by the other. Currently, barium enema is performed only rarely, having been replaced by colonoscopy and computed tomographic (CT) or magnetic resonance (MR) colonography. Although the colonographic studies are noninvasive, published reports in adults demonstrate diminished sensitivity and specificity for the detection of inflammation compared to colonoscopy.[143] In most circumstances, the child with suspected UC should still undergo an evaluation of the small bowel to help exclude the possibility of Crohn's disease. This can be done by upper gastrointestinal series with small bowel follow-through, CT or MR enterography, or capsule endoscopy depending on local availability and expertise with each of the modalities.

Abdominal ultrasonography and various scintigraphic techniques including technetium-99m-hexamethylpropyleneamine oxime (HMPAO)-labeled white cell scan can be used to assess the presence and extent of intestinal inflammation, although these studies are not used widely to establish the initial diagnosis. Overall, these modalities, along with CT or MR studies, are more useful in identifying complications associated with Crohn's disease than for UC.

Endoscopy

Colonoscopy allows accurate determination of the extent and distribution of colitis through direct visualization and biopsy of the affected segments. UC is characterized by diffuse inflammation, which begins at the anal verge and progresses proximally to a variable degree. Although rectal sparing is generally associated with Crohn's disease, untreated children can have rectal sparing at initial colonoscopy yet subsequently evidence typical UC.[68,144,145] In mild UC, the rectal and colonic mucosa appears erythematous, the normal vascular markings are lost, and there is increased friability evidenced by petechiae or contact hemorrhage (see Figure 45-1A). With more active disease, exudate, ulcerations and marked hemorrhage are evident (see Figure 45-1B,C). Skip lesions, aphthous ulcerations, and significant ileal inflammation are indicative of Crohn's disease. All children who undergo endoscopy should be biopsied, because the histologic appearance can often help differentiate among acute self-limiting colitis, Crohn's disease, and UC.[71]

Although UC is described as an inflammatory disease confined to the colon, endoscopic studies can reveal inflammation of the proximal gastrointestinal tract. A pattern of focally enhanced gastritis is seen in 21% of children with UC, and 50% can have features of chronic gastritis.[146] These observations require that clinicians do not automatically exclude the possible diagnosis of UC in a child with colitis who is shown to have endoscopic or histologic gastritis. Similarly, children with UC can also have discontinuous disease, with concomitant diffuse distal colitis and cecal or periappendiceal inflammation.[67]

Capsule endoscopy has been shown to be of benefit when there is some doubt in the diagnosis of UC versus Crohn's disease. Although a negative capsule study does not confirm a diagnosis of UC, detection of clear-cut ulceration in the small bowel disease can be helpful in confirming a diagnosis of Crohn's.[147]

DIFFERENTIAL DIAGNOSIS

The differential diagnosis is summarized in Table 45-4. Most can easily be excluded by history, physical examination, laboratory evaluation, or endoscopy and biopsy. In contrast to adults, neoplastic disease, ischemia, and radiation-induced injury are rarely significant diagnostic concerns in the child or adolescent.

MEDICAL THERAPIES

Because curative medical therapy does not exist, current treatment remains symptomatic and supportive. Treatment aims include the suppression of symptoms and the control of unavoidable complications. In many cases, UC and Crohn's disease respond to the same therapeutic modalities, and the reader may wish to review Chapter 44 for additional details of the various pharmacologic agents discussed later.

The treatment of children and adolescents presents the challenge of promoting normal growth and sexual development while controlling disease symptoms. Current treatment options at times promote one goal while hindering another. Therapy, therefore, may require striking a balance between potentially conflicting effects. Therapeutic options are listed in Table 45-5. Many of the data supporting the use of these medications have been extrapolated from adult studies. The following discussion focuses on aspects of treatment that have been shown to be particularly effective in the pediatric population.

TABLE 45-4. Differential Diagnosis of Ulcerative Colitis in Children

Enteric infection
  Salmonella
  Shigella
  Campylobacter
  Aeromonas
  Yersinia
  Enterohemorrhagic *E. coli*
  Entamoeba histolytica
  *Giardia lamblia**
  Cytomegalovirus†
  Norovirus
Pseudomembranous (postantibiotic) enterocolitis
  Clostridium difficile
Carbohydrate intolerance*
  Lactose
  Sucrose
  Nondigestible carbohydrates (sorbitol, xylitol, mannitol, maltitol)
Vasculitis
  Henoch-Schönlein purpura
  Hemolytic-uremic syndrome
Allergic enterocolitis‡
Hirschsprung's enterocolitis‡
Eosinophilic gastroenteritis
Celiac disease*
Laxative abuse*
Neoplasms
  Juvenile polyp‡
  Adenocarcinoma
  Intestinal polyposis
Immunodeficiencies‡

Modified from Park S-D, Markowitz JF. Ulcerative colitis (pediatric). In: Johnson L, ed. Encyclopedia of Gastroenterology. New York: Academic Press; 2004:400-408, with permission.
*Watery, nonbloody diarrhea.
†Primarily during flares of disease activity, especially in patients on immunomodulatory therapy.
‡Primarily in the young child.

TABLE 45-5. Medical Therapeutic Options in Ulcerative Colitis

Nutritionals

Appropriate dietary intake (with or without food supplements)
Short-chain fatty acids
n-3 fatty acids (fish oils)

Anti-inflammatories

Corticosteroids
    Prednisone, prednisolone, hydrocortisone
    Budesonide
5-Aminosalicylates
    Sulfasalazine
    Olsalazine
    Mesalamine
    Balsalazide

Immunomodulators

6-Mercaptopurine
Azathioprine
Ciclosporin
Tacrolimus
Methotrexate

Biologics

Infliximab

Nutritional Therapy

Although nutritional therapies have a role as primary treatment in Crohn's disease, UC is less amenable to nutritional interventions. Elimination diets rarely result in significant improvement in symptoms and can promote inadequate nutritional intake in the child who finds the elimination diet prescribed unpalatable or too restrictive. Similarly, although "bowel rest" can ameliorate symptoms in Crohn's disease of the small bowel, it is often ineffective in UC, possibly because the colonocyte derives energy from the fecal stream in the form of short-chain fatty acids. In addition, because growth failure is a much more frequent and dramatic problem in Crohn's disease than in UC, the nutritional therapy of growth failure becomes more central to the treatment of the former illness. Therefore, nutritional interventions in UC are generally adjunctive to other treatments. In UC, an adequate dietary intake promotes normal growth and prevents catabolism, thereby enhancing the effect of other treatment modalities.[148] Nutritional support can successfully be accomplished by a number of approaches, including dietary supplementation and enteral or parenteral nutrition.

The therapeutic use of short-chain fatty acids may represent one area where a "nutritional" intervention can offer benefit as primary therapy in UC. Adults with UC have been shown to have impaired butyrate metabolism. Similarly, fecal concentrations of n-butyrate are raised in children with inactive or mild UC, suggesting impaired utilization of this metabolic fuel.[54] A number of placebo-controlled trials of short-chain fatty acid or butyrate enemas have demonstrated limited improvement in symptom score and endoscopic appearance in actively treated adult subjects. The combination of 5-aminosalicylate (5-ASA) treatment and butyrate enemas has also been shown to be beneficial.[149] An additional study in adults has reported decreased mucosal hyperproliferation after short-chain fatty acid or butyrate enemas, suggesting that such treatment might have a role in decreasing the risk of colonic cancer in patients with UC.[150] More recent studies have explored the possibility that fecal butyrate concentrations can be effectively increased in patients with UC by adding specific dietary fibers such as oat bran[151] or a prebiotic such as germinated barley foodstuff[152] in an attempt to enhance the growth and metabolism of enteric butyrate-producing bacteria.

The oral supplementation of n-3 fatty acids derived from fish oil has also received some attention. Initial studies suggested that early relapse of UC could be delayed by supplementing the diet with 5.1 g/day of n-3 fatty acids, although relapse rates after 3 months were comparable to those in placebo-treated controls.[153] Similarly, n-3 fatty acids provided no, or only modest, steroid-sparing effect compared with placebo in the treatment of acute UC.[154] Only a single small pediatric trial has been reported. Compared with pretreatment values, children with UC in remission who were supplemented orally with purified eicosapentaenoic acid for 2 months had decreased leukocyte and rectal production of leukotriene B_4.[155] Whether this was clinically important could not be determined. Although no child relapsed during the study, there was no control group with whom clinical response could be compared. Clearly, further studies are necessary before the usefulness of this therapy in UC can be fully assessed.

Corticosteroids

Corticosteroids appear to down-regulate multiple steps in the inflammatory cascade that results in UC.[156,157] The initial use of corticosteroids as treatment for children with UC was largely extrapolated from studies in adults. Pediatric treatment regimens have evolved through empiric use and clinical experience, rather than controlled clinical trial. Prednisone, methylprednisolone, and hydrocortisone are the agents most frequently used. Commonly prescribed dosages are comparable to those prescribed for children with Crohn's disease. Oral doses greater than 40 mg of prednisone are rarely necessary for efficacy and can be associated with significant toxicity. Oral corticosteroids are well absorbed, although occasional children with poor absorption or corticosteroid resistance may benefit from intravenous bolus or continuous infusion dosing. When fulminant disease requires hospitalization for intravenous corticosteroid therapy, prospective pediatric data demonstrate that clinical features including the frequency of stools and the presence of nocturnal stools on day 3 and day 5 can predict the success or failure of therapy.[158] Because there are now reasonable medical alternatives to an extended course of intravenous corticosteroid (see later discussion), such observations strongly argue for limiting the use of intravenous corticosteroid to no more than a week when significant symptom improvement is not seen during that period of time. Rectal corticosteroids are particularly beneficial in children with severe tenesmus and urgency, but many children have difficulty retaining enema formulations, so that foam-based treatments or suppositories may be preferable in selected individuals.

The decision to use corticosteroids must be balanced by their potential adverse effects. A wide spectrum of complications occasionally occurs (Table 45-6). More important, systemically active corticosteroids can interfere with linear bone growth, even in the face of adequate dietary intake.[159] Alternate-day dosing minimizes these effects while maintaining reduced disease activity[160-162] and appears to have no deleterious effect on bone mineralization in children.[163] However, in patients who have not completed their linear growth and whose disease activity cannot be controlled by alternate-day dosing regimens,

TABLE 45-6. Side Effects of Corticosteroid Therapy

Cosmetic
  Moon facies
  Acne
  Hirsutism
  Striae
  Central obesity
Metabolic
  Hypokalemia
  Hyperglycemia
  Hyperlipidemia
  Systemic hypertension
Endocrinologic
  Growth suppression
  Delayed puberty
  Adrenal suppression
Musculoskeletal
  Osteopenia
  Aseptic necrosis of bone
  Vertebral collapse
  Myopathy
Ocular
  Cataracts
  Increased intraocular pressure

the anti-inflammatory effects of daily corticosteroids must be weighed against the coincident suppression of linear growth.

Topically active corticosteroids such as budesonide have the potential to provide anti-inflammatory activity to the gut without systemic toxicity because of their high first-pass metabolism.[164] These agents may offer particular advantages for the treatment of children if they prove to be minimally growth suppressive, but adequate pediatric studies in UC have yet to be reported. In adults, the enema formulation of budesonide is as effective as rectal mesalamine[165] and rectal prednisolone or hydrocortisone[166,167] in the treatment of left-sided and distal colitis. A budesonide rectal foam is also as effective as a hydrocortisone foam in adults with proctosigmoiditis, and 52% of previous rectal mesalamine failures responded to the budesonide foam.[168] In adults, budesonide enemas (2 mg) are associated with fewer abnormal adrenocorticotropic hormone (ACTH) stimulation test results than rectal hydrocortisone (100 mg).[167] Multiple courses of rectal budesonide are safe and effective for recurrent flares of UC.[167] Data on the effect of oral budesonide in UC are limited. A single study in adults with active extensive and distal UC demonstrated that oral budesonide (10 mg) delivered as a controlled-release preparation was as effective as oral prednisolone (40 mg), but did not suppress plasma cortisol levels.[169] Additional studies are required to determine whether the current oral formulation, which is designed to deliver active budesonide to the ileum and right colon, will be an effective therapy in children with UC.

Corticosteroid resistance remains a difficult problem for many patients. Although only 21% of a small pediatric UC cohort demonstrated no response to an acute course of corticosteroid, a complete response was seen in only 57% at 1 year, whereas 14% were steroid dependent and 29% required colectomy.[170] A large North American multicenter registry reported that 50% of children were responsive to an initial course of corticosteroid, but 45% were steroid dependent at 1 year.[171] A number of different mechanisms appear to result in corticosteroid resistance, including IL-2-induced inhibition of glucocorticoid receptor activity and decreased intracellular glucocorticoid levels due to overexpression of the multidrug resistance gene 1.[172] Therapeutic strategies designed to overcome these factors are under investigation. In preliminary trials, adults with corticosteroid-resistant UC responded dramatically to treatment with either daclizumab or basiliximab, anti-IL-2 receptor monoclonal antibodies that block the lymphocyte IL-2 receptor and prevent IL-2–induced inhibition of the glucocorticoid receptor.[173-175] Subsequent placebo-controlled evaluations of both agents, however, did not demonstrate benefit,[176] and it is not clear that either of these agents will be further investigated in the management of children with active or fulminant UC.

5-Aminosalicylates

It is postulated that the 5-ASA drugs (sulfasalazine, mesalamine, olsalazine, balsalazide) exert local anti-inflammatory effects through a number of different mechanisms. These include inhibition of 5-lipoxygenase with resulting decreased production of leukotriene B_4, scavenging of reactive oxygen metabolites, prevention of the up-regulation of leukocyte adhesion molecules, and inhibition of IL-1 synthesis.[157,177] Because 5-ASA is rapidly absorbed from the upper intestinal tract on oral ingestion, different delivery systems have been used to prevent absorption until the active drug can be delivered to the distal small bowel and colon. Sulfasalazine (Azulfidine) links 5-ASA via an azo bond to sulfapyridine. Bacterial enzymes in the colon break the azo linkage, releasing 5-ASA to exert its anti-inflammatory effect in the colon. Because the sulfapyridine moiety causes most of the untoward reactions to sulfasalazine and is thought to have no therapeutic activity, newer agents have been designed to deliver 5-ASA without sulfapyridine. Olsalazine (Dipentum) links two molecules of 5-ASA via an azo bond, and balsalazide (Colazal, Colazide) links 5-ASA via an azo bond to an inert, nonabsorbed carrier. A number of other delayed release preparations (Asacol, Asacol-HD, Claversal, Mesasal, Salofalk, Apriso) prevent rapid absorption of 5-ASA (also known generically as mesalamine) by coating it with pH-sensitive resins. Another preparation (Pentasa) coats microgranules of mesalamine with ethylcellulose, releasing it in a time-dependent fashion. Still another preparation utilizes a novel matrix system (Lialda) to deliver high concentrations of 5ASA to the colonic mucosa. Uncoated mesalamine is also available as a rectal suppository (Canasa, Salofalk) or enema formulation (Rowasa). Unfortunately, no liquid formulation of oral 5ASA is commercially available in the United States, and only the azo-bond formulations can be extemporaneously compounded into a suspension. Similarly, the coated formulations cannot be crushed or broken, limiting their use to children who are able to swallow pills intact.

Overall, the 5-ASA drugs have been shown to be effective in controlling mild to moderate UC in adults in 50 to 90% of cases, and effective in maintaining remission in 70 to 90%.[178,179] In addition, chronic treatment with a 5-ASA medication has been shown to be a chemopreventative therapy, decreasing the risk for the development of UC-associated colon cancer.[107] However, despite extensive studies in adults, few pediatric studies exist. Clinical experience with sulfasalazine in children with UC has generally mirrored the adult experience.[180] One pediatric study made a direct comparison of the efficacy of sulfasalazine and olsalazine.[181] In this study, 79% of children with mildly to moderately active UC treated with sulfasalazine (60 mg/kg daily) improved clinically, compared with only 39% of those treated with olsalazine (30 mg/kg daily). Several smaller open-label or double-blind pediatric trials, and one larger retrospective analysis of 10 years' clinical experience with Eudragit-coated 5-ASA preparations in children, have reported therapeutic benefits in active UC as well as in active Crohn's colitis and active small-bowel Crohn's disease.[182-185] Dosing regimens in children have by and large been extrapolated from studies in adults, such that many physicians prescribe between two and four divided doses throughout the day. The high pill burden of some of the 5-ASA formulations as well as the frequent dosing regimens can result in poor adherence to a prescribed treatment regimen, a problem that occurs frequently and can be associated with poor clinical outcomes.[186] Higher potency oral formulations have been developed for adult use, and although these preparations have not been evaluated in children, studies in adults suggest that high-dose, once-daily dosing may be comparable, or even superior, to more traditional split-dose regimens.[187]

Adverse reactions to all of the 5-ASA preparations have been described, requiring discontinuation of treatment in 5 to 15% of cases. The more serious complications reported in children have included pancreatitis, nephritis, exacerbation of disease, and sulfa- or salicylate-induced allergic reactions. Although some toxicities (e.g., headache) to sulfasalazine have been attributed to slow acetylation of the drug, a recent study has demonstrated no association between N-acetyltransferase 1 or 2 genotype and efficacy or toxicity from either mesalamine or sulfasalazine.[188]

Antibiotics

There is little role for antibiotics in the primary therapy of active UC. Based on experience in adults, metronidazole is occasionally used for the treatment of mild to moderate UC or the maintenance of remission in the 5-ASA-intolerant or -allergic patient.[189] A controlled trial of ciprofloxacin as an adjunct to corticosteroids in adults with active UC demonstrated no benefit compared with placebo.[190] No pediatric studies exist.

Immunomodulators

6-Mercaptopurine and Azathioprine

Despite the surgically curable nature of UC (see later discussion), many parents and physicians are reluctant to perform colectomies in children, even those with severely active UC. As a consequence, immunomodulators are increasingly being used therapeutically. The most commonly prescribed agents are 6-mercaptopurine (6-MP) and azathioprine.[191] These purine analogues have long been thought to inhibit RNA and DNA synthesis, thereby down-regulating cytotoxic T-cell activity and delayed hypersensitivity reactions. More recent studies suggest that the thiopurines act by inhibiting an enzyme, *rac-1*, in T-cells resulting in increased apoptosis of these immunologically active cells.[192]

Clinical experience in children with UC has mirrored adult studies, demonstrating that 6-MP and azathioprine can act as steroid-sparing agents and induce and maintain remission in 60 to 75% of patients.[193-195] Onset of action is delayed, with a mean time to response of 4.5 ± 3.0 months.[195] In adults with UC achieving complete remission with 6-MP, 65% maintain continuous remission for 5 years if they remain on the medication, compared with only 13% of those who electively discontinue 6-MP after induction of remission.[196] These data are comparable to those from an earlier study using azathioprine in which 64% of adults maintained on azathioprine after induction

of remission remained well at 1 year, compared with only 41% of those switched to placebo after remission induction.[197] No comparable pediatric data have been published. Finally, studies have shown that azathioprine and 6-MP are effective agents for maintaining long-term remission induced by intravenous ciclosporin in both children and adults with severe UC.[198,199]

As maintenance drugs, the long-term safety profile of these therapies is especially important. At a 6-MP dose of 1.0 to 1.5 mg/kg daily, adverse reactions requiring discontinuation of treatment such as allergic reactions, pancreatitis, or severe leukopenia occur in less than 5% of pediatric patients.[200] The recognition of patients with subnormal or absent thiopurine methyltransferase (TPMT) activity (the major inactivating enzyme for both azathioprine and 6-MP), by screening for either TPMT genotype or enzyme activity before initiation of therapy, can reduce but not eliminate the potential for severe leukopenia.[201] Ongoing assessment of 6-MP and azathioprine metabolites can also identify subjects at risk for either leukopenia or hepatotoxicity.[202] Concern remains concerning the potential for these agents to increase the risk of cancer, especially lymphoma. It is now generally accepted that in patients with IBD, thiopurine therapy increases the risk of lymphoma three- to fourfold. Despite this, absolute risk is estimated to be only 3 to 4 per 10,000. Whether these risks require a reevaluation of the use of these treatments is currently a topic of ongoing debate.[203]

Calcineurin Inhibitors (Ciclosporin and Tacrolimus)

Ciclosporin and tacrolimus (FK506) are potent inhibitors of cell-mediated immunity. Both agents bind to their respective intracellular receptors (immunophilins). The resulting drug-immunophilin complex inhibits the action of another intracellular mediator, calcineurin, which in turn inactivates the genes responsible for the production of IL-2 and IL-4.[204] As a consequence, T cell, and to a lesser extent B cell, function is impaired.

The use of these agents for the treatment of severe UC in children has had mixed results. Initial response rates, defined as avoidance of imminent surgery and discharge from the hospital, of 20-80% have been reported with either oral or intravenous ciclosporin.[205,206] Responses generally occur within 7-14 days of initiating treatment, but relapses requiring colectomy occur within 1 year in 70 to 100% of initial responders during or after discontinuation of ciclosporin.[205,206] Addition of 6-MP or azathioprine to the therapeutic regimen once ciclosporin has induced remission results in long-term remission in 60-90% of patients.[199]

Oral tacrolimus can also be used to treat children with fulminant colitis. An open-label pediatric experience demonstrated that 69% of treated subjects initially avoided surgery and were discharged from hospital after tacrolimus was initiated. Despite addition of 6-MP or azathioprine, however, only 38% of the initial cohort avoided colectomy after 1 year.[207]

Tremors, hirsutism and systemic hypertension are the most common toxic effects of ciclosporin and tacrolimus that have been described in children with IBD. However, isolated reports of *Pneumocystis jirovecii* pneumonia, lymphoproliferative disease, and serious bacterial and fungal infection merit careful monitoring in all children treated with ciclosporin, especially those treated in combination with corticosteroids and 6-MP or azathioprine. Prophylaxis against *Pneumocystis* is necessary during the phase when ciclosporin or tacrolimus is used in conjunction with corticosteroids and 6-MP.

Other Immunomodulators

Methotrexate has been used with beneficial effects in a few children with severe Crohn's disease, but published pediatric experience in UC is lacking. Although studies in adult patients with UC suggest that methotrexate can provide benefit in the induction and maintenance of remission, a double-blind trial demonstrated no benefit compared with placebo for either indication.[208]

Infliximab

The chimeric anti-TNF-α monoclonal antibody infliximab is FDA approved for the treatment of both children and adults with Crohn's disease, and for the treatment of adults with UC. Two multicenter, placebo-controlled trials (ACT I and ACT II) demonstrated a 60 to 70% response rate in adults with moderately active UC to induction with 3 doses of infliximab over 6 weeks. Clinical response was maintained to 1 year in 45% of subjects receiving maintenance infusions every 8 weeks.[209] Open-label studies in hospitalized adults with steroid-refractory UC have also demonstrated excellent short-term responses, with 76% of patients discharged home without colectomy, and 62% remaining colectomy-free with maintenance infliximab or following introduction of a thiopurine.[210] Response and remission are associated with improved quality of life, ability to work, and overall productivity.[211] To date, no controlled clinical trials have been reported in children with UC, although one has recently completed enrollment. However, open-label experience in children appears to confirm the adult experience. Data from a single U.S. center identified a short-term response in 82% of children and sustained improvement in 62%, with most requiring repeated infliximab infusions.[212] Similar findings are reported from an open-label experience in Italy (18 of 22 [82%] acute response, 12 of 22 [55%] in remission at 1 year, 7 of 22 [32%] with colectomy by 1 year).[213] However, response may be influenced by prior therapy. In a small single-center retrospective evaluation, among children with either new-onset UC unresponsive to 5 to 10 days of intravenous steroids or chronic but non-steroid-dependent UC undergoing an acute exacerbation, infliximab induced long-term remission in 12 of 16 patients (75%), and only 2 (12.5%) required colectomy. By contrast, only 3 of 11 (27%) children with chronic, steroid-dependent UC achieved long-term relief of symptoms after infliximab.[214]

The most common adverse reactions are minor infusion reactions and increased risk of infection, although more severe delayed infusion reactions, anaphylaxis, reactivation of latent tuberculosis, demyelinating disease, and drug-induced lupus can occur.[215] Significant concern has also been raised about the possible development of malignancy, especially lymphoma.[216] In particular, a rare, usually fatal lymphoma, hepatosplenic T-cell lymphoma, has been noted in both Crohn's disease and UC patients treated with infliximab and a concomitant thiopurine.[217] This may be a particular problem for adolescents and young adults, the recognition of which has led to a new, but as yet untested, treatment paradigm among many pediatric gastroenterologists to utilize monotherapy with infliximab rather than combination therapy with a thiopurine whenever possible.

Other Biologics

Given the proven efficacy of infliximab, additional anti-TNF agents are undergoing trials in UC. As seen in Crohn's disease, adalimumab has been shown to rescue some adult patients with active UC who had lost response to or been intolerant of infliximab, avoiding colectomy in about half of the small population studied.[218] However, improved understanding of the pathophysiology of UC has resulted in the definition of numerous new potential targeted therapies. None, however, are currently FDA approved for treatment of UC, and in some cases the molecules are not yet FDA approved for any indication. Preventing white blood cell recruitment and invasion into the colonic tissue through blockade of adhesion molecules is one such approach. Natalizumab (Tysabri), an α4 integrin antagonist commercially available under a restricted-access program for multiple sclerosis and Crohn's disease, has shown benefit in a small preliminary study of adults with active UC.[219] The drug has been associated with the development of fatal progressive multifocal leukoencephalopathy (PML), however, and likely will not be further developed as a treatment for UC. Another more gut-specific anti–adhesion molecule therapy, vedolizumab (MLN02), an IgG1 monoclonal antibody directed against the β7 integrin, has also been shown to be of benefit for induction of remission in one trial of adults with moderately active UC.[220] It is hoped that the more gut-specific target of vedolizumab will result in a decreased risk of PML and other systemic infections. Alicaforsen represents another approach to anti–adhesion molecule therapy. This agent is an antisense inhibitor of intercellular adhesion molecule 1 and has shown benefit for the treatment of mild to moderate left-sided UC when given as an enema preparation in some but not all trials reported to date.[221,222]

Additional anticytokine therapies are also being developed. Monoclonal antibodies directed against IL12, IL23, and IL17 may hold promise as treatments for UC as well as Crohn's disease.[223] An early study with visilizumab, a humanized IgG(2) monoclonal anti-CD3 antibody, has been shown to induce a clinical response in a Phase I/II trial in adults with severe corticosteroid refractory UC.[224] A recent placebo-controlled trial of visilizumab was halted, however, when trends for increased toxicity without evidence of clinical benefit were identified during an interim analysis. Similarly, despite responses during an open-label clinical trial, the IL2 receptor antagonist daclizumab did not demonstrate efficacy in a placebo-controlled trial in adults with severe UC.[176]

Probiotics, Prebiotics, and Synbiotics

These approaches to therapy attempt to decrease UC activity by changing the bacterial flora. Probiotics are preparations that contain viable, nonpathogenic bacteria normally found within the gut microflora. Prebiotics stimulate the preferential growth of the probiotic organisms by providing appropriate substrates. Synbiotic preparations combine both prebiotics and probiotics. These related approaches to treatment are reported to decrease secretion of pro-inflammatory cytokines including interferon-γ, TNF-α, and interleukin-12, to interfere with the adherence of more proinflammatory organisms to the colonic epithelium, and to increase production of the anti-inflammatory cytokine IL10.[225]

Various probiotic organisms have been investigated as UC treatments. Sixty-eight percent of adults with mild to moderate UC entered remission after 4 weeks of treatment with *Saccharomyces boulardii*.[226] Similarly, 53% of adults with active mild to moderate UC were in remission, and another 24% had a partial response to 6 weeks of treatment with VSL#3, a commercially available proprietary mixture of probiotic bacteria.[227] This same probiotic preparation has been shown to induce a combined remission/response rate of 61% in children with mild to moderately active UC.[228] Used in conjunction with standard medical treatments, VSL#3 has also been shown to induce remission in 93% of children compared to 36% of those treated with a placebo plus standard treatments.[229] *Escherichia coli* strain Nissle 1917 has also been shown to be equivalent to mesalazine for the maintenance of remission in UC.[230]

Prebiotic treatment using bifidogenic growth stimulator increases the concentration of the probiotic bifidobacteria in the intestine,[231] as does bifidobacteria-fermented milk.[232] In both studies, patients with mildly active UC experienced clinical benefit. Similarly, synbiotic therapy utilizing a combination of *Bifidobacterium longum* and Synergy 1 (a proprietary growth substrate) has been shown to improve posttreatment sigmoidoscopy scores.[233]

Leukocyte Apheresis

Studies in children as well as adults have demonstrated the efficacy of leukocyte apheresis for the nonmedicinal treatment of severe UC. Treatment involves passing blood from a patient over an extracorporeal filter that acts as a selective adsorptive column. Two different columns have been investigated as treatments for UC, the Adacolumn and the Cellsorba column. Each column has somewhat different filtration properties, such that it appears that results from the two systems may ultimately prove to be somewhat different. The treated blood is reinfused, depleted of granulocytes, monocytes, and activated platelets. Studies on the effects of apheresis suggest a number of potential mechanisms of action, including reduction in reactive oxygen species-producing granulocytes, reduction of activated platelets, changes in lymphocyte populations, and decreases in circulating proinflammatory cytokines.[234]

Apheresis has been shown to effectively reduce corticosteroid requirements in adults with steroid-dependent UC, resulting in both clinical and endoscopic improvement.[235] It has also been beneficial in the treatment of adults with toxic megacolon.[236] Two small Japanese studies in children reported clinical improvement without significant toxicity, as did a somewhat larger report from Scandanavia[237] and one from Spain.[238] This approach appears to be quite safe. By 2005, a review of 11,428 apheresis sessions performed for a wide variety of non-UC indications reported few adverse effects, with difficulty obtaining venous access (3.1%) and hypotension (1.6%) being the most common.[239]

Colon Cancer Prophylaxis

Because the goals of treatment for UC include prevention of complications in addition to control of inflammation, the potential of medical therapy to prevent colitis-associated cancer has become the focus of intense interest. Epidemiologic and case-control studies have suggested that treatment with an aminosalicylate is associated with a decreased rate of dysplasia and colon cancer.[240] Although the mechanism of action for this benefit is not entirely clear, one recent study has documented that these agents can suppress expression of a colorectal cancer-associated protein, thereby inducing gene-level changes in several critical carcinogenic pathways.[241] Preliminary studies have also suggested that chronic folate supplementation might provide a degree of chemoprevention through suppression of

DNA hypermethylation.[242] The effect of other medications used for the treatment of UC, including 6-MP and infliximab, on prevention of colon carcinogenesis are less clear.

SURGERY

UC is a surgically curable condition, and within 5 years of diagnosis intractable or fulminant symptoms result in 19% of children and adolescents undergoing colectomy (see section on Prognosis).[10] Indications for surgery in UC are summarized in Table 45-7. Curative surgery requires total mucosal proctocolectomy. Although proctocolectomy and ileostomy result in a healthy patient with no risk of future recurrence, few children or parents readily accept the option of a permanent ileostomy. Most instead opt for restorative surgery, which allows the child to continue to defecate by the normal route.

Because it is often difficult to distinguish definitively between fulminant UC and Crohn's colitis before the operation, many centers perform a staged procedure in the child with active colitis who requires surgery. Initially subtotal colectomy and ileostomy are performed, followed at a later date by restorative surgery if the colectomy specimen confirms a diagnosis of UC. The most commonly performed restorative surgery is currently the ileal pouch–anal anastomosis (IPAA) (Figure 45-5). The continent ileostomy (Kock pouch) is rarely, if ever, performed in children, given the success of IPAA. Summaries of pediatric surgical experience document that IPAA utilizing an ileal J-pouch (or less commonly a W- or S-pouch) results in fewer daytime and nocturnal bowel movements, and less fecal soiling, than an ileoanal anastomosis without a pouch.[243-247] Anorectal function is well preserved in children, and postoperative fecal soiling is unusual.[245] In fact, pouch function remains acceptable in most patients over 20 years of follow-up, although stool frequency and rates of daytime incontinence increase somewhat.[248] When growth retardation is evident before surgery, significant increases in height velocity can be expected after surgery.[249]

Stricture of the ileoanal anastomosis and small bowel obstruction are the most common postoperative complications of IPAA.[250,251] Pouchitis is a common late complication, occurring in nearly 50% of cases.[250,251] Data in adults suggest that patients who are pANCA positive, as well as those with PSC and those with backwash ileitis before colectomy, have a greater risk for developing pouchitis.[252] Pouchitis generally responds to treatment with metronidazole, ciprofloxacin, 5-ASA, or corticosteroids.[245,246,250] Reports also suggest that probiotic therapy can control or even prevent pouchitis.[253] At times, however, chronic and intractable complications occur, including the development of inflammatory and/or fistulizing disease indistinguishable from Crohn's disease.[254] In many of these cases, therapy with immune modifiers or anti-TNF agents can control

Table 45-7. Indications for Surgery in Ulcerative Colitis

Failure of medical therapy
   Intractable symptoms
   Drug toxicity
Persistent hemorrhage requiring transfusion
Perforation
Toxic megacolon
Low- or high-grade dysplasia
Carcinoma

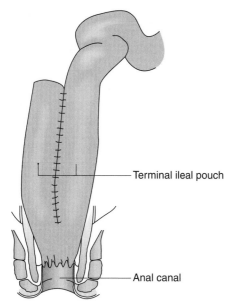

Figure 45-5. Ileal J-pouch–anal anastomosis (IPAA) – restorative surgery for ulcerative colitis.

the disease and salvage the pouch.[255] Unfortunately, at times therapy is unsuccessful, ultimately leading to pouch failure, requiring resection of the pouch in 8.6% of cases.[250]

COURSE AND PROGNOSIS

The course and prognosis of UC in children based on clinical experience derived after 1975 has been reported.[10] Seventy percent of children can be expected to enter remission within 3 months of initial diagnosis, irrespective of whether their initial attack is characterized as mild, moderate, or severe, and 45 to 58% remain inactive over the first year after diagnosis.[7] However, 10% of those whose symptoms are characterized as moderate or severe can be expected to remain continuously symptomatic. Over the ensuing 7- to 10-year intervals, approximately 55% of all patients have inactive disease, 40% have chronic intermittent symptoms, and 5 to 10% have continuous symptoms. These data are similar to those reported for adult populations.[256-258] Colectomy is required in 5% of all children within the first year after diagnosis, and in 19 to 23% by 5 years after diagnosis.[10,60] However, these rates rise to 9% and 26%, respectively, in the subgroup of children initially presenting with moderate or severe symptoms.[10] Overall these rates appear comparable to those recently reported in a Swedish pediatric population treated between 1961 and 1990,[258] and lower than those from older U.S. data that revealed colectomy rates of nearly 50% by

5 years after diagnosis in children presenting between 1955 and 1964, and 26% in those presenting between 1965 and 1974.[56] Clinical practice has changed significantly since the mid-1990s, with greater numbers of children with moderate-to-severe UC being treated with immune modulators and anti-TNF therapies. Although the acute effects of these therapies have been described in children, it is not yet clear whether such therapies are making a difference in colectomy rates.

Children with proctitis or proctosigmoiditis appear to follow a somewhat more benign course. More than 90% are asymptomatic within 6 months of diagnosis. In any given year of follow-up, 55% remain asymptomatic and less than 5% have continuously active disease.[61] In contrast to adults, however, proximal extension of disease occurs frequently, so that within 3 years of initial diagnosis as many as 25% of children may demonstrate signs of proximal extension. This rate of proximal extension may increase up to 70% over the course of follow-up.[60-62] Colectomy may eventually be required in 5% of patients.

REFERENCES

58. Gower-Rousseau C, Dauchet L, Vernier-Massouille G, et al. The natural history of pediatric ulcerative colitis: a population-based cohort study. Am J Gastroenterol 2009;104:2080–2088.

67. North American Society for Pediatric Gastroenterology, Hepatology, and Nutrition; Colitis Foundation of America, Bousvaros A, Antonioli DA, Colletti RB, et al. Differentiating ulcerative colitis from Crohn disease in children and young adults: report of a working group of the North American Society for Pediatric Gastroenterology, Hepatology, and Nutrition and the Crohn's and Colitis Foundation of America. J Pediatr Gastroenterol Nutr 2007;44:653–674.

107. Triantafillidis JK, Nasioulas G, Kosmidis PA. Colorectal cancer and inflammatory bowel disease: epidemiology, risk factors, mechanisms of carcinogenesis and prevention strategies. Anticancer Res 2009;29:2727–2737.

158. Turner D, Walsh CM, Benchimol EI, et al. Severe paediatric ulcerative colitis: incidence, outcomes and optimal timing for second-line therapy. Gut 2008;57:331–338.

171. Hyams J, Markowitz J, Lerer T, et al. Pediatric Inflammatory Bowel Disease Collaborative Research Group. The natural history of corticosteroid therapy for ulcerative colitis in children. Clin Gastroenterol Hepatol 2006;4:1094–1096.

203. Cucchiara S, Escher JC, Hildebrand H, et al. Pediatric inflammatory bowel diseases and the risk of lymphoma: should we revise our treatment strategies? J Pediatr Gastroenterol Nutr 2009;48:257–267.

209. Rutgeerts P, Sandborn WJ, Feagan BG, et al. Infliximab for induction and maintenance therapy for ulcerative colitis. N Engl J Med 2005;353:2462–2476.

217. Mackey AC, Green L, Leptak C, Avigan M. Hepatosplenic T cell lymphoma associated with infliximab use in young patients treated for inflammatory bowel disease: update. J Pediatr Gastroenterol Nutr 2009;48:386–388.

See expertconsult.com for a complete list of references and the review questions for this chapter.

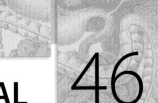

CHRONIC INTESTINAL PSEUDO-OBSTRUCTION

46

Paul E. Hyman

Chronic intestinal pseudo-obstruction (CIP) is a rare, disabling disorder characterized by repetitive episodes or continuous symptoms and signs of bowel obstruction, including radiographic documentation of dilated bowel with air-fluid levels, in the absence of a fixed, lumen-occluding lesion.[1] CIP is a clinical diagnosis based on phenotype, not pathology or manometry. Common signs are abdominal distention and failure to thrive. Common symptoms are abdominal pain, vomiting, and constipation or diarrhea. The term *CIP* is applied to different conditions that vary in cause, severity, course, and response to therapy (Table 46-1). Examples of genetic heterogeneity in CIP include, but are not limited to, a spectrum of abnormal gastric, small intestinal, and colonic myoelectric activity, contractions, and matrix proteins as well as histologic abnormalities in nerve, muscle, and cells of Cajal. Although these diseases have distinctive pathophysiologies, they are considered together because of clinical and therapeutic similarities.

ETIOLOGY

CIP may occur as a primary disease or as a secondary manifestation of other conditions that transiently (e.g., hypothyroidism, phenothiazine overdose), or permanently (e.g., scleroderma, amyloidosis) alter bowel motility (Table 46-2).

Most congenital cases are both rare and sporadic, possibly representing new mutations. That is, there is no family history of pseudo-obstruction, no associated syndrome, and no evidence of other predisposing factors such as toxins, infections, ischemia, or autoimmune disease. In some cases, chronic intestinal pseudo-obstruction results from a familial inherited disease. There are reports of autosomal dominant[2,3] and recessive[4-6] neuropathic and dominant[7-9] and recessive[10,11] myopathic inheritance patterns. In the autosomal dominant diseases, expressivity and penetrance are variable; some of those affected die in childhood, but those less handicapped are able to reproduce. An X-linked recessive form of neuropathic pseudo-obstruction has been mapped to a locus, Xq28.[12]

CIP may result from exposure to toxins during critical developmental periods in utero. A few children with fetal alcohol syndrome[13] and a few exposed to narcotics in utero have neuropathic forms of pseudo-obstruction. Presumably, any substance that alters neuronal migration or maturation might affect myenteric plexus development and cause CIP.

Children with chromosomal abnormalities may suffer from CIP. Children with Down syndrome have a higher incidence of Hirschsprung's disease than the general population and may have abnormal esophageal motility[14] and neuronal dysplasia in the myenteric plexus. Rare children with Down syndrome have a myenteric plexus neuropathy so generalized and so severe that they present with CIP. Children with neurofibromatosis, multiple endocrine neoplasia type IIB, dysautonomic syndromes, and other chromosome aberrations may suffer from neuropathic constipation. Children with Duchenne's muscular dystrophy sometimes develop CIP in the terminal stages of life. Esophageal manometry and gastric emptying are abnormal in asymptomatic patients with Duchenne's dystrophy, suggesting that the myopathy includes gastrointestinal smooth muscle.[15]

Acquired CIP may be a rare complication of infection from cytomegalovirus[16] or Epstein-Barr virus.[17] Immunocompromised children and immunosuppressed transplant recipients seem at higher risk than the general population. Acquired CIP might result from myenteric plexus neuritis caused by persistent viral infection or an autoimmune inflammatory response.[18] With celiac disease,[19] Crohn's disease, and the chronic enterocolitis associated with Hirschsprung's disease, some patients develop dilated bowel and symptoms related to effects of inflammatory mediators on mucosal afferent sensory nerves or motor nerves in the enteric plexuses. Other rare causes of CIP associated with inflammation include myenteric neuritis associated with anti-neuronal antibodies[20] and intestinal myositis.[21]

PATHOLOGY

Histologic abnormalities appear in muscle or nerve or, rarely, both.[22] Rarely, CIP is caused by a systemic disease of matrix proteins. CIP may be associated with absent c-kit positive cells of Cajal.[23] Histology is normal in about 10% of cases that are studied appropriately. In such cases there may be an abnormality in some biochemical aspect of stimulus-contraction coupling, such as ion channels or mitochondrial energy production. Mitochondrial disorders are associated with a subset of those affected.[24]

When laparotomy is imminent for a child with CIP, there must be timely communication between the surgeon and pathologists. A laparotomy is not indicated for biopsy alone,[25] perhaps because a pathologic diagnosis usually does not alter management or outcome. When surgery is indicated (e.g., for colectomy, cholecystectomy, or creation of an ileostomy), there should be a plan to obtain a full-thickness bowel biopsy specimen at least 2 cm in diameter. Tissues should be processed for routine histology, histochemistry for selected neurotransmitters and receptors, special stains for Cajal cells, electron microscopy, and silver stains.

Muscle disease may be inflammatory but more often is not. In light microscopy of both familial and sporadic forms of hollow visceral myopathy, the muscularis appears thin. The external longitudinal muscle layer is more involved than the internal circular muscle, and there may be extensive fibrosis in the muscle tissue. By electron microscopy there are vacuolar degeneration and disordered myofilaments (Figure 46-1).

Neuropathic disease is examined with silver stains of the myenteric plexus[26,27] and routine histologic techniques. The presence of neurons in the submucous plexus of a suction biopsy eliminates Hirschsprung's disease but is inadequate for the evaluation of other neuropathies. There may be maturational arrest of the myenteric plexus (Figure 46-2). This

hypoganglionosis is characterized by fewer neurons, which may be smaller than normal. Maturational arrest can be a primary congenital disorder or occur secondary to ischemia or infection. Changes can be patchy or generalized.

Inflammatory infiltrates of eosinophils or lymphocytes in myenteric ganglia are associated with CIP.[28,29]

Intestinal neuronal dysplasia[30] is a histologic diagnosis defined by (1) hyperplasia of the parasympathetic neurons and fibers of the myenteric (and sometimes submucous) plexus, characterized by increases in the number and size of ganglia, thickened nerves, and increases in neuron cell bodies; (2) increased acetyl cholinesterase-positive nerve fibers in the lamina propria; (3) increased acetylcholine esterase-positive nerve fibers around submucosal blood vessels; and (4) heterotopic neuron cell bodies in the lamina propria, muscle, and serosal layers. The first two criteria are obligatory. Children with CIP associated with neuronal dysplasia may have disease that is limited to the colon or disseminated. Other children may have neuronal dysplasia associated with prematurity, protein allergy, chromosome abnormalities, multiple endocrine neoplasia (MEN) IIB, and neurofibromatosis; however, intestinal neuronal dysplasia is an occasional incidental finding in bowel

TABLE 46-1. Features of Chronic Intestinal Pseudo-obstruction in Pediatric Patients

Onset
  Congenital
  Acquired
  Acute
  Gradual
Presentation
  Megacystis-microcolon intestinal hypoperistalsis syndrome
  Acute neonatal bowel obstruction, with or without megacystis
  Chronic vomiting and failure to thrive
  Chronic abdominal distention and failure to thrive
Cause
  Sporadic
  Familial
  Toxic
  Ischemic
  Viral
  Inflammatory
  Autoimmune
Area of involvement
  Entire gastrointestinal tract
  Segment of gastrointestinal tract
  Megaduodenum
  Small bowel
  Colon
Pathology
  Myopathy
  Neuropathy
  Absent neurons
  Immature neurons
  Degenerating neurons
  Intestinal neuronal dysplasia
  Ganglionitis: eosinophilic or neutrophilic
  No microscopic abnormality

TABLE 46-2. Causes of Chronic Pseudo-obstruction in Children

Primary pseudo-obstruction
  Visceral myopathy: sporadic or familial
  Visceral neuropathy: sporadic or familial
Secondary pseudo-obstruction: related or associated recognized causes
  Muscular dystrophies
  Scleroderma and other connective tissue diseases
  Postischemic neuropathy
  Postviral neuropathy
  Generalized dysautonomia
  Hypothyroidism
  Diabetic autonomic neuropathy
  Drugs: anticholinergics, opiates, calcium channel blockers, many others
  Severe inflammatory bowel disease
  Organ transplantation
  Amyloidosis
  Chagas' disease
  Fetal alcohol syndrome
  Chromosome abnormalities
  Multiple endocrine neoplasia IIB
  Radiation enteritis

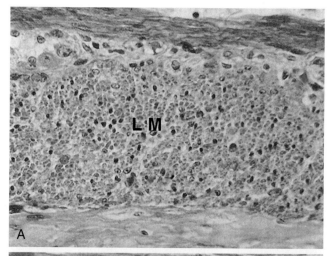
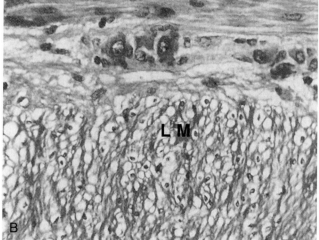

Figure 46-1. Visceral myopathy. (**A**) Longitudinal muscle cut in cross section from the small intestine of a control infant. (**B**) Longitudinal muscle from an infant with visceral myopathy shows classic vacuolar degeneration. Note the normal neurons in the myenteric plexus above the longitudinal muscle. ×136. Courtesy Michael D. Schuffler.

specimens examined for reasons unrelated to motility. Intestinal neuronal dysplasia correlates poorly with motility-related symptoms.[31] Thus, a pathologic diagnosis of intestinal neuronal dysplasia neither predicts clinical outcome nor influences management.

CLINICAL FEATURES

Presentation

More than half of the affected children develop symptoms at or shortly after birth. A few cases are diagnosed in utero, by ultrasound findings of polyhydramnios and megacystis and marked abdominal distention (Figure 46-3). Intestinal malrotation is common in both neuropathic and myopathic congenital CIP. Of children who present at birth, about 40% have an intestinal malrotation. In severely affected infants, symptoms of acute bowel obstruction appear within the first hours of life. Less severely affected infants present months later with constipation, vomiting, diarrhea, and failure to thrive. A few patients have megacystis at birth and insidious onset of gastrointestinal symptoms over the first few years. More than three-quarters of the children develop symptoms by the end of the first year of life, and the remainder present sporadically through the first two decades.

Abdominal distention and vomiting are the most common features (75%). Constipation, episodic or intermittent abdominal pain, and poor weight gain are features in about 60% of cases. Diarrhea is a complaint in one third. Urinary tract smooth muscle is affected in those with both neuropathy and myopathy, about 20% of CIP patients. Often these children are severely affected at birth and are described by the phenotype *megacystis-microcolon intestinal hypoperistalsis syndrome*.[32]

The clinical course is characterized by relative remissions and exacerbations. Many are able to identify factors that precipitate deteriorations, including intercurrent infections, general anesthesia, psychological stress, and poor nutritional status.

The radiographic signs are those of intestinal obstruction, with air-fluid levels (Figure 46-4), dilated stomach, small intestine and colon, or microcolon in those studied because of obstruction at birth.[33] There may be stasis of contrast material placed into the affected bowel, so it is prudent to use a nontoxic, isotonic, water-soluble contrast. Children who feel well still show radiographic evidence of bowel obstruction. The

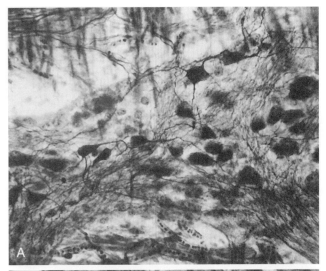

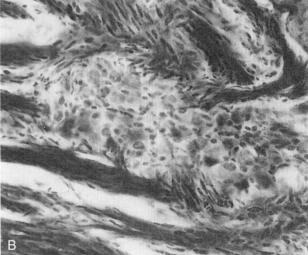

Figure 46-2. Maturational arrest of myenteric plexus. (**A**) Ganglionic area of myenteric plexus from the small intestine of a control infant. Note the numerous argyrophilic neurons and axons. (**B**) Ganglionic area of myenteric plexus from the small intestine of an infant with chronic intestinal pseudo-obstruction caused by maturational arrest. Note the absence of argyrophilic neurons and axons. The ganglion is filled with numerous cells, which are probably glial cells and immature neurons. ×544. *Courtesy Michael D. Schuffler.*

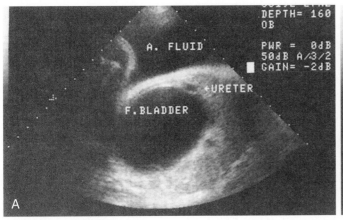

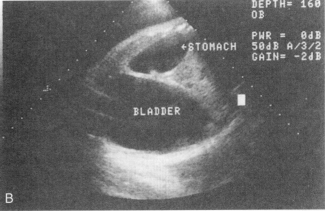

Figure 46-3. Ultrasound of infant with pseudo-obstruction diagnosed in utero. There is polyhydramnios as well as distention of the stomach and urinary bladder. *Courtesy Radha Cherukuri.*

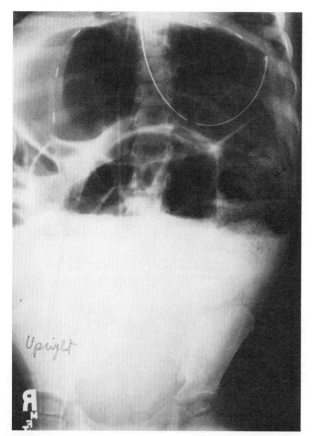

Figure 46-4. Upright abdominal radiograph in a 4-year-old boy with hollow visceral myopathy. Note bowel dilatation and air-fluid levels, central venous catheter in the inferior vena cava, and antroduodenal manometry catheter in the stomach and duodenum.

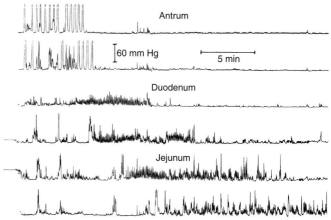

Figure 46-5. Phase 3 of the migrating motor complex (MMC), the marker for small intestinal neuromuscular health.

greater problem arises when children develop an acute deterioration. Radiographs demonstrate the same patterns of bowel obstruction that are seen when the child feels well. In children who previously had surgery, it can be difficult to discriminate between physical obstruction related to adhesions and an episodic increase in symptoms.

Diagnosis

An incorrect diagnosis of CIP results from misdiagnosis of infant and toddler victims of pediatric condition falsification, formerly known as Munchausen's syndrome by proxy.[34] Well-meaning clinicians inadvertently cocreate disease as they respond to a parent's symptom fabrications by performing tests and procedures, including parenteral nutrition support, repeated surgery, and even small bowel transplantation.[35] Preteens and adolescents with disabling abdominal pain may have a functional disorder and a comorbid psychiatric illness that do not respond to conventional management strategies and may be confused with CIP.[36]

Diagnostic testing provides information about the nature and severity of the pathophysiology. Manometry is superior to radiography to evaluate the strength and coordination of contraction and relaxation in the esophagus, gastric antrum, small intestine, colon, and anorectal area.

In affected children, scintigraphy demonstrates delayed gastric emptying of solids or liquids and reflux of intestinal

contents back into the stomach. Dilated bowel loops predispose to bacterial overgrowth, so breath hydrogen testing may reveal elevations in fasting breath hydrogen and a rapid increase in breath hydrogen with a carbohydrate meal.

Esophageal manometry is abnormal in about half those affected. In children with myopathy, contractions are persistently low amplitude but coordinated in the distal two thirds of the esophagus. Lower esophageal sphincter pressure is low, and sphincter relaxation is complete. When the esophagus is affected by neuropathy, contraction amplitude in the esophageal body may be high, normal, low, or absent. There may be simultaneous, spontaneous, or repetitive contractions. Relaxation of the lower esophageal sphincter may be incomplete or absent.

Antroduodenal manometry findings are always abnormal. However, manometry is often abnormal in partial or complete small bowel obstruction. Although the manometric patterns of true obstruction differ from those of pseudo-obstruction in adults,[37,38] such a distinction was not possible in children we have studied. Antroduodenal manometry should not be used to differentiate true bowel obstruction from CIP. Manometry should be done after a CIP diagnosis is established, to determine the physiologic correlates for the symptoms, to assess drug responses, and for prognosis.[39-41] Contrast radiography (e.g., enteroclysis or small bowel enema) and, as a last resort, exploratory laparotomy are best for differentiating true obstruction from pseudo-obstruction.

As in the esophagus, intestinal myopathy causes low-amplitude coordinated contractions and neuropathy causes uncoordinated contractions. The abnormalities in pseudo-obstruction are commonly discrete and easily interpreted by eye. They contrast markedly with normal features of antroduodenal manometry (Figure 46-5).

In most cases the manometric abnormality correlates with clinical severity of the disease. For example, children with total aganglionosis have contractions of normal amplitude that are never organized into migrating motor complexes (MMCs), fed patterns, or even bursts or clusters of contractions but are simply a monotonous pattern of random events. Children with such a pattern are dependent on total parenteral nutrition (TPN). More than 80% of children with MMCs are nourished enterally, but more than 80% of children without MMCs require partial or total parenteral nutrition.

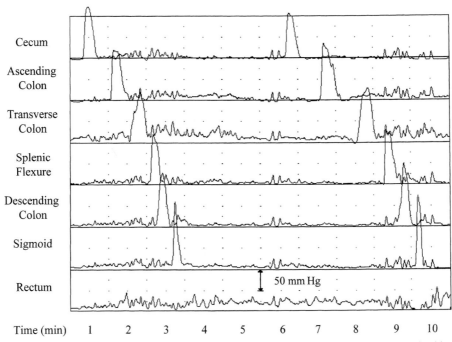

Figure 46-6. High-amplitude propagating contractions are a marker of colonic neuromuscular health.

Colonic manometry is abnormal in colonic CIP.[42] The normal features of colon manometry in children include (1) high-amplitude propagating contractions (phasic contractions stronger than 60 mm Hg amplitude propagating over at least 30 cm; Figure 46-6); (2) a gastrocolic response (the increase in motility that follows a meal); and (3) an absence of discrete abnormalities. With neuropathic disease, contractions are normal or reduced in amplitude, but there are no high-amplitude propagating contractions or gastrocolic response. With myopathy, there are usually no colonic contractions.

There are several pitfalls with intestinal and colonic manometry. In dilated bowel, no contractions are recorded and manometry is not diagnostic. Recordings filled with respiratory and movement artifacts from an agitated, angry, crying patient are uninterpretable. Acute pseudo-obstruction is usually associated with ileus, so that an absence of contractions may not reflect the underlying abnormality. Manometry is most helpful when performed in a cooperative patient at a time when the patient is feeling well.

Anorectal manometry is usually normal in CIP. The recto-inhibitory reflex is absent only in Hirschsprung's disease and in some patients with intestinal neuronal dysplasia.

TREATMENT

Nutrition Support

The goal of nutrition support is to achieve normal growth and development with the fewest complications and the greatest patient comfort. Motility improves as nutritional deficiencies resolve and worsens as malnutrition recurs.

Overall about one third of affected children require partial or total parenteral nutrition. One third require total or partial tube feedings and the rest eat by mouth. TPN is the least desirable means of achieving nutritional sufficiency because of the potential for life-threatening complications. In the absence of enteral nutrients, the gastrointestinal tract atrophies. Without enteral nutrients, the postprandial rise in trophic gastrointestinal hormones does not occur, and bile stasis and liver disease develop.[43] TPN-associated cholelithiasis[44] and progressive liver disease are important causes of morbidity and mortality in children with CIP. The minimal volume, composition, and route of enteral support required to reverse or prevent the progression of gastrointestinal complications have not been determined. Every effort should be extended to maximize enteral nutritional support in parenteral nutrition-dependent children.

Continuous feeding via gastrostomy or jejunostomy may be effective when bolus feedings fail. Most children with visceral myopathy and a few with neuropathy have an atonic stomach and almost no gastric emptying. In these children, a feeding jejunostomy may be helpful for the administration of medications and for drip feedings.[45] Care must be taken to place a jejunostomy into a normal-diameter bowel loop.

Drugs

Bethanechol, neostigmine, metoclopramide, and domperidone have not been useful. Cisapride has been helpful in a minority of children. Cisapride's mechanism of action is to bind to serotonin receptors on the motor nerves of the myenteric plexus, facilitating release of acetylcholine and stimulating gastrointestinal smooth muscle contraction. Cisapride is most likely to improve symptoms in children with MMCs and without dilated bowel.[40] Cisapride increases the number and strength of contractions in the duodenum of children with CIP but does not initiate the MMC in patients without it or inhibit discrete abnormalities.[46] Cisapride has been withdrawn from the commercial marketplace in much of the world because of concerns related to rare fatal cardiac arrhythmias. Cisapride overdose, or simultaneous administration of macrolide antibiotics or antifungal agents, is associated with an increased risk of ventricular arrhythmias. Janssen Pharmaceutica continues to manufacture cisapride and provide it at no cost to clinicians for individuals who meet criteria for and agree to a research protocol. A trial of cisapride is appropriate for every child with pseudo-obstruction related to hypomotility. It will not work for those with reduced inhibitory tone and too many disorganized contractions. For children on TPN, a cisapride trial should be initiated when there is no acute illness and no malnutrition, coincident with initiation of enteral feedings. Liquid suspension, 1 mg/mL, or tablet, 5 or 10 mg, is administered at 0.1 to 0.3 mg/kg per dose three or four times daily. Side effects include gastrointestinal complaints and irritability and are observed in about 5% of children. The addition of an acetylcholinesterase inhibitor such as neostigmine or physostigmine may improve the response to cisapride in some patients.

Erythromycin, a motilin receptor agonist, appears to facilitate gastric emptying in those with neuropathic gastroparesis by stimulating high-amplitude 3-min antral contractions, relaxing the pylorus, and inducing antral phase 3 episodes in doses of 1 to 3 mg/kg intravenously[47] or 3 to 5 mg/kg orally. Erythromycin does not appear to be effective for more generalized motility disorders.

Octreotide, a somatostatin analogue, given subcutaneously, induces small-intestinal phase 3–like clustered contractions and suppresses phase 2. However, the clusters may not propagate, or may propagate in either direction. Intestinal transit and absorption are best during phase 2. Thus somatostatin does not seem effective for generalized motility disorders.

Antibiotics are used for bacterial overgrowth. Bacterial overgrowth is associated with steatorrhea, fat-soluble vitamin malabsorption, and malabsorption of the intrinsic factor–vitamin B_{12} complex. It is possible that bacterial overgrowth contributes to bacteremia and frequent episodes of central venous catheter-related sepsis and to TPN-associated liver disease. Further, bacterial overgrowth, mucosal injury, malabsorption, fluid secretion, and gas production may contribute to chronic intestinal dilatation. Chronic antibiotic use may result in the emergence of resistant strains of bacteria or overgrowth with fungi. Thus, treating bacterial overgrowth must be considered on an individual basis. Often clinicians use a rotating schedule of antibiotics.

Excessive gastrostomy drainage may result from retrograde flow of intestinal contents into the stomach or from gastric acid hypersecretion. Gastric secretory function or gastric pH should be tested before beginning antisecretory drugs. Histamine H_2-receptor antagonists or proton pump inhibitors may be used to suppress gastric acid secretion. Tolerance develops with antihistamines after a few months of intravenous use,[48] so the drug should be given orally when possible. When a drug is added to TPN, gastric pH should be assessed at regular intervals to monitor drug efficacy. Induction of achlorhydria is inadvisable because it promotes bacterial overgrowth.

Constipation is treated with oral polyethylene glycol solutions, suppositories, or enemas. Oral enteral lavage solutions often cause abdominal distention because of delayed small bowel transit. For constipation and small bowel disease, cecostomy or appendicostomy may simplify management by bypassing the small bowel. If colon manometry shows no colon contractions, the most efficient course is ileostomy and colon resection. An ileostomy takes the resistance of the anal sphincter out of the system and facilitates flow of chyme from the higher pressures from gastric contractions to the absence of pressure at the stoma.

Acute pain is best treated by decompressing distended bowel. Opioids are rarely needed if the bowel is promptly decompressed. It is appropriate to consider nonsteroidal anti-inflammatory agents (e.g., ketorolac) and epidural anesthetics as alternatives to, or in combination with, systemic opioids. Opiates disorganize motility and increase fluid absorption.

Chronic pain is a problem in children with CIP and is common in adolescents who have autoimmune or inflammatory disease and progressive loss of intestinal function. Pain consists of a nociceptive component and an affective component. Patients with chronic pain benefit from a multidisciplinary approach including attention to gastrointestinal disease for the nociceptive component and mental health assessment and treatment for the affective pain component. Multiple modalities for pain relief are useful: cognitive behavioral therapy, massage, relaxation, hypnosis, psychotherapy, yoga, and drugs all have shown positive effects. Drugs that reduce afferent signaling, improving chronic visceral pain, include the tricyclic antidepressants, clonidine, and gabapentin.[49] Opioid use is inadvisable, because opioids disorganize intestinal motility, tolerance to opioids develops rapidly, and opioid withdrawal can simulate the pain of acute CIP.

Surgery

One of the management challenges in CIP is the evaluation and reevaluation of newborns and children with episodic acute obstructive symptoms. Although most acute episodes represent CIP, it is important to intervene with surgery when there is a true bowel obstruction, appendicitis, or another surgical condition. Many children with episodes of acute CIP undergo repeated exploratory laparotomies. It is important to avoid unnecessary abdominal surgery in children with CIP for several reasons: (1) They often suffer from prolonged postoperative ileus; (2) adhesions create a diagnostic problem each time there is a new obstructive episode; (3) adhesions following laparotomy may distort normal tissue planes and make future surgery riskier in terms of bleeding and organ perforation; and (4) each new pain experience activates sleeping nociceptors, leading to hyperalgesia. After several laparotomies turn up no evidence of mechanical obstruction, the surgeon may choose a more conservative management plan for subsequent episodes, including pain management, nutritional support, and abdominal decompression.

Gastrostomy was the only procedure that reduced hospitalizations in adults with CIP,[50] and the experience with children is similar. Gastrostomy provides a quick and comfortable means of evacuating gastric contents and relieves pain and nausea related to gastric and bowel distention. Continued "venting" may decompress distal regions of small bowel. Gastrostomy is used for feeding and administration of medication. Gastrostomy placement should be considered for those receiving parenteral nutrition and for children who will need tube feedings longer than 2 months. In many patients, endoscopic gastrostomy placement is ideal. In those with contraindications to endoscopic placement, surgical placement is appropriate.

CIP is a relative contraindication for fundoplication. After fundoplication, symptoms can change from vomiting to repeated retching.[51] Vomiting is reduced by venting the gastrostomy. Acid reflux is controlled with antisecretory medication.

Results of pyloroplasty or Roux-en-Y gastrojejunostomy to improve gastric emptying in CIP have been poor; gastric emptying remains delayed. Pyloroplasty and pyloric dilation failed to improve gastric emptying.[52] Small bowel resections or tapering operations may provide relief for months or even years; however, other areas of bowel gradually dilate and symptoms recur. Botulinum toxin also failed to improve gastric emptying.[53]

Ileostomy decompressed dilated distal small bowel and removed the high-pressure zone at the anal sphincter. Transit of luminal contents is always from a high-pressure zone to a lower-pressure one. In CIP patients with gastric antral contractions but no effective small bowel contractions, bowel transit improves with the creation of an ileostomy because of the absence of resistance to flow at the ostomy site.

Prolapse is common after enterostomy. Prolapse is a recurring problem that does not resolve after stomal revision. Each prolapse episode should be treated in a similar manner. The surgeon must use every conservative measure to return the prolapsed segment to the abdomen, from warm bath to general anesthesia. Unless the bowel loses viability there should be no surgery. The risk is that prolapses recur, resections mount up, and the child is left with a short failed intestine instead of a long one.

Colectomy is sometimes necessary in severe congenital pseudo-obstruction to decompress an abdomen so distended that respiration is impaired. In general, colon diversions are inadvisable because of a high incidence of diversion colitis.[54] Subtotal colectomy with ileoproctostomy cures rare children with CIP confined to the colon. Typically these children are able to eat normally and grow, but they are unable to defecate spontaneously. They differ from children with functional fecal retention in that their stools are never huge or hard, there is no retentive posturing, the history of constipation begins at birth, and there are often extrarectal fecal masses. Colon pathology may show neuronal dysplasia, maturational arrest, or no diagnostic abnormality, but colon manometry is always abnormal, without high-amplitude propagating contractions or a postprandial rise in motility index. Before colectomy for constipation, antroduodenal manometry is advisable to determine whether the upper gastrointestinal tract is involved. Abnormal antroduodenal manometry is a relative contraindication to colectomy because upper gastrointestinal symptoms appear after colon resection. A cecostomy using a small "button" ostomy appliance for regular infusion of colonic lavage solution has not been effective for severe colonic CIP. The abdomen distends, but the colon does not empty.

Failed medical management may signal a need for total bowel resection. Rarely, a mucosal secretory disorder complicates management. Several liters of intestinal secretions drain from enteric orifices each day. When secretions cannot be controlled with loperamide, anticholinergics, alosetron, antibiotics, steroids, or somatostatin analogue, it may be necessary to resect the entire bowel to avoid life-threatening electrolyte abnormalities and nutritional disturbances caused by volume losses. Total bowel resection may reduce episodes of bacterial transmigration across dilated bowel to eliminate repeated life-threatening central venous catheter infections. Total bowel resection should be considered alone or in combination with small bowel transplantation. Small bowel or combined liver-bowel transplants have the potential to cure. Outcomes in children with CIP are similar to outcomes in children undergoing transplantation for short bowel syndrome or intractable diarrhea.[55]

OUTCOMES

The quality of life for surviving children with CIP and their families is reduced compared to others with chronic disease.[56,57] The factors responsible for reduced quality of life in CIP were chronic pain and the caretaker's time commitment for participating in their child's medical care. We improve the quality of life for these patients by addressing these issues with collaborations from pain management clinicians including mental health professionals.

Parents looking for cures may find stem cell transplantation intriguing. Several groups are looking at the role that stem cells may have in correcting enteric nerve and smooth muscle abnormalities.[58]

REFERENCES

1. Connor FL, Di Lorenzo C. Chronic intestinal pseudo-obstruction: assessment and management. Gastroenterology 2006;130:529–538.
22. Krishnamurthy S, Schuffler MD. Pathology of neuromuscular disorders of the small intestine and colon. Gastroenterology 1987;93:610–639.
34. Hyman PE, Bursch B, Beck D, et al. Discriminating pediatric condition falsification from chronic intestinal pseudo-obstruction in toddlers. Child Maltreat 2002;7:132–137.
56. Mousa H, Hyman PE, Cocjin J, et al. Long term outcome of congenital intestinal pseudo-obstruction. Dig Dis Sci 2002;47:2298–2305.

See expertconsult.com for a complete list of references and the review questions for this chapter.

47 NEONATAL NECROTIZING ENTEROCOLITIS

Sabine Iben • Ricardo Rodriguez

Necrotizing enterocolitis (NEC) is the most common gastrointestinal emergency in the neonatal intensive care unit (NICU). It is primarily a disease of prematurity, with only 10% of affected infants born after 36 weeks of gestation.[1] NEC contributes significantly to short- and long-term morbidity as well as mortality of preterm infants. It is estimated that between 14% and 43% of all causes of intestinal failure are the result of sequelae of NEC.[2] Although the pathogenesis of the disease was first described more than 30 years ago,[3] the mortality rate for NEC has decreased minimally. Despite decades of vigorous research efforts, many unanswered questions remain. A number of potential contributing factors have been identified; however, the precise etiology of this multifactorial, complex disease process remains elusive. Preventive measures have been of limited success, and therapy is mostly supportive, consisting of medical stabilization and efforts to prevent progression of the disease.

EPIDEMIOLOGY

Despite significant advances in neonatal intensive care, necrotizing enterocolitis is associated with a high morbidity and mortality. It is estimated that $5 billion is spent annually in the care of patients with NEC and the morbidity associated with it.[4]

NEC affects about 1 to 5% of all newborns admitted to neonatal intensive care units, with an incidence of 7 to 14% in very low-birth-weight infants.[1,5] It is noteworthy that a significant intercenter variability has been reported. The only consistent epidemiologic precursors of NEC are prematurity and enteral alimentation,[6] although other risk factors have been identified. According to the data from the Vermont-Oxford Network encompassing about 2/3 of all extremely low-birth-weight (ELBW) infants born in the United States, the risk of NEC increases with lower gestational age and is as high as 12% in ELBW (501 to 750 g) compared to 3.3% in infants with birth weights between 1251 and 1500 g.[7] Because the number of ELBW infants treated in NICUs is relatively small, the majority of cases occur in the category of 30 to 32 weeks of gestation. Data from the National Institute of Child Health and Human Development (NICHD) Neonatal Research Network in three time periods from 1987 to 2000 show no change over time, with an incidence of 6-7% among infants with a birth weight less than 1500 g.[5] There is no consistent association between gender, socioeconomic status, or seasonal variability and the occurrence of necrotizing enterocolitis.

NEC is primarily a disease of the convalescent preterm infant with a peak incidence at 2 to 3 weeks postnatal age when the newborn has recovered from the acute period and is enterally fed. Earlier initiation of enteral feedings is associated with an earlier onset of NEC, which may account for the fact that

NEC occurs significantly earlier in more mature infants than in extremely preterm infants, as illustrated in Figure 47-1. In infants who have never been fed, NEC may be associated with maternal chorioamnionitis and intrauterine exposure to cytokines.[8] In general, cases of NEC are sporadic, although some centers have reported episodic outbreaks that occur more commonly in crowded nurseries. The vast majority of affected newborns are preterm (PT) infants; however, 10% of cases occur in full-term (FT) babies. Full-term infants tend to develop the disease earlier, at a mean age of less than 5 days,[9] and are more likely to have predisposing factors.[8,10,11] Some of the risk factors implicated include a history of abnormal antenatal Doppler studies,[12] gastroschisis, perinatal hypoxia, multiple gestation, history of umbilical artery catheter, polycythemia, sepsis, and congenital heart disease, all of which could potentially compromise intestinal blood flow. In a retrospective chart review by Ostlie et al.,[9] predisposing factors were lacking in 38% of NEC cases in FT infants, although most cases occur in the ICU setting.[11] Term infants who develop NEC are generally formula-fed, and the need for surgical intervention or survival does not seem to differ significantly from preterm infants.[11]

The reported incidence of NEC in infants with congenital heart disease is 3.3 to 6.8%, which is 10- to 100-fold higher than rates described for the entire late preterm/term newborn population.[13] In infants with congenital heart disease, NEC generally presents before surgical repair and is usually associated with anomalies that result in compromised mesenteric blood flow, such as left-sided obstructive lesions. Episodes of low cardiac output, shock, and cardiopulmonary bypass also represent significant risk factors. Independent of the anatomical defect, the presence of a left-to-right shunt at the level of the ductus arteriosus with a persistent diastolic flow reversal in the descending aorta (diastolic steal) and mesenteric hypoperfusion are postulated as the main pathogenic mechanisms.[14]

In recent years, epidemiologic data have emerged suggesting that interventions and therapies frequently used in the care of preterm infants may also be associated with an increased incidence of NEC. Particularly, the administration of prolonged courses of antibiotics resulting in altered microbial colonization and selection of pathogenic organisms seems to have a detrimental effect, potentially increasing long-term morbidity and mortality.[15] Other interventions implicated as risk factors include packed red blood cell transfusions[16,17] and respiratory support with continuous positive airway pressure (CPAP).[18] H_2 receptor antagonists frequently used for treatment of suspected gastrointestinal reflux in the NICU may also increase the infant's risk for the development of NEC by impairing a natural defense mechanism against bacterial overgrowth.[19]

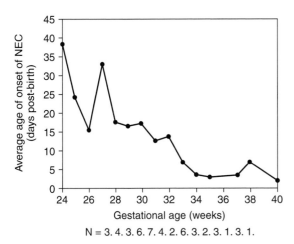

Figure 47-1. Necrotizing enterocolitis in babies over a 3-year period. Horizontal axis shows number of infants at increasing gestational ages. Vertical axis shows the postnatal age of onset of necrotizing enterocolitis. This graph demonstrates that there is an inverse relationship between age of onset and gestational age. From Neu (2005),[93] with permission.

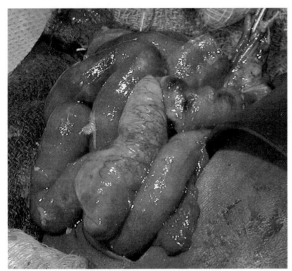

Figure 47-2. Intraoperative photograph of necrotizing enterocolitis demonstrating dilated bowel loops with areas of pneumatosis, bowel wall ischemia, and necrosis. Courtesy J. DiFiore, MD, and O. Soldes, MD.

PATHOLOGY

The characteristic gross pathologic features of NEC are signs of ischemia and patchy necrosis typically of the distal small intestine as well as the hepatic and splenic flexures of the colon (Figure 47-2). Involvement of both the small and large intestine is present in about 44% of cases, whereas 26% have only colonic compromise, and in 30% lesions are limited to small intestine.[20] The severity of bowel wall necrosis ranges from a small localized mucosal necrosis of a bowel segment to transmural necrosis of the entire small intestine and colon. In cases of fulminant presentation, the entire gastrointestinal tract may be involved, which is referred to as NEC totalis. Other pathologic findings include the presence of gastrointestinal bleeding, peritonitis, intestinal distension, pneumatosis intestinalis, and portal venous gas. Intra-abdominal fluid collection or a pneumoperitoneum, the latter indicating the presence of intestinal perforation, may also be found.

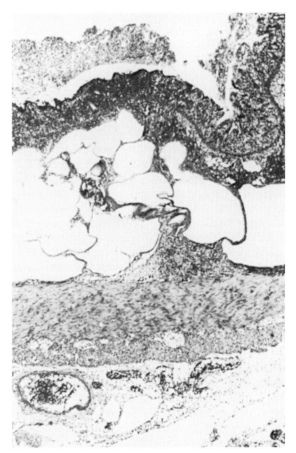

Figure 47-3. Microscopic evidence of severe submucosal gas-filled cysts (pneumatosis intestinalis) in a preterm infant with NEC. Note the marked hemorrhage throughout the bowel wall and the inflammatory exudate on the surface of the mucosa. Hematoxylin-eosin stain, ×56. Courtesy Beverly Dahms, MD.

Classical microscopic features (Figure 47-3) include areas of ulceration of the mucosa and submucosa in association with full-thickness necrosis, thrombosis of blood vessels, and a prominent influx of inflammatory cells (macrophages, neutrophils, and monocytes) into the submucosal layer. Coagulation necrosis, suggestive of an ischemic insult, is generally the predominant finding. Inflammatory changes and evidence of intestinal cell apoptosis are also characteristic microscopic features. Interestingly, in a series of pathologic observations, reparative changes including epithelial regeneration and granulation tissue fibrosis were reported in two thirds of cases.[20] In-situ hybridization studies in intestinal tissue from NEC patients demonstrated increased matrix metalloproteinase (MMP) mRNA expression, indicating an up-regulation of many members of the MMP family including MMP-1, 3 (stromelysin-1), 7, 12, and 24.[21,22] These zinc-dependent endopeptidases capable of degrading extracellular matrix have been shown to play a key role in tissue damage. In conjunction with stromelysin up-regulation, an increased transcription of TIMP-1, a natural tissue inhibitor of metalloproteinases, was also described, suggesting an active feedback loop to counteract ongoing tissue destruction. Interleukin (IL)-1β and tissue necrosis factor (TNF)-α, both important inflammatory mediators in NEC, stimulate the production of MMPs, whereas TNF-α down-regulates TIMP-1. These data indicate that TNF-α plays a crucial role in tissue destruction in patients with NEC. In pathologic specimens of patients undergoing intestinal resection for NEC, intestinal cell apoptosis and expression of the inducible isozyme of nitric oxide synthase (iNOS) have been demonstrated, as well as increased tissue transcripts for TNF-α, interleukins 8 and 11, and decreased interferon (IFN)-γ.[23-25,26]

PATHOGENESIS

The medical syndrome of NEC is well recognized; however, its pathogenesis remains poorly understood. Because of the multifactorial origin of the disease and the inherent limitations in experimental models, attempts to develop early diagnostic tools and preventive measures have been largely unsuccessful. Several animal models for the study of NEC have been developed. These experimental models yield pathologic and cytokine profiles similar to those observed in human newborns; however, they fail to reproduce the intrinsic and complex aspects of prematurity, thus limiting to some degree the extrapolation of results to clinical NEC.[27] The roles of factors involved in regulation of epithelial function, cytokine production, bacterial colonization, protective and toxic effects of nitric oxide (NO), intestinal mucosal restitution, and immaturity of protective mechanisms as contributors to the initiation and/or progression of NEC continue to be explored. The influence of genetics on the individual susceptibility to the development of NEC is still emerging. Recent studies have shown that a carrier state of genetic polymorphisms may be associated with perinatal morbidity, including NEC.[28] The identification of a genetic marker with high sensitivity and specificity for the prediction of NEC could potentially lead to the implementation of effective preventive measures.

A generally accepted hypothesis of the pathophysiology of NEC involves an initial insult, such as ischemia, contributing to loss of intestinal barrier integrity. Once formula feedings are introduced, they serve as substrate for bacterial proliferation. Pathogenic enteric organisms then invade the injured mucosa, promoting the production of proinflammatory cytokines.[3] Infants, particularly those born prematurely, may have a reduced ability to counterregulate this surge in proinflammatory mediators, leading to additional injury, eventual breach of the mucosal barrier, and bacterial translocation. A systemic inflammatory reaction syndrome (SIRS) results in a clinical picture of septic shock.

Ischemic Injury

Ischemic injury is thought to play a central role in the cascade of events leading to the development of NEC. Several investigators have used animal models of NEC that rely on the induction of intermittent ischemia and reperfusion of the intestine, typically through temporary occlusion of the blood supply to the small intestine. Although such models may provide valuable information regarding the biology of intestinal ischemia reperfusion injury, it is noteworthy that a clear ischemic/reperfusion injury is often absent or very remote in patients in whom NEC develops during the convalescence phase of their hospitalization.

Neonatal asphyxia, recurrent episodes of hypoxia-bradycardia, systemic arterial hypotension, patent ductus arteriosus, congenital heart disease, and polycythemia are some of the mechanisms that may lead to intestinal ischemia. In states of hypoperfusion, the "diving reflex" is activated as a protective mechanism to ensure adequate blood supply to vital organs, including the brain and the heart, while shunting blood away from the splanchnic circulation, thus worsening gut ischemia. Ischemic injury of the intestinal mucosa ensues, followed by activation of the inflammatory cascade, reperfusion injury, and gut barrier dysfunction with bacterial translocation and the systemic effects associated with it. Basal intestinal vascular resistance is maintained by a dynamic balance between constrictor (ET-1) and dilator (NO) stimuli, and in newborns this balance favors NO-dependent vasodilation, leading to a low vascular resistance ensuring adequate blood flow to the rapidly growing intestine. Disruption of intestinal endothelial cell function could alter this balance favoring ET-1-dependent vasoconstriction and thus lead to significant intestinal ischemia. Doppler studies of the superior mesenteric artery in premature infants who later developed NEC demonstrated a high resistance pattern suggestive of abnormal intestinal blood flow in these patients.[29] Interestingly, decreased resistance to blood flow was found in patients with established NEC. It has been postulated that this apparent discrepancy may actually represent a biphasic response of the mesenteric vessels, with an initial phase (high resistance to flow/ischemic injury), followed by rebound hyperemia (low resistance to flow/reperfusion injury), due to the release of inflammatory mediators.[29] It is possible that alterations in the autoregulation of intestinal blood flow, mediated by a balance between vasoconstrictor and vasodilator molecules, may play a role in the development and progression of NEC. In addition, intestinal tissue removed from infants with NEC demonstrates abnormalities in expression and regulation of these important vasoactive mediators.[30]

Gut Barrier

In mature animals, the intestine has many physical barriers to bacteria, including peristalsis, gastric acidity, proteolytic enzymes, intestinal mucus, cell surface glycoconjugates, and tight junctions between intestinal epithelial cells. These protective mechanisms limit the bacteria microenvironment to the gut lumen and prevent attachment and translocation across the intestinal epithelium.[31] However, experimental data demonstrate that pathogenic organisms adhere to and translocate across the intestine to a greater extent in immature compared to mature animals. Abnormal peristaltic activity and hypomotility in immature infants may increase bacterial adherence, allowing for bacterial overgrowth. In the NICU, the use of narcotics for sedation and pain management may accentuate this phenomenon. In preterm infants, the repertoire of cell surface glycoconjugates, which serve as adhesion sites for a variety of microbes, have a different pattern of carbohydrate residues. This functional difference may in part account for differences in bacterial colonization patterns in these infants. Colonization of the intestine by commensal microorganisms is a key step in intestinal maturation and maintenance of the gut barrier. Alternatively, colonization with pathogenic organisms may trigger an inappropriate reaction by the immature intestine with activation of the inflammatory cascade, which promotes disruption of the gut barrier resulting in NEC. Human defensins (or cryptidins) produced and secreted from Paneth cells protect against bacterial translocation; however, this mechanism is impaired in premature infants, particularly those with NEC. Trefoil factor peptides (TFF1-3) are part of the protective mechanism operating in the intestinal mucosa and play a fundamental role in epithelial protection, repair, and restitution. These secreted peptides have been identified in a site-specific pattern in the gastrointestinal mucosa, and their expression has been shown to be up-regulated in early stages of mucosal repair. A study by Lin et al.[32] demonstrated that TFF3 mRNA and protein expression is deficient in immature rats. Impaired mucosal regeneration in part due to failure of up-regulation of trefoil factor peptide expression may contribute to the pathogenesis of NEC.[33] Tight junctions between epithelial cells maintain the semipermeable properties of the intestinal epithelium, limiting the passage of bacteria and other macromolecules. Immaturity in the composition and function of the tight junctions through the interactions of structural proteins (claudins and occludins) may explain the increased permeability of the immature intestine. Furthermore, changes in expression of genes coding for these structural proteins have been described during the lesional and reparative phases of NEC.

In premature infants, there is immaturity of the functional barrier that limits growth of bacteria, the immunologic host defense mechanism, and various biochemical factors involved in gut barrier protection. It is known that the numbers of intestinal B and T lymphocytes are decreased in neonates and do not approach adult levels until 3 to 4 weeks of life. Newborns also have reduced levels of secretory IgA in salivary samples, presumably reflecting decreased activity in the intestine. Furthermore, the intestinal lamina propria is devoid of IgA secreting cells, rendering the newborn more susceptible to infection on the mucosal surface. Enteral administration of a formulation containing 73% IgA and 26% IgG was associated with a significant decreased incidence of NEC, though a recent meta-analysis showed no difference.[34,35]

Bacterial Colonization

The role of bacterial colonization in the pathogenesis of NEC has long been recognized. In utero, the intestinal tract is free of bacteria, but it becomes rapidly colonized during the first days of life. Mode of delivery and type of enteral feedings affect the timing and patterns of colonization. Infants delivered vaginally have earlier colonization with both *Bifidobacterium* and *Lactobacillus*, whereas infants delivered by cesarean section can have colonization with these beneficial organisms delayed by up to 30 days.[36,37] After birth and during the first week of life, the normal breast-fed newborn gut is colonized by predominantly protective anaerobe bacteria including lactobacilli and bifidobacteria. In formula-fed infants, similar amounts of *Bacteroides* and *Bifidobacterium* are found with minor components of the more pathogenic *Staphylococcus*, *Escherichia coli*, and *Clostridium*.[38,39] In contrast, the preterm infant's gut is exposed to a flora with a predominance of potentially pathogenic gram-negative species, with a lesser degree of bacterial diversity and fewer protective anaerobe species. The use of broad-spectrum antibiotics during the immediate neonatal period may select a population of resistant organisms, aggravating this situation. In the presence of other risk factors, alteration of the intestinal microbiome may set the stage for the later development of NEC. Despite the description of outbreaks of NEC in some nurseries, no single specific organism can be identified as the etiologic agent for NEC.[40] *Klebsiella*, *E. coli*, *Clostridium* species, and *Staphylococcus epidermidis*, as well as a variety of viruses and fungal species, have all been isolated from patients with NEC. Particular interest has been placed on a relatively new organism, *Enterobacter sakazakii* (ES). ES causes sepsis and meningitis in low-birth-weight infants and has been identified in the hospital environment in association with infant bottle brushes and food preparation equipment. Ingestion of ES-contaminated infant formula has been implicated in cases of necrotizing enterocolitis.[41,42] In vitro and in vivo studies suggest that ES adheres to the enterocyte and promotes cell necrosis and apoptosis in a dose-dependent manner. In 2002, the U.S. Food and Drug Administration (FDA) published a warning regarding the presence of ES in baby formula.[43]

Feedings and NEC

The contribution of different feeding practices to the pathogenesis of NEC has been extensively studied. Timing of introduction of feeds, type, volume, and rate of advance have all been subject of clinical studies. Experimental data suggest that introduction of feeds is important to establish intestinal barrier function. In a rat model, starvation reduces gut mucosal barrier function; conversely, early feeds improved intestinal mucosal growth in piglets.[44,45] In a recent study, infants who were never fed and developed NEC were more likely to rapidly progress to severe disease.[46] It is possible that the early introduction of breast-milk feedings prepares the intestinal barrier to better deal with noxious stress later on.

In four randomized controlled trials, rapid advancement of enteral feeds was associated with a shorter time to full feeds and more rapid attainment of birth weight without an increased incidence of NEC.[47,48] These results are tempered by another trial where rapid progression of enteral feeds was associated with NEC.[49]

Breast milk or donor breast milk are preferred for initiation of enteral alimentation for preterm infants when available. In a recent study, a protocol of enteral feedings containing at least 50% of human milk in the first 14 days of life was associated with a sixfold decrease in the incidence of NEC.[50] Interestingly, the benefits of breast-milk feedings may follow a dose-related beneficial effect on the risk of NEC and mortality.[51] Besides the well-known immunologic properties in breast milk, the presence of other factors such as epithelial growth factor (EGF), erythropoietin, insulinlike growth factor (IGF), and the anti-inflammatory cytokine IL-10 may account for its protective effects. The currently available data support the promotion of breast milk as the initial nutrient of choice for the premature infant. It is well known that feeding practices vary among centers, but in general, judicious introduction of gut-priming feeds followed by a slow rate of advancement with close attention paid to feeding intolerance seems to be the preponderant approach.[52] The effects of other enterally administered supplements (e.g., vitamins, iron, fortifiers) on the incidence of NEC are unclear.

Abnormal Inflammatory Response

The modulation of the inflammatory response seems to be developmentally regulated, and it requires an appropriate balance between pro- and anti-inflammatory signaling in order to maintain a healthy intestinal homeostatic environment.

The inability of the premature newborn to distinguish and respond appropriately to commensal and pathogenic microorganisms and the aberrant regulation of other mediators such as platelet activating factor (PAF) lead to a proinflammatory environment that could contribute to the pathology seen in NEC. Human fetal intestinal epithelial cells demonstrate an exaggerated production of inflammatory cytokines in response to pathogenic and commensal bacteria, as well as to endogenous inflammatory mediators such as TNF-α and interleukin. Several proinflammatory cytokines that mediate inflammatory cell recruitment through activation and amplification of the immune response in local host defense have been implicated in NEC, including TNF-α, IL-1β, IL-6, IL-8, IL-12, and IL-18.[53] Anti-inflammatory cytokines modulate the host's inflammatory response; a lack of up-regulation of these molecules to counteract the effects of proinflammatory mediators results in more severe tissue injury. Both anti- inflammatory cytokines, IL-4 and IL-10, have been implicated in NEC.[54]

Lipopolysaccharide (LPS), which is a principal component of the outer cell wall of gram-negative bacteria, recognizes and binds to Toll-like receptor 4 (TLR4). Circulating LPS is increased in patients with NEC, which inhibits epithelial restitution and initiates inflammatory signaling cascades within the enterocyte including activation of the transcription factor nuclear factor (NF)-κB. NF-κB proteins activate transcription of a wide variety of genes important in inflammatory and immune responses. In the resting state, NF-κB dimers are bound in the cytoplasm to inhibitory κB (IκB) proteins. By activation of an IKKinase, NFκB is freed to translocate to the nucleus, where it triggers gene transcription. An autoregulatory feedback loop exists in which NF-κB activation leads to IκBa synthesis, which in turn can terminate the NF-κB response. However, it has been shown that immature enterocytes have increased NF-κB activity associated with decreased baseline expression of IκB isoforms. In addition, there is more rapid I degradation and delayed resynthesis of IκBa in immature enterocytes. These data suggest that the increased inflammatory cytokine production in the immature intestine may result from the combined effect of (1) increased NF-κB activity and translocation to the nucleus because of decreased IκB expression and (2) decreased inhibition of NF-κB due to an accelerated degradation and delayed resynthesis of IκBa.[55]

The pathogenesis of NEC is complex, and our understanding of it is still incomplete. Multiple pathogenic mechanisms affecting the premature infant, such as perinatal ischemia, feedings and bacterial colonization, and inflammation, converge into a final common pathway leading to intestinal barrier failure, tissue damage, and organ system failure (Figure 47-4). Increasing our understanding of the mechanisms involved in NEC through well-designed clinical and basic research will allow us to develop and implement interventions aimed at early diagnosis and prevention. Currently, introduction of enteral feedings with breast milk is the most readily available way to decrease the incidence of the disease.

CLINICAL MANIFESTATIONS

The early stages of NEC present with nonspecific signs that may occur in an otherwise stable preterm infant or may represent alternative pathologies such as sepsis (Table 47-1). Temperature instability, lethargy, and apneic spells may precede abdominal symptoms. The majority of preterm infants develop NEC during their convalescent phase, generally while on or close to full enteral feeds.[56] A sudden increase in gastric residuals or episodes of emesis, which may be bilious or nonbilious, is suggestive of a disease process. The abdominal examination may reveal decreased or absent bowel sounds, distention, and tenderness. Although the presence of occult fecal blood is nonspecific,[57] a grossly bloody stool in a high-risk infant is suggestive of necrotizing enterocolitis and is the most common presenting sign in term infants.[13]

Abdominal distention may rapidly progress and be accompanied by abdominal skin discoloration. As the disease evolves, the infant may develop cardiovascular instability and respiratory failure. Endotracheal intubation and mechanical ventilation may be necessary because of either severe apnea or significant

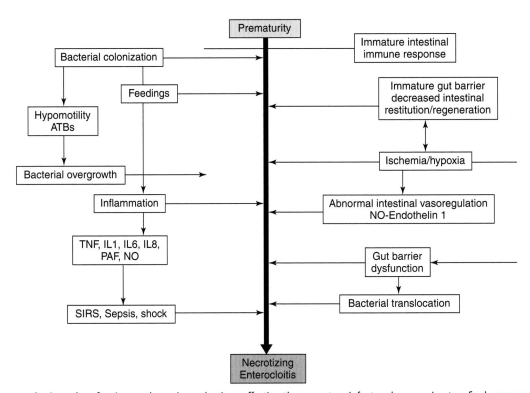

Figure 47-4. The complex interplay of various pathogenic mechanisms affecting the premature infant and converging to a final common pathway leading to NEC.

TABLE 47-1. Presentation of Necrotizing Enterocolitis

Clinical Signs and Symptoms
Apnea and bradycardia
Lethargy
Temperature instability (need to increase environmental temperature)
Abdominal distention/tenderness/guarding
Discoloration of abdominal skin
Bloody stools (grossly or occult)
Tachycardia
Hypotension
Poor perfusion
Respiratory failure

Laboratory Findings
Increased WBC count with or without left shift
Neutropenia
Coagulation abnormalities – DIC (↑ PT/PTT, ↓ Fibrinogen)
Anemia
Thrombocytopenia or thrombocytosis (less common)
Increased inflammatory markers (C-reactive protein)
Hyperglycemia
Electrolyte abnormalities/hyponatremia
Acidosis (metabolic and/or respiratory)

Radiographic Findings
Dilated bowel loops with "stacked" appearance
Thickened bowel walls
Fixed bowel loops
Pneumatosis intestinalis
Portal venous air
Free intra-abdominal air
Ascites
Gasless abdomen

Intraoperative Findings
Pneumatosis intestinalis
Intestinal inflammation
Bowel ischemia
Bowel necrosis
Perforation

DIC, disseminated intravascular coagulation; PT, prothrombin time; PTT, partial thromboplastin time; WBC, white blood cell count.

abdominal distention compromising pulmonary function. A significant increase in intra-abdominal pressure may lead to decreased venous return to the heart and thus contribute to hypotension and tachycardia. The infant may develop features of SIRS with evidence of cardiac dysfunction and septic shock, culminating in multiorgan system failure and death. The severity and progression of the disease are variable. Approximately one half of infants with NEC will recover fully with bowel rest and antibiotics, whereas up to 40% will develop severe disease requiring urgent surgical intervention.[58] An observational cohort study by Moss et al.[46] found that the median and mean time interval from the diagnosis of NEC to severe disease resulting in surgical intervention were 1 and 6 days, respectively. The highest risk for bowel perforation is during the first 72 hours after diagnosis.[4] Furthermore, 63% of the patients required surgical intervention within the first 2 days, 80% within the first week.[46] Symptoms of bowel perforation and peritonitis include marked abdominal distention with inability to ventilate, erythematous or blue discoloration of abdominal skin, and clinical deterioration. Laboratory findings consist of neutropenia or neutrophilia, thrombocytopenia, increased inflammatory markers (C-reactive protein), electrolyte imbalances, and abnormal coagulation panel consistent with disseminated intravascular coagulation (DIC) (see Table 47-1). A progressive decrease in absolute granulocyte counts and thrombocytopenia suggest increasing severity of disease. Persistent metabolic acidosis and refractory thrombocytopenia may indicate intestinal necrosis and the need for surgical exploration. Some patients will rapidly progress to shock, DIC, multisystem organ failure, and death despite maximized medical and/or surgical therapy. Unfortunately, at the present time there are no early clinical or laboratory markers available to identify patients at risk for rapid progression.[4]

To classify the severity of disease, Bell's staging criteria[5,59] as modified by Kliegman (Table 47-2) may be used. Stage I is nonspecific; symptoms may be present with the sepsis syndrome without intestinal involvement. Stage II is NEC as diagnosed by the presence of pneumatosis intestinalis in addition to systemic symptoms with increasing severity as outlined previously. Stage IIIA is defined by severe involvement with cardiorespiratory instability and stage IIIB by the presence of bowel perforation. Bell's classification has been used widely in research to stratify infants according to severity of disease.

DIAGNOSIS

The diagnosis of NEC rests on clinical and radiologic findings. However, clinical symptoms can be nonspecific. An abdominal x-ray is indicated if there are abnormal findings on physical examination. Characteristically, plain abdominal films may show signs of ileus with nonspecific dilated, "stacked" bowel loops in the early stages. Later, a thickened bowel wall may be appreciated. The development of a fixed loop on serial x-rays may be an ominous sign indicating bowel necrosis. The pathognomonic radiographic feature of NEC is pneumatosis intestinalis (Figure 47-5), which may be diffuse or localized and has a mottled appearance or may present as curvilinear translucencies within the bowel wall. Intramural gas is more commonly present in the distal small bowel and colon and is therefore most commonly seen in the right lower quadrant. In the absence of other symptoms, an otherwise normal bowel gas pattern with areas of mottled appearance predominantly in the left lower quadrant is more consistent with impacted stools rather than pneumatosis intestinalis. Infants who present with portal venous gas (Figure 47-6) are generally more severely affected and more likely to require surgical intervention.[60] "Medical NEC" becomes "surgical NEC" when there is evidence of bowel perforation. Because the risk of bowel perforation is higher during the first 24 to 48 hours of the disease process,[4] serial films should be obtained to assess for the presence of free air. Intestinal perforation can be diagnosed best in cross-table lateral or left lateral decubitus radiographs (Figure 47-7). Free air in the abdominal cavity is better visualized in these views because air rises to the top and is often seen above the liver shadow. In anteroposterior views of the abdomen, the visualization of the falciform ligament or football sign indicates the presence of a pneumoperitoneum. Usually, contrast studies are not necessary for diagnosis of NEC and may be indeed contraindicated because of the high risk of perforation.

Gray-scale and Doppler ultrasonography have been used to aid in the diagnosis of NEC. Sonographic findings may include fluid collections, increased bowel wall echogenicity, portal venous gas, bowel wall thinning or thickening, and intramural gas.[61-63] Doppler interrogation may be particularly useful to evaluate intestinal blood flow. Although some studies have found a good correlation with later bowel perforation, sensitivity and specificity are operator dependent[61]; thus, this method is not widely used in the United States.

TABLE 47-2. **Modified Bell's Staging Criteria for Neonatal Necrotizing Enterocolitis**

	Stage	Systemic Signs	Intestinal Signs	Radiologic Signs	Treatment
IA	Suspected NEC	Temperature instability, apnea, bradycardia, lethargy	Raised pre-gavage residuals, mild abdominal distention, emesis, guaiac-positive stool	Normal or intestinal dilation; mild ileus	NPO, antibiotics for 3 days pending cultures, gastric decompression
IB	Suspected NEC	Same as IA	Bright red blood from rectum	Same as IA	Same as IA
IIA	Definite NEC, mildly ill	Same as IA	Same as IA and IB plus diminished or absent bowel sounds ± abdominal tenderness	Intestinal dilation, ileus, pneumatosis intestinalis	Same as IA plus NPO, antibiotics for 7-10 days if examination is normal in 24-48 hours
IIB	Definite NEC, moderately ill	Same as IIA plus mild metabolic acidosis and mild thrombocytopenia	Same as IIA plus definite abdominal tenderness ± abdominal cellulitis, or right lower quadrant mass, absent bowel sounds	Same as IIA ± portal vein gas ± ascites	Same as IIA plus NPO, antibiotics for 14 days, NaHCO₃ for acidosis, volume replacement
IIIA	Advanced NEC, severely ill, bowel intact	Same as IIB plus hypotension, bradycardia, severe apnea, combined respiratory and metabolic acidosis, DIC, neutropenia, anuria	Same as IIB plus signs of generalized peritonitis, marked tenderness, distention and abdominal wall erythema	Same as IIB, definite ascites	Same as IIB plus as much as 200 mL/kg fluids, fresh frozen plasma, inotropic agents, intubation, ventilation therapy, paracentesis; surgical intervention if patient fails to improve with medical management within 24-48 hours
IIIB	Advanced NEC, severely ill, bowel perforated	Same as IIIA, sudden deterioration	Same as IIIA, sudden increased distention	Same as IIB plus pneumoperitoneum	Same as IIIA plus surgical intervention

From Kliegman R. Necrotizing enterocolitis. In: Burg FD, Ingelfinger JR, Wald ER, eds. Gellis & Kagan's Current Pediatric Therapy, 15th ed. Philadelphia: WB Saunders; 1996 pp. 217–220, with permission.
DIC, disseminated intravascular coagulation; NPO, *nil per os.*

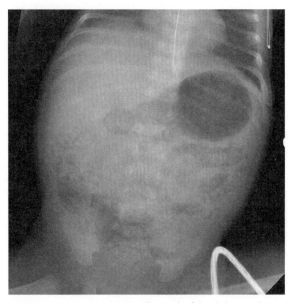

Figure 47-5. Anteroposterior (AP) radiograph of the abdomen demonstrating extensive pneumatosis intestinalis and paucity of bowel gas.

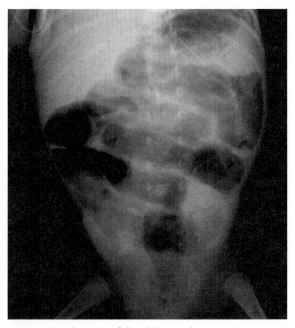

Figure 47-6. AP radiograph of the abdomen demonstrating pneumatosis intestinalis and portal venous gas. An abnormal abdominal gas pattern with distended, stacked loops of bowel is also present. Courtesy Stuart Morrison, MD.

The differential diagnosis of NEC is very limited, and in the presence of characteristic clinico-radiologic findings, the diagnosis is relatively straightforward. An entity sometimes confused with NEC is spontaneous intestinal perforation (SIP), which tends to occur earlier. Patients with SIP typically present with pneumoperitoneum within the first week of life, with few, if any, antecedent clinical symptoms or prodrome of systemic illness as is characteristic of NEC. SIP is associated with the use of glucocorticoids and indomethacin but not with aggressive enteral feeding, because many cases occur before feedings are introduced. Furthermore, the histopathology of SIP is more consistent with hemorrhagic necrosis rather than the typical coagulation necrosis seen in NEC.[64]

Prematurity is the only clearly identifiable risk factor for NEC. It is in this population that finding an early marker for the

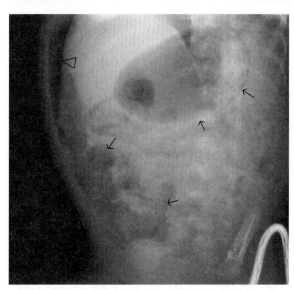

Figure 47-7. Left lateral decubitus radiograph demonstrating pneumo-peritoneum with air over the liver (arrowhead). There is also extensive pneumatosis intestinalis involving the gastric wall (arrows). Courtesy Stuart Morrison, MD.

disease would be desirable, because it may translate into better outcomes. Fecal calprotectin is regarded as a marker of intestinal inflammation and has been used in the adult population to follow the activity in inflammatory bowel disease. Joseffson et al.[65] studied a population of premature infants to establish reference values for fecal calprotectin l and found significantly elevated concentrations in infants with NEC concurrent with the time of radiologic diagnosis.

PREVENTION

The most effective way to decrease the incidence of NEC is to prevent premature birth. Antenatal interventions aimed at improving neonatal outcomes may also contribute to lower rates of NEC. One of such measures is the administration of antenatal steroids to mothers at risk for premature delivery. Antenatal corticosteroids, widely used for their beneficial effect on pulmonary maturation, have been linked to a reduced incidence of NEC via similar induction of intestinal maturity.[66]

Encouraging mothers to provide breast milk for optimal nutrition should start at the first encounter. Enteral feeding containing at least 50% of mother's milk in the first 14 days of life is associated with a sixfold decrease in the odds of NEC.[67] There is conflicting information about similar benefits of donor's milk.[68,69] Early initiation of gut stimulation feeds strengthens host defenses, potentially decreases bacterial overgrowth, and results in better feeding tolerance at the time of advancement without increasing the incidence of NEC.[70] Centers that are using feeding protocols with an advance of 10 to 20 mL/kg/day report a lower incidence of NEC[71] compared to centers with a nonstandardized feeding approach.

Currently the most promising preventative strategy, other than exclusive feeds with maternal breast milk, involves the use of probiotics and prebiotics. The most commonly used probiotic agents have been *Bifidobacterium*, *Lactobacillus*, and *Streptococcus*, which are components of commensal microflora. Probiotics have the potential to affect many aspects of the pathway leading to NEC, including protection against mucosal injury,

promoting a more favorable bacterial colonization, activating general intestinal immune defenses, and modulating intestinal inflammation. Clinical trials[72] show a consistent decrease in the incidence of NEC in treated infants. Recent meta-analyses[73,74] concluded that there was a significant reduction in NEC and in overall mortality with the use of probiotics. Although none of the controlled trials has reported significant adverse effects, there are reports of systemic infections with *Lactobacillus* in adults and children. There are also considerable variations in doses, timing of administration, and range of species used in the available studies. Additional studies are needed to establish the best and safest treatment strategy. Therefore, at this point probiotics are not widely used in the United States. The use of heat-killed, probiotic DNA or proteins rather than live microorganisms has been suggested as a means to control the microbial load and decrease the risk of sepsis while preserving the potential beneficial effects.[75]

Because of concern of altering microbial colonization, judicious use of intravenous antibiotics and H_2 receptor antagonists should be exercised. Oral antibiotics (vancomycin, gentamicin) have been used in an attempt to minimize intestinal colonization with pathogenic organisms and have been shown to decrease the incidence of NEC.[76] This strategy has not been widely adopted because of the potential emergence of multiresistant organisms.

Endothelial growth factor (EGF) is a mediator of gut homeostasis and plays an important role in intestinal repair. Breast milk is the main source of EGF in the postnatal period. In an animal model, enteral supplementation with EGF decreased the incidence and severity of NEC.[77] Currently, no randomized, controlled trials have been performed in preterm infants, and experts have expressed concerns about potential adverse effects.

Certain nutrients (glutamine, arginine, omega-3 fatty acids) counteract proinflammatory activation and promote intestinal barrier function, proliferation, and healing.[78] Although glutamine supplementation decreased the incidence of sepsis and mortality in adults, it did not show any effect on the incidence of NEC or any other important outcome measures in preterm infants.[79] In the only randomized, double blinded placebo-controlled trial of administration of oral arginine to premature infants, Amin et al.[80] reported a significant reduction in the incidence of all stages of NEC, but further studies are needed to confirm these results.

MANAGEMENT

The comprehensive management of babies with NEC requires a profound knowledge of neonatal physiology and the application of the basic principles of neonatal intensive care. The participation of a multidisciplinary team including neonatologists, pediatric surgeons, radiologists, gastroenterologists, nurses, respiratory therapists and other ancillary personnel is paramount in achieving a successful outcome. Maintenance of thermoregulation, initial assessment, and stabilization of cardiorespiratory function (airway, breathing, and circulation) and fluid resuscitation should be the immediate goals of therapy. Bowel rest and decompression are instituted by placement of a large-bore gastric catheter (Sump) to low intermittent suction. The patient should be kept nil per os (NPO), usually for a period of 10 to 14, days while optimizing parenteral nutrition. Careful attention to fluid balance and correction of acid-base abnormalities is of utmost importance.

Colonization with pathogenic gram-negative organisms and bacterial translocation are precursors to sepsis. However, positive blood cultures are obtained in only about 30% of patients with NEC.[81] Broad-spectrum antibiotics with adequate gram-negative and anaerobic coverage should be initiated, generally a semisynthetic penicillin (ampicillin or piperacillin/tazobactam) plus an aminoglycoside (gentamicin/amikacin) + clindamycin. In our institution, piperacillin, tazobactam, and gentamicin are used. Recommended length of antibiotic therapy is 10 to 14 days, even for patients with negative cultures. This approach is solely based on clinical experience. Dependable vascular access is necessary for fluid resuscitation, and placement of an arterial line may aid in continuous blood pressure monitoring. Glucose infusion rates may have to be decreased because of glucose intolerance. Hypotension can be attributed to loss of vascular tone due to vasoactive mediators, capillary leak syndrome, and third-spacing into the intestine. Patients with hemodynamic instability frequently require multiple fluid boluses and generous maintenance fluids. Vasopressors are commonly initiated if hypotension persists in spite of fluid resuscitation. In premature infants with catecholamine-resistant hypotension, secondary relative adrenal insufficiency should be suspected and the administration of stress-dose hydrocortisone considered.[82]

Indications for surgical intervention are generally failure of medical management, free intra-abdominal air, or suspected bowel necrosis. Worsening metabolic acidosis, inability to ventilate, persistent skin discoloration, protracted hypotension, persistent thrombocytopenia, or fixed bowel loops on x-ray[6] may lead to surgical intervention. Surgical options include bedside placement of a Penrose drain with or without irrigation or open laparotomy. The surgical approach is aimed at the removal of necrotic bowel and proximal diversion with the goal to preserve any bowel that appears viable. A second-look procedure may be indicated after 24 to 48 hours to reevaluate questionable viable bowel. In cases of pannecrosis, outcome is often extremely poor despite aggressive surgical intervention.

Treatment with a bedside drain has been advocated for the smallest patients thought to be at highest risk for anesthesia and laparotomy. This treatment option was first described in the 1970s in a small series in which three of five infants with bowel perforation survived after drain placement.[83] Because this procedure can be performed at the bedside, it has been used primarily as a temporary measure with the goal to stabilize the patient for further surgical treatment later on. Some surgeons have advocated it as the primary surgical intervention for the more unstable patients. Two randomized controlled trials have been published comparing drain placement with laparotomy, but neither showed a difference in mortality or length of stay.[84,85] The question of superiority of one procedure over the other remains unanswered. There could be a theoretical advantage of drain placement avoiding the significant release of proinflammatory cytokines that occurs with anesthesia and surgery. To date, the only data available evaluating cognitive outcomes at 18 months appear to favor open laparotomy, nonetheless with generally poor outcomes in both groups.[86] A major concern with this study is that patients were not randomized at enrollment and infants with both diagnoses, SIP and NEC, were included. As a result, smaller and more unstable patients were treated with peritoneal drains per surgeon's preference, introducing significant bias.

Enteral feedings are typically reintroduced after 10 to 14 days of fasting with a slow advance protocol to reach full feeds over a period of 7 to 10 days. Feeding intolerance after NEC is common and may be due to the development of malabsorption, dysmotility, or intestinal strictures. Use of hydrolyzed or elemental formulas is often necessary on reintroduction of enteral feeds. Strictures occur in 30% patients with a history of NEC regardless of initial medical or surgical therapy.[87] The most commonly affected areas include the terminal ileum, the splenic flexure, and the junction of the descending and sigmoid colon. Patients generally present with feeding intolerance, abdominal distention, gastrointestinal bleeding, and/or persistent thrombocytopenia while generally not appearing ill. Because of the high incidence of strictures in this population, some advocate routine contrast studies before initiation of feeds.

OUTCOME

The mortality rate after surgical intervention approaches 20 to 50%,[1,58] and a significant proportion of the survivors will suffer long-term morbidity including growth failure and gastrointestinal and neurodevelopmental sequelae. About half of NEC-associated in-hospital deaths occur during the first 3 weeks of hospitalization and 70% during the first 6 weeks.[1]

Long-term gastrointestinal morbidities related to NEC include malabsorption and failure to thrive because of loss of absorptive surface due to short bowel syndrome (SBS) or dysfunctional bowel. The incidence of SBS in very-low-birth-weight infants with NEC is as high as 8% and is associated with growth failure at 18 to 22 months.[88] Other complications are related to long-term use of parenteral nutrition, including catheter-related bloodstream infections, cholestasis, and liver failure.[2]

Significant neurologic morbidity may occur in neonates surviving NEC. This seems to be the case especially in those neonates requiring surgical interventions compared to medically treated patients or premature infants without NEC.[89-91] In addition, an increased incidence of late periventricular leukomalacia or white matter injury (a lesion also associated with a surge of proinflammatory mediators and neurodevelopmental impairment) has been noted.[56,90,92]

Despite significant improvements in neonatal intensive care, NEC remains as a leading cause of morbidity and mortality in the premature population. Future research should be geared toward early diagnosis and prevention.

REFERENCES

1. Holman RC, Stoll BJ, Curns AT. Necrotising enterocolitis hospitalisations among neonates in the Unites States. Paediatr Perinat Epidemiol 2006;20:498–506.
6. Guner YS, Chokshi N, Petrosyan M, et al. Necrotizing enterocolitis—bench to bedside: novel and emerging strategies. Semin Pediatr Surg 2008;17:255–265.
13. McElhinney DB, Hedrick HL, Bush DM, et al. Necrotizing enterocolitis in neonates with congenital heart disease: risk factors and outcomes. Pediatrics 2000;106:1080–1087.
27. Sodhi C, Richardson W, Gribar S, et al. The development of animal models for the study of necrotizing enterocolitis. Dis Models Mech 2008;1:94–98.
31. Anand RJ, Leaphart CL, Mollen KP, et al. The role of the intestinal barrier in the pathogenesis of necrotizing enterocolitis. Shock 2007;27:124–133.
72. Barclay AR, Stenson B, Simpson JH, et al. Probiotics for necrotizing enterocolitis: a systematic review. J Pediatr Gastroenterol Nutr 2007;45:569–576.
89. Hintz SR, Kendrick DE, Stoll BJ, et al. Neurodevelopmental and growth outcomes of extremely low birth weight infants after necrotizing enterocolitis. Pediatrics 2005;115:696–703.

See expertconsult.com for a complete list of references and the review questions for this chapter.

DISORDERS OF THE ANORECTUM: 48
FISSURES, FISTULAS, PROLAPSE, HEMORRHOIDS, TAGS

Marian D. Pfefferkorn • Joseph F. Fitzgerald

The anal sphincter consists of an inner ring of smooth muscle, the internal anal sphincter, the intersphincteric space, and an outer ring of skeletal muscle, the external anal sphincter. The internal sphincter is an involuntary muscle that maintains anal tone. It is in a continuous state of partial contraction and relaxes in response to rectal distension. The external sphincter is a voluntary muscle extending from the puborectalis and levator ani muscles that provides short-term augmentation of anal pressure to postpone defecation. The transitional and columnar epithelium of the rectum is separated from the squamous epithelium of the anus by the dentate line, which is located in the midportion of the anal canal (Figure 48-1). Anal crypts are located at the dentate line, and anal glands are found at the base of these crypts.

ANAL FISSURE

Anal fissure is a split in the skin of the anus. The passage of a hard stool commonly causes anal fissures; however, a history of constipation preceding the onset of an anal fissure is obtained in only one of four cases, and diarrhea is a predisposing factor in 4 to 7% of patients.[1] Fissures are usually located in the anterior or posterior midline. Other processes, for example infectious or inflammatory, should be entertained when the fissure is positioned laterally.[2] Blood is often seen on the surface of the stool, on the toilet tissue, or even dripping from the anus. There may be severe anal pain associated with the fissure, especially during defecation.

Physical examination of the patient in a lateral decubitus position involves gently parting the buttocks and stretching the anal skin laterally. An acute fissure is a superficial split in the anoderm with sharply demarcated edges. Induration at the edges of the fissure may be seen when the fissure is chronic (Figure 48-2). A skin tag may be present. Rectal examination using the fifth finger in an infant younger than 3 years, or the index finger in an older child, should be performed gently.

Most acute anal fissures heal with conservative therapy. The inciting factor, whether constipation or diarrhea, should be corrected. The presence of fecal material within the fissure inhibits healing; hence, it is ideal to instruct the caregivers to clean the child's anus after every stool. The application of a local anesthetic is unnecessary. Dietary bran supplements and warm sitz baths have been shown to be superior to topically applied local anesthetic or hydrocortisone cream in the treatment of an acute anal fissure, with healing in 87% after 3 weeks.[3]

Chronic fissures are unusual in children who have no underlying predisposing factors, such as inflammatory bowel disease or immunodeficiency (Figure 48-3). In adults, chronic fissures may not respond to conservative treatment and may require lateral internal sphincterotomy. Local injection of botulinum toxin and topical application of nitrates or calcium channel blockers are therapies under investigation.[4-8] A systematic review of medical therapy for anal fissure showed no significant advantage of glyceryl trinitrate or botulinum toxin over placebo.[9] Nifedipine and diltiazem did not differ from glyceryl trinitrate in efficacy. Surgery was more effective than medical therapy in curing chronic fissures.

RECTAL PROLAPSE

Rectal prolapse is the abnormal protrusion of one or more layers of the rectum through the anus. Mucosal or partial prolapse is less serious and less pronounced[10] (Figure 48-4). A complete rectal prolapse (procidentia), consisting of all layers of the rectal wall, frequently requires manual reduction.[10] Rectal prolapse is usually detected by the child's parents and is urgently brought to medical attention; however, it has often spontaneously reduced by the time the child is examined by medical personnel.

Rectal prolapse occurs most commonly under 4 years of age and may relate to the following anatomical considerations: the vertical course of the rectum along the straight surface of the sacrum and coccyx, the low position of the rectum in relation to other pelvic organs, the increased mobility of the sigmoid colon, the relative lack of support by the levator ani muscle, the loose attachment of the redundant rectal mucosa to the underlying muscularis, and the absence of Houston's valves in about 75% of infants under 1 year of age.[11,12] Prolonged straining during toilet training or with constipation is a frequent cause in children.[13,14] Acute and chronic diarrhea, intestinal parasites, and malnutrition are other common etiologies.[14-16] During malnutrition, the lack of ischiorectal fat resulting in decreased perirectal support may predispose to rectal prolapse. In underdeveloped countries, this may be further aggravated by chronic diarrhea from enteric infections.[12] Rectal prolapse has been reported in up to 19% of 605 patients with cystic fibrosis.[17,18] Rectal prolapse in these patients was often transient and usually resolved at 3 to 5 years of age, or following the institution of pancreatic enzyme replacement therapy.[17] There have been reports of rectal prolapse occurring with juvenile polyps (Figure 48-5), inflammatory polyps, lymphoid hyperplasia, solitary rectal ulcer, meningocele, pertussis, and Ehlers-Danlos syndrome.[19-23] Often, no underlying cause for the rectal prolapse is identified.[14,16]

The diagnosis is primarily historic, although it is prudent to screen patients for intestinal parasites and cystic fibrosis. Conservative management of rectal prolapse involves manual

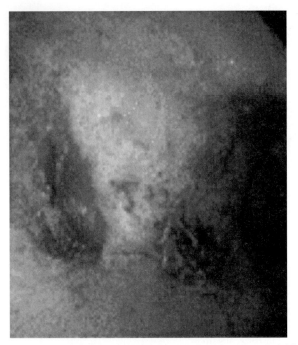

Figure 48-1. Schematic diagram of the perianal region. Reproduced from Sandborn et al. (2003),[28] with permission.

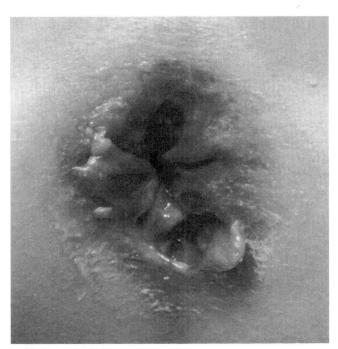

Figure 48-3. Crohn's disease–associated anal fissures with undermining of the edges.

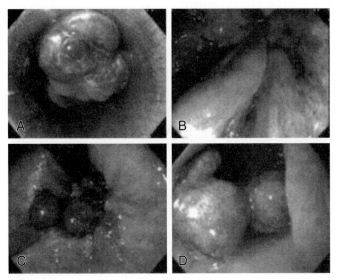

Figure 48-2. Large, indurated, chronic fissure associated with Crohn's disease.

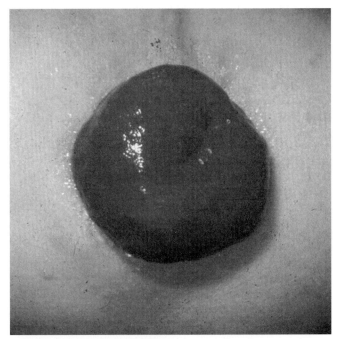

Figure 48-4. Mucosal prolapse. Photo courtesy Frederick Rescorla, MD.

reduction and treatment of the primary inciting factor. The parents should be trained to use disposable gloves and lubricating jelly to promptly reduce a prolapse whenever it occurs. If rectal prolapse becomes recurrent and persistent, the authors' approach has been to schedule the patient for examination under anesthesia to exclude an anatomic lead point for the prolapse, such as a polyp. If none is found, prolapse can be treated with submucosal injection of a sclerosant, such as 5% phenol in almond oil, 50% dextrose, 25% saline, or 1% sodium morrhuate.[13,15,24,25] Resolution of rectal prolapse was reported in 91 of 100 children who were treated with rectal submucosal injection of 5% phenol in oil.[26] Indications for surgical management are rare in children, but may include the development

of mucosal ulceration with bleeding (solitary rectal ulcer), irreducible prolapse, no improvement with conservative treatment, and rectal prolapse longer than 3 cm[27] (Figure 48-6).

FISTULAS

A perianal fistula is a chronic track of granulation tissue connecting two epithelium-lined surfaces, whereas a sinus track is a track of granulation tissue that is open only at one end.[28] A small perianal pustule or infected anal gland may spread to

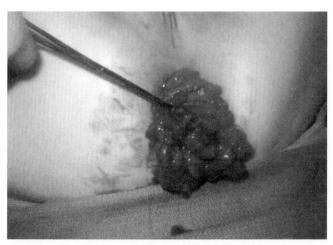

Figure 48-5. Prolapsed rectal juvenile polyps. Photo courtesy Frederick Rescorla, MD.

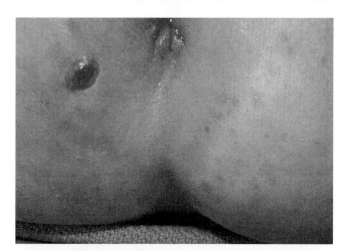

Figure 48-7. Fistula-in-ano. Photo courtesy Frederick Rescorla, MD.

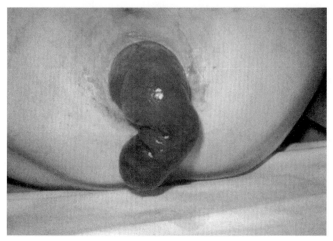

Figure 48-6. Necrotic rectal prolapse. Photo courtesy Frederick Rescorla, MD.

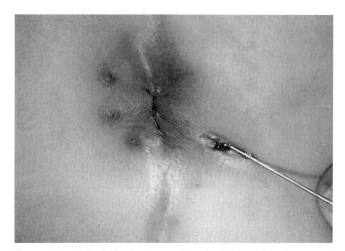

Figure 48-8. Multiple fistulas-in-ano. A probe is inserted in the external opening of one fistula. Photo courtesy Frederick Rescorla, MD.

the intersphincteric space and result in a fistulous abscess in infants and young children with a diaper rash.[29] A fistulous abscess becomes a fistula when it ruptures. At least 50% of perianal abscesses recur as fistulas.[29] A recent study of management of perianal abscess in infants younger than 12 months of age suggests that conservative therapy (local hygiene, sitz baths, and systemic antibiotics) without surgical drainage is effective and may be more beneficial in preventing the occurrence of fistula formation.[30] Of 140 patients, 83 abscesses were surgically drained and 53 were not drained. A fistula-in-ano developed in 50 of the surgically drained group compared to only 9 in the latter group. In a review of 36 patients older than 2 years of age (2.3 to 13 years old) presenting with perianal abscess, no associated pathology was noted in 35 and only 1 was eventually diagnosed as having Crohn's disease.[31] All patients received systemic antibiotics with needle aspiration of the abscess in 26, incision and drainage in 4, and local care in 6. Only 4 patients subsequently developed a fistula-in-ano; 2 had undergone needle aspiration, 1 incision and drainage, and 1 conservative therapy. The authors concluded that drainage of perianal abscess along with antibiotic therapy is effective with a low rate of evolution to fistula-*in-ano* in children older than 2 years of age. Most fistulas-*in-ano* originate below the dentate line[32] (Figure 48-7). The internal opening in infants is radially opposite the external

opening, unlike in adults where it is often in the posterior midline (Goodsall's rule). The earliest sign of a perianal abscess is an indurated tender area that may occur at any site around the anus. When the abscess ruptures, it discharges pus and/or blood. It may heal temporarily, only to recur with the next episode of inflammation. Once detected, management should include immediate drainage except in patients with known or suspected Crohn's disease, in whom management may be more complex, as outlined later.[33] Abscesses do not generally need to be cultured unless they persist or recur within days of drainage. The abscess cavity can be loosely packed to encourage hemostasis, or a catheter may be placed within the abscess cavity. Sitz or tub baths are initiated, along with analgesics, stool softeners, and dietary fiber supplementation. Antibiotics may be used as an adjunctive therapy to incision and drainage when there is extensive cellulitis, or in the presence of immunosuppression, valvular heart disease, and diabetes.[30]

When a fistula is present, a probe can be inserted into the external opening (Figure 48-8). The probe is passed out of the internal opening, and the fistula is then unroofed by incising down onto the probe. After surgery, the area needs to be kept clean with soap and water until it heals.[28]

The more complex forms of abscess and fistula are rarely encountered in children, but may be a complication of

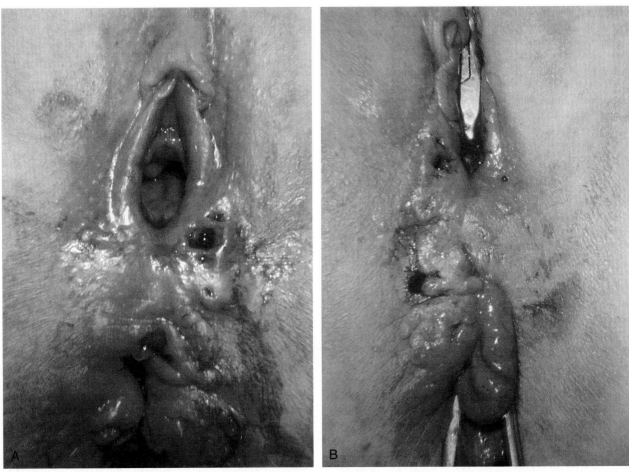

Figure 48-9. (**A**) Perineal fistula associated with Crohn's disease. (**B**) Rectovaginal fistula.

inflammatory bowel disease (IBD), especially Crohn's disease (Figures 48-9A,B). The American Gastroenterological Association Clinical Practice Committee published a technical review on perianal Crohn's disease in 2003.[28] It recommends physical examination of the perianal area to identify any perianal disease, and endoscopic examination to determine any rectal inflammation. Fistulas are then classified as either simple or complex. A simple fistula is low, has a single external opening, and has no pain or fluctuation to suggest a perianal abscess; there is also no evidence of rectovaginal fistula or anorectal stricture. A complex fistula is high, may have multiple external openings, and may be associated with a perianal abscess, rectovaginal fistula, anorectal stricture, or active rectal disease. Examination under anesthesia (EUA), endoscopic endoanal ultrasonography (EUS), fistulography, computed tomography (CT), and pelvic magnetic resonance imaging (MRI) are additional diagnostic modalities that may be needed to classify some fistulas accurately. Of these, EUA, with or without EUS, has been the most accurate in detecting and correctly classifying perianal fistulas, sinuses, and abscesses.

Medical treatment of perianal fistulas in Crohn's disease includes antibiotics, azathioprine/6-mercaptopurine, infliximab, adalimumab, ciclosporin, and tacrolimus.[28] Surgical treatment is determined by the presence or absence of macroscopic evidence of inflammation in the rectum and the type and location of the fistula. A treatment algorithm for managing patients with Crohn's perianal fistulas has been proposed (Figure 48-10).[28]

HEMORRHOIDS

Small asymptomatic hemorrhoids found incidentally on perianal examination are not uncommon in children. Symptomatic hemorrhoids are unusual in the pediatric age group, but may occur with chronic straining associated with constipation, as a result of an anal infection spreading to the hemorrhoidal veins, with underlying Crohn's disease, or with portal hypertension. Symptoms include bleeding, prolapse, discomfort/pain, fecal soiling, and pruritus (Figure 48-11).

The anal canal is lined by three fibrovascular cushions of submucosal tissue suspended by a connective tissue framework.[34] A venous plexus fed by arteriovenous communications is present within each cushion. Loss of the connective tissue supporting the cushions leads to their descent. Straining with the passage of hard stools produces an increase in venous pressure and engorgement, and hard stools alone produce a mechanical insult to the cushions. Hemorrhoids are classified as external, internal, or mixed. External hemorrhoids originate from the external hemorrhoidal venous plexus below the dentate line; internal hemorrhoids originate from the internal hemorrhoidal venous plexus above the dentate line. Hemorrhoids are also classified according to the degree of prolapse.[35] The prolapsed cushion has an impaired venous return resulting in dilation of the plexus and venous stasis. Inflammation occurs with erosion of the cushion's epithelium, resulting in bleeding. First-degree hemorrhoids protrude into the anal canal but do not prolapse.

Perianal fistula

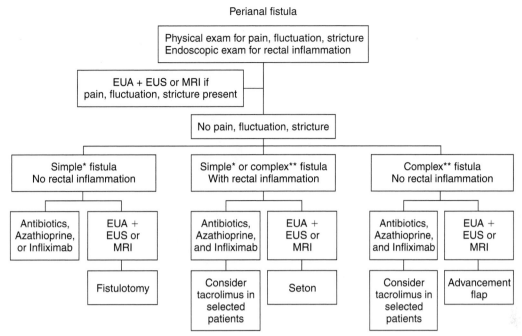

Physical exam for pain, fluctuation, stricture
Endoscopic exam for rectal inflammation

EUA + EUS or MRI if
pain, fluctuation, stricture present

No pain, fluctuation, stricture

Simple* fistula No rectal inflammation	Simple* or complex** fistula With rectal inflammation	Complex** fistula No rectal inflammation

| Antibiotics,
Azathioprine,
or Infliximab | EUA +
EUS or
MRI | Antibiotics,
Azathioprine,
and Infliximab | EUA +
EUS or
MRI | Antibiotics,
Azathioprine,
and Infliximab | EUA +
EUS or
MRI |

| | Fistulotomy | Consider
tacrolimus in
selected
patients | Seton | Consider
tacrolimus in
selected
patients | Advancement
flap |

Figure 48-10. Treatment algorithm for patients with Crohn's disease with a perianal fistula. *A simple fistula is low, has a single external opening, and is not associated with perianal abscess, rectovaginal fistula, anorectal stricture, or macroscopically evident rectal inflammation. **A complex fistula is high and/or has multiple external openings, perianal abscess, rectovaginal fistula, anorectal stricture, or macroscopic evidence of rectal inflammation. EUA, examination under anesthesia; EUS, endoscopic anorectal ultrasonography; MRI, pelvic magnetic resonance imaging. Reproduced from Sandborn et al. (2003),[28] with permission.

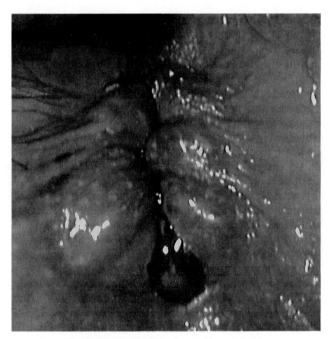

Figure 48-11. Bleeding external hemorrhoids.

Second-degree hemorrhoids prolapse on straining and reduce spontaneously. Third-degree hemorrhoids prolapse on straining and require manual reduction. Fourth-degree hemorrhoids are prolapsed and irreducible.

Asymptomatic hemorrhoids require no treatment. Conservative management of symptomatic hemorrhoids includes avoidance of straining with defecation and providing relief of constipation by increasing fluid and fiber intake and/or prescribing a stool softener. Warm-water sitz baths without soap or other irritating agents may alleviate symptoms. Patients should be advised to manually reduce prolapsed hemorrhoids during periods of exacerbation. Topical ointments or enemas containing local anesthetics and mild astringents or steroids may provide short-term symptomatic relief, but there is no evidence to support their long-term use.[34,35] Prolonged use may cause skin sensitization, and rectal absorption may lead to systemic side effects.

Thrombosed external hemorrhoids may be relieved with cooling packs. Within 48 to 72 hours, a thrombosed hemorrhoid may be excised with its overlying skin under general anesthesia.[36]

Several anoscopic and endoscopic therapies can be offered when patients do not respond to medical therapy. These include injection sclerotherapy, rubber band ligation, thermocoagulation (BICAP probe, heater probe, infrared coagulator), and electrocoagulation.[37,38] Sclerotherapy is indicated for grade I and II symptomatic internal hemorrhoids. Infrared coagulation is well tolerated with significantly less postoperative pain and fewer complications; however, it was less effective than banding and surgical hemorrhoidectomy.[39] The efficacy of bipolar and heater probe coagulation was equivalent with a 6.2% recurrence of bleeding at 12 months.[40] Heater probe treatment achieved hemorrhoid reduction and control of bleeding in a shorter period than bipolar coagulation (76.5 versus 120.5 days); however, postoperative pain was more severe with the former. Application of a small rubber band around the base of an internal hemorrhoid causes ischemic necrosis and sloughing of hemorrhoidal tissue, with ulceration resulting in fibrosis and obliteration of the submucosal tissue (Figure 48-12). Endoscopic banding is highly effective with nearly 90% cure rates and a relapse rate of only 3 to 9%.[39,41]

Surgical therapy is indicated if conservative measures fail. Surgical hemorrhoidectomy is the definitive treatment for

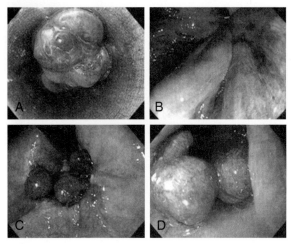

Figure 48-12. Grade III internal hemorrhoids before (**A**) and on retroflexion (**B**) and after standard rubber band ligation (retroflexion, **C**, and end-on views, **D**).

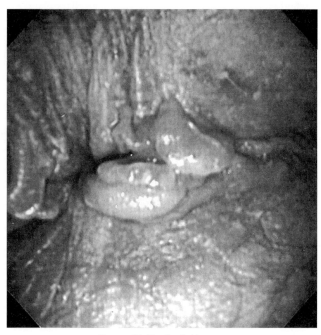

Figure 48-13. Anal skin tags.

symptomatic hemorrhoids. It is the primary treatment for acute or recurrent thrombosis, grade IV hemorrhoids, and hemorrhoids associated with significant rectal prolapse, or for complications (perianal abscess, fistula, or fissure).[42] Successful surgery removes a substantial amount of the hemorrhoidal plexus, and it can be effective for long periods, up to and beyond 10 years. Surgical procedures, however, are associated with substantial postoperative pain, and patients typically cannot return to usual activities for 2 to 4 weeks after surgery. Stapled hemorrhoidectomy is a newer technique that may be applicable to adolescents. A circular stapler removes excess anal mucosa. Several studies in adults have shown improvement in pain, faster return to work, and low rates of complications. In a series of 3711 adults, complications were few: bleeding 4.3%, pain requiring admission 1.6%, stricture 1.4%, abscess 0.03%, and recurrence 0.3%, and anastomotic dehiscence 0.08% of patients.[43]

TAGS AND MISCELLANEOUS CONDITIONS

An anal skin tag is usually asymptomatic and may be a remnant of a healed anal fissure or previously thrombosed external hemorrhoid (Figure 48-13). Anal tags that cause chronic pruritus or problems with hygiene can be excised when they are not associated with IBD.[2] Excision should be avoided for tags associated with Crohn's disease.

Hypertrophied anodermal papillae can evert during (and after) defecation; this is an annoyance, but rarely requires surgical management (Figure 48-14).

Perianal cellulitis due to group A β-hemolytic streptococcal infection occurs more frequently in children than in adults.[44] Examination of the perianal area reveals a well-demarcated, erythematous rash surrounding the anal opening (Figure 48-15). It is often associated with pain, pruritus, and bleeding, without fever and other systemic symptoms. Treatment with an oral antibiotic against streptococcus is effective.[45]

The solitary rectal ulcer syndrome commonly presents with rectal bleeding (Figure 48-16). Other symptoms include obstructed defecation, rectal pain, mucorrhea, prolapsing tissue, and fecal incontinence.[46] Evaluation of patients with video-defecography, with or without dynamic MRI of the pelvis, may

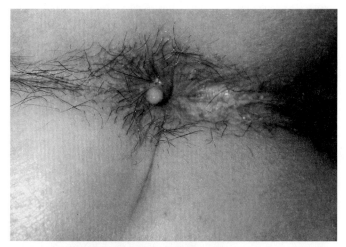

Figure 48-14. Hypertrophied anodermal papilla. Photo courtesy Frederick Rescorla, MD.

reveal either recto-rectal intussusception or anorectal redundancy with a scarcity of mesorectal fixation. Medical therapy includes the use of fiber supplements, stool softeners, steroid enema, mesalamine enema, or sucralfate enema. Anorectal biofeedback therapy may help facilitate ulcer healing in patients who are found to have pelvic dyssynergia.[47] Patients who are refractory to medical therapy may require surgical intervention (anterior resection with rectopexy or stapled transanal rectal resection).

Enterobius vermicularis (pinworm) infestation affects pediatric patients prevalently and commonly presents with anal pruritus. The most common physical finding of enterobiasis is excoriated perianal skin, which may be complicated by a secondary bacterial infection. Dead parasites or eggs deposited in the perianal area and other ectopic sites may also cause abscesses and granulomas.[48]

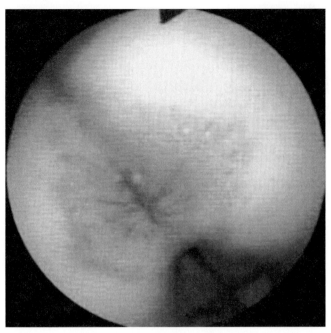

Figure 48-15. β-Streptococcal anusitis.

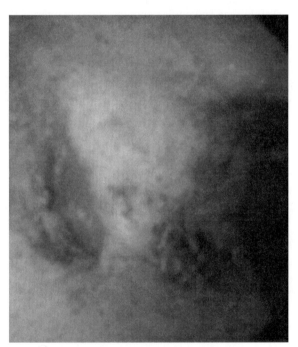

Figure 48-16. Bleeding solitary rectal ulcer.

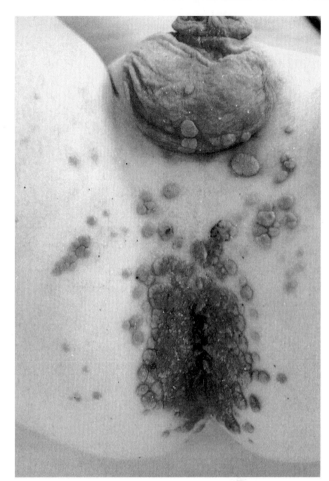

Figure 48-17. Condyloma acuminata. Photo courtesy Frederick Rescorla, MD.

A human papillomavirus (HPV) causes anogenital warts called condyloma acuminata (Figure 48-17). There has been an increase in the number of reported cases of anogenital warts in children since the 1980s.[49] Most HPV infections are subclinical and asymptomatic, and benign skin lesions are the most common manifestations.[50] They can, however, cause other problems including functional impairment, discomfort, and psychologic distress; malignant transformation is a concern.[51] Transmission of HPV occurs by direct sexual contact and raises the concern of sexual abuse in children. HPV may also be passed transplacentally to the fetus or during the passage of an infant through an infected birth canal. Nonsexual transmission may result from autoinoculation of HPV lesions on the hands. Fomites have also been implicated.[52] The usual therapeutic options include podophyllin, cryotherapy, curettage, and electrocautery.

REFERENCES

9. Nelson R. A systematic review of medical therapy for anal fissure. Dis Colon Rectum 2004;47:422–431.
12. Siafakas C, Vottler T, Andersen J. Rectal prolapse in pediatrics. Clin Pediatr 1999;38:63–72.
30. Christison-Lagay E, Hall H, Wales P, et al. Nonoperative management of perianal abscess in infants is associated with decreased risk for fistula formation. Pediatrics 2007;120:e548–e552.
31. Serour F, Gorenstein A. Characteristics of perianal abscess and fistula-in-ano in healthy children. World J Surg 2006;30:467–472.
46. Ortega A, Klipfel N, Kelso R, et al. Changing concepts in the pathogenesis, evaluation and management of solitary rectal ulcer syndrome. Am Surg 2008;74:967–972.
47. Rao S, Ozturk R, De Ocampo S, et al. Pathophysiology and role of biofeedback therapy in solitary rectal ulcer syndrome. Am J Gastroenterol 2006:613–618.

See expertconsult.com for a complete list of references and the review questions for this chapter.

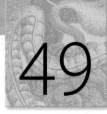

49

NEOPLASMS OF THE GASTROINTESTINAL TRACT AND LIVER

Karen F. Murray • Laura S. Finn

In contrast to the adult population, neoplasms of the gastrointestinal (GI) tract are uncommon in children. Furthermore, the symptoms leading to their diagnosis are usually nonspecific and may be erroneously attributed to a chronic underlying GI condition. Having an understanding of chronic conditions from which neoplasms can arise is important; however, most encountered neoplasms will be unanticipated, and the ability to arrive at a prompt and correct diagnosis can be crucial to the survival of the patient. Consequently, this chapter reviews the most common GI neoplasms encountered in childhood.

NEOPLASMS OF THE LUMINAL GASTROINTESTINAL TRACT

The GI tract is a relatively common site for involvement by childhood cancers, with approximately 5% of childhood cancers presenting in this organ system. Primary GI cancer in the pediatric population is rare, however. When neoplasms do arise from the GI tract, the presenting symptoms are variable and relatively nonspecific. The symptoms or signs may include abdominal pain, abdominal distention, vomiting, a palpable mass, anemia, GI bleeding, or weight loss. Neoplasms are also found at surgery for intussusception, bowel obstruction, or perforation, as well as incidentally during a surgical or radiologic procedure for other reasons. Definitive diagnosis usually requires a biopsy for histopathologic examination and possibly immunotyping and cytogenetics, depending on the tumor.

Neoplasms of the GI tract can be divided into categories based on their tissue of origin (Table 49-1). The most commonly encountered tumors in children arise from the lymphoid or epithelial tissues. Mesenchymal tumors are less frequent. Both benign and malignant tumors can be found within all of these categories. In the following sections we discuss the most commonly encountered neoplasms within these categories: their epidemiology, pathology, molecular biology, prognosis, and treatment.

NEOPLASMS OF LYMPHOID ORIGIN

The gastrointestinal tract is a lymphoid tissue-rich organ system, beautifully adapted to respond in a stimulatory or repressive fashion to recognized luminal antigens. Although there is lymphoid tissue throughout the GI tract, in the form of lymphoid follicles or scattered T and B lymphocytes in the lamina propria, they are particularly prominent in the ileum where they aggregate into Peyer's patches, well-organized germinal follicles of B lymphocytes with T lymphocytes in the interfollicular zones.

Lymphonodular Hyperplasia

Lymphonodular hyperplasia (LNH) is a common condition that can affect children of all ages. Its peak ages of occurrence are in early childhood and adolescence, as these are times of developmental lymphoid proliferation. Males more commonly than females usually present with right lower quadrant abdominal pain, diarrhea, intussusception, or gastrointestinal bleeding. Endoscopy reveals patchy exaggeration of lymphoid nodules in the large and small bowel, at times distorting the overlying mucosa into prominent folds. Histologically there is reactive hyperplasia with prominent germinal center formation, but no disruption in the normal lymphoid architecture or cellular pleomorphism (Figure 49-1). Assuming that acute management of symptoms is unnecessary, this condition is usually benign with no specific therapy required and an excellent prognosis.

In the setting of primary immunodeficiencies (hypogammaglobulinemias), however, LNH may occur with associated diarrhea, malabsorption, and chronic intestinal infections such as giardiasis. In adults, this lesion complicates primary hypogammaglobulinemia in approximately 20% of patients.[1] The presence of intestinal lymphomas of either the B- or T-cell type is now well described adjacent to hyperplastic nodules in some of these patients.[2,3]

Lymphoma

The gastrointestinal tract is the most common site of primary extranodal lymphomas. Primary gastrointestinal lymphomas are defined as tumors originating from the mucosa-associated lymphoid tissue and contiguous lymph nodes, where the main bulk of the disease is located in that particular region of the gastrointestinal tract (i.e., stomach, ileum, etc.). Lymphoma accounts for approximately 15% of all small bowel malignancies in individuals from North America and Western Europe. In people under the age of 20 years, lymphoma, the most common malignant neoplasm of the GI tract, is almost universally non-Hodgkin's lymphoma.[4-6] In children under 15 years of age, however, lymphoma is the third most common malignant neoplasm and accounts for 10% of all neoplasms.[7,8] The gastrointestinal distribution differs between adults and children. Whereas 40 to 50% of primary GI lymphomas occur in the

TABLE 49-1. Pediatric Gastrointestinal Tumors

Tissue of Origin	Tumor	Most Common GI Sites
Lymphoid	Lymphonodular hyperplasia	Ileum, colon
	Lymphoma	Ileum, appendix, colon
Epithelial	Carcinoid	Appendix
	Adenocarcinoma	Colon
Mesenchymal	Leiomyoma/ leiomyosarcoma	Colon
	Gastrointestinal stromal tumor	Stomach, small intestine
	Primitive neuroectodermal tumor	Small intestine
	Schwannoma/malignant nerve sheath tumor/ neurofibroma	Small intestine
	Hemangioma/vascular malformation	All levels
	Lipoma	Colon

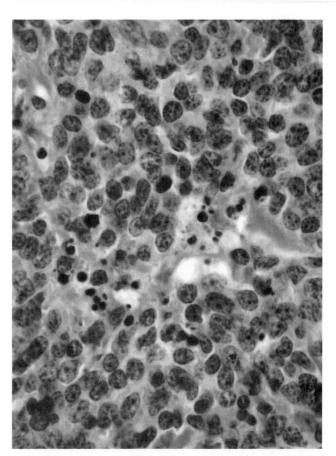

Figure 49-2. Burkitt's lymphoma. Sheets of monotonous intermediate-sized lymphoid cells have nondiscrete nucleoli. Abundant apoptotic nuclear debris is present centrally. (*See plate section for color.*)

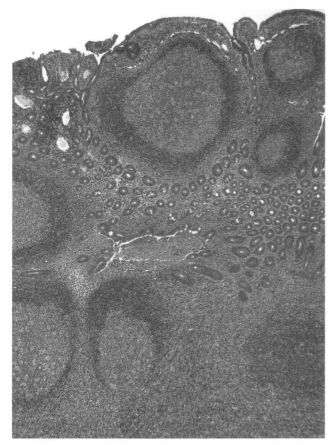

Figure 49-1. Lymphonodular hyperplasia. Numerous reactive germinal centers distort the normal villous architecture of the small bowel. (*See plate section for color.*)

stomach of adults, the most common sites in children are the terminal ileum, appendix, and cecum, with the frequency decreasing distally such that 10 to 20% occur in the colon.

Some 80% of primary intestinal non-Hodgkin's lymphomas are of B-cell origin,[4] collectively classified by the World Health Organization (WHO) as precursor or mature B-cell lymphomas,

or proliferations of uncertain malignant potential, as are seen in secondary immunodeficiency states.[9] In this same population, or in those individuals immunosuppressed by medications, Epstein-Barr virus (EBV) associated B-cell lymphoma can be a complicating development in their care.[10,11] EBV is also tightly linked to Burkitt's lymphoma in equatorial Africa, but there is a much weaker association in patients from North America. Celiac disease is associated with a variety of small bowel neoplasms, but the most common is T-cell lymphoma (70%). The mean age of presentation in the setting of celiac disease is in the fifth decade, with the jejunum being the most common location.[12] No pediatric cases have been reported.

Diagnosis usually requires surgical biopsy of a mass lesion; however, many lymphomas of the GI tract can be diagnosed through endoscopic biopsies if the lesion involves mucosa or submucosa. Rapid ascertainment of tumor distribution with abdominal computed tomography (CT), bone scan, lumbar puncture, and bone marrow aspirate is required, and consultation with an oncologist is mandatory.

The most common lymphoma arising in the pediatric gastrointestinal tract is Burkitt's lymphoma, which most frequently involves the ileocecal region where it presents as an abdominal mass or as the lead-point for intussusception. Burkitt's lymphoma is a highly aggressive tumor, composed of sheets of mitotically active monomorphic medium-sized cells with scanty cytoplasm and round to oval nuclei containing small nucleoli. Within the sheets there is apoptotic debris and numerous macrophages, producing a "starry-sky" appearance (Figure 49-2). The lymphoma

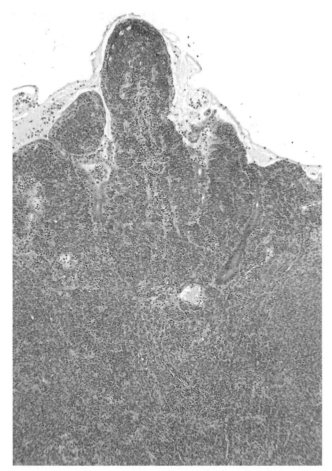

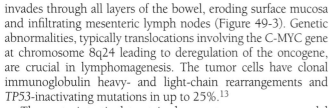

Figure 49-3. Burkitt's lymphoma. The neoplastic lymphoid cells diffusely infiltrate the mucosa, overrunning the epithelium. Contrast with the benign lymphoid reaction in Figure 49-1. (*See plate section for color.*)

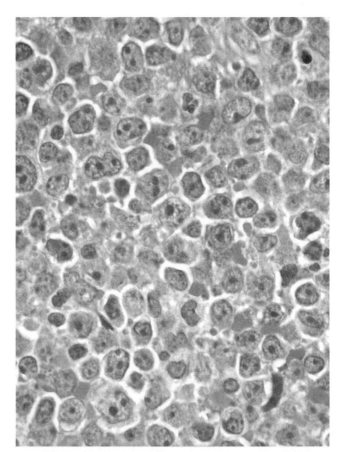

Figure 49-4. Diffuse large-cell lymphoma. Sheets of large, immunoblastic cells have prominent nucleoli; the tumor cells can diffusely infiltrate the bowel wall, similarly to Burkitt's lymphoma. (*See plate section for color.*)

invades through all layers of the bowel, eroding surface mucosa and infiltrating mesenteric lymph nodes (Figure 49-3). Genetic abnormalities, typically translocations involving the C-MYC gene at chromosome 8q24 leading to deregulation of the oncogene, are crucial in lymphomagenesis. The tumor cells have clonal immunoglobulin heavy- and light-chain rearrangements and *TP53*-inactivating mutations in up to 25%.[13]

The gastrointestinal tract is the most common extranodal site for diffuse large B-cell lymphoma (DLBCL), which develops in the pediatric ileocecal region, like Burkitt's, or commonly the stomach in adults, where it may result from secondary transformation of a less aggressive lymphoma. This latter phenomenon is virtually unheard-of in children, given the exceedingly low incidence of extranodal marginal zone B-cell lymphoma of mucosa-associated lymphoid tissue ("MALT" lymphoma) that is associated with *Helicobacter pylori* infection. DLBCL in the gastrointestinal tract is indistinguishable from those arising within lymph nodes. The intestinal architecture is often destroyed by medium to large cells with vesicular nuclei and typically prominent nucleoli (Figure 49-4). Most cases have clonal rearrangement of the immunoglobulin heavy and light chain genes and display often complex but not specific cytogenetic abnormalities. *BLC2* gene translocation (t(14;18)) occurs in 20 to 30% of adult cases but has not been described in pediatric DLBCL.[14] Abnormalities involving the *BCL6* protooncogene localized to the 3q27 region are identified in more than 30% of adult cases

TABLE 49-2. Staging of Non-Hodgkin's Lymphoma in Children

Stage	Description
A	Single extra-abdominal site
B	Multiple extra-abdominal sites
C	Intra-abdominal
D	Intra-abdominal with multiple extra-abdominal sites
AR	Intra-abdominal with more than 90% of the tumor surgical resected

of DLBCL, but extensive investigations have not been carried out in childhood DLBCL.[15]

Treatment of GI lymphoma is largely chemotherapy based, augmented with radiation therapy. Surgical resection is limited only to the rare circumstance of focal disease. The length and type of chemotherapeutic intervention depends on the extent of disease (Table 49-2) but generally requires systemic therapy as well as intrathecal delivery of agents to prevent or treat involvement in the cerebrospinal fluid. The most commonly employed chemotherapeutic agents include cyclophosphamide, doxorubicin, vincristine, prednisone, and intrathecal methotrexate. The best prognosis is with stage A and B lymphoma (greater that 90% long-term survival),[16,17] with stage AR having an equally favorable prognosis. Involvement with unresectable abdominal tumor carries a less favorable prognosis. With large tumor burden, the potential for tumor-lysis syndrome due to rapid cell turnover and consequent release of uric acid, potassium, and phosphorus into the bloodstream must be anticipated with the initiation of therapy.

NEOPLASMS OF EPITHELIAL ORIGIN

Neoplasms of epithelial origin include carcinomas as well as tumors derived from neuroendocrine elements. This group of tumors includes adenocarcinomas and carcinoids, which are uncommon in childhood but cause significant morbidity and mortality when they occur.

Carcinoma of the Colon

Colorectal cancer is the second leading cause of death in the United States,[18] with an average lifetime risk, equal in men and women, of 6%. Most colon cancer occurs in older adults, with only 1 to 4% occurring in individuals under 30 years of age.[19] Despite this infrequency, however, carcinoma of the colon is the most common primary solid malignancy of the GI tract among children, occurring in less than 0.1 cases per million children under 20 years of age and 0.7 cases per million among children 10 to 19 years of age.[20] The youngest reported case was in a 9-month-old female infant.[21]

Some 70 to 80% of adult colon cancer is sporadic, with environmental factors playing a significant role in its development. Overall, the incidence is higher among developed countries in northwestern Europe, the United States, and Canada, compared with Asia and Africa. Furthermore, immigrants acquire the incidence of their adopted country, assuming that their diet similarly changes. The exact reason for this has not been elucidated; however, high-fat, low-fiber diets have been implicated. Environmental factors are not the only contributor, because 10 to 20% of cases are in individuals with at least two first-degree relatives with the cancer but no obvious inheritance pattern.

In some families there is an autosomal dominant inheritance pattern to the development of colon cancer in the absence of any predisposing polyposis syndromes. Lynch syndrome I is characterized as an autosomal dominant pattern to the development of colon cancer only, whereas in Lynch syndrome II there is development of colon adenocarcinoma and extracolonic cancers that may involve the female genital tract, breast, and pancreas. These patients may develop multiple primary tumors, do so at a younger age, and have a high rate of subsequent tumors.[22] Pediatric cases have been described with this inheritance pattern.[23]

The possible development of colon cancer as a complication of an underlying bowel condition fosters angst in both the patient and the care provider. However, predisposing diseases such as inflammatory bowel disease and hereditary polyposis syndromes account for only 2% of the total cases of colon cancer. In children, however, 10% of those with colon cancer have an underlying condition of colitis or polyposis.[24] The polyposis syndromes and their relative risk to the development of GI cancer are discussed elsewhere in this volume. Underlying colitis of a duration of 10 years increases the cumulative risk of colorectal cancer by approximately 0.5 to 1% per year, with an overall increased relative risk of 20 in individuals with ulcerative colitis (UC) compared with the general population. The age of colitis onset is not important, but more extensive colon involvement increases the risk,[25] as does having primary sclerosing cholangitis. In contrast to sporadic colorectal carcinomas, those developing from underlying colitis can be multifocal and develop frequently from flat mucosa rather than adenomas, most likely contributing to their early mean occurrence in the fourth decade of life. The risk of developing colorectal cancer in subjects with colitis due to Crohn's disease (CD) is thought recently to be as high as with UC.[25a] Additionally, patients with CD do have an increased risk of small bowel cancer; their risk of anorectal cancer does not appear to be significantly elevated, however, but data remain conflicting. Furthermore, whereas the carcinoma develops in areas inflamed or previously inflamed in UC, those that develop in the setting of CD may do so in grossly normal intestine,[26] however, most have either adjacent or distant dysplasia.[27] In addition to the risk factors outlined previously for UC, smoking is an important variable leading to increased risk of colon cancer in Crohn's colitis.

The clinical presentation in children with colon cancer is similar to those of other GI neoplasms. Children report vague abdominal pain in approximately 95% of cases with less frequent reports of altered bowel habits (17 to 32%) and rectal bleeding (14 to 23%). Physical findings most commonly include an abdominal mass in 59% and abdominal distention in 48%, with emaciation and anemia found in less than 25%.[8,28-30] The infrequency of physical findings and the vagueness of symptoms probably contribute to the relative lengthy median time (2 to 6 months) between the onset of symptoms and diagnosis.[31,32] Hence, malignancy should be considered in the differential diagnosis of chronic abdominal pain.

The diagnosis of GI carcinoma starts by including its possibility in the differential of vague abdominal complaints. Depending on the presenting symptoms, the mass lesion may be found at endoscopic evaluation or by abdominal CT or magnetic resonance imaging (MRI). Consequently, if the etiology of persistent abdominal symptoms has not been forthcoming, an abdominal CT or MRI is an appropriate method of assessment. Definitive diagnosis is made by histologic evaluation of tissue. Laparotomy is generally required and is mandatory for proper staging with sampling of regional lymph nodes. Because the mainstay of therapy is surgical resection, careful attempts at complete, radical resection with primary anastomosis, without seeding of the peritoneum and viscera, is of greatest prognostic value to the subject. The staging evaluation is then completed with a CT of the chest and a bone scan (Table 49-3).

Mutational inactivation of the *APC* (*adenomatous polyposis coli*) gene in colon epithelial cells is thought to be the inciting event of most carcinomas. Patients with familial adenomatous polyposis (FAP) are at an increased risk for colon cancer because of their germline mutation in *APC*; by contrast, somatic mutations in *APC* are seen in sporadic colon carcinoma. Tumor progression results from mutations in other genes including activation of *c-myc* and *ras* oncogenes and inactivation of additional suppressor genes such as *DCC* (deleted-in-colorectal-carcinoma) and *TP53*.[33,34] These features of chromosomal instability, plus aneuploid DNA, typify tumors in the distal colon. Genetic instability allows for a "mutator phenotype" characterized by microsatellite instability, specifically, somatically acquired variations in the length of short, repetitive nucleotide sequences in DNA, resulting from either inherited or acquired mutations of DNA mismatch-repair genes (for example, *hMLH1, hMSH2,* and *hPMS2*).[35] High-frequency microsatellite instability is characteristic of carcinomas arising in

TABLE 49-3. Modified Dukes Classification of Colorectal Carcinoma

Stage	Description
A	Tumor confined to the bowel wall
B	Tumor extension to the serosal fat but without lymph node involvement
C	Lymph node involvement
D	Distant metastases

the hereditary nonpolyposis colorectal cancer (HNPCC) syndrome due to germline mutations of mismatch repair genes. Microsatellite instability appears frequently in colon carcinoma from young patients, though the genetic defects responsible are often not inherited but acquired.[36,37]

Colon carcinoma may be exophytic, endophytic, or diffusely infiltrative; proximal colon tumors more commonly seen in children tend to be exophytic. By definition, carcinoma requires invasion through the muscularis mucosa. Well- or moderately differentiated tumors are gland forming with progressive architectural complexity. The columnar epithelial cells have hyperchromatic enlarged nuclei and often prominent nucleoli; nuclear polarization is lost with increasing tumor grade (Figure 49-5). Poorly differentiated adenocarcinomas have little to no gland formation but infiltration by small cellular clusters or anaplastic cells. Compared with sporadic colorectal cancer that show chromosomal instability, tumors in HNPCC or with acquired mutations of DNA mismatch-repair genes are more often poorly differentiated, with an excess of mucoid and signet-cell features, accompanied by a modest inflammatory infiltrate, and often occur in the right colon (Figure 49-6).

The prognosis of children with colorectal carcinoma is poor, with some reported 5-year survival rates as low as 2 to 5%.[38] Most patients have evidence of distant metastases at the time of surgery; the few long-term survivors of colorectal carcinoma in childhood and adolescence have had Dukes stage B at surgery. The biggest reason for the more devastating prognosis in children with this condition is that the most common histology is an aggressive poorly differentiated mucin-producing cell type that represents fewer than 15% of cases in adults.[31,39,40] The delay in diagnosis due to the vague presenting symptoms and the uncommon frequency of the diagnosis also contributes to the poor prognosis.

Treatment is primarily surgical resection. When the tumor mass is unresectable, preoperative radiotherapy has been used with some success to reduce the tumor burden to one that is resectable.[39] Primary and adjuvant chemotherapy in the setting of metastatic disease has not been beneficial. Commonly employed drugs include vincristine, methyl-CCNU, and 5-fluorouracil.

Carcinoma of the Stomach

Few cases of gastric carcinoma have been reported in childhood, with most malignancies in the stomach being lymphoma or more rarely sarcomas. The symptoms are again nonspecific but include abdominal pain, nausea, anorexia, vomiting, weight loss, and hematemesis.[41-43] Most commonly because of an erroneous diagnosis of benign gastric tumor, there is a mean delay of 2.7 months from the onset of symptoms to diagnosis.[42]

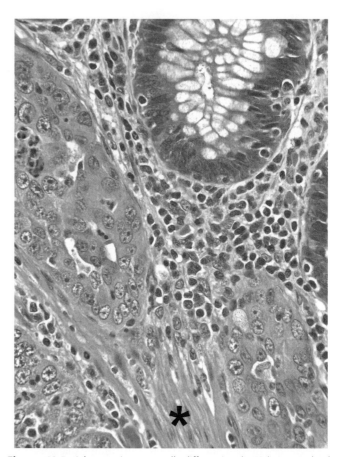

Figure 49-5. Adenocarcinoma, well differentiated. Malignant glands with complex architecture invade the muscularis (*) and are composed of crowded large epithelial cells with prominent nucleoli. By contrast, the overlying normal glands have a regimented nuclear polarization and obvious goblet cells. (*See plate section for color.*)

Diagnosis is usually made at endoscopy, with CT further defining the extent of disease presurgically. Resection is again the primary therapy, with adjuvant therapy typically modeled after that used in colorectal carcinoma.

Carcinoid

Carcinoid tumors are well-differentiated neoplasms of the diffuse endocrine system and arise from cells of endodermal origin in the GI epithelium. These cells synthesize a variety of GI peptides and hormones, and consequently the tumors that result from them may secrete a variety of physiologically active substances, resulting in the carcinoid syndrome. More commonly, however, these tumors are hormonally inactive.

Carcinoid tumors are uncommon. In a large autopsy series, they were found in 1 to 2% of people and account for a similar percentage of clinically evident GI neoplasms in adults.[44] As in adults, childhood carcinoid tumors are most commonly found in the appendix (40% in adults), but have been found in all parts of the GI tract including the small intestine, pancreas, and biliary system and in Meckel's diverticulum and GI duplications.[45-47]

Although most carcinoids are found incidentally in adults, children usually present with acute appendicitis[48,49] where the tumor may or may not have played an obstructive role in its development. Ileal and colonic lesions are more likely to present

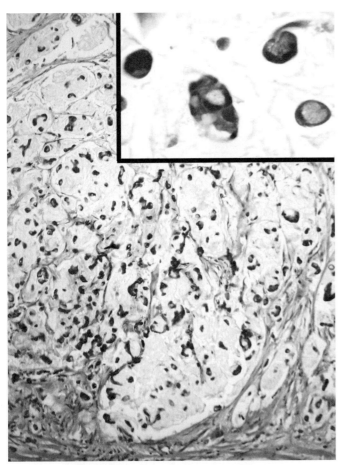

Figure 49-6. Adenocarcinoma, poorly differentiated (signet-ring cell carcinoma). Malignant epithelial cells float in pools of mucin. A "signet-ring" cell is created by a large mucin vacuole that fills the cytoplasm and displaces the nucleus (inset). (*See plate section for color.*)

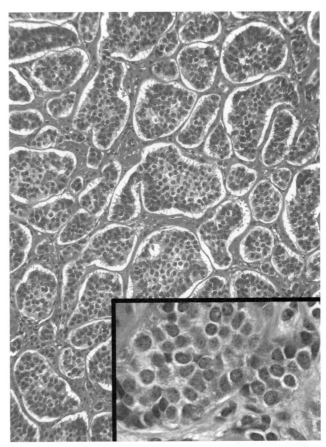

Figure 49-7. Carcinoid tumor. Fibrous stroma surrounds numerous well-demarcated islands of tumor cells. Uniform cells with faintly granular cytoplasm and round, bland nuclei that contain finely stippled chromatin are characteristic features of endocrine cell neoplasms (inset). (*See plate section for color.*)

as a palpable mass because of their increased size (90% over 2 cm) and to be metastatic at diagnosis.[50] Presentation of the tumor with symptoms attributable to the carcinoid syndrome is rare in children, with only a few reports in the literature.[47,51] As in adults, this syndrome is most common with metastatic tumors in the liver from a small bowel primary. Hormonal activity in carcinoid tumors results in the secretion of GI peptides and hormones including serotonin, 5-hydroxytryptophan, histamine, prostaglandins, catecholamines, and bradykinins. Resultant symptoms may include diarrhea, bronchoconstriction, edema, and flushing. Bradykinin may additionally induce fibrogenesis both locally and in the heart, resulting in the reports of valvular stenosis.[52]

Most carcinoid tumors are solitary and sporadic without predisposing factors. Loss of heterozygosity at the MEN-1 gene locus is significantly associated with gastrin-producing tumors arising in the duodenum and upper jejunum within the setting of multiple endocrine neoplasia.[53] Periampullary somatostatin-producing tumors occur in neurofibromatosis type 1.[54]

The majority of appendiceal endocrine tumors are found incidentally as firm whitish masses in the distal end; more proximal tumors may produce obstruction that results in appendicitis. The usual appearance of a carcinoid tumor in the appendix and elsewhere is that of multiple well-demarcated rounded or insular islands of closely packed cells with peripheral palisading that are separated by fibrotic stroma. The tumor

cells are uniformly bland and have round nuclei with finely stippled ("salt and pepper") chromatin that are surrounded by a moderate amount of lightly eosinophilic granular cytoplasm (Figure 49-7). Their neuroendocrine features can be confirmed by silver impregnation techniques or immunohistochemical staining for generic endocrine cell markers such as chromogranin A and PGP 9.5. The tumors arise in the mucosa, but the bulk of the mass often occupies the muscular walls and can extend into the mesoappendix.

Diagnosis is usually made on finding the tumor mass at surgery. In the unusual circumstances of carcinoid syndrome, the urine level of 5-HIAA (5-hydroxyindoleacetic acid), a major metabolite of serotonin, may be diagnostically elevated, especially on a 24-hour urine specimen (greater than 30 mg is indicative of carcinoid syndrome).[55] Foods rich in serotonin and certain drugs may artificially alter the results. Computed tomography of the abdomen is useful in localizing mass lesions and can identify any hepatic metastases, but GI contrast radiographic studies miss most GI carcinoids.

Surgical resection is the mainstay of therapy for carcinoid tumors. When the tumor mass is less than 2 cm in diameter, an appendectomy is sufficient,[48,49,56] but for larger tumors a right hemicolectomy is recommended. Any tumor without distant metastases should be completely resected.[57] Patients with symptoms attributable to the carcinoid syndrome may get symptomatic relief with long-acting somatostatin analogues, such as octreotide,[58,59] and proton-pump inhibitors are useful in treating the gastric acid hypersecretion resultant from gastrin-producing duodenal carcinoids (gastrinomas).[59] Octreotide alone or in combination with interferon alpha may also provide antiproliferative affects to control tumor growth, in 50% of patients, but tumor regression is less common.[59] Chemotherapeutic agents have not been found useful in the treatment of slowly growing carcinoids. For nonresectable liver tumors, cryotherapy has been used to provide transient symptomatic relief in carcinoid syndrome but does little to improve long-term survival.[60] Transcatheter arterial chemoembolization of liver metastases, however, has resulted in long-term palliation and may prove to be the treatment of choice in this situation.[61]

The prognosis of individuals with carcinoid tumors is good. Appendiceal tumors have a low chance of nodal or liver metastasis (4%) and a 5-year survival of 89% with surgical resection only. Colonic and ileojejunal tumors have much higher chances of local or distant metastasis (55% and 70%, respectively) but still have 5-year survivals of 75% and 68%, respectively.[62] The presence of distant metastases significantly worsens the prognosis compared with localized tumors only, but even in this situation there are long-term survivors, some for decades after the diagnosis, because of the slow rate of tumor growth.

NEOPLASMS OF MESENCHYMAL ORIGIN

Neoplasms arising for mesenchymal tissues are extremely rare and even more uncommon during childhood. Included in this group of tumors are vascular tumors (Figure 49-8), those arising from smooth muscle, and those of stromal cell origin. Primitive neuroectodermal tumors (Figure 49-9) and schwannomas arising from the GI tract would also be considered in this category.

Smooth Muscle Origin

Tumors arising from smooth muscle may originate from the muscularis mucosa or muscularis propria. The average age at diagnosis is the fourth to fifth decades, but they have been observed at all ages. Symptoms are usually minimal with those arising from the muscularis mucosa, however, those arising from the muscularis propria are frequently larger at presentation and have often ulcerated through the overlying mucosa resulting in hemorrhage, pain, or obstruction.

Smooth muscle tumors in the gastrointestinal tract are identical to those that occur in more common locations. Typically beginning as intramural lesions, they expand as well circumscribed spherical or sausage-shaped masses toward the lumen or mediastinal or peritoneal cavities. Benign smooth muscle tumors, leiomyomas, consist of interlacing bundles of bland spindled cells with cigar-shaped nuclei and a moderate amount of eosinophilic cytoplasm. Their smooth muscle origin is confirmed by demonstrating smooth muscle actin and desmin expression; these tumors are negative for CD34 and CD117 (C-Kit). Malignant tumors, leiomyosarcomas, have increased cellularity and mitotic activity compared to their benign counterparts.[63,64] Epstein-Barr virus associated smooth muscle tumors in children infected with the human immunodeficiency virus (HIV) not infrequently involve the gastrointestinal tract.[65]

Diagnosis is usually made incidentally during radiographic, endoscopic, or surgical evaluation of unrelated symptoms.

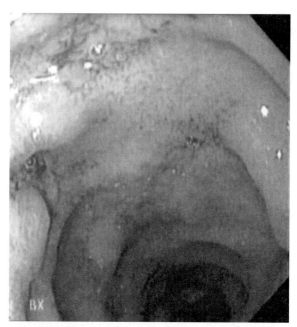

Figure 49-8. Intestinal vascular lesion. Endoscopic view of the duodenum with diffuse infiltration by a vascular lesion, composed of interdigitating capillary-sized vessels, in a 14-year-old boy who presented with gastrointestinal bleeding. (*See plate section for color.*)

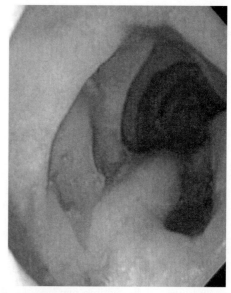

Figure 49-9. Primitive neuroectodermal tumor of the duodenum, endoscopic view. (*See plate section for color.*)

The mainstay of therapy is surgical resection; however, extensive local spread is possible with both benign and metastatic tumors, making complete resection difficult and leading to a high incidence of local recurrence. Survival is variable, and both local and distant metastases have occurred years after the primary resection.[66-68]

Stromal Cell Origin

GI stromal tumors (GISTs) arise from the intestinal wall, mesentery, omentum, or retroperitoneum.[69] The Finnish Cancer Registry estimates the incidence of these tumors to be roughly 4 per million, although the true incidence is not known. They are rare in childhood; the peak prevalence is in the fifth and sixth decades, although pediatric cases have been described.[70] Some 60 to 70% of the tumors arise in the stomach, 20 to 30% in the small intestine, and less than 10% from the remainder of the GI tract, omentum, mesentery, and retroperitoneum.

Stromal cell tumors may be derived from the interstitial cells of Cajal of the autonomic nervous system, as they usually express the transmembrane tyrosine kinase receptor CD 117(C-Kit proto-oncogene protein), in contrast to leiomyomas and leiomyosarcomas.[71] Staining for CD 117 is frequently necessary, because these tumors can have deceptively heterogeneous morphology. Most of the tumors also show immunopositivity for CD34.[72] These unique features have revolutionized the diagnosis of GIST. What in the mid-1990s became known as GISTs were generically classified as "stromal tumors" after the advent of immunohistochemistry in the 1980s demonstrated a lack of smooth muscle differentiation; before that they had been erroneously regarded as smooth muscle tumors, earning appellations such as "cellular leiomyomas" or "leiomyoblastomas." About 85 to 90% of GISTs have mutually exclusive mutations in one of two closely related receptor tyrosine kinases, KIT (75 to 80%) and platelet-derived growth factor receptor alpha polypeptide, PDGFRA (~8%).[73] Such mutations are likely sufficient for transformation, but progression from benign to malignant GIST is characterized by sequential acquisition of chromosomal deletions at 14q, 22q, 1p, and 9p and gains at 8p and 17q. Although pediatric GIST express KIT at levels comparable to adult GIST, only about 15% of pediatric tumors harbor activating mutations in KIT or PDGFA, and they progress to malignancy without acquiring large-scale chromosomal abnormalities.[74]

The histopathology of GISTs typically falls into one of three categories: spindle cell type (70%), epithelioid type (20%), or mixed.[72] The spindle cell type is composed of uniform plump eosinophilic cells arranged in short fascicles and whorls, whereas nests of moderately sized round cells with clear to eosinophilic cytoplasm constitute the epithelioid type (Figures 49-10, 49-11). Criteria for malignancy are disputed, but larger, mitotically active tumors and those that arise in the small bowel carry a higher risk of aggressive behavior including peritoneal cavity or hepatic metastases.

Primary treatment is surgical, with chemotherapy reserved for metastatic or unresectable tumors. Although standard chemotherapeutic agents are ineffective, imatinib mesylate, a selective inhibitor of tyrosine kinase, has been shown to reduce tumor size in 54.7% and 69.4% of cases and reliably achieves disease control in 70 to 85% of patients with advanced tumors.[75,76] The estimated median overall survival time with imatinib therapy exceeds 36 months in all large clinical studies. Alternative kinase inhibitors, such as sunitinib, were recently approved for treatment of imatinib-resistant tumors.[73]

Because imatinib mesylate has only been used in the treatment of stromal cell tumors in recent years, the long-term survival with this therapy has not yet been realized. The 5-year survival with surgical resection alone is 20 to 78%.

NEOPLASMS OF THE LIVER

Hepatic tumors make up only 1 to 4% of pediatric solid tumors, and most of these are metastatic lesions from an extrahepatic site. Five primary hepatobiliary tumors occur uniquely in childhood,

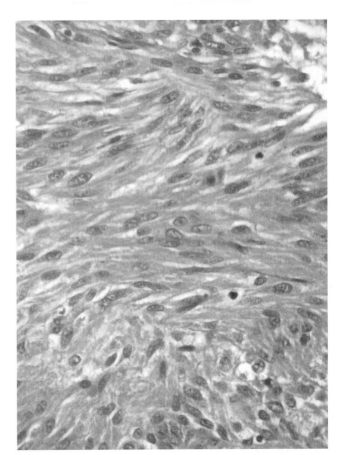

Figure 49-10. Gastrointestinal stromal cell tumor (GIST). Interlacing fascicles of plump cigar-shaped cells with tapered ends form the spindle cell GIST. (*See plate section for color.*)

however, including hepatoblastoma, infantile hemangioendothelioma, mesenchymal hamartoma, undifferentiated embryonal sarcoma, and embryonal rhabdomyosarcoma of the biliary system. Of these tumors, infantile hemangioendotheliomas usually occur in the first 6 months of life and 90% of hepatoblastomas in the first 5 years of life (68% in the first 2 years), with these two tumors representing roughly 80% of liver tumors in children under the age of 2 years. In contrast, undifferentiated embryonal sarcomas are most commonly encountered in school-aged children.[77] In this section, we review the most common pediatric primary liver tumors; a complete list may be found in Table 49-4.

Hepatoblastoma

The first case of hepatoblastoma was described in 1898,[78] and this tumor is now known to be the most common pediatric liver malignancy, accounting for 1% of all pediatric malignancies with an incidence of 0.5 to 1.5 cases per million children under the age of 15 years in Western countries.[79]

Patients usually present when family members notice an enlarging abdomen or when an irregular mass in the right upper quadrant is palpated on a routine physical examination. The mass is usually nontender. Accompanying anorexia, weight loss, nausea, vomiting, or abdominal pain is less commonly observed, and jaundice is uncommon (5%).[77]

Diagnosis is made with a combination of radiographic and laboratory tests. CT or MRI can be helpful in defining the size

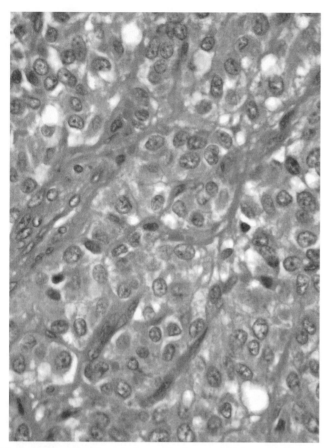

Figure 49-11. Gastrointestinal stromal cell tumor (GIST). Nests of medium-sized epithelioid cells with a moderate amount of eosinophilic cytoplasm form the epithelioid GIST. (*See plate section for color.*)

TABLE 49-4. Pediatric Primary Liver Neoplasms

Tumor	Most Common Age at Presentation
Hepatoblastoma	<5 years, most <2 years
Infantile hemangioma	<6 months
Hepatocellular carcinoma	>5 years
Fibrolamellar variant of hepatocellular carcinoma	2nd decade
Focal nodular hyperplasia	2nd decade
Mesenchymal hamartoma	Most <2 years
Undifferentiated embryonal sarcoma	5 to 10 years
Nodular regenerative hyperplasia	All ages
Hepatocellular adenoma	All ages
Angiosarcoma	All ages
Embryonal rhabdomyosarcoma	<5 years
Teratoma	<1 year

TABLE 49-5. Children's Cancer Study Group/Pediatric Oncology Group Hepatoblastoma Postoperative Staging System

Stage	Description
I	Complete resection of tumor
II	Microscopic residual tumor
III	Macroscopic residual tumor
IV	Distant metastases

and distribution of the mass and can identify features that distinguish it from other liver tumors. The finding of speckled calcifications is well described and found in roughly 50% of cases.[80] At diagnosis, approximately 20% of tumors have metastasized, most commonly to the lungs.[81] The most diagnostically useful laboratory finding seen with hepatoblastomas is a significant elevation in serum α-fetoprotein (AFP), which is present in approximately 90% of cases. The extent of AFP elevation correlates with tumor size or presence of metastases and its decrease, with tumor clearance after therapy. AFP levels are helpful in monitoring recurrence. The 10% of hepatoblastomas that do not have elevated AFP levels tend to be of small-cell undifferentiated histology and carry a poor prognosis.[77,82] Recent analysis confirms that having even a minor component of tumor with small-cell undifferentiated histology confers an adverse outcome. Some of these tumors have been shown to lack expression of the INI-1 protein, a characteristic feature of the malignant rhabdoid tumor.[83] Confirmation of the diagnosis and documentation of the histologic features require a biopsy.

Multiple scoring systems, preoperative and postoperative, have been developed over the years to predict prognosis. The simplest of these, the Children's Cancer Study Group/Pediatric Oncology Group staging system, has a highly significant predictive value for survival (*p* = 0.0009) (Table 49-5).

Hepatoblastomas are derived from undifferentiated embryonal tissue and do not have a characteristic chromosomal anomaly, although trisomies of chromosomes 20, 2, and 8 are frequent.[84] These tumors are associated with some familial conditions such as Beckwith-Wiedemann syndrome and familial adenomatous polyposis, as well as with trisomy 18. Hepatoblastomas are typically a single mass and involve the right lobe in slightly more than half of cases. Their gross appearance varies tremendously and is dependent on the proportion of mesenchymal elements. Most commonly, hepatoblastomas contain purely "fetal" epithelial cells, which are uniform, small to medium cuboidal cells that resemble fetal hepatocytes and are arranged in trabeculae. They may be mixed with "embryonal" epithelial cells that are smaller than their fetal counterparts and have an increased nuclear-to-cytoplasmic ratio. Embryonal cells often cluster into pseudorosettes or tubules.[85] A biphasic pattern produced by the mixture of fetal and embryonal epithelial cells is a pathognomonic feature of hepatoblastoma and helps to distinguish it from hepatocellular carcinoma (Figure 49-12). Almost half of hepatoblastomas have mesenchymal elements, notably osteoid-like and cartilaginous tissues. In some cases, hepatoblastomas are designated as "teratoid" when heterologous tissues are abundant and include muscle, melanin pigment, and squamous or mucinous epithelium. A rare "small cell undifferentiated" variant is made up of tumor cells that are indistinguishable from other "small round blue cell" tumors of childhood and are characterized by small, discohesive, undifferentiated cells with minimal cytoplasm and round nuclei that lack conspicuous nucleoli and do not form acini.[86] Cure of hepatoblastoma occurs only with complete surgical resection.[87] Early research showed that presurgery treatment with cisplatin and doxorubicin successfully shrinks the tumor mass and enhances its delineation from healthy liver parenchyma, optimizing surgical resection.

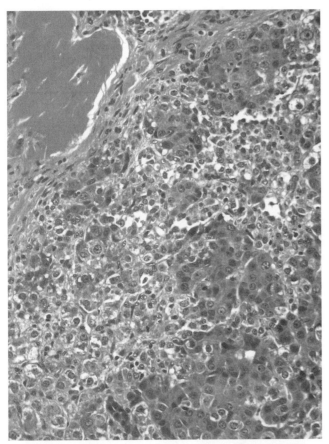

Figure 49-12. Hepatoblastoma. Trabeculae of hepatocyte-like cells resembling the fetal liver (lower right) mingle with the smaller "embryonal" cells (center); this biphasic pattern helps distinguish a primary liver tumor as hepatoblastoma. Homogenous eosinophilic osteoid-like material is a common mesenchymal element (top left). (*See plate section for color.*)

The current 5-year survival of children with hepatoblastoma is 75%,[88,89] leaving 25% who will die of the disease and are the current focus of treatment research.

Hepatic Hemangioma

Like their cutaneous counterparts, hepatic vascular lesions have been plagued with the overlapping nondiscriminatory use of various terms such as hepatic hemangioma; cellular, cavernous, or capillary hemangioma; infantile hemangioendothelioma; and arteriovenous malformations. The unfortunate use of the widely accepted term "infantile hemangioendothelioma" should be avoided to prevent confusion with "epithelioid hemangioendothelioma," a malignant tumor with metastatic potential. Hepatic hemangiomas are the most common benign liver tumors that occur in children, and based on more recent analysis, they can be classified into three subtypes: focal, multifocal, and diffuse.[90] Approximately 30% of them occur in the first month of life, with the majority of the remainder being diagnosed in the first 6 months of life; focal lesions are often asymptomatic but may be detected antenatally on routine ultrasound, after which they undergo rapid spontaneous involution.[90,91]

Given the vascular nature of these lesions, anemia is common (50%), and 10 to 15% of patients have congestive heart failure at presentation, particularly those with multifocal

lesions[90-92]; most patients have recognizable abdominal enlargement. Diffuse lesions are extensive and may nearly replace the liver parenchyma; these children often have serious clinical complications of massive hepatomegaly that results in respiratory compromise, abdominal compartment syndrome, multiorgan system failure, and, rarely, severe hypothyroidism.[93] Less common signs and symptoms include jaundice (20%), thrombocytopenia, failure to gain adequate weight, fever, and intra-abdominal/intrahepatic hemorrhage.[94,95] Although there are a number of extrahepatic anomalies or syndromes that have been associated with hemangiomas of the liver, the most frequent is cutaneous hemangiomas, which are more common in patients with multifocal rather than solitary hepatic lesions.

The diagnosis is usually suggested by radiographic evaluations. Ultrasound reveals hypoechoic, hyperechoic, or complex lesions as well as multifocality. CT and MRI can better delineate the details of the lesions and detect extrahepatic foci.[90] Selective angiography can then identify the major feeding vessels.[96,97]

Approximately half of lesions are solitary and range from less than 1 cm to 13 cm. Multifocal lesions may number from 2 to more than 25 and frequently involve large portions of both liver lobes.[90,98] Recent discovery of "hemangioma-specific markers" has led to new concepts about the nature of hepatic vascular lesions.[99] Focal hemangiomas typically have extensive central hemorrhage or infarction with focal calcifications and a peripheral spongy appearance. Histologically, the central zones contain large, tortuous, thin-walled channels with dense fibrous stroma. The outer portion is characterized by capillary-sized vessels lined by plump endothelium; entrapped hepatocytes and bile ducts are common, and neighboring hepatic sinusoids may be dilated (Figure 49-13). Whereas some observers have regarded these lesions as vascular malformations, many believe they represent the hepatic counterpart of the so-called cutaneous "rapidly involuting congenital hemangiomas."[90,100,101] By contrast, the multifocal lesions extensively involve the liver with reddish nodules ranging from a few millimeters to 3 cm. The cellular nodules contain closely packed capillaries with plump endothelium surrounded by pericytes; they are immunoreactive for Glut-1, an erythrocyte-type glucose transporter protein.[99] Mitotic activity can be prominent in regions of greatest cellularity and diminishes in areas of regression as vascular channels become more obvious.

Treatment depends on the severity of extrahepatic symptoms. Asymptomatic patients with focal or multifocal disease, without cardiac failure or significant shunting, should be observed and undergo serially ultrasounds to document regression. Medical treatment with diuretics alone or in combination with α-interferon or steroids has been used to hasten spontaneous regression in patients with hemodynamically significant shunting.[90-92] Patients in congestive heart failure or with large shunts should be considered for early embolization or undergo surgery when the lesion is resectable.[90,102] Infants with diffuse hepatic hemangiomas are at greatest risk for death and often have a poor response to pharmacologic therapy alone; they may benefit from orthotopic liver transplantation.[90,103-106]

The survival of infants is excellent, with rates of 70 to 92% to at least 2 years using surgery or other treatments.[95,107] Most deaths that occur are in young infants with diffuse lesions, who present with congestive heart failure and jaundice.[77,95]

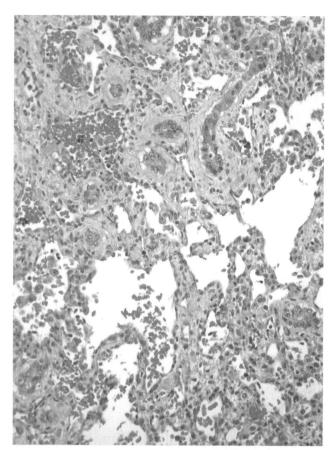

Figure 49-13. Hepatic hemangioma. Slightly ectatic vascular spaces are lined by plump endothelial cells and contain erythrocytes. Scattered hepatocytes and bile ducts may be entrapped (top). (*See plate section for color.*)

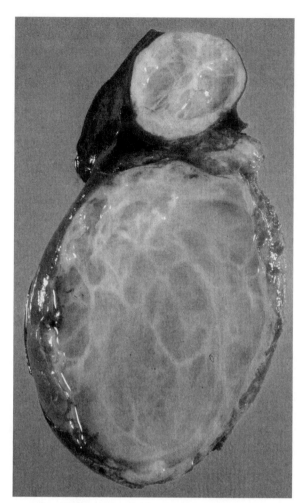

Figure 49-14. Mesenchymal hamartoma. The bisected multiloculated mass has fibrous septa dividing the lesion into cysts that contain viscous clear fluid. A thin rim of liver parenchyma is noted (upper left). (*See plate section for color.*)

Mesenchymal Hamartoma

Mesenchymal hamartomas of the liver are benign tumors that usually present with an enlarged abdomen from ascites accumulation in the first 2 years of life.[108-110]

Ultrasonographic (US), CT, or MRI imaging can define the location of the mass and generally is able to distinguish this tumor by its fluid-filled multicystic parenchyma (Figure 49-14) from hepatoblastomas or infantile hemangiomas, the other liver tumors that commonly occur in this age group. The well-circumscribed tumor is composed of a mixture of loose mesenchyme, bile ducts, hepatocyte cords, and blood vessels. Proposed etiologies have included developmental anomalies, biliary obstruction, and segmental ischemia, but recurring abnormalities involving chromosome band 19q13 corroborate a neoplastic origin.[111,112]

Surgical resection is the treatment of choice, with an excellent expected prognosis.[77]

Undifferentiated Embryonal Sarcoma

Undifferentiated embryonal sarcomas of the liver occur in children between 5 and 10 years of age, are derived from very primitive mesenchymal cells, and account for 9 to 13% of childhood hepatic tumors.[113-115] The oncogenesis of undifferentiated embryonal sarcoma remains uncertain, but reports of chromosome 19q13 abnormalities and development within mesenchymal hamartoma suggest a link between the two lesions.[116]

As with the other hepatic tumors developing in this age group, the most common presenting sign is abdominal enlargement or a mass, but fever, vomiting, and weight loss may also occur.[117] Diagnosis requires a biopsy to differentiate this tumor from other malignant tumors of the liver. By US these tumors are solid; however, CT and MRI sometimes suggests a cystic quality.

The majority of tumors are in the right lobe and typically measure 10 to 20 cm.[85] Tumor cells are stellate to spindled and often have markedly pleomorphic or bizarre giant nuclei. They are loosely or compactly arranged within abundant myxoid stroma that may focally become more fibrous. A characteristic and helpful diagnostic feature is the presence of numerous eosinophilic globules in tumor cells and extracellularly (Figure 49-15). Immunohistochemical and ultrastructural analyses have demonstrated limited differentiation along various lines including fibroblastic, rhabdomyoblastic, and leiomyoblastic; however, lack of immunoreactivity for the muscle-specific marker myogenin helps to distinguish this tumor from rhabdomyosarcoma.[118,119]

The prognosis of children with undifferentiated embryonal sarcomas is poor; however, recent advances in preoperative chemotherapy followed by surgical resection has improved the long-term survival to as high as 70%.[117,120,121]

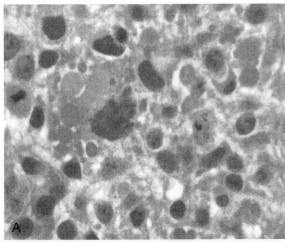

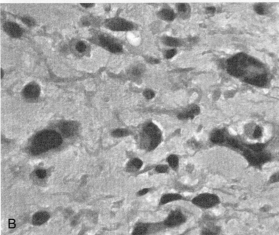

Figure 49-15. Undifferentiated embryonal sarcoma. Marked pleomorphism is characteristic, and cellular density is variable. Scattered atypical hyperchromatic multinucleated cells are sporadically distributed within abundant myxoid stroma (bottom). Another more cellular tumor has abundant eosinophilic hyaline globules (top). *(See plate section for color.)*

Embryonal Rhabdomyosarcoma of the Biliary Tree

Rhabdomyosarcomas are the most common sarcomas in children, but those involving the biliary system are rare, accounting for only 1% of liver tumors. Unlike rhabdomyosarcoma at other sites, biliary rhabdomyosarcoma have exclusively embryonal or botryoid histology, and patients are significantly younger (average age 3.5 years) at presentation, typically with jaundice in as many as 80% of cases.[122-124]

Although laboratory values are nonspecific and simply reflective of biliary ductal obstruction, CT, MRI, or US can localize the mass lesion to the intrahepatic or more commonly the extrahepatic ductal system.

Primary therapy of surgical resection is successful in fewer than 50% of cases because of local extension of the tumor into the liver, other intra-abdominal organs, or lymphatic metastasis. Current treatment recommendations, including initial surgery limited to biopsy for diagnosis and staging, followed by chemotherapy and radiotherapy, increased the 5-year survival to 66%.[122]

REFERENCES

5. North JH, Pack MS. Malignant tumors of the small intestine: a review of 144 cases. Am Surg 2000;66:46–51.
26. Greenstein AJ, Sachar DB, Smith H, et al. Patterns of neoplasia in Crohn's disease and ulcerative colitis. Cancer 1980;46:403–407.
63. Miettinen M, Kopczynski J, Makhlouf HR, et al. Gastrointestinal stromal tumors, intramural leiomyomas and leiomyosarcomas in the duodenum. A clinicopathologic, immunohistochemical and molecular genetic study of 167 cases. Am J Surg Pathol 2003;27:625–641.
77. Stocker JT. Hepatic tumors in children. Clin Liver Dis 2001;5: 259–281.
90. Christison-Lagay ER, Burrows PE, Alomari A, et al. Hepatic hemangiomas: subtype classification and development of a clinical practice algorithm and registry. J Pediatr Surg 2007;42:62–68.

See expertconsult.com for a complete list of references and the review questions for this chapter

OTHER DISEASES OF THE SMALL INTESTINE AND COLON

Elizabeth Gleghorn • Sabina Ali

HENOCH-SCHÖNLEIN PURPURA

Henoch-Schönlein purpura (HSP) is an acute leukocytoclastic vasculitis that affects mostly children. Of affected children, 75 to 90% are less than 10 years old,[1,2] although the reported age range is 6 months to 86 years.[1] Heberden described the palpable purpuric lesions in 1801. The combination of purpura and arthritis was described by Schönlein in 1899; Henoch added the descriptions of gastrointestinal (GI) disease and kidney lesions in 1874 and 1899.[3] The American College of Rheumatology established diagnostic criteria in 1990. Two of these four must be present: (1) age less than 20 years at onset, (2) palpable purpura, (3) bowel angina (pain, ischemia, or bloody diarrhea), or (4) histologic evidence of leukocytes in the walls of arterioles or venules. Presence of two or more criteria gives 87.1% sensitivity and 87.7% specificity for HSP.[4] If the rash is absent or atypical, sepsis, polyarteritis nodosa, systemic lupus erythematosus, and Wegener's granulomatosis could be considered.[1]

Clinical Presentation

The rash, purpuric or urticarial (Figure 50-1), is the hallmark of the disease. It usually occurs on the extensor and dependent areas of the body. The rash can also manifest as edema or hemorrhagic edema, especially in the youngest children.[5] Other manifestations may precede the rash. Arthritis occurs in 60 to 84% of cases. It involves noticeable swelling, usually in the knees and ankles.[6] The pain may be debilitating, but the arthritis does not cause articular damage. Renal disease occurs in 20 to 100% of children.[1,6] It ranges from hematuria with or without proteinuria to nephritis/nephrosis to rapidly progressive crescentic glomerulonephritis. Renal disease presents the greatest risk of long-term heath problems. The vasculitis may present with cerebral symptoms, commonly headache but also coma, seizures, paresis,[1] blindness,[6] or cerebral hemorrhage.[3,6] Guillain-Barré syndrome, parotitis, and carditis have also been reported.[1,6] Pulmonary findings include interstitial edema and loss of diffusing capacity as well as pulmonary hemorrhage. Scrotal edema and pain can imitate testicular torsion.[1] Priapism and other penile lesions have been reported.[3]

Gastrointestinal disease occurs in 65 to 76% of patients.[1,6] Edema and hemorrhage of the bowel wall lead to severe colicky *abdominal pain*. The ultrasound correlation of uncomplicated pain shows mural thickening and hemorrhage. Plain films may show dilated thickened bowel loops.[7] Contrast radiology, when used, shows thickened mucosal folds and small barium flecks, presumably in small ulcers (Figure 50-2). Endoscopic findings include ulceration, erythema, edema, hematoma-like protrusions, and petechiae.[8,9] In 14 to 36% of patients, the rash may occur later in the course than the GI manifestations, leading to diagnostic difficulties. Pain consistent with appendicitis can occur before the rash and lead to "unnecessary" appendectomy. Vasculitis and hemorrhage of the abdominal wall musculature can occur, leading to severe pain that can be difficult to diagnose.[7]

Intussusception, with areas of hemorrhage and edema acting as the lead point, develops in 4 to 5% of cases. Intussusception associated with HSP, in contrast to the usual early childhood presentation, occurs in the small bowel 58% of the time and at an average age of 6 years.[7] Paralytic *ileus* or pseudo-obstruction can occur, most likely secondary to ischemia. On occasion this has necessitated parenteral nutrition support, but it is usually transient.[7] Ischemia can clearly lead to *infarction* and necrosis of the bowel wall. Spontaneous *perforation* can occur, most commonly in the small intestine. Late *strictures* and *fistulas* can result from the bowel wall damage. Minor *bleeding* occurs in about 50% of large series with hematemesis, melena or heme positive stool. Severe GI bleeding is reported in 5%. If combined with the bleeding tendency of renal failure, this can be life threatening.[1]

Pancreatitis can occur with vasculitis and hemorrhage.[7,10] This can occur at any time in the course. Symptoms and laboratory findings are typical for pancreatitis of any cause and can mimic acute abdomen. Gallbladder involvement, with hydrops or necrosis, has been reported but is rare.[7]

Epidemiology

Estimates for the incidence of HSP range from 13.8 to 22.1 per 100,000.[1,3] Boys are more often affected than are girls. Most patients are between 4 and 7 years of age, with the peak being 5 years.[9] HSP is more frequent from late fall through spring. It is often reported after viral or bacterial infections such as *Staphylococcus aureus*[11]; clearly it is not any particular pathogen but a nonspecific immune stimulus.[2,3] Medications have also been causally associated with HSP, probably from nonspecific stimulation of the immune cascade.[9] Recurrent disease, often with abdominal pain, may occur in 3 to 40%, usually within the first year.[6] Renal disease is usually detected within the first 3 to 6 months.[12] Of all children with HSP, 1 to 5% progress to end-stage renal disease over time,[1,3,12] whereas up to 18% may have mild renal impairment. Those without early renal disease usually remain well, whereas those with severe renal disease at onset, severe abdominal pain, or very long persistence of rash seem more likely to have kidney damage.[1,3,12-14] Women who

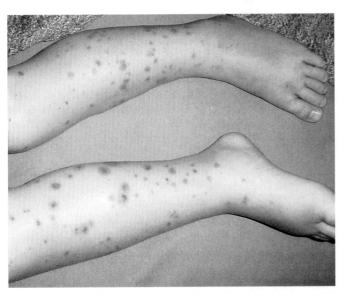

Figure 50-1. Palpable purpura on the back and legs of a 4-year-old with abdominal pain.

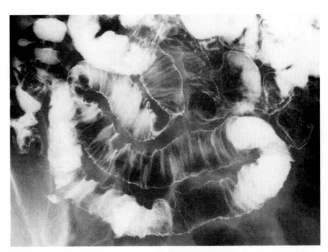

Figure 50-2. HSP characteristic protrusions into the lumen represent intramural purpura that can cause intussusception or bleeding.

had HSP are especially likely to display renal symptoms when pregnant. Thus, all girls who had HSP should be carefully monitored during pregnancy.[3,14]

The disease does occur in adults but more rarely, with an incidence of about 2 in 1,000,000. The male:female ratio is equal, and there is no obvious seasonality in adult cases. Nephritis occurs in 20 to 40% and end-stage renal disease in 10 to 20%.[2] HSP may account for 5 to 15% of all end-stage renal failure.[1]

Etiopathogenesis

HSP is a disorder of the inflammatory cascade, leading to pathologic inflammation of blood vessels. There is probably an inciting immune stimulus, perhaps infectious. It most commonly involves abnormalities in IgA, with elevated serum IgA, circulating IgA-containing immune complexes, and usually IgA deposition in blood vessel walls and in the kidney mesangium.[1,2,15] Factors that increase pathologic immune activation increase patient susceptibility to HSP.

Increased incidence has been described with mutations of the familial Mediterranean fever gene,[16] with HLA-B35,[2] with certain polymorphisms of interleukin 1 receptor antagonists,[17] or with impaired regulation of pro- and anti-inflammatory cytokines.[18] Overall, aberrant glycosylation of IgA 1 subclasses seems to lead to increased formation of immune complexes that are more likely to deposit in the kidney.[2] Understanding this phenomenon and its genetic substrate may ultimately help identify persons who are likely to develop renal disease. Abnormal nailfold capillaroscopy persisted 16 months after diagnosis in one study, a finding implying ongoing autoimmune activation in all patients.[19] Clearer understanding of the prognosis and possible therapy in HSP depends on further elucidation of the immune mechanisms.

Management

Management depends on recognition of the characteristic features of HSP and then monitoring for complications. If the rash and other extraintestinal features are absent, ultrasound and occasionally contrast radiography can be helpful, although the findings may simply be edema. Biopsy of the endoscopic lesions may show characteristic leukocytoclastic vasculitis.[8] It is accepted that glucocorticoids will lessen the severity or duration of abdominal pain as well as the rash and the arthritis.[20,21] A recent study showed that steroids begun at diagnosis would decrease the incidence of severe gastrointestinal complications.[13] No benefit was demonstrated for kidney disease. In usual clinical practice, steroids are begun at 1 mg/kg/day and continued for a week, then tapered slowly. Most immunoactive medications have been used, from prednisone through cyclosporine, methotrexate, thalidomide,[22] and plasmapheresis.[2] Treatment is escalated when simple steroid therapy seems insufficient or the disease is prolonged. It is important to remember that steroids can mask catastrophic intra-abdominal events. Some authorities recommend ongoing ultrasound surveillance.[20,21] However, because significant surgical lesions occur in only 2 to 6% of patients,[23] it would seem more rational to follow patients clinically and perform imaging, either abdominal plain film or ultrasound, for only the most worrisome patients. A combination of anti-inflammatory therapy to decrease the vasculitis and direct endoscopic or surgical intervention may be necessary to treat intussusception, perforation, and massive GI bleeding.[6] Repeat courses of steroids, colchicine,[24] rituximab,[25] or other immunomodulators have been used for refractory recurrent illness.

The most vexing question of HSP is whether therapy can prevent or modify the long-term renal consequences. The issue is clouded by lack of controls and the fact that those with abdominal pain are both more likely to be treated with steroids and more likely to suffer renal disease.[12] More aggressive therapy with cyclophosphamide, angiotensin-converting enzyme (ACE) inhibitors, dipyridamole, warfarin, or combinations may have greater effect, but there are no randomized trials. The use of fish oil supplements or tonsillectomy is not supported by the literature.[12]

ACRODERMATITIS ENTEROPATHICA

The autosomal recessive disorder acrodermatitis enteropathica (AE) was recognized as a zinc deficiency in the mid-1970s by Barnes and Moynahan.[26] Investigation of the inherited disease and its clinical imitators has helped illuminate the complicated biologic role of zinc. Primary AE occurs mostly in formula-fed infants or in children weaned from the breast. The full-fledged disease includes a characteristic acro-orificial rash, alopecia, and diarrhea. Lesions at the corners of the eyes and mouth and in the perineum can rapidly spread to a weeping desquamation and superinfection. Poor weight gain, stunting, susceptibility to infection, sepsis, and even death can occur. Response to large (5 to 10 mg/kg/day) oral doses of zinc is apparent in less than a week.[27] The need for zinc supplementation is lifelong because the underlying defect is profoundly depressed zinc absorption. Breast-milk zinc is much more bioavailable than zinc in formula or cow's milk,[28] which leads to the typical weanling onset of the disease. Zinc deficiency can also occur because of zinc-deficient diets or those with large amounts of phytates and other compounds that interfere with zinc absorption.[27,28] Abnormal zinc losses can occur in diarrhea with Crohn's disease, celiac disease, and cystic fibrosis and in urine in some liver diseases, diabetes mellitus, sickle cell disease, nephritis, and any disease with high metabolic stress. The requirement for zinc in severe illness or tissue repair, such as premature infants, postsurgical patients, or those with multiple episodes of infection, may outstrip the dietary supply and lead to acquired AE symptoms, which may be subtle.[28] Conditions blamed on mild to moderate zinc deficiency include short stature, poor appetite, abnormalities of the immune system (especially T-cell function),[29] a variety of skin and nail conditions, behavioral problems including irritability and withdrawal, delayed sexual maturation or impaired reproductive performance, eye lesions, and delayed wound healing.

The original reported cases of inherited AE had low plasma zinc levels. However, this is not universal. Plasma zinc concentrations are not always representative of actual zinc status. Levels below 60 µg/dL may occur in moderate to severe zinc deficiency but can also occur in stress, infection, or pregnancy.[28] Alternatively, symptoms of zinc deficiency, and response to zinc therapy, may occur in children with normal serum or plasma zinc levels. Alkaline phosphatase levels may be depressed in zinc deficiency and are often used as a surrogate test. However, this is not at all specific or sensitive, because other conditions may change alkaline phosphatase levels. Hair zinc has been suggested as a diagnostic tool but is unreliable in young children and in severe disease with arrest of hair growth. Urine zinc is insensitive. Response to therapy remains the best diagnostic tool.[28]

Pathobiology

Zinc has three major roles in physiology.[27] It is a catalyst in more than 100 zinc metalloenzymes, involved in every major enzyme classification.[28] These include alkaline phosphatase, alcohol dehydrogenase, carbonic anhydrase, and DNA polymerase. Zinc has a vital structural role. "Zinc fingers," which are zinc-complexed conformations of nuclear DNA binding proteins, are the most frequent binding motif for transcription factor proteins[28] and are essential to all gene expression. Zinc stabilizes polysomes during protein synthesis and stabilizes the biomembranes of circulating cellular elements.[30] It is an essential component of all tissues in organisms from viruses to mammals.[27] Zinc has a regulatory function, binding to and releasing from zinc-dependent proteins.[27] The essential involvement of

zinc in these basic processes of life explains the long list of disorders of zinc deficiency.

The defect in primary AE has been localized to 8q24.3 by homozygosity mapping.[31,32] This gene encodes a protein that is a member of the ZIP family of metallotransporters.[31] ZIP4 appears to be abnormal in congenital AE.[31] Several different mutations in SLC39A4 have been found in different AE families.[33] Normal ZIP4 appears to be up-regulated in conditions of low zinc availability, either by increased transcription or by increased expression on the cell membrane.[31] ZIP4 appears to function in the upper small intestine, where zinc absorption occurs. Rarely, breast milk is actually deficient in zinc, implying the uncommon occurrence of an abnormal ZIP protein in the breast,[28] a clinical phenotype represented by the lethal milk (lm) mutation in mice.[27]

HEMOLYTIC UREMIC SYNDROME

Hemolytic uremic syndrome (HUS) consists of a microangiopathic hemolytic anemia with some degree of thrombocytopenia and uremia. In children, 90% of cases of this syndrome follow a diarrheal illness, often with blood in the stool. Most of these cases occur in children under the age of 5 years, with an incidence of 1 to 3 per 100,000 children.[34] This type, called D+ HUS by most writers, is of course more interesting to gastroenterologists. The cause of this syndrome is usually a Shiga-like toxin. In the United States, most of the cases are due to enterotoxigenic Escherichia coli type O157:H7.[35] Other E. coli strains have been identified, more frequently in other countries but probably accounting for 25% of cases in the United States.[35] Other bacteria and viruses have also been linked to this disorder. Nondiarrheal HUS may be caused by bacterial infections in other locations or by other causes of increased thrombotic tendency, such as pregnancy, certain drugs, and inherited susceptibility. These "endemic" cases tend to have more severe consequences than the "epidemic" postdiarrheal form. Between 276 and 736 new cases of HUS occur in the United States each year, leading to 24 to 63 patients needing chronic dialysis or transplant.

Pathogenesis

Causal bacteria for D+HUS attach to enterocytes via the intestinal adherence factor intimin. This causes effacement of villi and induces water and electrolyte efflux, causing the early watery diarrhea. A Shiga-like toxin, also called verocytotoxin, causes the major symptoms of this illness. The toxin binds via its B subunits to galactose disaccharides in Globotriaosylceramide (GB3) receptors in the membranes of glomerular, colonic, and cerebral epithelial or microvascular endothelial cells, renal mesangial and tubular cells, platelets, and monocytes. Subjects vary in the amount of GB3 receptors that are present in different tissues. This may account for some of the variability in susceptibility to gastrointestinal, kidney, and nervous system disease.[37] Binding stimulates secretion of cytokines and chemoattractants and also activates platelets. The toxin is internalized into the cell. The A subunit enzymatically binds to ribosomes, ending protein synthesis and eventually causing cell death. Damage to vascular endothelial cells in the susceptible tissues leads to localized clotting, intravascular hemolysis, and platelet trapping. Microangiopathic damage is seen first in the intestine and later in the kidney. There is direct cellular damage as well.

Clinical Presentation

The usual clinical prodrome for D+ HUS is an acute gastroenteritis with vomiting, abdominal pain, fever, and watery diarrhea. In about 70%, bloody diarrhea follows. Diarrhea can last for weeks. Hemolysis and uremia occur within 5 to 14 days of the initial illness.[38] The child is pale, lethargic, sometimes jaundiced, and oliguric. In 10%, a seizure will herald the uremia.[38] There is intravascular hemolysis, burr cells, elevated plasma hemoglobin and hyperbilirubinemia, and negative Coombs' test. Platelets usually fall to 20 to 100,000, whereas the white count may be elevated. HUS occurs in 8 to 31%[35] of patients who are infected with E. coli 0157:H7. Death or end-stage renal disease occur in about 12% of patients with diarrhea associated HUS, and 25% of survivors exhibit long-term renal disease.[39] HUS is the most common cause of acute renal failure in children in many countries. Not surprisingly, the severity of disease at presentation predicts the seriousness of long-term renal problems.

Imaging studies and gross pathology demonstrate mucosal and submucosal hemorrhage and edema in the intestine (Figure 50-3). Barium enema may show spasm and ulceration. Both small and large intestine may be involved, although the colon suffers the majority of the significant damage. Ten percent have rectal prolapse. There may be jaundice, petechiae, purpura, and lethargy. Ulcerative colitis, Crohn's disease, intussusception, and appendicitis may be considered early in the course of the illness. The acute nature of the illness and the usual young age of the patients make inflammatory bowel disease less likely. There are surgical complications in 2 to 7%, including intussusception, severe colitis, sigmoid volvulus, rectal prolapse, and intestinal perforation. The surgical literature points out that perforation occurs after 10 days of illness in most cases.[40] Colitis usually resolves, but colectomy or colostomy has been required in up to 2% of cases. There have been reports of late stricture formation in 3%.[38] Other gastrointestinal complications include elevated transaminases in 40% and elevated lipase or amylase in 20%. Ongoing diabetes mellitus can occur in 8%.[38]

Cultures should be performed in cases of serious bloody diarrhea and D+HUS. E. coli such as O111:H- in Australia and O26:H11 in Germany have caused the syndrome. The verocytotoxin for HUS is plasmid encoded, allowing for transfer to other E. coli or even other species. This Shiga toxin should be sought where testing is available, because of the public health

implications.[34] The major reservoir for E. coli 0157:H7 is cattle, for which it is normal flora, colonizing 1 to 44% of beef cattle awaiting slaughter.[34] One meatpacking plant can send food all over the United States. Therefore, outbreaks can be widespread. Ground meat, in which the pathogen can be mixed throughout the entire lot, is the most likely to spread infection. Larger solid cuts of meat are more easily sterilized in the usual cooking process. A very interesting approach to reducing the burden of colonization is to alter feeding practices for beef cattle. A marked decrease in fecal E. coli was noted when hay rather than grain was fed for 5 days before slaughter. Health care professionals are increasingly aware of unusual sources of E. coli transmission, such as raw vegetables and juices, as well as lakes and pools. The incidence of the illness is higher in the summer months, corresponding to higher colonization in cattle and presumable higher exposure to environmental water sources and raw vegetables.

It is generally accepted that antibiotic treatment of the initial diarrhea should be withheld because it may increase the likelihood of HUS. In vitro, fosfomycin has been shown to increase release of verocytotoxin from E. coli.[41] However, whether this occurs in a clinically meaningful fashion is not clear. Antibiotic treatment did not seem to increase the risk of HUS in the 1993 Jack-in-the-Box outbreak and actually seemed protective in an outbreak in Japan in 1996.[36] It is not obvious that antibiotics would be helpful in treating the colitis, in which the damage may have already occurred. It has been shown that antibiotic therapy does not shorten the diarrheal illness. Thus, except for rare cases of sepsis, it seems safer to not treat.[35,38,42] Physicians considering antibiotics for nonbloody diarrhea in children should consider the possible prodrome relationship before treating. A randomized prospective study of this question is unlikely to occur because of the numbers needed and the ethical dilemmas involved.

RADIATION ENTERITIS

Radiation therapy is a very effective agent for the treatment of malignancy. In pediatric oncology, it is used for leukemia, intracranial malignancy, Wilms' tumor, sarcoma, and preparation for bone marrow transplant, among other indications.[44] Children are more susceptible to the acute effects of radiation therapy, because more of their tissues are actively growing. The intestine is quite sensitive to radiation, also because of rapid cell turnover. Radiation injury occurs through free radical formation from water in the irradiated tissue.[44] The free radicals disrupt DNA, leading to cell death as replication proceeds. The therapeutic goal is to cause more damage to tumor tissue than to healthy tissue. However, the therapeutic dose range, which maximizes tumor cell death, is often close to the toxic dose range for the tissue.[44] Complications of radiation to the intestine occur acutely, and in a more chronic phase, within the next year or even delayed for a decade or more.[44-47]

The acute consequences of radiation to the abdomen are visible as a sequence of histology changes. Damage to the small intestine is obvious in the first 12 hours. Over the first week, cell loss exceeds the mitotic ability of the crypt cells to regenerate new cells. The villi of the small intestine shorten and disaccharidases are lost. Edema and inflammation follow, leading to loss of absorptive capacity.[46] Bile salt malabsorption leads to choleretic diarrhea. Damage to the rectum is similar. Crypt abscesses in the rectum may contain a high proportion of eosinophils,

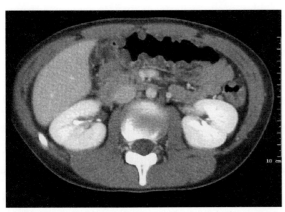

Figure 50-3. HUS Edema of the bowel wall produces the characteristic thumbprinting.

suggesting a localized allergic-type response, although the target is unclear.[46]

Intravenous nutrition is now routinely used to support the child through mucositis, diarrhea, and anorexia. In one early study, 70% of children subjected to radiotherapy exhibited diarrhea and vomiting during the course of radiation; 30% of these were severe enough to require intervention to maintain fluid and electrolyte balance. Half of children had weight loss.[45] There is abdominal pain, bloating, and tenesmus. Radiographic studies may show dilatation of bowel loops, wall edema, and loss of normal motility. Patients are empirically treated with lactose restriction or hypoallergenic diet, proton pump inhibitors, bile acid binding resins, loperamide, and probiotics. Hydrophilic stool softeners, steroid enemas, and sitz baths are used for proctitis. Kinsella showed normalization of tests of malabsorption after 1 year,[46] whereas others showed that most patients had permanent late alterations in bowel habit even though they did not voice any complaints.[48,49] Some authors feel that patients who had more severe symptoms early on are more likely to have late complications.

Donaldson et al.[45] described subacute damage in 11% of radiated children in the 2 to 12 months after therapy. These children presented with obstructive symptoms of vomiting and diarrhea as well as radiographic evidence of obstruction. There was an inflammatory infiltrate in the intestine with lymphangiectasia and villus atrophy. Exuberant fibrosis and adhesions caused the obstruction; vascular damage was not mentioned.

Later complications of radiation therapy are a consequence of ischemia. There is an obliterative endarteritis and fibrosis leading to ulceration, necrosis, perforation, and stricture.[46] Of patients with these problems, 85% present within 2 years, but the remainder may exhibit symptoms 15 or more years later.[47] Proctitis with tenesmus and bleeding is the major symptom in 75%. The diagnosis is made on endoscopy, which shows erythema, edema, friability, and often numerous telangiectasias.[44] There may be deep ulceration. Alternatively, the mucosa may be thin, translucent, and clearly exquisitely fragile.[46] Bleeding tends to be difficult to treat but self-limiting in about 80% of adults. In adults, a transfusion requirement predicts a low rate of remission and substantial mortality. Treatment for proctitis includes enemas of 2 g sucralfate suspended in 4% methylcellulose, hyperbaric oxygen, and use of an argon laser for coagulation of the telangiectasias.[50] In adult patients, ulcers are also treated with instillation of a 4% solution of formaldehyde directly into the rectum or application with gauze sponges. Studies show no evidence that mesalamine or steroids are helpful either orally or rectally.[50] Surgical exclusion of the rectum for severe bleeding is more effective than diversion, but all surgical procedures are subject to high complication rates. Better results are obtained when it is possible to use nonirradiated bowel for any anastomosis or stoma formation.[44]

Other late consequences of radiation stem from bowel fibrosis, which causes stricture formation. Fistulization and perforation are less common. Bacterial overgrowth may occur in the relatively stagnant loop, leading to irritant diarrhea, vitamin B_{12} loss, and destruction to villi with accompanying disaccharidase deficiency and loss of intraluminal bile salts due to deconjugation and early reabsorption. Malabsorption of sugars and fat leads to diarrhea and fat-soluble vitamin deficiency. The scarred intestine may have abnormal motility, leading to rapid intestinal transit, or perhaps to ileus or a functional motility disorder.[49] Therapy should be directed at the most likely cause of the

symptoms and carried out systematically. Empiric medication and diet change are the same as in acute radiation reaction but may need to be continued indefinitely. Nutritional supplementation may be crucial. If strictures cause only low-grade symptoms, surgery should be avoided. The same problems occur with attempted anastomosis of radiated bowel. Damage to the bowel and later consequences are increased by several different factors, some of which can be modified.[44] Normally the intestine, except for the rectum, is constantly moving during the application of radiation. This diminishes the point exposure time of any one segment and decreases damage. Bowel that is fixed by previous inflammation or surgery is less mobile and therefore more vulnerable. It is possible to place a polyglycolic acid mesh sling to raise the small bowel out of the range of pelvic irradiation, thus preventing much of the damage.[51] Certain chemotherapeutic drugs, such as 5-fluorouracil, doxorubicin, actinomycin D, and methotrexate, increase the risk of enteritis.[46] Newer treatment protocols may avoid using these agents or may time the dosing to allow maximal recovery of normal tissue while causing maximal damage to tumor cells.[43] Advances in radiation therapy technique permit targeting of therapy directly to small areas. Doses can be scaled to the size of individual children. There is new research into medications that protect normal tissues from radiation (amifostine or Ethylol, among others) and into techniques that preferentially sensitize tumor cells to the radiation.[42] There is some evidence for prophylaxis with sulfasalazine[52] and from the use of probiotics[53] at the time of the radiation. Once fully developed and implemented, these techniques will help prevent a large proportion of radiation damage to the intestine.

MALAKOPLAKIA

Malakoplakia is a rare and poorly understood chronic inflammatory process that seems to occur mostly in the setting of some type of immunodeficiency.[54] Michaelis and Gutmann and their mentor, Hanesmann, described it almost simultaneously in the early 1900s.[55,56] About 75% of the cases involve the genitourinary tract, with about 200 described in the intestine.[57] The disorder presents as friable yellow plaques or polypoid lesions on the mucosa of the gastrointestinal tract, sometimes with narrowing or stricturing of the colon. Fistulas can occur. There can be bleeding, pain, or obstructive symptoms. The plaques can grow very large and can present as an abdominal or rectal mass (Figure 50-4). Anemia, elevated erythrocyte sedimentation rate, leukocytosis, night sweats, and fatigue can be present.[57] Large masses concentrate gallium in nuclear medicine scanning.[54] The most common site of involvement in the gastrointestinal tract is the rectum, with the sigmoid and right colon being less common. Most examples of malakoplakia occur in middle age, but there is a small peak in childhood.[57]

The diagnosis of malakoplakia is made by the characteristic pathology. Abnormal phagocytic macrophages (von Hansemann cells) can be shown on electron microscopy to contain lysosomes swollen with partially degraded bacteria. Michaelis-Gutmann bodies, lamellated basophilic collections of calcified mucopolysaccharides and lipids that are similar to bacterial cell walls, must be evident in the lysosomes to substantiate the diagnosis[54] (Figure 50-5).

The ultramicroscopic appearance of the lesion hints at the pathogenesis of the problem, which is still poorly understood. There seems to be defective bacterial killing, whether because of

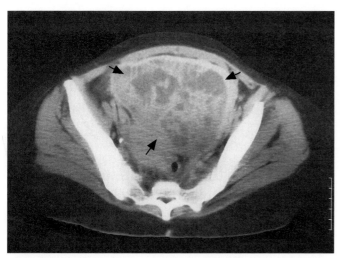

Figure 50-4. Malakoplakia: a large inhomogeneous mass with internal septa and peripheral enhancement seen on computed tomographic scan with intravenous contrast.

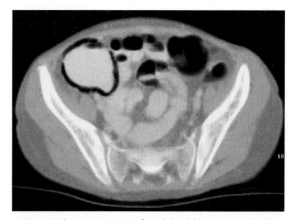

Figure 50-5. Light microscopy of malakoplakia: xanthogranulomatous inflammation in an area of malakoplakia, showing clear phagocytic cells (von Hansemann cells) surrounding dense black dots (Michaelis-Gutmann bodies).

a primary disease state or because of immunosuppressive medication. In many of the cases, *E. coli* was cultured. *Mycobacterium tuberculosis*, *Proteus*, and *Klebsiella* have also been cultured, whereas many lesions do not yield any organisms despite the fragments of bacteria therein.[54] The disease has been reported in patients taking prednisone or azathioprine. In these cases, withdrawal of the medications led to resolution. Other patients have had hypogammaglobulinemia, IgA deficiency, acquired immunodeficiency syndrome, or neoplasm.[57] One patient was found to have a selective defect in killing *Proteus* and *Salmonella*.[55] It has been theorized that deficient cyclic guanosine monophosphate (cGMP) in the macrophage could lead to deficient fusion of lysosomes with phagosomes containing bacterial products.[54,57] Overall, this could lead to incomplete bacterial killing and ongoing inflammation. There is substantial mortality in the adult series, up to 80% of untreated patients and 15% for all cases.[54] Therapy with a cholinergic agent, bethanechol, to increase cGMP, has occasionally been helpful. Ascorbic acid is thought to be synergistic with this therapy, by changing cGMP ratios. More frequently, therapy with trimethoprim-sulfamethoxazole or quinolones, antibiotics that are internally concentrated by macrophages, results in cure of the lesion. Surgical removal of large mass lesions may aid cure.[54]

BEHÇET'S SYNDROME

Behçet's disease is a chronically recurring inflammatory disorder of unknown cause. It occurs most frequently along the ancient Silk Route, which extends from the Far East through the middle East to the Mediterranean, the trade route taken by Marco Polo on his voyage to Cathay. The prevalence of Behçet's syndrome in Western countries is low: 0.64 per 100,000 in the United Kingdom and 0.12 to 0.33 per 100,000 in the United States. It is more common in Japan, Korea, China, Saudi Arabia, and Iran (13.5 to 20 cases per 100,000) but is rare in Japanese immigrants to the United States.[58] The disease has been reported in to occur in clusters in families, up to 15% in the Middle East but only 2 to 5% elsewhere. It is more common in females in the Far East and in males in the Middle East. Monozygotic twin pairs have been reported, both concordant and

discordant. Both environment and genetics are clearly important in the epidemiology of the illness.[59]

Behçet's is a vasculitis that causes lesions in many different organ systems. There are no pathognomonic findings, so the diagnosis depends on the presence of major and minor manifestations as defined by the International Study Group for Behçet's Disease. In some patients, the interesting phenomenon of pathergy can help make the diagnosis. The manifestations may occur over the course of years. The condition is quite rare in children, in part because the diagnostic symptoms may not appear rapidly enough to meet the definition until the child is older. Gastrointestinal disease is more common in children than in adults, whereas ocular disease is much less common.[58]

Oral ulcers, occurring in 70 to 90% of subjects with Behçet's, are painful round lesions with a sharp erythematous border, covered with a yellow pseudomembrane. These occur on the buccal and labial mucosa, the tongue, and the gingiva. The ulcers heal in 7 to 14 days without scarring; recurrence of lesions is the norm. This may be the first symptom of Behçet's but also can occur in up to 10% of normal persons. *Genital ulcers,* of similar frequency, occur on the vulva, the scrotum, and the penis. They are painful, deeper, and more serpiginous than the oral lesions. They heal within 2 weeks with scarring and also can recur periodically.[58]

Ocular lesions are usually the most serious problem in Behçet's disease in adults, occurring in 80% of patients. Only 20% of children develop this manifestation of the disease. Symptoms include pain, blurring, photophobia, floaters, tearing, and redness. Uveitis can be recurrent and eventually leads to scarring of the iris and glaucoma. Occlusive vascular disease causes painless decrease in visual acuity. Hypopyon, inflammatory cells layering out in the anterior chamber, is a visible characteristic, but can also occur in spondyloarthropathy.[58] There are a number of different skin lesions associated with Behçet's. Erythema nodosum, pseudofolliculitis, acneiform nodules, and migratory thrombophlebitis occur.[58]

Minor criteria include gastrointestinal disease, arthritis, and neurologic disease. *Intestinal symptoms* include nonspecific pain, vomiting, diarrhea, flatulence, or constipation. There can be more serious disease, with bloody diarrhea, perforation, and fistulas. The radiographic signs are thickened folds, mucosal ulcerations, deformation of bowel loops, and fistulas. The gut disease resembles ulcerative colitis histologically but can occur in the ileum (25%) and the esophagus (12%). Granulomata are absent, but differentiating from the classic inflammatory bowel diseases can be difficult. The bowel lesions are deeper than in ulcerative colitis, and the ulcers seem more isolated than in Crohn's disease. Gastrointestinal involvement varies in different geographic populations, being rare in patients in Turkey and in white patients in the West, but occurs in up to 15% of patients in Japan.[58] *Arthritis* in Behçet's is usually nondestructive, involving the large joints. Acneiform lesions and arthritis seem to occur together in the same patient with the same severity and timing.

Neurologic disease, occurring in up to 20% of Behçet's patients, can be useful in differentiating this from other inflammatory bowel diseases. Acute aseptic meningitis or meningoencephalitis may occur early on but is more frequent 5 years or more into the illness. There are brainstem symptoms and motor problems as well as personality changes. Cranial nerve palsies, pseudotumor cerebri, thromboses, and seizures can occur. Irreversible damage and dementia can evolve in 30% of affected patients. Magnetic resonance imaging shows typical multiple high-intensity focal lesions in the brainstem, white matter, and basal ganglia.[58]

Diffuse vascular disease can cause serious problems in Behçet's, including thrombophlebitis, large vessel aneurysms, infarction, and organ failure. Coronary vasculitis and valvular disease can occur. Dyspnea, cough, chest pain, and hemoptysis can result from pulmonary vasculitis.[58] Pathergy is a characteristic reaction to sterile needle disturbance of the skin, joint, or eye. A hypersensitivity reaction occurs at the needle track, causing a papule or pustule, synovitis or panophthalmitis, lesions filled with activated neutrophils.[58,59]

Etiopathogenesis

Behçet's disease may more accurately be described as a syndrome[59] because of the lack of homogeneity in its manifestations and even in its treatments. The disease is frequently associated with HLA-B51 in the Silk Route countries, up to 80% in Asian patients and 55% in Japan. Japanese carriers of HLA-B51 have a relative risk of 6.7 for Behçet's but only a 1.3 risk in the United States. HLA-B51 seems to be associated with a high prevalence and severity of eye and neurologic disease in Asia, but severe disease does occur without it. Other manifestations vary with geography. Intestinal involvement is common in the Far East but not the Middle East. Pathergy is frequent in the Mediterranean but not Europe. Some treatments are effective for female but not male patients, whereas others help some symptoms and exacerbate others.[59]

Behçet's disease seems to be a disease of cells rather than of circulating factors.[59] Neutrophils and lymphocytes function abnormally in Behçet's syndrome. Neutrophils are excessively active, leading to tissue injury through release of tumor necrosis factor, interleukin-1β, and interleukin-8. Lymphocytes home specifically to abnormal self proteins derived from heat shock proteins. These self proteins are present in the affected tissues of Behçet's patients, but not unaffected persons. These proteins seem to resemble bacterial heat shock proteins but are different from the abnormal heat shock proteins or rheumatoid arthritis.[58] Vasculitis is found near all of the characteristic lesions. Endothelial cells and platelets are activated. Despite the tendency for thrombosis, circulating thrombophilic factors are normal.[60] Behçet's has also been associated with microbial infections, but no one organism is found in all subjects. Instead it seems that cross-reactivity to self may be an important mechanism in this as in many similar diseases. However, some syndromes that commonly accompany other autoimmune diseases, such as Raynaud's phenomenon and autoantibodies, are absent in Behçet's.[59]

Therapy

Treatment depends on the type of involvement. Medications are usually those directed against autoimmune reactions. Treatment of the most serious lesions in the eyes, the gut, the nervous system, and those causing large vessel disease takes precedence.[58]

Colchicine, steroids, azathioprine, chlorambucil, and cyclophosphamide are used for ocular lesions. Unfortunately, 10 to 25% of patients still progress to blindness. Cyclosporine is also used, but has a declining response over time. Interferon alpha 2a has been used with greater success, but data are limited. Gastrointestinal disease can be treated like Crohn's disease with salicylates and steroids. Disease can be recurrent. Acute neurologic disease responds to corticosteroids whereas chronic disease may be refractory. Large-vessel pulmonary disease can be fatal if hemoptysis begins; steroids, antiplatelet drugs, and, sometimes and with caution, anticoagulants are used.[58,59,61] Because of the involvement of tumor necrosis factor, thalidomide, infliximab, and other tumor necrosis factor (TNF) antagonists have been used in a few cases with success.[62,63] This would seem to be the obvious choice in severe neurologic or ocular disease.[58,59]

TYPHLITIS

Also known as neutropenic enterocolitis and ileocecal syndrome, this ulcerating disease of the intestine occurs in patients who are profoundly neutropenic from chemotherapy for malignancy or from other drug therapy. It has also occurred in acquired immunodeficiency syndrome, in aplastic anemia, or from leukemia itself.[61,64] Typhlitis has been most often described in children, perhaps because their chemotherapeutic regimens have traditionally been very intense. Some authors suggest that adults are experiencing an increasing incidence as their therapeutic regimens are made more toxic. Postmortem series from large pediatric oncology services collecting cases up to the 1990s documented typhlitis in 10 to 24% of autopsied children.[65] Early series allow a crude estimate of overall incidence to be 5% of all pediatric patients treated for leukemia.[65,66] Case fatality rates for this problem seemed high in the beginning; cases were often recognized clinically because of complications that necessitated surgery. Operation was attempted but was often unsuccessful because the children were already moribund. Since then, greater awareness of the symptom complex has enabled clinicians to suspect the illness in its early presentations. More accurate imaging has most likely expanded the discovery and allowed earlier, more effective therapy.[66-68]

Symptoms of typhlitis include abdominal pain, which may be diffuse, localized to the right lower quadrant, or may be absent, most likely due to concomitant corticosteroid therapy. There is usually fever, abdominal distention, nausea, and vomiting. Constipation may occur, but diarrhea is more common. There may be gross blood in the stool. In most cases, chemotherapy was given 2 to 4 weeks before the onset of typhlitis.[66,68,69] The absolute neutrophil count is usually less than 500 per liter. Plain films may show thumbprinting of the colon, a dilated fluid-filled cecum, a soft tissue mass in the right lower quadrant, pneumatosis, or absence of air in most of the colonic lumen. Barium enema is now felt to be contraindicated but would show ileus, small bowel obstruction, and "nonfilling" of the colon. Ultrasound has given way to routine abdominal CT scan, which may demonstrate edema of the colon, inflammation surrounding the colon and in the mesenteric fat, and sometimes pneumatosis.[61,65,67,70] The differential diagnosis includes appendicitis, perforation from other cause, and volvulus or intussusception. It is not clear that any particular chemotherapeutic regimen is more likely to give rise to this complication.[67,70]

Autopsy and surgical findings show dilatation, edema, and hemorrhage of the bowel, with frank necrosis sometimes evident. The cecum alone may be involved, but other portions of the bowel, including appendix, ileum, ascending colon, or sporadic involvement of any portion of the intestine, can be seen in varied combinations.[70] Ulceration and diffuse necrotizing loss of the mucosa is seen. There is little inflammatory infiltrate, and leukemic infiltrate is not usually seen. Fungal or bacterial forms are frequently seen in the necrotic tissue. Blood cultures are positive for bacteria in 70 to 80% of patients and for fungus in about 30%. Bacteria include *Pseudomonas*, *S. aureus*, *E. coli*, and α-*Streptococcus*.[61,65,66,69]

The pathogenesis of typhlitis is unclear. Many of the chemotherapeutic regimens cause ileus as well as damage to the gastrointestinal mucosa. In combination with leukopenia or the immunoincompetence of leukemic cells, bacterial invasion of the bowel wall can occur. Subsequent toxin production could lead to further bowel wall damage and vascular compromise.[65,70] The cecum may be more vulnerable because of its watershed location, as in neonatal necrotizing enterocolitis, in some ways a similar situation.

Therapy of typhlitis begins prospectively with vigilance for the symptoms of fever and pain. Prompt CT scan or perhaps ultrasound may reveal suspicious findings. The patient is placed on bowel rest, often with nasogastric suction. Parenteral nutrition is usually started and antibiotics are begun if not already used. Immunosuppressants should be weaned if possible. Antifungal therapy is often started if fever does not decrease in 2 to 3 days. Filgrastim (GCSF) is given, based on the observation that regaining a leukocyte count to greater than 1000/L correlated with survival.[61,65,68,69] Laparoscopy should be performed when there is clinical suspicion of necrosis or CT evidence of perforation. Mortality in the early series was 50% or greater.[61,68] With earlier recognition and more effective therapy, mortality is falling below 10%.[61] Because repeated courses of chemotherapy often bring on repeated bouts of typhlitis, prophylactic colectomy has been recommended for children who have suffered this once and need further cytotoxins.[65] However, this advice does not seem to reflect usual clinical practice.

MICROSCOPIC COLITIS

Microscopic colitis is the overarching name for lymphocytic colitis (LC) and collagenous colitis (CC), disorders clinically characterized by copious watery, nonbloody diarrhea and cramping abdominal pain. These occur most often in middle-aged women and are uncommon in children. There are case series showing lymphocytic colitis in children with regressive autism, although the characteristic symptom of profuse diarrhea was not always reported.[71,72] A child with neurologic

disease developed lymphocytic colitis after carbamazepine.[73] Classic LC/CC was seen in a small case series in which recovery occurred over the course of a year.[74] A third series showed similar patients evolving into more classic inflammatory bowel disease.[75] The largest case series showed 20 pediatric patients over about 15 years.[76] Similar to the adult series, up to 30% of children with celiac disease also have LC/CC.[77] All series emphasize the dictum that tends to distinguish pediatric from adult endoscopists: systematic biopsies throughout the entire colon are indicated in children when nonspecific symptoms of diarrhea prompt endoscopy, even if the mucosa is grossly normal.[78]

Endoscopic findings are minimal to absent. Biopsies show an inflammatory infiltrate in the lamina propria. Lymphocytes predominate over plasma cells, mast cells, and eosinophils. Lymphocytes also infiltrate the crypts and the surface epithelium and should account for more than 10 to 25% of surface epithelial cells.[78] Subepithelial type I or type III collagen layers vary in thickness in both of these conditions. There may be marked variation in an individual patient. Biopsy findings of these diseases are sparse and discontinuous, adding to the difficulty of characterizing the findings in individual patients as well as in compiling meaningful case series.[79] Thus, there is controversy as to whether these are truly distinct diseases. Etiology is also unclear. Various medications, including nonsteroidal anti-inflammatory medications, and autoimmune conditions are associated with the biopsy findings in adults.

In childhood as in adulthood, therapy for these diseases is unclear. Celiac disease should be excluded, although treatment with a gluten-free diet has not shown efficacy for microscopic colitis. Possible causal medications should be stopped. Budesonide seems to be the most effective therapy for microscopic colitis, whereas other therapies (probiotics, mesalamine, bismuth) need further investigation.[80]

EHLERS-DANLOS SYNDROME

Ehlers-Danlos syndrome is a group of heritable diseases of collagen formation. The vascular type of EDS is characterized by mutations in the COL3A1 gene on chromosome 2q31, which leads to synthesis of abnormal type III procollagen molecules that are not secreted normally out of the cell. This type of collagen is widespread in the body, present in skin, blood vessels, bowel, and solid organs. Lack of this collagen leads to thin, tight skin, easy scarring, excessive mobility of joints, frequent breakage of blood vessels, and easy bruising. Rupture of large blood vessels is common. Patients frequently die of vascular complications before the end of their fifth decade. Further symptoms outside the gastrointestinal tract include aneurysm and fistula formation, diaphragmatic hernia, joint dislocation, cardiac abnormalities, and hypospadias. Pregnancy can end in uterine rupture. Fetuses with the syndrome may be premature and of low birth weight.[80]

EDS is inherited in an autosomal dominant fashion, but almost half of cases appear to be new mutations.[81,82] Characteristic features of this type are a thin face, narrow pinched nose, thin lips, prominent eyes, asthenic habitus, easily visible vessels, and hands that appear elderly in childhood. The symptoms may be subtle in early childhood, and a dangerous complication may be the first sign.[82,83] Diagnosis depends on awareness of the physical findings, a possible family history of vascular rupture, and the culture of skin fibroblasts. These cultured cells secrete reduced quantities or abnormal variants of type III collagen. mRNA sequencing will show an abnormal gene.[81] Ultrastructural examination of involved tissues will show reduced amounts of type III collagen and broken and fragmented elastic fibers.[82]

The major intestinal complication of this disorder is spontaneous perforation of the bowel. The most common location of perforation is the colon, especially the sigmoid. Multiple perforations are not uncommon. Sutures easily rip out of repaired tissues; wound infection and poor healing is common.[81,82] It is recommended that emergency surgery for perforation should consist of exteriorization of the perforation or resection and end colostomy with closure or mucous colostomy of the distal portion.[81] Many children who had closure of the bowel had recurrent perforation.[81,84] Therefore, permanent colostomy is recommended.[81,84,85] Other gastrointestinal symptoms include constipation, diverticulosis, gastrointestinal bleeding, and perhaps dysmotility.[85]

PNEUMATOSIS INTESTINALIS

This interesting condition was first described in 1730 by DuVernoi and documented in humans by Bang in 1730.[86] This sign has an ominous meaning to most pediatricians, based on its frequent occurrence in moribund premature infants with necrotizing enterocolitis. However, the condition is much more widespread and less dangerous overall than is commonly appreciated.[87-91]

Intraluminal gas in the intestine may be detected on plain abdominal radiography, by ultrasound, endoscopically, and even found incidentally on histology.[92] It is best visualized by computed tomography[88] (Figure 50-6). It may be associated with a wide variety of nonintestinal conditions as well as intra-abdominal illnesses and is even seen in healthy children (Table 50-1). Not all instances of pneumatosis intestinalis are dangerous, and most do not require operation.[89,91,93,94] The underlying illness, if any, the precipitating event, and the clinical course dictate the management.

There are several different possible theoretical mechanisms to explain gas entry into the abdominal wall.[87,89,93] The mechanical theory suggests that gas dissects into the bowel wall under pressure. This could occur with pulmonary obstructive disease, violent coughing, trauma,[93] or vomiting. In these situations, air could travel through lymphatics or vessels to the abdomen. This is supported by analysis of intramural gas showing composition consistent with alveolar air in some patients.[86]

Not all cysts contain this composition, however. Gas could also be forced from the bowel lumen into the walls if there is intestinal obstruction from any cause, or if there is an increase in intraluminal pressure from endoscopy or trauma. Another possibility would be intraluminal bacterial action that produces a great increase in the partial pressure of hydrogen or methane. The excess gas may diffuse into the bowel wall passively. This could occur as a result of any cause of carbohydrate malabsorption. In some cases, such as short bowel syndrome, the gas in the wall is indeed high in hydrogen.[86] Children with short bowel syndrome may have pneumatosis that fluctuates with the level of carbohydrate in their diet.[87] A bacterial invasion theory suggests that gas-forming bacteria enter the bowel wall under conditions of infection or inflammation, such as necrotizing enterocolitis or graft-versus-host disease colitis. The presence of high levels of breath hydrogen in some of these patients supports this theory as well. However, the cysts are usually sterile, and bacteria are not usually found on histologic examination. The intramural gas may again represent increased intraluminal gas forcing its way through microscopic rents in the tissue.[86] Most cases of pneumatosis can theoretically fit into one or a combination of these mechanisms.

There are several reviews of pneumatosis in children.[87,90,91] Short bowel syndrome, organ and bone marrow transplant, intestinal dysmotility, congenital heart disease, and toxicity from iron ingestion were common associated illnesses, perhaps reflecting in part the specialties of the reporting institutions. Healthy children also made up a considerable portion of the reported cases.[87] The inciting events were frequently infectious enteritis, noninfectious colitis, or ischemia.[87] Symptoms most commonly noted were abdominal distention, bloody diarrhea, vomiting, and lethargy.[86,87,91] Poor outcome and the need for surgical intervention were associated with more serious underlying disorders that increased the risk of multisystem disease and bowel necrosis. These disorders included decompensated

TABLE 50-1. Conditions Associated With Pneumatosis Intestinalis[86,87,89,91,93]

Healthy child
Asthma
Pulmonary fibrosis
Cystic fibrosis
Chronic obstructive pulmonary disease
Pyloric stenosis
Peptic ulcer
Intestinal obstruction
Intestinal pseudo-obstruction and other motility disorders
Inflammatory bowel disease
Celiac disease
Hirschsprung's disease
Jejunoileal bypass
Endoscopy (with or without biopsy)
Enteric tube placement (needle catheter jejunostomy)
Collagen vascular disease
Organ and bone marrow transplant
Graft-versus-host disease
Acquired immunodeficiency syndrome
Medications: prednisone, lactulose, cancer chemotherapy
Iron overdose
Decompensated heart disease
Gastroschisis
Short bowel syndrome
Closed abdominal trauma
Intestinal surgery

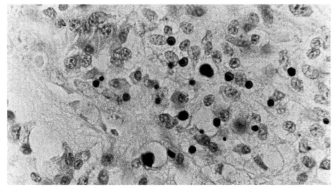

Figure 50-6. Pneumatosis intestinalis. Bowel wall is outlined by a black rim of air.

heart disease and transplant status, as well as iron toxicity.[87,91] Poor outcome was also associated with acidosis, hypotension, and portal venous gas.[87,91] Some children with pneumoperitoneum or portal venous gas did not require surgery and recovered with supportive care.[88,90] A review in adults suggests that patients with clinical signs of bowel obstruction or ischemic bowel require surgery, whereas those without metabolic acidosis can be observed. An elevated amylase also seemed to suggest a less favorable outcome.[94] Surgery, most often resection of an infarcted or perforated section of bowel, is indicated if there is steady deterioration, increased abdominal pain and rebound, and free air.[86,87,91]

Pneumatosis intestinalis may be an incidental finding. Rarely, crepitation may be felt in the abdomen or on rectal examination; air blebs may simulate polyps on rectal examination or endoscopy.[92] There may be abdominal distention or pain. Symptoms usually relate to the underlying disease. On rare occasions, the air blebs may cause pain or obstruction.[92] Treatment for pneumatosis itself may be indicated for mechanical problems. Treatment for the underlying disease may help decrease pneumatosis and prevent its recurrence. Conservative therapy includes placing the bowel at rest, using suction, and giving antibiotics (metronidazole, ampicillin, or ciprofloxacin).[92] Oxygen may be administered at moderate to high concentrations (40 to 100%) to achieve moderate to high partial pressure of oxygen (200 to 300 mm Hg[86,92]). Hyperbaric oxygen has been used. Some children receive no treatment and recover rapidly.[87]

SOLITARY RECTAL ULCER SYNDROME AND COLITIS CYSTICA PROFUNDA

Solitary rectal ulcer syndrome (SRS) is probably underdiagnosed in both children and adults because it is not always recognized as a distinct entity. This syndrome seems to result from disordered defecation.[92,95,96] There is a very high incidence of rectal prolapse, either obvious or occult. Prolapse may result from persistent contraction of the puborectalis muscle, keeping the anal canal closed with very high intrarectal pressure. The external anal sphincter may fail to relax, again leading to high pressure. Another mechanism is excessive perineal descent, so that the anterior rectal wall protrudes into the anal canal. Each of these mechanisms has been observed in some adult patients on defecography or manometry.[96] The dysfunction leads to straining to stool, pressure necrosis of the anal mucosa, or congestion and traction of the submucosal vessels.[92] Self-induced trauma due to digital removal of stool has also been described with this syndrome.[92,96]

The end result of this process is pressure necrosis of the bowel wall. The endoscopic appearance of SRS often belies the singularity implied by its name.[92] There frequently may be several shallow round or serpiginous ulcers with a thin erythematous rim. They range from 0.5 to 5 cm. The lesions are most often seen on the anterior wall but may be circumferential.[97] They are located 5 to 15 cm from the anal verge.[96] Early in the evolution of the lesion, or in a healing phase, there may be only erythema and edema. Less commonly, polypoid lesions may be found. These polypoid structures may themselves prolapse.[97]

Madigan and Morson described the characteristic histologic picture of SRS in 1969.[96] The features include obliteration of the lamina propria by fibromuscular proliferation of the muscularis mucosa, streaming of muscle fibers and fibroblasts between contorted branching crypts, thickening of the muscularis mucosa, and diffuse collagen infiltration of the lamina propria.[92] Orientation of the muscle fibers perpendicular to the lamina propria is pathognomonic.[97] The diffuse fibrosis in these cases differs from the focal fibrosis of inflammatory bowel disease or ischemia.[77] Some patients also have colitis cystica profunda (CCP), with submucosal cysts in the muscularis propria or even serosa.[92,96] The cysts may have benign colonic epithelium lining or may have no lining. It is postulated that these cysts result from translocation of surface epithelium into the deeper mucosal layers under pressure.[96] As many as 54% of patients with CCP have rectal prolapse, further strengthening the association of these two entities.[92]

Patients with these two syndromes have variable symptoms. Probably 25% are asymptomatic. Up to 89% have rectal bleeding, which rarely is profuse enough to require transfusion.[92] There may be mucorrhea, diarrhea, constipation, incontinence, proctalgia, abdominal pain, and tenesmus. There may be actual obstruction of defecation by the prolapse.[92,96]

Therapy for solitary rectal ulcer is poorly defined. Conservative therapy may be more effective in children, especially those in whom the lesion is polypoid rather than ulcerative.[96] This medical therapy includes stool softening, bowel retraining in positions to decrease straining, and reassurance. Corticosteroids, salicylates, and sucralfate have been tried, and probably each is useful for some patients. Local electrocautery, caustics, and antibiotics have been used.[92] Rectopexy tends to be the most successful. Simple excision of the lesion is not successful.[92,98] Success with surgery ranges from 65 to 94%, with most series in the lower range. Thus surgery should be reserved for those with intractable and disabling symptoms. Total diversion of the fecal stream can be used for the most symptomatic.[92,98]

AMYLOIDOSIS

Deposition of amyloid, an amorphous substance, is an infrequent consequence of a variety of inflammatory diseases (Table 50-2.) Exactly how inflammation causes this deposition is not completely clear, but the molecular nature of amyloid has been thoroughly explored. Amyloid exists as a beta-pleated sheet of long nonbranching fibrils 7.5 to 10 nm in diameter. The pleating accounts for its pathognomonic birefringence when stained with Congo red. Most of the fibrils in gastrointestinal disease are of two types. AL (amyloid light chains, derived from immunoglobulin light chains) are found in monoclonal B cell proliferation. AA (amyloid-associated protein made by the liver) deposits in tissues of persons affected with infectious and noninfectious inflammation. AA amyloid is also called secondary amyloidosis.

TABLE 50-2. Diseases Associated With Amyloid Deposition[57,96]

Tuberculosis
Bronchiectasis
Chronic osteomyelitis
Rheumatoid arthritis (3%)
Cystic fibrosis
Glycogenosis
Ankylosing spondylitis
Inflammatory bowel disease
"Skin popping" narcotics (chronic infection)
Familial Mediterranean fever
Hemodialysis (beta 2 microglobulin not removed by dialysis membrane)
Diabetes mellitus type 2

Amyloid deposits first around the blood vessels of the intestine but later infiltrates the submucosa, muscularis, and subserosa. The consequences of this are changes in motility and possibly ischemia. Clinically, amyloidosis of the intestine may be silent or may manifest as irregular contours of the bowel that do not change function. Other radiographic signs include dilatation,[96] granularity, 3- to 4-mm nodules, and polypoid lesions measuring up to 10 mm. Endoscopically visible lesions occur in the duodenum in 75% and in the colon of 54% of patients. Deep biopsies containing submucosa demonstrate a higher percentage of involvement.[57]

Poor motility, obstruction and pseudo-obstruction, abdominal pain, nausea, and vomiting may occur. There may be malabsorption, diarrhea, and weight loss. Occasionally there is bleeding, even massive hemorrhage, due to ischemia. Ischemic perforation may occur.[96] Therapy for the underlying disease may decrease the deposition of amyloid, and rarely the deposits themselves may shrink. If therapy is not successful, nutrition support and even parenteral nutrition may be necessary. Severe ischemic disease may necessitate resection.[57]

INTESTINAL GRAFT-VERSUS-HOST DISEASE

Allogeneic bone marrow transplantation (BMT) remains the treatment of choice for a number of malignant conditions. Graft-versus-host disease (GVHD), the primary complication of allogeneic BMT, remains the major limitation to this therapeutic approach. Barnes et al. first described GVHD in mice.[99] In 1966, Billingham proposed three conditions required for the development of GVHD: The graft must contain immunologically competent cells, the host must possess important transplant alloantigens that are lacking in the donor graft so that the host appears foreign to the graft, and the host itself must be incapable of mounting an effective immunologic reaction against the graft.[100]

Acute GVHD consists of dermatitis, enteritis, and hepatitis occurring within the first 100 days, but typically within 30 to 40 days, following a BMT. Chronic GVHD usually develops after 100 days, which presents as an autoimmune-like syndrome consisting of impairment of multiple organs or organ systems.[101]

Diagnosis of GVHD relies on synthesis of clinical and laboratory findings in the appropriate clinical context and, importantly, exclusion of other causes of organ dysfunction. The gut is the third organ system involved in GVHD after skin and liver but is frequently the most severe and difficult to treat. Manifestations are variable, but the most common presenting symptoms are nausea, vomiting, anorexia, and secretory diarrhea. In severe cases, GI bleeding, protein-losing enteropathy, or ileus may be seen.[102] The plain radiographic findings of intestinal GVHD include air fluid levels, bowel wall thickening, a gasless abdomen, bowel dilatation, and ascites. Ultrasonography shows multiple, fluid-filled, dilated bowel loops.[103] The CT findings include abnormal bowel wall enhancement, and this correlates histopathologically with mucosal destruction and its replacement by a thin layer of granulation tissue.[104] Bowel wall thickening may involve any part of the small or large bowel, but

this is less severe than that found in patients with typhlitis or pseudomembranous colitis. The common extraintestinal findings of intestinal GVHD include ascites and engorgement of the mesenteric vessels; these findings are more pronounced adjacent to the thickened bowel loops. The abnormal findings that represent periportal edema and abnormal enhancement of the gallbladder and urinary bladder wall may also occur.[105] Because differentiation of intestinal GVHD from infective enteritis is critical for proper patient treatment, tissue sampling via biopsy is often required for confirmation. The histological hallmark of acute GVHD in the GI tract is epithelial cell apoptosis, originally described as crypt cell degeneration and later determined by ultrastructural examination to represent apoptotic cell death.[106] In GVHD, apoptosis is more prominent in the regenerative compartment of the gland or crypt.[107] When well developed, these apoptotic cells contain intracytoplasmic vacuoles filled with nuclear dust and other debris and have been described as "exploding crypt" cells.[108] In mild cases, apoptotic bodies may be the only morphologic clue to GVHD; in more severe cases, cystic dilatation of glands or crypts lined by regenerative epithelium, crypt abscesses, and frank epithelial destruction are seen. Wireless capsule endoscopy (WCE) is a noninvasive technology allowing for complete small bowel evaluation, and has been successfully used in the diagnosis of occult bleeding and inflammatory bowel disease. More recently it has been used to assess gastrointestinal (GI) GVHD. It is a useful tool to diagnose GI GVHD in both the acute and chronic setting, especially for documenting small bowel involvement. It is well tolerated and less invasive than endoscopy. It will not eliminate the need for invasive procedures such as endoscopy, because a biopsy must still be obtained for histopathologic diagnosis.[109]

Despite vigorous GVHD prophylaxis, 10 to 50% of the patients still develop significant acute GVHD. Steroids, with their potent antilymphocyte and anti-inflammatory activity, are the gold standard for treatment of GVHD.[110] Monoclonal antibodies have been increasingly used for treatment.[110,111]

REFERENCES

25. Donnithorne KJ, Atkinson TP, Hinze CH, et al. Rituximab therapy for severe refractory chronic Henoch-Schönlein purpura. J Pediatr 2009;155:136–139.
27. Maverakis E, Fung MA, Lynch PJ, et al. Acrodermatitis enteropathica and an overview of zinc metabolism. J Am Acad Dermatol 2007;56:116–124.
39. Garg AX, Suri RS, Barrowman N, et al. Long-term renal prognosis of diarrhea-associated hemolytic uremic syndrome: a systematic review, meta-analysis, and meta-regression. JAMA 2003;290:1360–1370.
52. Zimmerer T, Bocker U, Wenz F, Singer MV. Medical prevention and treatment of acute and chronic radiation induced enteritis – is there any proven therapy? A short review. Z Gastroenterol 2008;46:441–448.
80. Chande N, MacDonald JK, McDonald JW. Interventions for treating microscopic colitis: a Cochrane Inflammatory Bowel Disease and Functional Bowel Disorders Review Group systematic review of randomized trials. Am J Gastroenterol 2009;104:235–241; quiz 4, 42.
101. Ferrara JL, Deeg HJ. Graft-versus-host disease. N Engl J Med 1991; 324:667–674.

See expertconsult.com for a complete list of references and the review questions for this chapter.

APPENDICITIS 51

Michael G. Caty • Sani Z. Yamout

Acute appendicitis is one of the most common surgical conditions afflicting children and adults. Approximately 250,000 cases occur annually in the United States, with the highest incidence in patients 10 to 19 years old. The lifetime risk of developing appendicitis has been estimated at 8.6% for males and 6.7% for females, with a lifetime risk of undergoing an appendectomy estimated at 12% for males and 23% for females.[1] Appendiceal perforation in the pediatric population is more common than in adults, occurring in up to 50% of patients. In children less than 5 years of age, the perforation rate is 65%, and in those less than 2 years of age, the rate is 95%.[2]

A thorough understanding of this common surgical condition is important for all health care providers, who should be able to recognize and promptly refer patients with possible appendicitis for further evaluation to avoid complications related to a delay in diagnosis.

EMBRYOLOGY AND ANATOMY

The development of the appendix begins during the eighth week of gestation. The appendix, which initially projects from the apex of the cecum, is progressively displaced medially toward the ileocecal valve.[3] Lymph nodes begin to develop by the seventh month of gestation and continue to proliferate until puberty, after which they start to regress.[4] In the adult, the appendix varies in length, but averages about 8 cm; it is relatively longer and narrower in children. It has its own mesentery, called the mesoappendix, which contains the appendicular artery, a branch of the ileocolic artery, which arises from the superior mesenteric artery (Figure 51-1). The ileocolic vein drains blood from the cecum and appendix and enters the superior mesenteric vein to drain into the portal vein.

PATHOPHYSIOLOGY

The etiology of appendicitis was initially outlined in 1939 by Wangensteen and Dennis in their paper "Experimental Proof of the Obstructive Origin of Appendicitis in Man."[6] Appendicitis is initiated by obstruction of the appendiceal lumen. When the lumen of the appendix becomes obstructed, the flow of normal mucosal secretions is inhibited. This leads to increased intraluminal pressure and compromised venous drainage, which leads to ischemic breakdown of the mucosa. Simultaneously, luminal bacteria, typically *Escherichia coli*, *Bacteroides fragilis*, *Pseudomonas aeruginosa,* and *Clostridium* species, proliferate and traverse the appendiceal wall. This sequence of events results in an acute infection, gangrene, and ultimately perforation.

As the inflammatory process progresses, the omentum as well as adjacent loops of bowel may surround the inflamed area. If the disease progresses to perforation, these surrounding structures act as barriers that wall off the infection and frequently prevent free perforation and instead result in the formation of an inflammatory mass (phlegmon) or abscess. The formation of a phlegmon or abscess is central to the success of nonoperative management of perforated appendicitis, which is discussed later. On the other hand, free perforation with diffuse peritonitis occurs when the appendix perforates before it is sufficiently isolated by surrounding tissue.

HISTOLOGY

The appendix is composed of the same four layers as the rest of the intestine: the mucosa, submucosa, muscularis propria, and serosa. The mucosa is made of a surface layer of epithelial cells, a loose connective tissue layer known as the lamina propria, as well as the muscularis mucosa that separates the mucosa from the submucosa. The epithelial surface contains a combination of columnar cells with basally located nuclei, mucus-secreting goblet cells, and absorptive cells. In addition, the epithelial surface contains Paneth cells, which harbor lysozyme-containing granules and are thought to contribute to the intestinal defense system against bacteria, as well as neuroendocrine cells. These neuroendocrine cells are the origin of the carcinoid tumor, which is the most common appendiceal neoplasm. The lamina propria, just underneath the surface epithelial layer, contains the crypts of Lieberkühn as well as lymphoid follicles with germinal centers. The next layer is the submucosa, which contains a rich network of blood vessels, lymphatics, and nerves. The network of ganglion cells and Schwann cells found within this layer is known as Meissner's plexus. The next layer is the muscularis propria, which consists of two layers of smooth muscle. The muscle fibers of the inner layer are arranged in a circular fashion, whereas the fibers of the outer layer are arranged longitudinally. Another neural network, known as Auerbach's plexus, lies between these muscle layers. The outermost layer of the appendiceal wall, the serosa, is made up of a band of fibrous tissue with an overlying layer of cuboidal mesothelial cells.

CLINICAL PRESENTATION

Early diagnosis is vital to improving outcome and avoiding the morbidity associated with appendiceal perforation. Although laboratory and radiologic studies are useful aids in making the diagnosis, the key components are the history and physical examination.

The "typical" presentation of periumbilical pain that migrates to the right lower quadrant is a reflection of the progression of inflammation and pain from visceral to somatic pathways. Initially the contraction of the appendix against an obstructed lumen results in activation of visceral afferent fibers that enter the spine at the level of T10, causing a vague pain that is referred to the periumbilical area. As the inflammation becomes

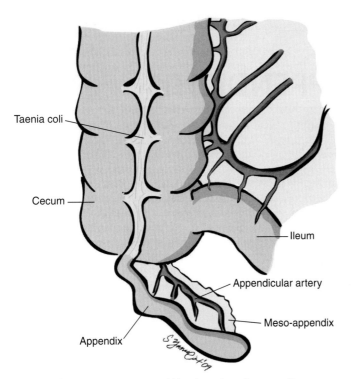

Figure 51-1. Location and blood supply to the appendix.

TABLE 51-1. **Pediatric Appendicitis Score (PAS) System**

Finding	Score
Symptoms	
Migration of pain	1
Anorexia	1
Nausea/emesis	1
Signs	
Tenderness in right lower quadrant	2
Cough/percussion/hopping tenderness	2
Fever > 38° C	1
Laboratory Studies	
WBC > 10,000 cells/mL	1
Polymorphonuclear neutrophilia > 7500 cells/mL	1

transmural and reaches the parietal peritoneum, the peritoneal somatic afferent pain fibers become involved. This causes pain that localizes to the vicinity of the appendix, which is usually at McBurney's point. This point is located in the right lower quadrant, two thirds of the distance between the umbilicus and anterior superior iliac spine. Localized pain may also occur in the right upper quadrant, the right flank, or the suprapubic area, depending on the location of the appendix in the abdomen. If the patient has malrotation or situs inversus, pain may occur in the epigastrium or left lower quadrant. If the appendix is close to the bladder, the inflammation may result in symptoms similar to those of a urinary tract infection.

Nausea and vomiting are common findings associated with appendicitis. The persistent obstruction of the lumen, which initially causes abdominal pain, ultimately results in dilation of the appendix and serosal stretching, which causes nausea and vomiting. Thus nausea and vomiting that occur before the onset of pain are unlikely to be secondary to appendicitis. Anorexia is also a common symptom, although somewhat less frequent in the pediatric population. Diarrhea can also occur with appendicitis, especially in younger children. If perforation occurs, the resulting decompression of the appendiceal lumen may transiently relieve symptoms.

The clinician should attempt to define the duration of illness by inquiring about vague symptoms that may precede pain. "When was the last time you felt perfectly fine?" is a question that can help clarify the duration of symptoms. The risk of appendiceal perforation increases substantially after 36 to 48 hours of symptoms.

Appendicitis in infants presents its own set of unique difficulties. The diagnosis is frequently delayed because of the inability to obtain an adequate history; this partly accounts for the increased incidence of appendiceal rupture, with subsequent increased morbidity and mortality. Common signs in infants with appendicitis include irritability, lethargy, fever, anorexia, and vomiting. In addition to the increased risk of perforation, infants are also at an increased risk to develop generalized peritonitis after perforation. This is thought to be due to the diminished ability of the body to contain a perforation in this population.[7-9]

PATIENT EVALUATION

The goals of patient evaluation are to promptly identify patients with appendicitis while avoiding unnecessary delays and excessive use of imaging studies. Delayed diagnosis may result in appendiceal perforation, whereas the incorrect diagnosis of appendicitis results in unnecessary surgery and potential postoperative complications.

A thorough history and physical examination remain central to the diagnosis of appendicitis. Unfortunately, both may be less reliable in younger children, which renders the use of imaging studies more frequent in this patient population. The onset, duration, and progression of abdominal pain are important factors to consider. Pain secondary to appendicitis is usually gradual in onset and persistent; classically, it begins in the periumbilical region and progressively localizes to the right lower quadrant. Physical findings include right lower quadrant tenderness, right lower quadrant pain with palpation of the left lower quadrant (Rovsing's sign), and right lower quadrant pain with extension of the right hip (psoas sign) or internal rotation of the flexed right thigh (obturator sign). Despite this relatively constant point of maximal tenderness, and depending on the location of the appendix, it is possible for tenderness to occur anywhere in the abdomen, including the left side in cases of malrotation or situs inversus.

In an attempt to improve the physician's diagnostic accuracy in cases of appendicitis, Samuel identified eight features of appendicitis and incorporated them into a Pediatric Appendicitis Score (PAS).[10] Patients are given scores based on points allotted to any positive findings (Table 51-1). Goldman et al. prospectively validated the PAS and noted that patients who had a score of 2 or lower and were discharged without further investigation (computed tomographic scan, ultrasonography, or hospital observation) had only a 2.4% chance of having appendicitis, whereas those who had a PAS of 7 or higher and were taken to the operating room without further studies had a 96% chance of having appendicitis. As for the patients with scores between 3 and 6, Goldman et al. recommended further evaluation with imaging studies or hospital observation.[11] Although the PAS seems to be a helpful addition to the algorithm of abdominal pain evaluation, it is not commonly used in clinical practice.

DIAGNOSTIC TESTS

The importance of the early diagnosis of acute appendicitis has led to attempts at defining the role of blood tests, specifically the white blood cell (WBC) count and C-reactive protein (CRP), as well as imaging studies in making the correct and prompt diagnosis. This is of particular importance in the pediatric population, where patients are more likely to have an atypical presentation and physicians may need to rely on additional tests to help make the diagnosis.

The WBC is usually elevated in patients with appendicitis, particularly in the presence of perforation.[12] Unfortunately, up to 20% of these patients have a normal WBC count. The role of CRP, an acute-phase reactant with a short half-life, in the work-up of appendicitis is similarly unclear, given that most conditions mimicking appendicitis involve inflammation and thus an elevation in CRP.[13] The literature is full of conflicting reports of the utility of CRP, when used alone or in conjunction with WBC counts, in the diagnosis of acute appendicitis.[13-15] A recent study looking at the role of WBC and CRP in the evaluation of abdominal pain noted that when both these values are normal for age, there is less than a 5% possibility that a patient has acute appendicitis.[15]

A urinalysis may help clarify the etiology of the abdominal pain. Although the finding of abnormal WBC and RBC counts in the urine may reflect an inflammatory process near the bladder or ureter, the presence of bacteria should raise the concern for the possibility of a urinary tract infection as the cause of abdominal pain.

Imaging Studies

Whereas the diagnosis of appendicitis may be straightforward in children who present with a classic history and physical examination findings, atypical presentations can result in diagnostic uncertainty, leading to delayed treatment. It is in these cases that imaging studies play a central role. The main aim of imaging studies is to expedite the identification of the cause of abdominal pain, define the extent of the disease in perforated appendicitis, and reduce the rates of perforation and unnecessary operations.[16]

Plain radiographs of the abdomen are generally unnecessary and contribute little to the evaluation of patients suspected to have appendicitis, unless small bowel obstruction is suspected. Some findings on abdominal radiographs that may suggest appendicitis include the presence of a fecalith, scoliosis, a focally dilated loop of bowel in the right lower quadrant (sentinel loop), focal loss of the right psoas shadow (psoas sign), and bowel obstruction.[17]

Computerized tomography (CT) is an accurate imaging modality used for diagnosing appendicitis. The reported sensitivity of helical CT is between 90% and 100%, and its specificity is between 91% and 99%.[18,19] Typical appendiceal CT protocols include 5-mm sections with both intravenous and oral contrast agents.[18] Intravenous contrast helps identify the inflamed appendix, which is especially helpful in patients with early appendicitis and a paucity of mesenteric fat. Oral contrast material, when present in the entire lumen of the appendix,

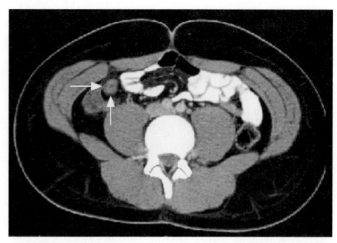

Figure 51-2. Abdominal CT scan demonstrating a thickened appendix (arrow) adjacent to the cecum.

rules out appendicitis. Oral contrast also helps differentiate a loop of bowel from a fluid-filled abscess in the vicinity of the appendix when perforated appendicitis is suspected. On CT scan, a normal appendix should appear as a contrast- or air-filled tubular structure. The wall should be less than 2 mm thick, and surrounding fat should appear homogenous with no stranding. The findings in appendicitis vary based on the severity of the disease. In early appendicitis, the appendix appears as a fluid-filled tubular structure with a thickened wall and a diameter between 7 and 15 mm, with adjacent fat stranding (Figure 51-2). CT findings that may be seen in perforated appendicitis include abscess formation or an inflammatory mass (phlegmon) as well extraluminal air in the area of the appendix.[18]

Graded compression sonography, the ultrasound (US) technique used to evaluate the appendix, is another radiologic technique available to the physician. With gradual compression sonography, sequential pressure is applied to the abdominal wall with the ultrasound probe. This displaces normal loops of bowel and identifies an abnormal appendix, which is seen as a fluid-filled, noncompressible structure larger than 6 mm in diameter (Figure 51-3). A fecalith, if present, appears as a bright, echogenic structure with posterior acoustic shadowing. The reported sensitivity of US is between 75% and 90%, and the specificity between 86% and 100%.[18]

The choice between US or CT varies between institutions, as the accuracy of ultrasound is somewhat operator dependent.[18,20] Doria et al., in a recent meta-analysis, noted that CT scans have a significantly higher sensitivity than US (94% versus 88%, respectively), and thus CT scans may decrease the rate of missed appendicitis.[21] Ultrasound offers the advantages of being fast, noninvasive, and inexpensive; it uses no ionizing radiation and can better delineate gynecological pathology. It also has the advantage of requiring no patient preparation or use of intravenous or oral contrast. On the other hand, CT scans are not operator dependent, have a higher sensitivity, and can better delineate the extent of disease in perforated appendicitis.[16]

MANAGEMENT OPTIONS

The treatment of simple appendicitis is primarily operative, using either an open or laparoscopic approach. The former involves a right lower quadrant incision placed over the point

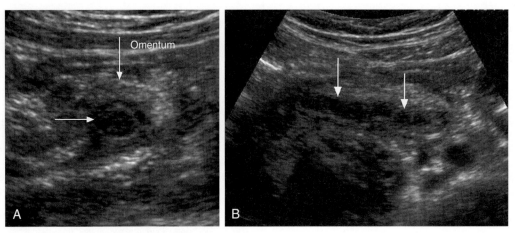

Figure 51-3. (A) Abdominal sonogram demonstrating a thickened appendix (arrows) surrounded by omentum. **(B)** Abdominal sonogram demonstrating a noncompressible appendix.

of maximal tenderness, which usually coincides with McBurney's point. The appendix is then delivered though the incision and resected. The main advantages of the open approach are that it is quick and inexpensive.[22] The main disadvantage is that the limited incision makes exploration of the entire abdomen difficult. This causes a dilemma when a normal appendix is encountered and the surgeon must search for other causes of abdominal pain, which may require him/her to extend the incision to improve exposure.

Kurt Semm first described the laparoscopic approach to an appendectomy in 1980. The most notable advantage to this approach is that it allows for a thorough evaluation of the peritoneal cavity; this is particularly useful in the face of an uncertain diagnosis preoperatively or a normal-appearing appendix intraoperatively.[23] Other reported advantages over the open approach include the ability to copiously irrigate the peritoneal cavity, less postoperative pain, decreased rate of wound infections, shorter hospital stay, and faster recovery time.[22,23] It is important to note that the advantage of the laparoscopic approach is still debatable and the choice of operation should be based on the surgeon's experience and preference.

The treatment of perforated appendicitis is more controversial. Operative management of perforated appendicitis is associated with a high rate of complications, up to 58% compared to 15% with nonoperative therapy.[24,25] Thus operative management should be avoided when possible, particularly in the presence of a large inflammatory mass or abscess, both of which may increase the risk for bowel injury, appendiceal stump leakage, need for more extensive intestinal resection, and wound infection. Despite the higher complication rate, operative management is generally mandatory in patients with free perforation and generalized peritonitis and those with intestinal obstruction. A safer option for the treatment of perforated appendicitis in the stable patient is nonoperative management with antibiotics and, if indicated, abscess drainage. This approach is successful in the vast majority of patients.[26] Although it is generally accepted that nonoperative management is safer, controversy exists over the type, duration, and method of antibiotic administration. Another point of contention in the nonoperative management of appendicitis is the need for an elective appendectomy (interval appendectomy) after resolution of the infection.

Antibiotics should target enteric organisms regardless of intra-abdominal culture results.[27] Antibiotics are used to decrease postoperative infectious complications such as wound infections and intra-abdominal abscess formation. The type and duration of administration of antibiotics vary between institutions. Some examples of antibiotic regimens used include intravenous ampicillin/gentamicin/metronidazole or clindamycin, ceftriaxone/metronidazole, ceftazidime/clindamycin, and meropenem.[28-30] The duration and method of administration also vary between institutions. Some protocols call for 10 to 14 days of intravenous antibiotics to be completed at home after insertion of a peripherally inserted central (PIC) line; others involve switching patients to oral antibiotics on discharge, whereas still others stop antibiotics once patients are afebrile and their WBC normalizes. Our institution is currently performing a randomized prospective trial to compare 10 days of intravenous antibiotics to sequential intravenous/oral antibiotics in an effort to decrease the resources required for PIC line placement and home administration of intravenous antibiotics.

Interval appendectomy, another controversial subject in the pediatric surgical literature,[31] involves the elective removal of the appendix 6 to 8 weeks after successful nonoperative management of perforated appendicitis. The 2-month delay is necessary in order to allow for the intra-abdominal inflammatory process to resolve and adhesions to soften, facilitating the removal of the appendix. Recent studies that cite a low recurrence rate of appendicitis (5%)[32] as well as a considerable rate of postoperative complications with an interval appendectomy[26] have prompted some surgeons to reconsider the need for an interval appendectomy. One identifiable risk factor for recurrence of appendicitis is the presence of a fecalith, which is reported to be associated with a 71% rate of recurrence.[33] Until long-term follow-up studies clarify the consequences of a retained appendix in children after an episode of appendicitis, we routinely offer patients the option of an interval appendectomy, particularly in the presence of a fecalith.

DIFFERENTIAL DIAGNOSIS

The clinical presentation of appendicitis can mimic many different conditions; conversely, many different conditions can present like appendicitis (Table 51-2). This is particularly true in children, who frequently present with an atypical history and physical examination findings.

TABLE 51-2. **Differential Diagnosis of Appendicitis**

Infant
    Abdominal trauma – child abuse
    Gastroenteritis
    Intussusception
    Pneumonia
    Urinary tract infection
    Meckel's diverticulitis
Child
    Constipation
    Gastroenteritis
    Henoch-Schönlein purpura
    Hemolytic uremic syndrome
    Meckel's diverticulitis
    Mesenteric adenitis
    Omental torsion
    Ovarian torsion
    Pneumonia
    Urinary tract infection
    Crohn's disease
Adolescent
    Constipation
    Crohn's disease
    Gastroenteritis
    Meckel's diverticulitis
    Mesenteric adenitis
    Mittelschmerz
    Omental torsion
    Ovarian cyst rupture
    Urinary tract infection

Acute gastroenteritis is a frequent cause of abdominal pain. Typically, the child presents with vomiting, diarrhea, fever, and generalized abdominal pain. These symptoms are usually self-limited and resolve within 48 hours. The pattern of diarrhea helps distinguish gastroenteritis from appendicitis. Children with gastroenteritis have watery diarrhea early in their illness. Diarrhea associated with perforated appendicitis presents at least 3 to 4 days after the onset of illness and is attributed to the effects of pelvic inflammation on the colon.

Mesenteric adenitis is a condition where enlarged mesenteric nodes, located in the region of the terminal ileum, are associated with nausea, fever, and abdominal pain. Mesenteric adenitis, which is usually associated with an upper respiratory tract infection, is often indistinguishable from acute appendicitis. This diagnosis should only be made after other conditions are excluded. A CT scan shows significant adenopathy in the absence of appendiceal inflammation.

Gynecologic conditions must be included in the differential diagnosis of appendicitis. The typical female patient with a tubo-ovarian abscess has had multiple sex partners and often has a history of recurrent episodes of pelvic pain. She will have cervical tenderness on pelvic examination, often with vaginal discharge and adnexal enlargement. Lower abdominal pain may also occur with an ovarian cyst that is either ruptured or hemorrhagic. Torsion of an ovary, ovarian cyst, or ovarian tumor may also cause acute and intense pain. An ectopic pregnancy must be considered in any female after menarche. The classic presentation is abdominal pain, vaginal bleeding, and amenorrhea, and the diagnosis can be made with a pregnancy test and pelvic ultrasound.

Meckel's diverticulitis may be impossible to differentiate from acute appendicitis. Operative exploration is usually indicated in either condition, and preoperative distinction is unnecessary.

Intussusception, whether idiopathic or secondary to a pathologic lead point, is another cause of abdominal pain. Idiopathic intussusception usually occurs in children under 2 years of age and frequently follows a viral illness that causes enlargement of the lymphoid tissue in the distal ileum (Peyer's patches). On the other hand, the majority of patients over 5 years old with intussusception have a pathologic lead point. Children with intussusception may present with intermittent abdominal pain or "fussiness." The child appears normal between these attacks. "Currant jelly" stools are almost pathognomonic of intussusception and represent the sloughed mucosal lining mixed with stool. Occasionally, the only sign at presentation is lethargy. Physical examination may reveal a sausage-shaped mass in the right side of the abdomen. The diagnosis, and often treatment, can be accomplished with air-contrast enema reduction under radiologic guidance.

Several common medical conditions may also present in a fashion similar to acute appendicitis. Constipation can present with abdominal pain, vomiting, and fever. Abdominal plain films can suggest this diagnosis. Right lower lobe pneumonia may also cause right lower quadrant abdominal pain. The typical patient would also have symptoms of coughing, tachypnea, and pleuritic chest pain, as well as fever and leukocytosis. A chest radiograph would confirm this diagnosis. A urinary tract infection can cause lower abdominal pain, fever, and dysuria. Laboratory studies may reveal leukocytosis, and a urinalysis is key to making this diagnosis.

Henoch-Schönlein purpura may also cause abdominal pain. This syndrome typically occurs several weeks after a streptococcal infection. Usually the child will also have joint pains, purpura, and nephritis.

Crohn's disease can mimic appendicitis. The most common location of disease involves the terminal ileum. There is usually a history of weight loss, fever, vomiting, and diarrhea. Abdominal pain may occur in the right lower quadrant or periumbilical location.

COMPLICATIONS

The type as well as rate of complications depends on whether one is dealing with simple or perforated appendicitis. The most common postoperative complication after an appendectomy is a wound infection. This typically presents with pain, erythema, and fluctuance or drainage from the wound. The treatment of a superficial wound infection entails opening the wound to allow drainage. The wound infection rates are 3% and 8% in simple and perforated appendicitis, respectively.

Major complications, which include the development of a postoperative intra-abdominal abscess and adhesive small bowel obstruction (SBO), are more common with perforated appendicitis than simple appendicitis, with a rate of 6.7% and 1.7%, respectively.[12] Studies report various rates of postoperative abscess formation in children after perforated appendicitis; this is partly related to different definitions of perforation. When perforated appendicitis is strictly defined by the presence of a hole in the appendix, as opposed to the mere presence of purulent fluid in the pelvis, the rate of postoperative abscess formation in simple and perforated appendicitis is 0.8% and 18%, respectively.[34] The development of an intra-abdominal abscess should be suspected when patients fail to improve postoperatively and continue to have an elevated temperature, diarrhea or delayed return of bowel function, and/or leukocytosis. A CT scan of the abdomen and pelvis should be obtained to confirm the diagnosis. Treatment of an intra-abdominal abscess consists of the administration of antibiotics and, when indicated, percutaneous drainage under radiologic guidance.

Adhesive postoperative SBO is another potential complication of appendectomy. The rate of SBO seems to depend on the operative approach used. When an open appendectomy is performed, the postoperative SBO rate is 4.5%. This is significantly higher than the SBO rate of 1.0% when the laparoscopic approach is used.[35] In addition, SBO is more common in the setting of perforated appendicitis.[36] Although most cases of postoperative SBO resolve spontaneously with bowel rest and gastric decompression, operative intervention is occasionally required.

CHRONIC APPENDICEAL PAIN

Some of the unexplained recurrent abdominal pain in children may be attributed to chronic appendiceal pain. Although the terms used to describe chronic appendiceal pain can be confusing, chronic appendiceal pain is as a broad category that includes three different conditions: chronic appendicitis, recurrent appendicitis, and appendiceal colic. Chronic appendicitis is, as its name implies, chronic inflammation of the appendix.[37,38] Recurrent appendicitis refers to the situation where an episode of appendicitis resolves spontaneously and then is followed by another episode. These two conditions are rare.[39] The most frequent cause of chronic appendiceal pain is appendiceal colic. Appendiceal colic is a condition believed to result from intermittent obstruction of the appendiceal lumen, resulting in chronic intermittent right lower quadrant pain. The majority of patients are females (75%), and half of them have a history of at least one prior visit to the emergency department for their abdominal pain before the diagnosis is made. Characteristically, imaging studies do not show signs of appendicitis. For this diagnosis to be made, patients must have recurrent intermittent abdominal pain, postprandial exacerbation of the pain, and right lower quadrant tenderness when examined during an acute episode. Of patients who meet these criteria, 98% will have resolution of symptoms with an appendectomy.[37]

REFERENCES

2. Stevenson RJ. Appendicitis. In: Azizkhan RG, Weber TR, editors. Operative Pediatric Surgery. New York: McGraw-Hill; 2003. p. 671–689.
11. Goldman RD, Carter S, Stephens D, et al. Prospective validation of the pediatric appendicitis score. J Pediatr 2008;153:278–282.
12. Pearl RH, Hale DA, Molloy M, et al. Pediatric appendectomy. J Pediatr Surg 1995;30:173–178; discussion 178–181.
23. el Ghoneimi A, Valla JS, Limonne B, et al. Laparoscopic appendectomy in children: report of 1,379 cases. J Pediatr Surg 1994;29:786–789.
34. St Peter SD, Sharp SW, Holcomb III GW, Ostlie DJ. An evidence-based definition for perforated appendicitis derived from a prospective randomized trial. J Pediatr Surg 2008;43:2242–2245.

See expertconsult.com for a complete list of references and the review questions for this chapter.

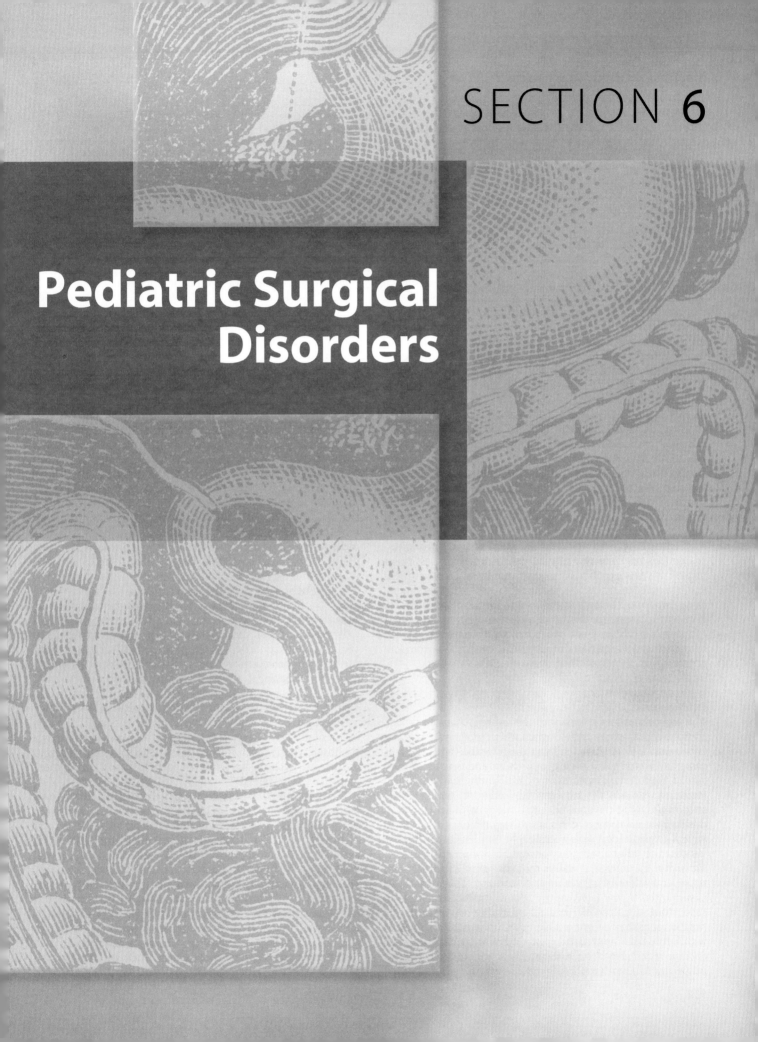

SECTION 6

Pediatric Surgical Disorders

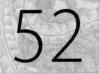

52 INTUSSUSCEPTION IN INFANTS AND CHILDREN

David K. Magnuson

Intussusception is a curious anatomic condition characterized by the invagination of one segment of the gastrointestinal tract into the lumen of an adjacent segment and distal propagation within the bowel lumen. The advancing tube of proximal intestine is referred to as the *intussusceptum*, whereas the distal recipient intestine is referred to as the *intussuscipiens*. Although any segment of the gastrointestinal tract may be involved, more than 80% of cases in infants and children are *ileocolic* – the invagination of the ileum into the colon. The intussusceptum usually extends to the hepatic flexure but may advance to the rectum and even prolapse through the anus. Isolated small intestinal and colonic intussusceptions occur less commonly. Retrograde intussusception has been reported in rare circumstances: duodenogastric intussusception related to the manipulation of gastrostomy tubes or the presence of duodenal polyps, retrograde jejunojejunal intussusception following repair of duodenal atresia, and gastroesophageal intussusception after forceful vomiting.[1-3]

Whatever the location and extent, the great majority of intussusceptions result in two distinct clinical problems: complete obstruction of the proximal intestine, and the progressive vascular compromise and eventual infarction of the intussusceptum. These two factors are largely responsible for the morbidity associated with intussusception. Diagnostic and therapeutic measures should therefore be approached with a sense of urgency, because the consequences of intestinal obstruction and ischemia progress rapidly in infants and children.

PATHOPHYSIOLOGY

The pathogenesis of intussusception is believed to be related to unbalanced forces created when a normal peristaltic wave encounters a focal abnormality in the intestinal wall. In some cases, the abnormality is clearly definable and is referred to as a "lead point." Early theories proposed that the lead point projected into the peristaltic stream and was simply pulled downstream, dragging the intestinal wall along with it. However, this hypothesis did not explain the vast majority of cases in which no pathologic lead point could be identified. In these instances of "idiopathic" intussusception, lymphoid hyperplasia within the intestinal wall is thought to produce the functional equivalent of a pathologic lead point. This hypothesis is supported by the fact that the majority of idiopathic intussusceptions are ileocolic, and that the terminal ileum is the richest repository of gut-associated lymphoid tissue (GALT) within the gastrointestinal tract. When a peristaltic wave encounters an area of intestinal wall with different mechanical properties (due to lymphoid hyperplasia or a pathologic lead

point), the imbalance of contractile forces causes the wall to kink or buckle, creating an infolding of the wall that extends circumferentially around the bowel wall until the entire wall is involved. This invaginated rim of intestinal wall initiates the intussusception and becomes its apex, propagating distally within the lumen.[4]

This model satisfactorily explains the occurrence of intussusception in certain disease states that are not associated with either lead points or lymphoid hyperplasia, including postoperative intussusception and cystic fibrosis. In postoperative intussusception, disorganized peristalsis results in the juxtaposition of contracting and noncontracting regions of the intestine where peristaltic waves meet akinetic bowel. In cystic fibrosis with mucoviscidosis, inspissated putty-like secretions adhere to the intestinal wall and alter its mechanical properties, resulting in focal areas of altered compliance and elasticity. Intussusception can also occur in conditions characterized by purely functional disturbances in intestinal motility, including neonates with central nervous system hypoxia and children with systemic inflammatory response associated with major burn injury.[5,6]

Once the intussusceptum advances distally, the mesenteric vascular supply to the intussusceptum is angulated and compressed at the point where it enters the intussuscipiens. Initially, this produces venous outflow obstruction and leads to venous congestion and edema, generating a vicious cycle of venous hypertension, swelling, and ischemia. Mucosal slough leads to the passage of blood, desquamated epithelium, and mucus – the classic "currant jelly" stool. Progressive ischemia results barrier dysfunction, leading to endotoxemia and a systemic inflammatory state characterized by increased levels of circulating cytokines.[7] Arterial inflow is eventually compromised, and infarction extends from the intussusceptum to the intussuscipiens, culminating in perforation, peritonitis, and shock.

This sequence of events applies to ileocolic intussusceptions; other types of intussusception may have a different natural history. Isolated small-intestinal intussusceptions may indeed progress to infarction, but the increased use of ultrasonography and computed tomography (CT) has documented asymptomatic small intestinal intussusceptions that reduce spontaneously.[8] Fetal intussusception has been detected on prenatal ultrasonography and has been proposed as one cause of jejunoileal atresia in neonates.[9,10] Resorption of the infracted intussusception in the sterile intrauterine environment accounts for the atresia and mesenteric defect. Fetal intussusception may also lead to perforation and meconium peritonitis.[11] A documented case of jejunal atresia with connecting fibrous cord was associated with the presence of a residual intussusceptum in the bowel lumen distal to the atresia, suggesting that the obliterated cord of tissue bridging the atretic gap in this atresia may have been the remnant of a fetal intussusception.[12] This provides an alternative "nonvascular" hypothesis for the etiology of some intestinal atresias.

ETIOLOGY

Only 10% of intussusceptions in childhood are associated with a pathologic lead point, the incidence of which varies with age.[13,14] In patients younger than 2 years, lead points are identified in less than 4% of cases.[15] Above 2 years, lead points are found in as many as one third of patients; above 4 years, the reported incidence is as high as 57%, and in adults the incidence exceeds 90%.[16,17] In the 90% of children with no structural abnormality, the presumed etiology is lymphoid hyperplasia in the vast majority of cases.[18,19]

No infectious agent has been proven to cause this disease, although epidemiologic studies in hospitalized patients have suggested an association with adenovirus.[20] Recent widespread vaccination of infants with tetravalent rhesus-human rotavirus vaccine resulted in increased rates of intussusception, leading to withdrawal of the vaccine from the market.[21] New vaccines (attenuated human and human-bovine) have been shown to be effective and not increase the incidence of intussusception. Studies performed to provide baseline data for vaccination safety studies have provided interesting data regarding global discrepancies in the incidence of intussusception in infants.[22] The reported number of intussusceptions per 100,000 infant-years was 18 in India, 30 to 70 in developed Western countries (Europe, United States, Australia), 165 in Japan, and 302 in Vietnam. The incidence of intussusception did not appear to be linked to actual rotavirus infection.

The use of antibiotics in infants and young children has been proposed as another etiologic factor for intussusception.[23] Oral administration of antibiotics is associated with the development of mesenteric adenitis in an animals, presumably by altering the natural gut flora and compromising the mucosal barrier.[24] A more recent prospective study supports this association and suggested that both lymphoid hyperplasia and altered motility may be factors that link antibiotic usage to increased risk for intussusception in infants.[25]

The most common pathologic lead point in children of all ages is a Meckel's diverticulum (Figure 52-1). Almost any process that results in a structural abnormality of the bowel wall has been described as a pathologic lead point (Table 52-1)[26-30] Duplication cysts, ectopic pancreatic and gastric rests, vascular anomalies, inverted postappendectomy stumps, and anastomotic suture lines have all been implicated as lead points in intussusception. Neoplastic lead points include intestinal polyps, Peutz-Jeghers hamartomas, carcinoids, leiomyomas and leiomyosarcomas, intestinal related Kaposi's sarcoma, and lymphomas (particularly Burkitt's lymphoma). Other causes include Crohn's disease, posttransplant lymphoproliferative disease, and submucosal hemorrhage associated with idiopathic thrombocytopenic purpura, hemophilia, leukemia, Kasabach-Merritt syndrome, and anticoagulation therapy. Two conditions more commonly associated with intussusception, cystic fibrosis and Henoch-Schönlein purpura (HSP), are discussed later.

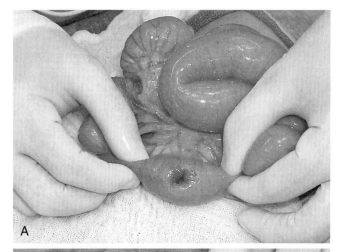
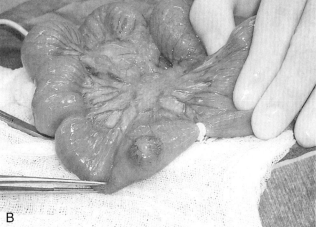

Figure 52-1. Surgically reduced ileocolic intussusception secondary to Meckel's diverticulum as lead point. (**A**) Inverted diverticulum as lead point. (**B**) Everted diverticulum in normal orientation. (*See plate section for color.*)

CLINICAL PRESENTATION

Approximately 60% of intussusceptions occur within the first year of life, with a peak incidence between 6 months and 1 year of age.[13,31] The remaining 40% of cases in the pediatric population are distributed more or less evenly between the second year of life and later childhood. As described previously, the majority of cases within the first 2 years of life are idiopathic and likely related to lymphoid hyperplasia. Conversely, the majority of cases in patients older than 2 years are associated with a pathologic lead point. There is a male predominance of about 3:1. Institutions from different geographic regions report inconsistent seasonal variations, and no pattern emerges when data from these institutions are grouped together.

Children with intussusception present with an acute bowel obstruction. In fact, intussusception ranks as one of the leading causes of mechanical small bowel obstruction in children, accounting for more than 50% of cases in some series.[32] Infants with intussusception usually are previously healthy and present with an acute onset of abdominal pain. The pain is typically severe, colicky, and intermittent. Pallor and diaphoresis are commonly described. These episodes may last for several minutes and are separated by variable periods of relief lasting from 30 minutes to several hours. During these quiescent periods, infants often exhibit a worrisome degree of lethargy and

TABLE 52-1. Relative Incidence of Pathologic Lead Points in Childhood Intussusception

Type of Lead Point	Number of Cases						
	Ref. 15	**Ref. 26**	**Ref. 28**	**Ref. 29**	**Ref. 30**	**Ref. 41**	**Total (n = 179)**
Meckel's diverticulum	27	6	14	7	12	7	73 (40.8)
Intestinal polyps	12	2	8	1	8	3	34 (19.0)
Duplication cyst	4	4	5	2	3	1	19 (10.6)
Lymphoma	5	1	1	6	3	1	17 (9.5)
Henoch-Schönlein purpura		2	1		6		9 (5.0)
Lymphoid hyperplasia				5	1		6 (3.4)
Cystic fibrosis		2			4		6 (3.4)
Appendiceal disease/mucocele			1	2	2	1	6 (3.4)
Carcinoid	2						2 (1.1)
Ectopic pancreatic tissue				2			2 (1.1)
Neutropenic colitis					2		2 (1.1)
Celiac disease		1					1 (0.6)
Leiomyoma				1			1 (0.6)
Leukemia		1					1 (0.6)

Reproduced from Navarro and Daneman (2004),[26] with permission of Springer Science and Media.
Values in parentheses are percentages.

somnolence. This altered mental state accompanying intussusception may be the most alarming aspect of the clinical presentation. The pattern of colicky pain alternating with periods of profound lethargy should alert the examiner to the possibility of intussusception. In one study, 17% of patients admitted for intussusception had clinically significant neurological findings, including lethargy, hypotonia, and a fluctuating level of consciousness.[33] These patients tend to be younger and present with a more acute course of illness. An association with poorer outcome or with complications related to bowel ischemia and perforation was not found.

Other findings include a history of vomiting, the passage of grossly bloody stools with mucus (currant jelly stools), the presence of occult blood on digital rectal examination, and the presence of a palpable abdominal mass. Initially the vomiting is reflexive and nonbilious, but eventually becomes bilious as the mechanical obstruction becomes clinically manifest. The abdominal mass is usually felt in the right upper quadrant. In rare cases, the intussusceptum can be felt on digital rectal examination or may even be seen prolapsing from the anus, in which case it must be distinguished from a simple rectal prolapse by the presence of a sulcus between the anus and the intussusceptum. Nonbloody diarrhea, resulting from evacuation of the distal gastrointestinal tract before the onset of mucosal slough, occurs in 10% of patients.[34]

The presence of certain signs and symptoms has a well-defined predictive power.[13] Pain and vomiting each occur in over 80% of cases, a palpable abdominal mass in 55 to 65%, and occult or gross rectal bleeding in 50 to 60%. However, the classic triad of paroxysmal pain, vomiting, and passage of currant jelly stools occurs in less than one third of patients. Certain combinations of these findings can increase diagnostic accuracy.[35] The combination of pain, vomiting, and a palpable right upper quadrant mass has a positive predictive value (PPV) of 93%. The addition of rectal bleeding to this triad increases the PPV to virtually 100%. Some retrospective studies, however, have failed to identify patterns of clinical predictors that have sufficient accuracy to allow for the exclusion of the diagnosis on clinical grounds alone.[36]

Infants with advanced intussusception may present with a more dramatic clinical picture. Obtundation, abdominal distention, peritonitis, dehydration, metabolic acidosis, and hypotension occur when ischemia of the involved bowel has occurred. These patients require nasogastric decompression, systemic antibiotics, aggressive resuscitation, and possibly airway control and ventilatory support concurrent with an expeditious diagnostic evaluation. The rare occurrence of intussusception in the premature neonate is usually misdiagnosed as necrotizing enterocolitis, the correct diagnosis usually being made only at laparotomy. Most of these patients do not have pathologic lead points yet require resection for advanced disease.[37]

DIAGNOSTIC WORK-UP

Although most infants and children presenting with acute abdominal complaints undergo plain abdominal radiography, the diagnostic value of plain x-rays in the diagnosis of intussusception is low for most practitioners.[38] Despite this, there are certain radiographic findings that, when present, help to suggest the diagnosis of intussusception. The presence of a soft-tissue mass in the right upper quadrant or epigastrium is suggestive of intussusception and is present in 25 to 60% of cases (Figure 52-2).[39] This is particularly true if the soft tissue mass exhibits the characteristic appearance of two concentric circles of soft tissue density representing the intussusceptum and intussuscipiens, respectively. Other indirect signs such as a paucity of gas in the right iliac fossa are not sufficiently reliable to be of much help in further directing the work-up (Figure 52-3). Occasionally, the only plain radiographic finding is a small bowel obstruction. Any infant or child who has a plain abdominal radiograph consistent with a mechanical small bowel obstruction, and who does not have either a palpable hernia or a history of prior surgery, should be considered to have an intussusception until proven otherwise.

Definitive diagnostic studies include noninvasive modalities such as ultrasonography and CT; invasive studies such as contrast enema are highly accurate and may also be therapeutic. The decision to evaluate a child by noninvasive means before

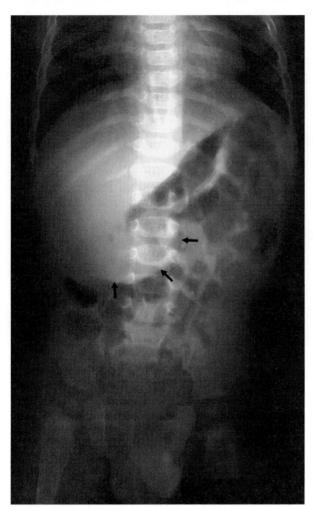

Figure 52-2. Plain abdominal radiograph demonstrating a soft tissue mass in the right upper quadrant. From Vasavada P. Ultrasound evaluation of acute abdominal emergencies in infants and children. Radiol Clin North Am 2004; 42:445-456, with permission.

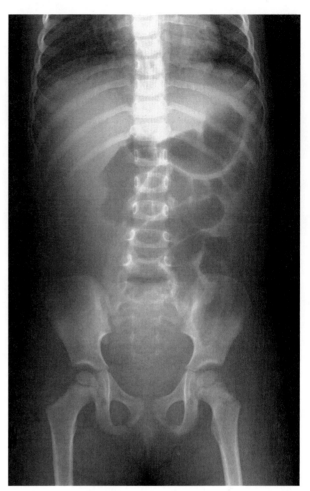

Figure 52-3. Plain abdominal radiograph exhibiting indirect signs of intussusception, including paucity of gas in the right lower quadrant, displacement of the small intestine, and abrupt cutoff of gas in the transverse colon.

contrast enema must be based on certain considerations. If the diagnosis of intussusception is strongly suspected on the basis of rigorous diagnostic criteria and the child is an acceptable candidate for nonoperative treatment, proceeding directly to contrast enema without prior ultrasonography or CT is a reasonable approach and eliminates the delay caused by multiple imaging studies. Alternatively, if the diagnosis is less certain, or if certain features of the presentation make surgical intervention preferable in the event that the diagnosis of intussusception is confirmed, noninvasive screening can decrease the expense, discomfort, and exposure to radiation associated with unnecessary contrast enemas in a large number of children.[40] Retrospective studies document that more than 60% of children suspected of having intussusception and subjected to barium enema on the basis of nonrigorous clinical criteria have normal study findings.[41]

Ultrasonography has emerged as the "gold standard" for noninvasive imaging of intussusception. The characteristic cross-sectional appearance of the intussusception is that of a "target" or "doughnut" (Figure 52-4); in the longitudinal view, a "pseudo-kidney sign" is seen (Figure 52-5). These findings are extremely reliable and reproducible, allowing the accurate diagnosis of intussusception even in less experienced hands.[42] In multiple reports, the positive and negative predictive values

of ultrasonography approach 100%.[43-45] Ultrasonography has the additional advantages of detecting small bowel intussusceptions and lead points, avoiding ionizing radiation, and maintaining superior patient comfort. Reduced blood flow in the intussusceptum assessed by color Doppler sonography has been shown to be highly predictive of irreducibility or irreversible ischemia (Figure 52-6).[46]

CT can be highly accurate in the diagnosis of intussusception, although it offers little advantage over ultrasonography to justify the additional expense and exposure to radiation. Although CT is not commonly used as a primary diagnostic modality for intussusception, unsuspected intussusceptions are occasionally demonstrated on abdominal CT performed for other indications. The diagnostic accuracy of CT in this setting is quite high.[47] One potential advantage of CT over ultrasonography in the diagnosis of intussusception is its uniform availability – ultrasonography is more user dependent, and continuously available expertise is costly. This cost may be mitigated by training nonradiology staff to perform targeted sonographic studies in the emergency room setting, as is currently done for blunt abdominal trauma in some institutions.[48] On the other hand, the performance of tomographic imaging is not operator dependent, requires only existing technical support, and produces

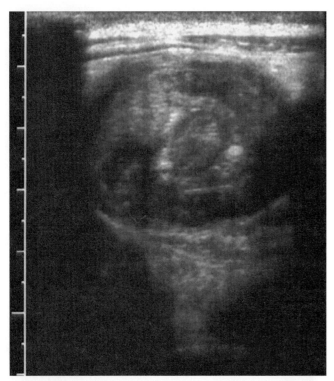

Figure 52-4. Sonographic image of intussusception in the transverse section demonstrating the echodense intussusceptum within the echolucent intussuscipiens. Note the bright mesenteric vessels on end, running along the intestinal wall.

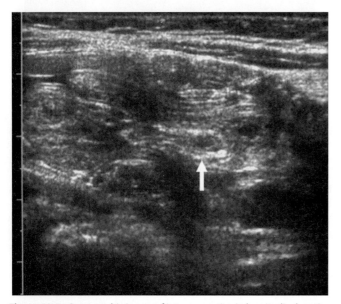

Figure 52-5. Sonographic image of intussusception in longitudinal section demonstrating the "pseudo-kidney" sign. From Vasavada P. Ultrasound evaluation of acute abdominal emergencies in infants and children. Radiol Clin North Am 2004; 42:445-456, with permission.

images that are easily interpreted by emergency-department personnel and can be digitally transferred to an available radiologist. As protocols become faster, more focused, and less expensive and require less radiation, CT may replace ultrasonography for the imaging of intussusception, much as it has done for acute appendicitis.

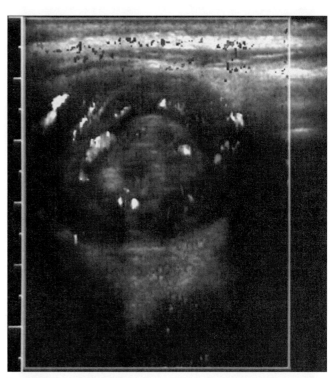

Figure 52-6. Transverse Doppler sonogram of reducible intussusception demonstrating intact blood flow. From Vasavada P. Ultrasound evaluation of acute abdominal emergencies in infants and children. Radiol Clin North Am 2004; 42:445-456, with permission.

THERAPEUTIC OPTIONS

Once the diagnosis is clear, the intussusception must be reduced in the safest and most expeditious manner – any delay increases the likelihood of complications. Strategies for reduction include nonoperative and surgical techniques. The choice of technique is dictated by the condition of the child and factors that predict the probability of complications such as perforation and presence of pathologic lead points. Peritonitis, pneumoperitoneum, and physiologic instability are absolute contraindications to nonoperative reduction, and patients with these features should be resuscitated and explored surgically.

Image-Guided Pressure Reduction

The application of positive intraluminal pressure to the intussusceptum, while imaging its retrograde movement out of the intussuscipiens, is the most common therapeutic approach to this disease. Hirschsprung advocated the use of an enema to reduce intussusception in 1876 and presented a large series of successful attempts in 1905. Following the introduction of diagnostic barium enema techniques after the turn of the 20th century, the use of barium enema for the controlled, monitored reduction of intussusception was reported in the late 1920s and adopted in Scandinavia and South America. This approach was introduced in the United States in 1939 and was widely adopted after publication of a standardized technique by Ravitch and McCune in 1948.[49] Subsequently, the use of barium enema reduction became universal in its application and is reported to be successful in 50 to 85% of cases (Figure 52-7).

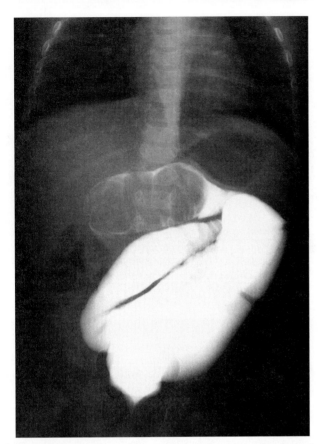

Figure 52-7. Hydrostatic reduction of ileocolic intussusception by barium enema. This intussusceptum was encountered in the transverse colon.

Children treated by hydrostatic reduction should have intravenous access established and fluid resuscitation completed before the attempt. Patients with more significant vomiting, abdominal distention, or signs of systemic toxicity should also have a nasogastric tube placed and receive broad-spectrum antibiotics. Hydrostatic reduction by gravity feed with 60% barium suspension should be limited to a column height of 100 cm, generating a retrograde pressure of 100 to 120 mm Hg. Pressures greater than this were found by Ravitch to be capable of reducing a gangrenous intussusceptum, resulting in perforation. Water-soluble agents may also be used, although they require a higher fluid column in order to generate comparable pressures because of their lower specific gravity. The intussusceptum is subjected to the enema pressure for 3 to 5 minutes, and progress is monitored fluoroscopically. Several attempts may be required to reduce the intussusception fully. Complete reduction is demonstrated when contrast flows past the ileocecal valve and fills the terminal ileum, although retrograde reflux of contrast into the terminal ileum is not mandatory, and its absence is not an indication for surgical exploration.[50] After successful reduction, fluid resuscitation is continued and feedings are withheld for 12 to 24 hours while the child is observed for complications of reduction or early recurrence. In asymptomatic patients, immediate discharge from the hospital and outpatient follow-up appear to be equally safe.[51,52]

Pneumatic reduction of the intussusception using air and fluoroscopic guidance has supplanted hydrostatic reduction as the preferred nonoperative strategy in most pediatric institutions.[53] The advantages of using air as opposed to barium for pressure reduction include increased efficacy, improved cleanliness and patient acceptance, faster procedure time, less average radiation dose, and the avoidance of barium contamination of the peritoneal cavity when the rare perforation event occurs. Success rates of 75 to 95% have been reported, exceeding those for barium reduction.[54-56] With pneumatic reduction, air is introduced at a constant pressure of 120 torr, which is more easily and precisely controlled than barium. It is likely that the enhanced success rates for air enema reduction compared with barium are related to the perception that perforation is less catastrophic with air, allowing a more aggressive approach.

Routine air enema reduction requires exposure to radiation. A recent large series of more than 6000 consecutive cases of intussusception from China documented the efficacy of pneumatic reduction without imaging guidance of any kind.[57] Uncomfortable with the notion of unmonitored reduction, radiologists are now exploring the use of ultrasonography to monitor reduction without radiation. Initial reports of ultrasonographically guided pneumatic reduction have documented its feasibility and a successful reduction rate of 92 to 95%.[58,59] Although air reduction under sonographic guidance is effective, recent experience with saline reduction has also yielded excellent results.[60,61] As with air, perforation of the colon with saline does not lead to complicated peritonitis. Saline reduction is preferred by some to air reduction when using sonographic monitoring, as the saline-filled colon transmits a better sonographic image than does an air-filled colon and allows for better detection of pathologic lead points.[62] Some radiologists use a very dilute solution of water-soluble contrast agent so that complete reduction can be documented by plain radiography, demonstrating contrast refluxing in the terminal ileum. Published success rates for saline enema range from 70 to 90%, exceeding those for barium enema reduction.[63,64] It appears that air is a slightly more effective agent than fluid (barium or saline) when reducing intussusceptions, regardless of whether fluoroscopy or ultrasonography are used for monitoring.[65] The recent report of an intussusception reduction during colonoscopy offers a unique radiation-free, monitored solution.[66]

Failure to achieve complete reduction after three or four attempts usually mandates surgical exploration. In a stable patient with incomplete reduction, however, some surgeons and radiologists advocate repeated attempts at hydrostatic or pneumatic reduction after a rest period of 2 to 3 hours.[67] If the radiologist feels the reduction was complete but reflux of contrast into the terminal ileum was prevented by edema at the ileocecal valve, close observation may be undertaken if the child is stable. Follow-up imaging by ultrasonography to confirm reduction may be possible if saline or air has been used, or the majority of the barium has been evacuated.

Historically, certain features identifiable at presentation were thought to be relative contraindications to image-guided pressure reduction, as they predict a low probability of successful reduction, a high probability of perforation, or the presence of a pathologic lead point requiring surgical resection. These factors include premature and neonatal age group, age greater than 2 years, duration of symptoms greater than 48 hours, radiographic evidence of a small bowel obstruction, isolated small intestinal (e.g., jejunoileal) intussusception defined by noninvasive imaging, and multiple recurrences. Some of these relative contraindications have been modified or refuted by objective data.[68-73] Studies of success rates for either air or liquid pressure reduction have shown that successful nonoperative reduction is less common in the presence of clinically significant intestinal obstruction, prolapse of the intussusceptum through the anus, and age greater than 3 years. The data are conflicting as to whether or not duration of symptoms is an independent predictor of treatment failure. Despite a lower probability of success in these conditions, the probability of perforation or other treatment-related complication was not increased, and it is now thought that virtually all clinically stable patients presenting with intussusception should be given a trial of image-guided pressure reduction.

One remaining relative contraindication to nonoperative reduction is the presence of a sonographically defined pathological lead point at initial diagnosis. Ultrasound is accurate at detecting pathological lead points at the leading edge of the intussusceptum in about two thirds of cases, and their presence predicts both an increased failure of pressure reduction and the ultimate need for surgical exploration.[61] Many of these lead points in older patients are either neoplastic or fixed abnormalities such as Meckel's diverticulum. Burkitt's lymphoma represents a special case of intussusception. Roughly 20% of patients with Burkitt's lymphoma initially present with intussusception.[74] This subgroup of patients with Burkitt's lymphoma tend to present with earlier-stage disease, and resection at the time of initial treatment is usually complete. This allows for a less intensive and more effective course of adjuvant chemotherapy. Although intussusceptions caused by neoplastic lead points are usually not reducible, reports of successful reductions in the presence of lymphoma make it mandatory to obtain serial postreduction ultrasounds in older patients who undergo successful nonoperative reduction.

Surgical Management

Despite the wide variety of effective nonoperative options for infants and children with intussusception, surgery remains a common therapeutic mainstay for the 10 to 50% of infants in whom pressure enema reduction fails, for children with pathologic lead points, and for the 0.5 to 1% of patients with perforation during reduction. The traditional open operation is usually performed through a transverse incision in the right lower abdomen, although small-intestinal intussusceptions can be managed through a limited midline incision. Once the peritoneal cavity has been entered and explored, the involved intestine is externalized and inspected (Figure 52-8). Obvious perforation or infarction mandates resection without an attempt at manual reduction.

If no absolute indications for resection are encountered, reduction is attempted by carefully and gradually compressing the bowel just distal to the apex of the intussusceptum and gently pushing it retrograde until reduction is accomplished. The intussusceptum is never pulled out of the intussuscipiens, because traction injuries are common in the compromised bowel. Irreversible ischemic injury may be apparent only after successful manual reduction. Failure of manual reduction usually indicates a gangrenous intussusceptum. Resection of any pathologic lead point is also mandatory. In cases of Burkitt's lymphoma, a thorough abdominal survey should be carried out, including complete inspection of peritoneal membrane, liver, spleen, mesentery, and retroperitoneal nodes and the collection of ascetic fluid. Regardless of the reason for resection, primary anastomosis is usually recommended over the creation of an enterostomy unless the resection involves unprepared colon in a compromised patient.

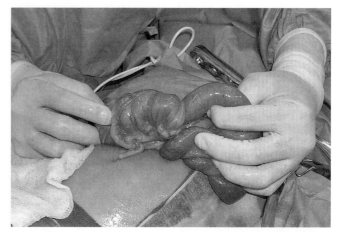

Figure 52-8. Intraoperative photograph of an ileocolic intussusception through the ileocecal valve. The absence of ischemic changes predicts successful manual reduction. (*See plate section for color.*)

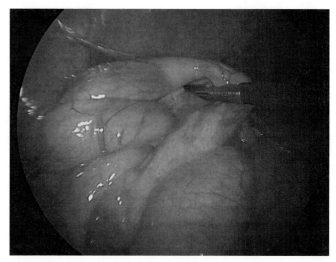

Figure 52-9. Laparoscopic reduction of ileocolic intussusception. (*See plate section for color.*)

Ileocecopexy, previously advocated to prevent recurrence, has been abandoned as unnecessary. Most surgeons, however, still perform an incidental appendectomy at the time of operation in order to avoid diagnostic confusion in the future due to the placement of an incision in the right lower quadrant, although no evidence can be found to support this practice. On the other hand, the presence of a fresh appendiceal stump may discourage reasonable attempts at hydrostatic reduction in the event of a recurrent intussusception in the early postoperative period.

Considerable experience with the use of minimally invasive surgical techniques in the treatment of intussusception has accumulated.[75,76] Laparoscopy may be beneficial in the occasional infant with idiopathic intussusception who fails pressure enema reduction, and in cases where complete reduction by nonoperative means is uncertain (Figure 52-9). When possible, laparoscopic reduction is equally safe when compared to open surgery and is associated with reduced times to feedings and shorter hospitalization.[77,78] Minimally invasive techniques are not as useful in managing an unreduced intussusception due to a pathological lead point because of the need for bowel manipulation and resection. Initial laparoscopy may be helpful in these cases as a diagnostic maneuver and in mobilizing the bowel, allowing the definitive procedure to be carried out through a small extension of the umbilical laparoscopic port site.[79] Conversion from laparoscopic to open surgery is more common in patients with pathological lead points and in those who present with a longer duration of symptoms.[80]

Observation

The finding of unsuspected intussusceptions on abdominal ultrasonography and CT has led some to question the necessity of intervention in asymptomatic patients.[81] The majority of these intussusceptions are limited to the small intestine (Figure 52-10), and many are associated with HSP. Close observation, nasogastric decompression, frequent physical examinations, and serial ultrasonography when necessary can identify those patients who go on to spontaneous resolution. The rare occurrence of intussusception in the premature neonate is another situation best managed expectantly. The intussusceptions are typically confined to the small intestine, are diagnosed by bedside ultrasonography, and are often misdiagnosed as necrotizing enterocolitis.[82] Persistence of symptoms or signs of systemic toxicity, however, indicates an urgent need for prompt surgical exploration. Pressure enema reduction and surgery can ultimately be avoided in a large number of these patients. The use of systemic corticosteroids to reduce lymphoid hyperplasia has been proposed to decrease the likelihood of recurrence in patients successfully managed by observation alone.[83]

RECURRENCE

Recurrence after either nonoperative or surgical reduction of intussusception is well recognized. After pressure enema reduction, recurrence rates range from 5 to 11% in most centers, but have been reported to be as high as 21%. Recurrence rates after surgical management are reported to be less than 4%. Approximately half of recurrences present within the first 3 days, many within the first 12 to 24 hours. In patients with a single recurrence, a repeat attempt at nonoperative reduction is justifiable, because pathologic lead points are ultimately found in less than 10% of these patients.[84] In patients with multiple recurrences, however, laparoscopy or surgical exploration is warranted to identify and remove the anticipated lead point. In infants with multiple episodes of reducible intussusception due to lymphoid hyperplasia, presumptive treatment of food allergies by dietary restriction may prevent further symptomatic episodes.[85]

SPECIAL CONSIDERATIONS

Postoperative Intussusception

Postoperative intussusception (POI) is uncommon in children of all ages, occurring in less than 1% of abdominal operations, and accounts for approximately 5 to 15% of all cases of intussusception.[86,87] Although no specific surgical procedure has been identified as a risk factor for POI, there may be an association between POI and certain procedures: fundoplications for gastroesophageal reflux, appendectomy, and intestinal

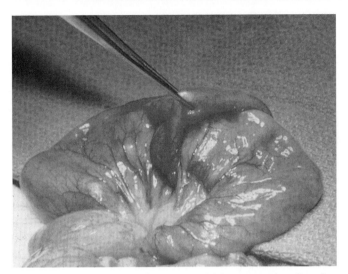

Figure 52-10. Small intestinal (enteroenteric) intussusception. (*See plate section for color.*)

resection.[88-91] Relatively high incidences of 2 to 3% have been reported for POI in association with Ladd's procedure for malrotation and with laparotomies for major tumor resection.[92-94] The causes of intussusception in these patients are various and may be related to inverted appendiceal stumps, anastomotic suture lines, disordered peristalsis following a prolonged ileus, and the absence of intestinal and mesenteric fixation found in malrotation. In addition, POI can occur after operations outside of the abdomen, including thoracic and neurosurgical procedures.

In the patient with delayed return of bowel function after surgery, differentiating POI from prolonged postoperative ileus or early postoperative adhesive bowel obstruction can be a significant challenge. Unlike most adhesive bowel obstructions, the mean time from surgery to obstruction is 5 to 10 days, rather than the 14 to 21 days more typically found for adhesive obstructions.[95] Unlike prolonged ileus, the majority of children with POI experience an initial return of bowel function before exhibiting signs of acute obstruction. Otherwise, the clinical appearance of POI may be indistinguishable from other causes of postoperative obstruction. Grossly bloody or currant-jelly stools are absent.

The majority of POIs are small intestinal in location, and therefore not amenable to nonoperative reduction. Patients suspected of experiencing POI should be evaluated by ultrasonography. If an ileocolic POI is present, an attempt at hydrostatic or pneumatic reduction is reasonable. The presence of a fresh appendiceal stump or other suture line may be a strong relative contraindication to pressure enema reduction; certainly, the use of barium should be avoided. In cases of postoperative enteroenteric intussusception, surgery is necessary and is successful in 90% of cases.[89,91,95]

Henoch-Schönlein Purpura

HSP is a diffuse autoimmune vasculitis that occurs in a variety of clinical settings. Approximately 75% of children with HSP have a history of an antecedent infection, frequently streptococcal pharyngitis or upper respiratory illness. Patients with HSP exhibit clinical signs of diffuse microvascular hemorrhage. A purpuric rash, often on the lower extremities, is

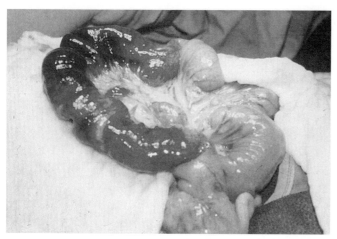

Figure 52-11. Intramural hemorrhage in small intestine secondary to Henoch-Schönlein purpura. (*See plate section for color.*)

common. Multifocal submucosal hemorrhage throughout the gastrointestinal tract is also seen in a large proportion of patients and is associated with intussusception, which results from hemorrhage-induced alterations in bowel-wall mechanics (Figure 52-11).[96]

Abdominal complaints are common among children with HSP, occurring in approximately 40- to 80% of all patients.[97-100] The vast majority of these patients experience severe, colicky abdominal pain, and a significant number also develop nausea, vomiting, and overt gastrointestinal hemorrhage. Understandably, the diagnosis of intussusception is considered in a large number of patients with HSP and this constellation of clinical signs. The onset of abdominal pain precedes the appearance of the purpuric rash in up to one third of patients, confounding the diagnosis further.

Intussusception is the most common gastrointestinal complication of HSP and has been documented by ultrasonography, contrast enema, or surgical exploration in at least 5 to 10% of affected children.[101,102] It is likely, however, that the actual percentage of patients with HSP who develop intussusception is much higher. Serial sonographic examination in children with HSP documents findings consistent with intramural hemorrhage in virtually all patients, and the presence of intussusception in as many as one third of patients.[103,104] It is recognized that 60 to 90% of intussusceptions related to HSP are limited to the small intestine. A significant number of enteroenteric intussusceptions (especially HSP-related intussusceptions) have been found to reduce spontaneously without developing complications.[105,106]

It is generally accepted that many of the intermittent painful episodes experienced by children with HSP are caused by self-reducing enteroenteric intussusceptions, leading to a more conservative management plan in these patients. Close clinical observation by an experienced surgeon can usually detect those patients with HSP who have persistent, nonreducing intussusceptions and require surgical exploration. The sonographic measurement of an enteroenteric intussusceptum more than 3.5 cm in length predicts a high probability of surgical intervention.[107] The administration of corticosteroids to increase the likelihood of spontaneous reduction and reduce the need for surgical intervention has been reported, but has not been studied prospectively.[108]

Cystic Fibrosis

Children with cystic fibrosis represent a special group of patients at risk for intussusception, which occurs in 1 to 2% of affected individuals.[109,110] Cystic fibrosis is a genetic disease characterized by dysfunctional chloride transport across epithelial cells, resulting in the production of thick, viscous secretions that obstruct the ductal systems of solid organs as well as the lumen of the intestinal tract. These secretions can become densely adherent to the intestinal wall, altering peristalsis and precipitating intussusception. Ultrasonography of asymptomatic patients with cystic fibrosis has documented the presence of unsuspected, self-reducing enteroenteric intussusceptions in 4% of patients.[111]

In addition to the pulmonary manifestations of cystic fibrosis, which are associated with most of the morbidity and mortality attendant on the disease, gastrointestinal symptoms and complications occur in over 50% of patients. The most common acute gastrointestinal complication of cystic fibrosis in children is the distal intestinal obstruction syndrome (DIOS) in which thick, inspissated secretions block the terminal ileum, producing a mechanical bowel obstruction. This syndrome is analogous to meconium ileus in the neonate with cystic fibrosis, and is often referred to as meconium ileus equivalent (MIE). These patients present with acute, colicky abdominal pain, abdominal distention, vomiting, and the radiographic appearance of an acute small bowel obstruction. On examination, many of these patients have a palpable right lower quadrant mass. The diagnostic overlap between DIOS and intussusception is obvious.

Distinguishing DIOS from intussusception at the outset is crucial, as the treatment for DIOS involves antegrade administration of a large volume of a hyperosmotic solution such as polyethylene glycol in order to flush the meconium-like plug out of the ileum and into the colon. Such treatment might easily precipitate an abdominal crisis in a patient with intussusception. As there is no reliable clinical feature that can differentiate intussusception from DIOS, sonographic examination of the abdomen should be performed promptly in patients with severe pain, systemic toxicity, or bloody stools. If ultrasonography documents intussusception, the treatment options are essentially the same as for other varieties of intussusception: hydrostatic, pneumatic, or surgical reduction. The success rate for hydrostatic reduction is sufficiently high to recommend it for most patients with cystic fibrosis and ileocolic intussusception. The safety of conservative observation and supportive measures in patients with cystic fibrosis and symptomatic enteroenteric intussusceptions has not been studied by any prospective trial, and surgical exploration and reduction should still be considered the current standard of care in these patients.

REFERENCES

13. Stringer MD, Pablot SM, Brereton FJ. Pediatric intussusception. Br J Surg 1992;79:867–876.
27. DiFiore JW. Intussusception. Semin Pediatr Surg 1999;8:214–220.
28. Ein SH. Leading points in childhood intussusception. J Pediatr Surg 1976;11:209–211.
45. Hryhorczuk AL, Strouse PJ. Validation of US as a first-line diagnostic test for assessment of pediatric ileocolic intussusception. Pediatr Radiol 2009;39:1075–1079.
49. Ravitch MM, McCune RM. Reduction of intussusception by hydrostatic pressure: an experimental study. Bull Johns Hopkins Hosp 1948;82:550–568.

61. Bai YZ, Qu RB, Wang GD, et al. Ultrasound-guided hydrostatic reduction of intussusceptions by saline enema: a review of 5218 cases in 17 years. Am J Surg 2006;192:273–275.

70. Simanovsky N, Hiller N, Koplewitz BZ, et al. Is non-operative intussusception reduction effective in older children? Ten-year experience in a university affiliated medical center. Pediatr Surg Int 2007;23: 261–264.

72. Somme S, To T, Langer JC. Factors determining the need for operative reduction in children with intussusception: a population-based study. J Pediatr Surg 2006;41:1014–1019.

74. Gupta H, Davidoff AM, Pui CH, et al. Clinical implications and surgical management of intussusception in pediatric patients with Burkitt lymphoma. J Pediatr Surg 2007;42:998–1001; discussion 1001.

77. Bailey KA, Wales PW, Gerstle JT. Laparoscopic versus open reduction of intussusception in children: a single-institution comparative experience. J Pediatr Surg 2007;42:845–848.

79. Fraser JD, Aguayo P, Ho B, et al. Laparoscopic management of intussusception in pediatric patients. J Laparoendosc Adv Surg Tech A 2009;19: 563–565.

88. West KW, Stephens B, Rescorla FJ, et al. Postoperative intussusception: experience with 36 cases in children. Surgery 1988;104:781–787.

107. Munden MM, Bruzzi JF, Coley BD, Munden RF. Sonography of pediatric small-bowel intussusception: differentiating surgical from nonsurgical cases. AJR Am J Roentgenol 2007;188:275–279.

See expertconsult.com for a complete list of references and the review questions for this chapter.

53 INGUINAL HERNIAS AND HYDROCELES

Anthony Capizzani • Peter F. Ehrlich

A hernia can be defined as a communication between two structures or cavities that do not normally communicate. A hydrocele is a fluid collection in the tunica vaginalis or processus vaginalis. Hydroceles can be communicating, where fluid flows between the peritoneal cavity and the scrotum and the hydrocele will change in size, whereas a noncommunicating hydrocele has a fixed size because there is no connection between the cavities (Figure 53-1).

Hernias can result in structures passing through cavities and becoming wedged in a space. Inguinal hernia contents can include bowel, bladder, or gonads, which can result in pain, incarceration, and strangulation if the structure is trapped. Hernias can present at any age. However, the highest incidence of hernias occurs in the first year of life and has been reported to be between 1 and 5% in full-term infants and up to 25% in preterm children.[1-3] Boys are affected six times more often than girls.[4]

An inguinal hernia presents clinically as a mass in the groin and/or labia and scrotum (Figure 53-2). The main differential diagnosis includes inguinal hernia, femoral hernia, communicating hydrocele, and noncommunicating hydrocele. Hernias can be either unilateral or bilateral. An inguinal hernia can be either direct or indirect (congenital) hernia. The distinction is based on the relationship to the epigastric artery (Figure 53-3). In children, 99% of hernias are indirect. An indirect hernia is a patent continuation of the peritoneum through the inguinal canal along the spermatic cord lateral to the inferior epigastric vein. A direct hernia originates medial to inferior epigastric vessels and protrudes directly through the posterior wall of the inguinal canal. A femoral hernia is medial to the femoral vessels and inferior to the inguinal ligament. In children, an indirect hernia is not typically associated with muscle weakness. Thus, repair of the floor of the inguinal canal is not necessary.

Bassini[5] in 1887 was credited as the first to describe an inguinal hernia repair using a high ligation of the hernia sac in combination with anatomic repair. In 1899, Ferguson[6] modified this to include an incision of the external oblique fascia to improve surgical exposure. In 1950, Potts et al.[7] recommended simple high ligation and removal of the hernia sac for routine hernia repair. In children, high ligation has become the standard of care.

PATHOGENESIS

An indirect inguinal hernia occurs when the processus vaginalis fails to close. The processus vaginalis is an extension of the peritoneum that accompanies the descending testicle. This membrane surrounds the testis and gubernaculum. The processus gives rise to the tunica vaginalis and normally obliterates after the testicles descend. Communication occurs between the abdominal cavity and inguinal canal/scrotum when the processus fails to close, creating a potential hernia.

Testicle descent is a complex process controlled by both mechanical and hormonal factors.[8] The testicle initially develops in the abdomen adjacent to the kidney and then descends into the scrotum. Transabdominal descent takes place when the testicle moves from the urogenital ridge to the inguinal region between 12 and 17 weeks' gestation. Inguinoscrotal descent through the inguinal canal to the scrotum occurs in the last trimester. As the testicle descends, it drags a tongue of peritoneum with it (processus vaginalis). Prematurity may interrupt this process. Therefore it is not surprising that inguinal hernias are more frequent in premature infants. The left testicle descends first, followed by the right; thus, indirect inguinal hernias are more common on the right.

Not all children with patent process vaginalis will present clinically with an inguinal hernia.[9,10] Autopsy studies demonstrate that the people can have a patent processus vaginalis and be asymptomatic.[9] In addition, with the advent of laparoscopy (e.g., during an operation for appendicitis), a patent process can be detected without prior clinical knowledge of an inguinal hernia. Why only some children with a patent processus develop clinical symptoms of a hernia or hydrocele is not yet clear.

CLINICAL PRESENTATION

Hernias and hydroceles are diagnosed by a thorough history and physical examination. A hernia or a communicating hydrocele will present as an intermittent groin or scrotal mass. In young children, they are often noticed when a parent changes a diaper, during a bath, or at a medical examination. Older children may discover a mass themselves after strenuous activity. During physical examination, a key finding is whether the inguinal mass is intermittent or persistent when distinguishing between a hernia and a noncommunicating hydrocele. A noncommunicating hydrocele is typically confined to the scrotum. It will not change in size, has a bluish hue when the child cries, and is asymptomatic. Communicating hydroceles fluctuate in size, becoming less prominent at night when the child is sleeping.

When children present to a surgeon, it is quite common for the clinical examination to be normal or for the parent to arrive stating, "My doctor thinks my child may have a hernia." In this situation the authors look for important features to confirm the diagnosis. We assess for a distinct history of an intermittent swelling or mass. Second, we assess whether the mass goes

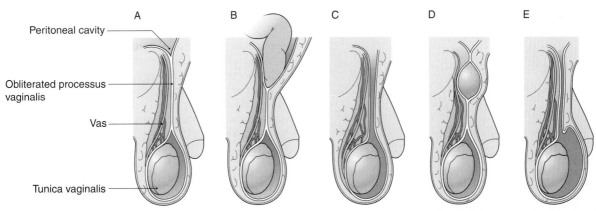

Figure 53-1. Spectrum of anatomic abnormalities of the processus vaginalis. (**A**) Normal anatomy. (**B**) Inguinal hernia. (**C**) Complete hernia. (**D**) Hydrocele of the cord. (**E**) Communicating hydrocele.

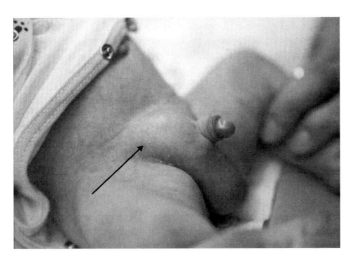

Figure 53-2. Typical appearance of a child with a hernia. The black arrow points to the mass.

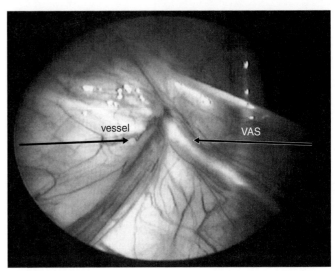

Figure 53-3. The relationship of the anatomic structures (vas deferens and epigastric vessels) to the left internal ring.

from the inguinal region toward the scrotum or labia. We will ask whether the referring health professional actually saw or reduced a groin mass, and in some cases we call the referring physician directly. If we do not get that history and a hernia/hydrocele cannot be found on careful physical examination, we do not make a diagnosis but will reassess at a second visit.

On physical examination, the clinician should examine the testicles, scrotal size, and both groins to assess symmetry. If a groin mass is present, easily palpable, and reducible, the diagnosis is easy. In other situations, examination can be facilitated by placing the child in an upright position or by encouraging straining or coughing. In young children, examination techniques include instructing the child to "blow up a balloon" to increase abdominal pressure in order to enhance a possible hernia defect. It is important to palpate both testicles within the scrotum, because an undescended or retractile testis may often pose as a groin mass. If a mass is detected, an attempt to reduce it should be made. While doing this procedure, it is important to keep in mind the anatomic relationship between the internal ring and external ring. The internal ring is cephalad, lateral, and posterior to the external ring. A common mistake made by clinicians is to try to reduce the hernia by directly pushing the mass into the abdomen. This will not work and frequently

causes pain. In order to reduce a hernia successfully, gentle pressure is applied bimanually in a cephalad and posterior direction and will result in a sudden reduction of an inguinal hernia (Figure 53-4).

In females, a hernia sac may contain either bowel or an ovary. On physical examination, bowel is softer and tends to glide back into the peritoneal cavity, whereas an ovary feels hard, like a nut, and tends to "pop" back into the abdominal cavity when reduced.

Transillumination is the trademark of a hydrocele. If the fluid goes away, it is a communicating hydrocele. A noncommunicating hydrocele will transilluminate and feels like a small balloon, and the whole structure can be palpated between both hands. In addition, most of these are also in the scrotum and asymptomatic.

A challenging examination point is distinguishing between an incarcerated hernia and a hydrocele of the cord, particularly in premature or neonatal infants. Both conditions may transilluminate and may be irreducible. However, a hydrocele of the cord is otherwise asymptomatic as opposed to an incarcerated hernia, which is generally tender and associated with intestinal symptoms. Another way to differentiate these two entities in the neonate is to perform a digital rectal examination and feel

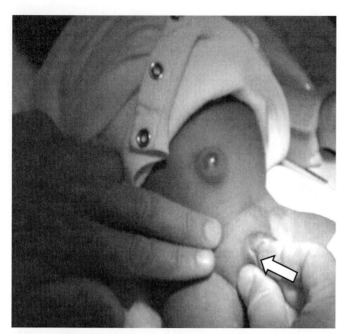

Figure 53-4. Proper technique in reducing an inguinal hernia.

for the internal ring. With an incarcerated hernia, a mass can be palpated traveling through the internal ring. If the clinician is unable to distinguish an incarcerated hernia from a hydrocele, surgical exploration is recommended.

MANAGEMENT

Inguinal hernias or communicating hydroceles should be repaired after the diagnosis is made. A communicating hydrocele is a de facto hernia (see Figure 53-1); the difference is the size of the patent processus vaginalis. In a communicating hydrocele, the size of the processus only allows fluid through at clinical presentation. Nevertheless, closure is required because of the potential risk of incarceration. The majority of noncommunicating hydroceles in infancy resolve spontaneously during the first year of life. If the hydrocele has not resolved by 1 year of age, we recommend reassessing the child. If the hydrocele shows signs of resolution, we would follow for another year. If a mass still persists at that time, then surgical repair should be recommended on an elective basis. Although hydroceles cause no real problems, they can grow quite large and cause significant discomfort as the child grows. In addition, if a hernia is found when a child is in the hospital for an unrelated illness, herniorrhaphy is best deferred until the primary problem is resolved. Premature infants have a 25% risk of having a hernia, and often hernias are detected while in the hospital.[2] Premature infants are also at high risk for respiratory complications due to surgery. Confounding this known respiratory compromise, premature infants also have the highest risk of incarceration. Therefore, avoiding an emergent operation is most desirable. Several studies have addressed the question of timing and anesthetic technique for premature infants with hernias.[12-15] Based on the evidence, repair is often deferred until just before discharge from the neonatal intensive care unit, and if possible, repair is performed under caudal or spinal anesthesia so that the patient can be closely observed postoperatively for apnea and bradycardia.

Hernias are repaired to avoid incarceration. Incarceration occurs when a segment of intestine becomes trapped in the hernia sac. Incarceration may result in a small bowel obstruction, vascular compromise to the bowel, and strangulation with ischemic necrosis. Erythema and edema overlying a tender groin mass are suggestive of strangulation and are an emergent indication for an operation. Rowe and Clatworthy[16,17] found that incarceration was most common in the first 6 months of life, with 71% of incarnated hernias requiring operative reduction in children younger than 1 year. In addition, their data demonstrated that two thirds of children with an incarceration required surgical reduction. To facilitate reduction in the child with an incarcerated hernia, it is often helpful to place the child in a head-down position for 30 minutes before attempting reduction. Sedation is also used to facilitate hernia reduction. If sedation is required, we admit the patient and fix the hernia urgently. If the there is concern about bowel viability, the surgeon should perform a diagnostic laparoscopy followed by a hernia repair.

Surgical repair of hernias and hydroceles is normally performed as an outpatient procedure with general anesthesia. Anatomic landmarks are the anterior superior iliac crest, the symphysis pubis, and the inguinal ligament. A transverse skin incision is made within a skin crease midway between the symphysis pubis and anterior iliac crest. Scarpa's fascia is identified and incised, and the external oblique aponeurosis is identified. The external ring is opened to expose the inguinal canal. The cremasteric muscle is gently separated, exposing the hernia sac cord structures. The hernia sac is always anterior and medial to the vas deferens and vascular structures. Careful observation of the sac is performed to ensure that it is empty and with no component of a sliding hernia. Then the hernia sac is gently dissected away from the structures of the cord and back to the internal ring, where it is ligated and amputated. In females, the round ligament and sac are divided distally before a high ligation. A similar procedure is performed for a hydrocele. The distal portion of the hydrocele should be excised carefully to prevent a recurrence. In a child with an associated undescended testicle, orchiopexy must be performed in conjunction with the hernia repair. Sliding hernias are rare in children and may include the appendix, bladder, salpinx, or Meckel's diverticulum (Littre's hernia) as part of the hernia sac. In this situation, the structure must be carefully dissected away from the wall of the sac before high ligation. When performing surgery for incarceration, the entrapped viscera should be carefully inspected for signs of ischemic necrosis and, if none are found, subsequently reduced. In most cases, if an incarcerated hernia is successfully reduced manually before surgery, it is unnecessary to inspect the intestine at the time of the subsequent hernia repair.

A controversy exists over the issue of routine contralateral exploration and more recently of peritoneoscopy of the opposite side to look for bilateral hernias. Routine contralateral exploration avoids a second operation with its associated cost and risk of anesthesia. The major disadvantages of routine contralateral exploration include the possibility of a technical mishap. Older studies[18-20] have reported a high incidence up to 50 to 60% of contralateral inguinal hernia or patent processus vaginalis when routine contralateral groin exploration is carried out. Based on this reported high incidence, for many years routine contralateral hernia repair was justifiable in any healthy infant or child with a unilaterally apparent hernia.[21]

Other studies have questioned these findings and recommendations.[22] In 2006, Ein et al.[23] published a series of 6361 hernia repairs with 35-year follow-up. An opposite-side hernia developed in only 5%, 95% within the first 5 years. Furthermore, only 0.7% presented with an incarceration. The authors concluded that routine contralateral groin exploration is not indicated in any situation. A recent paper with 5095 children used logistic regression to predict metachronous hernia (MH).[24] Predictors of developing a MH included a left-sided hernia (OR = 2.2, CI = 1.7 to 2.8; P < 0.0005) and age less than 6 months (OR = 0.39, CI = 0.25 to 0.59; P < 0.0005). Gender, history of incarceration, prematurity, or ventriculoperitoneal shunt were not associated with MH development. This paper does not advocate routine contralateral exploration.

The use of laparoscopy/peritoneoscopy has been advocated as a quick, safe method to evaluate the contralateral side for a patient process vaginalis.[25,26] However, a patent process vaginalis does not inevitably lead to hernia formation.[9,27,28] Thus, even when contralateral exploration is restricted to patients with a patient processus, at least five of six operations are unnecessary.

COMPLICATIONS

Complications for any surgical procedure relate to the technical aspects, elective or urgent conditions, patient characteristics, and anesthetic complications. The overall preoperative complication rate for elective hernia repairs is reported to be between 1 and 2%. This rate can increase significantly in patients requiring an emergent operation secondary to an incarceration. Recurrences have been reported between 1 and 2%, 96% within 5 years.[23,24] Injuries to the vas deferens or the vascular bundle supplying the testicle are the two most serious complications. If the testicle is pulled out of the scrotum and not replaced, this could result in an undescended testicle. A postoperative scrotal hydrocele or hematoma can occur. In most instances, this will resolve spontaneously, but in some instance it will not and can be quite large.[29] Hernia recurrence and injury to structures within the sac also can occur. The most common problems following an elective hernia repair are local wound infection or a foreign body reaction secondary to the stitches. This latter problem will present often 2 to 3 weeks following surgery. Wound infections and suture material reactions respond to conservative therapy with topical antibiotics. If an emergent operation is required for incarceration, the complication rate is increased. Gender-specific complications for incarcerated inguinal hernia repair include testicular atrophy (males) secondary to decreased testicular blood supply from the incarcerated bowel and ovarian atrophy (females) secondary to an incarcerated ovary with torsion.

The incidence of postoperative complications is higher in the premature infant, especially respiratory complications.[12] Postoperative apnea caused by immaturity of the diaphragm or the intercostals muscle or abnormal responses to hypoxia and hypercapnia are not uncommon in premature infants. Many centers have gestation age limits for who can and cannot go home following surgery.[30] Those less than 50 weeks tend to be kept overnight for 24 hours on an apnea and bradycardia monitor. Premature infants who still have respiratory issues and are greater than 50 weeks' gestation may also need to be monitored longer following surgery, and the decision should be made on a case-by-case basis.

REFERENCES

8. Hutson JM, Hasthorpe S. Testicular descent and cryptorchidism: the state of the art in 2004. J Pediatr Surg 2004;40:297–302.
17. Rowe MI, Clatworthy HW. Incarcerated and strangulated hernias in children. A statistical study of high-risk factors. Arch Surg 1970;101:136–139.
22. Surana R, Puri P. Is contralateral exploration necessary in infants with unilateral inguinal hernia? J Pediatr Surg 1993;28:1026–1027.
23. Ein SH, Njere I, Ein A. Six thousand three hundred sixty-one pediatric inguinal hernias: a 35-year review. J Pediatr Surg 2006;41:980–986.
25. Holcomb III GW, Miller KA, Chaignaud BE, et al. The parental perspective regarding the contralateral inguinal region in a child with a known unilateral inguinal hernia. J Pediatr Surg 2004;39:480–482.

See expertconsult.com for a complete list of references and the review questions for this chapter.

54

MECKEL'S DIVERTICULUM AND OTHER OMPHALOMESENTERIC DUCT REMNANTS

Brendan T. Campbell

A Meckel's diverticulum is located along the antimesenteric border of the distal ileum and may contain rests of ectopic tissue. It is the most common congenital anomaly of the alimentary tract, with an estimated prevalence of 2% in the general population.[1] The embryologic development of a Meckel's diverticulum is believed to result from the incomplete obliteration of the vitelline (omphalomesenteric) duct that results in an outpocketing of ileum proximal to the ileocecal valve.[2] Individuals with a Meckel's diverticulum may develop symptoms from infancy through adulthood that include intestinal obstruction, gastrointestinal bleeding, acute intra-abdominal inflammation, Littre's hernia (inguinal hernia with a Meckel's diverticulum in the hernia sac), or umbilical anomalies.[2,3]

Meckel's diverticulum was initially described by the German surgeon Wilhelm Fabricius Hildanus in 1598, but it was the German comparative anatomist Sir Johann Friedrich Meckel who described its embryologic origin in 1809.[4] Meckel's diverticulum garners substantial attention in the medical literature, but is not unique to humans. It is frequently identified in pigs, horses, and geese and is occasionally described in other mammals.[5,6]

Most data on Meckel's diverticulum and its clinical sequelae come from case reports and single-institution case series. For all that is written about this anomaly, very few good data about its natural history and epidemiology exist. The Pediatric Health Information System (PHIS) database collects administrative data from 43 children's hospitals in the United States. A query of 2008 data from this database identified 853 patients less than 18 years of age who had Meckel's diverticulectomies. These data confirm that Meckel's diverticula are found twice as often in males (male:female, 2.3:1). Forty-two percent of Meckel's diverticulectomies are performed in children less than 2 years of age, and the remainder of cases are evenly distributed among children 2 to 17 years of age.

EMBRYOLOGY AND ANATOMY

The vitelline duct acts as a communicating tract between the embryonic yolk sac and its primitive midgut during early human development. During the eighth week of gestation, the vitelline duct is normally obliterated as the placenta replaces the yolk sac as the primary source for fetal nutrition.[7] A Meckel's diverticulum develops when incomplete obliteration of the vitelline duct occurs between the fifth and seventh week of gestation.

The vitelline duct receives its blood supply from paired vitelline arteries. As alimentary tract development proceeds, the left

vitelline artery involutes and the right vitelline artery becomes the superior mesenteric artery. The blood supply of a Meckel's diverticulum, therefore, arises directly from the midgut mesentery. Failure of obliteration of the vitelline duct produces several gastrointestinal anomalies, the most common of which is a Meckel's diverticulum. Other related anomalies include a vitelline fistula, which occurs when the vitelline duct remains patent, forming a direct connection between the umbilicus and the ileum. This may result in fecal discharge from the umbilicus. Alternatively, both ends can develop into fibrous cords while the midportion forms a vitelline cyst. Finally, a fibrous cord can extend from the Meckel's diverticulum to the umbilicus. This structure may form a fixed point around which bowel loops may become entangled, resulting in a bowel obstruction (Figure 54-1).

A Meckel's diverticulum is a true diverticulum that contains all three layers of the bowel wall. The location of this anomaly along the antimesenteric border of the distal ileum is variable, but it is usually located within 100 cm of the ileocecal valve.[8] The average length of a Meckel's diverticulum is about 3 cm. The length can range from 1 to 26 cm, but most are 1 to 5 cm long.[9] Besides normal ileal mucosa, up to 60% of these diverticula contain ectopic tissue, which is most commonly gastric or pancreatic, but may occasionally contain duodenal or colonic mucosa[10] (Figures 54-2 and 54-3).

CLINICAL PRESENTATION

The wide range of clinical presentations associated with Meckel's diverticulum frequently makes establishing a diagnosis challenging until surgical exploration is undertaken. Presenting symptoms related to a Meckel's diverticulum vary with age. The most common presentation during the newborn period is intestinal obstruction. Children older than 2 years of age with a Meckel's diverticulum are more likely to present with asymptomatic lower gastrointestinal (GI) bleeding. Children in this age group can also present with intestinal obstruction, which can be caused by volvulus around a fibrous band that extends from the Meckel's diverticulum to the undersurface of the umbilicus, intussusception with the Meckel's diverticulum acting as the lead point, internal hernia from bands arising from the Meckel's diverticulum, and prolapse of intestine through a patent vitelline fistula (Figure 54-4).

Meckel's diverticulitis is another type of presentation in this age group. Meckel's diverticulitis is usually clinically indistinguishable from acute appendicitis. Obstruction of

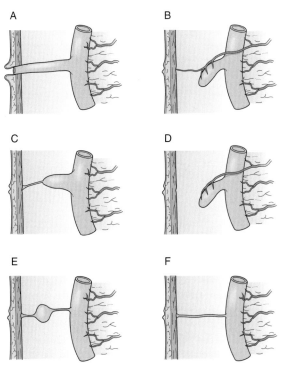

Figure 54-1. Some of the more common residual congenital abnormalities that result from the embryonic yolk sac. (**A**) Patent omphalomesenteric duct representing a communication from the terminal ileum to the umbilicus. (**B**) Meckel's diverticulum with a patent right vitelline artery as blood supply to the Meckel's diverticulum and a residual of the vitelline artery illustrated as a cord to the undersurface to the umbilicus. (**C**) Meckel's diverticulum with a cord connecting the tip of the Meckel's diverticulum to the undersurface of the umbilicus. The cord (band) represents the distal residual of the omphalomesenteric duct. (**D**) Typical appearance of a Meckel's diverticulum with persistence of the vitelline artery. (**E**) Involution of the proximal and distal ends of the omphalomesenteric duct with residual cord or band and central preservation of the omphalomesenteric duct, resulting in a mucosa-lined cyst. (**F**) Intraperitoneal band from the ileum to the undersurface of the umbilicus representing involution without resolution of the omphalomesenteric duct.

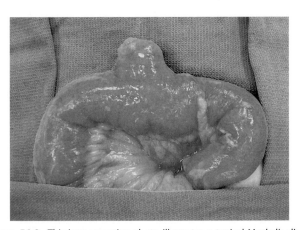

Figure 54-2. This intraoperative photo illustrates a typical Meckel's diverticulum arising along the antimesenteric border of the terminal ileum.

the diverticulum produces distal inflammation, necrosis, and occasionally perforation. Materials that have been demonstrated to cause obstruction in these surgical specimens include fishbones, phytobezoars, enteroliths, gallstones, and bullets.[11]

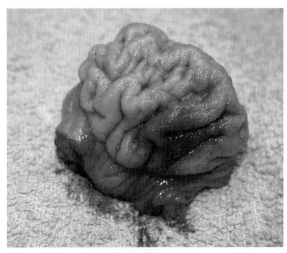

Figure 54-3. Surgical specimen opened demonstrating gastric rugae grossly with resultant bleeding from the adjacent ileal mucosa.

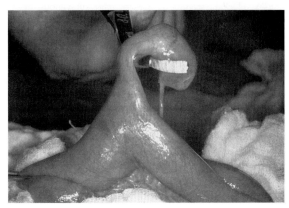

Figure 54-4. This intraoperative picture illustrates a Meckel's diverticulum with a band that can form a fixed point around which bowel loops can twist, resulting in a bowel obstruction.

Gastrointestinal neoplasms may arise from a Meckel's diverticulum, but this is uncommon in children. Case reports describe a wide variety of tumors arising from Meckel's diverticula, but carcinoid tumors are the most frequently reported.[12]

DIAGNOSIS

Given the diversity of presentations that can occur with a Meckel's diverticulum, the diagnostic work-up should be tailored to the clinical circumstances of each individual patient. In the absence of lower GI bleeding, the clinical diagnosis of a symptomatic Meckel's diverticulum preoperatively is often not possible. Whenever evidence of a bowel obstruction or an acute abdomen exists, prompt surgical consultation is indicated.

Routine history and physical examination are important and may provide information that is valuable such as bloody or tarry stools, feculent drainage from the umbilicus, or symptoms that can be attributed to chronic iron-deficiency anemia.

Plain films are valuable screening studies and may reveal obstruction, free intraperitoneal air, or, on rare occasions, enteroliths. Abdominal ultrasound and computed tomographic (CT) scans can identify intestinal obstruction, inflammatory changes, and abscess formation, but these tests cannot

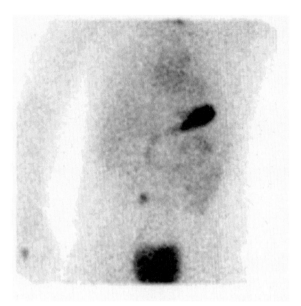

Figure 54-5. Meckel's scan at 60 minutes after intravenous injection of technetium-99m pertechnetate. Uptake of tracer is demonstrated in the stomach and bladder, as well as the Meckel's diverticulum in the right lower quadrant. Image courtesy Ronald J. Rosenberg, MD, Jefferson Radiology, PC.

discriminate between a Meckel's diverticulum and intestinal loops. When a Meckel's diverticulum leads to intussusception, ultrasound can readily identify a target sign and a pseudokidney sign and help establish the diagnosis.[13] The three findings most commonly associated with Meckel's diverticulum on CT scan are isolated small bowel obstruction, intussusception with small bowel obstruction, and an inflammatory cystic mass.[14]

Technetium-99m pertechnetate scintigraphy, more commonly referred to as a Meckel's scan, is the best way to screen patients with lower GI bleeding or other symptoms suspicious for Meckel's diverticulum. Technetium-99m pertechnetate is avidly taken up by parietal cells of gastric mucosa and permits the noninvasive detection of ectopic gastric tissue. A Meckel's diverticulum with rests of gastric mucosa, can be detected with high specificity and a positive predictive value of nearly 100%[15] (Figure 54-5).

A Meckel's scan is performed after intravenous injection of ^{99m}Tc pertechnetate. Serial images of the abdomen are obtained over 60 minutes. A positive study demonstrates activity in the ectopic gastric mucosa concurrently with the activity seen in the stomach. A Meckel's diverticulum may appear anywhere in the abdomen, but it is most commonly identified in the right lower quadrant. Occasionally, the kidneys, ureters, or bladder may be mistaken for a Meckel's diverticulum, but activity in these structures usually appears after activity is seen in the stomach.[15]

Pharmacologic provocation with cimetidine, pentagastrin, and glucagon has been shown to increase the sensitivity of Meckel's detection, but its role in clinical practice has not been clearly defined, and it is not needed to obtain high-quality images.[16,17] The location of a Meckel's diverticulum makes it difficult to identify using traditional contrast studies and endoscopy. Although there have been reports of Meckel's diverticula being diagnosed by wireless video capsule endoscopy, this type of testing is generally not recommended.[18]

Patients with a high clinical suspicion for the diagnosis of Meckel's diverticulum and a negative Meckel's scan should be considered candidates for diagnostic laparoscopy given that a Meckel's scan has a relatively low sensitivity and because laparoscopy when performed by a pediatric surgeon with minimally invasive skills is a very safe and sensitive means of screening patients for Meckel's diverticulum and other intra-abdominal pathology.[19]

TREATMENT

Whenever a symptomatic Meckel's diverticulum is identified, either preoperatively or intraoperatively, it should be removed. Diverticulectomy or segmental small bowel resection including the diverticulum should be performed. It is important to remove all of the ectopic gastric tissue to prevent rebleeding episodes. The standard of care at most tertiary centers with pediatric surgical expertise would be a laparoscopic approach with either extracorporeal or intracorporeal resection. The indications for minimally invasive approaches to intra-abdominal pathology continue to expand, and this should be the preferred approach in cases of diagnostic uncertainty, positive Meckel's scan, intussusception, and Meckel's diverticulitis.[1,20]

Younger children (especially those younger than 5 years) with suspected Meckel's diverticulum should be referred to centers with pediatric subspecialty expertise that routinely take care of children with these types of problems.[21] There is considerable evidence that children undergoing higher risk surgical procedures have improved outcomes if care is provided by pediatric subspecialists and at hospitals that have a high case load of patients with the same condition.[22]

What to do with an incidentally discovered Meckel's diverticulum at the time of surgery for another condition is controversial. There are no good data to guide clinical decisions in this situation. For all that has been written about Meckel's diverticulum, very little is known about the natural history of this entity.[23] Often-cited previous papers on this subject are retrospective and outdated and should not be used to guide clinical decision making in the modern era.[24-26] Most pediatric surgeons would recommend removal of an incidentally discovered Meckel's diverticulum in stable pediatric patients because their life expectancy is long and the risk of surgical complications is extremely low.[23] There are some situations, however, such as damage control procedures for trauma, where resection of an incidentally discovered Meckel's diverticulum may not be practical.[27]

SUMMARY

Key facts about Meckel's diverticulum can be remembered by its association with the number 2: 2% of the population harbors a Meckel's diverticulum, men are afflicted twice as often as women, children less than 2 years of age are more apt to develop symptoms, it generally resides 2 feet from the ileocecal valve, its average length is 2 inches, and it may contain two types of ectopic tissue.

The most important factor to remember about Meckel's diverticulum is to consider it as a possibility in the differential diagnosis of any patient presenting with bowel obstruction, lower GI bleeding, or intra-abdominal inflammation. The index of suspicion should be highest when children less than 2 years of age present with intestinal obstruction and no prior history of abdominal surgery.

REFERENCES

7. Yahchouchy EK, Marano AF, Etienne JC, et al. Meckel's diverticulum. J Am Coll Surg 2001;192:658–662.

19. Swaniker F, Soldes O, Hirschl RB. The utility of technetium 99m pertechnetate scintigraphy in the evaluation of patients with Meckel's diverticulum. J Pediatr Surg 1999;34:760–775.

21. Surgical Advisory Panel. Guidelines for referral to pediatric surgical specialists. Pediatrics 2002;110:187–191.

22. Kizer KW. The volume-outcome conundrum. N Engl J Med 2003;349:2159–2161.

23. Behrns KE. Meckel diverticulum: "Too" much chatter. South Med J 2004;97:1029–1030.

25. Cullen JJ, Kelly KA, Moir CR, et al. Surgical management of Meckel's diverticulum: an epidemiologic, population-based study. Ann Surg 1994;220:564–568; discussion, 568–569.

26. St-Vil D, Brandt ML, Panic S, et al. Meckel's diverticulum in children: a 20-year-review. J Pediatr Surg 1991;26:1289–1292.

See expertconsult.com for a complete list of references and the review questions for this chapter.

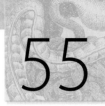

55 HIRSCHSPRUNG'S DISEASE

Peter Mattei

Hirschsprung's disease (HD) is a disorder of distal intestinal motility that is the result of a congenital absence of ganglion cells in the myenteric plexuses of the rectum and distal colon. This causes constipation that is often severe and a clinical picture consistent with a distal pseudo-obstruction characterized by enlargement of the normally ganglionated proximal colon (megacolon). Surgical resection of the aganglionic segment of bowel and reconstruction with normal proximal bowel is the treatment of choice and is associated with overall excellent results in the majority of patients.

EPIDEMIOLOGY AND GENETICS

The incidence of HD is approximately 1 in 5000 live births.[1] In approximately 85% of cases, aganglionosis is limited to the rectum and distal sigmoid colon; it involves a significantly longer portion of the remainder of the colon and distal ileum in 15% of patients. Aganglionosis can rarely involve the entire large and small intestine. Overall, HD occurs more frequently in boys, with a ratio of nearly 4 to 1, but in patients with total colonic aganglionosis, the ratio is approximately 2 to 1. Fewer than 10% of affected individuals have a relative with the disease, except for those with total colonic involvement, nearly one third of whom will have a positive family history.[2]

Although the etiology of HD is not known, there are clues to suggest that there is a significant genetic basis.[3] Heredity patterns are not straightforward and appear to involve multiple mutations at different sites on the genome.[4] In fact, mutations identified in patients with HD can be mapped to at least nine different loci, including the RET proto-oncogene. This variation appears to account to some degree for the variation in associated anomalies.[5] Other anomalies are found in nearly one third of patients with HD[3]: Trisomy 21 affects up to 5% of patients with HD.[6] Congenital heart disease occurs in approximately 5% of patients without trisomy 21 and nearly one half of those with trisomy 21. HD also occurs in association with other disorders of neural crest development such as Waardenburg-Shah syndrome,[7] Ondine's curse,[8] multiple endocrine neoplasia (MEN) 2,[9] neurofibromatosis,[10] and neuroblastoma.[11] Rarely, HD forms part of specific genetic syndromes such as Smith-Lemli-Opitz.[3,12]

PATHOPHYSIOLOGY

Aganglionosis results in a lack of receptive relaxation in the affected segment of bowel, creating a pseudo-obstruction. When this occurs in the rectum and distal colon as it does in HD, the result is a functional obstruction clinically manifest as constipation. Normal peristalsis depends on adjacent portions of the intestine contracting and relaxing in sequence. An intestine that cannot relax does not allow propagation of the peristaltic wave.

Nor does it serve as an effective reservoir, perhaps explaining the fact that the rectal vault is usually empty in patients with HD. Instead, the normal bowel becomes dilated proximal to the aganglionic segment, as it might in the presence of a true mechanical obstruction. Thus, the typical HD bowel pattern includes normal-appearing distal colon, dilated proximal colon (megacolon), and a tapered or funnel-shaped transition zone in between.

Ganglion cells originate in the neural crest and come to reside within the myenteric plexuses (Auerbach and Meissner) of the intestinal wall in early embryonic development where they differentiate into ganglion cells (Figure 55-1). The foregut is populated first; the cells then proceed distally along the entire length of the bowel, arriving at the level of the distal colon and rectum last. HD results from the incomplete caudal migration of neural crest cells along the intestinal tract, such that the proximal bowel is normally ganglionated but some portion of the distal portion remains aganglionated.[13] Where this migration stops is variable; consequently, patients differ with respect to the length of rectum and colon that is involved.

As an integral component of the enteric nervous system, ganglion cells inhibit local smooth muscle activity via a mechanism that is mediated by nitric oxide,[14] which allows normal receptive relaxation of the bowel. In addition, the absence of reflexive inhibitory activity at the level of the anal sphincter results in loss of the rectosphincteric reflex, an important component of defecation in which the anal sphincter relaxes in response to stimulation of the rectum by the arrival of a stool bolus. This forms the basis for anal manometric studies that are sometimes used to confirm the diagnosis.

Hirschsprung-associated enterocolitis (HAEC) is an acute and sometimes recurrent diarrheal illness that occurs only in children with HD. It occurs less frequently after the age of 2 years, but can affect even those who have undergone definitive surgical repair. The etiology is not known, and understanding of the pathophysiology remains incomplete. Bacterial overgrowth due to stasis probably plays a role in the pathogenesis; however, infants with other forms of mechanical or functional obstruction almost never develop true enterocolitis. There are clearly other factors that specifically place children with HD at risk for this potentially lethal illness. Possibilities include a specific immunodeficiency or mucosal barrier defect that is associated with the absence of ganglion cells.[15]

CLINICAL PRESENTATION

Hirschsprung's disease typically presents in infancy but can present at any age, including occasionally in adults. The hallmark of the disease is constipation, but there are several recognizable patterns of initial presentation. The first is the healthy-appearing newborn infant who fails to pass meconium

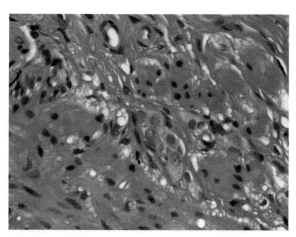

Figure 55-1. Ganglion cells within the myenteric plexus of the rectum. (Hematoxylin and eosin.)

TABLE 55-1. Causes of Severe Constipation by Age Group

Age Group	Differential Diagnosis
Newborn	Intestinal atresia/stenosis Meconium plug syndrome Intestinal duplication Small left colon syndrome Meconium ileus Imperforate anus Incarcerated hernia Intestinal volvulus
Toddler/school age	"Functional" constipation Milk-protein allergy Intestinal neuronal dysplasia Sacral agenesis Tethered cord Rectal duplication Pelvic tumor
Adolescent/adult	Functional constipation Dietary constipation Intestinal pseudo-obstruction Chagas disease

in the first 48 hours of life, which should always raise the suspicion of HD. The second is the newborn infant who develops abdominal distention and feeding intolerance within the first day or two of life, often accompanied by bilious emesis. Though the differential diagnosis also includes intestinal atresia, meconium ileus, and meconium plug/small left colon syndrome, HD is also in the differential diagnosis. Some infants with HD initially stool normally, especially if they are breast-fed,[16] and then develop severe constipation either when weaned to formula or table food: any child with constipation who requires rectal stimulation, suppositories, or enemas to evacuate should be evaluated for HD, especially if the history of constipation begins before attempts at potty training. Finally, the rare child with HD will present with an acute diarrheal illness, HAEC, rather than constipation. The clinical picture resembles a severe gastroenteritis, including vomiting, diarrhea, and abdominal distention and pain. Sometimes there is a history of constipation, but this is not always the case. These children can become extremely ill very quickly, with the rapid onset of severe dehydration, lethargy, and overwhelming sepsis. A low index of suspicion and aggressive management is necessary to avoid a lethal outcome.

Interestingly, there appears to be no correlation between the length of the aganglionic segment and the severity of the clinical presentation: some infants with total colonic aganglionosis have mild constipation, whereas others with short-segment disease can have severe obstipation. Although it is important to consider the diagnosis of HD in any child with constipation, children with mild symptoms that respond well to dietary changes or gentle laxatives are unlikely to have the disease. Similarly, older children with encopresis and soiling are much more likely to have functional constipation than HD.

DIFFERENTIAL DIAGNOSIS

Constipation is an extremely common complaint. Most cases can be classified as idiopathic or functional and are usually successfully treated with dietary changes, modification of toilet training technique, or mild stool softeners. Severe constipation is defined somewhat subjectively, but a more extensive evaluation should be considered for children who routinely go more than 2 days without a bowel movement, have a great deal of difficulty passing their stool, or cannot spontaneously defecate

without extraneous influence in the form of suppositories, enemas, or digital disimpaction.

The differential diagnosis of severe constipation depends on the age of the patient (Table 55-1). In newborns, failure to pass meconium in the first 48 hours of life, especially if associated with feeding intolerance, bilious emesis, or abdominal distention, requires consideration of other congenital intestinal anomalies that fall into the category of neonatal bowel obstruction: meconium plug, meconium ileus, or intestinal atresia. One should also consider imperforate anus, incarcerated hernia, volvulus, and intestinal duplication cyst. Meconium plug syndrome is a mechanical distal colonic obstruction that results from inspissated meconium and thick mucus. In the majority of cases, the cause is unknown and there are no long-term sequelae. However, it can be the harbinger of a more serious condition, specifically cystic fibrosis or HD, and may also be associated with small left colon syndrome, which commonly occurs in infants of diabetic mothers. A water-soluble contrast enema is therapeutic, allowing passage of the meconium plug and complete relief the obstruction. Meconium ileus is also caused by inspissated meconium, but the site of obstruction is the ileum. It is nearly always associated with cystic fibrosis. Water-soluble contrast enema is the initial treatment of choice, as it confirms the diagnosis, revealing a small unused colon (microcolon) and ileal pellets of hard meconium, and is sometimes successful in relieving the obstruction. Intestinal atresia most commonly occurs in the ileum or jejunum, though rare cases of colonic atresia have been reported. Contrast enema is sometimes necessary to confirm the diagnosis, but surgical repair is always required. A careful physical examination should exclude the diagnosis of imperforate anus, though in some patients a perianal fistula may be present and can be mistaken for an anal opening. Finally, children with partial sacral agenesis can have severe constipation, presumably due to poor development of associated muscles or nerves in the pelvis.

Children with HD who are breast-fed will occasionally do well initially, presumably because of the light consistency of the stool. Constipation might then develop when they transition to formula or solid food.

Toddlers who develop constipation are usually diagnosed with functional constipation or withholding behavior due to the pressures of toilet training. Although children with HD classically have a history of constipation from birth, the diagnosis should be considered in any child with severe constipation, even if it develops beyond the newborn period. Children with functional constipation sometimes require mechanical assistance (suppositories, enemas) to have a bowel movement and will often demonstrate frequent soiling of their underpants or frank incontinence (encopresis). On physical examination, their rectal vault is usually filled with a large amount of hard stool. Children with HD, on the other hand, very rarely develop fecal incontinence, and on examination the rectum is essentially normal and nearly always empty. Nevertheless, some older children or adolescents with what otherwise appears to be more typical severe constipation should undergo a work-up to exclude the diagnosis of HD.

Constipation in young children can also be due to dietary causes such as milk-protein allergy,[17] neurologic causes such as an unrecognized tethered cord, or true mechanical causes such as a rectal duplication cyst. Children with pelvic tumors such as neuroblastoma or sacrococcygeal teratoma can also sometimes present with the chief complaint of constipation. Finally, a child with one of the much less common types of intestinal pseudo-obstruction can present with severe constipation at an older age. Intestinal neuronal dysplasia is similar to HD in that it is caused by dysfunction of intestinal ganglion cells but is much less completely understood and difficult to treat. It can also occur in association with HD.[18] Syndromes associated with chronic intestinal pseudo-obstruction, an example of which is hollow visceral myopathy, can initially present much like HD.[19] Finally, though rarely seen in the United States, acquired enteric ganglionopathy (Chagas disease) can cause severe constipation; however, most patients also have significant esophageal dysmotility.[20]

DIAGNOSIS

The diagnosis of HD cannot be confirmed with certainty on the basis of history and physical examination alone. On physical examination, the child is typically well nourished and asymptomatic, although older infants and children with the disease can be malnourished. The abdomen is sometimes distended and tympanitic to percussion but can be unremarkable. There is often stool palpable in the lower abdomen and left lower quadrant. Though some experienced pediatricians and surgeons believe that digital rectal examination in patients with HD is notable for a characteristic hypertonicity, this is clearly very subjective and not sufficient to make the diagnosis. Likewise, an explosive bowel movement upon removal of the examining finger has been taught for many years to be a classic sign of HD. However, because the sensitivity and specificity of this sign appear to be poor, it cannot be used to confirm or exclude the diagnosis with any degree of certainty. Although history and physical examination findings might suggest the diagnosis of HD, further testing is always necessary to confirm or exclude the diagnosis.

In the past, anorectal manometry was used at some centers as the first diagnostic study in children beyond the newborn period who were thought to have HD.[21] A balloon is inserted into the rectum and a pressure transducer is placed within the anus. Normally, when the inflated balloon exerts pressure on the walls of the rectum, there should be a measurable decrease in the muscle tone of the anal sphincter. Individuals with HD lack this reflex relaxation. The test is considered somewhat reliable but very difficult to administer and interpret, especially in children at the extremes of size and age. Today, it is mainly used as a research tool at centers with considerable experience and occasionally in children who are thought to have "ultrashort segment" HD (also known as internal anal sphincter neurogenic achalasia, IASNA), in which the anal sphincter is involved but the diagnosis is otherwise impossible to confirm by biopsy.

The first diagnostic test recommended is usually the contrast enema. In newborns with a clinical picture of obstruction, it very useful as a diagnostic tool, and for conditions such as meconium plug or meconium ileus, it can also be therapeutic. Barium suspension is still often used, but because children with HD can have a great deal of difficulty clearing inspissated barium, it is usually preferable to use a water-soluble contrast agent. In normal individuals, the rectum is always larger in diameter than the sigmoid colon. The diagnosis of HD is suspected if the anterior-posterior diameter of the mid-rectum is less than that of the descending colon (Figure 55-2). The diagnosis is further supported by the combination of dilated proximal bowel and narrow or normal-appearing distal colon, separated by a tapered or funnel-shaped "transition zone."[22] A distinct transition may not be apparent in children with total colonic aganglionosis[23] or ultrashort-segment HD. Finally, some radiologists do not consider the diagnostic work-up to be complete until a radiograph is taken 24 hours after barium enema, as failure to evacuate all of the contrast within this time is considered further evidence of HD.

If the contrast enema is normal or otherwise nondiagnostic, the work-up for HD is usually considered to have been complete. However, there are some situations in which the clinical suspicion remains high or the enema is considered unreliable or equivocal. Furthermore, even when the contrast enema reveals what is considered to be a classic picture of HD, further confirmation is required before surgical intervention is undertaken.

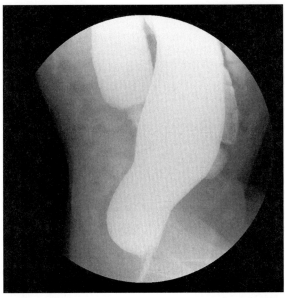

Figure 55-2. Contrast enema in two newborn patients with Hirschsprung's disease. Note the transition zone as the more dilated proximal colon tapers down to a narrower distal colon at the rectosigmoid junction.

In each of these situations, rectal biopsy to look for ganglion cells is considered a more definitive test.

Rectal biopsy can be performed in one of several ways. In children under 4 to 6 months of age, suction rectal biopsy is the procedure of choice: It is painless and can be performed safely at the bedside or in the office. It is also rapid and quite accurate, though it requires an experienced pathologist to review the histopathology. There are several commercially available devices, most of which are based on the same principle.[24] The smooth end of the instrument has a small side hole and a sharp blade that can slide back and forth just inside the opening. It is important to note that the very distal portion of the rectum normally lacks ganglion cells, so the biopsy must be taken at least 2 to 3 cm above the dentate line. After it is inserted into the rectum, suction is applied with a large syringe, which draws the mucosa into the lumen. The blade is then advanced, harvesting a small piece of tissue. This is usually repeated until two or three adequate samples are obtained. An adequate sample contains submucosa, which is visible as whitish tissue that has a firm consistency, distinguishable from the mucosa, which is red or pink and much more delicate. The technique is generally quite safe; however, bacteremia and bleeding may occur. Bowel perforation can occur if the device is advanced above the level of the peritoneal reflection, especially in very small infants, but this is extremely uncommon.[25]

An adequate suction rectal biopsy specimen must include the submucosa, which is examined using standard histopathologic techniques for the presence of ganglion cells. When ganglion cells are not seen, the diagnostic accuracy of the study is increased by finding hypertrophied nerve trunks (Figure 55-3). The accuracy of the technique may also be improved by staining for acetylcholinesterase, the level of which is markedly increased in patients with Hirschsprung's disease.[26]

Suction rectal biopsy is felt to be very accurate and, in most centers, is the standard approach to the diagnosis of HD. However, in children over the age of approximately 6 months and in those in whom suction rectal biopsy has been performed but is inconclusive, open rectal biopsy may be necessary. This is performed in the operating room under general anesthesia. A full-thickness biopsy is usually performed and, because it provides the opportunity to examine both myenteric and submucosal

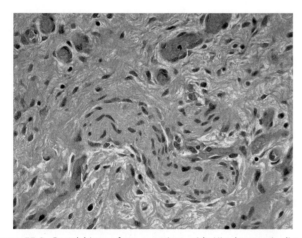

Figure 55-3. Rectal biopsy from a patient with Hirschsprung's disease. Ganglion cells were not identified. Hypertrophied nerves are clearly visible, which confirms the diagnosis of Hirschsprung's disease. (Hematoxylin and eosin.)

plexuses for the presence of ganglion cells, it is considered the diagnostic gold standard. It is also generally very safe and produces minimal if any postoperative discomfort.

TREATMENT

Most children with HD are candidates for definitive surgery, which involves removal of the aganglionic segment of colon and rectum, and the creation of a neorectum using proximal normally ganglionated bowel. Three operations have been developed since operative repair became feasible in the 1950s and 1960s (Figure 55-4). The decision as to which operation to perform is based principally on the training and preference of the surgeon and sometimes based on the clinical characteristics of the patient. The operations have been studied extensively, and each has produced similar excellent results.

Swenson developed the first successful operation to treat HD in the 1950s,[27] and Swenson's is still the standard to which all new operations for HD are compared. It is still the preferred approach by many pediatric surgeons around the world. The basic principles of the operation are to resect the aganglionic colon and rectum down to the anus (the dentate line) and to pull the normally ganglionated colon down to the anus, where a circumferential anastomosis is created transanally. The operation has been modified somewhat in that it now usually includes an internal sphincterotomy, but the underlying principles remain the same.[28] Although today it has been replaced for the most part by the other two available operations, the long-term results published by its many proponents (including Dr. Swenson himself[29]) suggest that it is an excellent operation for the treatment of this disease.[30]

The second operation to become popular was developed by Duhamel in 1960[31] and modified by Martin in 1967.[32] The Duhamel-Martin operation is different from the others in that the aganglionic rectum is retained and becomes part of the neorectum. The aganglionic colon above the rectum is resected, the ganglionated colon is brought down to the anus behind the native rectum, and a side-to-side anastomosis is created between the two by using a gastrointestinal stapling device to obliterate the common wall between the two. The stapling device is placed through the anus and is designed to seal the two portions of bowel with a secure line of staples and to cut between the two staple lines to divide the common wall, thus creating a single common lumen. Retaining the native rectum is thought to maintain normal sensory and innervation of the rectum and pelvic organs. Meanwhile, the normal colon placed in apposition to the immotile native segment provides the propulsive action to evacuate the rectum. Martin's modification included using much less length of rectum and colon (less stasis) and the trimming of the blind upper pouch of the native rectum to prevent a diverticulum in which stool could accumulate. This operation is still performed today with some frequency, especially for reoperations and other unusual circumstances, but also in many cases as the first operation. Its principal drawback is that it is difficult to perform in newborn infants as a primary procedure (without a temporizing colostomy), which is more and more the trend in this day and age. Nevertheless, the long-term results are overall quite good.[33]

The most commonly performed operation for the treatment of HD today is the Soave endorectal pull-through operation. It was first described by Soave in 1964[34] and modified by Boley in 1967.[35] In the this operation, rather than removing the entire

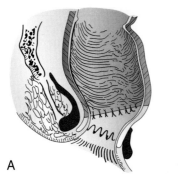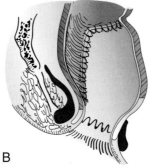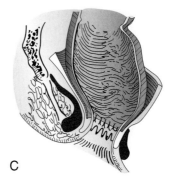

A   B   C

Figure 55-4. The three most commonly performed operations for Hirschsprung's disease: (**A**) Swenson's operation: The aganglionic rectum is removed and the normally ganglionated proximal bowel is pulled through and anastomosed at the dentate line. (**B**) Duhamel-Martin operation: The aganglionic rectum is preserved, the normally ganglionated proximal bowel is brought down behind the native rectum, and the wall between the two is obliterated with a stapling device to create a single common lumen. (**C**) Soave-Boley operation: The mucosa and submucosa of the distal rectum is removed, preserving the outer muscle layer, and the proximal ganglionated bowel is delivered through the muscle cuff and sutured just above the dentate line.

rectum, the muscular outer layer of the rectum is preserved, for the purpose of trying to preserve normal sensory function and to avoid injury to the other nerves of the pelvis. In effect, the mucosa and submucosa are removed, leaving the muscle layers intact. The ganglionated colon is then pulled through this "cuff" of muscle (which is split in the posterior midline) and anastomosed just above the dentate line. The normal colon is thus enclosed circumferentially by the musculature of the native rectum. The recommended length of retained muscular cuff is getting shorter, as is the recommended length of the normal mucosa that is retained above the dentate line, leading some to suggest that there is currently very little difference between the Swenson and Soave operations as they are performed today.

In the past, all children with HD initially underwent a diverting colostomy performed at the distalmost level of normal ganglionation, referred to as a "leveling" colostomy. Definitive surgery was usually felt to be safe after 3 to 6 months, depending on the child's growth and the presence of comorbidities. This was considered mandatory in order to allow the dilated proximal bowel to return to normal caliber, and for the child to be large enough for the operation to be performed safely. Leveling colostomies are rarely performed today, because the diagnosis of HD is being made earlier and surgical techniques have been refined to allow operations to be performed in the newborn period. There are also several very good minimal-access surgical techniques available. these include laparoscopic-assisted operations[36] and the transanal primary pull-through.[37-40] Using these approaches, the operation can be performed almost entirely transanally. The pull-through operation itself is always a version of one of the three traditional operations, and it is important for the surgeon to adhere strictly to the basic principles of the standard operation, but thus far the results from these minimally invasive operations appear to be quite good.

Eighty-five percent of individuals with HD have so-called *short-segment* disease, meaning that the aganglionic segment includes only the rectum and some variable length of distal sigmoid colon. These are the patients whose long-term results are the best after having undergone one the three procedures described. In general, the longer the aganglionic segment, the less likely the patient will be a candidate for a primary pull-through operation and the less optimal the long-term results. In extremely rare cases, the entire intestinal tract lacks

ganglion cells. These patients were formerly treated with the longitudinal intestinal myomectomy procedure[41] but today are more likely to be treated by small bowel transplantation.[42] When the entire colon (and usually a short segment of the ileum) is involved, this is referred to as *total colonic aganglionosis*. These patients are usually managed using a modification of one of the three basic operations, but the results are generally not as good compared to those achieved with short-segment disease.[43] At the other extreme is the controversial concept of *ultrashort-segment* disease, in which only the internal sphincter is affected by aganglionosis.[44,45] In these patients, rectal biopsy is, by definition, normal. Anal manometry might therefore be the only way to confirm the diagnosis.[46] Patients given the diagnosis of HD as adolescents or adults are difficult to manage because of the significant anatomic and physiologic effects of years of chronic colonic dilatation and laxative abuse.[47] A leveling colostomy is almost always needed for several months to allow the bowel to return to a more normal diameter before definitive surgery can be performed safely.

Hirschsprung-Associated Enterocolitis

Hirschsprung-associated enterocolitis (HAEC) is a severe infectious colitis that is peculiar to children with HD and can occur even after definitive surgery for the disease. Children who present with signs and symptoms suggestive of enterocolitis must be treated urgently and with extreme vigilance. The classic picture includes abdominal distention and diarrhea that is often described as "explosive." Patients often also have fever, lethargy, and/or vomiting. The stool sometimes contains obvious blood or mucus, and parents frequently describe it as intensely malodorous. Infants especially can progress rapidly to dehydration, obtundation, and shock. On physical examination, the child might have an explosive bowel movement immediately after digital rectal examination. The important thing to remember is that the initial clinical clues to the diagnosis can be subtle and nonspecific. Therefore any child with HD who presents with a clinical picture that suggests gastroenteritis or a viral syndrome should be aggressively evaluated for the possibility of enterocolitis.

Primary treatment of the child with enterocolitis includes intravenous hydration, broad-spectrum antibiotic therapy (including coverage for anaerobic bacteria), and rectal irrigation with normal saline to help evacuate stool from the rectum and distal colon. The child is not fed initially and should be monitored closely for signs of sepsis. Mortality was formerly quite high,[48] but more recent studies report that the current mortality rate is minimal, although deaths still occasionally occur.[49] Parents and pediatricians must be trained to identify the early signs of enterocolitis and to send any patient with even mild symptoms to the emergency department for evaluation. There should be a low threshold to admit the patient to the hospital for observation and empiric therapy.

Treatment of HAEC should continue for 3 days to 2 weeks, depending on illness severity. Potential complications include colonic perforation and overwhelming sepsis, but surgical intervention, in the form of diverting colostomy or ileostomy, is rarely needed. Some surgeons recommend empiric prophylactic saline rectal irrigations in all patients with HD for 1 year after definitive surgery.[50] This appears to reduce the risk of HAEC, but it is labor intensive and difficult for many families to perform on a routine basis.

RESULTS OF SURGICAL THERAPY

Overall, the results of surgical therapy for HD are very good, with most children being able to defecate regularly and to grow normally.[51] Nevertheless, there is a significant minority of children who have ongoing issues, mostly related to persistent constipation, anastomotic stricture, or problems with toilet training, or recurrent enterocolitis.[52,53] Overall, mortality varies but is less than 5% in most studies, but significantly higher in patients with trisomy 21 and total colonic aganglionosis.[51] Most are treated effectively with an individualized bowel regimen, usually best managed by experts who specialize in severe constipation in a multidisciplinary clinic that includes experienced surgeons, gastroenterologists with expertise in gastrointestinal motility, and dedicated nurse practitioners.

Patients with recurrent constipation after definitive surgery should be evaluated for "recurrent" HD.[54] This is somewhat controversial, in that it is not clear how a congenital disease can recur in the true sense of the word. Nevertheless, it is clear that there are those who are documented to have ganglion cells in the segment of bowel that was pulled through (on the basis of biopsies performed at the time of the operation), but who now lack ganglion cells on repeat full-thickness biopsy some time after the operation. Theories include erroneous biopsy, the possibility that it was the transition zone that was pulled through, and that ganglion cells can die and thus disappear after surgery, presumably due to ischemia or surgical handling. Some of these patients have mild recurrent disease that can be managed medically with a bowel regimen. Patients with intractable constipation require surgical therapy in the form of myomectomy[55] or another pull-through operation.[56]

Complications are common but usually easily managed. Anastomotic leaks are extremely rare, but are known to occur from time to time, usually due to ischemia of the distal segment, excessive tension, or a technical error. A stricture may develop at the anastomosis, but this is usually easily treated with anal dilatation, which might need to be repeated several times over the course of several months before it heals properly.[57] Fecal incontinence is rare and is usually the result of recurrent constipation and subsequent overflow incontinence

or technical error.[58] Frank neurogenic incontinence appears to be quite rare, but is more common in children with associated trisomy 21, sacral agenesis, or tethered cord. In many cases, a poor functional result cannot be easily explained on the basis of a technical complication or obvious physiologic problem and appears instead to be related to some other factors related to the disease itself but that remain incompletely understood.

It is probably best to think of HD as a systemic disease and the operation as palliative rather than curative. Many patients report significant ongoing issues related to bowel habits in the long term that affect their quality of life.[59] Ongoing problems can continue, and these patients should be followed periodically throughout childhood and even into adolescence to be sure that bowel function is as close to normal as possible and that the child is maintaining normal growth and development.

SUMMARY

Hirschsprung's disease is a congenital intestinal pseudo-obstruction that always involves the rectum and a variable portion of the colon, usually resulting in severe constipation. The cause is unknown, though there is increasing evidence that it is at least partially determined by genetic factors. The defining feature of the disease is the inability to demonstrate the presence of ganglion cells within the myenteric plexuses of the affected colon and rectum. Although it can present at any age, including in adulthood, the disease more commonly presents in infants who have failed to pass meconium within 48 hours of birth or who develop severe constipation very early in life. Rarely, it can present acutely with enterocolitis, an acute diarrheal illness that can cause life-threatening complications.

Derived from the neural crest, ganglion cells migrate down the entire length of the intestinal tract, starting in the proximal bowel and working their way toward the rectum during development. Hirschsprung's disease results when this cranial-caudal migration fails to progress beyond a certain point (the transition zone), leaving the distal colon and rectum without ganglion cells. An important part of the enteric neural network, ganglion cells appear to mediate bowel wall relaxation, which is critical for the propagation of a peristaltic wave. Aganglionic bowel thus remains contracted, resulting in a type of pseudo-obstruction.

The diagnosis is supported by findings on contrast enema, in which the proximal normal bowel appears dilated (megacolon) while the distal aganglionic bowel appears essentially normal. The diagnosis is confirmed by the demonstration of ganglion cells on rectal biopsy. The primary treatment is one of several operations that involves removal of the affected bowel and creation of a neorectum with more proximal ganglionated colon. Nowadays, patients rarely require a temporary colostomy before definitive surgical repair and instead are often considered candidates for primary repair in infancy. Minimally invasive techniques are also available in many centers. The outcomes of surgical therapy are generally good, but there are some patients who continue to have constipation or complications of their surgery, including stricture, recurrent aganglionosis, and episodes of enterocolitis requiring treatment. Overall, the majority of children with Hirschsprung's disease are able to grow normally and live happy and healthy lives.

REFERENCES

3. Stewart DR, von Allmen D. The genetics of Hirschsprung disease. Gastroenterol Clin North Am 2003;32:819–837, vi.

13. Iwashita T, Kruger GM, Pardal R, et al. Hirschsprung disease is linked to defects in neural crest stem cell function. Science 2003;301:972–976.

29. Swenson O. Hirschsprung's disease: a review. Pediatrics 2002;109:914–918.

36. Georgeson KE, Cohen RD, Hebra A, et al. Primary laparoscopic-assisted endorectal colon pull-through for Hirschsprung's disease: a new gold standard. Ann Surg 1999;229:678–682; discussion 682–683.

38. Langer JC, Seifert M, Minkes RK. One-stage Soave pull-through for Hirschsprung's disease: a comparison of the transanal and open approaches. J Pediatr Surg 2000;35:820–822.

49. Wang JS, Lee HC, Huang FY, et al. Unexpected mortality in pediatric patients with postoperative Hirschsprung's disease. Pediatr Surg Int 2004;20:525–528.

See expertconsult.com for a complete list of references and the review questions for this chapter.

IMPERFORATE ANUS 56

Alberto Peña • Marc A. Levitt

The term *imperforate anus* is a misnomer that is commonly used to refer to a spectrum of anorectal malformations, ranging from a benign defect that requires a minor operation and results in an excellent prognosis to complex malformations with a high incidence of associated defects requiring sophisticated and specialized surgical procedures. Since the mid-1980s, significant advances have been achieved in the field of pediatric surgery that allow for a better anatomic reconstruction of these defects, preserving other important pelvic structures. Yet, at least 30% of all patients born with these defects still have fecal incontinence even after a technically correct surgical repair, and another 30% have other functional defecation problems, mainly constipation and varying degrees of soiling.[1,2] We have made great strides in the anatomic reconstruction, but are still challenged in consistently obtaining an excellent functional result. These malformations occur in about 1:4000 to 1:5000 newborns.[3-5] The chance of having a second child affected by this type of defect is about 1%.[6-9]

CLASSIFICATION AND DESCRIPTION OF DEFECTS

A classification presented here (Table 56-1) is based on therapeutic and prognostic facts as well as the frequency of associated defects. It was designed to help the clinician increase the index of suspicion and to establish therapeutic priorities.

Perineal Fistula

In this defect, the rectum opens into the perineum anterior to the center of the sphincter, into a usually stenotic orifice. In male patients, the perineum may exhibit other features that help in recognition of this defect, such as a prominent midline skin bridge (known as "bucket-handle" malformation) or a subepithelial midline raphe fistula that looks like a black ribbon because it is full of meconium (Figure 56-1). These features are externally visible and help in the diagnosis of a perineal fistula. This is the most benign of anorectal defects. Fewer than 10% of these children have an associated urologic defect, and 100% of them achieve bowel control after proper treatment.[1,2]

Interestingly, this group of patients suffers from the highest incidence of constipation, a disorder that should not be underestimated, as discussed later in this chapter. The operation to repair these malformations is a relatively simple anoplasty; it usually is performed during the neonatal period without a protective colostomy. Even when this is considered a relatively easy procedure, there is a risk of provoking an urethral injury in male patients. Therefore, this operation should always be performed with a urethral catheter in place.

Rectal Atresia/Stenosis

In this rare defect, the patient is born with a normal-looking anus externally, but an attempt to take the rectal temperature discloses an obstruction located 1 to 2 cm above the mucocutaneous junction of the anus. The sphincter mechanism in these patients is normal, as is the anal canal. Associated defects are almost nonexistent except for presacral mass, which must be screened for. The prognosis is excellent, and 100% of these patients achieve bowel control.[1,2,10] The repair involves an operation called a posterior-sagittal anorectoplasty (PSARP), which can be done at birth, with or without a diverting colostomy.

Imperforate Anus Without Fistula

In these cases, the rectum ends blindly, without a fistula, approximately 1 to 2 cm above the perineum, usually at the level of the bulbar urethra. The sacrum and sphincter mechanism are usually good, and about 80% of these patients achieve bowel control after the main repair.[1,2,10,11] Approximately 50% of patients with this defect have Down syndrome. Conversely, 95% of patients with Down syndrome who have anorectal malformations have this specific type.[11] With or without Down syndrome, children with this defect have a good functional prognosis. This malformation can be repaired primarily at birth, without a colostomy, provided the surgeon has enough experience and the baby is in good condition. The distal rectum, although not connected to the urinary tract, is intimately attached to the urethra, and great care must be taken not to injure it.

Vestibular Fistula

This is the most common defect in female patients. The rectum opens into the vestibule of the female genitalia, which is the mucosa lined area outside the hymen (Figure 56-2). The rectum and vagina share a very thin common wall. The sacrum and sphincters are usually of good quality. Approximately 95% of these patients achieve bowel control after surgery,[1,2,10] and 30% of them have associated urologic defects.[12]

This malformation can also be repaired primarily, without a colostomy, provided the patient is in good health and the surgeon has experience in the management of newborns with these defects. Approximately 5% have an associated gynecologic anomaly, either a vaginal septum or absence of the vagina, and a vaginoscopy is performed at the time of the planned reconstruction to assess this.[13]

TABLE 56-1. **Classification of Anorectal Malformations**

Males	Females
Cutaneous (perineal fistula)	Cutaneous (perineal fistula)
Recto-urethral fistula	Vestibular fistula
Bulbar	Imperforate anus without fistula
Prostatic	Rectal atresia
Recto-bladder neck fistula	Cloaca
Imperforate anus without fistula	Complex malformations

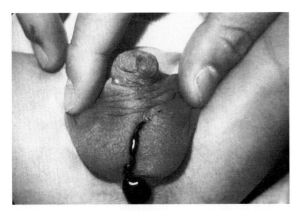

Figure 56-1. Perineum of a male patient with a perineal fistula. The meconium can be seen under a very thin layer of epithelium.

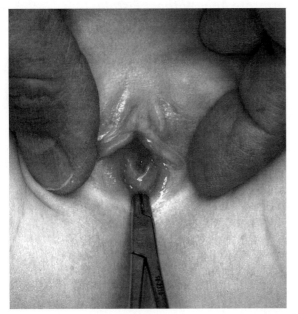

Figure 56-2. Perineum of a female patient with a rectovestibular fistula.

Rectourethral Fistula

This is by far the most common defect in male patients. The rectum communicates with the posterior urethra through a narrow orifice (fistula). This fistula may be located in the lower posterior urethra (bulbar fistula) (Figure 56-3) or in the upper posterior urethra (prostatic fistula) (Figure 56-4). Of patients with rectourethral bulbar fistula, 85% achieve fecal continence after the main repair, but only 60% of those with rectoprostatic fistula do so.[1,2,10] About 30% of patients with bulbar urethral

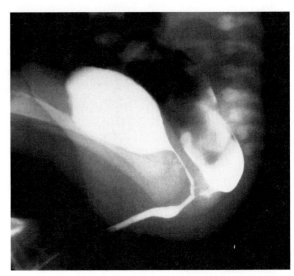

Figure 56-3. Colostogram of bulbar fistula. From Holcomb, GW, and Murphy, JP, eds. Ashcraft's Pediatric Surgery, 5th ed. Philadelphia: Elsevier; 2010.

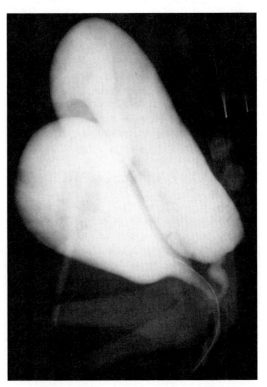

Figure 56-4. Colostogram of prostatic fistula.

fistula and 60% of patients with rectoprostatic fistula have associated urological defects.[12] The quality of the sacrum usually is good in the former case but frequently is abnormal in the latter. Most of these patients must receive a colostomy at birth. Patients with rectourethral bulbar fistula can be repaired at birth without a previous protective colostomy, provided the baby is in good condition and the surgeon has enough experience.

Recto-bladder Neck Fistula

This is the highest defect seen in male patients. The rectum opens into the bladder neck (Figure 56-5). Some 90% of these patients have significant associated urologic defects.[12] Only

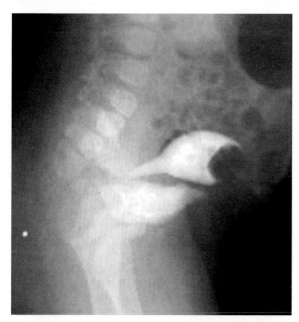

Figure 56-5. Colostogram of recto-bladder neck fistula.

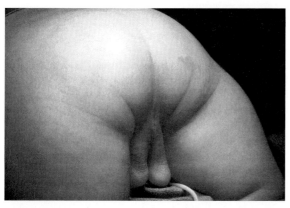

Figure 56-6. Perineum of a patient with a recto-bladder neck fistula. These patients with very high defects have a flat bottom, no perineal groove, and frequently a bifid scrotum.

15% achieve bowel control after the main repair.[1,2,10] The sacrum usually has poor quality. In these patients, the repair includes a posterior-sagittal approach plus a laparotomy or a laparoscopy to reach a very high rectum. The perineum in these patients is usually flat, meaning that they do not have the normal midline groove and one cannot see an anal dimple (Figure 56-6).

Cloaca

This is by far the most complex problem seen in female patients (Figure 56-7). This defect is defined as a malformation in which rectum, vagina, and urethra are fused together into a single common channel that opens into a single orifice in the perineum[14] (Figures 56-7 and 56-8). The prognosis varies depending on the quality of the sacrum and the length of the common channel. Most patients with a common channel longer than 3 cm require intermittent catheterization after the main repair in order to empty the bladder. About 50% of these patients have voluntary bowel movements.[10,15] On the other hand, if the common channel is shorter than 3 cm, 20% of the

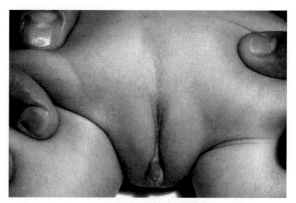

Figure 56-7. Perineum of a patient with a cloaca showing single perineal orifice.

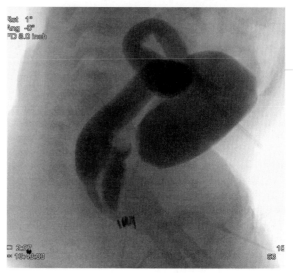

Figure 56-8. Cloacogram.

patients require intermittent catheterization to empty the bladder and about 70% have voluntary bowel movements.[10,14,15]

Ninety percent of patients with cloaca have an associated urologic problem.[12] This may represent a serious urologic emergency that the clinician should recognize early in life, in order to detect and treat an obstructive uropathy.

More than 40% of cloacas also have hydrocolpos, which is a very distended, tense, giant vagina that may compress the opening of the ureters at the trigone, provoking bilateral megaureters.[14-16] A significant number of these patients also have vesicoureteral reflux. At birth, these patients require the opening of a colostomy and drainage of the hydrocolpos when present. Rarely, some sort of urinary diversion to take care of the obstructive uropathy is also needed. After 2 to 4 months of life, they undergo a complex operation during which the three main structures (the rectum, vagina, and urethra) are separated and placed in their normal location. Patients suffering from cloacas with a common channel shorter than 3 cm require an operation done posterior-sagittally, and it is not usually necessary to open the abdomen. In doing this procedure, a maneuver called total urogenital mobilization is performed[17] (Figure 56-9), which facilitates the procedure, and therefore this type of malformation can be repaired by most general pediatric surgeons. On the other hand, a cloaca with a common channel longer than 3 cm

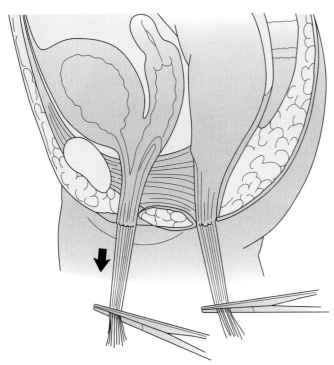

Figure 56-9. Illustration of total urogenital mobilization. Modified with permission from Peña (1997).[17]

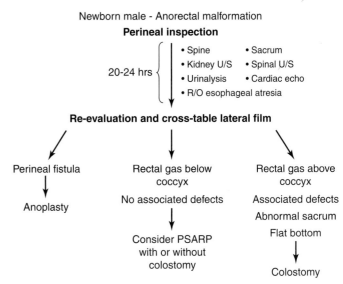

Figure 56-10. Decision-making algorithm for male newborns. Adapted from Peña and Levitt (2005).[13]

requires not only the posterior-sagittal approach but also a laparotomy and a series of decision-making steps that require a significant amount of experience. These malformations should be repaired by specialized surgeons in centers with much experience in this area.[15]

ASSOCIATED DEFECTS

The most common defects associated with anorectal malformations are urologic. The frequency of these associations varies with each defect as has already been described.[1,2] The next most common associated defects are those of the spine and sacrum. The quality of the spine and sacrum has a direct impact on the prognosis for bowel and urinary control. A very hypoplastic sacrum, absent sacrum, or associated spinal problem such as tethered cord or myelomeningocele correlate directly with poor fecal and urinary incontinence.

Another group of patients have gastrointestinal defects, including esophageal atresia, duodenal atresia, or other kinds of atresia in the intestinal tract. Approximately 30% of all patients suffer from some sort of cardiovascular defect, but only 10% require surgery. The other 20% usually represent patent ductus arteriosus, atrial or ventricular septal defects, or defects with no hemodynamic implications.

EARLY MANAGEMENT AND DIAGNOSIS

When a child is born with an anorectal malformation, two main questions must be answered within the first 24 hours of life:
1. Does the infant have an associated defect (most likely urologic or cardiac) that endangers his or her life and requires immediate treatment?
2. Does the infant need a colostomy, or can the malformation be repaired in a primary way without a colostomy?

These two questions must be answered in this order. The higher and more complex the anorectal defect, the greater the chance of a dangerous associated defect. Figures 56-10 and 56-11 show decision-making algorithms used in the early management of these newborns.

All infants with anorectal malformations should have an abdominal and pelvic ultrasound examination during the first hours of life. This simple test can exclude hydronephrosis, megaureters, and hydrocolpos. If the patient has any of these conditions, further urologic evaluation may be required. An echocardiogram can also be performed. The perineum must be meticulously evaluated, because it provides a series of clues that help to answer the second question. The presence of a midline groove with two well-formed buttocks and a conspicuous anal dimple (Figure 56-12) is a good prognostic sign indicating that the patient probably has a low type of malformation. One should always look for the presence of a perineal fistula, which sometimes is extremely small. On the other hand, a flat bottom (no midline groove and absence of an anal dimple) occurs in infants with high defects (see Figure 56-6). An ultrasound of the lower spine done in the first few days of life can rule out the presence of tethered cord, or other spinal problems that are associated with a higher type of anorectal malformation with poor prognosis.[18]

When a child is born with an anorectal malformation, the abdomen is not distended. During the following 18 to 24 hours, the abdomen becomes distended and the intraluminal pressure of the bowel significantly increases, forcing the meconium through the lowest part of the rectum, which is surrounded by the sphincter mechanism. One can expect that the meconium will pass through a fistula, usually after 18 to 24 hours. The golden rule in the early diagnosis of these children is to wait at least 18 to 24 hours before making a decision. Male infants need a urinalysis to look for traces of meconium. A piece of gauze placed on the tip of the penis may filter the meconium when the infant voids, making the diagnosis of a rectourinary fistula, which is an indication to open a colostomy in most cases. A tiny perineal fistula may remain unnoticed and after 18 to 24 hours a drop of meconium may become evident. A patient with meconium on the perineum, evidence

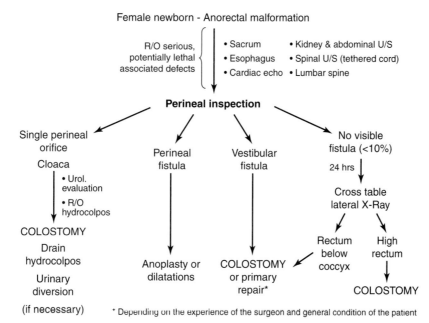

Female newborn - Anorectal malformation

R/O serious, potentially lethal associated defects
- Sacrum
- Esophagus
- Cardiac echo
- Kidney & abdominal U/S
- Spinal U/S (tethered cord)
- Lumbar spine

Perineal inspection

Single perineal orifice — Cloaca
- Urol. evaluation
- R/O hydrocolpos

COLOSTOMY
Drain hydrocolpos
Urinary diversion
(if necessary)

Perineal fistula → Anoplasty or dilatations

Vestibular fistula → COLOSTOMY or primary repair*

No visible fistula (<10%) → 24 hrs → Cross table lateral X-Ray → Rectum below coccyx / High rectum → COLOSTOMY

* Depending on the experience of the surgeon and general condition of the patient

Figure 56-11. Decision-making algorithm for female newborns. Adapted from Peña and Levitt (2005).[13]

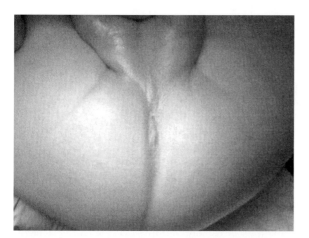

Figure 56-12. Perineum of a patient with a rectourethral fistula. The patient has a perineal groove, well-formed buttocks, and an anal dimple.

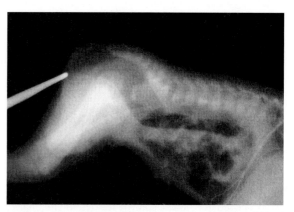

Figure 56-13. Cross-table lateral film. From Holcomb GW, and Murphy JP, eds. Ashcraft's Pediatric Surgery, 5th ed. Philadelphia: Elsevier; 2010.

of a perineal fistula, can be treated with an anoplasty, without a colostomy.

In about 5% of patients, a perineal fistula cannot be found. There is no evidence of a cloaca, no evidence of vestibular fistula, and no meconium in the urine. In such cases, the patient may have an imperforate anus without fistula. To confirm this, a cross-table lateral film with the child prone and the pelvis elevated is taken with a radiopaque marker placed on the anal dimple. The location of the rectum full of gas can be radiologically demonstrated, and the distance between the rectum and the perineum can be measured. A primary approach without a colostomy can be considered when the image of the rectum with gas is seen below the coccyx (Figure 56-13).

Recently, the pediatric surgical community has shown a tendency to operate on more and more anorectal malformations primarily, without a protective colostomy. The rationale is to try to avoid the three-stage approach (colostomy, main repair, and colostomy closure), decreasing the number of operations to one. We agree with this tendency with the specific purpose of

decreasing the trauma to the patient. However, the colostomy is still the safest way to avoid complications during the repair of anorectal malformations. We believe that every surgeon should make an individual decision concerning colostomy or primary repair, based on the general condition of the patient, the infrastructure of the hospital where the surgeon works, and his or her own personal experience in the management of these children.

MAIN REPAIR

Anoplasty

An anoplasty is an operation performed with the patient in prone position and the pelvis elevated. A newborn does not require bowel preparation. The operation takes about 1 hour but requires many meticulous and delicate maneuvers to avoid damage to important continence structures, as well as injury to the urethra in male patients.

An older child with an untreated perineal fistula usually presents with fecal impaction and megasigmoid. These patients require a full bowel preparation before the operation, and after the procedure also need parenteral nutrition and fasting 7 to 10 days to avoid passage of stool and potential infection.

Posterior Sagittal Anorectoplasty

Most anorectal malformations can be repaired by using a posterior-sagittal approach between the buttocks. The rationale behind this operation is that the entire sphincter mechanism can be divided in the midline to avoid nerve damage. An electric stimulator is used to determine the precise limits of the sphincter. The goal of the operation is to separate the rectum from the genitourinary tract, to dissect it enough to reach the perineum, and to place it within the limits of the sphincter mechanism. Sometimes the rectum is so dilated that some degree of tapering is needed to achieve this goal. In 10% of male patients, it is necessary to open the abdomen or to perform a laparoscopic procedure in addition to the posterior-sagittal approach to reach a rectum that is located extremely high in the abdomen (recto-bladder neck fistula).[1,2,10] In such cases, the rectum can be mobilized with a laparotomy or laparoscopy. The posterior-sagittal incision can be done with the patient supine and the legs elevated. The surgeon creates a path immediately behind the urinary tract, through which the rectum is pulled. About 40% of female patients born with a cloaca also need a laparotomy to reach a very high rectum, a very high vagina, or both. In these cases, the operation is called posterior sagittal ano-recto-vagino-urethroplasty which is a very specialized and delicate operation that has a goal of anatomic reconstruction of the rectum, urethra, and vagina.[15]

FUNCTIONAL SEQUELAE

Elements Required for Bowel Control

Bowel continence involves three main elements: anal canal and rectal sensation, sphincters, and colonic motility.[19]

Anal Canal and Rectal Sensation

Sensation needed for bowel control resides in the anal canal, from a few millimeters above the pectinate line to the anal verge. In that area, it is possible for the patient to discriminate between gas, liquid, and solid contents and even to discern changes in temperature.[20] Another type of sensation that resides in the rectum and is elicited when the rectum is distended (which likely stretches the voluntary muscles that surround the rectum) is called proprioception. The rectal mucosa has no sensation; the proprioception receptors reside in the voluntary muscle that surrounds the rectum.[21,22]

Sphincters

The sphincters are represented by a funnel-like voluntary muscle structure that inserts in the middle portion of the pelvic rim and extends all the way down to the skin surrounding the rectum and anus and a thickening of the circular layer of the smooth muscle in the lowest part of the intestine. The individual must detect the presence of stool and then use the sphincters to contract and, at the appropriate time, relax.

Rectosigmoid Motility

Under normal circumstances, the rectosigmoid acts like a reservoir. It catches all the solid stool that comes from the rest of the colon. Once a day or every other day, depending on the person's habit, the rectosigmoid starts to empty by pushing the fecal contents toward the anal canal. The contact of the rectal contents with the anal canal gives the person the necessary information to note the nature of the rectal contents. Depending on the surrounding social circumstances, the person may elect to relax the voluntary sphincter or to contract it. Once the decision is made to empty the rectosigmoid, the voluntary sphincter is relaxed and the next wave of peristaltic contraction empties the rectosigmoid.

Children with anorectal malformations have deficiencies in all three of these main elements of bowel control. The sensation that resides in the anal canal exists only in those with anorectal malformations in which an anal canal is present. There is only one specific defect with that characteristic; it is called rectal atresia and occurs in only 1% of all cases.[1,2] These patients have a normal-looking anus with an atresia located 1 to 2 cm above the anal verge. All other patients with anorectal malformations are born with no anal canal or with a very abnormal one. Therefore, one cannot expect very precise discrimination in these children. They have different degrees of proprioception, usually good enough to be toilet trained. The presence of a solid piece of stool moving in the rectum is perceived by the patient in a rather vague manner, but it is strong enough to give the signal to defecate. Liquid stool is more difficult to sense.

The internal sphincteric mechanism in children with anorectal malformations is a matter of debate and, in addition, there is no scientific evidence that such a structure exists or is preserved after the surgical repair of these defects. Functional and pharmacologic studies of the distal end of the rectum (fistula) in specimens of patients suffering from anorectal malformations attempting to demonstrate the presence of an internal sphincter have yielded ambiguous results.[23] The voluntary sphincter mechanism has various degrees of hypodevelopment in children with anorectal malformations. In very severe cases of high defects, there is basically no trace of the sphincter, whereas in patients with perineal fistula, the sphincter is essentially normal. Finally, rectosigmoid motility in children with anorectal malformations is usually abnormal. If the surgical technique includes preservation of the rectosigmoid, these children usually experience constipation, which is the clinical manifestation of rectosigmoid hypomotility. They do not have the capacity to empty the rectum an efficient way but rather keep passing small amounts of stool throughout the day. The severity of this disorder varies from minimal to very severe, the latter resulting in fecal impaction.

Patients for whom the operative technique included resection of the rectosigmoid do not have a reservoir. They have a tendency to pass more liquid stools constantly day and night, which is the worst type of incontinence. This resulted from the use of endorectal and abdomino-perineal techniques, which are very rarely used today.

Fecal Incontinence

The most feared sequela in children with anorectal malformations is fecal incontinence. At least 30% of all children with these defects have this devastating problem.[1,2,19]

The general goals in the management of children with anorectal malformations are to anatomically reconstruct all malformations, to monitor the patients on a long-term basis taking care of their functional disturbances, and to provide the optimal circumstances for them to maintain bowel control if possible. For those patients who were born with a poor-prognosis type of defect, a bowel management program must be provided so that they can stay artificially clean and socially accepted.[24,25] Some patients who were born with a defect that has a good prognosis reach 3 years of age and still do not have bowel control. In these cases, the bowel management program is provided on a temporary basis, and every year during the summer vacation, the child is again given the opportunity to become toilet trained.

The bowel management program used for children with fecal incontinence consists of teaching the family to clean the colon once a day with an enema. The type and quality of the enemas vary, depending on the type of colon that the patient has.

The bowel management program is implemented over a period of 1 week. The contrast enema performed at the initiation of the program provides a clue to the volume and type of enema that the patient requires. A nurse teaches the parents how to clean the colon. It is a process of trial and error to determine the precise enema that works.

Fecally incontinent constipated patients require a large enema to stay completely clean, 24 hours per day. The fact that they are constipated is beneficial because it helps them to remain clean in between enemas. The saline enema may need to be combined with glycerin, soap, or phosphate to make it stronger. There is another group of patients who have fecal incontinence and a tendency to diarrhea. Often they were operated on with a technique that included resection of the original rectosigmoid. The main challenge in their bowel management is to keep the colon quiet between enemas. The colon is easy to clean because it is not dilated, and yet liquid stool that comes from the cecum moves very fast to anus and in a few hours, the patient passes stool again. Therefore, in this group of patients, the emphasis is on a constipating diet and administration of medication to decrease colonic peristalsis, such as loperamide and pectin. In our experience, this bowel management program has been successful in 95% of cases.[24,25]

Once the patient responds to the bowel management program and remains completely clean for 24 hours, the patient and family are offered an operation called the Malone procedure (continent appendicostomy),[26,27] which consists of connecting the appendix to the umbilicus so as to be able administer enemas through it in an antegrade fashion. A one-way valve mechanism is created between the appendix and the cecum to avoid stool leakage and allow catheterization. The patient can self-administer an enema while sitting on the toilet. This operation is favored by patients who want to gain some independence and do not like to receive rectal enemas from their parents. For those patients who have lost their appendix for whatever reason, one can create a new appendix from the wall of the cecum. This operation is called a continent neo-appendicostomy.[27]

Soiling

Some 70% of all patients who were born with anorectal malformations have voluntary bowel movements, but almost 50% of them still soil their underwear occasionally. Evaluation of these patients, including a contrast enema, usually reveals that they have chronic fecal impactions. In other words, the soiling often represents overflow pseudoincontinence. Use of laxatives and bulking agents may help to eliminate this type of soiling in most patients. When the soiling is significant enough to interfere with the social life of the patient, then it is preferable to implement the bowel management program with a daily enema as previously described.

Constipation

Constipation is the most common problem in children with anorectal malformations who have undergone an operation in which the original rectum was preserved. The rectosigmoid in these patients behaves like an excessively large reservoir that does not have the capacity to empty as well as in a normal individual. Constipation is a self-aggravating and self-perpetuating disorder. If the rectum is not emptied every day by some mechanism, it accumulates stool and becomes larger (megarectum), resulting in decreased or ineffective peristalsis. This provokes more constipation, creating a vicious cycle. The worst final sequela from constipation is overflow pseudoincontinence. This occurs in severely constipated children (i.e., those with chronic impaction). They constantly pass small amounts of stool as an overflow phenomenon. Sometimes patients who are born with a benign anorectal defect with good functional prognosis do not achieve fecal continence, simply because they have overflow pseudoincontinence secondary to chronic fecal impaction.

The problem of constipation correlates directly with the degree of rectal dilatation that the patient had originally. Some malformations include more severe megarectum than others. The lower the defect, the greater the megarectum and the worse the constipation. Patients with higher defects (and therefore poorer prognosis for functional bowel control) have less constipation.[2] Other factors, such as the type of colostomy, also influence the degree of megarectum. A loop colostomy sometimes allows the passage of stool from the proximal to the distal colon, provoking a megarectum, and for that reason is contraindicated. Patients with transverse colostomies develop a more severe megarectum and more constipation. Patients who are born with perineal fistulas and are not treated early in life develop a very severe megarectum and may eventually have overflow pseudoincontinence. Every effort should be made at prevention, but when a megarectum is present, the patient should receive enough laxatives to empty it every day.

Urinary Incontinence

Male patients with anorectal malformations almost never have urinary incontinence unless they have an absent sacrum, a severe dysplastic sacrum, a spinal anomaly, or nerve damage occurring during the main repair of the malformation.[2,28] Female patients who are born with a cloaca frequently have the incapacity to empty the bladder and require a program of intermittent catheterization. Leakage of urine because of lack of bladder neck tone is very unusual in patients with anorectal malformations. Rather, these patients have an atonic type of megabladder. Only 20% of patients born with a cloaca with a common channel shorter than 3 cm require intermittent catheterization; 70% of those with a common channel longer than 3 cm require this to remain clean and dry.[2,14,15]

REFERENCES

9. Falcone RA, Levitt MA, Peña A, Bates MD. Increased heritability of certain types of anorectal malformations. J Pediatr Surg 2007;42:124–128.

10. Levitt MA, Bischoff A, Breech L, Peña A. Rectovestibular fistula – rarely recognized associated gynecologic anomalies. J Pediatr Surg 2009;44: 1261–1267.

13. Peña A, Levitt MA. Imperforate anus and cloacal malformations. In: Ashcraft KW, Holcomb GW, Murphy JP, editors. Pediatric Surgery. 4th ed Philadelphia: Elsevier; 2005, Saunders. p. 496–517.

16. Levitt MA, Peña A. Pitfalls in the management of newborn cloacas. Pediatr Surg Int 2005;21:264–269.

25. Bischoff A, Levitt MA, Bauer C, et al. Treatment of fecal incontinence with a comprehensive bowel management program. J Pediatr Surg 2009;44:1278–1284.

See expertconsult.com for a complete list of references and the review questions for this chapter.

ABNORMAL ROTATION AND FIXATION OF THE INTESTINE

Thomas T. Sato

Normal intestinal growth and development follows a stereotypical pattern of mesenteric rotation and subsequent intestinal fixation to the body wall during fetal life. The term *malrotation* has been widely used to describe the various disorders of abnormal intestinal rotation and fixation.[1] Clinically apparent abnormalities of intestinal rotation and fixation are encountered on an infrequent basis. The major life-threatening problem associated with abnormal intestinal rotation and fixation is the potential for the intestine to twist upon its mesenteric axis, giving rise to a surgical condition known as midgut volvulus. Given the relatively unpredictable nature of midgut volvulus and the catastrophic consequences of total intestinal necrosis, clinicians must maintain a high index of suspicion for malrotation with volvulus in any infant or child with bilious emesis. In a symptomatic infant or child with midgut volvulus, prompt diagnosis and surgical intervention is essential for prevention of intestinal necrosis. Because the presence of intestinal malrotation is a risk factor for midgut volvulus, most pediatric surgeons also recommend prophylactic, operative intervention in the incidentally diagnosed, asymptomatic infant or child as well.

EMBRYOLOGY

Critical embryologic events occur during normal intestinal fixation to the developing body wall. Normal intestinal fixation requires sequential growth, elongation, and rotation of the intestine beginning as early as the fifth week of gestation and is illustrated in Figure 57-1. Three distinct events must occur for normal intestinal fixation. The first stage involves herniation of the primary intestinal midgut loop into the base of the umbilical cord, where it remains until the 10th week of gestation. The axis of the midgut loop is the vascular pedicle of the superior mesenteric artery (SMA). The SMA axis divides the midgut into prearterial and postarterial segments, with the omphalomesenteric duct located at the apex of the midgut loop. This loop rotates 180° counterclockwise so that the proximal prearterial half of the loop passes posterior to the SMA. The prearterial segment gives rise to the proximal duodenum, which normally lies to the right of midline. The more distal prearterial segment passes posterior and to the left of the SMA, becoming the third and fourth portions of the duodenum. The distal duodenum is normally fixed to the left of the aorta at the ligament of Treitz, having rotated 270° counterclockwise from its original position. The jejunoileal segment undergoes substantial elongation to form the remainder of the small intestine. The embryonic postarterial segment, which gives rise to

the cecum and right colon, also undergoes growth and elongation with 270° counterclockwise rotation. Therefore, although the cecum is initially positioned to the left, the normal rotational pattern places the cecum anterior and ultimately to the right of the SMA before attaching to the posterior wall of the right iliac fossa.[2]

The second important state of midgut rotation and fixation is reduction of the extracelomic gut, occurring between weeks 10 and 12 of gestational age. At this point in fetal development, the duodenojejunal junction has passed posterior to the SMA and the midgut has rotated 180° counterclockwise. The small intestine initially remains to the right side of midline, and the cecum and ascending colon are still anterior to the SMA on return of the intestine to the abdominal cavity. Many common abnormalities of intestinal fixation occur as a result of arrested development during this 2-week period.

The final stage of midgut development is fixation of the intestine to the posterior body wall, occurring after the 12th week of gestation. Normal points of fixation include the cecum in the right iliac fossa and the duodenojejunal junction at the ligament of Treitz (Figure 57-2). The normal small bowel mesentery is therefore fixed to the posterior body wall with a broad base extending from the ligament of Treitz to the cecum. This broad-based mesenteric attachment normally prevents torsion of the intestinal mesentery around its vascular supply. In contrast, abnormalities of intestinal rotation may cause the base of the mesentery to lack broad-based attachment or poor fixation to the posterior body wall. The lack of intestinal fixation, along with a narrow vascular pedicle, produces an anatomic predisposition that may lead to volvulus.

ANATOMY

The normal embryologic sequence for intestinal rotation and fixation can be interrupted at any developmental stage, producing a diverse spectrum of rotational and fixation abnormalities. There are a number of distinct congenital anomalies strongly associated with abnormalities of intestinal rotation and fixation secondary to persistent midgut herniation from the abdominal cavity during fetal development. These anomalies include congenital diaphragmatic hernia and congenital abdominal wall defects such as omphalocele and gastroschisis. Therefore, an associated anomaly in patients diagnosed with intestinal malrotation is quite common.[3] Several conditions associated with an increased rate of intestinal malrotation are listed in Table 57-1.

Although abnormalities of intestinal malrotation and fixation are often described under the general term *malrotation*, specific

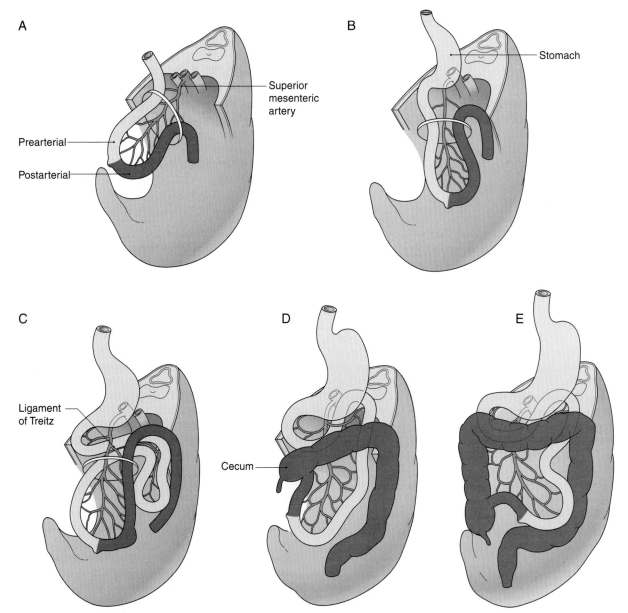

Figure 57-1. Normal intestinal rotation of the duodenum, small intestine and cecum from the fifth gestational week (**A**) through completion by the 12th gestational week (**E**).

anatomic conditions are further characterized in the following subsections.

Nonrotation

This is a relatively common anomaly characterized by incomplete counterclockwise rotation of the midgut around the SMA. Instead of the normal 270° arc, rotation is either absent or arrested before exceeding 90° (Figure 57-3). The small intestine resides on the right side of midline, the colon resides on the left, and the cecum is displaced anteriorly and midline. The duodenojejunal junction is to the right of midline and is more caudal and anterior in position. Nonrotation carries a significant clinical risk of midgut volvulus because the small bowel mesenteric vascular pedicle is very narrow at its base. Duodenal obstruction may also occur as a result of peritoneal attachments fixing the cecum to the posterior body wall. These peritoneal

attachments, also known as Ladd's bands, pass anterior and lateral to the distal duodenum. Duodenal obstruction secondary to Ladd's bands is treated with division of the abnormal cecal attachments crossing the duodenum.

Incomplete (Mixed) Rotation

This abnormality of intestinal rotation is characterized by arrest of normal rotation at or near 180° rather than the normal 270° (Figure 57-4). Instead of rotating posterior and left of the SMA, incomplete rotation of the prearterial segment leaves the duodenojejunal junction to the right of midline. The cecum does not complete counterclockwise passage anterior to the SMA and, therefore, the incompletely rotated cecum usually resides in the upper abdomen just to the left of the SMA. Similar to nonrotation, abnormal fixation of the cecum to the right posterolateral body wall by Ladd's bands places the duodenum

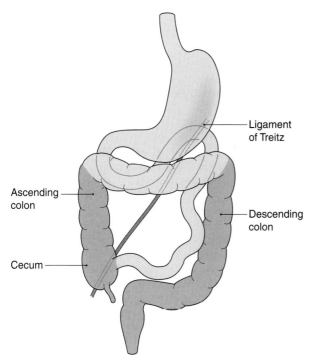

Figure 57-2. Normal fixation of the midgut mesentery to the posterior body wall with the duodenojejunal segment at the ligament of Treitz and the cecum in the right lower quadrant. The shaded portions of the colon are extraperitoneal.

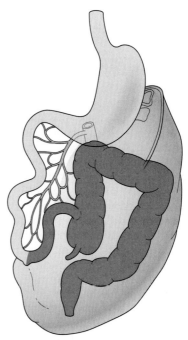

Figure 57-3. Nonrotation. The small intestine, including the duodenojejunal junction, resides in the right side of the abdomen with the cecum and colon on the left.

TABLE 57-1. **Clinical Conditions Associated With Intestinal Malrotation**

Asplenia/polysplenia/heterotaxy syndrome[4,5]
Atrial isomerism[6]
Congenital diaphragmatic hernia
Duodenal, jejunoileal atresia[3,7]
Esophageal atresia/tracheoesophageal fistula[8,9]
Gastroschisis/omphalocele
Hirschsprung's disease, intestinal pseudo-obstruction[3]
Intussusception[10]

at risk for compression or obstruction. In addition, the mesenteric vascular pedicle is narrow and places the entire midgut at risk for volvulus.

Reversed Rotation

This is a rare condition with sporadic case reports in the literature.[11,12] Instead of the normal counterclockwise rotation, the proximal segment of the developing midgut rotates in a 90° clockwise arc, resulting in the cecum and transverse colon passing posterior to the SMA, while the duodenum passes anterior to the SMA. Duodenal or colonic obstructive symptoms caused by reversed rotation are often chronic in nature and may be difficult to diagnose.

Mesocolic Hernia

Congenital mesocolic hernias are exceedingly rare. These anomalies are caused by lack of fixation of either the right or left mesocolon to the posterior body wall. Small intestine can become incarcerated in the potential mesocolic space, causing small-intestinal obstruction from an internal hernia.[13]

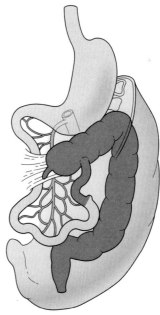

Figure 57-4. Incomplete rotation. The small intestine, including the duodenojejunal junction, resides in the right side of the abdomen, whereas the cecum has partially rotated and lies anterior to the duodenum. Ladd's bands from the posterior abdominal wall may compress and obstruct the duodenum.

A right-sided paraduodenal hernia is associated with nonrotation of the proximal midgut segment; paraduodenal hernia is characterized by entrapment of small intestine posterior to the right colon and cecum. Small bowel entrapment into a left mesocolic hernia may occur despite normal colonic and cecal position. A left mesocolic hernia is usually associated with a hernia sac, with the neck of the sac adjacent to the inferior mesenteric vein along with peritoneal bands extending to the posterior body wall. Mesocolic hernias are difficult to diagnose and may present as either chronic gastrointestinal symptoms or acute bowel obstruction in the absence of previous abdominal operation.

CLINICAL PRESENTATION

Abnormalities of intestinal rotation are historically estimated to be present in approximately 1 to 2% of the total population. However, the true incidence of intestinal malrotation is difficult to define given the spectrum of anatomic variation and the propensity for the majority of these abnormalities to remain asymptomatic. Data from a population-based birth defect registry in Hawaii demonstrated an identified case rate of 2.86 cases of malrotation per 10,000 live births and fetal deaths.[14]

Many children with asymptomatic malrotation will be incidentally diagnosed by upper gastrointestinal contrast studies performed for other clinical reasons. Symptomatic malrotation is usually encountered in the clinical setting of duodenal obstruction or midgut volvulus. Duodenal obstruction occurs as a result of Ladd's bands causing extrinsic compression and obstruction of the distal duodenum as they pass anterior to the duodenum. Older infants and children with symptomatic duodenal obstruction may present with bilious emesis associated with gastric and proximal duodenal distention. Newborn infants may present with bilious emesis without abdominal distention secondary to partial duodenal obstruction. A paucity of small bowel gas may be seen on plain abdominal films.

Midgut volvulus should be considered in the differential diagnosis of any infant or child presenting with bilious emesis. A prospective audit of 63 consecutive neonates with bilious emesis demonstrated a surgical cause of intestinal obstruction in 24 (38%), with four of the infants having intestinal malrotation.[15] The clinical outcome of midgut volvulus is time dependent, and this is the fundamental reason why signs and symptoms of intestinal obstruction in an infant or child must be pursued on an aggressive, emergent basis until definitive diagnosis is made. Delay in diagnosis or definitive treatment will lead to intestinal vascular ischemia and subsequent strangulation of the entire small intestine. Initial symptoms may be subtle and limited to irritability and feeding intolerance with progressive bilious emesis. Guaiac-positive stool associated with bilious emesis should be considered indicative of mechanical small bowel obstruction until proven otherwise. Late clinical findings include progressive abdominal distention and the development of peritonitis. Systemic symptoms and signs of metabolic acidosis, coagulopathy, hypotension and shock reflect the progression of untreated bowel ischemia and infarction. Systemic features are generally considered to represent poor prognostic factors for small bowel salvage and overall survival.

More than 50% of symptomatic intestinal rotational abnormalities are discovered within the first month of life, and approximately 90% occur in children less than 1 year of age.[16,17] Symptomatic infants and children require emergent diagnosis, operative exploration, and definitive correction. Older children and adults may also present with acute symptomatic volvulus, but they may also have a history of vague, recurrent, and chronic abdominal pain associated with episodic symptoms of intestinal obstruction. Although volvulus from malrotation occurs more commonly in the neonate and infant, older children and adults with malrotation may present with volvulus in an unpredictable manner.[18,19] Symptomatic intestinal malrotation presenting outside of the neonatal period may be characterized by intermittent abdominal pain, recurrent episodic emesis, and malnutrition associated with failure to thrive.[20] Chronic diarrhea or malabsorptive symptoms may be found.[21] Regardless of age at diagnosis, operative treatment of malrotation can be life-saving in the setting of volvulus and may prevent a life-threatening situation in the asymptomatic individual.[22]

DIAGNOSIS

Diagnostic imaging evaluation generally begins with plain abdominal radiography. Classic radiographic findings with malrotation include gastric and proximal duodenal distention with a paucity or absence of small bowel gas due to partial duodenal obstruction. The plain film alone may not differentiate malrotation from duodenal atresia or stenosis in a neonate; this is an important clinical distinction given the emergent need for intervention in the setting of volvulus versus the relatively elective repair of duodenal atresia.[23] In most instances of suspected duodenal obstruction with concern of malrotation, an upper gastrointestinal series is a definitive imaging study (Figure 57-5). Malrotation with volvulus typically produces incomplete duodenal obstruction with a "corkscrew" or "coiled spring" appearance of contrast passing into the distal duodenum and proximal jejunum. Duodenal atresia and stenosis may occur anywhere within the duodenum, but is more commonly proximal than obstruction observed with malrotation with volvulus. Complete absence of small bowel gas and a "double-bubble" appearance on plain abdominal film is typical of duodenal atresia, whereas diminished but discernable distal gas is characteristic of duodenal stenosis or malrotation with incomplete obstruction.

Other more subtle radiographic findings consistent with a diagnosis of malrotation include duodenal redundancy and incorrect position of the duodenojejunal junction, particularly in a location to the right of midline and inferior to the pylorus.[24] A classic finding of malrotation observed with contrast enema is cecal malposition to the midline or left of the vertebral column. However, the reported sensitivity and specificity of gastrointestinal contrast studies in the diagnosis of malrotation varies, with false-positive rates as high as 15%.[25]

Recent interest in ultrasonographic diagnosis of malrotation has led to emerging case series reporting sensitivity and accuracy in detecting malrotation. Ultrasonography relies, in part, on the relationship of the SMA to the superior mesenteric vein; normally, the superior mesenteric vein is to the right of the SMA on transverse sonograms. Abnormal position of the superior mesenteric vein either ventral or to the left of the SMA is associated with malrotation.[26] In addition to inversion of the mesenteric vessels, the ultrasonographic presence of duodenal dilation with tapering has been reported to have a sensitivity of 89% and a specificity of 92% in the detection of volvulus.[27] However, a normal relationship of the SMA and the SMV does not exclude the presence of asymptomatic malrotation.[28] Finally, helical CT scan imaging in the setting of malrotation with volvulus has been described as demonstrating a "whirlpool" sign from the twisted duodenojejunal junction. Regardless of the modality, several important points in the diagnostic work-up of malrotation include:

- Symptomatic malrotation with or without volvulus is more common in the neonate and infant, but can occur at any age.
- If malrotation with volvulus is suspected clinically, aggressive resuscitation along with emergent radiologic studies and surgical consultation are indicated.

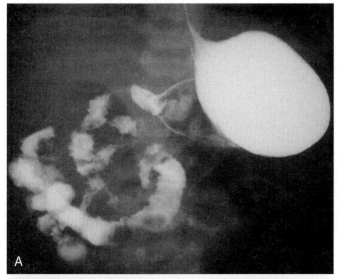

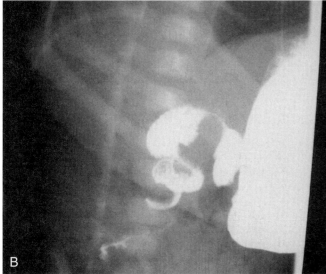

Figure 57-5. (A) Upper gastrointestinal contrast study demonstrating intestinal malrotation (nonrotation) without volvulus. **(B)** Contrast study in a neonate demonstrating intestinal malrotation with vovulus. Note the "corkscrew" appearance of contrast in the proximal jejunum. Courtesy Jack R. Sty, MD, and Thomas T. Sato, MD, Children's Hospital of Wisconsin.

- In a symptomatic infant or child, radiographic evidence of malrotation alone is enough to warrant emergent exploration.
- It may be difficult to differentiate the presence or absence of volvulus radiologically, and the absence of definitive radiographic evidence should not defer operative intervention if clinical suspicion is high.

TREATMENT

The management of symptomatic malrotation is operative regardless of age at presentation. Emphasis should be placed on the expedient assessment, resuscitation, and preoperative preparation of a symptomatic infant or child so that radiologic confirmation can be followed promptly by laparotomy. In the presence of confirmed or suspected volvulus, emergent laparotomy is warranted, because even minimal delay may cause further injury to the compromised intestine. The critical surgical

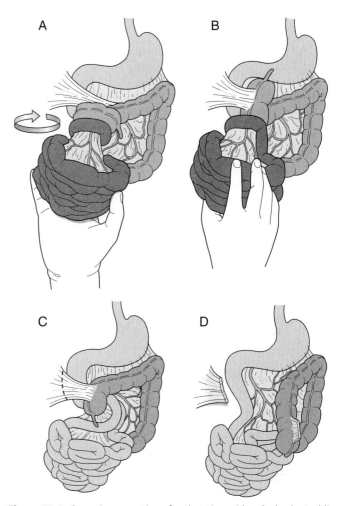

Figure 57-6. Operative correction of malrotation with volvulus by Ladd's procedure. **(A, B)** Reduction of volvulus. **(C, D)** Division of cecal attachments (Ladd's bands) to the body wall.

issue is to intervene before irreversible ischemic injury causes intestinal infarction.

Operative repair of malrotation with or without volvulus is performed by Ladd's procedure.[29] This operation includes several important maneuvers, including:
- Delivery of the entire midgut and inspection of the vascular mesentery
- Reduction of the volvulus, if present, and evaluation of intestinal viability
- Division of Ladd's bands
- Broadening the base of the mesenteric vascular pedicle
- Appendectomy, given the abnormal position of the cecum
- Return of the gastrointestinal tract with the small intestine in the right abdomen and the large intestine in the left abdomen

This operation involves delivery and reduction of the volvulus, if present. The base of the mesenteric vascular pedicle is broadened by dividing the peritoneal bands that tether the cecum as well as congenital adhesions around the base of the SMA (Figure 57-6). Broadening the mesenteric pedicle reduces the risk for recurrent volvulus. Mesenteric fixation via cecal or duodenal suture plication to the body wall has been largely abandoned.[30] It is presumed that one mechanism by which Ladd's procedure reduces the rate of subsequent volvulus is via formation of intra-abdominal adhesions that reduce the mobility of the broadened mesenteric vascular pedicle. Postoperative small bowel obstruction secondary to intra-abdominal adhesion formation is reported in approximately 10 to 24% of patients undergoing Ladd's procedure.[31]

Any abnormal peritoneal attachments (Ladd's bands) between the cecum and the posterior body wall are divided, relieving any present or potential extrinsic duodenal obstruction. An extensive Kocher maneuver is performed, mobilizing the entire duodenum and dividing all anterior, lateral, and posterior duodenal attachments. The patency of the duodenum should be demonstrated in a newborn with passage of an intraluminal tube or insufflation with air; this will exclude the presence of coexistent duodenal atresia. Given the abnormal position of the cecum, an appendectomy is performed.

Midgut volvulus causing complete intestinal infarction often involves the entire small intestine just distal to the duodenojejunal junction to a point approximately halfway in the transverse colon. Intestinal infarction of this magnitude, if not immediately fatal, is survivable only with resection of all infarcted intestine and either diverting enterostomy or enterocolic anastomosis. This unfortunate situation requires long-term total parenteral nutritional support and leads to substantial morbidity, and in many cases predictable death in the short or long term. Midgut volvulus associated with intestinal necrosis is treated by preservation of as much intestinal length as possible. If bowel viability is uncertain during initial exploration, a planned second-look procedure 24 to 48 hours later may be useful in determining the ultimate extent of irreversible intestinal injury.

Whether or not to perform Ladd's procedure in the asymptomatic infant or child remains controversial and subject to individual surgeon bias. In a large retrospective case series of 447 infants diagnosed with malrotation, the outcome of 331 neonates with malrotation associated with either congenital diaphragmatic hernia ($n = 111$) or abdominal wall defects ($n = 220$) was reported.[32] Seventy-seven of these infants underwent Ladd's procedure. Some 1.2% of surviving infants with abdominal wall defects (2 of 172) and 2.9% of surviving infants with congenital diaphragmatic hernia (1 of 34) untreated for malrotation ultimately developed midgut volvulus. In this study, the risk of midgut volvulus in untreated patients with malrotation was relatively low and thought to be a consequence, in part, of intra-abdominal adhesion formation from previous neonatal laparotomy. Compared to elective operations for malrotation without volvulus, there appears to be increased morbidity (delayed diagnosis, higher postoperative complication rate) in adults requiring emergent operations for symptomatic malrotation.[33,34] Given the unpredictable nature of midgut volvulus from malrotation, and the potential catastrophic consequences of total intestinal injury with volvulus, most pediatric surgeons perform an elective Ladd's procedure on asymptomatic infants and children as a preventive measure.

Performance of laparoscopic Ladd's procedure for malrotation without volvulus has been demonstrated to be feasible and may help to reduce time to enteral feeding and length of hospital stay.[35-38] Early experience with laparoscopic Ladd's procedure emphasized the utility of laparoscopy in the diagnosis and treatment of abnormal intestinal rotation and fixation in infants and children without volvulus. This approach has been adopted by most major pediatric surgical centers with advanced laparoscopic expertise. The performance of laparoscopic Ladd's procedure in the setting of volvulus is less commonly practiced, as there are inherent operative risks from peritoneal insufflation with carbon dioxide on a hemodynamically compromised infant. In addition, the intestine may be quite distended and fragile from transient ischemia, making it difficult to reduce the volvulus without formal laparotomy. The long-term recurrence rate of volvulus following laparoscopic Ladd's procedure remains unknown. There has been some concern that a laparoscopic approach may not produce the same extent of intra-abdominal adhesion speculated to play a role in prevention of recurrent volvulus following an open Ladd's procedure.

The surgical management of internal hernias from mesocolic hernia, paraduodenal hernia, or reversed rotation must be individualized. General principles include reduction of the incarcerated viscera, evaluation of the mesenteric pedicle with establishment of a broad vascular pedicle, and elimination of the potential space via division of the abnormal peritoneal attachments or, in the case of a left mesocolic hernia, resection or obliteration of the hernia sac.

COMPLICATIONS, RESULTS, OUTCOME

With accurate diagnosis and treatment, results of operative correction of abnormalities of intestinal rotation and fixation should be excellent, and in the absence of intestinal necrosis, life expectancy should be unrelated to the intestinal malrotation. Given the propensity for other coexisting, potentially life-threatening, anomalies such as congenital diaphragmatic hernia to be present with malrotation, overall survival may not be equivalent to that of an age-matched cohort. Long-term outcome is substantially less favorable in infants with intestinal necrosis at the time of exploration, and extensive intestinal resection can be anticipated to create short bowel syndrome with the potential consequences of recurrent sepsis and progressive liver failure.

A technically complete Ladd's procedure makes recurrent volvulus and recurrent duodenal obstruction distinctly unusual. No long-term randomized clinical trials have compared open and laparoscopic procedures in the treatment of intestinal malrotation. Complications reported with the surgical management of intestinal malrotation are reflective of operative intervention in a fragile neonatal population and include systemic inflammatory response syndrome, infection, pneumonia, feeding difficulties, and small bowel obstruction. Adhesive small bowel obstruction following neonatal laparotomy is reported to occur in 1 to 15% of patients.[39] The incidence rate of small bowel obstruction following Ladd's procedure is probably higher (10 to 24%).[31] Return of gastrointestinal function may be delayed, particularly in the presence of volvulus; prolonged nasogastric decompression along with total parenteral nutritional may be required.[40] Some infants and children may have persistent postoperative emesis, diarrhea, or feeding intolerance with intestinal motility patterns that mimic neuropathic intestinal pseudo-obstruction.[41] It remains unclear whether the intestinal motility defect is a cause or consequence of the observed intestinal malrotation.

Historic case series have demonstrated improved overall survival rates over the past 30 years, with highest mortality rates in infants less than 1 month of age with multiple congenital anomalies, or volvulus with intestinal gangrene at exploration.[42] Reported perioperative mortality rates in infants and children treated surgically for malrotation over the past 30 years range from 2.9% to 28% and depend on the age of the child and the extent of intestinal ischemia and necrosis.[32,43,44]

SUMMARY

Abnormalities of intestinal rotation and fixation are infrequent but important pediatric gastrointestinal conditions. The presence of midgut volvulus is heralded by feeding intolerance and bilious emesis in the neonate; in this setting, a high index of suspicion and a low threshold for emergent radiologic and surgical consultation is warranted. Older children may present with more vague chronic symptoms of intermittent emesis, pain, and diarrhea. A diagnosis of midgut volvulus requires emergent surgical intervention. A diagnosis of intestinal malrotation without volvulus is an indication for surgical consultation and careful consideration of operative intervention as a prophylactic measure to reduce the risk of volvulus.

REFERENCES

16. Andrassy RJ, Mahour GH. Malrotation of the midgut in infants and children: a 25-year review. Arch Surg 1981;116:158–160.
28. Lampl B, Levin TL, Berdon WE, Cowles RA. Malrotation and midgut volvulus: a historical review and current controversies in diagnosis and management. Pediatr Radiol 2009;39:359–366.
29. Ladd WE, Gross RE. Abdominal Surgery of Infancy and Childhood. Philadelphia: Saunders; 1941.
32. Rescorla FJ, Shedd FJ, Grosfeld JL, et al. Anomalies of intestinal rotation in childhood: analysis of 447 cases. Surgery 1990;108:710–715.
38. Fraser JD, Aguayo P, Sharp SW, et al. The role of laparoscopy in the management of malrotation. J Surg Res 2009;156:80–82.
44. Ford EG, Senac Jr MO, Srikanth MS, et al. Malrotation of the intestine in children. Ann Surg 1992;215:172–178.

See expertconsult.com for a complete list of references and the review questions for this chapter.

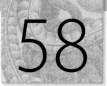

58

SMALL AND LARGE BOWEL STENOSIS AND ATRESIAS

Marjorie J. Arca • Keith T. Oldham

Within the gastrointestinal tract, the term *atresia* refers to the lack of continuity within a segment of bowel due to an anatomic obstruction. *Stenosis* refers to a partial obstruction within the lumen of the intestine. A congenital stenosis typically results from an intraluminal membrane with a small opening, which allows some passage of enteric contents.

DUODENAL STENOSIS AND ATRESIA

Calder first described duodenal atresia as a cause of intestinal obstruction in 1733.[1] However, it was not until 1916 that Ernst reported the first survivor of this anomaly.[2] By 1931, there were 250 cases of duodenal atresia reported in the literature with only nine survivors.[3,4] Current long-term survival rates for duodenal atresia are 86 to 90%, with operative mortality rates of 4%,[5] most related to associated anomalies, particularly various forms of congenital heart disease.

Embryology

A popular, although unproven, concept offered to explain the genesis of duodenal atresia is the failure of recanalization of the duodenal lumen, a theory first espoused in 1902 by Tandler.[6] Early in the fourth week of gestation, the duodenum develops as the caudal portion of the foregut and the cranial segment of the midgut. These parts of the foregut and midgut grow rapidly and project ventrally. The junction of these two regions is just distal to the origin of the bile ducts. During the fifth and sixth gestational weeks, the duodenal lumen is reduced or obliterated by rapidly proliferating epithelial cells. By the end of the embryonic period, vacuolization of these cells and recanalization of the duodenum normally yields a patent lumen. The second portion of the duodenum is the last to recanalize.

During the third week of embryonic development, the liver, gallbladder, and biliary duct system develop, initially as a ventral bud from the most caudal segment of the foregut. The pancreas arises from both the dorsal and ventral pancreatic buds and is composed of endodermal cells arising from the caudal part of the foregut. The larger dorsal anlage appears first. The dorsal bud gives rise to most of the pancreas. The ventral bud develops near the entry of the bile duct into the duodenum. When the duodenum rotates clockwise to assume its adult C-shape, the ventral pancreatic bud is carried dorsally with the bile duct. The ventral bud ultimately fuses with larger dorsal anlage to become the uncinate process and the inferior part of the head of the pancreas.

Familial intestinal atresia and syndromic associations for duodenal atresia have been described.[7] Recently, fibroblast growth factor 10 has been found to regulate normal duodenal development; its absence results in failure to develop duodenal continuity in the mouse.[8] Duodenal atresia has been reported in infants of mothers who have taken simvastatin or lovastatin,[9] although the mechanism is not known.

Incidence

The incidence of congenital duodenal obstruction in the United States is approximately 1 in 6000 live births.[10] In Finland, congenital duodenal obstruction is reported in 1 in 3400 births.[10] Intrinsic duodenal obstruction comprises about two thirds of patients' pathology. Accounting for the remainder, annular pancreas, preduodenal portal vein, or Ladd's bands may cause extrinsic duodenal obstruction, although annular pancreas is commonly associated with underlying duodenal atresia.

Children with duodenal atresia often have associated anomalies. These commonly include trisomy 21, cardiac anomalies, and intestinal rotational anomalies. About 7 to 8% of babies with trisomy 21 have duodenal anomalies. Congenital foregut anomalies such as preduodenal portal vein or annular pancreas can be seen in patients with intrinsic duodenal obstruction.

Clinical Presentation

Improvements in ultrasonography have improved the rates of antenatal diagnosis of congenital duodenal obstruction in developing countries. About 30 to 59% of infants with congenital duodenal obstruction demonstrate polyhydramnios on antenatal ultrasonography.[4,10] Early in the third trimester, a dilated, fluid-filled stomach and duodenum may be evident on ultrasound.

A newborn with duodenal atresia typically has onset of vomiting within hours of birth and is not able to tolerate feeds. Because 85% of affected neonates have a postampullary site obstruction, the emesis is most often bile-tinged. The abdomen is not distended because of the proximal level of obstruction. An abdominal radiograph usually shows a "double-bubble sign" (Figure 58-1), with a large amount of air within the stomach and a smaller amount of air within the proximal duodenum, but a gasless abdomen otherwise.

Infants with duodenal stenosis may tolerate some enteral nutrition because the obstruction is incomplete. On abdominal radiographs, these patients will have some air distal to the duodenal bubble, thus making it difficult to differentiate from infants with malrotation and midgut volvulus. Some children with duodenal stenosis or web may be diagnosed at months or even years of age when an upper gastrointestinal contrast study is performed to evaluate suspected gastroesophageal reflux, vomiting, or failure to thrive.

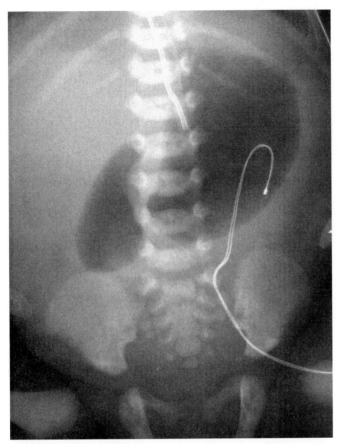

Figure 58-1. Plain radiograph demonstrating the "double-bubble" sign associated with duodenal atresia. There is a gastric air collection and a duodenal air pocket. It is important to note that there is no distal gas. The presence of air in the distal small bowel in a patient with a "double-bubble sign" is worrisome for malrotation with volvulus.

Classification (Figure 58-2)[11]

In type I duodenal atresia, there is usually a mucosal membrane, typically occluding the lumen of the duodenum. Sometimes, a small fenestration is present in the membrane, which allows passage of some enteric contents and air. A common variant of this problem is a "wind-sock anomaly," where the origin of the membrane is located a few centimeters proximal to the distal apex of the web. The "wind-sock" appearance likely results from antegrade peristalsis and can be a source of anatomic uncertainty to the occasional pediatric surgeon. The papilla is almost always adjacent to or traverses the medial wall of the membrane. Type II duodenal atresias have a fibrous cord connecting the two atretic ends of the duodenum. The most rare type of duodenal atresia, the type III anomaly, consists of separated blind ends, with the mesentery missing between the ends. Type III atresias may be associated with congenital biliary anomalies.

Treatment

An orogastric tube is placed to decompress the stomach. Intravenous fluids and antibiotics are administered. An echocardiogram should be performed in patients with duodenal atresia before repair. Patients with duodenal atresia and trisomy 21 carry a relative risk of 2.61 of having congenital cardiac anomalies.[12] Up to 23% of patients with duodenal atresia and normal karyotype have congenital heart disease.[12]

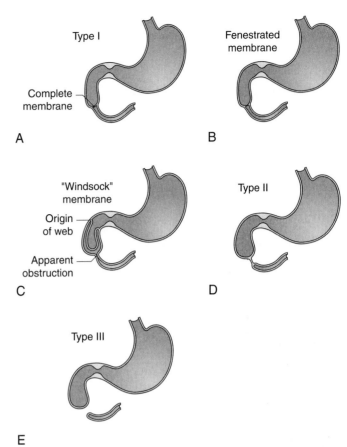

Figure 58-2. Classification of duodenal atresia. Type I atresia (**A**) has an intact mucosal membrane; (**B**) demonstrates a diaphragm with a small fenestration, allowing partial passage of enteric contents, and (**C**) demonstrates a wind-sock anomaly where the diaphragm is elongated and terminates beyond its origin. Type II atresia has a fibrous band connecting the two blind ends (**D**). Type III atresia has completely separate blind ends (**E**). Type III atresias may be associated with anomalous hepatobiliary anatomy. From Magnuson and Schwartz (1997).[11]

The usual operative approach is through a supraumbilical transverse abdominal incision. A rotational anomaly is corrected if present. Ladd's procedure is discussed in detail in Chapter 57 on malrotation. The hepatic flexure of the colon is mobilized medially. The presence of an annular pancreas or a preduodenal portal vein is noted. The lateral attachments of the duodenum are freed, fully mobilizing the organ anterior. In general, transverse duodenotomy is performed just proximal to the apparent point of obstruction. This can be subtle or difficult to localize in the circumstance of partial obstruction. Once the duodenum is open, the location of the papilla may be defined by compressing the gallbladder and identifying the site where bile empties into the duodenum. A proximal transverse to distal longitudinal (Kimura's diamond shape) anastomosis[13] or a side-to-side anastomosis is performed, bypassing the point of obstruction, and is generally the best reconstructive option, although this must be individualized based on specific anatomic findings. A small rubber catheter should be passed distal to the anastomosis to rule out a second duodenal obstruction, which may be present in 1 to 3% of patients.

In patients with the wind-sock variant, an orogastric tube is passed through the pylorus to assist in determining the origin and the level of the obstructing membrane. With distal traction, an indentation in the proximal dilated part of the duodenum may be identified and will correspond with the base of the membrane. The initial duodenotomy should be placed just proximal to the base. The web may be excised laterally, because the papilla is typically intimately associated with the medial aspect of the web. The duodenotomy is then closed. If the location of the ampulla and its relationship to the web (wind sock) are difficult or impossible to ascertain, then bypass of the obstruction is the appropriate and safest operative approach.

Structures such as an anterior duodenal portal vein or an annular pancreas should be left alone. The duodenal obstruction should be bypassed using a duodenoduodenal or duodenojejunal anastomosis. Patients with associated malrotation should undergo Ladd's procedure.

At the time of operation, the surgeon may decide that the ectatic proximal segment of the duodenum is sufficiently dilated that it is likely to remain dysfunctional postoperatively. In such cases, an antimesenteric tapering duodenoplasty may be performed. The routine addition of a duodenoplasty to duodenal atresia repair issue remains a point of controversy in the surgical community.

Recently, laparoscopic approaches to repair of duodenal atresia have been reported. Data from small, retrospective reports have shown that the minimally invasive technique can be safe and effective.[14]

An orogastric tube is left in place. Feeding is started when gastrointestinal function is reestablished. Some series have advocated feeding after a contrast study confirms patency and anastomotic integrity at 7 days. Operative mortality for neonates with duodenal atresia is approximately 4%; mortality is highest in the population with complex cardiac anomalies.[10]

Long-term follow-up of patients with duodenal atresia reveals a 12% rate of late complications including reflux, peptic ulcer disease, duodenal dysmotility, or anastomotic failure.[15] In a series of 169 patients, 16 children underwent revision of their initial repair. Late deaths (6%) were attributable to complex cardiac malformations, central nervous system bleeding, pneumonia, anastomotic leak, and multisystem organ failure.

SMALL BOWEL ATRESIA

Embryology

In 1912, Spriggs hypothesized that anatomic accidents, such as vascular occlusion, may cause atresia of the small intestine. Subsequent experimental and clinical experience indicates that intrauterine vascular insults related to volvulus, internal hernia, or gastroschisis have resulted in intestinal atresias. Animal models of intestinal atresia have confirmed that local vascular compromise, subsequent intestinal necrosis, and intestinal resorption are a cause of intestinal atresia.[16,17]

Incidence

Small bowel atresia is reported to occur in about 1 in 4000 to 5000 live births.[18] Jejunoileal atresia is associated with gastroschisis, omphalocele, meconium ileus, and cystic fibrosis. Male and female infants appear equally affected.

Clinical Presentation

Jejunoileal atresia is associated with maternal polyhydramnios in 24% of patients and is more prominent with a more proximal level of obstruction. Dilated echogenic bowel may also be appreciated on prenatal ultrasound.

Abdominal distention is more pronounced in more distal lesions. Often a dilated loop of intestine is appreciable on physical examination, although this may take a number of hours to develop. Bilious emesis is seen earlier and more often in infants with more proximal obstructions. Jaundice is seen in more than 30% of babies with jejunal atresia and 20% with ileal atresia. This is believed to result from delay in the maturation of the glucuronyl transferase enzyme in the absence of normal enteral feedings. Cholestasis was found to resolve in all survivors of patients with jejunoileal atresia.[19] Therefore, selective evaluation and expectant management have been advocated.

In abdominal radiographs of infants with proximal intestinal atresia, there are few dilated bowel loops and air-fluid levels (Figure 58-3). The more distal atresias tend to have more dilated intestine on radiograph. A dominant dilated loop of intestine may be present. A contrast enema usually shows a microcolon in patients with small-intestinal atresia, although this is nonspecific. This study may also aid in establishing the diagnosis of meconium plug or Hirschsprung's disease.

Classification (Figure 58-4)[18]

Grosfeld et al.[20] and Touloukian[21] have modified an intestinal atresia classification proposed by Martin and Zerella[22] to yield an anatomic system in use today. Type I intestinal atresia has an intraluminal diaphragm in continuity with the muscular layers of the proximal and distal segments. In type II atresias, fibrous bands separate the ends of the two relevant segments. Type IIIa atresias are characterized by a V-shaped mesenteric defect and intestinal discontinuity. Type IIIb atresias have an extensive mesenteric defect, with the distal ileum receiving its entire blood supply retrograde via the ileocolic or right colic artery. In this circumstance, the distal intestine coils itself around the artery, giving rise to descriptive terms such as "apple-peel" or "Christmas tree" deformity. This type of anomaly is often associated with particularly small distal bowel and a significant loss in overall bowel length.[23] Type IV atresias are composed of multiple atresias within the length of the small bowel, and sometimes these require multiple anastomoses to preserve bowel length.

Treatment

Preoperative care is similar for that of duodenal atresia. Gastric decompression, intravenous fluid resuscitation, and antibiotic administration are required. It is important to remember that the dilated proximal segment can serve as a fixed point, around which the bowel can volvulize. Prompt abdominal exploration is required and is generally performed through a transverse supraumbilical incision. The entire bowel is eviscerated and the point(s) of obstruction identified. It is imperative to explore the distal intestine for the presence of other atresias. A small-caliber rubber catheter may be introduced into the distal segment and the remaining intestine flushed with saline for this purpose. Colonic patency is confirmed either by inserting a rectal tube and filling the colon intraoperatively or a preoperative contrast enema.

The surgeon must determine the length of the functional intestine. If the baby has adequate length of bowel, then the bulbous proximal intestine may be resected to perform an end-to-end anastomosis between two ends of bowel with relatively equal sizes. However, if the bowel length is limited, a tapering enteroplasty should be considered to preserve as much bowel

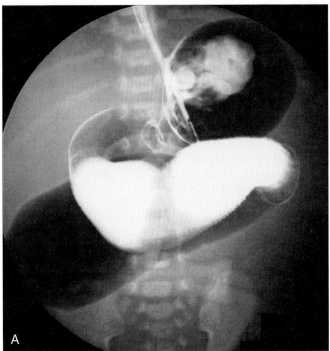

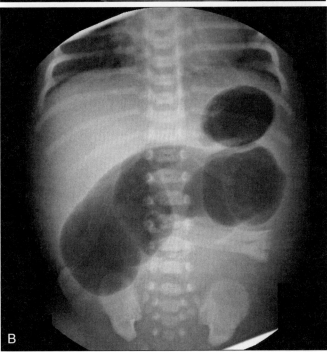

Figure 58-3. (**A**) Plain abdominal radiograph in a baby with jejunal atresia. (**B**) A contrast study demonstrates the blind end in the same baby.

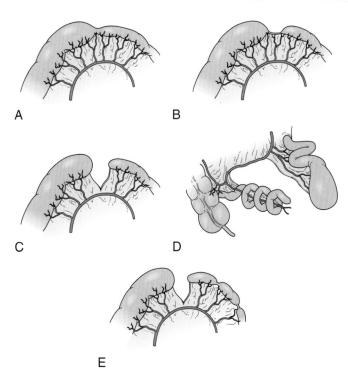

Figure 58-4. Classification of small-intestinal atresia. (**A**) Type I atresia has an obstructing membrane with musculoserosal continuity. (**B**) Type II atresia has a fibrous band between the two atretic ends. (**C**) Type IIIA is characterized by two blind intestinal ends with no intervening mesentery. (**D**) Type IIIB (apple peel atresia) is characterized by a bulbous proximal small intestine, which is usually foreshortened. The distal, small-caliber intestine is wrapped around the ileocolic artery. (**E**) Type IV atresia has multiple segments of atretic bowel. Adapted from Grosfeld (1986).[18]

small-intestinal atresia is dependent on the length of residual functional small bowel.[27] At least 40 cm of small intestine without an ileocecal valve or 20 cm with an ileocecal valve is considered necessary for adequate long intestinal adaptation, although these must be considered generalizations only.[28] Postoperatively, an orogastric tube is left in place until intestinal motility resumes. The infant's diet is then slowly advanced to goal volume. A child with short bowel syndrome requires complex postsurgical care that is discussed elsewhere in this text.

COLONIC ATRESIA

Embryology

Similar to jejunoileal atresia, colonic atresia is thought to occur because of vascular compromise of a colon segment in utero. This happens after the midgut has returned into the celomic cavity between the 10th and 12th week of gestation.[29] Although atresias may occur anywhere along the length of the colon, they are more likely to occur in the vascular watershed areas of the hepatic flexure.[29] As in duodenal atresia, the lack of fibroblast growth factor 10 has been identified in the animal model of colonic atresia without mesenteric vascular obstruction.[30]

Incidence

The incidence of colon atresia is approximately 1 in 20,000 live births, and it is the least common of all intestinal atresias.[31] There is a 2% incidence of Hirschsprung's disease in patients with colon atresia[32]; therefore, this possibility should be ruled

length as possible.[24] In patients with a short dilated segment with inevitable short bowel syndrome, serial transverse enteroplasty (STEP) procedures should be considered as part of the surgical armamentarium in the neonatal period for increasing the surface area for digestion and absorption.[25]

Reported operative mortality rates are about 1%.[10] In preterm infants (less than 37 weeks' gestation), there is an 87% survival.[26] Term infants have a 98% survival. A late mortality of 11% has been described, and is highest in patients with short bowel syndrome.[26] The prognosis for patients with

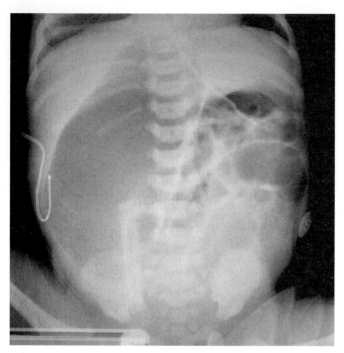

Figure 58-5. Plain abdominal radiograph in a baby with colonic atresia.

out with a suction rectal biopsy before reestablishing intestinal continuity in patients with colon atresia. Jejunal-ileal atresia, cardiac anomalies, and abnormalities of the musculoskeletal system have been reported to coexist with this entity.

Clinical Presentation

Prenatal ultrasound of a fetus with colonic atresia may show an enlarged loop of intestine or colon that is larger for gestational age, but one cannot reliably localize the site of obstruction. Infants with colonic atresia or stenosis usually have no acute problems at birth but develop a distended abdomen within 24 to 48 hours (Figure 58-5). They may require mechanical ventilation secondary to the distention. Failure to pass meconium is typical, but some infants may pass a small amount of mucus per rectum. Plain abdominal radiographs show multiple distended small intestinal loops. In neonates, it is difficult to differentiate between small and large intestine on abdominal radiographs, thus making the distinction between distal ileal obstruction and colonic obstruction difficult or impossible.

Contrast radiography with isotonic contrast agent may establish the diagnosis of colonic atresia or stenosis. This study is important in evaluating patients for other causes of distal obstruction such as meconium plug syndrome, Hirschsprung's disease, or small left colon syndrome. Therefore, it is routinely recommended in the clinical setting of neonatal distal bowel obstruction.

Treatment

After resuscitation, gastric decompression, and administration of intravenous antibiotics, exploratory laparotomy is performed. The most common finding in colon atresia is two blind-ending segments of colon with no intervening mesentery. Historically, surgical correction often involved staged procedures, initially with the creation of a functioning colostomy and a distal mucous fistula. In this scenario, the dilated proximal colon is allowed to decompress and the luminal diameter reduce to roughly normal size before an ileocolostomy or a colocolostomy is performed months later. However, resection of the dilated segment and primary anastomosis to establish intestinal continuity is a reasonable surgical option in children without perforation, short gut, hemodynamic compromise, or medical contraindications. Primary establishment of intestinal continuity is common in contemporary pediatric surgical practice.[33] Regardless, patency of the distal segment should be evaluated either preoperatively or intraoperatively. If a primary anastomosis is performed, it is imperative to make sure that the distal segment has normal ganglion cells using either suction or open rectal biopsy.

Operative mortality for colon atresia is low.[10]

SUMMARY

Intestinal atresia is an important cause of bowel obstruction in the newborn period. Advancements in neonatal anesthesia, intensive perioperative management, and parenteral nutrition have improved the survival and outcomes of these patients. Although surgical correction can be technically complex, it is generally possible today. Higher rates of morbidity and late mortality are still observed in patients with concurrent anatomic anomalies of other systems, especially congenital heart disease and those who have short gut syndrome.

REFERENCES

8. Kanard RC, Fairbanks TJ, De Langhe SP, et al. Colonic atresia without mesenteric vascular occlusion. The role of the fibroblast growth factor 10 signaling pathway. J Pediatr Surg 2005;40:313–316.
10. Dalla Vecchia LK, Grosfeld JL, West KW, et al. Intestinal atresia and stenosis: a 25-year experience with 277 cases. Arch Surg 1998;133:490–497.
15. Escobar MA, Ladd AP, Grosfeld JL, et al. Duodenal atresia and stenosis: long-term follow-up over 30 years. J Pediatr Surg 2004;39:867–871; discussion 867-871.
26. Walker K, Badawi N, Hamid CH, et al. A population-based study of the outcome after small bowel atresia/stenosis in New South Wales and the Australian Capital Territory Australia, 1992-2003. J Pediatr Surg 2008;43:484–488.
31. Oldham K, Arca M. Atresia, stenosis and other obstructions of the colon. In: Grosfeld JL, O'Neill Jr JA, Fonkalsrud EW, Coran AG, editors. Pediatric Surgery. 6th ed. Philadelphia: Mosby-Elsevier; 2006.

See expertconsult.com for a complete list of references and the review questions for this chapter.

NEWBORN ABDOMINAL WALL DEFECTS

59

Danny C. Little • Shane D. Lewis

HISTORICAL BACKGROUND AND TERMINOLOGY

Ambrose Pare[1] recorded the first description of omphalocele during the 16th century emphasizing the serious nature of the condition and the poor prognosis. Gastroschisis was subsequently described by Calder in 1733.[1] Traditionally, nomenclature has included many confusing terms such as epiomphaschisis and hologastroestroschisis. In 1953, Moore and Stokes[1] established the present day classification, distinguishing omphalocele from gastroschisis on the basis of the site of the umbilical cord, the presence or absence of a covering sac, and the appearance of eviscerated bowel (Table 59-1).

The first known child to survive with an omphalocele was treated nonoperatively in 1751. Subsequently, various topical regimens have been recommended. In 1899, Ahlfeld[1] described treatment with alcohol dressings. In 1957, Grob[1] described the use of 2% aqueous solution of merbromin as a topical agent, producing a dry crust on the sac with a granulating surface beneath. Gradual epithelialization occurred over many weeks.

Surgical cures of omphalocele were first reported in 1803 and 1806.[1] Except for small defects, most of the early surgical attempts were unsuccessful. In 1887, Olshausen[1] described mobilization of abdominal skin flaps to cover the sac. This method was not adopted until 1948, when Gross[1] reported this technique to close three giant omphaloceles. Skin flap closure necessitated future repair of the resultant, and often quite challenging, ventral hernia. However, adoption of this technique was a major advance in the survival of infants with omphaloceles.

Watkins[1,2] performed the first successful surgical repair of gastroschisis in 1943. Watkins enlarged the existing 1-inch defect to 2 inches, just 30 minutes following delivery. The viscera were placed in the abdominal cavity and sprinkled with sulfanilamide crystals, and the wound was closed with interrupted sutures. The infant was started on atropine on the fourth day due to vomiting and on lactic acid milk on day 6. By the 16th day, the baby was discharged to home, and at 30 days follow-up the baby was gaining weight and appeared normal except for a bulging umbilicus.[2] Other surgeons during the 1940s and 1950s used drastic measures to reduce abdominal volume and close the defect utilizing partial hepatectomy, splenectomy, and bowel resection,[1] usually leading to the death of the baby. Izant[1] in 1966 recommended manual stretching of the abdominal wall to enlarge the cavity. In 1967, Schuster[1] reported a new technique that revolutionized surgical management. He noted that in children with omphaloceles, the

rectus muscles approximate each other behind the eviscerated mass. Furthermore, skin flap closure did little to alter intra-abdominal forces or stimulate the growth of the abdominal cavity. The resulting huge ventral hernias were just as difficult to repair as the original omphalocele. By attaching sheets of prosthetic material to the abdominal fascia, the intra-abdominal forces could be altered, favoring gradual enlargement of the abdominal cavity. Schuster used sheets of mesh that were sewn to lateral margins of the defect. The mesh was sutured together under tension, and the skin closed. Subsequent operative maneuvers involved reopening the skin and excising redundant mesh as the abdominal cavity grew until the mesh could be completely removed.

In 1968, Gilbert[1] reported a modification of Schuster's technique utilizing reinforced sheets of silicone that were sutured to the abdominal fascia and left to protrude from the wound. To improve on this technique, Allen and Wrenn[1] in 1969 used silicone sheets to construct a silo around the eviscerated mass. Gradually, the silo was reduced until closure of the fascia was achieved. For the past 40 years, this technique has played a prominent role in the management of abdominal wall defects, replacing other approaches from the previous 200 years.

Despite successful surgical treatment before the 1970s, many infants died from starvation as a result of prolonged ileus. In 1971 Filler[1] first reported using total parenteral nutrition (TPN) to provide nutrition for five infants with ruptured omphalocele and gastroschisis. Today, TPN remains a vital part of the standard management of infants with abdominal wall defects.

EMBRYOGENESIS DICTATES THE TYPE OF DEFECT

Closure of the body wall begins at 2 weeks' gestation and results from growth and longitudinal infolding of the embryonic disk. The cephalic fold forms the thoracic and epigastric wall. The caudal fold contributes the hindgut, bladder, and hypogastric wall. The lateral folds form the lateral abdominal walls. These four folds meet in the midline to form the umbilical ring, which is usually fully developed by the fourth week. During the sixth week, growth of the midgut causes a physiologic herniation of the gut out through the umbilical ring. The midgut then rotates as it reenters the abdominal cavity so that the small intestine and colon come to lie in their correct anatomical positions. The intestine migrates to its normal intraperitoneal location by the end of the 10th week of development. Because this process does not occur in cases of omphalocele and gastroschisis, these patients always have malrotation.

TABLE 59-1. Clinical Findings in Infants With Abdominal Wall Defects

Factor	Omphalocele	Gastroschisis
Location	Umbilical ring	Lateral to cord
Size of defect	2.0-10.0 cm	Small (4.0 cm)
Umbilical cord	Inserts in sac	Normal insertion
Sac	Present (amnion and peritoneum)	None
Contents	Liver, bowel, etc.	Bowel, stomach
Bowel appearance	Normal	Matted, foreshortened exudate
Malrotation	Present	Present
Small abdominal cavity	Present	Present
Postoperative alimentary function	Normal	Prolonged ileus
Associated anomalies	Common (50-67%)	Unusual (10% atresia of gut)

The embryogenesis of omphalocele remains controversial. Duhamel[1] suggested that failure of body wall morphogenesis of the cephalic fold would result in an "epigastric omphalocele." These infants have an omphalocele associated with cleft sternum, anterior diaphragmatic hernia, possible ectopia cordis, congenital heart defects, and absence of a portion of the pericardium. This group of anomalies, first described in 1958, is now recognized as the pentalogy of Cantrell. With a small omphalocele or hernia into the umbilical cord, the umbilical ring is only slightly widened. These defects probably represent failure of the intestine to return completely after its normal period of extracolonic development. Failure to form the caudal fold results in hypogastric omphalocele. Both the somatic and splanchnic layers of the fold are affected so that there may be agenesis of the hindgut, exstrophy of the bladder or cloaca, and a fistula between the intestine and bladder. If only the lateral folds fail to develop, the umbilical orifice remains widely open, resulting in a centrally located omphalocele allowing for prolapse of the liver, stomach, spleen, ovaries, small intestine, and colon.

The embryogenesis of gastroschisis is more controversial. Duhamel[1] proposed that gastroschisis was caused by failure of differentiation of embryonic mesenchyme of the lateral folds, which is supported by de Vries's study[1] of serial sections of human fetuses in the Carnegie collection. Involution of the right umbilical vein results in the mesenchymal defect at the junction of the body stalk with the body wall.

FACTORS THAT MAY CAUSE THE DEFECT

Etiologic factors causing omphalocele or gastroschisis have not been conclusively identified in humans. These anomalies may be experimentally induced in rats by folic acid deficiency,[1] administration of salicylates,[1] hypoxia,[1] carbon monoxide, protein-zinc deficiencies,[3] and even increased surface water levels of atrazine and nitrate,[4] which are common agricultural fertilizers. In addition, vasoconstricting medications such as pseudoephedrine, phenylpropanolamine, and ephedrine and nicotine increase the risk of gastroschisis and intestinal atresia.[5] Familial cases of both defects have been reported and major chromosomal anomalies are associated with 10 to 38% of cases

of omphalocele.[6,7] Some cases of omphalocele and gastroschisis may be genetically determined. Obtaining an accurate family history enables the physician to provide recurrence risk counseling in the rare event of familial or syndromic cases. However, providing specific information to families regarding the risk to future pregnancies must be done cautiously until additional studies clarify the genetic and environmental roles.

A CHANGING EPIDEMIOLOGY

The Centers for Disease Control and Prevention estimates that the combined incidence of omphalocele and gastroschisis is approximately 1 in 2000 live births in the United States. In the past, omphalocele was clearly the most common condition; however, the global incidence of gastroschisis is increasing, as noted in reports from Utah,[8] California,[1] Sweden,[1] Finland,[1] Tennessee,[9] New Zealand,[10] and Spain.[11] The incidence of omphalocele remains virtually unchanged.

The incidence of gastroschisis is inversely related to maternal age,[12] being most common in young mothers with low gravidity.[8,13,14] Although both conditions are associated with lower gestational age, prematurity is more common in gastroschisis.[11] Infants have lower birth weight than normal babies of the same gestational age. Gastroschisis infants are often smaller than omphalocele newborns. These observations suggest that abdominal wall defects may be related to prenatal care of the mother. This supposition is reinforced by reports indicating that periconceptional use of multivitamins is associated with a 68% reduction in nonsyndromic omphalocele.[15]

No racial or geographic associations have been observed for either condition. A slight male predominance (1.5:1) is reported for omphalocele but not for gastroschisis.[13] Omphaloceles have occurred in consecutive children, in twins, and in different generations of the same family.

A SPECTRUM OF DEFECTS

Congenital Hernia of the Cord (the Very Small Omphalocele)

Congenital hernias of the umbilical cord should be no larger than 4 cm in diameter, and the sac should contain only a few bowel loops. Careless cord clamping can cause injury to the intestine. Hernias of the cord should be differentiated from larger omphaloceles because the intestine is easily reduced, surgical closure is simple, and excellent results are expected (Figure 59-1A). If left untreated, these small hernias of the cord may gradually reepithelialize (cutis navel). Unlike their larger counterparts, these smaller omphaloceles have traditionally been regarded as isolated defects. However, Ladd's recent report indicates an association with other gastrointestinal anomalies including Meckel's diverticulum and intestinal atresia.[16]

Omphaloceles

An omphalocele is an umbilical ring defect, varying in size from a small, easily treated, condition to a "giant" omphalocele requiring special care (Figure 59-1B). The eviscerated contents are contained within a sac consisting of a translucent avascular membrane composed of peritoneum, Wharton's jelly, and amnion. The umbilical cord is inserted directly onto the sac. The abdominal wall defect varies from 4 to 12 cm and usually contains stomach and loops of large and small intestine. The liver remains extraperitoneal in 48% of cases.[17] Giant omphaloceles have a massive sac that contains most of the abdominal viscera, including the liver, spleen, bladder, gonads, and entire intestinal tract as well as a small underdeveloped peritoneal cavity. Successful management in these cases is challenging and associated with higher morbidity.

The omphalocele sac may rupture in utero, during labor (4% of cases),[6] or after birth (Figure 59-2A). Prenatal rupture of the sac has been reported to occur in 10 to 18% of cases.[18,19] With early disruption, the eviscerated intestine may be covered by thick matted exudate. Gastroschisis may have a similar appearance, but a prenatally ruptured omphalocele can be differentiated by its midline position, abnormal insertion of the umbilical cord, and presence of sac remnants (Figure 59-2B).

Gastroschisis

In gastroschisis, the small smooth-edged opening is located to the right of the umbilical cord (see Figure 59-2B). Rare cases of left-sided gastroschisis have been reported.[20] The size of the defect may be dangerously small but usually varies from 3 to 5 cm. The stomach as well as the small and large intestine are herniated, but the liver is rarely involved. Evisceration of the gallbladder, uterus, fallopian tubes, urinary bladder, testes, and ovaries has been reported.[21] The extruded intestine has an abnormal, matted appearance and may be at risk for vascular compromise (see Figure 59-2B). The abdominal musculature is normally developed, and the underdeveloped abdominal cavity is usually larger than that seen is cases of omphalocele. Associated anomalies are rare. Clinical differences between omphalocele and gastroschisis are summarized in Table 59-1.

ASSOCIATED ANOMALIES (THE MAJOR DETERMINANT OF MORBIDITY AND MORTALITY)

Congenital anomalies are frequently associated with omphalocele. Cardiovascular anomalies are encountered in at least 20% of patients.[22] Tetralogy of Fallot (33%) and atrial septal defects

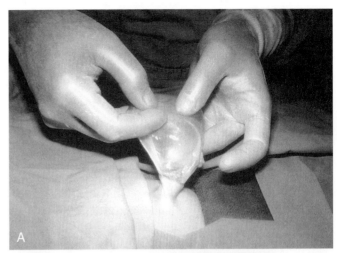

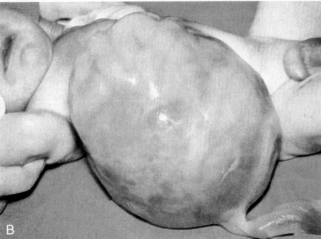

Figure 59-1. (**A**) Congenital hernia of the cord; a very small omphalocele that is easily reduced and repaired by primary closure of the fascia. (**B**) A giant omphalocele, difficult to close, place in a silo, or cover with skin flaps; associated with much higher morbidity and mortality.

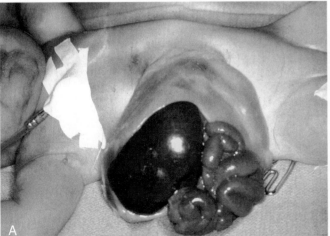

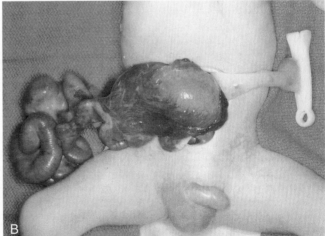

Figure 59-2. (**A**) An infant with a ruptured omphalocele with a large defect; liver is present; the umbilical cord is distorted, and remnants of the sac remain. (**B**) A gastroschisis presenting to the right of a normal-appearing umbilical cord; the bowel is covered with exudate, and a portion appears to be experiencing vascular compromise.

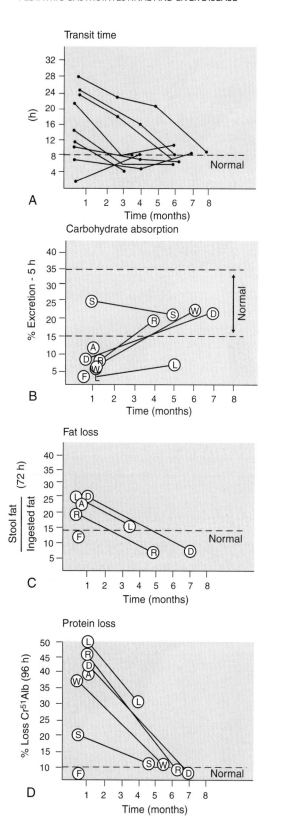

Figure 59-3. (A-D) Initial changes in transit, carbohydrate, protein, and fat absorption in relationship to time in abdominal wall defect patients.

Omphalocele may be associated with trisomies 3,[23] 13, 14, 15, 18, or 21. Beckwith-Wiedemann syndrome is found in approximately 12% of patients. These infants have enlarged tongues, large and rounded craniofacial features, and visceromegaly and are prone to develop hypoglycemia, presumably caused by hyperplasia of the pancreatic islet cells.

Genitourinary anomalies may be associated with omphalocele as part of the syndrome of bladder exstrophy or hindgut agenesis in cases of hypogastric omphalocele. Renal malrotation has been documented in cases of omphalocele.[24] Cryptorchidism is associated with both omphalocele and gastroschisis.

Lower midline syndrome consists of hypogastric omphalocele, cloacal exstrophy, possible duplication of the colon and/or appendix, imperforate anus, colonic atresia, sacral anomalies, myelomeningocele, hydro- or diastematomyelia, and skeletal or limb deformities. This syndrome is very rare and requires sophisticated multidisciplinary management to avoid excessive morbidity. Pentalogy of Cantrell consists of an epigastric omphalocele, diastasis recti, central midline diaphragmatic hernia, distal sternal cleft, pericardial defect, anterior displacement of the heart, and congenital heart disease. Again, individualized management is required.

Other associated anomalies include musculoskeletal abnormalities, cleft palate, Rieger's syndrome, hydrocephalus, pulmonary hypoplasia, and respiratory distress. Prune-belly syndrome is associated with omphaloceles. Abnormalities of the intestinal tract occur with both omphalocele and gastroschisis. Malrotation occurs in all cases of omphalocele and gastroschisis. Lack of intestinal fixation and a narrow mesentery leads to an increased risk of midgut volvulus; however, following surgery, postoperative adhesions significantly lessen this risk. Intestinal atresia, Meckel's diverticulum, and intestinal duplication may be encountered and are especially common in cases of gastroschisis (10 to 15%).[21] The eviscerated intestine is thickened, inflamed, edematous, and matted together, often appearing congested and ischemic. The mesentery is also thickened and short. The length of intestine in most cases of gastroschisis is foreshortened (mean 70 cm), but this is not necessarily of clinical importance because it seems to reverse spontaneously as the inflammation and edema resolve.[25] Irving's[1] postoperative radiographic studies have confirmed the early return to near normal length. Prolonged ileus with delayed transit has been demonstrated in both omphalocele and gastroschisis and particularly when exudate is present.[25] The period of dysfunction usually lasts 20 to 30 days.[19] Studies have documented decreased carbohydrate, fat, and protein absorption. Transit and absorption patterns usually return to normal within 6 months (Figure 59-3).[25]

The severity of intestinal macroscopic damages may be related to the length of time for which the intestine is exposed to amniotic fluid. Gastrointestinal function returns sooner in patients with fewer exudative changes, as is more commonly seen in premature infants. Intestinal wall inflammation is usually less severe in ruptured omphalocele than in gastroschisis. Alteration in amniotic fluid composition with the onset of fetal renal function may contribute to the deleterious effect on the exposed intestine.[25] In fetal lambs with gastroschisis, atrophy of myenteric ganglion cells can be observed, resulting in disordered peristalsis.[26] Moreover, decreased blood flow may be responsible for the changes in "motility" and absorption. Intestinal compression at the neck of the defect results in edema and ischemic damage. In an in utero fetal model, a ligature placed

(25%) are most common. Congenital heart disease is more common with epigastric omphaloceles and may be associated with a diaphragmatic hernia and sternal defect. More than half of patients with omphalocele and congenital heart disease have multiple congenital anomalies or a specific syndrome.[22]

around the herniated bowel causing constriction resulted in bowel dysmotility.[27] It appears that both constriction and ischemia of the intestine as well as exposure to amniotic fluid contribute to the intestinal changes.

PRENATAL MANAGEMENT

Prenatal diagnosis allows for rational decisions regarding such issues as timing, location, and method of delivery as well as risk to the mother, termination of the pregnancy, and parental counseling. If the defect is associated with other severe anomalies, moral, religious, and ethical questions may arise, including discussion regarding termination of the pregnancy. Antenatal diagnosis of anterior abdominal wall defects, though very useful for planning and prenatal counseling, has not proven to have an impact on outcomes including birth weight, gestational age at birth, time to full feeding, requirement for ventilator support, length of stay, or mortality.[28,31] However, there remains a natural benefit for the family and their understanding. The clinician may find it helpful to show families pictures of abdominal wall defects and management in order to best prepare families.

Unborn infants with abdominal wall defects should be monitored by serial ultrasonography to detect intrauterine growth retardation. Prenatal diagnosis allows for appropriate referral to a tertiary care center to plan for the delivery and the surgical care of the newborn.

Gastroschisis and omphalocele may be detected by an elevated maternal serum alpha-fetoprotein (MSAFP) but must be differentiated from other fetal abnormalities, especially spina bifida. Omphalocele may be distinguished from gastroschisis by determining the ratio of acetylcholinesterase to pseudocholinesterase in the amniotic fluid[29] and by appearance on ultrasound.

Ultrasound has become a standard component of prenatal care. Ultrasonography allows for detection of abdominal wall defects after the bowel returns to the peritoneal cavity at the 10th week of gestation. Infants with omphalocele are distinguished from those with gastroschisis by a membranous sac and liver protruding from the abdomen. Children with gastroschisis are characterized by the presence of loops of intestine floating freely in the amniotic fluid. Fetal echocardiography should be performed to detect cardiac defects. In a recent study, 15% of gastroschisis babies and 45% of omphalocele infants had congenital heart disease.[30] This information is critical to advise the parents and prepare the medical team for delivery.

Doppler ultrasonography can be used to evaluate visceral blood flow to the bowel. In cases of gastroschisis, the ultrasonographic appearance of the intestine may be related to the clinical outcome. In addition, polyhydramnios may be a predictor of bowel complications such as atresia or obstruction.[31] In one series, small intestinal dilatation and wall thickening were associated with intestinal atresia or stenosis.[32] Though secondary gastrointestinal changes identified via prenatal ultrasonography have historically been identified as possible predictors of postnatal outcomes that could aide in the accuracy of prenatal counseling as well as identify patients who may benefit from closer fetal surveillance, a recent review suggests that such correlation does not exist.[33] The appearance of the intestine on ultrasonography is not an indication for early delivery of the child.

Amniocentesis

Amniocentesis and chromosomal analysis may be considered to detect abnormalities that commonly occur. Amnio-exchange may reduce inflammation in the exposed gastroschisis by reducing gastrointestinal waste in the amniotic fluid.[34] Luton's publication described transabdominal amniotic fluid drainage. Beginning at 30 weeks' gestation, approximately 900 mL amniotic fluid would be removed and replaced with an equal amount of warm normal saline. This procedure was repeated every 2 to 3 weeks. No adverse incidents were identified, and significant improvement was noted in degree of intestinal exudate, duration of ventilation, and length of stay in the neonatal intensive care unit (NICU).[34] Although a novel idea, amnio-exchange is not practiced routinely.

Cesarean Section Versus Vaginal Delivery

Large omphaloceles may cause obstructed labor or liver injury, necessitating C-section. Several years ago these anecdotal reports led to proposals that cesarean section was the preferred method of delivery. Cameron set the precedence in 1978 describing elective cesarean section for a prenatally diagnosed omphalocele.[35] Lenke and Hatch[1] claimed that babies with gastroschisis delivered by cesarean section have less intestinal edema, were easier to repair, and had shorter hospital stays with lower mortality.

However, numerous recent studies have concluded that cesarean section is unwarranted. Bethel, Carpenter, Davidson, and Kirk[1] have concluded that cesarean section does not confer any advantage with regard to survival or other neonatal postoperative parameters. A meta-analysis of existing studies dealing with the mode of delivery was recently completed by Segal et al. and confirmed these findings.[36] Although medical and legal issues may understandably influence obstetric care, there are currently no prospective, well-controlled studies that support the contention that cesarean section provides an additional measure of safety for babies with abdominal wall defects.[37]

INITIAL MANAGEMENT AFTER DELIVERY

Resuscitation should begin immediately. An orogastric tube is inserted to prevent vomiting and aspiration, to improve ventilation, to decrease intestinal distention, and to facilitate visceral reduction. Newborns with signs of respiratory distress should undergo immediate endotracheal intubation. Fluid resuscitation must be initiated promptly to avoid hypothermia. An intravenous line should be placed, preferably in an upper limb because inferior vena caval compression may occur during reduction. However, catheters inserted into the lower limbs and advanced into the inferior vena cava may be useful in determining the intra-abdominal pressure. A 6-French Foley catheter should be inserted into the bladder to monitor urine output and intravesicular pressure. Hematocrit, serum electrolytes, blood glucose, and arterial blood gas values should be obtained soon after birth to guide resuscitation.

Although normal neonates require limited maintenance volumes for the first few days of life (60 to 80 mL/kg per day), infants with abdominal wall defects experience abnormal fluid losses particularly with gastroschisis and ruptured omphalocele. The resulting metabolic acidosis may last several days.

The previously described intestinal changes result in substantial water, electrolyte, and protein losses. Atmospheric exposure of the intestine results in increased insensible fluid and heat losses. Initial fluid resuscitation should consist of rapid bolus infusion of 20 mL/kg of isotonic crystalloid solution. Tradition has maintained that solutions low in electrolytes are most appropriate for infants; however, this is not true for infants with omphalocele or gastroschisis. The rate of infusion should be guided by the clinical condition of the baby as determined by pulse rate, mean arterial blood pressure, and urine output. Infusion of D_5 0.5 NS at two to three times maintenance requirements is usually necessary. Babies with eviscerated intestines have abnormally low levels of immunoglobulin and are probably at greater risk for developing infection. Despite attempts to maintain sterility, contamination of the intestine is inevitable and broad-spectrum antibiotics should be administered as well as vitamin K in anticipation of the surgical procedure.

Once fluid resuscitation has begun, attention should be directed to the herniated intestine and avoidance of hypothermia. If the intestine is contained within a sac, it should be left intact. In some cases of gastroschisis, it may be apparent that the defect is so small that it is causing vascular compromise of the intestine. In these cases, the physician should immediately enlarge the defect. This may be quickly accomplished by applying a straight hemostat superior to the defect in the midline and then dividing the tissue. Occasionally, gastroschisis loops of intestine will require untwisting to restore circulation. The infant should be placed on the side with the organs arranged to avoid injury or vascular compromise. The gastroschisis should be covered by encircling the torso of the infant in sterile gauze and clear plastic wrap to reduce the evaporative loss of heat and fluid and to allow for frequent examination (Figure 59-4). More recently, "bowel bags" have been developed that allows the neonate's lower extremities and abdominal wall defect to be placed inside (Figure 59-5). A drawstring then secures the bag around the lower chest. Hypothermia is a frequent and serious problem that can be avoided by placing the infant under a radiant heater immediately after birth and maintaining the infant in a heated incubator or infant care island.

After initial resuscitation, the infant should undergo careful evaluation for associated anomalies. Episodes of cyanosis, absence of the xiphoid, or cleft sternum should alert the clinician to the possibility of a cardiac or diaphragmatic defect. Chest radiographs may be helpful in identifying associated cardiac anomalies, diaphragmatic defects, or aspiration. If trisomy 13 or 18 is confirmed, the prognosis is poor, and consultation with the parents is advisable before further treatment is undertaken. Discussions with the family and ethics committee may be helpful in defining the most appropriate course.

Although surgical procedures are not especially difficult, intraoperative judgment and postoperative expertise are major determinants of good outcome. Transfer of these infants to an appropriate tertiary care center is always recommended. Heated incubators should be used to prevent hypothermia. A secure intravenous fluid infusion should be continued, and qualified personnel should accompany the infant.

SPECIFIC MANAGEMENT OF THE DEFECT

Initial management of the defect may be operative or nonoperative. Surgical treatment of omphalocele and gastroschisis is similar and should take into account the size of the defect, the eviscerated mass, gestational age, birth weight, and the presence of other anomalies. The goal is to achieve closure of the

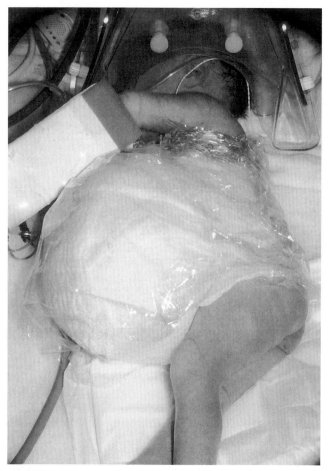

Figure 59-4. Infant recently born with abdominal wall defect wrapped in dry gauze and covered with plastic wrap to protect from contamination and avoid fluid and heat loss. Before wrapping bowel, one must inspect the bowel; untwist the mesentery, if necessary; and then place the baby on his or her side to facilitate blood flow return.

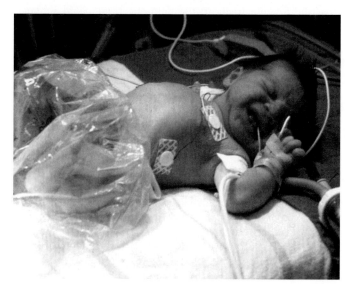

Figure 59-5. Newborn with abdominal wall defect that has been secured in preformed bowel bag with drawstring.

defect as soon as possible, avoid complications, and shorten hospital stay. Nonoperative topical treatment of omphalocele is occasionally indicated and may be helpful when transportation to a tertiary care facility is impossible or when ethical issues are encountered. Topical treatment of gastroschisis is not appropriate.

Nonoperative Treatment

Nonoperative treatment of omphaloceles is associated with a significant risk for infection, sac rupture during the gradual epithelialization phase, and prolonged hospitalization. In addition, the infant is left with a large ventral hernia that must be repaired later (Figure 59-6A,B). However, nonoperative management may be indicated in infants who have other life-threatening conditions, thoracic hypoplasia, severe cardiac lesions, or chromosomal syndromes. Silver sulfadiazine has become the favored topical treatment. Two percent merbromin solution for topical application to the omphalocele sac[38] can result in toxic mercury levels necessitating monitoring of serum mercury levels. Alternative topical agents include 0.5% silver nitrate solution, 70% alcohol, or biologic dressings. Regardless of which agent is selected, the skin will gradually grow up and around the defect. Improved surgical therapy and NICU care have relegated topical therapy to a secondary role.

General Principles of Surgical Management

Before proceeding with operative care, it is imperative to ensure that the infant has received adequate fluid resuscitation and is not hypothermic or acidotic. There is no advantage in rushing to the operating theater. Heat loss during the procedure should be prevented by placing the infant on a neonatal warming unit, wrapping the head and limbs, and increasing the ambient temperature of the room.

Surgery is performed under general anesthesia with muscle relaxation. Bacterial contamination can be reduced by thorough cleansing of the exposed intestine with povidone-iodine solution, which is washed off with warm sterile saline solution. Rectal irrigation with warm saline will evacuate bulky meconium from the intestine. A Foley catheter is inserted once the sterile field has been established.

An intact omphalocele sac should be excised while avoiding injury to adherent liver. Amnion that is clearly adherent to the liver should be left in place. The hepatic veins may be elongated and can kink with excessive torsion. Usually, the defect will be enlarged to allow adequate inspection and reduction of the intestine. Ladd's bands may be present in association with malrotation and should be divided to preclude duodenal obstruction; however, a formal Ladd's procedure with appendectomy is not required. In gastroschisis, inspection of the intestine may be difficult because of the covering inflammatory peel, which should not be removed because considerable blood loss or inadvertent intestinal perforation may occur. Often the bowel will appear abnormal and may suggest the presence of an intestinal atresia; however, more often than not, the edematous bowel has lumen continuity. Obvious atretic areas may be detected. If primary closure is feasible and areas of intestinal atresia are encountered that are not excessively matted, the bowel may be resected and primary anastomosis accomplished without undue risk.[14] However, if inflammation of the intestine is severe, it may be prudent to leave the segment of atresia in situ and plan for delayed repair in 4 to 6 weeks when the inflammation has resolved. Some authors have advocated the use of temporary exteriorizing ostomies for atresias, whereas others have suggested that an intestinal anastomosis in these babies may be complicated by an increased risk of a postoperative stricture.[39,40] However, we believe that, because of the risk of infection, exteriorization of the intestine is unnecessary and unwise. When a silo is used, the atresia may be repaired when the edema has partially resolved. A primary anastomosis can be safely performed at the time of final fascial closure.[41]

After the intestine has been inspected, a diaphragmatic hernia should be excluded. If the liver is herniated in the omphalocele, careful division of the diaphragmatic attachments allows for easier reduction. The liver has an abnormal globular shape,

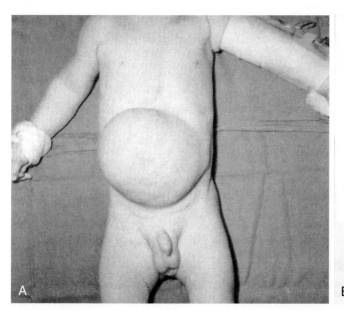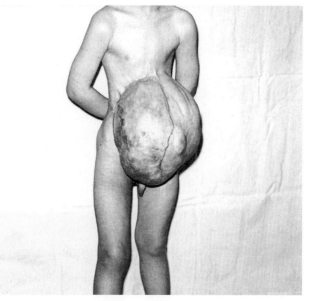

Figure 59-6. **(A)** Infant treated by skin flap closure with resultant large ventral hernia. **(B)** Child with same treatment in which hernia has enlarged and loss of domain has occurred. The peritoneal cavity has become relatively smaller.

and it may be difficult to reduce the organ to the normal anatomical position. Care must be taken not to injure elongated hepatic veins, obstruct the stomach, or compress the inferior vena cava during reduction of the liver. Acute bradycardia or hypotension may be signs of decreased preload from vascular obstruction.

The decision whether to repair the abdominal wall defect by primary fascial closure or to utilize a staged repair is a critical one. No consensus exists regarding the optimal approach. For hernias of the cord or small omphaloceles, primary closure is clearly preferred and is associated with the fewest complications. For larger defects, the degree of visceroabdominal disproportion often makes it difficult to reduce the viscera in one stage without causing hemodynamic or respiratory compromise. Historically, one of the immediate problems facing the surgical team at the conclusion of the operation was achieving safe extubation of the patient. For this reason, infants were allowed to breathe spontaneously during surgery. Muscle relaxants were not used. This concern dictated the use of the staged silo approach during the late 1960s and 1970s. With improved postoperative ventilator care, primary closure has been accepted as appropriate management for babies born with abdominal wall defects. Currently, for giant omphaloceles, various closure techniques have been described including the use of human acellular dermis (AlloDerm) as a primary abdominal fascial substitute,[42] tissue expanders,[43] and bovine pericardial patches.[44]

To Close or Stage Considerations

When to close the defect as opposed to using a silo remains one of the most important considerations. The anesthetist must monitor airway resistance, pulmonary compliance, and hemodynamic status and should alert the surgeon if visceral reduction causes respiratory, metabolic, or hemodynamic compromise. Intra-abdominal pressure may be measured during closure of all abdominal wall defects. Intravesicular and inferior vena cava pressures closely correlate with intra-abdominal pressure.[45] The indirect measurement of intra-abdominal pressure should not exceed 20 mm Hg. Intraoperative measurement of intra-abdominal pressure, central venous pressure, or cardiac index should reliably predict success or failure of primary operative repair. In contrast, heart rate, blood pressure, and systemic vascular resistance are not reliable indicators. Alternatively, the surgeon may follow peak inspiratory pressure as the fascia is closed. In most instances, the surgeon will also have to rely on his or her clinical experience.

Primary Closure Guidelines

Primary closure has historically been the goal because it is associated with an excellent outcome.[46] Muscle relaxants during the operation are necessary to achieve safe primary closure. Older publications suggested that newborns treated by primary closure had a shorter hospital stay compared to staged silo closure as well as improved survival, reduced risk of sepsis, and less intestinal dysfunction.[47] Transient edema of the lower limbs is common and is not usually associated with any morbidity. With primary closure, the loops of intestine are carefully returned to the abdominal cavity, with care taken to orient the mesentery correctly and to avoid vascular compromise. The fascia is approximated with interrupted suture, and the skin is closed with absorbable subcuticular suture. Stretching the abdominal wall may render an incision unnecessary. With gastroschisis, a portion of the umbilical cord is preserved. The remaining skin can be encircled and gathered around the cord remnant. The cosmetic results, as depicted in Figure 59-7A, have been excellent. Years later, the uninformed clinician may not recognize that the patient has had an operation (Figure 59-7B).

Respiratory compromise can be avoided by monitoring the intraoperative airway pressure. As a guide, airway pressure should not exceed 25 mm Hg. Although it is possible to overcome respiratory problems encountered during the primary closure, other consequences of a "tight" closure may occur. Cardiac output may be reduced and corrected by intravascular volume expansion, ionotropic agents, or both. Renal blood flow and glomerular filtration rate can be dramatically reduced

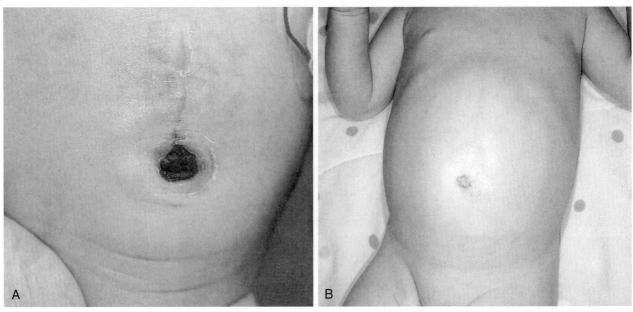

Figure 59-7. **(A)** Immediate postoperative appearance of a baby with upper midline incision and use of umbilical cord umbilicoplasty, forming a near normal appearance of the abdominal wall. **(B)** Older child following primary closure of gastroschisis; note that there is no incision and the neo-umbilicus appears relatively normal with an excellent cosmetic appearance.

and may not be restored by fluid volume replacement. Intra-abdominal pressures that exceed 20 mm Hg may cause renal vein thrombosis and renal failure. If the pressure exceeds this level, the baby should be returned to the operating room, the fascia opened, and a silo applied.

Silo Closure Guidelines

This method has been widely adopted and is associated with low morbidity and mortality.[48] Silo closure avoids manipulation of the abdominal wall, intestinal milking of meconium, and the use of high-pressure postoperative ventilation, mitigating the risk of pulmonary barotrauma. Recent reviews advocating the use of the silo have noted an association with a decreased incidence of abdominal compartment syndrome, better bowel motility, and fewer complications.[49,50] In addition, a recent prospective multicenter randomized controlled trial revealed that the routine use of a preformed silo produces similar outcomes to primary closure yet produces fewer days on the ventilator.[51]

If staged silo closure is chosen for treatment, Silastic sheeting may be used to construct the silo, or a preformed silo can be used. All skin is saved and not sutured to Silastic sheeting. A closed silo is then constructed around the intestine by stapling or suturing the sheet to itself (Figure 59-8A). The silo should be perpendicular to the defect, and the walls kept parallel to avoid a constriction at the base of the silo where the prosthesis joins the abdominal wall (see Figure 59-8A). After the silo is applied, it should be wrapped in sterile, thick gauze bandages to protect the silo and prevent evaporation and contamination. Some surgeons favor completely wrapping the silo, whereas others opt to keep the top free from gauze and thus allow a window to frequently inspect the bowel. When the infant is returned to an

open incubator, the apex of the silo should be suspended from the overhead warming lights to prevent it from tilting over and to allow gravity to encourage reduction (Figure 59-8B). Prefashioned silos have been increasingly favored in the past few years (Figure 59-9A). They have become the preferred method because they are applied quickly in the NICU, avoid suturing to the abdominal wall, and do not require anesthesia.

POSTOPERATIVE MANAGEMENT

Infants with large defects require postoperative ventilation until the abdominal wall relaxes and edema resolves sufficiently to allow for adequate spontaneous respiration. Arterial blood gas values should be carefully monitored, and the respiratory rate, inspired oxygen, peak airway pressure, and tidal volume should be adjusted as necessary to maintain optimal ventilation and oxygenation. A decrease in urine output may represent decreased preload from vena cava compression or increased intra-abdominal pressure. Fluid resuscitation should be aggressive. If a fluid challenge fails to improve renal function, reoperation to relieve intra-abdominal pressure and application of a silo may be required to avert serious renal damage.

Fluid Management

Even if preoperative and intraoperative fluid resuscitation has been vigorous, postoperative fluid requirements are much higher for babies with abdominal wall defects. These infants require as much as 312 mL/kg or as little as 83 mL/kg in the first 24 hours of life to support tissue perfusion as determined by muscle pH studies. A mean fluid volume of 146 ± 35 mg/kg may

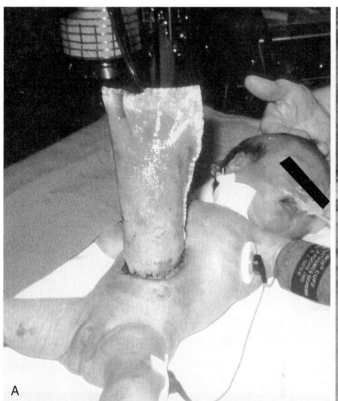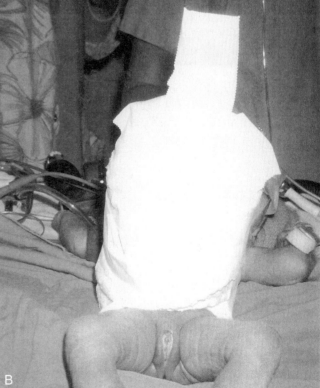

Figure 59-8. (**A**) Newborn requiring placement of bowel within a "constructed" silo; bowel loops and exudative fluid are visible. (**B**) Silo covered with thick dry gauze dressings; suspension avoids kinking of the silo and facilitates effects of gravity.

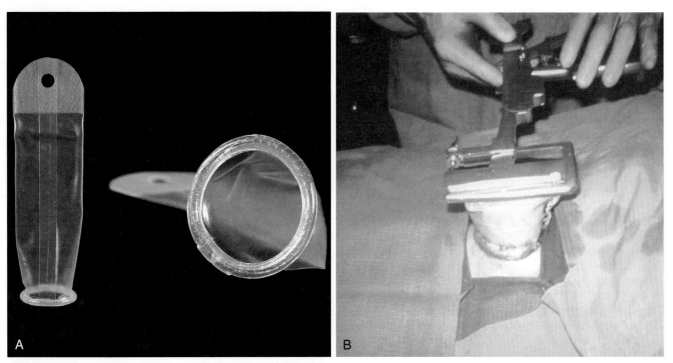

Figure 59-9. (**A**) Preformed silo with spring coil at base opening; easy to place bowel in silo and quick to insert beneath the fascia; avoids time-consuming attachment to the abdominal wall. (**B**) Depicts the use of the stapling device to sequentially and safely reduce the size of the silo.

be required for the first day.[52] The requirements for the first, second, and third days after surgical repair, respectively, may vary as follows: 160.7 mL/kg on the first day, 125.4 mL/kg on the second day, and 141.5 mL/kg on the third day. Frequent bedside evaluation is crucial. Urinary output should be used to adjust the actual volumes administered. Postoperative fluid requirements for infants with gastroschisis and babies with silos may be higher compared with patients with omphalocele and primary closure patients throughout the first postoperative week.

Delay in the return of intestinal function must be anticipated. Parents are best informed of this expectation right after surgery. Prokinetic agents such as erythromycin have not proven effective in randomized trials at speeding return of intestinal function.[53] The orogastric tube should be left in position and frequently aspirated to keep the intestine decompressed. Parenteral nutrition will be necessary for all infants. During the period of prolonged ileus, trophic feedings to facilitate intestinal recovery have been well established as safe and effective.[54] TPN is best started early in anticipation that intestinal motility will not return immediately. Delivery of 100 to120kcal/kg with frequent monitoring of prealbumin levels is usually sufficient. Patients with ruptured omphalocele or gastroschisis are most likely to require prolonged TPN. Insertion of a central venous catheter or PICC line is beneficial. Catheter-related sepsis and liver disease are complications of TPN therapy. Blood cultures should be obtained if fever is detected, and the central catheter should be removed if there are signs of infection. Some surgeons defer insertion of TPN catheters for several days to minimize the chance of contamination induced by the initial operative procedure. Liver enzyme values should be monitored to evaluate liver function. Oral feeding should not be started until orogastric aspirates are negligible and stools are passed. Because infants with these disorders often have some degree of malabsorption, it is advisable to begin feeding with semielemental or predigested formulas.

Infants with silo closure are at risk for dehydration owing to loss of fluid around the silo. Septicemia, although possible, is not likely. As the abdominal wall relaxes and the edema resolves, the contents of the silo should be reduced every 12 to 24 hours, with care being taken not to cause excessive elevation of intra-abdominal pressure. Slow, gradual reduction is favored because overly aggressive attempts often lead to silo dislodgement. Manipulation of the silo must be done under strict aseptic conditions. Each time the viscera are reduced, the silo volume must be adjusted accordingly. This can be done by suturing the sac, using umbilical tape, or applying a stapling device (Figure 59-9B). Usually within a week, complete reduction of the gastroschisis is achieved, and the infant may be returned to the operating theater for removal of the prosthesis and final closure of the defect (Figure 59-10). Silo reduction of omphaloceles often takes longer.

ALTERNATIVE METHODS OF CLOSURE

Gross's skin flap closure techniques have assumed a secondary role. This technique may still be useful when a prosthesis is not available, when premature separation of the silo occurs, or when the surgeon determines that fascial closure is dangerous. Although Gross originally advised leaving the omphalocele sac intact, most surgeons today advise removing the sac to inspect the viscera. Barlow[1] recommended the application of an external bandage silo to reduce the giant omphalocele for several days before operation is undertaken. Jona suggested that the effects of gravity and time may be sufficient to reduce the bowel within a silo while avoiding the potential complications of abdominal compartment syndrome or respiratory compromise.[55] Hendrickson recommended sequential bedside clamping without a prosthesis as a useful alternative to silo or skin flap closure for omphalocele.[56] In 1990, Klein[1] reported the treatment of infants with abdominal wall defects utilizing dura to close the abdominal wall. Saxena recommended this

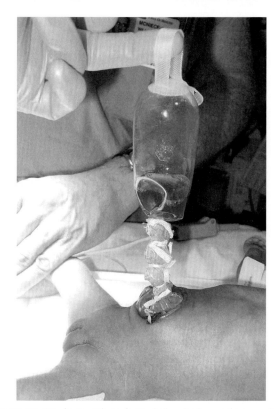

Figure 59-10. Newborn with preformed silo who has undergone daily silo reductions. Daily progress has been secured with umbilical tape. The newborn is now ready for definitive fascial closure.

method for cases of giant omphalocele when a silo is not available or skin flaps would not cover the defect.[57] Meddings[1] recently reported the use of polyglactin mesh to achieve closure of the abdominal wall. Yazbeck[1] reported use of a polyamide mesh that was glued to the abdominal wall and reduced by segmental infolding of the mesh. Hong[1] suggested sequential reduction of the intact sac to reduce giant omphaloceles. Bax[1] and DeUgarte[58] reported a new concept using tissue expanders that are placed into the peritoneal cavity for several days. After the expander is progressively enlarged and sufficient volume is achieved, the expander is removed and the abdomen is closed. With so many options, there is no clear consensus on how best to approach the newborn with a giant omphalocele.

EXPECTED MORTALITY

Until the 1960s and 1970s, omphalocele and gastroschisis were associated with a very high mortality rate. The advent of parenteral nutrition and staged methods of closure in the late 1970s contributed to improved survival. The size of the defect and the presence of herniated liver appear to have no influence on mortality. In cases of omphalocele, babies weighing less than 2500 g have a higher rate of mortality. In cases of gastroschisis, the mortality rate is not related to birth weight. Multiple congenital anomalies continue to be the major cause of death in omphalocele patients, and mortality rates have not improved over the past several years. In contrast, the overall survival rate for patients with gastroschisis markedly improved to 90% during the last several decades. Prematurity, intestinal complications, and sepsis associated with parenteral nutrition have been the major contributors to mortality.[1]

TABLE 59-2. Possible Postsurgical Complications

Early	Intermediate	Late
Respiratory distress	Inguinal hernia	Growth delay
Wound infection	Gastroesophageal reflux	Low IQ
Postsurgical ileus	Cryptorchidism	Malpositioned
Dehydration	Ventral hernia	viscera
Enteric fistula	Small intestinal	Atypical
Necrotizing enterocolitis	obstruction	appendicitis
Gastric outlet	Malrotation with	Intestinal
obstruction	obstruction	obstruction
Malabsorption	Necrotizing enterocolitis	
Lower limb swelling	Gastric outlet	
Renal vein thrombosis	obstruction	
Premature separation	Malabsorption	
of silo		

In general, there is a gratifying trend toward improved survival and simpler procedures. In the future, morbidity and mortality will most likely be determined by associated anomalies, prematurity, and unexpected postsurgical complications.

INCREASING HOSPITAL COSTS

Patient care continues to be the paramount concern. However, the cost of hospital care is becoming an increasing concern. The average cost of hospitalization has been reported as US$123,000.[59] Room charges contributed to 43% of total costs. Additional costs included physician fees collected (15%), respiratory care (10%), supplies (10%), pharmacy (6%), lab (4%), operating room charges (4%), and other (8%). Cost per day was nearly US$2700. Significant cost differences between staged repair (US$154,000) and primary repair (US$93,800) were noted. Cost for babies with gastrointestinal complications averaged US$219,200 versus US$83,800 for those without such complications. There was strong correlation between hospital costs, the use of the NICU, and overall length of stay.[59] Clearly every effort should be made to use methods that minimize the risk of complications and at the same time avoid overuse of the neonatal intensive care unit.

POSTOPERATIVE COMPLICATIONS

Postoperative complications can be divided into early, intermediate, and late (Table 59-2). Whichever method of closure has been used, high-volume bilious aspirates and failure to pass stool may suggest obstruction. The radiographic appearance of dilated intestine may mimic intestinal obstruction. In fact, radiographs may appear abnormal for several months postoperatively. However, mechanical obstruction is relatively uncommon, and these signs usually indicate prolonged postoperative ileus. If there is clinical suspicion of obstruction, upper gastrointestinal radiographic contrast studies are helpful. These studies are usually delayed for at least 1 month postoperatively, given that most clinicians are unlikely to reexplore a newborn before that. Moreover, water-soluble contrast examination of the colon may actually help to evacuate meconium, provide information regarding the distal small intestine, demonstrate sites of obstruction, and stimulate peristalsis. Occasionally, sites of atresia or obstruction due to Ladd's bands will be missed at the time of the initial operation. However, the abdomen should only be reexplored if there is definite radiographic evidence of mechanical obstruction. Intestinal obstruction may occur months or years after the original operation and can be related to intraperitoneal adhesions or malrotation. However, such adhesions do not seem to be a common long-term problem.

One of the most problematic complications has been the development of postoperative necrotizing enterocolitis.[60] During the past few years, this complication has contributed to approximately 20% of the deaths at one institution. Management consists of orogastric tube decompression, antibiotics, and physiologic support. Operative intervention is reserved for patients with physiologic deterioration or perforation.

Enteric fistulas may develop at the site of inadvertent intestinal injury, unrecognized areas of ischemia, or atresia. Compression of intestinal loops by tight closure or erosion due to contact with suture may cause intestinal injury and lead to fistula formation. Perforation of intestine in a silo is possible. Moreover, a fistula may develop if a primary anastomosis fails. Fistulas without distal obstruction often close spontaneously, and therefore a period of observation and TPN may be warranted. If further complications develop, reoperation and exteriorization may be desirable.

Development of inguinal hernia after closure of the defect has been reported and is presumably caused by increased intra-abdominal pressure. In one series, inguinal hernias occurred in 14% of patients with omphalocele and 2% of patients with gastroschisis.[18] Ventral hernias occur in infants who are treated by skin flap closure or by nonoperative measures. In addition, because the fascial closure is sometimes done under considerable tension, hernias may occur along the closure line and necessitate repair. Small hernias may heal spontaneously. Late secondary hernia repairs in older children may require staged closure or the use of prosthetic materials.

Increased intra-abdominal pressure may also lead to gastroesophageal reflux.[14,17] Nissen fundoplication should be considered. Conversely, low intra-abdominal pressure during fetal development may contribute to the increased incidence of cryptorchidism, which is seen frequently in male infants with abdominal wall defects.[24]

LATE MORBIDITY AND QUALITY OF LIFE

Long-term problems related to intestinal function are uncommon. As noted, absorption of carbohydrate, protein, and fat may be abnormal at birth and in the early postoperative period. This may result from a combination of bowel dysmotility and bacterial overgrowth. Families may note irritability, abdominal distention, and foul-smelling stools. Occasionally bowel "decontamination" will be required with a 7-day course of oral antibiotics. The authors counsel families that these findings and the associated radiographic abnormalities may be present up until 6 months of life. At that point intestinal function has usually returned to normal. Predigested formulas should be considered initially. Berseth[1] studied 22 survivors of omphalocele and gastroschisis. Fecal fat excretion and serum chemistry were normal in all patients at 3 years of age. However, at 1 year of age, these patients were between the 3rd and 15th percentile for weight and height and by 10 years of age, no child demonstrated a height or weight above the 50th percentile.

The cause of poor growth is unclear, although it must be remembered that many patients with gastroschisis have low birth weight, and failure to attain normal growth may be caused by underlying prenatal factors or associated anomalies. Berseth[1]

found that one third of their patients had IQs of less than 90. Intellectual impairment seemed to be related to the length of hospital stay. The authors concluded that this complication might be related to prematurity, low birth weight, and other nongastrointestinal neonatal complications.

Koivusalo[61] reviewed 57 patients, aged 17 years or older, with congenital abdominal wall defects. With the exception of rheumatoid arthritis, the prevalence of acquired disease in abdominal wall defect patients was comparable to that in the general population. A number of patients had concerns related to the abdominal scar (37%); 51% appeared to have disturbances best characterized as functional gastrointestinal disorders. Most important, overall quality of life and education levels of these patients were similar to those of the general population.[61]

In his review, Zaccara[62] focused on possible long-term physiologic limitations of children with abdominal wall defects. Following the Bruce protocol for children, 18 children ranging in age from 7 to 18 years with previous abdominal wall defects underwent stress treadmill testing with a stepwise workload increase until exhaustion. Ergometric data were compared with the normal pediatric population. Parameters included exercise time, maximal oxygen consumption, heart rate, systolic blood pressure, and forced vital capacity. These patients exhibited normal cardiopulmonary function with no abnormalities detected at rest or exertion.[62] No limitation to motor performances should exist for these patients.

Finally, malposition of the abdominal viscera may cause problems. Gastric outlet obstruction caused by displacement of the spleen or other organs has been documented.[63] The previously eviscerated globular liver may be misdiagnosed as an epigastric abdominal mass and is more susceptible to traumatic injury.[63] Finally, the associated malrotation may create a diagnostic dilemma if the child develops appendicitis later in life, because the cecum may not reside in the right lower quadrant. For this reason, some surgeons will remove the appendix if it can be safely done during the original operation and if no associated genitourinary anomalies requiring bladder augmentation are present.

REFERENCES

16. Kumar HR, Jester AL, Ladd AP. Impact of omphalocele size on associated conditions. J Pediatr Surg 2008;43:2216–2219.
28. Murphy FL, Mazlan TA, Tarheen F, et al. Gastroschisis and exomphalos in Ireland 1998-2004. Does antenatal diagnosis impact on outcome? Pediatr Surg Int 2007;23:1059–1063.
50. Schlatter M, Norris K, Uitvlugt N, et al. Improved outcomes in the treatment of gastroschisis using a preformed silo and delayed repair approach. J Pediatr Surg 2003;38:459–464.
51. Pastor AC, Phillips JD, Fenton SJ, et al. Routine use of a Silastic spring-loaded silo for infants with gastroschisis: a multicenter randomized controlled trial. J Pediatr Surg 2008;43:1807–1812.
53. Curry JI, Lander AD, Stringer MD, et al. A multicenter, randomized, double-blind, placebo-controlled trial of the prokinetic agent erythromycin in the postoperative recovery of infants with gastroschisis. J Pediatr Surg 2004;39:565–569.
61. Koivusalo A, Lindahl H, Rintala RJ. Morbidity and quality of life in adult patients with a congenital abdominal wall defect: a questionnaire survey. J Pediatr Surg 2002;37:1594–1601.

See expertconsult.com for a complete list of references and the review questions for this chapter.

STOMAS OF THE SMALL AND LARGE INTESTINE

60

Michael W. L. Gauderer • Daniel F. Saad

Enterostomies play an important role in the management of numerous gastrointestinal conditions in the pediatric age group. Indications for such stomas comprise a broad spectrum ranging from decompression for congenital to acquired bowel obstructions, from diversion for neonatal intestinal perforations to abdominoperineal trauma, from foregut access for long-term enteral feedings to hindgut access for antegrade enemas. Pediatric stomas differ from those in adult patients in many aspects, including the criteria for the selection of the most appropriate type, the importance of technical precision in the placement, the specialized age-related care, growth, and the consideration of the psychologic needs of the child. Because of this, a team approach is highly desirable in the management of these patients.

HISTORICAL NOTE

The word *stoma* comes from the Greek *stomoun* (to provide with an opening or mouth). The history of intestinal stomas is long and colorful.[1] Indeed, the concept of treating intestinal obstruction with exteriorization of the colon dates back to the eighteenth century, and among the first survivors were children with imperforate anus.[2] However, despite a few early successes, the use of stomas in the large intestine and later in the small intestine in children evolved slowly. With the advent of modern pediatric surgical practice and survival of children with conditions that were formally likely to be fatal, the need for stomas increased. Enterostomal construction techniques, initially developed for adults,[1,3] were modified and adapted for pediatric patients. Early approaches focused on newborns with congenital intestinal obstruction.[4-7] These were followed by new techniques combining proximal decompression with distal feeding for neonates with high intestinal atresia.[8-10] A number of other special, child-oriented stomas of the small and large intestine were introduced next.[11-19] In the past couple of decades, in great part because of the increased incidence of foregut dysmotility, new procedures aimed at providing postpyloric feeding access continue to be developed and evaluated.[11,14,16,20] In addition, the advent of minimally invasive techniques provides new and exciting opportunities for the creation of feeding as well as venting, decompressing, and irrigating stomas.[21-28]

Several factors have contributed to the safety, effectiveness, and ease of care of pediatric stomas. Paramount among these is the advent of enterostomal therapy, which has evolved into a specialty in its own right.[29-31] The knowledge and experience derived from enterostomal care has led to the creation of child-specific appliances in a wide variety of types and sizes, as well as better tolerated biomaterials and sophisticated management techniques. Another important development has been the creation of nonmedical support systems and organizations for ostomates.[32] Along with this is the availability of a significant number of publications for parents, caregivers, and teenage patients.[33-36] Greater awareness and acceptance of ostomates, as well as the recognition of their needs and rights among the lay population, has also helped to improve their quality of life.[37] On the physician's side, understanding of stomal physiology and of specialized enteral and parenteral nutrition, as well as the diagnosis and management of stoma-related complications, has further improved care and outcome.[29,38,39] Although surgeons and gastroenterologists caring for children are continuously developing and evaluating alternatives to stomas,[40] the creation, management, and closure of these accesses to the intestinal tract continue to occupy a substantial portion of their practice.[41]

CHILD WITH A STOMA

An enterostomy in a child is a major disruption of normality and frequently leads to significant psychologic trauma for the child and parents.[42] Most intestinal stomas in the pediatric age group are temporary, and correction of the underlying problem often leads to closure of the diverting opening. In instances of noncorrectable and crippling pathologic conditions of the intestines, a permanent well-functioning stoma contributes to an improved quality of life.[37]

Despite many advances related to enterostomies, their placement, care, and closure are associated with a surprisingly high rate of both early and late complications.[43-53] These facts present the surgeon, the gastroenterologist, the enterostomal therapist, the nurses, the parents and the child with major challenges. Therefore, when the need for a stoma arises, the best results are achieved by carefully evaluating the child's pathologic condition and health status, weighing the pros and cons of diversion, planning ahead (for closure) whenever possible, and considering both construction and takedowns as major interventions. In addition to the well-defined guidelines for stomal placement established for adult patients, such factors as anatomic and physiologic differences, delicate structures, growth, and physical and emotional maturity need to be considered. It must always be kept in mind that the quality of life of a patient with a stoma is largely related to the quality of that stoma.

TYPES OF INTESTINAL STOMA AND THEIR APPLICATIONS

Depending on their primary purpose, enterostomas can be divided into four basic types.

1   Administration of Feeding, Medication, or Both (Figure 60-1)

The access can be done indirectly, *without entering the small bowel wall*, using nasojejunal or gastrostomy-jejunostomy tubes.[55] This approach works well if used for a limited number of days or a few weeks. However, catheter plugging as well as dislodgement through accidental removal or displacement back into the stomach is common, restricting this modality largely to short-term use.

For long-term use, *direct access through the small bowel wall* is preferred. The options are needle-catheter jejunostomy,[11] tunneled catheter jejunostomy,[16] placement of a T tube,[13] or a button.[14] In addition, in selected patients, a direct percutaneous endoscopic jejunostomy or a laparoscopically assisted jejunostomy[21] may be used, obviating the need for a laparotomy. Because of mechanical problems, particularly leakage, some surgeons use an isolated jejunal loop brought directly to the abdominal wall in the Roux-en-Y manner.[20] In this latter modality, the distal (feeding) limb can be made to exit through the abdominal wall and be catheterized intermittently, or the limb can remain under the abdominal wall and be accessed by means of a skin-level device such as a button.

2   Proximal Decompression and Distal Feeding (Figure 60-2)

Here, too, the access can be done *without entering the small bowel wall*, as with a gastrostomy-jejunostomy combination.[55] An early classic example of this arrangement is the use of a gastrostomy along with a transpyloric, transanastomotic feeding tube in newborns with duodenal atresia.[9] Presently the combination gastrostomy button–transpyloric feeding tube is commonly used in children with gastric dysmotility or complex gastroesophageal reflux. A variant of this setup, but *entering the bowel wall*, can be used in children with jejunal atresia and a very dilated proximal bowel. The decompressing catheter is

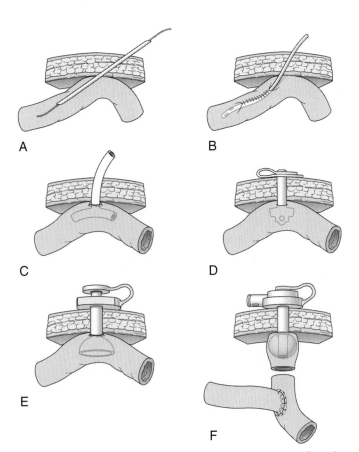

Figure 60-1. Diagram of select feeding jejunostomies. (**A**) Needle catheter.[11] (**B**) Tunneled catheter.[16] (**C**) T tube.[13] (**D**) Button.[14] (**E**) Direct percutaneous endoscopic jejunostomy converted to a skin-level device.[52] (**F**) Roux-en-Y feeding jejunostomy with a balloon-type skin-level device.[20] Adapted from Gauderer (1998).[84]

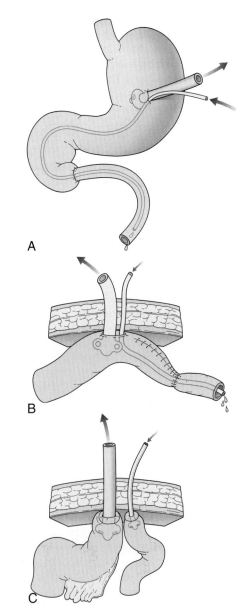

Figure 60-2. Diagram of selected feeding-decompressing jejunostomies. (**A**) Classic gastrostomy-jejunostomy arrangement for children with duodenal atresia.[9] (**B**) Similar arrangement for high jejunal atresia.[8] (**C**) Temporary decompression-feeding using catheters when primary anastomosis is unsafe and intestinal exteriorization is undesirable.[10] Adapted from Gauderer (1998).[84]

placed in the dilated, commonly tapered (and often hypo-peristaltic), segment and a second, smaller tube advanced either transanastomotically or directly into the narrower distal bowel.[8] A third option is the placement of a large decompressing tube in the proximal bowel and a smaller feeding tube into the distal bowel's proximal end when a primary anastomosis is unsafe and intestinal exteriorization is undesirable or impossible following an intra-abdominal catastrophe leading to bowel resection.[10]

3   Access for Antegrade Irrigation

The appendix or other specially modified colonic conduit can be brought *through the abdominal wall* for intermittent catheterization.[19] Long-term access can also be established by means of a device such as a catheter, a T tube, or a skin-level button-type device implanted in a *nonexteriorized segment* of colon.[13,14,17,26]

4   Decompression, Diversion, or Evacuation (Figure 60-3)

This is the largest group and comprises the most commonly used types of stoma.[1,2,41] The bowel can be exteriorized as an *end stoma* with a single opening,[3] a *double-barrel* opening,[6] or a *loop stoma*.[7] Variations include end-to-side anastomosis with a distal vent for irrigation, or the reverse type, side-to-end with a proximal vent.[5] Additional types include open or closed loops accessed with large

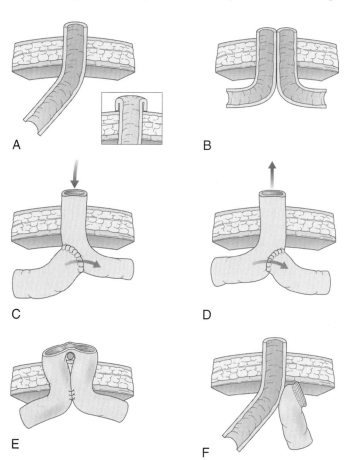

Figure 60-3. Examples of decompressing, diverting and evacuating stomas. **(A)** End-stoma (insert shows typical maturation). **(B)** Double-barrel stoma.[6] **(C)** End-to-side anastomosis with distal vent for irrigation.[4] **(D)** Side-to-end anastomosis with proximal vent.[5] **(E)** Loop-stoma.[7] **(F)** End-stoma with closed subfascial distal intestine. Adapted from Gauderer (1998).[84]

catheters or occluding valve-type devices allowing controlled egress of liquid or semiliquid stools.[1,38] Further variants comprise special stomas, such as a catheterizable pouch.[56]

The *exit* of an enterostomy through the abdominal wall can be handled in several ways (Figures 60-4 and 60-5).

Proximal Stoma

The bowel segment may be brought out *through the laparotomy incision, through a separate incision, with proximal and distal limbs close to each other* or with *both openings* apart. The patient may require multiple stomas and, at times, variations of the foregoing.

Distal Stoma

The intestine may be exteriorized as a *mucous fistula adjacent to*, or *separate from*, the proximal stoma. It may also be *closed and replaced into the abdominal cavity*. As a variant to this approach, a catheter may be placed into the closed distal segment for subsequent access for irrigation or contrast studies.

INDICATIONS FOR ENTEROSTOMIES IN CHILDREN

Stomas of the small and large intestine, whether temporary or permanent, are used in the management of a wide variety of surgical and nonsurgical conditions in neonates, infants, and children. Their primary uses are described next.

Jejunostomies

Direct access to the proximal small bowel is primarily an alternative to a gastrostomy, which is the preferred route for long-term enteral alimentation.[55] The majority of patients requiring a feeding jejunostomy are neurologically impaired children, usually with complex medical problems associated with foregut dysmotility. At times, both a gastrostomy and a jejunostomy are required (Figure 60-6). In addition, jejunostomies can be useful in the care of patients with acute surgical problems benefiting from early enteral nutrition, such as major trauma or burns, and in children needing long-term supplemental feedings (e.g., cystic fibrosis). Various types of exteriorized jejunal segments were once used in the management of children with biliary atresia, primarily in an attempt to reduce ascending cholangitis. However, this approach is no longer used, in part because of secondary problems such as bleeding from stomal varices associated with portal hypertension,[57] and because the stomas can add possible problems at the time of a future liver transplantation. On the other hand, the use of a segment of intestine interposed between the gallbladder and the abdominal wall for partial drainage of bile has been helpful in the management of children with certain cholestatic syndromes (Figure 60-7).[18,58] Stomas are also used in the monitoring of the intestinal graft in patients with small bowel transplantation. As with other segments of the intestine, exteriorization or tube decompression is clearly indicated after jejunal resection when peritonitis or severe ischemia is present.

Ileostomies

These more distal small bowel stomas are widely used when primary anastomosis is impossible or unsafe. Typical indications include neonatal necrotizing enterocolitis[41,59] or other adverse

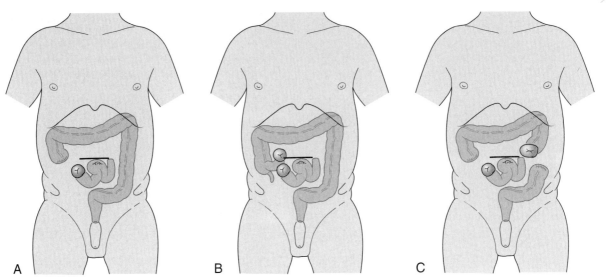

Figure 60-4. Example of options for the management of infants after intestinal resection. (**A**) Exteriorization of proximal intestine through a counterincision and closure of distal intestine beneath the abdominal wall. (This is our preferred arrangement.) (**B**) Same procedure as in (**A**), *with* exteriorization of proximal end of distal intestine through the wound edge. (**C**) Arrangement after resection of two intestinal segments. Adapted from Gauderer (1998).[84]

intra-abdominal events (Figure 60-8). Ileostomies are essential in the management of neonates with certain types of distal intestinal obstruction, such as long-segment Hirschsprung's disease, complex meconium ileus, and gastroschisis with atresia (Figure 60-9). Ileostomies are used extensively in the management of ulcerative colitis and familial polyposis as temporary, protective or, at times, permanent stomas[3,29,60] (Figures 60-10, 60-11, and 60-12). Less common indications include other forms of inflammatory bowel disease and rare manifestations of colonic dysmotility.[29]

Appendicostomies, Tube Cecostomies, and Tube Sigmoidostomies

The main indication for these interventions is to provide access sites for antegrade intestinal irrigation in children with complex anal sphincter and hindgut problems (Figure 60-13), as well as those with myelodysplasia.[1,17,19,26,27]

Colostomies

Stomas of the large bowel have the longest history, and extensive experience with these enterostomies has accrued.[1,2,29] Although modern pediatric surgical practice has led to a decrease in the use of preliminary colostomies in selected children with conditions such as Hirschsprung's disease,[40] diversion of the fecal stream is essential in the management of several congenital and acquired pathologies such as high forms of imperforate anus,[41,61] complex pelvic malformations, and colonic atresia. In addition, colostomies have a place in the care of patients with colonic, anorectal, and anoperineal trauma[62] and malignant conditions.[50]

Urostomies

Exteriorized segments of ileum or colon have been utilized as conduits in the management of urinary tract pathologies, although these external diversions are seldom used today. However, the mobilized appendix, interposed between the bladder and the abdomen, is still used in children with various urinary dysfunctions to provide a catheterizable conduit to the urinary bladder.[12,63]

CHOICE OF ENTEROSTOMY

Feeding Jejunostomy

Various approaches for constructing a feeding jejunostomy are now available.[14,21,23] The "open" placement through a small, left upper quadrant incision (see Figure 60-6) permits unequivocal identification of the stoma site in the proximal jejunum, as well as secure attachment of the bowel to the abdominal wall.[14] The laparoscopic approach is a good alternative.[21] Direct percutaneous jejunostomies are difficult in small children because of limitations imposed by the endoscopic equipment. The technique is, however, applicable to older patients.[23] Because conventional tunneled straight catheters can be difficult to immobilize or replace, our preference is for a T tube for infants and small children (because these do not obstruct the narrow lumen) (see Figure 60-6), and a button[14] or a nonballoon skin-level device[64] for older pediatric patients. These devices are replaceable as an office procedure. An alternative for long-term jejunal access, purported to have fewer problems with peristomal leakage, is the more complex approach constructing a Roux-en-Y.[20,65] However, because of the changes in the position of the bowel, this method has the potential for serious complications such as volvulus and internal hernias with intestinal obstruction.[66]

Ileostomy

In neonatal necrotizing enterocolitis or other major intra-abdominal events requiring intestinal resection, we prefer to bring a single end stoma out through a counterincision (see Figure 60-4A). A more expedient alternative is to bring the proximal intestine through the end of the incision (see Figures 60-4B,C and 60-8). However, with this approach, wound complications tend to be more common, and if the stoma must remain for a prolonged period of time and the

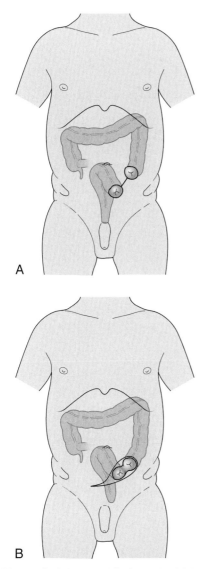

A

B

Figure 60-5. Diagram depicting sigmoid colostomies. (**A**) Separated stomas. The proximal intestine is at the upper end of the incision and the mucous fistula at the lower one. (**B**) Loop colostomy. The intestine is exteriorized over a rod, skin bridge, or simply with sutures (our preference). The circumscribing comma-shaped incision is used for takedown and pull-through procedures. Adapted from Gauderer (1998).[84]

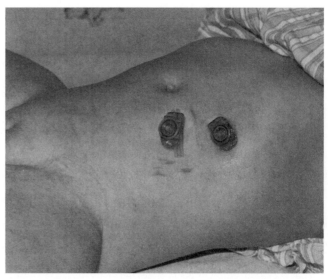

Figure 60-6. Neurologically impaired child with both a gastrostomy and feeding jejunostomy. The jejunostomy was placed using a small laparotomy. The gastrostomy was placed previously using the percutaneous endoscopic technique.[55] The small crossbar under the jejunostomy was placed for temporary immobilization and removed. Both skin-level devices are of the changeable external-valve type.[64]

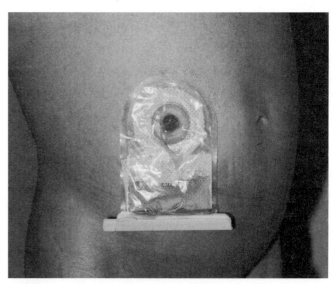

Figure 60-7. An 11-year-old child with Alagille syndrome, 2 months after cholecystoappendicostomy.[18] Note the bile-filled one-piece infant-type pouch.

child gains weight, the fold created by the laparotomy incision may interfere with fitting of the stoma appliance (see Figure 60-8). With a healthy distal intestine and anticipated downstream patency, we close the distal limb and place it intra-abdominally adjacent to the proximal stoma. Otherwise, exteriorization as a mucous fistula is prudent. The use of a loop stoma rather than an end stoma is an alternative in which the intact mesentery provides maximal perfusion.[67] A double-barrel stoma is another option.[6,59] To save as much intestine as possible, the placement of multiple stomas may be necessary (see Figure 60-4C).

In children with ulcerative colitis or familial polyposis, the enterostomal principles are similar to those established for adult patients. Choices for a temporary protective diverting ileostomy include a simple loop, an end loop, and an end stoma, with the closed end under the fascia[60] (see Figures 60-11 and 60-12).

Appendicostomy, Tube Cecostomy, or Tube Sigmoidostomy

The choice of antegrade enema depends on the type of colonic pathology being managed. With normal peristalsis, either the right[17,19] or the left[26] colon may be chosen for the access. However, if dysmotility is a concern, access to the right colon is indicated. If the appendix is present, it is exteriorized with or without interposition of a valve by either an "open" or a laparoscopic approach. If the appendix is not available, the wall of the cecum may be fashioned into a conduit that is then brought to the skin level. Bringing the stoma out at the umbilicus has cosmetic advantages. Either the appendix or the conduit so constructed is then catheterized to instill the enema fluid. A simpler technique, when there is no appendix, is the

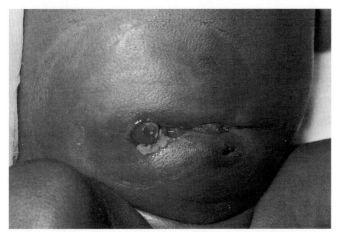

Figure 60-8. Two-month-old premature baby, 6 weeks after bowel resection for severe neonatal necrotizing enterocolitis. Because of the tenuous status during operation, the proximal ileal segment was brought out through the lateral portion of the incision rather than through a counterincision, which is our preferred approach (see Fig. 60-4**A**). Notice the slight retraction of the stoma, the undesirable crease formed by the incision following weight gain (rendering pouch application more difficult), and the presence of granulation tissue around absorbable sutures at the fascial level. To control leakage, a paste was placed in the "groove" adjacent to the stoma to allow for proper fit of the pouch.

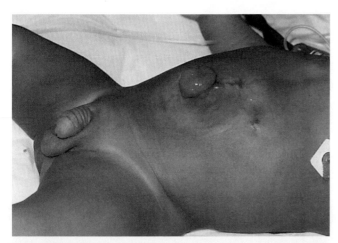

Figure 60-9. Two-month-old baby with gastroschisis and bowel atresia, before stoma closure with reestablishment of bowel continuity. Because of the large size of the exposed bowel, a silo pouch was needed for its reduction. At the time of the abdominal wall closure, at 1 week of age, the end of the distended atretic bowel was brought out through the incision, at the umbilical level. Because short gut syndrome was suspected, a gastrostomy (since removed) was added.

placement of a skin-level device.[17] For patients with normal colonic motility, our preference is for access to the left colon by means of a sigmoid irrigation tube[26] (see Figure 60-13).

Colostomy

Most colostomies fall into three categories: right transverse, left transverse, and sigmoid.[1,2,7,24] The significant physiologic and anatomic differences among these three segments must be taken into consideration when choosing the site for the stoma.

For infants with high imperforate anus, the high sigmoid is the preferred site for exteriorization.[61] The main advantages are firmer stools with less tendency for skin excoriation, less

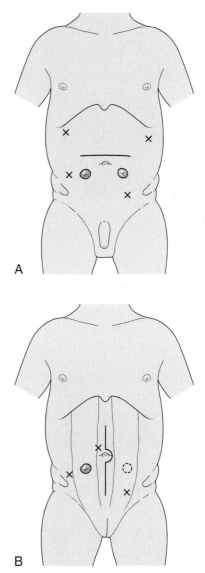

Figure 60-10. Diagram showing ideal sites for stomas. (**A**) Infant. The end stoma can be brought out through a counterincision in the lower right or left quadrant. The sites marked with an X are unsuitable because they are too close to the rib cage, the anterior superior iliac spine, the flank, or the groin. (**B**) Older child or adolescent. The best site for the stoma is in the mid-rectus abdominis in the right lower quadrant. The opposite side is an alternative. Areas marked with an X are unsuitable. Adapted from Gauderer (1998).[84]

tendency for prolapse, less surface for urine absorption in male children with rectovesical fistula, and the possibility of evacuation of distal sigmoid meconium during the initial procedure. In addition the surgeon is better able to identify the correct site, using the pelvic peritoneal reflection as a guide. A further advantage is that there are no scars in the epigastrium. However, if the low- or mid-sigmoid is exteriorized, there may be interference with the blood supply as well as insufficient bowel length for the future pull-through.[53,61] If the transverse colon is exteriorized, there is always adequate bowel length for a pull-through; the intestine is easy to mobilize and has a smaller diameter and no meconium. However, the disadvantages of the transverse colon colostomy are far greater: the stools are looser and skin maceration and dehydration more common, and there is a higher prolapse rate and a greater absorptive surface for urine in the distal limb.[43,53] In addition, adequate evacuation of meconium

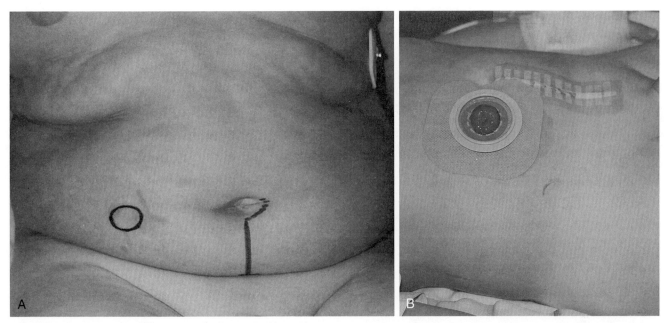

Figure 60-11. Eight-year-old boy with intractable ulcerative colitis that failed to respond to aggressive medical management including steroids, azathioprine, and infliximab. He underwent total abdominal colectomy and ileostomy as a preliminary stage to ileoanal anastomosis. (**A**) Bringing the already anesthetized patient into a sitting position confirmed the adequacy of the stoma site away from major abdominal folds. The ileostomy site had been determined several days before the procedure. At that time, the boy was asked to wear a two-piece pouch using the selected site as a guide. (**B**) Skin barrier with flange (two-piece pouching system) applied to the matured ileostoma at the completion of the colectomy.

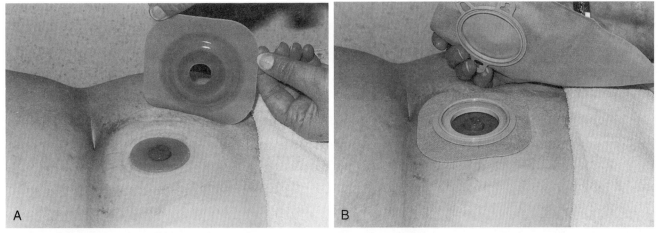

Figure 60-12. (**A**) Overweight 17-year-old girl following total abdominal colectomy for severe ulcerative colitis. Because of weight gain, the stoma is now in a depression on the right lower quadrant. To allow proper fit of the pouch, a soft, adherent disk is placed before the application of the skin barrier with flange. (**B**) The pouch, ready to be snapped onto the flange.

is nearly impossible. Our preference is for a high sigmoid loop colostomy. However, many surgeons prefer separation of the stomas, particularly in boys.[53,61] Advantages of separation are less contamination of the urinary tract and lower rate of prolapse, most notably of the distal limb. Disadvantages include a longer incision, greater potential for wound problems, and greater difficulty when applying a stoma device in small neonates.

In children with Hirschsprung's disease, the best site for a colostomy is the dilated segment that contains normal ganglion cells found immediately proximal to the transition zone. A loop colostomy is usually chosen because of its simplicity in construction and takedown.[7] Because most transition zones are in the sigmoid colon, this lower left quadrant stoma is taken down at the time of the definitive corrective operation (see Figure 60-5B). When separation of the stomas is chosen, the distal intestine should not be oversewn in Hirschsprung's disease if the aganglionic segment is long, because mucus cannot be appropriately evacuated or washed out. Although similar data are not available in children, properly constructed loop colostomies are fully diverting in adults.[68]

TECHNICAL ASPECTS

Feeding jejunostomies are generally placed in the left upper abdomen, slightly above the level of the umbilicus, not so cephalic as to interfere with a possible gastrostomy (see Figure 60-6). To minimize leakage (the most common problem with jejunostomies), catheters should be brought out through a counterincision, and excessive tension on immobilizing crossbars must be avoided to decrease the chance for bowel wall or skin ischemia.

Decompressing ileostomies are usually made to exit in the right lower quadrant. Figure 60-10A illustrates both appropriate and undesirable stoma exit sites in neonates, infants, and small children (e.g., those with necrotizing enterocolitis). Figure 60-10B demonstrates the correct exit sites in older children or adolescents (e.g., those with ulcerative colitis or familial polyposis).

Incisions in the lower quadrants should be avoided in patients who may eventually have long-standing or permanent stomas because such incisions can create an uneven surface that interferes with pouch adherence. It is essential to mark the site

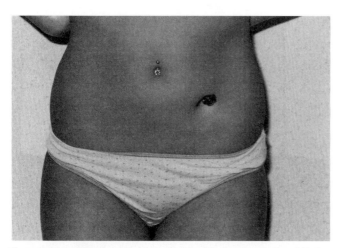

Figure 60-13. A 16-year-old girl 7 years after placement of a sigmoid irrigation tube.[26] She had been unable to evacuate without enemas since early infancy. Rectal biopsies were normal. Colonic transit of radiopaque markers and anal manometry confirmed the diagnosis of pelvic floor dysfunction with complications of acquired megarectum and increased rectal sensitivity threshold. The patient had failed to respond to laxative, prokinetic, and biofeedback therapy. She irrigates herself every 2 to 3 days with 600 to 900 mL tap water and has no stooling-related difficulties. The skin-level device[64] was changed twice.

of the stoma, as well as possible alternatives, on the abdominal wall before any incision is made. This planning is desirable in both elective and emergency settings. For elective long-standing stomas, the best location is marked the day before the operation (see Figure 60-11). The exit site should be located over the convex midportion of the rectus muscle, away from the incision, umbilicus, bony prominences, and skin folds. Depending on the size of the child, ileostomies must be at least 1 to 2 cm above the skin level to allow proper pouch immobilization. The preferred colostomy site is the left lower quadrant (Figures 60-5 and 60-14). The guidelines for the placement are similar to those for the ileostomies. The most common problem, particularly in newborns, is that the stoma is placed too caudally, close to the inguinoabdominal skin folds. When the infants raise their legs, the resulting folds tend to lift the edges of the stoma appliance, leading to leakage. Colostomies need not protrude as much as ileostomies, but if there is minimal or no rim it is difficult to keep the pouches in situ.

STOMA CARE

Proper perioperative and long-term care of an enterostomy is essential.[29,31,33-35,69] Parents, as well as older children, must be carefully taught by a committed team and reassured before leaving the hospital as well as during the follow-up visits. For certain age groups, ostomy dolls can be of help in the teaching process.[33] A large variety of stoma appliances are commercially available, including disposable and reusable pouches for all ages and sizes, even the smallest premature infants. Skin barriers, adhesives, powders, vented pouches, and odor-control solutions are among the products that facilitate the care of today's ostomate.[31-38,69]

Properly fitted appliances should remain in place for several days; 3 days is a reasonable expectation. There are two basic types of pediatric appliance: the one-piece pouching system in which the adhesive skin barrier is already attached to the pouch (see

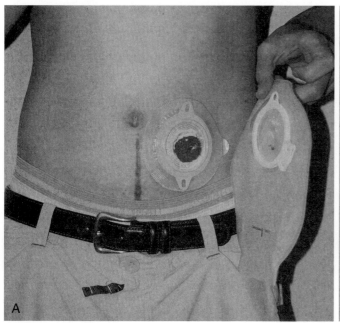
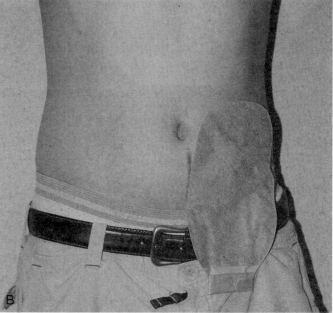

Figure 60-14. (A, B) Seventeen-year-old boy with previously undiagnosed Hirschsprung's disease, 4 months after resection of most of his massively dilated sigmoid. Because of the size of the remaining bowel, a temporary end stoma was placed. In these pictures, the patient demonstrates the use of a typical two-piece pouching system. Although the flange of the skin barrier has loops for a belt, this additional securing is not usually needed (the vertically oriented position of the loops makes this point).

Figure 60-7), and the two-piece system in which the adhesive barrier is separate from the pouch (see Figures 60-11B, 60-12, and 60-14). In the latter, the pieces snap together with a flange. Because of the holding power of contemporary adhesive skin barriers, additional fixation with tape or belts is usually not needed. The skin barrier is cut to the proper stoma size with the help of a template provided with the pouches. Because some infants with a sigmoidostomy have fairly firm stools, an occasional parent may choose to forego the use of a pouch. However, if skin breakdown sets in, the problem is harder to correct. In less affluent countries, creative, inexpensive alternatives to a pouch have been used.[70] In addition to instructions provided by the physicians, nurses, and enterostomal therapist, parents are encouraged to contact one of the enterostomal societies and make use of the extensive available educational material. Although "continent stomas" using special intra-abdominal intestinal pouches, magnetic caps, short balloon catheters, and other forms of intraluminal occlusion have been attempted,[38] there is limited experience with such operations or devices in the pediatric age group.

Moniliasis remains a common problem in the parastomal skin, and local antifungal medication should be used at the earliest sign of irritation. With skin excoriation, the area is exposed to air and a synthetic barrier is applied. To accelerate the process, a hair dryer can be very useful. Mild stomal bleeding is usually self-limiting. Control of granulation tissue around the mucosa-skin interface in the early postoperative stages can be done with judicious application of silver nitrate. Remaining sutures may be the cause and should be removed. We do not routinely dilate stomas and only occasionally irrigate the distal intestine. Malfunctioning stomas generally require early takedown or revision before more serious complications set in. Dietary and pharmacologic manipulations are helpful in changing stool consistency. Children with high (proximal) ileostomies must be monitored carefully to prevent electrolyte imbalance and insufficient nutrient absorption.

REESTABLISHING INTESTINAL CONTINUITY

Timing of enterostomy closure varies widely depending on the underlying condition, health status of the child, and the presence or absence of stoma-related complications. Unnecessary delays in the reestablishment of bowel continuity tend to increase morbidity and should be avoided.[51,71-74] The more proximal the stoma, the earlier it should be closed to decrease complications. Children who undergo stoma placement with resection of ischemic intestine must have a preoperative contrast study of the distal segment to rule out the presence of strictures or complete luminal obstruction. Reestablishment of small bowel continuity generally does not require intestinal preparation. Takedown of a colostomy is preceded by antegrade intestinal irrigation, supplemented by conventional enemas. Although we routinely administer perioperative intravenous antibiotics, we do not use intraluminal antibiotic solutions. The children are fed as soon as intestinal function returns.[75]

COMPLICATIONS OF ENTEROSTOMIES AND THEIR MANAGEMENT

Problems related to the construction, care and closure of stomas in the small and large intestines are numerous and common (Table 60-1). Naturally these can lead to significant morbidity and occasional mortality. Analysis of pediatric series

TABLE 60-1. Common Complications of Enterostomas

Prolapse
Stricture
Retraction
Wound separation, dehiscence
Wound infection, postoperative sepsis
Parastomal hernia
Intestinal wall separation or perforation with catheter change
Exteriorization of wrong intestinal segment or end
Intestinal obstruction (adhesion, internal hernia)
Intestinal torsion and ischemia
Fistula formation
Perforation by feeding or irrigating catheter
Poor appliance fitting and leakage
Psychologic trauma
Skin excoriation, moniliasis, dermatitis
Mucosal excoriation and bleeding
Granulation tissue of mucosa-skin interface
Variceal bleeding with portal hypertension
Electrolyte imbalance
Acidosis (caused by urine absorption in the distal loop of intestine)
Fecal impaction (in the distal loop of intestine)

reveals complication rates that often reach and sometimes exceed 50%.[41,43,44,46-54,71] In addition, stoma revision or early takedown is frequently necessary. Complications of enterostomies used for enteral alimentation are often accentuated by the patient's underlying disease, particularly in malnourished, debilitated, neurologically impaired children.[49] Overall, feeding jejunostomies have a much higher complication rate than gastrostomies.[55] Evacuating stomas of the small intestine are associated with a higher morbidity than colostomies because they are compounded by fluid, electrolyte, and absorption losses.[45,46,67] Transverse colostomies are more prone to complications than are sigmoid stomas* (Figure 60-15). In several series, divided colostomies have been preferred over loop colostomies.[51,53,61]

Among the more serious mechanical complications are prolapse, stricture, and retraction.[41,44,47-49,51] The incidence of prolapse in children's stomas exceeds 20% and is more common if the distal loop is exteriorized.[41,44,47-49,51,53] Stomal prolapse may be categorized into minor and major forms. Minor prolapse is associated with protuberant, edematous stoma that is still functional. Major prolapse is heralded by cyanotic, dusky edematous protruding bowel that may totally occlude the stomal orifice. Minor prolapse is usually amenable to nonsurgical techniques aimed at decreasing bowel edema and manual reduction. The application of table sugar, ionized salt crystals, and hypertonic saline injections has been shown to effectively diminish bowel wall edema osmotically, thereby aiding manual reduction of minor stomal prolapses.[76,77] Major prolapse requires prompt attention, and general anesthesia is often needed for intestinal reduction. Temporizing measures for control of prolapse include purse-string-type suture techniques[78] or the placement of sutures through the reduced intestinal segment, anchoring it to the abdominal wall[28,79] (Figure 60-16). Pledgets must be used to prevent the sutures from cutting through the tissues. Stricture, if mild, may respond to dilation. However, if evacuation is decreased and the proximal intestine begins to dilate, revision is advisable. This procedure is usually possible by incising all layers around the strictured stoma and bringing out healthy, at times dilated, bowel. The opening should not be excessive, though, because this might lead to prolapse. If the problem is

*References 41, 44, 47, 51, 53, 54.

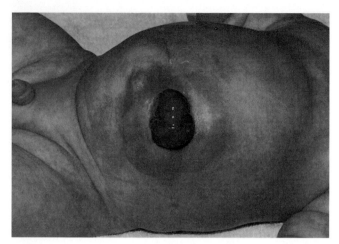

Figure 60-15. Four-month-old boy who had a sigmoid loop colostomy as an emergency procedure for severe Hirschsprung's enterocolitis at 5 weeks of age. The child had to be resuscitated aggressively following an arrest at an outlying hospital. To shorten the operating time for this very ill child, the bowel was brought out through the edge of the laparotomy incision. In this picture a partial prolapse is seen. The stoma was subsequently taken down and the child underwent a successful endorectal pull-through.

more complex or a parastomal hernia is present, the pathology is best addressed through a separate incision. Retraction of an end stoma may lead to skin-level stricture and obstruction. It also results in poor fitting of the appliance. Retraction of a loop stoma interferes with proper evacuation and leads to filling of the distal intestinal loop with stool. Stomal bleeding is a rare but serious complication in the pediatric population. Bleeding may be associated with long-term parenteral nutrition with resultant liver dysfunction. Subsequent collateral varices develop between the portal and systemic circulations and may result in vulnerable mucosal vessels around the stomas. Frequent bleeds may result in significant drops in hemoglobin levels. Most of these hemorrhages are amenable to direct pressure, suture ligation of offending vessel(s), or application of hemostatic substances. Tranexamic acid, an anti-fibrinolytic amino acid, has been associated with stabilization of formed clots and reduced rebleeding.[81,82] Other topically applied, degradable hemostatic agents include Surgicel or Gelfoam.[83]

Stoma takedown and bowel reanastomosis is also associated with a high rate of complications, most notably wound infection, dehiscence, fistula formation, and intestinal obstruction.[51,59,72,74] Among the various factors contributing to this morbidity are poor timing, inadequate bowel preparation, technical errors, and shortcuts. As expected, malnourished, debilitated, anemic patients and those on steroids are at greatest risk for complications. These contributing factors should be corrected before reestablishment of intestinal continuity is planned.

OSTOMY TRENDS

Innovative, less invasive surgical techniques are increasingly being applied to provide access to the small and large intestine for the creation and the take-down of stomas placed for feeding[22,23] as well as evacuation.[17,26] Newer, better tolerated, long-term skin-level enteral access devices or "buttons" continue to add safety and facilitate care.[84] Prompt attention to stoma complications, as well as early closure of very proximal enterostomies, has contributed to decrease short and long-term morbidity.[44-54] Several traditional indications for stoma formation, especially colostomies, have

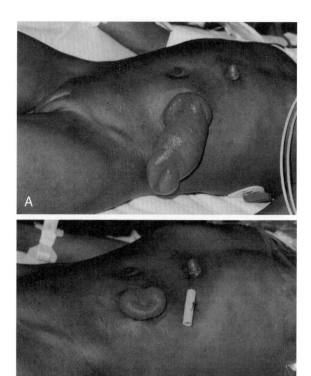

Figure 60-16. Seven-year-old girl with developmental delay, failure to thrive, and pathologic aerophagia. A gastrostomy was placed for feeding and venting to help with the management of her severe air swallowing. The aerophagia eventually led to massive bowel distention, particularly the colon, which measured over 12 cm in diameter. Following the exclusion of the diagnosis of aganglionosis and after multiple other conservative measures failed, an end sigmoid colostomy was placed. Once the abdominal girth and colonic diameter decreased, the bowel prolapsed **(A)**. Following reduction in the operating room, the prolapsed bowel segment was anchored to the abdominal wall with two latex tube segments, one inside the bowel lumen and the other one on the skin surface, held in place by a heavy monofilament suture.[79] In addition, a purse-string suture, using the same material, was placed around the ostomy to narrow the opening.[78] **(B)** Eventually both sutures and the bolsters could be removed.

changed with the advent of recent pediatric surgical advances. Because of the still very significant complication rate of colostomies in infants,[53,85] alternatives continue to be developed.

REFERENCES

1. Cataldo PA. History of stomas. In: MacKeigan JM, Cataldo PA, editors. Intestinal Stomas: Principles, Techniques, and Management. St. Louis, MO: Quality Medical Publishers; 1993. p. 3–37.
22. Raval MV, Phillips JD. Optimal enteral feeding in children with gastric dysfunction: surgical jejunostomy vs image-guided gastro-jejunal tube placement. J Pediatr Surg 2006;41:1679–1682.
26. Gauderer MWL, DeCou JM, Boyle JT. Sigmoid irrigation tube for the management of chronic evacuation disorders. J Pediatr Surg 2002;37:348–351.
41. Millar AJ, Lakhoo K, Rode M, et al. Bowel stomas in infants and children: a five-year audit of 203 patients. S Afr J Surg 1993;31:110–113.
48. Nour S, Beck J, Stringer MD. Colostomy complications in infants and children. Ann R Coll Surg Engl 1996;78:526–530.
53. Pena A, Migotto-Krieger M, Levitt MA. Colostomy in ano-rectal malformations: a procedure with serious but preventable complications. J Pediatr Surg 2006;41:748–756.

See expertconsult.com for a complete list of references and the review questions for this chapter.

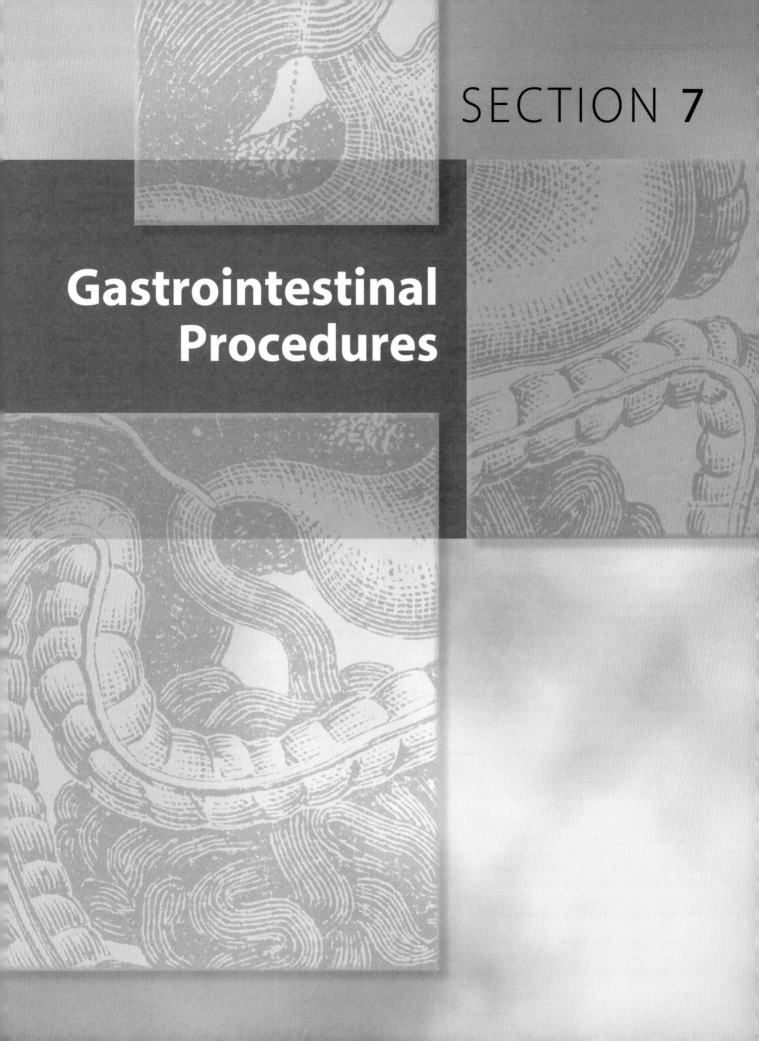

SECTION 7

Gastrointestinal Procedures

61 ESOPHAGOGASTRODUODENOSCOPY AND RELATED TECHNIQUES

Marsha Kay • Robert Wyllie

The earliest gastrointestinal endoscopies were performed in the late 1880s using rigid instruments, looking initially at the esophagus and rectum. The semiflexible gastroscope was developed in the early 1930s by Schindler and Wolf utilizing a series of short-focal-length lenses and a semiflexible tube.[1] Fiberoptic endoscopes representing a significant advance in endoscopy were popularized in the late 1960s and early 1970s, based on the principle of total internal reflection of light along cylindrical glass rods coated with a material of low refractive index. As light enters one end and strikes the interface between the highly refractive glass and the low refractive index of the glass coating, it is advanced by a series of internal reflections and emitted at the opposite end of the rod. Its position is maintained by maintaining the same relative position of each rod at both ends of the endoscope. With the advent of fiberoptic endoscopes came the availability of both tip control and biopsy capability. The first small-diameter instrument used for esophagogastroduodenoscopy (EGD) in a child was a fiberoptic bronchoscope.[2]

Gastrocameras were used for still photographs in the late 1940s, but video endoscopy has been developed over the past three decades, with the first mass-produced video instruments introduced in the 1980s. Currently, video endoscopes have all but replaced fiberoptic endoscopes for EGD, endoscopic retrograde cholangiopancreatography (ERCP), and colonoscopy. Present-day trainees are unlikely to have used or even seen a fiberoptic endoscope, with the exception of some endoscopes still utilized for endoscopic ultrasonography (EUS). Dedicated pediatric video endoscopes with a narrow instrument diameter and preserved optic clarity are now widespread in their availability with instrument outer diameters in the range of 5 to 6 mm. These small-caliber endoscopes have found widespread application for both children and adults and are now being used with increased frequency in adults undergoing unsedated endoscopic procedures.

Pediatric gastrointestinal endoscopists are able to perform almost all of the endoscopic techniques of their adult counterparts. At the same time, they are developing unique applications of these techniques for pediatric patients. The advantage of pediatric gastrointestinal endoscopists is familiarity not only with age-related physiology but also with the spectrum of disease in pediatric patients. The referring physician and endoscopist should be familiar with the risks and benefits of endoscopy and those clinical situations in infants and children in which it is most likely to be useful.

PERSONNEL

Specially trained pediatric endoscopy assistants are an important component of the endoscopy team. Procedure anxiety can be diminished by an assistant who has previously met the child and parent(s), explained the procedure, and greeted them in the endoscopy suite. The same person can hold and reassure the child throughout the procedure. A second assistant is typically needed to help obtain and process tissue during the procedure and assist with other equipment. Specially trained child life personnel can also be utilized to reduce procedure-related anxiety. Psychologic preparation before endoscopy has been shown to reduce procedure-related anxiety, improve patient cooperation, decrease autonomic nervous system stimulation during the procedure, and reduce the amount of medication required.[3]

Physicians performing endoscopy on infants and children should have completed a pediatric gastroenterology fellowship or have experience with pediatric gastrointestinal diseases and adequate training in pediatric endoscopy. Guidelines for the minimal number of procedures to establish competency have been established by the North American Society for Pediatric Gastroenterology, Hepatology and Nutrition and the American Society for Gastrointestinal Endoscopy.[4-8] Intravenous sedation should be used only by physicians competent in the administration of drugs and resuscitation in children. Levels of sedation must be carefully and continuously assessed. There is a continuum from conscious sedation to deep sedation to general anesthesia. Physicians administering sedation should be familiar with the definitions of these three levels of sedation and appropriately credentialed for sedation administration, with appropriate equipment and personnel available for monitoring and resuscitation.[9]

FACILITIES

Routine endoscopy in infants and children is typically performed in an outpatient setting using parenteral sedation. Large series have reported on the efficacy and safety of this type of sedation with combined minor and major complication rates of less than 0.5 to 9% for both EGD and colonoscopy and major complication rates usually less than 0.5% depending on the series and how adverse events were defined.[10,11] Occasionally it is necessary to perform endoscopy at the hospital bedside or in an operating room. In many institutions, anesthesiologists are utilized to administer sedation for more invasive or therapeutic procedures such as foreign body removal (see Chapter 19), placement of percutaneous tubes (gastrostomy or cecostomy), dilation of strictures and pneumatic dilation, variceal band ligation, and therapeutic endoscopy for gastrointestinal bleeding. Some endoscopists may also prefer the assistance of an anesthesiologist for younger patients or those in whom cooperation may be impaired. Some pediatric centers utilize pediatric anesthesiologists to provide sedation for the majority of their procedures. To date, an advantage of one form of sedation over another has not been demonstrated.

The endoscopy suite should be equipped with instruments to monitor blood pressure, pulse rate, and oxygen saturation. Pediatric resuscitation equipment including emergency medications and reversal agents, intravenous fluids, appropriately sized endotracheal tubes and laryngoscopes, oxygen, and resuscitation bags should be available. Newer methods of noninvasive monitoring such as capnography are being evaluated primarily in the operating room setting and, if found to be helpful, may be adapted for use with procedures being performed utilizing conscious sedation.

EQUIPMENT

Almost all endoscopes currently utilized are video endoscopes. Upper gastrointestinal endoscopes may also be divided on the basis of their angle of viewing: either forward or side viewing. Currently, side-viewing endoscopes are used only for ERCP and will be discussed in that context.

The video endoscope, an adaptation of the earlier fiberoptic instrument, is composed of a control handle that is attached to an insertion tube with a charge coupled device (CCD) located at its distal tip behind the objective lens.[12] The objective lens focuses a miniature picture on the surface of the CCD. The pattern of light falling on the CCD is converted to an array of electrical charges, transforming the optical image into an electronic representation. The charges developed in the CCD are "read" and processed to reproduce the image ultimately being transmitted to a video processor for display on a television monitor.[12] Images are "colorized" by different color imaging systems such as RGB (red, green, blue) sequential imaging system or color chip imaging technology. Each of the systems has advantages, descriptions of which are beyond the scope of this text. Differential color imaging systems are currently being used in adults as an alternative to chromoendoscopy. These are discussed later in the chapter, in the section on special endoscopic techniques.

The control section of the endoscope is attached via a universal cord to a light, water, suction, and electrical source. On the control handle, dials control the up-down and right-left angulation of the instrument tip. Lateral to each dial is a locking mechanism that increases the resistance to turning the dial. On the proximal shaft of the endoscope, there are two valves. The more proximal valve is for suction, and the distal one controls air and water. Air is insufflated through the endoscope by lightly occluding the distal button. Firmly pushing down on the button provides a stream of water for irrigation through the endoscope. The control handle contains additional buttons to freeze or alter the image on the video screen. Parts or all of the procedure can be recorded for image storage or later review on digital video recorders.

Further down the endoscope is a channel with a biopsy valve, through which can be passed various instruments including biopsy forceps, cytology brushes, needles for sclerotherapy or injection, guidewires, coagulation probes, heater probes, polypectomy snares, and other instruments. The endoscopic field can be irrigated manually by using a blunt-ended needle attached to a syringe and manually flushing the channel. The rate of irrigation that can be achieved by this method is greater than the rate achieved by occluding the button on the endoscope. Irrigation pumps are also available. If the air button does not function properly during endoscopy, air can also be injected with a syringe via this channel to avoid switching endoscopes in midprocedure. At the endoscope tip are various openings: an air-water outlet (for lens cleaning), the objective lens, a light guide, and an instrument channel for suction and biopsy forceps. Large-diameter therapeutic instruments may contain an auxiliary water channel or a second suction/instrument channel, or both. The tip of the endoscope has a certain degree of angulation possible in an up or down, right or left direction. The flexible portion of the endoscope is the "working length" of the instrument. Equipment such as a friction fit adaptor or hood has been developed to attach to the endoscope tip. The friction fit adaptor is used primarily to deploy bands for esophageal variceal ligation but can also be used in the treatment of esophageal meat impactions. The endoscopic hood is used primarily to assist with endoscopic mucosal resection (EMR), a newer technique that has been developed primarily in adult patients for resection of large mucosal lesions including dysplastic epithelium or carcinomas.

There are three main types of small-bowel enteroscopes. The first is the push-type enteroscope, which represents a modification of the pediatric colonoscope with an increased working length. The second type of small-bowel endoscope is the passive enteroscope, also known as the Sonde-type small intestinal fiberscope. It is of much smaller diameter than the push-type enteroscope and is a forward-viewing instrument with a balloon cuff located at the scope tip to facilitate advancement of the scope by peristalsis into the small intestine. Most small-bowel enteroscopies are currently performed using the push-type endoscope. Recently single and double balloon endoscopes have been developed to allow for examination and treatment of lesions identified in the more distal small bowel. The advantage of push-type endoscopes and balloon enteroscopes is that they have a working channel to perform therapeutic procedures such as polypectomy, biopsy, injection, or coagulation. The balloon enteroscopes allow for more distal small bowel examination and are now starting to be utilized for pediatric patients. Video capsule endoscopy is another technique that competes with small bowel enteroscopy as a method to examine the small bowel distal to the ligament of Treitz. Although capsules are not currently able to be read in real time and do not allow for tissue sampling or endoscopic therapy, future modifications of this technology may allow for these types of advancement, increasing the utility of this technology. Balloon enteroscopy and capsule endoscopy are discussed in more detail in Chapter 64.

The most important issues related to pediatric endoscopy equipment are the diameter and length of the insertion tube, the degree of tip angulation, and the depth of field. In term infants, the esophagus measures only 4 to 6 mm in diameter and 9 to 10 cm in length.[2] Some of the earliest EGDs were performed using small-diameter bronchoscopes with an insertion tube diameter of 5 mm. However, the tubes were too short to allow adequate visualization of the small bowel. Despite theoretical concerns of trauma, perforation, or airway compression, early pediatric endoscopists found that they could safely and effectively examine a neonate's digestive tract with an instrument of 7 mm in diameter without complication, because of the distensibility of the esophagus. Newer gastrointestinal endoscopes have a 5- to 6-mm outer diameter with a 2-mm instrument channel, and side-viewing endoscopes have an outer diameter in the range of 7 to 8 mm. Standard upper endoscopes have an external diameter in the range of 8.0 to 9.8 mm with a 2.4- to 2.8-mm channel. Therapeutic channel scopes have an outer diameter in the range of 11.3 to 13.2 mm with an instrument channel of 3.2 to 3.7 mm, and in the larger scopes dual channels up to 3.8 mm in diameter.

INDICATIONS

The indications for gastrointestinal endoscopy vary with the age of the patient. The need for upper endoscopy in neonates and infants is usually suggested by physical signs reported by parents or other observers, which include dysphagia, vomiting, hematemesis, melena, hypotension, respiratory distress, abnormal posturing, or anemia. With toddlers and older children, the history is of greater importance in identifying gastrointestinal disorders. The sensitivity of gastrointestinal endoscopy in establishing a diagnosis varies with the indication for the procedure (Table 61-1).

The yield of upper endoscopic examination in pediatric patients differs with the age of the child and the indication for the procedure. Younger patients with specific complaints such as failure to thrive and weight loss appear to have an increased incidence of pathology on endoscopic examination compared with older children with nonspecific abdominal pain. In addition, endoscopies performed for gastrointestinal bleeding are more likely to identify a cause than procedures for nonspecific complaints. Endoscopy can be performed for diagnosis of gastroesophageal reflux (GER), eosinophilic esophagitis and gastroenteritis, celiac disease, and small bowel enteropathy; evaluation of graft-versus-host disease and surveillance for Barrett's esophagus, polyposis syndromes, or following transplantation including evaluation for posttransplant lymphoproliferative disease (PTLD); therapy, as in stricture dilation,

foreign body removal, percutaneous endoscopic gastrostomy (PEG) insertion, pyloric dilation, pneumatic dilation, catheter placement, stent insertion, or gastroplication; or a combination of diagnosis and therapy, such as evaluation and treatment of gastrointestinal bleeding, including that from acid peptic disease and variceal sources, or in evaluation of injury following a caustic ingestion.[13-15] Current guidelines and standards of practice should be followed in terms of the yield of endoscopy.[8,13] New endoscopic techniques continue to be developed, will be applied increasingly to pediatric patients, and are discussed at the end of this chapter.

CONTRAINDICATIONS

Absolute contraindications to gastrointestinal endoscopy include suspected perforation of the intestine and peritonitis in a toxic patient. There are several relative contraindications, including patients who are severely neutropenic or have bleeding disorders and children with a recent history of bowel surgery. In addition, patients with connective tissue disease, especially Ehlers-Danlos and Marfan syndromes, are at increased risk of perforation during endoscopy.[16] Other relative contraindications include partial or complete bowel obstruction and aneurysm of the abdominal and iliac aorta. In all endoscopic procedures, the clinician and endoscopist must determine whether the potential information or therapeutic intervention outweighs the risk of the procedure (Table 61-2).

ANTIBIOTIC PROPHYLAXIS

The incidence of bacteremia after gastrointestinal endoscopy varies according to the patient's underlying medical problem and the procedure performed: EGD 0 to 8% (mean 4.4%), colonoscopy 0 to 25% (mean 4.4%), sclerotherapy 0 to 52% (mean 14.6%), endoscopic variceal ligation 1 to 25% (mean 8.8%) , esophageal dilation 12 to 22%, and ERCP 6.4 to 18%.[17] Certain bacteria are more likely to be the cause of bacteremia after a procedure. These include *Escherichia coli*, *Bacteroides*, *Pseudomonas*, *Veillonella*, and *Peptostreptococcus*, especially after a lower gastrointestinal procedure.[18] However, other bacteria may be more virulent and more likely to cause endocarditis, especially *Streptococcus viridans* and enterococcus.[19] Prophylaxis is directed by the frequency and virulence of the anticipated organisms that may be encountered during the procedure.

The actual incidence of bacterial endocarditis following gastrointestinal procedures is quite low, with fewer than 20 cases

TABLE 61-1. Indications for Esophagogastroduodenoscopy

Acid peptic disease
Suspicion of mucosal inflammation (including infection); biopsy, brushing, and cytology examination
Acute epigastric or right upper quadrant pain
Hematemesis or melena
Dysphagia or odynophagia
Caustic ingestion or foreign-body ingestion
Recurrent vomiting
Following solid organ, bone marrow or stem cell transplant to assess for GVHD or PTLD
Therapeutic intervention
  Injection, coagulation, or ligation of a bleeding lesion
  Stricture dilation or dilation of gastric outlet obstruction
  Pneumatic dilation
  PEG/PEJ
  Catheter placement
  Foreign body removal
  Endoscopic lesion resection
  Endoscopic therapy for GER

GER, gastroesophageal reflux; GVHD, graft-versus-host disease; PEG, percutaneous endoscopic gastrostomy; PEJ, percutaneous endoscopic jejunostomy; PTLD, posttransplant lymphoproliferative disease.

TABLE 61-2. Contraindications to Endoscopy in Infants and Children

Absolute Contraindications
Suspected bowel perforation
Acute peritonitis

Relative Contraindications
Bleeding disorders and/or impaired platelet function
Neutropenia
Patients with increased risk of bowel perforation, including:
  Connective tissue disorders (Ehlers-Danlos and Marfan syndromes)
  Toxic dilation of the bowel
  Partial or complete intestinal obstruction
  Recent bowel surgery

reported. Antibiotic recommendations are based on a combination of procedure-related risk of bacteremia and patient risk and should be reassessed periodically as new data and guidelines become available.[17,20,21]

Patients at high risk for infective endocarditis are those with prosthetic heart valves, including bioprosthetic and homograft valves; a previous history of bacterial endocarditis; a surgically constructed systemic pulmonary shunt or conduit; those who have had a cardiac transplant with cardiac valvuloplasty; and those with complex cyanotic congenital cardiac malformations, including single-ventricle states, transposition of the great arteries, and tetralogy of Fallot.[17] If indicated, prophylaxis is usually given before the procedure, but is no longer repeated 6 to 8 hours after the procedure except in the case of PEGs or other special procedures as indicated in current guidelines.

Intermediate-risk patients include most other congenital cardiac malformations, acquired valvular dysfunction (e.g., rheumatic heart disease), hypertrophic cardiomyopathy, mitral valve prolapse with valvular regurgitation, and/or thickened leaflets.

The most current recommendations are that antibiotic prophylaxis solely to prevent infective endocarditis is no longer recommended before endoscopic procedures except as specified elsewhere in this document. For patients with established gastrointestinal (GI) tract infection in which enterococci may be part of the infecting bacterial flora, such as in cases of cholangitis and with one of the previously listed cardiac conditions associated with highest risk of adverse outcome from endocarditis, amoxicillin or ampicillin should be included in the antibiotic regimen for enterococcal coverage. Vancomycin may be substituted for patients allergic or unable to tolerate amoxicillin or ampicillin (Table 61-3).

Antibiotic prophylaxis may be useful for prevention of infection related to some endoscopic procedures, before placement of prosthetic devices and in specific clinical scenarios. The current guidelines are complex and subject to continual update and revision and should be reviewed.

Antibiotic prophylaxis is recommended for all patients before PEG placement. Thirty minutes before PEG placement, parenteral coverage with cefazolin or an equivalent antibiotic is indicated. Additional doses of antibiotics are required following PEG placement.

Antibiotic prophylaxis should be considered for all patients undergoing ERCP for known or suspected biliary obstruction in which there is a possibility of incomplete biliary drainage, and antibiotics should be continued following the procedure. In the case of ERCP, antibiotics should be directed against biliary flora including enteric gram-negative organisms, enterococci, and possibly *Pseudomonas* species. Antibiotics should also be continued postprocedure even if complete biliary drainage is achieved in cases of posttransplant biliary strictures. Antibiotic prophylaxis is also recommended before ERCP in patients with communicating cysts or pseudocysts and before transpapillary drainage of pseudocysts.

Although uncommonly performed in pediatrics, antibiotic prophylaxis is recommended before EUS with fine-needle aspiration (FNA) of cystic lesions along the GI tract. Because of the risk of cyst infection, antibiotics are also continued for 3 to 5 days following the procedure. Prophylaxis is not recommended for EUS FNA of solid lesions in the upper GI tract, and there is no recommendation for EUS FNA of lower GI tract solid lesions.[17]

Other special patient populations include those with a prosthetic joint or orthopedic prosthesis, synthetic vascular grafts, or other nonvalvular cardiac devices in whom antibiotics are not recommended, and patients with gastrointestinal hemorrhage, in whom antibiotics are generally recommended. In patients with cirrhosis, especially those with ascites or with GI bleeding, antibiotics are strongly recommended starting at admission (intravenous [IV] ceftriaxone or oral norfloxacin in adults if allergic or intolerant to ceftriaxone). In patients following transplantation or other immunocompromised patients undergoing high-risk procedures, prophylaxis should be considered on a case-by-case basis except as otherwise specified.[17,20]

PREPARATION

Esophagogastroduodenoscopy

Preparation for upper gastrointestinal endoscopic procedures involves a period of fasting except in emergency situations. Infants less than 6 months of age are not fed for 2 to 4 hours before endoscopy, and children over 2 years of age fast for 6 to 8 hours. Studies have suggested that a shorter period of pre-endoscopy fasting may be possible.[22] Although fasting for milk and solids for 6 to 8 hours, depending on patient age, before endoscopy is still required, it may be possible to decrease the pre-endoscopy fasting interval for clear liquids to 2 to 3 hours, especially for younger children.[23] Current fasting guidelines should be followed.[9] Some patients may require longer than standard fasting intervals because of their underlying conditions. These include patients with achalasia with delayed esophageal (and in some cases gastric) emptying, patients with delayed gastric emptying, and those with other motility issues.

SEDATION AND MONITORING

Sedation is used in most pediatric patients not only to minimize discomfort but also to provide amnesia for the procedure. This helps to prevent the child from becoming fearful of contact with the physician, which is especially important in pediatric patients with chronic conditions that may require repeated procedures. Most pediatric endoscopists have replaced general anesthesia with intravenous sedation for routine upper and lower endoscopy. General anesthesia may be required for

---

TABLE 61-3. Regimen for Endocarditis Prophylaxis

1. Amoxicillin 2.0 g by mouth (adult) or 50 mg/kg by mouth (child) 60 min before procedure. Alternative for those unable to take by mouth: ampicillin 2.0 g IV or IM (adult) or 50 mg/kg IV or IM (child) within 30 min before procedure
2. *For patients who are penicillin allergic:* Clindamycin 600 mg by mouth (adult) or 20 mg/kg by mouth (child) 1 h before procedure. Alternatives: cephalexin or cefadroxil 2.0 g by mouth (adult) or 50 mg/kg (child) 1 h before procedure; azithromycin or clarithromycin 500 mg by mouth (adult) or 15 mg/kg by mouth (child) 1 h before procedure
3. *For patients who are penicillin allergic and unable to take by mouth:* Clindamycin 600 mg IV (adult) or 20 mg/kg IV (child) within 30 min before procedure. Alternatives: cefazolin 1.0 g IV or IM (adult) or 25 mg/kg IV or IM (child) within 30 min before procedure; vancomycin 1.0 g IV (adult) or 10-20 mg/kg (child)
4. *PEG prophylaxis:* Parenteral cefazolin (or an antibiotic with equivalent coverage) 30 min before the procedure; additional doses following the procedure may be indicated

Data from Hirota et al., 2003.[20] IM, intramuscular; IV, intravenous; PEG, percutaneous endoscopic gastrostomy.

therapeutic procedures such as foreign body removal, dilation, or PEG placement, or in patients in whom cooperation is not anticipated. A variety of regimens have been tried in pediatric patients, although there are few comparative trials. Most pediatric endoscopists use a combination of a benzodiazepine such as midazolam and a narcotic such as meperidine for conscious sedation. A variety of other agents, such as fentanyl, ketamine-midazolam, and, more recently, propofol administered by an anesthesiologist and considered a sedative anesthetic, have also been used in pediatric patients.[24-29] Oral midazolam premedication before conscious sedation with a combination of a benzodiazepine and a narcotic has also been reported to be beneficial in improving both patient and parent satisfaction.[25] In selected highly motivated pediatric patients, unsedated endoscopy has been successful.[30]

When used together, meperidine 1 to 2 mg/kg body weight to a maximum of 100 mg is administered by slow infusion followed by midazolam 0.1 to 0.2 mg/kg body weight. The dose of midazolam is titrated according to the patient's level of consciousness, but rarely exceeds 5 mg as a total dose. Meperidine is usually given first to decrease the discomfort at the site of injection associated with intravenous midazolam. Younger children may require more midazolam per kilogram of body weight. Occasionally, it may be necessary to administer additional amounts of these medications during the procedure.

Transient reactions at the site of medication administration are not unusual and include cutaneous erythema distal to the site of injection not associated with clinically significant thrombophlebitis. Other reactions include coughing and a characteristic taste with meperidine infusion. In a prospective evaluation of this method of sedation in 100 pediatric endoscopic procedures at the Cleveland Clinic, approximately 50% of the patients had generalized cutaneous flushing, and urticaria without audible wheezing developed in 12 children. Rechallenge with the same sedative in two patients did not result in a more severe reaction.[31] Endoscopy in neonates may be performed with or without sedation, depending on the indication for the procedure. Sedation is helpful if the procedure will last more than a few minutes or interventional endoscopy is anticipated.

General anesthesia is necessary when a patient is uncooperative, requires a lengthy or complicated procedure, or has extenuating medical problems. Increasingly propofol (2,6-diisopropylphenol) has been administered primarily by pediatric anesthesiologists for sedation for pediatric procedures. It is classified as an ultrashort acting hypnotic agent that provides sedative, amnestic, and hypnotic effects with no analgesic properties. It rapidly crosses the blood-brain barrier and causes a depression in consciousness likely related to potentiation of the γ-aminobutyric acid A receptor in the brain.[32] It is contraindicated in patients with propofol allergy or hypersensitivity to eggs or soybeans. It is metabolized primarily in the liver. Dose reduction is required in patients with cardiac dysfunction and in those with decreased clearance of the drug. Onset of action is rapid following injection.[32] It is highly effective at inducing sedation and provides excellent amnesia for the procedure.[29] In addition, the pharmacokinetics of this agent allow for rapid patient awakening once the agent is turned off. There are limited pediatric trials that compare this agent to standard endoscopist-administered sedation of a narcotic and benzodiazepine. A recent nonrandomized pediatric trial suggests that there is no advantage of this agent in

terms of procedure time or time to patient discharge, especially in healthy patients undergoing diagnostic upper endoscopy.[29] In addition, propofol administration appears to be associated with a higher likelihood of endotracheal intubation during or before the endoscopic procedure.[29] However, further study is indicated to determine whether anesthesiologist-administered propofol offers other advantages in selected pediatric patients undergoing endoscopy.

During the endoscopic procedure, arterial oxygen saturation and electrocardiographic tracings are routinely monitored. Patients aged less than 1 year, compared with patients more than 1 year of age and those with underlying cardiopulmonary disease, have a greater tendency for decreased mean oxygen saturation with endoscopy.

Oxygen desaturation during sedation may occur without clinically apparent signs and symptoms. For this reason, pulse oximetry should be monitored during endoscopy. Neurologically impaired patients often have gastrointestinal problems that require endoscopy. Sedation in these patients can be unpredictable, and respiratory depression is more common. The dosage of meperidine is therefore reduced to 0.5 to 1.0 mg/kg body weight, and the dosage of midazolam, if this drug is used, is titrated very slowly. Careful and attentive monitoring of the cardiopulmonary status is essential. Medication dosages are also reduced in patients who have undergone a recent weight loss where the volume of distribution may be altered. These include patients with inflammatory bowel disease, malignancy, and anorexia nervosa. A number of other adverse effects, including respiratory depression, pulmonary edema, allergic reactions, arrhythmias, hypotension, paradoxical reactions, and hallucinations, have been reported following a variety of sedation regimens.[27,33] Endoscopists should counsel patients and their families based on the specific known risks associated with their preferred sedation regimen.

Naloxone is indicated only for narcotic-induced respiratory depression, because its use is usually associated with marked irritability in infants and young children. Flumazenil (Mazicon) is a intravenous benzodiazepine antagonist that competitively blocks the effects of benzodiazepines on γ-aminobutyric acid pathway-mediated inhibition in the central nervous system.[34] Experience is limited with this agent; side effects with administration include facial erythema, dizziness, hyperexcitability, seizures, and serious cardiac arrhythmias. Because its half-life is shorter than that of benzodiazepines, resedation after reversal of benzodiazepine sedation may occur, and patients should be monitored accordingly. Routine administration after endoscopy appears to be of questionable benefit in pediatric patients.[35] Recommended doses for intravenous sedation medications and reversal agents are indicated in Table 61-4.

ANATOMY

Esophagogastroduodenoscopy

The esophagus is located posterior to the trachea in the neck. It ranges in diameter from 4 to 6 mm and in length from 9 to 10 cm in the term infant, to a length of approximately 25 cm in the adult.[2] It begins distal to the cricoid cartilage and ends at the cardiac orifice of the stomach.

The esophagus opens with swallowing, unlike the trachea, which is always open except with vocal cord movement. The esophageal opening appears lateral and posterior to each side of the trachea with swallowing. The trachea is easily distinguished

TABLE 61-4. Recommended Doses for Intravenous Sedation Medications and Reversal Agents

Medication	Dose	Maximum total dose	Onset (min)	Duration of Action
Benzodiazepines				
Midazolam	0.05-0.4 mg/kg	≤5 years: 6 mg >5 years: 10 mg	1-5	1-5 h IM 20-30 min IV
Diazepam	0.1-0.3 mg/kg	10 mg	5-30	30-60 h
Narcotics				
Meperidine	1-2 mg/kg	100 mg/dose	5-15	3-5 h IM 2-3 h IV
Fentanyl	1-5 µg/kg	100 µg	1-5	0.5-1 h
Antagonists				
Flumazenil	0.01 mg/kg	0.2 mg/dose or 1.0 mg total	1-2	20-60 min
Naloxone	0.1 mg/kg	2 mg/dose or 10 mg total	2-5	20-60 min

Data from Nowicki and Vaughn (2002),[27] with permission.

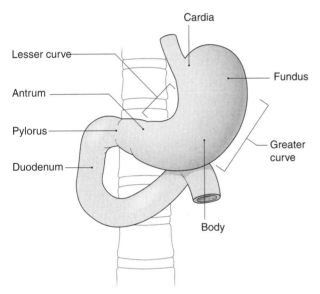

Figure 61-1. Endoscopic anatomy of the stomach and duodenum.

from the esophagus by the presence of bilateral vocal cords on its anterolateral aspects and, if intubated, by the circular tracheal rings along its length.

The esophagus is narrowed at four locations: (1) at the level of the cricopharyngeus, (2) where the esophagus is crossed by the aortic arch, (3) where it is crossed by the left mainstream bronchus, and (4) at the lower esophageal sphincter. Of these, the regions just below the cricopharyngeus and just above the lower esophageal sphincter are often the sites where foreign bodies lodge after ingestion. The lower esophageal sphincter plays an important role in certain diseases, such as achalasia and GER.

The stomach is usually located beneath the diaphragm and, in an adult, is approximately 40 cm distal to the incisors. The right aspect of the esophagus is in continuity with the lesser curvature of the stomach, whereas the left margin of the esophagus joins the greater curvature (Figure 61-1). The gastric rugae are most prominent along the greater curvature. The area of the stomach where the esophagus enters is known as the gastric cardia. The portion of the stomach above the junction of the esophagus and stomach is known as the fundus; it is also the most posterior aspect of the stomach. The majority of the stomach is known as the body of the stomach. On occasion, the

esophagogastric junction is located above the diaphragm, representing a hiatal hernia. Along the lesser curvature of the stomach is the incisura. This notch divides the body of the stomach from the gastric antrum. The pylorus is the muscular junction between the stomach and the small intestine. The pyloric canal is 2 to 3 cm in length in the adult. The diameter of the pyloric opening may vary according to patient age and size and may be affected or altered in certain disease states.

The most proximal portion of the small intestine is the duodenum. The average duodenal length in a full-term infant is 5 cm.[36] The duodenal bulb is an expanded region immediately distal to the pylorus. The duodenum then forms a C-shaped loop and, from the endoscopist's point of view, turns posteriorly and to the right for 2.5 cm in the older child and adult, then inferiorly for 7.5 to 10 cm (descending portion), then anteriorly and to the left for approximately 2.5 cm, finally connecting to the jejunum at the level of the ligament of Treitz. When it joins the jejunum, it turns abruptly forward.

The common bile duct and pancreatic duct enter the duodenal wall obliquely and join together in the ampulla of Vater, which opens into the descending portion of the duodenum via the duodenal papilla. The papilla is usually located approximately 8 to 10 cm distal to the pylorus in adults. The pancreatic duct may also empty via an accessory pancreatic duct, which is usually located proximal to the major duodenal papilla. The duodenum, unlike the jejunum or ileum, does not have a mesentery.

The jejunum and ileum form a series of loops attached to the posterior abdominal wall via a mesentery. In a newborn, the average small intestinal length is 266 ± 56 cm.[37] In adults, the jejunum represents the proximal 2.5 m and the ileum represents the distal 3.5 m of the small bowel. Although the point of transition is often unclear, the jejunum is initially located in the left upper and left lower quadrants. Intraluminally, the jejunum is characterized by large thick folds, large villi, and a luminal diameter of approximately 4 cm. The ileum is thinner walled than the jejunum, with an inner diameter of 3.5 cm, smaller villi, and an increased amount of lymphoid tissue compared with the jejunum.

TECHNIQUE

The endoscope is usually held in the left hand. The thumb is used to turn the large dial; the index finger and sometimes the middle finger are used to control the suction, air, and water valves; and the remaining fingers hold the control handle. The insertion tube is held in the right hand. The lateral wheel, which controls right and left tip deflection, is usually manipulated with the right hand by endoscopists with smaller hands, but may be controlled by either the left hand or the right hand in endoscopists with larger hands. The instruments used via the biopsy channel include needles for injection, biopsy forceps, cytology brushes, foreign-body retrieval instruments, polypectomy snares, probes for cautery, and syringes for irrigation and are usually inserted with the right hand. Before initiating a procedure, the suction and air channels should be checked to ensure proper functioning.

Upper Endoscopy

The endoscopist usually stands on the patient's left during performance of EGD. After sedation in the supine position, the patient is turned to the left lateral decubitus position with the neck flexed downward in preparation for the procedure. Patients undergoing endoscopy under general anesthesia are usually left in the supine position rather than being placed in the lateral decubitus position for ease of airway management. Before insertion of the endoscope into the oral cavity a bite block is placed in the mouth of the nonintubated patient. The endoscope dials are placed in a neutral position. Some operators prefer to lock the right-left dial during esophageal intubation. The endoscope is guided through the bite block over the tongue to the back of the oropharynx by directing the endoscope tip posteriorly and somewhat laterally to the trachea; lateral motion is obtained by right and left torque on the shaft rather than by turning the dial. Some individuals use their forefinger to direct the tip and blindly advance the instrument. As the patient swallows, the cricopharyngeus relaxes and the esophagus, located posteriorly to the trachea and between the pyriform sinuses, can be intubated under direct vision. If the patient is unwilling or unable to swallow after the tip of the instrument is positioned at the esophageal inlet, gentle pressure will usually ease the tip through the cricopharyngeus into the proximal esophagus. The position of the endoscope during this procedure usually makes the patient gag, and if the instrument cannot be passed expeditiously, it should be withdrawn.

After intubating the esophagus, the instrument is advanced down the esophageal lumen while simultaneously examining the mucosa for any lesions. The mucosa is examined as the instrument is inserted to avoid misinterpreting mucosal changes caused by passage of the endoscope. The esophagus is examined for evidence of inflammation, ulcerations, furrowing, varices, hernias, and strictures. The location of the lower esophageal sphincter should be noted. The transition between squamous esophageal and gastric columnar mucosa is called the "Z line." At this point, the mucosa changes from a pale pink to a deep red. The diaphragmatic constriction of the lumen should be noted within 2 cm of the squamocolumnar junction unless a hiatal hernia or Barrett's esophagus is present.

When the stomach is entered, suction is utilized to remove any residual gastric secretions. After the gastric secretions are removed, air is insufflated to separate the gastric rugae. The endoscope is then advanced while torquing to the right. This can be accomplished by applying pressure to the shaft or by the endoscopist twisting to the right; torque can also be achieved by dropping the handle to the right or left, depending on the desired direction of torque. The endoscope is advanced along

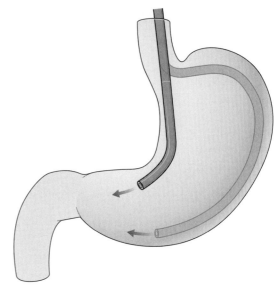

Figure 61-2. Advancement of the endoscope to the duodenum by filling the loop of the greater curvature.

the lesser curve toward the pylorus, but it is usually necessary to fill the greater curvature with the endoscope before cannulating the pyloric canal (Figure 61-2).

The pylorus appears as a small opening with radiating folds around it. Periodic antral waves may pass to the pylorus, changing its location and the size of the canal opening. The pylorus is entered by nudging the tip of the endoscope up to the opening and then directly cannulating the pyloric canal.

The duodenal bulb should be examined on endoscope insertion rather than during withdrawal because of possible mucosal changes caused by passage of the instrument. After examination of all four quadrants, the scope is advanced to the posterior aspect of the bulb, where the duodenum takes a sharp right and downward turn. The instrument is advanced using the dials and shaft torque, usually down and to the right followed by an upward spin of the dial, bringing the tip into the descending duodenum. Once the lumen of the descending duodenum is seen, a straightening maneuver is performed. This consists of pulling the endoscope slowly backward while maintaining the lumen in view. This reduces the loop along the greater curvature of the stomach and usually, paradoxically, advances the endoscope into the distal duodenum (Figure 61-3). The duodenal mucosa, including ampulla of Vater, is examined while withdrawing the endoscope.

After adequate examination of the antrum, pylorus, and duodenum, the endoscope is retroflexed to look for lesions in the gastric cardia and fundus (Figure 61-4). With the instrument looking toward the pylorus and located proximal to the incisura, the tip is deflected until the proximal stomach comes into view. The endoscope is then progressively withdrawn, bringing the cardia closer to the instrument tip while distending the cardia and fundus with air (Figure 61-5). Patients often burp during this maneuver, and cooperative children under conscious sedation may be instructed to try to hold the air in the stomach. The endoscope is then rotated 180° in each direction by torquing the insertion tube in a clockwise or counterclockwise manner.

The instrument is then straightened, the remainder of the gastric mucosa is examined, and biopsies, if necessary, are

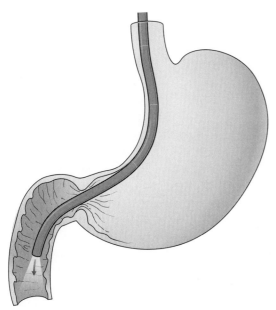

Figure 61-3. Duodenal straightening maneuver that paradoxically advances the endoscope into the distal duodenum by scope withdrawal.

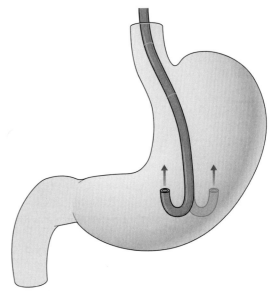

Figure 61-5. Examination of the gastric cardia and fundus by retroflexion, scope withdrawal, and rotation.

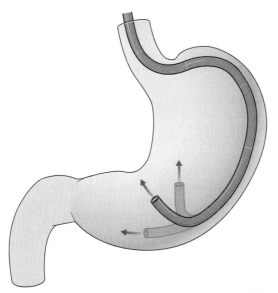

Figure 61-4. Examination of the antrum and incisura by upward deflection of the endoscope tip.

performed. The endoscope is then withdrawn. Immediately before its leaving the stomach, air is aspirated from the stomach. The esophageal mucosa is once again examined. The endoscope is usually withdrawn rapidly in children when the level of the larynx is reached in order to increase patient comfort and diminish gagging.

BIOPSY TECHNIQUE

Histopathologic evaluation of the gastrointestinal tract is helpful in differentiating infectious, inflammatory, and malignant processes. Tissue biopsy is routinely obtained from suspicious lesions during endoscopic examination, and in many centers routine endoscopic biopsy is performed at designated sites,

because clinically significant disease may be present with macroscopically normal appearing mucosa. Recent advances in our understanding of the pathogenesis of disease, such as the relationship of *Helicobacter pylori* and peptic ulcer disease, indicate that tissue biopsy may be indicated even when the source of gastrointestinal bleeding, from a duodenal ulcer for example, is apparent. Numerous techniques and devices have been designed to obtain tissue samples. A variety of pinch biopsy forceps are available that are coordinated in size with endoscopic channel diameter. Standard-size biopsy forceps are fenestrated with a needle so that two sequential biopsies may be performed without removing the forceps from the endoscope. "Spiked" forceps that fit through a 2.0-mm channel are not yet available. Fine-needle biopsy may have an advantage when biopsy material from submucosal lesions is sought. Suction biopsy, which has been adapted to the endoscope, is designed to obtain deeper samples, and jumbo biopsy forceps are also available. Larger biopsy specimens may also be obtained with a turn and suction technique. Multiple biopsy specimens improve the diagnostic yield, but the size and location of the biopsies are probably more important. Brush cytology or other combinations of techniques can increase diagnostic yield. Snare excision is usually reserved for large polyps. For a more detailed discussion, see Chapter 66.

The technique of biopsy varies according to the lesion to be biopsied. To perform a routine biopsy, the closed pinch biopsy forceps are advanced through the biopsy channel to a point just past the tip of the endoscope; they are then opened immediately adjacent and perpendicular to the lesion if possible. This angulation may be difficult to achieve in the esophagus, small bowel, and terminal ileum. The open forceps are then advanced and closed, and the tissue removed through the endoscope. The depth of biopsy is determined by the lesion being sought and the application force of the forceps. There is an ideal distance at which to obtain endoscopic biopsies. Biopsies obtained too close or too far away may be of insufficient size, or associated with mucosal trauma or shear injury.

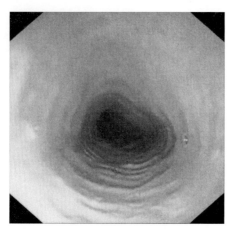

Figure 61-6. Rings of the proximal and midesophagus in a patient with eosinophilic esophagitis. (*See plate section for color.*)

Esophagus

Reflux esophagitis is traditionally diagnosed by clinical criteria. Endoscopy and biopsy are indicated in patients refractory to therapy. Biopsy increases the diagnostic yield compared with visual examination alone. There is a high rate of interobserver variability in the diagnosis of milder forms of esophagitis when "erythema and edema" are the only diagnostic findings. There is a greater uniformity of diagnosis when esophageal erosions are present. Prolonged pH probe and impedance monitoring appears to be the current "gold standard" for the diagnosis of GER and is discussed elsewhere in the text.[38] Numerous eosinophils found in the esophagus can be due to reflux esophagitis or due to eosinophilic esophagitis (Figure 61-6). The two conditions are distinguished by histologic findings, clinical course, and response to therapy.[39-41] Midesophageal endoscopic biopsies demonstrating an increased number of intraepithelial eosinophils or eosinophilic microabscesses are particularly helpful in establishing the diagnosis of eosinophilic esophagitis. The finding of the highly specialized columnar epithelium of Barrett's esophagus necessitates multiple biopsies obtained in a serial and directed manner to screen for dysplasia or adenocarcinoma. Fungal and viral (cytomegalovirus, herpes simplex virus) esophagitis occurs in both immunocompromised and immunocompetent hosts. Biopsy, cytology, and cultures aid in the diagnosis.[42] Malignant tumors of the esophagus are diagnosed by biopsy in the majority of cases. The addition of brush cytology increases the diagnostic yield in cancerous lesions, and EUS is frequently used to stage lesions. Although exceedingly uncommon, adenocarcinoma of the esophagus has been reported in adolescent patients.

STOMACH

The base of gastric ulcers is not routinely biopsied because ulcerating gastric malignancies are rare in pediatric patients. Biopsies should be obtained from the edge rather than the base of the lesion to look for *H. pylori,* but biopsies may be relatively contraindicated if a visible vessel is present. Complications include perforation and bleeding.

Gastritis secondary to drug administration does not usually require biopsy. Gastritis and duodenitis due to nonsteroidal inflammatory drug use may be significant even in otherwise healthy patients and can be associated with the presence of

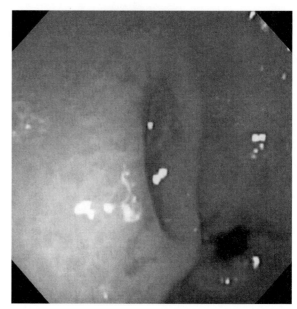

Figure 61-7. Endoscopic appearance of gastric PTLD in a 1-year-old following liver transplantation on tacrolimus immunosuppression. Note the large characteristic raised lesion with central umbilication proximal to the pylorus. The lesion was positive for Epstein-Barr virus (EBV) by in-situ hybridization. (*See plate section for color.*)

gastric or duodenal erosions.[43] Generalized gastritis especially in the setting of a nodular-appearing mucosa may suggest the diagnosis of *H. pylori* infection, confirmed by Giemsa staining or urease testing of antral biopsies.[44] Gastric biopsy may also aid in the diagnosis of idiopathic granulomatous gastritis, Crohn's disease, eosinophilic gastroenteritis, sarcoidosis, and Ménétrier's disease.

Gastric neoplasia, although uncommon in pediatric patients, may appear as an ulcerative, polypoid, or submucosal deformity, or as thickened gastric folds. Gastric malignancies presenting in the pediatric age group include gastrointestinal stromal tumors (GISTs), which may present with GI bleeding, and post-transplantation lymphoproliferative disease (PTLD), which may present with bleeding in addition to a variety of other presentations discussed in detail in Chapter 78.[45,46] PTLD lesions can be single or multiple, have a characteristic appearance, and can be found in the stomach, small bowel, or colon (Figure 61-7).

Pinch biopsy is the preferred technique for ulcerative or small polypoid lesions. Adenomas or hyperplastic polyps of 1.0 cm or more in size should be removed if feasible. Snare polypectomy in the stomach is associated with an increased risk of gastric perforation. Submucosal saline injection may be an important adjuvant technique in this circumstance and is discussed in Chapter 62. Gastric polypectomy should only be performed by practitioners with adequate experience in this technique, and polypectomy should not be performed if submucosal expansion of the lesion is suspected. Submucosal deformities may be evaluated by deep biopsies from a single site, with or without fine-needle aspiration. EUS examination may assist with evaluation of the submucosal extent of disease in worrisome lesions such as GISTs.[45]

Small Intestine

Endoscopic pinch biopsy of the small bowel is helpful in the diagnosis of celiac disease, intestinal lymphangiectasia, and Crohn's disease. Multiple directed specimens obtained from the descending duodenum or the more distal bowel have replaced capsule biopsy, with comparable accuracy, increased patient comfort, and decreased risk of complications. Characteristic endoscopic findings of celiac disease in children include scalloping of folds, loss of folds, visible vasculature, and a mucosal mosaic pattern, especially in the duodenal bulb. This mosaic pattern may be more evident when chromoendoscopy is used.[47,48] However, the most common mucosal appearance in celiac disease is normal mucosa, emphasizing the need for endoscopic biopsy to establish this diagnosis. Intestinal lymphangiectasia in the duodenum and jejunum is often characterized endoscopically by a change in the appearance of the mucosa to white. Specific findings include diffuse whitish mucosa, scattered white spots, white nodules 3 to 8 mm in size with sharply demarcated margins, and submucosal elevations.[49]

Jumbo forceps (open diameter 9 mm) or the turn and suction technique allows for larger small-bowel specimens. Distal biopsies can be obtained using small-caliber colonoscopes or dedicated enteroscopes. This technique may be especially useful for lesions that characteristically have a patchy distribution. Biopsy of macroscopically normal tissue may occasionally establish the diagnosis and allows for determination of disaccharidase levels if appropriate.

Small bowel parasitic infection may be identified by direct observation or pathologic identification of removed worms. Aspiration of duodenal contents and histologic examination can identify parasites such as *Giardia lamblia* or *Strongyloides*, which may not produce visible mucosal changes.[50] Duodenal tumors are rare and can be biopsied with either the forward- or side-viewing endoscopes. With increasing number of pediatric solid organ transplantations being performed, PTLD is occurring with an increased frequency in children and may involve the small intestine in addition or without gastric involvement.

THERAPEUTIC ENDOSCOPY

During the early years of gastrointestinal endoscopy, endoscopic examination was primarily a diagnostic tool. As technology advanced and procedural skills developed, the endoscope became a therapeutic instrument. Endoscopes have been used in children to remove foreign bodies and polyps; to insert tubes, catheters, and stents into various organs; and to stop bleeding lesions. For detailed discussions, the reader is also referred to Chapters 14, 19, 62, 63,64, 65, and 76.

Acute gastrointestinal hemorrhage is an indication for therapeutic endoscopic intervention, but emergent gastrointestinal endoscopy is associated with an increased risk of complications.[51] This includes a risk of aspiration of gastric contents and a higher risk associated with sedating an actively bleeding patient or a patient with decompensated cardiopulmonary or hepatic function.[51] Upper gastrointestinal lesions that may be amenable to endoscopic therapy include ulcers with evidence of active bleeding, oozing from beneath a clot overlying an ulcer (sentinel clot), or an ulcer with a visible vessel at its base that is not actively bleeding but appears as a red, blue, or white plug.[52] These same lesions have a high rate of rebleeding, approximately 50%, compared with an incidence of 10% or less of rebleeding with other lesions, including those with an overlying clot without oozing or flat spots.

Bleeding from esophageal varices can also be treated by endoscopic sclerotherapy, band ligation or a combination of the techniques.[53-57] Therefore, ongoing therapy to ablate distal esophageal varices is usually undertaken after the initial bleeding episode has resolved but in some cases prophylactic endoscopic band ligation is performed in patients who cannot tolerate, have a contraindication to or fail to respond to β-blockade[58] (see Chapter 76).

Diffuse mucosal bleeding from duodenitis or gastritis is usually not responsive to endoscopic interventions. The exception to this is gastric antral vascular ectasia amenable to treatment with the argon plasma coagulator.[59] Lesions that may be treatable with endoscopic therapy include bleeding lesions, angiomata, and polyps.

There are five well-established types of therapeutic intervention for acute gastrointestinal bleeding: injection; coagulation or thermal therapy including the recently developed argon plasma coagulator (APC); laser therapy; endoscopic hemostatic devices; and ligation therapy. The specific techniques used depend on equipment availability and experience of the endoscopist. The techniques appear to have roughly equivalent efficacy, but some lesions are more amenable to a particular type of therapy.[52]

Therapeutic endoscopy is most easily accomplished using a two-channeled therapeutic scope so that therapy (injection, coagulation, etc.) may be accomplished via one channel and simultaneous suction or irrigation may be performed using the second channel to keep the field in view. Unfortunately, therapeutic endoscopes are of a large diameter compared with standard pediatric endoscopes and often cannot be used in the pediatric patient. Therapeutic endoscopy may still be performed using a single-channel scope, but depending on the modality used, this may be technically more difficult.

INJECTION

Injection therapy is used for both variceal and nonvariceal bleeding. A variety of sclerosants are available for esophageal sclerotherapy. The respective agents act as tissue irritants that cause vascular thrombosis and endothelial damage leading to endofibrosis and vascular obliteration when injected into or adjacent to blood vessels.[60] Most of the sclerosants are fatty acid derivatives, synthetic chemicals, alcohols, or sugars. Each agent also has unique properties based on its composition. Volumes of injection vary by agent. Current guidelines should be followed when performing esophageal sclerotherapy in pediatric or adult patients.[60] The technique of esophageal sclerotherapy for varices is discussed elsewhere in the text (see Chapter 76). Nonvariceal injection therapy is usually performed by injecting a sclerosing agent at three to four sites around an exposed bleeding vessel (Figure 61-8). Maximal volumes of sclerosant have been established in adults to minimize the risk of ulcer extension or perforation. Maximal volumes of sclerosants in pediatric patients have not been studied; however, maximal adult volumes should not be exceeded.[52] Complications including perforation may occur with volumes of injection even less than the recommended maximum volumes. Table 61-5 lists the most commonly used solutions, their concentrations, and estimated maximal volumes. Several general principles should be noted. First, except under unusual circumstances, injection therapy should be confined to a single solution (single agent or a combination agent) during a given injection episode. Utilizing two sequential solutions may increase the risk of complication with smaller volumes of sclerosant than would be required by using a single agent alone. Second, the injection site (into vessel vs. surrounding vessel vs. submucosal) is specific for certain agents. Without appropriate clinical trials, changing the site of injection is probably hazardous. Third, the risks with injection therapy include increased bleeding, rebleeding, bowel ischemia, and perforation. Fourth, precise volumes of injection are required. Injections that involve smaller volumes may be more technically difficult. Fifth, although submucosal injection has been used to assist in resection of colonic polyps, optimal volumes of injection of a number of agents have not been established for the large bowel.

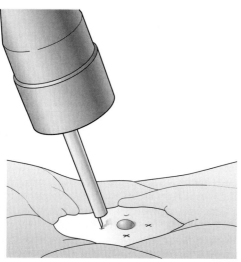

Figure 61-8. Injection circumferentially around a visible vessel in an ulcer base. Injection is performed at three to four sites around the exposed vessel.

THERMOCOAGULATION

A second method of establishing hemostasis is thermocoagulation, utilizing the heater probe, monopolar or bipolar, also known as multipolar coagulators (MPEC) (Table 61-6). The heater probe is composed of polytetrafluoroethylene (PTFE)-coated hollow aluminum cylinders with an inner heater coil and a maximum internal temperature. The probe is water perfused to prevent tissue adherence, an advantage over monopolar coagulation, and heat is delivered via conduction to the tissue. There are small-diameter (2.4 mm) and large-diameter (3.2 mm) probes. The patient should be positioned so that the blood flows away from the ulcer base if possible. The probe is passed through the therapeutic channel, and coagulation is performed by tamponading the bleeding vessel by direct firm pressure using the heater probe and then coagulating the vessel (Figure 61-9). Coagulation is usually performed in adults by two to four 30-J pulses in succession.[61] Coagulation should be around the bleeding point first, and then directly on it. In studies of adult patients, the greatest success appears to be with firm tamponade on the ulcer bleeding point or nonbleeding visible vessel, and four pulses for a total of 120 J in succession before the probe position is changed.[61,62] This technique, however, may increase the risk of complications when applied to other types of lesion, specifically Mallory-Weiss tears or angiomata, that occur in areas with a thinner gut wall.[61]

ELECTROCOAGULATION

There are two main types of electrocoagulation probes, monopolar and bipolar. In monopolar coagulation, a continuous or intermittent current is passed via the tip or side of the probe.

TABLE 61-5. **Sclerosants for Nonvariceal Bleeding**

Solution	Concentration	Volume/No. of Injections/Location	Maximum Volume	Comments
Hypertonic saline–epinephrine combination	3.6% saline + 1:20,000 epinephrine or 7.2% saline + 1:20,000 epinephrine[a]	3 mL/3-4 injections at base of bleeding vessel 1 mL/3-4 injections	9-12 mL	Repeat prophylactic injections if visible vessel present 24-48 h after first hemostasis for lesions with extensive fibrosis*
Epinephrine with normal saline	1 mL 1:1000 epinephrine + 9 mL normal saline	0.5-2.0 mL injected in multiple sites around bleeding vessel and into bleeding point itself	10 mL	Range 1.5-10 mL, mean 4.1 mL; larger volumes in range for spurting vessels
Epinephrine followed by polidocanol	5-10 mL 1:10,000 epinephrine, 5 mL 1% polidocanol	Inject epinephrine into the submucosa directly around blood vessel to achieve hemostasis by compression/vasoconstriction, then obliterate vessel with polidocanol	Epinephrine 5-10 mL Polidocanol 5 mL	May substitute bipolar coagulation or Nd:YAG laser for polidocanol
Thrombin in normal saline	100 IU thrombin in 3 mL normal saline	Inject into bleeding vessel, 10-15 mL total volume	10-15 mL	
Absolute ethanol	98% dehydrated ethanol	0.1-0.2 mL/injection at 3-4 sites surrounding bleeding vessel and 1-2 mm away from vessel	0.6-1.22 mL total	Inject via tuberculin syringe *slowly* (0.2 mL/3 s); extension/perforation significant risk if maximum volume exceeded; may be technically more difficult to control volume
Epinephrine with normal saline for submucosal injection[†]	1 mL 1:1000 epinephrine + 9 mL normal saline	1.0-2.0 mL per injection injected in multiple sites (3-4) around the polyp to be raised up	30 mL	Goal is lack of vascular markings within injection site

Adapted from Sugawa (1989),[51] with permission.
*3.6%/0.005% epinephrine prepared by combining 1 part of solution A (20 mL 15% NaCl solution and 1 mL 0.1% epinephrine) to 3 parts of solution B (20 mL distilled water, with 1 mL 0.1% epinephrine). 7.2%/0.005% prepared by combining equal parts (1:1) of solutions A and B.
[†]From Waye (2001).[135]

TABLE 61-6. **Thermocoagulation**

Method	Site	Setting	Application time	No. of Applications	Technique	Notes
Heater probe	Upper GI tract	30 J		2-4	Firm tamponade, then coagulate around bleeding point, then on it	Decreased setting/time of application in colon or thinner gut wall
Monopolar	Upper GI tract	Mid-range	1-2 s/pulse		Directly on vessel <1 mm in diameter; circumferentially around vessel >1 mm in diameter	Perforation likely in colon
Bipolar/ multipolar	Upper GI tract	15-25 W	2 s/pulse or Up to 14-s pulse	Multiple Single	Firm tamponade, then coagulate	Difficult angulation in lesser curve or deformed duodenum
Argon plasma coagulator	Upper GI tract	40-50 W 0.8 l/min	0.5-2 s	Multiple	Operative distance 2-8 mm	Paint confluent or near-confluent areas; avoid tissue contact with probe tip; surface should be free of liquid

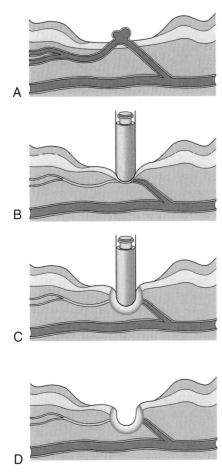

Figure 61-9. Coaptive coagulation utilizing the heater probe. (**A**) Visible vessel in an ulcer base. Note vessel is not an end artery. (**B**) Tamponade with probe initially. (**C**) Coagulation after tamponade. (**D**) "White footprint" at coagulation site.

The current is conducted to the patient's ground plate. The current is converted to high-temperature heat at the tissue contact point, which coagulates the tissue, causing collagen contraction and vessel shrinkage. For vessels less than 1 mm in diameter, the electrode is placed directly on the vessel, and pressure is applied directly on the vessel to coapt it. With larger vessels, the coagulating current is placed circumferentially around the vessel until bleeding stops. Usually a midrange setting is used for 1 to 2 seconds per pulse at a distance of 2 to 3 mm from the

vessel. This is because an artery in an ulcer base may bleed from either side if it is not an end artery; therefore, a ring of tissue must be treated around the bleeding point to ensure adequate hemostasis. The aim is to achieve hemostasis of the underlying artery and not the overlying clot. There are two main problems with monopolar coagulation. The first is that the depth of the burn is very difficult to regulate, and perforation is possible. The second problem is that there is a moderate amount of electrode adherence to the underlying tissue at the treated site and therefore poor visibility, especially in nonirrigated systems. A third technical problem is the need to clean the tip of the probe as the coagulum accumulates during electrocoagulation.

Currently bipolar or multipolar coagulation is the most popular method with endoscopists. Unlike monopolar coagulation, a grounding plate is not required. Current is transmitted from one electrode on the probe to another, and energy is delivered when any pair of electrodes is in contact with the bleeding target. The MPEC (multipolar) probe has six points through which current can be passed; contact between any two is sufficient. This has the advantage of allowing for tangential contact.[63] The maximal temperature achieved with this method is significantly less than that of monopolar coagulation or the Nd:YAG laser, causing less tissue injury and having greater efficacy for vessels less than 2 mm in diameter. Two sizes of probe are available: 2.3 and 3.2 mm. As with the heater probe, the correct technique is to compress the bleeding vessel first, then to coagulate. Forceful application of the larger probe appears to increase hemostatic bond strength and the area and depth of coagulation.[64] The greatest depth of coagulation is usually achieved with a low to midrange setting (15 to 25 W) as increased wattage settings are not associated with increased energy delivery.[65] Pulses should be applied as short, multiple pulses (2 seconds in duration) or a single long pulse of up to 14 seconds in duration.[64] The longer, lower-voltage pulse is thought to work by increasing the depth of coagulation and surface area treated by decreasing tissue desiccation.[66] In adults, a total of up to 40 seconds of electrocoagulation is required.[64] Modest tamponade is necessary to achieve hemostasis when the MPEC probe is applied to a bleeding vessel. Failure to tamponade may result in failure to achieve hemostasis.[66] Increased bleeding after MPEC has been reported in cases with a visible vessel; usually this bleeding is controllable with further MPEC coagulation, but on occasion surgery has been required.

Multipolar electrocoagulation appears to be as effective as the heater probe in terms of hemostasis, incidence of rebleeding, transfusion requirement, and need for emergency surgery. Several studies report a hemostasis rate in the 90% range for both modalities.[64] Multipolar electrocoagulation also appears to be as efficacious as the laser at a marked reduction in cost. The angulation of the probe, or use of a MPEC electrode compared with a laser, does not appear to affect the rebleeding rate. However, poor angulation along the lesser curvature of the stomach or in a deformed duodenum may make pressure application more difficult.

MPEC therapy of angiodysplasia, which occurs predominantly in the colon, and use of hot biopsy forceps for coagulation is discussed in more detail in Chapter 62. Perforation has been reported at an increased rate with hot biopsy forceps use in the upper gastrointestinal tract, both in the stomach (secondary to increased gastric thickness, limiting tenting of the mucosa) and in the duodenum and ileum (secondary to thinness of the bowel wall and variable depth of penetration).[67] Another complication of the hot biopsy forceps application is major hemorrhage; the etiologies of this complication are discussed in Chapter 62. Hemorrhage may be immediate or delayed for up to 1 week after biopsy and may not respond to conservative therapy.

Results of comparative trials of injection, coagulation, and heater probe therapy vary according to the method used; however, in many studies the different techniques are of comparable efficacy given established volumes of injection, thermocoagulation settings, appropriate indications, and times of application.[63] Injection therapy in the setting of peptic ulcer disease has been shown to decrease the rate of rebleeding, the transfusion requirement, the need for emergency surgery and the length of hospital stay. Similar results have been noted in trials comparing MPEC, heater probe, and Nd:YAG laser therapy, with higher costs noted for laser therapy.[63] A systematic review of 49 contemporary trials encompassing more than 4000 adult patients with peptic ulcer bleeding and high-risk lesions has demonstrated that although all endoscopic therapies are superior to pharmacotherapy alone in these high-risk patients, thermal therapies or endoscopic clips, discussed in further detail later, alone or in combination appear to be the optimal method to prevent rebleeding.[68] Other studies have also demonstrated the benefit of combination therapy compared to injection therapy alone.[69]

In some circumstances, one method of achieving hemostasis may be technically easier than other techniques. With MPEC probes, the depth of coagulation is limited to 2 mm, which limits their use with larger vessels. However, the probes have a built-in wash system, aiding visibility in cases of brisk bleeding compared with injection therapy. The choice of therapeutic endoscopic technique depends to a significant extent on the training of the endoscopist and equipment availability. If the technique is properly performed, the results are similar using injection or thermal coagulation. Certain lesions, based on their anatomic location or briskness of bleeding, may be more amenable to one method than another. Equipment portability may also be an issue, with injection therapy and coagulation techniques such as the heater probe or multipolar probe, or even the argon plasma coagulator, being significantly more portable than laser techniques. Complication rates may vary among the techniques, with perforations and rebleeding being reported after monopolar, MPEC, laser therapy, and APC application.[63] Injection therapy is rarely associated with perforation unless nonstandard volumes of injection are used.[63] Similarly,

hemostatic clips (discussed later), when properly applied, are rarely associated with the development of complications.

Argon Plasma Coagulation

The APC was initially used for surgery, both open and laparoscopic, with endoscopic applications after 1991. It is a noncontact method delivered via the accessory channel of the endoscope. The major benefit of this technique is that it is a quick method of therapy deliverable over a large treatment area. The principle of APC is that high-frequency monopolar current is conducted to target tissues *through* ionized argon gas (argon plasma). Argon gas passes through the coagulation probe with an electrode at its tip. The foot switch activates the electrode. Electrons flow through the channel of electrically activated ionized argon gas from the probe to the tissue.[70] The arrival of the current density at the tissue surface results in coagulation. The grounding pad completes the circuit. The principles of APC are discussed in detail in Chapter 62.

Current probes have an outer diameter of 2.3 or 3.2 mm. Therapy is performed for hemostasis of superficial vascular ectasias such as watermelon stomach (gastric antral vascular ectasia), also known as GAVE, for hemostasis of peptic ulcers, and for tissue ablation. Settings vary significantly by indication. In adults, superficial vascular lesions are typically treated by low power (40 to 50 W) and gas flow rates (0.8 L/min) with an operative distance between the tissue and the probe of 2 to 8 mm.[70] Closer contact is used with lower power settings to allow for contact between the plasma and the targeted tissue. Application times are in the range of 0.5 to 2.0 seconds. Similar settings have been reported in a pediatric series.[71] The technique is to paint confluent or near-confluent surface areas. Use of a two-channel endoscope, if possible, allows for aspiration of argon gas. If the probe tip contacts the bowel wall, it becomes similar to a grounded monopolar probe (discussed previously) and may result in deep tissue injury. The surface to be treated needs to be clear of liquid and blood; if not, coagulated film develops and the tissue beneath may not be adequately treated, limiting the usefulness of this technology in patients with active bleeding. In the treatment of gastric vascular ectasia lesions, including those due to portal hypertensive gastropathy, a particularly challenging source of chronic GI blood loss in adults, APC application has been associated with success rates in the range of 86% (range 81 to 90%) in terms of reducing rebleeding rates and transfusion requirement with a low procedural complication rate.[59]

Endoscopic Hemostatic Devices Including Bands and Clips

Band Ligation

Band ligation was initially utilized for the management of esophageal variceal hemorrhage starting in the late 1980s. Endoscopic variceal ligation (EVL) is the treatment of choice for control of variceal hemorrhage in appropriately sized pediatric patients and for variceal obliteration in secondary prophylaxis, that is, in patients who cannot tolerate or have a contraindication to β-blocker use and those who do not have an adequate drop in hepatic venous pressure gradient in response to β-blocker therapy.[58] Multiple randomized controlled trials and a meta-analysis in adults comparing esophageal sclerotherapy to EVL report the superiority of EVL in several major outcomes.

These include recurrent bleeding, local complications including ulceration and stricture formation, time to variceal eradication, and patient survival. However, esophageal variceal recurrence appears to be more frequent following EVL than sclerotherapy.[58] In pediatric patients, the size of the band ligator/friction fit adaptor may limit use of EVL in patients aged 4 years or younger, and sclerotherapy may be the primary modality of therapy in these younger or smaller patients. Indications and technique of EVL and sclerotherapy are discussed in more detail in the chapter on portal hypertension.

This technique has subsequently been used for the management of bleeding gastric and intestinal varices, Dieulafoy lesions, bleeding Mallory-Weiss tears, angiectasias including GAVE, and duodenal ulcers.[63,72] Band ligation is most effective for bleeding lesions in nonfibrotic tissue. Typically, after a diagnostic endoscopy to identify the source of bleeding, the endoscope is withdrawn. The ligating device, composed of a control handle and attached adaptor, is loaded via the biopsy channel, and a friction fit adaptor with the ligating bands is placed at the end of the endoscope (usually a standard-size adult upper endoscope). Ligation kits contain a variable number of bands, but typically multiband ligators are utilized. After passage of the endoscope to the desired location, suction is applied to draw the lesion to be ligated into the friction fit adaptor at the end of the endoscope.[56] The bands are deployed by rotation of the ligating control handle while in the locked position. Positional adjustments and inspection for continued evidence of bleeding can be made between subsequent band deployments. In the case of a bleeding lesion such as a Dieulafoy lesion, only a single band may need to be deployed. Because the presence of more bands on the friction fit adaptor limits the endoscopic view, some pediatric gastroenterologists choose to deploy some of the bands outside the patient before endoscope insertion to improve the field of view. Band ligators are currently not available for smaller pediatric-size endoscopes.

Hemostatic Clips

Originally developed in the 1970s for deployment through the endoscope, endoclips have significantly increased in popularity and ease of use in the past 5 to 10 years.[73] Originally the clips were designed to be placed on a deployment device that could be reused, and deployment of the clip resulted in the need to remove and reload the device after each clip application. This technique was cumbersome and time consuming. More recently, clips have been developed that are preloaded and designed for single use, although single-use clips are typically more costly than the multiuse deployment devices. Hemoclip application requires an endoscope with a 2.8-mm channel. Preloaded clips are available in different lengths, allowing use with both upper endoscopes and colonoscopes. Rotatable clips and clips that can be reopened several times before final deployment are also available. Endoscopic clipping is used primarily for endoscopic hemostasis, but has also been applied for binding tubes or catheters to the gastrointestinal wall (stent, feeding tube, manometry catheter); closure of fistulas, leaks, and perforations; and marking anatomic landmarks for subsequent therapy or surgery.[73,74] Lesions amenable to clip application for hemostasis include gastric and duodenal ulcers with high-risk stigmata, Mallory-Weiss tears, and Dieulafoy's lesion. Endoclip application for ulcer bleeding is associated with a high primary hemostatic rate (85 to 100%), depending on the series, and a low recurrent bleeding rate (2 to 20%).[73] Currently endoscopic

clipping of ulcers with high-risk stigmata as a monotherapy is thought to be as effective as a variety of combination therapies (combination of injection and coagulation techniques) in achieving primary hemostasis and reducing the rebleeding rate and need for surgery of these high-risk lesions.[68,75] Ulcers most amenable to endoclip therapy include those with small arteries and those not located on the difficult areas for endoscopic therapy: the proximal posterior wall of the stomach, high on the lesser curvature of the stomach, and the posterior duodenal wall. Clips have also been used for lower gastrointestinal bleeding as discussed in Chapter 62.

Endoclips are deployed by the following technique, although the specifics vary by manufacturer. After passage through the endoscope channel, the stopper on the clip is removed and the cylinder is pulled back, exposing the clip. The slider is slowly pulled back, opening the clip to its maximum width. The clip is pressed against the lesion; a small amount of suction is applied before deployment, allowing the lumen to collapse; and the slider is quickly pulled back. This closes the clip and deploys it. Some clips require an additional step to dislodge the clip from the application device. Typically more than one clip is deployed in a single endoscopic session. The first clip is placed on the bleeding point, and subsequent clips may be placed around the bleeding point to occlude the submucosal vessel (opposite to the technique of heater probe application).[73] Some lesions can be closed by sequential application of clips in a zipper-like fashion. The clips dislodge spontaneously after application and have not been associated with long-term sequelae. Caveats of clip application include tangential application and suction immediately before closure when possible to capture more tissue within the prongs, use on lesions that are pliable enough with enough soft tissue on either side of the prongs, and ideal use for vessels less than 2 mm in size.[75] Significant benefits of clipping include the avoidance of thermally induced ulceration, and the fact that clipping does not exacerbate bleeding in the setting of clotting abnormalities.[75] This modality therefore may be particularly advantageous in cardiology or oncology patients with bleeding from high-risk lesions with reduced numbers of platelets or platelet dysfunction due to their disease process or medication use (Figure 61-10A,B).

Endoloops

Endoloops are utilized primarily for the management of potential or actual postpolypectomy hemorrhage and are discussed in Chapter 62. Detachable loops have also been used in the management of gastric varices.[63] Loops are deployed through the biopsy channel.

Laser Photocoagulation

Laser photocoagulation is another modality occasionally used to achieve endoscopic hemostasis. There are two main types of laser: the argon and the Nd:YAG laser. The argon laser's usefulness is limited because of light absorption by surrounding red blood. Clinically, the argon laser is used primarily for right-sided colonic lesions. When compared with the Nd:YAG laser, it has a lower power and depth of tissue penetration.

The Nd:YAG laser is the most popular laser used in endoscopy. The laser admits a continuous wave of infrared light of wavelength 1064 nm with a power up to 100 W. This light is transmitted via a 600-μm glass fiber in a 2.5-mm PTFE catheter passed down the endoscope biopsy channel. Carbon dioxide

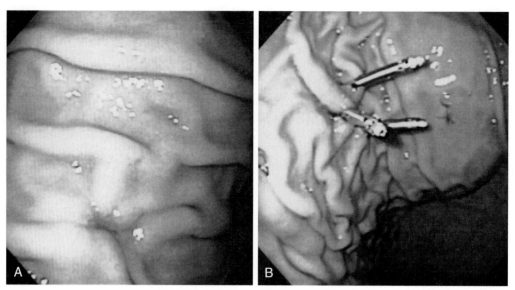

Figure 61-10. Endoscopic clipping of a gastric Dieulafoy lesion in a teenage patient following cardiac surgery on aspirin and antiplatelet therapy. The patient presented with a massive upper GI bleed with ongoing hemodynamic instability despite transfusion. (**A**) The clips were applied sequentially to approximate the edges of the lesion which terminated the bleeding episode. (**B**) (*See plate section for color.*)

is passed coaxially along the catheter to clear blood from the bleeding site and to keep the fiber tip cool and free from debris. A filter is attached to the eyepiece to prevent reflected laser light from entering the endoscopist's eye. The intense laser light is directed to coagulate tissue circumferentially around the bleeding site. Contact and noncontact applications are possible.[63] The current recommendation for adults is to deliver 0.5-second pulses, at 80 W of energy, from a distance of 1 cm, and at least 2 to 3 mm away from visible arterial segments for upper gastrointestinal lesions.[76]

Lasers have been used in the small bowel for congenital vascular lesions as well as superficial vascular lesions, including angiodysplasia, telangiectasia, and arteriovenous malformations. Asymptomatic, nonbleeding angiodysplasias are usually not treated. One problem after laser photocoagulation of a lesion is that the histologic diagnosis is difficult to confirm.

Like the heater probe, laser therapy can also provoke bleeding, which can usually be stopped with further laser coagulation.[76] In addition, there is an increased chance of full-thickness perforation of the gut wall. Application of the laser in the colon is discussed in Chapter 62. There is a long learning curve associated with use of the laser, and this modality should be used only by experienced operators. Currently the laser seems to offer little advantage over other coagulation techniques, and because of its increased cost and decreased portability, the other modalities are likely to predominate in the foreseeable future.

STRICTURE DILATION

Esophageal strictures in children can occur as a result of a variety of conditions including GER, eosinophilic esophagitis, scleroderma; following caustic ingestion, drug injury, repair of esophageal atresia, or radiation therapy; or as a consequence of sclerotherapy. They may also be idiopathic.[77]

Esophageal dilation can be performed with a variety of instruments, but only endoscopic dilation is discussed in this section. The advantage of endoscopic dilation is the ability to visualize the stenotic area, estimate its size, select an appropriately sized

dilator, and, if necessary, pass a guidewire beyond the stenotic area. Dilation techniques can be divided into those performed using the endoscope itself, those performed over a wire (OTW), and those using through the endoscope dilators (TTS).

Savary-Gillard dilators are among the most frequently used types of dilator. They are hollow bougies of plastic-coated polyvinyl ranging in size from 5 to 15 mm (15 to 45 Fr). The tip is tapered and flexible, and the shaft is more rigid. Endoscopy is initially performed to the level of the stenosis, or beyond the stenosis if possible. A flexible-tip guidewire is then advanced via the biopsy channel through the stricture under direct observation. When it passes the stricture, the endoscope is removed while the wire is kept in place by advancing it as the endoscope is withdrawn. Typically a wire with a spring-coiled tip is utilized. The wire is advanced into the gastric antrum if possible, for example, in patients with esophageal stricture. The coil at the tip of the wire helps to reduce the incidence of perforation due to the wire. The lubricated bougie is then threaded over the guidewire, which is held taut. Serial dilations are performed by progressively increasing the bougie size according to the amount of resistance encountered. The dilators should be checked for blood following each dilation. Strictures typically need to be dilated over several sessions rather than on a single occasion. The guidewire must be held in place in between application of serial bougies in order to avoid slippage.

In a large French-American series, larger-diameter dilations could be performed using the Savary system than with the Eder-Puestow dilating system. There was no statistically significant difference in the incidence of complications between the two methods.[78] The occurrence of esophageal perforation may relate more to the reason for dilation (e.g., caustic ingestion or malignancy versus peptic stenosis) than the dilating method used. Also, the success of dilation may relate to the indication. Dilating congenital stenosis is usually more effective than dilating achalasia or postsurgical stenosis.

Endoscopic balloon dilation may also be performed utilizing TTS balloon dilators. After visualizing the stricture, these types of balloon can be passed through an endoscope with a

2.8-mm channel under direct vision. These single-use dilators have an inflatable balloon at their tip. The balloon is inflatable to a preset maximum diameter and pressure. If the pressure is exceeded, the balloon ruptures, reducing the risk of esophageal perforation. Inflation exerts only radially directed forces as opposed to the shearing longitudinal forces that occur with conventional bougienage (Savary-Gillard or Maloney dilators). The balloon dilator is positioned through the endoscope with or without the use of a guidewire. The balloon is inflated with water or, occasionally, Gastrografin, and held in inflation for 30 to 90 seconds, then deflated.[79] Usually two or three inflations are performed per endoscopic session, with repositioning of the balloon in between inflations. In addition, balloon size can be increased for subsequent dilations in the same session if indicated. Sessions are repeated over several weeks or months with progressively larger-diameter balloons. This technique has been utilized for esophageal atresia with postoperative strictures and is especially useful for strictures of recent onset. Endoscopically directed hydrostatic balloon dilation has also been reported in obstructive gastroduodenal Crohn's disease. Successful endoscopic guided OTW balloon dilation of esophageal strictures has been reported in recessive dystrophic epidermolysis bullosa, a condition associated with proximal esophageal strictures and an increased vulnerability of the esophageal mucosa to minor injury.[80,81]

Balloons that can be inflated to three distinct diameters have been developed and are now widely available. These balloons exert a high degree of radial vector force at each of the different standardized pressures, but are still designed to rupture if preset pressures are exceeded. They represent a potential cost saving to the patient if progressive serial diameter dilations are performed on the same day, and may decrease the time of the endoscopic procedure because of decreased need to exchange balloons during the procedure.

Intralesional steroid injection of peptic and caustic esophageal strictures has been reported as an adjuvant to endoscopic dilation. Small volumes (0.25 to 1.0 mL per injection) of triamcinolone acetonide (Kenalog 10 mg/mL; Bristol Meyers Squibb Princeton, NJ, USA) are injected in four quadrants of the narrowest stricture segment. The efficacy of triamcinolone appears to be based on its interference with collagen synthesis and subsequent scar formation.[79] This technique has been associated with increased efficacy of dilation and longer symptom-free intervals between endoscopic dilations.[82] Topical application of mitomycin C, an antiproliferative agent, has been tried for pediatric patients with refractory esophageal strictures; this agent may be associated with an increased risk of complications, and a larger experience is required before this can be recommended.[83,84]

Esophageal dilation can also be performed by passage of progressively larger endoscopes. This is usually performed for esophageal strictures with a luminal diameter in the range of 6 to 8 mm. Typically a gastroscope with an outer diameter of 5 to 6 mm is passed initially across the stricture. Subsequently gastroscopes with an outer diameter of 8 to 9 mm can be passed under direct endoscopic vision using careful steady pressure. Perforation is a potential complication of this technique, and the endoscopist must use judgment as to appropriate dilating diameter and the amount of pressure to be exerted, as with any endoscopic technique. The advantage of serial endoscopic dilation compared with OTW dilation is that the length of the stricture can be carefully visualized and assessed, irregularities of

the stricture such as shelves can be identified, the direction of the dilating force can be more directly controlled, and bleeding or excessive trauma is identified immediately.

Eosinophilic esophagitis has been identified as a cause of esophageal strictures and ringed esophagus. This condition and its management are discussed elsewhere in the text. This condition can be associated with short or long esophageal strictures and/or diffuse narrowing of the esophagus. Dilation of strictures associated with this condition may require special precautions. The esophagus in this condition appears to be especially susceptible to shear injury, and longitudinal tears of the esophagus have been reported following endoscopy without dilation and after small-diameter dilations.[85,86] Strictures in this condition may occur throughout the length of the esophagus, and there is a higher incidence of proximal strictures compared with reflux-related strictures, which are more typically distal. TTS balloon dilation under direct endoscopic vision may be one method to manage these proximal esophageal strictures effectively, which may be endoscopically challenging.

SMALL BOWEL ENTEROSCOPY

There are three primary techniques of small bowel enteroscopy currently applicable to pediatric patients. In children, this procedure is used primarily for the evaluation of gastrointestinal bleeding of unknown origin. It may occasionally be indicated for small bowel biopsy, although this can usually be accomplished utilizing the standard upper endoscopes.

This procedure is also utilized for jejunal polypectomy and can be used in conjunction with open or laparoscopic surgical procedures as a method of evaluating the distal small bowel. Additional indications include evaluation of extent of inflammatory bowel disease or polyposis syndromes, including surveillance, evaluation of lymphoma or lymphangiectasia, graft assessment after small bowel transplant, dilation of strictures, and directed tube placement such as percutaneous jejunostomy (PEJ) placement (discussed later) and nasojejunal tube placement.[87]

The most popular type of small bowel endoscopic examination in children is push enteroscopy. The limitation of this technique is that the angulation of the duodenum dissipates the propelling force transmitted to the shaft of the endoscope and subsequently creates a large loop in the stomach and duodenum. Gastroduodenal loops can occasionally be reduced by use of a straightening tube, but are more often reduced by endoscopic techniques of withdrawal and torque similar to those utilized in colonoscopy. This type of enteroscopy is performed with either a sterilized pediatric colonoscope or a special push-type enteroscope. Both of these endoscopes have a larger diameter than standard pediatric gastroscopes, limiting their usefulness in infants and small children. These endoscopes do, however, have a biopsy channel, and angulation of the tip is possible. Therefore, therapeutic interventions such as biopsy, injection, coagulation, and polypectomy are possible. The exact extent of evaluation is variable, based on patient size and anatomy, but distances of 120 to 180 cm beyond the ligament of Treitz have been visualized with this technique, and full examination to the terminal ileum may be possible using a combined enteroscopic-operative advancement technique.[87] After the scope is fully inserted, glucagon may be administered to decrease intestinal peristalsis. The lumen is visualized primarily on scope withdrawal, combining air insufflation and slow withdrawal of the scope. This technique is useful to detect a diffuse lesion and the causes of small bowel bleeding, especially arteriovenous malformations.

The second type of small bowel endoscopy is passive, using a Sonde-type enteroscope passed intranasally. These instruments have a balloon at the tip and, when it is inflated, bowel peristalsis acts to pull the endoscope through the small bowel. This procedure may take 12 to 24 hours. Compared with the push-type enteroscopes, the Sonde scope has a much narrower diameter for greater patient comfort. It has no tip control for angulation, however, and no biopsy channel. As with the push-type enteroscope, the lumen is visualized using glucagon paralysis on scope withdrawal. Sonde small bowel enteroscopy has decreased significantly in popularity compared with push enteroscopy, and with the development of video capsule endoscopy and balloon enteroscopy will likely become obsolete.

In July 2004 a double-balloon small bowel enteroscope was released for clinical use in the United States. This scope used a combination of balloon inflation and deflation, and use of a small bowel overtube for visualization of the distal small bowel. The scope can also be passed via the rectum for evaluation of the proximal ileum. The scope has a working channel through which biopsies and other procedures can be performed. Subsequently a single-balloon enteroscope has also been developed. This type of endoscope may offer therapeutic advantages compared with the other methods of small bowel endoscopy and wire capsule endoscopy, and its use in pediatric patients is discussed in detail in Chapter 64.

WIRELESS CAPSULE ENDOSCOPY

Wireless capsule endoscopy has largely replaced passive small bowel enteroscopy as a method to evaluate the distal small bowel between the ligament of Treitz and the distal ileum. It is discussed in detail in Chapter 64.

The capsule may be swallowed, or in younger or smaller patients who are unable to swallow the capsule, it can be deployed into the duodenum endoscopically utilizing a "through the endoscope channel" capsule delivery device (AdvanCE, US Endoscopy, Mentor, OH, USA.) This device may increase the likelihood of small intestinal visualization in patients with impaired or delayed gastric emptying.

Potential indications for wireless capsule endoscopy are similar to those discussed previously for small bowel enteroscopy and include evaluation of gastrointestinal bleeding of unknown origin, evaluation of extent of inflammatory bowel disease or polyposis syndromes, evaluation of medication-induced mucosal injury (including nonsteroidal anti-inflammatory drugs), evaluation of suspected lymphoma or lymphangiectasia, and graft assessment after small bowel transplant or suspected graft-versus-host disease. Current limitations of the technique include capsule size, particularly in small patients; failure of capsule passage at several potential locations, including the pylorus, areas of anatomic narrowing such as strictures, and the ileocecal valve; failure of the capsule to completely image the small bowel within the available battery life in patients with impaired motility; time delay between imaging and image evaluation; time required to evaluate the images; lack of ability to perform therapy or obtain biopsies of abnormalities detected; and lack of ability to direct the capsule to desired areas of image acquisition.

The presence of strictures or other obstructions in the intestinal tract is currently a contraindication to the use of capsule endoscopy. Capsules have become impacted at the site of strictures, and have required endoscopic or surgical removal. A lactose-based patency capsule without recording capabilities but with radiologic markings is currently available and can be administered to patients with suspected anatomic narrowing to determine whether the standard capsule device is likely to become lodged.

PERCUTANEOUS ENDOSCOPIC GASTROSTOMY

The first report of successful PEG tube placement was in 1980 by Gauderer, Ponsky, and Izant.[88] PEG tube insertion is one of the unique endoscopic procedures that originated in pediatric patients, was subsequently popularized in adults, and was later reintroduced in children by pediatric gastroenterologists. Although initially developed by surgeons, it is now performed at an equal or greater frequency by adult and pediatric gastroenterologists. Despite many similarities in the indications and some technical aspects of the procedure between children and adults, there are also significant differences in the indications, limitations, and technical aspects of the procedure.

Indications

PEG tubes are appropriate in any pediatric patient who requires a gastrostomy tube (G tube) and does not require an open surgical procedure at the same time as the gastrostomy tube placement. Patients undergoing a simultaneous fundoplication, pyloroplasty, or pyloromyotomy would in all likelihood not derive additional benefit from placement of a PEG tube versus a surgical gastrostomy at the time of surgery. PEG tube placement does not interfere with subsequent fundoplication, pyloroplasty, or pyloromyotomy in patients who may have reflux or gastric emptying issues unresponsive to medical or endoscopic therapy. Benefits of PEG tube insertion versus surgical gastrostomy include reduced procedure time with reduced cost, smaller incision, shorter length of hospital stay, potentially decreased incidence of severe GER in the postoperative period, and decreased incidence of postoperative complications including wound infection, dehiscence at operative site, bowel obstruction, pain, atelectasis, and impaired mobility. Contraindications are limited. Placement of a PEG tube should not be attempted if there are patient factors that would interfere with successful transillumination of the gastric wall and identification of the indentation performed during the procedure, or if there is a suspicion that the anterior gastric wall is not opposed to the abdominal wall, as in the case of an intervening colon or other abdominal organ. As with any endoscopic procedure, the patient should be medically stable to undergo the procedure; airway protection and management is imperative, and the endoscopist should be willing to abort the procedure if it is not progressing as anticipated. This may be due, for example, to positioning of the colon between the stomach and the anterior abdominal wall. This problem may often not be identified before surgery and may necessitate conversion to an open procedure. PEG tubes may be more difficult to place, should be placed with increased caution, and may require additional pre-procedure evaluation in patients with the following conditions: ascites or peritoneal dialysis; scoliosis or spine abnormalities; small size; ventriculoperitoneal shunt; prior abdominal surgery; congenital abnormalities such as situs inversus, hepatomegaly, or splenomegaly or other abdominal masses; patients with small laryngeal or tracheal size or compromise, or ventilatory issues.

Patients undergoing peritoneal dialysis (PD) appear to have a high rate of significant complications associated with PEG placement. These include peritonitis, which may be bacterial or fungal; wound infections; need for PD catheter replacement; conversion to hemodialysis; and death.[89] Therefore, PEG may be relatively contraindicated in patients on PD, and if it is performed, careful attention to antibiotic and antifungal prophylaxis is required.

PEGs can be placed for medication administration, feeding administration, gastric decompression, or a combination of these reasons. The preprocedure evaluation may vary based on the indication. For example, in a well-nourished, neurologically impaired child who is having the PEG tube placed for medication administration only, a preoperative evaluation for reflux may not be indicated. In the same child who has severe vomiting and failure to thrive, additional testing including 24-hour pH or impedance probe testing may be indicated before surgery to determine whether he or she is a candidate for a simultaneous antireflux procedure. Open gastrostomy does not reduce the incidence of severe postoperative GER in neurologically impaired children compared with PEG placement, and is associated with a higher likelihood of severe reflux requiring a fundoplication (odds ratio 6-7:1).[90] Potential contributing factors include alteration of the angle of His and reduced lower esophageal sphincter pressure by an open gastrostomy. In many centers, evaluation before PEG includes upper gastrointestinal radiography to exclude malrotation and, if possible, to identify whether a portion of the stomach is located below the rib cage. In patients who are having PEGs placed for feeding, a trial of nasogastric feedings (usually outpatient) for approximately 10 days before placement of the PEG tube may offer a functional preoperative evaluation of GER. Patients who are intolerant of nasogastric feeds can undergo additional evaluation for an antireflux procedure. Patients who tolerate the feedings generally gain weight and improve their nutritional status before the anesthetic and operative procedure.

Technique

In most pediatric centers, two physicians perform PEGs; one physician performs the endoscopic portion of the procedure and the other performs the abdominal portion. The physicians may be two pediatric gastroenterologists, a pediatric gastroenterologist and a pediatric surgeon, or an interventional radiologist. Insertion of a PEG tube should be considered an advanced endoscopic procedure with a higher rate of associated complications than standard endoscopy. Patients should be nil per os before the procedure. Administration of preoperative antibiotics with good coverage for skin flora and two additional peri/postoperative doses has been shown to decrease the incidence of postoperative wound infection.[20,21,91] The abdomen should be prepped and draped in a sterile fashion. Frequently the procedure is performed utilizing a general anesthetic or sedation provided by a pediatric intensivist. Deep sedation has been used successfully for this procedure.

The endoscopist will pass the appropriately sized endoscope and fill the greater curvature of the stomach without intubating the pylorus. Initially, excessive air insufflation should be avoided because this may distend the small bowel loops and interfere with the gastric impression. The other physician, who

is "sterile" throughout the procedure, then performs finger indentation to identify an impression along the anterior gastric wall, preferably away from the gastric cardia and located near the junction of the gastric body and antrum (Figure 61-11). The optimal indentation is perpendicular to the anterior gastric wall to avoid entering the stomach inferiorly, as this may increase the risk of entering the colon or its mesentery. The indentation should allow enough space for tube insertion away from the costal margin, because tubes too close to the ribs can be associated with significant pain. After identification of a good impression, the sterile physician will inset a 25- or 21-G needle attached to a syringe, usually filled with 1% lidocaine solution to test the tract identified by the gastric indentation. This needle should pass into the stomach under the direct vision of the endoscopist in the same length as the anticipated internal length of the PEG tube. Failure to see passage of the needle into the stomach when it is inserted to its hub suggests that repositioning of the PEG site is necessary or that there is an intervening organ such as colon or bowel mesentery. Lidocaine for local anesthesia is usually injected with needle withdrawal. Some endoscopists will watch for bubbling of air in the syringe of the needle with insertion. Visualized air bubbling before the endoscopist seeing the needle in the stomach may indicate an intervening loop of bowel, and can result in complications as described later.

After a good site has been identified, the sterile physician makes a small incision in the anterior abdominal wall at the site of catheter insertion. This is usually transverse and should be through the skin, large enough to allow passage of the PEG tube but not so large that suturing would be required. On occasion, this incision needs to be extended during the pull aspect of the PEG. Too small an incision, and therefore too tight a catheter, increases the risk of postoperative wound infection and development of granulation tissue. Under direct endoscopic vision, the sterile physician then repeats the angiocatheter insertion, using the same technique but with a larger (14 G) cannula/catheter that will accommodate passage of the guidewire. As soon as the catheter is visualized in the stomach, the endoscopist passes biopsy forceps or a snare through the biopsy port in order to grasp the guidewire, which the sterile physician is simultaneously passing via the cannula through the anterior abdominal wall. The sterile physician should hold the catheter carefully at all times until the endoscopist secures the guidewire. Once the guidewire is secured, the procedure can almost always be completed safely, but accidental dislodgment of the cannula before guidewire insertion can result in a free perforation or other complication. For smaller endoscopes with a 2.0-mm channel, guidewires are grasped utilizing small forceps. For standard endoscopes with a 2.8-mm channel, the guidewire can be grasped using standard forceps, foreign-body forceps such as alligator or rat tooth forceps, or a polypectomy snare. On occasion, a portion of the cannula is seen in the stomach, but not enough that the endoscopist feels comfortable with the length of the cannula in the stomach, or the cannula may be seen coming up through the lower esophageal sphincter into the esophagus in very small patients or across to the posterior gastric wall. The endoscopist can use very gentle endoscopic traction to reduce tenting of the gastric wall on the cannula, which will allow advancement of the cannula safely into the stomach without through-and-through placement. Additional air insufflation *immediately* before catheter puncture may also help when the gastric indentation is not optimal. After the endoscopist grasps

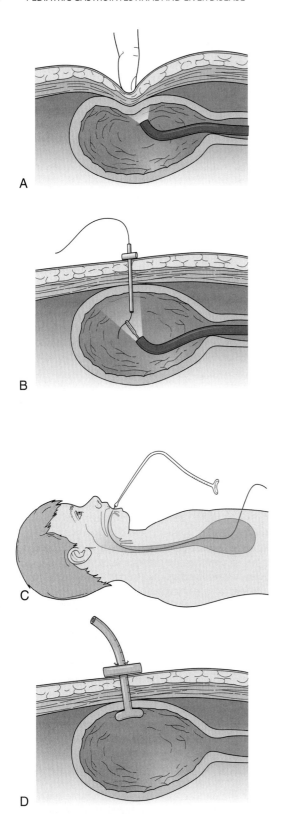

Figure 61-11. PEG placement. (**A**) Finger indentation is performed to identify the optimal position. (**B**) After trochar introduction through the anterior abdominal wall, a suture or guidewire is passed through the trochar and grasped with a snare or forceps. (**C**) The PEG is positioned by pulling the tube through the stomach and into position. (**D**) The PEG catheter may be secured to the anterior abdominal wall with an external bolster. From George and Dokler (2002),[134] with permission.

the guidewire, the guidewire and endoscope are withdrawn through the esophagus and out of the mouth.

After withdrawal, the endoscopist attaches the PEG catheter to the guidewire. The endoscopist then guides the catheter down the patient's mouth and into the esophagus while the sterile physician is pulling the catheter gently though the anterior abdominal wall. There may be some resistance when the guidewire catheter knot reaches the abdominal wall. In this case, slightly extending the incision may help pull the catheter through the wall, and circular rotation of the guidewire with steady traction by the sterile physician will facilitate this maneuver. In the off-chance that the guidewire breaks as it is coming through the abdominal wall, hemostats can be used to bring the guidewire and catheter though the abdominal wall. Care should be taken to avoid pulling too hard as the catheter is coming though the abdominal wall, especially in small, malnourished, or immunocompromised patients, as there have been reports of pulling the catheter entirely through the abdominal wall. The endoscopist will verify the position of the PEG tube and the length to the skin. An excess length to the skin (i.e., 5 to 6 cm) should raise the possibility that something may be trapped between the stomach and the anterior abdominal wall. An external bumper secures the PEG, leaving room for swelling in the immediate perioperative period. The incision is dressed with antibiotic ointment, and additional intravenous antibiotics are administered in the postoperative period, usually for two further doses. The tubes can generally be used within 6 to 24 hours.

Indications of a potential problem and when to abort include:
- Failure to identify a good gastric impression
- Excess angiocatheter length without seeing the tip in the stomach, or air bubbling in the needle syringe without seeing the needle tip in the stomach
- Gastric varices or significant ulceration
- Identification of stool at any point during the procedure.

Conversion of a PEG procedure to an open gastrostomy may occur in 2% of procedures or more.[92] Catheters are not changed until at least 6 weeks after the PEG procedure, and preferably after 2 months to allow the tract to mature.[93] Percutaneous replacement of PEG tubes following accidental dislodgment has been reported within a couple of weeks of placement. Catheters can be changed by traction removal or endoscopically, where the catheter is cut and retrieved like a foreign body.[92] The cut and await passage technique has resulted in intestinal obstruction, impaction, and perforation. Endoscopic visualization of placement of the new gastrostomy button at the time of initial conversion from a PEG tube is helpful. If the button is placed in the tract but is not visualized in the stomach, there may be a false tract, a portion of the colon or small bowel may have been trapped between the PEG tube and the abdominal wall, and the button may be located in the colon, small bowel, or mesentery. Surgical consultation is appropriate at this point.

Multiple complications have been reported in the literature after PEG placement. Rates in the literature vary, but are generally in the range of 5 to 30%.[92] Some are preventable with appropriate antibiotic prophylaxis, good endoscopic/percutaneous technique, and recognition by the physicians performing the procedure that things are not going well with a decision to abort the procedure and proceed with open gastrostomy. Some complications may be unavoidable because of patient anatomy or underlying disease. Reported minor complications include cellulitis, uncomplicated pneumoperitoneum, tube defects or disconnection, GER, granulation tissue, or pain at the insertion site. Major complications include gastrocolic fistula, gastroileal fistula, gastro(colo/ileal)cutaneous fistulas, placement of catheter through the liver, duodenal hematoma, complicated pneumoperitoneum, aspiration, peritonitis, and catheter complications, including migration, buried bumper syndrome, partial gastric separation, catheter/bumper impaction if not retrieved, ventriculoperitoneal shunt infection, gastric perforation, or death.[93] Late complications include gastrocolic fistula, gastroileal fistula, catheter migration/buried bumper syndrome/partial gastric separation, gastric ulceration, cellulitis, fasciitis, gastric perforation, catheter migration or other catheter-related complications, bronchoesophageal fistula (following removal), and aortic perforation (following cut and pass catheter removal).[93]

PERCUTANEOUS ENDOSCOPIC JEJUNOSTOMY (PEJ)

Direct PEJ has also been reported and is indicated in patients prone to aspiration, with complete or partial gastric or duodenal obstruction, or gastric motility disorders. Because of the smaller jejunal size and its variable position, the technique is technically more difficult than PEG. The procedure is performed utilizing a push enteroscope, which is advanced into the jejunum up to 24 inches distal to the ligament of Treitz in adult-size patients. The endoscope tip is used to transilluminate the abdominal wall in a 2- to 3-cm area. The second physician uses direct fingertip pressure to identify a discrete intrajejunal indentation to the endoscopist. Placement is similar to the PEG technique just described. Catheter size is limited because of the narrower jejunal lumen, and feeding schedules are modified accordingly. In some instances a PEJ tube may not be able to be placed because of inability to appose and transilluminate a jejunal segment adjacent to the abdominal wall. Theoretical problems with PEJ insertion include increased technical difficulty, including maintenance of correct jejunal position, and risk of needle entry into the abdomen either directly or through the posterior jejunal wall secondary to diminished luminal size. This technique may prove to be especially difficult in pediatric patients because of the reduced diameter of the intestinal lumen. As with PEG procedures, prophylactic antibiotics are administered routinely.

POLYPECTOMY

Polyps may be encountered outside of the colon, including the esophagus, stomach, and small bowel. Small bowel polyps are generally amenable to snare removal. Small bowel enteroscopy as discussed in Chapter 64, either alone or intraoperatively, can be used for resection of larger small-bowel polyps in patients with Peutz-Jeghers syndrome or other conditions presenting with polyps of the small intestine.[94]

Gastric polyps may be subclassified into fundic gland polyps, hyperplastic polyps, adenomas, inflammatory fibroid polyps, Peutz-Jeghers polyps, or juvenile polyps.[95] Hot biopsy forceps should generally not be used to remove polyps in the stomach or at any location where adequate tenting of the mucosa is not possible. Patient grounding is always required with any form of monopolar coagulation. Gastric polyps may be more amenable to snare removal with or without a submucosal injection technique, although caution should be exercised to avoid associated perforation.[95] Other polypoid lesions in the stomach include xanthomas, pancreatic heterotopia (pancreatic rest), gastrointestinal stromal tumors, and carcinoids as well as various gastric malignancies. Routine "polypectomy" of these lesions should not be performed, but endoscopic biopsies may be indicated in some cases to aid in the diagnosis. Specific management may include observation only, surveillance, or resection based on the specific lesion identified.[95]

Esophageal polyps are rare in pediatric patients, although esophageal squamous papillomas may occur near the squamous columnar junction.[96] These polyps are typically benign in the pediatric patient, and they can be diagnosed and usually removed if indicated using cold biopsy techniques. Larger esophageal lesions should be approached with caution, because esophageal cancers can occur in pediatric patients, including those with and without predisposing conditions. Cold biopsy of suspicious lesions is probably the safest technique for pediatric endoscopists. Lesions suspicious for cancer should undergo evaluation according to adult-based protocols including EUS with tissue sampling (discussed later) if indicated.

SPECIAL ENDOSCOPIC TECHNIQUES

Pyloric Balloon Dilation

With advances in endoscopic equipment and accessories such as the development of controlled radial expansion (CRE) through-the-scope (TTS) balloons have come new applications of older endoscopic techniques. Endoscopic pyloric balloon dilation (PBD) represents a modification of techniques used for esophageal stricture dilation. Initially reported in 2001 in pediatric patients, this technique has been successfully used by other centers.[97,98] The primary indication for this procedure is delayed gastric emptying. PBD is performed by passage of a CRE TTS balloon through the endoscopic channel. The balloon is positioned across the pylorus and under direct endoscopic vision is inflated to a controlled pressure for a period of time, usually 60-90 seconds. Inflation pressures vary based on balloon size. Several inflations are typically used in a single endoscopic session, often of progressively larger balloons. Patients may need to undergo more than one session depending on their response to therapy.[98] Outer diameters of balloons used are typically in the range of 10 to 16 mm in adult-sized pediatric patients, but therapy should be individualized for the patient, and smaller balloons are used in younger patients. Depending on the etiology of delayed gastric emptying or the procedure indication, symptom resolution may be seen in 27 to 68% and symptomatic improvement may be seen in 26 to 57% of patients.[97,98] Response to PBD can also be used to assess likelihood of response to surgical pyloroplasty.

Endoscopic Therapy for Achalasia

Pneumatic dilation has long been considered the "gold standard" for nonoperative management of achalasia. Dilators were positioned fluoroscopically and dilation was performed until obliteration of the "waist" was identified. Patients often required several dilation procedures, resulting in a cumulative radiation exposure for the patient and for physicians performing the procedure. Balloon dilation using Rigiflex dilators (dilators that maintain a similar pressure and diameter along the entire length of the balloon) can be performed under direct endoscopic vision or with fluoroscopic guidance.[79] When performed endoscopically, the dilator is advanced across the lower esophageal sphincter over an endoscopically placed guidewire, which is usually positioned in the antrum. Positioning of the dilator can be monitored by simultaneous endoscopy with the scope positioned adjacent and proximal to the balloon during dilation.[79] This allows for direct visualization of obliteration of the "waist" and early recognition of mucosal or deeper injury during the dilation procedure. Serial inflations of 60 to 90 seconds in duration are usually performed. Dilation is usually initiated with 30-mm outer-diameter balloons and advanced over subsequent sessions to balloons of 40-mm outer diameter, based on patient size and response.[79]

Placement of Motility Catheters

There have been significant recent advances in the area of gastrointestinal motility. Antroduodenal motility procedures to evaluate patients with conditions such as chronic intestinal pseudo-obstruction are becoming increasingly common in pediatric centers with a special interest in gastrointestinal motility and are discussed in Chapter 65. Unlike rectal motility, in which catheter placement is straightforward, antroduodenal motility requires the monitoring catheter to be placed in the small intestine. Many centers use endoscopy for initial catheter placement. For antroduodenal motility, a standard EGD is performed. The catheter can be advanced adjacent to the endoscope under direct endoscopic vision or with the aid of forceps across the pylorus and into the small intestine. A loop of suture can also be attached to the end of the catheter. The loop is the grabbed with endoscopic forceps, and the catheter can then be guided to its position in the small intestine. Care must be taken not to pull back the catheter when the endoscope is removed.

Endoscopic Therapy for Gastroesophageal Reflux

A number of endoscopic techniques have recently been developed in adults to assist with the management of GER. These techniques are in various stages of development. Some are currently being evaluated in comparative trials to determine the optimal long-term therapy with a high rate of efficacy and low risk of complications, whereas others have been tested and subsequently withdrawn from clinical use because of lack of efficacy or unacceptable complications. Techniques that have been reported in adults include full-thickness plication, endoscopic suturing/endoluminal gastroplication (Endocinch), implantation of polymethyl methacrylate (PMMA) microspheres or a nonresorbable biocompatible polymer (Enteryx) and radiofrequency energy delivery to the gastroesophageal junction (Stretta).[99-104] The latter two products (Enteryx and Stretta) have been withdrawn from the U.S. market because of complications and lack of demonstrated efficacy. The only technique reported to date in pediatric patients is endoluminal gastroplication, which has been performed in 17 pediatric patients with symptoms of GER dependent on or refractory to proton pump inhibitor therapy. Patients undergoing this treatment had a significant improvement in heartburn, regurgitation, nausea score, and reflux quality of life, and a significant reduction in median reflux index and DeMeester scores and a decrease in proton pump inhibitor use.[105,106] Complications of the procedure in pediatric patients included bleeding necessitating transfusion.[105] Of the patients undergoing the procedure, 29% needed

at least one additional procedure within 3 years of follow-up. Other significant complications were not reported at the 3-year follow-up, although some patients needed to resume antireflux medications.[106] A number of other complications of the various anti-GER procedures have been reported in adults, and further evaluation is likely required before recommendation of these procedures in pediatric patients.

Esophageal Stent Placement

Although used for several years in adults primarily as a palliative procedure to relieve dysphagia associated with esophageal cancer, endoscopic placement of esophageal stents has recently been reported in pediatric patients. Indications for placement relate primarily to failure of endoscopic dilation to control a patient's symptoms from a stricture. Concerns about placing stents in children have related to tissue ingrowth into the stent, and lack of appropriately sized stents designed for small pediatric patients. Recent series have reported success of short-term (less than 14-day) serial stent placement utilizing stents designed for the tracheobronchial tree placed utilizing a combination of endoscopic and fluoroscopic guidance. These stents are self-expanding and can also be removed following collapse of the top of the stent by grasping the purse-string suture utilizing endoscopic forceps.[77] Tissue ingrowth, stent migration, dysphagia, respiratory distress, need for repeated dilations, and some difficulties related to stent removal have been reported. In addition, perforation and hemorrhage are known complications of self-expanding metal stents. There is also a case report of placement of a biodegradable esophageal stent in a 10-year-old child following caustic ingestion.[107] Further advancements are required in these techniques and equipment availability before widespread application can be recommended for pediatric patients.

Endoscopic Closure of Fistulas

Endoscopic closure of fistulas in children has been reported utilizing two techniques primarily, endoscopic clipping and endoscopic injection of fibrin glue. Teitelbaum et al. reported closure of two gastrocutaneous fistulas using a combination of MPEC coagulation and metal clip application.[108] Multiple clips may need to be applied to a gastrostomy tube site in a sequential zipper-like fashion to close the defect, and cautery may not be required to achieve fistula closure. In our experience, reopening of the gastrostomy tract may occasionally occur once the clip "falls off," which may occur a year or more following clip application; this may be treated with clip reapplication. Endoscopic obliteration of a recurrent tracheoesophageal fistula and obliteration of an esophagobronchial fistula have been reported in children using injection of Histoacryl or fibrin glue.[109,110]

Endoscopic Mucosal Resection

Endoscopic mucosal resection (EMR) is an emerging endoscopic technique that allows for mucosectomy or mucosal resection without surgery. Resection levels are typically into the middle or deeper layers of the submucosa when performed. Four types of EMR are performed: inject and cut; inject, lift, and cut; cap-assisted EMR; and EMR with ligation.[111] Injection is used in a similar fashion to saline-assisted polypectomy (discussed in Chapter 62) to increase the safety of the procedure while allowing for a complete mucosal injection. EMR is often performed using the adjunctive technique of chromoscopy to allow for identification of lesion margins. Indications for this type of procedure are primarily cancer related in adults (esophageal, gastric, or colonic carcinoma). Additional potential indications include resection of Barrett's esophagus with high-grade dysplasia, diagnosis and resection of submucosal tumors with low potential for metastases, and resection of small carcinoid tumors found incidentally.[111] Unique pediatric indications for this procedure have not yet been established. Reported complications include pain, bleeding, perforation, and stricture formation. Endoscopic clipping may be used at the time of EMR because of the potential perforation risk with this technique.

ENDOSCOPIC ULTRASONOGRAPHY

EUS is typically performed using specialized radial endosonographic endoscopes or curvilinear echoendoscopes if FNA or fine-needle injection (FNI) for cytopathology are indicated. It is a highly specialized procedure and requires advanced training to ensure safe performance and correct interpretation of findings. EUS allows the endoscopist to differentiate gut wall layers, differentiate solid versus cystic lesions, determine the origin of subepithelial lesions and intramural vascular structures, and evaluate extraluminal structures. In addition, tissue sampling of suspicious lesions can be performed. Although previously reported in pediatric patients,[112] the largest pediatric EUS series to date is of 38 patients undergoing evaluation at two adult tertiary care centers over a 7-year period.[113] The primary indications for evaluation were known or suspected pancreaticobiliary disease (63%), evaluation of gastric masses (15%), and mediastinal mass/lymph node evaluation (13%). EUS appears to be helpful for these select indications in children and may aid in the diagnosis for example of GIST lesions or chronic pancreatitis. Both false positive and false negative results including on FNA are possible in children, and findings on EUS should be interpreted in the context of the clinical picture and other imaging results.

CHROMOENDOSCOPY AND NARROW BAND IMAGING

Differential color imaging systems are currently being used in adults as an alternative to chromoendoscopy. Chromoendoscopy is the topical application of stains or dyes at the time of endoscopy to enhance tissue characteristics. The procedure is safe and inexpensive. This technique is used to distinguish dysplastic from nondysplastic epithelium or to determine the margins of suspicious lesions by highlighting surface topography and mucosal irregularities.[114] Specific stains used include Lugol's solution, methylene blue, toluidine blue, crystal violet, indigo carmine, Congo red, phenol red, and acetic acid. Although helpful in identifying conditions such as Barrett's esophagus, esophageal cancer, gastric cancer, colon polyps and cancers, especially in the case of flat lesions, and dysplasia in ulcerative colitis (UC), there is a lack of standardization of techniques and significant interobserver variability.[114]

Currently available commercial endoscopic differential color imaging systems include narrow-band imaging (NBI) (Olympus Medical Systems, Tokyo, Japan) and multiband imaging (MBI) (Fujinon, Saitama, Japan). These are real-time, on-demand techniques used to enhance the visualization of the vascular network and surface texture of the mucosa in order to improve tissue characterization, differentiation, and diagnosis.[115] These imaging systems are easier to use than chromoendoscopy and are built into many endoscopes already available in the pediatric endoscopy suite and activated by pushing a button on the endoscope control handle or computer keyboard. Enhancement of particular mucosal features occurs because of selective light transmittance accomplished by optical filtering in NBI and software-driven processing in MBI.[115] Blood and blood vessels, especially capillaries, are highlighted, allowing for differentiation of Barrett's esophagus and colon polyps, for example, from normal tissue. One day unique pediatric applications of these imaging systems may be identified.

CONFOCAL LASER MICROSCOPY (ENDOMICROSCOPY)

This is a new technique that allows high-resolution tissue imaging with magnification approximately 1000-fold, allowing for "real-time" histologic evaluation during endoscopic procedures. The principle behind this is tissue examination with a low-power laser with subsequent detection of the fluorescence light reflected from the tissue through a pinhole, resulting in a dramatic increase in spatial resolution. This allows for histologic evaluation of the superficial epithelial layers.[116] Confocal microscopy is currently performed with a dedicated endoscope or via a miniprobe passed via the endoscope accessory channel. Initial applications appear to be in the evaluation of dysplastic or suspicious lesions in patients with precancerous conditions such as Barrett's esophagus or ulcerative colitis. Potential applications are real-time biopsy or removal of concerning lesions with a reduction in the number of "random" biopsies required. Depending on equipment development and advances in the technique, this technique may be applied in the future for pediatric patients with similar indications.

NEW TECHNIQUES

Several other new techniques have been reported. Okamatsu et al. performed a successful endoscopic membranectomy on a 60-day-old infant with trisomy 21 syndrome and a congenital duodenal membrane, and Torroni et al. reported the same procedure in three children ranging in age from 4 months to 66 months.[117,118] Beeks et al. reported partial resection of a duodenal web in a 15-month-old utilizing hot biopsy forceps.[119]

COMPLICATIONS

Esophagogastroduodenoscopy

As with any procedure, the benefits of the endoscopic procedure and the diagnostic information obtained should outweigh the relative risk to the patient. Endoscopic complications can be classified into four types: sedation related, procedure related, those associated with therapeutic interventions, and those related to the patient's underlying disease or reason for endoscopy. In some cases, the cause of the complication may be multifactorial or remain indeterminate. When reviewing risks of various endoscopic procedures it is important to identify patient- and procedure-related factors that may increase the risk of the procedure (e.g., increased risk of sedation in a child with cyanotic congenital heart disease or cystic fibrosis). Limited studies are available that have assessed the risk of complications of endoscopy, especially in pediatric patients. In a large retrospective series of 2711 upper and lower endoscopies in pediatric patients primarily utilizing conscious sedation, minor complications occurred in 0.3% of patients, including oxygen desaturation that responded to narcotic reversal and medication-related urticaria.[10] In the same series, one patient had a major complication (1 of 1653, rate of 0.06%), which was a guidewire-related perforation. In a large pediatric series reviewing the efficacy of intravenous midazolam and fentanyl for conscious sedation in 1578 GI procedures, approximately 25% of patients experienced adverse events as defined in the study. Respiratory adverse effects occurred in 9% of patients; the majority were mild, with only 0.2% of patients experiencing apnea. Other adverse events reported in the series were hypotension (8%), hypertension (3%), skin rash, agitation, and vomiting during recovery (5%). Adverse events in that series responded to conservative treatment. No intubation or sedation reversal was required.[11] A recent cross-sectional database report of complications occurring following EGD from 13 facilities between 1999 and 2003, which reviewed 10,236 procedures performed in 9234 pediatric patients, gave an immediate complication rate of 2.3% associated with EGD.[120] The most common complications in that series were hypoxia (1.5%) and bleeding (0.3%). In that series, higher complication rates were noted in the youngest age group, in patients with higher ASA classes, in female patients, in patients receiving IV sedation, and in procedures performed in the presence of a fellow. Because of the methodology of data collection, the overall complication rate and specifically complications related to administration of general anesthesia may have been underestimated in that series.[120] Another recent pediatric series comparing intravenous endoscopist-administered sedation to anesthesiologist administration of propofol in 329 patients reported an immediate complication rate of 2.0% for primarily diagnostic procedures.[29]

In a 30-day telephone follow-up survey of 393 children undergoing EGD under general anesthesia at a single center, 42% reported a complication or adverse event, although only 6% sought medical advice regarding their symptoms.[121] In that series the vast majority of adverse events were minor, such as sore throat or hoarseness, fatigue, cough, or headache, and were thought to be related to anesthesia rather than the procedure; no major complications were reported.[121] The American Society for Gastrointestinal Endoscopy (ASGE) reviewed 21,011 gastrointestinal endoscopies to determine the relative rate of drug-related complications.[122] In a group consisting primarily of adult patients, the overall medication complication rate was 13.5 per 1000 procedures; of these, 5.4 per 1000 represented serious cardiac or respiratory complications, with a fatality rate of 0.3 per 1000 procedures. Patients at highest risk for medication-related complications were those who received narcotics, were undergoing an emergent or urgent procedure, or were undergoing colonoscopy. The medication dosage did not correlate with the complication rate.[122] In a recent retrospective review of the adult CORI (Clinical Outcomes Research Initiative) database, more than 300,000 endoscopic procedures were reviewed to determine complication rates and contributing factors. In that series approximately 97% of the cases were performed utilizing conscious sedation.[123] There were unplanned events in 1.4% of procedures and unplanned cardiopulmonary events in 0.9% of procedures. There were 39 deaths in the series (rate of 11/100,000 or 0.01%), the majority of which were due to cardiopulmonary causes. Increasing patient age, increase in ASA

classification, higher doses of meperidine, use of supplemental oxygen, inpatient status, nonuniversity practice sites, and trainee involvement were significant predictors of unplanned cardiopulmonary events.[123] The possible mechanisms of some of the associations that are not intuitive are discussed in the manuscript. For example, supplemental oxygen is not considered harmful per se but may result in the delay of detection of hypercapnia and hypoxemia, emphasizing the need to monitor the effectiveness of pulmonary ventilation, not just pulse oximetry readings alone. Although this is an adult study, some of the risk factors (ASA class, inpatient status, oxygen use) likely can be translated to pediatric patients in whom response to sedation is likely more unpredictable. In a very large prospective series from Germany, most of the adverse effects associated with diagnostic endoscopy were attributable to medication use.[124] In that series of more than 190,000 endoscopies, the overall complication rates were low for EGD, colonoscopy and polypectomy (0.009%, 0.02% and 0.36% respectively). The overall complication rate for procedures performed by gastroenterologists in that series was 1 per 5155 procedures (0.019%).[124]

A number of mechanical complications have been reported after upper gastrointestinal endoscopy. In the 1974 ASGE survey, the major complication rate was 1.32 per 1000 upper endoscopies, including infection, perforation, bleeding, cardiopulmonary complications, and death.[125] In the same series, esophageal dilation was associated with a much higher complication rate, ranging from 4.25 per 1000 cases using mercury bougies, to 6.1 per 1000 using metal olives, and up to 18.1 per 1000 when pneumatic or mechanical dilation was performed. Recent series have reported lower complication rates with wire-guided polyvinyl dilators or balloon dilators.[126] Strictures following caustic ingestion are associated with a higher rate of perforation at the time of dilation compared with other benign strictures. Despite the age of the 1974 series, large series prospectively reporting complication rates of diagnostic endoscopies are infrequent.[126]

Intramural duodenal hematoma resulting in complete bowel obstruction and necessitating blood transfusion has been reported after duodenal biopsies in children. Contributing factors include the fixed third portion of the duodenum, the rich submucosal vascular plexus, lack of a well-developed serosal layer in the retroperitoneum, and variations of biopsy technique.[127,128] Significant bleeding following diagnostic endoscopy with biopsy has been reported in children who have undergone a bone marrow transplant or hematopoietic stem cell transplant. The endoscopic procedure is usually performed to evaluate for GVHD or infection. Bleeding may be significant and result in hematoma formation in the duodenum or elsewhere.[127] Complications may include need for transfusion, pancreatitis, or duodenal obstruction secondary to hematoma with need for hyperalimentation and need for repeat endoscopy for therapeutic intervention.[129] Thrombocytopenia or abnormal platelet function may confer an increased risk of complications in these conditions, and caution should be exercised when performing endoscopic therapy in patients with these conditions.

Spontaneous bowel perforation has been reported in patients with Ehlers-Danlos syndrome type 4.[16] These patients may theoretically be at higher risk for perforation during or after gastrointestinal endoscopy.

Serious complications have also been reported after therapeutic injection for bleeding. Full-thickness gastric necrosis has been reported after injection of 12 mL 5% ethanolamine oleate (a sclerosant) into and around a benign actively bleeding ulcer,[130] and following injection of a combination of 4 mL 1% polidocanol and 8 mL 1:10,000 epinephrine solution in a small posterior gastric ulcer.[131] Complications have also been reported after endoscopic laser therapy with an Nd:YAG laser with coaxial carbon dioxide, including free perforation, pneumoperitoneum (thought to occur because of dissection of high-pressure carbon dioxide gas through a laser-induced mucosal erosion and subsequent rupture of the gas-filled bleb), and delayed massive hemorrhage following laser coagulation of angiodysplasia.

There have been two cases of fatal air embolism reported in pediatric patients who had undergone a Kasai procedure for biliary atresia and who were undergoing upper gastrointestinal endoscopy under general anesthesia. The first occurred in a 4-month-old baby undergoing endoscopy to determine the etiology of a diminished stomal bile output. Air apparently was infused into the bed of the porta hepatis, and the authors proposed that, under pressure, this air dissected across diseased liver tissue into a large hepatic vein.[132]

A second similar case was reported in a 10-year-old girl who, also after a Kasai procedure, developed a stricture at the anastomotic site with a stone above it. Under general anesthesia, she underwent an endoscopic procedure to remove the stone and dilate the stricture through a percutaneous jejunal loop. The patient developed circulatory collapse and died from a massive air embolus.[133] Because the mechanism of death in these two cases is not entirely clear, extra caution is required in endoscopic procedures involving an exteriorized loop in a patient who has undergone a Kasai procedure. PEG-related complications were discussed earlier, and complications related to foreign bodies, caustic ingestions, and therapy for varices are discussed in other chapters.

REFERENCES

8. Standards of Practice Committee ASGE, Lee KK, Anderson MA, Baron TH, et al. Modifications in endoscopic practice for pediatric patients. Gastrointest Endosc 2008;67:1–9.
9. American Academy of Pediatrics. American Academy of Pediatric Dentistry, Cote CJ, Wilson S, Work Group on Sedation. Guidelines for monitoring and management of pediatric patients during and after sedation for diagnostic and therapeutic procedures: an update. Pediatrics 2006;118:2587–2602.
10. Balsells F, Wyllie R, Kay M, Steffen R. Use of conscious sedation for lower and upper gastrointestinal endoscopic examinations in children, adolescents, and young adults: a twelve-year review. Gastrointest Endosc 1997;45:375–380.
11. Mamula P, Markowitz JE, Neiswender K, et al. Safety of intravenous midazolam and fentanyl for pediatric GI endoscopy: prospective study of 1578 endoscopies [see comment]. Gastrointest Endosc 2007;65:203–210.
17. Stan Asge, Banerjee S, Shen B, Baron TH, et al. Antibiotic prophylaxis for GI endoscopy. Gastrointest Endosc 2008;67:791–798.
52. Kay MH, Wyllie R. Therapeutic endoscopy for nonvariceal gastrointestinal bleeding. J Pediatr Gastroenterol Nutr 2007;45:157–171.
66. Laine L, Long GL, Bakos GJ, et al. Optimizing bipolar electrocoagulation for endoscopic hemostasis: assessment of factors influencing energy delivery and coagulation. Gastrointest Endosc 2008;67:502–508.
75. Anastassiades CP, Baron TH, Wong K. Endoscopic clipping for the management of gastrointestinal bleeding. Nat Clin Pract Gastroenterol Hepatol 2008;5:559–568.

See expertconsult.com for a complete list of references and the review questions for this chapter.

62

COLONOSCOPY, POLYPECTOMY, AND RELATED TECHNIQUES

Marsha Kay • Robert Wyllie

The development of the colonoscope followed that of upper panendoscopes. Rigid proctoscopes were developed in the late 1800s, and fiberoptic techniques were adapted to visualize the sigmoid and descending colon in the 1960s. In the 1970s the colonoscope was lengthened with four-way tip deflection, allowing for modern-day colonoscopic techniques.

The first mass-produced video instruments were introduced in the 1980s and 1990s. Dedicated pediatric video colonoscopes with a narrow instrument diameter and preserved optic clarity are now widespread in their availability. These small-caliber endoscopes have found widespread application for both children and adults and are now being used with increased frequency in adults undergoing unsedated endoscopic procedures.

PERSONNEL, SEDATION, AND ANTIBIOTIC PROPHYLAXIS

The personnel, facilities, sedation and monitoring requirements, and antibiotic prophylaxis regimens for colonoscopy in pediatric patients are discussed in Chapter 61 on esophagogastroduodenoscopy. Colonoscopy is technically more challenging than esophagogastroduodenoscopy, especially in pediatric patients. Individuals performing colonoscopy in children should be specifically trained to do so and have met the standard of current training guidelines.[1]

EQUIPMENT

Colonoscopes are similar in construction to the upper endoscopes, with different diameters, instrument lengths, range of tip bending, and fields of view. In the past several years, colonoscopes of variable stiffness have been developed to decrease loop formation and assist with loop reduction. Although they are available for use in pediatric patients, variable stiffening of the endoscope should not be used to replace good endoscopic technique with the primary emphasis on minimal loop formation and rapid loop reduction.

The most important issues related to pediatric endoscopy equipment are the diameter and length of the insertion tube, the degree of tip angulation, and the depth of field. Colonoscopy in infants and young children is usually performed with instruments designed for upper endoscopy because of their smaller diameter. Polypectomy snares can be passed via an upper endoscope with a 2.8-mm channel. Colonoscopy in normally developed children over 3 to 4 years of age can usually be performed with a colonoscope designed specifically for pediatric patients. Pediatric colonoscopes, including those with variable stiffness capabilities, have a distal end with an outer diameter in the range of 11.3 to 11.6 mm with a 3.2- to 3.8-mm channel, compared with an outer diameter of 12.8 mm for adult colonoscopes. (Endoscope information courtesy of Olympus America Inc., Melville, NY, and Pentax Precision Instrument Corporation, Orangeburg, NY.)

INDICATIONS

The indications for colonoscopy vary with the age of the patient. The need for colonoscopy in neonates and infants is usually suggested by physical signs reported by parents or other observers, which include hematochezia, melena, hypotension, or anemia. With toddlers and older children, the history is of greater importance in identifying gastrointestinal disorders. The sensitivity of gastrointestinal endoscopy in establishing a diagnosis varies with the indication for the procedure (Table 62-1).

The major indications for colonoscopy in infants and children include rectal bleeding, unexplained diarrhea, and abdominal pain with abnormal growth, weight loss, or other constitutional symptoms. Colonoscopy is also performed to investigate abnormalities suspected on barium enema, small-bowel follow-through, or computed tomography. Colonoscopy is typically the first line of investigation for patients with suspected mucosal disease, and barium enema is rarely performed for this indication. If inflammatory bowel disease (IBD) is suspected, colonoscopy can provide visual evidence of the nature and extent of disease, and biopsies obtained at the time of the procedure may define the nature of the underlying inflammation. Terminal ileal intubation and biopsy is especially important in the diagnosis of IBD and in the evaluation of known IBD. Infectious colitis may be difficult to distinguish visually from IBD of recent onset, both visually and histologically, especially in patients less than 10 years of age[2,3] (Figure 62-1A,B). Crohn's disease involving only the colon may also present with a focal active colitis pattern of injury similar to that seen with infection. Some patients may require follow-up endoscopic examination with biopsy to look for evidence of chronicity before establishing a firm diagnosis of IBD. Colonoscopy is also indicated in the postoperative setting in patients with IBD to evaluate a stoma to look for evidence of Crohn's disease, to examine "out of circuit" bowel, and to evaluate the pouch for pouchitis or dysplasia in patients following ileal pouch anal anastomosis.[4]

Visualization and biopsy of the terminal ileum may be helpful in the diagnosis of infectious ileitis. In some infections, such as ileocecal tuberculosis, colonic schistosomiasis, and amebiasis, stool cultures are usually negative, but colonoscopy with biopsies may identify the etiologic organism on biopsy specimens or cytologic brushing.

Lymphonodular hyperplasia of the colon, although not an indication for colonoscopy, may be a cause of painless rectal bleeding identified at endoscopy. Thinning of the surface epithelium over the protruding lymphatic tissue with subsequent trauma from the passage of fecal material is thought to lead to ulceration and hematochezia. Prominent lymphatic nodules can be found throughout the large and small bowel. They appear as smooth, round, 2- to 4-mm nodules with normal overlying mucosa. Occasionally larger nodules may have central umbilication or overlying erosion. This nodular lymph node tissue is thought to represent a self-limiting response to antigenic stimulation and does not require any additional evaluation or therapy.

In children with suspected polyps, colonoscopy is both diagnostic and therapeutic. In diseases associated with an increased rate of malignancy, such as ulcerative colitis, Crohn's disease, or familial adenomatous polyposis and other polyposis syndromes, colonoscopic surveillance for dysplastic changes is usually performed at regular intervals. Colonoscopy has been reported for the diagnosis and evaluation of smooth muscle tumors in children with acquired immune deficiency syndrome. These lesions may appear as a submucosal nodule with central umbilication.[5] Colonoscopy is usually not indicated in children complaining of chronic abdominal pain or constipation with unremarkable physical examinations and laboratory studies. However, changes of mucosal prolapse in patients with chronic constipation may on occasion be noted at endoscopy

(Figure 62-2). Colonoscopy or more typically flexible sigmoidoscopy is use in the evaluation of suspected acute graft-versus-host disease (GVHD) following hematopoietic stem cell transplant.

Indications for therapeutic colonoscopy include polypectomy, therapy for gastrointestinal (GI) bleeding including bleeding following polypectomy, vascular ablation, retrieval of a foreign body, placement of a percutaneous cecostomy, and colonic decompression in toxic megacolon. Colonoscopy with therapeutic intervention for vascular lesions can eliminate the need for surgery in some cases. The types of lesion encountered include cavernous hemangiomas and small telangiectasias. Syndromes associated with vascular lesions in the gastrointestinal tract include Osler-Weber-Rendu, CREST syndrome (calcinosis cutis, Raynaud phenomenon, sclerodactyly, and telangiectasis), dyschondroplasia (Maffucci's syndrome), blue rubber bleb nevus syndrome, diffuse neonatal hemangiomatosis, Turner's syndrome, and pseudoxanthoma elasticum.

Colonic strictures can also be dilated through the endoscope using through the channel controlled external diameter balloon dilators. Intussusception has been identified and reduced during colonoscopy, but air-contrast reduction remains the procedure of choice. Colonoscopy has been used as an alternative to surgery to direct colonic Gastrografin administration in patients with cystic fibrosis and distal intestinal obstruction syndrome refractory to medical therapy.[6] Only practitioners with adequate experience should undertake technically advanced therapeutic endoscopic procedures.

CONTRAINDICATIONS

Absolute contraindications to gastrointestinal endoscopy include suspected perforation of the intestine and peritonitis in a toxic patient. There are several relative contraindications, including patients who are severely neutropenic or have bleeding disorders and children with a recent history of bowel surgery. In addition, patients with connective tissue disease, especially Ehlers-Danlos and Marfan syndromes,

TABLE 62-1. Indications for Colonoscopy

Gastrointestinal hemorrhage
Chronic diarrhea
Suspected inflammatory bowel disease
Cancer surveillance
   Inflammatory bowel disease
   Polyposis syndromes
Therapeutic intervention
   Polyp removal
   Foreign-body removal
   Decompression of toxic megacolon
   Dilation of stricture
   Cautery or injection/ablation of bleeding lesion
   Percutaneous cecostomy
   Stricture dilation

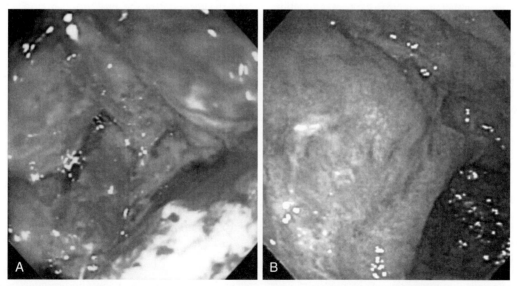

Figure 62-1. Endoscopic appearance of the colonic mucosa in a pediatric patient with acute infectious colitis due to *Escherichia coli* O157:H7 infection (**A**) compared to the mucosal appearance of ulcerative colitis (**B**). Although both are characterized by marked friability, hemorrhage, and superficial erosions, the infectious process lacks some of the typical features seen in chronic IBD. In addition to clinical and laboratory features, endoscopic biopsy may help to distinguish the two conditions. (*See plate section for color.*)

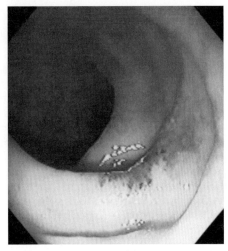

Figure 62-2. Endoscopic appearance of the rectum in a patient with mucosal prolapse. Note localized friability due to repetitive prolapse with an otherwise normal mucosal appearance. (*See plate section for color.*)

TABLE 62-2. Bowel Preparation Using PEG-ELS Oral Solutions

Weight of Child (kg)	Volume (mL) Each 10 Min Until Passage of Clear Fecal Effluent	Maximum Volume (mL)
<10	80	1100
10-20	100	1600
20-30	140	2200
30-40	180	2900
40-50	200	3200
>50	240	4000

Adapted from Bines and Winter (1991),[82] with permission.

are at increased risk of perforation during endoscopy.[7] Toxic dilation of the bowel carries an increased risk of perforation during colonoscopy, although the procedure may relieve the distention. Other relative contraindications include partial or complete bowel obstruction and aneurysm of the abdominal and iliac aorta. In all endoscopic procedures, the clinician and endoscopist must determine whether the potential information or therapeutic intervention outweighs the risk of the procedure.

PREPARATION

In addition to a period of preprocedure fasting, colonoscopy can be accomplished successfully only if the colon is free of fecal debris. Large amounts of stool compromise the ability to negotiate the curves of the large bowel and prohibit complete visualization of the mucosa. Stool adherent to the lens often requires additional maneuvering and added air-water insufflation to clear the field of vision. Liquid stool can be aspirated through the suction channel but increases the examination time.

Many bowel preparations have been utilized successfully to cleanse the colon. The method depends on the age and cooperation of the child and the individual experience of the examiner. In infants who are totally breast- or bottle-fed, adequate preparation can usually be obtained with the use of small-volume enemas and substituting clear liquids for breast- or bottle-feeding for 12 to 24 hours. In older children and adolescents, the best preparation is usually obtained with the use of colonic lavage solutions that contain a nonabsorbable solution of polyethylene glycol and electrolytes (PEG-ELS), which causes an osmotic diarrhea.[8] The risk of dehydration is minimal because of the limited transmural flux of sodium and water. To be effective, a large volume of solution must be ingested over a relatively short period of time. In adolescents of adult size, the usual regimen is 240 mL every 10 min until the fecal effluent is clear. This often requires 3 or 4 liters of solution. Smaller volumes are recommended for younger children (Table 62-2). Occasionally, nasogastric administration may be necessary. The rate of nasogastric administration is 20 to 30 mL/min, or 1.2 to 1.8 L/h in an older child or adolescent. Appropriate volume reductions can be made for infants and smaller children.

Oral cleansing solutions are effective in over 95% of the patients who drink adequate amounts of the fluid. An occasional patient may experience presumed allergic reactions manifested as dermatitis, urticarial, and rhinorrhea.[9] Combination regimens have been evaluated in adults using bisacodyl in addition to PEG-ELS. Addition of bisacodyl may allow for a reduction in the volume of PEG-ELS required, or allow for the use of split-dose regimens.[10] Split-dose regimens of PEG-ELS have recently been determined to be more effective compared to a standard 4 liter preparation administered the evening before colonoscopy.[11] Nonabsorbable polyethylene glycol without electrolytes has been reported as an effective bowel-cleansing regimen in children.[12,13] Minor electrolyte changes may be noted with this regimen. Initially this regimen involved ingestion of the PEG without ELS solution over several days. Recently use of a single-day preparation of this type of solution has been reported, primarily in abstract form.[14] Although likely to improve compliance because of increased palatability, clinical trials in pediatric patients will be necessary to determine the safety, efficacy, and dose recommendations of this agent for pediatric patients before widespread use.

If the child cannot comply with a large-volume lavage preparation, most endoscopists use an alternative regimen of clear liquids for 48 to 72 hours, accompanied by magnesium citrate or milk of magnesia one or two nights before the procedure with or without saline enemas administered the night before and the morning of the procedure to clear any residual stool (Table 62-3).

Oral sodium phosphate is an alternative regimen, available in both liquid and tablet form. The cathartic action of oral sodium phosphate is due to its osmotic properties. Oral sodium phosphate solutions are generally safe and effective in patients without significant comorbid conditions.[11,15,16] Aphthous ulceration of the colon has been observed following sodium phosphate bowel preparation. However, the cathartic effects of oral sodium phosphate may result in significant hypovolemia.[17] There are a number of case reports of serious adverse effects, related primarily to inappropriate dosing or noncompliance with the prescribed regimen of medication dilution or administration of additional fluids.[18,19] In addition, acute phosphate nephropathy followed by chronic renal insufficiency in patients with normal precolonoscopy renal function has been reported following oral sodium phosphate preparation.[11] Extra caution must be used in patients vulnerable to minor shifts in intravascular volume or transient increases in serum phosphate levels.[11,17,19] This regimen is contraindicated in patients with renal disease, megacolon, bowel obstruction, ascites, or congestive heart disease. Because of reported significant adverse effects with oral sodium phosphate regimens, significant caution must

TABLE 62-3. Alternate Bowel Preparation Regimens (Non-PEG to Electrolyte)*

Product	Dose	Duration	Maximum	Additional Comments	Side Effects(Noninclusive)	References
PEG (Miralax)	1.5 g/kg daily divided bid or tid	4 days	102 g/day (adult)	± Normal saline enema. Clears day before. Mixing beverage: patient choice	Nausea, abdominal pain, vomiting, mild electrolyte changes (K, CO_2, BUN)	12
Magnesium citrate	1 oz per year of age	Evening before procedure	10 oz	± Saline enema		
Magnesium citrate with X-prep	Age 2-5 years: 4 oz magnesium citrate and 2.5 oz X-prep Age >5 years: 6 oz magnesium citrate and 2.5 oz X-prep	1 dose on day before colonoscopy				8
Bisacodyl (Dulcolax)	Age 2-5 years: 5 mg Age 5-12 years: 10 mg Age ≥ 12 years: 15 mg	Each day for 2 days before colonoscopy		Fleet enema on morning of colonoscopy. May be associated with inadequate mucosal visualization		8

*Clear liquids for 24-48 hours required in association with the above preparations. BUN, blood urea nitrogen.

be exercised with utilization of these products in both pediatric and adult patients, and the most current FDA and manufacturer's recommendations should be followed.[11] A variety of other regimens with variable efficacy have been reported in children, including use of a combination of bisacodyl tablets, sodium phosphate enemas, and a clear liquid diet.[20]

ANATOMY

The small intestine and transverse and sigmoid colons are attached to mesentery and shift positions freely (Figure 62-3). Their excursion during a procedure is limited by the length of bowel and length of their attachment. Disease processes, masses, prior surgical procedures, or adhesions may influence their configuration or limit their mobility. The ascending colon and descending colon are relatively fixed in the retroperitoneum. The rectum is also relatively fixed as it passes through the pelvic connective tissue, with only a short segment free within the peritoneal cavity.

From the endoscopist's point of view, the anus is first intubated, then the rectum courses posteriorly to the coccyx and follows the gentle angle of the sacrum to the peritoneal reflection. Three "valves of Houston," two on the right and the middle one on the left, are encountered. These are crescentic, or semilunar, folds and are due to tension by the longitudinal muscle fibers of the teniae coli. The colonic assume a more circular pattern in the sigmoid and descending colon, and a characteristic triangular pattern in the transverse colon.

The sigmoid colon is attached to a mesentery and is relatively mobile. The descending colon is usually straight and ends at the splenic flexure, which forms an acute angulation with the transverse colon, turning abruptly to the right and anteriorly. The hepatic flexure forms the distal margin of the transverse colon and forms another abrupt, but inferior and posterior, angle with the ascending colon. The transverse colon has a variable configuration and is suspended on a mesentery between the two fixed flexures. The ascending colon is fixed in the retroperitoneum and is relatively straight, ending in the mobile cecum.

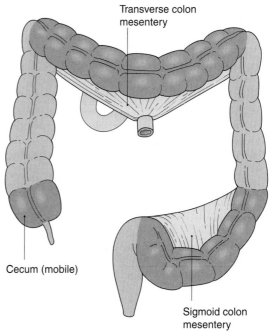

Figure 62-3. Mesenteric attachments of the colon. Mobile areas are darkened.

At the pole of the cecum, the tenia fuse to cause a marked cecal haustration, often forming a "crow's foot" or "Mercedes Benz" sign. The appendiceal orifice is usually a crescentic opening slightly to the left of the midline (Figure 62-4). Occasionally it may appear as a tubular diverticulum. The postappendectomy opening appears identical unless the appendiceal stump has been inverted.

The ileocecal valve lies proximal to the cecal pole on the prominent ileocecal fold. It usually cannot be directly visualized but is recognizable by a slight irregularity of the fold, with the ileum passing obliquely downward from its cecal opening. The ileum is characterized by the circumferential valvular

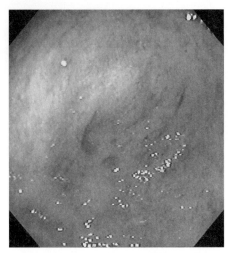

Figure 62-4. Typical appearance of the appendiceal orifice at colonoscopy. (*See plate section for color.*)

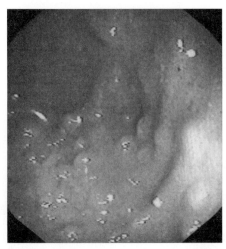

Figure 62-5. Lymphonodular hyperplasia of the terminal ileum. Note glistening mucosa and nodularity without erosions, which is characteristic. (*See plate section for color.*)

conniventes and a predominance of lymphoid tissue, especially in younger children (Figure 62-5).

TECHNIQUE

The endoscope is held in the left hand for right-handed individuals. The thumb is used to turn the large dial; the index finger and sometimes the middle finger are used to control the suction and air and water valves; and the remaining fingers hold the control handle. The insertion tube is held in the right hand. Some endoscopists advocate holding the insertion tube in the fingers like a pencil, rather than in the hand like a tennis racquet.[21] The lateral wheel, which controls right and left tip deflection, is usually manipulated with the right hand by endoscopists with smaller hands, but may be controlled by either the left hand or the right hand in endoscopists with larger hands. The instruments used via the biopsy channel include needles for injection, biopsy forceps, cytology brushes, foreign-body retrieval instruments, polypectomy snares, probes for cautery, and syringes for irrigation, and these are usually inserted with the right hand. Before initiating

a procedure, the suction and air channels should be checked to ensure proper functioning.

Colonoscopy

Colonoscopy is traditionally performed in the left lateral decubitus position with the knees bent. Patients who are receiving a general anesthesia may have the procedure performed in the supine position. A lubricant is usually applied to the tip of the instrument before insertion into the anus. In patients with active perianal disease, lubrication with viscous lidocaine may relieve some discomfort. It is usually necessary to reapply lubricant during the procedure, as the lubricant tends to dry as the endoscope is serially advanced and withdrawn. The endoscopist may mistake the increased resistance secondary to poor lubrication as coming from the more proximal colon.

The anus is inspected visually, examining for fissures, fistulas, or skin tags, and the instrument is inserted into the anus and advanced into the rectum. The anal canal is 2 to 3 cm long (in the older child and adolescent) and is angled toward the umbilicus. The instrument is inserted until there is an abrupt decrease in resistance, indicating that the tip has passed from the anal canal into the rectal ampulla. Following insertion, the scope tip usually comes to rest near the anterior wall of the rectum, because the junction of the rectum and anal canal forms an angle of approximately 90°. If the lumen is not in view, a small puff of air or withdrawing the endoscope a few centimeters will usually locate the lumen. Negotiating the colon is similar to the examination of the duodenum. Rather than simply "pushing," the instrument should be subtly advanced using the dials for tip deflection, and the techniques of air insufflation and suction, rotation or torquing of the insertion tube, external pressure applied to the abdomen, and changing the position of the patient. The elastic nature of the colon allows it to become long and tortuous when it is stretched by the colonoscope. Alternatively, it can be telescoped onto the instrument with little stretching by experienced endoscopists. The fundamentals of colonoscopy are[21,22]:

- Advance the endoscope under direct observation
- Use as little air as possible while maintaining adequate visualization
- Avoid forming loops; when loops are formed, reduce them as quickly as possible
- Pull back and telescope the bowel onto the colonoscope whenever possible

The most prominent landmarks in the rectum are the fixed "valves of Houston." These folds are accentuated haustral markings, and the lumen will veer toward the side of the fold. The endoscope is advanced with a series of short movements, jiggling motions, or torquing technique, depending on the skill and preference of the examiner. The junction of the rectum and sigmoid usually presents the first major problem and opportunity to form a loop. If the endoscopist simply advances the instrument, the force of the colonoscope is transmitted to the wall of the colon, with progressive distention of the bowel and its mesentery; the patient usually experiences pain, and the examiner feels increasing resistance to forward motion. This is often accompanied by the failure of the tip to advance despite insertion of the colonoscope. Paradoxical movement may occur when the tip recedes as the instrument is advanced and a larger loop is formed.

Early colonoscopes with limited tip deflection and fields of view required a "slide by" technique, as the lumen could not

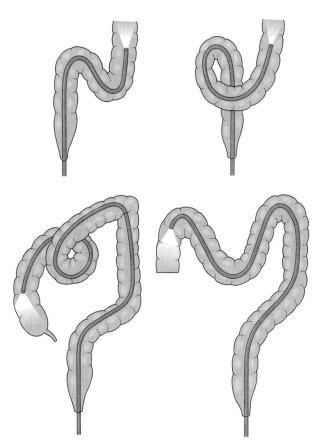

Figure 62-6. Common loops: "N" loop, alpha loop, gamma loop, and "U" loop.

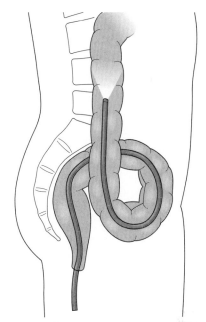

Figure 62-7. Lateral view of common loops.

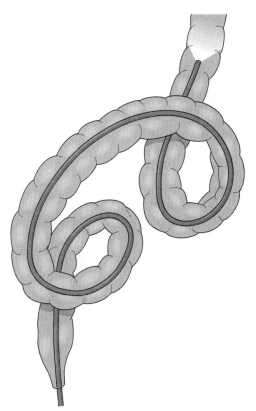

Figure 62-8. Double-alpha loop of the sigmoid colon.

always be kept in view. The instrument was advanced while the endoscopist had only a red field of view as the mucosa moved past the tip of the instrument. Advancement was halted when the mucosa was no longer slipping past the instrument tip or the mucosa took on a whitish hue, suggesting that compression of the bowel wall by the colonoscope was decreasing perfusion to the mucosa.

The instruments currently available reduce some of the technical difficulties, and the instrument should be advanced under direct visualization and not by the "slide by" technique. The skillful negotiation of the rectosigmoid junction is the key to successful colonoscopy. The experienced endoscopist will anticipate many of the potential problems. Several loops may be formed in the sigmoid colon. Names have been given to various configurations as they were seen under the fluoroscope with the patient positioned in the anterior posterior position (Figure 62-6). The alpha loop resembles the Greek letter α and may occur in either a normal or reversed configuration. The most common loop is the "N" loop, which is shaped like the letter N. Each of these loops has a similar appearance when viewed from the lateral position. The sigmoid colon is usually directed upward and then forms a caudad-directed convex loop in the anterior-posterior plane and a second cephalad convex loop with an oblique orientation to the anterior-posterior plane (Figure 62-7). Less common loops such as the double alpha loop can occur in a forward or backward orientation (Figure 62-8). Regardless of the anatomy in the individual patient, the endoscopist is unaware of the anatomy unless fluoroscopy or another form of scope position tracking is used during the procedure. Because it is rarely needed to complete the procedure and exposes the patient, physician, and equipment to radiation, the experienced endoscopist will anticipate the potential problems rather than utilizing fluoroscopy. Endoscopes with electromagnetic coils built into the endoscope insertion tube or special coils that can be passed via the endoscope channel are now available that allow for real-time three-dimensional computer rendering of the endoscope (and therefore the loop) configuration. (Information courtesy of Olympus America.)

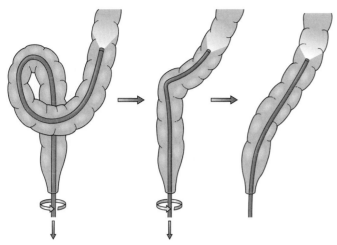

Figure 62-9. Alpha loop. Note initial posterior, then anterior, configuration of the sigmoid colon. Clockwise torque and scope withdrawal allows reduction of the loop and straightening of the sigmoid colon.

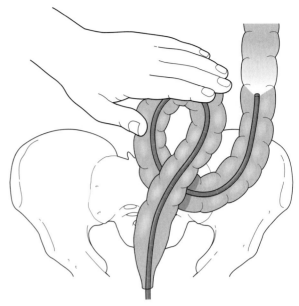

Figure 62-10. Anterior abdominal pressure may facilitate scope advancement by increasing resistance to loop formation.

Additional monitoring equipment is required for utilization of these colonoscopes, and the increased insertion tube diameter of the scopes with built-in coils compared to standard pediatric colonoscopes and associated costs have limited widespread utilization of this equipment to date in pediatric patients.[23] This technology may be more useful in the training setting and has not yet been shown to reduce procedure time or increase terminal ileal intubation rates in pediatric patients.[23]

Advancing the endoscope through the sigmoid colon should be a smooth and coordinated procedure. This often involves torquing the instrument along its shaft with the right hand and using the left hand to control the tip deflection. Repeated backward and forward motions are usually needed to telescope the colon onto the instrument. As the tip of the instrument reaches a bend, the dials or a combination of dials and torque are used to rotate the tip around the bend into the lumen. Withdrawing the instrument will often straighten the loop and allow advancement to the next bend. To reduce an alpha loop, the scope is withdrawn so the tip lies just distal to the rectosigmoid junction and then is rotated 180° (Figure 62-9). Failure of "one to one" movement, increasing patient discomfort, and increased resistance to insertion of the endoscope are usually signs of loop formation. Repeated attempts at loop removal are often necessary to traverse the sigmoid colon. In an occasional patient, it may be necessary to push through the loop and then reduce it after the instrument reaches the more proximal colon. Hand pressure by an assistant on the anterior abdominal wall may be beneficial during this maneuver (Figure 62-10). This should be done with caution only by an experienced endoscopist.

Alpha sigmoid loops, with the endoscope advanced into the distal descending colon, can be reduced by rotation (usually clockwise) and withdrawal. N loops can usually be removed with simple withdrawal. Occasionally an N loop has to be converted to an alpha loop for reduction to be successful. This can be done by withdrawal and counterclockwise rotation. The conversion usually allows the endoscope to be advanced to the level of the descending colon, as most of the forward force on the N loop is directed at the apex of the loop and the forces in the alpha loop are more radially distributed. This permits advancement of the instrument despite the presence of the alpha loop. When the instrument reaches the descending colon, the loop

can be reduced. Attempted examination of the proximal colon is usually limited if there is a residual sigmoid loop.

There is no anatomic demarcation between the sigmoid and descending colon, but there is a tendency for the descending colon to be slightly smaller in diameter and to contain residual fecal debris because of its dependent position. Often a long tunnel view may be obtained, and if the sigmoid loops have been reduced, the endoscope can usually be advanced to the level of the splenic flexure without difficulty. A straight sigmoid colon is essential for successful maneuvering around the splenic flexure. Expert endoscopists have counseled to "master the left colon" as the key to successful colonoscopy with "time spent in the left colon saving twice as much time beyond the splenic flexure."[21] Paradoxical motion is often noted as the endoscope is advanced into the transverse colon. The configuration and forces resemble those of the N loop in the sigmoid colon. To reduce this tendency, the patient is often rotated from the left lateral to the supine position. Clockwise rotation of the endoscope may also be helpful. The relationship of the transverse colon and splenic flexure also varies with respiration. Deep sustained inspiration in the cooperative child may decrease the acute angle of the splenic flexure and allow easier passage of the endoscope. If the endoscopist is unsuccessful, the instrument should be withdrawn to ensure reduction of a sigmoid loop that may not have been reduced or one that may have reformed during maneuvers to negotiate the flexure (Figure 62-11). Multiple attempts by trial and error may be necessary to advance the instrument into the transverse colon.

The transverse colon is characterized by triangular haustral folds (Figure 62-12). The endoscope can usually be advanced without difficulty to the hepatic flexure, which is easily identified by the bluish discoloration of the outer wall caused by its close approximation to the liver. Occasionally a U-shaped loop is formed; this requires reduction before attempted negotiation of the hepatic flexure (see Figure 62-6). If the transverse colon is redundant, a gamma loop may form. Reduction of this loop is difficult because rotational forces are poorly transmitted and the loop is usually large. Reduction is less difficult if the

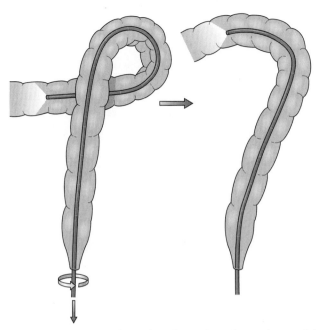

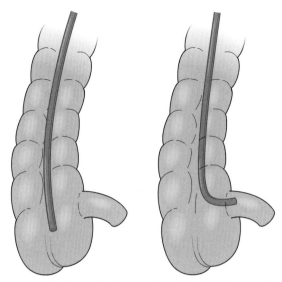

Figure 62-13. The ileocecal valve is intubated by tip deflection rather than *en face*.

Figure 62-11. Reduction of the splenic flexure loop after intubation of the transverse colon. Without straightening, further advancement of the endoscope is difficult and uncomfortable.

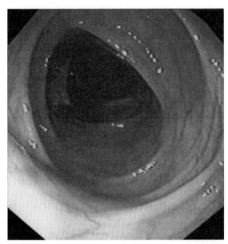

Figure 62-12. Normal colonic mucosal appearance of the transverse colon. Triangular shape of the folds is typical of this area. (*See plate section for color.*)

instrument can be advanced into the ascending colon and then withdrawn to reduce the loop.

The fixed position of the splenic flexure acts as a fulcrum while trying to negotiate the hepatic flexure. Suctioning in the region of the hepatic flexure usually draws the mucosa to the tip of the endoscope, and subsequently the tip can be maneuvered around the flexure into the ascending colon. If the flexure cannot be negotiated, withdrawal, manual rotation of the insertion tube, suctioning, manual compression of the abdominal wall, and/or sustained deep inspiration may be attempted to facilitate passage. If these measures fail, it may still be possible to advance the endoscope, but the patient usually experiences some discomfort. Rotation of the patient from the left lateral position to a supine or right lateral decubitus position may also facilitate scope advancement from the hepatic flexure in to the ascending colon. Reduction of sigmoid looping is key to successful negotiation of the hepatic flexure.

To advance the endoscope into the ascending colon, the tip of the instrument is usually turned into the lumen with the dials. Additional procedures such as withdrawal and rotation may be necessary if paradoxical movement is encountered. Deep inspiration may be effective in "pushing" the instrument into the ascending colon. After the tip is aligned with the lumen, suctioning will also collapse the cecum toward the tip of the instrument. If there have been any difficulties with the cleansing of the colon, they are most likely to become apparent in the ascending colon. Multiple washings of the mucosa and lens may be necessary to allow full examination of the mucosa. The cecum can be recognized by the typical anatomic landmarks of the triangular folds and the appendiceal orifice. With video endoscopes, the tip of the instrument can often be identified in the right lower quadrant as it transilluminates the anterior abdominal wall. The ileocecal valve can be identified on the lateral surface of the prominent ileal fold as a slight irregularity of the valve contour. Occasionally the valve can be directly intubated, but usually it must be approached indirectly. The tip of the endoscope is brought to a position parallel to the valve, and the dials are used to deflect the tip 90° toward the valve (Figure 62-13). The maneuver is designed to catch the proximal lip of the valve with the tip of the endoscope. If the maneuver is successful, the lumen of the ileum will open, and adjustment of the tip will advance the instrument several centimeters. Several attempts may be needed to achieve success. Rotating the patient and suctioning the air from the cecum to draw the valve opening closer to the endoscope may be helpful. The mucosa of the ileum is easily identified by the presence of valvula conniventes and lymphoid aggregates, which appear as submucosal 2- to 4-mm mounds of tissue with normal overlying mucosa. The presence of lymphoid aggregates in adults has been associated with immunoglobulin A deficiency, but is normal in children and even adolescents; the amount tends to decrease with advancing age. If the valve cannot be cannulated and pathologic evaluation is needed, the forceps can sometimes be gently advanced through the valve and biopsy material obtained.

Examination of the mucosa and therapeutic procedures such as polypectomy are conducted principally as the instrument is withdrawn. All areas must be routinely examined, paying special attention to the areas behind folds. Observation of areas around flexures may not be adequate if the scope slips back rapidly, and the instrument may have to be advanced back through areas not well visualized. Observation of the distal rectum requires a retroflexed maneuver for complete examination. This is done by turning the dials to their maximum deflection in the midrectum. The endoscope is then slowly rotated to obtain an unobstructed view. The scope must be straightened before removal from the anus.

Colostomies and ileostomies can usually be examined as long as the openings are large enough to admit the tip of the instrument. In some cases, an upper endoscope is more appropriate in size for stomal examination. Depending on the stomal size, an appropriate scope should be chosen after a finger has been inserted into the opening. The length of bowel that can be examined is usually dependent on whether adhesions have formed. Advancement of the instrument around flexures in the bowel again involves repeated advancement, withdrawal, and torque of the insertion tube. Ileoscopy of the allograft after transplantation is typically performed using an instrument designed for upper endoscopy with antibiotic prophylaxis, but usually without sedation.[24] In the immediate postoperative period, the endoscope is advanced only 5 to 10 cm with minimal air insufflation to avoid anastomotic trauma. Subsequently the endoscope can be advanced further with both random and directed endoscopic biopsies. Indications for small bowel ileoscopy after transplantation include routine surveillance, fever, bacteremia, increased stoma output, diarrhea, and bleeding.[24] In addition to detection of rejection, this technique is helpful for detection of infection such as Epstein-Barr virus and cytomegalovirus, and posttransplantation lymphoproliferative disorder.[24]

Flexible Proctosigmoidoscopy

Routine flexible proctosigmoidoscopy is useful in some pediatric patients. In compliant, usually older children with a chronic illness such as ulcerative colitis, routine office examination to assess the extent and severity of disease when the history is in doubt or before initiating topical therapy for localized disease is useful. Examinations can be performed routinely with the same instruments that are used for full colonoscopy. Examination using either short (35 cm) or long (60 cm) flexible instruments in adults has produced similar pathologic yields. No comparable information is available for the pediatric population, but when it is necessary to sedate pediatric patients for their comfort, it is usually appropriate to be prepared to perform a full colonoscopic examination. If pathology is encountered that is compatible with the patient's symptoms and therapeutic options do not rest on establishing the extent of the disease, the procedure can be terminated without attempting to examine the entire colon. Flexible sigmoidoscopy with biopsy is frequently performed in the infant with rectal bleeding with suspected cow's milk or soy protein allergy. Use of a small-diameter upper endoscope in the range of 5 to 6 mm and the brief nature of the examination often allow the procedure to be performed without sedation.

Anoscopy and Rigid Proctosigmoidoscopy

Anoscopy and rigid proctosigmoidoscopy are infrequently used procedures in the pediatric patient. Most pediatric gastroenterologists and their patients prefer flexible instruments when

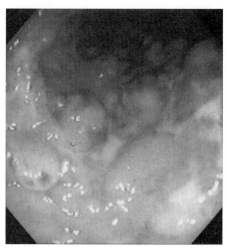

Figure 62-14. Endoscopic appearance of Crohn's colitis involving the transverse colon. Note marked nodularity, mucosal erosions, and overlying exudate in contrast to the appearance in Figure 62-12. (*See plate section for color.*)

examination is required. The anoscope, however, remains a useful office instrument for better visualization of the anal canal and identification of sources of bleeding. In addition, pediatric surgeons will occasionally use this type of instrument.

BIOPSY TECHNIQUE

The technique of endoscopic biopsy is reviewed in detail in Chapter 61. Colonoscopy allows the endoscopist to obtain biopsy material and collect specimens for culture from the distal small bowel and colon. Histopathologic examination is useful in the differentiation of infectious, inflammatory, and malignant processes. Guidelines have outlined the general indications for colonoscopy and biopsy in patients with colonic polyps and inflammatory bowel disease.[25-29] Visual evidence of a suspicious lesion warrants histopathologic evaluation, and most pediatric gastroenterologists routinely biopsy normal tissue including the terminal ileum if inflammatory bowel disease is suspected. Methods for obtaining tissue include snare excision, forceps biopsy, hot biopsy forceps, needle biopsy, and brushings for cytology. Needle biopsy and brush cytology are utilized mainly in the adult population to enhance the yield in patients with suspected colorectal malignancy. Additional screening tests for colorectal malignancy including fecal DNA testing are being studied in adults.[25] Flow cytometry of colonoscopically obtained tissue has recently been used as part of a dysplasia screening protocol in adolescent patients with long-standing ulcerative colitis or Crohn's disease.[30] Needle biopsy has the theoretical advantage in ulcerated lesions of providing histologic material not only from the surface but also from areas deeper within the lesion. Needle biopsy may be useful in submucosal lesions that are difficult to access by biopsy forceps and may be performed using EUS. In most diseases involving pediatric patients, the forceps for pediatric-size instruments or standard forceps provide adequate tissue for mucosal evaluation.

Endoscopy and biopsy can be useful in the diagnosis of infection and in the diagnosis and management of IBD (Figure 62-14). Biopsy specimens (one or two per site using routine forceps) obtained during the acute phase of a bloody diarrheal illness may differentiate acute self-limiting colitis from an initial or recurrent attack of chronic ulcerative colitis. During the resolving phase of acute self-limiting colitis, histologic changes may mimic those of Crohn's disease. Bacterial cultures may be obtained during the procedure by the attachment of a "trap" to the suction equipment that gathers fecal effluent. Colonic biopsy has also been shown to be helpful in human immunodeficiency virus-infected patients with chronic unexplained diarrhea, and it appears to be superior to flexible sigmoidoscopy in this patient population.[31]

Terminal ileal examination may be useful in the diagnosis of Crohn's disease and in the differentiation of Crohn's disease from lymphonodular hyperplasia. Ileal visualization and biopsy may occasionally be useful in patients with infectious ileitis.

Ulcerative colitis and Crohn's disease are predisposing risk factors for the development of colorectal cancer.[32] Routine colonoscopy is usually initiated after 7 to 8 years in patients with colitis due to ulcerative colitis or Crohn's disease.[30] Biopsies should be taken from any suspicious areas, and serial biopsies should be taken from representative areas of the bowel for detection of dysplasia. Typically a total of 36 to 40 specimens are taken from 10 sites throughout the colon for dysplasia screening.

Biopsies from macroscopically normal mucosa may be useful in the diagnosis of disease. Collagenous colitis or lymphocytic colitis, both with associated chronic diarrhea, may present with macroscopically normal mucosa but characteristic histologic abnormalities.[33] Other diseases, such as amyloidosis, inflammatory bowel disease, "microscopic colitis in children," and chronic schistosomiasis, have been diagnosed by biopsy of the colon when the mucosa has been macroscopically normal. Complications after biopsy may include perforation and bleeding. For a more detailed discussion, see the section on complications.

THERAPEUTIC COLONOSCOPY

Initially colonoscopy was primarily a diagnostic tool. As technology advanced and procedural skills developed, colonoscopy, like upper endoscopy, has become increasingly therapeutic. Colonoscopy has been used to remove polyps or foreign bodies; to control bleeding from polyps, polypectomy sites, and other sources; to dilate strictures; to gain access to the GI tract in the case of percutaneous cecostomy placement; and to place various tubes such as colonic motility catheters. The general risks and relative merits of therapeutic endoscopy are discussed in Chapter 61.

Acute gastrointestinal hemorrhage is an indication for therapeutic colonoscopy, but as with upper endoscopy, emergent colonoscopy is associated with an increased risk of complications.[34] Colonic lesions treatable with endoscopic therapy include bleeding ulcers, angiomata, polyps and bleeding polyp stalks, an adherent clot in a diverticulum, or an ulcerative lesion that is resistant to washing, with fresh blood nearby and no other visible lesion in the colon. [35]As with upper gastrointestinal tract disease, diffusely bleeding colonic lesions generally cannot be controlled successfully by endoscopic intervention. The exception is radiation proctitis, which is amenable to treatment by the argon plasma coagulator discussed later.

There are five well-established types of therapeutic intervention for acute gastrointestinal bleeding: injection, coagulation or thermal therapy including the argon plasma coagulator (APC), laser therapy, endoscopic hemostatic devices, and ligation therapy. The specific techniques used depend on equipment availability and experience of the endoscopist. The techniques appear to have roughly equivalent efficacy, but some lesions are more amenable to a particular type of therapy. [35]

Therapeutic endoscopy is most easily accomplished using a two-channeled therapeutic scope so that therapy (injection, coagulation, etc.) may be accomplished via one channel and simultaneous suction or irrigation may be performed using the second channel to keep the field in view, or alternatively with a scope with a single larger therapeutic channel. Unfortunately, therapeutic colonoscopes are significantly larger in diameter compared with standard pediatric colonoscopes and often cannot be used in the pediatric patient. Therapeutic endoscopy may still be performed using a single-channel scope, but depending on the modality used may be technically more difficult.

INJECTION

Injection therapy is used for lower GI bleeding from a variety of sources.[36] However, the most common etiologies of lower GI bleeding in pediatric patients differ significantly from those in adults and are particularly different from the sources in most elderly patients. As a result, colonic injection therapy as a therapeutic modality is used comparatively less in children than in adults. Injection therapy is usually performed by injecting a typically hemostatic or rarely sclerosant agent at three to four sites around an exposed bleeding vessel. Maximal volumes of agents for injection have been established in adults to minimize the risk of perforation and other complications. Maximal volumes in pediatric patients have not been studied; however, maximal adult volumes should not be exceeded. Complications including perforation may occur with volumes of injection even less than the recommended maximum volumes or with injection of a sclerosant in the thinner colonic wall. Chapter 61 outlines the principles of endoscopic injection therapy. Caveats of injection in the colon include use of epinephrine in normal saline as the primary hemostatic agent (final concentration of epinephrine 1:10,000), avoidance of sclerosant injection, lower volume of injection, and use of adjuvant therapies such as clipping in combination with injection.[37] Injection in the colon, if four quadrant, is typically performed behind (i.e., proximal to) the lesion first in order to avoid obscuring the view by lifting the site away from view (Figure 62-15). Although submucosal saline injection has been used to assist in resection of colonic polyps, optimal volumes of injection of many other agents have not been established for the large bowel. When used as part of combination therapy, injection is often performed first to clear the field of active bleeding before clip application or thermal therapy.

THERMOCOAGULATION: HEATER PROBE, MULTIPOLAR PROBES, AND HOT BIOPSY FORCEPS

A second method of establishing hemostasis is thermocoagulation, utilizing the heater probe or monopolar or multipolar coagulators (Table 62-4). The composition, mechanism of action, and settings of the heater and multipolar probes are discussed in Chapter 61. Probe settings should be modified appropriately in the colon, which has a significantly thinner wall compared to the stomach, for example. The heater probe may be used to treat colonic bleeding. Heater probe application may be associated with an increased risk of complications in areas with a thinner gut wall, and therefore the number of joules per pulse should be reduced, especially in right-sided colonic lesions.[38]

There are two main types of electrocoagulation probes: monopolar and bipolar. Monopolar probes require patient grounding. There are two main problems with monopolar coagulation. The first is that the depth of the burn is very difficult to regulate, and perforation is possible. This is especially true in the colon, where deep necrosis, perforation, and delayed massive bleeding have been reported with monopolar electrocoagulation. The second problem is that there is a moderate amount of electrode adherence to the underlying tissue at the treated site and therefore poor visibility, especially in nonirrigated systems. A third technical problem is the need to clean the tip of the probe as the coagulum accumulates during electrocoagulation.

Currently bipolar, also known as multipolar, coagulation is the most popular method with endoscopists. Unlike monopolar coagulation, a grounding plate is not required. Two sizes of probe are available: 2.3 and 3.2 mm. As with the heater probe, the correct technique is to compress the bleeding vessel first, then to coagulate. This is known as coaptive coagulation.

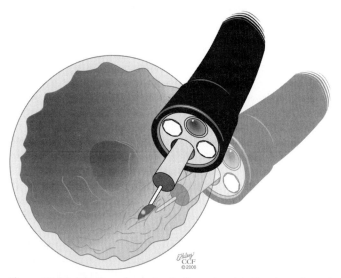

Figure 62-15. Injection of a lesion in the colon; injection is performed behind the lesion first and then distally in order to avoid lifting the lesion to be treated away from the endoscopic view. Adapted from Ref. 35 with permission.

Coaptive coagulation results in the tissues being physically apposed during heating. This is essential to achieve coagulation of large vessels 1 mm or more in diameter and is the optimal technique for smaller diameter arteries. Forceful application to a midrange force of the larger probe appears to increase hemostatic bond strength and the area and depth of coagulation.[39,40] The greatest depth of coagulation is usually achieved with a low to midrange setting (15 to 25 W). This is because at higher watt settings there is an earlier rise in impedance resulting in less energy delivery. Pulses should be applied as short, multiple pulses (2 seconds in duration) or a single long pulse of up to 10 seconds in duration.[39,40] The longer, lower-voltage pulse is thought to work by increasing the depth of coagulation by decreasing tissue desiccation. In adults, a total of up to 40 seconds of electrocoagulation may be required.[39] Increased bleeding after bipolar coagulation has been reported in cases with a visible vessel; usually this bleeding is controllable with further bipolar coagulation and adjuvant use of injection therapy, but on occasion surgery has been required.[40]

Angiodysplasia, predominantly of the colon, has been treated successfully by endoscopic electrocoagulation. Hemorrhagic proctocolitis with recurrent bleeding after radiation therapy has also been successfully treated with a bipolar probe at a power setting of 5 W with short 2-second pulses by coagulating at multiple bleeding sites. Late rebleeding has been reported and was treated successfully by repeat electrocoagulation. In some cases, surgery is still required. Use of the argon plasma coagulator discussed later in the chapter has been particularly effective in the therapy of radiation proctitis.

A further coagulation technique used primarily in the colon is the hot biopsy forceps. This technique combines the principles of endoscopic biopsy and monopolar electrocoagulation. The lesion to be biopsied is grasped in the jaw of insulated biopsy forceps, including polyps of up to 5 mm in size. The forceps are used to tent the mucosa upward away from the colonic muscular layer (Figure 62-16). A brief electrocoagulating current passes through the forceps to the mucosa and sometimes the submucosa, producing coagulation at its base, while preserving the histologic integrity of the specimen. The unit is set on coagulation, at a setting of 10 to 15 W for 1 to 2 seconds in the cecum and ascending colon, and up to 15 to 20 W for 2 seconds in the left colon. Higher settings or longer application times have been associated with an increased risk of perforation, especially in the right colon with perforation rates in the range of 0.05%, less than that associated with snare polypectomy but

TABLE 62-4. Thermocoagulation

Method	Site	Setting	Application Time	No. of Applications	Technique	Notes
Heater probe	Colon	15 J	2-3 s/pulse	2-4	Firm tamponade, then coagulate around bleeding point, then on it	Decreased setting/time of application in colon or thinner gut wall
Bipolar/multipolar	Colon	5-15 W	2 s/pulse	Multiple		
Argon plasma coagulator	Colon	40-50 W 0.8 L/min	0.5-2 s	Multiple	Operative distance 2-8 mm	Paint confluent or near-confluent areas; avoid tissue contact with probe tip; surface should be free of liquid
Hot biopsy forceps	Cecum and ascending colon Left colon	10-15 W 15-20 W	1-2 s 2 s		Tent mucosa away	Polyps ≤5 mm in size

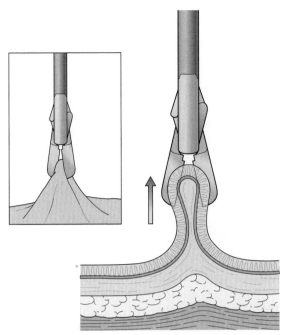

Figure 62-16. Insulated hot biopsy forceps. The mucosa is tented away from the colonic wall before electrocoagulation. From Wadas and Sanowski, Complications of the hot biopsy forceps technique. 1988; 34(1): 32-37,[41] with permission, copyright of the American Society for Gastrointest Endosc.

greater than that of routine colonoscopy.[41] For lesions greater than 5 mm, snare polypectomy is the preferred technique.

Another complication of the hot biopsy forceps is major hemorrhage, which may occur in 0.41% of cases.[41] This is especially likely if the forceps are not held perpendicular to the mucosa. Short-circuiting of the current has been reported between the forceps tip and the noninsulated portion of the forceps with massive hemorrhage, if the forceps are held at an angle of 15° or less to the bowel wall.[42] Hemorrhage may be immediate or delayed for up to 1 week after biopsy and may not respond to conservative therapy.

Results of comparative trials of injection, coagulation, and heater probe therapy vary according to the method used; however, in many studies the different techniques are of comparable efficacy given established volumes of injection, thermocoagulation settings, appropriate indications, and times of application.[43]

In some circumstances, one method of achieving hemostasis may be technically easier than other techniques. With the BICAP probe, the depth of coagulation is limited to 2 mm, which limits its use with larger vessels. However, it has the advantage of a built-in wash system, aiding visibility in cases of brisk bleeding compared with injection therapy. The choice of therapeutic endoscopic technique depends to a significant extent on the training of the endoscopist and equipment availability. If the technique is properly performed, the results are similar using injection or thermal coagulation. Certain lesions, based on their anatomic location or briskness of bleeding, may be more amenable to one method than another. Equipment portability may also be an issue, with injection therapy and coagulation techniques such as the heater probe or multipolar probe, or even the argon plasma coagulator, being significantly more portable than laser techniques, which as a result have fallen out of favor. Complication rates may vary among the techniques, with perforations and rebleeding being reported after monopolar and multipolar coagulation, laser therapy, and APC application.[43] Injection therapy is rarely associated with perforation unless nonstandard volumes of injection are used or if a sclerosing agent is injected in to the colonic wall.[43] Similarly, hemostatic clips (discussed later), when properly applied, are rarely associated with the development of complications.

Argon Plasma Coagulation

The APC method was initially used for surgery, both open and laparoscopic, with endoscopic applications after 1991. It is a noncontact method delivered via the accessory channel of the endoscope. The major benefit of this technique is that it is a quick method of therapy deliverable over a large treatment area. The principle of APC is that high-frequency monopolar current is conducted to target tissues *through* ionized argon gas (argon plasma). Argon gas passes through the coagulation probe with an electrode at its tip. The foot switch activates the electrode. Electrons flow through the channel of electrically activated ionized argon gas from the probe to the tissue.[44] The arrival of the current density at the tissue surface results in coagulation. The grounding pad completes the circuit. If electrical energy is not discharged by arcing to nearby tissues, there is no ignition, and therefore activation of the foot switch causes insufflation of inert argon gas only. The depth of coagulation using this technique is dependent on the generator power setting, flow rate of argon gas, duration of application, and distance between the probe tip and target tissue. The arc contacts the tissue closest to the electrode (keeping in mind that this is a noncontact technique); therefore *en face* or tangential coagulation is possible. Following thermal coagulation, a thin, superficial, electrically insulating zone of desiccation develops, and also a steam layer from boiling of tissue. Both result in a limitation of carbonization and depth of coagulation. After desiccation, electrical resistance of the treated area increases, prompting the current to move to another area of lower resistance for subsequent treatment. With prolonged treatment or application, carbonization, vaporization, and deep tissue injury may occur. Contact of the probe tip with the colonic wall may result in inflation of the colonic submucosa with argon gas, resulting in pneumatosis and potentially extraintestinal gas.[43]

Current probes have an outer diameter of 2.3 or 3.2 mm. Therapy in the colon is performed for hemostasis of superficial vascular ectasias, following polypectomy for resection of residual adenoma if cancer is of concern, for coagulation for postpolypectomy bleeding, for tissue ablation, and for radiation enteritis and proctitis.[37,44-48] APC therapy for vascular ectasias may offer an advantage versus other thermal methods, especially if they are multiple or diffuse. Settings vary significantly by indication. In adults, superficial vascular lesions are typically treated by low power (30-45 W) and gas flow rates (0.8-1 L/min), and an operative distance between the tissue and the probe of 2 to 8 mm.[37,44] Closer contact is used with lower power settings to allow for contact between the plasma and the targeted tissue. Application times are in the range of 0.5 to 2.0 seconds. Similar settings have been reported in a pediatric series.[49]

The technique of APC is to paint confluent or near-confluent surface areas. Use of a two-channel endoscope, if possible, allows for aspiration of argon gas. If the probe tip contacts the bowel wall, it becomes similar to a grounded monopolar probe (discussed previously) and may result in deep tissue injury. The surface to be treated needs to be clear of liquid and blood; if not, coagulated film develops and the tissue beneath may not be

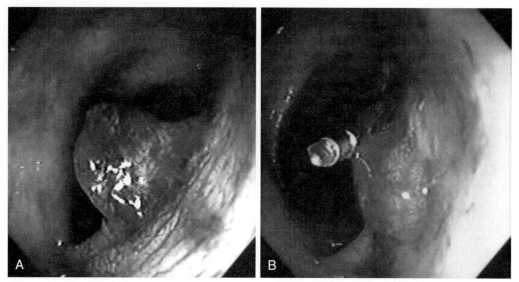

Figure 62-17. Juvenile polyp stalk that bled following snare polypectomy. Stalk was initially injected with epinephrine to achieve hemostasis (**A**) and clip was then applied to stalk after injection to achieve permanent hemostasis. (**B**) (*See plate section for color.*)

adequately treated, limiting the usefulness of this technology in patients with active bleeding. For vascular lesions, before APC application, partially collapsing the colonic lumen while keeping the lesions in view may help avoid excessive air insufflation that may result in colonic wall thinning and perforation following therapy. Whitening of tissue is the endpoint of therapy.[37] Radiation proctitis is best treated in short bursts of coagulation that result in superficial ablation. Because of poor healing of tissues in the previously irradiated rectum, treatment-induced deep ulcerations should be avoided. [37]

Endoscopic Hemostatic Devices Including Bands and Clips

Band Ligation

The technique of band ligation is discussed in more detail in Chapter 61. Band ligation has been used for the management of bleeding colonic varices, Dieulafoy lesions, bleeding hemorrhoids, angiectasias, and polypectomy sites.[43] Band ligation is most effective for bleeding lesions in nonfibrotic tissue. In the case of a discrete bleeding lesion, only a single band may need to be deployed. Caution must be exercised with band ligation in the colon to avoid full-thickness entrapment of the bowel in the cap, which may result in necrosis and perforation.[37]

Hemostatic Clips

The development, characteristics, and technique to deploy endoclips are discussed in detail in Chapter 61. Endoscopic clipping in the colon is used primarily for endoscopic hemostasis, but has also been applied for closure of fistulas, leaks, and perforations and for marking anatomic landmarks for subsequent therapy or surgery.[50,51] Colonic lesions amenable to clip application for hemostasis include hemorrhoids, diverticular bleeding, solitary rectal ulcer syndrome, bleeding following biopsy, and, most commonly, for bleeding polypectomy stalks or for bleeding at the site of resected sessile polyps.[43] Clipping may be performed in conjunction with injection therapy for postpolypectomy bleeding (Figure 62-17A,B). Some endoscopists will apply clips prophylactically following polypectomy in high-risk patients such as those on anticoagulation therapy. To

date this has only been studied in adults. Sequential clip application has been used to close postpolypectomy defects identified at the time of the procedure unless the defects are large in diameter.[52] Clips work well for pliable lesions that can be captured within the open prongs, which have a width span of 11 to 12 mm and for mucosal defects 1 to 1.5 cm or less in size.[37] All clip types require enough tissue capture on either side of the prongs for adequate grasping, but rotatable clips may currently offer an advantage in the colon if there is difficulty accessing a particular lesion. Clips are ineffective for hemostasis of vessels within a large hard fibrotic base and in some cases may precipitate significant bleeding due to trauma to the vessel.[37] Clipping may be particularly effective for bleeding in the setting of clotting abnormalities because clip placement results in minimal to no tissue injury as compared to thermal methods.[52]

As with upper tract application, the first clip is placed on the bleeding point and subsequent clips may be placed around the bleeding point if required. The clips dislodge spontaneously after application and have not been associated with long-term sequelae.

Endoloops

Endoloops are utilized primarily for the management of potential or actual postpolypectomy hemorrhage. They are deployed through the biopsy channel and are placed either before placement of the standard polypectomy snare or following polypectomy to the transected stalk to reduce the rate of postpolypectomy hemorrhage. Detachable loops work mechanically as a ligating device but are not capable of electrocautery.

When placed before polypectomy, if placed too tightly they may result in inadvertent transection of the polyp stalk with resultant bleeding (due to the lack of cautery); if placed too loosely, bleeding can occur following polypectomy. Correct placement is indicated by change in the color of the polyp head without transection. Loop placement before snare polypectomy can also be associated with entanglement of the loop within the polypectomy snare.

Loop placement on a polyp stalk after polypectomy may be complicated by difficult placement due to retraction of the stalk. One method to overcome this technique is the lift and ligate technique using a two-channel scope, where the stalk is lifted by forceps from one channel and ligated using a detachable snare from the second channel.[53] When using this technique, the loop is placed first around the stalk but not tightened; the forceps are then used to lift the stalk, and the endoloop is tightened.

Laser Photocoagulation

Laser photocoagulation is another modality occasionally used to achieve endoscopic hemostasis. There are two main types of laser: the argon and the Nd:YAG laser. The argon laser's usefulness is limited because of light absorption by surrounding red blood. Therefore, to use the argon laser, overlying blood must be eliminated with a coaxial air jet. Clinically, the argon laser is used primarily for right-sided colonic lesions. When compared with the Nd:YAG laser, it has a lower power and depth of tissue penetration.

The Nd:YAG laser is the most popular laser used in endoscopy. The laser admits a continuous wave of infrared light of wavelength 1064 nm with a power up to 100 W. This light is transmitted via a 600-µm glass fiber in a 2.5-mm polytetrafluoroethylene catheter passed down the endoscope biopsy channel. Carbon dioxide is passed coaxially along the catheter to clear blood from the bleeding site and to keep the fiber tip cool and free from debris. A filter is attached to the eyepiece to prevent reflected laser light from entering the endoscopist's eye. The intense laser light is directed to coagulate tissue circumferentially around the bleeding site. Contact and noncontact applications are possible.[43] Lasers have been used for congenital vascular lesions (hereditary hemorrhagic telangiectasia, blue rubber bleb nevi syndrome) as well as superficial vascular lesions, including angiodysplasia, telangiectasia, and arteriovenous malformation in the colon. Asymptomatic, nonbleeding angiodysplasias are usually not treated. One problem after laser photocoagulation of a lesion is that the histologic diagnosis is difficult to confirm.

Like the heater probe, laser therapy can also provoke bleeding, which can usually be stopped with further laser coagulation.[54] In addition, there is an increased chance of full-thickness perforation of the gut wall. Application of the laser in the colon requires modification of both technique and power settings. The thermal effects of a laser beam on tissue vary according to the power density (the amount of energy converted to heat at the point where the laser beam strikes tissue) and the size of the contact area. Although the power setting and exposure time can be preset, movement, especially in the right colon, and varying wall thickness, especially the thin ascending colon, can change the exposure time required to produce perforation. Instead of coagulating tissue, vaporization of tissue can occur.

There is a long learning curve associated with use of the laser, and this modality should be used only by experienced operators. Currently the laser seems to offer little advantage over the heater probe, multipolar probe, or APC, and because of its increased cost and decreased portability, the other modalities are likely to predominate in the foreseeable future.

STRICTURE DILATION

The equipment available for and technique of balloon dilation are discussed in Chapter 61. For colonic strictures proximal to the rectum, the majority of dilations are performed using TTS balloon dilators. After visualizing the stricture, these types of balloon can be passed through an endoscope with a 2.8-mm channel under direct vision. As with upper tract lesions, usually two or three inflations are performed per endoscopic session, with repositioning of the balloon in between inflations. Sessions are repeated over several weeks or months with progressively larger-diameter balloons. This technique has been used for postoperative or inflammatory strictures and is especially useful for strictures of recent onset. Cicatricial anastomotic strictures of the colon have been dilated with air-and-water-filled balloons or with a mechanical dilator (e.g., Savary dilator) placed over an endoscopically directed guidewire. Intralesional steroid injection of strictures has been reported as an adjuvant to endoscopic dilation. Small volumes (0.25 to 1.0 mL per injection) of triamcinolone acetonide (Kenalog 10 mg/mL; Bristol Meyers Squibb, Princeton, NJ, USA) are injected in four quadrants of the narrowest stricture segment. The efficacy of triamcinolone appears to be based on its interference with collagen synthesis and subsequent scar formation.[55] This technique has been associated with increased efficacy of dilation and longer symptom-free intervals between endoscopic dilations.[56] Recently, intralesional injection of infliximab (Centacor, Malvern PA, USA) has been reported to aid in the management of colonic strictures in adult patients with Crohn's disease.[57]

PERCUTANEOUS CECOSTOMY

Recently, percutaneous cecostomy (PEC) and percutaneous colostomy of the left colon have been reported.[58,59] These techniques were developed to assist in the management of intractable constipation in children. After placement, the PEC tube is used to administer antegrade continence enemas and represents a modification of the surgical approach to this problem introduced by Malone et al. in 1990. After bowel preparation, prophylactic antibiotic administration (metronidazole and gentamicin, or cefotaxime and metronidazole) and a sterile skin preparation, colonoscopy is performed to the cecum. The bowel is transilluminated, a small incision is made, and a trocar is passed into the cecum under direct vision, using a technique similar to PEG placement as described in Chapter 61. For left-sided tube placement, tubes have been placed at the junction of the descending and sigmoid colon.[59] The guidewire is passed, grasped via a snare passed via the colonoscope, and pulled out through the anus. A 12- to 20-Fr pull-type PEG tube is attached to the wire, and subsequently the PEG tube is pulled in a retrograde fashion through the colon and out through the anterior abdominal wall. The position of the PEC tube in the cecum or alternate location is verified endoscopically.[58] PEC tubes are flushed in the postoperative period, usually starting 24 hours after surgery, and subsequently can be used for antegrade enema administration of standard concentration solutions. Prophylactic antibiotics are typically administered for 24 hours. After development of a mature tract, tubes can be changed to a low-profile device. Complications of this procedure include granulation tissue formation, local or generalized infection, dislodgment of the tube, misplacement of the tube, pain, pressure necrosis, and abdominal distention.[58,59]

POLYPECTOMY

The rationale for colonoscopy for suspected polyps in adults is based on the assumption that cancers arise from preexisting adenomas or neoplastic polyps. Screening has been suggested for patients as they enter higher-risk age groups, for those with a family or personal history of colonic cancer, and for those who have an underlying disease process that would make them more susceptible to the development of carcinoma. Most polyps in the pediatric population are simple juvenile polyps and have no premalignant potential. The majority are pedunculated with a moderate to long stalk. Mucosa adjacent to the juvenile polyp may have a characteristic appearance known as "chicken skin mucosa," a result of mucosal lipid-laden macrophages; this is a benign condition in children.[60] Recently, however, a greater frequency of adenomas has been identified in pediatric patients. In addition, an increasing percentage of pediatric patients are recognized to have more than one polyp at the time of colonoscopy.[61] Juvenile polyps or adenomas, when multiple, recurrent, or associated with extraintestinal abnormalities in pediatric patients, may occur as part of a polyposis syndrome. With advances in genetic testing, these syndromes have been further characterized and are discussed in more detail elsewhere in the text. Up to one third of patients with simple juvenile polyps develop an iron deficiency anemia and require polypectomy to prevent ongoing blood loss.

Before polypectomy, the patient must be cleansed of fecal debris. A poorly prepared colon limits visualization and increases the technical difficulty of the procedure. Excessive fecal debris or the use of certain gavage solutions such as mannitol places the patient at risk for explosion during attempted polypectomy.[62] The patient's risk of bleeding should be assessed by history, and studies such as a complete blood count, coagulation profile, and blood typing may be indicated.

Diminutive polyps of 5 mm or less in diameter are typically removed with biopsy forceps. Use of hot biopsy monopolar forceps or routine forceps biopsy followed by coagulation, if necessary, allows for histologic evaluation. If lesions are too numerous for removal, representative samples should be obtained. Cold snare technique should be avoided in pediatric patients.

Large polyps (more than 5 mm in diameter) are usually removed with snare electrocautery. The minimal channel diameter for current polypectomy snares is 2.8 mm; therefore, the current minimum endoscope outer diameter for polypectomy is in the range of 9.0 mm. The snare is inserted into the endoscope with the wire loop retracted. The endoscope tip should be stabilized before advancing the polypectomy snare. The polyp, and therefore the snare, is optimally positioned in the 5 to 7 o'clock position.[63] Only the amount of snare necessary fully to encompass the polyp should be extended. The polyp is then lassoed and the sheath maneuvered to the stalk (Figure 62-18). The endoscopist should ensure that the snare encompasses only the polyp head and stalk, and that normal bowel is not within in the snare.

Because most polyps in pediatric patients are pedunculated with a moderate to long stalk, the snare should be positioned to perform electrocautery closer to the polyp head rather than close to the bowel wall or base of the polyp stalk. This allows for grasping of the stalk and coagulation if postpolypectomy bleeding occurs. This is in distinction to adenomas in the adult patient, where carcinoma in situ may be suspected and the endoscopist is trying to achieve as complete a resection as possible. The head of the polyp should be lifted off the mucosa before electrocautery; contact between the polyp head and opposing mucosa should be avoided to prevent a mucosal burn on the opposite colonic wall. The shaft of the snare should

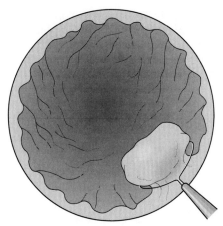

Figure 62-18. Snare polypectomy of a pedunculated polyp. After ensnarement, the loop is advanced to the polyp neck before closure, in order to allow sufficient length to resnare a bleeding polyp stalk and avoid thermal injury to the bowel wall.

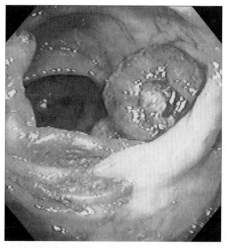

Figure 62-19. Head of a resected and coagulated juvenile polyp. Note the whitish area in the center of the polyp representing the area of coagulation. (*See plate section for color.*)

be approximated to the polyp head as the endoscopist closes the polypectomy snare, bringing the distal aspect of the snare toward the polyp head. To remove large polyps of 2 cm or more in size, piecemeal resection may be necessary. After the head is reduced in size, it is usually possible to snare the stalk and safely remove the remainder of the polyp.

After the polyp has been snared, a current is passed through the snare, which is slowly closed by the assistant. Rapid closure results in bleeding from vessels in the stalk that have been amputated but not coagulated. Most endoscopists use a combination of coagulation and cutting settings for snare polypectomy. Use of cutting current alone, particularly with vascular juvenile polyps, is likely to result in significant postpolypectomy bleeding. Coagulation current alone without cutting may also be effective because of the cutting properties of the snare. Lower settings are typically used in the right side of the colon compared with the left. As the polyp coagulates, there is a whitish discoloration of the polyp (Figure 62-19).

Large or broad-based polyps must be removed with care (Figure 62-20). Transection of the polyp close to the bowel wall risks perforation. The colonic wall is thin, in the range of

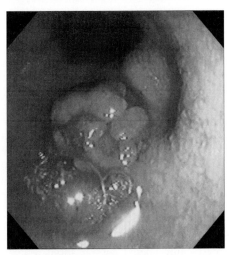

Figure 62-20. Large right-sided sessile polyp in a patient with long-standing Crohn's disease. (*See plate section for color.*)

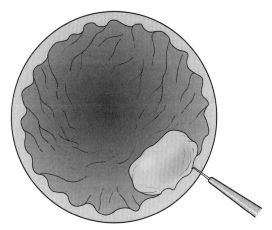

Figure 62-21. Saline-assisted polypectomy of a large sessile polyp. Saline is injected submucosally to elevate the polyp before application of electrical current.

1.7 to 2.2 mm, especially on the right side.[63] Submucosal injection of saline (saline-assisted polypectomy) can be used to elevate the polyp onto a submucosal saline cushion, allowing for safer resection[63,64] (Figure 62-21). Sterile normal saline or hypertonic saline with epinephrine is typically injected to raise a sessile polyp before cautery, increasing the distance between the base of the polyp and the serosa. If the polyp is large, injection should initially be performed behind the polyp (proximally) in order to avoid obscuring the view of the polyp by lifting it away. This may require three to four injections of 1 mL or more per injection. Signs of a good submucosal injection include raising of the polyp and lack of vascular markings within the injection site.[64] If there is no submucosal bleb, the injection needle may have penetrated the serosa and may require repositioning. Care should be taken to avoid snaring submucosal tissue. In the case of large sessile polyps, the endoscopist must assess the risk of polypectomy and the nature of the information to be gained before deciding whether the polyp should be removed endoscopically or surgically. Often segmental resection or multiple biopsies of sessile or broad-based polyps remove adequate tissue for pathologic differentiation. Occasionally large polyps may need to be reduced in multiple

sessions for complete obliteration. Rarely, cancers may present as intraluminal lesions that mimic polyps in pediatric patients. In these cases endoscopic resection of the lesion may be hazardous because of intramural extension or increased vascularity of these lesions. Therefore in the case of polypoid lesions with an irregular appearance, endoscopic biopsy to determine tissue type and adjuvant imaging may be beneficial before attempted endoscopic resection to reduce the risk of uncontrollable bleeding or perforation.[65]

When multiple polyps are encountered, the most proximal should be removed first so that subsequent passage of the endoscope will not precipitate hemorrhage over the base of an already amputated polyp. In the patient with large numbers of polyps, representative polyps should be removed or biopsied for pathologic analysis. In patients with familial adenomatous polyposis, there are too many polyps typically present to biopsy or remove all of them. Larger polyps should be biopsied or removed for histologic analysis. Dysplasia screening in this condition is discussed elsewhere in the book.

After amputation, polyps should be retrieved. Small polyps can be suctioned through the endoscope and the polyp retrieved in a trap. Large polyps can usually be retrieved with the snare, with standard or foreign-body forceps such as the Pentapod forceps, or by using the Roth retrieval net.[66] If the endoscopist is unable to retrieve the polyp, the patient can be given an enema or the parents can be asked to strain the stool and submit the tissue for later analysis.

Ancillary equipment should be available before starting polypectomy, including needles for injection of saline or epinephrine. In addition to epinephrine injection, detachable polypectomy loops and hemostatic clips are useful for postpolypectomy bleeding. Detachable polypectomy loops should be used with caution because of the possibility of inadvertent transection or inadequate hemostasis.[67] Sterile India ink can be injected for tattooing if the polyp site needs to be marked for future surgical or endoscopic procedures. This tattooing is permanent and should be used for limited indications.[68,69]

SPECIAL ENDOSCOPIC TECHNIQUES

Placement of Motility Catheters

There have been significant recent advances in the area of gastrointestinal motility. Colonic motility procedures to evaluate patients with conditions such as chronic intestinal pseudoobstruction are becoming increasingly common in pediatric centers with a special interest in gastrointestinal motility and are discussed elsewhere in the text. Unlike rectal motility, in which catheter placement is straightforward, colonic motility procedures require the monitoring catheter to be placed in the cecum. Many centers use endoscopy for initial catheter placement. Colonic motility catheters are usually placed after a standard colonoscopy. Once the colonoscope is in the cecum, a guidewire is advanced via the endoscope channel to the cecum. The colonoscope is withdrawn, taking care to advance the guidewire in equal increments with scope withdrawal so that the guidewire stays in the cecum; overadvancement of the guidewire should be avoided because of the risk of perforation. After the endoscope has been removed, the motility catheter is advanced over the guidewire to the cecum. The wire is withdrawn, the catheter secured in place, and monitoring can be initiated once the effects of anesthesia have worn off. Colonic motility catheter placement is facilitated by performing a relatively "loopless" colonoscopy, allowing for "one to one" movement of the catheter over the wire. Abdominal radiography is typically performed before the motility procedure to verify catheter placement.

Endoscopic Mucosal Resection

Endoscopic mucosal resection (EMR) is an emerging endoscopic technique that allows for mucosectomy or mucosal resection without surgery. Resection levels are typically into the middle or deeper layers of the submucosa when performed. The types of EMR are discussed in Chapter 61. Colonic indications for this type of procedure are primarily cancer related in adults. Additional potential indications include resection of small carcinoid tumors found incidentally.[70] Unique pediatric indications for this procedure have not yet been established. Reported complications include pain, bleeding, perforation, and stricture formation. Endoscopic clipping is often used at the time of EMR because of the potential perforation risk with this technique.

Third-Eye Retroscope

One of the recently developed tools used primarily to increase polyp detection is known as the third-eye retroscope (Avantis Medical, Sunnyvale, CA). This is a disposable colonoscope accessory and accompanying equipment that allows for examination of the haustral folds from the retroflexed view at the time of colonoscope withdrawal. The catheter is placed via the endoscope channel after the colonoscope is fully inserted. A special cap device is required at the end of the colonoscope to allow for normal functioning of the colonoscope and to lock the catheter in place in its retroflexed position.[71] When the catheter is inserted, the endoscopist is able to see two simultaneous views, the standard forward image from the colonoscope and the retroflex view from the third-eye device. If a polyp or other lesion is identified, the third-eye device is removed, a polypectomy or biopsy is performed, and then the device can be reinserted to examine the remainder of the mucosa with endoscope withdrawal. The primary advantage of this device appears to be improved adenoma detection in adult patients, and in limited adult studies addition of the third-eye device has increased the polyp detection rate in the range of 9 to 13%.[71] To date this device has not been studied in pediatric patients but may have a pediatric indication for patients with polyps or polyposis conditions that are associated with an increased risk of dysplasia and in the evaluation of children with GI bleeding of obscure origin.

COMPLICATIONS

Sedation-, procedure-, and patient-related endoscopic complications are discussed in Chapter 61.

Sedation complications during colonoscopy are similar to those reported during upper gastrointestinal tract examination. A large single-center pediatric series looking at sedation-related complications in pediatric patients receiving intravenous sedation for 2711 endoscopic procedures demonstrated sedation-related complications at a rate comparable to or lower than that reported in adults with oxygen desaturation responding to bag mask ventilation in 2 of 2366 patients (0.08%), medication-related urticaria in 3 of 2366 (0.13%), and no major

cardiopulmonary complications.[72] Another large prospective pediatric single-center series of intravenous sedation revealed a 0.2% rate of serious sedation-related complications (apnea) and a 0.7% rate of desaturation for longer than 20 seconds; in that series no cardiopulmonary resuscitation or sedation reversal was required.[73] In a large recent retrospective multicenter database study of colonoscopy procedures in children, immediate cardiopulmonary complications occurred in 0.4% of children, with the most common complication in this group being hypoxia.[74] In that series, the incidence of hypoxia was significantly higher in the patients undergoing colonoscopy under intravenous sedation compared to those having the procedure during general anesthesia. However, there are significant methodological limitations in terms of how the data were collected, the comparability of the groups, and the completeness of data about a given complication. Therefore, generalities about the incidence of sedation-related complications as a function of type of sedation cannot be drawn from that study.

Several series have demonstrated a correlation between the frequency of technical complications during colonoscopy and the experience of the endoscopist. Gastroenterologists treating adults have their highest complication rates during the first 50 to 100 colonoscopic procedures.[75] In addition, if incomplete examination (i.e., failure to reach the cecum or terminal ileum) is considered a complication, incomplete examination is significantly more likely when procedures are performed by an individual with less experience.[1,76]

Bleeding after colonoscopy is usually minimal but may follow mucosal biopsy or polypectomy. Bleeding following a diagnostic procedure has been reported in 0.008 to 0.17% of procedures in adults and is likely as rare in children.[74] Patients undergoing colonoscopy or sigmoidoscopy follow hematopoietic stem cell transplantation appear to be at higher risk of bleeding following endoscopic biopsy.[77] Thrombocytopenia may be a risk factor that is associated with a higher rate of post-biopsy bleeding in these patients.[77]

Bleeding following polypectomy is uncommon, but may occur in 0.26 to 2.5% of patients depending on the series.[74,78,79] Techniques to reduce the risk of postpolypectomy bleeding were discussed previously.[78] In adults, increased polyp size and hypertension have been associated with an increased risk of postpolypectomy bleeding, which may be delayed.[77]

Perforation is the most serious complication of colonoscopy in children. It is usually related to polypectomy and successfully managed with surgical intervention. The risk of perforation, based primarily on series of adult patients, is increased in patients with severe active colitis, strictures, diverticula, large polyps, and adhesions due to prior surgery. The risk ranges from 0.06 to 0.3%.[78,80] Some centers attempt to manage small perforations of the rectum and distal sigmoid colon conservatively.[78,81] Clinically silent diastatic tears have been reported in children, but are thought to be unusual. Advanced endoscopic procedures such as percutaneous cecostomy are likely to be associated with a higher complication rate, and further studies are indicated.

REFERENCES

1. Kay M, Piccoli DA, Barth B, et al. NASPGHAN guideline for training in endoscopy and related procedures. J Pediatr Gastroenterol Nutr. In press.
11. Mamula P, Adler DG, et al. *ASGE* Technology Committee, Colonoscopy preparation. Gastrointest Endosc 2009;69:1201–1209.

35. Kay MH, Wyllie R. Therapeutic endoscopy for nonvariceal gastrointestinal bleeding. J Pediatr Gastroenterol Nutr 2007;45:157–171.

37. Wong K, Baron TH. Endoscopic management of acute lower gastrointestinal bleeding. Am J Gastroenterol 2008;103:1881–1887.

52. Anastassiades CP, Baron TH, Wong K. Endoscopic clipping for the management of gastrointestinal bleeding. Nat Clin Pract Gastroenterol Hepatol 2008;5:559–568.

73. Mamula P, Markowitz JE, Neiswender K, et al. Safety of intravenous midazolam and fentanyl for pediatric GI endoscopy: prospective study of 1578 endoscopies.[see comment]. Gastrointest Endosc 2007;65:203–210.

See expertconsult.com for a complete list of references and the review questions for this chapter.

63

ENDOSCOPIC RETROGRADE CHOLANGIOPANCREATOGRAPHY

Atif Saleem • Mounif El-Youssef • Todd H. Baron

Endoscopic retrograde cholangiopancreatography (ERCP) is a combined endoscopic and radiologic procedure used for both diagnostic, but more important, therapeutic interventions within the pancreatic and biliary tree. During the procedure, fluoroscopy is utilized to assist in performance, and radiographic images are obtained and stored for documentation and clinical use. Initially introduced as a diagnostic procedure, the use of ERCP in children has mirrored that of adults and has shifted from a predominately diagnostic procedure to a therapeutic one.[1,2] This is due to the technological advancements in complementary, noninvasive diagnostic imaging tools. Nonetheless, ERCP can still provide valuable diagnostic information in selected cases.

Increased experience over the past 10 years with the use of ERCP by dedicated endoscopists in tertiary care centers has resulted in a high success rate in the performance of diagnostic and therapeutic procedures.[3,4] Optimal performance of ERCP requires skilled endoscopists familiar with the equipment and techniques accumulated from frequent procedures. With the infrequent use of ERCP in children, pediatric gastroenterologists have rightly relied on experienced colleagues in adult and pediatric gastroenterology for this procedure.[5]

PANCREATICOBILIARY IMAGING METHODS

Several imaging modalities are available for the diagnosis of pancreaticobiliary disease. Appropriate selection of imaging technique depends on the underlying pathologic process.

Ultrasonography (US) has the advantages of being inexpensive, portable, well tolerated in patients of all ages, and readily available. US is the method of choice for diagnosing gallstones at any age. It is helpful in detecting and estimating the degree of biliary and pancreatic ductal dilation or in detecting pseudocysts, but may fail to provide accurate information in and around the distal common bile duct and head of pancreas due to overlying bowel gas.

Abdominal computed tomography (CT) is also useful for evaluating the degree and level of biliary obstruction. It provides superior imaging of the pancreatic parenchyma and presence of pancreatic ductal obstruction as compared to ultrasound. However, CT often fails to detect gallstones because of their similar density to the surrounding bile. It has good sensitivity and specificity for the detection of bile duct stones.

Magnetic resonance cholangiopancreatography (MRCP) has become extremely useful for imaging the bile ducts and pancreatic ducts. It is noninvasive and can provide information about the patient's anatomy and the presence of obstruction, stricture, neoplasm, or injury following trauma.[6,7] MRCP can be a valuable tool in diagnosing primary sclerosing cholangitis (PSC) and can

demonstrate intra- and extrahepatic bile ducts.[8] Disadvantages of MRCP include the need for sedation in younger or uncooperative patients and contraindication in patients with metallic implants.

Percutaneous transhepatic cholangiography (PTC) is an invasive procedure that also has diagnostic accuracy, but because of its invasiveness is reserved for therapeutic intervention. Access to the biliary tree is achieved by passing a needle through the liver and into an intrahepatic duct. This can be facilitated by the use of CT or ultrasonography. Dilation of the biliary tree facilitates biliary access. Although imaging of the pancreatic duct is generally not achieved unless an abnormally long pancreaticobiliary junction is present, on occasion pancreatic duct filling occurs even in normal pancreaticobiliary anatomy in the absence of distal bile duct obstruction. Because almost all therapeutic interventions following PTC require an external drain that is poorly tolerated by children, PTC is generally reserved for those cases when access to the duodenum is not possible or when biliary cannulation or traversal of a guidewire across an obstruction fails. Complications of PTC include bleeding and bile leakage at the entry site into the abdomen with resultant bile peritonitis.

Endoscopic ultrasonography (EUS) is largely a diagnostic tool for evaluation of gastrointestinal diseases in adults; however, there is limited experience using EUS in children. EUS, like ERCP, requires additional advanced endoscopic training and is typically performed by specially trained adult gastroenterologists. Tissue can be obtained by passing a needle under direct ultrasound guidance into areas of interest, such as lymph nodes and masses (fine needle aspiration or FNA). The role of EUS in pediatric patients[9] with pancreaticobiliary disorders has been studied both retrospectively[10,11] and prospectively.[12] EUS and EUS-guided FNA were found to be feasible and safe and to significantly alter subsequent management in the majority of children in the limited pediatric series reported to date.

EUS is also a useful modality that offers the precise evaluation of portal hypertension in orthotopic liver transplantation (OLT) candidates.[13] EUS displays abnormal vessels that develop in the circulation called "deep varices" that have a high risk of bleeding in patients with cirrhosis and are not detected with routine ultrasonography.

INDICATIONS FOR ERCP

The primary indication for ERCP in neonates and young infants is the evaluation of cholestasis where the diagnosis is not established by other modalities.[14-16] Although liver biopsy has a very high sensitivity and specificity for the diagnosis of neonatal cholestasis, it is complemented by ERCP in cases where biliary ductular abnormalities are noted on imaging studies. Diagnostic and/or therapeutic biliary indications for

ERCP in children older than 1 year and in adolescents include obstructive jaundice, high clinical suspicion of or known choledocholithiasis, suspected primary sclerosing cholangitis in the setting of inflammatory bowel disease when MRCP is non-diagnostic, treatment of bile ductal leaks after blunt abdominal trauma[17] or cholecystectomy, treatment of anastomotic biliary strictures and leaks following liver transplantation, and for the evaluation and treatment of abnormal imaging studies (US, CT, or MRCP). Pancreatic indications for ERCP in children include nonresolving acute pancreatitis, idiopathic recurrent pancreatitis, and symptomatic chronic pancreatitis[18,19]; evaluation of persistently increased levels of pancreatic enzymes; evaluation of abnormal imaging studies; treatment of pancreatic pseudocysts and pancreatic ascites; and evaluation and treatment of pancreatic ductal leaks from blunt abdominal trauma.[20] Table 63-1 outlines the indications for ERCP.

CONTRAINDICATIONS TO ERCP

Relative contraindications to ERCP are coagulation disorders that are severe or uncorrectable. An international normalized ratio (INR) of approximately 1.5 is considered the cutoff value for safe performance of biliary sphincterotomy. Absolute contraindications to ERCP include inability to obtain informed consent; cardiovascular, respiratory and neurological instability; luminal perforation; and esophageal, gastric, or duodenal obstruction precluding passage of the duodenoscope to the level of the papilla. Surgically altered anatomy of the gastroduodenal and/or pancreaticobiliary tract (e.g., Roux-en-Y choledochojejunostomy with orthotropic liver transplantation) may make ERCP difficult or impossible to perform. However, newer endoscopes may make ERCP possible in selected cases.[21,22]

PREPARATION FOR ERCP

A well-equipped endoscopy suite with fluoroscopy and a multitude of necessary endoscopic accessories is required to perform ERCP. Equipment for monitoring vital signs, oxygen saturation, and medications and equipment for resuscitation are absolutely essential. Occasionally ERCP is done in an operating room, and the same equipment is needed. Pediatric endoscopy assistants and specially trained nurses are required for assistance in handling accessories such as guidewires and catheters. One team member, usually an RN, should be present whose sole purpose is monitoring the patient and administration of medication. More often, a pediatric anesthesiologist is available to ensure proper, adequate sedation and airway control to optimize the smooth performance of the procedure.

Assistants who are familiar with ERCP goals, anatomy, and types of accessories as well as how to use the accessories and to inject contrast are absolutely critical for ensuring procedural success.

Preparation for ERCP is the same as for upper gastrointestinal endoscopy except for the administration of antibiotic prophylaxis in selected cases and the potential need for preprocedural laboratory work.[23] Antibiotic prophylaxis for cardiac conditions is given according to the current guidelines of the American Heart Association for children with congenital and rheumatic heart disease.[24,25] Antibiotics are also administered to prevent infectious complications of cholangitis or pancreatic abscess formation from injection of contrast material into potentially inadequately drained spaces, such as in those with

TABLE 63-1. Indications for ERCP: Evaluation and/or Therapy for the Following

Congenital Anomalies*
Biliary atresia vs. neonatal hepatitis
Alagille syndrome and paucity syndrome
Congenital hepatic fibrosis
Caroli's disease and Caroli's syndrome
Biliary strictures
Choledochal cyst
Treatment of pancreas divisum
Diagnosis of annular pancreas
Cystic dilation of the pancreatic duct (pancreatocele)

Acquired Diseases
Treatment of benign biliary strictures
Removal of bile duct stones
Treatment of biliary complications after liver transplantation
Diagnosis and treatment of primary sclerosing cholangitis
Biliary obstruction due to parasitic infestation
Parasitic infestation: *Ascaris*
Diagnosis and treatment of sphincter of Oddi dysfunction
Diagnosis and treatment of pancreatic trauma
Treatment of acquired immune deficiency syndrome cholangiopathy
Treatment of chronic pancreatitis
Drainage of pancreatic pseudocysts

*Initial presentation may not be at birth or in infancy.

biliary obstruction in whom inadequate drainage is anticipated (primary sclerosing cholangitis, hilar obstruction) and those with pancreatic pseudocysts.[26]

Current guidelines should be followed for children with a valvular prosthesis, vascular graft material, and indwelling catheters, or status following organ transplant, and in immunosuppressed patients. A period of fasting precedes sedation and intubation with the endoscope as per published guidelines.[27]

An intravenous line is placed for sedation and administration of glucagon or other antiperistaltic agents such as atropine or glucagon to facilitate cannulation of the papilla. The primary goals of most sedation regimens for pediatric endoscopic procedures are to ensure a patient's safety, comfort, and cooperation continuously throughout the procedure. Secondary and often desirable goals of sedation are to affect periprocedural amnesia, maximize procedural efficiency, minimize recovery times, and maintain cost-effectiveness. Premedication can be administered to sedate the child, minimize discomfort, and induce amnesia. Anesthesia support is most often used in children undergoing ERCP because it is a complex procedure and requires the patient to remain relatively motionless.[28]

There are two main types of sedation for pediatric endoscopy: general endotracheal anesthesia (GETA) and intravenous (IV) sedation. Intravenous sedation can be administered by the endoscopist (moderate sedation) or an anesthesia team member (monitored anesthesia care or MAC).

In general,[29] the most common IV sedation regimens used for pediatric endoscopy administered by gastroenterologists combine a narcotic analgesic (e.g., meperidine or fentanyl) with a benzodiazepine (diazepam or midazolam). Narcotics produce analgesia while benzodiazepines provide for anxiolysis and amnesia.

For sedation best practices, children undergoing GI endoscopy should also be classified in accordance with guidelines defined by the American Society of Anesthesiologists (ASA) to identify patients who will be best served by GETA.[30] Patients can be divided into age groups as follows: younger than 6 months, older than 6 months, school-aged (4 to 11 years), and adolescents. Infants younger than 6 months may have little anxiety and tend to sedate easily. Infants older than 6 months who have developed "stranger anxiety" may be more easily sedated if parents remain next to them during induction. School-aged children manifest "concrete thinking" and may be surprisingly difficult to sedate because of higher anxiety levels than may be appreciated. In mature older children, moderate sedation can be safely achieved using a combination of narcotic and a benzodiazepine. Use of pharyngeal spray to anesthetize the pharynx is not required, but can be used at the operator's discretion. Sedation for endoscopy is discussed in greater detail in Chapter 61.

TECHNIQUE OF ERCP

Standard adult side-viewing endoscopes (duodenoscopes) are used in children older than 1 year of age and in adolescents. Commercially available specialized smaller diameter video pediatric side-viewing instruments are available for use in infants less than 1 year of age.[31] The disadvantages of such small-caliber endoscopes are the decrement in optics and the small working channel diameter, which limits the use of accessories and stents.

The patient is placed in the prone or supine position (based on endoscopist and anesthesia preference) to allow ideal fluoroscopic views of the pancreaticobiliary tree. After adequate sedation, a plastic bite-block is inserted between the teeth, and intubation of the esophagus is done "blindly" because of the side-viewing nature of the endoscope. After the endoscope is guided into the descending duodenum, the papilla is brought into close position so the desired target duct may be cannulated from an *en face* position. A catheter is manipulated into the papilla, and contrast material is injected to outline the duct(s) of interest (biliary and/or pancreatic duct). Care must be taken to remove any air in the contrast syringe, because introduction of air into the ducts will appear as rounded filling defects and mimic stones.[32] Some endoscopists prefer to use diluted contrast for detection of bile duct stones.

Special tapered-tip cannulas should be available for pediatric patients and for cannulation of the accessory (minor) papilla if necessary. Most endoscopists use a sphincterotome instead of a cannula as a primary bile duct cannulation device because it has the ability to be bowed, increasing the likelihood of cannulating the biliary tree. Selected fluoroscopic images are saved, and therapeutic maneuvers are performed as required.

After removal of the endoscope, placing the patient in the supine position or in the right lateral decubitus position facilitates filling of the upper hepatic ducts by gravity. Spot images may be obtained without the endoscope in the field to ensure full visualization. Cholangioscopy can be performed using very small-caliber endoscopes passed through the working channel of the duodenoscope,[33-35] but applications for diseases in children are limited and the smaller caliber bile ducts often prevent passage.

BILIARY DISORDERS

Diagnosis of Biliary Atresia and Neonatal Hepatitis

Neonatal cholestasis is defined as prolonged conjugated hyperbilirubinemia that occurs in the newborn period. It results from diminished bile flow and/or excretion. The neonatal liver is susceptible to a wide variety of injuries, but the histologic reaction

is characteristic but nonspecific. Liver biopsy may demonstrate cholestasis, giant cell transformation, inflammation, hepatocellular necrosis, extramedullary hematopoiesis, fibrosis, and bile duct proliferation. Proliferation of bile ducts on liver biopsy is typical for biliary atresia,[36] but percutaneous liver biopsy may result in insufficient tissue for diagnosis, and early biopsy may not be diagnostic.

The findings on biopsy of several cholestatic liver diseases may overlap in early infancy.[37] The differential diagnosis of idiopathic neonatal obstructive cholangiopathy is critical in the first weeks of life because early performance of a hepatoportoenterostomy in patients with biliary atresia is known to reduce morbidity and mortality.[38,39]

Exclusion of infectious, metabolic and other causes of prolonged cholestasis in the newborn will leave 70 to 80% of patients with conjugated hyperbilirubinemia without an identified etiology. The key differentiation in these patients is between extrahepatic biliary atresia and neonatal hepatitis, which account for the vast majority of cases.[40,41] These conditions are discussed in greater detail in Chapters 17, 68, and 69.

Extrahepatic biliary atresia (BA)[42] is rare, occurs in one in 10,000 to 20,000 births, and is characterized by inflammation of bile ducts leading to progressive obliteration of the extrahepatic biliary tract leading to cirrhosis and hepatic failure. Biliary atresia represents the most common indication for pediatric liver transplant, representing more than 50% of cases in most series. Biliary atresia at the time of birth has a very poor prognosis, usually associated with other congenital defects and is also called embryonal BA. Without treatment, patients with biliary atresia will ultimately develop cirrhosis, and rapid identification of this condition is necessary because the success rate of establishing bile flow declines after 2 months of age. Increased age at surgery has a progressive and deleterious effect on the results of the Kasai operation until adolescence.[43] These findings provide a basis for early recognition of biliary atresia to reduce the need for liver transplantation in infancy and childhood.

None of the currently available tests or combinations is 100% reliable in diagnosing biliary atresia.[44-47] Laparotomy with intraoperative cholangiography and wedge hepatic biopsy has been considered the best available method to establish the presence or absence of BA. If BA is identified, a Kasai procedure can be performed. The chief disadvantage of this approach is that some infants with neonatal hepatitis will undergo surgery to exclude BA, whereas others with diseases such as arteriohepatic dysplasia (Alagille syndrome)[48] will undergo hepatoportoenterostomy but remain cholestatic. More recently, cholangiography has been performed laparoscopically with or without liver biopsy in the diagnosis of BA and is another way to obtain cholangiography. Finally, PTC can also provide a diagnosis of BA.

ERCP is a direct method of establishing a diagnosis of biliary continuity but requires an experienced endoscopist and is associated with complications, some of which can be life-threatening. However, in expert hands, ERCP can be safely performed even in the smallest infants.[49] Cholangiographic features of BA are illustrated in Figures 63-1 through 63-4.

One large series was recently published in which ERCP was performed in 140 consecutive patients less than 6 months of age (mean age 60 days, weight 4 kg) with suspected extrahepatic cholestasis over a 7-year period.[50] ERCP diagnosis was correlated with intraoperative findings. ERCP excluded BA in 34 (25%) but failed in 18 newborns (13%) for technical reasons. No severe complications occurred. Exploratory laparotomy was

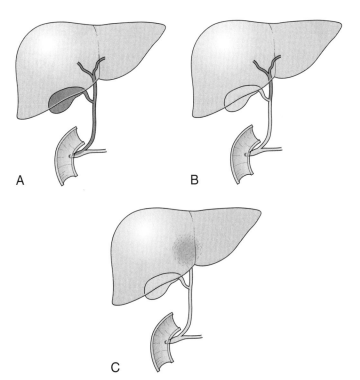

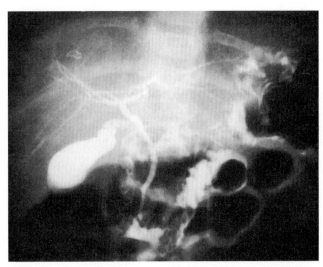

Figure 63-2. Neonatal hepatitis in a 41-day-old infant. A normal biliary tree is observed.

Figure 63-1. Schematic representation of the radiologic findings at ERCP in biliary atresia. In type 1 (**A**) there is no visualization of biliary tree. Type 2 (**B**) involves opacification of the distal common duct and gallbladder without visualization of the main hepatic duct. Type 3 (**C**) is divided in two subtypes: in Type 3a (shown) there is visualization of the distal common duct, the gallbladder and a segment of the main hepatic duct with biliary lakes at the porta hepatis; and in Type 3b both hepatic ducts are seen with biliary lakes.

performed in 106 (75%) patients and revealed BA in 80 (75% of the operated patients). Thus, the sensitivity of ERCP for diagnosing biliary atresia was 92% with a specificity of 73% and suggests that although ERCP is not a substitute for noninvasive imaging, it has the potential to avoid unnecessary surgery in almost 25% of cases. Hence, some recommend ERCP before exploratory laparotomy in all patients with suspected biliary atresia. The approach to BA and use of ERCP differs from center to center, but ERCP is feasible and safe[51,52] in the evaluation of neonatal cholestasis when other imaging modalities are inconclusive. In addition, despite the expanding role of MRCP, ERCP may still have a role in the multidisciplinary work-up of these patients, especially in those with an atypical presentation and in those with a nondiagnostic evaluation before surgery. One major drawback in patients with BA is that an inability to visualize the biliary tree may be due to technical reasons as well as complete obliteration of the bile duct, thus rendering a negative study inconclusive.

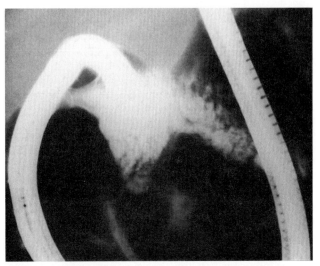

Figure 63-3. Pancreatogram of biliary atresia type 1 with acinarization. No opacification of the biliary tree is seen despite several maneuvers to opacify the common duct.

CHOLEDOCHOLITHIASIS

Common bile duct stones rarely occur in infants and children. Symptomatic choledocholithiasis, usually associated with cholelithiasis, is the predominant indication for ERCP in children (Figure 63-5). Laparoscopic cholecystectomy is now commonly performed in children for treatment of symptomatic cholelithiasis. ERCP is performed preoperatively when patients present with cholangitis and pancreatitis and when there is a high clinical suspicion of choledocholithiasis based on symptoms and imaging studies. ERCP is performed in the early postoperative

period when bile duct stones are identified by intraoperative cholangiography and/or cannot be removed intraoperatively by laparoscopic methods. Finally, ERCP is performed in the post-cholecystectomy patient who presents with choledocholithiasis.

Black pigment stones are usually found in children with hematological conditions that favor biliary pigment cholelithiasis, whereas light-colored cholesterol stones are more typical in adults.[53]

Conditions associated with the presence of stones include biliary tract malformations such as choledochal cyst, chronic liver disease, hemolysis, and progressive familial intrahepatic cholestasis type 3 (PFIC3). Bile duct stones may occur without any known predisposing conditions[54] and may be identified incidentally when imaging of other organ systems is performed. Asymptomatic neonatal cholelithiasis may resolve spontaneously, and even asymptomatic choledocholithiasis[55] can resolve without the need for aggressive intervention.[56] However, the risk of untreated choledocholithiasis, even in an asymptomatic patient, warrants stone removal because bile duct stones may become impacted in the distal common bile duct, resulting in

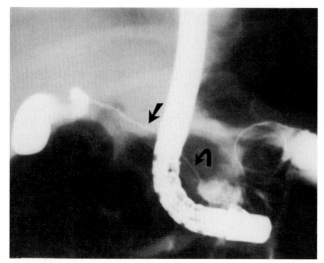

Figure 63-4. Biliary atresia type 2. A distal, narrowed, and irregular common bile duct is seen (curved arrow). The cystic duct is wider than the common duct (straight arrow). The gallbladder is normal. No opacification of the main hepatic ducts or the intrahepatic ducts is seen.

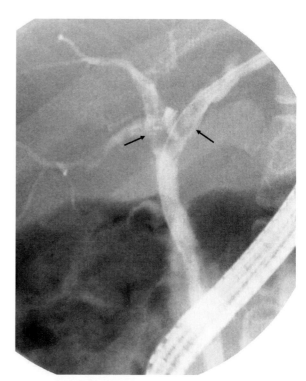

Figure 63-5. A 16-year-old with choledocholithiasis. ERCP shows filling defects (stones) in the intrahepatic system just above the biliary bifurcation (arrows).

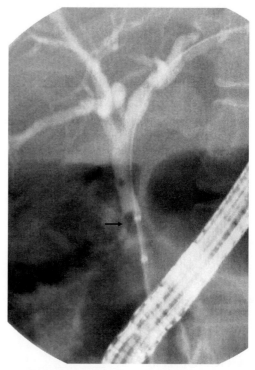

Figure 63-6. Same patient as Figure 63-5 following sphincterotomy and balloon sweeping of the duct. The filling defects at the bifurcation are no longer visible. The balloon is inflated (arrow).

clinical and biochemical obstructive jaundice and/or pancreatitis, even in infants. In the setting of cholangitis, urgent ERCP should be undertaken.

In patients with suspected choledocholithiasis, ultrasonography and MRCP[57,58] are useful for diagnosis, but ERCP allows for stone extraction. Bile duct stones are most commonly removed by incising the biliary sphincter (endoscopic biliary sphincterotomy)[59] using electrosurgical generators. Passage of retrieval balloons or baskets into the bile duct allows withdrawal of the stones into the duodenum (Figure 63-6). Endoscopic sphincterotomy with stone removal using balloons and/or baskets is effective in over 90% of patients. Balloon dilation of the biliary sphincter (sphincteroplasty) rather than sphincterotomy might seem to be an appealing alternative in young children because the long-term effects of sphincterotomy performed in childhood are unknown,[60] though the risk of pancreatitis is higher.[61]

CHOLEDOCHAL CYST

A choledochal cyst is a malformation of the biliary tract characterized by abnormal dilation (fusiform, saccular types) of the biliary tree.[62] Often they are accompanied by an anomalous pancreaticobiliary union (APBU).[63,64] However, APBU may also be found incidentally without cystic changes in the bile duct or in association with acute recurrent pancreatitis.[65]

The etiology remains obscure, and it is speculated that an anomalous connection of the pancreatic and bile ducts is a factor in the development of a choledochal cyst, with biliary dilatation following reflux of activated pancreatic secretions,[66] and that the cyst may be acquired.

Choledochal cyst is often an incidental finding. The classic triad of intermittent abdominal pain, jaundice, and a right upper quadrant abdominal mass is found in the minority of patients.

Choledochal cysts are classified according to the method proposed by Todani et al.[67] (Figure 63-7). Type 1 choledochal cyst is the most common and accounts for 90% of all choledochal cysts.[68] Congenital cystic dilation of the common bile duct is seen, and the terminal common bile duct is frequently narrowed as it enters the duodenum. Type I cysts vary in size

and shape. Type II is a rare congenital diverticulum of the common bile duct and does not produce jaundice.

The term *choledochocele* is applied to a type III cyst that is limited to the small intraduodenal segment of the common bile duct that herniates into the duodenal lumen. The clinical presentation is intermittent cholangitis and/or pancreatitis. This cyst has no premalignant potential and is essentially cured with ERCP and biliary sphincterotomy.[69]

Caroli's disease is classified as type IVA biliary cystic dilation with multiple intrahepatic and extrahepatic cysts; type IVB is cyst in the extrahepatic duct system only. Solitary liver cysts make up a type V lesion.[70]

Choledochal cysts have the potential for development of primary bile duct cancer (cholangiocarcinoma). Therefore, complete surgical excision of the cyst with the formation of a Roux-en-Y biliary enteric anastomosis is recommended and should be performed as early as possible to prevent complications. Long-term follow-up is required for surveillance for late complications and for cancer, particularly in type IV and V choledochal cysts where complete excision is not possible.

ERCP and MRCP are of value in outlining these cysts and their relationship to both ductal systems, and in detecting anomalous union of the duct.[71,72] These studies allow the surgical approach to be planned. Ultrasonography and CT do not provide the same quality of anatomic details, but can provide information about size, contour, position, and the presence of stones.

BILIARY STRICTURES

Primary Sclerosing Cholangitis

Primary sclerosing cholangitis (PSC) is a chronic, insidious cholestatic liver disease of uncertain etiology, characterized by inflammation and progressive obliterative intrahepatic and/or extrahepatic bile duct fibrosis.[73] It may lead to cirrhosis, end-stage liver disease, cholangiocarcinoma, and the need for liver transplantation. In children, the incidence of PSC is reported to be 0.23 cases per 100,000 person-years compared with 1.11 cases per 100,000 person-years in adults.[74] Sclerosing cholangitis in children is commonly associated with chronic inflammatory bowel disease (ulcerative colitis and Crohn's disease) and is

the most common hepatic complication of primary immunodeficiency disorders. Patients with PSC may present with clinical features that are indistinguishable from autoimmune hepatitis, and distinction is made during cholangiography.[75]

Liver histology can suggest the presence of large duct obstruction in PSC but cannot provide a specific diagnosis, as can ERCP. The accuracy of ERCP to diagnose PSC in children is the same as in adult patients. Characteristic radiographic findings include diffuse strictures of the intrahepatic or extrahepatic biliary tree, or both (Figure 63-8).

MRCP[76,77] has been shown to be a useful noninvasive method of evaluating the ductal system for strictures. The typical picture is one of the subtle, diffusely irregular intrahepatic ducts of alternating thin and thick caliber. Symptomatic patients, that is, those with frequent recurrent cholangitis or with progressive jaundice, may harbor a so-called dominant stricture and often demonstrate dramatic clinical improvement following ERCP with stricture dilation and short-term stent placement.

Balloon dilation and/or stenting of dominant biliary strictures in the setting of PSC may improve the observed 5-year survival rate significantly compared to that predicted from the Mayo risk scoring system. These data suggest that repeated endoscopic attempts to maintain biliary patency may improve the survival of patients with PSC and dominant strictures, though most data are derived from adult series.[78-80]

Post Liver Transplantation Strictures

Biliary strictures following pediatric liver transplantation may be assessed with MRCP. However, the biliary tree may be inaccessible for ERC because in infants and young children, as well as in those with PSC, choledochojejunal or hepaticojejunal anastomoses are usually performed during whole organ transplantation. However, the use of pediatric colonoscopes and balloon

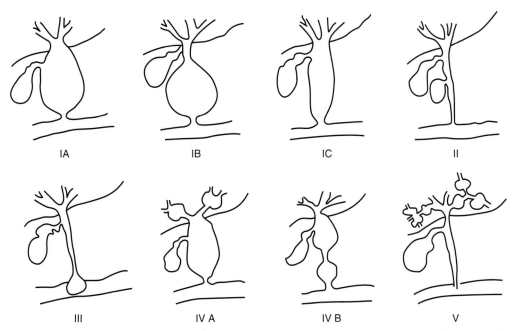

Figure 63-7. Choledochal cysts classification as described by Todani. Type IA: Saccular dilatation involving all or most of the extrahepatic bile duct. Type IB: Saccular dilatation involving a limited segment of the bile duct. Type IC: Fusiform dilatation involving all or most of the extrahepatic bile duct. Type II: Isolated diverticulum protruding from the wall of the common bile duct or joined to the common bile duct by a narrow stalk. Type III: Also known as choledochocele. Cystic dilatation of the intraduodenal portion of the common bile duct. Type IVA: Multiple dilatations of the intrahepatic and extrahepatic bile ducts. Type IVB: Multiple dilatations involving only the extrahepatic bile ducts. Type V: Also known as Caroli's disease. Multiple dilatations limited to the intrahepatic bile ducts.

enteroscopes[81,82] allows the hepaticojejunostomy (HJ) to be reached in most patients. Older children and adolescents often undergo transplantation with duct-to-duct anastomosis, which is managed as in adult liver transplant patients using standard duodenoscopes (Figure 63-9A,B). Strictures at the biliary enteric anastomoses are usually due to ischemia and may require surgical or radiologic intervention.

Strictures are definitely diagnosed and treated with PTC or ERCP.[83] Anastomotic strictures after duct to duct anastomosis are managed the same way as in adult patients at ERCP using dilation and stent therapy.[84-88]

BILIARY LEAKS

Biliary leaks occur in children with laceration of the liver after blunt abdominal trauma and also after cholecystectomy or other biliary surgery.[89-91] ERCP can be safely performed to confirm the source and to treat the leak by transpapillary stent placement with or without sphincterotomy (Figure 63-10A,B).[92,93] ERCP may also be helpful in identifying severity of ductal injury and need for surgery.[94] The diameter of biliary stent placed is determined by the ductal diameter. Therapeutic ERCP procedures like endoscopic sphincterotomy with stenting or nasobiliary drainage are effective in management of bile leaks following blunt abdominal trauma.

UNUSUAL BILIARY INFECTIONS

Human immunodeficiency virus (HIV) associated cholangiopathy has been described in children.[95] As in adults, the biliary abnormalities include irregularities of contour and caliber of the intrahepatic and extrahepatic ducts and papillary stenosis. The changes may result from concomitant infection with opportunistic organisms such as cytomegalovirus and *Cryptosporidium parvum*.

Parasitic Infections of the biliary tract are a common cause of biliary obstruction in endemic areas.[96,97] Tropical and subtropical countries have the highest incidence and prevalence of these infections. Radiologic imaging may show intrahepatic ductal dilatation. ERCP can be used diagnostically and therapeutically.[98] Endoscopic extraction of biliary ascariasis can be performed without sphincterotomy using wire guide baskets.[99,100]

BILIARY DYSKINESIA

Biliary dyskinesia[101,102] is a broad term for dysmotility of the gallbladder, termed gallbladder dyskinesia (GBD) and dysfunction of the sphincter of Oddi. Sphincter of Oddi dysfunction (SOD) is further subdivided into biliary SOD and pancreatic

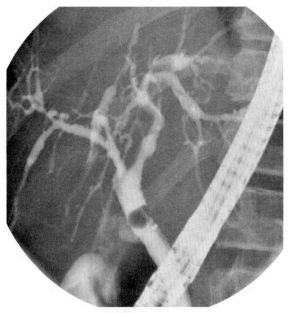

Figure 63-8. Cholangiogram showing changes of primary sclerosing cholangitis. Diffuse intrahepatic strictures and irregular bile ducts are seen.

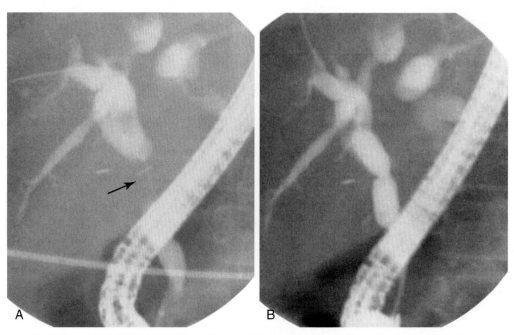

Figure 63-9. A 14-year-old girl transplanted for autoimmune hepatitis at age 9 with duct-to-duct biliary anastomosis. (**A**) Cholangiogram shows severe anastomotic biliary stricture (arrow). (**B**) Endoscopic balloon dilation shows waist at the level of the stricture. A stent was placed with good result.

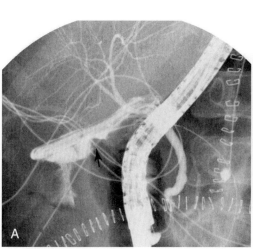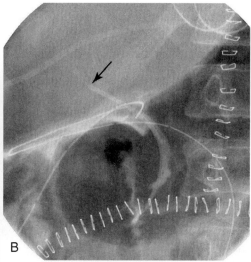

Figure 63-10. Bile leak following liver transplant with duct-to-duct biliary anastomosis. (**A**) Cholangiogram shows leak at the cystic duct (arrow). (**B**) Radiograph following endoscopic stent placement across the leak site (arrow denotes proximal end of stent).

SOD. GBD and biliary SOD cause typical biliary colic in the absence of gallstones (or postcholecystectomy), whereas pancreatic SOD typically presents with recurrent pancreatitis[103] or intermittent abdominal pain. GBD and SOD are uncommon in children. Sphincter of Oddi dysmotility is sometimes considered in children with unexplained biliary colic-like pain.

Manometric studies of the sphincter of Oddi during ERCP can be performed in the investigation of biliary dyskinesia. A water-perfused catheter with a pressure transducer is passed into the bile duct, and pressures are recorded during pull-through maneuvers. Normal values have been established in adults.[104] Although no normal manometric values have been established for children, some experts apply adult normal data and perform interventions such as biliary sphincterotomy when basal pressures exceeds 40 mm Hg (as is done in adults).

Combined biliary and pancreatic (dual) sphincterotomy is effective in relieving symptoms in a subgroup of children with SOD.[105,106] Improvement of abdominal pain following sphincterotomy has been reported in small numbers of patients, but no controlled outcome data exist for children.[105] The risk of post-ERCP pancreatitis is higher in patients with known or suspected SOD, and prophylactic pancreatic stents are often used.[107]

PANCREATIC DISORDERS

Congenital Malformations

Variants of the pancreatic duct system have been studied in autopsy series. The most common variant is pancreas divisum, occurring at a frequency of 3 to 10%.[108]

Pancreas divisum results from the failure of the dorsal and ventral pancreatic ducts to fuse. There is controversy in the literature at to whether pancreas divisum is a cause of pancreatitis. The most convincing data suggest that it is a cause of acute recurrent pancreatitis, though its role in chronic abdominal pain and chronic pancreatitis is unclear. Clinical recurrent pancreatitis has been found in pediatric patients with pancreas divisum without and with pancreatic duct stones.

MRCP and endoscopic ultrasound can be diagnostic of pancreas divisum[109-111] but ERCP is considered the gold standard to confirm the diagnosis. Cannulation of the major papilla

shows a short duct of Wirsung (ventral pancreas) that quickly tapers and arborizes (Figure 63-11A). Cannulation of the minor papilla is necessary to demonstrate the complete dorsal pancreatic ductal system (Figure 63-11B). Treatment is recommended only for patients with documented acute recurrent pancreatitis. Pancreas divisum patients with well-defined bouts of pancreatitis are more likely to benefit from endoscopic minor papillotomy than those without symptom-free intervals between "attacks" and those with pain that is not associated with elevated pancreatic enzymes.[112,113]

Endoscopic minor papilla sphincterotomy is the treatment of choice. Surgical sphincteroplasty of the minor papilla is indicated if endoscopic treatment fails and reendoscopy confirms persistent stenosis.

Although endoscopic treatment of pancreas divisum is performed in patients with disabling symptoms of chronic pancreatitis and includes dilation of strictures, removal of stones, and stent placement, this therapy is not performed specifically to treat pancreas divisum but rather to alleviate ductal obstruction. These maneuvers lead to clinical improvement in approximately 75% of children.[114,115]

Annular pancreas is an uncommon congenital anomaly, sometimes found incidentally. It is a ring of pancreatic tissue surrounding the duodenum that may cause symptoms and can present from the newborn period to advanced age.

In the pediatric age group, annular pancreas manifests with duodenal obstruction. Other features can include peptic ulceration, pancreatitis, and obstructive jaundice. Congenital anomalies are more common in children with annular pancreas (pancreatic divisum, Down syndrome, or cardiac and intestinal anomalies).[116]

Treatment involves bypassing the obstructed segment of duodenum by creating a duodenoduodenostomy or laparoscopic gastrojejunostomy.[117]

Acquired Disorders

Pancreatitis complicating ascariasis infestation occurs uncommonly in children living in endemic areas. *Ascaris lumbricoides* can cause biliary obstruction and result in obstructive jaundice

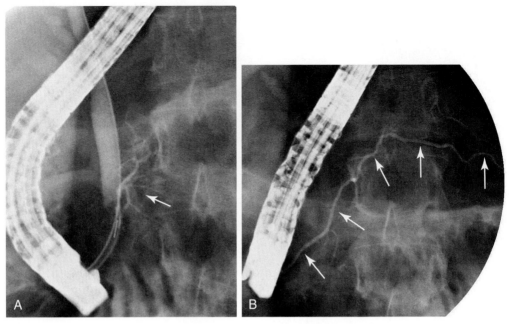

Figure 63-11. Pancreas divisum in a young girl. (**A**) Injection of contrast into major papilla fills bile duct and normal ventral pancreas (arrow). (**B**) Injection of contrast into minor papilla fills normal dorsal pancreatic duct, which fills to the tail. (Arrows outline the entire main pancreatic duct.)

and pancreatitis. These worms may be removed from the pancreaticobiliary tree with a tripod snare and other special instruments.[118,119] Drug therapy is administered concomitantly.

Sphincter of Oddi dysfunction of the pancreatic sphincter is also thought to be a potential cause of recurrent pancreatitis. In a retrospective review of 128 ERCP studies in children older than 1 year, nine patients underwent sphincter of Oddi manometry. Correlation was found between patients with anomalous pancreaticobiliary union, recurrent pancreatitis, and abnormal sphincter function. In another series ERCP was performed 34 times in 22 patients. Nine of these included sphincter manometry with abnormal results, leading to sphincterotomy in four patients. There was a significant reduction in the frequency and severity of pain after intervention.[120]

Dual endoscopic sphincterotomy of the pancreatic and common duct sphincters may reduce episodes of acute recurrent pancreatitis. However, the safety and efficacy of sphincter of Oddi manometry and sphincterotomy in the pediatric population with recurrent pancreatitis requires further study.

Abdominal Trauma

Motor vehicle accidents and other causes of blunt or penetrating trauma may cause pancreatic ductal disruption in children. Delayed recognition is not uncommon, because injuries to the body and tail of the pancreas may be clinically indolent. The pancreas is positioned over the spine; its location makes the organ vulnerable to injury by blunt abdominal trauma, which may fracture or sever the pancreatic duct. CT and magnetic resonance imaging (MRI) can suggest pancreatic rupture. Traumatic pancreatitis and its sequelae are associated with significant morbidity and mortality. Diagnosis with subsequent therapy should be accomplished as soon as possible to improve outcome. Patients with normal findings on ductography are treated conservatively.

ERCP is diagnostic for pancreatic duct laceration, showing extravasation of contrast material at the point of disruption.

Endoscopic transpapillary stent placement can produce rapid clinical and chemical improvement[121-124] and allow nonsurgical management of these patients.[125]

Pancreatic Pseudocysts

Pancreatic pseudocysts may be a result of acute or chronic pancreatitis and trauma (including postsurgical).[126] Endoscopic drainage is effective in most patients but is undertaken based on symptoms and not by size alone. Spontaneous resolution of large pseudocysts is known to occur. Endoscopic drainage, an alternative to percutaneous and surgical management, can be performed using a transpapillary or transmural approach. Transpapillary drainage is achieved by placing stents within the main pancreatic duct, whereas transmural drainage is achieved by passing large-bore stents through the gastric or duodenal wall into the pseudocyst (Figure 63-12A,B). Experience in children is limited to case reports and small series.[127,128]

Long-term outcome after successful endoscopic drainage of pancreatic pseudocysts is variable and is determined by the extent of pancreatic ductal damage after acute pancreatitis, degree of underlying chronic pancreatitis, and underlying etiology of pancreatitis.[129]

Acute Pancreatitis

Gallstones are uncommon in children and are a rare cause of pancreatitis. Trauma, infections, and idiopathic causes are the commonest etiological factors. Imaging plays a crucial role in the diagnosis of acute and chronic pancreatitis in children.[130,131] ERCP is rarely indicated in the setting of acute pancreatitis. If gallstones are present, they are managed by laparoscopic cholecystectomy with or without ERCP.[132]

As in adults, ERCP is most helpful in the setting of acute biliary pancreatitis when there is evidence of choledocholithiasis and biliary obstruction with cholangitis. Endoscopic biliary sphincterotomy and stone removal produce rapid improvement

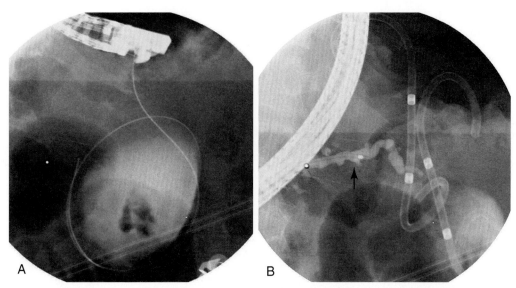

Figure 63-12. Endoscopic transmural pseudocyst drainage in a 16-year-old. (**A**) Following transgastric puncture, a guidewire is coiled inside an infected pseudocyst. (**B**) Radiograph after two stents have been passed through the gastrostomy into the pseudocyst. A pancreatogram was also obtained (arrow).

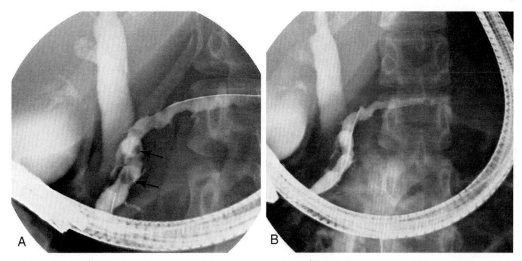

Figure 63-13. Endoscopic removal of pancreatic duct stones. (**A**) Pancreatogram shows filling defects (arrows) within a dilated pancreatic duct with changes of chronic pancreatitis. (**B**) Pancreatogram following pancreatic sphincterotomy and stone extraction using a balloon catheter.

without necessarily improving the pancreatitis because of improvement in cholangitis.

Chronic Pancreatitis

Recurrent episodes of pancreatitis may be caused by anomalies and abnormalities of the pancreatic and biliary ducts[133,134] and can be defined precisely by ERCP, but MRCP and endoscopic ultrasound are now used for diagnosis. ERCP is reserved for therapeutic maneuvers such as placement of a pancreatic duct endoprostheses and pancreatic stone extraction (Figure 63-13A,B). A longer follow-up period will be necessary to determine whether endoscopic success produces long-standing clinical improvement.

COMPLICATIONS OF ERCP

When performed by expert endoscopists, ERCP in children has a low complication rate comparable to that seen in adults. Complications include those related to sedation, pancreatitis, perforation, bleeding (following sphincterotomy), and infection

(cholangitis and infection of pancreatic pseudocyst). In general, infection is uncommon if adequate drainage is achieved, in either the bile duct or pancreas. The risk for ERCP-related complications in children is not well established because reported series include small numbers of patients. Reported complication rates range from 0 to 11%, with pancreatitis being the most common complication, as seen in the adult population.[135]

Interestingly, no major complications have been reported following ERCP in several series of neonates and young infants with neonatal cholestasis.

Prophylactic placement of small-caliber, temporary pancreatic duct stents has been shown to diminish the risk of post-ERCP pancreatitis in high-risk adult patients.[136] Data on the use of such stents in children are lacking.

SUMMARY

The diagnostic approach to disorders of the pancreaticobiliary system in children is through clinical evaluation combined with noninvasive imaging studies. Because ERCP is an invasive procedure, its diagnostic role has been replaced by high-quality CT, MRCP, and endoscopic ultrasound. ERCP is now used almost exclusively as a therapeutic tool, though it has some role in the diagnosis of biliary atresia in selected patients and centers. ERCP is not as commonly used in pediatric patients as in adult patients and is usually performed by specially trained adult gastroenterologists. Advanced training and continuing experience in ERCP are needed beyond general endoscopic competence. Increasingly, some pediatric gastroenterologists are undergoing specialized training in order to perform ERCP in pediatric patients. Careful patient selection and knowledge of available local skills and alternative methods will influence utilization and referral for ERCP in pediatric patients.

REFERENCES

1. Fox VL, Werlin SL, Heyman HB. Endoscopic retrograde cholangio-pancreatography in children. Subcommittee on Endoscopy and Procedures of the Patient Care Committee of the North American Society for Pediatric Gastroenterology and Nutrition. J Pediatr Gastroenterol Nutr 2000;30:335–342.
2. Pfau PR, Chelimsky GG, Kinnard MF, et al. Endoscopic retrograde cholangio-pancreatography in children and adolescents. J Pediatr Gastroenterol Nutr 2002;35:619–623.
4. Cheng CL, Fogel EL, Sherman S, et al. Diagnostic and therapeutic endoscopic retrograde cholangiopancreatography in children: a large series report. J Pediatr Gastroenterol Nutr 2005;41:445–453.
50. Petersen C, Meier PN, Schneider A, et al. Endoscopic retrograde cholangiopancreaticography prior to explorative laparotomy avoids unnecessary surgery in patients suspected for biliary atresia. J Hepatol 2009;51:1055–1060.
105. Varadarajulu S, Wilcox CM. Endoscopic management of sphincter of Oddi dysfunction in children. J Pediatr Gastroenterol Nutr 2006;42:526–530.
127. Haluszka O, Campbell A, Horvath K. Endoscopic management of pancreatic pseudocyst in children. Gastrointest Endosc 2002;55:128–131.
129. Sharma SS, Maharshi S. Endoscopic management of pancreatic pseudocyst in children-a long-term follow-up. J Pediatr Surg 2008;43:1636–1639.
135. Varadarajulu S, Wilcox CM, Hawes RH, Cotton PB. Technical outcomes and complications of ERCP in children. Gastrointest Endosc 2004;60:367–371.

See expertconsult.com for a complete list of references and the review questions for this chapter.

CAPSULE ENDOSCOPY AND SMALL BOWEL ENTEROSCOPY

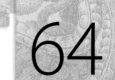

64

Brad Barth

Small bowel capsule endoscopy (CE) was introduced in 2001 as a noninvasive means of obtaining high-quality, color endoscopic images from the duodenum to the cecum. Soon thereafter, CE challenged traditional studies as the preferred method of examining the small bowel mucosa in adults. Early studies suggested superior lesion detection when compared to push enteroscopy[1-4] and small bowel follow-through or enteroclysis[5-8] in the evaluation of obscure gastrointestinal bleeding (GIB) and small bowel involvement of Crohn's disease (CD). Since those initial reports, CE has become a widely used tool in both adult and pediatric-aged patients for a number of indications including inflammatory disorders of the small bowel such as CD and celiac disease, obscure GIB, polyposis syndromes, unexplained growth failure, abdominal pain, and vascular anomalies. Diagnostic yield has been found to be superior to both small bowel follow-through and standard endoscopic investigation in the evaluation of children with suspected small bowel disease.[9] As of September 2009, CE had been approved by the Food and Drug Administration for use in children 2 years of age and older.

EQUIPMENT

The history of the development of the small bowel capsule is fascinating and has been well documented.[10] Although several companies now produce CE equipment, most clinical and research experience involves the PillCam SB by Given Imaging[11] (Yoqneam, Israel). This system uses a 26-mm by 11-mm capsule containing among other things a transmitter, battery, light source, and camera, which takes two pictures per second over a span of approximately 8 hours. The images are transmitted by radiotelemetry to a recording device worn by the patient[12] (Figure 64-1). A computer workstation is then used by the provider to download and review images and to create a report. A similar system called Endocapsule is produced by Olympus[13] using a capsule of identical size (Olympus America Inc, Center Valley, PA). Unfortunately, as of this writing no significantly smaller capsule is available.

PERFORMANCE OF CE STUDY

Compared with other methods of small bowel examination including radiographic evaluation, push enteroscopy, and over-tube or balloon-assisted enteroscopy, CE is easily performed. In our institution's experience, the capsule can be swallowed by children as young as 6 years of age. However, success of voluntary ingestion may depend more on maturity level and confidence of the child than chronologic age, because many older children and teenagers fail or refuse to swallow the capsule. In patients unable to swallow the capsule, endoscopic placement across the pylorus is fairly routine.

Patient Preparation

Debate continues over what type of preparation is superior before CE study. Standard instructions often include nothing by mouth for 12 hours before capsule ingestion. Then, 2 hours after capsule ingestion, the patient may take clear liquids. Four hours after ingestion, the patient may have a light meal. However, a recent meta-analysis has shown that bowel preparation with a purgative such as polyethylene glycol the day before the procedure,[14] and possibly with simethicone just before capsule ingestion,[15] improves visualization of small bowel mucosa. However, these preparations have not shown a beneficial effect on rate of complete examination or transit time. All reports on the effects of bowel preparation have been in adult patients; the ideal preparation for children, and its positive or negative effects, remains unknown.

Ingestion Versus Endoscopic Placement

Before performing capsule endoscopy studies in children, a fundamental question that must be answered is whether the patient will be able to voluntarily ingest the capsule. A swallowed capsule is preferable and tends to provide cleaner images, as capsule placement in small patients frequently causes mucosal trauma and self-limited bleeding that can confound the study interpretation. As mentioned previously, patients as young as 6 years of age have successfully swallowed the capsule, but children over the age of 8 will more reliably succeed. Seidman et al. have proposed a trial with candy such as large jelly beans before the study date to predict success.[16]

If a capsule cannot be swallowed, endoscopic placement across the pylorus is usually not a difficult procedure. This has been reported in children using polypectomy snares and Roth Net (US Endoscopy, Mentor, OH) to advance the capsule,[16,17] and a simple capsule delivery device for use with standard gastroscopes (AdvanCE, US Endoscopy, Mentor, OH) is now commercially available. Successful use of this device has been reported in a series of nine children from 4 to 8 years old.[18]

Endoscopic capsule placement can be performed with patients in the supine position, but passage through the posterior pharynx may be facilitated by a left lateral position. Following esophageal intubation, the next difficulty may be encountered when advancing the capsule through the pylorus. If significant resistance is encountered, careful balloon dilation of the pylorus to a diameter of 11 mm or greater is possible, or a small dose of glucagon will likely lead to pyloric relaxation, permitting passage. Another option is to gently pass a pediatric colonoscope or therapeutic endoscope across the pylorus just before passing the capsule to achieve dilation of the entire upper gastrointestinal (GI) tract. In cases where the capsule cannot pass the pylorus, it should not be deposited in the stomach, because the chances of it entering the duodenum without assistance are low. After the release of the capsule in the duodenum, it may be helpful to push the capsule as far distally as possible using the endoscope to prevent retrograde migration into the stomach. Prokinetic agents such as erythromycin or metoclopramide may be beneficial as well in preventing retrograde migration after endoscopic placement.

Image Review

Diagnostic review of capsule endoscopy studies is technically uncomplicated, and the software is well designed and user friendly. Formal recommendations do not yet exist regarding credentialing and competence for pediatric gastroenterology, but American Society for Gastrointestinal Endoscopy recommendations include completion of a gastrointestinal endoscopy training program, competence in upper GI endoscopy and colonoscopy, and either formal training in capsule endoscopy during GI fellowship or completion of a hands-on capsule endoscopy course with review of the first 10 capsule studies by an experienced capsule endoscopist.[19]

Physician review of capsule endoscopy studies can be time consuming, and the question has been raised whether the time required makes economic or practical sense.[20] Viewing practices certainly vary among physicians, but early studies reported small bowel viewing times of 34 to 120 minutes in adults.[2,3,5] It has been recommended that novice viewers read studies at an image rate of no higher than 12 to 15 frames per second, with experts reading at rates of up to 20 frames per second.[12]

INDICATIONS

There are a number of indications for small bowel CE in children. These include evaluation of small bowel mucosa for evidence of Crohn's disease, occult GIB, celiac disease, polyps and tumors, and graft-versus-host disease (GVHD). Other indications include evaluation of unexplained growth failure, abdominal pain, and protein-losing enteropathy or intestinal lymphangiectasia (Figure 64-2). These indications have primarily been described in retrospective case series and will be discussed individually.

Crohn's Disease

Capsule endoscopy is frequently used in the evaluation of suspected CD and has been shown to detect small bowel inflammation in patients with otherwise normal evaluations[5,6] (Figure 64-3). In adult patients, CE has been compared to enteroclysis, small bowel follow-through, and CT scan and found to be superior in establishing the presence and extent of small bowel inflammation in patients with known or suspected CD.[21-23] Based on several retrospective series, capsule endoscopy has been effective in the evaluation of suspected CD in children as well[9,24-26] and has been recommended by the North American Society for Pediatric Gastroenterology, Hepatology and Nutrition as an appropriate procedure when CD of the small bowel is strongly suspected but cannot be detected by other modalities.[27]

Differentiation of CD from ulcerative colitis remains clinically challenging at times, but one finding that is useful in this differentiation is significant small bowel mucosal inflammation. Cohen et al. retrospectively concluded that CE may lead to reclassification of inflammatory bowel disease (IBD) from ulcerative colitis or IBD unclassified to definitive CD.[28] Capsule endoscopy may also prove useful as a noninvasive way to document mucosal healing in CD and to monitor for postoperative recurrence proximal to surgical anastomoses. The use of CE as first-line evaluation of the small bowel in patients with suspected CD has been discussed but remains controversial;

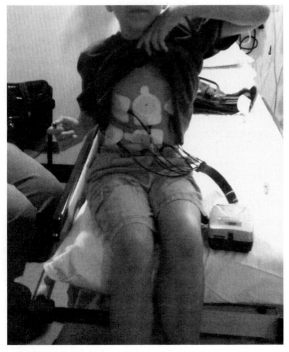

Figure 64-1. A 9-year-old boy with Crohn's disease preparing to undergo small bowel capsule endoscopy study.

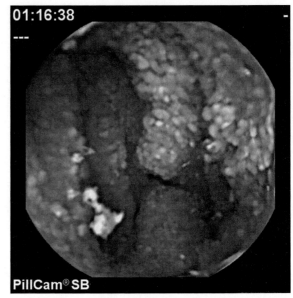

Figure 64-2. Dilated lacteals and focal bleeding in the mid small bowel seen on capsule endoscopy of an 8-year-old girl with protein-losing enteropathy and edema. (*See plate section for color.*)

however, it is clear that CE in children can be useful in the diagnosis and classification of IBD and may help to improve outcomes by facilitating appropriate choices of therapy.

Occult Gastrointestinal Bleeding

Soon after the introduction of small bowel CE, it became clear that the color images it provided were superior to radiographic evaluation in cases of suspected small bowel bleeding. Subsequently, it was determined that CE had higher diagnostic yield when compared to push enteroscopy,[2,3] likely due to its ability to view a greater length of small bowel mucosa. Based on these results, CE has become the first line of evaluation in adult patients with suspected small bowel bleeding when a lesion has not been identified by EGD or colonoscopy. No prospective studies have been performed in children, but case reports and small retrospective series support the use of CE in pediatric populations for this indication, reporting diagnostic yields of 62 to 100%.[9,29-32]

Celiac Disease

Traditional upper GI endoscopy with multiple duodenal biopsies, in conjunction with serologic evaluation, remains the standard approach for the diagnosis of celiac disease in children. However, recent literature has suggested that the use of small bowel biopsy as a gold standard for diagnosis of celiac disease has significant limitations such as poor acceptance of endoscopy in asymptomatic patients, patchy mucosal changes that could lead to false negative results, and the possibility of more severe villous atrophy in the proximal jejunum, not reachable by standard upper GI endoscopy.[33] Studies have not been performed in children, but a meta-analysis of three adult studies involving 107 patients revealed a sensitivity of 83% and specificity of 98% when CE was used to evaluate the proximal small bowel in patients with suspected celiac disease.[34] This analysis concluded that routine use of CE in the diagnosis of celiac disease could not be justified. However, in cases where standard endoscopy is refused or not possible, diagnosis is especially challenging, or patients are not

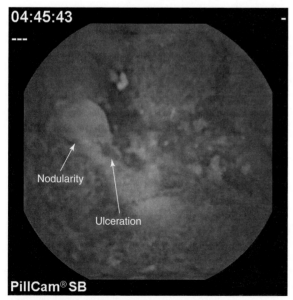

Figure 64-3. Capsule endoscopy image showing jejunal ulceration, exudates, and nodularity in a child with Crohn's disease. (*See plate section for color.*)

responding to appropriate therapy, CE could be considered as an option to view the more distal small bowel mucosa.

Polyposis

Children with polyposis syndromes such as Peutz-Jeghers syndrome, juvenile polyposis syndrome, and familial adenomatous polyposis are at risk of developing polyps in the small bowel. These polyps can predispose patients to complications ranging from bleeding to bowel obstruction to neoplastic transformation. Several studies have demonstrated the utility of CE in identifying polyps in the small bowel,[35-37] and small blinded comparisons to barium follow-through have favored CE for this indication.[38-40] One small pediatric trial showed that 90% of polyposis patients preferred CE to barium follow-through.[38] In summary, CE shows promise as a method of evaluating the small bowel in children with polyposis syndromes while avoiding exposure to radiation.

Graft-Versus-Host Disease

GVHD causes significant morbidity and mortality in patients undergoing stem cell transplantation, and the small intestine is a common site that requires investigation. Standard evaluation when GI symptoms are present includes endoscopy with biopsy,[41] but several groups have found CE to be useful as a low-risk, noninvasive alternative that allows visualization of a greater portion of the small bowel.[42-45] In fact, Neumann et al.[44] found that CE detected three cases of GVHD that would have been missed by standard endoscopy alone. However, three cases of GVHD were diagnosed on biopsy alone after normal-appearing upper endoscopy. Several weaknesses associated with this approach include the high prevalence of vomiting in patients with GVHD, making CE less likely to be successful, and the inability of CE to take biopsies. The lack of histologic specimens could result in failure to diagnose opportunistic infections or the misattribution of ulcerations found at CE as being due to GVHD rather than being due to other causes such as nonsteroidal anti-inflammatory medication usage.

Unexplained Growth Failure

Moy and Levine reported a series of seven patients who underwent CE following grossly and histologically normal upper GI endoscopy and colonoscopy in the evaluation of unexplained growth failure.[46] Four of these patients were found to have jejunal erosions or ulcerations, leading to therapy for Crohn's disease and subsequent weight gain.

Recurrent Abdominal Pain

The role of endoscopic evaluation in children with recurrent abdominal pain (RAP) is controversial. Shamir et al. performed CE in 10 children with RAP, hypothesizing that intestinal lesions beyond the reach of an endoscope may be responsible for patient symptoms.[47] All patients subsequently underwent standard upper GI endoscopy with biopsies. Capsule endoscopy in three patients revealed gross evidence of gastritis not seen by EGD, but detected on biopsy. All three subsequently responded to proton pump inhibitor therapy. In addition, evidence of ileocecal CD was found in a fourth patient by capsule endoscopy. Several months later this patient developed classic clinical signs of CD. Arguelles-Arias et al. performed CE in 16 children with chronic abdominal pain.[48] Significant findings were seen in the ileum of one patient suggestive of small bowel CD. Although CE is possibly helpful in rare, isolated cases, routine use of CE in children with abdominal pain without other symptoms cannot be supported based on these findings.

Protein-Losing Enteropathy/Intestinal Lymphangiectasia

Gastrointestinal protein loss can be a challenging clinical problem. CE has been used to diagnose and determine the extent of lymphangiectasia,[9,49] yielding positive results in patients following normal upper GI endoscopy due to the potentially patchy distribution of the disease.

LIMITATIONS

The limitations of small bowel CE are apparent, and the true sensitivity of CE studies remains unknown. The greatest limitation is the inability to obtain tissue samples for histologic evaluation. In addition, the clinician reading CE images is at the mercy of variations in gastrointestinal motility that can greatly affect the amount of mucosa that is actually seen. Other limitations include incomplete small bowel transit, luminal debris impairing visualization, inadequate bowel distention, rapid transit through portions of the bowel, and inability to steer or deflect the field of view.[50,51]

Another significant limitation of CE in a pediatric population is the large size of the capsule. Although inability to swallow the capsule can easily be overcome by endoscopic placement, the ability of the capsule to traverse a child's GI tract can be limited by the size of the upper esophagus, pylorus, bowel lumen, and ileocecal valve. Publications have reported CE in children as young as 18 months[52] and as small as 12 kg,[30] and at our center successful CE has been performed in children as small as 9 kg.

CONTRAINDICATIONS AND COMPLICATIONS

There are few absolute contraindications to performing CE in pediatric or adult-sized patients. In 2006 the American Society for Gastrointestinal Endoscopy listed the presence of known or suspected stricture, bowel obstruction or pseudo-obstruction, presence of pacemaker or other implanted electromedical device, swallowing disorder, and pregnancy as contraindications to CE study.[53] However, with the exception of pseudo-obstruction and pregnancy, these could be considered relative contraindications. In patients with known strictures where surgery is planned, CE could help surgeons identify clinically significant lesions. Safe and effective CE has been reported in patients with pacemakers as well, including one child,[54,55] although telemetry should be considered for the duration of the study.

The primary complication associated with CE in children is capsule retention, or failure to naturally excrete the capsule. Atay et al. reported a series of 207 pediatric patients undergoing CE study for various indications.[56] The capsule retention rate was 1.4% which is similar to rates reported in larger adult series. All three patients in this series who suffered capsule retention had known Crohn's disease, and all had a body mass index below the 5th percentile for age. Thus, known Crohn's disease and BMI less than the 5th percentile should be considered red flags for potential CE retention.

There is no recommendation as to how long a retained capsule may safely remain in the GI tract, and the longest reported period a capsule has been retained in an adult is 38 months.[57] However, complications such as perforation, impaction, and fracture of the capsule requiring laparotomy have been reported.[58-60] Prevention of capsule retention is difficult, if not impossible. And, with the exception of known Crohn's disease, in the majority of patients, small bowel contrast series has repeatedly been shown to be ineffective in identifying lesions predisposing to capsule retention. The Patency System, or Agile Capsule (Given Imaging Ltd, Yoqneam, Israel), is a biodegradable capsule of identical size to the video capsule that may be useful in determining the safety of performing CE in adults and children. Failure of the patency capsule to traverse the GI tract should be considered a relative contraindication to capsule endoscopy.

Other potential complications include emesis related to capsule ingestion, aspiration of video capsule,[61] and equipment failure, which may not be evident until review of the images is attempted.

ENTEROSCOPY

Introduction

Although capsule endoscopy has revolutionized diagnostic examination of the entire length of the small bowel, its inability to biopsy or perform therapeutic interventions when lesions are detected remains a significant limitation. However, new techniques such as balloon and spiral enteroscopy now allow fairly low-risk and reliable access to the jejunum and ileum where biopsies and standard endoscopic therapies such as polypectomy, foreign body or retained video capsule removal, stricture dilation, and hemostasis can be performed. These innovative techniques often allow deep intubation of the small intestine without the need for surgical assistance and can be performed safely in an outpatient setting.

Push Enteroscopy

Historically the most popular type of small bowel endoscopic exam, push enteroscopy involves the gradual advancement of a specially designed, long enteroscope with a standard working channel as deeply as possible into the small intestine. Alternatively, a pediatric colonoscope is often used. The primary limitation of push enteroscopy is that sharp angulation of the duodenum dissipates the propelling force transmitted to the endoscope, resulting in loop formation in the upper GI tract.[62] Reducing these loops is difficult, and they significantly affect depth of intubation. True depth of insertion is difficult to measure and varies greatly among patients and examiners, but 120 to 180 cm beyond the ligament of Treitz is possible using standard push enteroscopy.[63] Sonde enteroscopy is currently considered obsolete and will not be discussed in this chapter.

Balloon Enteroscopy (Push and Pull Enteroscopy)

Double-Balloon Enteroscopy

First described in 2001,[64] and commercially available since 2003, double-balloon enteroscopy (DBE) (Fujinon Inc, Saitama, Japan) allows evaluation and therapy of the jejunum and ileum in adults and children. The principle involved is that an overtube with an inflated balloon can anchor and shorten the intestine when retracted, while straightening the bowel yet to be examined, allowing deep advancement of the enteroscope and preventing undesired looping (Figure 64-4). Thus, the force of insertion is transmitted to the tip of the enteroscope. The bowel that has already been viewed is "telescoped" on the overtube so no further stretching occurs.[65] The "second" balloon is located at the tip of the enteroscope and is intermittently inflated to anchor the scope and prevent slippage while the overtube is gradually advanced. Well-organized, concentric rings should be created as the endoscope traverses the small bowel, signifying successful deep enteroscopy (Figure 64-5). Using this technique, complete small bowel viewing from duodenum to cecum, or by a combined antegrade and retrograde approach can at times be achieved, although the rate of complete examination varies by reporting author and geographic origin of the series. The overtubes used for diagnostic and therapeutic DBE have outer diameters of 12.2 and 13.2 mm, respectively.

Double-balloon enteroscopy and capsule endoscopy have been compared in adults, and a meta-analysis suggests that the two techniques have a comparable diagnostic yield in the evaluation of small bowel disease, including obscure GI bleeding.[66] However, Nakamura et al. found that the entire small bowel could be viewed 90% of the time by CE compared to only 62% of the time by DBE.[67] Although there have been reports of lesions missed by CE and detected by DBE,[68,69] it is likely that CE provides a more complete exam of the entire length of small bowel. Given its noninvasive qualities, CE should be considered the first line of endoscopic evaluation for portions of small

bowel not viewed by standard upper endoscopy and ileocolonoscopy when urgent therapeutic techniques are not indicated.

Successful DBE has been reported in children. Leung performed DBE in 15 patients under 20 years of age, five of whom were less than 10 years old.[70] Indications included GI bleeding, recurrent abdominal pain, Crohn's disease, and suspected stricture. Liu et al. reported successful DBE in 31 children aged 3 to 14 years with a reported diagnostic rate of 77.8%.[71] Lin et al. reported successful DBE and small bowel polypectomy in a small series of children aged 8 to 19 years.[72]

Indications for DBE in children are identical to those in adults and include biopsy, evaluation and treatment of small bowel bleeding, polypectomy, and stricture dilation (Figure 64-6). Furthermore, DBE can be used to intubate the Roux-en-Y limb and obtain access to the biliary tree after hepatoenterostomy in adults and children.[73,74]

Single-Balloon Enteroscopy

The technique of single-balloon enteroscopy (SBE) is quite similar to that of DBE in that a 13.2-mm outer diameter overtube with a balloon at the distal end is used to shorten and straighten the small bowel, allowing deep intubation and biopsy or therapeutic maneuvers (Figure 64-7). In contrast to DBE, there is no balloon on the tip of the enteroscope. Indications for SBE are identical to those for DBE, including histologic evaluation of suspected small bowel Crohn's disease (Figure 64-8). Concerning patient size, successful SBE has been reported in a 37-month-old, 13.5-kg toddler with occult GI bleeding and an abnormal capsule endoscopy study.[75] It is generally thought that the depth of insertion is slightly less using SBE compared to DBE, but this has not been formally evaluated in children.

Spiral Enteroscopy

Another method of performing deep enteroscopy involves an overtube with a flexible spiral at the tip (Figure 64-9). When rotated, the spiral on the overtube pleats, straightens, and

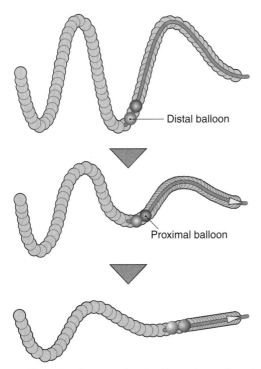

Figure 64-4. Illustration demonstrating the effects of overtube reduction on the bowel. Note in the middle image the small bowel pleating as the overtube is reduced in the direction of the small arrow. The most distal balloon (labeled) at the tip of the enteroscope helps to anchor the scope and prevent slippage. The more proximal balloon (labeled) is attached to the overtube and pulls the intestine when the overtube is retracted. In the bottom image, the bowel proximal to the balloons has shortened, while the bowel distal to the scope and overtube has straightened, facilitating deeper insertion. Adapted with permission from Yamamoto H, Kita H. Double-balloon endoscopy: from concept to reality. Gastrointest Endosc Clin North Am 2006;16:352.

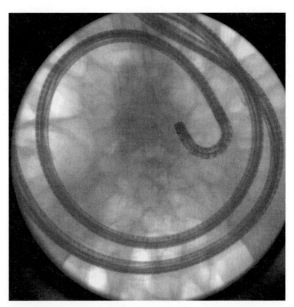

Figure 64-5. Intraprocedural fluoroscopy image demonstrating organized concentric ring formation of the enteroscope and overtube. This configuration is important for successful deep intubation of the small bowel.

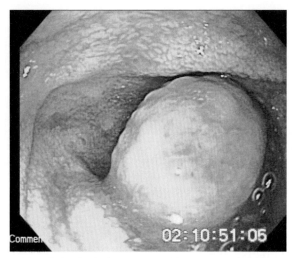

Figure 64-6. Ileal polyp before snare resection using single-balloon enteroscopy in a 14-year-old girl with juvenile polyposis syndrome. (*See plate section for color.*)

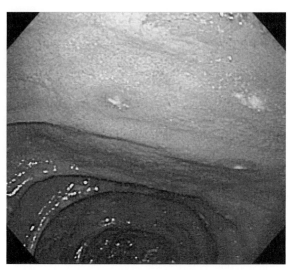

Figure 64-8. Retrograde single-balloon enteroscopy image demonstrating scattered, focal, aphthous ulcers in the proximal ileum of a child with Crohn's disease. (*See plate section for color.*)

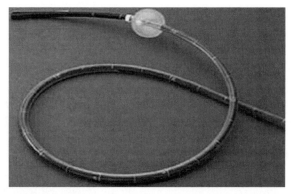

Figure 64-7. Single-balloon enteroscopy overtube with enteroscope. From Pasha SF, Leighton JA. Enteroscopy in the diagnosis and management of Crohn disease. Gastrointest Endosc Clin North Am 2009;19:435.

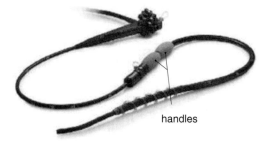

handles

Figure 64-9. Spiral overtube and enteroscope. The handles are used to rotate the overtube, allowing the soft spiral portion to act as a "corkscrew," leading to rapid, deep small bowel intubation as the intestine is retracted. Akerman PA, Cantero D. Spiral enteroscopy and push enteroscopy. Gastrointest Endosc Clin North Am 2009;19:358.

retracts the small bowel using an action similar to that of a corkscrew, leading to rapid and easy advancement of the enteroscope. Although spiral enteroscopy appears to be the simplest and most affordable method of deep enteroscopy (no equipment is required other than the overtube), the 16-mm diameter of the overtube plus spiral currently makes this technique impractical for most pediatric patients.

COMPLICATIONS

Potential complications of enteroscopy include those common to any endoscopic procedure, specifically bleeding, perforation, and sedation- or anesthesia-related problems. A large retrospective multicenter study of DBE complications reported a major complication rate of 0.9%, including perforation (0.4%), bleeding (0.2%), and pancreatitis (0.2%) in adults.[76] Perforation was more likely to occur with a transanal or retrograde approach and in patients with surgically altered anatomy where adhesions may have impeded retraction of the bowel onto the overtube. A perforation in a 46-month-old boy with Peutz-Jeghers syndrome has been reported following DBE and small bowel polypectomy.[77] Sore throat, abdominal

discomfort, and postoperative nausea are the only reported complications in the three reported pediatric series.[69-71]

INTRAOPERATIVE ENTEROSCOPY

Intraoperative enteroscopy reliably accesses the entire small bowel by passing an endoscope throughout the lumen to the cecum either via a surgically created enterotomy or by mouth. This technique requires the assistance of a surgeon and has the advantage of assured success and the ability to immediately treat any bleeding or perforation associated with the procedure. The obvious disadvantage is the invasive nature of the procedure and likelihood of prolonged postoperative ileus. Laparoscopically assisted intraoperative enteroscopy has been reported but is technically challenging.

CONCLUSION

Technological advances in the 21st century now allow detailed and safe endoscopic examination and therapy of the entire small bowel in children as well as adults. Capsule endoscopy and deep enteroscopy complement each other well and should be considered valuable tools in the evaluation and management of children with suspected or confirmed diseases of the small bowel.

REFERENCES

5. Costamagna G, Shah SK, Riccioni ME, et al. A prospective trial comparing small bowel radiographs and video capsule endoscopy for suspected small bowel disease. Gastroenterology 2002;123:999–1005.

9. Thomson M, Fritscher-Ravens A, Mylonaki M, et al. Wireless capsule endoscopy in children: a study to assess diagnostic yield in small bowel disease in paediatric patients. J Pediatr Gastroenterol Nutr 2007;44:192–197.

29. Guilhon de Araujo Sant' Anna AM, Kubois J, Miron M, et al. Wireless capsule endoscopy for obscure small-bowel disorders: final results of the first pediatric controlled trial. Clin Gastroenterol Hepatol 2005;3:264–270.

52. Fritscher-Ravens A, Scherbakov P, Bufler P, et al. The feasibility of wireless capsule endoscopy in detecting small intestinal pathology in children under the age of 8 years – a multicenter European study. Gut 2009;58:1467–1472.

70. Leung Y. Double balloon endoscopy in pediatric patients. Gastrointest Endosc 2007;66:s54–s56.

71. Liu W, Xu C, Zhong J. The diagnostic value of double-balloon enteroscopy in children with small bowel disease: report of 31 cases. Can J Gastroenterol 2009;23:635–638.

See expertconsult.com for a complete list of references and the review questions for this chapter.

65

GASTROINTESTINAL MOTILITY PROCEDURES

Leonel Rodriguez • Samuel Nurko

The gastrointestinal (GI) tract has evolved specific mechanisms to allow ingestion of nutrients, their transport for digestion and absorption, and finally the expulsion of unused portions. This aboral propulsion of gastrointestinal contents is orchestrated by the complex interaction between the gastrointestinal muscle and the enteric, peripheral, and central nervous systems and is discussed elsewhere in the text. Each area of the gastrointestinal tract has a specific motility pattern that allows it to perform its necessary function. In children, these patterns have been well characterized for the esophagus, gastric antrum, duodenum, jejunum, ileum, colon, and anorectum.[1]

Gastrointestinal transit can be evaluated by many different techniques (markers, radionuclide testing, etc.). However, the evaluation of gastrointestinal motility can only be performed with the use of manometric studies, which are designed to show the contractile events of the organ that is being studied. This allows the understanding of gastrointestinal physiology and the pathophysiology of motility disorders. The main focus of this chapter is on those manometry tests that have been designed to study gastrointestinal motility.[1]

GASTOINTESTINAL MOTILITY STUDIES

Gastrointestinal motility is assessed by identifying and characterizing intraluminal pressure changes detected by the introduction of specially designed catheters in the lumen of the organ that is being studied. The intraluminal pressure is then transmitted and recorded. In general, intraluminal pressure can be evaluated with water-perfused or solid-state systems.[1] Many pediatric laboratories use water-perfused systems, in which the catheter is connected indirectly to a computer by a series of transducers. The catheters have predetermined openings that allow the recording of different segments. The catheters are perfused with a pneumohydraulic pump at a predetermined rate, and pressure changes in the orifices are transmitted to pressure transducers with the use of low-compliance capillary tubing. On the other hand, solid-state catheters have strain-gauge pressure transducers; the information is captured by digital recording systems and is downloaded into computers for analysis. The main advantage of the solid-state catheter is that it does not involve perfusion and allows the performance of prolonged ambulatory studies. The main limitations have been the cost and the larger caliber of the catheters, although recent years have seen the technical development of much smaller catheters.

There are important differences in the performance of manometric studies in children when compared to adults. These include the different ages of the studied patients, as there may be developmental changes; a paucity of studies in normal controls; and technical difficulties inherent to studying children. The lack of normal controls has been the most important limiting factor for the establishment of normal motility patterns in children, although in recent years more studies performed in children without a motility disorder have been reported.[2] This lack of control information can make the interpretation difficult and may potentially lead to overinterpretation of the findings. Performing studies in children requires a certain level of cooperation, because motility patterns are difficult to interpret when there is significant artifact. Young and uncooperative patients may require sedation[1]; there are studies that report no effect of midazolam on esophageal motility,[3] and others that show that chloral hydrate,[1] midazolam, and certain agents used for general anesthesia have no effect on the rectoanal inhibitory reflex.

Recently, a pediatric task force and a group of experts of the American Neurogastroenterology and Motility Society (ANMS) established minimum standards for the performance of manometric studies in children and adults.[1,4]

ESOPHAGEAL MANOMETRY

Esophageal manometry is the gold standard for the diagnosis of primary motor disorders of the esophagus (Table 65-1).[5,6] The most common indication in children is dysphagia with no evidence of anatomic obstruction.[1]

Normal Anatomy and Physiology

There are three functional regions of the esophagus: the upper esophageal sphincter (UES), the esophageal body, and the lower esophageal sphincter (LES). The UES is composed of striated muscle that relaxes in response to swallows and remains closed in between swallows by tonic stimulation of somatic nerves. It is asymmetric, with greater resting pressure values in the anteroposterior axis.[5] The UES measures 0.5 to 1 cm at birth and increases in length to 3 cm in the adult.[7] UES resting pressure in adults varies from 40 to 193 mm Hg,[5] and we have reported a mean pressure of 116 ± 9.6 mm Hg in healthy children.[2]

The esophageal body is composed of both striated (in the upper third) and smooth muscle. The resting pressure is usually lower than intragastric pressure and varies with respiration. Primary peristalsis occurs after swallowing,[5,7] normally progresses at a speed of 2 to 4 cm/s, and has a typical duration of 4 seconds (Figure 65-1).[8] The typical contraction pressures of peristaltic waves are between 35 and 180 mm Hg. Limited information

TABLE 65-1. Manometric Findings in Esophageal Motility Disorders

Upper Esophageal Sphincter (UES) Achalasia

Incomplete or delayed UES relaxation in relationship to pharyngeal contraction

Lower Esophageal Sphincter (LES) Achalasia

Absence of esophageal peristalsis*
Incomplete or abnormal LES relaxation
Increased LES pressure
Elevated intraesophageal pressure as compared to intragastric pressure

Incompetent LES

LES resting pressure < 10 mm Hg

Diffuse Esophageal Spasms

Repetitive, simultaneous (nonperistaltic) contractions, at least 20% of wet swallows
Periods of normal peristaltic sequences
Alterations in the contraction waves (repetitive, increased duration and amplitude), although there are patients who can have normal amplitude
A normal LES in most patients, although incomplete LES relaxation or a hypertensive sphincter have been described

Nutcracker Esophagus

Increased distal peristaltic amplitude (180 mm Hg)
Increased distal peristaltic duration (>6 s)

Ineffective Esophageal Motility

Low-amplitude contractions (<30 mm Hg)
Triple peaked waves, spontaneous isolated contractions, retrograde contractions
Prolonged contractions (>6 s)
Aperistalsis or nontransmitted contractions (during >20% of wet swallows)
Simultaneous contractions (>30% of wet swallows)

*Required to make the diagnosis.

is available in healthy children; in our studies, the mean contraction amplitude in the upper esophagus was 60.7 ± 9.5 mm Hg and in the lower esophagus 94 ± 3.3 mm Hg, with a mean duration of contractions of 3.5 ± 0.1 seconds.[2] Peristaltic characteristics need to be evaluated during wet swallows. Secondary peristalsis occurs in response to luminal distention, and tertiary contractions consist of spontaneous and usually simultaneous nonperistaltic contractions.

The LES is tonically contracted and its resting pressure varies based on series. Some authors have reported a value of 22 ± 5 mm Hg[9]; others have reported 15 ± 2 mm Hg[10] and 29 ± 2 mm Hg[11]; and we have reported a mean LES pressure of 24 ± 2 mm Hg.[2] In adults, LES pressure varies from 10 to 45 mm Hg.[12] LES relaxation usually occurs with swallowing, and it has also been reported to occur transiently not associated to swallowing known as transient lower esophageal sphincter relaxations (TLESR). TLESRs are thought to be the main pathophysiologic mechanism in the development of gastroesophageal reflux disease (GERD).[10,12] The most accurate way to measure LES pressure and function is with the use of a sleeve, which straddles the LES. However, accurate measurements for clinical use can also be obtained with regular perfused unidirectional pressure ports. The measurement of LES pressure is always performed relative to intragastric pressure. Different methods used to measure basal lower esophageal sphincter pressure include either midrespiratory or end-expiratory points. Midexpiratory pressure is the mean pressure at the midpoint of amplitude of the phasic respiratory component, whereas the end-expiratory pressure is when the tonic component is used alone.[5]

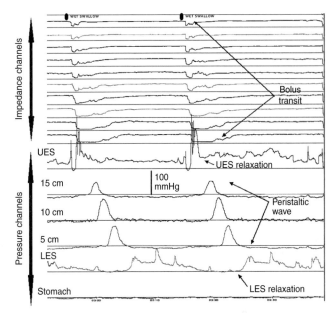

Figure 65-1. Normal esophageal manometry. This represents a combined manometry and impedance study. The upper 10 channels represent impedance measurements, while the lower 6 channels represent pressure measurements. A normal response to wet swallows can be observed. There are UES and LES relaxations, followed by normal esophageal peristalsis. The impedance channels show a normal progression of a saline bolus. UES, upper esophageal sphincter; LES, lower esophageal sphincter.

Before the Procedure

Medications known to affect motility (e.g., prokinetics, anticholinergics, narcotics) are held for at least 48 hours before the procedure, and children fast for 4 to 6 hours, depending on their age and the need for sedation.

Catheter Placement

The manometry catheter is usually placed nasally, although it can be placed orally as well, particularly in premature infants. In older children, nasal topical anesthesia with topical cocaine or viscous lidocaine is frequently used.

Procedure

There is no standardized protocol to perform esophageal manometry in children. The pediatric task force of the AMS recommends the use of the slow pull-through technique.[1] This consists of the introduction of the catheter into the stomach, and its slow withdrawal until the different esophageal segments are identified. After the catheter is in position, and baseline measurements are recorded, responses to swallowing are observed. If possible, a swallowing marker should be used, although, particularly in young children, careful observation and manual recording are often employed. Swallows of water (wet swallows) at room temperature (approximately 1 mL in infants and 3 to 5 mL in older children) are necessary for peristaltic evaluation,[1] as they result in a more consistent peristaltic response than those occurring with saliva.[8] In a typical study, 10 separate wet swallows are evaluated.[13] In young children and infants, gently blowing air in the child's face (the Santmeyer reflex) may induce swallowing.[14] The amplitude, duration, and peristaltic characteristics of the esophageal contractions are then measured.[14] The UES is usually evaluated at the end of the study, although with the advent of high-resolution manometry it can be done simultaneously. The UES relaxes to baseline, and the relationship between pharyngeal contractions and UES relaxation is determined. The clinical utility of UES/pharyngeal measurements is not well established in children. Even though UES measurements can be obtained, it is not clear that manometric findings are sensitive enough to have a clear impact on patient management.[5] The role of provocative tests during esophageal manometry has not been evaluated in children, so their use is not currently recommended.

The use of high-resolution manometry (see later discussion) is simplifying and revolutionizing the performance of esophageal manometry in children, as it allows a single intubation that will measure the whole esophageal length, without the need for a pull-through (Figure 65-2).

Interpretation

Normal Motility

LES pressure varies from 10 to 45 mm Hg in adults. LES relaxation needs to be coordinated for more than 90% of wet swallows and complete, with a drop to intragastric pressure. Normal peristaltic variants include failed peristalsis in 4 to 15%[8] and double-peak contractions in adult controls.[8] Normal peristalsis is considered present when at least 70% of wet swallows are normal. Based on simultaneous manometric, videofluoroscopic and impedance studies, an esophageal contraction less than 30 mm Hg is now considered hypotensive and is used to separate effective from ineffective peristalsis[5,812,15]; any contraction higher than 180 mm Hg is considered hypertensive.[5,8]

Indications and Clinical Utility

Esophageal manometry is indicated to assess esophageal function in children and adolescents with dysphagia, odynophagia and chest pain of noncardiac origin.[1] Esophageal motility is the gold standard for diagnosing primary motility disorders (see Table 65-1).

Primary Esophageal Motility Disorders

Esophageal motility is gold standard in the diagnosis of achalasia.[1] Manometric findings characteristic of achalasia include esophageal body aperistalsis (hallmark of the disease), elevated LES resting pressure, incomplete or absent LES relaxation (some show normal relaxation), and higher esophageal intraluminal pressure compared to intragastric pressure[16,17] (Figure 65-3). It has been reported that esophageal manometry also provides quantitative information about the severity of the achalasia and the response to medical treatment.[1] The utility of esophageal motility in the evaluation of the symptomatic child after achalasia treatment has also been shown.[18] Esophageal manometry also aids in the diagnosis of other esophageal motility disorders, including diffuse esophageal spasm and nutcracker esophagus. The term *ineffective esophageal motility* is used to describe abnormal manometric findings (including aperistaltic, repetitive, or multipeaked contractions; low-amplitude contractions; intermittent segmental contractions; and prolonged contraction duration[8]) that do not fit the criteria for a defined primary esophageal motility disorder.[19]

Gastroesophageal Reflux Disease

Manometry is not indicated in the routine evaluation of GERD, but it may be helpful when the diagnosis is not clear and a primary motility disorder is being considered[5] in patients who have not responded to medical therapy, before a fundoplication, when a severe underlying motility disorder is suspected, and to locate the LES before the placement of a pH/impedance probe. Preoperative manometry in patients with GERD has not predicted postoperative outcome[5,20] Preoperative esophageal manometry may have a role evaluating children with scleroderma or tracheoesophageal fistula,[21,22] in which fundoplication may create or aggravate a functional obstruction.

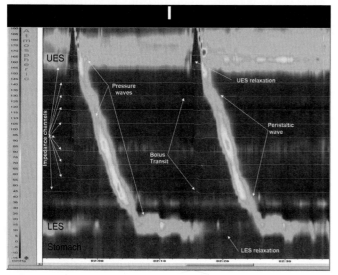

Figure 65-2. Normal high-resolution manometry. Contour plot obtained with the use of high-resolution manometry and impedance in a healthy child. The colors represent different pressure intensity, as can be seen in the scale. A normal response to wet swallows can be observed. There are UES and LES relaxations, followed by normal esophageal peristalsis. The impedance channels in white show a normal progression of a saline bolus (bolus transit).

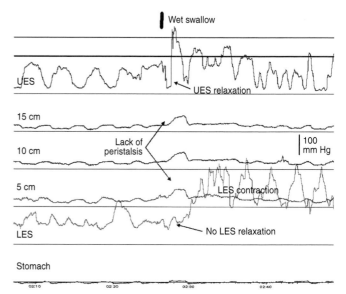

Figure 65-3. Manometric findings in achalasia. Esophageal manometry of a child with achalasia. There is normal UES relaxation, a lack of LES relaxation, with a paradoxical contraction after swallowing, lack of esophageal peristalsis, and a high baseline esophageal pressure.

Connective Tissue Disorders

Esophageal manometry may be useful in confirming the diagnosis of connective tissue diseases,[1,12] particularly scleroderma, which shows the most defined esophageal abnormalities.[23,24] Other connective tissue disorders also have motor alterations in the esophagus, including juvenile localized scleroderma,[25] systemic lupus erythematosus, and those with mixed connective tissue disease.[26]

Chest Pain

Esophageal manometry should not be routinely used as the initial test,[12] but rather when other tests do not provide a clear explanation. Most patient show ineffective esophageal motility and only a minority show achalasia or diffuse esophageal spasms.[12] In a large study of esophageal manometry in 154 children, in 45 patients with chest pain or dysphagia (with frequent history of food impaction) not associated with GERD, manometry showed abnormal findings in 30 (67%), achalasia in 12, pseudo-obstruction in 3, diffuse esophageal spasm in 1, dysmotility after tracheoesophageal fistula repair in 1, and ineffective motility in 13 patients.[19]

Newer Techniques to Perform Esophageal Manometry

Prolonged Manometry Studies

A recent clinical application of esophageal manometry is the performance of prolonged ambulatory monitoring of esophageal pressures.[27] We have reported reference values for healthy children.[2] Manometry is performed with a solid-state catheter that has pressure transducers and, usually, one or two pH electrodes allowing for correlation of symptoms with both motor events and acid reflux. The primary indication of prolonged esophageal manometry is in the evaluation of patients with noncardiac chest pain,[27,28] because it allows the demonstration of associated esophageal events (either motor or acid reflux) related with the pain symptoms.[27] It may be also used to define pathophysiology of esophageal motor disorders in GERD,[29] tracheoesophageal fistula,[30] or eosinophilic esophagitis.[31]

Multichannel Intraluminal Impedance Combined With Manometry

This technique permits the simultaneous evaluation of esophageal motility and bolus transit (see Figure 65-1).[15,32-36] The advantage is that it provides an objective measurement of esophageal transit and how it correlates with motility events. Values for normal adults have been established,[15,32,35,36] and the technique has been validated with the simultaneous use of manometry, videoesophagram, and impedance.[35] The test can be done with either liquid or viscous swallows, and recently it has been shown that the transit of viscous material is slower.[15,32,33,35,36] Normal bolus transit in healthy individuals occurs in at least 80% of liquid and 70% of viscous swallows when solid-state catheters are used[15] and in 70% of liquid and 60% of viscous swallows when perfused catheters are utilized.[36] Preliminary findings in children have shown that the technique is feasible.[33] This technique has shown that manometric evaluation demonstrating ineffective peristalsis may underestimate the true rate of bolus clearance.[32,33,35,36] (The combined used of manometry and impedance has shown that approximately 97% of normal peristaltic swallows have normal bolus transit, but also that almost half of manometrically ineffective peristalsis is associated with normal liquid transit.[15]) In children, preliminary information has shown that effective bolus clearance by impedance is present in 75% of swallows that had ineffective peristalsis.[33] Adult patients with achalasia and scleroderma seem to have abnormal bolus transit time with every swallow. Almost all patients with normal esophageal manometry, nutcracker esophagus, poorly relaxing LES, hypertensive LES, and hypotensive LES have normal bolus transit, whereas 51% of those with ineffective esophageal motility and 55% of those with diffuse esophageal spasm also have normal bolus transit.[13] These results indicate that the addition of impedance testing and the study of bolus transit may provide a more accurate diagnosis as compared to esophageal manometry alone.[32,33,35,36] However, recently high-resolution manometry with impedance has become available and will probably supplant the use of simple solid-state manometry with impedance (see Figure 65-2).

High-Resolution Manometry

The most recent advance in the study of esophageal physiology is the use of high-resolution manometry (HRM) (see Figure 65-2).[37] This is achieved by increasing the number of recording sites and decreasing the spacing between them, allowing a better definition of the intraluminal pressure environment without spatial gaps and with minimal movement-related artifacts.[37,38] The software to analyze the data has been also been greatly improved, making it appear as a space-time continuum that can be displayed as isobaric contour plots. The advantages of isobaric contour plots are multiple, but the most evident is that they provide a seamless, dynamic representation of peristalsis at every axial position within and across the esophagus.[37,38] HRM has evidenced that the esophageal body has distinctive pressure segments and that esophageal peristalsis is the result of an orchestrated sequential chain of events composed by contractions of those pressure segments.[39,40] HRM predicts the presence of abnormal bolus transport more accurately than conventional manometry, and it identifies clinically important motor dysfunction not previously detected by either manometry or radiography.[41,42] The exact role that HRM will play in the evaluation of esophageal motor disorders still needs to be defined, and the only reports in children currently have evaluated only developmental and anatomical features of esophageal motility.[39,40] In the largest report to date, Staiano et al.[39] described the findings in 40 children from age 1 day of life to 14 years. They found three distinctive segments of peristalsis, similar to those found in adult studies. Recently impedance measurements have been added to HRM catheters, allowing the simultaneous measurement of both pressure and impedance changes (see Figure 65-2). This new technology will probably serve as a substitute for the esophageal function testing mentioned earlier. There is no question that HRM has greatly simplified the performance of esophageal motility testing in children, as it requires only one intubation, without the need to do a pull-through. However, it is not clear whether it will change the diagnostic accuracy as compared with standard manometry.

ANTRODUODENAL MANOMETRY

Antroduodenal manometry measures the intraluminal pressure of the antrum and duodenum,[1,4,43] providing information of the contraction patterns of the upper gastrointestinal tract. Manometry tests may not be useful in patient management when there is a known underlying cause of dysmotility,[1] but they may be important in the study of selected children and adults with unexplained, severe upper gastrointestinal dysfunction, or when there is a discrepancy between the clinical impression and the severity of the patient's condition. As is true of most tests in children, the utility of antroduodenal manometry has been limited by the lack of normal data in healthy controls,[44] and extrapolation of normal values has been obtained from patients referred for antroduodenal motility who later were considered as normal.[45] Some studies in adults report no difference in the frequency of abnormal manometric patterns between healthy and symptomatic patients,[46] resulting in a debate about what constitutes a significant abnormality, so one must pay close attention during interpretation of the study to avoid overinterpretation of the findings.[1,47]

Normal Physiology

Antroduodenal motility has very characteristic patterns in both the fasting state and after a meal.

Fasting Motility

During fasting, the stomach and small bowel show a cyclic pattern, known as the migrating motor complex (MMC) (Figure 65-4).[45] This cyclic activity is divided into three phases. Phase I is characterized by motor quiescence and seems to be predominant in the antrum. Phase II has irregular contractions with varied amplitude, is the longest in duration, and is predominant in the duodenum and jejunum. Phase III consists of regular rhythmic peristaltic contractions that start proximally and migrate down to the ileum with decreasing velocity of propagation and increased duration. As a cycle is fading on reaching the ileum, a new one starts in the antrum. Phase III contractions in the antrum occur at a rate of 3 per minute and 9 to 12 per minute in the small bowel. In adults, phase I lasts from 12 to 20 minutes, phase II lasts from 30 to 130 minutes, and phase III lasts from 3 to 15 minutes,[43,48] with a large variation in cycle duration between individuals and within the same individual.[43] There are no established standards for normal duration of the cycle in children, but the duration of the MMC seems to be shorter than

in adults[44,48] with the phase III propagation velocity increasing with age; overall cycle length shows no age-dependent variation. In children without upper gastrointestinal symptoms, the phase III contractions are present in most during fasting and induced in the remainder with erythromycin.[49] Phase III occupies around 3%, phase I about 10% and phase II roughly 87% of recording time.[45] The presence of phase III activity is a marker of neuroenteric integrity,[1,4,44,48] and its absence is abnormal.[1,4,44,48] Because one third to one half of the activity front may commence distal to the stomach, the absence of antral phase III is not necessarily abnormal.[43,50] Because even some normal adult subjects may have no phase III activity during stationary studies, this finding may have limitations in the interpretation of suspected neuropathic disorders.[46,51] Data from 24-hour ambulatory studies show that adult volunteers have at least one or more MMCs per 24 hours, so they can provide more definitive evidence of normal enteric nervous system function.[51]

Postprandial Motility

After a meal ingestion, the fasting pattern is interrupted by the fed pattern characterized by irregular contractions of various amplitudes, which are strong and repetitive in the antrum and similar to the phase II of the MMC in the duodenum (Figure 65-5).[1] An antral motility index has been used to evaluate both the frequency and the amplitude of these contractions, usually over 2 hours, and the calculation is derived from measurements of the prepyloric area. It is usually calculated automatically by the equipment software or manually with this formula: ln(amplitude × number of contractions + 1), with a normal value being 13.67 to 15.65 (5th to 95th percentile).[43] The characteristics of the fed pattern vary with the type, composition, and amount of nutrients. Liquid nutrients decrease the amplitude of antral contractions and generate an irregular movement in the small bowel, whereas solid foods produce high-amplitude contractions in the antrum and a pattern similar to that of liquids in the small bowel.

Before the Procedure

The patient should be fasting overnight and stop medications that can affect motility for at least 48 hours before the test.

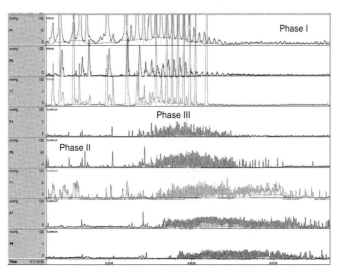

Figure 65-4. Normal antroduodenal motility during fasting. Antroduodenal manometry tracing during fasting in an 8 year old child. The tracing shows a migrating motor complex (MMC). The three phases of the MMC can seen.

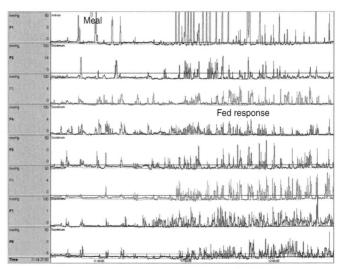

Figure 65-5. Normal Antroduodenal response to feeding. Antroduodenal manometry tracing that shows the normal response to feeding.

Equipment

Small bowel motility tests can be performed with solid-state pressure transducers, impedance sensors, or perfused catheters.[1] The configuration of the catheters can be customized, but the minimum recommended recording ports include one in the antrum and three in the small bowel.[1] The distance for duodenal and jejunal ports varies according to the age of the patient, with a range from 3 to 10 cm between ports. In children a distance of 3 cm and in adolescents a distance of 5 cm is sufficient. Continuous monitoring is important in patients undergoing studies using perfused systems to avoid fluid overload, particularly in infants and small children.[52] The perfusion rates usually vary from 0.1 to 0.4 mL/min per port. The perfusion rates for the study of premature and young infants should be decreased, and some units have reported perfusion rates as low as 0.01 to 0.02 mL/min.[52,53] Most adult laboratories use distilled water, but most pediatric centers use 0.2 to half-normal saline or oral hydration solutions[1,54] to avoid hyponatremia. We recommend saline solutions over oral hydration solutions to avoid clogging of the system from glucose residues and bacterial growth from the carbohydrate content of the oral hydration solutions.

Catheter Placement

The catheter is introduced nasally or through an existing gastrostomy, jejunostomy, or ileostomy and advanced with endoscopic or fluoroscopic assistance into the small bowel, ideally beyond the angle of Treitz but most importantly across the antroduodenal junction.[43] The position of the catheter needs to be checked during the performance of the test to ensure the correct position across the antroduodenal junction. This can be achieved by looking at the manometric patterns, but at times radiography or fluoroscopy may be needed. One adult study reported that on average up to five adjustments of tube location may be needed, particularly in the postprandial period, to ensure accurate antral recordings.[43] It is preferable to avoid anesthesia and sedation for placement, as the effects of most anesthetics and sedatives on antroduodenal motility recordings have not been evaluated. It has been suggested that sedation with midazolam (2 to 5 mg, or 0.05 to 0.2 mg/kg) followed by reversal with intravenous flumazenil (0.2 to 0.4 mg) does not result in appreciable change in motility recordings. In children the use of either sedation or general anesthesia is frequently necessary, particularly when catheters are being placed endoscopically. To avoid possible confounding effects of the sedation or anesthesia, in most centers the study is performed the day after the catheter has been placed.

Study Procedure

The optimum duration of the test is not known. Most centers use 3 to 4 hours of fasting followed by 2 hours postprandially,[43,51] and some authors advocate the use of prolonged ambulatory studies. The pediatric task force of the ANMS recommended at least 3 hours of fasting (or two migrating motor complexes [MMCs]) and at least 1 postprandial hour.[1] Some have shown an increased diagnostic accuracy with prolonged studies,[51] but at the expense of more frequent catheter displacements, potentially limiting the evaluation of the postprandial activity of the antrum.[43] After recording the fasting phase, the patient is given a standardized meal over 30 to 60 minutes to stimulate fed motility pattern, and the postprandial phase is recorded for 60 minutes. The AMS task force recommends that the type and size of the meal should be adjusted according to the patient's age and preference (at least 10 kcal/kg or 400 kcal; more than 30% of kilocalories from lipids).[55] The task force also recommends administering the meal by mouth or intragastrically if possible. In general, for those children who cannot eat solid food, most authors have used 5 to 10 mL/kg,[55] or 20 cal/kg.[56] In adults, the meal has been standardized to be at least 400 kcal.[43] The solid or liquid meal should be balanced and typical of an average U.S. diet, with 20 to 25% fat, 20 to 25% protein, and 50 to 55% carbohydrate.[43]

In patients in whom the normal MMC is not observed during the fasting phase, a dose of intravenous erythromycin is given over 30 minutes.[1,57] Erythromycin at doses of 1 to 3 mg/kg acts as a motilin receptor agonist,[45,58] increasing antral motility and inducing phase III of the MMC in adults and children, particularly in those with spontaneous phase III during fasting compared to those without fasting MMC. The same effect is seen in full-term neonates[58] and in premature infants older than 32 weeks.[59] Erythromycin at higher doses induces a higher level of antral motility but also is associated with greater side effects, and there is no difference noted for inducing phase III of the MMC.[57] Some authors have suggested shortening the study time by eliminating the fasting phase and substituting in the administration of erythromycin,[48] but the utility of this approach has not been validated. The ANMS pediatric task force recommended the use of erythromycin 1 mg/kg over 30 minutes if no MMC is recorded during fasting.[1] For those in whom no MMC is noticed in the small bowel during fasting and during erythromycin infusion, a dose of octreotide is given subcutaneously to induce phase III activity in the small bowel.[60-62] The effect of octreotide on the antrum is variable; most often it results in decreased antral activity, unless the patient has been pretreated with erythromycin.[60-62]

Interpretation

Data interpretation is usually performed by visual inspection,[1] typically by identifying certain patterns with limited quantitative features.[43] A recent pediatric multicenter study showed an excellent interobserver agreement in differentiating normal from abnormal, specifically when objective findings such as the number and measurements of phase III of the MMC during fasting were used. Other findings were not as reproducible.[63]

Manometric Diagnosis by Antroduodenal Manometry

Normal Motility

One of the most important contributions of the antroduodenal motility may be the demonstration of normal motility (see Figures 65-4 and 65-5) in patients with apparent intestinal failure,[1,4,47] indicating other etiologies, including factitious disorders.[64]

Chronic Intestinal Pseudo-obstruction

The most important use of the study is to diagnose (or rule out) and subsequently classifying chronic intestinal pseudo-obstruction (CIPO). This condition can be subclassified into neuropathic disorders (Figure 65-6), which are characterized

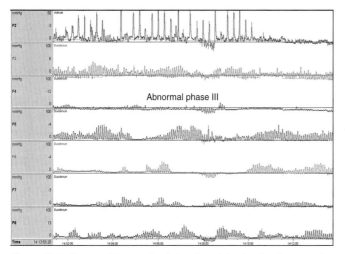

Figure 65-6. Neuropathic pseudo-obstruction. Antroduodenal manometry tracing that shows a disorganized migrating motor complex (MMC). The figure shows an abnormal phase III that is disorganized, simultaneous, and does not have normal progression.

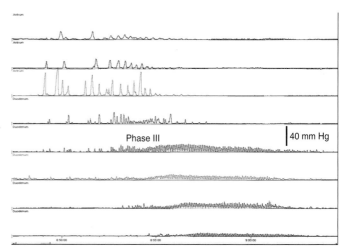

Figure 65-7. Myopathic pseudo-obstruction. Antroduodenal motility tracing that shows the presence of a normal migrating motor complex (MMC) that has abnormal reduced amplitude.

by antral hypomotility, absence of phase III activity, abnormal propagation of phase III of MMC, bursts and sustained uncoordinated pressure activity (hypercontractility), and a lack of a fed response[65]; and myopathic disorders (Figure 65-7), characterized by low-amplitude contractions of less than 20 mm Hg[66] that are usually less than 10 mm Hg, depending on the luminal diameter (low because of dilatation).[43] Studies evaluating the correlation of histology and manometry with outcomes in children have reported that a low-amplitude phase III motility index below 10 kPa/min correlates with poor outcomes, including dependence on total parenteral nutrition or death. Therefore, this type of study not only is useful in diagnosing the etiology of pseudo-obstruction, but also may be important in predicting outcome.[67]

Postprandial Antral Hypomotility

A reduced motility index of postprandial distal antral contractions correlates with impaired gastric emptying of solids from the stomach[68] (Figure 65-8). This is frequently seen in patients with gastroparesis.

Mechanical Obstruction

Patterns seen in unrecognized mechanical obstruction include postprandial clustered contractions (more than 30 minutes' duration) separated by quiescence or simultaneous prolonged (longer than 8 seconds) or summated contractions.[1,4,69] A report in neonates describes a new pattern consisting of high-amplitude, retrograde, prolonged contractions.[70]

Rumination

Antroduodenal manometry may be useful to distinguish between rumination and vomiting by showing simultaneous contractions or R waves with the regurgitation episode.[1]

Indications and Clinical Utility

Antroduodenal motility is used to study the pathophysiology and to diagnose the presence or absence of gastrointestinal motility disorders. Antroduodenal manometry is indicated for patients with unexplained upper gastrointestinal problems

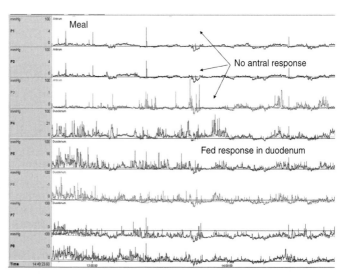

Figure 65-8. Antral hypomotility. Antroduodenal manometry showing the lack of an antral fed response in a child with gastroparesis. Note the normal fed response in the duodenum, and the lack of response in the antrum.

or symptoms suggestive of upper gastrointestinal dysmotility, mainly to confirm or exclude chronic intestinal pseudo-obstruction or a motility disorder.[49] A normal study indicates that a motility problem is not the likely cause of the symptoms.[1,4,43] The presence of phase III of the MMC is considered a hallmark of neuroenteric integrity. In general, findings are considered abnormal if there is abnormal propagation or configuration of the MMC, uncoordinated intestinal bursts of phasic pressure activity sustained over 30 minutes, uncoordinated intestinal pressure activity, or failure of the meal to produce a fed pattern. Different manometric patterns allow a classification of abnormalities into neuropathic (see Figure 65-6) or myopathic (see Figure 65-7) problems,[1,4,71] which are defined based on qualitative changes.[1] Some patterns have been associated with upper gastrointestinal motility disorders when compared to patients without motility disorders. These include absence of phase III of the MMC, abnormal migration of phase III, short intervals between phase III episodes, persistent low-amplitude contractions, and sustained tonic-phasic contractions.[44] However, other findings such as short or prolonged phase III, low amplitude of phase III in a single recording site, and clusters of contractions or prolonged propagating contractions during phase II are not more frequent in patients than in controls.[44]

Antroduodenal manometry may also be useful to study the effects of medications and the tolerance for enteral feedings in patients with motility disturbances. In premature infants, the antroduodenal motility study may help to establish readiness to start enteral feedings, or the best way to feed them. Studies have shown that continuous infusions produce better motor responses than bolus feedings and full-strength formula triggers adult-like motor activity.[52,72] In children, the absence of MMCs serves as an indicator of poor response to enteral feedings.[56] Other authors have reported the use of antroduodenal manometry to evaluate feeding intolerance in children with developmental delay,[73] mitochondrial diseases,[71] a history of neonatal ECMO use (extracorporeal membrane oxygenation),[70] celiac disease,[74] feeding refusal in medically fragile toddlers,[75] and following fundoplication.[55]

Future

With the introduction of high-resolution manometry, another door has opened to improve the evaluation of the antroduodenal motility. A study including 12 healthy adult volunteers demonstrated the feasibility and utility of HRM to identify the pyloric region.[76] We anticipate that the use of this technique will provide valuable information, particularly if impedance is added to the system so that transit can be evaluated as well. Evaluation of gastric emptying time and gastrointestinal transit as well as gastrointestinal motility is also now possible with wireless technology in the form of a capsule. The capsule is able to record pressure, temperature, and pH measurement data in both elapsed and real time. The device has FDA approval for use in adults, and studies to validate its use in adults are now underway. If it proves to be accurate, the use of an ingested capsule to assess gastric and small bowel motility may well become a noninvasive technique for use in the evaluation of children in whom dysmotility is suspected.

COLONIC MANOMETRY

Evaluation of colon motility by means of measurement of intraluminal pressure has been performed successfully in pediatric patients for many years, but no prospective evaluations of outcomes have been obtained. Despite that, it is considered a valuable tool in selected patients with intractable constipation.[1]

Normal Physiology

In the colon, unlike the stomach and small bowel, there is no interdigestive cyclic motor activity. Colonic motility is characterized by the presence of irregular alterations of quiescence with nonpropagating and propagating contractions. The motility of the colon in the fasting state is characterized by low-amplitude (5 to 50 mm Hg), nonpropulsive, segmental contractions with rare peristaltic movements.[77] Segmental nonpropagating contractions are more common in toddlers than infants.[57] Colonic propagated contractions are classified according to their amplitude as low-amplitude propagating contractions (LAPCs) or high-amplitude propagating contractions (HAPCs).[77] HAPCs are defined as contractions of at least 60 to 100 mm Hg (may reach more than 200 mm Hg), lasting 10 seconds and propagating for at least 30 cm (Figure 65-9). HAPCs originate in the proximal colon and migrate distally more than 95% of the time, usually stopping or decreasing in amplitude in the distal sigmoid colon.[77] LAPCs are propagated contractions of less than 40 mm Hg of unknown physiologic or clinical significance, but some believe they may help in transporting stools and the passage of flatus.[77]

Postprandial colonic motility is characterized by segmental contractions associated with an increase in tone that may last up to 3 hours, and in children HAPCs have been described.[1,78-81] This response is influenced by the meal content, with fat and carbohydrate stimulating and protein inhibiting colonic activity[77] (Figure 65-10).

Before the Procedure

Even though preparation may alter colonic motility, studies of colonic motility are difficult to perform in unprepared colons. In fact, most studies include a bowel cleanout with an oral

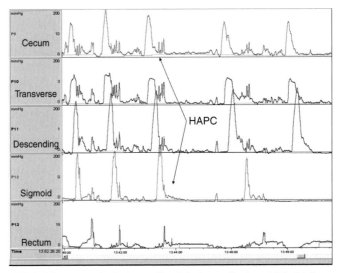

Figure 65-9. Normal colonic motility. Colonic motility in a child with functional constipation. Note the high-amplitude propagating contractions (HAPCs) that resulted after bisacodyl administration.

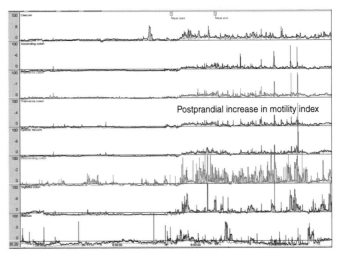

Figure 65-10. Normal postprandial colonic motility. This colonic motility shows the normal postprandial increase in the motility index.

balanced electrolyte solution[77] the day before the procedure, and preferably no enemas are given on the day of the study. Also, medications that can influence motility should be stopped for at least 48 hours before the study.

Equipment

Most centers use perfusion catheters, as the placement requires endoscopy and/or fluoroscopy. The recording ports spacing varies according to the size of the patient, usually 5 to 15 cm. The equipment used and the perfusion methodology are similar to those described under antroduodenal manometry.

Catheter Placement

The catheter is usually placed during colonoscopy after reaching the right colon. In most cases, a guidewire is placed into the colon and the colonoscope is withdrawn with the guidewire left in position. A motility catheter is then fed over the wire with fluoroscopy assistance to avoid coiling of the catheter and also to prevent the guidewire from losing its position so far as possible. In some cases, cooling the catheter may prevent coiling, as it makes it firmer. The final position of the tube is checked by fluoroscopy.[1,4,57,79,80] The catheter can also be dragged with the colonoscope during the colonoscopy and placed directly into the desired location. A recent study reported the successful placement of the catheter with fluoroscopy alone, with the disadvantage of longer radiation exposure compared to the use of colonoscopy with fluoroscopy.[82] Another advantage of using a colonoscopy is that it permits evaluation of the colonic mucosa. Colonoscopy is usually performed under general anesthesia, and the study performed the next day. When intravenous sedation with benzodiazepines is used for the colonoscopy, the study may be performed on the same day, after recovery from the sedation.[56]

Study

The study typically lasts from 4 to 8 hours, and recently some authors have reported the utility of a 24-hour study[83] The study starts with a fasting recording for 2 hours followed by a meal given over 30 to 60 minutes. From adult studies we know that a high-calorie (1000 kcal) meal stimulates colonic motility in healthy subjects,[79,80] but a 350-kcal meal does not. In children a combined liquid and solid meal (at least 20 kcal/kg, with fat providing more than 30% of the energy) has a similar effect.[79] In patients in whom a normal HAPC is not observed during fasting or after a meal, a dose of bisacodyl is given through the colonic motility catheter. The usual dose is 0.2 mg/kg, and it can be given as a single dose or can be repeated after 20 to 60 minutes. There is no evidence that single versus double dosing makes a difference in the quantity and quality of HAPCs. Intracolonic bisacodyl can be administered to shorten the duration of the motility study in ill children or in those who cannot eat.[81] HAPCs induced after bisacodyl are similar in amplitude, duration, propagation velocity, and sites of origin and extinction compared with normally occurring HAPCs.[81] The effect of intrarectal bisacodyl is similar to that of intracecal bisacodyl, except for a delay of 10 minutes in onset.[81] A study combining antroduodenal and colonic manometry has showed that erythromycin lacks a prokinetic effect on the colon[84] despite

some authors reporting its clinical utility in the treatment of constipation.

Interpretation

Normal Patterns

Interpretation is done mostly by visual inspection, with attention to identifying the change in motility index after a meal and the presence of spontaneous, meal-induced, or bisacodyl-induced HAPCs. The postprandial response to a meal (see Figure 65-10) and the presence of HAPCs (see Figure 65-9) have been associated with preservation of the enteric nervous system. Patterns of colonic motility in healthy children have not yet been established. Most information is obtained from studies of children referred for the evaluation of neuropathy, constipation, or nonulcer dyspepsia.[78-80,85]

Gastrocolonic Response

This is usually determined by visual inspection, but a motility index can also be calculated for the period of 30 to 60 minutes before and 30 to 60 minutes after ingestion of the meal as described earlier in the section on antroduodenal manometry. In the postprandial period, one HAPC is usually followed by others 3 to 4 minutes later.[78-80,85] Some authors have shown an inverse correlation between the number of HAPCs and chronologic age, with HAPCs being more frequent during fasting and in the first 30 postprandial minutes in younger patients.[56]

HAPCs

Response to bisacodyl administration is the easiest measure to evaluate and probably the most important part of the test. Therefore, in certain cases it may not be necessary to study colonic motility after a meal. However, further validation of this recommendation is needed. A recent study showed that another possible method to elicit propagated colonic contractions is the intraluminal distention of the colon; the response, however, is not as consistent as the contractions elicited with bisacodyl.[86] Abnormal propagation of the HAPCs may indicate a segmental motility disorder (Figure 65-11), and absent motility and lack of postprandial response may indicate severe neuropathy (Figure 65-12).

Indications and Clinical Significance

The main indication for colonic motility is in the evaluation of selected patients with intractable constipation to assist in differentiating between functional constipation and colonic pseudo-obstruction[1,81]; to characterize the relationship between motor abnormalities and symptoms, particularly when a colectomy is being considered[87]; and to evaluate persistent symptoms following surgery.[1,88]

As with most motility procedures in children, information obtained from colonic motility needs to be considered in the context of a lack of normal controls in children, and physicians must also weigh the potential effects of colonic preparation on the test results.[1] Some have reported the utility of colonic manometry to differentiate between myopathy and neuropathy,[1,80] but a recent study failed to show a correlation between manometric and histologic findings.[89] In another study, children with neuropathy were differentiated from those with functional fecal retention by the absence of HAPCs and a lack of increase in the postprandial motility index.[79] In young

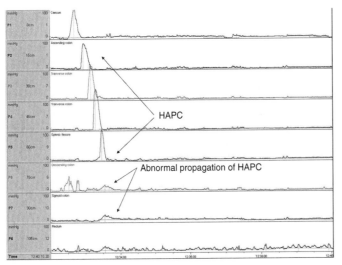

Figure 65-11. Segmental colonic abnormality. Colonic motility tracing in a child with severe constipation. There is a lack of propagation of the high-amplitude contraction (HAPC) into the distal colonic segments.

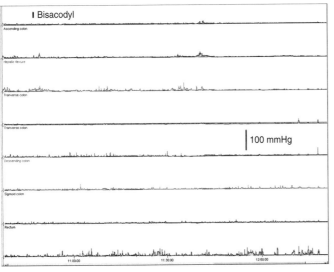

Figure 65-12. Severe colonic neuropathy. Colonic motility tracing in a child with severe intractable constipation. There are no high-amplitude contractions (HAPCs) in response to bisacodyl.

children, the lack of HAPCs may also be a sensitive marker of neuromuscular disease.[78-80,85]

Constipation

Colon manometry is also useful to differentiate children with functional constipation from those with more severe chronic constipation associated with neuropathies or myopathies. Children with functional constipation have an increase in motility index postprandially (see Figure 65-10) and are more likely to show HAPCs (see Figure 65-9) than children with colonic neuropathies (see Figures 65-11 and 65-12).[79] We have also demonstrated that colon manometry predicts long-term response to daily use of bisacodyl.[90] Previous studies have suggested that colonic motility may help detect abnormal colonic segments that require surgical resection (see Figure 65-11).[87,91] However, the data are limited, and until prospective studies are completed, caution should be observed before manometry is used as the only factor that dictates a colonic resection. It has also

been suggested that colon manometry can help predict which patients will have good results to antegrade colonic enemas[88] and to assess the improvement of colonic dysmotility after long-term use of antegrade colonic enemas.[92] In adults, colonic motility does not seem more accurate than transit studies and pelvic floor evaluation in discriminating subgroups of chronic constipation.[77] It is possible that colonic motility may be more useful in the pediatric population.[1,4]

Chronic Intestinal Pseudo-obstruction

Colon motility is abnormal in the majority of patients. In the neuropathic type the motility shows abnormal basal activity and absence of HAPCs and gastrocolic response. In the myopathic type, the study shows no contractions. CIPO patients with constipation show no significant gastrocolonic response, and 75% have no HAPCs.[80]

Hirschsprung's Disease

Colonic motility is also useful in understanding the pathophysiology of postoperative symptoms and for guiding the management of patients with Hirschsprung's disease. Four motility patterns have been reported in these patients: HAPCs migrating through the neorectum in patients with fecal soiling, normal colonic manometry in patients with functional fecal retention, absence of HAPCs or persistent simultaneous contractions in children with constipation, and normal colonic motility in patients with constipation and a hypertensive internal anal sphincter. Treatment that is guided by the results of the motility study may result in a significant improvement in global and emotional health as well as in the frequency of bowel movements and abdominal pain.[91]

Imperforate Anus

Colonic manometry is also a valuable tool in the evaluation of postoperative fecal incontinence in patients with a repaired imperforate anus. A study showed that patients with incontinence had HAPCs propagating into the neorectum 80% of the time. Internal anal sphincter resting pressure was low in 60% of cases, with normal relaxation in the same proportion. The treatment was changed based on the results of the study, which resulted in improvement of fecal incontinence in 45% of patients.[93] In our experience, manometry is also useful in defining the etiology of fecal incontinence in cases where left or total colon dysfunction is seen, confirming constipation as the etiology of the incontinence.

Outcome

Overall, colon manometry may prove to be useful in the evaluation and management of children with defecation disorders. In a large retrospective study of children with defecation disorders, which included 150 colonic manometry studies, the most common indications for the procedure were lower GI symptoms (68%), persistent symptoms after corrective surgery in Hirschsprung's disease (14%), evaluation of CIPO (11%), and evaluation before considering closure of a diverting ostomy (7%). Normal colonic motility was found in 38% of children, left colon dysmotility was found in 17%, and total colonic dysmotility in the rest. Based on the results of the study, treatment changes were recommended in 93% of patients, resulting in symptom improvement in 78% and worsening in 4%; parental satisfaction with therapy was 88%.[87]

We have recently reported our own experience with very similar results.

Future

The wireless capsule (mentioned earlier), which is designed to evaluate gastric emptying time and gastrointestinal transit as well as gastrointestinal motility, may also prove to be useful in the evaluation of colonic transit as well as the detection of high-amplitude colonic contractions. Currently it is being evaluated as a tool to study total gastrointestinal transit, including colonic transit in adults. Further studies will be needed to validate that indication.

ANORECTAL MANOMETRY

Anorectal manometry is the most frequently performed motility test in children. The main indications are the evaluation of the rectoanal inhibitory reflex, which is absent in internal anal sphincter achalasia[94,95] and in Hirschsprung's disease,[1,54,95,96] and the evaluation of fecal incontinence from various etiologies, such as myelomeningocele and imperforate anus.[54]

Normal Anorectal Anatomy and Physiology

The most important function of the anorectal complex is the maintenance of fecal continence. Intra-anal pressure is a combination of both internal and external anal sphincter interaction, with the former providing about 75% of the total pressure.[97] The internal anal sphincter (IAS) is composed of smooth muscle in constant tone.[98] The external anal sphincter (EAS) and the muscles of the pelvic floor also maintain continuous tone. The rectoanal inhibitory reflex (RAIR) (Figure 65-13) consists of a reflex relaxation of the IAS and transient contraction of the EAS when stools distend the rectum[98] and returns to baseline when the rectum accommodates to the distention. This transient and simultaneous contraction of the EAS allows time for the IAS to recuperate, thereby avoiding incontinence. The relaxation of the IAS is independent of the spine and is absent when the inhibitory effect of the ganglion cells is not present.[99] Further rectal distention with increasing volumes results in nonrecovery of the IAS.

Before the Procedure

In older patients, an enema is usually given the night before the study; when a fecal impaction is present, a bowel cleanout may be needed. Medications known to affect anorectal function (opiates, prokinetics, anticholinergics) are stopped 48 hours before the test. Small children and infants requiring sedation will need to receive nothing by mouth for 4 to 6 hours before the procedure.

Equipment

Most centers use water-perfused catheters with ports at different levels of the longitudinal and radial axis[1,99-102] and a balloon attached to the distal segment and inflated to produce rectal distention. Usually, this balloon is made of latex, and care should be taken when the test is performed in children who may be latex allergic, in which case a latex-free balloon should be substituted. Solid-state catheters have also been used, but

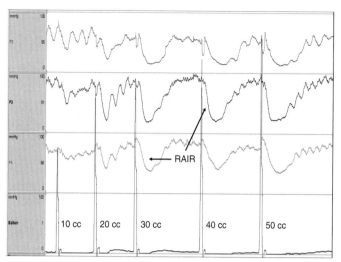

Figure 65-13. Normal anorectal manometry. Anorectal manometry tracing that shows the presence of the rectoanal inhibitory reflex (RAIR) after balloon distention. The lower channel shows the balloon distention. The upper three channels reflect the measurements obtained in the high-pressure zone of the anal canal. There is a normal dose-response curve, with a progression in the degree of relaxation as the balloon volume is increased.

they are much more expensive. Some adult centers use the Shuster balloon, a double-balloon catheter, rarely used in children because of its large size. Recently, some have reported the use of micromanometric techniques, with the use of sleeve sensors, in the evaluation of anal sphincters in the newborn,[103] including very low-birth-weight babies.[104]

Procedure

The study can be performed either by the stationary, slow pull-through or stationary pull-through technique.[105] In children, the stationary pull-through technique is the most commonly used. The probe is inserted completely in the rectum and then pulled back until the high-pressure zone is identified (intra-anal pressure). The balloon is then inflated sequentially at different volume levels to elicit the RAIR[1,99-102,106] (see Figure 65-13). The minimum amount of air required to elicit a relaxation is determined (referred to as the threshold of relaxation). The amount of relaxation is influenced not only by the volume, but by the speed of the inflated balloon, as well as by rectal resting volume and compliance. The volume necessary for constant relaxation, which is the minimal amount of air that is necessary to produce a complete sustained relaxation of both the IAS and the EAS, is determined by adding air progressively until either there is constant relaxation or the patient has reached the critical volume.[98] Besides measuring the resting pressure of the anal canal, the patient is also asked to squeeze at each station. The squeeze pressure is then measured as the maximum pressure obtained above anal resting pressure.[1,100] In cooperative unsedated children, sensation information is obtained[1]; the smallest volume of balloon distention felt by the patient defines the sensation threshold.[1,99-102,106] The threshold of sensation is usually determined with the use of a rectal balloon that is inflated with a handheld syringe. Air is rapidly injected and then immediately withdrawn. The type of inflation (speed, phasic versus continuous), the size and shape of the balloon, and the distance of the balloon to the anal verge all can affect the threshold of sensation. The lowest volume to elicit urge to defecate[1,99,100,106] and the volume associated with sensation of pain (maximum tolerable volume) are also obtained, although there is no clear role for those values in clinical practice.[98] The responses of the IAS to long balloon distentions are also quantified. The relaxed sphincter usually recovers before the balloon is deflated, and abnormalities in this response may indicate neuropathy. Compliance is measured as the ratio of pressure to volume at several distending volumes, although measurements are usually inaccurate unless a barostat is being used.[88] Increased compliance is the most prominent feature in patients with functional constipation,[107] and decreased compliance is associated with an increase in stool frequency, rapid transit of stool in the rectum, and increased risk of fecal incontinence.[98] Anorectal manometry is also useful in evaluating the dynamics of defecation. During push effort, normally the rectal pressure increases and the external anal sphincter pressure decreases. In pelvic floor dyssynergia or anismus, the EAS resting pressure fails to relax or actually increases.[108,109] Some suggest it is not as accurate as defecography, as the agreement in adults when manometry shows anismus is 36%; when manometry is normal, defecography is also normal in 88%.[110] Similar information is not available in children.

Interpretation

The main indication of the study is to evaluate the presence of RAIR, but also to evaluate the rectal sensation thresholds, squeeze pressures, rectal compliance, and push effort. False-negative test results probably represent artifacts, such as probe migration, passage of flatus or feces, or relaxation of the EAS. These artifacts can be prevented by ensuring an empty rectum before the study, ensuring correct position of the probe, and monitoring closely for probe movement, because displacement of the probe away from the high-pressure zone may be interpreted as relaxation. False-positive manometries may be due to a variety of reasons including immaturity of ganglion cells, distended rectum leading to a high relaxation threshold, technical errors in which the relaxation zone is missed, or the presence of feces in the anorectum.[111]

Normal Values

Normal values for anorectal manometry in adults are published.[98,112] The length of the anal canal ranges from 2.2 to 4.0 ± 1.0 cm in women and from 2.8 to 4.0 ± 1.0 in men. Anal resting tone varies from 49 ± 3 to 58 ± 3 mm Hg in women and from 49 ± 3 to 66 ± 6 mm Hg in men. Maximum squeeze ranges from 90 ± 9 to 159 ± 45 mm Hg in women and from 218 ± 18 to 238 ± 38 in men. The threshold for IAS relaxation varies from 14 ± 1 to 25 ± 2 mL, and the threshold for sensation varies from 12 ± 1 to 17 ± 9 mL.[98,112] Anal pressure and rectal compliance measurements are both highly reproducible within healthy subjects on separate days, whereas sensory thresholds are reproducible to a variable degree dependent on the intensity of the stimulation and the perception being assessed.[100]

Normal values have been reported in children, mainly from patients undergoing anorectal manometry and later found to have functional constipation. Some authors have reported a mean normal anal resting pressure ranging from 57 ± 10 mm Hg[106] to 67 ± 12 mm Hg,[113] maximum squeeze pressure ranging from 118 ± 42 mm Hg[106] to 140 ± 52 mm Hg,[113] anal length around 3.3 ± 0.8 cm,[113] threshold to produce relaxation (RAIR) ranging from 5 ± 1 mL[106] to 11 ± 5 mL,[113] the threshold of rectal sensation ranging from 5 ± 2 mL[106] to 14 ± 7 mL,[113] volume of constant relaxation of 104 ± 49 mL,[113] and a critical

volume of 101 ± 39 mL.[113] A recent study done in 90 healthy children showed high-pressure zone or anal canal length was 1.67 ± 0.34 cm in neonates, 1.86 ± 0.6 cm in infants, and 3.03 ± 0.52 cm in children. The mean resting pressure of the anal canal was 31.07 ± 10.9 mm Hg in neonates, 42.43 ± 8.9 mm Hg in infants, and 43.43 ± 8.79 mm Hg in children. The mean threshold volume to elicit RAIR was 9.67 ± 3.6 for neonates, 14.0 ± 9.5 for infants and 25.0 ± 11.6 mL for children.[114]

Indications and Clinical Significance

The main indication for anorectal manometry is to evaluate the presence of the RAIR (see Figure 65-13) to exclude internal anal sphincter achalasia and Hirschsprung's disease (Figure 65-14) in children with constipation.[1]

Constipation

The main indication for the test is to evaluate the presence of RAIR, which excludes Hirschsprung's disease[111] and obviates the need of more invasive testing such as a rectal biopsy.[99] Absence of an RAIR indicates the presence of a nonrelaxing IAS (see Figure 65-14), which most likely represents Hirschsprung's disease, but a confirmatory rectal biopsy is necessary.[99,113] An anorectal manometry showing absent RAIR and presence of ganglion cells and normal acetylcholinesterase staining on a rectal biopsy establishes the diagnosis of IAS achalasia, also known as ultrashort-segment Hirschsprung's disease.[94,95,115,116] This condition can be treated with intrasphincteric injections of botulinum toxin.[94,95,116]

The accuracy of the study for the diagnosis of Hirschsprung's disease varies with age[111,117]; it seems to be more accurate in older children,[118] with an accuracy of 90 to 100%, and less accurate in neonates.[1,99,101,111,118,119] The largest study reported an inaccurate diagnosis in 26% of newborns and 71.4% of premature infants.[111] This and other studies confirm the impression that accuracy increases with age. Multiple studies have confirmed the high sensitivity and specificity of suction rectal biopsy in the diagnosis of Hirschsprung's disease, but some authors have reported that the diagnostic sensitivity and

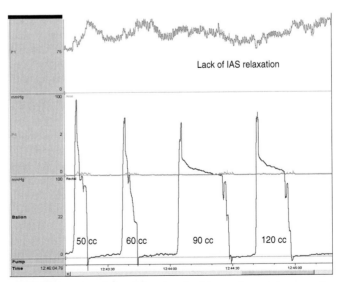

Figure 65-14. Nonrelaxing internal anal sphincter. Anorectal manometry tracing of a child with Hirschsprung's disease. There is a lack of internal anal sphincter relaxation after balloon distention.

specificity are not significantly different from those obtained with barium enema and/or anorectal manometry.[120,121] However, a systematic review found that rectal suction biopsy was the most accurate test to diagnose Hirschsprung's disease, with anorectal manometry having a sensitivity of 91% and a significantly lower specificity.[120] Changes in resting and squeeze pressures, as well as abnormal sensation on manometry, are found inconsistently in patients with constipation and do not seem to have major clinical implications.[1,122-124] Abnormal sensation has also been described in children with functional constipation,[1,122-124] but it is not known if the abnormality represents a primary problem or if it is simply secondary to the megarectum. Findings on anorectal manometry have been reported to correlate with clinical symptoms in patients with constipation. Specifically, there is a positive correlation between soiling and the volume threshold to elicit the RAIR and the urge to defecate.[125]

Postoperative Hirschsprung's Disease

Besides suggesting the diagnosis, anorectal manometry is also useful in the evaluation of persistent symptoms of fecal incontinence or constipation after corrective surgery for Hirschsprung's disease.[1,96] The presence of RAIR in postoperative patients is variable; in most studies it does not correlate with outcome.[96] There seems to be a positive correlation between functional outcome and anal resting pressure.[126] Patients with obstructive symptoms and a normal or high-pressure, nonrelaxing anal sphincter may benefit from IAS myectomy[127] or injection of botulinum toxin.[95,116,128]

Pelvic Floor Dyssynergia (Anismus)

Another use of anorectal manometry in children with constipation is the evaluation of pelvic floor dyssynergia.[122] Although its significance is controversial, it has been suggested that its presence is associated with lower response rates to therapy.[109,129] Biofeedback has been attempted to improve function[122,130] but does not seem to have a sustained long-term effect.[122] On the other hand, recent studies in adults document the utility of biofeedback in the treatment of adult patients with dyssynergia.[131] The reason for this discrepancy has not been elucidated.

Fecal Incontinence

Anorectal manometry allows some discrimination between patients with and without fecal incontinence.[1,132,133] Squeeze pressure measurement seems to have greater sensitivity than resting anal canal pressure.[132,134] Abnormal sensation is also reported in patients with fecal incontinence,[133] and the most important component of biofeedback training for fecal incontinence is an improved ability to detect rectal distention.

Imperforate Anus

Anorectal manometry is useful to evaluate intrarectal pressure and sensation and the function of the voluntary muscles,[1,132,133] as patients with this condition show lower squeeze pressures and sensation abnormalities.[133] It is also used to detect dysfunction that may respond to biofeedback.[1,54,131-133]

Spinal Neuropathy

Anorectal manometry has been able to show distinctive changes that vary according to the level of the spinal lesion,[135] and we have also seen the presence of IAS muscle spasms in children with tethered spinal cord. Further prospective studies are needed to evaluate the utility of anorectal manometry in the detection of spinal cord abnormalities.

SUMMARY

The study of gastrointestinal motility in children has taken a primary role in the evaluation of children with suspected motility disorders, and its clinical indications are becoming better defined, particularly for esophageal, antroduodenal, colonic, and anorectal manometry. The performance of pediatric manometry requires knowledge about age-related developmental changes of the GI tract, and an understanding of the technical challenges posed by performance of these studies in children. Recent advances have allowed the study of younger and smaller patients, and new, specially designed instruments have had a major impact in the manometric study of children. Manometry is useful for the diagnosis of primary motility disorders, can be useful in some cases in which the motility alterations are secondary to other illness, and can demonstrate the presence of normal motility in children with unexplained symptoms. Physicians must exercise caution to avoid overinterpretation of the manometric findings, as in many instances there are no normal controls available in children, and not all manometric findings may have clinical importance.

REFERENCES

1. DiLorenzo C, Hillemeier C, Hyman P, et al. Manometry studies in children: minimum standards for procedures. Neurogastroenterol Motil 2002;14:411–420.
4. Camilleri M, Bharucha AE, di Lorenzo C, et al. American Neurogastroenterology and Motility Society consensus statement on intraluminal measurement of gastrointestinal and colonic motility in clinical practice. Neurogastroenterol Motil 2008;20:1269–1282.
35. Imam H, Shay S, Ali A, Baker M. Bolus transit patterns in healthy subjects: a study using simultaneous impedance monitoring, videoesophagram and esophageal manometry. Am J Physiol Gastrointest Liver Physiol 2005;288:G1000–G1006.
39. Staiano A, Boccia G, Miele E, Clouse RE. Segmental characteristics of oesophageal peristalsis in paediatric patients. Neurogastroenterol Motil 2008;20:19–26.
79. Di Lorenzo C, Flores AF, Reddy SN, Hyman PE. Use of colonic manometry to differentiate causes of intractable constipation in children. J Pediatr 1992;120:690–695.
89. van den Berg MM, Di Lorenzo C, Mousa HM, et al. Morphological changes of the enteric nervous system, interstitial cells of Cajal, and smooth muscle in children with colonic motility disorders. J Pediatr Gastroenterol Nutr 2009;48:22–29.
112. Rao SS, Hatfield R, Soffer E, et al. Manometric tests of anorectal function in healthy adults. Am J Gastroenterol 1999;94:773–783.
114. Kumar S, Ramadan S, Gupta V, et al. Manometric tests of anorectal function in 90 healthy children: a clinical study from Kuwait. J Pediatr Surg 2009;44:1786–1790.
120. de Lorijn F, Kremer LC, Reitsma JB, Benninga MA. Diagnostic tests in Hirschsprung disease: a systematic review. J Pediatr Gastroenterol Nutr 2006;42:496–505.

See expertconsult.com for a complete list of references and the review questions for this chapter.

GASTROINTESTINAL PATHOLOGY 66

Robert E. Petras

Histopathologic interpretation of endoscopic gastrointestinal biopsy specimens is a major focus for this chapter and requires adequate clinical information as well as sufficient tissue. The clinical history should include appropriate medication history and any known illnesses that may have associated gastrointestinal findings. The clinical history can alert the pathologist to perform appropriate special studies in addition to the standard hematoxylin and eosin staining. Precise identification of the biopsy site enables the pathologist to provide the most accurate and definitive diagnosis. This is most evident in the diagnosis of inflammatory bowel disease (IBD).

In the absence of granulomas, the distinction between ulcerative colitis and Crohn's disease is based on the distribution of the colitis. Specifically, the presence or absence of rectal involvement as well as documentation of diffuse disease (ulcerative colitis) versus skip lesions (Crohn's disease) requires the gastroenterologist to submit separate, labeled containers with biopsies from each region of the colon. The endoscopist should attempt to obtain the largest possible piece of tissue. Multiple biopsies for each site often provide the best information. If special studies such as culture for microorganisms, electron microscopy, or flow cytometry are required, communication with the laboratory before biopsy is recommended. Standard histopathologic evaluation is best performed on tissue immediately placed in fixative. The resulting "final diagnosis" may require review if additional clinical findings are obtained.

ESOPHAGEAL BIOPSY

Gastroesophageal Reflux

Gastroesophageal reflux disease (GERD) describes a symptomatic clinical condition related to reflux of gastric and/or duodenal contents into the esophagus that usually presents with pyrosis (heartburn), acid regurgitation, and dysphagia.[1] The term *reflux esophagitis* refers to a subset of patients, usually with symptoms of GERD, who show endoscopic and/or histologic manifestations of inflammation within squamous and/or gastric cardia type mucosa. Many consider esophagogastroduodenoscopy with biopsy the prudent initial evaluation of patients with symptoms of GERD. It quickly excludes other conditions in the clinical differential such as infective esophagitis and "pill esophagitis."

The endoscopic changes described with GERD are seen more often in severe cases and include erosions, ulcers, and stricture. Biopsy specimens are generally obtained to confirm reflux, to rule out infection or to establish a diagnosis of Barrett's esophagus. Erosive lesions are often sampled to rule out *Candida* species and herpes virus infection. Approximately one third of patients with reflux have endoscopically normal or only slightly hyperemic esophageal mucosa; however, endoscopic biopsy specimens show characteristic histologic changes (see later discussion).[2] Though debated, some investigators consider

histologic evaluation of biopsy specimens the "gold standard" in the diagnosis of GERD and reflux esophagitis.[3]

Histologic Changes—Squamous Mucosa

Well-oriented normal esophageal squamous mucosa demonstrates a basal cell layer that is usually one to three cells thick. These basal cells can be discerned by their smaller size and their more basophilic cytoplasm compared with normal surface squamous cells. The cytoplasmic appearance of basal cells and their relative lack of glycogen can be highlighted with a periodic acid-Schiff (PAS) stain. Lamina propria papillae are present, but make up only one half of the total epithelial thickness.[4,5]

Biopsy specimens from endoscopically demonstrable lesions in GERD (erosions, ulcers) show acute inflammation of the mucosa and lamina propria. Exudates containing neutrophils and eosinophils often overlie an erosion or an ulcer with an inflamed granulation tissue base. Acute inflammation is fairly specific but insensitive for reflux esophagitis.[5,6] Many patients with clinical symptoms and the acid abnormalities of GERD, as measured by intraesophageal pH probes, have an endoscopically normal-appearing esophagus or show only minimal esophageal changes such as hyperemia. Although acute inflammation may be lacking, many patients show characteristic squamous mucosal changes of reflux consisting of hyperplasia (lamina propria papilla greater than 67% of the thickness of the squamous mucosa) and an increase in the basal cell layer (more than 15% of the squamous mucosal thickness).[5-7] These abnormalities are often accompanied by increased numbers of intraepithelial eosinophils and lymphocytes[5,6,8-11] (Figure 66-1). The squamous mucosa adjacent to ulcers and erosions can show striking regenerative features, with basal cells occupying the full thickness of the squamous mucosa and papillomatosis that may mimic squamous carcinoma or dysplasia.

Histologic Changes—Glandular Mucosa

Several investigators have suggested that the presence of gastric cardia-type mucosa in the esophagus at or near the squamocolumnar junction may be metaplastic, and that inflammation of this metaplastic gastric cardia-type mucosa (so-called "carditis") correlates strongly with GERD.[12,13] In contrast, other investigators have concluded that this "carditis" is a manifestation of gastric *Helicobacter pylori* infection.[14,15]

The author believes that these apparent disparate viewpoints can be reconciled based on methodologic differences and inherent biases within these studies, and that, depending on the patient population and biopsy location, both schools of thought may be correct. Biopsy specimens from the stomach, even millimeters below the squamocolumnar junction, reflect disease processes of the stomach. Therefore, inflammation and intestinal metaplasia in that area correlate with *Helicobacter pylori* infection. However, "carditis" at the esophagogastric junction or

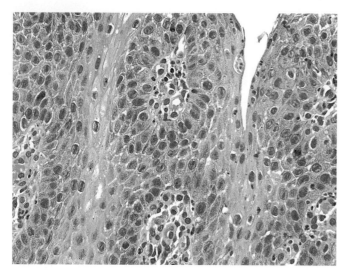

Figure 66-1. Esophageal squamous epithelial changes of reflux. In addition to papillomatosis, an increase in the squamous basal cell layer, and increased intraepithelial lymphocytes and eosinophils, surface neutrophils are also present. (*See plate section for color.*)

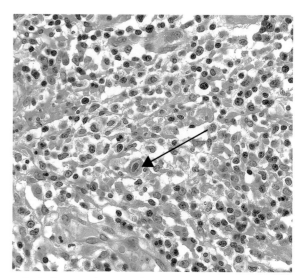

Figure 66-2. Cytomegalovirus inclusion found in ulcer base (center). The infected mesenchymal cell shows cellular enlargement. The nucleus contains a large basophilic inclusion body with surrounding halo and preservation of the nucleolus. (*See plate section for color.*)

above is characteristic of patients with gastroesophageal reflux as demonstrated by symptoms and manometric and pH probe abnormalities, and it probably comprises more than 90% of the gastric carditis seen in practice.

Differential Diagnosis

Infectious Esophagitis

Herpetic esophagitis typically occurs in immunosuppressed patients, for example, those with acquired immune deficiency syndrome, those receiving chemotherapy, and following bone marrow transplantation.[16] Endoscopically, ulcers occur that are typically described as shallow and "punched out" with adjacent normal-appearing squamous mucosa. Biopsy specimens demonstrate an ulcer base that is relatively bland in terms of acute inflammation but may have prominent aggregates of larger mononuclear cells.[16] The diagnostic epithelial changes are found in the adjacent squamous mucosa with giant cell formation, ground-glass nuclei, and eosinophilic intranuclear (Cowdry type A) inclusions.[17,18] Infection can be confirmed with immunohistochemical stains. Occasional multinucleated squamous epithelial giant cells without viral inclusion may occur as part of reflux esophagitis and should not be confused with herpetic infection.[19]

Inclusions of cytomegalovirus (CMV) can be seen in the base of some esophageal ulcers. The role played by CMV as a primary etiologic agent may be difficult to prove. CMV inclusions typically affect mesenchymal cells such as fibroblasts, smooth muscle, and endothelial cells and usually spare the epithelium[20,21] (Figure 66-2). Immunostains for CMV are also available.

Esophagitis due to *Candida* species usually presents endoscopically as brownish-white plaques with exudate that has been described as "cheesy." *Candida* esophagitis often occurs in patients with other debilitating illnesses such as immunosuppression, diabetes mellitus, and long-term antibiotic therapy. The diagnosis of *Candida* esophagitis requires the identification of budding yeast and pseudohyphae, usually within the inflammatory exudate. Their identification is certainly enhanced by using special stains for fungi. The author recommends the routine use of the Alcian blue–PAS combination stain for all

esophageal biopsy specimens because it is a useful fungal stain, it highlights the basal cell layer, it vividly decorates signet ring cell adenocarcinoma, making it easier to identify, and it can be used to verify the specialized columnar epithelium (intestinal metaplasia) of Barrett's esophagus.

Allergic (Eosinophilic) Esophagitis

Symptomatic and histologic reflux esophagitis occurs in children.[22] One should, however, be wary of diagnosing reflux esophagitis in the presence of large numbers of eosinophils because many of these cases represent "allergic (eosinophilic) esophagitis," a condition that may be related to eosinophilic gastroenteritis.[23-25] Children with allergic esophagitis usually present with dysphagia or "food-catching" and often have an "allergic history." Endoscopic erosions or ulcers are seldom seen, but many patients exhibit longitudinal esophageal furrows, rings, stenosis, or small white vesicles or plaques.[26] Esophageal pH probe studies typically show normal or borderline acid levels in these children, and the symptoms of allergic esophagitis usually do not respond to acid suppression therapy. The most useful histologic criteria to differentiate allergic esophagitis from reflux esophagitis are large numbers of intraepithelial eosinophils (15 or more per high-magnification field), intramucosal eosinophilic aggregates, and superficial eosinophils[23] (Figure 66-3). The American Gastroenterological Association Institute and the North American Society of Pediatric Gastroenterology, Hepatology and Nutrition have reported consensus recommendations for the diagnosis of eosinophilic esophagitis that include (1) feeding intolerance and symptoms of reflux, (2) 15 eosinophils or more per high-magnification field, and (3) exclusion of other disorders, especially reflux.[27] That said, the author believes that reflux can and often does coexist in patients with eosinophilic esophagitis. Patients with allergic esophagitis may respond to dietary therapy, drugs that stabilize mast cells, and corticosteroids.[27]

"Pill Esophagitis"

Esophageal injury can occur with prolonged direct mucosal contact with medicinal tablets or capsules, even in therapeutic doses.[28,29] Symptomatic "pill esophagitis" has been associated

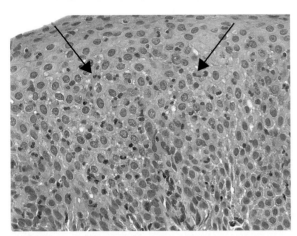

Figure 66-3. Eosinophilic esophagitis. Sections show squamous papillomatosis, a marked increase in the squamous epithelial basal cell layer, and numerous intraepithelial eosinophils leukocytes. (*See plate section for color.*)

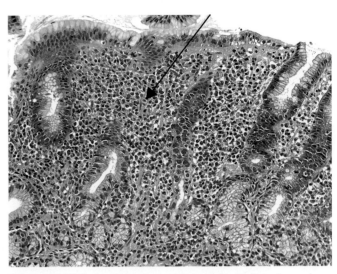

Figure 66-4. *Helicobacter pylori*–associated gastritis. Sections show a dense chronic inflammatory cell infiltrate of the lamina propria associated with some acute inflammation. (*See plate section for color.*)

with odynophagia (pain on swallowing) or the feeling of a "lump in the throat." Patients frequently take pills with little or no water. Endoscopic erosions and ulcers are found in more proximal locations of the esophagus (versus GERD), often in areas of external esophageal compression such as near the arch of the aorta or near the left atrial appendage, especially in patients with cardiomegaly. The histology of "pill esophagitis" is nonspecific.

Barrett's Esophagus

Barrett's esophagus, the eponym given to columnar epithelium-lined esophagus, is acquired through chronic gastroesophageal reflux and occurs rarely in children. The American College of Gastroenterology (ACG) defines Barrett's esophagus as an endoscopic change in esophageal epithelium of any length proved by biopsy to contain intestinal metaplasia.[30]

Endoscopy remains the mainstay in the diagnosis of Barrett's esophagus.[31] In general, the color (orange-red) and appearance (velvety) of Barrett's epithelium as seen through the endoscope is similar to that of normal gastric mucosa. Barrett's epithelium can appear as circumferential or tonguelike extensions of orange-red mucosa into the tubular esophagus. Occasionally, Barrett's epithelium can present as an island of orange-red mucosa entirely surrounded by the more pale pink to gray-white squamous epithelium of normal esophagus. Because other conditions can sometimes mimic Barrett's esophagus endoscopically, the endoscopist's impression must be confirmed histologically.[30,31]

Specialized columnar epithelium (incomplete intestinal metaplasia) is the distinctive epithelial type considered diagnostic for Barrett's esophagus.[30,31] Specialized columnar epithelium can occur in a flat or villous configuration and consists of goblet cells and columnar cells. The goblet cells contain mucin that stains positively with both PAS and Alcian blue at pH 2.5. The columnar cells between goblet cells most often resemble gastric foveolar epithelium, or rarely intestinal absorptive cells.

Barrett's esophagus is encountered only rarely in children undergoing upper endoscopy, with an estimated prevalence of 0.02 to 0.5%. These patients often have comorbidities that predispose to severe reflux, such as neurologic impairment, chronic lung disease, repaired esophageal atresia, or treated intrathoracic malignancy.[32] Dysplasia or carcinoma complicating Barrett's esophagus in children is even rarer. Guidelines have been proposed for surveillance endoscopy with biopsy in children with Barrett's esophagus.[32]

STOMACH BIOPSY

Endoscopy and biopsy in children is used to establish a diagnosis of gastritis and to look specifically for *Helicobacter pylori* infection, eosinophilic gastroenteritis (see later discussion), or Crohn's disease.

H. pylori is responsible for up to 70% of cases of chronic gastritis and can be found in the stomachs of more than 90% of children who have a duodenal ulcer.[33] *H. pylori* infection is easily diagnosed in endoscopic biopsy specimens. Typical patterns of inflammation include chronic inflammation of antral mucosa (chronic antral gastritis) and lymphoplasmacytic infiltration of the lamina propria adjacent to gastric pits (chronic superficial gastritis) in gastric body type mucosa (Figure 66-4); either pattern can be associated with acute inflammation. The organisms can be seen on routine hematoxylin and eosin-stained sections, but identification is enhanced by use of special techniques such as Giemsa (Figure 66-5), Steiner, Warthin-Starry, or immunohistochemistry. The comma-shaped bacilli are typically encountered in the mucous layer overlying gastric foveolar epithelium. The principal differential diagnostic consideration is acute erosive gastritis/reactive gastropathy, often referred to as chemical-type gastritis because of its association with bile reflux, steroid use, and nonsteroidal anti-inflammatory drugs (NSAIDs). The gastric mucosa of erosive gastritis/reactive gastropathy may be erythematous with areas of erosion or ulcer. Histologically, mucosal erosions and/or fibromuscular change in the lamina propria are seen; both can be associated with loss of mucin in the foveolar epithelium and foveolar hyperplasia.

Gastric inflammatory lesions of Crohn's disease usually occur in association with Crohn's disease lesions elsewhere in the gastrointestinal tract. Granulomatous inflammation can be seen; however, focally enhanced chronic active gastritis seen in the absence of *H. pylori* is a pattern more often seen in patients with Crohn's disease.[34]

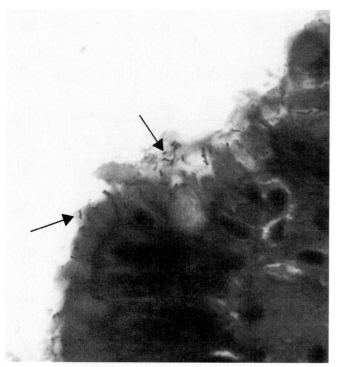

Figure 66-5. *Helicobacter pylori*–associated gastritis, Giemsa stain. Note the curved bacilli within the mucous layer. (*See plate section for color.*)

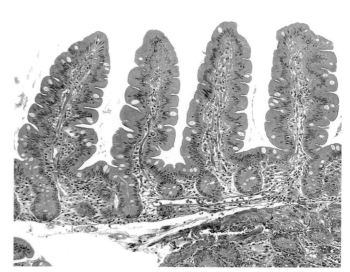

Figure 66-6. Normal small-bowel mucosa. The villi are long and slender. The ratio of villus:crypt length is approximately 4:1. Enterocyte nuclei are basilar in location and evenly aligned. Occasional intraepithelial lymphocytes are present. (*See plate section for color.*)

Ménétrier's-type gastritis with foveolar hyperplasia and protein loss has been described in children in whom it is usually associated with CMV infection. Unlike Ménétrier's disease of adults, the pediatric lesion is usually self-limiting.[35]

SMALL INTESTINAL BIOPSY

Specimen Procurement and Processing

Endoscopic small bowel biopsy is often required to evaluate malabsorption.[36] Proper interpretation of the specimen requires examination of optimally oriented intestinal villi. Multiple specimens should be obtained and fixed in 4% formaldehyde solution and processed routinely. Three to four step-section slides are obtained, with one stained with Alcian blue–PAS, and the rest routinely stained with hematoxylin and eosin.

Normal Small Intestinal Histology

The ratio of villus:crypt length approximates 3:1 to 5:1.[37] Inflammatory cells, including plasma cells, are normally present in the lamina propria. Intraepithelial lymphocytes are present in a ratio of approximately 20 lymphocytes per 100 enterocytes. A brush border should be discernible on the enterocyte. Enterocyte nuclei should be basilar in location and evenly aligned. Identification of four normal villi in a row usually indicates that the villous architecture of the whole biopsy specimen is normal[37,38] (Figure 66-6). This does not mean that biopsy specimens with fewer than four aligned normal villi should be considered inadequate for evaluation, because even one normal villus in a proximal small bowel biopsy specimen rules out celiac sprue. Conversely, finding four normal villi in a row does not necessarily rule out focal lesions, although it almost always does.

Patterns of Abnormal Small Bowel Architecture

The small bowel mucosal responses to injury are limited, and recognition of a response pattern can be useful in differential diagnosis (Table 66-1). In this chapter, the term *severe villus abnormality* describes a flat intestinal mucosa in which no villi are seen or the villi are markedly shortened (villus:crypt length approximately 1:1). Usually, this change is diffuse, accompanied by epithelial lymphocytosis (30 to 40 or more intraepithelial lymphocytes per 100 enterocytes) and associated with crypt hyperplasia, evidenced by numerous mitotic figures. The term *variable villus abnormality* describes specimens in which the villi are either only focally flat or are less than flat (mild or moderate villus shortening). Many specimens in this category also show increased intraepithelial lymphocytes. These changes may be associated with features that suggest a specific diagnosis (e.g., numerous eosinophils, granulomas, parasites) or may be nonspecific.

Entities Associated With a Diffuse Severe Villus Abnormality and Crypt Hyperplasia

Celiac Sprue. Celiac sprue, also known as *gluten-induced enteropathy*, *gluten-sensitive enteropathy*, and *nontropical sprue*, is a major cause of malabsorption.[38,39] The pathogenesis of celiac sprue involves immunologic injury to the enterocyte associated with the ingestion of the protein gluten, which is found in cereal grains such as wheat, rye, and barley. Celiac sprue is clearly a human leukocyte antigen (HLA)-associated condition, primarily associated with the major histocompatibility complex class II alleles DQA1*0501 and DQB1*0201. This HLA-DQ2 allelic combination is found in 98% of patients with celiac sprue.[39] Patients with celiac sprue usually show a quick and dramatic clinical and histologic improvement following removal of gluten from the diet, and quickly relapse after its reintroduction.[40]

The severe villous abnormality of celiac sprue is associated with increased lymphocytes and plasma cells in the lamina propria and intraepithelial lymphocytosis (Figure 66-7). The

TABLE 66-1. **Patterns of Abnormal Small Bowel Architecture**

Pattern	Conditions
Entities usually associated with a diffuse severe villus abnormality and crypt hyperplasia	Celiac sprue Refractory or unclassified sprue Other protein allergies Lymphocytic enterocolitis
Entities usually associated with a variable villus abnormality and crypt hypoplasia	Kwashiorkor, malnutrition Megaloblastic anemia variable Radiation and chemotherapeutic effect Microvillus inclusion disease End-stage refractory or unclassified sprue
Entities usually associated with a nonspecific variable villus abnormality, usually not flat	Changes associated with dermatitis herpetiformis Partially treated or clinically latent celiac sprue Infection Stasis Tropical sprue Mastocytosis Nonspecific duodenitis Autoimmune enteropathy
Entities associated with variable villus abnormalities illustrating specific diagnostic changes	Collagenous sprue Common variable immunodeficiency Whipple's disease *Mycobacterium avium-intracellulare* complex infection Eosinophilic gastroenteritis Parasitic infestation Lymphangiectasia Abetalipoproteinemia Tufting enteropathy

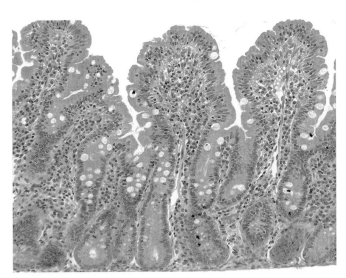

Figure 66-7. Severe villous abnormality typical of celiac sprue. The villus:crypt length is less than 1:1. Inflammatory cells are increased within the lamina propria. Numerous intraepithelial lymphocytes are also present. (*See plate section for color.*)

enterocyte nuclei lose their basilar alignment and become stratified. The histologic abnormality is most severe in the duodenum and gradually lessens distally. With gluten withdrawal, the abnormalities recede from distal to cephalad in the small intestinal mucosa. Thus, proximal small bowel biopsy specimens may remain abnormal for quite some time, even in patients showing marked clinical improvement. A pathologist does not make the diagnosis of celiac sprue. All that can be said is that the specimens contain a severe villus abnormality that is consistent with celiac sprue. Definitive diagnosis depends on demonstration of a suitable clinical presentation; compatible serologic tests (e.g., IgA-anti-endomysial antibodies, anti-tissue transglutaminase antibodies) and small bowel histology; and clinical and, ideally, histologic response to a gluten-free diet.[38-41]

The histologic differential diagnosis includes all entities that may cause at least a focal severe villus abnormality: immunodeficiency syndromes, protein allergies other than gluten, some cases of infectious gastroenteritis,[42] tropical sprue,[43] stasis,[44] IBD including Crohn's disease,[45] and nonspecific duodenitis. Clinicopathologic correlation is essential for proper diagnosis. All biopsy specimens should be evaluated carefully for plasma cells, because their absence in common variable immunodeficiency syndrome (CVID) is easy to overlook. Numerous neutrophils, cryptitis, and crypt abscess formation are usually not part of celiac sprue, and entities such as infectious gastroenteritis, Crohn's disease, nonspecific duodenitis, and stasis syndromes should therefore be considered.

The most common cause of unresponsiveness after implementing a gluten-free diet is that the diet is not really gluten free.[38] If dietary indiscretions are ruled out, patients may have refractory or unclassified sprue,[39] which may respond to the administration of corticosteroids. Refractory sprue can also be associated with cavitation of mesenteric lymph nodes and hyposplenism.[46] Persistent symptoms despite gluten withdrawal with small-bowel histologic improvement should be a clue to search for comorbidities that may cause diarrhea, such as pancreatic insufficiency, lactase deficiency, bacterial overgrowth, or coexisting IBD.[47]

Other Protein Allergies. Patients with allergic reactions to chicken, soy protein, milk, eggs, and tuna fish have been described and show a flat small-bowel mucosa similar to that seen in celiac sprue.[47-51] Definitive diagnosis depends on identifying the offending protein, showing a response to its withdrawal from the diet, and demonstrating recrudescence of symptoms and pathology with its reintroduction.

Entities Associated With a Variable Villus Abnormality and Crypt Hypoplasia

Marasmus and Kwashiorkor. Biopsy specimens from malnourished patients with marasmus (severe calorie and protein deficiency) and kwashiorkor (low protein but adequate caloric intake) have reportedly shown variable villus abnormalities associated with increased intraepithelial lymphocytes, sometimes indistinguishable from those of celiac sprue.[52-54]

Megaloblastic Anemia–Radiation and Chemotherapy Effect. Nutritional deficiency of folate and vitamin B_{12} may result in impaired epithelial cell replacement because of decreased DNA synthesis. Consequently, a variable villus abnormality with or without megaloblastic epithelial changes can be seen.[55,56] Because radiation therapy and chemotherapeutic agents inhibit DNA synthesis, the intestinal mucosal changes are similar to those in folate and vitamin B_{12} deficiency and are associated with decreased mitotic activity in the crypts. Chemotherapy and irradiation may also cause focal necrosis of epithelial cells (apoptosis) and increased numbers of chronic inflammatory cells within the mucosa and submucosa.[57,58]

Microvillus Inclusion Disease. Microvillus inclusion disease, which also includes patients classified as microvillus dystrophy, is an inherited autosomal recessive condition causing intractable diarrhea with steatorrhea in infants. It was first reported under the designation *familial enteropathy.*[59] Diarrhea persists despite total parenteral nutrition, and patients often require small bowel transplantation.[60] The entity should be recognized so that genetic counseling can be offered.[61] Small-bowel biopsy specimens show a severe villus abnormality with crypt hypoplasia. In general, the mucosal specimen may resemble celiac sprue, but intraepithelial lymphocyte levels are usually not increased. Transmission electron microscopy can establish the diagnosis by identifying abnormal microvillus structures at the luminal border of the enterocyte and apical intracytoplasmic inclusions lined by microvilli in the same cells.[62] The intracytoplasmic vacuoles can also be detected with PAS stain or with carcinoembryonic antigen (CEA) immunostaining.[63] Prominent surface enterocyte CD10 immunoreactivity is also described in microvillus inclusion disease.[64]

Entities Associated With a Nonspecific Variable Villus Abnormality

Many diseases are associated with nonspecific variable villus abnormalities that are usually not flat. Although most biopsy specimens showing this change are from patients with clinically latent or partially treated celiac sprue,[39,65] other conditions entering the differential diagnosis include dermatitis herpetiformis, tropical sprue, infectious gastroenteritis, stasis of small intestinal contents, Zollinger-Ellison syndrome, mastocytosis, duodenitis and peptic ulcer disease, and autoimmune enteropathy.[66]

The term *autoimmune enteropathy* has been applied to an intractable watery diarrhea syndrome occurring in infants that has been associated with circulating autoantibodies against intestinal epithelial cells.[67,68] The patients often have variable immunodeficiency and autoimmune phenomena such as juvenile-onset diabetes mellitus, rheumatoid arthritis, and hemolytic anemia.[69,70] The related IPEX syndrome refers to an X-linked immune dysregulation, polyendocrinopathy and enteropathy associated with a mutation of the FOXP3 gene.[71] The small bowel mucosa shows a variable villus abnormality that is often severe and resembles that of celiac sprue. Surface and crypt epithelial degenerative and regenerative changes occur, but many illustrated cases show few intraepithelial lymphocytes, a feature that may distinguish autoimmune enteropathy from celiac sprue. Some patients with autoimmune enteropathy have also had colitis. In some patients the associated colitis resembles lymphocytic colitis, whereas in others the endoscopic and histologic pictures are similar to that of ulcerative colitis.[72] Autoimmune enteropathy is usually severe and intractable, often requiring total parenteral nutrition. There have been scattered reports of favorable responses to tacrolimus,[72] cyclosporin,[73] and infliximab.[74]

Entities Associated With Variable Villus Abnormalities Illustrating Specific Diagnostic Changes

Collagenous Sprue. The term *collagenous sprue* describes the excessive subepithelial deposition of collagen associated with a severe villus abnormality noted in small-bowel biopsy specimens from some patients with malabsorption unresponsive to

gluten-free diet.[75] Although some patients with this finding have ultimately responded to a gluten-free diet,[76] many have followed a fulminant and generally fatal course.

Immunodeficiency Syndromes (Excluding Acquired Immune Deficiency Syndrome). Normal small-bowel morphology is often seen on routine light microscopy in selective IgA deficiency, although nodular lymphoid hyperplasia may also be present.[77] Decreased numbers of IgA-containing plasma cells can be demonstrated by immunocytochemical techniques, but these stains are not recommended for diagnosis.

Patients with CVID may have chronic diarrhea, malabsorption, and recurrent gastrointestinal giardiasis.[78,79] The morphology of small intestinal biopsy specimens may vary from normal to a severe abnormality mimicking celiac sprue.[78-82] In contrast to celiac sprue, plasma cells in CVID are decreased and IgA-containing plasma cells are absent. Occasionally in CVID, the mucosa demonstrates nodular lymphoid hyperplasia associated with absent or markedly reduced numbers of plasma cells. Giardiasis can be found with either histology. Nodular lymphoid hyperplasia without plasma cell changes may also be seen in asymptomatic patients without an immunodeficiency syndrome, especially in children, in whom it may be considered a normal finding. An injury pattern resembling acute graft-versus-host disease, with numerous apoptotic bodies deep in crypts, can also be seen in selective IgA deficiency and in CVID.[82]

Whipple's Disease. Whipple's disease, a chronic systemic illness with numerous gastrointestinal features such as diarrhea and malabsorption, is caused by *Tropheryma whipplei*, a rod-shaped microorganism.[83,84] The diagnosis of Whipple's disease is usually based on the identification of PAS-positive, diastase-resistant bacilli in small intestinal biopsy specimens. A polymerase chain reaction (PCR)-based test is also available but is rarely if ever needed for diagnosis.

Eosinophilic Gastroenteritis. The term *eosinophilic gastroenteritis* has been used to describe a collection of clinical syndromes that are usually seen in children or young adults and that have in common infiltration of the gastrointestinal tract by large numbers of eosinophilic leukocytes.[85,86] Infiltration primarily in the mucosa of the esophagus is associated with dysphagia and mucosal furrows or rings endoscopically (see earlier discussion). Mucosal involvement of the stomach and small intestine may cause abdominal pain with diarrhea and malabsorption, whereas eosinophils predominantly in the muscularis mucosae, submucosa, and muscularis propria are associated with obstruction. Ascites is a major manifestation when the eosinophils infiltrate the subserosa.[85-89]

The histologic diagnosis of eosinophilic gastroenteritis may be difficult. Infiltration of the submucosa, muscularis propria, and subserosal connective tissue by eosinophils is always abnormal and, when corroborated clinically, is diagnostic of eosinophilic gastroenteritis; however, this type of evaluation does, in general, require a resection specimen. The diagnosis of the mucosal pattern of eosinophilic gastroenteritis in biopsy specimens can be particularly challenging to the pathologist. Scattered intramucosal eosinophils are normal in the gastrointestinal tract, and their mere presence should not prompt a diagnosis of eosinophilic gastroenteritis. However, collections of eosinophils not associated with other inflammatory cells, groups of eosinophils associated with focal mucosal architectural distortion or injury (cryptitis, crypt abscesses), and infiltration of the muscularis mucosae and superficial submucosa by eosinophils are all abnormal and, in a corroborative clinical setting, are diagnostic of eosinophilic gastroenteritis (Figure 66-8). The mucosal involvement in eosinophilic gastroenteritis is notoriously patchy; therefore, if the clinical suspicion is great, multiple or additional biopsy specimens should be obtained.

Parasitic Infestations. A large number of parasites may infect the gastrointestinal tract, including *Giardia* (Figure 66-9), *Strongyloides*, *Capillaria*, *Cryptosporidium* species, *Microsporidia* species, and *Isospora* species.[66] Enteric parasites are discussed in greater detail in Chapter 40.

Intestinal Lymphangiectasia. Intestinal lymphangiectasia is characterized by focal or diffuse dilation of the mucosal, submucosal, and subserosal lymphatics that may be associated with protein-losing enteropathy, hypoalbuminemia, hypoproteinemic edema, and lymphocytopenia.[90,91] It can occur in a primary or secondary form. The primary form has a predilection for children and is caused by a congenital obstructive defect of the lymphatics.[91] Secondary lymphangiectasia is associated with many diseases, including retroperitoneal fibrosis, pancreatitis, constrictive pericarditis, primary myocardial disease, intestinal Behçet's disease, intestinal malignancy, Waldenström's macroglobulinemia, and sarcoidosis.[91,92] In both forms, the histologic

appearance of mucosal biopsy specimens is identical: dilated lymphatics located in otherwise normal tissue (Figure 66-10). Therapy includes treatment of underlying conditions, dietary manipulation, and, in some localized forms of lymphangiectasia, resection.[90] Focal lymphangiectasia can occasionally be seen in apparently normal individuals as well.

Abetalipoproteinemia. In abetalipoproteinemia, a condition inherited as an autosomal recessive trait,[93] patients are unable to synthesize apoprotein B. Therefore, fatty acids within intestinal absorptive cells can be reesterified to triglyceride but cannot be changed into chylomicrons for transport. As a result, fat accumulates in the absorptive cells. Biopsy specimens have a normal villus architecture. Enterocytes, however, have

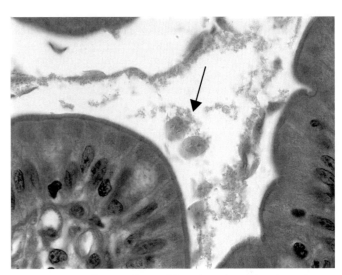

Figure 66-9. Giardiasis. In this small bowel specimen, the diagnosis rests on demonstration of the trophozoite in tissue section. Seen *en face, Giardia lamblia* is pear-shaped and demonstrates prominent paired nuclei. (*See plate section for color.*)

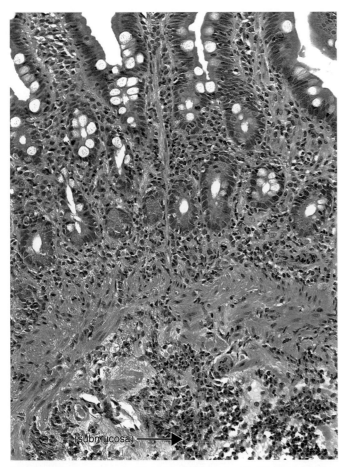

Figure 66-8. Small bowel with eosinophilic gastroenteritis. Note the large collection of eosinophils within the submucosa with lesser numbers infiltrating the muscularis mucosae and lamina propria. (*See plate section for color.*)

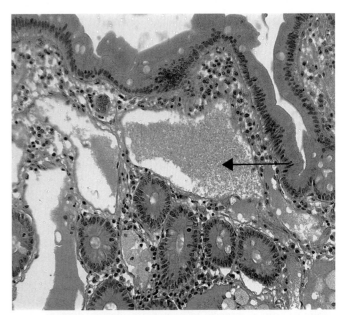

Figure 66-10. Intestinal lymphangiectasia. The primary and secondary forms appear identical in histologic sections, demonstrating dilated lymphatics located in otherwise normal mucosa. (*See plate section for color.*)

cytoplasm packed with droplets of lipid that appear optically clear or foamy. The changes are most prominent at the tips of the villi. This enterocyte vacuolization, although characteristic, is not pathognomonic, because similar vacuolar change has been described in megaloblastic anemia, celiac sprue, and tropical sprue.[94] I have occasionally observed it in patients with no apparent disease process.

Acrodermatitis Enteropathica. Acrodermatitis enteropathica is inherited as an autosomal recessive trait linked to a gene identified as SLC39A4. It manifests in children and has been linked to zinc deficiency. The patients are typically afflicted by cutaneous lesions (perioral and extremity skin lesions, alopecia, nail dystrophy), diarrhea, and malabsorption; they usually respond favorably to the administration of zinc sulfate.[95-97] Small bowel morphology varies, with some investigators reporting a severe villous abnormality similar to that in celiac sprue, which improved with zinc therapy, and others reporting normal or only minimally abnormal small intestinal mucosa by routine light microscopy. Ultrastructural changes that consist of rod-like, fibrillar inclusions in Paneth cells are considered diagnostic for acrodermatitis enteropathica.

Tufting Enteropathy. The term *tufting enteropathy* has been applied to a sometimes familial intractable diarrhea syndrome in children.[98-101] Symptoms usually begin in the neonatal period with the patient requiring total parenteral nutrition. Small-bowel biopsy specimens have demonstrated a variable villus abnormality that is usually not associated with epithelial lymphocytosis, as well as a distinctive surface epithelial appearance consisting of epithelial crowding, disorganization, and focal tufting. Abnormalities of basement membrane structure have been described.

INTERPRETATION OF COLONIC MUCOSAL BIOPSY SPECIMENS IN THE EVALUATION OF INFLAMMATORY BOWEL DISEASE

The pathologist plays an important role in the diagnosis and management of patients with colitis. Patterns of inflammation (chronic colitis, diffuse active colitis, focal active colitis, ischemic-type colitis, trauma change, and apoptotic colopathy) can be identified and may be helpful in assessing patients by creating a relevant differential diagnosis.

Chronic Colitis – Differential Diagnosis

Chronic colitis, the pattern of abnormality in chronic ulcerative colitis in remission (quiescent), includes mucosal atrophy and mucosal architectural distortion.[66,102,103] The luminal border is irregular. The number of crypts is decreased; in addition, the remaining crypts appear short (i.e., not touching the muscularis mucosae) and lose their parallel arrangement, appearing branched and budded. The goblet cell population is usually preserved. Inflammatory cells are typically only mildly increased in the lamina propria. Paneth cells may be present. Although almost all patients with this pattern of injury have ulcerative colitis, it can also be seen in healing Crohn's disease, ischemia, irradiation damage, chemotherapy effect, and chronic infections (e.g., tuberculosis, schistosomiasis).

Active Colitis–Differential Diagnosis

The term *active colitis* describes an inflammatory condition in which neutrophils are present in the lamina propria, within epithelial cells (cryptitis), or within crypt lumens (crypt abscesses). Included under this heading are[104,105]:
- Ulcerative colitis in an active phase
- Most examples of Crohn's colitis
- Infectious colitis/acute self-limiting colitis

Recognition of an inflammatory pattern coupled with clinical and endoscopic correlation allows a fairly specific diagnosis to be made in many patients.

Diffuse Active Colitis

Untreated ulcerative colitis in an active phase represents the prototypic diffuse active colitis. Biopsy specimens demonstrate a diffuse abnormality, meaning that changes are of approximately the same intensity in all areas of the tissue from a particular region (Figure 66-11). The luminal border of the mucosa is irregular.[103,106,107] Increased numbers of chronic inflammatory cells are present in the lamina propria. Cryptitis and crypt abscess formation are often prominent. Even in ulcerative colitis of extremely short overt clinical duration, some atrophy, branching, and budding of crypts are already apparent in many specimens. This crypt distortion and basal plasmacytosis (increased numbers of plasma cells in the lower fifth of the mucosa) are the most useful criteria to differentiate ulcerative colitis from

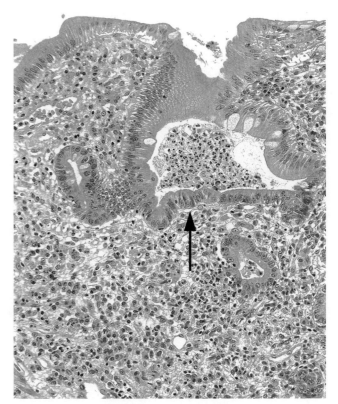

Figure 66-11. Ulcerative colitis in an active phase. Sections show diffuse architectural change, prominent lamina proprial plasmacytosis, and crypt abscess formation (arrow). (*See plate section for color.*)

infectious colitis/acute self-limiting colitis.[103-105] The most a pathologist can conclude from a biopsy specimen showing this pattern is that the changes are consistent with ulcerative colitis in an active phase, because the diffuse active colitis pattern has been described in some examples of Crohn's colitis and in some cases of documented infectious colitis, although these reports more likely represent infectious exacerbation of an underlying primary inflammatory bowel disease.

Focal Active Colitis

Focal active colitis is described as patchy distribution of inflammation with or without architectural change in a mucosal biopsy specimen.[66] Definitionally, some areas of the biopsy specimen must maintain an essentially normal appearance. The focal active colitis pattern is usually not seen with ulcerative colitis and, when present, suggests Crohn's colitis[108] or infectious colitis/acute self-limiting colitis[103-105,109] (Figure 66-12). However, the focal active colitis pattern can be seen in resolving ulcerative colitis under medical treatment,[107,110] and areas of previously inflamed colon and rectum in ulcerative colitis can return, with therapy, to an almost normal histologic appearance. The focal active colitis pattern has been described in some patients with ischemia and has been linked to NSAIDs and to bowel preparation itself.[108,109,111]

The definitive classification of IBD rests on clinicopathologic correlation. The pathologist should convey the histologic pattern of injury to the clinician, who then collates that information with the clinical history and data obtained from endoscopic, microbiologic, and radiologic examination. Through consideration of all this information, an accurate diagnosis can often be rendered.

Acute Ischemic-Type Change

The characteristic pattern of acute ischemic-type injury consists of hemorrhage into the lamina propria associated with superficial epithelial coagulative necrosis, with sparing of the deep portions of the crypts.[66] These changes may occasionally be associated with more extensive necrosis of superficial epithelium with inflammatory pseudomembrane formation.

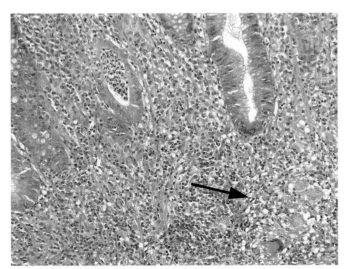

Figure 66-12. Colonic Crohn's disease showing focal active colitis with an intramucosal nonnecrotizing granuloma (arrow). (*See plate section for color.*)

Surprisingly, acute and chronic inflammatory cells (e.g., plasma cells) are typically few in number in ischemic-type damage, and this feature can be helpful in differentiating ischemic-type damage from primary IBD.

The differential diagnosis of acute ischemic-type damage is very wide and includes all causes of true ischemia such as inadequate perfusion, narrowing of blood vessels for any reason, obstructing lesions of the bowel, and bowel distention. Ischemic-type change is also associated with a wide variety of drugs including vasopressors, oral contraceptives, NSAIDs, and glutaraldehyde (used to clean endoscopes).[112-114] Some infectious agents, such as CMV, *Clostridium difficile*, *Clostridium septicum*, and the enterohemorrhagic *Escherichia coli*, typically cause ischemic-type damage.

Trauma-Type Change

Trauma-type histologic changes frequently coexist clinically with mucosal ulcers. The characteristic trauma-type histopathology is found in the mucosa adjacent to ulcers or in polypoid areas and consists of fibromuscular obliteration of the lamina propria associated with mucosal architectural distortion and capillary ectasia. The trauma-type histology can be seen in the solitary rectal ulcer syndrome, localized colitis cystica profunda, inflammatory cloacogenic polyp, and inflammatory cap polyposis and is a frequent finding in the vicinity of the ileocecal valve.[66]

Apoptotic Colopathies

Surface colonic epithelial apoptosis and karyorrhectic debris in the superficial lamina propria are commonly seen in mucosal biopsy specimens and are widely attributed to bowel preparation.[66] Apoptotic bodies in the deep crypts are rarely seen (fewer than 1 per 20 crypts) outside pathologic conditions. Increased deep apoptotic bodies are characteristic in ischemic-type damage, CMV infection, damage associated with mycophenolate mofetil (CellCept),[115] and chemotherapy or radiation. Although seen in association with a variety of injurious agents, apoptosis is the characteristic form of cell death in cell-mediated immune cytotoxicity as demonstrated in grade I graft-versus-host disease, other immune deficiency syndromes, and patients with thymoma.[82]

Specific Infectious Colitides

Common Bacterial Agents

Colitis can be caused by a host of bacteria, including *Campylobacter* species, *Salmonella* species, *Shigella* species, *Staphylococcus aureus*, *Neisseria gonorrhoeae*, *E. coli*, *Treponema pallidum*, *Yersinia* species, and *Mycobacterium* species. Although the colonic mucosal biopsy appearance in these infections can vary greatly (from essentially normal to lesions like those of idiopathic ulcerative colitis), a large number of specimens demonstrate the focal active pattern of injury outlined earlier that strongly suggests infectious colitis/acute self-limiting colitis.[66,104,105] The definitive diagnosis of infectious colitis requires laboratory documentation by culture, PCR identification on the paraffin block, or serologic analysis. In general, invasive organisms cause greater changes in morphology than those that produce their effect by toxins.

Histologic evaluation, although helpful in suggesting an infectious etiology, can only rarely suggest a specific agent. True granulomas can be seen in tuberculosis, syphilis, *Chlamydia* species infection, and *Yersinia pseudotuberculosis* infection. Microgranulomas are described in infection with *Salmonella* species, *Campylobacter* species, and *Yersinia enterocolitica*. Isolated mucosal giant cells, although nonspecific, have been described in *Chlamydia trachomatis* infection.[104,116] Identification of adherent organisms is characteristics of enteroadherent *E. coli* and spirochetosis[66] (Figure 66-13).

Hemorrhagic Colitis Syndrome

The clinical syndrome of hemorrhagic colitis is characterized by abdominal cramping, bloody diarrhea, and no or low-grade fever.[117] Patients typically demonstrate right-sided colonic edema, erosions and hemorrhage. Investigations of epidemic outbreaks have confirmed the association between hemorrhagic colitis and enterohemorrhagic *E. coli*, the most important of which is *E. coli* O157:H7.[117,118]

Symptoms in patients with hemorrhagic colitis characteristically present several days after ingestion of contaminated food—usually undercooked hamburger. In almost all patients the disease resolves spontaneously, but some cases can be complicated by the hemolytic uremic syndrome and thrombotic thrombocytopenic purpura.[118,119]

Most patients demonstrate focal necrosis of the superficial mucosa, associated with hemorrhage and acute inflammation, and preservation of the deep portion of the colonic crypts, an appearance similar to the pattern of injury described with acute ischemic colitis.[117] Some specimens have shown the focal active colitis pattern of injury (see the earlier discussion of focal active colitis) (Figure 66-14). Because routine stool culture media do not distinguish *E. coli* O157:H7 from other strains of *E. coli* normally present in the stool, physicians suspecting hemorrhagic colitis caused by enterohemorrhagic *E. coli* should specifically request that stools be screened for these organisms.

Antibiotic-Associated Colitis and Pseudomembranous Colitis

Toxin-producing *C. difficile* may cause some antibiotic-associated diarrheas but is more strongly associated with pseudomembranous colitis. Administration of any antibiotic that favors the growth of *C. difficile* can lead to pseudomembranous colitis.[120,121] Characteristic lesions occur only early in the disease. Endoscopically the surface of the mucosa contains focal plaquelike cream to yellow pseudomembranes[122]; some early lesions resemble aphthoid ulcers of Crohn's disease. Histologically, there is patchy necrosis of the superficial portions of the colonic crypts, not unlike that seen in ischemia, although true ischemia tends to show more extensive hyalinization of the lamina propria[123] (Figure 66-15). The affected crypts become dilated, and an inflammatory pseudomembrane exudes from the superficial aspects of the degenerating crypt in an eruptive or mushroom-like configuration. This pseudomembrane extends laterally to overlie adjacent virtually normal colonic mucosa. The karyorrhectic debris and neutrophils within the pseudomembrane often align in a curious linear configuration within the mucin. Very early lesions (as well as the mucosa between diagnostic lesions) can, on occasion, show the focal active colitis pattern of inflammation associated with infectious colitis/acute self-limiting colitis. With progression of disease, the plaques become confluent and the crypt necrosis becomes complete. At this point, pseudomembranous colitis becomes indistinguishable from ischemic colitis. Toxic megacolon and perforation can occur.

Viral Agents

Norwalk agent and rotavirus, common causes of viral gastroenteritis, are not known to cause morphologic changes in the colon. CMV and herpes simplex virus (HSV) may cause proctitis and colitis.

Specific Forms of Colitis

Eosinophilic Colitis/Proctitis

Infiltration of the large intestine by large numbers of eosinophils correlates with a variety of clinical syndromes. One variant is probably an extension of the eosinophilic gastroenteritis discussed previously. Peripheral eosinophilia is marked, and a history of atopy is common.[124-127] A second type, primarily in adolescents and adults, previously termed *allergic proctitis* is

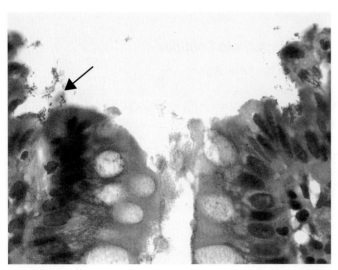

Figure 66-13. Enteroadherent *Escherichia coli*. Note the surface epithelial changes with adherent rod-shaped bacteria. (*See plate section for color.*)

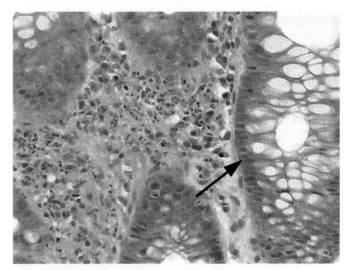

Figure 66-14. Infectious-type focal active colitis pattern of injury from a patient with culture-proved *E. coli* O157:H7 infection. Sections show a collection of lamina proprial neutrophils adjacent to a relatively normal colonic crypt (arrow). (*See plate section for color.*)

likely a form of ulcerative colitis.[128] Whenever large numbers of eosinophils are encountered in colonic biopsy specimens, this should prompt a thorough search for parasites, especially *Strongyloides* species.

The most common type of primary colorectal eosinophilic infiltrate is confined to the mucosa and occurs in infants and young children as a result of dietary-related (protein) allergy (allergic proctitis/colitis).[129,130] These children typically have rectal bleeding with or without diarrhea and many show peripheral blood eosinophilia. Colonic biopsy specimens may show increased numbers of eosinophils within the lamina propria, often accompanied by a mild focal active colitis. Precise biopsy classification may be difficult. In general, however, more than 60 eosinophils per 10 high-magnification fields and eosinophils in the muscularis mucosae or as the predominant cell in crypt abscesses are features suggestive of an allergic etiology.[130]

EVALUATION OF RESECTION SPECIMENS IN INFLAMMATORY BOWEL DISEASE

Once specific causes of enteritis and colitis have been ruled out, what is left is a group of diseases referred to as *idiopathic IBD*. IBD describes at least three entities: Crohn's disease, ulcerative colitis, and colitis of indeterminate type. Despite their nonspecific nature, the pathologic features of Crohn's disease and

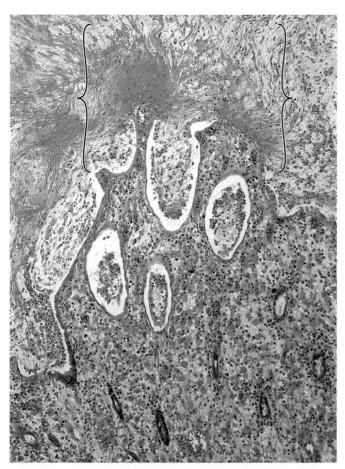

Figure 66-15. *Clostridium difficile*–associated pseudomembranous colitis. An inflammatory pseudomembrane exudes from dilated degenerating crypts in an erosive fashion. The karyorrhectic debris and neutrophils within the pseudomembrane tend to align in a linear configuration within the mucus. (*See plate section for color.*)

ulcerative colitis are sufficiently distinctive that they can usually be distinguished from each other and from other kinds of bowel inflammation.

Crohn's Disease and Ulcerative Colitis

The distributional features, gross appearance, and histologic characteristics of typical cases of Crohn's disease and ulcerative colitis have been well described;[131-134] the distinguishing features are summarized in Tables 66-2 and 66-3. In the colon, rectal sparing, skip areas of involvement, and preferential right-sided localization are gross features favoring Crohn's disease over ulcerative colitis. Discriminating microscopic features of Crohn's disease include nonnecrotizing granulomas, fissuring ulcers, and transmural inflammation. The granulomas, noted in 50 to 70% of patients, are generally poorly formed, few in number, and seen more often in Crohn's enteritis. The fissuring ulcers are lined by granulation tissue rather than neutrophils and extend into the deep submucosa, muscularis propria, or beyond. Transmural inflammation is usually in the form of lymphoid aggregates with a propensity to localize around lymphatic and blood vessels.

Colitis–Type Indeterminate

The term *colitis–type indeterminate* describes approximately 5 to 10% of operative specimens, almost always from patients with acute or severe clinical disease requiring urgent or emergent colectomy (fulminant colitis), in which pathologic features are ambiguous and do not permit precise separation of Crohn's disease from ulcerative colitis.[133,134] In fulminant colitis, fissuring ulcers and transmural inflammation (normally major criteria of Crohn's disease) may be seen in otherwise typical cases of ulcerative colitis. Although fulminant colitis with toxic megacolon is strongly associated with ulcerative colitis, many of such patients do, in fact, follow a clinical course indicative of Crohn's disease. A three-tiered classification system for primary IBD (ulcerative

TABLE 66-2. Distinguishing Gross Features of Crohn's Disease and Ulcerative Colitis

Feature	Crohn's Enteritis	Crohn's Colitis	Ulcerative Colitis
Serositis	Yes	Yes	No, except in fulminant colitis
Thick bowel wall	Yes	Yes	No, except when complicated by carcinoma
Stricture	Often	Sometimes	No, except when complicated by carcinoma
Mucosal edema	Yes	Yes	Usually no
Discrete mucosal ulcers	Yes	Yes	Usually no, except in fulminant colitis
Fat wrapping	Often present	Often present	Usually no
Fistula	Common	Sometimes	No
Distribution	Focal	Usually focal	Diffuse
Rectal involvement	No	Sometimes	Yes

TABLE 66-3. **Distinguishing Histologic Features of Crohn's Disease and Ulcerative Colitis**

Feature	Crohn's Enteritis	Crohn's Colitis	Ulcerative Colitis
Granulomas	Common	Sometimes	No
Fissuring ulcer	Common	Common	No, except in fulminant colitis
Transmural inflammation	Yes	Yes	No, except in fulminant colitis
Submucosal edema	Yes	Yes	Usually no
Submucosal inflammation	Yes	Yes	Usually no
Neuronal hyperplasia	Yes	Sometimes	Usually no
Thickening of muscularis mucosae	Yes, patchy	Yes, patchy	Yes, diffuse (in chronic mucosal ulcerative colitis)
Pyloric gland metaplasia	Common	Rare	Rare
Mucosal inflammation and architectural distortion	Focal	Usually focal	Diffuse
Paneth cell metaplasia	No	Yes	Yes

colitis, Crohn's disease, or colitis of indeterminate type) in colectomy specimens is used.[134] The definitive diagnosis of ulcerative colitis requires all of the following features:
- Diffuse disease limited to the large intestine
- Involvement of the rectum
- More proximal colonic disease occurring in continuity with an involved rectum (i.e., no gross or histologic skip lesions)
- No deep fissural ulcers
- No mural sinus tracts
- No transmural lymphoid aggregates or granulomas

The definitive diagnosis of Crohn's disease requires histologic verification, with the demonstration of transmural lymphoid aggregates in areas not deeply ulcerated or the presence of nonnecrotizing granulomas. In patients in whom the gross and clinical features suggest Crohn's disease (e.g., skip lesions, linear ulcers, cobblestoning, fat wrapping, terminal ileal inflammation), extensive histologic sampling should be done to find definitive histologic features of Crohn's disease.

Several studies have apparently concluded that indeterminate colitis clinically acts like ulcerative colitis. However, many more reports outline a pouch failure rate in indeterminate colitis (19%) that is intermediate between that seen with overt Crohn's disease (34%) and ulcerative colitis (8%).[134-137]

Lesions Associated With Surgical Procedures

Diversion Colitis/Defunctionalized Bowel

A rectum surgically placed out of circuit acquires histologic changes associated with defunctioning alone, regardless of the original reason for diversion.[138,139] The changes probably reflect a physiologic response to stasis and the loss of trophic factors in the feces, most notably short-chain fatty acids. The mucosa of the diverted segment appears erythematous, granular, and friable. Histologic changes include marked lymphoid hyperplasia with germinal center formation, usually accompanied by mild colitis with crypt abscess formation. The changes may be indistinguishable from follicular proctitis (ulcerative proctitis or localized ulcerative colitis). The mucosal lymphoid hyperplasia may be accompanied by lymphoid aggregates scattered in the deep submucosa, muscular wall, and perirectal adipose tissue. Because these changes may occur in diverted segments in patients without IBD, care must be taken not to base a diagnosis of primary IBD, especially Crohn's disease, solely on the histologic changes seen in such specimens.[139] In many patients, the rectum is placed out of circuit during an operation for IBD. In these instances, the rectum can show changes of both primary IBD and diversion colitis. The histologic changes in defunctioned rectums do not, in general, correlate with the original diagnosis or clinical outcome.[139]

Ileal Reservoirs (Pouches) and Pouchitis

For patients requiring total colectomy, several surgical operations have been developed that either create continence in an ileostomy (Kock's ileostomy) or preserve anal sphincter function and restore the continuity to the bowel (ileal pouch-anal anastomosis). These operations have in common the creation of a reservoir (pouch), which is formed by interconnecting loops of terminal ileum. These pouch procedures are contraindicated in patients with Crohn's disease because of increased morbidity (e.g., fistula and abscess).

Pouch complications include fistula, obstruction, incontinence, and anastomotic leaks.[140] Although many complications result from surgical and mechanical difficulties, and others relate to the development of primary inflammation in the pouch ("pouchitis"), some of these complicated cases likely represent pouch recurrence of initially undiagnosed Crohn's disease. These cases illustrate the pathologists' inability to reliably differentiate ulcerative colitis from Crohn's disease in severe colitis, even after examination of the colectomy specimen (see the earlier discussion of colitis – type indeterminate). Virtually all reports of surgical experiences with ileal pouch-anal anastomosis for presumed ulcerative colitis contain approximately 2 to 7% of patients in whom the actual diagnosis proved to be Crohn's disease.[134-137,141]

A late complication of pouch construction is the development of primary inflammation in the pouch with its associated clinical syndrome, pouchitis,[140,142] which affects almost one half of patients. Nausea, vomiting, malaise, fever, and abdominal cramping develop. There is increased effluent and stool from the pouch that may be watery, foul smelling, or grossly bloody; patients often become incontinent. Pouch bacterial ecology is often altered, and patients usually respond to antibiotics, suggesting a bacterial etiology. However, some patients require sulfasalazine, corticosteroids, immunomodulator therapy, or even pouch excision for management of pouchitis.

Pouch biopsy may be performed to confirm the presence of inflammation or to evaluate the possibility of Crohn's disease.[143] Biopsy specimens obtained from nondysfunctional pouches may show mild villus shortening and increased chronic inflammation with increased crypt mitoses, but, in the author's experience, most specimens appear similar to the normal terminal ileum. A few neutrophils in the surface epithelium and lamina propria are commonly seen. In contrast, pouches with pouchitis often have decreased epithelial cell mucin and decreased or absent lymphoid follicles. The most consistent findings in pouchitis have been ulcers with granulation tissue and patchy accumulations of neutrophils in the lamina propria, with cryptitis and crypt abscess formation.[143,144]

Many investigators report an inconsistent relationship between endoscopic and histologic changes in the pouch and patient symptoms. Therefore, many clinicians diagnose pouchitis solely on clinical grounds and reserve endoscopic examination with biopsy for those patients with refractory pouchitis or possible Crohn's disease. There are no reliable endoscopic or histologic criteria to differentiate most examples of pouchitis from new onset or recurrence of Crohn's disease in the pouch.

Although debated,[134,145] missed Crohn's disease is more likely to present as a late pouch fistula than as refractory pouchitis. However, refractory pouchitis has been seen in which pouch biopsy specimens contained granulomas or in which the excised pouch has shown major histologic criteria for Crohn's disease.[143] Invariably, the original pathology of the colectomy specimen was either missed Crohn's colitis or indeterminate colitis. Ulcers in the afferent limb of a pelvic pouch correlate with a diagnosis of Crohn's disease or with the use of NSAIDs in patients without Crohn's disease.[146]

Some investigators have identified histologic patterns of mucosal adaptation in pouches.[147-150] Approximately 60% of patients exhibit what has been called type A mucosa with normal small-bowel biopsy histologic appearance or only mild mucosal atrophy with no or minimal inflammation. The so-called type B mucosa, characterized by transient atrophy with temporary moderate to severe inflammation followed by normalization of the intestinal mucosa, is seen in 40% of patients. The type C mucosa with permanent persistent atrophy and severe inflammation occurs in approximately 10% of pouches. Colonic-type features have been reported at least focally in pouches of all types by routine morphology, mucin histochemistry, immunohistochemistry, lectin binding, or electron microscopy. This colonic-type metaplasia is most well developed in the type C mucosa, but is never complete. All pouches seem to retain mostly small-bowel properties regardless of mucosal type or the duration of the pouch.

DISORDERS OF INTESTINAL MOTILITY

Intestinal Pseudo-obstruction

Intestinal pseudo-obstruction is the term used to describe patients with signs and symptoms of intestinal obstruction in whom no mechanical obstructive lesion can be demonstrated.[151] Intestinal pseudo-obstruction may be caused by a heterogeneous group of lesions. In some cases, the condition is associated with a familiar disease or drug. The bowel obstruction is considered a local manifestation of the more generalized disease process or drug effect and, in general, the intestinal pathology is either unknown or nonspecific. In other cases, pseudo-obstruction is associated with a familiar disease in which pathologic changes can be seen in the intestine (e.g., scleroderma). Finally, there are several intestinal motility disorders in which the primary pathologic changes and clinical manifestations are gastrointestinal.

Visceral Myopathies

There are multiple variants of familial visceral myopathy that demonstrate differences in the mode of inheritance (autosomal dominant versus recessive), sites of involvement in the gut,

clinical symptoms, and extraintestinal manifestations. Visceral myopathies also occur in a sporadic form.[152]

The intestinal pathologic changes in many familial and sporadic hollow visceral myopathies are identical and consist of muscle cell degeneration, muscle cell loss, and fibrosis of the muscularis propria. The degenerative fibers appear swollen and rarefied. Collagen may encircle the residual muscle fibers in areas of muscle fiber dropout and impart a vacuolated appearance.[152-154] These changes are limited to, or more severe in, the external layer of the muscularis propria. The small intestinal mucosa may show changes associated with stasis; these include a variable villus abnormality with increased chronic inflammatory cells, occasionally mixed with acute inflammatory cells. Eosinophilic intracytoplasmic inclusions within smooth muscle cells can be seen in some forms of sporadic and familial visceral myopathies.[155,156]

Visceral Neuropathies

The visceral neuropathies form a complex group of unusual entities that vary in their pattern of inheritance (familial versus sporadic), the extent of intestinal and extraintestinal involvement, and the nature of the histopathologic changes in the intramural neural plexi of the gut. Many of the neuronal and axonal changes are subtle; with the exception of inflammatory neuropathies or, perhaps, familial neuropathies associated with intranuclear inclusions, they cannot be recognized in routine sections, and special silver-staining techniques are needed to demonstrate them.[157] Difficult and unusual cases should probably be referred for consultation to pathology departments with particular expertise in evaluating visceral neuropathies. Some sporadic cases demonstrate mononuclear inflammation in the myenteric plexus, and these can be identified by routine light microscopy alone and can be associated with circulating antibodies.[158-161]

An increasing role for the interstitial cells of Cajal as gut pacemakers and mediators of neurotransmission has been proposed. Interstitial cells of Cajal stain specifically with the tyrosine kinase receptor, c-kit. Immunohistochemistry for c-kit (CD117) and CD34 (which reacts with many c-kit receptors) represents a relatively easy way to study severe constipation and intestinal pseudo-obstruction. Streutker et al.[162] have described completely absent or markedly reduced numbers of interstitial cells of Cajal in intestinal pseudo-obstruction. Although these observations could be an epiphenomenon, they might form the basis of an alternate classification system for pseudo-obstruction.

Ceroidosis: The "Brown Bowel Syndrome"

Severe intestinal malabsorption, for whatever reason, can be associated with dark brown or orange-brown discoloration of the bowel wall,[163,164] owing to deposition of a granular material that has the characteristics of lipofuscin in the smooth muscle of the muscularis propria and, to a lesser degree, the muscularis mucosae. This excessive accumulation of lipofuscin is termed ceroidosis or the "brown bowel syndrome." Whether this pigment deposition adversely affects muscle function is debated.

Melanosis Coli

Melanosis coli is a condition in which macrophages filled with lipofuscin-like pigment are found within the lamina propria or deeper in the wall of the colon. They may be of such numbers as to impart a brown or black color to the colon. Melanosis coli has been associated with increased apoptosis, which is often linked to ingestion of purgatives of the anthracene group (cascara, sagrada, aloe, rhubarb, senna, frangula)[165,166] and is often seen in severely constipated patients.

Hirschsprung's Disease and Allied Conditions

Hirschsprung's Disease

Hirschsprung's disease (aganglionic megacolon) demonstrates a predilection for male patients. Approximately 90% of patients are first seen in infancy, usually with constipation, abdominal distention, vomiting, and delay of meconium stool; diarrhea may occur,[167,168] and some patients may even be affected by life-threatening enterocolitis. Hirschsprung's disease has been linked to inactivating mutations of the *RET* proto-oncogene.[169] Several cases of familial Hirschsprung's disease have been associated to mutations of the endothelin receptor B gene.[170] Other genes have been implicated as well.[171] In the typical clinical picture, the anus is normal; the anal canal and rectum are usually small and devoid of stool. In classic cases, these physical findings are confirmed by barium enema: The contrast material flows into an unexpanded distal segment, then passes through a cone-shaped area, and finally into the dilated proximal bowel. The pathologic change is aganglionosis. The narrowed distal segment shows complete absence of ganglion cells from both the submucosal and myenteric plexi, usually accompanied by hypertrophy of the muscularis mucosae and increased numbers

and size of nerves in the submucosa and between the muscle layers of the muscularis propria[172] (Figure 66-16). In the tapered or cone-shaped region, the number of ganglion cells may be decreased.

Historically, histologic diagnosis was made on full-thickness rectal biopsy specimens. However, this procedure requires general anesthesia and risks the development of stricture and perforation. Because the submucosal and myenteric plexi stop at about the same level in Hirschsprung's disease,[172,173] suction biopsy sampling of the mucosa and submucosa is considered the method of choice for the diagnosis. All rectal biopsy specimens for suspected Hirschsprung's disease should be serially sectioned throughout the block, and each section examined. If no ganglion cells are found, then some comment should be made concerning the adequacy of the specimen. Biopsy specimens devoid of ganglion cells, but in which the amount of submucosa is less than the thickness of the mucosa, should be considered as insufficient to diagnose Hirschsprung's disease.[172] If biopsy specimens contain epithelium of the anal canal, this specimen should be considered inadequate, because the anal canal and distal 2 cm of rectum typically are relatively hypoganglionated or aganglionated.

Many pathologists prefer to examine a frozen-section slide stained for acetylcholinesterase in addition to standard hematoxylin and eosin–stained sections.[174] In Hirschsprung's disease, the acetylcholinesterase stain demonstrates a marked increase in acetylcholinesterase-positive nerve fibers in the

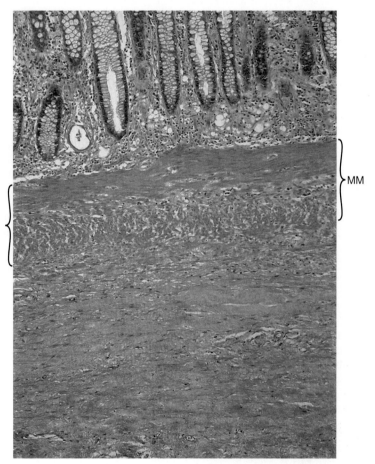

Figure 66-16. Biopsy specimen from patient with Hirschsprung's disease illustrating an absence of ganglion cells associated with marked hypertrophy of the muscularis mucosae. (*See plate section for color.*)

lamina propria and muscularis mucosae. The utility of this technique as an adjunct to diagnosis is debated. False-positive and false-negative reactions have been reported, and its use is a matter of personal preference.[172,175-177]

Occasionally, ganglion cells may be difficult to identify using light microscopy alone, especially in the neonate.[172] In such cases, a positive immunocytochemical reaction for neuron-specific enolase can be helpful in documenting ganglion cells.[178] Other immunostains such as cathepsin D and protein gene product (PGP) 9.5 can also decorate ganglion cells.[179] Frozen-section evaluation is often used as an adjunct to visual inspection to select the site for colostomy. However, use of frozen section to establish a primary diagnosis of Hirschsprung's disease is best avoided because of the high rate of interpretative errors.[180]

Long-Segment Hirschsprung's Disease

In 90% of patients with Hirschsprung's disease, the aganglionosis involves segments of colon less than 40 cm in length. The remaining cases demonstrate a longer aganglionic segment that may even extend into the small intestine.[152] Microscopically the hypertrophied nerve trunks of short-segment Hirschsprung's disease are absent, but the increased number of acetylcholinesterase-positive mucosal nerve fibers can be seen.[174]

Ultrashort-Segment Hirschsprung's Disease

Ultrashort-segment Hirschsprung's disease (segment smaller than 2 cm) reportedly exists but is probably impossible for a pathologist to document by routine hematoxylin and eosin staining of rectal mucosa and submucosa alone, because this segment of rectum is relatively hypoganglionated or aganglionated, even in normal individuals. Rectal manometry plays a premier role in the diagnosis of this lesion. Acetylcholinesterase nerve abnormalities similar to those of Hirschsprung's disease may complement that study.

Hypoganglionosis

Hypoganglionosis is regularly observed in the cone-shaped transition zone between normal and aganglionic bowel in Hirschsprung's disease.[152] Some authors believe that diffuse hypoganglionosis of the colon may give rise to megacolon similar to that observed in Hirschsprung's disease.[174,181] There is no accepted definition of hypoganglionosis; however, guidelines are offered by Meier-Ruge, suggesting that a decrease by a factor of 10 in the number of ganglion cells per centimeter of bowel compared with normal (40 to 80 myenteric plexus neurons per 100 cm of bowel) is diagnostic of hypoganglionosis.[174] In general, the condition has not been well characterized, and many reports lack quantitation.[152] Diverse abnormalities have been described by special silver stains in cases that would have been called hypoganglionosis by routine microscopy,[182] and some cases of hypoganglionosis may be similar to those reported as severe idiopathic constipation or cathartic colon.

Intestinal Neuronal Dysplasia (Hyperganglionosis)

Intestinal neuronal dysplasia is characterized by hyperplasia of myenteric plexi, increased acetylcholinesterase activity in nerves of the lamina propria and submucosa, and increased numbers of ganglion cells with formation of giant ganglions.[183,184] These giant ganglions typically contain more than 7 to 10 neurons (normal is 3 to 5), make up only 3 to 5% of all ganglions in a given case, and are usually not seen in the distal rectum. Occasionally,

ganglion cells may be found within the lamina propria.[181] The condition may give rise to signs and symptoms similar to those of Hirschsprung's disease. It may occur in a localized or disseminated form. Similar lesions, sometimes referred to as ganglioneuromatosis, may be observed in patients with von Recklinghausen's disease or the multiple endocrine neoplasia (MEN) syndrome type IIB.[152,184] Although some investigators diagnose intestinal neuronal dysplasia based on abnormal acetylcholinesterase staining in specimens containing ganglion cells, others believe that acetylcholinesterase staining alone cannot be relied on for the diagnosis.[185,186] Diagnostic criteria for intestinal neuronal dysplasia and even its existence are challenged[186] because 95% of infants so diagnosed experience normalization of gut motility within 1 year. Therefore, many of the observed abnormalities could be within normal range and, in general, the diagnosis should be reserved for florid pathologic cases.[187]

Other Related Conditions

In zonal aganglionosis or "skip-segment" Hirschsprung's disease, ganglion cells are found distal to one or more aganglionic segments.[187-189] The problem here is that a rectal biopsy specimen may yield ganglion cells despite an authentic, more proximal, Hirschsprung's-like aganglionic lesion. Immaturity of ganglion cells[152,174] and hypogenesis of the myenteric plexus[174] have also been reported to cause signs and symptoms similar to those of Hirschsprung's disease. Immunostains for bcl-2 may be helpful in detecting immature ganglion cells.[190]

GASTROINTESTINAL POLYPS AND POLYPOSIS SYNDROMES

Familial Adenomatous Polyposis

Familial adenomatous polyposis (FAP) is inherited as an autosomal dominant trait. Bussey[191] recognized that 100 or more colonic adenomas (recognized grossly) phenotypically identified patients with FAP and distinguished them from patients with multiple adenomas in whom inheritance was not seen (Figure 66-17). In typical FAP, hundreds to thousands of adenomas develop within the colon (Figure 66-18). The adenomas

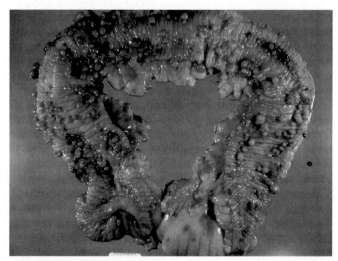

Figure 66-17. Resected colonic resection specimen from a patient with familial adenomatous polyposis. (*See plate section for color.*)

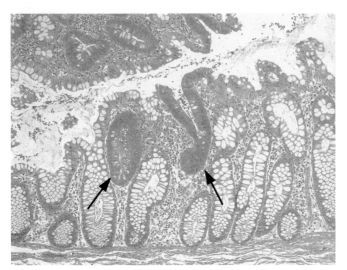

Figure 66-18. Familial adenomatous polyposis. Sections show tubular adenomas including one-gland adenomas (arrow) typical for the syndrome. (*See plate section for color.*)

Genetics of Familial Adenomatous Polyposis and Related Syndromes

The gene responsible for familial adenomatous polyposis (*APC* gene) has been localized to chromosome 5 (5q21-q22).[198,199] Mutation in most patients with FAP and its variants creates a stop codon resulting in a truncated protein product. Direct mutational analysis of the *APC* gene can be performed.[200] Localization of mutations within the *APC* gene locus correlates with phenotype. For example, germline mutations between codons 1250 and 1464 are associated with very large numbers of colonic adenomas, whereas mutations elsewhere, especially near the 5′ or 3′ end of *APC*, yield lesser numbers of colonic adenomas (see the later discussion of attenuated familial adenomatous polyposis).[192,201]

Gardner's and some Turcot's syndromes are variants of FAP. In Gardner's, in addition to colonic adenomas and upper gastrointestinal polyps, patients can exhibit a number of extraintestinal manifestation such as osteomas, epidermal inclusion cysts, other benign skin tumors, desmoid tumors of the abdomen/abdominal wall, fibrosis of mesentery, dental abnormalities, carcinoma of the periampullary region/duodenum, and carcinoma of the thyroid. Turcot's syndrome describes the association of colonic adenomas with tumors of the central nervous system.[202] Turcot's syndrome families with germline mutations of the *APC* gene develop a typical FAP colonic phenotype and often develop medulloblastomas. Other patients reported as having Turcot's syndrome have had mutations in DNA mismatch repair genes that are characteristic of the Lynch syndrome. The brain tumor in this group are usually classified as glioblastoma.

Mutations of the *APC* gene near the 5′ and 3′ ends may have fewer adenomas (fewer than 100), a tendency for the adenomas to be macroscopically flat, and a propensity for these adenomas to cluster in the right colon. These cases are now referred to as attenuated familial adenomatous polyposis.[192,201] As in typical FAP, these patients can develop fundic gland polyposis, duodenal adenomas, and periampullary carcinoma. The risk of colorectal carcinoma is increased in these patients, albeit to a lesser degree than in other forms of FAP, and the cancers tend to occur later in life.

Inherited variants of the base excision repair gene mutY homolog (*MYH*) have been associated with colorectal polyposis with an autosomal recessive mode of inheritance.[203,204] Cases phenotypically resemble FAP or attenuated FAP and are referred to as "MYH-associated polyposis" or "MAP."[203-205]

Juvenile Polyps and Juvenile Polyposis Syndromes

Juvenile polyps can occur in a sporadic form or be part of juvenile polyposis syndrome. In the sporadic form, juvenile polyps have their peak prevalence in children aged between 1 and 7 years. There is some evidence that juvenile polyps can regress, but they are certainly seen in adults. Sporadic juvenile polyps typically occur singly, although patients may have up to five, usually in the rectum. Juvenile polyps typically range in size from millimeters to 2 cm in size (Figure 66-19). As they are often attached only by a small pedicle, these polyps are particularly prone to autoamputation. Histologically, typical juvenile polyps consists of a hamartomatous overgrowth of the lamina propria accompanied by elongation and cystic dilation of crypts lined by nondysplastic colonic epithelium[206] (Figure 66-20). The inflammatory component of juvenile polyps can

begin to appear in the second decade of life and are surprisingly asymptomatic considering their usually large numbers. Symptomatic patients present with signs and symptoms of increased bowel motility and the passage of blood and/or mucus, which often heralds the onset of carcinoma. Two thirds of these so-called propositus cases present with carcinoma and nearly one half of them will have more than one carcinoma in the colon. This high risk of invasive cancer in symptomatic patients forms the basis for polyposis registries and the screening of asymptomatic kindred at risk for FAP.

Most patients are now diagnosed by DNA sequencing, and genetic testing is recommended for any individual with 10 or more colorectal adenomas detected over time.[192-194] In the absence of genetic testing, endoscopic screening beginning at age 10 is still useful to detect FAP.[192] All affected patients have adenomas within the range of the sigmoidoscope. It is therefore recommended that screening sigmoidoscopy begin at age 10 to 12 years, with reexamination every 2 years. The diagnosis of FAP must be confirmed with biopsy because lymphoid polyposis and hyperplastic polyposis can mimic FAP grossly and endoscopically. Once a diagnosis of FAP has been established, prophylactic proctocolectomy is recommended. Most investigators recommend sigmoidoscopy for mutation negative kindred at the age of 12 years, just in case the genetic test is erroneous. Thyroid examination and serum α-fetoprotein determination to screen for hepatoblastoma are recommended.

Regular upper endoscopy should be done. Gastric and duodenal polyps develop in 30 to 90% of patients with FAP.[195,196] The gastric lesions are usually fundic gland polyposis, whereas the duodenal polyps are usually adenomas. The incidence of duodenal adenomas in FAP increases with increasing age. There is a propensity for these to develop in the periampullary region. Adenomas everywhere are prone to proceed through the dysplasia-carcinoma sequence. The relative risk of duodenal/periampullary carcinoma is approximately 125 to 350 times that seen in the general population, and duodenal/periampullary carcinoma has become a major cause of morbidity and mortality in patients with FAP in the post–prophylactic colectomy era.[197]

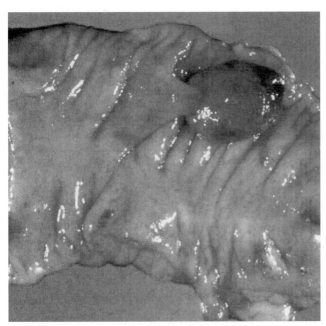

Figure 66-19. Resected colonic juvenile polyp. Note the spherical red polyp attached by an elongate pedicle. (*See plate section for color.*)

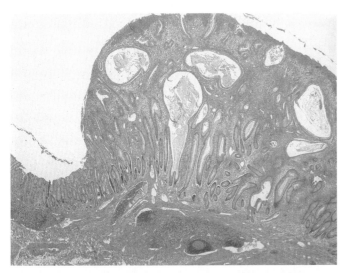

Figure 66-20. Juvenile polyp demonstrating edematous and inflammatory expansion of the lamina propria with colonic mucosal epithelial microcyst formation. (*See plate section for color.*)

be quite prominent, with neutrophils and lymphoid follicles in the lamina propria. Frequently, the distinction between juvenile polyps and inflammatory polyps of primary IBD cannot be made by histologic examination alone and requires clinical correlation. Sporadic juvenile polyps appear to have no malignant potential.[207]

Juvenile polyposis syndromes can be familial or nonfamilial and usually become clinically apparent within the first decade of life with painless rectal bleeding, prolapse, and iron deficiency anemia, or by passing an autoamputated polyp. A patient is considered to have juvenile polyposis syndrome if he or she has six or more juvenile polyps in the colon and rectum, has juvenile polyps throughout the gastrointestinal tract, or has any number of juvenile polyps in association with a positive family history.[208,209] In the nonfamilial form of juvenile polyposis

syndrome (approximately 30% of the total), patients frequently have associated anomalies, such as cardiac defects, hydrocephalus, malrotation, undescended testes, and skull abnormalities. The familial form usually lacks these extraintestinal manifestations. Inherited as an autosomal dominant trait with variable penetrance, familial forms of juvenile polyposis syndrome appear to be associated with an increased risk of colorectal carcinoma.[209] Prophylactic colectomy may be prudent in juvenile polyposis syndrome.

The number of polyps in juvenile polyposis syndrome typically ranges from a few dozen to several hundred. Phenotypically, juvenile polyposis syndrome appears to occur in three varieties: (1) polyps limited to the colon; (2) polyps limited to the stomach; and (3) polyps throughout the entire gastrointestinal tract.[210-212] The mucosal polyps found in the context of juvenile polyposis syndromes are often unusual histologically. In addition to typical juvenile polyps (described earlier), one can find juvenile polyps with unusual features in which there is much more epithelium than lamina propria. In addition, mixture polyps (juvenile polyps with areas of adenoma/dysplasia) are quite frequent.[209] A family showing an autosomal dominant inheritance of atypical juvenile polyps, adenomas, hyperplastic polyps, and polyps showing a mixture of all three types (hereditary mixed polyposis syndrome)[213] may be a variant of juvenile polyposis,[214] although some may be diagnosed as MAP.[215,216]

Two genes are linked to familial juvenile polyposis syndrome, *MADH-4* (18q21.1) and BMPR1A (10q22.3).[206,217,218] Juvenile polyps can be found in patients with other hamartomatous syndromes of the colon, such as intestinal ganglioneuromatosis/ganglioneurofibromatosis, although patients with these associations may be best diagnosed as PTEN syndrome (see later discussion).[219,220]

Patients can sometimes be managed with endoscopy and polypectomy (every 1 to 3 years); however, colectomy must be considered for patients with large numbers of polyps, polyps with dysplasia, or complications (e.g., bleeding). Upper endoscopy is also recommended in patients with juvenile polyposis syndrome.[206,221]

PTEN Hamartoma Tumor Syndrome (Ruvalcabas-Myhre-Smith Syndrome [Bannayan-Riley-Ruvalcabas Syndrome] and Cowden's Syndrome)

Ruvalcabas-Myhre-Smith Syndrome

The Ruvalcabas-Myhre-Smith syndrome consists of macrocephaly, intellectual impairment, unusual craniofacial appearance, pigmented macules on the penis, and hamartomatous polyps in the gastrointestinal tract. Patients may have lipomatosis and hemangiomas. The syndrome may be passed on in an autosomal dominant pattern.[221,222] The gastrointestinal polyps have been indistinguishable from juvenile polyps and, in rare instances, intestinal ganglioneuromatosis has also been described. The syndrome has been linked to mutations in the *PTEN* gene (10q22-q23).[221,223]

Cowden's Syndrome

Cowden's syndrome describes a multiple hamartoma syndrome in which patients have multiple orocutaneous hamartomas (e.g., facial trichilemmomas, mucosal papillomas), fibrocystic disease of the breast, an increased risk of breast carcinoma, thyroid abnormalities, and hamartomatous polyps in the stomach, small intestine, and colon. Consensus criteria for diagnosis have been developed and are reviewed annually by the National Comprehensive Cancer Network Genetic/Familial High-Risk Assessment panel.[221] Polyps of the gastrointestinal tract, when described, have often demonstrated an abnormal proliferation of the smooth muscle lamina propria and have generally resembled the polypoid variant of solitary rectal ulcer syndrome. Some have resembled juvenile polyps. Intestinal ganglioneuromatosis has also been described.[224] The gene (*PTEN*) for Cowden's disease has been mapped to chromosome 10 (10q22-q23).[221,225,226]

Intestinal Ganglioneuromatosis

Intestinal ganglioneuromatosis is defined as proliferation of ganglion cells, neuritis, and supporting cells that can affect any layer of the gastrointestinal wall.[222] These proliferations often present as mucosal polyps. Although these lesions can occur as an isolated phenomenon, the importance of intestinal polypoid ganglioneuromatosis is in recognizing the other settings in which it occurs, such as von Recklinghausen's disease (*NF-1* mutation), MEN type IIB (*RET* gene mutation), Cowden's syndrome (*PTEN* mutation), and tuberous sclerosis (TSC1 [9q34] or TSC2 [16p13] mutation).[221,227-229] Intestinal ganglioneuromatosis can coexist with juvenile polyps, but many of these patients are probably best classified as PTEN hamartoma syndrome.

Peutz-Jeghers Syndrome

Peutz-Jeghers polyps can be found throughout the gastrointestinal tract and are commonly seen as part of the Peutz-Jeghers syndrome.[230] The polyp itself is characterized by fairly normal epithelium and lamina propria lining an abnormal arborizing network of smooth muscle that represents hamartomatous overgrowth of the muscularis mucosae[230,231] (Figure 66-21). Peutz-Jeghers syndrome, usually inherited as

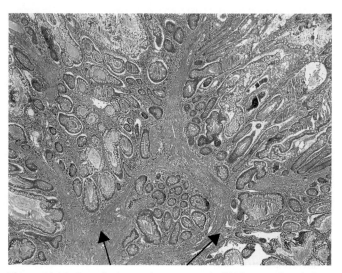

Figure 66-21. Peutz-Jeghers polyp composed of fairly normal epithelium and lamina propria lining an abnormal arborizing overgrowth of the smooth muscle of the muscularis mucosae. (*See plate section for color.*)

an autosomal dominant trait, is the combination of skin hyperpigmentation and Peutz-Jeghers polyps in the gastrointestinal tract. The pigmentation consists of clusters of black-brown freckles about the lips, the buccal mucosa, and the perianal and genital area. Pigmented areas can occasionally be seen on the fingers and toes. The spots appear in the first year of life and tend to fade toward middle age. The polyps usually number only in the dozens and are found throughout the gastrointestinal tract. However, there is a propensity for these polyps to form in the small intestine, where they often cause intussusception. There are rare kindred in which Peutz-Jeghers polyps have been limited to the large bowel. Cases of complicating gastrointestinal carcinoma have been reported.[232] Approximately 5% of females with Peutz-Jeghers syndrome have a peculiar ovarian tumor, namely sex cord tumor with annular tubules.[233] Males with Peutz-Jeghers syndrome occasionally have unilateral or bilateral Sertoli cell tumors of the testes.[234] The gene for Peutz-Jeghers syndrome has been linked to the STK11 gene on chromosome 19.[235]

Esophagogastroduodenoscopy, colonoscopy, and upper gastrointestinal series with small bowel follow-through are recommended in patients with Peutz-Jeghers syndrome, starting at the age of 8, although in some cases follow-up radiologic and endoscopic examinations are based on clinical course and symptoms. Testicular examination starting at age 10 years, pelvic examination, mammographic examination, and endoscopic ultrasonography of the pancreas are recommended.[236]

ACKNOWLEDGMENTS

The author acknowledges and thanks Michelle Guerin for secretarial assistance in preparing this manuscript.

REFERENCES

27. Furuta GT, Liacouras CA, Collins MH, et al. Eosinophilic esophagitis in children and adults: a systematic review and consensus recommendations for diagnosis and treatment. Gastroenterology 2007;133:1342–1363.
30. Wang KK, Sampliner RE, the Practice Parameters Committee of the American College of Gastroenterology. Updated guidelines 2008 for the diagnosis, surveillance and therapy of Barrett's esophagus. Am J Gastroenterol 2008;103:788–797.
41. Rostom A, Murray JA, Kagnoff MF. American Gastroenterological Association (AGA) Institute technical review on the diagnosis and management of celiac disease. Gastroenterology 2006;131:1981–2002.
102. Goldman H, Antonioli DA. Mucosal biopsy of the rectum, colon, and distal ileum. Hum Pathol 1982;13:981–1012.
134. Rudolph WG, Uthoff SMS, McAuliffe TL, et al. Indeterminate colitis: the real story. Dis Colon Rectum 2002;45:1528–1534.
140. Shen B, Remzi FH, Lavery IC, et al. A proposed classification of ileal pouch disorders and associated complications after restorative proctocolectomy. Clin Gastroenterol Hepatol 2008;6:145–158.
152. Krishnamurthy S, Schuffler MD. Pathology of neuromuscular disorders of the small intestine and colon. Gastroenterology 1987;93:610–639.
193. Galiatsatos P, Foulkes WD. Familial adenomatous polyposis. Am J Gastroenterol 2006;101:85–398.
221. Gammon A, Jasperson K, Kohlmann W, Burt RW. Hamartomatous polyposis syndromes. Best Pract Res Clin Gastroenterol 2009;23:219–231.
236. Giardiello FM, Trimbath JD. Peutz-Jeghers syndrome and management recommendations. Clin Gastroenterol Hepatol 2006;4:408–415.

See expertconsult.com for a complete list of references and the review questions for this chapter.

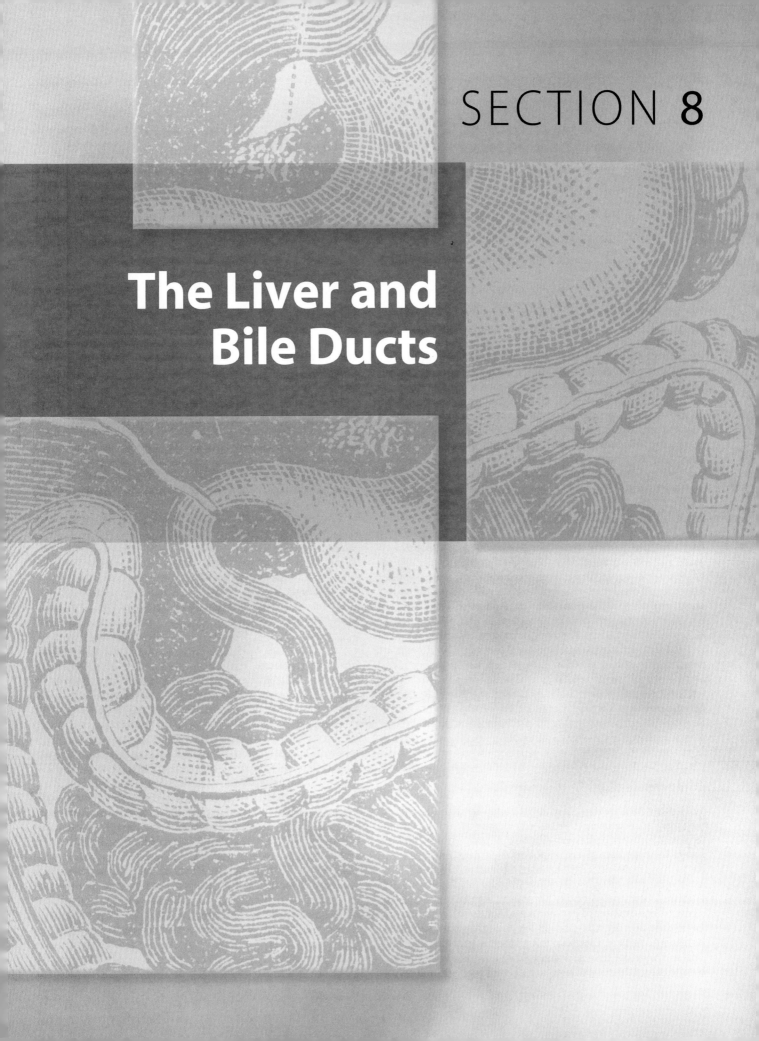

SECTION 8

The Liver and Bile Ducts

67

DEVELOPMENTAL ANATOMY AND PHYSIOLOGY OF THE LIVER AND BILE DUCTS

Valérie A. McLin • Nada Yazigi

The goal of summarizing the development of the hepatobiliary system in a clinical textbook is primarily to help physicians caring for patients with liver disease gain an appreciation of the efforts driving the study of cell-fate regulation both in vivo and in vitro for the purposes of developing cell-based therapies. Further, as several congenital liver diseases are developmental in origin (Alagille, ARPKD), understanding the developmental steps occurring before and after birth should aid in multiple clinical and diagnostic situations. Finally, it is commonly accepted that certain developmental paradigms are recapitulated in disease states and therefore lead to a better understanding of organ response to "injury."

EARLY DEVELOPMENT OF THE LIVER IN HUMANS AND OTHER VERTEBRATES

Early developmental paradigms are conserved across species. Much of what is understood about liver development today is derived from studies in vertebrate models, mostly the mouse. The liver and gallbladder are mostly derived from the endoderm, one of the three germ layers formed at gastrulation. The endoderm follows the same developmental paradigm as all germ layers by evolving from a multipotent tissue to a differentiated cell through the developmental steps of *competence*, *specification*, and *differentiation*, ultimately leading to morphogenesis. During development, liver progenitors undergo multiple cell-fate decisions that ultimately affect organ size, organization, and the capacity to regenerate (allocation of somatic stem cells). Several of the new findings in liver development since the last edition offer insight into these previously poorly characterized phenomena.

Competence

Very early signals, both from within the endoderm itself and from neighboring germ layers, "prime" the endoderm by "activating" its potential to become liver, gallbladder, pancreas, thyroid, or lungs. In other words, the endoderm becomes *competent*[1] to respond to signals directing it toward a liver fate (Figure 67-1A). Competence implies that endodermal cells have the ability to give rise to a restricted number of tissues in response to a given signal.[2,3] For example, a certain part of the anterior endoderm, rather than another, will develop the ability to form a liver bud in response to later, *specification* signals (see later discussion).[4] This is an area of intense study in different vertebrate models because of its direct relevance to directing cell fate in vitro for cell-based therapies: Cells must be in a "primed" developmental state to respond predictably to a soluble signal in vitro.[5] Mutations in genes regulating this very early phase of development are often lethal to the mouse embryo and accepted to have the same effect in humans. However, it is unclear if partial loss-of-function is compatible with a term delivery and postnatal life.

At a molecular level, *competence* occurs through the unraveling or opening of chromatin by transcription factors.[5] In the early, pre-hepatic endoderm, it has been shown that the presence of HNF1β, FoxA1, FoxA2, and GATA4 on the albumin promoter is required for the prehepatic endoderm to respond to inductive signals from the adjacent tissues[5] (Figure 67-2). Among these signals, it is now well established that Wnt signaling needs to be inhibited for foregut identity to be maintained and initiate the hepatic program.[6,7] More recently, it has been shown that hdac1 controls liver fate in a cell-autonomous fashion to direct the hepatic (and pancreatic) lineage in zebrafish.[8] The mechanism whereby these genes modify chromatin structure is still incompletely understood. By the third week of human gestation, cells in the anterior endoderm have acquired the *competence* for liver development to begin.[9]

Specification

The next important step in liver development occurs when the *competent* prehepatic endoderm receives fibroblast growth factor (FGF) signals from the adjacent precardiac mesoderm and bone morphogenetic protein (BMP) signals from the septum transversum (ST) mesenchyme, two populations of cells neighboring the endoderm.[1] In response to inductive signals, competent cells are specified to become liver (committed to a hepatic fate) (Figure 67-1B). Studies in the mouse have shown that, if the FGF signal is absent, the default fate for the prehepatic anterior endoderm is to form pancreatic tissue.[10] More recent investigations have revealed that it is more than just an on-off decision; in other words, it is not the presence or absence of the secreted FGF or BMP signal that regulates the fate of the endoderm, but rather the amount of signal. Indeed, the relative amount of FGFs regulates the fate of the anterior endoderm into lung, liver, and pancreas.[11] Likewise, by disrupting the location of the FGF source and thereby losing the inductive signal, the early liver diverticulum undergoes apoptosis.[12] Taken together, these findings illustrate the temporal and spatial complexity of cell fate decisions necessary to direct the early morphogenesis of different organs from the same tissue and highlight the challenges of "making liver in a dish."

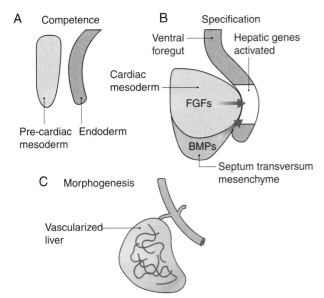

Figure 67-1. Schematic of very early vertebrate liver development. (**A**) Competence. (**B**) Specification; arrow indicates fibroblast growth factor (FGF) signaling from precardiac mesoderm to induce liver. (**C**) Morphogenesis; arrow represents bone morphogenetic protein (BMP) signaling from septum transversum mesenchyme. Adapted from Zaret K. Regulatory phases of early liver development: paradigms of organogenesis. Nat Rev Genet 2002; 3:499-512, with permission of Macmillan Magazines Ltd.[54]

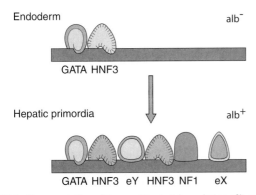

Figure 67-2. Representation of the combinatorial regulation of liver-specific genes by transcription factors. Adapted from Zaret (2001),[58] with permission.

Morphogenesis: Emergence and Growth of the Liver Bud

The liver bud emerges from two lateral domains and one small medial domain of progenitors found on the ventral midline of the early embryo (E8.25; S1-10).[13] In humans, the liver bud emerges at the beginning of the fourth week of gestation (day 22-3) (Figure 67-3).[14] First, the endodermal cells now specified to become liver start to divide and differentiate into columnar epithelial cells. In response to multiple signals, these hepatocyte precursors, called hepatoblasts, invade the ST mesenchyme, a loose tissue composed of a few cells and extracellular matrix separating the pericardium from the peritoneum. Invasion of the ST mesenchyme by hepatoblasts is a complex process involving numerous intercellular signals that results in both migration and proliferation of the hepatoblasts. In addition, as the hepatoblasts invade the ST mesenchyme, so do other cell types, including hematopoietic and endothelial precursors.

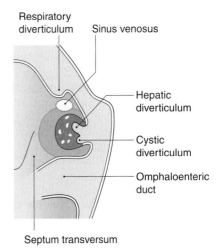

Figure 67-3. Midline section of the developing vertebrate embryo at the level of the anterior endoderm. Cranial (hepatic) diverticulum and caudal (cystic) diverticulum. Both are adjacent to the developing lung diverticula, consistent with a common anterior endodermal lineage. Modified from O'Rahilly, R, Muller F. The digestive system-the liver. In: O'Rahilly R, Muller F (1992) Human Embryology and Teratology, 2nd ed., with permission of John Wiley & Sons, Inc.

Cross-talk between the different cell types is crucial for normal liver development: in the absence of endothelial cells, for example, the liver bud fails to develop.[15]

At the molecular level, a complex network of transcription factors and signaling and extracellular-matrix molecules is essential for the onset and maintenance of liver morphogenesis. First, Hex and GATA-6 regulate the initial proliferation and maintain the differentiation of hepatoblasts.[16-19] In the absence of Hex and GATA-6, early but transient expression of early liver genes is observed (albumin, α-fetoprotein), meaning that early hepatic specification has occurred, whereas this is not the case in the absence of Prox1.[20] Second, an array of genes controls the hepatocytes' ability to delaminate and invade the septum transversum. Among these, Prox1 and Tbx3 contribute to the migration into the ST.[20,21] It is probable that these transcription factors act upstream of extracellular-matrix molecules and enzymes such as the metalloproteases[22] and molecules affecting cell shape and movement such as the integrins and cadherins.[23]

Growth and Size Regulation of the Liver Bud

After the early events of specification and budding, the hepatic anlage undergoes intense growth and architectural organization, while the hepatoblasts differentiate into hepatocytes and biliary epithelial cells. By the end of the sixth week of human gestation, the hepatic anlage resembles the adult lobulated structure.[9] Once again, multiple cell-fate decisions involving both the epithelial and mesenchymal components contribute to the determination of organ size and spatial organization into functional zones. These processes are not quite complete at birth and continue into the first 2 months of life. More important, a small proportion of hepatoblasts do not differentiate but retain their bipotentiality and may participate in the ability of the adult liver to respond to injury (see section on liver regeneration). In the rest of the hepatocyte cell mass, replication is low but sufficient to maintain an organ mass proportional to the size of the child.

Regulation of organ size depends on a tight balance between cellular proliferation and control of apoptosis, controlled both by cell-autonomous and paracrine signals. Multiple epithelial growth factors participate in hepatoblast proliferation and organ growth. These include hepatocyte growth factor, c-Met, JNK, TGF-β, and HDGF.[24-26] β-Catenin, best known for its role as the intracellular mediator of Wnt signaling, appears to be at the convergence of multiple signaling pathways (Wnts, FGFs, hepatocyte growth factor [HGF]) that promote liver growth and cellular proliferation.[27-29] Its role in liver growth is manifold. In liver-specific knockouts of β-catenin, liver size is compromised, consistent with its role in proliferation.[30-34] Its contribution to organ size and shape is also readily illustrated by the grossly impaired liver morphology in chick models where β-catenin loss of function in peripheral growth zones leads to altered gross hepatic structure and organ size.[35]

Liver size regulation is not only a cell-autonomous process. Rather, there are several examples of the mesenchyme-derived mesothelium secreting proliferative signals to the adjacent, developing parenchyma. The first is the β-catenin-dependent growth zones above. Another is the example of retinoic acid signaling between the mesothelium and its receptor in the parenchyma.[36] Finally, the mesenchymal homeobox transcription factor Hlx appears to be upstream of paracrine growth factors.[37] In the regulation of organ size, the logical corollary to cellular proliferation is limiting apoptosis. To this end, IκB kinase in the TNF pathway and c-Raf-1 in the Fas-L pathway are essential factors to protect the hepatoblasts from excessive apoptosis.[38,39]

The concept of a "dynamic transcriptional network" has been proposed to explain the increasing complexity of the growing liver bud, whereby a set of liver-enriched factors interact synergistically, creating increasing numbers of regulatory loops as development proceeds.[40] This attractive model offers an explanation for the multiple different temporal roles of liver transcription factors: for example, FoxA2 has an early developmental role (highlighted earlier) and a later metabolic role (detailed later). According to this model, the complexity and number of interactions between the different factors and regulatory molecules is threshold dependent and increases as development proceeds (Figure 67-4), activating and inhibiting genes in a timely fashion. Table 67-1 summarizes the phenotypes of the knockouts of some of the members of the "transcriptional network."

DEVELOPMENT OF THE BILIARY TREE

An important aspect of liver bud growth and differentiation is the developmental biliary tree beginning at the end of the second month of human gestation. It occurs simultaneously in two neighboring areas of the liver bud (see Figure 67-3):

- The hepatic (cranial) diverticulum: *hepatoblasts* give rise to intrahepatic bile ducts
- The cystic (caudal) diverticulum: *endoderm* gives rise to the extrahepatic biliary tree (gallbladder, common bile duct, and cystic duct).

As development proceeds and the intrahepatic biliary tree develops, the common bile duct, derived from the cranial bud, merges with the cystic duct, derived from the caudal bud. Anomalies in this crucial step, although not well understood, are commonly accepted to contribute to some of the congenital hepatobiliary disorders, such as choledochal cyst and biliary atresia, and to the pathogenesis of some rare conditions

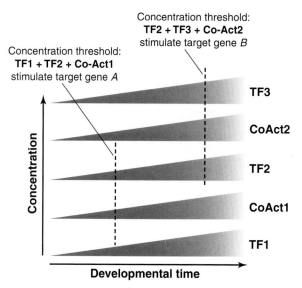

Figure 67-4. Time and threshold model governing the transcriptional control of liver development. Concentration of transcription factors and their partners increase over time. As these increase, increasing local concentrations can be achieved, allowing for increased regulation of gene expression. From Lemaigre (2009).[82]

TABLE 67-1.   Liver Phenotype of Hepatocyte Transcription Factor Knockout or Homozygous Null Mice

Gene	Phenotype
Hnf3β⁻/⁻ (FoxA2)	Embryonic lethal
Hnf3αα⁻/⁻ (FoxA1)	No liver phenotype
Hnf3γ⁻/⁻ (FoxA3)	50% reduction in expression of hepatocyte genes: tyrosine aminotransferase, PEPCK, transferrin. Compensatory increase in FoxA1 and FoxA2
FoxA1⁻/⁻ FoxA2⁻/⁻	No liver[87]
Hnf6⁻/⁻	Absence of gallbladder and abnormal differentiation of intrahepatic bile ducts, atretic hepatic vasculature
Hnf4α⁻/⁻	Diminished expression of pregnane X receptor, Hnf1 α, albumin, α-fetoprotein, apolipoproteins A1, A4, B, C3 and C2, PAH, erythropoietin, retinol binding protein
Hnf1 α⁻/⁻	Hepatic expression of PAH is totally absent in these mice. There is decreased expression of albumin, α₁-antitrypsin, and β-fibrinogen
C/EBPα⁻/⁻	Increased hepatocyte proliferation and decreased postnatal expression of glycogen synthase, glucose-6-phosphatase, and PEPCK. In the adult mouse there is also diminished expression of bilirubin UDP-glucuronosyltransferase and factor IX

Modified from Costa et al. (2001),[86] with permission.
PAH, phenylalanine hydroxylase; PEPCK, phosphoenolpyruvate carboxykinase; UDP, uridine diphosphate.

including spontaneous perforation of the common bile duct. A recent and important finding in understanding the origin of the extrahepatic bile ducts, and consequently an avenue to explore in deciphering the pathogenesis of biliary atresia, is the discovery that the extrahepatic biliary tree is derived from the same anterior endodermal progenitors as the ventral pancreas. Indeed, in a mouse model, the timing and quantity of transcription factor Sox 17, under the control of the Hedgehog effector Hes1, regulates the amount and location of extrahepatic

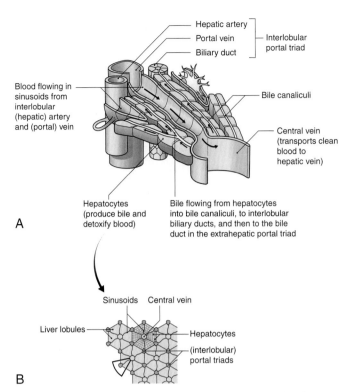

A

B

Figure 67-5. (**A**) Three-dimensional section across a liver lobule. The hepatocytes form rows, separated by the sinusoids, which flow from the portal trial to the centrilobular vein. The biliary pole of the hepatocyte drains into the canaliculi, which are oriented perpendicular to sinusoidal flow. (**B**) Cross-section across a vertebrate liver lobule, as seen in histologic sections. From Moore (1999),[9] with permission.

biliary lineage derived from the posterior ventral endoderm.[41] Although it was previously accepted that the extrahepatic biliary tree derived from the endoderm and caudal diverticulum, the ontologic relationship with the developing pancreas is a novel finding.

At the intrahepatic level, the most commonly accepted theory known as the *ductal plate theory*,[42,43] offers some insight into the pathogenesis of an array of conditions (known as "ductal plate malformations") including congenital hepatic fibrosis, Caroli's disease, Meckel's syndrome, and the recessive and dominant forms of polycystic kidney disease[43,44] (Figure 67-5). According to this model, bipotential hepatoblasts acquire characteristics similar to those of the cholangiocytes of the extrahepatic biliary tree when they come in contact with the mesenchyme surrounding the larger branches of the portal vein. This is the *formation of the ductal plate*. As the hepatoblast changes fate, morphologic changes are subtle, but cell identity can be traced by means of immunocytochemistry: hepatoblasts fated to become biliary epithelial cells (BECs) express cytokeratins, and hepatoblasts fated to become hepatocytes begin to express α-fetoprotein and albumin, as well as staining for glycogen.[45] As development proceeds, this continuous monolayer around the portal vein branches stratifies into a bilayer and then becomes fenestrated; this is known as *remodeling of the ductal plate* (Figure 67-6). Finally, only a few segments of the stratified biliary epithelial cells become bile ducts as they in turn *invade* the mesenchyme to become part of the functional unit called the portal triad. Both ductal plate formation and remodeling, and migration of the bile ducts into the mesenchyme, occur in a centrifugal fashion, starting at the hilum. More important,

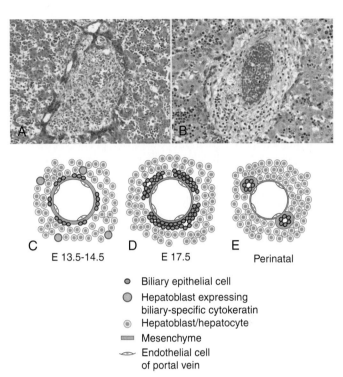

E 13.5-14.5   E 17.5   Perinatal

- Biliary epithelial cell
- Hepatoblast expressing biliary-specific cytokeratin
- Hepatoblast/hepatocyte
- Mesenchyme
- Endothelial cell of portal vein

Figure 67-6. Human fetal liver tissue at weeks 16 (**A**) and 20 (**B**). (**A**) Remodeling of the ductal plate. (**B**) Remodeling is almost complete. (**C-E**) Schematic illustration of the remodeling of the ductal plate in the mouse embryo. (*See plate section for color.*) From Lemaigre (2003),[44] with permission. Pictures courtesy Gail Deutsch, MD.

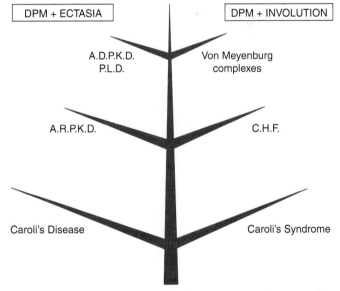

| DPM + ECTASIA | | DPM + INVOLUTION |

A.D.P.K.D.
P.L.D.

Von Meyenburg complexes

A.R.P.K.D.

C.H.F.

Caroli's Disease

Caroli's Syndrome

Figure 67-7. Schematic representation of the biliary tree and corresponding levels of ductal plate malformations. Diseases on the left-hand side of the figure are characterized by biliary structure dilatation; the right-hand side illustrates malformations characterized at least in part by involution of the ductal structures. ADPKD, autosomal dominant polycystic kidney disease; ARPKD, autosomal recessive polycystic kidney disease; CHF, congenital hepatic fibrosis; PLD, polycystic liver disease. From Desmet (2009),[83] with permission.

this process continues postnatally at the periphery of the organ, which should be considered when obtaining and interpreting the biopsies of very young infants. Desmet proposes that the level of the "remodeling error" dictates the disease phenotype (Figure 67-7).

Significant progress has been made on the molecular regulation of intrahepatic biliary development. The clinical relevance of this research is twofold: (1) to develop a better understanding of ductal plate malformations and (2) to comprehend the apparent difficulty of the liver to regenerate functional bile ducts in severe liver disease. Indeed, although hepatocyte regeneration has long been accepted as an example of organ regeneration in humans, the ducts rarely recapitulate a functional intrahepatic tree. Rather, a "neoductular" reaction whereby the hepatocytes bordering the portal triad adopt a biliary phenotype is seen in response to a liver insult (usually obstructive) and suggests that, in response to injury, the biliary program is at least in part reactivated.

The key concepts in which there have been notable advances in understanding the molecular control are the following: differentiation of biliary epithelial cells from the hepatoblast, timing of the differentiation, and mechanisms of bile duct formation. To date, it has been difficult to identify when the cholangiocyte becomes committed to its lineage. In the normal liver, it has been shown that the transcription factor SOX9 expressed at E11.5 is likely the earliest true marker of hepatoblast-to-cholangiocyte differentiation.[46] From these findings we now understand that to conserve a normal cholangiocyte-to-hepatocyte ratio, the onset of cholangiocyte differentiation must be tightly controlled. The transcription factor Tbx3 appears to regulate timing, and therefore number of cholangiocytes. In the absence of Tbx3, there is a premature (E9.5) expression of HNF-6, which acts as a sort of biliary master regulator gene.[21,47] Consequently, if the lineage decision is made early, each early biliary precursor gives rise to more generations of cholangiocytes, and the number of cholangiocytes is increased relative to hepatocytes. Following the initial ductal plate induction, there appears to be a second wave of cholangiocyte differentiation that also warrants temporal regulation: after the first cholangiocytes are apposed to the portal vein and acquire their characteristic shape and gene expression, a second population of undifferentiated hepatoblasts migrates toward the new biliary epithelium to form the ducts.[48] These findings are important for two reasons: first, they complement the ductal plate theory, and second, they highlight the progressive differentiation of the liver and the need for the maintenance of a pool of undifferentiated hepatoblasts.

Further, the development of the biliary tree is intimately linked to that of the hepatic vasculature. Indeed, ductal plates form only where there is a branch of the portal vein. Knockout studies in mice have shown that when genes affecting biliary development (*HNF6*, *HNF1β*, *Notch2*, and *Jagged1* in varying combinations) are absent, the resulting phenotype includes vascular defects affecting branches of the portal vein, or of the hepatic artery and its peribiliary capillaries.[44] It is not excluded that the *primum movens* in ductal plate malformations could be a defect in a mesenchymal protein, or in a vascular gene, which would lead to secondary biliary defects.

DEVELOPMENT OF THE HEPATIC VASCULATURE

Development of the hepatic vasculature mimics that of the bile ducts. At the *intrahepatic* level, there is evidence in vertebrate models that endothelial cells are required for liver induction and migration of the early hepatic epithelium into the ST mesenchyme.[49] These early endothelial cells go on to form the fenestrated lining of the hepatic sinusoids.[50] They participate

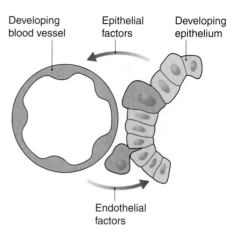

Figure 67-8. Diagrammatic representation of cross-talk between vascular endothelium and developing bile ducts. The Notch/Jagged pathway is known to participate in this process. Reproduced from Lammert E, Cleaver O, Melton D. Role of endothelial cells in early pancreas and liver development. Mech Dev 2003; 120:59-64, with permission.[49]

in the early organization of the liver into its structural unit, the lobule, by directing the migration of the hepatoblasts into cords[51] (Figure 67-8).

The *extrahepatic* vasculature is composed of the afferent portal vein and hepatic artery and the efferent hepatic veins. In all vertebrates, liver development is intimately linked to the yolk sac. It follows that the vitelline veins eventually form the portal vein.[51] At the hilum, the portal vein branches invade the mesenchyme in a centrifugal fashion, as they interact with neighboring mesenchyme and hepatoblasts. In the fetus, the portal vein is joined by the umbilical vein to form the portal sinus or ductus venosus. Most of the umbilical blood is directed toward the left lobe of the liver, with most of the mesenteric portal blood directed toward the right lobe (Figure 67-9). The clinical correlate is that most of the hematopoietic activity in the liver is localized to the right lobe, owing to low oxygen saturation. In utero, a large amount of the prehepatic blood flow is shunted directly to the suprahepatic veins by means of the ductus venosus. After birth, the first enteral feeding acts as trigger for this physiologic shunt to close.[52] Typically, the transition occurs slowly, and this should be considered in the care of premature infants in whom enteral feedings are often withheld in the first few days of life. Although the effect on the splanchnic vasculature of early enteral feedings in premature infants is unclear, there are reports of liver tumors or encephalopathy in older children that were associated with the persistence of a permeable ductus venosus.[53,54]

The liver has an intrahepatic lymphatic system, which begins to develop in the 15th week of human gestation. A vast network of extrahepatic lymphatics, mostly localized to the capsule, also exists. Their function becomes evident only when there is increased resistance to intrahepatic blood flow in diseased states.

THE FUNCTIONAL UNIT OF THE LIVER: THE HEPATIC LOBULE AND SINUSOIDAL SYSTEM

Mature hepatic function depends on a normally functioning sinusoidal system. Development of a normal hepatic vasculature and biliary tree, both intrahepatic and extrahepatic, allows the functional unit of the liver, the hepatic lobule, to perform its functions (Figures 67-5 and 67-10).

The hepatic lobule is a carefully orchestrated unit composed of radially arranged hepatocyte cords lined by fenestrated sinusoids. It is the product of the close interactions among vascular precursors, hepatoblasts, and mesenchyme during the early phases of development. It relies on *two substrate supply routes*, the hepatic artery and the portal vein, and *two metabolite exit routes*, the hepatic veins and the biliary system.

The structure of the lobule is such that it operates along several gradients. Anatomic specialization of hepatocyte function occurs postnatally through a mechanism leading to "enzymatic zoning" (zones 1, 2, and 3) from the portal triad to the central vein: hepatocytes express different enzymes according to their position along the portal to central axis. First, there is a sinusoidal concentration gradient from portal triad to central vein pertaining to oxygen saturation as well as to the concentration of any nutrient or xenobiotic transported through the portal vein. Second, there exists a cytosolic concentration gradient of both solutes and enzymes across the hepatocyte, as bile acids (and other biliary constituents) are synthesized and transported across the hepatocyte to the apical membrane to be exported via the canaliculus. Finally, there is a concentration gradient within the biliary tree, as both the composition and the concentration of bile change as it travels through the canaliculi and interlobular bile ducts toward the hilum of the liver.

Until recently, the molecular mechanisms controlling liver zonation were poorly understood. Progress in the last few years points to Wnt/β-catenin signaling as a crucial regulator of this postnatal event (Figure 67-11). The current model stipulates that a yet uncharacterized Wnt signal from the central vein endothelium promotes the activation of pericentral (PC) genes and the inactivation of periportal (PV) while a periportal Wnt inhibitor favors the transcription of PV genes in zone 1.[55-57] Because the ammonia detoxifying enzymes are PP enzymes (zone 1), one of the clinically significant points of these findings may be that in situations requiring active β-catenin signaling, nitrogen metabolism may be compromised. For example, the requirements of liver regeneration (β-catenin-dependent oval cell proliferation) are not compatible with the expression of ammonia-metabolizing enzymes. This may in part explain the hyperammonemia in acute liver failure and other situations of insufficient hepatic cell mass.

Whereas microscopically the *lobule* is recognized as the functional liver unit, surgeons consider the *segment* to be the macroscopically recognizable unit (Figure 67-12). As described previously, liver anatomy is defined by vascular and biliary development. The result is an organ composed of eight surgically divisible segments defined by vascular and biliary conduits. In partial hepatectomies or segmental liver transplants, dissection is performed according to this segmental anatomy.

FUNCTIONAL DEVELOPMENT OF THE LIVER

Although bile acids in immature form are synthesized as early as the end of the first trimester, metabolic functions of the liver mature slowly throughout gestation. Furthermore, the placenta and maternal liver perform many of the necessary functions in lieu of the fetal liver until birth. The loss of umbilical blood at birth acts as an inducer for many enzymes.[53] Nonetheless, the ontogeny of hepatic anabolic and catabolic enzymes is a long and complicated process with much interindividual variability. One might hypothesize that the hepatic-enriched molecular network is at the root of this variability. For example, the newborn does not metabolize drugs like the adult, nor is a fully mature hepatic metabolism reached before the end of the first year of life.[58] This

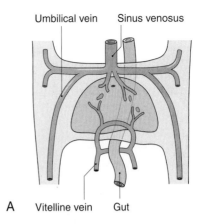

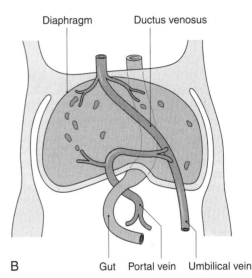

Figure 67-9. Frontal section through a developing human embryo at 6 weeks (**A**) and 10 weeks (**B**): venous system. (**A**) In the 6-week fetus, the vitelline veins carry blood from the yolk sac to the developing embryo. They have not fused on the midline yet and are not connected to the umbilical vein. (**B**) By 10 weeks' gestation, the vitelline veins have fused, becoming the portal vein, and the umbilical vein joins the portal system, forming the ductus venosus, supplying oxygenated blood to the liver and returning mixed blood to the heart via the inferior vena cava. The newly formed portal vein returns blood from the mesenteric tree to the liver (low oxygenation saturation). Adapted from Rappaport and Wanless, 1993.[84]

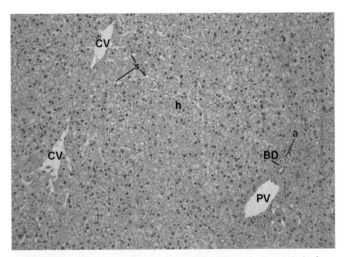

Figure 67-10. Microscopic functional unit of the liver: the liver lobule, from a mature child. a, Arteriole; BD, bile duct; CV, central vein; h, hepatocytes; PV, portal vein; s, sinusoids. (*See plate section for color.*)

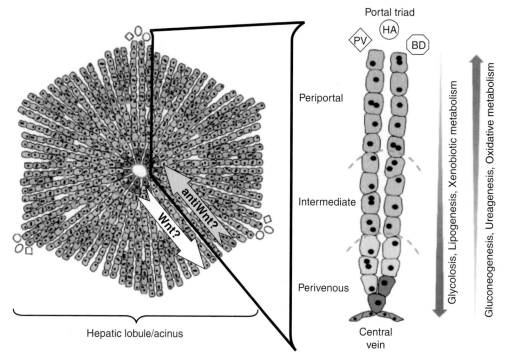

Figure 67-11. Schematic representation of the three different functional and concentric zones of the liver lobule and the putative contribution of the Wnt pathway in its zonal organization. The dark blue zone is periportal, whereas the red is centrolobular or pericentral. A central-to-portal gradient of Wnt ligands contributes to differential metabolic and structural gene expression, whereas Wnt antagonists likely are expressed in a reverse gradient offering a second level of gene expression control from the periportal area toward the center of the lobule. Modified from Burke and Tosh (2006).[57]

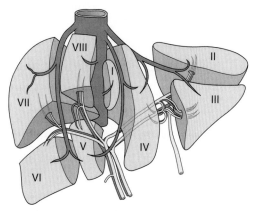

Figure 67-12. Division of the liver into segments as defined by Couinaud. This is the surgical anatomy used both in partial hepatectomy and in reduced-graft and living-related liver transplantation. Segmental anatomy is defined according to vascular and biliary branches. From Bismuth (1999),[85] with permission.

relative immaturity offers an explanation for why so many of the systemic insults in the newborn period result in abnormal liver function test results. The purpose of both the anatomic and physiologic development of the liver is to prepare the fetus for the drastic transition of parturition and extrauterine life.

LIVER AS A METABOLIC ORGAN

Much like the pancreas, liver functions can be divided into endocrine and exocrine, according to the exit route of its metabolites:

- *Endocrine* function implies secretion into the sinusoidal system
- *Exocrine* means secretion into the biliary system

Endocrine Liver

Carbohydrates

The transition to extrauterine life means that the fetus no longer has a continuous supply of glucose at a time when its metabolic demands are very high. Instead, it needs to rely on stores and the ability to synthesize glucose *de novo*. Thus, the fetal liver accrues a large amount of glycogen during the second half of gestation, which in turn it consumes postnatally. Similarly, the enzymatic pathways for gluconeogenesis reach functional levels by term. Consequently, premature infants are at risk for hypoglycemia for two reasons: insufficient glycogen accrual and immature gluconeogenesis enzymes.

As discussed earlier, an emerging theme in the understanding of liver development is the temporal regulation of genes. In other words, genes that are "used" for one purpose in very early liver development can be reactivated later in development for another mission. Such is the case of Foxa3, which participates in early cell-fate decisions in pancreas and liver specification. In adult Foxa3 –/– mice, fasting blood glucose is significantly lower than in fasted wild-type mice.[59] Evidence suggests that this effect is mediated by the GLUT2 transporter, which appears to be a main target for Foxa3.[59,60] Another example is HNF1α, which, when knocked out, leads to biliary development defects as well as deficiencies in glucose homeostasis[60] as well as in amino acid and fatty acid oxidation metabolism.

Protein

The main circulating and transport protein in the fetus is α-fetoprotein. Toward term, transcription and translation of albumin begins, although serum levels do not yet reach adult levels. During the first few months of life, α-fetoprotein levels drop under the control of transcriptional repressors,[61-63] as albumin levels rise. All of the other major secreted proteins are synthesized at the time of birth: coagulation factors, complement proteins, and apolipoproteins. A full year is required for many of these proteins to reach adult levels. The abundant serum protein albumin is such an example. The infant has about 60% of the circulating concentration of albumin of a 1-year-old child (2.5 versus 4 g/L). The clinical corollary is that this affects serum levels of unconjugated bilirubin in the neonate and of xenobiotics in the infant. Concurrently, intracellular enzyme concentrations and functions mature as the hepatocyte prepares for detoxification and conjugation.

Lipids

During the first few days of life, an additional metabolic pathway matures to meet the metabolic demands of the fetus: fatty acid oxidation and ketogenesis. Fatty acid oxidation allows the utilization of fats in breast milk transported to the liver by the portal system. Ketogenesis offers a substrate for cerebral metabolism and hepatic neoglucogenesis.

Coagulation Factors

The synthesis of this particular subset of vital circulating proteins has reached maturity by parturition. Most of these factors require vitamin K for their synthesis. Although the enzymatic pathways of the coagulation cascade are mature at birth, the newborn is at risk for a bleeding diathesis, because its gut is not yet colonized with vitamin K–producing bacteria; hence the universal recommendation for neonatal vitamin K administration.

Hormones

The liver also serves an endocrine function via the tight regulation of the half-lives of hormones such as insulin and the sex hormone estrogen. It is also an end-organ for insulin and glucagon. The liver responds to insulin by storing carbohydrates as glycogen and to glucagon, by initiating gluconeogenesis.

Exocrine Liver

Bile Acids

Of all the metabolic functions of the liver, its "exocrine" function is the longest in reaching maturity. First, at the onset of bile acid synthesis, rather than the functional adult-type bile acids, the developing hepatocyte produces "atypical" bile acids, which may act as trophic factors for the developing biliary tree. Second, overall synthesis is less abundant than that in the mature infant. Third, enteral and hepatic uptake of secreted and circulating bile acids is immature, and thus less efficient than in the adult. Finally, the ability of the hepatocyte to excrete bile acids into the canaliculus does not mature until well into the first year of life.[64,65] The biliary route is a major pathway for the excretion of metabolites; its immaturity in the first few months of life makes the neonate vulnerable to develop cholestasis in response to endobiotics or xenobiotics.

On a molecular level, a significant development has been the identification of the important role of the transcription factor FoxA2 in bile acid homeostasis. Indeed, not only do *FoxA2*–/– livers have an increased susceptibility to cholestasis, but *FOXA2* is down-regulated in human cholestatic livers,[66] suggesting a homeostatic role of this hitherto embryonic gene. These findings mirror those described earlier for glucose homeostasis. Developmental genes are reactivated in the adult liver to serve homeostatic functions, among others.

Cholesterol and Phospholipids

Bile acid metabolism is inexorably linked to cholesterol and phospholipid metabolism in humans. Bile acids are cholesterol metabolites. The liver is the main site of human cholesterol synthesis, which begins in utero. The rate-limiting step is hydroxymethylglutaryl coenzyme A (HMG-CoA) reductase, which is regulated by serum bile acid concentration from the enterohepatic circulation. Because bile acid composition varies through development and early extrauterine life, it is likely that HMG-CoA reductase function, and cholesterol synthesis, follow a similar pattern to that of other hepatic enzymes, not reaching mature levels until the end of the first year of life.

LIVER AS A FILTER

Finally, whereas most of the functions described previously can be described as "anabolic," the liver has multiple "catabolic" functions. Through its vast array of transferases and conjugation reactions, the liver, together with the kidney, is the main factor protecting the organism against harmful xenobiotics, such as medications, toxins, and bacteria derived from the gut via the portal circulation.

LIVER AS A HEMATOPOIETIC ORGAN

The liver is the major site of hematopoiesis in the fetus, beginning around the fourth to fifth weeks of gestation and peaking toward the early third trimester. The population of hematopoietic cells drops rapidly in the first 2 months of life.

LIVER AS AN IMMUNE ORGAN

The liver is accepted to play a crucial role in defending the body against enteric bacteria and bacterial toxins entering via the portal vein. To this end, the liver macrophages (Kupffer cells) are localized along the sinusoids and display specialized functions according to their position along the porto-to-central axis. Likewise, other cells of the innate and adaptive immune systems are dispersed throughout the liver respecting the form-and-function paradigm. Together, they contribute to the liver's role in the response to systemic infections and in the fight against autoimmune disorders and have conferred on the liver its recognition as a pivotal immune organ. The balance of this unique immune makeup likely explains the tolerogenic potential of the liver as well as its critical role in the systemic inflammatory cascade observed in situations of liver failure.[67] From a teleological perspective, it appears logical that the liver play a central role in immune tolerance and regulation because it serves as an interface between the organism and the environment. The clinical ramifications of the immune role of the liver are only beginning to be understood.

STEM CELLS AND LIVER REGENERATION

Developmental and stem cell biology jointly with the study of liver regeneration work together to develop alternate therapeutic modalities to cadaveric whole organ or cell transplantation for the treatment of diabetes and liver failure. The experimental importance of understanding how anterior endoderm gives rise to liver and pancreas progenitors is that adult hepatocytes cannot be maintained in culture without dedifferentiation occurring. Therefore, stem cells are the most attractive source of future therapeutic liver and pancreas cells; hence the need understand liver and pancreas development in vivo before making functional tissue in vitro. The purpose of discussing stem cells in this section is twofold: to understand their role in regeneration and to gain an understanding of experimental efforts to direct stem cells toward a hepatic fate in vitro.

Regeneration

It has been long known that the liver has a remarkable regenerative potential. Hepatectomy models in mice have shown that liver volume, although not structure, is restored after 2 weeks.[68] More recently, with the advent of both segmental and living-related liver transplantation, the use of volumetric imaging has shown that the donor liver doubles its volume in 7 days, and the recipient liver in 14 days.[68,69] It is liver volume, not structure, that is replaced. Liver regeneration is a heterogeneous process[70] that involves the recruitment of many different cells: hepatocytes, hepatocyte progenitors (or stem cells), endothelial cells, leukocytes, and stellate cells. In the mouse, the sequence of events begins by hepatocyte replication at 24 hours postinjury, followed by biliary epithelial cells and endothelial cells within 72 hours.[71,72] If the hepatocyte compartment is severely injured, oval cells take over. Liver regeneration is multifactorial, and this section focuses on the cell types and molecules currently under the most scientific scrutiny.

The term *stem cell* is used to describe cells involved in both tissue homeostasis and repair after damage. These somatic progenitor cells have two main characteristics: self-maintenance and multipotency.[73] In the liver, two populations of cells have been identified for their ability to regenerate: hepatic stem cells and oval cells.[74] *Hepatic stem cells* are pluripotent cells residing *in loco* in the canals of Hering, next to the peripheral small biliary ductules. Some of these CD34+ cells may be remnants from the days when the liver was a major hematopoietic organ; these cells may reacquire their hematopoietic potential or may adopt a hepatic fate.[73] *Oval cells*, which reside in the portal tracts, are also known as hepatocyte progenitor cells. They are conditional stem cells and the alleged progeny of organ-specific stem cells.[73] They have a modest proliferative capacity, which is initiated given the correct, permissive environment.[73] Cells with the same "hepatogenic" potential have also been isolated from the pancreas in certain experimental conditions, reflecting the common origin between liver and pancreas.[71,72] These cells have also been labeled "oval" cells. Oval cells can differentiate into hepatocytes, cholangiocytes, and abnormal ductular reactive cells.[71,72] These are the cells accepted to contribute to the nonspecific "ductular reaction" characteristic of cholestatic disease.

Although little is known regarding the reactivation of developmental pathways in these "progenitor" or "stem" cells as they repopulate an injured liver, it has been shown that hepatocytes, which are the first to respond to regenerative signals following injury, require *hepatocyte growth factor* signaling from the mesenchyme and reciprocally express HGF receptors, recapitulating the early steps of liver bud formation. Recently, the Notch/Jagged pathway was shown to confer regenerative potential to dividing hepatocytes in a mouse model of liver regeneration.[75] Mostly, *humoral factors* have been shown to play an important role in the onset of liver regeneration, namely the cytokines tumor necrosis factor (TNF)-α and interleukin-6 (IL-6),[76] and the subsequent activation of their downstream pathways.

Future studies in the field of liver regeneration and stem cell biology should aim to identify the cross-regulation between these different pathways.

A large body of literature[71-73] provides compelling evidence suggesting that hematopoietic precursors and hepatic precursors share cell surface markers, and thus probably a common lineage. Furthermore, it appears that certain cells derived from the bone marrow have the ability to migrate to the liver and may therefore also be an important source of hepatocyte precursors.[51,71-73] Thus, in addition to three in situ populations of cells capable of responding to regenerative stimuli, the liver also has a circulating pool of stem cells that appear to fuse with hepatocytes to participate in liver regeneration.[77-79] The current model for the relationship between hepatocyte precursors and their mechanism of action is illustrated in Figure 67-13.

In summary, the liver has three in situ compartments of possible stem cells: the hepatocytes themselves, the periportal oval cells, and the periductular organ specific stem cells. Current evidence suggests that each of these cells responds to different permissive conditions (different disease or injury) to acquire a hepatocyte or biliary phenotype, and that developmental pathways are reactivated in this process. In addition, the liver, like many other organs, has a circulating pool of stem cells derived from the bone marrow. As research in the field of stem cells progresses, clinicians undoubtedly will see this knowledge applied to the management of acute and chronic liver diseases.

Experimental Biology

The most recent advances in the manipulation of stem cells with a view to direct cell fate in vitro can be summarized as an effort along a continuum from human embryonic stem cells (hESCs) to endoderm to pancreas or liver (hepatocytes and cholangiocytes).

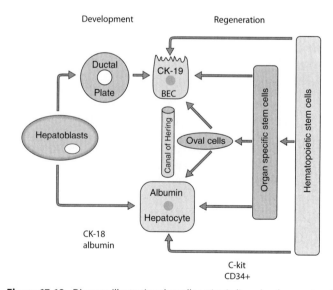

Figure 67-13. Diagram illustrating the cells active in liver development and regeneration. In development, the hepatoblast has the capacity to develop into biliary epithelial cells (BECs) or mature hepatocytes. Following an injury, the hepatocytes can regenerate. Oval cells, which lie adjacent to the canals of Hering, can generate both mature cell types. Other liver-specific stem cells, thought to reside close to the portal triad, also participate in liver regeneration. Finally, hematopoietic stem cells can home to the liver and fuse with BECs or hepatocytes, where they are believed to initiate regeneration. The characteristic markers expressed by the cells are indicated. Adapted from Di Campli et al.(2003).[71]

The most recent exciting advances made in the effort to direct stem cells toward endoderm is the identification of two novel molecules with an endoderm-inducing potential. First, the IDE1 and IDE2 compounds can transform ESC into definitive endoderm with a higher efficiency than the developmental signals Nodal and Activin A.[80] Not only is the efficiency of differentiation high, but the chemically induced endodermal cells are then susceptible to a pancreas-inducing regimen, also with a higher efficiency than previously reported.[80] With the pancreatic and liver lineages being so closely linked, one can only predict that the liver potential of the chemically induced endoderm is also promising. Likewise, another group has also succeeded in differentiating endoderm in vitro from ESC using FGFs,[81] and these endoderm-like cells can express pancreatic or liver markers.[81] We look forward to data concerning the therapeutic potential of these cells.

CONCLUSION

Understanding liver embryology is of importance to clinicians dealing with perinatal and childhood liver diseases. In particular, an appreciation for the molecular regulation of liver development highlights the research efforts of many aiming to generate endodermal organs "in a dish": for example, hepatocytes or pancreatic islet cells for the purposes of cell transplantation.

ACKNOWLEDGMENTS

VAM thanks M. G. Schäppi, D. C. Belli, C. A. Siegrist, K. Posfay-Barbe, and the members of the P. L. Herrera lab for their support.

REFERENCES

5. Cirillo LA, Lin FR, Cuesta, et al. Opening of compacted chromatin by early developmental transcription factors HNF3 (FoxA) and GATA-4. Mol Cell 2002;9:279–289.
10. Deutsch G, Jung J, Zheng M, et al. A bipotential precursor population for pancreas and liver within the embryonic endoderm. Development 2001;128:871–881.
54. Zaret KS. Regulatory phases of early liver development: paradigms of organogenesis. Nat Rev Genet 2002;3:499–512.
82. Lemaigre FP. Mechanisms of liver development: concepts for understanding liver disorders and design of novel therapies. Gastroenterology 2009;137:62–79.

See expertconsult.com for a complete list of references and the review questions for this chapter.

68 NEONATAL HEPATITIS

Scott Nightingale • Vicky Lee Ng

The term *neonatal hepatitis* originated in the 1950s when few etiologies of neonatal liver disease were identified, and pathologists recognized a characteristic histologic appearance of the neonatal liver in response to injury.[1] The term has since been used to refer to virtually all forms of liver dysfunction in the neonate presenting clinically as jaundice due to conjugated hyperbilirubinemia within the first 3 months of life, after structural or anatomic disorders of the biliary tree have been excluded. However, this term is misleading because it implies an infectious process involving the liver (such as the numerous forms of viral hepatitis), because hepatic inflammation may not be a predominant histologic feature, and because it is really a pathologic appearance rather than a diagnosis. A term proposed to circumvent these imprecisions is *neonatal hepatitis syndrome*, emphasizing the uniformity of the clinical phenotype caused by the conglomerate of infectious, genetic, toxic, and metabolic causative disease processes leading to impaired excretory function and bile secretion.[2] Advances in diagnostic technology have enabled identification of a host of discrete entities including inherited conditions such as the progressive familial intrahepatic cholestatic (PFIC) syndromes, bile acid synthetic defects, and more recently, citrin deficiency. As a result, the designation of *idiopathic neonatal hepatitis* continues to be used for neonatal liver disease for which no specific etiologic factor can be ascertained, after a thorough work-up using contemporary technology. As newer disease entities are characterized, these terms are likely to become less useful.[3]

Neonates have immature hepatic excretory functions, giving rise to a period of *physiologic* cholestasis.[4] Almost any insult to the neonatal liver thus results in further impairment of the excretory machinery, resulting in clinically significant cholestasis and a prominent conjugated hyperbilirubinemia. For this reason, *neonatal cholestasis* is often used to describe the spectrum of presentations of neonatal liver injury. For practical purposes, neonatal cholestasis is defined as a conjugated bilirubin fraction greater than 20% of the total serum bilirubin level.[5]

This chapter initially presents a diagnostic approach to the neonate with cholestasis. We then describe the more common infectious, endocrinologic, chromosomal, immunologic, and toxic etiologies that present with neonatal cholestasis. Finally, general principles of management of the cholestatic neonate are considered. Anatomic abnormalities including extrahepatic biliary atresia and each of the discrete inherited and metabolic entities leading to the common phenotype of pathologic cholestasis in the neonate are considered in subsequent chapters.

APPROACH TO THE INFANT WITH CHOLESTASIS

The Cholestasis Guideline Committee of the North American Society for Pediatric Gastroenterology, Hepatology and Nutrition (NASPGHAN) recommends all infants who are jaundiced at 2 weeks of age (or 3 weeks if breast-fed and with normal history and no pale stools or dark urine) be screened for cholestasis with measurement of fractionated serum bilirubin.[5] Disorders associated with cholestasis in the neonate are diverse, although the clinical presentation is similar, reflecting the underlying decrease in bile flow common to all the disorders. Early recognition of cholestasis in the infant and prompt identification of the treatable disorders such as sepsis, endocrinopathies (including panhypopituitarism and congenital hypothyroidism), and specific metabolic disorders (such as galactosemia, tyrosinemia type I, and inborn errors of bile acid metabolism) allow initiation of appropriate treatment to prevent progression of liver damage and, if possible, reverse damage that has already occurred. Table 68-1 outlines the wide variety of known etiologies. The commonest discrete etiologies encountered are biliary atresia, alpha-1-antitrypsin deficiency, infectious, and parenteral nutrition associated cholestasis.[6] Early recognition of diagnostic clues may assist in differential diagnosis. Awareness of the multiple clinical complications common to all disorders with prolonged cholestasis leading to early application of medical therapy will improve the ultimate outcome and quality of life for these patients.

Differentiation of extrahepatic obstruction (particularly biliary atresia) from intrahepatic etiologies is necessary both to identify disorders amenable to surgical intervention and to avoid the adverse outcomes reported with inappropriate surgery.[7] A stepwise and organized approach should be taken in the diagnostic evaluation of each cholestatic infant (Table 68-2), optimally involving close collaboration with radiology, surgical, and pathology colleagues.

Clinical Features

A number of clinical features may provide clues during evaluation of the infant with jaundice due to conjugated hyperbilirubinemia (Table 68-3), and thorough history taking and physical examination are mandatory. Liver disease should be suspected in a jaundiced infant whose urine is dark in color rather than light yellow or colorless. A history of persistently pale stools suggests extrahepatic obstruction such as caused by biliary atresia; however, acholic stools are not specific to this entity. Vomiting, poor feeding, lethargy, or irritability may indicate the presence of a generalized infectious process such as sepsis, or a metabolic condition such as galactosemia. The mother's antenatal history may be significant for infectious illness associated with congenital infection. She may have a history of cholestasis related to taking estrogen-based contraceptive medication, or of intrahepatic cholestasis of pregnancy. Both are associated with mutations of the genes encoding the bile salt export pump (BSEP) or canalicular phospholipid transporter multidrug resistance protein 3 (MDR3), that can be passed onto the

TABLE 68-1. Mechanistic Classification of the Etiologies of Neonatal Cholestasis

Impaired bile flow

Extrahepatic ducts
  Biliary atresia
  Choledochal cyst
  Spontaneous bile duct perforation
  Choledocholithiasis, biliary sludge
  Duct compression (may also be intrahepatic), e.g., hepatoblastoma, neuroblastoma, rhabdomyosarcoma, neonatal leukemia, systemic juvenile xanthogranuloma, Langerhans cell histiocytosis
  Bile duct stenosis
Intrahepatic duct obstruction/formation
  Alagille syndrome
  "Nonsyndromic paucity of interlobular bile ducts" e.g., Williams syndrome
  Cystic fibrosis
  Ductal plate malformations: congenital hepatic fibrosis, ARPKD, Caroli's disease; Ivermark, Jeune, Joubert, Bardet-Biedl syndromes
  Neonatal sclerosing cholangitis
Canalicular membrane transporters
  PFIC type 1, BRIC, Nielsen syndrome (familial Greenland cholestasis)
  PFIC type 2
  PFIC type 3
  Neonatal Dubin-Johnson syndrome
  Villin functional defect
  Overload of excretory mechanism capacity: ABO incompatibility with hemolysis
Hepatocyte tight junctions
  Neonatal ichthyosis–sclerosing cholangitis syndrome–claudin-1 protein
  Familial hypercholanemia due to TJP2 (zonulin-2) deficiency

Hepatocyte dysfunction

Bile acid synthesis
  1°: BASD
    3-oxo-Δ^4-steroid 5β-reductase deficiency
    3β-hydroxy-Δ^5-C27-steroid dehydrogenase/isomerase deficiency
    Oxysterol 7α-hydroxylase deficiency
    Familial hypercholanemia due to BAAT deficiency
  2°: organelle dysfunction
    Smith-Lemli-Opitz syndrome (cholesterol formation)
    Zellweger
    Peroxisomal disorders–Zellweger, infantile refsum, neonatal ALD
Infectious
  Bacterial: sepsis (endotoxemia, e.g., UTI, gastroenteritis)
  Listeria
  Syphilis
  TB
  Viral: herpes viruses: CMV, HSV, HHV-6
  Parvovirus B19
  Hepatitis A, B, C
  Enterovirus: coxsackieviruses, echoviruses, "numbered" enteroviruses
  Adenovirus
  Rubella
  HIV
  Paramyxovirus
Protozoal
  Toxoplasmosis
Toxic
  Parenteral nutrition associated liver disease
  Fetal alcohol syndrome
  Drugs–maternal amphetamines, anticonvulsants; infant antifungals

Endocrine
  Panhypopituitarism
  Hypothyroidism, cortisol deficiency
  McCune-Albright syndrome
  Donohue syndrome (leprechaunism)
Metabolic
  Alpha-1-antitrypsin deficiency
  Carbohydrate disorders
    Galactosemia
    Fructosemia (hereditary fructose intolerance)
    Glycogen storage disease type IV (Andersen disease)
Amino acid disorders
  Tyrosinemia type I
Lipid disorders
  Niemann-Pick disease type C
  Gaucher disease
  Cerebrotendinous xanthomatosis
  Farber's disease
  β-Oxidation defects: short- and long-chain acyl-CoA dehydrogenase deficiencies
Lysosomal storage disorders
  Niemann-Pick disease, type C
  Gaucher disease
  Farber disease
  Mucopolysaccharidosis VI (Maroteaux-Lamy syndrome)
  Mucolipidosis II (I-cell disease)
Urea cycle defects
  Citrin deficiency (formerly type II citrullinemia)
Metal metabolism
  Neonatal iron storage disease
Mitochondrial respiratory chain disorders
  Complex deficiencies
  Growth retardation, amino aciduria, cholestasis, iron overload, lactic acidosis, and early death (GRACILE)
Immune mediated:
  Neonatal lupus erythematosus
  Autoimmune hemolytic anemia with giant cell hepatitis
  Hemophagocytic lymphohistiocytosis
Hypoxic/ischemic/vascular
  Shock/hypoperfusion/hypoxia
  Budd-Chiari syndrome
  Cardiac insufficiency (congenital heart disease, arrhythmia)
  Multiple hemangiomata
  Sinusoidal obstruction syndrome
Miscellaneous/unclear mechanism
  ARC syndrome (arthrogryposis–renal tubular dysfunction–cholestasis; defective vacuolar protein sorting)
  Chromosomal: trisomy 18, 21
  Congenital disorders of glycosylation
  Hardikar syndrome
  Lymphoedema cholestasis syndrome (Aagenaes syndrome)
  Kabuki syndrome
  North American Indian childhood cirrhosis (defective cirhin protein–unknown function)
  Pseudo-TORCH syndrome
  "Idiopathic neonatal hepatitis"

Abbreviations: ALD, adrenoleukodystrophy; ARPKD, autosomal recessive polycystic kidney disease; BAAT, bile acid Coenzyme A: amino acid N-acyltransferase; BRIC, benign recurrent intrahepatic cholestasis; CMV, cytomegalovirus; HHV-6, human herpesvirus type 6; HIV, human immunodeficiency virus; HSV, herpes simplex virus; PFIC, progressive familial intrahepatic cholestasis; UTI, urinary tract infection.

infant resulting in progressive familial intrahepatic cholestasis (PFIC) types 2 and 3, respectively.[8,9] A parental history of gallstones may be significant, as this has also been associated with MDR3 mutations. Fatty acid oxidation disorders in the fetus have been associated with the development of acute fatty liver of pregnancy (AFLP) and, to a lesser extent, with preeclampsia accompanied by the syndrome of hemolysis, elevated liver enzymes and low platelets (HELLP).[10] A maternal history of thrombophilia has been associated with a fetal thrombotic vasculopathy resulting in severe neonatal liver disease including Budd-Chiari syndrome.[11] Maternal medication and drug history is also important, as amphetamine abuse,[12] anticonvulsant

TABLE 68-2. Diagnostic Evaluation of Neonatal Cholestasis

History and physical examination
  Includes family history, observation of stools, growth parameters, dysmorphic features, signs of fat-soluble vitamin deficiency
Confirm cholestasis and determine severity of liver disease and complications
  Fractionated serum bilirubin
  ALT, AST, alkaline phosphatase, GGT
  Prothrombin time/INR and serum albumin
  Glucose
  Fat-soluble vitamin levels: vitamins A, D, and E
Initiate investigation for conditions requiring prompt specific therapy
  Complete blood count
  Bacteriologic: culture urine, blood, ± CSF
  Virologic: viral cultures/PCR–urine, stool, blood ± CSF
  Serologic: HSV, CMV, HHV-6, hepatitis A, B, and C, enterovirus
  Urine reducing substances
  Galactosemia screen, erythrocyte galactose-1-phosphate uridyl transferase
  Cortisol, TSH, T4
  Chest radiograph
  Serum iron, ferritin
  Urine organic acids (including succinylacetone, succinylacetoacetate)
Investigate for more common causes not already excluded
  Alpha-1-antitrypsin level and phenotype
  Abdominal ultrasonography, including Doppler studies*
  Hepatobiliary scintigraphy with pharmacologic priming*
  Sweat chloride analysis
Investigate for less common causes not already excluded
  Serum bile acids
  Serum ammonia
  α-Fetoprotein
  Urine and plasma amino acids
  Cholesterol
  Skull, long bone (peroxisomal disorders) and spine radiography (Alagille)
  Ophthalmologic consultation–embryotoxon, retinal examination
  Cardiologic assessment including echocardiogram
  Liver biopsy for histology, electron microscopy, immunohistochemistry, viral culture
  Cholangiography: intraoperative, percutaneous, ERCP, MRCP
Other specific diagnostic tests if indicated
  Paracentesis and analysis of ascitic fluid if present (infection, bile)
  Endocrine stimulation testing, magnetic resonance imaging of brain
  Karyotype
  Very long-chain fatty acids
  Plasma acylcarnitines
  Isoelectric focusing of serum transferrin
  ANA, anti-Ro, anti-La antibodies
  Bone marrow examination
  Specific enzyme analysis in leukocytes or tissue (skin fibroblasts, muscle, liver)
  Genetic testing: cystic fibrosis, Alagille syndrome, PFIC disorders

Abbreviations: ALT, alanine aminotransferase; AST, alanine aminotransferase; CMV, cytomegalovirus; CSF, cerebrospinal fluid; ERCP, endoscopic retrograde cholangiopancreatography; GGT, gamma-glutamyltranspeptidase; HHV-6, human herpesvirus-6; HSV, herpes simplex virus; INR, international normalized ratio; MRCP, magnetic resonance cholangiopancreatography; PCR, polymerase chain reaction; TSH, thyroid stimulating hormone.
*Note: These imaging studies are best performed in a unit experienced with their use and interpretation in neonates. Ultrasonography may be one of the initial investigations as it may identify an anatomical cause for cholestasis, obviating the need for further extensive investigation.

TABLE 68-3. Potential Clues to Specific Etiologies

Racial background
  Amish: PFIC type 1, familial hypercholanemia
  Greenland Eskimo: Nielsen syndrome (familial Greenland cholestasis)
  North American Indian (Ojibway-Cree): North American Indian cirrhosis
  East Asian: Citrin deficiency
  Norwegian: Aagenaes syndrome (lymphedema cholestasis syndrome)
Family history
  Lung or liver disease: alpha-1-antitrypsin deficiency
  Lung disease: cystic fibrosis
  Congenital heart disease: Alagille syndrome
Maternal history of hepatobiliary problems
  Intrahepatic cholestasis of pregnancy: PFIC types 2 and 3
  Preeclampsia with HELLP: fatty acid oxidation disorders
Other maternal history
  SLE or Sjögren disease: neonatal lupus erythematosus
Dysmorphism
  Alagille syndrome
  Trisomies
  Micropenis–hypopituitarism
  Cleft palate–Kabuki syndrome, Hardikar syndrome
  Chubby cheeks–citrin deficiency
Neurologic abnormalities
  Niemann-Pick type C
  Septo-optic dysplasia (hypopituitarism)
  Congenital disorders of glycosylation
Early-onset severe liver dysfunction (synthetic dysfunction)
  Herpes simplex virus
  Neonatal iron storage disease
  Tyrosinemia type I
  Galactosemia
  Neimann-Pick C
  Hemophagocytic lymphohistiocytosis
  Mitochondrial respiratory chain dysfunction
  Bile acid synthetic disorders
Temporal association with dietary commencement/changes
  Galactosemia
  Fructosemia
Cholestasis/pruritus but anicteric
  PFIC type 2
  Bile acid synthetic disorders
  Familial hypercholanemia
Low or normal serum GGT
  PFIC type 1 or 2
  Bile acid synthetic disorders
  Endocrine causes
  Arthrogryposis–renal tubular dysfunction–cholestasis syndrome
  Lymphedema cholestasis syndrome (Aagenaes syndrome)
Renal disease
  Tyrosinemia type I
  Ductal plate malformation/fibrocystic diseases: congenital hepatic fibrosis, ARPKD
  Alagille syndrome
  Arthrogryposis–renal tubular dysfunction–cholestasis syndrome

Abbreviations: ARPKD, autosomal recessive polycystic kidney disease; GGT, gamma-glutamyl transpeptidase; HELLP, hemolysis, elevation liver enzymes and low platelets; PFIC, progressive familial intrahepatic cholestasis; SLE, systemic lupus erythematosus.

A temporal association of illness with ingestion of lactose- or fructose-containing feeds, or medications containing fructose, may suggest galactosemia or fructosemia, respectively.

It is important to review serial infant growth parameters. Small-for-gestational-age at birth and failure to thrive occurs with congenital infection and chromosomal abnormalities. Neonatal iron storage disease often begins in utero and intrauterine growth restriction is associated.[17] In contrast, infants with biliary atresia tend to have normal growth parameters at diagnosis. A number of characteristic dysmorphic syndromes

drugs,[13] and fetal alcohol syndrome[14] can all present with neonatal cholestasis. The early neonatal history may be significant for asphyxia causing hypoxic liver injury, prematurity, or gastrointestinal complications that required treatment with parenteral nutrition. Neonatal exposure to medications such as fluconazole[15] or micafungin[16] may cause cholestasis, whereas third-generation cephalosporin use can result in biliary sludge.

are associated with neonatal cholestasis, including trisomy 21, trisomy 18, Zellweger, Smith-Lemli-Opitz, and Alagille syndromes. Infants with citrin deficiency have a characteristic facial appearance with "chubby cheeks."[18] A cleft palate and a history of gastrointestinal or genitourinary obstruction suggests Hardikar syndrome.[19] Abdominal examination may reveal a palpable mass in the case of tumor or choledochal cyst. Splenomegaly suggests either early cirrhosis with portal hypertension, congenital infection, Niemann-Pick type C, or other lysosomal storage disease. Examination of the genitalia may reveal a micropenis or cryptorchidism, suggestive of panhypopituitarism. The skin should be examined for complications of cholestasis such as bruising, although xanthomatosis and scratch marks typically are not observed in the neonate. Ichthyosis may suggest neonatal ichthyosis sclerosing cholangitis (NISCH) syndrome, or be a clue to the arthrogryposis-renal-cholestasis (ARC) syndrome,[20] which may present without arthrogryposis.[21] Purpuric rashes occur with congenital infections such as cytomegalovirus (CMV), toxoplasmosis, and rubella. Infiltrative skin lesions occur with juvenile xanthogranuloma and Langerhans cell histiocytosis. The café-au-lait skin macules of McCune-Albright syndrome usually manifest beyond the neonatal period. Abnormalities of the cardiovascular system such as peripheral pulmonary stenosis are associated with Alagille syndrome and dextrocardia/situs inversus with the "embryonic" form of biliary atresia.[22] Cardiologic assessment including echocardiography can be helpful in detecting subtle anomalies. Neurologic abnormalities such as hypotonia, hyporeflexia, and ataxia may be due to vitamin E deficiency secondary to cholestasis, or associated with specific disease entities such as Niemann-Pick type C and peroxisomal and mitochondrial respiratory chain disorders. Signs of rickets such as rib rosary, flared metaphyses, or craniotabes suggest severe vitamin D deficiency secondary to cholestasis. Ophthalmologic examination may be helpful in revealing the persistent posterior embryotoxon of Alagille syndrome, retinal changes with septo-optic dysplasia (these infants may also display nystagmus), or cataracts with galactosemia or peroxisomal disorders.

Laboratory and Radiographic Evaluation

The goal of the optimal investigative approach to the cholestatic infant is to evaluate the severity of liver disease, assess for the presence of complications of chronic cholestasis, and provide a timely final diagnosis while minimizing risk to the infant in a cost-effective manner. Table 68-2 outlines a staged approach that excludes treatable life-threatening conditions early, then considers investigations relevant for more common conditions, and finally those investigations that either are more specialized or are targeted at specific conditions. In clinical practice investigations are initiated simultaneously, with clinical features and results of preliminary investigations steering further evaluation. The precise point of involvement of subspecialty support will vary depending on the case and local resources.

Standard liver biochemical tests include serum total and conjugated (direct) bilirubin, alanine aminotransferase (ALT), aspartate aminotransferase (AST), alkaline phosphatase (ALP), and γ-glutamyl transpeptidase (GGT). Elevated aminotransferase concentrations typically indicate primarily hepatocellular damage, whereas elevations of ALP and GGT indicate biliary tract injury or obstruction. Serum GGT is elevated in most cholestatic disorders including biliary atresia, Alagille syndrome, and alpha-1-antitrypsin deficiency.[23] A low or normal GGT level in the presence of a conjugated hyperbilirubinemia merits further work-up for rarer entities such as PFIC types 1 or 2 or primary bile acid synthetic defects,[24,25] although it may also be seen with endocrinologic causes for cholestasis (see Table 68-3). Serum glucose, albumin, and a coagulation profile provide an indication of the synthetic functional capacity of the liver and allow intervention for the serious complications of hypoglycemia and coagulopathy if present. Abnormal coagulation indices out of proportion to what would be expected for the degree of conjugated hyperbilirubinemia can be seen with severe vitamin K deficiency or may be an early indication of metabolic liver disease such as tyrosinemia type I or neonatal iron storage disease. Chronic cholestasis results in fat-soluble vitamin deficiency, and measurement of vitamin A, D, and E levels and prothrombin time/international normalized ratio (INR) are useful in screening for these complications.

As bacterial sepsis, severe viral infections, hypopituitarism, and metabolic conditions such as galactosemia and tyrosinemia type I can cause rapid deterioration and even death without prompt recognition and treatment, it is important that these conditions be among those excluded early in the diagnostic process. Thus, appropriate bacterial and viral cultures, serology, and molecular testing are important to consider early. Urine reducing substances can be tested at the bedside, and if positive can suggest galactosemia, but they may be falsely negative in a patient with galactosemia either not receiving lactose (e.g., fasting, on parenteral nutrition, or receiving a lactose-free formula) or vomiting excessively before assessment. Measurement of red blood cell galactose-1-phosphate uridyl transferase activity (with the proviso that the infant has not received a recent blood transfusion) is useful in this situation. Endocrinologic causes can be screened by measurement of thyroid-stimulating hormone, free T4, and cortisol levels. A chest radiograph is useful in the sepsis work-up, but also may provide other diagnostic clues such as dextrocardia associated with the embryonal form of biliary atresia, or the butterfly vertebrae of Alagille syndrome. Grossly elevated ferritin levels are seen with neonatal iron storage disease, typically over 1000 μg/L, but can exceed 100,000 μg/L.[26] Increased urinary succinylacetone is pathognomonic for tyrosinemia type I.

Biliary atresia, although not immediately life-threatening, is a common cause of neonatal cholestasis, has a better outcome if treated early with Kasai portoenterostomy, and should also be considered early. A combination of imaging and pathology assists with this diagnosis (see later discussion). Alpha-1-antitrypsin phenotype by isoelectric focusing is important, because serum alpha-1-antitrypsin levels may be normal in infants with liver disease due to alpha-1-antitrypsin deficiency.[27] α-Fetoprotein levels are normally high at birth and decline rapidly over subsequent weeks.[28] Excessively high levels in the setting of cholestasis are seen with malignancy such as hepatoblastoma and are characteristic of citrin deficiency. Sweat chloride testing may identify the infant with cystic fibrosis and should be considered early in populations with a high prevalence of this condition. Low or undetectable serum bile acid levels in the setting of other signs or symptoms of cholestasis suggest bile acid synthetic disorders. Hyperammonemia may be present with citrin deficiency, or in the setting of severe liver failure. Patterns of elevation of plasma amino acids can help distinguish citrin deficiency from other urea cycle disorders. Low serum cholesterol, especially in the cholestatic infant with dysmorphism or neurologic abnormalities, suggests a peroxisomal disorder. It can be significantly elevated in Alagille syndrome, but is nonspecific.

Among the available imaging modalities, ultrasonography is noninvasive and provides information about liver structure, size, composition, and vascular flow and therefore is best used as an initial imaging modality. Ultrasonography can delineate the external biliary anatomy and identify signs of obstruction such as duct dilatation, or abnormalities of the ducts themselves such as caused by a choledochal cyst or Caroli's disease. Extrinsic masses or tumors causing biliary compression may also be seen. A number of signs are associated with biliary atresia, including sonographic absence of the gallbladder, lack of visualization of extrahepatic ducts, and the "triangular cord sign." This latter sign reflects a fibrous cone of tissue at the porta hepatis and has been reported to have positive predictive values between 78 and 95% for biliary atresia.[29,30] It is proposed that combining this sign with gallbladder measurements can improve ultrasonographic accuracy in diagnosing biliary atresia[31,32]; however, because ultrasonography is very operator dependent, experience and care in the performance of the scan and interpretation of the images are required. Ultrasonography can also detect gallstones and biliary sludge and demonstrate complications of liver disease such as ascites or the development of intra-abdominal collateral vessels reflecting portal hypertension. Hepatobiliary scintigraphy using technetium-99m iminodiacetic acid derivatives has been used to differentiate nonobstructive causes of neonatal cholestasis from extrahepatic biliary atresia. Hepatic uptake and secretion into bile of intravenously administered iminodiacetic acid derivatives occur by carrier-mediated organic anion pathway and depend on the structure of the specific analog, the integrity of hepatocellular function, and biliary tract patency. Pretreatment with oral phenobarbital (5 mg/kg per day for 3 to 5 days) or ursodeoxycholic acid (20 mg/kg twice daily for 2 to 3 days) stimulates bile secretion and enhances the ability to detect biliary excretion of the isotope into the intestinal tract.[33,34] A negative result merely confirms the presence of severe cholestasis, but positive identification of radioactivity in the intestine establishes patency of the biliary tree. One study using planar imaging found sensitivity of 100% and specificity of only 74% for diagnosing biliary atresia.[35] More recently, a study using single photon emission computed tomography (SPECT) found that when combined with phenobarbitone stimulation, a sensitivity of 100% and specificity of 97% for biliary atresia could be achieved.[36]

Liver biopsy remains an important diagnostic tool for evaluating neonatal cholestasis. Tissue may be obtained via percutaneous needle biopsy, or as a wedge biopsy at the time of a laparoscopy/laparotomy performed for cholangiography or portoenterostomy procedure. Ductular proliferation and ductular bile plugs suggest extrahepatic obstruction such as with biliary atresia.[37] The histologic findings of nonobstructive causes of neonatal cholestasis are variable and often nonspecific. Giant cell transformation is a common response of the neonatal liver to any of a number of heterogeneous insults and occurs predominantly around central veins (Figure 68-1). Paucity of intralobular bile ducts may indicate Alagille syndrome, though in premature infants and term neonates within the first month of life interlobular ducts are still forming, and so experience in interpreting these biopsies is essential. The histologic assessment of the biopsy is enhanced with specialized processing

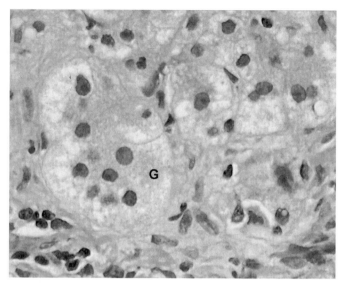

Figure 68-1. Multi-nucleated giant cell (G) transformation typical of neonatal hepatitis. (Hematoxylin-eosin, original magnification ×600.)

techniques, stains, and immunohistochemistry, which assist in the diagnosis of conditions such as alpha-1-antitrypsin deficiency and viral infections such as CMV. Electron microscopy may provide additional information such as the granular appearance of "Byler's bile" in PFIC type 1, or the presence of viral particles. Liver tissue may also be diagnostic when subjected to enzymatic testing such as with mitochondrial respiratory chain disorders.

Direct demonstration of the extrahepatic biliary passages via operative cholangiography is indicated when liver histopathology suggests extrahepatic bile duct obstruction and the results of hepatobiliary scintigraphy are consistent with such an interpretation. Traditionally this has been with direct cholangiography via percutaneous transhepatic cholangiography or cholecystocholangiography, or via operative cholangiography. Other less invasive options now utilized include laparoscopic cholangiography,[38] endoscopic retrograde cholangiography,[39,40] and magnetic resonance cholangiopancreatography.[41,42] The optimal cholangiographic study will depend on other differential diagnoses and institutional expertise, emphasizing the need for close collaboration among the physician, surgeon, and radiologist.

More specialized investigations are generally reserved for situations where clinical features or previous tests suggest a rare diagnosis, or when preceding investigations have not yielded a diagnosis. Endocrine stimulation testing or pituitary magnetic resonance imaging can confirm a diagnosis of hypopituitarism. Genetic studies include a karyotype to demonstrate trisomy 18 or 21, and specific gene testing where available for conditions such as Alagille syndrome, the PFIC conditions, and cystic fibrosis. Plasma acylcarnitine analysis can identify specific disorders of fatty acid oxidation. Very long-chain fatty acids are elevated with peroxisomal disorders. Isoelectric focusing of transferrin can diagnose most congenital disorders of glycosylation. On bone marrow examination, macrophages may have a "crinkled tissue paper" appearance with Gaucher disease or a foamy appearance with Niemann-Pick type C or Farber disease. Activity of specific enzymes can be tested on leukocytes, cultured fibroblasts, or tissue when confirming diagnoses of peroxisomal disorders, Niemann-Pick type C, glycogen storage disease type IV, or mitochondrial respiratory chain disorders.

CHOLESTASIS ASSOCIATED WITH INFECTION

Various bacterial, viral, and protozoal agents are associated with neonatal cholestasis, resulting from pre-, peri-, or postnatal infections.

Bacterial Infections

Extrahepatic bacterial infection, either generalized or localized, has long been recognized as a cause of conjugated hyperbilirubinemia in infants.[43] The mechanisms by which this occurs are being elucidated with increasing knowledge of the molecular mechanisms of bile acid processing and transport within the hepatocyte and their regulation by nucleic factors. Bacterial endotoxin and inflammatory cytokines released by activated Kupffer cells have been shown to reduce both basolateral and canalicular transport of bile acids.[44] These effects are mediated by alterations in the expression and function of hepatocyte nuclear receptors.[45] The transporters responsible for hepatocyte uptake of unconjugated bilirubin and excretion of conjugated bilirubin are also affected, although the conjugating machinery is not. The relatively immature bile acid transport mechanisms of newborns may make this group susceptible to developing clinically evident cholestasis during episodes of sepsis, though it is important to remember that the infant need not appear clinically very ill for this to occur.[46] The most common site for infection in these infants is the urinary tract, and *Escherichia coli* is the most common organism involved, although other sites and organisms have been reported.[43,44,46,47] Galactosemia is associated with increased risk of gram-negative sepsis and thus should be excluded in infants with liver disease and these infections.

Bacterial cultures of blood and urine obtained in a sterile fashion are an important part of the work-up of neonatal cholestasis. Cerebrospinal fluid cultures should also be considered. This should be followed by the immediate initiation of appropriate empiric antibiotic therapy in an infant suspected to have sepsis.

Congenital Syphilis

Congenital syphilis is caused by *Treponema pallidum*, contracted from an infected mother via transplacental transmission at any time during pregnancy or at delivery by contact with maternal secretions. At the time of infection, *T. pallidum* is liberated directly into the circulation of the fetus (spirochetemia). The clinical, laboratory, and radiographic abnormalities of congenital syphilis are a consequence of the inflammatory response to spirochetes induced in various body organs and tissues. The signs and symptoms of congenital syphilis are divided arbitrarily into early manifestations and late manifestations. Clinical features in the neonatal period may include a snuffly nose; hepatosplenomegaly; lymphadenopathy; mucosal lesions; painful bone and cartilage lesions; an erythematous, scaly maculopapular rash; and chorioretinitis. Thrombocytopenia and hemolytic anemia may also be present. Late manifestations tend to occur after age 2 years and include destructive bone lesions, a "saddle-nose" deformity, and Hutchinson teeth. Diagnosis involves confirming infection in the mother (if not already done) and comparing infant nontreponemal (venereal disease research laboratory, VDRL; rapid plasmin reagin, RPR) titers with those of the mother. Evaluation of the infant also includes a complete blood count (including platelet count), cerebrospinal fluid for cells, protein, and VDRL titer. If clinically indicated, radiography of chest and long bones, neuroimaging, auditory brainstem responses, eye examination, and liver function tests are also recommended.[48]

Neonatal liver disease has been associated with congenital syphilis.[49,50] Jaundice may either occur within the first day of life and mimic erythroblastosis fetalis, or present as later-onset jaundice. Hepatomegaly is the most common clinical sign in congenital syphilis and results mainly from extramedullary hematopoiesis.[51] A more fulminant presentation with subsequent hepatic calcification also has been reported.[52] Hypopituitarism as a complication of congenital syphilis has been reported.[53]

Liver biopsy is not necessary if a clear diagnosis of congenital syphilis is made. Histology may show a characteristic centrilobular mononuclear infiltrate with extensive fibrosis of the interstitia and of the portal triads surrounding the bile ducts and blood vessels and giant cell transformation. Bile duct paucity has been reported.[54] Silver stains or transmission electron microscopy may reveal spirochetes, most commonly in the space of Disse and between reactive mesenchymal cells. Gumma lesions, characterized by a central zone of necrosis surrounded by a dense infiltrate of lymphocytes, plasma cells, histiocytes, epithelioid cells, and giant cells, are seldom seen in early congenital syphilis.[55]

Treatment with 10 days of parenteral penicillin is recommended. For penicillin allergy, desensitization is preferred over use of alternative antibiotics.[48] Liver disease may be exacerbated by penicillin therapy before improving.[55,56] The liver disease often resolves slowly, even after apparently adequate therapy. There are no known long-term liver sequelae for infants adequately treated for congenital syphilis.

Perinatal Tuberculosis

Neonatal liver infection with *Mycobacterium tuberculosis* is very rare. Perinatal tuberculosis can be acquired by the infant (a) in utero by transplacental hematogenous spread via the umbilical vein from the infected mother, or by ingestion of infected amniotic fluid; (b) intrapartum by ingestion or inhalation of infected amniotic or maternal fluids, or by direct contact with maternal genital tract lesions; or (c) postnatally by ingestion or inhalation of material from an infectious source (which may not be the mother).[57] Maternal history may not be helpful, because most pregnant women with tuberculosis are asymptomatic.

Neonates typically present after 2 weeks of age with fever, hepatomegaly, and respiratory symptoms and are often initially treated for presumed bacterial sepsis.[58] Presentation with progressive liver dysfunction without pulmonary symptoms,[59] or as part of a multiorgan dysfunction, may also occur.[60] Liver histopathology is not necessary for diagnosis, but shows granulomatous hepatic lesions with or without caseation, surrounding giant cells and lymphocytes and epithelioid cells with tubercle bacilli.[60,61] Diagnostic testing includes the tuberculin skin test, chest radiograph, lumbar puncture, obtaining appropriate fluid or tissue for acid-fast bacilli staining, mycobacterial cultures, and/or polymerase chain reaction (PCR) testing. Specimens include cerebrospinal fluid, gastric fluid aspirates, ascitic fluid, tracheal aspirates, and lymph node or bone marrow biopsies. Because of the relative immaturity of their immune systems, the skin test result very rarely is positive in infants[62] and may indeed be negative in the mother[63] because of anergy associated with pregnancy. Therefore, examination for tubercle bacilli and mycobacterial cultures of appropriate body fluid specimens is essential. At present there is insufficient experience with interferon-gamma release assays in the diagnosis of perinatal tuberculosis.[58] Treatment of suspected perinatal tuberculosis should not be delayed pending the results of mycobacterial cultures and involves prompt commencement of isoniazid, rifampin, pyrazinamide, and an aminoglycoside such as amikacin.[48] Corticosteroids are added if tuberculous meningitis is also present. The prognosis is poor with disseminated extrapulmonary disease and with coexistent human immunodeficiency virus (HIV) infection, although successful treatment of perinatal tuberculosis involving the liver has been reported.[60]

Listeriosis

Listeria monocytogenes infection in the neonatal period causes severe illness and may have an early (within the first days of life) or late (after 1 week of age) onset.[64] Transmission of this gram-positive bacillus occurs via the transplacental route or at delivery from infected cervicovaginal secretions. In utero infections typically result in premature delivery. In contrast to the infant, maternal illness, which may include fever, flu-like symptoms, or diarrhea, is typically mild. Early infection is usually disseminated and characterized by multiple organ involvement.[65] Meningitis occurs with the late-onset form. Hepatic manifestations are always present in these critically ill infants.[65,66] Hepatosplenomegaly occurs with or without jaundice. Liver histopathology shows diffuse hepatitis or miliary microabscesses containing abundant gram-positive rods.[65,67] A severe early form of the infection may be accompanied by an erythematous rash with pale papules that are granulomatous histologically. Diagnosis is made by isolating the organisms from blood, meconium, cerebrospinal fluid, or the liver. Treatment is with ampicillin and an aminoglycoside such as gentamicin, although mortality remains as high as 30 to 50% despite therapy.[66,68]

Viral Infections

Cytomegalovirus

Cytomegalovirus (CMV) is a member of the Herpesviridae family and is a common congenital infection, with approximately 1 to 2% of all live-born infants infected in utero and excreting the virus at birth.[69] Transmission occurs in utero by transplacental passage of maternal bloodborne virus, at delivery by passage through an infected maternal genital tract, postnatally via maternal breast milk or saliva, or iatrogenically from transfusion of blood products.

For the 90% of neonates with congenital CMV infection that are asymptomatic, infection may not be detected, though up to 7.2% of these infants will later develop sensorineural hearing loss.[70] Typical clinical features in those with overt disease in the neonatal period include hepatomegaly, splenomegaly, jaundice, petechiae or purpura secondary to thrombocytopenia, pneumonia, microcephaly, chorioretinitis, and neurologic features such as poor feeding, hypotonia, or seizures due to cerebral calcifications. Hepatosplenomegaly is caused by mild hepatitis, a reticuloendothelial response to chronic infection, and extramedullary hematopoiesis.[71] CMV hepatitis is usually associated with a conjugated hyperbilirubinemia and mild elevation of liver transaminases, and hepatomegaly may persist for up to a year.[72] Although CMV hepatitis is usually mild, ascites,

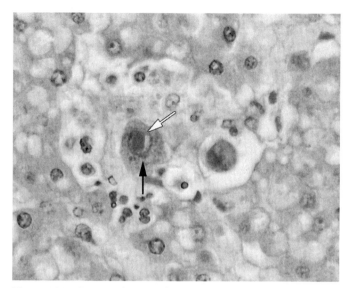

Figure 68-2. Cytomegalovirus infection. Enlarged hepatocyte contains basophilic granules in the cytoplasm (black arrow). Intranuclear inclusions are surrounded by a clear halo (white arrow). Both the nuclear and cytoplasmic inclusions represent closely packed virions. (Hematoxylin-eosin, original magnification ×600.)

bleeding diathesis, disseminated intravascular coagulopathy, secondary bacterial infections, and ensuing death have been reported.[73-75] Hepatic histopathology includes multinucleated giant cell transformation, large inclusion-bearing cells, cholestasis, cholangitis, and extramedullary hematopoiesis. The characteristic finding is an enlarged (endothelial, hepatocyte, or bile duct epithelial) cell containing basophilic granules in the cytoplasm and a swollen nucleus. An amphiphilic intranuclear inclusion is surrounded by a clear halo, resembling an owl's eye (Figure 68-2). Both nuclear and cytoplasmic inclusions represent closely packed virions.[76] Liver calcifications may also be found on imaging.

CMV infection should be excluded in all neonates with prolonged cholestasis. Isolation of the virus from tissue cultures or detection in urine, saliva, blood, cerebrospinal fluid, and tissue biopsies by culture or PCR all can be used to diagnose CMV infection. Assessment of extrahepatic involvement should be part of the routine work-up including fundoscopy, brain ultrasound, and computed tomographic (CT) scan and assessment of hearing by brainstem evoked potentials.

There is a benefit of intravenous ganciclovir treatment for infants with congenital CMV infection manifesting neurologic symptoms, in terms of reduced rates of hearing loss and possibly other developmental outcomes.[77,78] The toxicity of this treatment, which is given for 6 weeks, included neutropenia in almost two thirds of patients.[78] Although hepatomegaly and mild alteration in liver function test results may persist for several months after birth, severe chronic liver disease rarely occurs, and there is no evidence to support treatment unless neurologic features are present.

Herpes Simplex Virus

Neonatal herpes simplex virus (HSV) infection can manifest as a disseminated disease involving multiple organs, most prominently liver and lungs; localized central nervous system (CNS) disease; or disease localized to the skin, eyes, and mouth. Overall, HSV type 2 strains cause more infections in neonates than

HSV type 1 strains; however, HSV-1 was more common in a case series of patients with neonatal liver failure.[79] In the United States, the incidence of neonatal HSV infection is estimated to be 1:3200 live births.[80] Prematurity is a risk factor, with premature infants accounting for 40 to 50% of cases of neonatal herpes and having a greater likelihood of having a fatal outcome. Whether the increased frequency of prematurity among neonates with herpes indicates a greater propensity of mothers with genital herpes to deliver prematurely or a greater susceptibility of premature infants to HSV infection remains unknown. Transmission occurs during delivery via exposure to an infected maternal genital tract, by ascending infection, or postnatally from a parent or other caregiver (most often from a nongenital infection such as the mouth or hands). It is important to note that in most cases of neonatal HSV infection, the mother has no history or current evidence of herpetic genital lesions.[81]

HSV hepatitis presents as part of a generalized herpetic disease in the newborn infant and is usually fulminant. These infants manifest jaundice, hepatomegaly, conjugated hyperbilirubinemia and elevated transaminases, major abnormalities of blood clotting factors, and bleeding complications. At least 20% will not display the typical vesicular rash of cutaneous involvement.[81] Liver histopathology reveals generalized or multifocal hepatocyte necrosis and cholestasis with characteristic intranuclear acidophilic inclusion bodies representing the herpes simplex virions.[49,82]

Diagnosis of neonatal HSV infection is confirmed by viral culture of specimens from the skin (such as scrapings of the base of skin lesions if present), conjunctivae, oropharyngeal mucosa, stool, urine, and CSF. Rapid diagnosis can be achieved using detection of viral DNA by PCR, or from skin lesions by direct immunofluorescence or enzyme immunoassay. PCR testing of CSF and blood is positive in over 90% of infants with disseminated disease,[81] although lumbar puncture is not recommended in the setting of coagulopathy. Serology testing is of little value because of possible confounding by the presence of maternal IgG in the infant's serum. Liver biopsy is not usually necessary for diagnosis and indeed would be risky, given the coagulopathy that is often present in these infants.

Three weeks of treatment with parenteral acyclovir reduces mortality to 29% in disseminated disease,[83] as compared to historical data in which mortality was 85% with no antiviral treatment.[84] Successful liver transplantation for neonatal acute liver failure secondary to HSV has been reported.[82,85,86]

Congenital Rubella

Rubella virus is an enveloped RNA virus in the family Togaviridae. Although rubella usually is a mild, often subclinical disease affecting school-age children and young adults, congenital rubella syndrome is associated with multiple anomalies. These congenital malformations include ophthalmologic (cataracts, retinopathy, and congenital glaucoma), cardiac (patent ductus arteriosus and peripheral pulmonary artery stenosis), auditory (sensorineural hearing impairment), and neurologic (behavioral disorders, meningoencephalitis, and mental retardation). Additional features include growth retardation, radiolucent bone disease, hepatosplenomegaly, thrombocytopenia causing a purpuric rash, and the "blueberry muffin" lesions of hematopoiesis within the skin.

Hepatic manifestations range from jaundice, hepatosplenomegaly, and transient cholestasis to a late anicteric hepatitis.[87] Hepatosplenomegaly persists for longer periods of time and resolves after 12 months or longer.[49] Diagnosis of congenital rubella is made by the detection of rubella-specific IgM antibody in serum or oral fluid, viral isolation, or detection of viral RNA by PCR in nasopharyngeal swabs, blood, or body fluid.[88] Liver histology typically demonstrates giant cell hepatitis.[89] Infants with congenital rubella usually recover from the hepatitis, and most of their morbidity relates to structural heart disease and neurologic complications. Treatment for congenital rubella is supportive. Immunization of prepubertal females offers the best hope for prevention of this disease.

Enteroviruses

The nonpolio enteroviruses are single-stranded RNA viruses belonging to the family Picornaviridae and include coxsackie A and B viruses, echoviruses, and the "numbered" enteroviruses. Neonatal infection with coxsackieviruses and echoviruses can result from transplacental viral transmission, contact with infected secretions during birth, and human-to-human contact after birth. Coxsackieviral and echoviral infections in neonates result in a wide variety of clinical manifestations ranging from asymptomatic infection to fatal hepatitis, encephalitis, myocarditis, and disseminated intravascular coagulation. The most common manifestations are nonspecific, including fever, irritability, and lethargy, which leads to an evaluation for bacterial sepsis. Some infants display a maculopapular rash. Although enteroviral infections tend to occur most commonly in the winter and fall, there appears to be less seasonality in neonatal presentations.[90] There is often a history of recent maternal or other close contact illness.[91]

The viruses associated with severe hepatitis, often with hepatic necrosis, include echovirus 6, enterovirus 71, and coxsackieviruses B1-4.[92-94] Liver calcifications may develop in survivors of coxsackievirus B1 hepatitis.

Specimens providing the highest yield for virus culture are swabs or fluids obtained from the respiratory or gastrointestinal tract or from CSF. Diagnosis can also be made by detecting enteroviral RNA using reverse transcriptase PCR. Serology testing is of limited value because of low sensitivity resulting from a lack of a common antigen in so many antigenically different enteroviruses.[95]

Treatment is primarily supportive. Pleconaril is the most promising antiviral agent[96] and is currently being evaluated in a multicenter randomized double-blinded placebo-controlled trial. Intravenous immune globulin (IVIg) has been used for both postexposure prophylaxis and treatment, but no strong evidence for efficacy exists. In those neonates with severe hepatitis, mortality has been reported as 24 to 31% in larger series, and up to 71% if myocarditis is also evident.[92,97] Most survivors do not have residual hepatic impairment.

Hepatotropic Viruses

The hepatotropic viruses, hepatitis A (HAV), B (HBV), C (HCV), D (HDV), and E (HEV), cause hepatitis as their primary disease manifestation, but likely play a limited role in clinical neonatal disease. In infants, HAV and HBV infections are generally asymptomatic. Neonatal cholestasis resulting from vertical transmission of HAV infection has been reported.[98] HBV is vertically transmitted during pregnancy or delivery. Depending on the mother's e-antigen status, the risks of transmission can be reduced from up to 90% down to 1 to 10% with active and passive immunization of the newborn.[99] Most infected infants will become asymptomatic carriers, although rarely a fulminant hepatitis may occur.[100]

HCV can be transmitted perinatally, with some infected infants having mild to moderate elevation of aminotransferase levels,[101] and death from liver failure has been reported.[102] Perinatal transmission of HDV is uncommon and occurs in the presence of HBV transmission.[103] Vertical transmission of HEV may be common and has been reported as causing a high rate of icteric hepatitis, which may be fatal.[104] Hence, screening for the hepatotropic viruses in infants presenting with prolonged cholestasis remains in diagnostic algorithms. Chapter 75 provides further discussion of these viruses in older children and adolescents.

Human Immunodeficiency Virus

HIV infection in children causes a broad spectrum of disease and a varied clinical course. Acquired immunodeficiency syndrome (AIDS) represents the most severe end of the clinical spectrum. The established modes of HIV transmission include sexual contact; percutaneous or mucous membrane exposure to contaminated blood or other body fluids with high titers of HIV; mother-to-infant transmission before or around the time of birth; and breast-feeding. Children with HIV infection often develop liver disease, which may be as a result of cytopathic effects of the virus, opportunistic infections, or hepatotoxicity related to medications, or through metabolic derangements such as nonalcoholic fatty liver disease.[105] Clinical manifestations include failure to thrive, recurrent diarrhea, oral candidiasis, hepatitis, hepatomegaly, and splenomegaly, as well as generalized lymphadenopathy, parotitis, cardiomyopathy, nephropathy, central nervous system disease (including developmental delay), lymphoid interstitial pneumonia, recurrent invasive bacterial infections, opportunistic infections, and specific malignant neoplasms. Cholestatic hepatitis may be the first manifestation of HIV infection in young infants and has caused fatal liver failure.[106] Giant cell hepatitis has been reported in relation to vertically acquired HIV infection.[107] Antiretroviral agents used to prevent vertical transmission may also cause cholestasis in the neonate.[108]

Other Viruses

Human herpes virus (HHV)-6, the cause of childhood roseola infantum with fever and exanthem subitum, has been associated with cholestasis, neonatal hepatitis, giant cell transformation,[109] and fatal fulminant hepatitis.[110,111] There may be accompanying thrombocytopenia.[111] It has recently been shown that congenital infection results from chromosomal integration of the virus.[112] The histopathology is of a nonspecific lobular hepatitis with necrosis. Diagnosis is confirmed by serology, which may be negative in the acute phase, or PCR on body fluids and infected tissues.

Human parvovirus (B19 virus), the cause of erythema infectiosum in childhood, is thought to principally infect pronormoblastic erythroid cells, resulting in severe hemolytic anemia in the fetus with hydrops.[113] Many fetal organs, including the liver, are affected, and hepatocyte necrosis has been reported in fetuses and in newborn infants with parvovirus infection.[114,115] An acute severe hepatitis has been described in an older infant in association with parvovirus B19 infection.[116] Diagnosis of parvovirus B19 is confirmed by serology with detection of IgM and IgG in blood samples or by the detection of virus by PCR in blood or tissue samples.

Adenoviruses are DNA viruses, which most commonly infect the upper respiratory tract. Transmission is either perinatal during delivery or postnatal through contact with infected caregivers. Life-threatening disseminated infection occasionally occurs among young infants and immunocompromised hosts, with severe hepatitis and liver failure.[117,118] The pathology is similar to that seen in HSV infection, with widespread hepatocyte necrosis and intranuclear viral inclusion bodies. Diagnosis is confirmed by isolation of the virus from nasopharyngeal or pulmonary secretions or by detection of viral DNA by PCR in infected tissues, such as the liver and lungs.

Maternal varicella infection in the last 3 weeks of pregnancy can result in neonatal varicella infection, which generally occurs within the first 10 to 12 days of life. Illness is more severe if maternal infection manifests between 5 days before and 2 days after delivery.[119] Severe necrotizing hepatitis may occur as a feature of multisystem involvement that may include extensive skin lesions, pneumonitis, and meningoencephalitis.[119] Varicella acquired postnatally can also present with a severe hepatitis and has been associated with hemolytic anemia.[120] Treatment is with acyclovir, and zoster immunoglobulin is used to prevent severe disease in newborns whose mothers manifest infection late in pregnancy or shortly after delivery.

Transfusion-transmitted virus (TTV) is an unenveloped single-stranded DNA virus initially implicated as a cause of posttransfusion hepatitis. Initial reports suggested a possible role in neonatal hepatitis[121]; however, the role of TTV in contributing to liver disease has not been proven.[122]

Reovirus-3 has been proposed as a candidate virus serving as an etiologic agent for neonatal hepatitis as well as biliary atresia. Infection of weanling mice results in hepatic lesions similar to those observed in neonates with neonatal hepatitis. However, studies in humans using molecular techniques have yielded mixed results.[123,124]

Paramyxovirus infection has been attributed as the etiologic agent in a rare form of hepatitis termed *syncytial giant-cell hepatitis* affecting both children and adults.[125] In neonates, syncytial giant-cell hepatitis is associated with a severe hepatitis, with progression to chronic cholestasis and decompensated cirrhosis over the first year of life. Liver histology reveals both the hallmark syncytial-type giant cells replacing hepatocyte cords, most prominently in the centrilobular region, as well as severe acute and chronic hepatitis with bridging necrosis of hepatocytes, ballooning and dropout of hepatocytes, cholestasis, and small round cell inflammation within the lobule. Virus-like structures within giant cells resembling the nucleocapsids of paramyxovirus have been seen on electron microscopy. These giant cells are larger and of different morphology than the giant cells typically encountered in neonatal liver disease.[126] The putative virus from the paramyxoviruses family has not been subsequently identified since this entity was first described.

Parasitic Infections

Toxoplasmosis

Toxoplasma gondii is an obligate intracellular protozoan parasite that can cross the placenta and infect the fetus. Congenital infection occurs primarily as a result of maternal infection during pregnancy acquired by consumption of undercooked meat or direct contact with the feces of infected animals, particularly cats. IgM screening has documented the prevalence of congenital infection to range from 2 to 8 per 10,000 live births in developed nations.[127]

Most infants born with congenital *Toxoplasma* infection are asymptomatic in the neonatal period, with clinical signs and symptoms being present in only approximately 10 to 30% of infants.[69] The most characteristic clinical findings, referred to as the classic triad of congenital toxoplasmosis, include chorioretinitis, intracranial calcifications, and hydrocephalus. Other signs and symptoms include hepatosplenomegaly, jaundice, maculopapular rash, lymphadenopathy, and thrombocytopenia. Serum aminotransferase levels are elevated, and progressive liver dysfunction with ascites may occur. Liver histopathology features include nonspecific giant-cell hepatitis with focal necrosis associated with parasitized sinusoidal cells. Congenital toxoplasmosis has been reported in a newborn with severe pneumonitis, hepatitis, and disseminated intravascular coagulation.[128,129]

The diagnosis of congenital toxoplasmosis can be made prenatally by the detection of *T. gondii* in fetal blood or amniotic fluid, or from the placenta, umbilical cord, or infant peripheral blood via PCR. Serologic diagnosis can be made by IgM or IgA or persistent (over 12 months) IgG anti-*Toxoplasma* antibody tests determined in the infant's blood. Treatment with pyrimethamine and sulfadiazine prevents progression of organ damage.

SYSTEMIC CONDITIONS ASSOCIATED WITH NEONATAL HEPATITIS

Endocrinopathies

Conjugated hyperbilirubinemia has been associated with disturbance of the pituitary-adrenal axis. Hypoglycemia is often the initial manifestation of congenital anterior hypopituitarism. The associated prolonged neonatal cholestasis is typically accompanied by a normal serum GGT level.[130] Male infants may display micropenis and cryptorchidism. The resultant cholestasis is probably a secondary feature of an inadequate development of the hepatobiliary secretory apparatus from the absence of the trophic hormones modulating or stimulating bile canalicular development and bile acid synthesis, conjugation, and secretion. The presence of "wandering" nystagmus on physical examination suggests septo-optic dysplasia as seen with de Morsier's syndrome.[131] The diagnosis can be confirmed by assay of cortisol, growth hormone, and insulin levels or use of pituitary stimulation testing. A liver biopsy is typically not helpful, with nonspecific features of neonatal hepatitis. Replacement of cortisol and thyroid hormone results in resolution of the cholestasis.[132]

Isolated cortisol and thyroid hormone deficiencies can cause neonatal cholestasis.[133,134] Cholestatic liver disease has been reported in an infant with adrenal insufficiency following bilateral adrenal hemorrhage.[135] Iatrogenic hypothyroidism following iodinated contrast enema administration has resulted in cholestasis in premature infants.[136] There has been no clearly documented case of cholestasis secondary to isolated growth hormone (GH) deficiency, although animal studies support GH deficiency as a factor responsible for hepatic dysfunction.

Chromosomal Disorders

Neonatal hepatitis syndrome is reported in association with trisomy 17, trisomy 18, and trisomy 21 (Down syndrome).[137,138] Paucity of the intrahepatic bile duct in infants and children has been reported in Down syndrome.[138] The mechanisms underlying these associations remain unknown, though in some cases of Down syndrome, the cholestasis may be related to congenital hypothyroidism.[139]

Autoimmune Conditions

Neonatal lupus erythematosus (NLE) is an uncommon autoimmune disease caused by the passage of maternal anti-Ro (SS-A) or anti-La (SS-B) antibodies across the placenta. Affected organs include the heart, skin, and liver, as these are the fetal tissues that express the Ro and La antigens. The disease may present prenatally with fetal bradycardia, heart failure, and hydrops, or more commonly postnatally. The mother usually has either systemic lupus erythematosus (SLE) or Sjögren's disease, but this may be asymptomatic or undiagnosed.[140] The most striking manifestations are congenital complete heart block and a discoid lupus erythematosus rash, appearing either in the newborn period or weeks later.

A retrospective analysis of a United States NLE research registry revealed that 9% of newborns with NLE have some degree of hepatic involvement, and that liver disease may be the sole manifestation in some cases.[141] Other features may include hemolytic anemia, thrombocytopenia, or neutropenia.[142] The clinical spectrum of liver disease ranges from fatal liver failure to mild asymptomatic elevations of aminotransferases. Liver histology usually resembles giant cell hepatitis with ductular obstruction and extramedullary hematopoiesis. In fatal cases, liver pathology was consistent with the typical findings of neonatal hemochromatosis.[141]

Diagnosis is based on a maternal history of SLE or Sjögren's disease, typical clinical findings, and the presence of anti-Ro or anti-La antibodies in the serum of the neonate. Anti-nuclear antibody can be detected in some of the cases with hepatic involvement and might have a role in the pathogenesis of liver disease.[143] Congenital heart block requires treatment with a cardiac pacemaker, and the other manifestations generally resolve as levels of the maternally derived antibodies decline. Immunosuppressive treatment with prednisone may improve liver disease.

Hepatic Ischemia

The liver's metabolic activity is relatively constant and demands around 25% of cardiac output. The liver is unique in having two sources of oxygenated blood: one third via the hepatic arterial circulation and two thirds via the portal venous circulation, which has been partially deoxygenated in the intestine. Each compensate to some extent for impairment in the flow of the other. At the microscopic level, hepatic arterial blood mixes with portal venous blood rich in nutrients and hormones from the gastrointestinal tract. Under normal conditions, oxygen and nutrients in the blood decrease from periportal (zone 1) to pericentral (zone 3) areas. The low oxygen tension in the sinusoidal blood in zone 3 of the hepatic acinus makes pericentral hepatocytes in this zone relatively vulnerable to ischemic injury and necrosis.[144]

Hence, ischemic hepatitis, which clinically may mimic toxic or infectious hepatitis, occurs in association with chronic conditions such as congenital heart disease (for example, hypoplastic left heart syndrome and coarctation of the aorta, or congenital heart block), or with acute events such as asphyxia, septic or hypovolemic shock, cardiorespiratory arrest, prolonged seizures, cardiac bypass, or pericardial tamponade.[145,146] The hypotensive episode may not have been recognized clinically. Left-sided heart failure tends not to cause hepatic symptoms until hypotension or reduced cardiac output is present.[147,148] Up to one third of patients who have undergone the Fontan procedure have elevated serum bilirubin levels.[149]

Ischemic hepatitis related to an acute event is characterized by a marked and rapid elevation of serum transaminases within 24 to 48 hours after the initial insult, with a rapid decline by 3 to 11 days if perfusion and oxygenation are restored. Serum aminotransferase concentrations peak to 5000 to 10,000 U/L; alkaline phosphatase is usually normal. Hepatomegaly, jaundice, and coagulopathy are detected in up to 50% of affected patients. Elevations of serum creatine phosphokinase (CPK) and serum creatinine reflect hypotensive injury to other organs and are helpful indicators of global hypoperfusion. As the diagnosis is usually made on clinical and biochemical grounds, liver biopsy is usually not necessary. The prognosis depends primarily on the response of the underlying disorder to therapy. Because of the sensitive arterial supply to the bile ducts, ischemic damage may result in strictures and subsequent biliary cirrhosis.

Vascular occlusion may also result in ischemic hepatitis. Microthrombotic arterial occlusion occurs with disseminated intravascular coagulation (for example, with meningococcal sepsis), and venous outflow occlusion occurs with sinusoidal obstruction syndrome (formerly called hepatic veno-occlusive disease) or Budd-Chiari syndrome.[11,150]

Parenteral Nutrition

With increasing use of parenteral nutrition (PN) in premature infants and those with gastrointestinal anomalies or disease, parenteral nutrition associated liver disease (PNALD) is now a common entity in neonatal nurseries. PNALD develops in 40 to 60% of infants who require long-term TPN for intestinal failure.[151] Parenteral nutrition has been associated with a wide spectrum of adverse hepatobiliary consequences, from asymptomatic biliary sludge or stones related to reduced cholecystokinin stimulation of gallbladder contraction, to end-stage chronic liver failure. In infants, cholestasis is the primary form of PNALD, whereas in adults steatosis is the predominant hepatic response. These differences, and the fact that PNALD can manifest after a much shorter duration in infants than adults, relate to the immaturity of neonatal bile salt processing and transport machinery. The rate of progression of PNALD may vary from months to several years.

The pathogenesis of PNALD in infants remains ill defined; however, clues are provided by the clear risk factors that have been identified.[152] These include duration of PN therapy, prematurity, low birth weight, no or minimal enteral feeding, sepsis related to intravenous catheters or small bowel bacterial overgrowth, and a history of gastrointestinal surgery or short gut. Lack of enteral feeding leads to reduced gut hormone secretion, a reduction in bile flow, and biliary stasis. Endotoxin reduces bile acid uptake, processing, and excretion in the hepatocyte. Components of the PN infusate have been implicated in causing toxicity to the hepatocyte, with recent attention focusing on lipids (see later discussion). These infants are often ill, with many possible contributing factors to liver injury: for example, a premature infant with hypoxic-ischemic injury at birth, multiple episodes of sepsis, and necrotizing enterocolitis requiring intestinal surgery.

The morphologic changes of PNALD in infants are nonspecific and variable. Liver biopsy is not usually necessary to make the diagnosis, but may be required to exclude other possible diagnoses depending on clinical features and the results of other investigations. Hepatocyte and canalicular cholestasis without significant inflammation occurs early in the course. This is usually followed by a variable mixed inflammatory cell infiltrate in the portal tracts and subsequently progressive hepatic ultimately leading to biliary cirrhosis.[153] Severe fibrosis can be seen after 6 weeks of TPN.[154] Other histopathologic features include cholestatic rosettes formation, bile plugs, and steatosis.

Management and prevention strategies for PNALD include early enteral feeding, even if "trophic," and careful attention to the handling of venous catheters to reduce episodes of sepsis. The administration of ursodeoxycholic acid may improve bile flow and reduce gallbladder and intestinal stasis, and it can improve biochemical parameters; however, a beneficial effect on long-term outcomes in a prospective randomized trial is yet to be demonstrated.[155] Use of fish-oil based parenteral lipid solutions has shown promise in treatment of PNALD in case series[156,157] and is currently being evaluated in a randomized PNALD prevention trial.[158] It has been suggested that the benefit may derive from a reduced n6:n3 polyunsaturated fatty acid ratio resulting in reduced production of inflammatory mediators. Experimental evidence showing that phytosterols impair normal bile acid homeostasis suggests that the benefit may relate to avoidance of these products in soybean-derived lipids.[159] Routine monitoring of hepatic transaminases and synthetic function in all neonates receiving PN allows early detection and potential interventions. For patients who remain PN dependent with progressive liver failure, transplantation (usually combined with a small bowel graft) may be indicated.

IDIOPATHIC NEONATAL HEPATITIS

Idiopathic neonatal hepatitis (INH) continues to be a descriptive term and "default" diagnosis applied to infants with prolonged cholestasis for which no cause can be found, despite thorough work-up. The liver injury is highlighted by the presence of variable numbers of multinuclear giant cells, regarded as a nonspecific response of the neonatal liver to injury. INH has traditionally been categorized into familial and nonfamilial forms. The familial form (which probably represents a heterogeneous collection of undiagnosed or unrecognized genetic etiologies) is more likely to be progressive or recurrent than the nonfamilial form.

The overall prognosis in INH is difficult to estimate, because this is constantly changing as individual entities are identified. For example, alpha-1-antitrypsin deficiency and the PFIC disorders, which have different natural histories, were once considered under the same umbrella of INH. For this reason, one should be careful about using older literature to prognosticate a current infant labeled as having INH. In one relatively recent large series of cholestatic infants with no specific cause found, the cholestasis was found to be transient and recovery was observed with long-term follow-up.[160]

MANAGEMENT OF NEONATAL CHOLESTASIS

Management of the cholestatic infant has two main components: specific management related to individual entities and general principles applicable to all patients.[161] The former is

TABLE 68-4. **Medical Management of Neonatal Cholestasis**

Malabsorption/malnutrition
    Optimize caloric intake
    Feed fortification/ concentration
    Fat supplementation, giving 30-50% of total fat as MCT
    Enteral tube feeds or parenteral nutrition if necessary
Vitamin and micronutrients
    Monitor for fat-soluble vitamin deficiencies, and response to therapy
    Vitamin A: 5000-25,000 U/day*
    Vitamin D: 400 IU/day*
    Vitamin E: 15-25 IU/kg/day*
    Vitamin K: 2.5-5 mg/day*
    Water-soluble vitamin and trace elements: multivitamin providing at
        least 100% of recommended dietary allowance
Pruritus
    Medical therapy
        Ursodeoxycholic acid
        Cholestyramine
        Rifampicin
        Naloxone
    Surgical therapy
        Partial external biliary diversion
Ascites
    Sodium restriction
    Diuretic therapy: spironolactone, furosemide
    Consider antibacterial prophylaxis if peritonitis develops
    Therapeutic paracentesis
Portal hypertension and variceal hemorrhage
    Endoscopic sclerotherapy
    Surgical shunt procedure
    Liver transplantation
End-stage liver disease, severe refractory symptoms
    Liver transplantation

MCT, medium-chain triglyceride.
*Note: Doses provided are a guide only and will need to be adjusted based on monitoring response and vitamin levels.

discussed in the preceding sections on specific diseases and in subsequent chapters. The latter is outlined in Table 68-4 and discussed next.

Cholestasis results in decreased concentrations of bile acids and phospholipids in the small intestine, thus reducing micelle formation and hence absorption of long-chain fat and accompanying fat-soluble vitamins. Because neonates rely heavily on the calories obtained from dietary fat, its malabsorption can result in significant and early malnutrition with resulting poor growth. Other disease-related factors such as inflammation, ascites, or portal hypertension also contribute to malnutrition through reduced oral intake, impaired intestinal function, impaired substrate utilization, and increased energy expenditure. There may be associated pancreatic exocrine insufficiency, as associated with PFIC type 1 and Alagille syndrome, requiring enzyme replacement. Thus, early and aggressive nutritional management of the cholestatic infant is vital to optimize growth and development through what may be a chronic condition. Dietary fat in the form of medium-chain triglyceride (MCT), which is less dependent on micelle formation for absorption than long-chain fat, is supplemented. Specialized MCT-based formulas are also available for this purpose. Further nonfat calories may be added in the form of glucose polymers or by concentrating the milk formula. Close monitoring of growth parameters and anthropometry will enable the response to nutritional interventions to be monitored, with care to consider the impact that ascites or edema may have on weight measurements. Invasive measures such as enteral tube feeding or gastrostomy may be required if oral intake is insufficient. Parenteral nutrition may

be necessary if malabsorption or gut dysfunction prevents adequate digestion and absorption of enteral feeds. Nocturnal enteral feeding improves nutritional indices of children with chronic cholestatic disease.[162] Infants and young children with cholestatic liver disease require at least 130% of the caloric requirements of a healthy child, and so at least this amount of calories (and often more) must be provided to preserve and improve nutritional status.[163,164]

Fat-soluble vitamin deficiency is common in infants and young children with chronic cholestatic conditions.[165] This may occur early in neonatal cholestasis, and indeed may be a presenting feature. Catastrophic intracranial hemorrhage can result from a vitamin K–deficient coagulopathy.[166] Significant rickets with minimal trauma fractures occurs with vitamin D deficiency. Neurologic abnormalities such as ataxia, neuropathy, and retinopathy can result from vitamin E deficiency and may not reverse fully with correction. Vitamin A deficiency can cause impaired vision in the form of night blindness or corneal scarring. Human breast milk is low in vitamins D and K, and so breast-fed cholestatic infants are at particular risk of deficiency. Premature infants have reduced body stores of these vitamins and may manifest early. Serum levels of vitamins A, D, and E and coagulation indices such as prothrombin time or INR for vitamin K status are generally used to screen for deficiency and monitor response to therapy and avoid toxicity. Very high oral doses or parenteral doses of individual vitamins may be required. Little is known about water-soluble vitamin deficiency in neonatal cholestasis, though it is quite reasonable to administer a multivitamin in standard dose to these infants, remembering that many preparations also contain vitamin A.

Cholestasis usually results in elevated serum bile acid concentrations, which are associated with the development of pruritus. Young infants may not manifest with scratching but may instead be irritable. Precise mechanisms of cholestasis-related pruritus remain to be elucidated, and empirical therapy is often necessary for severe pruritus.[167] Ursodeoxycholic acid may be effective for pruritic symptoms by resolving or improving cholestasis, but its effects are inconsistent. Anion-exchange resins such as cholestyramine and colestipol are thought to bind pruritogens in the intestine, preventing reabsorption, and may be more effective if there is adequate biliary drainage to allow bile acids to reach the gut lumen. Hepatic cytochrome enzyme inducers such as rifampicin and phenobarbital may increase the metabolism of pruritogens and thereby enhance their removal. Antihistamines may be effective but are likely to sedate the infant rather than act mechanistically, because skin changes consistent with histamine-mediated effects are not typically found in cholestatic pruritus. Opiate antagonists such as naloxone and serotonergic agents such as sertraline have shown promise in adult studies, but experience in children is limited. Surgical measures such as partial external biliary drainage or ileal bypass procedures have been used in refractory situations where there remains some residual bile flow.

In some infants with cholestasis, progressive hepatic fibrosis and cirrhosis ultimately lead to the development of portal hypertension with sequelae of ascites and variceal hemorrhage. The medical management of ascites needs to consider patient comfort and the relative risk of peritoneal bacterial infection. Judicious use of sodium restriction and diuretic therapy may help control the accumulation of ascites. Refractory ascites with respiratory compromise is best managed by therapeutic paracentesis with concomitant administration of intravenous albumin. Portal hypertension and its attendant complications are discussed in Chapter 76. Treatment of complicated portal hypertension in young infants is challenging, because the safety and efficacy of medical treatment with nonselective beta blockers has not been proven, and endoscopic variceal ligation is not technically possible. Consideration for liver transplantation is usually necessary for these infants and for those with progressive liver failure. Early referral to a transplant center is important so that appropriate evaluation can be initiated.

A multidisciplinary team approach of care for these infants is important not only for optimization of medical and dietary management but also in providing support to the family.

SUMMARY

The past decade has seen further elucidation of molecular mechanisms of cholestasis, and with this has come the identification of newly described diseases resulting from specific genetic defects. Simultaneously, terms such as *idiopathic neonatal hepatitis* have become less meaningful. A timely and careful evaluation of potential causes of neonatal cholestasis is critical in identifying those conditions where specific therapeutic interventions can change their natural history.

ACKNOWLEGMENTS

We thank Dr. Ernest Cutz, Professor of Pathology, and Dr. Bo Ngan, Assistant Professor of Pathology, from the Department of Pathology and Laboratory Medicine at the Hospital for Sick Children and University of Toronto, for providing the photomicrographs.

REFERENCES

3. Balistreri WF, Bezerra JA. Whatever happened to "neonatal hepatitis." Clin Liver Dis 2006;10:27–53.
5. Moyer V, Freese DK, Whitington PF, et al. Guideline for the evaluation of cholestatic jaundice in infants: recommendations of the North American Society for Pediatric Gastroenterology, Hepatology and Nutrition. J Pediatr Gastroenterol Nutr 2004;39:115–128.
44. Chand N, Sanyal AJ. Sepsis-induced cholestasis. Hepatology 2007;45:230–241.
81. Kimberlin DW, Whitley RJ. Neonatal herpes: what have we learned. Semin Pediatr Infect Dis 2005;16:7–16.
152. Carter BA, Shulman RJ. Mechanisms of disease: update on the molecular etiology and fundamentals of parenteral nutrition associated cholestasis. Nat Clin Pract Gastroenterol Hepatol 2007;4:277–287.
161. Ng VL, Balistreri WF. Treatment options for chronic cholestasis in infancy and childhood. Curr Treat Options Gastroenterol 2005;8:419–430.

See expertconsult.com for a complete list of references and the review questions for this chapter.

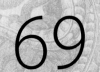

BILIARY ATRESIA AND NEONATAL DISORDERS OF THE BILE DUCTS

69

Giorgina Mieli-Vergani • Nedim Hadžić

Children with primary disorders of the bile ducts present early in life with classic signs of prolonged conjugated jaundice, pale stools, and dark urine. They represent an important group within the so-called neonatal cholestasis syndrome. Disorders of the bile ducts can be due to developmental anomalies, an inflammatory process, or genetic causes. If corrective surgical treatment is available, it should be instituted early in order to minimize the progression of chronic liver disease.[1]

SURGICALLY CORRECTABLE DISORDERS

Biliary Atresia

Biliary atresia (BA) is the most common surgically correctable liver disorder in infancy, affecting sporadically between 1 in 8000 (Far-East, Oceania) to 16,000 (Europe, North America) live-born infants.[2,3] It is characterized by complete obstruction of the bile flow due to progressive ascending destruction and obliteration of part or all of the extrahepatic biliary tree. The intrahepatic bile ducts become affected as well. Studies of bile duct remnants removed at surgery and from serial sectioning and reconstruction of surgical and necropsy liver specimens indicate that BA arises from a sclerosing inflammatory process affecting previously formed bile ducts.[4] Comparative anatomic studies have suggested that, at least in some cases, BA may be caused by failure of the intrauterine remodeling process at the hepatic hilum, with persistence of fetal bile ducts poorly supported by mesenchyme. As bile flow dramatically increases postnatally, bile leakage from these abnormal ducts may trigger an intense inflammatory reaction, with consequent obliteration of the biliary tree.[4] The extrahepatic ducts are primarily affected, whereas the intrahepatic bile ducts remain patent in early infancy but eventually also become inflamed and obliterated and eventually disappear.[5] Biliary cirrhosis with complications such as portal hypertension may develop at any time from 2 months of age; few unoperated children survive beyond 18 months of age.

Clinical Features and Diagnosis

Two forms of BA are described: (1) a more common (around 85 to 90% of cases) peri- or postnatal sporadic form ("acquired"), possibly virus related, and (2) a less common (around 10 to 15% of cases) fetal or embryonic form ("congenital"), with a high frequency of associated malformations. BA splenic malformation (BASM) syndrome is characterized by polysplenia or asplenia, various laterality defects such as abdominal or complete situs inversus, mediopositioned liver and intestinal malrotation, cardiac laterality defects, and positional abnormalities of the major abdominal blood vessels.[6,7] Intriguingly, BASM

syndrome is less commonly seen in the Far East and Asia, where BA is twice as common as in the rest of the world.[3] An increased incidence of maternal diabetes mellitus and female gender has been observed in the BASM syndrome.[6] Children with this syndrome appear to have an increased frequency of infections, possibly leading to their poorer long-term prognosis compared with classic BA, including after liver transplantation, although no formal defect in their humoral immunity has been identified.[8] It has also been suggested that the precarious blood supply to the biliary tree may be further jeopardized by their vascular abnormalities.[6]

Clinical features of BA are jaundice, pale stools, and dark urine presenting at or soon after birth.[8] As physiologic jaundice, characterized by unconjugated bilirubinemia, is common in neonates and most infants with BA have no major symptoms in the first few weeks of life, diagnosis is often delayed.[1] This is a particular problem for infants with the perinatal or "acquired" form of BA, whose stools may have some pigment in the first few weeks of life, before bile flow is completely obstructed (Figure 69-1).[1,9] Delayed diagnosis and surgical treatment carry a severe prognosis.[10-14] Age at surgical correction is inversely correlated with the medium-term (up to 20 years) survival with native liver.[14] Hence it is of paramount importance for health professionals attending young infants to check the color of the urine and stools of all jaundiced babies, irrespective of their general health or age, and refer those with dark urine and pale stools promptly to specialized hepatology centers. No satisfactory screening test is available for BA, though promising results using universal neonatal stool color cards have been recently reported from Taiwan.[15]

Physical examination and laboratory tests give little clue to the diagnosis of BA. Most of the affected infants have a mild degree of hepatomegaly and splenomegaly. Ascites or cutaneous signs of chronic liver disease are rarely detected in the early stages of the disease, when correct diagnosis is most important for effective surgical intervention. Biochemical findings are nonspecific, with levels of transaminases, γ-glutamyltranspeptidase (GGT), and alkaline phosphatase similar to those found in other forms of neonatal cholestasis. Coagulopathy, if present, is responsive to intravenous vitamin K. An ultrasound scan revealing an absent or abnormal gallbladder with an irregular wall[16] or, in older infants, the "triangular cord" sign[17] is suggestive of BA. However, a normal gallbladder or absence of the triangular cord sign do not exclude BA.[18]

Histologic examination of the liver by an experienced histopathologist leads to the correct diagnosis of BA in up to 90% of cases.[19] Typical histologic findings are edematous portal tracts with inflammatory changes, bile duct proliferation, and bile plugs (Figure 69-2A), but in very young babies these features can be much less obvious. Biliary radionuclide scans are only useful if isotope is demonstrated in the gut, thereby excluding BA and avoiding laparotomy. If the liver biopsy is ambiguous, but the stools remain acholic, endoscopic retrograde cholangiopancreatography (ERCP)[20,21] is indicated to assess the patency of the biliary system. Future improvements in sensitivity of magnetic resonance cholangiopancreatography (MRCP) may offer an additional noninvasive way of assessing the biliary tree in suspected BA.[22,23] If the cholangiography is not informative, an explorative laparotomy with intraoperative cholangiography is required, but should be undertaken by an experienced surgeon, because hypoplastic extrahepatic ducts caused by a severe intrahepatic cholestasis may be interpreted as atretic, leading to an unnecessary and possibly damaging operation.[24] The diagnosis of BA should always be confirmed by histologic examination of the excised biliary remnants (Figure 69-2B).

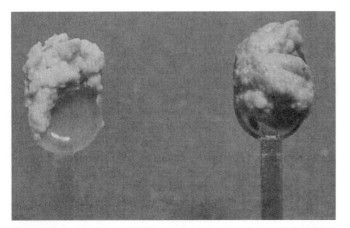

Figure 69-1. Acholic stool (left) strongly suggestive of a surgical problem during neonatal period. Children with biliary atresia can, however, have initially pigmented stools (right). (*See plate section for color.*) Reproduced from Francavilla R, Mieli-Vergani G. Liver and biliary disease in infancy. Medicine 2002; 30:45-47, with permission from The Medicine Publishing Company, Abingdon.

Etiopathogenesis

Studies of bile duct remnants removed at surgery and from serial sectioning and reconstruction of surgical and postmortem liver specimens indicate that BA is in most cases a sclerosing inflammatory process affecting previously formed bile ducts.[4,5] The cause of such inflammatory process remains unknown. It is conceivable that BA represents a common final phenotypic pathway of neonatal liver injury caused by diverse causes, including developmental, vascular, or infectious factors, which may act antenatally or within the first 3 months of life, in a genetically predisposed individual.[25] Though BA is not an inherited disorder, because identical twins are usually discordant for the disease and occurrence of BA within the same family is exceedingly rare,[26,27] it is possible that a genetic predisposition to an aberrant immune response against an exogenous agent and/or somatic mutations of genes regulating bile duct morphogenesis in fetal life are involved. Whatever the initiating event, as bile flow dramatically increases perinatally, bile leakage from the abnormal ducts is likely to trigger an intense inflammatory reaction, with consequent obliteration of the biliary tree. The detergent effect of the extravasated bile, however, cannot be the only explanation for the liver damage, because the disease can also progress in those patients in whom the Kasai portoenterostomy has achieved adequate bile flow. Proposed etiologic factors in BA include defective morphogenesis/genetic factors, vascular abnormalities, viral infection, exposure to toxins, and aberrant immune mechanisms.[25]

Genetic Factors/Defective Morphogenesis

A separate clinical and etiologic subgroup, named BA splenic malformation (BASM) syndrome, is believed to be caused by defective morphogenesis of the biliary tree.[6,7] A recessive insertional mutation in the proximal region of mouse chromosome 4 or complete deletion of the inversion (inv) gene in a murine model leads to anomalous development of the hepatobiliary system.[28] However, no consistent mutations in the INV gene were identified in patients with BA, including those with

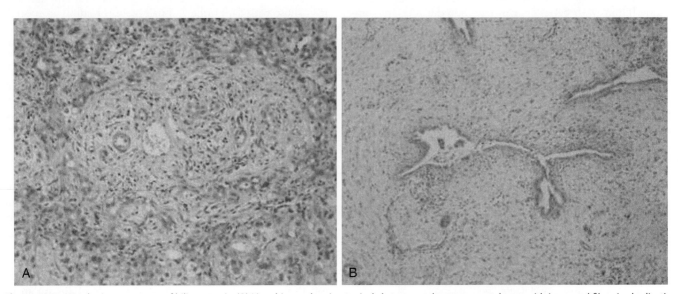

Figure 69-2. Histologic appearance of biliary atresia. (**A**) Liver biopsy showing typical changes – edematous portal tract with increased fibrosis, duplicating bile ducts, and cholestatic plugs (hematoxylin-eosin stain, ×250). (**B**) Bile duct remnant obtained at Kasai portoenterostomy showing fibrosis and occlusion of extrahepatic bile ducts (hematoxylin-eosin stain, ×125). (*See plate section for color.*) Reproduced from Francavilla R, Mieli-Vergani G. Liver and biliary disease in infancy. Medicine 2002; 30:45–47, with permission from The Medicine Publishing Company, Abingdon.

BASM syndrome, suggesting that the INV gene is unlikely to be involved in the fetal cases of BA.[29] CFC1, coding for the CRYPTIC protein, is another gene investigated in BA. Although the precise function of the CRYPTIC protein is unknown, it is believed to act as a cofactor in the Nodal pathway that determines left-right axis development, disturbed in the BASM syndrome.[30] Recently, a genetic mutation in exon 5 of the CFC1 gene, leading to the amino acid substitution Ala145Thr, was found in 5 of 10 infants with BASM syndrome.[31] It is conceivable that CFC1 heterozygous mutations predispose to BASM, but then a second genetic or environmental factor is necessary to produce the disease phenotype.

Histologic features similar to the inherited group of disorders termed *ductal plate malformation syndrome,* which include congenital hepatic fibrosis and Caroli syndrome, have been reported in fetal type BA,[32] suggesting that abnormalities in hepatocyte growth factor signaling during a critical period for mesenchymal/epithelial differentiation or other defects in intracellular adhesion molecule systems might be involved in the pathogenesis of this form of the disease. Of note, however, among 9 children with BA diagnosed in utero, only one had BASM syndrome and none had histologic appearances of "ductal plate malformation."[7]

Tan et al.[33] postulated that BA may derive from failure of the ductal plate structure remodeling between 11 and 13 weeks' gestation leading to the formation of an inadequate mesenchymal cuff around the developing hilar bile ducts, which could potentially be prone to rupture at the initiation of bile flow at 12 to 13 weeks' gestation.

Two recent studies report the presence of maternal microchimerism in children with BA. Hayashida et al.[34] demonstrate three times more XX-chromosome cells in males with BA compared with age-matched controls. Kobayashi et al.[35] confirm maternal microchimerism in male patients with BA and show maternal microchimerism in females with BA by demonstrating presence of maternal human leukocyte antigens (HLAs). They suggest that maternal microchimerism could be a potential causative factor in BA, as maternal cells could elicit an immune response similar to graft-versus-host disease.

Vascular Abnormalities

Intrahepatic and extrahepatic bile ducts receive their blood supply exclusively from the hepatic artery.[36] An arteriopathy affecting branches of the hepatic artery has been reported in patients with BA.[37] These observations have led to the proposal that a vasculopathy may be the cause of BA, though whether vascular problems are primary or secondary to bile duct damage remains to be clarified.

Viral Infection

The reported seasonal clustering of human BA cases[38] and experimental evidence of virus-induced BA have suggested a link between this disorder and exposure to viral agents.[39] An initial bile duct epithelial injury caused by viral infection would lead to a progressive immune-mediated inflammatory and sclerosing process resulting in damage and eventually obstruction of the bile ducts.[40] Several viruses have in turn been suggested in the pathogenesis of human BA, though published reports have been largely anecdotal and have given controversial results.[41-46]

Epidemiologic studies on reovirus and rotavirus, currently believed to be the most likely infectious agents involved in the pathogenesis of BA on the basis of experimental models, are also conflicting.[47] Interest in reovirus stems from the observation that infection in weanling mice causes bile duct and liver damage similar to that observed in BA,[48] with the lesions persisting after the virus or viral antigens are no longer detected. Search for reovirus antibodies, however, in infants with BA has been inconclusive,[49-51] possibly because of a high incidence of passively transferred maternal anti-reovirus immunoglobulin G. Studies in the liver tissue have also given discrepant results.[48,49,51-53]

The demonstration that in mice BA can be induced by rotavirus has elicited a strong interest in the possible role of this pathogen in the causation of the human disease. Rotavirus infection of newborn mice in the first 24 hours of life leads to jaundice, acholic stools, and hyperbilirubinemia by the end of the first week of life.[42] Progressive inflammation and obstruction of the extrahepatic bile duct is observed by 2 weeks of age, mimicking human BA.[54-56] In this animal model, which has been replicated in various laboratories, bile duct injury is associated with an initial CD4 T helper-1 (T_H1) immune response that through the release of interferon (IFN)-γ induces macrophages to produce tumor necrosis factor (TNF)-α and nitric oxide and immune activation persisting after viral clearance.[57] Mack et al.[58] have been able to provoke bile duct-specific inflammatory changes into naïve syngeneic severe combined immunodeficiency (SCID) mice by adoptively transferring T cells obtained from mice in which rotavirus had induced BA. Emergence of the bile duct lesions in the absence of virus in the recipients suggests that biliary epithelial cell-specific autoreactive T cells are generated in the course of rotavirus infection and cause biliary damage. Although this animal model suggests that BA could be the result of rotavirus infection, its role in the human disease remains uncertain.[54,56]

Toxins

Outbreaks of BA in lambs and calves in Australia, possibly related to a fungal or other environmental toxin exposure,[59] as well as the reported time and space clustering of BA cases in humans, have led to the proposal that an environmental toxin could be involved in its pathogenesis. However, to date no environmental agent, apart from viruses, has been clearly associated with BA in humans.

Immune Mechanisms

The presence of a portal tract mononuclear cell infiltrate in the liver biopsies of infants with BA has suggested a primary inflammatory process leading to bile duct obstruction.[60-62] The mechanism by which immune cells induce bile duct damage, however, is unclear. The currently favored immune pathogenic scenario[40,63] postulates that a viral or toxic insult to the biliary epithelium leads to the expression of new or altered antigens. In predisposed individuals, a peptide derived from these neoantigens would be presented to naive T lymphocytes by a professional antigen-presenting cell (APC), or directly by biliary epithelial cells that themselves express antigen-presenting HLA class I and II molecules. Of note, patients with BA have an increased number of resident liver macrophages – Kupffer cells, which can act as APCs.[64] Primed T_H1 lymphocytes would then orchestrate a damaging immune response, unfolding through the release of proinflammatory cytokines and recruitment of cytotoxic T cells, leading to progressive bile duct epithelial injury, fibrosis, and eventually occlusion of the extrahepatic bile ducts. No information is available as yet on the role of the recently described proinflammatory T_H17 cells.

Immune-mediated diseases are frequently associated with specific HLA molecules, which present peptide antigens to unprimed T lymphocytes. Several groups, therefore, have investigated a possible HLA predisposition to BA. Though an early report in a relatively small number of BA patients suggested that the possession of the allotype HLA-B12 (49% of BA patients versus 23% of control subjects) and haplotypes A9-B5 and A28-B35 could predispose to non-BASM BA in a European population,[65] other groups could not replicate these findings,[66] and a subsequent study from the same group using more sensitive molecular techniques in a larger number of patients (101 European children) failed to detect any HLA association.[67] An Egyptian study showed an increased frequency of HLA-B8 and DR3 in 18 children with BA, 10 having the B8/DR3 haplotype that is associated with autoimmune hepatitis, primary sclerosing cholangitis, and inflammatory bowel disease.[67a] Though the available data do not support a strong link between HLA and BA, larger studies in patients of different ethnicities are needed. While exploring the involvement in BA predisposition of immunologically relevant non-HLA molecules that have been associated with other immune-mediated liver diseases, Donaldson et al. found no difference in polymorphism prevalence in genes encoding the proinflammatory TNF-α and interleukin (IL)-1 and the anti-inflammatory IL-10 cytokines in 101 children with BA when compared to 96 geographically and ethnically matched adult controls.[67]

In keeping with a T_H orchestrated immune process, an abundance of CD4+ T lymphocytes has been described in the liver and extrahepatic bile ducts of BA patients.[68,69] These cells may have accumulated in the liver through the enhanced expression of adhesion molecules,[70] an event that may also explain the high number of natural killer (CD56+) cells among the inflammatory infiltrate.[70] DNA microarray techniques have shown up-regulation of T_H1 cytokine encoding genes, such as IFN-γ, and down-regulation of genes encoding T_H2 cytokines.[71] A possible T_H2 involvement in the pathogenesis of BA, however, is suggested by the finding in affected children of circulating autoantibodies, including anti-neutrophil cytoplasmic antibodies[72] and antibodies directed to alpha-enolase and vimentin.[73] There is also evidence that in BA biliary epithelial cells undergo an augmented rate of apoptosis[74] promoted by *de novo* expression of Fas ligand.[75] Bile drainage after portoenterostomy is reportedly better in patients with Fas ligand-negative biliary epithelial cells.[75]

Recently, an attempt has been made to map the sequential behavior of an array of soluble mediators of inflammation reported or assumed to be involved in the pathogenesis of BA, including adhesion molecules and pro- and anti-inflammatory cytokines, by prospectively studying 21 consecutive infants with BA at the time of Kasai portoenterostomy and serially thereafter for 6 months.[76] As controls, other neonatal cholestatic diseases and infants with no liver disease were investigated. No significant differences in the baseline cytokine levels were found between BA and normal controls; however, IL-2 and IL-10 were significantly higher in comparison with other cholestatic disease controls. Soluble intercellular adhesion molecule-1 (sICAM-1) levels were substantially higher in BA at baseline compared to the two control groups. Within the first 6 months after portoenterostomy, all plasma cytokine and adhesion molecule levels increased significantly, with the exception of IL-10, suggesting that the inflammatory process is progressive and involves both nonpolarized T_H and macrophage immune responses that are not ameliorated by portoenterostomy.[76] Among the circulating immune modulators investigated, sICAM-1 was the best

candidate plasma biomarker for BA severity, with total serum bilirubin level being significantly positively correlated with the sICAM-1 levels at 1, 3, and 6 months after the surgery. Moreover, a cutoff level of serum sICAM-1 of 1779 ng/mL at 1 month after Kasai portoenterostomy predicted the need for transplantation in the first year of life with 87% sensitivity and 92% specificity, suggesting that plasma sICAM-1 level could be used as a marker of disease progression and outcome in BA.[76]

Treatment

The treatment of BA is surgical. In 5 to 10% of infants with BA, the surgeon can identify a patent common bile duct containing bile and in continuity with intrahepatic bile ducts.[10] In these infants a biliary-intestinal anastomosis via a long Roux-en-Y loop may allow bile to drain satisfactorily. In the majority of patients, however, the proximal common hepatic duct is absent or completely obliterated up to the point at which it enters the liver, and at the porta hepatis is replaced by fibrous tissue. This tissue needs to be transected flush within the liver, and then a Roux-en-Y loop of jejunum is anastomosed around the fibrous edges of the transected tissue, forming a portoenterostomy (Kasai procedure) (Figure 69-3).[10] For surgery to be effective, the intrahepatic bile ducts must be patent at the porta hepatitis.[10] Later modifications of the Kasai procedure undertaken to reduce the risks of cholangitis are usually unsuccessful, unless there is a radiologically identifiable complication, amenable to a simple surgical correction.[77] Of note, these attempts could increase the operative risks during liver transplantation if this is required subsequently.

There are three macroscopic types of BA:
- Type I – affecting the distal part of the common duct
- Type II – affecting the common hepatic duct, but sparing the gallbladder and common bile duct
- Type III – affecting right and left intrahepatic ducts and the gallbladder

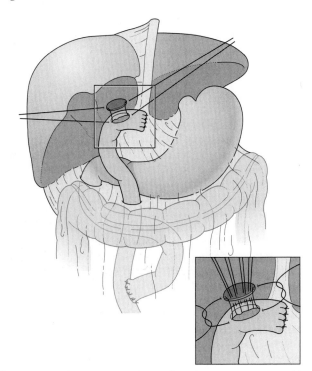

Figure 69-3. Schematic presentation of Kasai portoenterostomy with creation of jejunal Roux-en-Y loop.

The most common form is type III (85 to 90% of cases), which is often referred to as "uncorrectable"; surgical reconstruction (portoenterostomy) is most challenging in this variant.

After surgery the authors use phenobarbital at a dose of 5 to 7 mg/kg/day for long-term induction of the microsomal enzymes of the hepatocyte endoplasmic reticulum.[9] If the jaundice reappears, the dose could be doubled, following exclusion of a mechanical problem with the Roux-en-Y loop. All children should be supplemented with fat-soluble vitamins, which should be continued medium or long term according to resolution of jaundice. Choleretic treatment with ursodeoxycholic acid (UDCA, 15 to 25 mg/kg/day) could also be considered. If the portoenterostomy is performed by an experienced surgeon, good bile flow with normal serum bilirubin values can be achieved in more than 80% of children operated on by 60 days of age, but in only 20 to 30% with later surgery.[1,11-13] If bilirubin returns to normal, a 90% 15-year survival rate has been reported,[11] with a good quality of life into the fourth decade.[78] Up to 11% of children could be completely free of clinical and biochemical signs of liver disease after 10-year follow-up.[79] If the bilirubin level is not reduced, the rate of progression of cirrhosis is not slowed and survival beyond the second birthday is unusual. If partial bile drainage is obtained, development of end-stage chronic liver disease may be delayed, but liver replacement usually becomes unavoidable by puberty. A recent Japanese report on long-term follow-up of BA patients, all of whom underwent a Kasai portoenterostomy in the 1970s, quotes a native liver 20-year survival of 44%, but with significant morbidity, including recurrent cholangitis and gastrointestinal bleeding in 37% and 17% of patients, respectively.[80]

In view of the strong inflammatory component in the pathogenesis of BA, steroids have been in empirical use for many years.[81-83] Besides their immunologic and anti-inflammatory effects,[84] steroids can increase bile flow by inducing canalicular electrolyte transport.[85] There is, however, no solid clinical evidence that steroids are of benefit. Most published studies are retrospective and uncontrolled,[86,87] with only two being prospective and controlled: Davenport et al.[88] performed a randomized double-blinded, placebo-controlled trial of low-dose oral prednisolone in 71 children with BA, and Petersen et al.[89] used a high-dose steroid regimen to treat 20 consecutive patients after Kasai portoenterostomy and compared them with a historical control group. Neither study showed any difference in overall survival, liver transplant requirements, survival with native liver, or jaundice-free survival with native liver. Further and larger studies testing randomly different steroid doses and regimens are required to establish the possible beneficial effect of this mode of treatment.

An important postoperative complication of BA is cholangitis. This is seen in more than 50% of patients in the first 2 years after surgery, and a wide range of microorganisms could be implicated.[90] Cholangitis is characterized by fever, recurrence or aggravation of jaundice, and, frequently, clinical features of septicemia. Blood culture, ascitic aspirate, or liver biopsy to identify the organism responsible should precede intravenous antibiotic therapy, which is continued for 14 days if a pathogen is identified. Often, however, the diagnosis of cholangitis is not obvious, and unexplained fever may be the only symptom. Intravenous antibiotics are then started empirically, after taking a blood culture and assessing liver function, C-reactive protein level, and full blood count. If the fever responds to the antibiotics, these are continued for 5 days. Should the fever recur after stopping them, a liver biopsy is performed for histologic examination and culture. Amoxicillin and ceftazidime are currently the authors' initial choice pending in vitro sensitivities. Long-term prophylaxis with rotating antibiotics may be indicated for recurrent cholangitis.[12]

A degree of portal hypertension is present in almost all patients at the time of initial surgery. Approximately 50% of all survivors aged 5 years, even those with normal bilirubin levels, have esophageal varices, but only 10 to 15% have gastrointestinal bleeding. For these, variceal banding or injection sclerotherapy is the treatment of choice. In approximately 10% of patients in whom the serum bilirubin level returns to normal, intrahepatic cholangiopathy progresses and complications of biliary cirrhosis ultimately develop.[91] For these patients, and those with persistent jaundice, liver transplantation should be considered.[92] With 1-year survival rates approaching 90%, and 5-year survival rates of over 80%,[93,94] liver transplantation is now a standard therapeutic option, although it remains a formidable surgicomedical procedure. The recipient is likely to have one or more life-threatening complications in the perioperative or postoperative period. Lifelong immunosuppressive therapy is required, frequently resulting in chronic nephrotoxicity and increased risk of opportunistic and community-acquired infections and malignancies, all necessitating a close medical and surgical supervision. Most of the survivors have a good quality of life and attend school, although the long-term medical and psychologic effects of liver transplantation in childhood are as yet largely understudied.[95] The supply of donors of suitable size and blood group, even with an increased use of split grafts where one donor liver is used for two recipients (usually one child and one adult), remains a major limiting factor in liver transplantation. Segmental graft transplant from living relatives has given survival rates of 90% in infants in whom Kasai portoenterostomy was unsuccessful.[94] The results are better in children transplanted when heavier than 10 kg (or after the age of 1 year) and when the procedure is done electively.[93]

Liver transplantation in patients with BA should be complementary to portoenterostomy, except for infants in whom decompensated cirrhosis has developed because of delayed diagnosis. The combination of Kasai portoenterostomy followed by transplantation in case of failure has considerably improved the survival of children with BA. The reported 4-year actuarial survival rate with native liver is 51%, and an overall (with native liver and post liver transplant) 4-year actuarial survival rate is 89%.[13] The precise indications, timing, and optimal management of some of the intraoperative and postoperative problems, including the control of rejection, remain the subject of ongoing research.

Choledochal Cysts

Choledochal cysts are congenital dilations of the biliary ducts that may be associated with intermittent biliary obstruction (Figure 69-4). If the condition is unrecognized and uncorrected, the impaired bile outflow can lead to chronic hepatic injury, fibrosis, and, ultimately, biliary cirrhosis with ensuing portal hypertension. Choledochal cysts can present at any age, often with nonspecific abdominal symptoms and jaundice, but sometimes they are detected incidentally. Their occurrence is sporadic with an unexplained female prevalence. In the newborn period, the presentation may be indistinguishable from the syndrome of neonatal cholestasis, including BA. A cystic

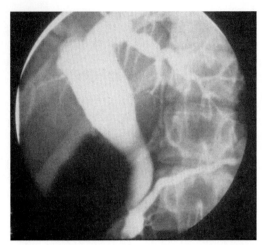

Figure 69-4. Percutaneous transhepatic cholangiography demonstrating a fusiform choledochal cyst affecting common, right, and left bile ducts.

echo-free mass demonstrated in the biliary tree by ultrasonography is strong evidence for this diagnosis. The intrahepatic bile ducts may be dilated because of the distal stasis. There are five types of choledochal cyst, affecting various segments of the biliary tree (Figure 69-5). The most difficult for surgical management is type V, the most proximal type, in which the intrahepatic ducts are primarily affected. Classically, cystic and fusiform macroscopic variants are described.

Choledochal cysts can be diagnosed prenatally on routine ultrasonography.[96] Children in whom a prenatal diagnosis of choledochal cyst is made should be referred promptly to a specialized pediatric hepatology center, as this can also be the mode of presentation of BA.[7,96] The suspected cyst can be confirmed by MRCP, but often ERCP or percutaneous transhepatic cholangiography (PTC) is needed. Percutaneous liver biopsy is contraindicated because of risks of biliary injury and peritonitis. Clinical examination of the abdomen should be restrained, as there is a risk of perforation. Radionucleotide scanning adds little to direct and indirect cholangiography.

Up to two thirds of children with choledochal cyst have a longer common pathway between the pancreatic and common bile ducts ("common channel").[97] This anatomic variant may give rise to a reflux of proteolytic pancreatic enzymes into the bile structures, possibly playing a role in the pathogenesis of choledochal cyst by facilitating the initial injury of the biliary mucosa.

Cholangitis, rupture, pancreatitis, and gallstones are important complications of choledochal cysts and may occur even in early infancy, whereas chronic cholecystitis and cholangiocarcinoma may be long-term complications if the cyst is not fully removed. The definitive treatment is, whenever possible, complete surgical removal of the choledochal cyst with biliary drainage via a Roux-en-Y loop (hepaticojejunostomy).[98] With adequate surgery, the long-term prognosis is good.[97]

Widespread use and improved quality of ultrasonography, both prenatally and postnatally, has led to increased detection of minor bile duct dilations early in infancy.[16] These dilations rarely, if ever, cause biochemical abnormalities, and further increase of the bile duct caliber on follow-up ultrasonography is exceptional. Whether they represent incidental findings or "forme fruste" of choledochal cysts remains to be established. UDCA is often used as a choleretic, with no documented evidence for its benefits.

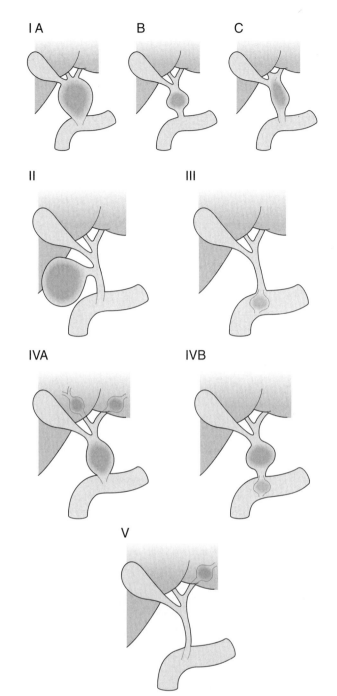

Figure 69-5. Schematic representation of different types of choledochal cyst.

Spontaneous Perforation of the Bile Duct

Spontaneous perforation of the bile duct at the junction of the cystic duct and common hepatic duct occurs when, for some unexplained reason, the common bile duct becomes blocked, usually at its distal end. Affected infants have mild jaundice, failure to gain weight, and abdominal distention due to ascites, which classically causes the development of bile-stained inguinal or umbilical hernias (Figure 69-6). The stools are white or cream in color, the urine is dark, and the biochemical markers of obstruction may be mildly abnormal. Paracentesis confirms the presence of bile-stained ascites.[99]

If operative cholangiography shows free drainage of contrast into the duodenum, the ruptured duct may be sutured, but

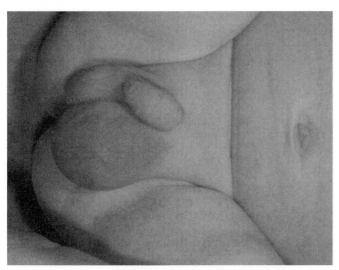

Figure 69-6. Green-yellow discoloration of scrotum and umbilicus due to intra-abdominal presence of bile following spontaneous perforation of the bile duct. (*See plate section for color.*)

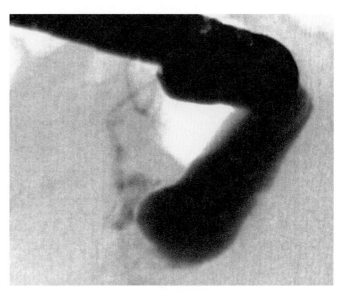

Figure 69-7. Endoscopic retrograde cholangiopancreatography demonstrating a patent biliary system in a 2-month-old infant with suspected biliary atresia.

more commonly it is necessary to establish cholecystojejunostomy drainage via a Roux-en-Y loop. With effective surgery, the prognosis is excellent.[99] Delay in instituting surgery may lead to peritonitis and septicemia and nutritional difficulties.

Neonatal Sclerosing Cholangitis

This condition is increasingly recognized as a result of the wider use of direct cholangiography (ERCP, PTC) in this age group.[20,21] The infants present with conjugated jaundice, hepatosplenomegaly, and dark urine, but, in contrast to BA, the stools are pigmented.[100] Affected children are usually not dysmorphic and have no associated extrahepatic anomalies. The histologic features are indistinguishable from those of large bile duct obstruction. Dynamic radionucleotide imaging can be helpful if it demonstrates the presence of contrast in the gut. ERCP remains a "golden" diagnostic standard, but requires a degree of technical expertise (Figure 69-7).[21]

Familial occurrence has been described.[101] The recent description of an association between neonatal sclerosing cholangitis and ichthyosis (NISCH syndrome), assigned to chromosome 3q27-q28, has pointed to lack of expression of one of the tight junction proteins – claudin-1 in the cholangiocytes.[102] Bile duct injury could be due to increased paracellular permeability and toxic effects of bile acids.

Medical treatment is restricted to the enhancement of choleresis with UDCA (20 to 30 mg/kg/day) and medical management of cholestasis with fat-soluble vitamin supplements and medium-chain triglyceride (MCT)-based milk formula. The response is variable, and some children need liver replacement because of the development of biliary cirrhosis during early childhood.

Paucity of Interlobular Bile Ducts (Alagille Syndrome, Intrahepatic Biliary Hypoplasia)

Paucity of interlobar bile ducts or Alagille syndrome (AGS) is a highly variable, autosomal dominant disorder that affects the liver, heart, kidneys, eyes, and skeleton with recognizable facial dysmorphic features, including triangular facies, prominent

quadrangular forehead, deep-set eyes with mild hypertelorism, and small pointed chin.[103-106] AGS is caused by mutations in *Jagged1* (JAG1), a ligand in the Notch signaling pathway.[107,108] This ubiquitous pathway is evolutionarily conserved and plays a role in cell fate determination. The prevalence of AGS is estimated at 1 in 70,000 live-born infants, though the recent advent of molecular testing with subsequent identification of mildly affected or asymptomatic individuals suggests that this is possibly an underestimation.[109,110]

AGS has conventionally been diagnosed in the presence of intrahepatic bile duct paucity on liver biopsy in association with at least three of the five major clinical features: cholestasis, cardiac disease (right-sided lesions; typically peripheral pulmonary stenosis), skeletal abnormalities (butterfly vertebrae and rib anomalies), ocular abnormalities (most commonly posterior embryotoxon), and characteristic facial features (Figure 69-8; Table 69-1).[104,105] Increased serum cholesterol levels support the diagnosis. AGS is frequently associated with short stature and renal and dental anomalies; pancreatic, bone, and vascular involvement have also been described.[106,111] Renal abnormalities have been reported in 19% of patients (Table 69-2).[111]

To date, more than 430 JAG1 mutations have been identified in more than 90% of clinically diagnosed probands.[112,113] In addition, mutations in NOTCH2 have also been demonstrated in a few patients with AGS who do not have JAG1 mutations.[110] With the advent of molecular screening identifying individuals carrying a mutation in JAG1, but with no or minimal clinical features, the traditional clinical criteria have been challenged.[114] It has been proposed that the name AGS remain in use for children with the liver involvement, whereas the broader term—JAG1 disease could be reserved for all carriers of the mutations, in whom clinical hepatic manifestations may not necessarily be present.[115]

An increased incidence of potentially life-threatening episodes of intracranial bleeding in AGS has been reported in some studies.[106] They are difficult to explain on the basis of typically unremarkable coagulation parameters and platelet count in AGS. One possibility is that the JAG1 mutation in the Notch signaling pathway may play a role in the integrity of vascular endothelium,

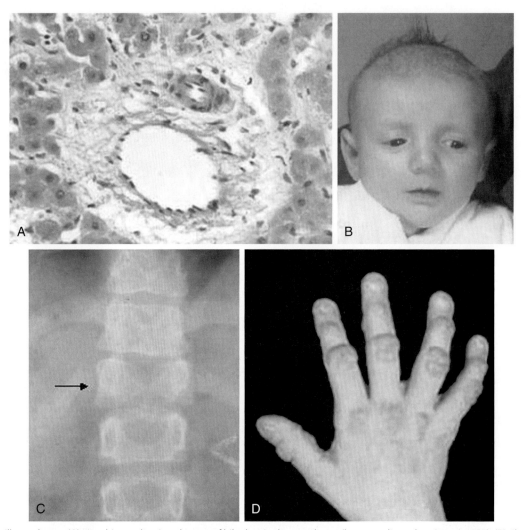

Figure 69-8. Alagille syndrome. (**A**) Liver biopsy showing absence of bile duct in the portal tract (hematoxylin and eosin stain, 320). (**B**) Classic facial appearance – triangular face, deep-set eyes, mild hypertelorism, prominent forehead, small pointed chin, low-set ears. (**C**) Typical appearance of a "butterfly" vertebra (arrow) on spinal radiography. (**D**) Disfiguring xanthomas on the hand. Reproduced from Francavilla R, Mieli-Vergani G. Liver and biliary disease in infancy. Medicine 2002; 30:45–47, with permission from The Medicine Publishing Company.

akin to association of the human NOTCH3 receptor defect and adult-onset cerebral autosomal dominant arteriopathy with subcortical infarcts and leukoencephalopathy (CADASIL).

The long-standing aberrant bile flow in AGS causes jaundice, pruritus, hypercholesterolemia, xanthomas, and failure to thrive. The severity of the cholestasis varies and mild cases may have pruritus only. The majority would have jaundice from the neonatal period, which in severe cases may persist but in others clears in late childhood or early adult life.[111]

The treatment is that of chronic cholestasis, with particular emphasis on the control of pruritus and adequacy of vitamin D, E, K, and A supplementation (Table 69-3). In spite of maximal nutritional support, which often includes overnight nasogastric feeding, the majority of children will remain thin and short for age.

The long-term prognosis is unknown, but some 15% may go on to develop cirrhosis and 5 to 10% die from liver disease.[106] In one series 25% of patients died from cardiac involvement or infection.[111] Liver transplantation has improved the overall outcome, although postoperative recovery may be additionally complicated by cardiac problems and long-term survival affected by added chronic calcineurin inhibitor-related renal impairment.[115,116] Although hypercholesterolemia could represent

TABLE 69-1.   Conditions Associated With Paucity of Bile Ducts

Alagille syndrome
Nonsyndromic paucity of bile ducts
α_1-Antitrypsin deficiency
Prematurity
Down syndrome
Chronic rejection after liver transplantation
Hepatic graft-versus-host disease
Drugs
Advanced phase of any chronic cholangiopathy
Idiopathic

a significant risk factor for cardiovascular disease, no difference was found in ultrasound-assessed intimal thickness between AGS and other forms of chronic cholestasis.[117]

Neonatal Gallstones

Cholelithiasis is an uncommon condition in children, but as a result of better ultrasonographic surveillance there is an increase in its detection.[118] In the neonatal age group, improved

TABLE 69-2. Extrahepatic Manifestations of Alagille Syndrome

Cardiac
  Peripheral pulmonary stenosis
  Tetralogy of Fallot
  Ventricular septal defect
  Atrial septal defect
  Aortic coarctation
  Pulmonary atresia
Skeletal
  Short stature
  Butterfly vertebrae
  Fused vertebrae
  Rib anomalies
  Spina bifida occulta
  Thin cortical bones
Ocular
  Posterior embryotoxon
  Axenfeld anomaly
  Optic disk drusen
  Shallow anterior chamber
  Microcornea
Vascular
  Renal artery stenosis
  Intracranial bleeding
  CNS malformations
Other
  Renal developmental abnormalities
  Renal tubulopathies
  Pancreatic exocrine and endocrine insufficiency
  High-pitched voice
  Microcolon

TABLE 69-3. Recommended Doses of Fat-Soluble Vitamin Supplements in Chronic Cholestasis

Vitamin	Dosage
D	Ergocalciferol 800 IU per day, cholecalciferol 10,000 IU/kg per month, or α-calcidol 100 ng/kg per day
K	Phytomenadione (Konakion) 1 mg daily
A	Retinol 2500 IU daily
E	α-Tocopherylacetate 100 mg/kg per day

survival of premature and small-for-gestational age children has led to an increased recognition of children with biliary sludge or "inspissated bile syndrome" following sepsis, exposure to total parenteral nutrition (TPN), dehydration, or prolonged use of diuretics. Some of these children present with clinical signs of obstructive jaundice, but the majority are asymptomatic.[119] Some may have an underlying hemolytic condition, dyslipoproteinemia, or a family history of gallstones. A female prevalence is not observed until adolescence.[118] It is important to exclude familial disorders of biliary transport, such as bile salt export pump (BSEP) deficiency and multidrug resistance (MDR) 3 deficiency, which may both present with infantile gallstones. It is noteworthy that about 50% of pediatric patients have black pigment stones.[120]

PTC with biliary drainage is an effective means of both diagnosis and treatment of infants with dilated intrahepatic ducts and common bile duct obstruction due to sludge or small stones.[119] Positive centrifugal pressure at cholangiography flushes the retained bile and improves the drainage. Formal biliary surgery can then be restricted to a limited number of patients, particularly those with underlying congenital anomalies and/or associated strictures of the bile ducts. UDCA is a valuable addition to the radiologic management.

The long-term natural history of asymptomatic gallstones and sludge in children is largely unknown.

Progressive Familial Intrahepatic Cholestasis Syndrome

Over the past decade, different types of progressive familial intrahepatic cholestasis (PFIC) syndrome, associated with a low or high GGT phenotype, have been characterized.[121] These autosomal recessive conditions can present with prolonged conjugated jaundice in infancy. GGT in the liver is normally bound to the canalicular membrane and to the biliary epithelium of cholangiocytes. Under cholestatic conditions, the detergent effect of the bile acids liberates GGT from the membrane. When this is combined with a poor bile flow, GGT leaks back into the circulation, where raised levels can be detected. In the absence of bile acids in the bile, even when there is a poor bile flow, GGT is not released and the serum levels remain normal. Therefore, in the presence of cholestasis, a normal serum level of GGT correlates well with low levels of biliary bile acids. The PFIC patients usually have low biliary but high serum levels of bile acids in the absence of a primary defect in bile acid synthesis.[121,122]

The original patients described with this phenotype were among the Old Order Amish in North America.[123] This condition has been termed Byler disease, according to the name of the original family. Byler disease, or FIC-1, represents a third of the patients with low-GGT PFIC and maps to chromosome 18.[124] The gene is termed *FIC1* and encodes FIC-1 or ABCB8 protein. These patients may present with infantile jaundice of variable severity. The *FIC1* gene is widely expressed, with only relatively low-level expression in the liver. The function of the ABCB8 protein is incompletely understood. Patients with FIC-1 disease often have extrahepatic manifestations. Expression of *FIC1* is particularly high in the small intestine and pancreas. Thus, children with FIC-1 disease may have pancreatic insufficiency, and many have a significant malabsorption, which is not improved and may be even worsened by liver transplantation and contributes to their typically short stature. A proportion will have abnormal sweat test and conductive deafness. The condition historically described as benign recurrent intrahepatic cholestasis (BRIC) and the clinically more severe Greenland Eskimo infantile cholestasis also map to the chromosome 18 locus and probably represent a different, milder phenotype of FIC-1 disease.[124,125] Histologically, these patients usually have features of a bland cholestasis with no major inflammatory features. The disease frequently progresses to end-stage liver disease in childhood. The outcome of transplantation, however, is not satisfactory owing to a number of problems not corrected by liver replacement, such as continuing malabsorption, rapid secondary fatty liver infiltration, and failure to thrive.[126] External or internal ("ileal bypass") diversion of biliary flow by preventing enterohepatic recirculation of the bile may represent one therapeutic option with unknown long-term outcome.[126,127] It is often used to control intractable pruritus.

A third of patients with low-GGT PFIC have an isolated defect in bile acid transport owing to deficiency of the BSEP. The condition maps to chromosome 2 and is due to mutations of the *ABCB11* gene.[128] These patients usually present in the first few months of life with a conjugated hyperbilirubinemia.

Initial histologic appearances are those of giant cell hepatitis. Immunohistochemical staining with anti-BSEP antibodies is negative, pointing to this diagnosis even in the absence of genuine clinical symptoms, such as pruritus, which are often not present in early infancy. The disease progresses and pruritus usually becomes a prominent problem toward the end of the first year. The rate of progression is variable and could result in end-stage liver disease between 2 and 10 years of age, or possibly even later. No treatment apart from transplantation has shown to be of benefit, and it is particularly noteworthy that these patients appear to be incapable of excreting UDCA.[129] Treatment with modest doses of UDCA, however, may have a beneficial effect by further suppressing endogenous bile acid production. As expression of the gene appears to be limited entirely to the liver, liver transplantation has proved to be curative. An important observation has been made recently when hepatocellular carcinoma[130] and cholangiocarcinoma[131] were described in a series of children with advanced liver disease secondary to BSEP deficiency. It has been suggested that the ones in possession of truncated mutations of BSEP polypeptide are at a higher risk to develop this serious complication.[130]

Appearances of bile at electromicroscopy could help differentiate between FIC-1 disease and BSEP deficiency. In BSEP deficiency the bile is amorphous, whereas in FIC-1 it has a coarse granular appearance ("Byler" bile) (Figure 69-9), which could be due to ongoing microvillus damage.[122] The genetic basis of the remaining third of the patients within the spectrum of low-GGT PFIC syndrome has not yet been clarified.

MDR3 deficiency is a form of high-GGT PFIC, resulting from mutations of the *ABCB4* gene.[132] *ABCB4* is a floppase type of lipid translocator, as it transfers phosphatidylcholine, the major lipid component of human bile, from the inner to the outer leaflet of the cholangiocyte membrane. Its absence results in bile devoid of phosphatidylcholine and phospholipids, which physiologically link simple bile salt micelles to form mixed micelles, defending the cell membrane from the highly detergent effect of the bile, which can cause considerable tissue damage.[133] Indeed, children with MDR3 deficiency histologically have marked portal inflammation and bile duct proliferation. Some patients, particularly those who have some residual protein function, show a good clinical response to UDCA, based on its effect in reducing the hydrophobicity of the bile.[134] The diagnosis is confirmed by low concentration of phospholipids in the bile, sampled at ERCP, or by mutation analysis.

In addition to cholestatic liver disease, MDR3 deficiency is now implicated in at least two other clinical syndromes: low phospholipid-associated cholelithiasis (LPAC) syndrome and intrahepatic cholestasis of pregnancy (ICP).[134] Patients with ABCB4 mutations can have cholesterol gallstones and intrahepatic microlithiasis, with limited effect of UDCA on the symptoms and dissolution of the stones. A considerable proportion of women with ICP are MDR3 deficient and will develop jaundice with severe pruritus toward the end of the pregnancy. There is increased chance for premature and stillbirths. UDCA when used in the third trimester can ameliorate the symptoms.[134] In contrast to most other forms of cholestasis, lipoprotein X is typically absent from serum of the patients with MDR3 deficiency.[133]

Preliminary data from a murine model showed that transplanted hepatocytes are capable of ameliorating the phenotype, suggesting that such transport defects in humans are potential candidates for hepatocyte transplantation or gene therapy.[135]

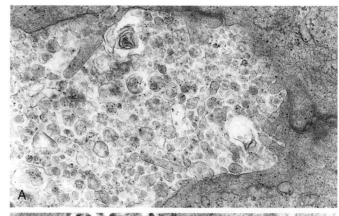
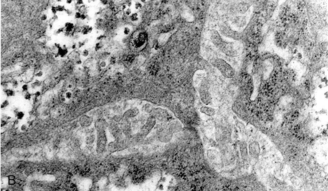

Figure 69-9. (A) Coarsely granular bile (Byler bile) seen in FIC-1 disease, with a normal canaliculus **(B)** normal, for comparison (electron microscopy, ×10,000).

Fibrocystic Liver Disease

This group of rare disorders includes three clinical entities: congenital hepatic fibrosis (CHF), Caroli disease, and Caroli syndrome.[136] Caroli disease is characterized by a cystic dilation of the intrahepatic bile ducts that can affect the entire liver or be segmental or lobar. The grossly dilated ducts could be detected with ultrasonography, computed tomography, PTC, ERCP, or, more recently, MRCP.[137] More commonly, the disease is associated with CHF and then termed Caroli syndrome.

The term *ductal plate malformation* (DPM) refers to the histologic changes seen in the liver of a heterogeneous group of genetic disorders in which segmental dilations of the intrahepatic bile ducts are associated with fibrosis (Table 69-4). They represent a merging spectrum of microscopic and/or macroscopic cystic lesions often associated with fibrocystic anomalies in the kidneys. Close histologic resemblance to an exuberant embryonal ductal plate supports the concept that an aberrant remodeling during organogenesis is the pathogenic mechanism common to these inherited disorders (Figure 69-10).[32,136]

Patients may present with an incidental finding of bile duct dilation or with symptoms of recurrent cholangitis at any time in life, but frequently in childhood, including the neonatal period.[138] Clinically, there is recurrent fever and abdominal pain with signs of systemic infection. When CHF is associated, portal hypertension is likely to be present. Complications include abscess formation, septicemia, and intrahepatic lithiasis.[139] Late development of hepatic malignancies has been reported in a few adult patients.[140,141] Autosomal recessive polycystic kidney disease (ARPKD) or some form of renal tubular ectasia is often

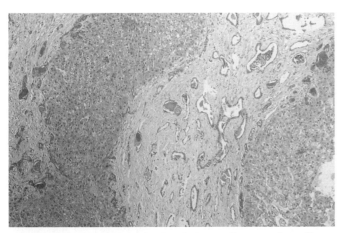

Figure 69-10. Liver biopsy in the ductal plate malformation; loose fibrous tissue containing small irregular bile ducts, some of them dilated and containing bile (hematoxylin-eosin stain, ×125). (*See plate section for color.*)

associated with Caroli syndrome. Recently, an interesting yet unexplained clinical association was described between CHF and carbohydrate glycoprotein deficiency type Ib.[142]

The gene for ARPKD has been identified and termed *PKDH1*. This gene is large, with 67 exons, and more than 120 different mutations have been described.[136] Some genotype-phenotype relationship appears to exist for severity of renal disease, with truncated mutations seen in more severe renal phenotypes with neonatal presentation. Fibrocystin is a protein present in the collecting ducts of the kidney and in the biliary epithelium. It is believed that fibrocystin expression is regulated by the *PKDH1* gene and that its absence could explain a link between renal and liver pathology.[143]

Morphologically, the liver contains rounded or lanceolated bile duct cysts, some with characteristic fibrovascular bridges across their cavity. Inspissated bile, soft and friable bilirubin calculi, or mucopus may be present in the lumen. Histologically, the cysts are lined by cubic or tall columnar epithelium, which may be ulcerated or focally hyperplastic. There is chronic and acute inflammation of the wall with fibrosis and, often, prominent mucus glands.[136] The lesion has to be distinguished from the pseudocystic lesions that develop secondary to a chronic obstructive cholangiopathy such as BA. In this situation inflammatory cholangiodestruction and the detergent power of extravasated bile operate to produce cystic cavities lined by inflamed granulation tissue and often filled with inspissated bile.

The severity of the renal lesions may overshadow the liver disease, as is observed in the early presentation of ARPKD. Conversely, portal hypertension with a typically preserved liver synthetic function may dominate the delayed clinical presentation as seen in CHF (Table 69-5).[139] The management is for complications of portal hypertension, as described elsewhere (see Chapter 76). Recurrent cholangitis may develop, especially when the cysts communicate with the biliary system. Complications of portal hypertension and cholangitis are the main presenting features in children.[139] A liver biopsy may not be always indicated in the presence of convincing clinical and ultrasonographic information because of the risk of introducing infection in an abnormal biliary system. Radiologic investigation with ultrasound and MRCP, a noninvasive technique that has reached the sensitivity levels of direct cholangiography (PTC and ERCP),[144] is essential for diagnosis.

TABLE 69-4. Syndromes Described in Association With Ductal Plate Malformation

Autosomal recessive (infantile) and autosomal dominant (adult)
  polycystic kidney disease
Nephronophthisis
Ivemark syndrome
Gruber syndrome
Jeune syndrome
Laurence-Moon-Biedl syndrome
Tuberous sclerosis
Ellis-van Creveld syndrome
Meckel syndrome
Senior-Loken syndrome

TABLE 69-5. Clinical Manifestations of Congenital Hepatic Fibrosis

Firm hepatomegaly
Abdominal distention
Splenomegaly/hypersplenism
Sudden gastrointestinal bleeding
Renal polycystic disease
Other vascular malformations

Caroli disease is managed with aggressive antibiotic therapy. Nonsurgical approaches such as percutaneous biliary drainage, extracorporeal shockwave lithotripsy, and transhepatic or endoscopic decompression have been attempted with unconvincing results. Segmental or lobar forms have been treated by partial hepatectomy.

Isolated or combined kidney and liver transplants have become available for children with polycystic liver and kidney disease.[145] Immunosuppression after isolated renal transplantation may lead to an increased number of episodes of cholangitis and worsening liver condition. Therefore, a combined liver-kidney transplant may be required in children with established end-stage renal failure and advanced chronic liver disease.

REFERENCES

13. Davenport M, De Ville de Goyet J, Stringer MD, et al. Seamless management of biliary atresia in England and Wales (1999-2002). Lancet 2004;363:1354–1357.
14. Serinet MO, Wildhaber BE, Broué P, et al. Impact of age at Kasai operation on its results in late childhood and adolescence: a rational basis for biliary atresia screening. Pediatrics 2009;123:1280–1286.
40. Sokol RJ, Mack C, Narkewicz MR, Karrer FM. Pathogenesis and outcome of biliary atresia: current concepts. J Pediatr Gastroenterol Nutr 2003;37:4–21.
97. Stringer MD, Dhawan A, Davenport M, et al. Choledochal cysts: lessons from a 20-year experience. Arch Dis Child 1995;73:528–531.
111. McDaniell R, Warthen DM, Sanchez-Lara PA, et al. NOTCH2 mutations cause Alagille syndrome, a heterogeneous disorder of the notch signaling pathway. Am J Hum Genet 2006;79:169–173.
130. Knisely AS, Strautnieks SS, Meier Y, et al. Hepatocellular carcinoma in ten children under five years of age with bile salt export pump deficiency. Hepatology 2006;44:478–486.
142. Nichues R, Hasilik M, Alton G, et al. Carbohydrate-deficient glycoprotein syndrome type 1b: phosphomannose isomerase deficiency and mannose therapy. J Clin Invest 1998;191:1414–1420.

See expertconsult.com for a complete list of references and the review questions for this chapter.

70 PEDIATRIC CHOLESTATIC LIVER DISEASE WITH GENETIC ETIOLOGY

Kathleen M. Loomes • Karan McBride Emerick

Cholestasis is defined as a pathologic state of reduced bile formation or flow. Most cholestatic conditions can be classified as either obstructive or hepatocellular in origin and result in the retention of substances normally excreted into the bile, such as bilirubin, bile acids, or cholesterol, with consequent cell injury. Obstructive cholestasis results from an anatomic or functional obstruction of the biliary system. This can be at the level of the large or extrahepatic bile ducts (i.e., biliary atresia or cholelithiasis) or smaller intrahepatic ducts (i.e., bile duct paucity associated with Alagille syndrome). Hepatocellular cholestasis results from impairment of mechanisms of bile formation and implies defective function of most or all hepatocytes. This chapter discusses the most common cholestatic diseases that have a defined genetic etiology. The function and distribution of the specific genes involved in any of these conditions will dictate whether a defect in the gene results in an isolated cholestatic liver disease (i.e., PFIC3) or a systemic disease (i.e., cystic fibrosis or Alagille syndrome). The diseases are categorized mechanistically according to where their associated genetic defect affects bile formation or flow.[1] Using the information from Chapter 3 regarding bile acid physiology as a background, the various necessary components of bile production may be divided into (1) bile acid production, (2) hepatocellular transporters that facilitate bile flow, and (3) membranes and organelles that participate in bile flow. In most clinical forms of hepatocellular cholestasis, the molecular mechanism is a result of impaired bile flow secondary to a defect in membrane transport, embryogenesis, mitochondrial function or bile acid biosynthesis (Table 70-1).

DEFECTS IN BILE ACID PRODUCTION

Bile Acid Synthetic Defects

Bile acid synthetic defect (BAD) diseases constitute the first general category of genetic cholestatic diseases in which the mechanism is impairment in bile acid production. The bile acids are produced in the hepatocyte and drive more than 60% of bile flow. They are synthesized from cholesterol by 14 enzymatic steps, all of which are coded for by a specific gene. There are seven known gene defects in this pathway, which are described in Chapter 3. These diseases cause hepatocellular cholestasis due to toxicity of retained abnormal bile acid intermediates and low production of normal bile acids with resultant insufficient bile flow for normal function. Progressive liver damage is then inevitable. Clinical presentation varies among the seven disorders; however, jaundice, cholestasis, elevated transaminases, fat-soluble vitamin deficiency associated with low GGT, and low serum bile acids are the hallmarks of the disease. Diagnosis

of BAD is made by testing the urine for normal and abnormal bile acid species by fast atom bombardment spectroscopy (FABS), which can identify the "fingerprint" of the inborn error by the pattern of bile acids present.

DEFECTS IN MEMBRANE TRANSPORTERS

The normal mechanisms of bile formation are described in Chapter 3. Specifically, bile formation is dependent on the interaction of the bile acid transporters and solute carrier systems on the basolateral membrane of the hepatocyte and the mostly ATP-dependent transporters (ABC transporters) located on the canalicular membrane (Figure 70-1). Bile flow begins at the basolateral membrane with uptake and exchange of solute from the portal blood, which does not require active transport. The basolateral transporters include the superfamily of organic ion transport proteins (OATPs), which allow organic anion uptake in exchange for bicarbonate or glutathione. The sodium-dependent taurocholate co-transporter (NTCP) transports only bile acids coupled with sodium. The MRP3(Abcc3) and MRP4(Abcc4) function as basolateral efflux pumps and are up-regulated under cholestatic conditions to export bilirubin conjugates (by the former) and bile acids and glutathione (by the latter). There are no described genetic disorders of cholestasis related to basolateral membrane transporters.

The canalicular membrane transporters reside in the canalicular membrane, which is rich in cholesterol and sphingomyelin (see Figure 70-1). This membrane is very metabolically active, containing many ATP-dependent solute transport proteins. It also houses ion and water exchangers, vesicle fusion proteins (i.e., SNAP or SNARE), skeletal proteins (i.e., villin) and tight-junction proteins. Of particular importance are FIC1(ATP8B1), which is an aminophospholipid translocase; the bile salt export pump (BSEP)(ABCB11), which mediates conjugated bile acid transport; and MDR3(ABCB4), a flippase of phosphatidylcholine. Defects in each of these transporters have been linked to inherited cholestatic diseases that were commonly identified as progressive familial intrahepatic cholestasis types I, II, and III respectively (Table 70-2).

Progressive Familial Intrahepatic Cholestasis (PFIC)

Our understanding of the family of conditions that make up PFIC and the genotypic and phenotypic differences among them is the result of functional and genetic mapping studies that have identified the genes and their functions over the past 15 years. Initially PFIC was clinically identified by the presence of hepatocellular cholestasis, low serum levels of γ-glutamyl transferase (GGT) activity and autosomal recessive inheritance. PFIC has now been redefined into five separate and distinct diseases with their own specific gene defects and distinct clinical profiles. Each of these genes codes for a canalicular transporter involved in bile export (see Table 70-2).

PFIC has evolved from its origins as a constellation of symptoms seen in the Amish who were descended from a single ancestor, Jacob Byler, when it was labeled "Byler's disease."[2] Subsequently, numerous phenotypically similar non-Amish patients were reported, and then the term *Byler syndrome* was used to describe these patients. Later, the term *PFIC* was applied to all Byler-like patients – however, the patients were sorted into two distinct subtypes: [low-GGT PFIC (PFIC-1 and PFIC-2) and high-GGT PFIC (PFIC-3)].[3] It is now the custom to refer to these diseases by their gene defect, that is, PFIC-1 as FIC1 disease; by

the PFIC nomenclature; or by the transporter defect (see Table 70-2) – ATP8B1(FIC1), ABCB11(BSEP), and ABCB4(MDR3).[4-6] Despite their genetic distinctness, there are many clinical similarities between the PFIC subtypes, especially between PFIC-1 and PFIC-2. PFIC is clinically characterized by chronic cholestasis that begins in early childhood and usually progresses to cirrhosis within the first decade of life.[7] The average age at onset is 3 months, and the disease may progress rapidly and result in cirrhosis during infancy or be slowly progressive with minimal scarring well into the teenage years. Pruritus is the dominant feature of cholestasis in the majority of patients. The pruritus is often misdiagnosed as skin disease because of the intense itching, which is unexplained; liver disease is not considered because of the disproportionately low level of jaundice in this condition. Patients begin to present with generalized mutilation of skin, usually most severe on the extensor surfaces of the arms and legs and on the flanks of the back, due to the disabling pruritus, which does not usually respond to medical therapies.[7]

Severe episodes of recurrent epistaxis, perennial asthmalike disease, and growth failure are common problems. PFIC patients are described as "stocky" because of a high prevalence of short stature (95% of patients have stature below the 5th percentile), with often normal weight for height.[7,8] Without treatment, there is often delayed onset of puberty and sexual development. Intellectually, these patients are equal to their peers if their pruritus is treated. Without treatment, their scholastic achievement can be compromised by inability to focus or concentrate and loss of sleep due to constant pruritus. Complications of cholestasis such as fat-soluble vitamin deficiencies are prevalent in untreated patients (discussed in Chapter 68). Most patients will develop hepatic fibrosis and eventually

TABLE 70-1. Inherited Cholestatic Diseases Listed According to Pathogenesis

Defect in	Cholestatic Disease
Membrane transport	Progressive familial intrahepatic cholestasis
	Benign recurrent intrahepatic cholestasis
	Cystic fibrosis
	ARC syndrome
	NISCH syndrome
Embryogenesis	Alagille syndrome
Bile acid biosynthesis	Disorders of BILE ACID Synthesis
Mitochondrial function	Mitochondrial hepatopathy
	Navajo, GRACILE
	Alpha1-antitrypsin deficiency

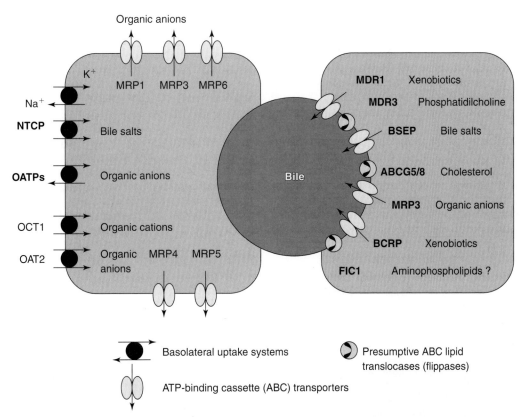

Figure 70-1. Schematic representation of the major hepatobiliary transporters. The ATP-binding cassette transporters are located primarily on the canalicular membrane, whereas the basolateral membrane contains the solute carrier systems.

cirrhosis, which is associated with the findings of hepatomegaly and sometimes splenomegaly. Unlike other cholestatic disease such as Alagille syndrome (AGS), PFIC patients do not develop xanthomas. In a recent clinical study comparing the presentation and course of PFIC-1 and PFIC-2 patients, several key differences were noted, which included that PFIC-2 (BSEP) patients exhibited more severe hepatobiliary disease compared to PFIC-1 (FIC-1) patients,[9] whereas PFIC-1 patients had greater evidence of extrahepatic disease with diarrhea, pancreatic disease, pneumonia, abnormal sweat tests, hearing impairment, and poor growth. Patients with PFIC-1 are more likely to have associated watery diarrhea, some of which is very severe. This secretory diarrhea may persist after liver transplantation.

Hallmark laboratory findings in PFIC-1 and -2 are low GGT and normal or near-normal serum cholesterol, but markedly elevated levels of serum bile acids. In contrast, the GGT in PFIC-3 is elevated. Other serum values of liver-related enzymes such as alkaline phosphatase, aminotransferases, bilirubin, and bile salts are not distinct from those seen in several other cholestatic disorders.[7]

The histopathologies of PFIC-1 and PFIC-2 are similar at the light microscopy level (Figures 70-2 and 70-3). Uniformly there is the presence of hepatocellular and canalicular cholestasis with pseudoacinar transformation consistent with cholate injury.[10] The presence of multinucleated giant cell transformation is most commonly seen in infancy and has been recently reported to be more commonly seen in PFIC-2 (BSEP-deficiency) than PFIC-1 (FIC-1 deficiency). Degeneration of bile ducts may be seen with apoptotic changes of biliary epithelium consisting of pyknotic nuclei (small and hyperchromatic) and attenuated cytoplasm and loss of duct lumina. Inflammation is absent. Bile duct paucity develops in 70% of older children as a consequence of these changes. In advanced fibrosis there may be bile ductules at the edge of the portal tract. Lacy lobular fibrosis typically develops early and progresses to portal to central bridging and eventually to cirrhosis (see Figures 70-2 and 70-3). The rate of progression of the fibrosis is highly variable, but correlates loosely to the severity of the clinical disease. The major distinguishing histological finding is seen at the level of electron microscopy with the presence of coarse granular bile in canalicular spaces of PFIC-1 patients, labeled "Byler's bile."[11,12] PFIC-2 patients have a more filamentous morphology to the bile seen in the canalicular spaces. PFIC -2 (BSEP disease) has been associated with multiple cases of gallstones and hepatocellular carcinoma.[13]

In PFIC-1 and -2 there is also an abnormal distribution both quantitatively and qualitatively of bile acids in serum and bile. Total serum bile acid concentrations are markedly elevated (usually above 200 μmol/L, normal less than 10) with a elevated ratio of chenodeoxycholic acid to cholic acid conjugates, usually greater than 10 to 1.[7] The total biliary bile acid concentrations are low (0.1 to 0.3 mmol/L, normal above 20) even in comparison to other cholestatic syndromes such as AGS, with a predominance of cholic acid conjugates.[14]

As indicated by its name, PFIC is a progressive disease that culminates in cirrhosis and end-stage liver disease in the majority of patients. Medical treatment has consisted of the usual supportive care of cholestatic disease with fat-soluble vitamin supplementation and the use of ursodeoxycholic acid (ursodiol, 20 to 30 mg/kg/day).[15] Although there is evidence that ursodiol may enhance bile flow, there is no evidence that it alters disease progression overall.

Surgical therapy consisting of the partial external biliary diversion (PEBD) has been used for the past two decades to treat PFIC and AGS.[16-18] PEBD involves the surgical placement of an enteric conduit between the gallbladder and the skin through which bile flow is partially diverted away from the enterohepatic circulation.[19] It typically results in an approximately 50% diversion of bile flow, which amounts to ~30 to 120 mL of bile per day that drains into the ostomy bag and is discarded.[19] PEBD has been effective in improving chronic cholestasis and its associated complications in both AGS and PFIC. PEBD has become a standard intervention for PFIC and can slow or halt the progression of liver disease in this condition, which usually progresses to cirrhosis and end-stage liver disease if untreated.[7,8,16,19-21] After diversion, the bile salt pool converts to predominantly cholic acid conjugates, which has been associated with histologic and clinical improvement of the liver disease.[14] PEBD may not always affect the natural progression of either AGS or PFIC, and at present no clinical parameters have been defined that predict patients who are likely to respond to biliary diversion procedure. Although PEBD has been shown in some cases to halt or reverse disease progression, it is generally ineffective in patients with established cirrhosis. Rare patients develop "watery" bile output after PEBD with severe electrolyte losses that need to be monitored and replaced. Twenty years of experience with PEBD and PFIC has demonstrated variable relief of pruritus, improvement in liver histology, improved growth, and improvement in bile acid content of bile.[14,16,20,22] A variation of PEBD is the limited ileal diversion, in which the distal 20 to 25% of the ileum is removed from the intestinal mainstream and made into a self-emptying blind loop, which results in loss of bile salts similar to PEBD. Ileal diversion is usually reserved for patients who have had a cholecystectomy, as it tends to become less effective over time.[21] In some cases, PEBD or ileal diversion does not significantly affect the progression to cirrhosis, and liver transplantation becomes necessary.[14,16,21,22]

PFIC-1: FIC1 Disease

The gene for PFIC-1 (Byler's disease), *FIC-1*, has been mapped to a 19 cM region of 18q21-q22 by the detection of a preserved haplotype in affected members of the Byler pedigree. FIC-1 codes for an ATP-binding cassette (ABC), which is an aminophospholipid translocase that flips phosphatidylserine and phosphatidylethanolamine from the outer to the inner layer of the canalicular membrane.[4]

PFIC-2: BSEP Disease

The PFIC-2 gene was located at chromosome 2q24.[4] It codes for an ABC bile salt transporter also called the BSEP.[23] The PFIC-2 gene is analogous to the rat sister gene of p-glycoprotein

TABLE 70-2. Progressive Intrahepatic Familial Cholestasis Genetics and Transporter Defects and Associated GGT Levels

	Locus	Gene	Defect	GGT
PFIC-1 BRIC-1	18q21-22	ATP8B1 FIC1	ATP-dependent amino-phospholipid transport	Normal
PFIC-2 BRIC-2	2q24	ABCB11 BSEP	ATP-dependent bile-acid transport	Normal
PFIC-3	7q21	ABCB4 MDR3	ATP-dependent translocation of phosphatidylcholine	High

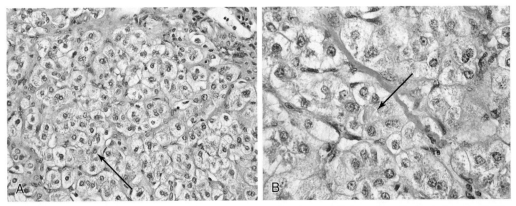

Figure 70-2. Liver histopathology in PFIC-1 (FIC1) disease with (**A**) hepatocyte-swelling hepatocellular and canalicular cholestasis, (**B**) bile canaliculi distended with thick bile. Images courtesy of Dr. Hector Melin-Aldana.

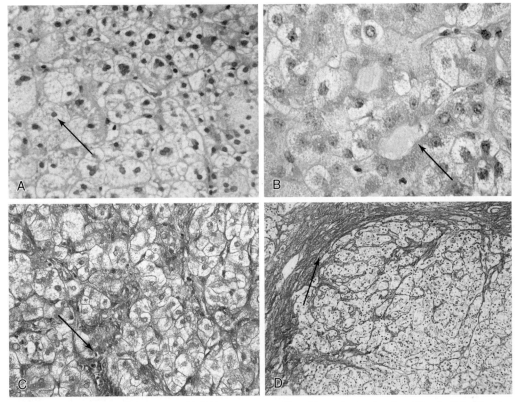

Figure 70-3. Liver histopathology in PFIC-2 (BSEP) disease with (**A**) hepatocyte swelling, (**B**) canalicular plugging, (**C**) pericellular fibrosis, and (**D**) formation of nodule in advanced disease. Images courtesy of Dr. Hector Melin-Aldana.

(S-PGP), which, in rats, has been shown to be important in bile salt transport. Studies of liver tissue from patients with mutation of BSEP have revealed lack of canalicular BSEP expression by immunohistochemistry (Figure 70-4).[24,25] This finding has clarified that PFIC-2 patients may have limited or no BSEP protein and therefore have a primary inability to transport bile salt.

PFIC-3, Multidrug Resistance Gene-3 (MDR-3) Deficient Disease

PFIC-3 is distinct from the previous two disorders primarily in that high serum GGT is present. This condition shares the pattern of the first two disorders in that it is familial, recessive, and begins as intrahepatic cholestasis in the first year and progresses toward hepatic failure in the first few years of life. A major distinction, besides the high GGT, is the histopathology,

which has more of an "obstructive" pattern.[6] Liver biopsies show expanded portal areas with proliferation of interlobular bile ducts plugged with bile. Analysis of PFIC-3 bile revealed very low concentrations of phospholipids and led to investigations of the human analogue of the Mdr-2 knockout mouse, which had a similar phenotype of no phospholipids in the bile and obstructive findings on liver biopsy. It was thereby discovered that PFIC-3 is due to mutations in an export pump of the ABC transporter family called multidrug resistance 3 (MDR-3) that is expressed on the canalicular membrane.[26,27] It functions in the translocation of phosphatidylcholine across the canalicular membrane. Mdr-2 deficient mice made transgenic by expression of the human homologue of mdr-2, MDR-3, recover function and excrete phospholipid in their bile.[27] This finding confirms the functional homology between the mouse

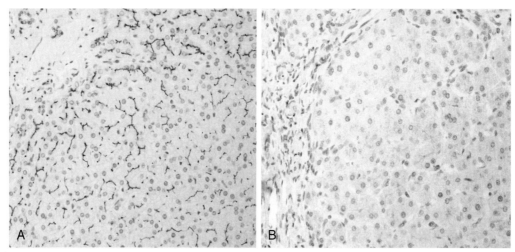

Figure 70-4. Hepatic immunohistochemical staining for BSEP expression reveals (**A**) normal expression in a control liver versus (**B**) no staining in the liver of a PFIC-2 (BSEP deficiency) patient. Images courtesy of Dr. Alex Kniseley.

and human genes and further suggests that phospholipid excretion is limited by the amount of MDR-3 or mdr-2 present. The MDR3 gene has been mapped to 7q21.[6] The absence of phospholipids in this condition is felt to destabilize the formation of micelles due to insufficient phospholipids to solubilize the cholesterol. The imbalanced micelles likely promote lithogenic bile with crystallized cholesterol, which could produce small bile duct obstruction.

There have been reports of several families with clinical and biochemical features consistent with PFIC who do not have mutations in FIC-1, BSEP, or MDR-3. Four children from an Amish kindred have recently been described with a defect in the sinusoidal uptake of bile salts. Therefore, there may be a wider spectrum of disease in PFIC yet to be described.[28]

Benign Recurrent Intrahepatic Cholestasis

The condition benign recurrent intrahepatic cholestasis (BRIC) presents very similarly to PFIC, with cholestasis, pruritus, low GGT, and high serum bile acids; however, the hallmark of this condition is intermittent episodes of cholestasis without progression to liver failure and later onset than PFIC.[29,30] Patients are totally asymptomatic both clinically and biochemically in between the episodes of cholestasis. BRIC shares the same locus with PFIC-1 (ATP8B1 mutation) and PFIC-2 [ABCB11 (BSEP)], but the mutations cause only partially impaired protein synthesis[31,32] (see Table 70-2). The cholestasis episodes have been treated by temporary biliary diversion using nasobiliary tube drainage of bile during the episode with some success in relieving the pruritus.[33] However, in select cases, surgical biliary diversion has also been used for cases of BRIC with frequent debilitating attacks, or when there appears to be progression to permanent cholestasis.[34] The clinically more severe disease identified as Greenland Eskimo infantile cholestasis is a seemingly also a variant of FIC1 disease.[35]

Hereditary Cholestasis With Lymphedema: Aagenaes Syndrome

Aagenaes syndrome is identified as a genetic form of cholestasis associated with lymphedema that is mapped to chromosome 15q.[36-38] It was initially reported in Norwegian patients;

however, subsequently there have been reports in Italian children, in Japanese children, and in siblings with French/German heritage. The inheritance appears to be autosomal recessive. Studies are underway to identify the gene locus for this disease using linkage disequilibrium.

Clinically, jaundice in the first weeks of life with acholic stools may be the first manifestation of the disease. Overall the cholestatic liver disease tends to improve with age such that bilirubin and aminotransferases may be normal by school age.[36] Cholestasis occurs episodically in older children with cholestatic periods lasting 2 to 6 months. The liver disease tends to be mild in most patients, but several older children and adults have progressed to cirrhosis.[36] Both puberty and pregnancy have been associated with transient increases in cholestasis.

The liver histopathology in early childhood shows massive giant cell transformation of hepatocytes and intracellular retention of bile pigment.[38] Patients in clinical remission may have liver morphology close to normal. Some patients may have bile plugs and a slight increase in portal fibrosis. Four of 26 patients reported by Aagenaes have developed biopsy-proven cirrhosis.[39] Treatment is that of cholestasis, with support of fat-soluble vitamins and choleretic agents. The lymphedema usually appears in the lower extremities early childhood and has been attributed to lymphatic vessel hypoplasia. The greater clinical problem tends to be the lymphedema, which can become disabling. Patients are offered physical therapy and restrictive wraps to limit the fluid accumulation and prevent skin breakdown.

Arthrogryposis Multiplex Congenita, Renal Dysfunction, and Cholestasis Syndrome

Arthrogryposis multiplex congenita, renal dysfunction, and cholestasis syndrome (ARC) is an autosomal recessive multisystemic disorder associated with germline mutations VPS33B that is mapped to 15q26.[40] In the largest study of ARC patients published, involving 66 patients, the most prevalent clinical features described were failure to thrive, the presence of neonatal cholestasis with low GGT, platelet dysfunction with high risk of hemorrhage with liver biopsy and spontaneous bleeding, renal tubular leak, and hypotonia with arthrogryposis. Less frequent clinical features include small for gestational age, dysmorphic features (lax skin, low-set ears, high arched palate, and crypt-orchidism), ichthyosis, metabolic acidosis, nephrogenic diabetes insipidus, recurrent infections, recurrent febrile illnesses, and diarrhea.[41] Survival beyond a year of age is unusual. If the patient survives infancy, cerebral manifestations including severe developmental delay, hypotonia, nerve deafness, poor feeding, microcephaly, and defects of the corpus callosum may become evident.[42]

VPS33B is a vacuolar sorting protein involved in the regulation of vesicular membrane fusion and protein sorting by interacting with SNARE protein on membranes such as the canalicular membrane. ARC patients have evidence of abnormal polarized membrane protein trafficking by immunostaining of renal and liver biopsies that show mislocalization of several apical membrane proteins in the liver and kidney (Figure 70-5).[40] In the zebrafish knockdown of the vsp33b ortholog, bile duct paucity and impaired intestinal lipid absorption were observed.[43] These findings phenocopied the digestive disease seen in ARC patients and suggest that VPS33B may play a role in primary bile duct development.[43] Inheritance is autosomal recessive.

Severe cholestasis may occur in association with arthrogryposis multiplex congenita and renal disease. The cholestatic liver disease is usually present at birth, and paucity of intrahepatic bile ducts and multinucleate transformation of hepatocytes are the predominant features.[40-42] Lipofuscin disposition has been described in several cases of ARC, and pigmentary change, bile duct paucity, and giant cell transformation may coexist in some patients. Patients with ARC rarely survive long enough to develop cirrhosis. Causes of death has been reported as infection, bleeding complications, or metabolic derangements.[42]

Neonatal Ichthyosis–Sclerosing Cholangitis Syndrome

Most human and animal cholestatic disorders are associated with changes in hepatocyte cytoskeleton and tight junctions (TJs). Neonatal ichthyosis–sclerosing cholangitis syndrome (NISCH) is identified in neonates by the presence of ichthyosis and sclerosing cholangitis. The liver histology reveals initially cholestasis that rapidly progresses to the classical fibrous obliteration of small bile ducts and "onion-skinning" periductal fibrosis (Figure 70-6).[44] NISCH is caused by a mutation in the *claudin-1* gene located on chromosome 3q27-q28.[44] Claudin-1 is a tight junction protein. In the liver, tight junctions separate bile flow from plasma and are composed of strands of claudins and occludin. This mutation results in total absence of the

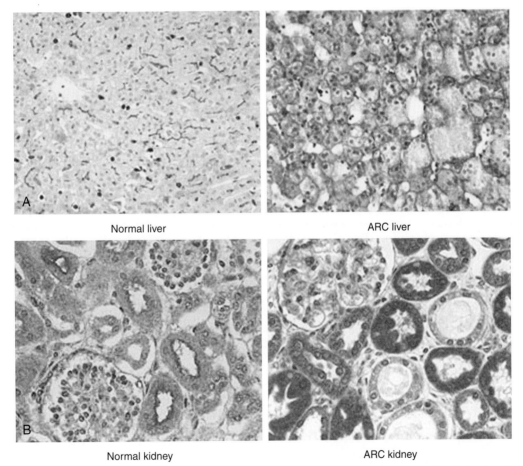

Normal liver — ARC liver

Normal kidney — ARC kidney

Figure 70-5. Immunostaining of liver and kidney biopsy samples from individuals with ARC. (**A**) Immunostaining with polyclonal antibody to CEA (original magnification, ×200). Formalin-fixed, paraffin-embedded liver from an individual with ARC from family ARC09. Distribution of CEA is markedly disturbed. In the age-matched control, marking for CEA is limited to the canalicular membrane. In the individual with ARC, CEA is seen in cytoplasm and at basolateral membranes as well. (**B**) Immunostaining with antibody to CD26 (original magnification, ×400). Formalin-fixed, paraffin-embedded kidney from an individual with ARC from family ARC01 and an age-matched control. Loss of brush-border accentuation is apparent in the individual with ARC. Reprinted with permission from Gissen P, Johnson CA, Morgan NV, et al. Mutations in VPS33B, encoding a regulator of SNARE-dependent membrane fusion, cause arthrogryposis-renal dysfunction-cholestasis (ARC) syndrome. Nature Genetics 36, 400-404 (2004).[40]

claudin-1 protein in the liver and skin of affected patients. The lack of the claudin-1 protein may lead to increased paracellular permeability between epithelial cells.

North American Indian Cirrhosis

North American Indian childhood cirrhosis (NAIC) is a nonsyndromic form of autosomal recessive cholestatic disease in Ojibway-Cree children from northwestern Quebec. It classically involves a child who had apparent transient neonatal jaundice who then progresses to biliary cirrhosis. The histopathological findings show bile duct damage and severe fibrosis. The condition has been mapped to chromosome a mutation in the *cirhin* gene, which is on chromosome 16q22.[45,46] Cirhin is found in embryonic liver, is predicted to localize to mitochondria, and has a structural motif.[46]

Cystic Fibrosis

Cystic fibrosis (CF) is fully described in Chapter 81. CF, however, deserves to be mentioned briefly here as an inherited disease of cholestasis that is known to be caused by a disorder of membrane transport. CF is due to a mutation in the gene *CFTR*, which codes for a chloride exchange channel that is expressed in tubular epithelium, particularly in the lung and biliary tract.[47-50] The mutated gene results in impaired chloride exchange, resulting in thickened secretions in the airways as well as the biliary system. The thickened secretions result in "inspissated bile," which lead to plugging of the small bile ducts and eventually biliary cirrhosis.[51-55]

DISORDERS OF EMBRYOGENESIS: ALAGILLE SYNDROME

Alagille syndrome (AGS; OMIM #118450), or arteriohepatic dysplasia, is an autosomal dominant disorder characterized by paucity of intrahepatic bile ducts, cholestasis, congenital heart defects, distinct facial appearance, and skeletal and eye anomalies. In addition, vascular system involvement and abnormalities of the kidney and pancreas are present in a significant number of AGS patients. Overall, the incidence of AGS is at least 1:70,000 live births, but the disease is likely underdiagnosed because of

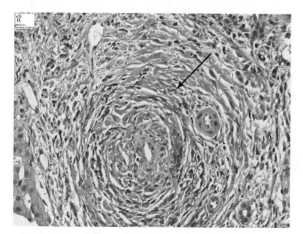

Figure 70-6. Histopathology of NISCH syndrome with "onion-skinning" of the periductal region similar to that seen in primary sclerosing cholangitis. Reprinted with permission from Hadj-Rabia S, Baala L, Vabres P, et al. Claudin-1 gene mutations in neonatal sclerosing cholangitis associated with ichthyosis: a tight junction disease. Gastroenterology 2004;127:1386–1390.

the variability in clinical presentation, even within the same family. Chronic cholestatic liver disease in AGS is a significant cause of morbidity, leading to significant pruritus, malabsorption, and xanthomas. In some patients, cholestasis improves over time, whereas in others it may progress to portal hypertension or liver failure. It is estimated that 20 to 40% of AGS patients will eventually require liver transplantation.[56-58] In 1997, mutations in the *JAG1* gene, which encodes a ligand in the Notch signaling pathway, were shown to cause AGS.[59,60] The discovery that *JAG1* is a disease gene for Alagille syndrome, a disorder with paucity of intrahepatic bile ducts as one of its major features, identified *JAG1* and the Notch signaling pathway as crucial for the development of liver, bile ducts, and other organs affected in this multisystem disorder. The advent of molecular testing for Alagille syndrome has led to improved insight into the spectrum of *JAG1*-mutation associated disease and has also advanced understanding of the role of the Notch pathway in organogenesis.

In their early report of arteriohepatic dysplasia, Watson and Miller suspected that the disorder was inherited in an autosomal dominant fashion.[61] It was later discovered that about 5% of patients carried cytogenetically visible deletions on chromosome 20, and studies of multiple patients and families with deletions and balanced translocations allowed narrowing of the critical region to a small area on chromosome 20p12.[62,63] In 1997, mutations in the *JAG1* gene, which encodes a ligand in the Notch signaling pathway, were shown to cause AGS.[59,60] With current techniques, *JAG1* mutations, 60% of which are *de novo*, can now be identified in as many as 94% of patients who meet clinical criteria for Alagille syndrome.[64] The majority of the mutations (72%) are protein-truncating, whereas about 15% occur in splice sites and 13% are missense mutations.[65] Despite the differences in *JAG1* mutation types, no genotype-phenotype correlation has been identified in AGS. In fact, related patients who carry the same mutation may have widely variable clinical phenotypes, suggesting that genetic modifiers may play a role. *NOTCH2* mutations have been identified in a small group of *JAG1*-negative individuals,[66] and a small percentage of AGS patients remain without a molecular diagnosis.

The Notch pathway is an evolutionarily conserved intercellular signaling mechanism involved in cell fate determination in multiple organ systems. The pathway was first described in *Drosophila*, where the Notch transmembrane receptor interacts with its ligands, Delta and Serrate, to govern cell differentiation.[67] To date, four Notch receptor genes have been identified in vertebrates (*Notch1*, *Notch2*, *Notch3*, and *Notch4*), which signal to five ligands (*Jag1*, *Jag2*, *Dll1*, *Dll3*, *Dll4*). It is generally accepted that the Notch receptors are activated by ligand binding to the extracellular domain. The intracellular domain is then proteolytically cleaved and translocated to the nucleus, where it interacts with nuclear proteins to activate a cascade of downstream transcription factors.[67]

JAG1 and the Notch receptor genes are widely expressed during development, especially in organs affected in Alagille syndrome, such as liver, heart, vasculature, and kidney. Multiple reports have demonstrated *JAG1* expression in vascular structures in the developing liver.[68-70] *JAG1* and *NOTCH2* are both expressed in the ductal plate during bile duct specification in embryonic liver.[69,71,72] *JAG1* is also expressed extensively in the developing heart, especially in the pulmonary artery, aorta, and developing valves, correlating with cardiovascular phenotypes in AGS.[73] Multiple mouse models have shed light on the critical roles of *JAG1* and *NOTCH2* in the development of the

TABLE 70-3.   Clinical Manifestations of Alagille Syndrome in Published Series

Feature, % (n)	Alagille,1987 (Ref. 74)	Deprettere,1987 (Ref. 139)	Hoffenberg et al.,1995 (Ref. 56)	Emerick et al.,1999 (Ref. 58)	Quiros-Tejeira et al.,1999 (Ref. 57)	Weighted %
Total patients	80	27	26	92	43	
Bile duct paucity	100 (80)	81 (22)	80 (20/25)	85 (69/81)	83 (34/41)	89
Cholestasis	91 (73)	93 (25)	100 (26)	96 (88)	100 (43)	95
Cardiac murmur	85 (68)	96 (26)	96 (24/25)	97 (90)	98 (42)	94
Vertebral anomalies	87 (70)	33 (6/18)	48 (11/23)	51 (37/71)	38 (12/32)	61
Facies	95 (76)	70 (19)	92 (23/25)	96 (86)	98 (42)	92
Ocular findings	88 (55/62)	56 (9/16)	85 (17/20)	78 (65/83)	73 (16/22)	80
Renal	73 (17/23)		19 (5)	40 (28/69)	50 (15/30)	44
Other						
Intracranial event or vascular anomaly			15 (4)	14 (13)	12 (5)	
Pancreatic insufficiency				41 (7/17)		
Growth retardation	50 (40)	90 (24)		87 (27/31)	86 (37)	71
Developmental delay		52 (14)		2 (2)		
Mental retardation	16 (13)			16 (15)		

organs affected in Alagille syndrome. Organ-specific expression patterns and Notch pathway functions are discussed in the sections on clinical manifestations.

In 1975, Alagille and colleagues published a case series of 15 patients with bile duct hypoplasia and characteristic features including distinctive facies, vertebral anomalies, cardiac murmur, and growth failure.[74] To this day, the clinical diagnosis of Alagille syndrome follows the same guidelines of bile duct paucity plus three of five clinical criteria including cholestasis, cardiac murmur or heart disease, skeletal anomalies, ocular findings, and characteristic facial features. With the advent of molecular diagnosis, it has become clear that not every individual carrying a damaging mutation in *JAG1* would be diagnosed with Alagille syndrome on a clinical basis. Kamath and colleagues studied 53 mutation-positive relatives of 34 AGS probands and found that only 21% had clinical features that would have led to a diagnosis of AGS.[75] Thirty-two percent had mild clinical features, and 45% did not meet clinical criteria. In stark contrast to the high penetrance of clinical features identified in studies of probands (Table 70-3), this study demonstrates the clinical variability in individuals carrying *JAG1* mutations. This information has led some investigators to suggest revising diagnostic criteria, taking into account family history and molecular testing.

Clinical Manifestations of Alagille Syndrome

Hepatic Manifestations of AGS

Neonatal Cholestasis. The most common clinical presentation of Alagille syndrome is neonatal cholestasis, which can be difficult to distinguish from other causes of obstructive cholestasis, especially biliary atresia. Typically the initial biochemical abnormalities consist of a conjugated hyperbilirubinemia, modestly elevated liver enzymes, and high alkaline phosphatase and GGT. Hepatomegaly is almost universally present. In the cholestasis evaluation, nuclear medicine scintiscan does not help to differentiate AGS from biliary atresia. In one report, 61% of AGS infants had no tracer excretion at 24 hours.[76] Liver biopsy may also be nondiagnostic in the neonatal period, because of evolution of bile duct paucity over time (Figure 70-7). In one large clinical study, paucity was present in 95% of biopsies after

6 months of age, but in only 60% of biopsies obtained earlier than 6 months.[76] If the liver biopsy shows features of bile duct proliferation suggestive of biliary atresia, intraoperative cholangiogram is required. Abnormalities of the intrahepatic and extrahepatic biliary tree are common at the time of cholangiogram, with the most frequent abnormalities being nonvisualization of the intrahepatic biliary tree or hypoplasia of the extrahepatic system.[76] In most published series, a small number of AGS infants have undergone the Kasai portoenterostomy, for a presumed diagnosis of BA at the time of cholangiogram. The Kasai operation is not indicated in Alagille syndrome, and most published reports suggest that these infants may have a worse hepatic outcome and be more likely to require liver transplantation.[56,57,76]

Chronic Cholestasis and Natural History. Chronic cholestasis is a nearly universal feature of AGS, which may be mild or severe. As in infancy, biochemical abnormalities typically include elevations in bilirubin and serum bile acid levels and a high GGT out of proportion to alanine aminotransferase (ALT) and aspartate aminotransferase (AST). Total protein and albumin are usually normal, as are indicators of synthetic function such as the ratio of prothrombin time (PT) to the international normalized ratio (INR) and partial thromboplastin time (PTT), in the presence of adequate vitamin K. As cholestasis progresses, the cholesterol level may rise to the thousands, with the appearance of skin xanthomas at levels over about 500 mg/dL. Xanthomas typically appear on the extensor surfaces of the fingers, the palmar creases, popliteal fossa, and inguinal creases. Depending on their location, xanthomas can be quite debilitating and can impair movement and function. Pruritus is usually not apparent in early infancy, but it will progress over the first few years of life in cases of significant cholestasis. The pruritus in AGS can be extremely severe, interrupting sleep and daily activities, and may require multiple medical interventions. In cases refractory to medical therapy, severe cholestasis, pruritus, and xanthomas may respond to biliary diversion.[18] A minority of AGS patients develop progressive liver disease leading to cirrhosis and portal hypertension. Hepatocellular carcinoma has also been reported rarely in this disorder and may occur in young children in the absence of cirrhosis.

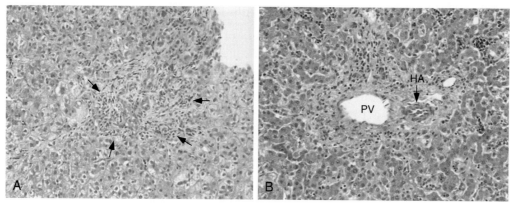

Figure 70-7. Histopathology of Alagille syndrome. (**A**) Proliferating bile ductules (arrows) in a portal tract in a liver biopsy from a 2-month old infant. (**B**) Liver biopsy done at age 6 years shows bile duct paucity, with a hepatic artery (HA) and portal vein (PV) branch within the portal tract, but absent bile duct. Photomicrographs courtesy Pierre Russo, MD.

The largest study of liver disease outcome in AGS is a report of 163 patients from France, 132 of whom presented with neonatal cholestasis and 31 of whom presented later with signs of cholestatic liver disease.[77] At the study endpoint, the patients who had presented with neonatal jaundice were much more likely to remain jaundiced, to have persistent pruritus and xanthomas, and to have ongoing hepatosplenomegaly.[77] Jaundice and cholestasis eventually resolved in the majority of patients with presentation in childhood, and in about 15% of the neonatal cholestasis group. Bile duct paucity in AGS appears to evolve during the postnatal period in many cases and is identified in only 60% of liver biopsies performed before 6 months of age.

In general, medical management of cholestasis in AGS is similar to that of other cholestatic disorders. Adequate nutrition is crucial; a high-calorie diet with a high proportion of fat from medium-chain triglycerides is recommended in the neonatal period. A detailed discussion of treatment of cholestasis is outside the scope of this chapter, but further information is provided in Chapter 68.

Liver Transplantation. Requirement for liver transplantation in AGS varies among the major clinical studies, ranging from 21%,[58] to 31%,[56] to 47% as reported by Quiros-Tejeira and colleagues.[78] In a study of liver disease outcome in 163 AGS children, the overall calculated survival with native liver was 51% at 10 years and 38% at 20 years.[77] The most common indications for liver transplantation in the AGS population were unremitting cholestasis leading to severe pruritus and xanthomata, recurrent and poorly healing bone fractures, end-stage liver disease, and portal hypertension with gastrointestinal bleeding.[56,58] Several retrospective studies have reported outcome of liver transplantation in AGS patients. One-year graft and patient survival have been reported as 87.5% and 91.7%, respectively, which is comparable to transplant outcomes for other diagnoses.[79] In a recent retrospective study utilizing the UNOS database, comparing transplant outcomes for AGS to biliary atresia, the AGS group had lower overall 1- and 5-year patient and graft survival and higher rates of graft failure than the BA group.[80] As would be expected, the Alagille syndrome patients also had higher rates of cardiac and neurologic complications leading to mortality posttransplant. In summary, liver transplantation can be accomplished successfully in AGS, with outcomes similar to other indications, but significant cardiac disease is a major cause of morbidity and mortality in this population, and a detailed cardiac evaluation is necessary even in the absence of severe structural heart disease.[81] Renal evaluation before transplantation is also advisable and may indicate that kidney-sparing immunosuppressive regimens should be used.

Cardiac murmur is a highly penetrant feature of AGS, with incidence ranging from 85 to 98% in major clinical studies (see Table 70-3). Overall, by far the most common abnormality is stenosis at some level in the pulmonary arterial tree, detected in 67% (49 of 73) of patients evaluated in a large study from the Children's Hospital of Philadelphia.[58] In this study, 22 of 92 patients (24%) had structural heart disease, with the most common structural lesion being tetralogy of Fallot (n = 10; 4 with associated pulmonary atresia). Other common heart lesions included ventricular septal defects, many of which were also associated with pulmonary atresia or pulmonic stenosis.[58] Mortality was dramatically higher in the group with structural heart disease compared to those without, with a predicted 20-year survival of only 40%.

The largest published study of cardiovascular phenotype in AGS is a retrospective analysis of 200 individuals with either a *JAG1* mutation or a clinical diagnosis of AGS. In this group, cardiovascular anomalies were identified by imaging in 75%, and 19% had a murmur consistent with peripheral pulmonic stenosis with either a normal echocardiogram or no imaging.[82] Of the patients with identified anomalies, 82% were right sided and 15% left-sided; 8% of patients had both right- and left-sided defects. The most common abnormality was stenosis or hypoplasia of the branch pulmonary arteries, with the most common structural anomaly being tetralogy of Fallot, present in 15%. Interestingly, a specific *JAG1* mutation has been associated with familial tetralogy of Fallot in the absence of hepatic or other AGS clinical manifestations.[83]

Skeletal Manifestations

Vertebral arch defects were identified in 8 of 15 patients (53%) in one of the earliest reports of the syndrome in 1975.[74] The typical finding of butterfly vertebrae seems to be one of the least penetrant features, reported in 33 to 87% of patients in the major case series (see Table 70-3). Other minor skeletal abnormalities identified in AGS patients include a decreased interpedicular distance in the lumbar spine, seen in 53% (23 of 43) of patients in a large study by Alagille and colleagues.[84] Shortened distal phalanges in the hands have also been reported.

Supernumerary digital flexion creases have been identified in 35% of AGS probands in one study, whereas they are found in only 1% of the general population.[85] Collectively, these musculoskeletal features may be useful in determining a clinical diagnosis of Alagille syndrome, but in general they are not clinically significant.

In contrast, risk of recurrent and poorly healing bone fractures in AGS patients is a significant source of morbidity in this population and may even become an indication for liver transplantation in severe cases.[56] AGS patients are recognized to have deficits in size-adjusted bone mass as measured by dual-energy x-ray absorptiometry (DXA).[86] In one report, AGS children were small for age and had decreased bone area and bone mineral content, adjusted for both age and height Z-score, when compared with controls.[86] In another recent study, the estimated incidence rate of femur fracture in AGS was 50 times that seen in the general population.[87]

Ocular Manifestations

Ocular abnormalities are extremely common in children and adults with AGS. The most well known ocular features are deep-set hyperteloric eyes and the finding of bilateral posterior embryotoxon. The latter finding was first noted in 1979 and has subsequently become a major feature of the disease.[88] Posterior embryotoxon is thought to represent a prominent thickened or hypertrophied Schwalbe's line that is anteriorly displaced, visible through a clear cornea as a sharply defined, concentric white line or opacity anterior to the limbus (Figure 70-8). Whereas it may be found in 90 to 95% of patients with AGS and is also found in parents of patients with AGS, it is present in the normal population at a frequency between 8 and 15%.[88,89] Other common ocular findings in AGS include posterior segment eye changes in 90% of patients, a variety of optic disk findings in 76%, anomalous retinal vasculature in 29%, alteration of the chorioretinal pigment in 76%, diffuse hypopigmentation of the fundus, and the presence of optic disk drusen on B scan. Despite the high prevalence of optic abnormalities in these patients, visual acuity does not appear to be adversely affected, and the changes do not appear to be progressive, although longitudinal studies will be required.

Facial Features

Characteristic facial features are a highly penetrant manifestation of Alagille syndrome, identified in 70 to 98% of patients in the major clinical studies (see Table 70-3). During childhood, the facies are typically described as triangular, with a broad forehead, deeply set eyes, a pointed chin, and a straight nose with a bulbous tip (Figure 70-9). In adulthood, the facial appearance becomes less triangular, and the chin becomes more angular and prominent (see Figure 70-9D). Characteristic facies can be difficult to identify during infancy, sometimes complicating the diagnosis in a cholestatic infant if other major features are absent.

Some authors have proposed that these facial features are not specific for the diagnosis of Alagille syndrome, but are in fact a result of chronic cholestasis, leading to the term *cholestatic facies*. In one study, North American or European hepatologists were only able to identify AGS patients with about 50% accuracy by examining facial photographs.[90] In a later study, Kamath and colleagues surveyed clinical dysmorphologists, who were able to distinguish between Alagille and non-Alagille individuals with a frequency of 79%.[91] The adult facies proved more difficult to recognize and were correctly identified only 67% of the time.

Renal Involvement in AGS

Renal anomalies occur in 40 to 50% of AGS patients, and renal involvement is now considered one of the major criteria for the diagnosis.[92] Reported structural abnormalities include solitary kidney, ectopic kidney, bifid renal pelvis, multicystic or dysplastic kidneys (unilateral or bilateral), and reduplicated ureters.[92,93] Functional abnormalities may include renal tubular acidosis, neonatal renal insufficiency, fatal juvenile nephronophthisis, lipidosis of the glomeruli, and tubulointerstitial nephropathy.[92,94] The most common glomerular

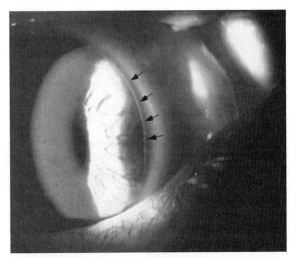

Figure 70-8. Posterior embryotoxon visible on slit lamp examination in a patient with Alagille syndrome. The finding appears as a prominent Schwalbe's line in the anterior chamber of the eye.

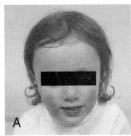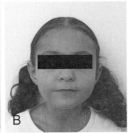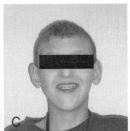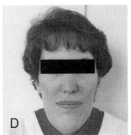

Figure 70-9. Characteristic facies in Alagille syndrome. Alagille facies in patients at age 2 years (**A**), 4 years (**B**), 14 years (**C**), and adult (**D**) show the evolution of the facial features over time. In childhood, the facial features consist of a broad forehead, widely spaced eyes, and pointed chin. In adulthood, the chin becomes more prominent and the face appears less triangular.

lesion in AGS is mesangiolipidosis, characterized by enlarged glomeruli secondary to an increase in the mesangial matrix and the presence of cells containing lipid droplets.[95] Renal insufficiency or failure may occur in childhood, adolescence, or adulthood and has been reported as the initial presentation of some unrecognized cases of AGS.[96,97] In addition to being a primary manifestation of the syndrome, renal issues may complicate the course of AGS patients who undergo orthotopic liver transplantation (OLT). In a long-term follow-up study of renal function in children undergoing OLT, the cumulative incidence of chronic renal insufficiency (CRI) varied significantly based on the classification of their pretransplant primary liver disease as being either associated with a risk of renal disease or not associated. The cumulative incidence of CRI at 10-year follow-up was 60% in patients whose liver disease was associated with a risk of renal involvement (including AGS) compared with an incidence of 17.5% in the group without.[98]

Vascular Involvement in AGS

In addition to pulmonary artery stenosis, noted as a hallmark feature of Alagille syndrome in the earliest reports, multiple case studies in the literature document other vascular anomalies in AGS, involving the aorta, renal arteries, and other vessels. One large recent study of 268 individuals with AGS found that 25 (9%) had a documented vessel abnormality (n = 16) or history of a vascular event.[99] The spectrum of cerebrovascular findings in this study included intracranial vessel aneurysms, internal carotid artery aneurysms, and moyamoya disease. In addition, other patients had evidence of systemic vascular anomalies including aortic coarctation, aortic aneurysms, and renal artery stenosis. Nine patients in this study had a significant intracranial event with no documented vessel abnormality; some of these events were accompanied by trauma or critical illness. Of the 11% mortality in this cohort of patients, 34% (10 of 29 patients) was due to noncardiac vascular events.

The cerebrovascular findings in AGS are particularly important in light of the fact that that intracranial bleeding is a major cause of morbidity and mortality in the AGS population. The incidence of intracranial events or vascular anomalies is significant, ranging from 12 to 15%[56-58] (see Table 70-3). In the large series by Emerick and colleagues, intracranial hemorrhage was documented in 13/92 patients (14%), with 31% of the incidents resulting in death.[58] Intracranial bleeding accounted for 25% of the overall mortality in this series. The majority of the events occurred with little or no antecedent trauma and in the absence of coagulopathy or thrombocytopenia. In 2005 Emerick and colleagues specifically investigated intracranial vascular abnormalities in 26 AGS patients.[100] Among asymptomatic patients, 5 of 22 (23%) had abnormalities of the cerebrovascular circulation demonstrated by MRA, and 2 others had evidence of prior ischemic events on imaging. In the 4 symptomatic patients, all had evidence of cardiovascular abnormalities (unilateral or bilateral internal carotid artery narrowing), new ischemic events, and prior infarcts. Overall, in both groups, the most common finding was unilateral or bilateral narrowing or nonvisualization of the ICA, consistent with moyamoya disease. Further studies are required to determine the optimum screening protocols for the cerebrovascular lesions in AGS. At this time, most would recommend a screening MRI/MRA as a baseline, and a low threshold for reimaging in the setting of even minor head trauma or the onset of any acute neurologic symptoms.

Growth, Nutrition, and Pancreatic Involvement

Growth failure has long been recognized as a feature of Alagille syndrome, with multifactorial etiology including genetic contribution, chronic cholestasis, fat malabsorption, congenital heart disease, and limited oral intake. In their study of 92 patients, Emerick and colleagues reported that length and weight were below the 5th percentile in the first 3 years of life in 87% of patients where growth information was available.[58] In other large clinical studies, growth retardation has been reported in a majority of the patients, ranging from 50 to 90% (see Table 70-3).

Specific studies of nutritional parameters in the AGS population have shown that height and weight z-scores are uniformly decreased in these patients.[101] Absolute values of resting energy expenditure (REE) were low in the AGS group, but when normalized for body weight, there was no change from controls, indicating that increased REE does not account for poor growth in these patients. Another study examined nutritional intake in AGS in relation to body mass. Despite the fact that physicians prescribed a high calorie diet, only 24% of the patients were consuming greater than 100% of the Recommended Dietary Allowance (RDA).[102] In that study, 96% of the patients had steatorrhea as measured by 72-hour fecal fat collection, but specific studies of pancreatic function were not done.[102]

Several reports exist of pancreatic involvement in AGS; however the pancreatic manifestations have not been studied systematically. In one study, pancreatic insufficiency was documented by either abnormal coefficient of fat absorption on fecal fat screening or abnormal pancreatic stimulation testing in 7 of 17 AGS patients (42%). There is also a report of one patient with severe failure to thrive and cystic dilatation of the pancreatic ducts.[58]

Notch Pathway and Development

There is evidence to suggest that the Notch pathway may be involved in bile duct branching and elongation during postnatal liver growth. Recent studies in tissue-specific knockout mouse models have shown a role for Notch signaling in biliary cell specification during formation of the ductal plate.[103] In addition, targeted deletion of *Jag1* or *Notch2* in the developing liver results in bile duct proliferation, abnormal bile duct remodeling, and hepatic fibrosis.[104-106]

JAG1 and the Notch pathway are crucial for normal cardiovascular development.[107,108] Consistent with the right-sided heart defects and branch PA stenosis observed in AGS, *JAG1* is expressed in the developing pulmonary arteries and cardiac outflow tracts.[73] Mice heterozygous for mutations in *Jag1* and *Notch2* demonstrate PA stenosis and VSD, as well with other features of Alagille syndrome.[72] Other heart-specific conditional Notch pathway mouse models have shown similar findings, recapitulating the clinical phenotypes seen in the human disease.

It is unclear whether genetic disruptions in Notch signaling may alter skeletal integrity and morphology. It is well established that *Jag1* is expressed in osteoblasts[109] and in the developing spine.[71] Interestingly, a polymorphism in human *JAG1* has recently been associated with an osteoporosis phenotype in a genome-wide association study.[110] Furthermore, genetic disruptions in Notch signaling in mouse models can result in altered bone development and decreased bone density.[111]

Some authors have proposed that the clinical features of Alagille syndrome are the result of a systemic vasculopathy.[99] Molecular studies and targeted mutations in mouse models have demonstrated that Notch signaling is crucial for normal angiogenesis and vascular development. Both *JAG1* and *NOTCH2* are widely expressed in vascular structures during development.[68,70,71,112] Mice homozygous for a *Jag1* null mutation die during embryonic development as a result of severely impaired vasculogenesis.[113] Interestingly, mice carrying *Jag1* mutations specifically targeted to endothelial cells demonstrate impaired vascular smooth muscle development resulting in embryonic lethality.[114] Similarly, *Notch2* mutations targeted to neural crest cells in mice result in narrowed aorta and pulmonary arteries due to decreased smooth muscle cell proliferation.[112]

DISORDER OF MITOCHONDRIAL FUNCTION

Mitochondrial disease can be due to a mutation in nuclear or mitochondrial encoded DNA. These changes can lead to respiratory chain disorders or limited disease. There is broad genetic and clinical heterogeneity among these conditions. Genetic conditions that cause cholestasis and involve known mitochondrial mutations or dysfunction are discussed here.

Navajo Neurohepatopathy

Navajo neurohepatopathy (NNH) is an autosomal recessive disease found in the Navajo tribe of the southwestern United States. The essential findings include hepatopathy, peripheral neuropathy, corneal anesthesia and scarring, cerebral leukoencephalopathy, failure to thrive, and recurrent metabolic acidosis and infections.[115,116] The disease has been separated into three forms according to age of onset: before 6 months is "infantile," between 1 and 5 years old is "childhood," and older is considered "classic." The infantile and childhood forms are associated with severe liver disease, development of cirrhosis, and death from liver failure. The classic form has a milder form of liver disease but progressive neuropathy. Using homozygosity mapping of affected families, a single missense mutation in the *MPV17* gene located on chromosome 2p24 has been demonstrated in these patients. Functional analysis of mutations performed in HeLa cells revealed that MPV17 is involved in mtDNA maintenance and the regulation of oxidative phosphorylation. When mutated, the MPV17 gene is known to cause a hepatocerebral form of mtDNA depletion.[116]

GRACILE Syndrome

GRACILE syndrome is named after the cardinal findings of the disorder, which include growth retardation, aminoaciduria, cholestasis, iron overload, lactic acidosis. and early death.[117,118] The clinical picture was described in 12 Finnish families in 2002. The infants uniformly were small for gestational age, had Fanconi's aminoaciduria, lactic acidosis, and hemosiderosis of the liver, and died by 4 months of age. Most patients develop fulminant lactic acidosis during the first day of life. The hemosiderosis of the liver is associated with increased serum ferritin, hypotransferrinemia with increased transferrin saturation, and free plasma iron. The condition is autosomal recessive and has been localized to mutations in the gene *BCS1L* located on chromosome 2q 33-37.[119] *BCS1L* encodes a mitochondrial protein that functions as a chaperone in the assembly of respiratory

chain complex III (cytochrome *bc1* complex). Several mutations in *BCS1L* have been described among patients studied from three different countries. Finnish patients had a homozygous missense mutation that caused a functionally detective BCS1L protein.[119] There was heterogeneity among Finnish, British, and Turkish GRACILE patients studied both in the mutations present and clinical manifestations. Clinically Finnish patients had marked hepatic iron overload but no decreased complex III activity, whereas the British and Turkish patients had severe neurological problems and complex III deficiency, which was more typical for mitochondrial respiratory chain defects.[119] The hepatic iron overload suggests a role for this gene in hepatic iron metabolism.

Alpha1-Antitrypsin Deficiency

Alpha1-antitrypsin (α1-AT) deficiency is the most common genetic cause of liver disease in childhood, affecting 1 in 1600 to 1 in 2000 live births.[120] It is the most frequent genetic diagnosis for which liver transplantation is carried out in children. The condition is autosomal codominant and is associated with a single amino acid substitution in the *SERPINA* gene on chromosome 14q31-32.2.[121] The gene mutation results in an abnormal tertiary structure of the α1-AT protein, which causes it to be mishandled such that instead of being secreted it is retained in the endoplasmic reticulum. There is an associated 80% reduction in serum levels of α1-AT. The mutation is associated with the development of destructive lung disease and emphysema and liver disease of varying severity depending on the degree of deficiency.[122]

The α1-AT protein is a secretory glycoprotein of the family of serine protease inhibitors called *serpins*. Its function is to inhibit destructive proteases and elastases released from neutrophils, and therefore the levels of α1-AT protein increase in response to tissue injury or inflammation. The α1-AT protein is predominantly derived from the liver but is also produced by a number of epithelial cell types including intestine and respiratory epithelia. The α1-AT protein binds directly to target proteases in an interaction that structurally rearranges it and allows it to inactivate the target protease. The gene mutations associated with α1-AT protein deficiency and clinical disease involve a single nucleotide substitution in the α1-AT gene that results in a single amino acid change of the variant protein, The changes in the Z variant allele are glutamate 342 to lysine and for the S variant are glutamate 264 to valine.[123] An 85 to 90% reduction in serum levels of α1-AT results for ZZ homozygotes and a 60 to 70% reduction for SZ compound heterozygotes. The classical form of the deficiency is constituted by homozygosity for the Z allele of α1-AT. Liver injury and carcinogenesis has also been observed in compound heterozygotes for the S and Z alleles, the so-called SZ phenotype. So, for the purposes of clinical diagnosis, the definition of α1-AT deficiency is low serum levels of α1-AT associated with a PI phenotype of ZZ or SZ, or genetic testing indicative of ZZ homozygosity of SZ compound heterozygosity.[124] The α1-AT phenotype is determined by isoelectric focusing or by agarose electrophoresis at acid pH.

Clinical disease of the lung and the liver in α1-AT deficiency has a wide spectrum based on genotype or Pi typing (specific alleles present).[123,125-129] From prospective population studies begun in Sweden in the early 1970s that have followed 180 infants with the ZZ or SZ genotype for over 30 years, only 8 to 10% of ZZ homozygotes and SZ compound heterozygotes develop clinically significant liver disease within the first 3 decades of life.[120] Autopsy studies have shown that the ZZ homozygous state is associated with a statistically significant increase in the incidence of cirrhosis and hepatocellular carcinoma. The prevalence of emphysema is not known, but homozygotes may not develop emphysema or even pulmonary function abnormalities altogether or at least until age 60 to 70 if they avoid cigarette smoking.[130]

Clinical manifestations of the disease usually begin with cholestatic jaundice in infants.[128,129] Conjugated hyperbilirubinemia with elevated transaminases and alkaline phosphatase may be associated with mild hepatomegaly. The disease in infancy is usually mild; however, about 10% of the deficient population have hepatosplenomegaly, ascites, and liver synthetic dysfunction in early infancy.[131,132] A small number have severe fulminant liver failure in infancy. The cholestatic pattern might mimic biliary atresia; however, the liver biopsy reveals paucity, not proliferation, of intrahepatic bile ducts. Frequently the liver disease associated with α1-AT deficiency may become evident in late childhood or early adolescence because of the presence of hepatosplenomegaly or evidence of portal hypertension.[128,129]

The etiology of the liver disease in α1-AT deficiency is postulated to be due to the retention of the mutant protein within the endoplasmic reticulum (ER) of liver cells, which initiates a series of events that are toxic and promote carcinogenesis.[122,133,134] The exact mechanism of liver cell injury is not known, but there is evidence for mitochondrial dysfunction, activation of mitochondrial and ER caspases, and activation of NF-κB-mediated inflammation. There is also evidence that cells damaged by accumulation of abnormal α1-AT protein may stimulate proliferation of less damaged cells and thereby fuel regeneration in the presence of tissue injury that results in adenomas and ultimately carcinomas.[135]

The liver histology of α1-AT deficiency reveals the misfolded protein as periodic acid-Schiff-positive (PAS-positive), diastase-resistant globules in the ER of hepatocytes (Figure 70-10). The inclusions are eosinophilic, round to oval, and 1 to 40 μm in diameter but are not pathognomonic of the disease.[128] They are most prominent in periportal hepatocytes. There is also characteristically hepatocellular necrosis, inflammatory cell

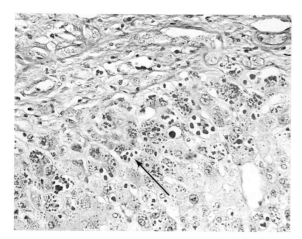

Figure 70-10. Histopathology of alpha1-antitrypsin deficiency with periodic acid-Schiff-positive, diastase-resistant globules in the endoplasmic reticulum of the hepatocytes.

infiltration, and periportal fibrosis, or cirrhosis. Bile ducts may be damaged, and paucity may also develop.

Lung injury in α1-AT deficiency appears to occur as a result of unrestricted proteolytic attack on the connective tissue of the lung.[125,136] Lung disease in the form of emphysema rarely presents before the third decade. Cigarette smoking markedly accelerates lung injury as a result of oxidative inactivation of residual α1-AT by phagocyte-derived active oxygen intermediates and possibly an overactivity of elastase that leads to the breakdown of the connective tissue matrix.[137]

The alpha1-antitrypsin phenotype should be determined in cases of neonatal hepatitis or unexplained chronic liver disease in older children, adolescents, and adults. Serum concentrations of AT can be used to screen for AT deficiency. Serum concentrations of AT may also be helpful together with the phenotype to distinguish individuals who are homozygous for the Z allele from SZ compound heterozygotes. In some cases phenotype determinations on the parents may be helpful in sorting out any confusion that arises from the combination of the AT level and phenotype.

The most important principle in the treatment of AT deficiency is avoidance of cigarette smoking. Smoking markedly accelerates the destructive lung disease that is associated with AT deficiency.[137] Clinical care of the liver disease is supportive as with all chronic liver diseases. Liver failure and cirrhosis is treated by orthotopic liver transplantation with survival rates and outcomes that are parallel to other conditions requiring transplantation. There are, however, reports of children with classical AT deficiency surviving with relatively normal overall life functioning for more than 10 to 15 years despite fairly significant liver dysfunction. Hence, timing of liver transplantation depends more on the overall life functioning of the affected child.

GENETIC CHOLESTASIS

The diagnosis of a genetic cholestatic disease relies on close scrutiny of the historical and clinical clues of the distinct causes. Vital information includes a very detailed family history that includes questions regarding cholelithiasis, fetal loss, early demise, episodes of jaundice, and history of liver diseases or liver tumors. Consanguinity is an important clue in all of the autosomal recessive conditions. The physical exam should focus not only on the liver findings but also on extrahepatic symptoms, such as the presence of dysmorphic features, failure to thrive, diarrhea, acidosis, neurologic or pulmonary symptoms, or presence of skin findings. Some of the most helpful laboratory values include assessment of high versus low GGT levels and the levels of serum bile acids. Clearly the light microscopy liver biopsy findings are critical and sometimes distinctive and diagnostic (Figure 70-11). However, additional clues may now be found histologically by looking for distinct electron micrograph changes or immunohistochemical stains (i.e., BSEP staining). Finally, there is genetic testing (commercial or research), which is now available for most of these conditions. Sequencing gene chips to perform high nucleotide sequence readout for the five most common genes associated with inherited syndromes of intrahepatic cholestasis (ATP8B1, ABCB11, ABCB4, JAG1, and SERPINA1) have been developed and require only 1 mL of blood.[138]

The study of genetic cholestatic diseases in children has recently benefited from the formation of national study consortia

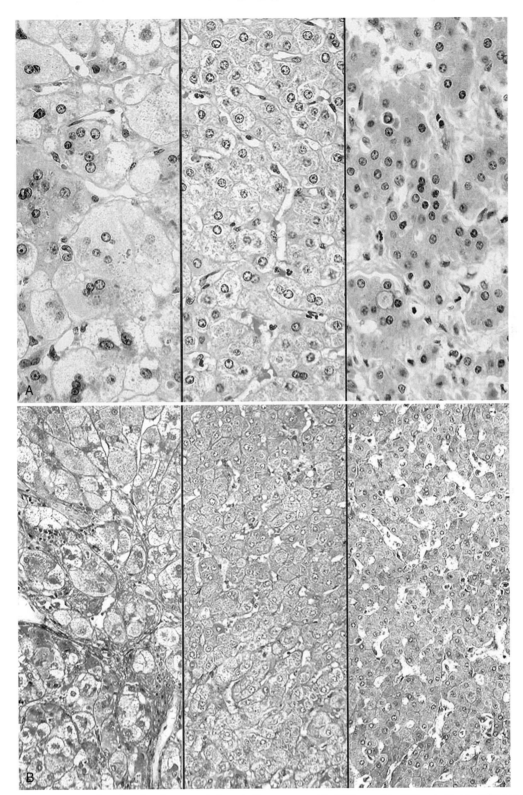

Figure 70-11. Comparative changes of liver histology between cholestatic diseases – panel 1 = PFIC, panel 2 = AGS, and panel 3 = biliary atresia. Part (**A**) shows the comparative differences in hepatocellular and cholestatic changes, and part (**B**) reveals marked differences in the pattern of fibrosis by trichrome staining. Images courtesy Dr. Hector Melin-Aldana.

funded by the NIDDK/NIH: the Biliary Atresia Research Consortia (BARC) and the Childhood Liver Disease Research and Education Network (ChiLDREN) (http://rarediseasesnetwork.epi.usf.edu/clic/index.htm). The diseases being studied by these groups include biliary atresia, α1-AT, Alagille, PFIC, bile acid synthesis defects, mitochondrial hepatopathies, and cystic fibrosis. These collaborations have already led to rapidly growing data and sample collections from patients with these rare disorders and have facilitated progress toward a more complete understanding of these disorders.

REFERENCES

3. Carlton VE, Pawlikowska L, Bull LN. Molecular basis of intrahepatic cholestasis. Ann Med 2004;36:606–617.
7. Whitington PF, Freese DK, Alonso EM, et al. Clinical and biochemical findings in progressive familial intrahepatic cholestasis. J Pediatr Gastroenterol Nutr 1994;18:134–141.
11. Thompson R, Strautnieks SBSEP. function and role in progressive familial intrahepatic cholestasis. Semin Liver Dis 2001;21:545–550.
12. van Mil SW, Klomp LW, Bull LN, Houwen RH. FIC1 disease: a spectrum of intrahepatic cholestatic disorders. Semin Liver Dis 2001;21:535–544.
38. Aagenaes O. Hereditary cholestasis with lymphoedema (Aagenaes syndrome, cholestasis-lymphoedema syndrome). New cases and follow-up from infancy to adult age. Scand J Gastroenterol 1998;33:335–345.
41. Gissen P, Tee L, Johnson CA, et al. Clinical and molecular genetic features of ARC syndrome. Hum Genet 2006;120:396–409.
44. Hadj-Rabia S, Baala L, Vabres P, et al. Claudin-1 gene mutations in neonatal sclerosing cholangitis associated with ichthyosis: a tight junction disease. Gastroenterology 2004;127:1386–1390.
49. Colombo C, Battezzati PM, Crosignani A, et al. Liver disease in cystic fibrosis: a prospective study on incidence, risk factors, and outcome. Hepatology 2002;36:1374–1382.
50. Farrell PM, Rosenstein BJ, White TB, et al. Guidelines for diagnosis of cystic fibrosis in newborns through older adults: Cystic Fibrosis Foundation consensus report. J Pediatr 2008;153:S4–S14.
58. Emerick KM, Rand EB, Goldmuntz E, et al. Features of Alagille syndrome in 92 patients: frequency and relation to prognosis. Hepatology 1999;29:822–829.
99. Kamath BM, Spinner NB, Emerick KM, et al. Vascular anomalies in Alagille syndrome: a significant cause of morbidity and mortality. Circulation 2004;109:1354–1358.
117. Fellman V. The GRACILE syndrome, a neonatal lethal metabolic disorder with iron overload. Blood Cells Mol Dis 2002;29:444–450.
127. Schmitt Jr MG, Phillips RB, Matzen RN, Rodey G. Alpha 1 antitrypsin deficiency: a study of the relationship between the Pi system and genetic markers. Am J Hum Genet 1975;27:315–321.
129. Perlmutter DH, Brodsky JL, Balistreri WF, Trapnell BC. Molecular pathogenesis of alpha-1-antitrypsin deficiency-associated liver disease: a meeting review. Hepatology 2007;45:1313–1323.

See expertconsult.com for a complete list of references and the review questions for this chapter.

MITOCHONDRIAL HEPATOPATHIES: DISORDERS OF FATTY ACID OXIDATION AND THE RESPIRATORY CHAIN

William R. Treem

Inherited mitochondrial disorders of fatty acid oxidation (FAO) and the mitochondrial respiratory chain (mtRC) both result in severe deficits in energy production. These disorders affect mitochondrial oxidative phosphorylation (OXPHOS) with subsequent decreased generation of ATP and failure of the maintenance of the intramitochondrial redox ratio (NAD^+:NADH). The consequence is profound dysfunction in organs with the highest demand for energy; muscle, brain, liver, heart, and kidney. In the liver, disruption of hepatocyte metabolic homeostasis, generation of injurious oxygen free radicals, and accumulation and export of potentially toxic metabolites to other organs are the result. Whereas clinical manifestations of respiratory chain (RC) disorders tend to be progressive, those of FAO are more likely episodic, evident during periods of fasting and catabolic stress. This chapter reviews the clinical features of those FAO and RC disorders primarily expressed as hepatopathies. Patients affected may present with hepatic steatosis and steatohepatitis, acute liver failure, and even cirrhosis with chronic liver failure. Multiorgan manifestations primarily affecting the brain, muscles, heart, kidneys, pancreas, and small intestine are often present but are not discussed here. The reader is directed to other reviews for more detail about extrahepatic manifestations.[1,2]

FAO DISORDERS

Mitochondrial FAO disorders comprise more than 20 distinct defects in the transport and metabolism of fatty acids (FA) in the mitochondria (Table 71-1). During prolonged fasting or catabolic stress, the inability to fully metabolize long-chain fatty acids (LCFA) leads to continued reliance on glucose metabolism with resulting hypoglycemia; decreased flow of electrons to the RC; a deficiency in intracellular energy that compromises other metabolic pathways; and the accumulation of toxic metabolites that further inhibit critical intracellular functions. These effects are evident not only in the tissues expressing the defective enzyme or transporter, but also in distant tissues such as the brain, as a result of the cumulative actions of both circulating toxic metabolites and energy deficiency.

The pediatric gastroenterologist will see these patients because of several clinical features including hypoketotic hypoglycemia and liver dysfunction; marked hepatomegaly with microvesicular and macrovesicular steatosis; hepatic failure with jaundice, coagulopathy, and marked elevations of aminotransferases; acute fatty liver of pregnancy in the mother of an affected infant; and, less commonly, pancreatitis, gastroesophageal reflux with poor feeding and failure to thrive, and "cyclic"

vomiting. These presentations may dominate the picture or be overshadowed by cardiomyopathy, hypotonia, and rhabdomyolysis, or even sudden cardiorespiratory arrest.

A high index of suspicion is required to diagnose FAO disorders in infants and young children who appear in the emergency room with a sudden decompensation labeled "possible sepsis" during a presumed viral illness. Critical clues in this window of diagnostic opportunity can easily be missed if urine and blood samples are not collected at the time of presentation, before cellular metabolism is modified by the introduction of large quantities of intravenous dextrose. In these cases, what is often absent (ketones) is just as important as what is present. Other pitfalls that prevent a timely diagnosis include ignoring a constellation of stereotypic but less dramatic findings such as mild acidosis and increases in the levels of creatine phosphokinase (CPK) and aminotransferases that may persist between metabolic crises.

PHYSIOLOGY OF NORMAL FAO

Adipose tissue triglycerides (TG) are the primary source of LCFA substrate for FAO during fasting conditions. The intramitochondrial β-oxidation of LCFA provides a significant proportion of the energy needed in heart and muscle much of the time, but during prolonged fasting (when glycogen stores have been depleted), FAO becomes the critical metabolic pathway to sustain energy production.[3] This pathway is activated by pancreatic secretion of glucagon in excess of insulin, which also provokes glycogenolysis, gluconeogenesis, adipose tissue lipolysis, and the release of amino acids and lactate from skeletal muscle. In extrahepatic mitochondria, complete oxidation of LCFA results in CO_2 production and is coupled to adenosine triphosphate (ATP) synthesis by supplying acetyl-coenzyme A (CoA) for the tricarboxylic acid (TCA) cycle and electrons for the mitochondrial respiratory chain. In the liver, LCFA are oxidized to acetyl-CoA, a substrate for the production of ketone bodies that are exported to extrahepatic tissues such as cardiac and skeletal muscle and even utilized by the brain when the supply of glucose is limited.[4] These adaptive mechanisms are designed to maintain blood glucose concentrations by allowing the consumption of alternative fuels by the bulk of body tissues, thereby preserving glucose for brain metabolism. Under conditions of adequate availability of glucose (the fed state), FA are repackaged into TG and stored in the hepatocyte or exported as lipoproteins.

In an adult man, FA provide 80% of caloric requirements after a 24-hour period of fasting.[5] During prolonged aerobic

TABLE 71-1. Inherited Disorders of Intramitochondrial Fatty Acid Oxidation

Disorder (Common Name)	Abbreviation	First Report (Year)
Plasma Membrane		
Long-chain fatty acid transporter defect		1998
Carnitine transporter defect	CT	1988
Carnitine Cycle		
Carnitine palmitoyl transferase I deficiency (liver-type CPT deficiency)	CPT I	1988
Carnitine-acylcarnitine translocase deficiency	CACT	1992
Carnitine palmitoyl transferase II deficiency (neonatal onset)	CPT II	1988
Carnitine palmitoyl transferase II deficiency (late-onset muscle disease)	CPT II	1973
β-Oxidation Cycle, Inner Mitochondrial Membrane		
Very-long-chain acyl-CoA dehydrogenase deficiency	VLCAD	1993
Acyl CoA dehydrogenase 9 deficiency	ACAD9	2007
Trifunctional protein deficiency (α-subunit)	TFP-α	1992
Trifunctional protein deficiency (β-subunit)	TFP-β	1996
Long-chain 3-hydroxylacyl-CoA dehydrogenase deficiency	LCHAD	1990
Electron transport flavoprotein dehydrogenase deficiency (glutaric aciduria IIC)	ETFDH	1985
Mitochondrial Matrix Enzymes		
Medium-chain acyl-CoA dehydrogenase deficiency	MCAD	1982
Short-chain acyl-CoA dehydrogenase deficiency	SCAD	1987
Electron transport flavoprotein, α-subunit (glutaric aciduria IIA)	ETF-α	1985
Electron transport flavoprotein, β-subunit (glutaric aciduria IIB)	ETF-β	1990
Riboflavin-responsive glutaric aciduria II		1982
Short-chain 3-hydroxyacyl-CoA dehydrogenase deficiency (muscle)	SCHAD	1991
Medium/short-chain 3-hydroxyacyl-CoA dehydrogenase deficiency (liver)	MCHAD/SCHAD (HAD)	1996
Medium-chain 3-ketoacyl-CoA thiolase deficiency	MCKAT	1997
Unsaturated Fatty Acids		
2,4-Dienoyl-CoA reductase deficiency		1990
Ketone Body Synthesis		
3-Hydroxy-3-methylglutaryl-CoA synthase deficiency	HMG-CoA synthase	1997
3-Hydroxy-3-methylglutaryl-CoA lyase deficiency	HMG-CoA lyase	1976

Adapted from Treem (2001).[1]

exercise, FAO accounts for 60% of muscle oxygen consumption. Cardiac muscle relies predominantly on FA metabolism under almost all conditions. Reliance on FAO is even greater in infants, who generate ketones earlier than adults during a fasting period.[6]

Reasons for this phenomenon include:
- The infant's large ratio of surface area:body mass increases the basal energy needed to maintain body temperature.
- The developing brain is highly dependent on glucose, and infants have a larger brain:body size ratio.
- The infant has decreased glycogen stores and muscle mass for glucose production.
- Enzymes involved in the gluconeogenic, glycogenolytic, and carnitine synthesis pathways are less active in infants. This increased reliance on effective ketogenesis for metabolic homeostasis during fasting renders infants particularly susceptible to disorders of FAO.

Studies in homozygous knockout mice lacking key enzymes in the β-oxidation pathway demonstrate the importance of FAO immediately after birth. Within 36 hours of switching from placental glucose-based nutrition to maternal breast milk with a high fat content, these mice suffer hypoglycemia and sudden death accompanied by hepatic steatosis, and acute necrosis of cardiac and diaphragmatic myocytes.[7]

Figure 71-1 summarizes the uptake and transport of LCFA into the hepatocyte, and subsequently across the mitochondrial membrane to enter the β-oxidation cycle, generating acetyl-CoA, which is converted to ketone bodies. Aside from providing substrate for ketogenesis, the maintenance of adequate levels of intramitochondrial acetyl-CoA is critical to activating the gluconeogenic pathway via the enzyme *pyruvate carboxylase*.[8] Low intramitochondrial acetyl-CoA levels contribute to hyperammonemia through an inhibition of the production of *N*-acetylglutamate, which is an allosteric activator of *carbamoyl phosphate synthetase*, the first enzyme in the urea cycle. Decreased availability of acetyl-CoA as a substrate for the TCA cycle will depress ATP production.

Although short- and medium-chain FA (C_4-C_{12}) diffuse freely across cell membranes, the uptake of saturated and unsaturated LCFA across the plasma membrane occurs by sodium-dependent active transport and is mediated by a family of tissue-specific fatty acid-binding transport proteins, some unique to the liver (FATP2) and others found in multiple tissues.[9] Inside the cell, FA are esterified to CoA by the enzyme *acyl-CoA synthetase*, located on the outer aspect of the mitochondrial membrane. The resulting acyl-CoA esters can serve as substrates for triglyceride, phospholipids and cholesterol ester synthesis, but under fasting conditions they are directed largely toward mitochondrial β-oxidation. Like other enzyme families in the FAO pathway, the *acyl-CoA synthetases* differ in their specificities with respect to the chain lengths of FA substrates. Their chain-length specificities are the basis for classifying them as *short-*, *medium-*, *long-*, or *very-long-chain acyl-CoA synthetases*.

Carnitine Cycle

After activation to their CoA esters in the cytoplasm, LCFA are shuttled across the mitochondrial membrane by entering the carnitine cycle. In order to traverse the inner mitochondrial membrane, which is impermeable to CoA esters, long-chain acyl-CoA esters must first be transesterified to carnitine by the liver-specific isoform of the outer mitochondrial membrane enzyme *carnitine palmitoyltransferase I (CPT I)* to yield long-chain acylcarnitines. There are three different isoforms of *CPT 1* with tissue-specific expression encoded by different genes.[10] Only deficiency of the liver type, *CPT 1A*, has been demonstrated in humans. *CPT I* is a key enzyme in the regulation of intramitochondrial FAO and is directly responsive to levels of malonyl-CoA, which rise during the fed state and suppress *CPT I* activity, and fall during fasting allowing increased enzyme activity and shunting of FA into the β-oxidation pathway. The activity, immunoreactive protein, mRNA, and transcription rate of *CPT I* are increased during high-fat feeding, starvation, and diabetes, and by glucagon, cyclic adenosine monophosphate (cAMP), aspirin, hypolipidemic drugs, and inflammatory cytokines.[11] A lipid-activated transcription factor, the peroxisome proliferators-activated receptor α (PPAR-α), plays a pivotal role in the cellular response to fasting, inducing the expression of key intramitochondrial enzymes in the FAO pathway, including *CPT1*.[12,13] The mitochondrial transport system is highly specific for the transport of straight-chain FA and restricts entry of branched-chain FA (pristinic, phytanic acid), which are oxidized in the peroxisomes. In contrast to LCFA (palmitate, oleate), medium- and short-chain FA (octanoate, butyrate) can traverse the mitochondrial membrane without esterification to carnitine.

Carnitine (β-hydroxy-γ-trimethylaminobutyric acid) is formed from lysine with *S*-adenosylmethionine specifically required as a methyl donor. The rate-limiting enzyme in the synthetic pathway is γ-*butyrobetaine hydroxylase*, found only in the cytosol of the liver and kidney. The activity of this enzyme in the livers of infants younger than 3 months is only approximately one tenth of that found in adults, making carnitine an essential nutrient during the neonatal period that must be supplied via breast milk or infant formula.[14] Later, rich sources of carnitine in the diet include dairy products and red meat. Strict vegetarians maintain normal carnitine levels, indicating that humans not only synthesize carnitine, but also effectively conserve it through renal tubular reabsorption.

Because the muscle and heart must take up carnitine synthesized and exported from the liver and kidney, and maintain concentrations of carnitine 20- to 40-fold higher than in the blood, the transport of carnitine across the plasma membrane must be mediated by an active transport mechanism. A recently cloned homolog of the organic cation transporter *OCTN1* (designated *OCTN2*) has sodium-dependent carnitine uptake properties, has been mapped to human chromosome 5q31.2-32, and is highly expressed in cultured human hepatoma cells.[15] Mutations in *OCTN2* have been identified in patients with systemic primary carnitine deficiency (PCD) and in mice with juvenile visceral steatosis. Carnitine transporters, like LCFA transporters, are tissue specific, and those found in skeletal and cardiac muscle have a much higher K_m for the interaction of carnitine with *CPT I* compared with the liver isoform of this enzyme.[16] Thus, defects in carnitine uptake have more severe consequences for cardiac and skeletal muscle than for other tissues.

Accumulating acylcarnitines in the plasma and urine reflect accumulating acyl-CoA esters within the mitochondria. During fasting, plasma acetyl-CoA rises, and the ratio of acetylcarnitine to free carnitine increases. However, in patients with FAO defects, the medium- and long-chain acylcarnitines excreted in the plasma and urine reflect the site of the metabolic block and are clues to the identification of the intramitochondrial defect. Detoxification of accumulating intramitochondrial acyl-CoAs by esterification to carnitine and transport out of mitochondria is crucial to the maintenance of the intramitochondrial free CoA pool on which many other intramitochondrial metabolic pathways depend.[17] If not transported out of the mitochondria, accumulating long-chain acyl-CoA esters inhibit specific

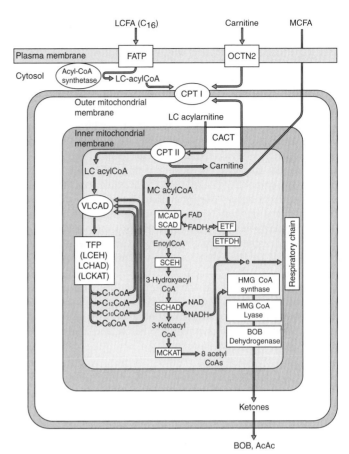

Figure 71-1. Pathway of hepatic mitochondrial fatty acid oxidation and ketogenesis showing steps for the oxidation of palmitate, a 16-carbon (C_{16}) long-chain fatty acid (LCFA). Note that eight-carbon medium-chain fatty acids (MCFA) enter the mitochondrion independent of the carnitine cycle. LCFAs are transported across the plasma membrane by a liver-specific LCFA-transporting polypeptide (FATP). Carnitine is supplied by a plasma membrane sodium-dependent carnitine transporter (OCTN2). On the outer mitochondrial membrane, carnitine palmitoyl transferase I (CPT I) is a major site of regulation that determines whether LCFAs are directed toward β-oxidation to ketones or to the resynthesis of triglycerides. LCFA-CoAs in the cytosol must first be transesterified to long-chain (LC) acylcarnitines by CPT I and then enter the carnitine cycle to be shuttled across the inner mitochondrial membrane. Once across the membrane, the acylcarnitine is reesterified to a LC acyl-CoA and enters the β-oxidation cycle. All the relevant enzymes for LC acyl-CoAs are bound to the inner mitochondrial membrane (VLCAD, TFP). At completion of the four reactions of the β-oxidation cycle, the LCFA has been shortened by two carbons, one molecule of acetyl-CoA has been generated for ketone body synthesis, and electrons have been transported to the respiratory chain via flavin-adenine dinucleotide (FAD) and nicotinamide-adenine dinucleotide (NAD). As the LCFA is shortened, β-oxidation proceeds via enzymes located in the mitochondrial matrix (MCAD, SCAD, HAD, MCKAT). Enzymes and transporters are circled. CACT, carnitine acylcarnitine translocase; CPT II, carnitine palmitoyl transferase II; VLCAD, very-long-chain acyl-CoA dehydrogenase; TFP, trifunctional protein; LCAD, long-chain acyl-CoA dehydrogenase; MCAD, medium-chain acyl-CoA dehydrogenase; HAD, medium-/short-chain 3-hydroxyacyl-CoA dehydrogenase; SCAD, short-chain acyl-CoA dehydrogenase; LCHAD, long-chain 3-hydroxyacyl-CoA dehydrogenase; LCEH, long-chain enoyl-CoA hydratase; LCKAT, long-chain ketothiolase; SCEH, short-chain enoyl-CoA dehydrogenase; MCKAT, medium-chain ketothiolase; HMG CoA, 3-hydroxy-3-methylglutaryl-CoA; AcAc, acetoacetate; BOB, β-hydroxybutyrate; ETF, electron transport flavoprotein; ETFDH, electron transport flavoprotein dehydrogenase; FADH2, reduced flavin-adenine dinucleotide; NADH, reduced nicotinamide-adenine dinucleotide. Adapted from Treem (2001).[1]

enzymes and transporters such as *adenine nucleotide translocase*, needed for the transport of ATP from the mitochondria to the cytosol, and *pantothenic acid kinase*, a major regulator of free CoA synthesis in the heart, liver, and kidney.[18]

After transesterification to carnitine, the resultant long-chain acylcarnitines are transported across the inner mitochondrial membrane by *carnitine-acylcarnitine translocase (CACT)*. At the interface of the inner membrane with the mitochondrial matrix, acylcarnitines are reesterified to regenerate acyl-CoA esters and free carnitine by *carnitine palmitoyltransferase II (CPT II)*. The reconstituted acyl-CoA is delivered into the mitochondrial matrix and enters the β-oxidation cycle while free carnitine is reshuttled back across the inner mitochondrial membrane for transesterification with another long-chain acyl-CoA. Each turn of the β-oxidation cycle results in the progressive cleavage of two carbon fragments from the original LCFA in the form of acetyl-CoAs that are then directed into ketone body synthesis. An important by-product of the β-oxidation cycle is the generation of electrons for the RC in the form of reduced flavin-adenine dinucleotide (FADH$_2$) and reduced nicotinamide-adenine dinucleotide (NADH). Transfer of these electrons to the mtRC yields ATP via oxidative phosphorylation and maintains the normal intramitochondrial redox state.

β-Oxidation Cycle

Figure 71-2 shows the four enzymes responsible for each turn of the β-oxidation cycle. Each of these enzyme activities is actually a family of enzymes with different chain-length specificities for FA composed of 4- to 24-carbon-atom backbones. Enzymes responsible for the β-oxidation of longer chain-length species are associated with the inner mitochondrial membrane, whereas those responsible for the metabolism of medium- and short-chain FA are located within the mitochondrial matrix. The metabolism of FA with more than 24 carbon atoms starts in the peroxisomes and can be continued there until the FA is reduced to eight carbons (medium-chain acyl-CoAs). However, certain characteristics of peroxisomal oxidation limit its ability to compensate for intramitochondrial FAO.[19] Electrons generated by peroxisomal oxidation are passed to oxygen forming hydrogen peroxide, instead of entering the mtRC, resulting in ATP generation. Also, peroxisomes lack a TCA cycle that, in mitochondria, is primed by acetyl-CoA from FAO.

The rate-limiting step in β-oxidation is the first reaction catalyzed by a family of flavin adenine dinucleotide (FAD)-dependent *acyl-CoA dehydrogenases*. *Very-long-chain acyl-CoA dehydrogenase (VLCAD)* is bound to the inner mitochondrial membrane and accepts acyl-CoAs ranging from C$_{24}$-CoA to C$_{12}$-CoA with palmitoyl-CoA (C$_{16}$) as the optimal substrate. The substrates for *long-chain acyl-CoA dehydrogenase (LCAD)* overlap with those of *VLCAD*. However, recent work suggests that *LCAD* is much less important in humans than was once thought.[20] Current thinking is that *LCAD* might play a major role in the metabolism of long branched-chain FA because, as opposed to *VLCAD*, it has high affinity for 2-methyl-decanoyl-CoA and 2-methylpalmitoyl-CoA. *Acyl CoA Dehydrogenase 9 (ACAD9)* is a recently described inner mitochondrial membrane enzyme with maximal activity for unsaturated long-chain acyl CoAs.[21] Despite significant overlap in substrate specificity, it appears that *VLCAD* and *ACAD9* are unable to compensate for each other in patients with deficiencies in either enzyme.[22] Located within the mitochondrial matrix are the other two *acyl-CoA*

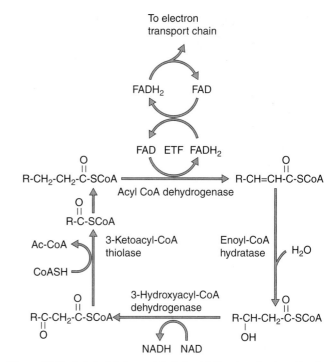

Figure 71-2. Spiral of fatty acyl-CoA β-oxidation in mitochondria. Acyl-CoA enters the spiral, whereupon acyl-CoA dehydrogenase inserts a double bond, forming an enoyl-CoA and transferring electrons to electron transfer flavoprotein (ETF). Enoyl-CoA hydratase adds water across the double bond to form 3-hydroxyacyl-CoA, which is oxidized by a nicotinamide-adenine dinucleotide (NAD)-linked 3-hydroxyacyl-CoA dehydrogenase to form a 3-ketoacyl-CoA. In the presence of free coenzyme A (CoASH), 3-ketoacyl-CoA thiolase cleaves the α-β bond to yield acetyl-CoA and an acyl-CoA moiety, now two carbons shorter, which can then reenter the spiral. FADH$_2$, reduced flavin-adenine dinucleotide. Adapted from Treem (2001).[1]

dehydrogenases, medium-chain acyl-CoA dehydrogenase (MCAD) with a broad chain-length specificity and optimal activity with C$_8$-CoA (octanoyl-CoA), and *short-chain acyl-CoA dehydrogenase (SCAD)*, which binds to C$_4$ and C$_6$ acyl-CoA esters.

For long-chain acyl-CoAs, the next three reactions of the β-oxidation cycle are catalyzed by the trifunctional protein (TFP) bound to the inner mitochondrial membrane. TFP is a hetero-octamer of four α- and four β-subunits encoded by two separate genes. On the α-subunit of this protein is encoded the *enoyl-CoA hydratase* activity and the NAD$^+$-dependent *long-chain 3-hydroxy-CoA dehydrogenase (LCHAD)* activity. The smaller β-subunit encodes the *long-chain 3-ketoacyl-CoA thiolase (LKAT)* activity.[23] Because of the complex association of the four α- and four β-subunits, mutations in either subunit may affect the intricate folding of the protein, rendering the entire complex unstable.

For medium- and short-chain acyl-CoAs, the relevant enzymes are located in the mitochondrial matrix rather than attached to the inner mitochondrial membrane, and they are synthesized as unrelated proteins and encoded by separate nuclear genes. These include a *short-chain enoyl-CoA hydratase (crotonase)*, a *medium-chain 3-hydroxy acyl-CoA dehydrogenase (HAD)*, and *medium-chain 3-ketoacyl-CoA thiolase (MCKAT)*. *Short-chain 3-hydroxyacyl-CoA dehydrogenase (SCHAD)* acts on a wide spectrum of substrates including steroids, cholic acid, and FA with a preference for short-chain methyl-branched acyl-CoAs. Patients previously characterized as having *SCHAD* deficiency variously presenting with hypoketotic hypoglycemia and hyperinsulinism, hepatic dysfunction, and cardiomyopathy actually have *HAD1* deficiency.[24] The intramitochondrial *short-chain ketothiolase (acetoacetyl CoA thiolase)* is active only with acetoacetyl-CoA and 2-methylacetoacetyl-CoA, which makes it indispensable for isoleucine degradation and important in ketone body metabolism, but suggests no role in FAO. Riboflavin (vitamin B_2) is the major precursor for flavin coenzymes including FAD, which is linked to all three *acyl-CoA dehydrogenases* and acts as an electron transporter to the mtRC. In experimental animals, riboflavin deficiency produces a rapid and selective decrease in FAO. Some patients with multiple *acyl-CoA dehydrogenase (MAD)* deficiency, due to a deficit in electron transfer flavoprotein (ETF), are responsive to treatment with large doses of riboflavin.[25]

In the liver, acetyl-CoA liberated by FAO is targeted toward ketogenesis. *3-Hydroxy-3-methylglutaryl-CoA (HMG-CoA) synthetase* combines one molecule of acetyl-CoA and one of acetoacetyl-CoA to form HMG-CoA. This is then cleaved by *HMG-CoA lyase* to yield a molecule of acetoacetate, which is in redox equilibrium with 3-hydroxybutyrate. Ketone bodies then enter the bloodstream and are taken up by tissues with a limited capacity to carry out β-oxidation, in particular the brain. There, acetoacetyl-CoA is cleaved into two molecules of acetyl-CoA that enter the TCA cycle.

EPIDEMIOLOGY AND GENETICS OF FAO DISORDERS

The FAO defects so far described exhibit autosomal recessive inheritance of nuclear encoded genes. It is estimated that FAO disorders affect approximately 1:10,000 in the general population, but exact incidence and prevalence data are lacking for most disorders owing to the lack of identification of a common mutation allowing for large-scale population screening.[26] Other factors that hamper an accurate assessment include the lack of large numbers of described patients for most of the FAO disorders, and the finding of multiple mutations responsible for the same phenotype.

An exception to the impediments described earlier and the best studied disorder is *MCAD* deficiency, in which homozygosity for a common point mutation accounts for approximately 80% of symptomatic cases; no other mutation has been found in more than 1% of the mutant alleles. Estimates of the prevalence of homozygosity for the common mutation in the general white population are approximately 1 in 12,000, but appear to be higher in the United States (1 in 9000) and the UK (1 in 6000).[27] Because about 10% of affected individuals are compound heterozygotes, with one allele carrying the common mutation and the other a less frequent mutation, the prevalence of *MCAD* deficiency is actually greater than these numbers suggest. In large neonatal screening programs, using tandem mass spectrometry to detect excess plasma octanoylcarnitine, the incidence is 1 in 13,600 live births in the United States, 1 in 12,600 in the UK, and 1 in 10,600 in Germany.[28] Other FAO disorders have a lower frequency of 1:20,000 to 1:100,000 live births.

The ability to determine the common mutation in *MCAD* deficiency using dried filter-paper blood spots to extract DNA has led to screening studies of gene mutation frequency in the general populations of various countries (the carrier state). Estimates range from as low as 1 in 68 in England, to 1 in 71 in Australia, about 1 in 100 in Denmark and the Netherlands, and approximately 1 in 107 in the United States.[29] Two recent studies of patients with *MCAD* deficiency revealed that 159 of 161 were white.[30] In most, their country of origin was either the British Isles or Germany. In contrast, the frequency of the carrier state for the common mutation in Italy is only 1 in 333; and in Japan, no carrier was identified in 500 Japanese neonates.[31] These data have led to the hypothesis that the common mutant allele for *MCAD* deficiency came from a small ancient population centered in Denmark or northern Germany, with subsequent spread to England, Ireland, and later to the United States and Australia.

A common mutation has also been found for isolated *LCHAD* deficiency. This single base-pair change in the α-subunit of TFP has been found to account for as many as 87% of the mutant alleles in a study from Europe, but only approximately 65% of the mutations in the United States.[32] An analysis of the frequency of this G1528C mutation in Finland revealed a carrier frequency of 1 in 240.[33] In the United States, a carrier frequency of approximately 1 in 175 has been found, and in the Netherlands, 1 in 680.[34]

A number of the nuclear genes encoding enzymes involved in the carnitine and β-oxidation cycles have been cloned, including genes for the *PCD*, *CPT I*, and *CPT II* deficiency, *VLCAD*, *MCAD*, and *SCAD* deficiency, and *LCHAD*, TFP, and *HAD* deficiency. This has led to the discovery of specific genetic mutations resulting in reduced enzyme activity, and the development of molecular probes to detect specific defects. Polymerase chain reaction–based assays are available commercially in a restricted number of laboratories to detect the common mutations in *MCAD* and *LCHAD* deficiencies. Because all of these disorders are autosomal recessive, study of the implicated enzyme activity in cultured skin fibroblasts from the parents of index cases shows approximately 50% of control values. Recently, patients with *HAD* deficiency have been described with only one mutation found in the *M/SCHAD* gene in synergy with mutations in other genes of the FAO pathway.[35] This raises the issue of the role of combined synergy of partial defects in FAO, and other host factors and/or environmental "stressors" in the pathogenesis of FAO disorders.

CLINICAL PRESENTATIONS OF FAO DISORDERS

Heterogeneous clinical presentations are the rule rather than the exception in FAO disorders (Table 71-2). In many patients, the presentation predominantly affects organs outside the usual purview of the pediatric gastroenterologist. These patients present as early as the first week of life with cardiomyopathy, arrhythmia, and even sudden infant death. They also may present later in childhood or adolescence with persistent hypotonia and developmental delay, or intermittent bouts of muscle pain, weakness, and rhabdomyolysis. Deficiency of *CPT II* is a good example of this phenotypic heterogeneity, with three different presentations including (1) a severe, rapidly fatal presentation in the perinatal period with dysmorphic features, hypoketotic hypoglycemia, acidosis, seizures, arrhythmias, hepatomegaly, nephromegaly, and cardiomyopathy; (2) an infantile presentation between 6 and 24 months with episodes of fasting-induced hypoketotic hypoglycemia, hepatic steatosis and steatohepatitis, and elevated muscle enzymes; and (3) the most common presentation in adolescence or adulthood with fasting-, exercise-, or stress-induced rhabdomyolysis and myoglobinuria.

TABLE 71-2. Clinical Manifestations of the Fatty Acid Oxidation Disorders

Organ or System	Clinical Manifestations
Liver	Hepatomegaly, steatosis (common); fibrosis, cirrhosis (rare)
	Aminotransferase 2-10 times normal (common); >1000 U/L (rare)
	Bilirubin level normal (common); moderately raised (rare)
	Coagulopathy (mild to moderate)
	Pruritus (rare); hepatic failure (rare)
Cardiac	Cardiomyopathy (hypertrophic and dilated)
	Congestive heart failure
	Cardiac arrhythmia
	Sudden infant death
	Increased CPK
Muscle	Hypotonic, weakness
	Muscle pain (exercise, stress)
	Rhabdomyolysis
	Increased CPK
Metabolic	Vomiting, lethargy, coma
	Encephalopathy
	Mild acidosis
	Increased lactate (LCHAD)
	Increased uric acid
Renal	Myoglobinuria
	Renal tubular acidosis (CPT1, CPT 2, MAD, LCHAD)
	Renal cysts, dysplasia (MAD, CPT 2)
Nonspecific	Failure to thrive
	Gastroesophageal reflux, vomiting
	Pancreatitis (CPT 2)
	Retinitis pigmentosa (LCHAD, long term)
	Peripheral neuropathy (LCHAD)
	Hypoparathyroidism (LCHAD)
	Acute fatty liver of pregnancy (LCHAD, HAD, CPT 1)
	Asymptomatic (MCAD)

Adapted from Treem (2000)[183]
CPK, creatine phosphokinase; CPT, carnitine palmitoyl transferase; LCHAD, long-chain 3-hydroxyacyl coenzyme A (CoA) dehydrogenase; MCAD, medium-chain acyl-CoA dehydrogenase; SCHAD, short-chain 3-hydroxyacyl-CoA dehydrogenase.

The existence of different tissue isoforms of some of the enzymes in the FAO pathway encoded by different genes is partially responsible for this heterogeneity. This section focuses on the hepatic manifestations of FAO disorders either as the primary presenting symptoms or in conjunction with findings in other organ systems. This multisystem presentation may be an important clue to the underlying ubiquitous metabolic nature of the illness.

Hypoketotic Hypoglycemia, Hepatomegaly, Liver Dysfunction, and Encephalopathy

These dramatic findings in a "previously healthy" child, usually in the first 2 years of life, will prompt a referral to the pediatric gastroenterologist for a Reye syndrome–like presentation or "hepatic failure." Diagnostic considerations will include severe viral hepatitis, galactosemia (on a lactose-containing diet), glycogen storage disease (type I, III), hereditary fructose intolerance (on a fructose- or sucrose-containing diet), hereditary

tyrosinemia type I, neonatal iron storage liver disease, mtRC defects, and erythrophagocytic lymphohistiocytosis. This presentation is most characteristic of carnitine uptake (PCD) and translocase (CACT) deficiencies; CPT II, VLCAD, and LCHAD deficiencies (all often in conjunction with cardiomyopathy); MCAD and MAD (ETF) deficiencies; and HMG-CoA lyase deficiency.

Most often, this presentation is preceded by what appears to be a routine viral infection or middle ear infection with fever and vomiting. The common denominator is poor oral intake over several days and development of a catabolic state. Less frequently, young infants present after weaning from the breast and fasting for longer periods through the night. The most likely symptoms at the time of presentation are lethargy, emesis, apnea and even respiratory arrest, and seizures. Physical findings generally include marked hepatomegaly without splenomegaly, hypotonia, and a gallop rhythm and poor perfusion if the heart is affected. Jaundice at the time of presentation is not common, thus contrasting these FAO disorders from fulminant viral, drug-induced, sepsis-induced, or ischemic hepatitis.[36] A family history of sudden infant death syndrome (SIDS), "Reye" syndrome, sudden cardiac decompensation, or early infant death from presumed "sepsis" or "liver failure" can be elicited in approximately one third of the patients.

Fasting hypoketotic or nonketotic hypoglycemia is a hallmark of most FAO disorders. Hypoglycemia is the result of hepatic glycogen depletion and impaired gluconeogenesis, and insulin levels are appropriately low. The one exception is HAD deficiency, where several patients have been described with hyperinsulinism responsible for their nonketotic hypoglycemia.[37] The observation that alterations in mental status precede overt hypoglycemia in some patients with FAO disorders has led to a search for accumulating neurotoxins (Figure 71-3). Mild to moderate hyperammonemia is often present (50 to 150 µM) and arises from urea cycle dysfunction due to diminished availability of N-acetylglutamate. In vivo animal studies and in vitro cellular studies have implicated medium-chain FA (octanoate), long-chain acyl-CoAs, and long-chain dicarboxylic acids as direct brain mitochondrial toxins and inhibitors of brain energy metabolism.[38] Infusion of octanoate into normal rabbits, at concentrations reached in the blood of patients with MCAD deficiency, results in coma, hyperammonemia, electroencephalographic changes, increased intracranial pressure, gross ultrastructural changes of brain mitochondria, and depression of intramitochondrial ATP production.[39] In LCHAD deficiency, the accumulating intermediates include long-chain 3-hydroxy fatty acids, 3-hydroxyacylcarnitines, 3-hydroxyacyl-CoAs, and 3-hydroxy-dicarboxylic acids. In high concentrations, these can injure cell membranes, potentiate free radical-induced lipid peroxidation, inhibit Na^+,K^+-ATPase, uncouple mitochondrial oxidative phosphorylation, and damage mitochondria.

Levels of aminotransferases are mildly increased (2- to 10-fold) in most patients. Bilirubin concentration is usually normal or only mildly elevated at the time of presentation. Although the clotting studies may be normal, at times the degree of coagulopathy appears incongruous with the mild increase in aminotransferases. Other accompanying abnormalities include mild to moderate increases in blood urea nitrogen (BUN), uric acid, and CPK. Acidosis, if present, is usually mild, with the exception of some cases of LCHAD, TFP, and MAD deficiencies, where significant lactic acidemia may be encountered.[40]

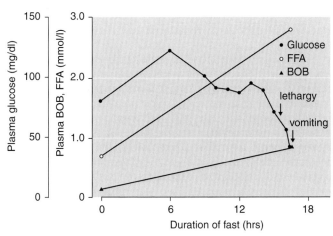

Figure 71-3. Consequences of prolonged fasting in a patient with MCAD deficiency. Normally, glucose concentration falls slightly and remains stable, while levels of ketones (β-hydroxybutyrate; BOB) rise steeply and free fatty acids (FFA) rise slightly and then stabilize. Here, because of the defect in FAO, glucose falls precipitously during a prolonged fast, with an inadequate ketogenic response and a marked rise in FFA levels. Note that lethargy and mental status changes precede actual hypoglycemia. In these disorders, the accumulations of toxic medium- and long-chain fatty acyl-CoAs and acylcarnitines mediate the central nervous system toxicity even before the hypoglycemia becomes critical. Adapted from Treem (2001).[1]

Dramatic increases in liver size often develop over the first 48 hours, even after intravenous dextrose has been provided and hypoglycemia ameliorated. The liver is brightly echogenic and homogeneous when examined with ultrasonography. Computed tomography (CT) shows a low-density liver characteristic of diffuse fatty infiltration. A liver biopsy performed at the time of the illness most often reveals diffuse macrovesicular steatosis. Some patients, particularly those with *MCAD* or *SCAD* deficiency, have only microvesicular fat accumulation, and these more subtle changes can escape notice without the help of special stains (Oil Red-O) or electron microscopy. More severe changes with portal infiltrates, bile duct proliferation, hepatic fibrosis, and even established cirrhosis have been noted in a minority of patients with *LCHAD* deficiency. Electron microscopy of liver tissue reveals an increase in the size and number of mitochondria, as well as markers of mitochondrial stress and damage manifested as swelling, irregular cristae, and paracrystalline arrays (Figure 71-4).

Fulminant Hepatic Failure

A minority of patients with FAO defects present with fulminant hepatic failure characterized by dramatic increases in aminotransferases (more than 20 times normal), profound coagulopathy, hyperammonemia, hypoglycemia, coma, and significant hyperbilirubinemia. Biopsies show significant confluent areas of hepatocyte necrosis and collapse. Although uncommon, this presentation has been described in patients with *LCHAD*, *CACT*, and *MCKAT* deficiencies.[41,42] Two patients with in vitro evidence of a defect of LCFA transport at the plasma membrane level have been reported with recurrent life-threatening episodes of acute liver failure that evolved into chronic severe liver disease necessitating transplantation.[43] At least one case of *ACAD9* deficiency has been described in a 14-year-old boy who presented with a Reye-like illness associated with aspirin use that progressed to liver failure, cerebral edema, and death.[22] A previously healthy 3-year-old child with *HAD* deficiency was

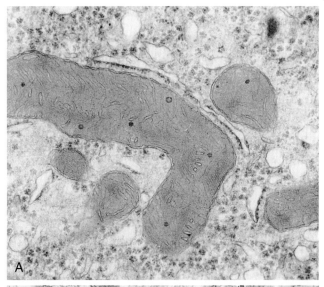

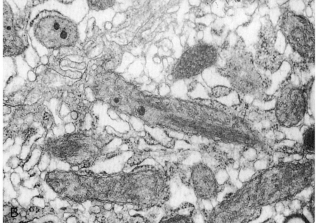

Figure 71-4. Electron micrographs of the liver from patients with (**A**) MCAD deficiency and (**B**) carnitine transport defect, showing the elongated giant mitochondria with linear crystalline arrays in the matrix. From Treem (2001).[1]

recently reported who presented with nonketotic hypoglycemia, hepatic failure, and encephalopathy and a liver biopsy showing centrilobular necrosis and periportal steatosis.[44] She underwent successful living-related donor liver transplantation.

Sudden Infant Death Syndrome

Recent studies have suggested that 1 to 5% of all cases of SIDS are due to abnormalities in FAO, including *MCAD*, *VLCAD*, *MAD*, and *LCHAD* deficiencies.[45] Various tissues and fluids are suitable for acylcarnitine or enzyme analysis postmortem in infants with SIDS, including swabbed urine from the bladder, bile accumulated in the gallbladder, vitreous humor, and frozen liver, skeletal, and cardiac muscle.[46] Postmortem skin biopsies yield skin fibroblasts that can still be grown in tissue culture for later examination. Some of these cases have been discovered when a subsequent sibling is diagnosed with an FAO disorder years after the SIDS case. The use of polymerase chain reaction (PCR) to amplify a small DNA fragment from genomic DNA in postmortem paraffin-embedded or formalin-fixed tissue stored for as long as 18 years has allowed the diagnosis of *MCAD* deficiency in a SIDS victim.[47] A family history of SIDS should always provoke a suspicion of the possibility of a defect in FAO in another child who later exhibits one of the clinical presentations described earlier.

Acute Fatty Liver of Pregnancy in Mothers Carrying Infants with FAO Defects

A number of published reports have established a link between acute fatty liver of pregnancy (AFLP) and FAO disorders, most notably *LCHAD* deficiency.[48-50] AFLP has an incidence of 1 in 13,000 deliveries and affects women of all ages and races.[51] The estimated prevalence of all TFP defects (including isolated *LCHAD* deficiency) is 1:38,000 pregnancies.[50] Women who carry a mutation in the α-subunit of TFP (thus reducing the synthesis of *LCHAD* by approximately 50%), and who are carrying a fetus affected by *LCHAD* deficiency, are at increased risk of developing AFLP in the last trimester of that pregnancy. Carrying an affected fetus appears to be a necessary condition for the development of AFLP, as these same women do not develop AFLP when carrying a heterozygous or completely unaffected fetus. A retrospective study of fetal genotypes and pregnancy outcomes in 83 pregnancies in 35 families carrying documented mutations of the α-subunit of TFP has shown that in 70% of the women, 20 pregnancies were complicated by AFLP; 2 by the syndrome of hemolysis, raised liver enzymes, and low platelets (HELLP syndrome); and 2 by preeclampsia.[52] In all of these pregnancies, the women carried *LCHAD*-deficient fetuses homozygous for the common G1528C mutation. Five pregnant mothers carrying fetuses with complete TFP deficiency and different mutations did not suffer pregnancy complications. Approximately 15% of women who carry fetuses with a mutation in the β-subunit of the TFP also develop AFLP or HELLP syndrome.[53]

Half of the affected pregnancies were also associated with premature delivery and intrauterine growth retardation, suggesting a key role for this enzyme in fetal development. Previously, it was thought that FAO did not play a significant role in fetal growth and metabolism during embryogenesis; but recent studies of human fetuses between 5 and 10 weeks' gestation indicate near-adult levels of expression of *VLCAD* and *LCHAD* mRNA in fetal heart, liver, neural retina, spinal cord, and kidney.[54] The presence of dysmorphic features, renal dysgenesis, and neuronal migration defects in infants with *CPT II* and *MAD* deficiencies similar to those seen in Zellweger syndrome, a disorder of peroxisomal FAO, suggests that FAO plays an important role in fetal development. Thus, a fetus affected by an FAO disorder could generate toxic by-products of this metabolically active pathway that cross the placenta and affect the maternal liver.

During the latter stages of a normal pregnancy, insulin resistance, increased activity of *lipoprotein lipase*, and inhibition of FAO lead to increased LCFA substrate flux through a relatively inefficient pathway.[55] As a result, hepatic synthesis of triglycerides, secretion of VLDL, and maternal plasma LCFA all increase significantly. Preeclampsia, a common precursor of AFLP, further exaggerates these imbalances and also results in a reduction of hepatic antioxidants. Women with preeclampsia have elevated levels of very-long-chain acylcarnitines, suggesting that relative insufficiency of mitochondrial FAO is associated with this condition.[56]

At least six enzymes of the FAO pathway are active in the normal human placenta, and their activity decreases during the second and third trimesters.[57] Cultured trophoblast cells oxidize palmitate and myristate in substantial amounts, indicating that the placenta utilizes LCFA as a significant metabolic fuel.[58] Early in gestation, the placenta contains levels of FAO enzymes comparable to those present in mature, FA-dependent tissues such as skeletal muscle. Contrary to the prevailing belief that glucose is the sole energy source in the placenta, these studies suggest that FAO is critical for normal growth and maturation of the placenta and for providing fuel for energy-consuming placental functions of ion, nutrient, and waste transplacental transport. Thus, under certain circumstances, the 50% reduction in *LCHAD* activity in both the maternal liver and the placenta, which is normally inconsequential to female carriers of *LCHAD* deficiency, may become critical and contribute to the development of AFLP. The placental unit, in addition to the affected fetus, could also be the source of the generation of liver-toxic metabolites (long-chain 3-hydroxyacyl CoAs) in the *LCHAD*-deficient heterozygous mothers carrying affected fetuses. It is estimated that this situation is responsible for approximately 20% of all cases of AFLP.[59] Recent case reports have now linked other fetal FAO disorders with AFLP, including *SCAD* and *CPT I* deficiencies.[60,61]

The clinical implications of this link between FAO disorders in the offspring and severe pregnancy complications in the mother are important to recognize. Because of the autosomal recessive nature of these disorders, the recurrence risk with subsequent pregnancies is 25%, and all subsequent pregnancies must be assiduously monitored. Also, all newborns surviving a pregnancy complicated by AFLP must undergo immediate testing to identify a FAO defect. Measures to prevent cardiac or liver decompensation should be put in place while awaiting the results.

DIAGNOSIS OF FAO DISORDERS

Fortunately, a number of signature metabolites in the urine and blood point to the presence of a defect in FAO (Table 71-3). These metabolites are most likely to be found at the time of presentation before substantial amounts of intravenous dextrose have been given to correct hypoglycemia and dehydration. The practice of obtaining extra urine and plasma and freezing it for later analysis in any patient presenting to the emergency room with a profile that fits the clinical scenarios just described may yield important diagnostic clues. This is critical because tissue enzyme analysis of liver, muscle or skin fibroblasts, or DNA analysis of known mutations is often delayed by technical limitations and laboratory availability.

Urine Organic Acids

Analysis of the urine organic acid profile is a powerful diagnostic tool. The presence of increased concentrations of dicarboxylic acids reflects the microsomal omega-oxidation of FA in the liver through the action of a cytochrome P450-linked mixed-function oxygenase (CYP4A). Dicarboxylic acids appear in the blood transiently as long-, medium-, or short-chain dicarboxylic acids for eventual excretion in the kidney. Peroxisomal metabolism of dicarboxylic acids explains how patients with defects in mitochondrial β-oxidation may excrete dicarboxylic acids with a shorter chain length than would be predicted by the position of the defect. Dicarboxylic acids are formed whenever there is increased flux through the β-oxidation spiral (i.e., diabetic ketoacidosis). They are also present in the urine of infants fed a formula high in medium-chain triglycerides (MCTs). However, in these normal infants the ratio of β-hydroxybutyrate:dicarboxylic acids when fasting is greater than 1, whereas the ratio is reversed in infants presenting with symptoms of most FAO disorders. In

TABLE 71-3.   Characteristic Urinary and Plasma Metabolites (During Fasting or Acute Illness)

Deficiency	Urinary Organic Acids	Plasma Acylcarnitine	Diagnostic Metabolites
MCAD	C_6-C_{10} DCA (saturated and unsaturated glycine conjugates)	Octanoylcarnitine	Phenylpropionylglycine (urine)
	Hexanoylcarnitine	Hexanoylglycine (urine)	
	Decenoylcarnitine	Octanoic acid (plasma)	
		cis-4-Decenoic acid	
VLCAD	C_6-C_{10} DCA C_{12}-C_{14} DCA $C_{12:1}$ DCA	Acetylcarnitine (low) $C_{14:1}$, C_{16}, $C_{16:1}$, $C_{18:1}$, $C_{18:2}$ acylcarnitines	$C_{14:1}$ acylcarnitine (plasma)
SCAD	C_6-C_{10} DCA, ethylmalonic, butyric	Butyrylcarnitine	Butyrylglycine
HMG-CoA lyase	Butyric, 3-hydroxymethylglutaric, 3-methylglutaric, 3-methylglutaconic, 3-hydroxyisovaleric	3-Methylglutarylcarnitine, 3-hydroxy-isovalerylcarnitine	3-Methylglutarylcarnitine
HMG-CoA synthase	Normal	Normal	Low β-hydroxybutyrate after fat load
ETF (mild)	C_6-C_{10} DCA, ethylmalonic		
ETF/ETF-DH (severe)	C_6-C_{10} DCA, glutaric, isovaleric	Glutarylcarnitine Octanoylcarnitine Butyrylcarnitine Isovalerylcarnitine	Glutarylcarnitine
LCHAD	C_6-C_{10} DCA, lactate	Acrylylcarnitine ($C_{3:1}$) C_{10}-C_{18} acylcarnitines (saturated and unsaturated)	C_{12}-C_{14} 3-hydroxy-DCA > C_6 DCA
C_6-C_{18} 3-hydroxy-DCA	C_{14}-C_{18} hydroxyacylcarnitine	C_{14}-C_{18} 3-hydroxyacylacarnitine (plasma)	
HAD	C_{6-14} 3-hydroxy-DCA, C_6-C_{10} DCA, ethylmalonic, 3-hydroxy glutarate	Butyrylcarnitine	
MCKAT	C_6-C_{12} DCA, lactic 3-hydroxy C_6-C_{14} DCA, 3-methylglutaconic		
Fatty acid transport	Minimal C_6-C_{12} DCA		High C_8-C_{18} FFA (plasma)
CPT II	Normal	Palmitoylcarnitine C_{18}, $C_{18:1}$, $C_{18:2}$ acylcarnitines	Very low free plasma carnitine; acylcarnitines 90% of total
CPT I	Normal 3-hydroxyglutaric, C_{12} DCA	Normal	Free plasma carnitine level raised; absent long-chain acylcarnitines
CT	Normal	Normal	Total plasma carnitine <5% of normal (very low)
CACT	Normal; nonspecific DCA	C_{16}, $C_{18:1}$ acylcarnitines	Very low free plasma carnitine; acylcarnitine 90% of total
2,4-Dienoyl-CoA reductase	Normal	$C_{10:2}$ acylcarnitine	

MCAD, medium-chain acyl-Co-A dehydrogenase; DCA, dicarboxylic acid; VLCAD, very-long-chain acyl-CoA dehydrogenase; SCAD, short-chain acyl-CoA dehydrogenase; HMG-CoA, hydroxymethylglutaryl coenzyme A; ETF, electron transport flavoprotein; LCHAD, long-chain 3-hydroxyacyl-CoA dehydrogenase; SCHAD, short-chain 3-hydroxyacyl-CoA dehydrogenase; MCKAT, medium-chain 3-ketoacyl-CoA thiolase; CPT, carnitine palmitoyl transferase; CT, carnitine transport; CACT, carnitine-acylcarnitine translocase; FFA, free fatty acids. From Treem (2001).

patients with the three most common FAO disorders (*MCAD*, *VLCAD*. and *LCHAD* deficiencies), a pattern of medium-chain dicarboxylic aciduria (adipic C_6 > suberic C_8 > sebacic C_{10}) with prominent unsaturated species ($C_{8:1}$ > C_8, $C_{10:1}$ > C_{10}) is observed during acute episodes. In *LCHAD* deficiency, C_6-C_{14} 3-hydroxydicarboxylic aciduria often predominates.

Although the presence of dicarboxylic aciduria is a useful sign in patients with defects in the β-oxidation spiral, this is not the case in patients with disorders involving transport of LCFAs into mitochondria via the carnitine cycle (*PCD*, *CACT*, or *CPT* deficiencies). These defects are proximal to the entry of FA into the β-oxidation cycle, and there is little or no accumulation of intermediates even though ketogenesis is impaired. Thus, the absence of dicarboxylic acids does not rule out a defect in FAO.

Other metabolites that appear in the urine of these patients are the glycine conjugates of acyl-CoA esters that can be detected using stable isotope dilution mass spectrometry. The advantage of this technique is that small amounts of acylglycines appear to be consistently excreted in children with certain defects in FAO, even when they are well.[62] This technique has been particularly useful for the recognition of patients with mild or intermittent biochemical phenotypes, such as some patients with *MCAD* or *MAD* deficiencies or with polymorphisms of the *SCAD* gene. Glycine conjugation is exclusively carried out in the mitochondria, with short- and medium-chain acyl-CoA esters acting as the preferred substrates. Therefore, the occurrence of glycine conjugates in a patient's urine reflects the intramitochondrial accumulation of acyl-CoA esters. This is the biochemical basis of the accumulation of suberylglycine, hexanoylglycine, and phenylpropionylglycine in the urine of patients with MCAD deficiency.

Plasma Acylcarnitine Profiles

Excessive long-, medium-, or short-chain acyl-CoAs that accumulate proximal to the metabolic block may be converted to acylcarnitines by chain length-specific *carnitine acyltransferases*.

Acylcarnitines are then transported out of the mitochondria into the plasma and are eventually filtered by the kidneys. They compete with free carnitine for renal tubular reabsorption and, because they have a higher affinity for the carnitine transporter, free carnitine will be excreted. This accounts for the low levels of total plasma carnitine and the higher fraction of acylcarnitine to free carnitine in most patients with FAO defects. The lowest total carnitine levels are found in PCD (0 to 5 μM, normal 25 to 50 μM), where the defective plasma membrane carnitine transporter expressed in the muscle, heart, kidney, and skin fibroblasts leads to severe urinary carnitine loss.[63] The only exception to low plasma carnitine is found in patients with CPT 1 deficiency, where disruption of the carnitine cycle at the outer mitochondrial membrane results in raised cytosolic and plasma carnitine.

Plasma acylcarnitine profiles are usually more informative than urinary levels because renal tubular absorption of long-chain acylcarnitines limits their appearance and detection in the urine. Also, under normoglycemic conditions, organic acids in the urine may revert to normal, but the plasma acylcarnitine profile remains abnormal. This, however, is not the case in PCD, where absence of carnitine transport limits the availability of carnitine to form esters with accumulating intramitochondrial acyl-CoAs. Other pitfalls in the interpretation of acylcarnitine profiles include the presence of certain medications that inhibit or overload the β-oxidation pathway such as valproic acid and propofol; the consumption of high MCT-containing formulas provoking formation of medium-chain acylcarnitines; or the presence of a defect in the mtRC with an acylcarnitine profile that mimics that seen in certain FAO disorders.[64] Sick premature infants receiving carnitine-free total parenteral nutrition may have marked renal wasting of carnitine and develop very low levels of total plasma carnitine even in the absence of any FAO disorder.

It is possible to analyze small amounts of plasma acylcarnitine conjugates of abnormal intermediates using fast atom bombardment mass spectrometry (FAB-MS) or, more recently, FAB using two mass spectrometry instruments in tandem (MS/MS).[65] Another recent technologic breakthrough is the use of electrospray ionization.[66] These techniques have been adapted to neonatal blood spots and have become the dominant method for state neonatal screening programs designed to detect FAO defects.

Plasma Free Fatty Acids and 3-Hydroxy Fatty Acids

When available, the measurement of total plasma free fatty acids (FFA) and β-hydroxybutyrate can signal a FAO disorder. Normal adaptation to prolonged fasting allows the increasing generation of ketones and the stabilization of plasma levels of FFA. However, when ketogenesis is disrupted, the ratio of β-hydroxybutyrate to FFA is reversed. Plasma LCFA and 3-hydroxy FA are found consistently in patients with LCHAD and TFP deficiencies even when they are asymptomatic. In other defects (VLCAD and MCAD deficiencies), the presence of long- or medium-chain FFA in the plasma reflects the localization of the enzymatic defect. Target compounds in the plasma must first undergo derivatization of hydroxyl and carboxyl groups and then analysis with gas chromatography/mass spectroscopy, which allows the simultaneous discovery of both FFA and 3-hydroxy fatty acids.[67]

Tissue Enzyme and Molecular Studies

Assays are available to measure the enzyme activity of virtually all the enzymes involved in FAO defects in various tissues, including the liver, muscle, lymphocytes, and skin fibroblasts, by determining specific substrate utilization rates. Skin fibroblasts are particularly useful as they can be cultured and kept alive indefinitely. Prenatal diagnosis is facilitated by chorionic villus sampling or amniocyte cultures. These tissues can also be incubated with radiolabeled LCFA of various chain lengths with measurement of the rate of labeled CO_2 or H_2O production, depending on whether the FA was labeled with ^{14}C or ^{3}H. An alternative technique involves incubation of the target tissue with labeled acylcarnitines.[68] Because of overlap with some of the mtRC defects, the result of in vitro acylcarnitine profiling requires further confirmation with enzymatic or mutational analysis.

Most of the genes encoding enzymes involved in the carnitine and β-oxidation cycles have been cloned. This has led to the discovery of specific genetic mutations responsible for the reduced enzyme activity in most of the known FAO defects and the development of molecular probes to detect specific defects. Certain commercial laboratories offer examination of DNA from white blood cells to detect the common mutations responsible for most cases of MCAD and LCHAD deficiency.

TREATMENT OF DISORDERS OF FAO

Management of Acute Illness

Management of acute episodes of metabolic decompensation with hypoketotic hypoglycemia, coma, hepatic steatosis, and liver dysfunction requires the rapid institution of intravenous dextrose, even when the blood glucose level is normal or only mildly reduced. The rate of glucose infusion should equal at least 10 mg/kg/min in infants to raise insulin levels sufficiently to inhibit FAO and block further release of FA from adipose tissue. Blood glucose levels should be maintained above 100 mg/dL (5.5 mmol/L). Drugs that inhibit FAO (e.g., valproate, salicylate and nonsteroidal anti-inflammatory drugs), and those that increase FFA release (e.g., epinephrine), should be avoided. Intravenous fat emulsions used in parenteral nutrition solutions and intravenous propofol should not be given. Propofol is a soybean emulsion that provides a medium- and long-chain triglyceride load to the patient. Scattered case reports of "propofol infusion syndrome" in children, characterized by metabolic acidosis, rhabdomyolysis, cardiac and renal failure, and the accumulation of intermediates of β-oxidation, mimic the phenotype of FAO and mtRC disorders.[69] Cold exposure leading to shivering thermogenesis with the liberation of FFA should be avoided and fever controlled.

In certain patients presenting with coma and profound liver dysfunction, there may be a role for exchange transfusion or continuous venovenous hemofiltration to remove toxic metabolites.[70] This is particularly true in defects primarily affecting LCFA oxidation where there is little renal excretion of toxic long-chain acylcarnitines or long-chain dicarboxylic acids. Anecdotal reports documenting the disappearance of toxic metabolites from blood and urine, and the resolution of coma, have suggested a therapeutic role for these interventions.

L-Carnitine therapy (100 mg/kg daily) is recommended either intravenously or via a nasogastric tube if there is no vomiting or diarrhea. It is potentially life-saving in patients with PCD, whose plasma carnitine levels are near zero. Large doses of carnitine will allow normalization of tissue carnitine levels in the liver and passive uptake of some carnitine into critically compromised tissues such as the myocardium. Its role in other defects is more controversial. Some investigators point to the increased concentrations of acylcarnitines in the urine and blood as evidence that exogenous carnitine supplementation is preventing the buildup of toxic long- and medium-chain acyl-CoAs in the mitochondria.[71] However, no controlled randomized trials have been conducted. Also, long-chain acylcarnitines are known to cause cardiac arrhythmias in animal models and could further impair the FAO pathway by substrate/product feedback inhibition.[72,73]

Preventive Measures to Reduce Fasting-Induced Metabolic Stress

Avoidance of fasting is the mainstay of therapy for disorders of FAO. In young infants, more than 6 hours of fasting may be sufficient to provoke metabolic decompensation. In older infants, longer episodes are required or repetitive days of poor oral intake and catabolic stress. Thus, the prompt administration of intravenous dextrose in the early stages of any illness with fever, vomiting, or diarrhea is mandatory even when there are no signs of dehydration. Waiting for the onset of hypoglycemia is a mistake, because at that time levels of FFA and toxic metabolites are already high. Glucagon injections have no effect because glycogen stores are already depleted at the time of hypoglycemia. Prolonged aerobic exercise and cold exposure are other potential precipitating factors provoking early mobilization of FFA. A high carbohydrate load before such activities is advisable.

Preventing overnight fasting in the well infant with some disorders of FAO may take the form of late night and early morning feeding, or the use of uncooked cornstarch at night similar to the treatment of infants and young children with glycogen storage disease type I. However, in infants with defects in LCFA oxidation (*VLCAD, LCHAD, CPT, CACT* or PCD), or in those with previous episodes of hypoketotic hypoglycemia and coma or cardiac decompensation, a more reliable preventive therapy is the placement of a gastrostomy tube and the institution of overnight feedings. In general, we recommend that patients with defects in the carnitine cycle and LCFA oxidation receive a high-carbohydrate, low-fat formula or diet with approximately 65% of the calories from carbohydrate, 15% from protein, and 20% from fat. Formulas high in MCTs are recommended because medium-chain fatty acids do not require an intact carnitine cycle for entry into the mitochondria. *MCAD-* and *SCAD-*deficient patients do not appear to require a special formula, and there is no clear evidence that restricting long-chain fats is necessary. In spite of these generally accepted recommendations, there is no consensus among metabolic dieticians on the optimum dietary management of patients with defects in FAO, and little evidence supporting the protocols currently in use.[74]

In addition to dietary restrictions, the addition of MCT supplements has been advocated. No controlled trials of MCT oil supplementation have been conducted. A recent survey of physicians caring for children with *LCHAD* deficiency suggested that a low-fat, MCT-supplemented diet reduced the incidence of hypoketotic hypoglycemia and improved hypotonia, hepatomegaly, cardiomyopathy, and lactic acidosis.[75] In 10 patients with *LCHAD* deficiency, a diet that provided approximately 10% of energy as dietary LCFA and 10 to 20% as MCTs, with 12% of energy coming from standard protein sources and 66%

from carbohydrate, resulted in the maintenance of normal levels of hydroxypalmitoleic, hydroxyoleic, and hydroxylinoleic carnitine esters and no episodes of metabolic decompensation. This diet should be supplemented with fat-soluble vitamins and vegetable oils to provide essential fatty acids.[76] MCT oil supplementation is contraindicated in patients with *MCAD, SCAD, MCKAT*, and *HAD* deficiencies.

Treatment of stable patients with FAO disorders with daily oral L-carnitine restores normal levels of plasma carnitine but does not correct the basic enzymatic defect. The administration of large doses of L-carnitine (100 mg/kg daily) results in increased excretion of octanoylcarnitine in patients with *MCAD* deficiency, and this has been taken as evidence of protection of the inner mitochondrial milieu from accumulating medium-chain acyl-CoA.[77] However, there have been no direct measurements of acyl-CoAs in tissue before and after treatment to support this hypothesis. In addition, studies in *VLCAD*-deficient mice show that carnitine supplementation does not raise plasma carnitine levels and increases the levels of potential toxic acylcarnitines present, thus raising controversy about this treatment.[78] There have been isolated published reports of small numbers of patients, primarily with LCFA oxidation defects, who appeared to be more tolerant of fasting and have reduced accumulation of plasma FFAs when supplemented with carnitine.[79] Most physicians caring for these patients supplement with L-carnitine to keep plasma levels within the normal range. However, recent studies in patients with *LCHAD* deficiency have found no correlation between carnitine supplementation and the levels of plasma hydroxyacylcarnitines or the frequency of metabolic decompensations.

Supplementation with riboflavin (300 mg/day) has been used in patients with *MAD, MCAD*, and *VLCAD* deficiency, with reductions in the excretion of abnormal urinary metabolites and modest increases in enzyme activity of *MCAD* in cultured skin fibroblasts before and after therapy.[80] Riboflavin (vitamin B2) is a major precursor for flavin coenzymes, including FAD, which is a cofactor for the *acyl-CoA dehydrogenases* that catalyze the first reaction in the β-oxidation cycle.

New and Experimental Therapies

Several promising therapeutic approaches are currently under investigation. The first involves supplying anaplerotic odd-chain triglycerides (in the form of triheptanoin oil) to treat cardiomyopathy and rhabdomyolysis in LCFA disorders.[81] β-Oxidation of triheptanoin results in the formation of both acetyl-CoA and propionyl-CoA. Propionyl-CoA is an efficient substrate for citric acid cycle intermediates, the restoration of which would be expected to increase ATP production and improve cardiac and skeletal muscle function. In three patients with *VLCAD* deficiency, this treatment led to clinical improvement, including the permanent disappearance of chronic cardiomyopathy, rhabdomyolysis, and muscle weakness. This therapy might also be effective in patients with deficiencies of *CPT I, CACT, CPT II, VLCAD*, and *LCHAD* but has not been tested.

Agonists of PPAR-α such as bezafibrate, fenofibrate, and clofibrate have been shown to increase *CPT I, CPT II*, and *MCAD* mRNA expression in fetal rat hepatocytes and hamster liver and muscle.[82,83] Bezafibrate raises *VLCAD* activity to near normal in human skin fibroblasts from patients with the late-onset myopathic form of *VLCAD* deficiency who retain some remaining enzyme activity.[84,85] Fenofibrate restores both *CPT II* activity and LCFA oxidation in fibroblasts and myoblasts from patients with the adult form of *CPT II* deficiency.[86,87] Another attractive target to up-regulate genes regulating enzymes of FAO is *stearoyl-CoA desaturase 1 (SCD1)*, the rate-limiting enzyme in the biosynthesis of monounsaturated fatty acids. *SCD1* knockout mice produce more ketones after a 4-hour fast than wild-type mice, and genes for key enzymes in the FAO pathway are up-regulated in these mice, including *VLCAD* and *CPT*.[88]

Gene therapy has successfully corrected biochemical abnormalities in *MCAD*-deficient cultured human fibroblasts and in an animal model of *VLCAD* deficiency.[89,90] Using a recombinant adenoviral vector that constitutively expressed the human *MCAD* protein, transfected human fibroblasts were shown to produce a 55-kDa protein colocalizing in mitochondria and demonstrated restoration of normal *MCAD*-catalyzed metabolism of octanoyl-CoA and a normal acylcarnitine profile. A recombinant adeno-associated virus expressing the human *VLCAD* gene administered via the tail vein to *VLCAD* knockout mice resulted in short-term gene expression in the liver and muscle and longer-term expression in the heart, as well as improvement in the maintenance of normoglycemia and the prevention of accumulating long-chain acylcarnitines.

RESPIRATORY CHAIN DISORDERS

Mitochondrial disorders of the RC (mtRC) are often difficult to identify because of wide variability in clinical presentation, severity, and age at presentation. "Classical" clinical features focus on the central nervous system and include well-described syndromes such as MELAS (mitochondrial encephalomyopathy with lactic acidosis and stroke-like episodes); LHON (Leber hereditary optic neuropathy); and NARP (neurogenic weakness ataxia with retinitis pigmentosa). However, systemic presentations of mitochondrial disorders include a wide range of symptoms and signs.[2] This is due to the far-reaching consequences of mitochondrial RC dysfunction, which include (1) cellular energy deficits secondary to reduced ATP synthesis; (2) increased dependence on glycolysis with increased lactate production; (3) intramitochondrial accumulation of reducing equivalents and an altered redox state; (4) impairment of the TCA cycle, β-oxidation cycle, and urea cycle; (5) increased generation of reactive oxygen species (ROS); and (6) opening of the mitochondrial permeability pore, releasing calcium, cytochrome c, and apoptosis factors into the cytosol.

This section focuses on inherited mtRC disorders that cause liver failure due to mutations in mitochondrial DNA (mtDNA) or, more commonly, in nuclear DNA. These mutations affect the activity or assembly of one or more RC components, or the overall production and maintenance of mtDNA, or both. Multiple examples exist of secondary mitochondrial hepatopathies mediated by increased ROS and acquired damage to the RC. Discussed in other sections, these include nonalcoholic steatohepatitis (NASH), ischemia/reperfusion injury, Wilson's disease, cholestatic liver diseases resulting in the accumulation of hydrophobic bile acids, and drug-induced hepatotoxicity with valproic acid, salicylates, nucleoside analogues, nonsteroidal anti-inflammatory drugs (NSAIDs), and other drugs.

MITOCHONDRIAL RC GENETICS AND BIOLOGY

Figure 71-5 summarizes the components, substrates, and products of the RC. The RC is composed of five multiheteromeric enzyme complexes embedded in the inner mitochondrial

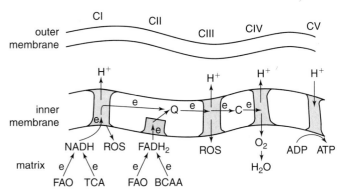

Figure 71-5. Electron transport pathway of the intramitochondrial respiratory chain with electrons (e) transported via NADH and FADH$_2$ after being generated by metabolism of fatty acids via FAO, pyruvate, and TCA cycle intermediates via the TCA cycle, and branched-chain amino acids (BCAA). Electrons are transported via four carrier complexes embedded in the inner mitochondrial membrane and two cofactors (coenzyme Q and cytochrome c) resulting in the active translocation of protons (H$_2$) out of the matrix and into the intermembrane space and generating a transmembrane proton (H$^+$) gradient. This gradient allows protons to flow back into the mitochondrial matrix and supplies the energy transduction for the synthesis of ATP molecules in complex V (APTase). During the oxidation process, electrons are transferred to oxygen forming reactive oxygen species (ROS) that must be reduced further to water.

membrane and two mobile electron carriers, ubiquinone (coenzyme Q) and cytochrome c. Electrons are donated to complexes I and II from various respiratory substrates generated by intramitochondrial pathways including NADH and FADH$_2$ from both the TCA cycle and the FAO cycle. They are then transferred down the electrochemical gradient of the RC by a series of sequential redox reactions, finally reducing molecular oxygen and generating two molecules of water. FAD and NAD$^+$ are regenerated, restoring the intramitochondrial redox state. The electron flow through the RC is coupled to the active translocation of hydrogen ions out of the mitochondrial matrix into the intermembrane space. This generates the proton gradient across the membrane that drives the influx of protons back into the mitochondrial matrix through complex V (*ATP synthase*), allowing the phosphorylation of ADP to ATP. This process is called oxidative phosphorylation (OXPHOS) and generates three ATP molecules for each NADH molecule oxidized.

The ROS superoxide is also generated during mitochondrial respiration at complex I and at the interaction of coenzyme Q (CoQ) with complex III. Normally, mitochondrial *manganese superoxide dismutase (MnSOD)* and *mitochondrial glutathione peroxidase* detoxify superoxide to water, but this detoxification process can be overwhelmed by the depletion of reduced mitochondrial glutathione or by a partial block in the flow of electrons within the RC. Accumulation of ROS damages RC protein and mtDNA and induces the mitochondrial permeability transition with loss of the transmembrane potential. The mitochondrial matrix then expands because of water accumulation, leading to the rupture of the outer membrane and the release of proapoptotic proteins from the intermembrane space into the cytosol. Cytochrome c is also released, further depleting the mitochondrial RC. Induction of the mitochondrial permeability transition can result in either apoptosis or necrosis, depending on the number of unpermeabilized residual mitochondria still capable of generating ATP.[91]

Mitochondrial DNA (mtDNA) is a separate genome derived exclusively from the unfertilized ovum. It is a double-stranded closed circular DNA with 16,569 base pairs encoding 37 genes including 2 ribosomal RNAs, 22 tRNAs, and 13 subunits of the RC including subunits of complexes I, III, IV, and *ATPase* (complex V). Great heterogeneity is the rule rather than the exception when considering mtDNA. From the outset, there is a variability of genomes per mature oocyte. Each mitochondrion contains 2 to 10 copies of the mtDNA, and each hepatocyte contains approximately 1000 copies of mtDNA. Somatic mutations occur 10 to 20 times more frequently in mtDNA compared to nuclear DNA because of the absence of protective histones, the lack of an effective excision and recombination repair system, and the constant exposure to ROS generated by OXPHOS in the RC. Both normal and mutant mtDNA can coexist in various proportions in a single cell, a condition called heteroplasmy that allows the persistence of lethal mutations. During cell division, the mitochondria segregate randomly, thus changing the ratio of normal to mutated mtDNA in daughter cells and determining the phenotype of the cell by the relative proportions of the two. The "threshold" of mutated mtDNA required for the phenotypic expression of dysfunction varies among various tissues and even among individuals, which accounts for the wide spectrum in clinical presentation even with the same genotype, and the plasticity of the phenotype with aging. Organs with a high cell turnover such as bone marrow, liver, and intestine may improve with time because cells with less mutated mtDNA have selective survival advantage. Interestingly, organs with low levels of cell replication, such as brain or muscle, appear to deteriorate progressively. Thus, it appears that earlier versus later organ expression is dependent on the tissue's mitotic rate and energy requirements.

Mutations in mtDNA only account for 10 to 15% of RC disorders in pediatric patients.[92] Nuclear DNA encodes the majority of subunits of the RC (more than 70 subunits), including all of complex II and the majority of subunits that compose complexes I, III, IV, and V. Nuclear DNA also encodes proteins that control transcription, translation, salvage, and repair of mtDNA. All of the proteins involved in these processes are translated in the cytosol and then translocated to the mitochondria. To date, more than 100 nuclear genes that result in mtDNA loss when defective have been identified in yeast.[93] But only a small number of nuclear genes that play a role in mtRC disorders resulting in pediatric liver disease have been identified. What is clear is that there is a two-way communication and coordination between the two genomes; that normal mitochondrial protein translation is primarily controlled by nuclear genes; and that abnormal translation can be due to either mutant mtDNA or nuclear DNA mutations that result in mtDNA depletion or disrupt the assembly and stability of RC components. This complex interaction between two genomes accounts for the varied modes of inheritance of the RC defects, including X-linked, autosomal recessive, autosomal dominant, maternal, sporadic, and unknown.

EPIDEMIOLOGY OF RC DISORDERS

The prevalence of inherited mtRC disorders is largely unknown. It is estimated that mtRC disorders of all types affect 1 in 20,000 children under 16 years of age.[94] However, the estimated prevalence in the general population is as high as 1 in 5000.[95] The male:female ratio appears to be approximately 1.5:1.[96] In Sweden, liver involvement was noted in 20% of children with mtRC encephalomyopathies.[97] Ten percent of 234 children with mtRC

disorders seen at a tertiary referral center in France exhibited liver dysfunction, and 50% of those presented with liver disease in the neonatal period.[98]

Inherited disorders of the mtRC may account for a significant proportion of cases of acute liver failure of unknown etiology, especially in infants less than 2 years of age. A recent prospective multicentered study of acute liver failure in 331 children from North America and Europe included 36 children (11%) with metabolic diseases.[99] In the children less than 3 years of age, metabolic disease accounted for 19% of the total number, and all 7 of the patients with mtRC disorders fell into this group, presenting between 1 week and 24 months of age. In Japan, a recent study of 8 infants less than 8 months of age at the time of a clinical presentation of idiopathic acute liver failure showed that 4 patients had mtDNA depletion syndromes with very low activities of complexes I, III, and IV.[100] Mitochondrial RC disorders should be added to the limited list of diseases including neonatal hemochromatosis, galactosemia, tyrosinemia 1, overwhelming viral hepatitis, and familial hemophagocytic lymphohistiocytosis that cause liver failure in the first weeks of life.

CLINICAL PRESENTATION

Prenatal abnormalities are reported in a large proportion of patients diagnosed with mtRC disorders, including most prominently intrauterine growth retardation in 25%, prematurity in 10 to 15%, and a variety of fetal abnormalities including polyhydramnios, hydrops, hypertrophic cardiomyopathy, cardiac rhythm abnormalities, ventricular septal defects, cataracts, and hydronephrosis.[101] Studies in human fetal tissues show that RC complexes are fully assembled and function between 11 and 15 weeks in heart, liver, muscle, brain, and kidney.[102] Although, infants and children with liver disease caused by inherited mtRC disorders have a heterogeneous presentation, they often manifest nonspecific symptoms in the first weeks of life.[103] Poor suck and feeding, vomiting, and failure to thrive are the most common findings. Intestinal dysmotility with abdominal distention, constipation, and diarrhea have also been documented in some patients.

Neonatal Liver Failure

Most infants presenting with early liver failure exhibit the following major clinical features: (1) onset in the first week of life, (2) transient hypoglycemia, (3) neurologic involvement with severe hypotonia and myoclonic seizures, and (4) a rapidly fatal course. However, it is important to note that some infants who present with neonatal liver failure have minimal or no neurologic findings at the time of presentation and have no abnormal findings using standard magnetic resonance (MR) or CT brain imaging.[104] The involvement of siblings of both sexes, the lack of affected parents, and the presence of consanguinity in many cases all point to a nuclear gene mutation with autosomal recessive inheritance. Biochemical evidence of liver synthetic failure (hypoglycemia, hypoalbuminemia, hyperammonemia, and coagulopathy) is always evident, even in the presence of relatively modest elevations of aminotransferases (2 to 20 times normal). Direct hyperbilirubinemia is common, in contrast to FAO disorders that affect the liver. Elevated tyrosine, phenylalanine, methionine, and markedly increased α-fetoprotein are nonspecific indicators of severe liver disease but may invite confusion with hereditary tyrosinemia. Key diagnostic features include an elevated plasma lactate concentration, an elevated molar ratio of plasma lactate to pyruvate (often more than 30 mol/mol with normal less than 20:1), and an increased ratio of β-hydroxybutyrate to acetoacetate, above 2.0 mol/mol. An elevated CSF lactate and lactate-to-pyruvate ratio may also be present and may be a more reliable indicator than plasma lactate in patients with neurologic symptoms.[105]

Liver biopsy specimens typically show microvesicular or, at times, macrovesicular steatosis. Hepatocellular and canalicular cholestasis, bile ductular proliferation, isolated hepatocyte necrosis, periportal and/or bridging fibrosis, cirrhosis, and iron deposition in hepatocytes and sinusoidal cells are present in varying proportions depending on the chronicity of the disease. Neonatal giant cell hepatitis has been reported in a few patients. Ultrastructural studies have revealed proliferation and crowding of mitochondria, dilated and distorted cristae, megamitochondria, dense accumulation of the mitochondrial matrix, and diminished prominence of matrix granules.[106,107] Mitochondrial proliferation is commonly observed in affected tissues of patients with mtRC disorders and is believed to be a compensatory mechanism triggered by the reduction in OXPHOS activity.[108]

Analysis of RC complex subunit activity in liver or muscle usually shows low activity of complexes I, III, IV (cytochrome c oxidase deficiency), and V. However, some patients have been reported in whom only liver tissue RC activity was informative at the time of presentation, with normal enzyme activity in muscle and skin fibroblasts. These findings emphasize the importance of analyzing the most severely affected organ. Even in infants with predominant neurologic involvement and minimal hepatic disease, liver biopsy can be revealing by showing RC enzyme deficiencies.[109] Liver failure usually progresses to death within weeks to months, although some infants have a more prolonged course.

Delayed-Onset Liver Failure

Several previously described disorders of delayed-onset liver failure have now been found to result from mtDNA depletion secondary to mutations in key nuclear genes. Infants with *Alpers-Huttenlocher syndrome* appear to be normal at birth and then present between 2 and 24 months of age with nonspecific symptoms of hypotonia, feeding difficulties, gastroesophageal reflux, failure to thrive, and ataxia. In some series, there is a strong male predominance.[110] Psychomotor regression, refractory mix-typed or myoclonic seizures, cortical blindness, and the onset of liver disease may occur spontaneously or be triggered by an intercurrent infection. Hepatic failure precipitated by influenza A or herpesvirus infection has been reported.[111,112] These cases suggest that evaluation for mtDNA depletion syndromes should be considered in patients with acute liver failure during infancy even if it appears to be triggered by a viral infection. Progressive neurologic deterioration may occur rapidly or may be less severe and occur later in the first decade. Most children will have elevated CSF lactate and lactate-to-pyruvate ratio, characteristic electroencephalographic findings, and low-density areas of atrophy in the occipital or temporal lobes.[113,114]

The administration of valproic acid in children with Alpers-Huttenlocher syndrome has been associated with marked deterioration to fulminant liver failure.[115,116] At times, progression of liver disease is insidious and only discovered by detecting persistently elevated aminotransferases while monitoring valproate levels. However, evidence of liver synthetic failure is often already present, with low serum albumin and elevated ammonia and prothrombin time indicative of a poor prognosis. Liver biopsies show microvesicular steatosis, mild inflammation, and focal hepatocyte necrosis until the disease progresses just before death, when there is rapid loss of viable hepatocytes without marked elevations of aminotransferases. This finding suggests that apoptosis, not necrosis, is the predominant pathway of hepatocyte cell death.[117] Typical findings at autopsy are micronodular cirrhosis, with marked loss of hepatocyte mass, steatosis, and bile ductular proliferation.

Navajo neurohepatopathy (NNH) is a sensorimotor neuropathy with progressive liver disease that has been described in full-blooded Navajo children with an incidence of 1:1600 live births.[118] It was originally thought of as a neurodegenerative disease characterized by weakness, hypotonia, areflexia, loss of sensation in the extremities, acral mutilation, corneal ulceration, loss of myelinated fibers in peripheral nerve biopsies, and progressive brain white matter lesions.[119] Subsequently, it was shown that liver failure was the dominant clinical feature in infants who died within the first 2 years of life with or without neurologic findings. Another subgroup of older children was also described with more slowly progressive liver disease and Reye syndrome–like episodes resulting in chronic cholestasis and cirrhosis.[120] Even in patients with the "classical" late neurodegenerative form, liver dysfunction and even cirrhosis is present. Liver histology demonstrates portal fibrosis or micronodular cirrhosis, micro- and macrovesicular steatosis, multinucleated giant cells, and cholestasis. Blood lactate levels and lactate-to-pyruvate ratios are often normal. These patients have now been shown to have a mitochondrial DNA depletion syndrome caused by mutations in MPV17, a nuclear gene that encodes for a mitochondrial inner membrane protein thought to be important in the maintenance of mitochondrial DNA.[121]

Pearson's marrow-pancreas syndrome was originally described in 1979 in four infants with severe macrocytic anemia, variable neutropenia and thrombocytopenia, vacuolation of erythroid and myeloid precursors, and ringed sideroblasts in the bone marrow.[122] Diarrhea and malabsorption with partial villous atrophy and pancreatic insufficiency associated with extensive pancreatic fibrosis and acinar atrophy develop early in childhood. Marked enlargement of the liver, hepatic steatosis, hemosiderosis, and cirrhosis associated with liver failure and death occur in some patients in by 4 years of age.[123] 3-Methylglutaconic aciduria, seen in other mtRC disorders, is also present in Pearson's syndrome and is thought to be a useful marker for this disorder.[124] Large (3500 to 5000 bp) deletions of mitochondrial DNA have now been shown in the majority of cases, with complex I of the RC the most severely affected.

Other clinical manifestations of Pearson's syndrome include renal tubular disease, patchy erythematous skin lesions, photosensitivity, diabetes mellitus, and the late development of pigmentary retinopathy, tremor, ataxia, proximal muscle weakness, and external ophthalmoplegia. These latter features are also found in Kearns-Sayre syndrome, a mitochondrial RC disease also characterized by a large (5 kb) mtDNA deletion.[125] The occurrence of Kearns-Sayre syndrome in patients with Pearson's syndrome who survive into later childhood is an example of the dependence of phenotypic expression on random partitioning of mutated mtDNA during cell division and alterations in the proportion of deleted mtDNA in various tissues over time.[126]

Supporting this hypothesis is the converse loss of the sideroblastic anemia of Pearson's syndrome with aging, often eliminating the need for red blood cell transfusions after the age of 2 years. Thus, the number of hematopoietic cells containing a high proportion of deleted mtDNA appears to decrease with time as a result of apparent selection of cells with normal mtDNA.

Hepatocellular carcinoma (HCC) has now been reported in several patients with mtDNA depletion syndromes who have survived early childhood, including a patient with NNH at age 11 years, two patients with DGUOK mutations, and two patients with deficiencies in mtRC complexes I, III, and IV of unknown etiology at age 6 and 7 years.[127-129] Significant reductions of RC enzymes and mtDNA are detectable in HCC accompanying cirrhosis of other causes, arguing that these changes may play a role in carcinogenesis.[130] Accumulation of ROS and other intermediate metabolites is thought to be oncogenic in hereditary tyrosinemia, and the same mechanisms may be in play in the pathogenesis of HCC in mtRC defects. Already elevated α-fetoprotein levels at the time of presentation make monitoring for HCC more difficult in these patients, and dictate that frequent imaging be utilized as well.

GENETICS OF MITOCHONDRIAL HEPATOPATHIES

As more is learned about the genetic underpinnings of inherited mitochondrial RC disorders, they are being classified as either those caused by mutations of mtDNA genes or those caused by mutations in nuclear genes that encode RC proteins, or encode enzymes and cofactors integral to the transcription, translation, or maintenance of mtDNA.[131] It is clear that most of the mitochondrial hepatopathies that affect children with presentations of early severe liver disease with or without other features are caused by nuclear DNA mutations and are inherited via an autosomal recessive pattern.[132] Nonmaternal inheritance is substantiated by the fact that introducing mitochondria derived from affected individuals into cells without mtDNA restores normal mtDNA levels.[133] These disorders result in marked depletion of otherwise nonmutated mtDNA and reductions in the activity of most complexes of the RC in the liver (Table 71-4). It is estimated that mtDNA depletion is the basis of approximately 50% of combined mtRC deficiencies in childhood.[134] Examples of nuclear gene mutations responsible for nonhepatic mtDNA depletion syndromes include thymidine kinase (TK) in myopathic mtDNA depletion syndrome, P53-ribonucleotide reductase subunit 2 in myopathic mtDNA depletion syndrome with renal tubular disease,[135] and TYMP encoding for *thymidine phosphorylase* in mitochondrial neurogastrointestinal encephalomyopathy (MNGIE).[136]

Mitochondrial nucleotides for mtDNA synthesis are formed by the salvage of deoxyribonucleosides catalyzed by four different *deoxynucleoside kinases*.[137] Two of them, *thymidine kinase1 (TK1)* and *deoxycytidine kinase*, are localized in the cytosol and their products must enter mitochondria to become available for mtDNA synthesis. The other two enzymes, *TK2 and deoxyguanosine kinase (dGK)*, are found inside mitochondria.[138] The substrate specificity of *TK2* permits the phosphorylation of pyrimidine substrates thymidine and deoxycytidine, and that of *dGK* the phosphorylation of purine substrates, deoxyguanosine and deoxyadenosine.[139]

Nuclear genes that affect the maintenance of mtDNA levels and have been implicated in mutations causing severe pediatric

liver disease secondary to mtDNA depletion include DGUOK encoding for *dGK*; POLG encoding for *DNA polymerase-γ*, and MPV17, whose gene product is currently unknown. DGUOK is the most frequently mutated gene in patients with early hepatocerebral mtDNA depletion syndromes, accounting for up to 50% of cases in some series.[128,134] It encodes for *dGK*, a protein of 260 amino acids that is active in all tissues investigated, with the highest abundance in muscle, brain, liver, and lymphoid tissues.[140] DGUOK mutations generally result in mtDNA content below 10% of controls in liver and in the reduction of enzymatic activities of RC complexes I, III, IV, and V but not complex II, which is solely encoded by nuclear genes. Deficiencies can be confined to the liver and not demonstrated in muscle, illustrating the tissue-specific nature of this disorder.[141] Genotype-phenotype correlation studies show that patients who harbor null mutations (nonsense, splice site, or frame-shift mutations producing truncated proteins) usually have early-onset hepatocerebral disease and die before 2 years of age. Patients carrying missense mutations usually have isolated liver disease without hypotonia, psychomotor retardation, or nystagmus and live into early childhood without the need for liver transplant.[112] Newborn screening reveals elevated plasma tyrosine or phenylalanine, likely indicating significant liver dysfunction already present at the time of birth.

Life-threatening mtDNA depletion syndrome can also result from the administration of nucleoside analogue reverse transcriptase inhibitors (NRTIs) such as zidovudine, didanosine, stavudine, and fialuridine in patients treated for human immunodeficiency virus (HIV) or chronic hepatitis B infections. These drugs require the same kinases (*dGK and TK2*) for their activation, thus competing with the natural nucleoside substrates and providing high levels of analogue dysfunctional nucleotides that can be incorporated into mtDNA by the relatively nonselective *mtDNA polymerase-γ*.[142] Depletion of mtDNA and reduction in RC electron transport further deplete the pyrimidine pool by impairing an enzyme critical for the *de novo* synthesis of pyrimidines, *dihydroorotate dehydrogenase*.

Mutations in the POLG1 gene, mapped to chromosome 2p13, have recently been shown to be the primary genetic cause of the Alpers-Huttenlocher syndrome, accounting for 87% of the cases in one recent large series.[143] POLG1 encodes for *mtDNA polymerase-γ (Pol γ)* that is essential for mtDNA replication and repair.[144] Pol γ is composed of an α subunit that contains *DNA polymerase, exonuclease,* and *deoxyribose phosphate (dRP) lyase* activities, and a β subunit that functions as a DNA binding factor. To date, more than 100 mutations in POLG have been found in patients with a broad clinical spectrum of mitochondrial diseases.[111] Most cases with severe disease onset in childhood are associated with at least one mutation in the linker region and one in the *polymerase* domain. The most common mutation found in 15 sequential probands presenting in early childhood with the clinical features of Alpers-Huttenlocher syndrome was the G1681A mutation in exon 7 (linker region) leading to an Ala467Thr substitution that accounted for 40% of the alleles and was present in 65% of the cases.[144] Recent in vitro data demonstrate that the A467Tmutant protein exhibits only 5% residual *polymerase* activity.[145] This mutation appears to be prevalent in control alleles of northern European populations (1:150 to 1:600 alleles) providing a reservoir for recessive disease.[110] Most affected patients are homozygous or compound heterozygous for mutations on two alleles with autosomal recessive inheritance. However, heterozygous alleles

TABLE 71-4.   Gene Mutations Responsible for Mitochondrial Respiratory Chain Disorders Presenting as Mitochondrial Hepatopathies

Clinical Presentation	Gene	Protein	Effect	Functions
Neonatal Liver Failure	*(nuclear gene)*			
	DGUOK	dGK	mtDNA depletion	nucleotide salvage for mtDNA synthesis
	POLG	pol-γ	mtDNA depletion	mtDNA replication and repair
	MPV-17	mt inner membrane protein	mtDNA depletion	mtDNA maintenance
	EFG-1	mt elongation factor	mtDNA translation	↓ complex I III IV V
	TRMU	5-methylaminomethyl - 2-thiouridylated methyltransferase	mt tRNA translation	thiolation of mt tRNA
	SCO1	copper chaperone of COX	↓ complex IV	transfers copper in complex IV
	BCS1L	assembly protein complex III	↓ complex III	catalyzes electron transfer to cytochrome c
Delayed-Onset liver Failure	*(nuclear gene)*			
Alpers-Huttenlocher	POLG	(see above)	(see above)	(see above)
	PEO 1	Twinkle helicase	mt DNA replication	
Navajo neurohepatopathy	MPV-17	(see above)	(see above)	(see above)
Pearson's syndrome	*(mt gene)*			
	5-kb mtDNA deletion		↓ complex I, III	

COX, cytochrome *c* oxidase.

have been found in some individuals with a family history consistent with autosomal dominant transmission.[110]

A related enzyme central to mtDNA replication called *Twinkle helicase* is encoded by the gene PEO1. Autosomal dominant mutations in PEO1 are responsible for progressive ophthalmoplegia in adults, but recently autosomal recessive mutations have been linked to hepatocerebral syndromes with features similar to Alpers-Huttenlocher syndrome.[146,147] However, these patients usually present with predominantly neurologic signs (spinocerebellar ataxia, hypotonia, athetosis, sensory neuropathy, hearing deficit, ophthalmoplegia, and epilepsy) that develop in early childhood, and milder manifestations of liver disease.

Mutations in MPV17, a gene mapped to chromosome 2p24, have recently been implicated in both NNH and hepatocerebral forms of mtDNA depletion with liver failure in non-Navajo infants.[121,127] In almost all non-Navajo patients, the presentation is dominated by liver failure with neurologic involvement absent or limited to generalized hypotonia with preserved cognitive development. The gene product of MPV17 is unknown but is thought to be localized to the inner mitochondrial membrane and involved in mtDNA maintenance. The knockout mouse model of MPV17 deficiency develops severe mtDNA in the liver, but a compensatory marked increase in mtDNA depletion transcription rate appears to prevent metabolic fragility, marked ultrastructural alterations, or liver failure. Knockout mice survive and later develop gray coats, cochlear degeneration, and focal segmental glomerulosclerosis.[148] This phenotype has not been duplicated in humans, possibly because it appears only late in mouse life.

The sequencing of MPV17 in six Navajo patients with NNH demonstrated the same homozygous disease-causing mutation in exon 2 in all patients, confirming a founder effect.[149] This homozygous R50Q mutation was found in another non-Navajo family from southern Italy, but different homozygous and compound heterozygous MPV17 mutations were responsible for mtDNA depletion in unrelated families from Morocco and Canada.[121] Three subsequent families of middle eastern, Mexican, and European descent were studied, and novel mutations were found associated with drastic reductions in liver mtDNA content to less than 5% of the mean of age and tissue-matched controls.[150] In two of the probands, the initial presentation was dominated by rapidly progressive liver failure in infancy in the absence of neurologic findings. Also, histochemical, ultrastructural, and RC activity studies of skeletal muscle were not informative in two cases whereas assays in liver tissue were more helpful.

Mutant mitochondrial elongation factor G1 (EFG1) is also responsible for a progressive hepatocerebral syndrome described in two siblings.[151] The nuclear gene EFG1 encodes a mitochondrial translation factor with a GTP-binding site. The EFG1 mutation appears to blunt GTP-binding activity with consequent loss of efficiency of mitochondrial translation. The patients were the children of consanguineous Lebanese parents and were characterized clinically by microcephaly, hypertonia, early profound metabolic acidosis with elevated lactate, liver failure evident in the first month of life, and death at 1 and 5 months of age. Reductions in activities of RC complexes I, III, IV, and V but normal levels of complex II were found in skin fibroblasts. Analysis of mtDNA by Southern blotting revealed no rearrangements or reduction in mtDNA levels; however, pulse labeling of the mitochondrial translation products with ^{35}S-methionine in skin fibroblasts showed a decrease in overall mitochondrial translation to approximately 20% of controls.

Mutations in human mt tRNA genes cause the common neurotropic mtRC disorders MELAS (mitochondrial encephalomyelopathy, lactic acidosis, strokelike symptoms), and MERRF (myoclonic epilepsy associated with ragged-red fibers). The transfer RNA methyltransferase U gene (TRMU) encodes *5-methylaminomethyl-2-thiouridylate-methyltransferase*, a sulfur-dependent enzyme responsible for thiolation of tRNA, which is critical for its cognate codon binding affinity. Mutations causing alterations in the codon-anticodon interaction affect the fidelity and efficiency of translation.[152] Thirteen unrelated infants from the Middle East have recently been described who presented with acute liver failure, lactic acidemia, and normal mtDNA content. Four died during the initial acute episodes. Mutations in the TRMU gene in these patients resulted in reduced thiouridylation levels of the mt tRNAs.[153]

Nuclear genes are also responsible for selective deficiencies of individual RC subunits. Mutations in the SCO1 gene, localized on chromosome 17p13.1m, have been found to cause a phenotype of neonatal-onset hepatic failure, lactic acidosis, and neurodevelopmental delay in two siblings.[154] SCO1 is involved in copper delivery to cytochrome c oxidase (COX, complex IV). BCS1L is a nuclear gene encoding proteins involved in the assembly of mtRC complex III. A mutation in BCS1L is associated with deficient activity of complex III in the liver, fibroblasts, and muscle in affected infants who present with hepatic failure, lactic acidosis, renal tubulopathy, and variable degrees of encephalopathy.[155]

DIAGNOSIS OF MITOCHONDRIAL HEPATOPATHIES

Although many features of inherited mitochondrial hepatopathies are nonspecific, the presence of certain clinical and histologic features should raise suspicions about the possibility of a mtRC disorder. Examples of scenarios that should provoke targeted investigations include (1) neonatal liver failure with or without neuromuscular dysfunction; (2) onset of liver dysfunction either spontaneously or provoked by a viral infection or medications such as valproic acid in a young child with chronic neurologic disease; (3) lactic acidosis; (4) hypoglycemia with ketosis; and (5) hepatic micro- or macrovesicular steatosis. Although neurologic dysfunction is often present, its absence should not preclude consideration of a mtRC disorder.

Table 71-5 summarizes laboratory determinations that support the diagnosis. Suggestive findings include a persistently elevated plasma lactate concentration (above 2.5mM) with an elevated arterial ratio of lactate:pyruvate above 20:1 and an elevated plasma ketone body ratio of β-hydroxybutyrate:acetoacetate greater than 2:1. Reduced reoxidation of NADH caused by impaired transfer of electrons from NADH to oxygen in the mtRC will drive the pyruvate produced by glycolysis toward lactate via anaerobic metabolism. However, raised levels of plasma lactate are absent in some patients or may only be intermittently present. Lactic acidemia is usually a feature of complex III or IV deficiencies or mtDNA depletion syndromes presenting as neonatal liver failure but may be relatively mild (2 to 5 mmol/L).[156] In general, it is not found in patients with Alpers-Huttenlocher syndrome or NNH. An elevated CSF lactate or lactate:pyruvate ratio can be more helpful in those settings, but may also be seen in other metabolic disorders, seizures, meningitis, encephalitis, and subarachnoid hemorrhage.[157]

In contrast to disorders of FAO, where prolonged fasting may provoke signature metabolites in the urine and plasma, a provocative test meal can be helpful in generating the lactate:pyruvate and ketone body ratios characteristic of the mtRC disorders. In the postprandial period, more NAD is required for adequate oxidation of glycolytic substrates, but in the presence of decreased NAD and increased NADH, pyruvate will be diverted to lactate. An oral glucose load (2 g/kg) as a test meal and pre and post measurements of lactate, pyruvate, ketone bodies, glucose, and FFA can clarify the picture. However, poor sample preparation or delayed processing may result

TABLE 71-5.   Screening Tests in Mitochondrial Hepatopathies.

Plasma lactate > 2.5 mmol/L
Plasma lactate:pyruvate ratio > 20:1 mol/mol
β-OH butyrate:acetoacetate ratio > 2:1 mol/mol
Increased lactate: pyruvate ratio after oral glucose load (2 g/kg)
Increased urine lactate, succinate, fumarate, malate, 3-methylglutaconic acid, 3-methylglutaric acid
Elevated CSF lactate:pyruvate ratio

Adapted from Treem and Sokal (1998).[2]

in spurious values because of the instability of pyruvate and acetoacetate compared with lactate and β-hydroxybutyrate.

The proximal renal tubular dysfunction present in some mtRC disorders may reduce plasma lactate and increase excretion of urinary lactate and other metabolites. In some cases, gas chromatography–mass spectrometry analysis of the urine will detect elevated lactate, TCA cycle intermediates (succinate, fumarate, malate), and 3-methylglutaconic or 3-methylglutaric acid. However, these metabolites may also be seen in patients with FAO disorders (SCAD, HAD). Because methionine is metabolized by hepatic mitochondrial decarboxylation, ^{13}C-labeled methionine breath tests have been used to measure mitochondrial metabolic function.[158] Reductions in $^{13}CO_2$ exhalation have been correlated with reduced mtDNA:nuclear DNA ratios in HIV-infected patients treated with nucleoside analogues that inhibit mtDNA polymerase-γ. To date, this methodology has not been utilized in patients with inherited mtDNA depletion syndromes.

Liver biopsy provides tissue for light microscopy and for special stains (oil red-O and immunostains for COX, NADH reductase, ATPase, and succinate dehydrogenase); ultrastructural characterization; mtRC enzyme analysis; and quantitative mtDNA and nuclear DNA measurements. The need for substantial tissue for RC analysis, and the presence of coagulopathy especially in young infants presenting with hepatic failure, dictates that an open surgical biopsy be considered in lieu of the percutaneous or transjugular approach. For enzyme measurements, fresh tissue must be frozen immediately and stored at –80° C.

Measurement of RC enzymes can be performed spectrophotometrically using specific electron acceptors and donors.[159] There is considerable variation in the absolute activity of each complex among individuals, but there is a constant ratio of RC enzymes to each other in all human tissues.[160] Thus, in these assays, each enzyme is compared with the activity of another enzyme in the electron transport chain. It is also compared with a non-RC mitochondrial enzyme (e.g., citrate synthase) to help detect a generalized mtRC deficiency, as would be the case in the mtDNA depletion syndromes. A more sensitive enzymatic assay involves analysis of mitochondrial-enriched fractions of liver or other tissues if this technique is available. In addition to liver tissue, other tissues such as muscle, peripheral blood lymphocytes, and cultured skin fibroblasts may be studied. But in patients with early-onset liver failure, analysis of these other tissues may not be revealing. Total nuclear DNA and mtDNA can be extracted from tissue with commercially available DNA isolation kits. The mtDNA copy number in various tissues is measured by real-time quantitative PCR with specific primers. A nuclear single copy gene is amplified with primers and used as a control.

TREATMENT OF MITOCHONDRIAL HEPATOPATHIES

Medical Therapy

Prophylactic measures include avoidance of medications that may enhance hepatotoxicity including most notably valproic acid, as well as nucleoside analogues, acetaminophen, tetracycline, barbiturates, salicylates, ibuprofen, and amiodarone. Vaccinations to prevent viral infections in the liver, including hepatitis A, B, varicella, and influenza, are important protective measures. Careful monitoring for the development of hepatocellular carcinoma is mandatory both pre- and post-liver transplantation.

At present, there are no tested, proven, effective medical therapies for inherited mtRC hepatopathies. Thus, recommendations for medical therapy are based on clinical experience and an emerging understanding of the pathophysiology of mtRC disorders. Small therapeutic trials have been reported, but most have been conducted in primarily myopathic forms of mtRC disorders.[161] Proposed medications fall into the categories of stimulators of mitochondrial respiration, promoters of electron transport, or scavengers of ROS (antioxidants).

Electron acceptors and cofactors include coenzyme Q10 (ubiquinone), idebenone (a CoQ analogue), thiamine, succinate, riboflavin, and menadione (vitamin K$_3$). The most studied is coenzyme Q (CoQ), an electron acceptor from complexes I and II of the RC, that receives electrons from NADH and FADH$_2$.[114] CoQ and idebenone increase OXPHOS activity in isolated hepatic and brain mitochondria and, when exogenously administered, have been effective in maintaining CoQ levels, suppressing lipid peroxidation, and increasing the survival rate in animal models of endotoxemia and ischemia-reperfusion injury.[2] Occasional patients with neurotropic mtRC disorders have been reported who have shown dramatic improvement in muscle strength, decreased incidence of strokelike episodes, and increase in cardiac function after CoQ supplementation.

Menadione (vitamin K$_3$) in conjunction with ascorbate (vitamin C) has been used to donate electrons to cytochrome c, thus avoiding upstream blocks in patients with mitochondrial myopathy secondary to complex II deficiency. Riboflavin is converted to flavin adenine dinucleotide (FAD), a cofactor for electron transport in complexes I and II and electron transfer flavoprotein (ETF). Treatment with riboflavin appears beneficial to a small number of patients with complex I deficiency. Both thiamine, a cofactor for NADH production by *pyruvate dehydrogenase*, and succinate, which enters the RC through complex II, have been given to patients with complex I deficiency. Dichloroacetate is proposed to treat lactic acidosis via stimulus of *pyruvate dehydrogenase* activity. Supportive treatments such as antioxidants (vitamin E, vitamin C) and L-carnitine to correct secondary carnitine deficiency have also been recommended. Unfortunately, these therapies are unlikely to improve the more severe ubiquitous dysfunction encountered in patients presenting in infancy and early childhood with inherited mtRC hepatopathies.

Several experimental medical therapies show promise. Two recent reports document the beneficial effect of uridine supplementation in a human hepatocyte cell culture exposed to stavudine and in a mouse model of zalcitabine-induced hepatotoxicity.[162,163] Both zalcitabine and stavudine are antiretroviral NRTI that interfere with mtDNA replication via their interaction with *mtDNA polymerase-γ*. Human hepatoma Hep2 cells treated with stavudine develop mtDNA depletion, increased generation of ROS, cell cycle arrest, and induction of caspase 3, all of which are reversed by uridine treatment. Mice treated with zalcitabine develop hepatic microvesicular steatosis, ultrastructural changes indicative of mitochondrial injury, mtDNA depletion, reduced *COX* activity, increased ROS, and increased hepatocyte apoptosis. Uridine replenished the nucleoside pool available for mtDNA synthesis through the pyrimidine salvage pathway, and its supplementation in the form of the uridine-rich dietary supplement mitocnol reversed all hepatotoxic abnormalities without apparent side effects. Uridine supplementation has also been shown to prevent muscle mtDNA depletion and toxicity and lactic acidemia in mice treated with Zidovudine, an inhibitor of *thymidine kinase*.[164] Human studies in patients with AIDS being treated with NRTI are underway and show promising initial results. No studies have yet been done in patients with inherited mtDNA depletion syndromes thought to be mediated by impairment of the nucleoside salvage pathways caused by POLG or MPV17 mutations.

Free nucleotide precursors enter mitochondria from the cytosol in the form of nucleotide monophosphates. Another strategy being studied is the supplementation of nucleotide monophosphates to stimulate mtDNA synthesis in patients with mtDNA depletion syndromes. MtDNA depletion can be prevented by supplementation of the purine precursors deoxyadenosine monophosphate (dAMP) and deoxyguanosine monophosphate (dGMP) to *dGK*-deficient fibroblasts.[165] Recent studies in human myotubes from patients with mtDNA depletion due to mutations in DGUOK and POLG1 have shown that dAMP/dGMP supplementation increased mtDNA copy number in DGUOK-deficient myotubes but not in those with POLG1 mutations.[166] In contrast, the pyrimidine substrate uridine did not produce an increase in mtDNA copy number.[2]

Induction of mitochondrial functional mass via pharmacologic or metabolic modulation has also been demonstrated in vitro. Transgenic expression of the human peroxisome proliferators activated receptor-γ (PPAR-γ) coactivator-α (PGC-1α) in mouse skeletal muscle stimulates enhanced OXPHOS activity per muscle mass.[167] Pharmacologic manipulation using the PPAR-α and PPAR-γ agonist bezafibrate produced similar results. When these manipulations were applied to a conditional knockout mouse model of *COX* deficiency in skeletal muscle, they resulted in an increased life span, a prolonged time with normal treadmill performance, restoration of normal muscle *COX* activity, and preservation of muscle ATP levels in COX10 knockouts expressing increased levels of PGC-1α or those treated with bezafibrate. These changes were the result of increased mitochondrial mass, because a reduction of *COX* activity in individual mitochondria to 20% of wild-type continued to be present in the transgenic or bezafibrate-treated animals. It is hypothesized that PGC-1α and bezafibrate result in increased biogenesis of all mitochondria, including those with competent RC activity, thus manipulating the number of metabolically competent cells through heteroplasmy and changing the threshold for phenotypic expression of the disorder.

Liver Transplantation

The multiorgan involvement in many of the mtRC disorders, and the observation that severe extrahepatic manifestations may not develop until after the initial liver-based presentation, have complicated the decision about offering liver transplantation. The overall experience of children with mtRC disorders undergoing liver transplantation shows a 48% survival rate, with 15 of 31 patients dying up to 24 months post transplant.[116,129,168-178] These include 17 patients transplanted with a diagnosis of a mtRC disorder, and the remainder with the diagnosis only confirmed after transplant or by postmortem examination. The causes of death were early postoperative multiorgan failure in 7 of 15, neurologic degeneration with respiratory complications in 5 of 15, and severe pulmonary hypertension in 3 of 15. Of the 16 surviving patients up to 8 years post transplant, only 2 have mild developmental delay. Thus, although the long-term reported survival posttransplant is significantly worse than other forms of liver disease, the quality of life in the survivors is acceptable. However, follow-up to date is relatively short, and unanticipated neuromuscular deterioration may occur in the future.

These data emphasize the need for proper selection of candidates for transplantation who do not have progressive extrahepatic organ dysfunction at the time of transplant and are unlikely to develop it later. Neither early age at onset nor gender is predictive of survival post liver transplantation. Genetic studies have thus far shown only partial correlations between genotype and phenotype. Different mutations can underlie the same phenotype, and different clinical phenotypes occur with the same mutation, even within a single family. Thus, knowledge of the genetic mutation responsible may not be helpful. The one exception may be detection of a POLG mutation, which is found in approximately 90% of patients with Alpers-Huttenlocher syndrome and would prompt an exhaustive search for any neuromuscular abnormalities. Clearly, the most important selection criteria are the presence or absence of significant neuromuscular (nystagmus, hypotonia, psychomotor retardation, seizures) or cardiovascular involvement. When present, these are an absolute contraindication to liver transplantation. Even minor neurologic problems, not attributable simply to developmental delay caused by chronic illness, are likely to predict neurologic deterioration after the surgery.[179] However, renal involvement is only a relative contraindication, with some series describing good outcomes in patients with renal tubulopathies.[180]

Standards for the extrahepatic evaluation of children with inherited mitochondrial hepatopathies have been advanced in the literature. A baseline evaluation, if time permits, includes a careful neurologic examination; an evaluation of renal function, muscle, and pancreatic enzymes; an electrocardiogram and echocardiogram; a fundoscopic examination and electroretinogram; a cranial CT scan; and a lumbar puncture with cerebrospinal fluid (CSF) analysis including lactate and pyruvate. Although an elevated ratio of CSF lactate to pyruvate has been interpreted as indicative of cerebral injury even with normal standard imaging of the brain, there have been such patients reported with good neurocognitive outcomes post transplantation.[128] Neuroimaging using MRI and MR spectroscopy has recently been proposed as a more sensitive method for detecting subtle neurologic deficits.[181] However, even patients with no obvious symptoms and a normal MRI have suffered neurologic deterioration post liver transplant. Specific symptoms such as diarrhea and malabsorption would dictate a small bowel biopsy and possible secretin stimulation test to evaluate for both villous atrophy and pancreatic exocrine insufficiency. If there is a high degree of suspicion for the possibility of a mtRC disorder, a muscle biopsy will often be done at the same time as a liver biopsy and skin biopsy in order to obtain multiple tissues for measurement of RC enzyme activity.

REFERENCES

1. Treem WR. Inborn defects in mitochondrial fatty acid oxidation. In: Suchy F, Sokal E, Balistreri W, editors. Liver Disease in Children. 2nd ed Philadelphia: Lippincott Williams & Wilkins; 2001. p. 735–785.
12. Leone T, Weinheimer C, Kelly D. A critical role for the peroxisome proliferators-activated receptor alpha (PPAR-α) in the cellular fasting response: the PPARα-null mouse as a model of fatty acid oxidation disorders. Proc Natl Acad Sci USA 1999;96:7473–7478.
41. Saudubray J, Martin D, DeLonlay P, et al. Recognition and management of fatty acid oxidation defects: a series of 107 patients. J Inherit Metab Dis 1999;22:488–502.
50. Ibdah J, Bennett M, Rinaldo P, et al. A fetal fatty-acid oxidation disorder as a cause of liver disease in pregnant women. N Engl J Med 1999;340:1723–1731.
68. Sim K, Hammond J, Wilcken B. Strategies for the diagnosis of mitochondrial fatty acid B-oxidation disorders. Clin Chim Acta 2002;323:37–58.
90. Merritt JL, Nguyen T, Daniels J, et al. Biochemical correction of very long-chain acyl-CoA dehydrogenase deficiency following adeno-associated virus gene therapy. Mol Ther 2009;17:425–429.
121. Spinazzola A, Viscomi C, Fernandez-Vizarra E, et al. MPV17 encodes an inner mitochondrial membrane protein and is mutated in infantile hepatic mitochondrial DNA depletion. Nat Genet 2006;38:570–575.
132. Lee WS, Sokal RJ. Mitochondrial hepatopathies: advances in genetics and pathogenesis. Hepatology 2007;45:1555–1565.
150. Wong LJC, Brunetti-Pierri N, Zhang Q, et al. Mutations in the MPV17 gene are responsible for rapidly progressive liver failure in infancy. Hepatology 2007.
155. DeLonlay P, Valnot I, Barrientos A, et al. A mutant mitochondrial respiratory chain assembly protein causes complex III deficiency in patients with tubulopathy, encephalopathy and liver failure. Nat Genet 2001;29:57–60.
160. Chretien D, Rustin P. Mitochondrial oxidative phosphorylation: pitfalls and tips in measuring and interpreting enzyme activities. J Inherited Metab Dis 2003;26:189–198.
162. Lebrecht D, Vargas-Infante YA, Setzer B, et al. Uridine supplementation antagonizes zalcitabine-induced microvesicular steatohepatitis in mice. Hepatology 2007;45:72–79.
166. Bulst S, Abicht A, Holinski-Feder E, et al. In vitro supplementation with dAMP/dGMP leads to partial restoration of mtDNA levels in mitochondrial depletion syndromes. Hum Mol Genet 2009;18:1590–1599.

See expertconsult.com for a complete list of references and the review questions for this chapter.

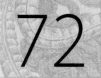

72

ABNORMALITIES OF HEPATIC PROTEIN METABOLISM

H. Hesham A-Kader • Fayez K. Ghishan

α_1-ANTITRYPSIN DEFICIENCY

The description of α_1-antitrypsin deficiency and its association with lung disease was reported 40 years ago by Laurell and Eriksson.[1] The association between α_1-antitrypsin deficiency and hepatic cirrhosis in children was initially identified in 1969 by Sharp and coworkers.[2] Since these original observations, it has become clear that α_1-antitrypsin deficiency is a relatively common genetic disorder, affecting one in 1600 to one in 2000 live births and resulting in liver disease in infants, children, and adults, as well as lung disease primarily in adults.[3]

Characteristics of the α_1-Antitrypsin Protein

α_1-Antitrypsin is a 52-kDa glycoprotein that is secreted by the hepatocytes and, to a minor extent, other tissues including lung epithelial cells, macrophages, renal tubular, and small intestinal epithelial cells.[4] The half-life of α_1-antitrypsin is approximately 4 to 5 days.[5] The function of α_1-antitrypsin protein is to inhibit chymotrypsin, pancreatic elastase, skin collagenase, renin, urokinase, Hageman factor/cofactor, and the neutral proteases of neutrophils.[6] α_1-Antitrypsin protein belongs to a large gene family of serine protease inhibitors referred to as serpins.[7, 8]

α_1-Antitrypsin is composed of 394 amino acids arranged into three β-sheets (A, β, and C), nine α-helices (A through I), and immobile inhibitory reactive center loop. The interaction between α_1-antitrypsin and proteases occurs by the formation of a 1-1 complex.[9] α_1-Antitrypsin protein is present in tears, duodenal fluid, saliva, nasal secretions, cerebral spinal fluid, pulmonary secretions, and mother's milk. α_1-Antitrypsin acts as an acute-phase reactant and increases in the setting of inflammation, neoplastic disease, and pregnancy. However, in patients with α_1-antitrypsin deficiency, these stimuli do not induce α_1-antitrypsin protein.[10]

Phenotyping of α_1-Antitrypsin

The serum level of α_1-antitrypsin in the plasma ranges from 100 to 200 mg/dL. This plasma level is determined by both α_1-antitrypsin gene alleles, which are codominantly inherited. Several techniques including protein electrophoresis on starch gels and isoelectric focusing have contributed to our understanding of the variation in α_1-antitrypsin.[11, 12] α_1-Globulins appear in this system as a series of characteristic bands of variable intensity. The α_1-antitrypsin variants included in an allelic system are called the Pi (protease inhibitor) system and are named based on their migration velocity in the starch-gel electrophoresis. Faster-moving protein complexes are identified by earlier letters in the alphabet, and the slowest-moving protein is labeled Z.

Thus, the variants of α_1-antitrypsin are labeled as M (medium), S (slow), F (fast), or Z (very slow).[13]

Three major categories of α_1-antitrypsin variants have been identified as useful clinical markers[14]:
1. Normal; this category includes the four more common M variants (M_1-M_4)
2. Deficient, those are characterized by the α_1-antitrypsin variants Z and S, and a number of less-frequent variants, such as M_{Malton}, $M_{Procida}$
3. Null, in which no detectable α_1-antitrypsin level is seen

There are currently at least 100 different alleles of α_1-antitrypsin that have been described. The normal allele is the PiM type with overall allelic frequency of 0.95. The next two most common alleles in the United States are PiS at 0.03 and PiZ at 0.01. Blacks have lower frequencies of these alleles. The highest prevalence of PiZ variant has been reported in Northern and Western European countries, peaking in Southern Scandinavia, Denmark, the Netherlands, the UK, and Northern France.[15] Table 72-1 depicts the relationship between Pi phenotypes and serum concentration of α_1-antitrypsin.

Genetics of α_1-Antitrypsin Deficiency

The gene encoding α_1-antitrypsin (SERPINA 1) has been cloned and is located on chromosome 14q31-32.2.[16-19] The α_1-antitrypsin gene is 12.2 kb in length and consists of seven exons, designated I_A, I_B, I_C, I (noncoding), and II, III, IV, and V (coding). Exons II through IV are translated into 52-kDa protein. The same gene is responsible for the α_1-antitrypsin production in the liver, lung, and macrophages. The first two exons (I_A, I_B) and a short 5' segment of I_C are included in the primary transcript in the macrophages, but not in hepatocytes.[20] The protein has three asparagine-linked branched oligosaccharide moieties. The basis for the genetic defect in the PiZ type of α_1-antitrypsin deficiency is the substitution of lysine for glutamic acid at position 342 from the carboxy terminus in the Z-type protein.[21,22]

Several mutations within the SERPINA1 gene have been found to cause deficiency. The prevalence of the three major α_1-antitrypsin variants (PiM, PiZ, and PiS) is reported as gene frequencies (the frequency of a variant in homozygotes). The highest prevalence of the PiZ variant has been recorded in European populations with a peak in Southern Scandinavia, Denmark, the Netherlands, UK, and Northern France.[23-25] Most recent surveys indicate that α_1-antitrypsin deficiency is also prevalent in populations in the Middle East and North Africa, Central and Southern Africa, and Central and Southeast Asia.[26] However, in Far East Asia, the gene frequency of α_1-antitrypsin

TABLE 72-1. Relationship between Pi Phenotypes and Serum Concentrations of α_1-Antitrypsin

Phenotype	Serum Concentration (%)
MM	100
MZ	60
SS	60
FZ	60
M-	50
PS	40
SZ	42.5
ZZ	15
Z-	10
–	0

deficiency is rather rare, especially in Japan and Far Eastern populations.[26]

Clinical Manifestations of α_1-Antitrypsin Deficiency

Liver Disease in Children

Neonatal cholestasis is the first manifestation of α_1-antitrypsin deficiency and is commonly seen in the first few weeks of life.[27,28]The affected babies are generally small for gestational age, and clinically, the liver is mildly enlarged. Acholic stools and dark urine may be seen. Biochemically, these patients have elevated conjugated bilirubin and mildly elevated serum aminotransferase levels. Alkaline phosphatase and γ-glutamyl transpeptidase are also elevated. The jaundice usually disappears during the second to the fourth months of life. Neonates may present with cirrhosis[29] or bleeding diathesis, including intracranial hemorrhage.[30]

The histological picture of the liver may be helpful in predicting the outcome of the liver disease. A picture similar to neonatal hepatitis, portal fibrosis with bile duct proliferation, or intrahepatic duct hypoplasia may be noted in the biopsies. Patients with portal fibrosis and bile duct proliferation appear to have worse outcomes.[31] However, the whole mark of the liver biopsy in these patients is the deposition of the PAS (periodic acid-Schiff) stain diastase resistant α_1-antitrypsin depositions in the periportal hepatocytes.[32]

The number of infants presenting with neonatal cholestasis was addressed in a large prospective study of 200,000 Swedish newborns in which 120 PiZ patients were identified.[33-35] Fourteen of the 120 PiZ infants had prolonged obstructive jaundice, and nine had severe clinical laboratory evidence of liver disease. Five patients had only laboratory evidence of liver disease. Eight other PiZ infants had minimal abnormalities in serum bilirubin and hepatic enzyme activity and variable hepatosplenomegaly. Approximately 50% of the remaining patients with PiZ had only abnormal aminotransferase levels. Follow-up studies of these patients at 18 years of age showed that more than 85% had persistently normal serum transaminase levels. Forty-eight patients with the phenotype PiSZ were identified in this study. None of these infants had clinical liver disease, but 10 of 42 patients at 3 months and 1 of 22 at 6 months of age had abnormal liver function tests.

In the United States, screening of 107,038 newborns had shown that 21 infants were found to have the phenotype PiZ.

Of the 18 infants followed, only one had neonatal cholestatic jaundice, and five had hepatomegaly and biochemical abnormalities or both. At 3 to 6 years of age, none of the children had evidence of hepatic cirrhosis.[36] Other reports indicate that patients with PiZ who present with neonatal cholestasis are more likely to develop serious liver disease in the future compared to those infants without a history of neonatal cholestatic jaundice.[37] The overall risk of death from liver disease in PiZ children during childhood is estimated at 2 to 3%. Boys are at higher risk compared to girls. Why some patients with PiZ have worse liver disease than others is not known. However, genetic and/or environmental factors may play a role.[38]

Liver Disease in Adults

Single case reports and retrospective studies have suggested that adult patients with PiZ are likely to develop liver disease and hepatocellular carcinoma.[39-41] Therefore, it does appear that α_1-antitrypsin deficiency should be considered in the differential diagnosis of any adult patient with abnormal liver function tests, liver cirrhosis, portal hypertension, or hepatocellular carcinoma. It is estimated that the risk of developing cirrhosis in adults with α_1-antitrypsin deficiency is about 10%.[42]

A retrospective study on 17 autopsied cases of α_1-antitrypsin deficiency identified in Sweden indicated a strong relation between α_1-antitrypsin deficiency, liver cirrhosis, and primary liver cancer.[39] However, the study suggests that male patients are the ones who are at higher risk of development of liver cirrhosis and hepatoma in α_1-antitrypsin deficiency.

The relationship between cirrhosis and partial deficiency or heterozygotic phenotype of α_1-antitrypsin has not been addressed on a larger scale in the literature. A number of case reports indicate the association of adult-onset liver cirrhosis with PiSZ.[43-45] In one study, there was an increased prevalence of phenotype MZ in patients with cryptogenic liver cirrhosis and with non-B chronic hepatitis.[46] However, in another prospective study, the heterozygote state occurred with approximately equal frequencies in patients with and without hepatobiliary disease.[47]

A subset (approximately 3 to 5%) of patients with cystic fibrosis (CF) develops severe liver disease with portal hypertension. It has been reported recently that the α_1-antitrypsin deficiency (SERPINA1) Z allele is a risk factor for liver disease in CF. Patients who carry the Z allele are at greater risk (odds ratio approximately 5) of developing severe liver disease with portal hypertension.[48]

In general, there is a suggestion that a partial deficiency of α_1-antitrypsin is more likely to predispose these patients to liver injury. What is clear is that patients with cirrhosis and α_1-antitrypsin deficiency are at risk of developing hepatocellular carcinoma. Indeed, Eriksson found six hepatomas in the nine cirrhotic adults who were phenotypically PiZ patients. Four of these tumors were hepatocellular carcinoma, and two were cholangiocarcinoma.[42, 48]

Liver disease has also been associated with several other allelic variants of α_1-antitrypsin deficiency, such as PiM_{Malton}, Pi_{FZ}, Pi_W, PiM_{Duarte}, and PiS_{iiyama}.[38]

Lung Disease

The development of lung disease in the pediatric patient is exceedingly rare, despite several reports that suggest that these patients do have increased respiratory infections. However, it is clear that adults who are smokers will most likely develop emphysema.[49,50] Autopsy studies indicate that approximately 60% of patients with PiZ develop clinically significant lung injury.

Pathophysiology of Liver Disease in α_1-Antitrypsin Deficiency

The mutation in PiZ α_1-antitrypsin leads to the deposition of globules of an amorphous material within the hepatocyte, particularly in the periportal areas. These globules, which have been shown to enlarge as the infant matures, are seen by positive PAS staining after treatment of the liver biopsy specimen with diastase. These globules are formed secondary to the accumulation of the mutated α_1-antitrypsin molecule and occur in the endoplasmic reticulum. Studies have suggested that the proper folding or assembly of the polypeptides is a prerequisite for their exit from the endoplasmic reticulum. Misfolding of the α_1-antitrypsin variants allows the protein to be retained. The substitution of glutamine 342 for lysine in the α_1-antitrypsin Z variant results in reducing the stability of the molecule in its monomeric form to a polymeric form by way of a mechanism termed loop-sheet insertion.[32,51,52]

It appears that the mutation in the PiZ α_1-antitrypsin that is located at the head of the strand 5A and at the base of the mobile reactive loop would open the β-sheet A between strands 3 and 5 to favor the incorporation of the reactive loop from a second α_1-antitrypsin molecule to produce the dimer, which then extends to form chains of loop-sheet polymers. The demonstration of spontaneous polymerization of the PiZ α_1-antitrypsin at 37°, whereas the normal M variant remains in its native confirmation, supported the observations by Lomas's group.[32] Thus, within the hepatocyte, the PiZ α_1-antitrypsin is degraded by both proteasomes dependent and independent pathways, and it appears that the clearing mechanism in those patients is inefficient.[52]

Indeed, this polymerization of the α_1-antitrypsin is not unique, as it does occur in other members of the serpin family, such as antithrombin, C1 inhibitor, and α_1-antichymotrypsin, to cause deficiency in the plasma level of these molecules, resulting in thrombosis, angioedema, and emphysema respectively. These serpin family disorders have been called conformational diseases.[53]

Not all patients with α_1-antitrypsin deficiency will develop liver disease. Therefore, other factors must be involved in the pathogenesis of the disease, including increased production or decreased degradation. A possible mechanism is the serpin-enzyme complex that is activated by α_1-antitrypsin -elastase complex or other inflammatory mediators. Defects in hepatic proteasome action or other mechanisms involved in removing abnormal protein from the endoplasmic reticulum may lead to excessive accumulation of abnormal α_1-antitrypsin in the hepatocytes. A possible mechanism is that susceptible individuals may have delayed intracellular degradation of the mutant protein, resulting from abnormalities in calnexin, a protein that interacts with the mutant α_1-antitrypsin protein in the endoplasmic reticulum. New therapeutic modalities such as the administration of chemical chaperones are aimed at targeting these mechanisms.[147-149]

Whereas liver injury results from retained alpha α_1-antitrypsin glycoprotein in the endoplasmic reticulum, the mechanism of lung injury is different. Lung damage occurs as a result of uninhibited proteolytic changes of the connective tissue secondary to low concentration of circulating α_1-antitrypsin.

Pathology of Liver Disease in α_1-Antitrypsin Deficiency

The hallmark of α_1-antitrypsin deficiency is the distinctive accumulation of PAS-positive, diastase-resistant globules in the endoplasmic reticulum in the periportal hepatocytes. These globules enlarge with increasing age. With hematoxylin-eosin staining, they appear as eosinophilic deposits in the cytoplasm of the hepatocytes. These globules have also been observed in heterozygous individuals.

The absence of liver disease in the few Pi-null individuals who have no deposits of these globules indicates that the deposition of the abnormal α_1-antitrypsin in the liver has a significant role in the pathogenesis of liver disease.[54] Electron-microscopy studies show that these amorphous deposits are primarily within the dilated rough endoplasmic reticulum.[55] Liver biopsies in neonates with α_1-antitrypsin deficiency have shown three morphological patterns of hepatic alteration, including hepatocellular damage with a picture compatible with neonatal hepatitis portal fibrosis with biliary duct proliferation and biliary duct hypoplasia.[31]

Diagnosis of α_1-Antitrypsin Deficiency

Circulating levels of α_1-antitrypsin is between 100 to 200 mg/dL. However, low serum level per se does not indicate the presence of α_1-antitrypsin deficiency, because this level could be low secondary to losses of α_1-antitrypsin in the gastrointestinal tract or in the lung. Therefore, determination of the α_1-antitrypsin phenotype by isoelectric focusing or by agarose electrophoresis at acid pH is indicated. α_1-Antitrypsin deficiency should be suspected in neonates with picture of neonatal hepatitis or in children and adults with unexplained chronic liver disease. Liver biopsies should be stained with PAS following diastase treatment to determine the presence of α_1-antitrypsin globules in the periportal hepatocytes.

Treatment of α_1-Antitrypsin Deficiency

The two major clinical problems in α_1-antitrypsin deficiency are emphysema and liver disease resulting in cirrhosis. Therefore, avoidance of smoking is the most important step in preventing the development of emphysema, because smoking accelerates the destructive lung disease. Once the patient develops cirrhosis, a liver transplant is the only viable option for these patients.[56] Replacement therapy of α_1-antitrypsin deficiency has been done in emphysema patients and found to be effective in raising the concentration of α_1-antitrypsin in the serum and in the lung.[57] The α_1-antitrypsin in the lung has been shown to be active in neutralizing the neutrophil elastases. A recombinant α_1-antitrypsin has been produced in *Escherichia coli* and in yeast and was noted to be functional as an elastase inhibitor.[58,59] However, because the recombinant α_1-antitrypsin lacks the carbohydrate side chain, this product is unstable with a short half-life.

Efforts to induce α_1-antitrypsin using danazol (isoxazole derivative of 17-ethinyl testosterone) have been show to increase serum levels of α_1-antitrypsin in only about 50% of deficient patients.[60] However, the potential hepatotoxicity has hampered the efforts to utilize danazol as a potential therapeutic agent. Moreover, whereas raising the level of α_1-antitrypsin in the serum has an effect on lung disease, it has no effect on liver disease. Novel therapies to inhibit the polymerization of the α_1-antitrypsin molecule or enhance its secretion[38] and gene therapy utilizing adeno-associated virus as vector are potential therapeutic targets in the future.[61]

Concordant results of prospective cohort studies suggest that augmentation therapy has efficacy in slowing the rate of decline of lung function in patients with moderate airflow obstruction and severe deficiency of α_1-antitrypsin. Although augmentation therapy is well tolerated, it does not satisfy criteria for cost-effectiveness.[145,146]

Few patients with metabolic defects of liver function have been treated with hepatocyte transplantation, including patients with urea cycle disorder, ornithine transcarbamoylase deficiency, Crigler-Najjar syndrome, and α_1-antitrypsin deficiency. Hepatocyte transplantation at this time is still considered an experimental procedure but may prove to be an effective therapeutic modality in the future for the treatment of patients with metabolic liver disease or as a bridge for those waiting for liver transplantation.[142]

TYROSINEMIA

Several genetic and acquired hepatic disorders can result in impaired degradation of the aromatic amino acid tyrosine (Table 72-2). The degradation of tyrosine (Figure 72-1) is catalyzed by a series of five enzymatic reactions yielding acetoacetate as well as the Krebs cycle intermediate fumarate. The complete pathway is expressed in only two cell types: the hepatocytes and renal proximal tubules, which contain sufficient quantities of the five enzymes required for tyrosine metabolism.

The most common cause of hypertyrosinemia is transient tyrosinemia of the newborn.[62,63] The condition results from immaturity of the liver and the enzymes involved in the degradation process. Transient tyrosinemia of the newborn, which used to be a common finding, is now a much more rare condition because of advanced neonatal management. Hypertyrosinemia and increased urinary excretion of tyrosine metabolites can result from hepatic dysfunction of any cause.

Although autosomal-recessive enzyme deficiencies have been reported for four of the five degradation reactions, elevated blood tyrosine level is not seen in all these conditions, and liver disease is seen in only one of these disorders, which is hereditary tyrosinemia type I (HTI).

Hepatorenal Tyrosinemia (Hereditary Tyrosinemia Type I)

Hepatorenal tyrosinemia, which is also referred to as hereditary tyrosinemia type I, was first reported by Sakai and Kitwaga in 1957[64-66] in a patient who developed progressive liver disease complicated with bleeding and coma resulting in death

at the age of 3 years. The patient also had rickets, which was resistant to vitamin D. In a report of seven patients, Gentz, Jagenburg, and Zetterstroem described the renal component of the disorder.[67] Neurological crises similar to porphyria led to the recognition that δ-aminolevulinic acid was excreted in large amounts.[68-70] Succinylacetone (SA) found in the urine of patients with tyrosinemia is an inhibitor of the synthesis of porphobilinogen from δ-aminolevulinic acid.[71]

Pathogenesis

The pathway for tyrosine metabolism is shown in Figure 72-1. Fumarylacetoacetate hydrolase (FAH), the last enzyme in the pathway, was identified by Lindblad et al.[72] as the defect leading to tyrosinemia. FAH deficiency leads to the accumulation of fumarylacetoacetate and maleylacetoacetate and their derivatives succinylacetoacetone (SAA) and succinylacetone (SA). Because fumarylacetoacetate and maleylacetoacetate usually initiate hepatocyte injury, maleylacetoacetate is more likely to lead to renal tubular dysfunction. SA is an inhibitor of the condensation of δ-aminolevulinic acid (δ-ALA) to porphobilinogen in heme synthesis, leading to accumulation of δ-ALA, which is neurotoxic.

Clinical Features

Acute and chronic forms of tyrosinemia are recognized, and both forms can be seen in the same family. Patients with the acute form present with hepatic dysfunction early in life, which

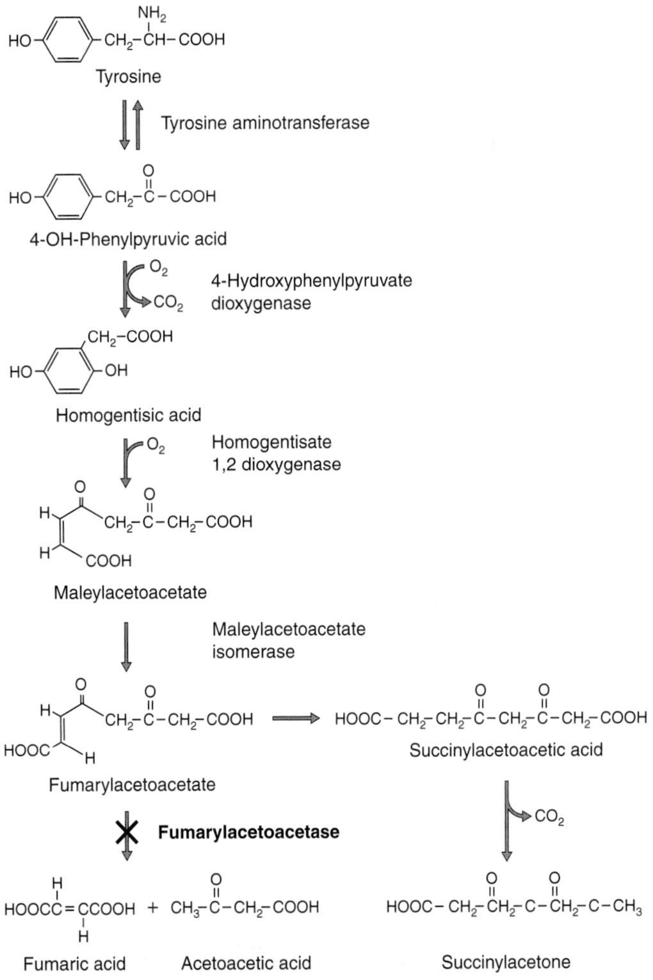

TABLE 72-2. Etiology of Elevated Blood Tyrosine Level

1. Transient tyrosinemia of the newborn
2. Hepatocellular dysfunction
3. Enzyme deficiencies in tyrosine metabolism
   Hepatorenal tyrosinemia (HTI)
   Oculocutaneous tyrosinemia (HT2)
4. OH-phenylpyruvate dioxygenase deficiency (HT3)
5. Hyperthyroidism
6. Scurvy

Figure 72-1. Tyrosine degradation.

is usually fatal during the first 2 years. Symptoms may include vomiting, diarrhea, hepatosplenomegaly, edema, ascites, bleeding diathesis, irritability, and jaundice. In a multicenter study, Van Spronsen et al.[73] showed that 25% of the patients presented during the first 2 years and that their 1- and 2-year survival rate was 38% and 29%, respectively. The earlier the onset, the worse the prognosis. The usual causes of death (35 of 47 deaths) were recurrent bleeding and liver failure. Hepatocellular carcinoma and neurological crisis were also major factors. On the other hand, the chronic form may be a continuation of the acute presentation or may start later during infancy or childhood with manifestations of chronic liver disease and renal tubular defects.

Neurological crises of pain and paresthesia are a result of peripheral neuropathy and are usually seen in patients presenting with the chronic form of the disease. The crises, which are usually precipitated by an infection, can be mistaken for porphyria. Symptoms may also include hypertonia, vomiting, and weakness.[73, 74] Paralysis may develop and progress to complete flaccid paraplegia requiring mechanical ventilation. The onset of neurological crisis is believed to be the result of the accumulation of SA blocking further metabolism of δ-ALA and is not necessarily associated with deterioration of hepatic function.

Hepatocellular carcinoma (HCC) can be seen in up to 37% of patients. The youngest reported patient was 33 months of age.[75] Detection of nodules with ultrasound and CT scan appears to be quite reliable because histological examination of livers of patients who underwent liver transplantation did not reveal carcinoma in patients who did not have nodules by those imaging modalities.[76] A significant rise of α-fetoprotein may herald the development of HCC. However, cancer can be seen in the face of normal levels.[76] Patients should be monitored by ultrasound, or CT scan, and α-fetoprotein on a regular basis.

Diagnosis

The diagnosis of tyrosinemia should be considered in any infant with neonatal liver disease and, later in life, in any child with undiagnosed liver disease or rickets. It is important that the diagnosis be made promptly in order to initiate medical treatment and prevent the evolution of hepatic fibrosis and cirrhosis. Patients with acute tyrosinemia often have evidence of impairment of hepatic synthetic function disproportionate to biochemical indices of liver injury. This is evidenced by hypoalbuminemia and marked coagulopathy, with only a mild to moderate rise in aminotransferase values. Hemolytic anemia and hypoglycemia may be present with a variable rise in total and direct bilirubin. The renal tubular dysfunction consists of Fanconi's syndrome with hyperphosphaturia, glucosuria, proteinuria, and aminoaciduria. Marked elevation of serum tyrosine is usually seen at levels higher than those seen in other liver disorders. Other features include hypermethioninemia, urinary excretion of phenolic acid by-products of tyrosine (p-hydroxyphenyllactic acid, p-hydroxyphenylpyruvic acid, and p-hydroxyphenylacetic acid), which can be screened for with nitrosonaphthol; SA and SAA in urine; and increased urinary excretion of δ-ALA.[102] Patients with the acute disease may have generalized aminoacidemia with a disproportionate elevation of serum levels of tyrosine and methionine, whereas later in life aminoacidemia is usually limited to tyrosine.

The presence of greatly increased amounts of α-fetoprotein, in the presence of normal levels of tyrosine in cord blood of affected infants, suggests that hypertyrosinemia may develop.

In the acute form, there is fatty infiltration of the liver; iron deposition; varying degrees of liver cell necrosis, which may be extreme; and fine diffuse fibrosis with formation of pseudoacini. Older children may exhibit gross multilobular cirrhosis, regenerative nodules and bile duct proliferation.[77,78]

Genetics and Prenatal Diagnosis

HTI is an uncommon inborn error of metabolism. The incidence of the disease is 1:100,000 to 1:120,000. However, the incidence is much greater in certain areas such as northern Europe and Quebec, Canada. The frequency of heterozygotes in the population of the Lac-Saint-Jean region in Quebec has been estimated to be about 7%.[79]

The human FAH cDNA has been cloned and mapped to chromosome 15.[80] The common mutations responsible for the clustering of cases in certain areas of the world have been identified.[81, 82] The IVS12+5G>A → a splice mutation, which is found in most cases of acute tyrosinemia in the HTI French Canadian cluster, also occurs in the chronic phenotype. Thus both clinical forms of HTI can result from the same mutation, and genetic heterogeneity is not a sufficient explanation for the clinical heterogeneity of the disorder.[83]

Prenatal diagnosis can be made by screening amniotic fluid for succinylacetone. However, false negative results have been reported.[84,85] FAH can be also screened in amniotic cells.[86] Diagnosis can be also made by direct mutation detection[87] and linkage analysis taking advantage of the presence of several intragenic polymorphic markers.[88,89] Newborn screening is performed in areas with high prevalence of the disorder such as the Canadian province of Quebec.

A mosaic pattern of immunoreactive FAH protein was found in livers removed from patients with HTI for transplantation was reported by Kvittingen et al.[90,91] Analysis for the tyrosinemia-causing mutations revealed that the immunonegative liver tissue contained the FAH mutations demonstrated in fibroblasts of the patients, whereas in the immunopositive nodules of regenerating liver tissue, mutation reversion was seen. The genetic mosaicism may explain the variability in the clinical manifestations of the disease, even within the same family. It is possible that patients with a larger mass of reverted hepatocytes may have the mild form of the disease. However, this remains to be further defined.

Treatment

Dietary restriction of phenylalanine and tyrosine has been the traditional treatment for patients with tyrosinemia. Dietary management has been shown to be effective for the renal tubular disease and the metabolic bone disease. However, there is no evidence that it prevents the development of cirrhosis or HCC.

NTBC (2-(2-nitro-4-trifluoromethylbenzoyl)-1,3-cyclohexanedione) belongs to a class of compounds developed in the 1980s as bleaching herbicides. During animal studies it was noted that rats treated with NTBC developed corneal ulceration, a hallmark of elevated tyrosine level in rats and humans. It was then found out that NTBC is an inhibitor of 4-hydroxyphenylpyruvate dioxygenase (HPD). In 1992 Lindstedt et al.[92] proposed that the inhibition of HPD by NTBC can prevent the accumulation of maleylacetoacetate and fumarylacetoacetate and their derivatives (SAA and SA).

Recently the results of treating more than 300 patients with NTBC were reviewed.[93,94] Marked hepatic improvement was seen in more than 95% of the patients. Renal functions also improved, and Fanconi's syndrome was avoided. A large number of patients have been on the drug more than 5 years (up to 9 years) without significant side effects. Typically NTBC is started at an oral dose of 1 mg/kg/day, and the dose can be adjusted depending on clinical response and biochemical parameters. It is important that patients on NTBC remain on a protein-restricted diet that is low in tyrosine and phenylalanine, because NTBC will increase the blood tyrosine level. Biochemical monitoring of plasma amino acids, blood, and urinary succinylacetone and liver functions is mandatory during therapy with NTBC. Recurrent ophthalmologic evaluation and hepatic imaging are also important. Measurement of α-fetoprotein is particularly important because a few late-treated patients developed HCC despite NTBC therapy.[94] Although NTBC is still an investigational drug, it can be obtained through research protocols in the United States, Canada, and Europe. Further follow-up is needed to assess the long-term effects and safety of NTBC therapy, taking into consideration the facts that some patients developed cancer despite therapy, that patients with HPD deficiency develop neurologic problems,[95,96] and that mental retardation is seen in 50% of tyrosinemia type II patients.[97]

Currently the mainstay treatment for patients with tyrosinemia with end-stage liver disease is orthotopic liver transplantation (OLT), normalizing FAH activity and correcting the metabolic derangement and hepatic function.[76] OLT is an effective treatment for tyrosinemia type I (TTI) with good quality of life. The current indications for OLT in TT1 are nonresponse to NTBC, risk of malignancy, and poor quality of life related to dietary restriction and frequency of blood[98] sampling. OLT also has a marked beneficial effect on the renal function with improvement in the tubular dysfunction.[99] However, patients with severe renal disease before OLT may continue to have borderline renal function and poor growth even after transplant.

UREA CYCLE DEFECTS

Catabolism of amino acids produces ammonia, which is a potent neurotoxin unless inactivated by the liver. Animal studies have shown that hyperammonemia is toxic to the immature nervous system, producing alterations in the level of consciousness. The neuropathologic changes involve the astrocytes and not the neurons, which suggests that the changes may be reversible.[100] However, repeated prolonged episodes of hyperammonemia can lead to permanent neurologic impairment.[101]

Detoxification of ammonia occurs through a series of reactions known as the Krebs-Henseleit or urea cycle (Figure 72-2). Besides converting ammonia into urea, the cycle produces arginine, which becomes an essential amino acid in all urea cycle defects except arginase deficiency. Five enzymes are involved in the formation of urea: carbamoyl phosphate synthetase (CPS), ornithine transcarbamylase (OTC), argininosuccinate synthetase (AS), argininosuccinate lyase (AL), and arginase. In addition, a sixth enzyme, N-acetylglutamate synthetase (NAGS), is also needed for the formation of N-acetylglutamate. Four enzymes operate in a cyclic manner using ornithine as a substrate, which is regenerated. On the other hand, CPS, which is produced by a series of enzymatic reactions, enters the cycle by combining with ornithine. The other nitrogen atom of urea is derived from aspartate, which combines with citrulline.

Clinical Features

Symptoms may start early in life or be delayed until late childhood or adulthood. Newborns may have rapid clinical deterioration resembling sepsis, usually after a few days of protein feedings. Symptoms include refusal to eat, vomiting, tachypnea, seizure, and lethargy progressing to coma. Increased intracranial pressure may be evident. Later in life, hyperammonemia may present with vomiting and multiple neurological abnormalities including irritability, mental confusion, ataxia, and combativeness, alternating with periods of drowsiness and coma. Delayed physical growth as well as development may be seen, and patients may elect to consume a low-protein diet in order to avoid the symptoms.

Diagnosis

Hyperammonemia is the characteristic feature of urea cycle defect. The degree of elevation in plasma ammonia varies according to the severity of the disorder and protein intake. Values up to 20 to 30 times normal may be seen during the neonatal period. Patients with late onset may have plasma ammonia levels around twice the normal values. A direct relation exists between the duration of the hyperammonemia and subsequent intellectual ability of the child.[101] However, there is no relation between the severity of hyperammonemia and later intelligence or neurologic development.[102]

Patients with CPS and OTC deficiencies do have specific abnormalities of plasma amino acids beside elevated alanine, glutamine, and aspartic acid secondary to hyperammonemia. Plasma citrulline level may serve as an initial screening tool in patients with urea cycle defects. Plasma citrulline, which is very

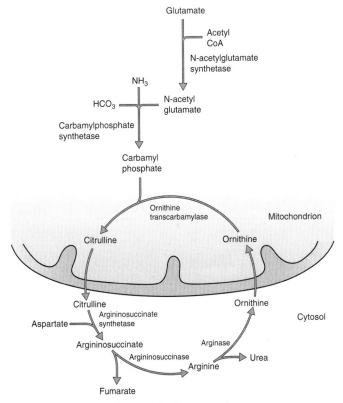

Figure 72-2. The urea cycle.

low in OTC and CPS deficiencies, exceeds 1000 μmol/L in AS deficiency (citrullinemia) and is usually in the range of 100 to 300 μmol/L in AL deficiency. Urinary orotic acid level may help to differentiate CPS and NAGS deficiencies, which are characterized by low orotic acid levels, from OTC deficiency, which is associated with high urinary orotic acid levels.

Serum transaminases are elevated during the acute exacerbations and may remain high between the episodes. Prothrombin time may be markedly prolonged. Respiratory alkalosis is transiently present in acute attacks. Hepatic histology is usually nonspecific and unremarkable.[102] However, fibrosis has been noted in patients with several disorders of the urea cycle.[103,104] Heterozygote OTC deficiency females may exhibit several histological abnormalities including steatosis, focal necrosis, and portal fibrosis.[103]

After the clinical condition stabilizes, the diagnosis should be confirmed by measurement of enzyme activity in an appropriate tissue (Table 72-3). Besides the liver, OTC is expressed in the intestinal mucosa, and therefore the diagnosis can be made by enzyme assays in duodenal and rectal biopsies.[105] However, the gold standard is measuring the enzyme activity in liver tissue in males with OTC deficiency, as the enzyme activity may be virtually absent.[106,107] Males with partial variants may have enzyme activity that ranges from 5 to 25% of normal.[108,109] In symptomatic heterozygous females, levels of activity range from 4 to 25% of normal.[107] Heterozygous mothers of affected children may have levels as high as 97% of normal activity. It has to be noted that the in vitro measurement of the enzyme activity may not accurately reflect the in vivo activity of the enzyme.

Differential Diagnosis

The differential diagnosis of hyperammonemia is summarized in Table 72-4. In the neonatal period it is important to differentiate transient hyperammonemia (THA) of the newborn (THN) from inborn error of metabolism, namely urea cycle defects and organic acidemias. Differentiation may be made using an algorithm suggested by Hudak and coworkers.[110] Neonates with THA were found to have lower weights and earlier gestational age. A rapid neurological deterioration is seen in patients with THN compared to those with urea cycle defects, in whom coma is seldom seen before the third day of life. THA is an ill-understood disorder. It has been suggested that decreased hepatic flow secondary to ductus venosus shunting[111] or transient platelet activation[112] may contribute to hyperammonemia.

In patients with later onset, the differential diagnosis is wider and includes an increasing range of organic acidurias such as fatty acid acyl CoA dehydrogenase deficiencies and isovaleric acidemias. The diagnosis of Reye's syndrome should be considered in the presence of hypoglycemia and coagulopathy.

Genetics and Prenatal Diagnosis

Individual deficiencies of the urea cycle enzymes have been observed with an estimated incidence of 1:25,000 to 30,000 newborns. All the enzymes for the urea cycle enzymes have been mapped, characterized and isolated with the exception of N-acetylglutamate synthetase. The gene for OTC is located on the X chromosome.[106,107] The disease, which is the most common form of urea cycle disorder, is expressed in an X-linked dominant pattern. Therefore, males with the defect are severely affected, whereas females may have heterogeneous manifestations due to inactivation of one X chromosome.

The cloning of the gene[113] and the characterization of its structure[114] have allowed the identification of a wide variety of mutations.[115-117] After the diagnosis is established, the carrier state of the mother should be determined. If the mutations are identified, they should be used for detection of heterozygosity. However, this procedure is usually impractical because of the wide variation of OTC deficiency. The most convenient investigation is the allopurinol test, which is an easier and safer test than protein or alanine loading. Allopurinol inhibits the decarboxylation of orotidine monophosphate (OMP). The accumulation of OMP results in increased urinary secretion of orotidine and orotic acid. The measurement of orotidine, rather than orotic acid, can increase the specificity of the test.[118] Prenatal diagnosis can be made by assay for TaqI cleavage[119] and for known mutations, which is less invasive than enzyme assay in fetal liver tissue.

The rest of the urea cycle enzyme disorders are inherited in an autosomal-recessive pattern, and prenatal diagnosis can be made for CPS deficiency using closely linked markers. The diagnosis can be also made by prenatal liver biopsy. The diagnosis of

TABLE 72-4. Differential Diagnosis of Hyperammonemia

Deficiencies of the urea cycle enzyme
  Carbamoyl phosphate synthetase deficiency
  Ornithine transcarbamylase deficiency
  Argininosuccinate synthetase deficiency
  Argininosuccinate lyase deficiency
  Arginase deficiency
  N-Acetylglutamate synthetase deficiency
Lysinuric protein intolerance
Organic acidemias
  Propionic acidemia
  Methylmalonic acidemia
  Isovaleric acidemia
  Glutaric acidemia type II
  Multiple carboxylase deficiencies
  3-Hydroxy-3-methylglutaric acidurias
  β-Ketothiolase deficiency
  Medium-chain fatty acid acyl CoA dehydrogenase deficiency
Systemic carnitine deficiency
Hyperammonemia-hyperornithinemia-homocitrullinemia syndrome
Transient hyperammonemia of the newborn
Severe systemic illness
Reye's syndrome
Liver failure

TABLE 72-3. Diagnostic Tests in Urea Cycle Defect

Disorder	Tissue Diagnosis	Urine Orotic Acid
Carbamoyl phosphate synthetase (CPS) deficiency	Liver	Normal
Ornithine transcarbamylase (OTC) deficiency	Liver	Very high
Argininosuccinate synthetase (AS) deficiency	Fibroblasts	High
Argininosuccinate lyase (AL) deficiency	Erythrocytes	High
Arginase deficiency	Erythrocytes	High
N-Acetylglutamate synthetase (NAGS) deficiency	Liver	High

ASA and citrullinemia can be made on chorionic villus biopsy. Arginase deficiency can be diagnosed using a fetal blood sample if molecular genetic studies are not informative.

Treatment

In the neonatal period, the immediate objective is to reduce the concentrations of ammonia and glutamine. All protein intake should be stopped and high energy supplied through glucose given intravenously or orally, if tolerated. Serum ammonia level above 400μmol/L needs urgent intervention with hemodialysis or exchange transfusion, which are much more effective than hemofiltration or peritoneal dialysis.[120]

Alternative pathways for nitrogen excretion have been possible through the development of compounds that can combine with amino acids and be excreted. The first compound introduced was sodium benzoate, which combines with glycine, generating hippurate, which is rapidly excreted. Therefore, for each mole of benzoate given, 1 mole of nitrogen is lost. The other compound is phenylbutyrate, which is metabolized by the liver, forming phenylacetate and then combines with glutamine to form phenylacetylglutamine. The excretion of phenylacetylglutamine results in the loss of 2 moles of nitrogen for each mole of phenylbutyrate given.

Nitrogen can be excreted in the form of citrulline and argininosuccinic acid in patients with citrullinemia and AS deficiency, respectively. However, the formation of these metabolites is limited because of the metabolic defect in these disorders. Therefore, arginine supplements may replenish ornithine supply, increasing the excretion of citrulline and argininosuccinic acid.

The long-term goals in patients with urea cycle disorders are to correct the metabolic derangement, yet provide a nutritionally complete diet in order to allow normal growth and development. These goals are sometimes difficult to achieve, especially in patients with severe disease. All patients should be maintained on a low-protein diet. It is important to know that the tolerance of protein may vary widely depending on the growth rate and the severity of the disorder. Mixtures of essential amino acids may provide adequate precursors for protein synthesis and at the same time minimize the nitrogen load to be excreted.

Patients with urea cycle disorders, except those with arginase deficiency, will benefit from an arginine supplement to replace that which is not synthesized. The aim is to keep arginine plasma level in the range of 50 to 150 μmol/L. Patients with severe OTC and CPS deficiencies may benefit from citrulline rather than arginine because it will excrete an additional nitrogen molecule.

Some patients with urea cycle disorders may need to be maintained on anticonvulsants. It is important to avoid sodium valproate, especially in patients with OTC deficiency, because it may precipitate fatal decompensation.[121]

Patients with urea cycle disorders should be monitored on a regular basis with measurements of plasma ammonia and amino acids, paying special attention to glutamine and essential amino acids. The goals are to keep plasma ammonia level below 80 μmol/L, plasma glutamine level below 800 μmol/L, and essential amino acids within the normal range.

Acute exacerbations can occur unpredictably as well as with fasting, intercurrent infections, anesthesia, or surgery. Patients with mild symptoms can be managed with reduced protein and high energy intake, whereas patients with severe episodes may need hospitalization and intravenous therapy.

Orthotopic liver transplantation is an alternative therapeutic modality for patients with severe urea cycle defects. It is usually reserved for patients with severe neonatal disease, such as CPS and OTC deficiencies. On the other hand, the decision to perform OLT in females with partial OTC activity is controversial. Factors to be considered include disease severity, failure of medical therapy, access to medical facilities with experience in the management of acute hyperammonemia, and social factors. Various reports have illustrated the preservation of cognitive function and prevention of neurologic decline in OTCD females who have undergone liver transplantation.[122,123]

Hepatocyte transplantation has been studied in experimental animals for more than 2 decades. The donor hepatocytes have been shown to correct the metabolic defects in liver function[124-132] and to provide temporary liver function in animal models of liver failure.[133-139] Hepatocyte transplantation has several advantages over OLT. Cell transplantation is a nonsurgical procedure and can be done on an outpatient basis in patients with metabolic liver disease, avoiding the high cost of hospitalization. Although the cost for long-term immune suppression is the same for hepatocyte transplantation and OLT, the initial cost of cell transplantation is estimated to be about 10% the cost of organ transplant. Hepatocytes can be genetically manipulated ex vivo as needed. The source of transplanted cells is usually organs that would be otherwise discarded. Therefore, hepatocyte transplantation can help relieve the current shortage of donor organs by making more organs available for the cases where cell transplant will not suffice.

Several patients with metabolic defects of the liver have been treated with hepatocyte transplantation.[140-142] A patient with OTC deficiency received 1 billion viable hepatocytes via the portal vein. His ammonia level normalized without medical therapy within 48 hours, and his glutamine levels returned to normal before discharge from the hospital. OTC activity that was zero before hepatocyte transplantation increased to 0.4 μmol/g/min 4 weeks after the transplant, which represents approximately 0.3 to 0.5% of normal OTC activity. However, the patient developed a hyperammonemic episode a few weeks after the transplant that did not respond to multiple intravenous boluses of scavengers. A repeated infusion of cryopreserved hepatocytes was given; however, the patient remained comatose and died with bronchopneumonia 43 days following the initial hepatocyte infusion. At autopsy, there was no evidence of portal vein thrombosis, portal hypertension, hepatic infection, or other complications related to hepatocyte transplantation.[142] In a recent report, four children with urea cycle defects received liver cell transplant, and all showed metabolic stabilization during observation periods of 4 to 13 months. However, one child with prenatally diagnosed ornithine transcarbamylase deficiency died after 4 months from a fatal metabolic decompensation.[143] Though cell therapy is not a permanent therapeutic option, bridging to liver transplantation may be substantially improved. These promising results suggest that hepatocyte transplantation has the potential to become an accepted therapeutic modality in patients with metabolic liver disease, including those with urea cycle defects.

In the future, other therapeutic options may include molecular manipulation, enzyme replacement, or gene transfer. A possible consideration for inherited metabolic disorders is the introduction of a normal allele of a gene into a cell that lacks its normal copy or has a defective copy. Strategies for genetic therapy may include gene replacement, where a functional gene replaces the defective gene in the proper location (homologous recombination), or gene augmentation, which involves the insertion of a normal gene into a cell that has a missing or defective gene without correcting the dysfunctional gene. These strategies may be applicable to recessive, single-gene disorders such as metabolic liver diseases in which the establishment of even low levels of enzyme activity may prevent the pathologic features associated with a defective or absent gene.

The prognosis in patients with urea cycle defects depends on several factors, including the age of the patient at diagnosis and the severity of the condition. Patients presenting with symptomatic hyperammonemia in the neonatal period usually have a poor prognosis despite aggressive medical therapy, and the majority of patients will suffer from long-term complications. On the other hand, patients who are treated prospectively may have a more favorable neurologic outcome. However, they require a lifelong medical regimen and may have handicaps that include impairment of development and recurrent episodes of hyperammonemia.[144]

REFERENCES

8. Carrell RW, Lomas DA. Alpha-1-antitrypsin deficiency. N Engl J Med 2002;346:45.

48. Bartlett JR, Friedman KJ, Ling SC, et al. Genetic modifiers of liver disease in cystic fibrosis. JAMA 2009;302:1076–1083.

92. Lindstedt S, Holme E, Locke E, et al. Treatment of hereditary tyrosinemia type I by inhibition of 4-hyroxyphenylpyruvate dioxygenase. Lancet 1992;340:813–818.

147. Burrows JA, Willis LK, Perlmutter DH. Chemical chaperones mediate increased secretion of mutant alpha I-antitrypsin (alpha I-AT) Z: a potential pharmacologic strategy for prevention of liver and emphysema in alpha I-AT deficiency. Proc Natl Acad Sci USA 2000;97:1796–1801.

149. Gooptu B, Lomas D. Conformational pathology of the serpins: themes, variations, and therapeutic strategies. Annu Rev Biochem 2009;78: 9.1-9.30.

See expertconsult.com for a complete list of references and the review questions for this chapter.

73

ABNORMALITIES OF CARBOHYDRATE METABOLISM AND THE LIVER

Shikha S. Sundaram • Estella M. Alonso

The liver is the central organ responsible for carbohydrate metabolism. The liver stores carbohydrates in the form of glycogen and synthesizes glucose through glycogen breakdown and gluconeogenesis. Glucose is an essential nutrient for the function of both the central nervous system and muscle. Disorders of carbohydrate metabolism may be acquired or inborn. This chapter highlights the molecular basis, clinical presentation, diagnosis, and therapy of the most common errors in carbohydrate metabolism. Nonalcoholic fatty liver disease, galactosemia, hereditary fructose intolerance, fructose 1,6-bisphosphatase deficiency, and glycogen storage disease are discussed.

NONALCOHOLIC FATTY LIVER DISEASE

Nonalcoholic fatty liver disease (NAFLD), the most frequent reason for chronically elevated aminotransferases among both adults and children in the United States, is a clinicopathologic condition characterized by abnormal lipid deposition in the absence of alcohol intake. NAFLD represents a spectrum of diseases, ranging from simple steatosis to steatosis in association with necroinflammation and fibrosis (nonalcoholic steatohepatitis, NASH) to cirrhosis.[1-3]

Hepatic steatosis is present in more than 60% of obese and 90% of morbidly obese adults.[4,5] Progression to NASH may occur in up 19% of obese and 50% of morbidly obese adults, with subsequent progression to fibrosis and cirrhosis in about 30%.[4-7] The exact prevalence of NAFLD in pediatrics is unknown. Elevated ALTs occur in 10 to 14% of adolescents in the United States. This likely underrepresents the true prevalence of NAFLD, which may occur despite normal aminotransferases.[8,9] Of note, 60% of adolescents with increased transaminases are either overweight or obese.[10] Studies using radiologic imaging estimate the prevalence of NAFLD as 18 to 53%, but also fail to identify all patients with NAFLD. A large pediatric autopsy study of NAFLD found a prevalence of 9.6% after adjusting for age, gender, and ethnicity, with a 38% prevalence in obese children.[11]

Most children with NAFLD are between the ages of 11.5 and 13.5 years, corresponding to a likely peak in pubertal insulin resistance. In pediatrics, males are more commonly affected (2:1) than females, suggesting that sex steroids may affect the development of NAFLD.[9,12,13] Ethnic variation also exists, with a relative paucity of NAFLD in African Americans, compared with whites and Hispanics.[5,14,15] Insulin resistance and type 2 diabetes mellitus, in particular, increase the likelihood of having an elevated ALT beyond that of obesity alone.[5,12,16] In addition, up to 75% of those with type 2 diabetes mellitus have fatty liver disease.[5,14] Type 2 diabetes mellitus is a key component of the metabolic syndrome, which includes hypertension, hyperlipidemia, and NAFLD. The metabolic syndrome may be present in up to 66% of children with biopsy-proven NAFLD.[17]

The etiopathogenesis of NAFLD and its progression to NASH are multifactorial (Figure 73-1). Central to the development of fatty liver disease is abnormal lipid homeostasis. Insulin resistance suppresses glycogenesis, promotes gluconeogenesis and glycogenolysis, and increases the release of free fatty acids from adipose tissue. Uptake of circulating free fatty acids by hepatocytes is unregulated, resulting in increased triglyceride synthesis and impaired free fatty acid oxidation, producing excess hepatocyte lipid.[18,19] Hyperinsulinemia may also increase hepatic triglyceride synthesis by overstimulating sterol regulatory element binding protein (SREBP)-1c.[20,21]

The progression to NASH may also in part be due to increased hepatocyte susceptibility to oxidative stress, through the generation of reactive oxygen species (ROS) formed by lipid peroxidation and peroxisomal β-oxidation. Numerous studies have demonstrated increased markers of oxidative stress in patients with NASH. The up-regulation of various cytochrome P450 systems, particularly CYP2E1 and CYP4A, also supports the role of oxidative stress in the pathogenesis of NASH. CYP2E1 and CYP4A are key enzymes responsible for microsomal lipoxygenation. Peroxisome proliferator activated receptor alpha (PPAR-α), a transcription factor that regulates microsomal and peroxisomal lipid peroxidation, may also contribute to the development of NASH through the formation of ROS.[22,23]

By-products of oxidative stress and lipid peroxidation are powerful chemoattractants of neutrophils and also stimulate hepatic stellate cells responsible for fibrosis. Oxidative stress also stimulates the release of inflammatory cytokines, including leptin and TNF-α. TNF-α, a proinflammatory and proapoptotic cytokine that promotes insulin resistance and is important in white blood cell recruitment, is increased in patients with NAFLD. Leptin is a regulator of body weight and energy expenditure. Leptin is crucial in preventing lipid accumulation in nonadipose tissue such as myocardial and skeletal muscle and liver.[23] Leptin likely has a role in the shunting of fat toward β-oxidation and away from triglyceride synthesis. In addition, adiponectin, an anti-inflammatory cytokine that typically inhibits fatty acid uptake, stimulates fatty acid oxidation and lipid export, and enhances insulin sensitivity, is decreased in NAFLD. Although much has been learned about

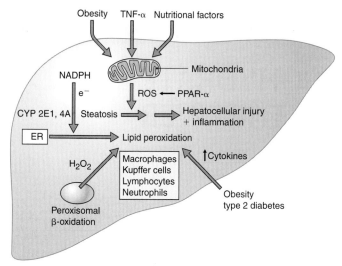

Figure 73-1. The etiopathogenesis of NASH. NADPH, reduced nicotinamide adenine dinucleotide phosphate; ER, endoplasmic reticulum; CYP, cytochrome; TNF-α, tumor necrosis factor alpha; ROS, reactive oxygen species. Adapted from Chitturi and Farrell (2001),[18] with permission from Thieme.

the pathophysiology of NAFLD and its progression to NASH and cirrhosis, many questions remain unanswered and are under active investigation.

Clinical Presentation

Most children with NAFLD are asymptomatic. Elevated transaminases or increased hepatic fat on abdominal imaging are often discovered during testing performed for unrelated reasons. The typical patient is overweight or obese, though NAFLD may occur in lean individuals. Patients may have complaints of fatigue, constipation, or mild abdominal pain that may be generalized or localized to the right upper quadrant. Physical exam may be normal, or demonstrate obesity (particularly central obesity), mild-moderate hepatomegaly, or acanthosis nigricans (a sign of insulin resistance).

Laboratory evaluation reveals mild to moderate elevations of serum aminotransferases, typically less than 1.5 times normal, with an ALT:AST ratio greater than 1.[24,25] Transaminase elevation cannot reliably confirm the diagnosis of NAFLD, nor predict the presence of fibrosis. Biopsy-proven NAFLD may occur with completely normal transaminases.[22] Total and direct bilirubin levels are typically normal, though GGTP and alkaline phosphatase may be mildly elevated in less than 50% of cases. Patients affected by NAFLD may also have hyperglycemia and hyperlipidemia, particularly hypertriglyceridemia.

A thorough evaluation and systematic exclusion of other etiologies of liver disease should also occur, including Wilson's disease (with a serum ceruloplasmin), alpha-1-antitryspin deficiency (using an alpha-1-antitryspin level and phenotype), viral hepatitis (using a hepatitis C antibody and hepatitis B surface antigen), and autoimmune hepatitis (with an anti-nuclear antibody, anti-smooth muscle antibody, and anti-liver kidney microsomal antibody). Low titers of elevated serum autoantibodies may occur in up to 3% of adults with NAFLD, though the prevalence in pediatrics is unknown. Care providers should also consider the potential for regular alcohol use as a cause of liver disease, particularly in adolescents.

Diagnosis and Treatment

Abdominal imaging may help to confirm hepatic fatty infiltration consistent with NAFLD. Abdominal ultrasound is widely used as it is relatively inexpensive, noninvasive, and easy to perform. Ultrasound, however, requires that at least 30% hepatic fat be present for detection, is not quantitative, and may be technically challenging to perform in patients with significant central obesity.[26] An abdominal computed tomographic (CT) scan may be also be used, but has the additional disadvantage of radiation exposure. Magnetic resonance imaging (MRI), though more costly, is more sensitive than other imaging modalities in detecting lesser amounts of fat and allows for more definitive hepatic fat quantification when performed using the modified Dixon technique or with magnetic resonance spectroscopy (MRS).[27,28] None of the currently available imaging modalities, however, allow differentiation of benign steatosis from NASH, or have the ability to grade the severity of inflammation or stage fibrosis.

Currently, liver biopsy is the only reliable method to assess the presence and extent of necroinflammation and fibrosis in NAFLD. Liver biopsy should be considered in patients who are a poor clinical fit for the just-described classic picture of NAFLD and in those who have a chronic hepatitis (elevated aminotransferases for greater than 3 to 6 months). Standard histologic assessment for NASH, including grading and staging of disease, may then occur. A three-tiered grading and staging system for NASH is widely used, based on a semiquantitative evaluation of multiple histologic features. The minimum criteria for NASH are (1) steatosis, with macrovesicular fat greater than microvesicular fat; (2) a mixed, mild lobular inflammation with scattered polymorphonuclear leukocytes and mononuclear cells; and (3) hepatocyte ballooning that is most apparent near steatotic liver cells.[29,30]

A unique histologic pattern of NASH has been observed in pediatrics. In this distinct pattern, referred to as type 2 NASH, inflammation and fibrosis are accentuated in the portal areas in contrast to the zone 3 injury typically observed in adults with NASH (type 1 NASH).[31] Type 2 NASH occurs in 28 to 51% of pediatric patients, type 1 NASH in 2.4 to 17% of pediatric patients, and an overlap pattern in 16 to 52% of pediatric patients.[31,32] Therefore, a spectrum of disease patterns likely exists in pediatric NASH.

Treatment of NAFLD focuses on slow, progressive weight loss through dietary modifications and exercise programs. Although the optimal diet for treating NAFLD is not well established, the importance of insulin resistance in the pathogenesis[36] of NAFLD suggests that low-glycemic diets may be beneficial.[33] Most patients, however, experience little success with this type of lifestyle modification. In adults, weight loss through bariatric surgery, both gastric bypass and laparoscopic adjustable gastric banding, has shown promise.[34,35] This treatment is extremely controversial, however, in pediatrics[37] and cannot be routinely recommended.

Given this common scenario, great interest lies in potential pharmacologic therapies for NAFLD. Both sibutramine (a serotonin and noradrenaline reuptake inhibitor) and orlistat (an enteric lipase inhibitor) resulted in weight loss and some improvement of NAFLD parameters in preliminary studies.[38-43] Small pediatric studies using metformin (a biguanide that improves hepatic insulin resistance) to treat NASH have shown improvements in aminotransferases and steatosis.[44-46]

A recent meta-analysis showed that NAFLD patients treated with metformin experienced normalization of aminotransferases and improved steatosis on radiologic imaging compared to those treated with dietary modifications alone.[47] Adequate long-term studies that include histologic assessment are lacking. Treatment with the thiazolidinediones pioglitazone and rosiglitazone, selective peroxisome proliferator-activated receptor gamma (PPAR-γ) agonists, improve liver biochemistries and histology, with steatosis affected more than inflammation, ballooning, or fibrosis.[44,48,49] These beneficial effects do not persist when medications are stopped.

Trials of antioxidants are also being made based on the role of oxidative stress in the pathogenesis of NAFLD. A small open-label pilot study of 11 pediatric patients with NASH treated with vitamin E for 2 to 4 months showed normalization of alanine aminotransferase (ALT).[50] Pilot trials in adults of N-acetylcysteine and betaine, a choline metabolite that increases S-adenosylmethionine levels, are also encouraging.[51,52] Ursodeoxycholic acid, a cytoprotective bile acid, is ineffective in normalizing aminotransferases or improving histologic parameters in NASH.[53,54] Adults treated with pentoxyfilline, a TNF-α inhibitor, also demonstrate improvements in aminotransferases, with some concurrent histologic improvements as well.[55,56]

GALACTOSEMIA

Galactosemia, an inborn error of galactose metabolism, is an autosomal recessive condition affecting 1 of 50,000 live births.[57] It is due to a cellular deficiency in one of three enzymes in the pathway of glucose-to-galactose conversion. The classic form of galactosemia, presenting with malnutrition, growth failure, and progressive liver disease, results from deficiency in galactose-1-phosphate uridyl transferase (GALT). A much more rare deficiency in uridine diphosphate galactose-4-epimerase results in a similar clinical presentation to GALT deficiency.[58,59] Last, galactokinase deficiency results primarily in cataract formation.[58] GALT is a 43-kDa protein encoded by a 4-kb gene on chromosome 9p13. A majority of patients with galactosemia have missense mutations, of which more than 150 have been identified.[60,61] The Q188R mutation, affecting 60 to 70% of whites, where arginine is substituted for glutamine, results in no enzymatic activity.[61,62] The milder Duarte variant (N314D mutation) involves a change from asparagine to aspartate, resulting in decreased enzymatic activity.[63]

Galactose is a monosaccharide derived from the hydrolysis of the milk sugar lactose. Lactose is converted to glucose and galactose by the enterocyte brush border enzyme lactase. Galactose is then transported across the enterocyte by a sodium-glucose/galactose transporter. Galactose is metabolized to glucose by a series of reactions that begin with the phosphorylation of galactose to galactose 1-phosphate (Figure 73-2). Galactose 1-phosphate is further converted to glucose 1-phosphate by GALT. In the absence of GALT, alternative pathways overproduce galactitol and galactonate, potentially toxic metabolites.[64]

Clinical Presentation

The clinical presentation of galactosemia varies from an acute illness with hypoglycemia, vomiting, diarrhea, and encephalopathy to a subacute illness. Patients most commonly present

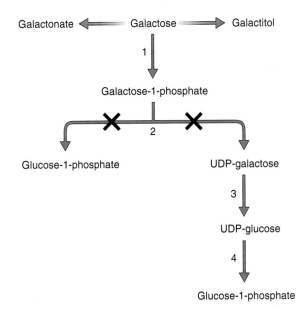

Figure 73-2. Galactose metabolism. Galactose is phosphorylated to galactose 1-phosphate, by galactokinase (1). This is then further converted to uridine diphosphate (UDP) galactose and glucose 1-phosphate by galactose-1-phosphate uridyl transferase (GALT) (2). UDP-galactose is converted to UDP-glucose by uridine diphosphate galactose-4-epimerase (3). UDP-glucose is converted to glucose 1-phosphate by uridine diphosphate glucose pyrophosphorylase (4). In the absence of GALT, galactitol and galactonate are overproduced.

with failure to thrive, weight loss, and emesis after the initiation of dietary lactose. Vomiting and diarrhea are almost universally present.[59] Patients may present with hypoglycemia and encephalopathy in the first few days of life or may present several days later with jaundice, ascites, hepatomegaly, splenomegaly, and liver failure.[65,66] Hemolytic anemia may also be observed. Cataracts may be present at birth if the mother ingested large amounts of dairy late in pregnancy or may develop postnatally, but may be difficult to detect without a slit lamp exam. Cataracts are formed because of increased oncotic pressure exerted by the accumulation of galactitol in the lens.[67] Levy et al. discovered a strong correlation between galactosemia and neonatal *Escherichia coli* sepsis.[68] Thus, the presence of *E. coli* sepsis in the neonate should prompt evaluation of galactosemia. Renal tubular dysfunction with albuminuria, aminoaciduria, and galactosuria can also occur.[59] Furthermore, patients may manifest increased blood and urinary galactose levels and hyperchloremic acidosis.[69]

Long-term prognosis is good for patients with early diagnosis and intervention. Acute symptoms and biochemical changes regress rapidly on withdrawal of lactose products. Long-term follow-up data of those treated show some variability. Growth and liver function revert to normal. Mental retardation is the most devastating result of toxicity. Intelligence, as measured by IQ, appears highly correlated with adequate dietary control. Some patients manifest residual defects in mental functioning despite dietary restrictions and normal IQ. These include speech and language delays, spatial and mathematic learning disabilities, short attention spans, abnormal visual perceptions, tremor, and ataxia.[70,71] In addition, there is a high incidence of postnatal hypergonadotropic hypogonadic ovarian failure. Pregnancy in affected females is rare.[72,73] Osteoporosis also commonly occurs in affected females, who may benefit from appropriate nutritional supplementation.[74]

These long-term complications may be the result of endogenous galactose synthesis.[75]

Diagnosis and Treatment

A diagnosis of galactosemia should be suspected in patients with any of the constellation of symptoms just described. The presence of urinary reducing substances in the absence of glucosuria is suggestive of galactosemia, but is neither very sensitive nor specific.[59] False negatives may occur with poor lactose intake or intermittent excretion of galactose. False positives may occur with severe liver disease and some medications. A diagnosis of galactosemia should be confirmed by quantitative measurement of GALT activity in red blood cells, which will be decreased.[59,69,76] Prenatal diagnosis is possible by measuring enzymatic activity of tissue or cells obtained by chorionic villus sampling or amniocentesis.[77] In the United States, most patients are detected through newborn screening programs.

Treatment of galactosemia is based on elimination of dietary galactose. In infants, this is achieved by feeding soy or protein hydrolysate formulas.[59] In older children and adults, dietary avoidance of dairy products, with special attention to food additives, is needed. Some concern exists regarding galactose toxicity from certain grains, fruits, and vegetables.[78] Controversy exists regarding safe or acceptable levels of galactose. In addition to dietary manipulation, close monitoring of neurodevelopment in children and yearly ophthalmologic exams to evaluate for cataracts are also recommended.[59]

HEREDITARY FRUCTOSE INTOLERANCE

Hereditary fructose intolerance is an autosomal recessive metabolic disorder occurring in approximately 1 in 20,000 live births. This disorder is caused by a deficiency of fructose-1,6-bisphosphate aldolase (aldolase B), one of a set of enzymes that converts fructose to intermediate constituents of the glycolytic-gluconeogenic pathway. These intermediary products are then further metabolized to glucose and glycogen (Figure 73-3). Aldolase B is the product of a 14.5-kb gene on chromosome 9q22.3 that encodes a 364-amino-acid polypeptide. It is expressed in the liver, kidney, and small intestine. More than 20 different mutations and five polymorphisms have been described.[79] Among people of northern European descent, the A149P allele is most common. The A174D allele is predominant in central and southern Europeans, whereas the N334K allele is predominant among those of central and eastern European descent.[80-82]

Fructose is transported into hepatocytes and intestinal cells via GLUT 5, a sodium-independent transporter. It is then phosphorylated into fructose 1-phosphate by fructokinase. Fructose 1-phosphate is cleaved by aldolase B into D-glyceraldehyde phosphate and dihydroxyacetone phosphate. These intermediates may then directly enter the glycolytic pathway or the gluconeogenesis pathway or become synthesized into glycogen (see Figure 73-2). Accumulation of fructose 1-phosphate results in hypoglycemia secondary to impaired glycogenolysis, as glycogen phosphorylase is inhibited, and impaired gluconeogenesis, as glyceraldehyde 3-phosphate and dihydroxyacetone phosphate cannot be converted. In addition, the formation and sequestration of large quantities of fructose 1-phosphate result in ATP and GTP depletion with impaired protein synthesis.[80,83]

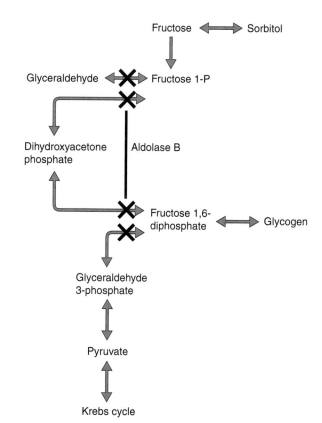

Figure 73-3. Fructose metabolism. Fructose is metabolized to glycogen or to components of the Krebs cycle. A deficiency in aldolase B, as in hereditary fructose intolerance, results in the accumulation of fructose 1-phosphate.

Clinical Presentation

Patients affected by this disorder remain completely asymptomatic unless they consume fructose-containing foods. Newborns fed breast milk do not manifest symptoms, as breast milk contains lactose (made of glucose and galactose). Symptoms, which occur as infants are weaned and either receive sucrose-containing formulas or begin baby foods, are related to the accumulation of fructose 1-phosphate in tissues where aldolase B is usually expressed. The most common symptoms are poor feeding and vomiting. Other gastrointestinal symptoms include diarrhea and abdominal pain. In addition, severe hypoglycemia with sweating, trembling, pallor, and metabolic acidosis can occur.[84,85] Irritability, apathy, and anuria/oliguria are also seen. A large fructose load may even cause seizures.[86] Chronic exposure to fructose leads to failure to thrive, signs of liver disease (hepatomegaly, splenomegaly, ascites, edema), and proximal renal tubular dysfunction (renal tubular acidosis, hypophosphatemia, and rickets).[84,85] Occasionally, affected patients remain undiagnosed into adolescence or adulthood because of self-imposed dietary restrictions.[84] These individuals develop aversions to fructose-containing foods, exhibiting unusual feeding behaviors such as eating the peel, but avoiding the fruit pulp.

Laboratory abnormalities are consistent with the affected organ systems. Patients may have elevations in liver transaminases, increased prothrombin times, hypoproteinemia, hypokalemia, and hypophosphatemia. Urine studies reveal increased reducing substances, proteinuria, amino aciduria, organic aciduria, and fructosuria. Patients may also have anemia and thrombocytopenia. Histology from liver biopsies shows steatosis with scattered hepatocyte necrosis and inter-lobular or periportal fibrosis. Electron microscopy reveals intracellular deposits of fructose 1-phosphate with polymorphous, electron-dense cytoplasmic inclusions in concentric membranous arrays.[85,86]

Diagnosis/Treatment

In the past, the definitive diagnosis of hereditary fructose intolerance required tissue enzyme assay on liver or small intestine samples.[87,88] Much more rarely, a diagnosis was made using an intravenous fructose tolerance test after several weeks of fructose withdrawal.[85,89] Recently, however, DNA mutation analysis has become commercially available as a diagnostic tool, alleviating the need to obtain a tissue specimen in the majority of patients.[90] Treatment of acutely ill patients consists of supportive care to correct metabolic derangements, hypoglycemia, and coagulopathy. The mainstay of long-term management is complete avoidance of fructose and sucrose. Sorbitol, converted by the body to fructose, should also be avoided. Special attention should be given to food additives and medications, as sucrose or sorbitol are often used as food additives, pill coatings, and medication suspensions.[80] Long-term abstinence from fructose results in reversal of organ dysfunction, normal intelligence, and catch-up growth. Hepatomegaly may, however, persist for years.[86,91]

FRUCTOSE-1,6-BISPHOSPHATASE DEFICIENCY

Fructose-1,6-bisphosphatase deficiency is an autosomal recessive disease that results in disordered gluconeogenesis. It is a genetically heterogeneous disorder that affects females more than males (1.5:1).[92] Parental consanguinity has been reported in several families. Fructose-1,6-bisphosphatase deficiency results in the inhibition of gluconeogenic substrates (Figure 73-4).[93] Therefore, normoglycemia depends on adequate glucose intake or degradation of hepatic glycogen. If glycogen stores are limited, as in newborns, or exhausted during fasting, hypoglycemia results and gluconeogenic precursors (lactate, glycerol, and alanine) accumulate. The enzyme deficiency is also present in liver, jejunum, and kidney tissue. Muscle levels, however, are normal as muscle fructose-1,6-bisphophatase is encoded by a different gene.[84]

Clinical Presentation

Fructose-1,6-bisphophatase deficiency should be suspected in newborns presenting with hypoglycemia, hyperventilation, and metabolic acidosis. Approximately half of affected patients will develop symptoms in the first 4 days of life. The remainder develop symptoms in the first few months of life. In addition to the symptoms just described, patients may have dyspnea or apnea, tachycardia, irritability, seizures, coma, hypotonia, or hepatomegaly. Later disturbances are often triggered by febrile illnesses with concurrent refusal to feed and emesis. Unlike hereditary fructose intolerance, patients do not develop an aversion to sweet foods. In addition, disturbances in liver function are rare and kidney function is normal. These patients do, however, have a reduced tolerance to fructose and sorbitol. This intolerance is less severe than in patients with hereditary fructose intolerance. Laboratory studies show elevations in blood and urine lactate,

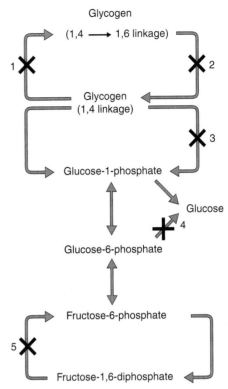

Figure 73-4. Glycogen metabolism. (1) Branching enzyme, deficient in glycogen storage disease (GSD) type IV; (2) debranching enzyme, deficient in GSD type III; (3) phosphorylase deficiency, defective in GSD type VI; (4) glucose-6-phophatase, deficient in GSD type I; (5) fructose-1,6-biphosphatase. Adapted from Ghishan FK, Ballew MP. Inborn errors of carbohydrate metabolism. In: Suchy FJ, Sokol RK, Balistreri WF, eds. Liver Disease in Children, with permission of Lippincott, Williams and Wilkins, 2001.[93]

ketones, alanine, and uric acid.[85] Histologic examination of liver biopsies shows fatty infiltration without fibrosis.[85]

Diagnosis/Treatment

Definitive diagnosis is established by observing a deficiency of fructose-1,6-bisphophatase in liver biopsy specimens. Whether this enzyme defect may be detected in leukocytes remains a matter of debate. Intravenous dextrose and sodium bicarbonate infusions are needed for the acute management of hypoglycemia and acidosis. In addition, fasting should be avoided, with careful attention to periods when children are febrile. Fructose and sucrose should be limited, though complete elimination is unnecessary.[84]

GLYCOGEN STORAGE DISEASE

Glycogen storage diseases (GSD) are caused by deficiencies of enzymes in the glycogenolytic pathways (see Figure 73-4).[93] Ten different types of glycogen storage disease have been reported, each with unique clinical features. Types I, III, IV, and VI primarily affect the liver. Glycogen production and breakdown are controlled by several factors through glycogen synthetase and phosphorylase. Both of these enzymes exist in active and inactive forms. After meals, sinusoidal glucose concentrations are high, allowing glucose to bind to phosphorylase. This changes the active enzyme to its inactive form, halting glycogenolysis. In addition, the active form of phosphorylase normally inhibits glycogen synthetase; the inactive phosphorylase allows glycogen synthesis to occur. During fasting, glucagon-mediated increases in cyclic AMP allow phosphorylase conversion from inactive to active, with subsequent glycogenolysis. High glycogen levels also allow glycogenolysis to occur by glycogen synthetase breakdown.[94]

Glycogen Storage Disease, Type I

Glycogen storage disease type I, glucose-6-phosphatase deficiency, was previously considered to be a single entity. It is now recognized that three distinct clinical forms exist: types Ia, Ib, and Ic. Glucose-6-phosphatase, located in the endoplasmic reticulum, catalyzes the terminal reaction of both glycogenolysis and gluconeogenesis (conversion of glucose 6-phosphate to glucose).[95] It is composed of a catalytic subunit and three distinct transport systems (Figure 73-5).[93] The catalytic subunit has six endoplasmic reticulum transmembrane domains.[57] There is a polypeptide stabilizing protein that transports glucose 6-phosphate, known as T1, two polypeptides responsible for phosphate transport (T2), and a glucose transporter (T3), also called GLUT-7.[95] Type Ia, the classic form of GSD, results from mutations in the catalytic subunit. The 12.5-kb gene for this entity is located on chromosome 17q21 and encodes a 357-amino-acid protein.[96] More than 30 distinct mutations have been identified in this gene, the most common being R83C and Q347X.[97] Type Ib GSD is caused by defects in the T1 translocase.[95] Normal phosphatase activity exists in fully disrupted microsomal preparations, but not in intact microsomal vesicles. The mutation for this disease is on chromosome 11q23.3.[98,99] The same genetic defect is seen in the liver, kidney, and leukocytes of affected patients.[100] Type Ic GSD is caused by a defective T2 translocase, encoded by the gene 11q23.3-24.2. Translocase 2 (T2) is a microsomal phosphate and pyrophosphate transport protein. These patients have impaired insulin secretion, as T2 is also located in the kidney and pancreas.[101,102]

Clinical Presentation

The clinical presentation of this disease can be quite varied. Type Ia GSD is considered the classic form of glycogen storage disease. It affects approximately 1 in 200,000 births. Patients commonly present with severe hypoglycemia and metabolic acidosis 3 to 4 hours after a feeding. Symptoms often begin after the first several weeks of life, when the interval between feeds increases and infants begin sleeping through the night, or when intercurrent illness disrupts feeds. Hypoglycemia is accompanied by a metabolic acidosis with increases in lactic acid, triglycerides, and uric acid. Some children present with failure to thrive because of peripheral starvation from lack of glucose, along with a protuberant abdomen and lordosis secondary to hepatomegaly. Untreated patients may develop failure to thrive, cushingoid facies, and delayed motor development. Social and cognitive development is not affected unless neurologic injury occurs from recurrent episodes of hypoglycemia.[95] Untreated patients may develop high serum triglycerides and moderate increases in cholesterol, phospholipids, free fatty acids, and apolipoprotein III. They may also develop xanthomas on the knees, elbows, and buttocks in adolescence. Impaired platelet function secondary to metabolic derangements may occur, resulting in epistaxis and oozing.[95] Liver transaminase elevations are typically mild and regress to normal as glucose levels stabilize. Liver histology shows only increased glycogen. Adolescent and adult patients may develop hepatic adenomas or carcinomas, nephrolithiasis,

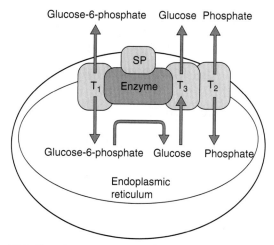

Figure 73-5. Hepatic microsomal glucose-6-phosphatase. Adapted from Ghishan FK, Ballew MP. Inborn errors of carbohydrate metabolism. In: Suchy FJ, Sokol RK, Balistreri WF, eds. Liver Disease in Children, with permission of Lippincott, Williams and Wilkins, 2001.[93]

nephropathy progressive renal dysfunction, and gouty arthritis.[103-108] Adenomas may occur in up to 75% of adolescents and adults with GSD type I and are thought to occur related to a metabolic imbalance.[109] Recent literature, however, suggests that there is no significant difference in the metabolic control of patients with and without adenoma development.[110]

Patients with type Ib GSD have similar symptoms to patients with type Ia GSD. In addition to these symptoms, patients with type Ib may have constant or cyclic neutropenia, with recurrent mild to severe bacterial infections. A majority of patients with GSD type Ib will also develop inflammatory bowel disease (IBD). IBD is underdiagnosed in this population and requires a high index of suspicion.[111,112] Patients with type Ic present with the classic symptoms of glycogen storage disease along with signs of impaired insulin secretion.

The metabolic consequences of GSD type I are profound. Hypoglycemia, secondary to an inability to mobilize glycogen, remains the predominant feature. Insulin levels are appropriately decreased, and glucagon levels are high, accompanying this hypoglycemia.[113] Lactic acidosis occurs as lactate generated during hepatic glycolysis cannot be converted to glucose.[114] Hyperuricemia also occurs because of de novo purine synthesis.[115] Hypophosphatemia is common during hypoglycemic episodes because glucose 6-phospate cannot be converted to glucose. Phosphate is trapped intracellularly, causing a shift of extracellular phosphate into the cell. Hyperlipidemia also occurs, with high serum triglycerides and moderate increases in cholesterol, phospholipids, and free fatty acids.[95] Based on these multiple risk factors, these patients are at increased theoretical risk of atherosclerosis development, though clinical studies have not confirmed this.[116,117] Abnormal platelet function, both aggregation and adhesiveness, causes recurrent oozing and epistaxis.[118]

Diagnosis/Treatment

The diagnosis of GSD type I should be considered in all children presenting with hypoglycemia and acidosis. Definitive diagnosis is made by assay of enzymatic activity of glucose-6-phophatase on liver biopsy specimens. Histologic exam of the liver shows hepatocytes filled with glycogen that is periodic acid-Schiff positive, diastase sensitive (Figure 73-6).

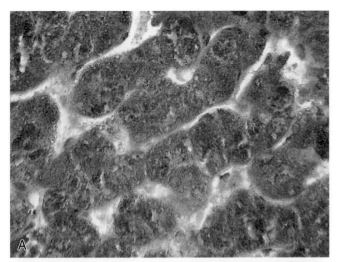

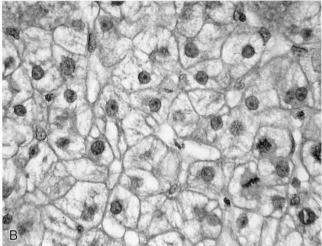

Figure 73-6. Type I glycogen storage disease. (**A**) Glycogen-filled hepatocytes seen on periodic acid-Schiff stain. (**B**) Plantlike mosaic pattern of hepatic lobules on hematoxylin-eosin stain. Courtesy of Dr. H. Melin-Aldana.

Management of patients with GSD type I requires a continuous dietary source of glucose to keep glucose levels greater than 70 mg/dL.[95] In infants, this can be accomplished by providing feedings every 2 to 3 hours while awake and at least every 3 hours while asleep.[95] It may be necessary to institute nocturnal nasogastric infusions of glucose.[119] When small frequent feedings or overnight nasogastric feedings are no longer feasible, raw cornstarch feedings may be used.[120,121] Cornstarch acts as a reservoir for glucose that can slowly be absorbed into the circulation and utilized as a glucose source for up to 6 hours. This therapy also restores hyperuricemia and hyperlipidemia to normal. Lipid-lowering agents are rarely needed.[95] Treatment with recombinant G-CSF has been important in managing patients with neutropenia.[122]

Liver transplant has been performed in select GSD type I patients because of multiple hepatic adenomas. More recently, liver transplant has been reported as a potential treatment for GSD type I patients with refractory metabolic derangements despite aggressive nutritional interventions, with excellent metabolic control achieved after transplant and good long-term outcomes.[123] In addition, with improved long-term survival of GSD type I patients, pregnancy has become an increasingly important issue among affected females. Recent data suggests that with careful monitoring and care by an experienced medical team, women affected by GSD can deliver healthy offspring.[124]

Glycogen Storage Disease Type III

Glycogen storage disease type III (GSD type III) is an autosomal recessive condition due to deficiency of the glycogen debranching enzyme. This enzyme is composed of two independent catalytic subunits on one polypeptide chain, oligo-1,4-1,4 glucantransferase and amylo-1,6-glucosidase. In order for glucose to be released from glycogen stores, glycogen phosphorylase and glycogen debranching enzyme must work together. The phosphorylase initially works on the outermost branches of the glycogen molecule. The transferase then moves glucose residues from one short outer branch to another. Finally, glucosidase works on the inner-chain 1,6 linkages. A lack of the debrancher enzyme results in accumulation of abnormal glycogen, called phosphorylase limit dextrin.[95] The 85-kb gene (AGL) for the debrancher enzyme is located on chromosome 1p21 and encodes a 268-kDa protein. The same gene encodes the debrancher enzyme in liver and muscle, but differential RNA transcription results in two separate isoforms.[125,126] GSD type III is further subdivided into IIIa, in which both liver and muscle are involved, and IIIb, involving only the liver.[127] In the United States, GSD type IIIa predominates.[95]

Clinical Presentation

Significant clinical heterogeneity exists among individual patients with GSD type III. Initially, symptoms in infants and young children appear very similar to GSD type I. They experience fasting hypoglycemia with a ketosis, hepatomegaly, hyperlipidemia, and growth retardation.[95] Patients typically have moderate increases in liver transaminases, though decreasing levels with a concomitant decrease in hepatomegaly have been reported beginning in puberty.[128] By 4 to 6 years of age, however, some patients may develop hepatic fibrosis with resultant splenomegaly and later develop liver failure.[129] Hepatocellular carcinoma also may occur in GSD type III patients, though much more rarely than in GSD type I.[130] Because gluconeogenesis remains intact and glucose can be cleaved from the outermost branches, GSD type III patients tolerate longer fasts than GSD type I patients. They are less likely to experience difficulty as long as they remain on the frequent feeding schedule typical of infants. They do not have difficulty when experiencing infections or stress.[95]

Those with GSD type IIIa have minimal muscle weakness in childhood. In the third to fourth decade, however, slow, progressive weakness of proximal and occasionally smaller distal muscles occurs.[95] Cardiac disease also develops because of limit dextrin accumulation in cardiac muscle. Some patients develop cardiomyopathy, whereas others manifest only subclinical disease with ventricular hypertrophy detected on echocardiogram or electrocardiogram.[131,132] The long-term prognosis for patients is variable, with some showing decreased hepatomegaly over time, whereas others develop fibrosis, cirrhosis, and worsening myopathy Patients with GSD type III also have abnormal bone mineral density, placing them at risk for potential fractures.[133]

Biochemically, patients with GSD type III have normal lactate and uric acid levels and less severe hyperlipidemia. In addition, they develop a more rapid ketonemia than those with GSD type I. Histologically, liver biopsy specimens have significantly increased glycogen content. Unlike in GSD type I, however, periportal septal fibrosis and a paucity of fat are seen on biopsy. Ultrastructural examination reveals small, lipid-filled vacuoles.[95,134]

Diagnosis/Therapy

Diagnosis of GSD type III is made by assaying the debrancher enzyme in liver or muscle tissue. An elevated level of creatinine phosphokinase can suggest muscle involvement, though it may be normal particularly in infants and young children.[95] Molecular analysis of the AGL gene using blood is now available commercially.[135] Therapy is aimed not only at preventing hypoglycemia, but also at achieving euglycemia. Similar to GSD type I, providing a continuous source of glucose using feedings of uncooked cornstarch is helpful in maintaining normoglycemia, achieving good growth, and decreasing transaminase elevation.[136] In patients with severe growth retardation or myopathy, a diet high in oligosaccharides and protein has been beneficial.[137] Because of the risk of hepatocellular adenomas, annual α-fetoprotein and ultrasound may be useful. Patients with myopathy should also have annual echocardiograms and electrocardiograms.[95] Liver transplants have been reported in three adult patients with GSD type III. One was transplanted for cirrhosis and hepatocellular carcinoma and two for liver failure.[138]

Glycogen Storage Disease Type IV

Glycogen storage disease type IV (GSD type IV) is an extremely rare condition, representing only 0.3% of all glycogenoses.[139] Also known as Andersen's disease or amylopectinosis, it is caused by a deficiency in the glycogen branching enzyme, α-1,4-glucan: α-1,4-glucan-6-glucosyltransferase. This enzyme usually creates branch points in the normal glycogen molecule. It is necessary for packing and degrading stored glycogen. Without this enzyme, a less soluble form of glycogen, similar to the plant starch amylopectin, accumulates. This glycogen is less soluble and has longer outer and inner chains, with fewer branch points.[139,140] GSD type IV is an autosomal recessive condition, due to a gene defect on chromosome 3p14.[141] The 3-kb cDNA encodes a 702-amino-acid protein.[141]

Clinical Presentation

Significant clinical variability exists among patients with GSD type IV. Patients with the classic form of the disease are normal at birth and then develop failure to thrive and abdominal distention with hepatosplenomegaly, followed by progressive liver failure and death by age 3 to 5.[139] Patients with a nonprogressive form of this liver disease have also been described.[127,142,143] Affected individuals may have concurrent abnormal neuromuscular development because of polysaccharide deposition. They may have neuronal involvement, severe hypotonia, and muscle atrophy at birth or present later in childhood with a progressive myopathy.[144] Cardiomyopathy and cardiac failure have been described secondary to myofibrillar damage resulting from cardiac amylopectin deposits.[145-147] Cardiac and neuromuscular symptoms may accompany or predominate the clinical picture.

Unlike other types of glycogen storage disease, hypoglycemia is rarely observed in GSD type IV.[142] Patients have a normal glycemic response to glucose, fructose, and galactose. In addition, their response to glucagon and epinephrine is most often normal.[148,149] Affected individuals have moderate elevations in hepatic transaminases and alkaline phosphatase. They have normal levels of both lactate and pyruvate, though their cholesterol may be slightly increased. As liver disease progresses, however, hypoglycemia and hypercholesterolemia became more prominent symptoms. Histologically, liver biopsy specimens may show both micronodular and macronodular cirrhosis. Hepatocytes contain strongly periodic acid-Schiff positive and partially diastase-sensitive deposits in the cytoplasm.[140] Ultrastructure evaluation by electron microscopy may show glycogen particles, amylopectin-like fibrils, and fine granular material.[139] Similar cytoplasmic deposits may be seen in cardiac, skeletal, and neurologic muscle.

Diagnosis and Therapy

The diagnosis of GSD type IV can be made prenatally using polymerase chain reaction (PCR)-based DNA mutation analysis. Diagnosis can also be made by evaluation of branching enzyme activity of cultured amniocytes or chorionic villi.[150,151] Glycogen branching enzyme deficiency can be demonstrated in liver biopsy specimens, erythrocytes, leukocytes, and fibroblasts.[152-154]

Liver transplantation is the only effective therapeutic modality currently available for GSD type IV patients.[140] This therapeutic modality is recommended only for individuals with progressive liver disease.[127] Some liver transplant recipients have improvement of abnormal glycogen in other affected organs such as heart or skeletal muscle after transplantation. This may be due to the development of systemic microchimerism that occurs after transplant, with lymphocytes and macrophages acting as migrating enzyme carriers.[139,155] Other patients, however, succumb to cardiac failure, despite successful liver transplantation.[156,157]

Glycogen Storage Disease Types VI and IX

Glycogen storage disease type VI and glycogen storage disease type IX are distinct, yet clinically similar disorders. GSD type VI is an extremely rare deficiency of glycogen phosphorylase, necessary to break down glycogen. The defect leading to this disorder occurs on chromosome 14.[158] GSD type IX is a more heterogeneous disorder, caused by a deficiency of phosphorylase kinase.[159] Phosphorylase kinase deficiency is the most common glycogen storage disease, representing 25% of all patients with a glycogen storage disease. Phosphorylase kinase is necessary to activate glycogen phosphorylase. It is composed of four subunits, encoded by different chromosomes. The α subunit is encoded by chromosome X, the β subunit by chromosome 16, the γ subunit by chromosome 17, and the δ subunit is a calmodulin.[160]

Clinical Presentation

There are several variations of GSD type IX, depending on the inheritance pattern and affected tissue. The most common subtype is X-linked and affects only the liver. The next most common group is an autosomal recessive variant that also only affects the liver. Several other exceedingly rare subtypes, all autosomal recessive, also exist. They affect liver and muscle together, isolated muscle, or heart.[160] GSD types VI and IX present with similar symptoms in infancy and early childhood. Most children have growth retardation, hepatomegaly, and a protuberant abdomen. Some children have slight motor developmental delay. They often have mild increases in triglycerides, cholesterol, and transaminases.[161] Metabolic acidosis is rare, and lactic and uric acid are normal. Hepatomegaly resolves around puberty, and final height is usually normal. Most adults are completely asymptomatic, despite a persistent enzyme defect.[95]

Diagnosis/Therapy

After an overnight fast, a glucagon stimulation test will show a normal glycemic response with increases in blood lactate. This will not, however, differentiate between phosphorylase and phosphorylase kinase deficiency.[162] Diminished phosphorylase kinase activity in erythrocytes can establish the diagnosis of liver and muscle disease. Normal activity, however, does not exclude these diagnoses. Therefore, study of enzymatic activity in tissue samples is ideal. Most patients require no specific therapy. Avoidance of prolonged fasting is recommended.[95,160]

REFERENCES

59. Walter JH, Collins JE, Leonard JV. Recommendations for the management of galactosaemia. UK Galactosaemia Steering Group Arch Dis Child 1999;80:93–96.

91. Mock DM, Perman JA, Thaler M, Morris Jr RC. Chronic fructose intoxication after infancy in children with hereditary fructose intolerance. A cause of growth retardation. N Engl J Med 1983;309:764–770.

95. Wolfsdorf JI, Holm IA, Weinstein DA. Glycogen storage diseases. Phenotypic, genetic and biochemical characteristics and therapy. Endocrinol Metab Clin North Am 1999;28:801–823.

120. Wolfsdorf JI, Keller RJ, Landy H, Crigler Jr JF. Glucose therapy for glycogenosis type 1 in infants: comparison of intermittent uncooked cornstarch and continuous overnight glucose feedings. J Pediatr 1990;117:384–391.

137. Slonim AE, Coleman RA, Moses WS. Myopathy and growth failure in debrancher enzyme deficiency: improvement with high-protein nocturnal enteral therapy. J Pediatr 1984;105:906–911.

See expertconsult.com for a complete list of references and the review questions for this chapter.

74 NONALCOHOLIC FATTY LIVER DISEASE

Anna Wieckowska • Ariel E. Feldstein

DEFINITION AND CAUSES

Nonalcoholic fatty liver disease (NAFLD) is an increasingly recognized form of chronic liver disease in both adults and children. It is a clinicopathologic entity defined as the presence of lipid deposition in hepatocytes in individuals who drink little or no alcohol. It ranges from hepatic steatosis (fatty liver), to nonalcoholic steatohepatitis (NASH – fatty changes with inflammation and hepatocellular injury or fibrosis), to advanced fibrosis and cirrhosis. The determination of the severity of the disease requires a liver biopsy with histologic evaluation. Studies have suggested that although fatty liver seems to be a benign condition, NASH may progress to fibrosis and lead to end-stage liver disease and hepatocellular carcinoma. NASH cirrhosis is now one of the leading indications for liver transplantation in the United States in the adult population. In children, the disease is mostly silent and is often discovered through incidentally elevated liver enzyme levels or abnormal findings on ultrasound. Although the natural history of NAFLD in pediatrics is not well defined, it is clear that a large proportion of patients present with fibrosis at diagnosis, and cirrhosis has been seen at young ages, as well as in adult patients with pediatric-onset NAFLD.[1,2] Because NAFLD is associated with obesity and insulin resistance, the epidemics of childhood obesity may one day make NAFLD the leading cause of liver disease in pediatrics, which will have serious implications for the future.[3]

PREVALENCE AND DEMOGRAPHIC PREDICTORS

Despite several recent advances, accurate epidemiologic data are lacking because of a lack of population-based studies and reliable noninvasive screening tools. The prevalence of NAFLD is affected by many factors, including genetics (predilection to alcohol abuse, gender) and environment, and is therefore difficult to define. In general, however, the risk of liver disease increases with the weight of the patient. From the available data, NAFLD is estimated to be present in one third of the general population in the United States. NASH seems to occur in approximately 3% of the population but may be found in more than 20% of obese individuals.[4] The increasing prevalence of childhood obesity in the United States is alarming, affecting 15% of children between 6 and 19 years of age, with an additional 30% considered overweight.[5] A large prospective study has shown that up to 50% of severely obese children have associated metabolic syndrome.[6]

Several studies used surrogate markers of NAFLD (elevated liver enzymes and ultrasound) to evaluate the prevalence of this condition in the pediatric population. American and Asian surveys report that approximately 3% and 3.2% of adolescents, respectively, have elevated serum alanine aminotransferase (ALT).[7,8] Utilizing liver ultrasound, a large study of schoolchildren in Japan showed the prevalence of NAFLD to be 2.6%.[9] Moreover, several studies in various countries have selectively examined the prevalence of NAFLD in groups of obese children and found that it may range from 23 to 77%.[10] Noninvasive techniques were used in these studies for diagnosis; thus, none was able to determine the relative proportion of hepatic steatosis versus more advanced forms of the disease such as NASH or cirrhosis. A recent large autopsy study found that 9.6% of the American population aged 2 to 19 years have NAFLD, and that figure increased to 38% among those who were obese.[11] Thus it appears that noninvasive methods to diagnose NAFLD may largely underestimate the prevalence of fatty liver in children.

Affected adults generally present between the fourth and sixth decades of life and are more frequently women (50 to 80%). Affected children mostly present in the pubertal age group and are predominantly male; there is a higher incidence in children of Hispanic origin. Several studies have hypothesized that hormonal changes during puberty are associated with increased serum insulin levels and insulin resistance, especially in boys, and thus a propensity for accumulation of fat in the liver.[12,13] Estrogens seem to be protective through their effect on reduction of apoptosis, lipid peroxidation, inflammation, and fibrosis, major mechanisms responsible of the progression of the disease. Several differences in ethnic predisposition to NAFLD and NASH have been seen. The highest rates of NAFLD and signs of liver damage on histology (higher grades of ballooning and Mallory bodies) are encountered in Mexican Americans as well as Asian Indians and Americans, probably because of higher rates of insulin resistance and increased visceral adiposity at equivalent BMI. African American patients have lower rate of NAFLD, NASH, and less severe fibrosis, suggesting a protective genetic or metabolic effect in this group. These differences may also be influenced by several environmental factors, including the type of diet, exercise choice, socioeconomic status, and living location.[1,3]

PATHOPHYSIOLOGY

Although major advances have been made, the pathogenesis of both NAFLD and NASH still remains incompletely defined. The development of NASH has been suggested to be the result of a two-hit process.[14] Hepatic steatosis represents the "first hit." In patients with NAFLD, hepatic lipid loading appears to be mainly determined by the availability of free fatty acids (FFA) from circulation. Other potentially important mechanisms include increased *de novo* lipogenesis from glucose, and decreased catabolism mainly through oxidation of FFA at the level of the mitochondria, or export of triglycerides (TG) from hepatocytes in the form of very low-density lipoproteins (VLDL). Insulin resistance and subsequent hyperinsulinemia typically associated with weight gain and obesity appears to be the key component of the "first hit" that results in hepatic steatosis. These changes have been postulated to result in an increased sensitivity to "second or multiple hits" that result in an inflammatory response and development of steatohepatitis. Experimental evidence increasingly suggests that the type of lipids accumulating in the liver may play a central role in disease progression to steatohepatitis and fibrosis. Triglyceride accumulation does not seem per se to be harmful to the liver and may even represent a protective mechanism that buffers the potential toxic effects of other lipids such as FFA. A surplus of FFA may enter deleterious pathways, resulting in an inflammatory response and progression of liver damage.[15] Oxidative stress, mainly caused by mitochondrial dysfunction and proinflammatory cytokines such as tumor necrosis factor, are believed to play an important role in the pathogenesis of NASH. In addition, adiponectin, an adipocyte-produced protein, is one of the attractive candidates for modulating liver injury. Adiponectin is secreted by adipocytes in inverse proportion to the BMI and metabolically acts to reduce body fat, improve insulin sensitivity, and decrease serum free fatty acid levels. Finally, hepatocyte apoptosis, an organized form of cell death, has been identified as a potential key component of the second hit involved in NAFLD progression.[16]

Although much progress has been made, further studies are needed to define the pathogenesis of NAFLD more clearly and explain the apparent interindividual variation in the susceptibility to progress to more advanced liver disease. Genetic factors have been suggested to play an important role in this variation, and several new candidate genes have recently been proposed. A familial aggregation study demonstrated that fatty liver was significantly more common in siblings (59%) and parents (78%) of overweight children with NAFLD, than in siblings (17%) and parents (37%) of overweight children without NAFLD.[17] A recent genome-wide association study conducted in a large cohort including Hispanics, African Americans, and European Americans found that an allele in patatin-like phospholipase 3 gene (PNPLA3) was strongly associated with increased hepatic fat levels and hepatic inflammation.[18]

NATURAL HISTORY

Several long-term longitudinal studies in both the United States and Europe have examined the outcome and prognosis of adult patients with NAFLD. Currently, there is only one available study with these characteristics addressing the course and natural history of the disease in children. At the time of initial biopsy, a substantial number of adult NASH patients may have advanced hepatic fibrosis, whereas 1 in 10 may show well-established cirrhosis. In addition, it is now recognized that a large proportion of patients with cryptogenic cirrhosis have burned-out NASH.[19] Available data suggest that the natural history of NAFLD seems to be determined by the severity of the histologic damage. A large study of 106 adult patients with pure steatosis without inflammation showed a benign clinical course, as only one patient developed cirrhosis over a median follow-up period of 9 years.[20] On the other hand, patients with NASH are believed to be at increased risk for advanced disease; progression of

fibrosis was seen in one third to one half of patients over a 3- to 5-year follow-up, and cirrhosis and its complications have been shown to occur in more than 9 to 20% of patients over the same period of time.[21-23] It is important to note that fibrosis may also regress in a number of patients. In addition, overall and liver-related mortality was also significantly higher in NAFLD patients than in the general population.[24]

In the pediatric population, cross-sectional studies have described cirrhotic-stage disease in children at diagnosis, and other reported cases of children with NAFLD who developed cirrhosis in early adulthood.[25] A recent study examined the long-term prognosis of children with NAFLD and compared their survival with the expected survival of the general population.[26] Sixty-six children with NAFLD with a mean age of 14 years were followed up for up to 20 years with a total of 409.6 person-years of follow-up. The metabolic syndrome was present in 19 (29%) children at the time of NAFLD diagnosis, with 55 (83%) presenting with at least one feature of the metabolic syndrome including obesity, hypertension, dyslipidemia, and/or hyperglycemia. Four children with baseline normal fasting glucose developed type II diabetes 4 to 11 years after NAFLD diagnosis. A total of 13 liver biopsies were obtained from 5 patients over a mean of about 5 years, showing progression of fibrosis stage in 4 children. During follow-up, 2 children died and 2 underwent liver transplantation for decompensated cirrhosis. The observed survival free of liver transplantation was significantly shorter in the NAFLD cohort as compared to the expected survival in the general U.S. population of the same age and sex, with a standardized mortality ratio of 13.6 (95% CI 3.8, 34.8). NAFLD recurred in the allograft in the 2 cases transplanted, with 1 case progressing to cirrhosis and requiring retransplantation. This study demonstrated for the first time that children with NAFLD may develop end-stage liver disease with the consequent need for liver transplantation during adolescence or early adulthood.

In addition to NASH cirrhosis being recognized as growing indication for liver transplantation, the disease is known to recur after transplantation in some cases.[26,27] The development of hepatocellular carcinoma has been reported in adult patients with onset of NAFLD in the pediatric age group.[28,29] Studies have described the prevalence of HCC in patients with NASH cirrhosis undergoing liver transplant to be more than 17%.[30] More important, NASH-related HCC has been increasingly reported in adults with noncirrhotic livers.[31]

Extensive epidemiologic studies have demonstrated that NAFLD may be associated not only with liver-related morbidity and mortality, but also with increased risk of obesity-related complications (dyslipidemia, hypertension, diabetes, sleep apnea, orthopedic complications) and cardiovascular and all-cause mortality in adults.[32] Finally, not only physical but also social and emotional parameters are affected in children with NAFLD. This was nicely shown in a recent large study suggesting that severely obese children are more likely to have impaired health-related quality of life than healthy children, with similar scores to those pediatric patients suffering from cancer.[33]

SIGNS AND SYMPTOMS

Most patients with NAFLD are asymptomatic, and the liver disease is often discovered incidentally when laboratory examination shows elevated liver enzyme levels. It is the most common cause of unexplained persistent elevation of liver enzyme levels after hepatitis and other chronic liver diseases have been excluded. The most common symptoms at presentation are malaise, fatigue, and right upper quadrant or diffuse abdominal discomfort. Hepatomegaly may be found on clinical exam in 33 to 55%, and acanthosis nigricans, a cutaneous marker of insulin resistance, has been described in about 30%. Children with NAFLD are usually obese and have associated features of metabolic syndrome (Table 74-1): insulin resistance in most patients, impaired glucose tolerance (10%) and type 2 diabetes (2%), and variable incidence of hyperlipidemia and hypertension at diagnosis. When cirrhosis appears, stigmata of chronic liver disease, such as spider angiomata, ascites, splenomegaly, hard liver border, palmar erythema, or asterixis, can be present.[10]

DIAGNOSIS

The diagnosis of NAFLD in children is most commonly made during further evaluation for elevated aminotransferases found on a routine checkup. NAFLD can also be identified incidentally on ultrasound or less frequently on liver biopsy done for other reasons. Many centers now screen for NAFLD in high-risk groups, especially those with features of the metabolic syndrome (obesity, diabetes, and hyperlipidemia).

Because NAFLD is a diagnosis of exclusion, a careful history, physical exam, and laboratory evaluation needs to be done, in particular in an atypical, nonobese patient. It is particularly relevant to inquire about excess alcohol consumption in adolescents. To exclude other known causes of fatty liver and elevated transaminases (Table 74-2) in young patients, several laboratory tests may be useful, including anti-hepatitis C antibody, hepatitis B serologies, autoimmune hepatitis serologies, serum ceruloplasmin, alpha-1-antitrypsin, and a screening for inborn errors of metabolism if indicated.

Primary noninvasive evaluation (laboratory and imaging tests) should be used as the first step to confirm the diagnosis of fatty liver disease, especially in the typical patient with characteristics of the metabolic syndrome. However, liver biopsy, the current gold standard for the diagnosis, is the only way to distinguish between NASH and hepatic steatosis and to determine the severity of liver damage and the presence and extent of fibrosis, as well as to rule out other diagnoses such as autoimmune hepatitis.

Laboratory Evaluation

In a patient with suspected NAFLD or NASH, useful baseline testing should include levels of transaminases (both AST and ALT), total and direct bilirubin, γ-glutamyl transpeptidase (GGT), fasting serum glucose, and insulin, as well as a lipid panel. Transaminases may range from normal to four to six times the upper limit of normal, but mild elevations are usually seen ranging between 1.5 and 2 times the upper limit of normal. In general, the ratio of AST to ALT is less than 1, but this ratio may increase as fibrosis advances. Liver enzyme levels may fluctuate over time and may be normal in a large proportion of children with NAFLD. Furthermore, normal aminotransferase levels do not exclude the presence of fibrosis or even cirrhosis.[34] Serum alkaline phosphatase and GGT levels may also be mildly abnormal. Given that the majority of patients with NAFLD have some components of the metabolic syndrome, serum levels of fasting cholesterol and triglycerides, as well as fasting glucose, should be verified. Insulin resistance can be determined by fasting insulin levels or by further studies if necessary (glucose challenge or glucose tolerance test). Albumin, bilirubin, and platelet levels are usually normal unless the disease has evolved to cirrhosis. Some patients with NAFLD may have low titers of autoimmune antibodies (antinuclear and anti-smooth muscle antibody), as well as an elevation of ferritin and transferrin saturation. The role of these markers is still unclear.

Imaging

The most commonly used imaging technique in the evaluation of a child suspected of having NAFLD is liver ultrasonography. The fatty overaccumulation in the liver produces a diffuse

TABLE 74-1. **The IDF Consensus Definition of Metabolic Syndrome in Children and Adolescents**

Age Group (Years)	Obesity (Waist Circumference)	Triglycerides	HDL-C	Blood Pressure	Glucose(mmol/L) or Known T2DM
6 to <10	≥90th percentile	Metabolic syndrome cannot be diagnosed in this age group, but further measurements should be made if there is a family history of metabolic syndrome, type 2 diabetes, dyslipidemia, cardiovascular disease, hypertension, and/or obesity.			
10 to <16 Metabolic syndrome	≥90th percentile or adult cutoff if lower	≥1.7 mmol/L (≥150 mg/dL)	<1.03 mmol/L (<40 mg/dL)	Systolic ≥130/ diastolic ≥85 mm Hg	≥5.6 mmol/L (100 mg/dL) (If ≥5.6 mmol/L [or known type 2 diabetes] recommend an oral glucose tolerance test)
16+ Metabolic syndrome	Use existing IDF criteria for adults, i.e.: Central obesity (defined as waist circumference ≥ 94 cm for Europid men and ≥ 80 cm for Europid women, with ethnicity specific values for other groups) plus any two of the following four factors: • Raised triglycerides: ≥ 1.7 mmol/L • Reduced HDL-cholesterol: <1.03 mmol/L (<40 mg/dL) in males and <1.29 mmol/L (<50 mg/dL) in females, or specific treatment for these lipid abnormalities • Raised blood pressure: systolic BP ≥ 130 or diastolic BP ≥ 85 mm Hg, or treatment of previously diagnosed hypertension • Impaired fasting glycemia: fasting plasma glucose ≥ 5.6 mmol/L (≥100 mg/dL), or previously diagnosed type 2 diabetes				

Adapted from the International Diabetes Foundation consensus definition of metabolic syndrome in children and adolescents (permission pending) (http://www.idf.org/webdata/docs/Mets_definition_children.pdf)

TABLE 74-2. Differential Diagnosis of Fatty Liver

Toxins	Alcohol, Ecstasy
Drugs	Amiodarone, methotrexate, prednisone, L-asparaginase, vitamin A, valproate
Autoimmune hepatitis	
Storage disorders	Alpha-1-antitrypsin deficiency, Wilson's disease
Metabolic disorders	Cystic fibrosis, galactosemia, fructosemia, cholesterol esterase (Wolman) disease, glycogen storage disease, mitochondrial and peroxisomal defects of oxidation of fatty acids, abetalipoproteinemia, and various syndromes
Syndromes associated with obesity/insulin resistance	Mauriac syndrome, lipodystrophies, Prader-Willi, Bardet-Biedl syndrome, hypopituitarism
Infections	Hepatitis C
Nutritional	Starvation, rapid weight loss, protein calorie malnutrition, celiac disease, total parenteral nutrition
Surgical	Gastrojejunal bypass

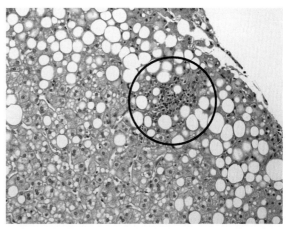

Figure 74-1. Histologic patterns of NASH in children. Representative microphotograph of a hematoxylin-eosin stained liver biopsy specimen from a child with NASH type 1 features (see text). Circle indicates an area of lobular inflammation. (Original magnification ×400.)

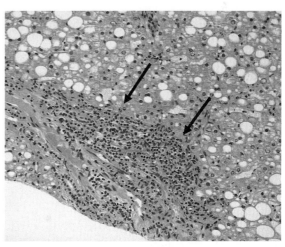

Figure 74-2. Representative microphotograph of a hematoxylin-eosin stained liver biopsy specimen from a child with NASH type 2 features (see text). Arrows indicate an area of portal inflammation. (Original magnification ×400.)

increase in echogenicity and vascular blurring. Unfortunately, ultrasound cannot rule out steatohepatitis or fibrosis, and its sensitivity drops sharply when the degree of steatosis decreases below 30%.[35] Both computed tomography and magnetic resonance imaging studies, especially the new technique of magnetic resonance spectroscopy, are more sensitive modalities for the quantification of steatosis. However, none of these imaging techniques has sufficient sensitivity and specificity for staging the disease, and they cannot distinguish between hepatic steatosis and NASH with or without fibrosis.

Liver Biopsy

Because the diagnostic accuracy of noninvasive diagnostic tools is low, liver biopsy is the gold standard for diagnosis of NAFLD and the grading of its severity: in other words, for distinguishing steatosis from steatohepatitis, and assessing the degree of fibrosis. Moreover, it is helpful in ruling out alternate etiologies involving steatosis, in particular hepatitis C, Wilson's disease, autoimmune hepatitis, and other metabolic liver disorders. In addition, histology permits the monitoring of disease progression and the response to therapy, because aminotransaminase levels may decrease during the course of the disease regardless of whether fibrosis progresses or improves.

NAFLD is histologically indistinguishable from liver damage resulting from alcohol abuse. The spectrum of abnormalities varies from isolated hepatic steatosis to NASH, in which steatosis is associated with mixed inflammatory cell infiltration and liver injury. Cell injury manifests by hepatocyte ballooning, Mallory hyaline, and acidophil bodies or apoptotic hepatocytes. Fibrosis and cirrhosis are increasingly reported in children.

Pediatric NASH can be a challenging diagnosis, as the histologic features differ from those commonly seen in adults.[36] The typical adult pattern (termed NASH type 1) is characterized by the presence of steatosis (mainly macrovesicular) with ballooning degeneration and/or perisinusoidal fibrosis (zone 3 lobular involvement), with the portal tracts being relatively spared (Figure 74-1). The pediatric type NASH (NASH Type 2) is described as the presence of steatosis along with portal inflammation and/or fibrosis in the absence of ballooning degeneration and perisinusoidal fibrosis (Figure 74-2). However, a large proportion of patients may have overlapping features of both type 1 and type 2 NASH.

Different populations of pediatric patients have shown variable distribution of the three types described earlier (Table 74-3).[36-38] Recently a multicenter clinicopathologic study evaluated 108 children from the United States and Canada with biopsy-proven NAFLD and showed similarly that although portal-based injury was seen in the majority of patients, it was associated with zone 3 pattern in most cases (overlap).[38]

Although type 2 has been associated with male sex, younger age, higher BMI, and nonwhite ethnic groups, it remains unclear whether these patterns differ in natural history, etiopathogenesis, prognosis, or response to treatments compared to patients with type 1 or overlap type.

In all pediatric reports, more than 60% of patients who had a biopsy for NAFLD had some stage of fibrosis, with stage 3 fibrosis as well as cirrhosis being described.

TABLE 74-3. Comparison of Histologic Features Between Three Major Pediatric Cohorts

	Number of Patients	Steatosis (%)	Type 1 NASH (%)	Type 2 NASH (%)	Overlap (%)
San Diego (36)	100	16%	17%	51%	16%
Rome (37)	84	16.7%	2.4%	28.6%	52.4%
Multicenter (38)	108	11%	7%	9%	73%

Several staging and grading systems have been developed in an attempt to standardize the histologic diagnostic criteria to be used for research and pre- and posttreatment comparison. The newest and most frequently used scoring system has recently been proposed by Kleiner et al. in adults.[39] The NAFLD activity score (NAS), ranging from 0 to 8, consists of the unweighted sum of scores for each of the following lesions: steatosis, lobular inflammation, and hepatocellular ballooning. An NAS score of 5 or more correlates well with a diagnosis of NASH, and scores of less than 3 are generally classified as non-NASH. NAS scores of 3 or 4 are considered borderline for a diagnosis of NASH. However, the scoring does not take into account the classical portal injury seen in pediatric patients and underestimates the scores in these patients, who are often classified as borderline NASH. There is a need for a more reproducible scoring system, perhaps a modified pediatric NAS incorporating portal inflammation into the scoring.

Despite the advantages of liver biopsy in the clarification of the diagnosis, evaluation of disease severity, and follow-up of the disease and treatment progression, its overall role in the evaluation of patients with NAFLD is unsettled, in large measure because of its risks and poor patient acceptance. In patients with risk factors for NAFLD (i.e., the metabolic syndrome), 3 to 6 months are often allowed for a trial of weight loss and for possible improvements in imaging studies and biochemical markers of liver disease. In the subset of patients most likely to have NASH or advanced disease (see predictors of the severity of the disease) and in those with an unclear diagnosis, a liver biopsy should be considered earlier.

Predictors of the Severity of the Disease

Because NAFLD may affect one third of the U.S. population and a large proportion of children, a reliable diagnostic test is necessary for screening and follow-up of patients. Liver biopsy is unacceptable for screening because of its invasive nature, and currently available noninvasive tests lack sensitivity and specificity for the detection of NASH and staging of fibrosis. Numerous groups have tried to identify clinical predictors, simple biologic tests, and imaging studies, as well as biomarkers able to detect more severe disease in patients with NAFLD.[40]

The adult literature suggests several clinical predictors, in particular older age, obesity, and type 2 diabetes mellitus, as well as AST/ALT ratio greater than 1, which may help to identify patients with more severe histologic disease.[41] One large prospective report in pediatric NAFLD identified increasing serum AST, γ-glutamyl transpeptidase, and higher titers of anti-smooth muscle antibody to be independent predictors of severity of NASH, and increasing concentration of serum AST, higher

white blood cell count, and lower hemoglobin concentrations to correlate with advanced fibrosis in children.[42] Several groups investigated such clinicopathologic correlates in pediatric NAFLD, but validation in larger cohorts as well as uniform reporting of results will be necessary before relying on these variables. Several scoring systems combining different variables have also been developed in the adult population.[43] Two of these multicomponent tests designed to detect more severe fibrosis have been tested in pediatric NAFLD and look promising: the Pediatric NAFLD Fibrosis Index[44] and the European Liver Fibrosis (ELF) score.[45] Numerous other biomarkers of inflammation, oxidative stress, apoptosis, and fibrosis are under investigation. Several radiologic techniques seem interesting for assessment of steatosis (computer tomography, magnetic resonance imaging, or magnetic resonance spectroscopy) as well as fibrosis (transient elastography). Transient elastography has been validated to assess liver fibrosis through tissue elasticity measured by ultrasound technology in several liver diseases and may be useful in NAFLD. More studies are needed to validate the existing markers and techniques and develop other accurate noninvasive predictors of disease severity in NAFLD.[40,43]

TREATMENT

Currently, therapeutic approaches are largely based on lifestyle modifications including diet and exercise. Although there is no medication yet proven to be effective for NAFLD treatment, there are a growing number of potential good drug candidates. Patients should avoid alcohol and other hepatotoxins. The overall goal is to improve the quality of life and reduce long-term liver morbidity and mortality, as well as cardiovascular complications. Because the prognosis of NASH depends in part on associated risk factors (obesity, insulin resistance, type 2 diabetes), these conditions have been the focus of treatment. Treatment strategies proposed for NAFLD in the adult and pediatric population have been based on the two-hit hypothesis, the first being fatty liver infiltration (linked to obesity and insulin resistance), and the second being factors such as oxidative stress, inflammation, and apoptosis.

Treatment of Obesity

Change in lifestyle, targeting gradual weight reduction and physical exercise, continues to be the gold standard of treatment for NAFLD in children as well as in adults.[46] Weight reduction has been widely studied in adults and has been shown to improve not only the biochemical parameters but also the liver histology.[47-49] Based on studies in adults, greater than 5% weight loss has been associated with significant improvement in liver histology. The relative efficacy of weight loss and degree of weight loss needed to induce histologic improvement in pediatric NAFLD is unknown, but rapid or sudden weight loss is not advised, because it may accelerate inflammation. In the context of evidence-based recommendations for NAFLD patients, advice is based on the pathologic mechanisms of disease progression, favoring nutrients that have beneficial effects on the metabolic syndrome parameters as well as on inflammation. Consumption of carbohydrates should be limited (especially a high-fructose, high-glucose diet) and low-glycemic-index foods prioritized. Saturated fats are limited in favor of monounsaturated fatty acids as well as polyunsaturated fatty acids (especially omega-3). Some proof-of-concept pediatric studies evaluating lifestyle dietary changes and weight loss showed improvement of serum AST and ALT as well as ultrasound liver brightness.[50,36] These markers are not reliable, however, for assessment of histologic severity. Although scant pediatric histologic studies suggest improvement or resolution of steatosis and inflammation on biopsy, more studies are needed to confirm this finding.[51]

Although no confirmatory studies exist in pediatric NAFLD, regular aerobic exercise, progressing in difficulty as fitness allows, has been advocated to reduce the risk of comorbidities associated with obesity. However, more realistically, the subjects should be encouraged to incorporate moderate activity into everyday life (e.g., climbing stairs, walking instead of taking the bus or car). Multidisciplinary management, including a consultation with a registered dietitian to assess quality of diet and measurement of caloric intake, is important. For compliance purposes, it is beneficial to encourage participation of other family members in dietary and lifestyle changes.

Pharmacologic treatment of obesity and associated NAFLD in children remains experimental. Several drugs have been studied in adults, including sibutramine, a serotonin reuptake inhibitor, and orlistat, producing fat malabsorption, both of which have been shown to improve liver enzyme levels and sonographic signs of fatty liver. Pediatric studies performed in obese adolescents (more than 12 years old) showed interesting weight-loss effects.[52,53] However, no studies assessed the direct effect on NAFLD.

Finally, bariatric surgery is now suggested for adolescents with a BMI of 40 kg/m^2 or above with a major comorbidity (diabetes, obstructive apnea, pseudotumor cerebri) or BMI of 50 kg/m^2 or above with or without major comorbidities.[54] Although adult studies suggest a significant improvement in histology after bariatric surgery in patients with NAFLD,[55,56] no such studies are yet available in pediatric patients with fatty liver.

Pharmacologic Therapy

Several pharmacologic agents, including drugs that improve insulin sensitivity, such as metformin, or glitazones (rosiglitazone, pioglitazone), lipid-lowering agents such as clofibrate, or gemfibrozil, hepatoprotective agents such as ursodeoxycholic acid (UDCA), and antioxidants such as vitamin E, betaine, or N-acetylcysteine, have been proposed as potential promising agents for the treatment of NASH in both adults and children. Unfortunately, most of the pediatric studies are small "proof of concept," open-label, uncontrolled trials. Moreover, histologic improvement is rarely evaluated with repeat follow-up biopsies in pediatric trials.

Insulin-Sensitizing Agents

NASH patients with diabetes are at higher risk of developing more aggressive disease. Several insulin-sensitizing agents such as peroxisome proliferator-activated receptor-gamma agonists (glitazones), as well as metformin, have been tested in adults with NASH and have been shown to improve insulin resistance, surrogate markers of fatty liver, and histology.[57,58] The major side effects of these type of drugs are expansion of adipose tissue and peripheral edema resulting in weight gain, but hepatotoxicity as well as cardiovascular effects have been described. Metformin has been shown to be safe and effective in the treatment of diabetes in children and is the only insulin-sensitizing agent thus far evaluated in the treatment of NAFLD in children.

Studies in pediatric NAFLD suggested improvement in serum ALT levels and reduction in hepatic steatosis as assessed by radiologic means.[59,60] A recent observational study confirmed positive histologic changes with metformin treatment.[61] A large multicenter double-blind, randomized controlled trial involving metformin in adults and children with NAFLD is ongoing.[62] At the present time, the routine use of these agents in nondiabetic subjects with NAFLD should be discouraged outside of clinical trials.

Hepatoprotective, Antioxidant Therapy

Several therapeutic agents thought to offer hepatocyte protection have been evaluated. Antioxidants have been hypothesized to decrease the oxidative stress and slow progression in NAFLD. A randomized controlled trial of vitamin E in adults showed improvement in transaminases and fibrosis.[63] Two pediatric studies with small number of NAFLD patients and no assessment in histology[64,65] suggested an improvement of liver enzymes but no change of liver brightness on ultrasound with vitamin E treatment. However, a recent RCT pediatric trial showed that the addition of vitamins E and C to a dietary weight loss program was not associated with a greater histologic or biochemical improvement as compared to placebo.[51] A phase 3 clinical trial is underway in adults and pediatric patients.[62]

Although several small adult studies suggested a benefit of ursodeoxycholic acid in the treatment of NASH, the preponderance of evidence in the literature is against its efficacy. Two adult randomized controlled trials showed contradictory results, the first showing that ursodiol with vitamin E may improve ALT and hepatic steatosis[66] and the second failing to demonstrate superiority of ursodiol over placebo on liver biochemistry and histology improvement.[67] Moreover, a pediatric study showed the lack of therapeutic benefit of ursodiol when used alone or in addition to diet and exercise in children.[68]

Other Therapies

The literature concerning lipid-lowering medication for NAFLD treatment is sparse. Reports have demonstrated improvement in transaminase levels with different classes of drugs, but there is a lack of histologic follow-up in most of these studies. Betaine, N-acetylcysteine, carnitine, and omega-3 polyunsaturated fatty acid supplementation have shown promising effects, but larger trials are needed.

Thus, current literature supports the use of nonpharmacologic approaches target to weight loss through lifestyle modifications as the mainstay of treatment for children with NAFLD. Specific therapies such as insulin-sensitizing, antioxidant, or hepatoprotective medications are promising targets (Table 74-4), but all of these interventions will require future

TABLE 74-4. Potential Therapeutic Approaches for Nonalcoholic Fatty Liver Disease in Children

Strategy	Treatment
Weight loss	Caloric restriction, exercise; sibutramine, orlistat; weight reduction surgery
Insulin-sensitizing agents	Metformin; peroxisome proliferator-activated receptor-gamma agonists also known as thiazolidinediones (rosiglitazone, pioglitazone)
Antioxidants	N-Acetylcysteine, vitamin E, betaine
Other	Omega-3, carnitine

evaluation in carefully controlled randomized clinical studies before any recommendation can be adopted.

Liver Transplantation

In patients with decompensated cirrhosis, liver transplantation should be considered. Coexisting conditions (e.g., morbid obesity, severe complications of diabetes, cardiac disease) and fear of intraoperative and posttransplantation complications have been reported to be key factors that preclude transplantation candidacy in many of these patients. In children the experience is very limited, and as in adults, NAFLD has been shown to recur in the liver allograft and may progress to steatohepatitis and cirrhosis.[26,27]

PREVENTION AND SCREENING

Because of the consequences of the disease, detection of NAFLD in high-risk groups, including obese children and those with evidence of insulin resistance or other components of the metabolic syndrome, is extremely important. However, screening remains complicated by the limited accuracy of available noninvasive diagnostic tools. Basic laboratory evaluation of liver enzyme levels may point to the diagnosis, but it cannot rule out NAFLD if normal. Moreover, imaging techniques have poor sensitivity for mild to moderate grades of steatosis and do not differentiate hepatic steatosis from NASH. Liver biopsy, the only reliable mean to clearly diagnose NASH and assess disease severity, cannot be applied as a general screening tool and should be used in carefully selected patients. In this context, reliable noninvasive techniques for diagnosis of NAFLD as well as detection of progressive liver disease are urgently needed.[43] The second issue is the lack of clearly established treatment for NAFLD, emphasizing the primordial importance of prevention and treatment of obesity and its complications including the aggressive management of the metabolic syndrome (diabetes, hyperlipidemia, and hypertension).

CONCLUSION

An underestimated condition in the past, pediatric NAFLD and NASH is now the most common cause of liver disease, affecting between 2 and 9% of children. Its incidence is predicted to rise with the increase in pediatric obesity and metabolic syndrome (insulin resistance, hyperlipidemia, and hypertension). Hepatic steatosis is the most common form of NAFLD and seems to be a benign condition. In contrast, nonalcoholic steatohepatitis or NASH may progress to advanced fibrosis and cirrhosis. The diagnosis of NAFLD is often made after incidentally finding elevated liver enzyme levels or by clinical suspicion in patients with obesity or diabetes. Laboratory results or imaging examinations may suggest the diagnosis. However, at present, only a liver biopsy can differentiate hepatic steatosis from NASH, and reliable noninvasive diagnostic techniques are needed. Lifestyle modifications, particularly weight loss, have been shown to be beneficial. Several specific therapies, including insulin-sensitizing, antioxidant agents and hepatoprotective medications, appeared to be promising, but large, randomized, confirmatory clinical trials are lacking, especially in the pediatric population. Research efforts are very important as there is still much to be learned concerning the pathogenesis of NAFLD, its natural history, and the difference between adult and pediatric disease. The understanding of the mechanisms involved in NAFLD progression may lead to potentially novel diagnostic and therapeutic strategies for this condition.

REFERENCES

1. Roberts E. Pediatric non-alcoholic fatty liver disease (NAFLD): a "growing" problem? J Hepatol 2007;46:1133–1142.
3. Loomba R, Sirlin CB, Schwimmer JB, et al. Advances in pediatric nonalcoholic fatty liver disease. Hepatology 2009;50; 4282-293.
26. Feldstein AE, Charatcharoenwitthaya P, Treeprasertsuk S, et al. The natural history of nonalcoholic fatty liver disease in children: a follow-up study for up to 20 years. Gut 2009;58:1538–1544.
36. Schwimmer JB, Behling C, Newbury R, et al. Histopathology of pediatric nonalcoholic fatty liver disease. Hepatology 2005;42:641–649.
38. Carter-Kent C, Yerian LM, Brunt EM, et al. Nonalcoholic steatohepatitis in children: A multicenter clinicopathological study. Hepatology 2009;50:1113–1120.
39. Kleiner DE, Brunt EM, Van Natta M, et al. Design and validation of a histologic scoring system for nonalcoholic fatty liver disease. Hepatology 2005;41:1313–1321.

See expertconsult.com for a complete list of references and the review questions for this chapter.

ACUTE AND CHRONIC HEPATITIS

75

Rima Fawaz • Maureen M. Jonas

Hepatitis is defined as inflammatory liver injury regardless of cause. Discoveries in the field of molecular biology, microbiology, metabolism, and immunology have greatly expanded the viral "hepatitis alphabet" and our understanding of many of these infectious and inflammatory diseases. New questions have also been raised, and the body of information has become more complex.

This chapter describes acute and chronic hepatitis caused by viruses that affect the liver (the "hepatotropic" viruses) as well as autoimmune hepatitis and nonalcoholic fatty liver disease, also known as nonalcoholic steatohepatitis (NASH). Other causes of hepatitis (e.g., chemical and nonviral infectious agents) are listed, to provide the reader with a comprehensive differential diagnosis.

EVALUATION OF THE CHILD WITH HEPATITIS

Hepatitis in pediatric patients has a diverse number of causes and can present with a variety of signs and symptoms. The evaluation may be divided into the assessment of the clinical presentation, serologic testing and imaging, and histopathologic examination. A list of the most common differential diagnoses of hepatitis in childhood is provided in Table 75-1.

Clinical Presentation

Some children with hepatitis are asymptomatic and the disease is discovered fortuitously during investigations for unrelated illness or during a routine well-child examination. This would be a typical presentation for chronic hepatitis B or C. Some present with the typical signs and symptoms of hepatic damage, such as jaundice, abdominal pain, and malaise. Still other children may present with signs of cirrhosis or hepatic failure. Among these extremes lies a spectrum of presentations.

A detailed history in a child with hepatitis should include an effort to determine the possible etiologic agent, such as exposure to hepatotoxic drugs, or mode of transmission, such as intravenous drug use or a family history of inherited or acquired liver disease. A complete physical examination should look for scleral, mucosal, or cutaneous icterus, hepatosplenomegaly, ascites, edema, clubbing, petechiae, ecchymosis, spider angiomas, and mental state changes. Nonhepatic causes of aminotransferase elevation, such as congestive heart failure or myopathy, should be considered.

Serologic Testing and Imaging

Blood tests have become the basis on which the diagnosis of hepatitis and the determination of its cause are made. Often the history and clinical examination will provide important clues and guidelines in the choice of appropriate tests. Imaging studies such as ultrasonography or computed topography are valuable tools in the evaluation of patients with liver dysfunction. However, they must be ordered judiciously and are not indicated in all patients.

Histopathologic Examination

Histologic examination of liver tissue is an important adjunct in the evaluation of children with hepatitis. It is not required in all patients, especially for those with acute hepatitis in whom the etiologic diagnosis is known and expected to have a good prognosis. However, in cases when the etiology and/or the outcome are uncertain, examination of liver tissue may be critical in the determination of diagnosis and prognosis.

HEPATOTROPIC VIRUSES

Hepatitis A
Biology and Pathogenesis

The virus responsible for hepatitis A (hepatitis A virus [HAV]) is a 27-nm, nonenveloped, spherical virus with a single-stranded RNA genome, a member of the Picornaviridae family.[1] Humans are the only natural host, although some primates can be experimentally infected.[2] Hepatitis is the result of direct cytolytic and immune-mediated effects of HAV.[3]

Epidemiology

Hepatitis A is widespread and can be found throughout the world. The reported incidence of hepatitis A in the United States has been steadily declining, with the lowest incidence ever recorded in 2007, approximately 3000 symptomatic cases.[4] However, if underreporting and asymptomatic infection are taken into account, an estimated 25,000 new infections occurred in 2007.[4] HAV is primarily spread by the fecal-oral route. The disease may be acquired from direct fecal contact (e.g., day-care centers) or indirectly through ingestion of contaminated water or food. There is no carrier state or chronic infection.

High rates of HAV infection have been associated with low socioeconomic status, both in the United States and in other countries.[5,6] In developing nations, under poor living conditions, HAV, like other enteroviral infections, is a childhood disease. In these countries, 92% to 100% of 18-year-olds have serologic evidence of past infection.[6] In developed countries the disease is acquired at a later age (20% by age 20, 50% by age 50 in the United States). As the disease is more severe in older patients, it poses a greater health problem in developed countries.[2,5,6]

Favorable conditions for endemic infections include crowding, poor sanitation, and poor personal hygienic practices. Specific risk factors reported to the CDC in 2007 included contact

TABLE 75-1. Causes and Differential Diagnosis of Hepatitis in Children

Infectious

Hepatotropic viruses
    HAV
    HBV
    HCV
    HEV
    HDV
    Hepatitis non-A-E viruses
Systemic infection that may include hepatitis
    Adenovirus
    Arbovirus
    Coxsackievirus
    Cytomegalovirus
    Enterovirus
    Epstein-Barr virus
    "Exotic" viruses (e.g., yellow fever)
    Herpes simplex virus
    Human immunodeficiency virus
    Paramyxovirus
    Rubella
    Varicella zoster
    Other
Nonviral liver infections
    Abscess
    Amebiasis
    Bacterial sepsis
    Brucellosis
    Fitz-Hugh-Curtis syndrome
    Histoplasmosis
    Leptospirosis
    Tuberculosis
    Other

Autoimmune

Chronic autoimmune hepatitis
Other (e.g., systemic lupus erythematosus, juvenile rheumatoid arthritis)

Metabolic

Alpha1-antitrypsin deficiency
Glycogen storage disease
Tyrosinemia
Wilson's disease
Other

Toxic

Iatrogenic/drug induced (e.g., acetaminophen)
Environmental (e.g., pesticides)

Anatomic

Choledochal cyst
Biliary atresia
Other

Hemodynamic

Shock
Congestive heart failure
Budd-Chiari syndrome
Other

Nonalcoholic Fatty Liver Disease

Idiopathic
Sclerosing cholangitis
Reye's syndrome
Other

with an infected person (8% of cases), homosexual activity (6%), foreign travel (18%), contact with children attending a day-care center (5%), and illicit drug use (1%). In 50% of cases no risk factor was reported.[4] Recognized high-risk locales include households with infected individuals, prisons, military camps, residential facilities for the disabled, and day-care centers.

Day-care centers are likely settings for transmission, especially if they have a large proportion of young children with orocentric behaviors or those not yet toilet trained. Under these conditions, the disease usually comes to medical attention from an infected adult staff member or an infected older household contact rather than the asymptomatic day-care vector.[7,8]

Historically there were geographic variations in the incidence of HAV in the United States.[9] However, over the past decade with widespread childhood vaccination, the rates in the West have been approximately equal to those in other regions of the United States.[4]

Clinical Course and Outcomes

The clinical and serologic course of a typical HAV infection is shown in Figure 75-1. The average incubation period is 28 days (range, 14 to 49).[10,11] Fecal shedding may occur for 2 to 3 weeks before and for 1 week after the onset of jaundice. It is during this period and while the patient is asymptomatic that viral transmission is most likely. Serum aminotransferase elevations may persist for several months and rarely for as long as a year.[2]

The clinical expression of HAV infection is age dependent, and there are no pathognomonic clinical signs that allow differentiation from other forms of acute hepatitis. Examination may be remarkable for jaundice, evidence of dehydration, and a mildly enlarged, tender liver. Occasionally, splenomegaly is noted. Serum aminotransferase values usually peak around the time that jaundice occurs. These values are often 20 to 100 times the upper limit of normal, and decrease rapidly within the first 2 to 3 weeks, although minor elevations may persist for months. Hyperbilirubinemia most often resolves within 4 weeks. Infants and toddlers are more likely to be asymptomatic ("anicteric hepatitis"), whereas the majority of adults will develop clinically evident hepatitis.[7,8,12] Only 1 of 12 young children develops jaundice,[13] and children are more likely than adults (60% versus 20%) to have diarrhea, often leading to the mistaken diagnosis of infectious gastroenteritis. Asymptomatic HAV infection among children facilitates transmission to adult contacts who are more likely to experience symptomatic and severe infection. The outcome of hepatitis A infection in general is excellent. There are no reported cases of chronic infection. Most complications are rare, and the fatality rate from fulminant hepatitis in children younger than 14 years of age is 0.1%, as compared with 1% in adults older than 40.[2,14] The complications and extrahepatic manifestations of HAV infection are outlined in Table 75-2.[15-25]

Diagnosis

The diagnosis of HAV infection is confirmed by specific serologic markers. A positive anti-HAV test indicates acute infection, immunity from past infection, passive antibody acquisition (e.g., transfusion, serum immune globulin infusion), or vaccination. The diagnosis of acute or recent HAV infection in the presence of a positive anti-HAV requires determination of anti-HAV IgM. Anti-HAV IgM is present at the onset of disease but persists for only 3 to 12 months. Detection of HAV antigen in stool and HAV-RNA in stool, liver, and sera of infected individuals are not commercially available tests, but these are rarely required for the diagnosis.[26] Serologic markers of HAV infection are described in Table 75-3.

Passive Immunoprophylaxis

Serum immune globulin can be given before exposure (e.g., travelers to endemic areas) or after exposure to an index case. The most frequent example of the latter occurs in the day-care

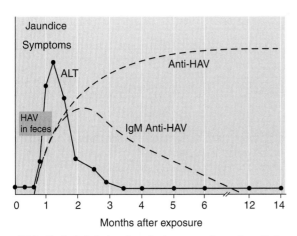

Figure 75-1. Typical clinical and serologic course of symptomatic hepatitis A. From Hoofnagle and Di Bisceglie (1991),[26] with permission.

TABLE 75-2. Complications of HAV Infection

Complication	Comments	Reference
Prolonged jaundice	May last 12 weeks; pruritus is frequent	16
Relapse	3–20% of cases; most often a single benign episode	17, 18
Meningoencephalitis		19, 20
Arthritis/rash		21, 22, 23
Cryoglobulinemia		22
Pancreatitis		24
Autoimmune hepatitis	Rare	23, 25
Fulminant hepatitis	0.1% in children	26

setting or in household contacts. The recommended dose is 0.02 mL/kg body weight given as soon as possible but no more than 2 weeks after exposure. Exact dosing and administration regimens are provided elsewhere.[27]

Active Immunoprophylaxis

In 1995, the United States became the 41st country to license a vaccine for HAV. Two preparations are currently available, both made from formalin-inactivated virus grown in culture.[28] Dosages are prescribed in proprietary unit measurements for pediatric and adult formulations. The recommended schedule is two injections 6 to 12 months apart, and 99% of children develop protective levels of antibody. The vaccine is safe, with no serious complications having been reported. The most frequent side effects reported in children are pain and tenderness at the injection site. Routine hepatitis A immunization is currently recommended for all children 1 year of age and older.[29,30] Persons traveling to regions of endemic infection and those who belong to groups at high risk of acquiring HAV (see epidemiology of HAV) should also be immunized. Vaccines should replace serum immune globulin for use in preexposure cases and may be active in interrupting epidemics. It may be reasonable in such situations to use both active and passive immunization. The impact of this vaccination strategy has been dramatic. The incidence of HAV has been falling since 1998, commensurate with the increasing use of widespread vaccination.[4]

TABLE 75-3. Serologic Markers of HAV Infection

Virus	Marker	Definition	Significance
HAV	Anti-HAV	Total antibodies to HAV	Current or past infection
	Anti-HAV-IgM	IgM antibody to HAV	Current or recent infection

Hepatitis B

Biology and Pathogenesis

Despite a reduction in newly acquired hepatitis B virus (HBV) infections since the mid-1980s, HBV remains an important cause of liver disease in the United States. HBV is a 42-nm-diameter spherical virus[31] and is a member of the hepadnavirus family (hepatotropic DNA viruses). It is the only member of this family capable of infecting humans and nonhuman primates.

The structure of the intact virus (the Dane particle) is double-shelled. The external shell, or envelope, expresses "the Australia antigen," the hepatitis B surface antigen (HBsAg). An inner shell termed the *core* or *nucleocapsid* expresses a second antigen, hepatitis B core antigen (HBcAg). The presence of a viral shell has been associated with the development of chronicity and carcinoma.[32] Inside the core resides the viral genome, a reverse transcriptase (DNA polymerase), and a third antigen, hepatitis B e antigen (HBeAg). The significance of these antigens is described in Table 75-4.

The HBV genome is a double-stranded DNA circle with a unique single-stranded area. It is 3200 nucleotide bases in length.[32] Viral replication, in a fashion similar to retroviruses, involves reverse transcription of an intermediate RNA template.[33] Although there is only one serotype, there are 8 genotypes, A through H, that vary by 8% at the nucleotide level over the entire genome,[34] and multiple subtypes. Genotype predominance varies with geographical location.[35,36] There are important pathogenic and therapeutic differences among the genotypes. Genotype C is associated with more severe liver disease than genotype B[37] and genotype D with more severe liver disease than genotype A.[38] Genotypes C and D are less responsive to interferon therapy than types A and B.[39,40] Mutations of the HBV genome have been described and may determine outcomes such as the development of a fulminant course, latency, or response to treatment.[41-43] Several types of mutants have been described: pre-core and core promoter mutants that have abnormal expression of the core protein, and pre-S/S mutants.[44]

Pre-core mutant HBV results from a single point mutation causing a premature stop codon. This typically develops at a late stage of chronic HBV infection, after natural HBeAg seroconversion. This variant is responsible for "e-minus" HBV infection in which HBeAg is absent, anti-HBe is found, and hepatitis B viral DNA (HBV DNA) remains detectable. HBeAg negative infections are associated with a more severe course and outbreaks of fulminant hepatitis.[44,45] The pre-S1, S2, and S genes are responsible for envelope protein synthesis, including HBsAg. Mutations in these genes have been found in chronically HBV-infected persons who are HBsAg negative. This has raised concerns regarding safety and screening of blood supplies. These individuals have detectable HBV-DNA, HBeAg, and anti-HBs antibody.[43,46] The clinical significance of HBV mutations in pediatric liver disease is unclear because pediatric reports are rare.[47,48] It is likely that these mutations do not

TABLE 75-4. Serologic Markers of HBV Infection

Marker	Definition	Method	Significance
HBsAg	Hepatitis B surface antigen	RIA/EIA	Ongoing HBV infection
Anti-HBS	Antibody to HBsAg	RIA/EIA	Resolving or past infection Protective immunity Immunity from vaccination
HBeAg	Nucleocapsid-derived Ag	RIA/EIA	Active infection, active viral replication
Anti-HBe	Antibody to HBeAg	RIA/EIA	Cessation of viral replication, or development of replicating precore mutant
HBV DNA	HBV viral DNA	PCR	Active infection Loss indicates resolution
HBcAg	Core Ag of HBV		Can be detected in liver only Sensitive indication of replication
Anti-HBc IgM	Antibody to HBcAg	RIA/EIA	Recent infection

EIA, electroimmunoassay; PCR, polymerase chain reaction; RIA, radioimmunoassay.

appear commonly in childhood because they represent a late stage of HBV, often seen after decades of infection.

Although HBV can infect other organs, such as the spleen, kidneys, or pancreas, its replication has been demonstrated only in the liver.[49,50] Replication produces not only complete viruses but also smaller 22-nm spherical and variable-length (50 to 1000 nm) filamentous particles. These latter particles are rich in HBsAg and are thought to be incomplete viral coats. All three forms can be detected in the blood.

Clinical expression of HBV is polymorphic and thought to be determined by the body's immune response to infection rather than a direct cytotoxic effect of the virus. The factors that determine a specific response, whether it is viral eradication, chronic persistent infection, or fulminant hepatitis, are incompletely defined.

Study of the pathogenesis of chronically acquired HBV infection is ongoing. It is thought that neonates are predisposed to chronic HBV infection as a result of their immature immune systems. This is supported by the observation that these children most often demonstrate little, if any, hepatic inflammatory injury. It has been shown that the passive transplacental transfer of anti-HBc IgG may interfere with the recognition of HBcAg on the hepatocyte surface by cytotoxic T-cells.[51] Additionally, two studies have shown that in both humans and transgenic mice, HBeAg crosses the placental barrier and may induce immune tolerance.[52,53] This tolerance is achieved through neonatal T-cell unresponsiveness to HBeAg and HBcAg, because these antigens share amino acid sequences.

Epidemiology

HBV is a major health problem throughout the world: an estimated 350 million people are chronically infected, with 250,000 deaths annually attributed to this virus.[54] In the United States, however, the incidence has declined steadily since 1985.[4] The true incidence of childhood infection is unknown because 85 to 90% of infections in this age group are asymptomatic.[55] In addition, surveillance is done for new infections, but does not detect asymptomatic perinatally acquired infections, the most common scenario in children.

The development of chronic infection is the most important consequence of HBV acquisition in childhood.[56] Ten percent of acute infections across all age groups will become chronically infected. However, even though children younger than age 5 represent only 1% to 3% of all new HBV infections in the United States, they account for 30% of all chronic infections.[55,57] The epidemiology of hepatitis B is strongly influenced by age, geographic location, and mode of transmission.

A 1985 study by McMahon and associates[58] followed 1280 seronegative Eskimos in an endemic area of Alaska for 5 years. The results show that age of infection is inversely related to likelihood of asymptomatic infection and to the development of chronicity. These results have been confirmed by others and underline the significant influence of age on the epidemiology of HBV infections.[55,59,60] Age at the time of initial infection is believed to be the most important factor affecting prevalence. In areas where prevalence rates are high, the disease is acquired perinatally or at a very young age. Chronically infected individuals represent a persistent reservoir for infection and contribute significantly over their life spans to the maintenance of high endemicity. In areas of low endemicity, the infection is acquired in adulthood and is less likely to become chronic and generate high prevalence rates.

Hepatitis B virus has a worldwide distribution, but prevalence rates vary significantly from areas of high endemicity, mainly in developing countries, to areas of low endemicity in developed countries[55] (Figure 75-2). Small pockets of high prevalence exist and may be associated with ethnic minorities (e.g., Alaskan Yupik Eskimos). In a mobile society it is important to recognize these geographic differences because it is not unusual to care for patients emigrating from areas of high endemicity. In the United States, chronic HBV infection is predominantly seen in immigrants from endemic parts of the world. It is likely that targeted screening of high-risk populations will be effective in identifying subjects who are at risk for complications of long-term HBV infection such as hepatocellular carcinoma (HCC), as well as susceptible individuals who are at risk of acquisition and thus most likely to benefit from vaccination.[61] Furthermore, prevalence of HBV genotypes varies in different regions of the United States. There is a strong correlation between HBV genotypes and ethnicity. These genotypes may account for the heterogeneity in disease manifestations among patients with chronic HBV.[35,62]

There are no environmental reservoirs (e.g., food, water) for HBV. There are no natural animal reservoirs, and humans are the principal source of HBV infection. The traditional route of transmission is parenteral, through contaminated transfused blood products or needles for intravenous drug use. Transmission may also occur percutaneously or transmucosally from exposure to blood or other contaminated body fluids. Although HBsAg has been found in virtually every body fluid (e.g., feces, bile, breast milk, sweat, tears, vaginal secretions, urine), only blood, semen, and saliva have been shown to contain infectious HBV particles.[63]

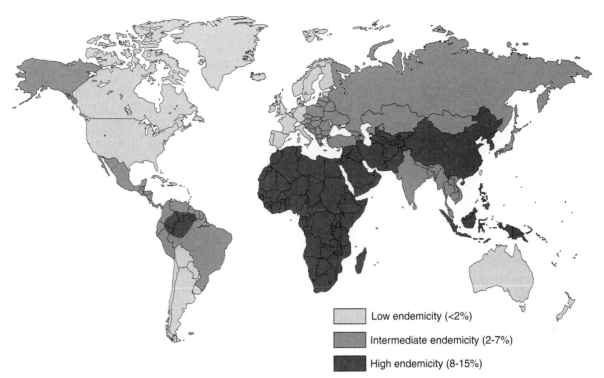

Figure 75-2. Geographic distribution of hepatitis B. (Adapted from Margolis HS, Alter MJ, Hadler SC: Evolving epidemiology and implications for control. Semin Liver Dis 1991;11:84-92, with permission.)

Transmission from infected human bites has been documented, whereas transmission from feces has not.[64,65] The lack of fecal-oral transmission and the types of close contact required for transmission probably explain the infrequent appearance of epidemics.

The route of acquisition within the pediatric population can be divided into three relevant age groups: perinatal, infancy-childhood, and adolescent-young adult.

Each year in the United States, 22,000 HBsAg-positive mothers give birth. Selective prenatal testing, based on the identification of known risk factors, is difficult and has shown an unacceptably low sensitivity (below 50%).[55,66] The failure of selective prenatal screening prompted recommendations for universal HBV screening of all pregnant women to identify at-risk newborns. The risk of perinatal or vertical transmission can be further defined by the mother's full serologic profile: mothers who are HBeAg positive have the highest rates of transmission (70 to 90%), whereas infants of mothers who are HBsAg positive but HBeAg negative are at lower risk (10 to 67%).[67-69] The presence of anti-HBe antibody in an HBsAg-positive mother does not always confer safety on her child: even though in most instances it signifies resolving disease, it may in rare cases predispose the newborn to fulminant hepatitis.[70-73] Acute maternal infection during the third trimester carries the highest risk of perinatal transmission.[59] In utero infections are rare but have been described.[74] Perinatal acquisition is thought to occur during the birthing process because infection in newborns cannot be detected serologically for the first 1 to 3 months. It is postulated that during birth the infant comes into contact with infected maternal body fluids, although whether the virus crosses through the infant's mucosal membranes, intestinal tract, or minor skin abrasions is still not known.

Infants and children who do not become infected perinatally remain at high risk of infection during the first 5 years of life.[75-77] This risk has been estimated in Asian children at 60% if the mother is HBeAg positive and 40% if she is HBeAg negative.[75] Transmission in these instances was found to occur horizontally between children within the family.[77] HBsAg can be detected in breast milk, but whether infection can be transmitted through ingested breast milk or from swallowed maternal blood from injured nipples is unclear.[73]

Available data suggest that the risk of HBV transmission within the day-care setting, either between children or between caregivers and children, is low.[78-80] Current recommendations are that HBV-infected children be allowed to attend day care unless they have other medical conditions or behaviors that would increase the risk of transmission.[79]

In 2007, the incidence of acute HBV in children was the lowest ever recorded since 1966 at 0.02/100,000 population in children under 15 years of age and 0.9/100,000 in people 15 to 24 years of age.[4] In 52% of the cases, no data were available. However, among the 48% with a reported exposure, 55% were from sexual contact and 15% from intravenous drug use. The male-to-female ratio in adolescents is equal, but in adults there is a slight male predominance.[4]

The epidemiology of HBV infection allows the identification of high-risk groups, which are listed in Table 75-5.

Acute HBV Infection

Clinical Course. The clinical expression of acute HBV infection depends on the age at acquisition. The clinical course of a typical icteric, self-limited, acute HBV infection is portrayed in Figure 75-3. The incubation period ranges from 28 to 180 days (mean 80), after which the patient may develop a prodrome consisting of fever, anorexia, fatigue, malaise, and nausea. Also during this period the child may present with immune-mediated extrahepatic manifestations, including migratory arthritis, angioedema, or a maculopapular or urticarial rash. Papular acrodermatitis of childhood, or Gianotti-Crosti syndrome, may

TABLE 75-5. Groups at High Risk for HBV Infection

Age	Group
<11 years	Children of HBsAg-positive mothers (especially ages 0-5 years)
	Children of immigrants from highly endemic areas
	Adoptees from highly endemic areas
	Minority inner-city children
	Household contacts of HBV carriers
	Institutionalized children
>11 years	Immigrants from highly endemic areas
	Sexually active adolescents, especially if multiple partners
	Intimate contacts of HBV carriers
	Intravenous drug abusers
	Homosexual males
	Prisoners
	Occupational exposure (e.g., health care)
	Travelers to highly endemic areas

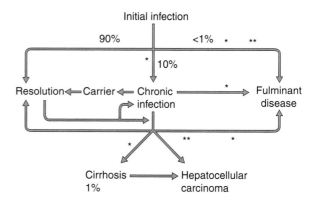

Figure 75-4. Potential outcomes of hepatitis B across all age groups.

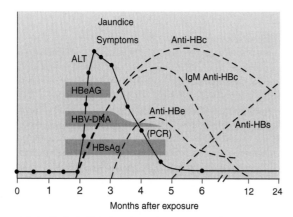

Figure 75-3. Typical clinical and serologic course of symptomatic acute hepatitis B. From Hoofnagle and Di Bisceglie (1991),[26] with permission.

become evident during this period. The syndrome includes a characteristic "lenticular, flat, erythematopapular" rash of the extremities, face, and buttocks and lymphadenitis associated with hepatitis.[81] It can be associated with other viral infections and is reported rarely in North America.[82] This syndrome is thought to be the result of circulating immune complexes.

After 1 to 2 weeks, most of the prodromal symptoms subside and clinically evident hepatitis develops, including, in many cases, jaundice, hepatosplenomegaly, and pruritus. Intense fatigue is a common complaint during this period. Symptoms may persist for 1 to 2 months, longer in a minority of patients.

Outcomes. The potential outcomes of an acute HBV infection are outlined in Figure 75-4. The complications that may result from acute infection with HBV include fulminant hepatitis or development of chronic infection. Any child with an acute fulminant HBV infection or a biphasic course should be investigated for concomitant HDV co-infection.

Chronic HBV Infection

Chronic infection with HBV is defined as the presence of HBsAg in the serum for at least 6 months. It should be characterized as HBeAg positive or negative, with or without detectable HBV

DNA, and with normal or raised levels of alanine aminotransferase (ALT). The inflammatory activity and degree of fibrosis are important histopathologic descriptors.

Terms such as "asymptomatic" or "healthy carrier state" are discouraged. "Inactive carrier state" refers to a patient who is HBsAg+ and HBeAg-, has a normal ALT, and has circulating HBV DNA less than 100,000 copies/mL. Resolved HBV is indicated by normal ALT, absence of HBsAg, and the presence of anti-HBc (with or without anti-HBs) in serum.[83]

Clinical Course. Chronic HBV infections in children may present clinically in a variety of ways. Often it is detected during the screening of asymptomatic children of HBV-positive mothers or other close household contacts. Other times the fortuitous discovery of raised aminotransferase levels in a child evaluated for an unrelated illness may lead to the diagnosis. Rarely, the initial presentation of this infection may be signs of well-established cirrhosis and end-stage liver disease, or even hepatocellular carcinoma. Finally, chronic HBV infection should be included in the differential diagnosis of any child with hepatomegaly, jaundice, or other signs of liver disease. Hepatitis D virus superinfection should be suspected in any patient with stable, chronic HBV infection whose condition deteriorates suddenly.

Outcomes. Cirrhosis, liver failure, or hepatocellular carcinoma will develop in approximately 15 to 40% of infected patients.[84] The natural history of chronic HBV infection in children has been partially defined. In a Chinese study of 51 asymptomatic HBsAg-positive children followed for up to 4 years (mean 30 months), persistently high levels of viral replication were found but were associated with mild and stable liver disease.[85] Over the study period, 7% cleared HBeAg but all continued to be HBsAg positive. In contrast, an Italian study observed 76 HBsAg-positive children for up to 12 years (mean 5 years).[86] Of this population, 70% lost serologic evidence of viral replication, with most of these (92%) developing normal ALT. Five patients became HBsAg negative. These results are more favorable than those of the earlier Chinese study but may reflect confounding variables, such as different epidemiologic backgrounds. Other pediatric reports have described a 10 to 14% annual seroconversion rate from HBeAg to anti-HBe, progression of liver disease over a longer follow-up period, and reactivation of viral replication after conversion to anti-HBe status in some chronically infected children.[87-90] It is difficult, owing to the number of variables, to compare these studies and draw broad conclusions.

Several studies in children with chronic HBV infection have shown cirrhosis in 3 to 5% of initial liver biopsy specimens.[86,91,92] In chronically infected adults with cirrhosis, the estimated 5-year survival rate is 50%.[93] In HBV-infected individuals with persistently normal aminotransferases, risk of developing cirrhosis is low, albeit higher than that in the HBV-negative population.

Hepatocellular Carcinoma

It has been estimated that as many as 570,000 new cases of HCC occurred worldwide in 2000,[94] and it is generally felt that the incidence is increasing. The majority of cases are associated with chronic HBV. This is an important sequela from the pediatric perspective, not only because it is a major cause of childhood malignancy in certain parts of the world such as Asia,[95] but also because the initial HBV infection in most patients with HCC occurred in childhood. Risk factors for the development of HCC include chronic infection with HBV, long duration of infection, male gender, the presence of cirrhosis, and family history of HBV-associated HCC.

The higher incidence of HBsAg positivity in the mothers than in the fathers of patients with HCC suggests that primary infection occurs perinatally or in early infancy.[96] This and other observations imply that the mean duration from primary infection to the development of HCC is 35 years.[97] However, reported cases in children, some as young as 8 months, raise the issue of different oncogenic mechanisms.[98] A study following 426 children with chronic HBV infection revealed that in 6250 person-years, two boys developed HCC. Both had e antigen seroconversion in early childhood and cirrhosis. Early e antigen seroconversion and/or cirrhosis may be risk factors for the development of HCC.[99]

Extrahepatic Manifestations

Circulating immune complexes including HBsAg/anti-HBs complexes are reported to be responsible for extrahepatic manifestations of chronic HBV. Essential mixed cryoglobulinemia, polyarteritis nodosa, and glomerulonephritis have been described in association with chronic infection[100-103] and may even be the presenting signs of HBV.

Diagnosis of Acute and Chronic Hepatitis B

HBsAg is the first serologic marker to appear and may be detected within 1 to 2 weeks after exposure. It precedes the development of symptoms by an average of 4 weeks.[104] The presence of HBsAg indicates ongoing infection. Qualitative but not quantitative methods are used by most clinical laboratories because the amount of antigen does not correlate with disease activity or with the presence of an acute or chronic infection.[26] Some symptomatic patients may have self-limited, acute HBV infection without detectable HBsAg. These patients, up to 9% in some studies, have other detectable markers of infection.[104] HBeAg appears virtually simultaneously, peaks, and then declines in parallel with HBsAg. It usually disappears before HBsAg. Adult patients who remain persistently positive for HBeAg for more than 10 weeks are likely to become chronically infected. HBeAg indicates a high level of viral replication

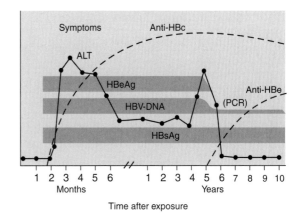

Figure 75-5. Typical clinical and serologic course of chronic hepatitis B. From Hoofnagle and Di Bisceglie (1991),[26] with permission.

and infectivity. Most patients with nondetectable HBeAg have resolving, minimal, or no active liver disease.[26] Pre-core mutants of HBV do not express HBeAg; they may be responsible for a more severe course and, in some cases, fulminant disease. Serum aminotransferase levels become raised but are nonspecific. They begin to increase just before the development of symptoms and then peak (sometimes 20 or more times higher than normal), with the development of jaundice.

The diagnosis of chronic HBV infection is based on the persistence of appropriate markers for at least 6 months or on detection of these markers in a child who on initial presentation has historic or physical evidence of long-standing infection. This information is summarized in Figures 75-3 and 75-5 and Tables 75-4 and 75-6.

The third marker of infection is HBV-DNA, which appears with HBsAg, peaks with the onset of symptoms, and then declines. Anti-HBc is the last serologic marker to appear. It can usually be detected 3 to 5 weeks after the appearance of HBsAg but before the onset of symptoms, and it persists for life. The presence of anti-HBc indicates ongoing or past infection. Anti-HBc does not appear after HBV vaccination and, in the presence of anti-HBs, is therefore helpful in distinguishing immunity due to vaccination from that due to natural infection.

Anti-HBs indicates resolving or past infection or successful immunization with vaccine and confers protective immunity. In the majority of patients with self-limited infection, it can be detected only after HBsAg becomes undetectable. In a minority of patients with serum sickness-like symptoms, anti-HBs may appear before the onset of clinical symptoms.[105,106] A "window" of variable duration has been described in some patients, during which HBsAg has disappeared and anti-HBs cannot yet be detected.[104] The determination of anti-HBc may be helpful in these instances.

Antibody to HBeAg (anti-HBe) appears after HBeAg becomes undetectable and persists for 1 to 2 years after the resolution of hepatitis. The markers of HBV and their interpretation are summarized in Table 75-4.

Treatment

Acute HBV. There are very few data regarding the treatment of acute HBV infection. The vast majority of affected individuals recover fully without treatment. Lamivudine may be useful in treating patients with severe acute hepatitis B[107,108] and fulminant hepatic failure due to exacerbation of chronic hepatitis B. In one study, 24 patients with exacerbation of chronic

TABLE 75-6.   Guidelines for the Serologic Diagnosis and Staging of HBV Infections*

HBsAg	HBeAg	Anti-HBs	Anti-HBc	Anti-HBe	Interpretation
+	±	–	–	–	Early acute disease or carrier state
+	±	–	+	–	Acute disease, chronic disease, or carrier state
+	–	–	+	–	Late acute disease or carrier state
+	–	–	+	+	Early resolution or "e-minus" disease
–	–	–	+	–	Early resolution or "window" period
–	–	+	+	+	Resolution
–	–	+	+	–	Immunity from past infection
–	–	+	–	–	Immunity from HBV vaccine

*Exceptions are described in the text.
HBV-DNA is of limited usefulness in this context except in specific circumstances (see text).

hepatitis B infection and fulminant hepatic failure were treated with lamivudine, 100 mg daily. Eight patients survived without transplantation.[109]

Chronic HBV. The goals of treatment of chronic HBV include cessation or decrease in viral replication and normalization of aminotransferases and liver histopathology, as well as prevention of cirrhosis and HCC. None of the medications currently licensed in the United States fulfills these goals for all children. For this reason, appropriate patient selection is critical so that those children who are most likely to benefit from therapy are identified. Children to be treated must display evidence of chronic HBV infection, that is, detectable serum HBsAg for at least 6 months, and evidence of active viral replication, that is, HBeAg and/or HBV DNA. In addition, children most likely to respond to treatment are those with consistently abnormal ALT values. Before starting treatment, a liver biopsy is helpful to establish the extent and stage of liver disease and to rule out any other potential disease processes. "Background rates" of seroconversion must also be considered in making a decision regarding whom and when to treat. There are currently three licensed medications for treatment of chronic HBV infection in children in the United States: interferon alfa (IFN-alfa), lamivudine, and adefovir, although the last is approved only for use in adolescents.

Since the first report in 1976 of treatment with pharmacologic doses of interferon, a number of studies in adults using mainly IFN-alfa have been published. They used a variety of treatment regimens in terms of dosage, length of treatment, and inclusion of adjuvant therapies, such as "steroid priming."[110] The greatest effectiveness was achieved at doses of 5 to 10 MU three times a week. Most studies define a favorable response to therapy as the sustained loss of HBeAg and HBV-DNA and normalization of aminotransferases. In many patients who eventually clear HBeAg and HBV-DNA, a transient increase in serum aminotransferase levels may occur between the first and third months of treatment. It is thought that this increase corresponds to activation of the host immune response and early clearance of HBV-DNA. Approximately half of the "responders" will eventually clear HBsAg and acquire anti-HBs.

In adults, predictors of a beneficial response to treatment include elevated serum aspartate aminotransferase levels and low HBV-DNA levels.[111] Other positive predictive factors include a short duration of infection, histologically active disease, and immunocompetence.[110] Our understanding of the benefits of IFN-alfa in the treatment of adults with chronic HBV infection is best summarized in a report by Wong et al.[112] In this meta-analysis of 15 previously published randomized and controlled trials, the authors showed that 36% of 498 treated patients lost HBV-DNA and 32% lost HBeAg as compared with 16% of 339 controls who lost HBV-DNA and 12% who lost HBeAg.

The results of therapy in 330 children have been reported in eight separate pediatric trials.[113,114] Comparison of the study parameters among these studies has shown a great degree of variability. These parameters have included choice of the study population (European or Chinese children), IFN dosage regimen (range, 3 to 10 MU/m² subcutaneously, thrice weekly), and duration of therapy (range, 12 to 48 weeks). In the studies from Europe, 36% of treated children (n = 124; range, 20 to 50%) lost HBeAg as compared with 14% of controls (n = 92; range, 9 to 25%). These results are comparable to those found in adults. In Chinese children the response rate was much lower: 9% of 72 treated children versus 5% of 42 controls. Genetic factors, the presence of mutant strains, perinatally acquired disease, and a long duration of infection in these Chinese children have all been postulated to justify these striking differences. The poorer response rate of Chinese children to IFN therapy is not well understood, but this may be an artifact of inclusion of a large number of children with normal ALT values. In Asian children with consistently abnormal ALT values, response rates may be similar to those of Western children.[115,116]

Children rarely need to discontinue IFN-alfa therapy because of side effects. Almost all children have an initial and transient influenza-like syndrome (fever, myalgia, headache, arthralgia, and anorexia). Starting at a low dose and increasing over a week to the recommended dose of 6 MU/m² can ameliorate these side effects. Other side effects include bone marrow suppression, especially neutropenia. Changes in personality and irritability are reported more frequently in children than adults. These changes are reversible on withdrawal of treatment. Other reported side effects are febrile seizures and markedly increased levels of aminotransferases.

Lamivudine is an orally administered nucleoside analogue. A clinical trial in children showed that the rate of virologic response after 52 weeks of treatment was higher among children who received lamivudine than among those who received placebo (23% versus 13%, p = 0.04). Lamivudine therapy was well tolerated and was also associated with higher rates of seroconversion from hepatitis B e antigen to hepatitis B e antibody, normalization of ALT levels, and suppression of HBV DNA.[117] As with IFN, children with higher ALT values have a higher likelihood of virologic response to lamivudine. Response rates to lamivudine are independent of previous IFN-alfa therapy.

Adverse events to lamivudine are very rare. However, the long-term use of lamivudine is limited by the rapid and frequent development of viral resistance. This has made lamivudine a less attractive option as newer antivirals have become available.

Adefovir dipivoxil is an orally administered nucleotide analogue, FDA approved for children 12 years of age and older. A clinical trial in children for 48 weeks revealed that adefovir dipivoxil was superior to placebo in achieving HBV DNA below 1000 copies/mL and normal ALT in the 12 to 17 year age group (23% versus 0%).[118] This effect was not seen in younger children. As with IFN-alfa and lamivudine, higher ALT and lower HBV DNA at baseline were associated with higher response rates. Adefovir dipivoxil was safe and well tolerated in children and adolescents. Adverse events were mild and no renal toxicity was noted. In adults, genotypic resistance to this drug is estimated to be around 20% after 5 years of therapy.[119] Resistance develops faster in patients with prior lamivudine resistance.[120] The optimal duration of therapy for adolescents has not been clearly defined.

Passive Prophylaxis

A detailed discussion of HBV immunoprophylaxis was provided several years ago by the Centers for Disease Control and Prevention (CDC).[80] Hepatitis B serum immune globulin (HBIG) is prepared from pooled plasma. It has a high titer of anti-HBS (higher than 1:100,000). Its protective value is excellent when given as soon as possible after exposure and persists for 3 to 6 months. Its benefit is doubtful, however, when given more than 7 days after exposure. HBIG is indicated for single instances of exposure, such as needlestick accidents, sexual contact, and perinatal exposure. It has also been proven valuable in the prevention of HBV recurrence after liver transplantation.[121] HBIG should be given with HBV vaccine in cases of repeated or prolonged exposure, such as in health care employees, intimate household contacts, and neonates of infected mothers.

Active Prophylaxis

The first vaccine against hepatitis B was prepared from human plasma of chronic HBV carriers and released in the United States in 1982. It has since been replaced by recombinant vaccines prepared by introducing an HBsAg gene containing plasmid into baker's yeast (*Saccharomyces cerevisiae*). Recommended schedules involve three intradeltoid injections over a 6-month period. HBV vaccine is also found in combination with a vaccine for *Haemophilus influenzae* type b. HBV vaccine is considered very safe; rare complications include anaphylaxis and Guillain-Barré syndrome.[80] The vaccine induces the production of anti-HBs, and the vaccine manufacturers report protective titers in 95 to 99% of healthy children who receive the full schedule of injections.

Initial immunization policies in the United States targeted individuals at high risk, such as newborns of seropositive mothers, illicit drug abusers, and homosexual males. However, it became apparent that this strategy was ineffective in reducing the incidence of hepatitis B, and in 1991 the CDC issued new recommendations.[122] This three-part strategy recommends prevention of mother-to-infant transmission through prenatal testing of all pregnant women, universal vaccination of all infants and children by age 11, and immunization of adolescents and adults in high-risk groups such as teenagers with multiple sexual partners and homosexual males. The long-term effectiveness of HBV vaccine, even in those who have lost detectable anti-HBs, does not support the administration of late booster doses.

A mass hepatitis B vaccination program, conducted by the government of Taiwan, was started in 1984. The success of this program has led to a decline in hepatitis B carrier rates among children in Taiwan from 10% to less than 1%. Furthermore, the mortality rate of fulminant hepatitis in infants and the annual incidence of childhood HCC have also decreased significantly. This is considered a remarkable success story in public health.[123]

Hepatitis C

A third form of infectious hepatitis, not due to hepatitis A or B ("non-A, non-B hepatitis" [NANB]), was first recognized epidemiologically in 1974 and was linked to transfused blood products in 1975.[106,124] In 1989, the cloned complementary DNA (cDNA) of RNA recovered from chimpanzees infected with posttransfusion NANB hepatitis was isolated.[125] This cDNA and its expressed antigen were linked etiologically to posttransfusion NANB hepatitis through the development of an antigen-antibody assay[126]; this long-suspected virus is called the hepatitis C virus (HCV). The immunologic assay against HCV (anti-HCV) allowed the demonstration that HCV was the major cause of posttransfusion NANB and sporadic NANB hepatitis.[127]

Biology and Pathogenesis

It has been suggested based on its physical properties and similarity to other viruses that HCV be considered a new genus within the flavivirus family. HCV is a 55-nm-diameter lipid-enveloped virus with a 33-nm inner nucleocapsid. The genome is a linear, single-stranded, positive-sense RNA approximately 9400 nucleotides in length. Translation of the genome results in three structural and four nonstructural proteins.

The HCV genome is highly susceptible to mutations, and comparison of different isolates has shown nucleotide sequence variation confined to specific areas. This has led to the identification of six major genotypes and a number of subtypes based on major and minor genomic differences.[128,129] Genotype determination is relevant for epidemiology and response to therapy. Mapping of the geographic distribution of the known genotypes shows that genotypes 1 (a and b) and 2 are the most prevalent genotypes in North America and western Europe.[128,130] This may have clinical significance for the development of effective vaccines. Type 1 has been shown to be particularly resistant to antiviral therapy.[128,130]

More than 80% of infected individuals develop chronic HCV. Chronic HCV is not the consequence of the direct destruction of hepatocytes by the virus. Rather, it results from an intermediate immune response that is vigorous enough to induce hepatic cell destruction and fibrosis but not enough to eradicate the virus.[131]

Epidemiology

The distribution of HCV is worldwide, and the prevalence rates appear to be evenly distributed, ranging from 0.3% to 1.5% when assessed among adult volunteer blood donors.[132] In the United States, HCV is associated with 40% of cases of chronic liver disease. Approximately 12,000 deaths each year in the United States are attributed to hepatitis C.[4] Only a small proportion of HCV-infected individuals are children, and there are few, if any, manifestations of this infection during childhood. The incidence of HCV-associated disease has been declining since 1989, corresponding to the development of the first serologic screening tools.

Bortolotti and coworkers have shown that anti-HCV prevalence rates in children with NANB hepatitis were 60 to 65% in children with thalassemia, 59 to 95% in those with hemophilia, and 52 to 72% in survivors of leukemia.[133] As the transmission of HCV via transfusion of blood and blood products has been virtually eliminated, these rates have substantially decreased in developed countries.

Although infection with HCV is far less common on a worldwide basis than infection with HAV or HBV, its propensity to become chronic has resulted in HCV becoming a major cause of chronic hepatitis. In the United States, it is responsible for most cases of chronic viral hepatitis and a large proportion of cases of chronic liver disease and cirrhosis. Most HCV-infected children develop chronic hepatitis, and although rare, cirrhosis and end-stage liver disease can occur during childhood.

There does not appear to be an epidemiologically relevant reservoir for HCV other than humans. The typical route of transmission is parenteral. Transmission may be divided into percutaneous (e.g., blood transfusions, intravenous drug use), and nonpercutaneous (e.g., intrafamilial and sexual routes).

Historically, the transmission of HCV has been associated with the transfusion of blood and blood products. With the advent of routine blood screening for HCV antibodies (1991 in most countries), transfusion-related HCV has almost disappeared. Transmission from blood products such as factor concentrates and immunoglobulin preparations has also decreased because of improved inactivation procedures. Perinatal transmission has become the major route of HCV acquisition in childhood.[134]

The proportion of cases attributable to intravenous drug use has been increasing and may be as high as 60% of new HCV infections.[135] This is due in part to the declining risk of transmission from blood products but also to the increasing frequency of drug abuse. The prevalence of anti-HCV among intravenous drug abusers ranges from 60 to 90%.[132] Intravenous drug abuse in mothers also imposes a significant risk to their children: in one study this association was found in 6% of pediatric HCV cases.[136]

Occupational exposure in health care professionals occurs from percutaneous transmission of contaminated blood in instances of accidental needlestick. The risk of infection from a single needlestick from an HCV-RNA-positive patient is 10%, and the disease is usually symptomatic.[137] Skin tattooing has become increasingly popular among adolescents and has been associated with the transmission of HCV.[138]

Nonpercutaneous transmission is the term used to describe cases that cannot be attributed to percutaneous transfer of HCV, such as perinatal and sexual transmission, intrafamilial and occupational spread, and sporadic infections in which no mode of transmission can be found. Transmission of HCV through body fluids other than blood has not been confirmed. Several studies have failed to detect the presence of HCV-RNA in the semen, saliva, urine, stool, or vaginal secretions of patients with chronic HCV infection, leaving uncertainty surrounding the mechanism of transmission in cases of nonpercutaneously transmitted infection.[139,140]

Acute HCV

Clinical Course. Acute hepatitis due to HCV appears to be an uncommon presentation in childhood; this implies that the majority of initial HCV infections in children are asymptomatic. When it presents acutely, it cannot be distinguished on clinical grounds from other forms of viral hepatitis. The incubation period is 4 to 8 weeks. Acute self-limited disease is the outcome in 15% to 50% of adults[26,141]; the percentage of resolving disease in children is unknown. Some individuals infected with HCV experience multiple episodes of acute hepatitis. Results of primate experimentation have shown that "relapse" may be the result of reinfection with a different strain of HCV or lack of complete protective immunity resulting in reinfection (or reactivation) with a homologous strain.[142,143]

Outcomes and Complications. Evolution of acute HCV to fulminant hepatitis is rare, but co-infection with other hepatotropic viruses (e.g., HBV) may accelerate progression.[137,144] The most common complication of primary infection with HCV is the development of chronic infection.

Chronic HCV

Clinical Course. The characteristics and evolution of HCV infection were retrospectively studied in 224 children with HCV at seven European centers.[145] Of 200 children followed for a mean of 6.2 years, only 12 (6%) achieved sustained viremia clearance and normalization of the ALT level. Older adolescents and young adults had a significantly higher rate of fibrosis than did younger children. Extrahepatic manifestations were rare. HCV is a mild disease in most children, independent of the source of infection. HCV infection may, however, cause significant morbidity and mortality later in life due to chronic inflammation and hepatic damage. Progressive liver disease and cirrhosis requiring transplant has been reported during childhood[146] and, more recently, hepatocellular carcinoma in two adolescents.[147] This highlights the importance of identifying, children with HCV, implementing routine follow-up, and being vigilant for liver-related complications. No pediatric studies to date have evaluated the effect of treatment on outcomes of cirrhosis or HCC.

Diagnosis of Acute and Chronic HCV

Virus-specific serology is required for the accurate diagnosis of HCV infection. The serologic course of HCV disease is shown in Figure 75-6. Serum aminotransferase levels begin to rise with the development of symptoms and jaundice. They rise rapidly and then decline in a fashion that may be either monophasic and rapid or multiphasic with wide fluctuations and a more protracted course. The multiphasic pattern may portend more severe disease or progression to a chronic state.[132,137] Assays for the detection of HCV antigens are not available, owing to the low concentrations of virus in the blood; diagnosis depends on the detection of antibodies to viral proteins (anti-HCV) and the viral genome (HCV-RNA) (Table 75-7).

A third-generation enzyme-linked immunosorbent assay (ELISA) test detects antibodies to multiple, immunodominant, structural, and nonstructural proteins of HCV. A positive anti-HCV indicates current or past infection. A negative anti-HCV does not exclude infection in its early stages, nor does it exclude past infection because it may disappear in patients whose disease has resolved. False-positive results are seen in patients with autoimmune disorders. HCV-RNA is the earliest detectable marker in the blood of patients with hepatitis C. It can be detected during the incubation period, before the development of symptoms. It is detected by the polymerase chain reaction (PCR), which can detect as few as 1 to 10 molecules of nucleic acid.[26] PCR testing for HCV-RNA is the primary method

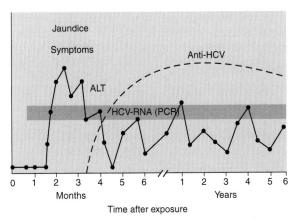

Figure 75-6. Typical clinical and serologic course of symptomatic acute hepatitis C. From Hoofnagle and Di Bisceglie (1991),[26] with permission.

TABLE 75-7.   **Serologic Markers of HCV Infection**

Virus	Marker	Definition	Method	Significance
HCV	Anti-HCV	Antibody to multiple HCV antigens	ELISA	Current or past HCV infection
	HCV-RNA	HCV viral RNA	PCR	Active infection

ELISA, enzyme-linked immunosorbent assay.

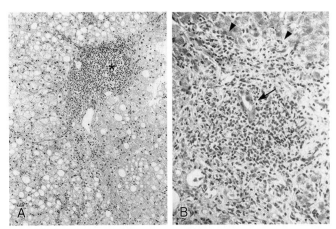

Figure 75-7. Histologic findings of HCV infection. Photomicrograph of the liver from a child with chronic hepatitis C. The characteristic histopathologic lesions include portal lymphoid aggregates or follicles (asterisk), sinusoidal lymphocytes, and steatosis (**A**). Necrosis and inflammation are usually mild. At higher power (**B**), the typical bile duct injury is seen (arrow). Interface hepatitis (arrowheads) is present in this case.

available for direct assay of the presence of HCV, which is the most reliable measure of active infection[148]; this may be the only test to detect early acute hepatitis C or infection in individuals who cannot mount an antibody response (e.g., immunocompromised patients). Persistence of HCV-RNA beyond 6 months indicates chronic infection, and its loss correlates with resolved disease. Quantification of HCV-RNA is helpful primarily in determining response to therapy.

Histologic features of chronic hepatitis C in children[149-152] are similar to those reported in adults and include portal inflammation with formation of lymphoid nodules, bile duct injury, and varying degrees of steatosis (Figure 75-7). Necrosis and inflammation are usually mild, but fibrosis is common and appears to progress with increasing age and duration of infection.

Treatment

Acute HCV. Treatment of acute hepatitis C in adults with either interferon alfa-2b or peginterferon alfa-2b prevents chronicity in nearly all cases when therapy is initiated within 3 months of exposure independent of hepatitis C genotype.[153,154] There are no studies that report treatment of children with acute HCV infection.

Chronic HCV. All patients with chronic HCV are potential treatment candidates. Treatment is recommended in patients with detectable HCV RNA and at least moderate inflammation with bridging or portal fibrosis on biopsy. However, even children with less advanced liver disease may be considered for treatment to prevent progression if they are at least 3 years of age and have no contraindications to therapy.

Combination therapy with pegylated interferon-alfa and ribavirin, a nucleoside analogue, is now the standard of care in adults. The indicator of response to therapy is sustained virologic response (SVR), defined as absence of viremia 6 months

after the end of treatment. The most important predictor of SVR is genotype, just as in adult patients. The SVR rate for genotype 2 and 3 infections approach 80 to 90%, versus 50 to 60% for genotype 1. Other predictors of SVR include short duration of infection, low HCV-RNA concentration, and absence of cirrhosis.[155] Contraindications to IFN include decompensated cirrhosis, illicit drug use, alcohol use, autoimmune disease, and other medical or severe neuropsychiatric conditions. Because ribavirin induces hemolytic anemia,[156] contraindications include renal failure (it is renally excreted and not removed by dialysis), anemia, hemoglobinopathies, and severe heart disease. IFN causes flulike symptoms early in the course of treatment. Depression, thyroid dysfunction, and neutropenia are also common.

Combination therapy with interferon-alfa 2b (Intron-A) and ribavirin (Rebetol) was approved in the United States for use in children as young as 3 years of age in 2003 after demonstrated safety and efficacy,[157] and peginterferon-alfa2b (PEG-Intron) with ribavirin in 2008. Peginterferon has been proven to be safe and efficacious in pediatric trials. Two small open-label trials from Europe using combination therapy with peginterferon and ribavirin in children showed comparable efficacy to that seen in adults.[158-160] An open-label multicenter study of peginterferon-alfa 2b and ribavirin demonstrated a 55% SVR rate in children with genotype 1 or 4, or genotype 3 with high viral load defined at more than 600,000 IU/mL, after 48 weeks of therapy. Of children with genotype 2 or those with genotype 3 and less than 600,000 IU/mL, 96% had SVR after 24 weeks of treatment.[161] A trial comparing peginterferon-alfa2a with ribavirin to peginterferon-alfa2a with placebo clearly demonstrated the advantage of using ribavirin, especially to prevent relapse, in children[162] just as had been seen in adults. The current recommendation is 24 weeks of combination therapy for children with genotypes 2 or 3 and 48 weeks for those with genotype 1 HCV. Because it appears that early virologic response, a drop in viremia of at least 2 $\log_{10}$ by week 12, may be a good predictor of likelihood or ultimate SVR, it seems prudent to stop treatment in those children who do not achieve this milestone. The role of longer-duration therapy in children who are slow virologic responders has not been explored.

Hepatitis D

The hepatitis D virus (HDV), a small defective RNA virus, is dependent on HBV and can cause simultaneous infection ("co-infection") in individuals with HBV or superinfection in individuals with chronic HBV. Superinfection by HDV leads to acute hepatitis and causes progression to liver cirrhosis in a significant proportion of HBsAg carriers. The diagnosis is made by detection of anti-HDV in serum. A PCR-based assay for direct viral detection is sometimes available. Although HDV has been shown to have a direct cytopathic effect on liver cells, this alone is inconsistent with the existence of a well-described HDV carrier state.[163,164] Immune-mediated mechanisms of hepatocyte injury are also suspected. The outcomes for both the acute and chronic forms of HDV infection are more severe than for HBV alone. The mortality rate from acute HDV infections ranges from 2 to 20%, as compared with less than 1% from acute HBV infections.[165] Cirrhosis may develop rapidly, within 2 years, in 15% and in 70 to 80% over the long term, as compared with 10% in chronic hepatitis B.[165] The only agent that has had a beneficial effect in HDV infection is IFN-alfa. HDV is more common in Europe than in North America. A recent review summarizes progress in understanding the pathobiology of the virus, epidemiology, clinical features, and therapeutic challenges of HDV infection over the past 30 years.[166] There are currently no recommendations regarding the treatment of chronic HDV infection in children.

Hepatitis E

Epidemic non-A, non-B hepatitis was first confirmed as a distinct entity in 1982, and the responsible viral particles were identified in fecal material.[167,168] The causative agent of epidemic NANB hepatitis was named hepatitis E virus (HEV) in 1988, and the complete genome was sequenced, with the subsequent development of diagnostic tests in the early 1990s.[169] The most common diagnostic tool is the assay for anti-HEV, but the quality of this assay varies around the world. Hepatitis E affects mainly adults, but isolated childhood infections have been reported.[170] It is considered a waterborne illness in developing countries and is spread from animal vectors, most commonly swine, in industrialized countries. The incubation period is about 40 days. The clinical illness resembles that of hepatitis A, with acute icteric hepatitis in the majority of instances. It is typically self-limited, with no chronic infections reported, but the overall mortality rate is 1 to 4%. There is a high mortality rate in pregnant women, up to 20%. Transmission of the virus to the fetus is common, with significant morbidity. Chronicity is not a feature. Multiple genotypes have been described, and the seroprevalence of anti-HEV in the United States is highest in areas that are large producers of swine. A recent comprehensive review has been published.[171]

Hepatitis Non-A-E

In one study of 79 patients with posttransfusion-associated hepatitis, 10 (13%) failed to show evidence for any of the known hepatitis viruses.[172] It is clear that other, as yet unidentified, agents may be responsible for clinically evident hepatitis. Consequently, it can be expected, especially with further refinements in molecular biology techniques, that the "hepatitis alphabet" will continue to expand, as will our knowledge of infectious hepatitis.

Epstein-Barr Virus

Epstein-Barr virus (EBV) is a gamma herpesvirus in the family of Herpesviridae. It is the principal cause of infectious mononucleosis, but it is also responsible for significant disease in immunocompromised patients such as children with the acquired immunodeficiency syndrome (AIDS) or those who have undergone organ transplantation. EBV has been linked to the development of tumors and lymphoproliferative disorders, especially in immunosuppressed posttransplant patients.

Infectious mononucleosis in otherwise healthy children is generally a mild disease.[173] In addition to generalized symptoms of malaise, fatigue, pharyngitis, and nausea, hepatitis is common, with hepatomegaly found in 10 to 15%. Serum aminotransferase levels are elevated in 80% of children, but jaundice becomes apparent in less than 5%. Major symptoms typically persist for 2 to 4 weeks and then gradually recede.[174] The prognosis is generally excellent, and once the diagnosis is established, the hepatic component need only be followed clinically. Diagnosis is strongly suspected based on clinical findings of exudative pharyngitis, lymphadenopathy, hepatosplenomegaly, and peripheral atypical lymphocytosis. The diagnosis is confirmed by the detection of heterophil and/or EBV-specific antibodies. EBV, like other herpesviruses, establishes a persistent latent infection after the primary illness. Fulminant hepatitis due to EBV is rare, and chronic hepatitis is not reported.

Cytomegalovirus

Cytomegalovirus (CMV) is the largest of the herpesviruses, with a diameter of 200 nm. Infection with CMV can be acquired by intrauterine, perinatal, intrafamilial, or sexual transmission as well as by transfusion or organ transplantation.[175] CMV DNA persists after primary infection, and multiple reactivations can occur; these are normally controlled by the host cell-mediated immune response. In immunocompetent individuals, the primary infection and subsequent reactivations are generally asymptomatic but may be responsible for an infectious mononucleosis-type picture with mild hepatic involvement.

From a pediatric perspective, congenital CMV infections and infections in immunocompromised children are especially important. In these circumstances a severe and/or chronic condition can ensue. Newborns with congenital CMV frequently have hepatic involvement, with hepatosplenomegaly in 60%, jaundice in 67%, and purpura in 13%.[176] The degree of jaundice is attributed to both the hepatitis and hemolytic anemia. The hepatitis may persist but rarely progresses to cirrhosis.[175]

The prototypical CMV infection in immunocompromised children occurs in those children who have received an organ transplant. The source of infection may be the grafted organ, transfused blood products, or reactivation of latent infection. The CMV infection may cause hepatitis, which, in the liver transplant patient for example, may be difficult to distinguish from rejection or vascular compromise of the graft. In these children the infection may become persistent and even lead to liver failure.[177]

Diagnosis is best established by isolation of CMV from urine, saliva, biopsy tissues, or other body secretions. Total antibodies against CMV may also be assayed, but results may be confounded in the multiply transfused child and in the neonate from circulating "foreign" IgG antibodies. Antibodies directed against CMV may be helpful in diagnosing a primary infection by determining the presence of IgM and seroconversion from IgM to IgG; PCR to detect the CMV genome may be helpful. In the presence of hepatitis, and when clinically indicated, characteristic intranuclear inclusion bodies can be found on histologic examination of liver biopsy specimens. CMV hepatitis may be treated with ganciclovir or valganciclovir. CMV-specific immunoglobulin preparations may be appropriate adjunctive therapy in selected clinical settings.

AUTOIMMUNE HEPATITIS

Definition and Classification

In children there are four forms of chronic hepatitis in which damage likely results from an autoimmune mechanism: autoimmune hepatitis (AIH), autoimmune sclerosing cholangitis overlap syndrome, *de novo* autoimmune hepatitis after liver transplantation, and a form of AIH that thus far seems unique to the pediatric population, the syndrome of postinfantile giant cell hepatitis associated with autoimmune hemolytic anemia.[178] AIH, which has been described since the early 1950s, is a chronic necroinflammatory hepatitis of unknown etiology. It is characterized histologically by dense mononuclear and plasma cell infiltrates in the portal tracts and serologically by autoantibodies targeted against nonspecific, liver-specific, or other organ-specific antigens.

Two main types of AIH have been described: type I or classic (AIH-I) and type II or anti-LKM-1 autoimmune hepatitis (AIH-II). The distinction is made according to differing profiles of circulating autoantibodies (Table 75-8). A third type of autoimmune hepatitis, characterized by antibodies against soluble liver antigens, has been proposed (AIH-III),[179] but has not been universally accepted, and many include this third type as a subset of AIH-I.[180] An overlapping syndrome between AIH and sclerosing cholangitis has been reported in both children and adults.[181,182] In fact, one study showed that 40% of patients with sclerosing cholangitis had clinical, biochemical, immunologic, and histologic features that are indistinguishable from those of AIH.[183] In the AIH associated with Coombs-positive hemolytic anemia, none of the typical autoantibodies are present.[178]

Pathogenesis

A proposed conceptual framework for the pathogenesis of AIH involves a genetically predisposed individual exposed to an environmental agent. This agent triggers an autoimmune response targeted against liver antigens and results in a chronic hepatic necroinflammatory response, leading to fibrosis and cirrhosis.[180]

The search for predisposing genetic factors has focused on the major histocompatibility complex on chromosome 6, and in particular on the HLA-DR region. Susceptibility to AIH has been linked to two histocompatibility genes: DR3 and DR4. It has been shown that the association with HLA-DR3 predisposes to more severe disease, which appears at an earlier age and results more frequently in liver transplantation.[184] A partial deficiency of the complement component C4, which is coded at the HLA-DR3 locus, has been described in some children with AIH. C4 plays a role in virus neutralization, and this type

TABLE 75-8. Classification of Autoimmune Hepatitis (AIH)

Type	Characteristic Autoantibodies	Occasionally Present Autoantibodies
I. Classic AIH	Anti-nuclear	Anti-mitochondrial
	Anti-smooth muscle	Anti-soluble liver antigen
	Anti-actin	Anti-liver-pancreas protein
	Anti-asialoglycoprotein receptor	Anti-neutrophil cytoplasmic
II. Anti-LKM-I AIH	Anti-LKM-I	Anti-liver cytosol*
	Anti-liver cytosol-I	Anti-nuclear*

of deficiency may lead to the development of autoimmunity.[185] One study reported regulator gene mutations in a series of children with type 2 AIH.[186]

The environmental triggers presumed to initiate autoimmune hepatitis are unknown, but several viral candidates have been proposed based on reported evidence. These include rubella, Epstein-Barr virus, and the hepatotropic viruses A, B, and C.

The target antigen for AIH-I has not been identified, and none of the diagnostic autoantibodies for AIH-I appear to be pathogenic. Anti-LKM-1 antibodies recognize the cytochrome mono-oxygenase P450IID6 expressed on hepatocyte membrane surfaces, and this protein is the pathogenic autoantigen in AIH-II.[179]

Clinical Course and Outcomes

AIH affects both children and adults, with two peaks of incidence at 10 to 20 and 45 to 70 years of age.[185] AIH-I represents 80% of all cases in adults.[179] AIH-II usually affects children and young adults. AIH was originally described as a disease of young women, but more reports have identified a broad age range. Half of the patients with AIH present between 10 and 20 years of age. Its course can be particularly severe and rapidly progressive. Cases of fulminant hepatitis in young children have been ascribed to AIH.[187]

Although AIH may present acutely, it always becomes chronic and it is not necessary to wait 6 months to confirm chronicity.[185] The clinical features are heterogeneous and cover the spectrum from asymptomatic patients in whom hepatitis is an incidental biochemical finding to patients with fulminant hepatitis and liver failure.[188] The differential diagnosis between AIH, acute viral hepatitis, and other acute or chronic liver disorders may not be straightforward.[189] There may be no correlation with the clinical findings, or lack thereof, and the often severe histologic lesion seen on liver biopsy.[188]

The clinical course in adults has been well described and may be benign in some cases.[179,188] This does not appear to be the case for AIH presenting in childhood. A 20-year experience in 52 children with a median follow-up of 5 years has been reported.[190] The results indicated that AIH-II presents at an earlier age, with a more severe initial presentation, including fulminant hepatitis, and a poorer response to immunosuppressive therapy (Table 75-9). Long-term outcome in both groups, however, appears to be similar. A significant number of associated

TABLE 75-9.   Characteristics, Clinical Course, and Outcomes in 52 Children with Autoimmune Hepatitis (AIH) Followed for a Median of 5 Years

	AIH-I	AIH-II
Demographics		
No. patients (%)	32 (62)	20 (38)
Females (%)	24 (75)	15 (75)
Age at diagnosis (range)	10 years (2-15)	7 years (0.3-19)
Initial Presentation		
Acute hepatitis (%)	16 (50)	13 (65)
Insidious onset (%)	12 (38)	5 (25)
Hepatosplenomegaly (%)	15 (47)	8 (40)
Cirrhosis on biopsy (%)	18/26 (69)	5/13 (38)
Fulminant hepatitis (%)	1 (3)	5 (25)
Response to Immunosuppressive Therapy		
Initial remission (%)	31 (97)	13 (65)
Stopped after 3 years (%)	6 (19)	0 (0)
Liver transplant	2 (19)	2 (65)
Deaths	1 (19)	2 (65)

From Gregorio et al. (1997),[190] with permission.

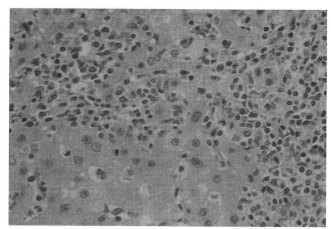

Figure 75-8. Histologic findings in autoimmune hepatitis. High-power micrograph of the liver from a child with autoimmune hepatitis demonstrating severe necroinflammatory hepatocellular injury and dense portal triad mononuclear cell infiltrates that include plasma cells. Parenchymal collapse is also common.

immune-related disorders have been found in patients and/or their first-degree relatives (21% and 40%, respectively), including inflammatory bowel disease, thyroiditis, and nephritis. Bilirubin level and prothrombin time at initial presentation appeared to be good predictors of outcome. Similar results in children with AIH were reported in two studies,[191,192] but cirrhosis was present on biopsy in a larger proportion of patients (up to 89%), emphasizing the severity of this disease in the pediatric population.

Adults with AIH frequently have other autoimmune disorders, but these are less common in children. Although type I patients frequently are seropositive for ANA, true SLE rarely coexists with AIH. Nonhepatic immunologic disorders are more common in type II than type I AIH (40% versus 17%), and organ-specific autoantibodies, such as anti-thyroid, anti-islet cell, and anti-parietal cell, are common (30%). Most of the concurrent immune disorders are clinically apparent, and routine testing is not indicated, but thyroid disease may be subtle in presentation, and periodic thyroid function testing should be considered in these individuals.

Diagnosis

The diagnosis of AIH in childhood must take into consideration clinical features, histologic findings, and the detection of autoantibodies. A severe presentation with deep jaundice, dark urine, and coagulopathy along with accompanying immune-related disorders (e.g., thyroiditis, ulcerative colitis) may be important diagnostic clues, allowing the differentiation from other liver diseases with which it may be easily confused. Liver biopsy is critical to establish the diagnosis. A histologic picture of severe necroinflammatory hepatocellular injury and dense portal triad mononuclear cell infiltrates including plasma cells with parenchymal collapse is helpful in differentiating AIH from viral or drug-induced hepatitis (Figure 75-8). In addition, AIH in older children and adolescents should be distinguished from the acute or chronic hepatitis presentation of Wilson's disease. A diagnostic scheme for the diagnosis of AIH in adults and children has

been proposed.[193] Although in some instances the diagnosis is straightforward, problems with the proposed systems have been identified, especially in individuals with cholestatic liver disease or fatty liver disease, and in some pediatric patients.[194]

Delineation of a patient's autoantibody profile is important for diagnostic, typing, and prognostic purposes. Patients with AIH-I typically present with circulating anti-nuclear, anti-smooth muscle, and/or anti-actin antibodies. Although anti-actin antibodies are more specific than anti-smooth muscle antibodies, testing for them is not performed in most clinical laboratories. In AIH-II, antibodies against liver-kidney microsome-1 (anti-LKM-1) are characteristically present. A large proportion of adult anti-LKM-1 patients will be positive for markers of HCV infection. This association is rare in children and most likely represents a reactivity different from the one found in AIH-II.[185,195] In some patients with AIH-II, anti-liver cytosol-1 antibodies can be present alone or with anti-LKM-1. Several pediatric patients with this profile and asymptomatic disease have been described.[196] Other antibodies not routinely sought but sometimes found in both AIH-1 and AIH-2 include anti-soluble liver antigen and anti-asialoglycoprotein-receptor autoantibody.[197,198]

Autoantibodies can be found in low titers in adults with a variety of non-autoimmune disorders. In children who are healthy or who have non-autoimmune diseases, however, this is rare, and the presence of autoantibodies even in low titers is sufficient for the diagnosis of AIH.[185] Some patients with all the features of autoimmune hepatitis but without detectable autoantibodies have been reported, and are labeled as having "seronegative AIH" or "cryptogenic cirrhosis."[180]

Since its initial description, hyperproteinemia and hyperglobulinemia have been described in association with AIH. The hyperglobulinemia may lead to false-positive screening results for hepatitis C, but more specific HCV testing (see hepatitis C) and detection of non-organ-specific and liver-specific autoantibodies should lead to the correct diagnosis.

Overlap Syndromes

Several overlap syndromes, in which features of more than one autoimmune hepatobiliary disease occur concurrently or consecutively, have been described. Some of these syndromes are classified in the group "autoimmune cholangiopathy." In children, the most problematic diagnostic issue is the distinction between PSC and AIH, with or without concurrent ulcerative colitis.[181,182] Histologic features of either or both may be present, and macroscopic bile ducts may or may not be affected. ANA and/or ASMA may be detected. For this reason, some authors recommend cholangiography in children who present with hepatitis, Hypergammaglobulinemia, and autoantibodies.

Treatment

Chronic AIH generally responds to immunosuppressive therapy, of which corticosteroids have become the mainstay. Immunosuppressive therapy for AIH can be divided into two phases: (1) induction of remission and (2) maintenance of remission. There are no widely accepted guidelines for initial dosage and withdrawal of immunosuppressive agents. One pediatric regimen begins with prednisolone, 2 mg/kg/day (maximum 60 mg) and is gradually decreased over a period of 4 to 6 weeks to the minimum dose capable of maintaining normal aminotransferase levels.[185] If excessive doses of corticosteroids are required to maintain normal aminotransferase levels or if the child does not achieve remission, then azathioprine at a dose of 0.5 mg/kg/day is started. Based on the patient's response and presence or lack of drug-induced toxicity, the dose of azathioprine may be increased to 2 mg/kg/day. 6-Mercaptopurine, a related purine analogue, can be substituted for azathioprine at a lower dose and, in some cases, has facilitated induction of remission when azathioprine has failed.[199] Results of this treatment protocol are shown in Table 75-9. The time necessary to achieve normalization of aminotransferases can be prolonged. In this protocol, normalization was reached after a median of 0.5 year (range, 0.2 to 7) in AIH-I and 0.8 year (range, 0.2 to 3.2) in AIH-II.[185]

Immunosuppressive therapy may be withdrawn in some patients, allowing a prolonged "disease-free" period. This is usually attempted when a liver biopsy shows minimal or no inflammatory changes after at least 1 year of normal aminotransferases. Withdrawal of therapy is preferably not attempted during or after puberty and within 3 years of diagnosis.[200] Most children will require indefinite chronic, low-maintenance doses of corticosteroids and a purine analogue, alone or in combination, to maintain remission. Alternate-day or pulsed corticosteroid regimens have been disappointing.[180]

Forty percent of children will have at least one episode of relapse while on treatment, and many will progress to cirrhosis.[185] The risk of relapse is greater if prednisone is administered on alternate days. Poor indicators of response to therapy include cirrhosis at initial biopsy, diagnosis at a young age, long duration of disease, and presence of the HLA-B8 or DR3 phenotype.[180] Empiric nonsteroidal treatments including ursodeoxycholic acid, cyclosporine, methotrexate, mycophenolate mofetil, and tacrolimus have been used in limited studies to treat recalcitrant disease or corticosteroid intolerance.

Of alternative agents, the greatest experience to date has been with cyclosporine. A pilot, multinational, multicenter, clinical trial of cyclosporine involving 32 children with autoimmune hepatitis was published in 1999.[201] Cyclosporine was administered alone for 6 months, followed by combined low doses of prednisone and azathioprine for 1 month, after which cyclosporine was discontinued. Of 30 patients, ALT levels normalized in 25 by 6 months and all had normal levels by 1 year of treatment. Longer-term follow-up (median 29 months) of 84 children on the same protocol revealed normalization of aminotransferases in 94% of patients, with remission obtained in 79% of patients at 7 months. The presence of both hyperbilirubinemia and portal hypertension at diagnosis were predictors of delay in remission.[202]

Limited data are available regarding other therapies. In some children with refractory AIH there seems to be a role for mycophenolate mofetil (MMF).[203,204] Budesonide, a synthetic glucocorticoid with a high first-pass metabolism by the liver, has been used with some success in a few cases,[205-207] but discordant results have also been published.[208]

Patients with AIH who have failed medical therapy or who presented initially with end-stage liver disease have been referred for liver transplantation with success. The disease may recur after transplantation despite aggressive immunosuppression or several years after grafting when immunosuppression is reduced.[180] Although liver transplantation may be undertaken in children with AIH, the recurrence rate is higher than that reported in adults,[209] and recurrence does not always respond to treatment. In addition, *de novo* AIH is sometimes seen in children after liver transplantation for an unrelated disease.

NONALCOHOLIC FATTY LIVER DISEASE

Introduction and Definitions

The epidemic of obesity in adults, children, and adolescents has many significant consequences for the health of the population. The high prevalence of obesity has led to the recognition and characterization of types of chronic liver disease previously thought to be uncommon and limited to selected adult patients. This group of disorders is called nonalcoholic fatty liver disease (NAFLD) when alcohol is excluded as the etiology. NAFLD is increasingly recognized in children and adolescents and has become the most common form of chronic liver disease in this population. Fatty liver, also referred to as hepatic steatosis, refers to accumulation of fat in the parenchymal cells of the liver. NAFLD represents a spectrum of types and severity of hepatic steatosis. When the steatosis is accompanied by necroinflammation and varying degrees of fibrosis, this more severe form of the disease is called nonalcoholic steatohepatitis (NASH). NAFLD should be distinguished from microvesicular steatosis of the liver, which is seen in a variety of inherited or acquired disorders that have a final common pathway of defective oxidation of free fatty acids. NAFLD is a histologic diagnosis: it may be associated with or caused by a variety of underlying diseases or drugs (Table 75-10). Progression of NASH to chronic liver disease with significant fibrosis and cirrhosis is well documented. NASH is now thought to be responsible for much of the noninfectious end-stage liver disease in the United States.

Histologic Features

Although liver biopsy may not be indicated in every child who is obese, has abnormal aminotransferases, and shows clinical evidence of insulin resistance (see later discussion), histology is required for the definitive diagnosis of NAFLD. Once the histologic lesion has gone beyond simple steatosis, the liver disease is classified as NASH. The primary defining features of NASH in adults include macrovesicular steatosis, parenchymal lymphocyte-predominant inflammation, and ballooning hepatocyte degeneration (Figure 75-9). Other features observed with variable frequency include perisinusoidal fibrosis (predominantly in zone 3, the hepatocytes around the central veins), Mallory's

TABLE 75-10. Causes of NAFLD and NASH

Acquired metabolic conditions
  Obesity
  Diabetes mellitus
  Rapid weight loss
  Total parenteral nutrition
  Acute starvation
Genetic metabolic conditions
  Wilson's disease
  Hereditary tyrosinemia
  Abetalipoproteinemia
Surgical procedures
  Jejunoileal bypass
  Gastroplasty
  Extensive small bowel resection
Drugs/toxins
  Glucocorticoids
  Amiodarone
  Synthetic estrogens
  Isoniazid
  Others
Miscellaneous
  Small bowel bacterial overgrowth

Adapted from Reid AE. Nonalcoholic steatohepatitis. Gastroenterology 2001; 121:710-723. Copyright 2001 AGA.

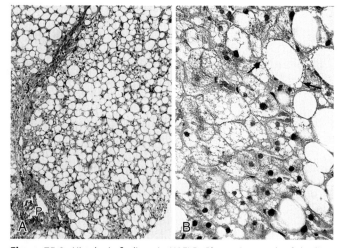

Figure 75-9. Histologic findings in NAFLD. Photomicrograph of the liver in NASH. (**A**) At low power, large lipid droplets can be seen in many of the enlarged hepatocytes. Bridging fibrosis and some inflammation in the portal areas are also noted. (**B**) At higher magnification, the large lipid vacuoles are seen to be compressing the cellular organelles and nuclei to the periphery of the hepatocytes (arrows).

hyaline, glycogenated nuclei, lipogranulomas, steatonecrosis, and iron accumulation. These findings in children are designated as "type1" NASH. "Type2" NASH, which is more common in children, is characterized by macrovesicular steatosis with portal inflammation and/or fibrosis, generally without lobular inflammation. Children with advanced fibrosis tend to have the "type 2" NASH pattern and to be younger and more obese.[210] It is not known whether the pattern of NASH evolves as children grow.

The extent of fibrosis varies considerably, but fibrosis has been found in a higher prevalence of pediatric patients with NASH at presentation, compared with adults.[211] Well-established cirrhosis is found on initial biopsies in 7 to 16% of adult patients with NASH.

Prevalence and Risk Factors

The prevalence of NAFLD in the general population is not known because the majority of affected individuals are asymptomatic and there is no reliable surrogate screening. Autopsy studies and studies of general populations have demonstrated rates of approximately 20% for NAFLD and 2 to 3% for NASH, but rates are substantially higher in obese and diabetic subjects. In a study of nonalcoholic adult patients referred for evaluation of abnormal aminotransferases, in whom no other etiology could be identified, NASH was found at biopsy in 26%.[212]

Prevalence rates for children and adolescents are not available because there are no large series of liver biopsies for abnormal aminotransferase values. However, an estimate of the magnitude of NAFLD in childhood was made from data gathered in the NHANES cycle III database (1988-1994).[213] Abnormal ALT values were noted in 1.5% of adolescents of normal weight, in 5% of the overweight, and in 9.5% of the obese. When children referred to obesity programs are studied, the prevalence of ALT abnormality increases to 12 to 25%, and the presence of fatty liver increases to 53%.[214] A children's autopsy study in the United States revealed the overall prevalence of NAFLD to be 9.6%, increasing with age (0.7% for ages 2 to 4 years versus17.3% for ages 15 to 19 years).[215]

Risk factors for NAFLD in adults include obesity, type 2 diabetes mellitus, dyslipidemia, and metabolic syndrome. In the pediatric study, the most prominent risk factor for NAFLD was obesity (38%), but race was also a strong predictor, with Hispanics having the highest risk and African Americans having the lowest.[215] In all reports of NAFLD in children, boys outnumber girls in a 2:1 ratio.[216]

Pathogenesis

The pathogenesis of NAFLD has not been completely elucidated. Fat deposition in the liver occurs when the degree of lipogenesis is greater than the rate of lipolysis. This may result from delivery of fatty acids to the liver in greater amounts than is needed for the processes of mitochondrial oxidation for energy and synthesis of necessary lipids and phospholipids. This mechanism might explain the hepatic steatosis in obesity, acute starvation, excessive dietary fat intake, and total parenteral nutrition. Alternatively, decreased use of fatty acids within the liver, by either disturbed mitochondrial oxidation or decreased synthesis, might also cause fat accumulation.

It is becoming clear that insulin resistance is a critical factor in the generation of NAFLD. Insulin promotes retention of triglyceride in hepatocytes. It has been demonstrated repeatedly that most patients with NAFLD or NASH have raised insulin levels or insulin resistance even in the absence of obesity or hyperglycemia. This association has been noted in children as well.[217]

The first inciting factor in the development of NAFLD and NASH is the accumulation of triglycerides in hepatocytes. It is now generally accepted that a "second hit" is necessary once hepatic steatosis is established, to promote progression to hepatocellular injury associated with inflammation and then fibrosis (Figure 75-10). The resultant hepatocyte damage may then stimulate the influx of inflammatory cells, initiating an inflammatory cytokine cascade and leading to further tissue injury.

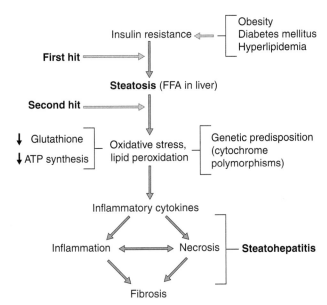

Figure 75-10. Two-hit hypothesis of NASH. Current understanding of the pathogenesis of hepatic steatosis and NASH. Insulin resistance associated with a variety of conditions causes accumulation of free fatty acids in hepatocytes, the "first hit" of hepatic steatosis. A "second hit" injury caused by or associated with steatosis and mediated through lipid peroxidation causes release of inflammatory cytokines. The resultant inflammation and cell necrosis stimulate fibrogenesis, leading to the full-blown picture of steatohepatitis.

Clinical Features

NAFLD and NASH are asymptomatic in the majority of patients. Symptoms such as fatigue, malaise, and vague right-upper-quadrant pain may be more common in adolescents. In most patients, NAFLD is discovered when hepatomegaly or abnormal ALT concentration is detected on routine testing or evaluation for another problem. Hepatomegaly, although sometimes difficult to appreciate owing to obesity, is present frequently, and not all patients have abnormal ALT values. Obese young adults with a high degree of abdominal-wall fat are more likely to have NAFLD. Acanthosis nigricans, commonly found on the neck and axillae of children and adolescents with insulin resistance, is found in 50% of children with NASH.[217,218] Ultrasonography may reveal a granular-appearing, echogenic liver that is difficult to penetrate.

Laboratory findings in NAFLD and NASH are nonspecific. Typically, AST and ALT levels are increased two- to fivefold, although higher levels are sometimes seen. The ALT is usually higher than the AST value. Some children have hyperlipidemia. Bilirubin, albumin, and prothrombin time values are normal until the very latest stages of disease.

Natural History

The natural history of pediatric NAFLD is unknown. Hepatic steatosis alone may have a benign or indolent course for many years. Once inflammation and tissue damage develop, progressive liver disease often ensues. In particular, the findings of inflammatory infiltrates and hepatocyte balloon degeneration suggest a high likelihood of progression to fibrosis and cirrhosis.[219]

The frequency with which NASH progresses to end-stage liver disease is unknown. A population based study in the United States found that NAFLD patients had a slightly higher mortality than the general population, associated with advanced age, impaired fasting glucose, and cirrhosis.[220] Similar results were reported in a more recent study.[221] In pediatrics there are no published longitudinal outcome studies of NAFLD. However, instances of advanced liver disease and cirrhosis have been described during childhood and adolescence.[222,223] NAFLD and NASH must be recognized as potential causes of serious liver disease in this population.

Treatment

All overweight or obese children and adolescents should undergo ALT testing and physical examination for hepatomegaly. Those with abnormalities should undergo diagnostic testing to exclude other causes of liver disease. If none is found, a trial of weight loss should be recommended; if successful, and ALT becomes normal, then perhaps no intervention is warranted. If unsuccessful, or if signs of more advanced liver disease are present, abdominal imaging and liver biopsy should be considered. The optimal treatment for NAFLD and NASH has not been determined. Treatment may not be necessary for simple steatosis because the natural history is benign, but at least from preliminary data it seems that most children and adolescents with fatty liver have some inflammation and fibrosis. It is important to determine, even in overweight children, if the steatohepatitis is secondary to another liver disease, such as Wilson's disease, chronic hepatitis C, inborn errors of metabolism, or hepatotoxic medications, because specific therapies are available.

Treatment may be directed at the underlying medical condition, if possible. Improvement in ALT levels and hepatic histopathology has been described with weight reduction in obese individuals. In a series of 33 obese children with NAFLD, liver tests became normal in all children who lost weight on a restricted calorie and exercise regimen, and ultrasonographic findings of hepatic steatosis improved significantly or normalized in children who lost at least 10% of body weight.[214] The optimal rate and degree of weight loss for improvement in hepatic histology has not been established. Therapy aimed at treatment of underlying diabetes mellitus or hyperlipidemia, common coexisting disorders with obesity, may be helpful in overall patient health, but efficacy in treatment of NAFLD has not been proven.

Pharmacologic therapies that have been attempted for NAFLD or NASH include ursodeoxycholic acid,[224] lipid lowering agents (clofibrate, gemfibrozil), betaine,[225] N-acetylcysteine, vitamin E,[226] and insulin-sensitizing agents (metformin,[227] thiazolidinediones[228]). Currently there are no conclusive data to support the use of pharmacological therapies for NAFLD in children, and it is advised only in the context of clinical trials.

At a minimum, it seems prudent to advise lifestyle changes achieved through diet and regular physical activity, and, in those with significant insulin resistance or diabetes mellitus, insulin-sensitizing agents may be considered.

TREATMENT OF HEPATITIS

Treatment of Acute Hepatitis
Acute-Phase Supportive Care

General supportive measures for acute hepatitis include adequate rest and diet, although these have not been studied in children. It is reasonable to advocate a balanced diet that prevents weight loss, dehydration, and nutritional deficiencies. Strict bed rest is generally not required, but permitted levels of activity should take into account the child's general condition. The return to normal activities and school requires knowledge of the child's clinical status, the type of hepatitis (including mode of transmission and duration of infectivity), and local health regulations. For example, most school-age children with acute HBV infection can return to school as soon as they are physically able because they pose little threat of transmission.[229] Young children with HAV infection, regardless of their general condition, however, should not return to day-care centers until their period of viral shedding has ended, which is 1 week after the onset of symptoms.[30]

Measures must also be undertaken to reduce the risk of spread of infectious hepatitis during the period of infectivity. These include education directed toward the child's caregivers and contacts, reporting to local health authorities when required, and active and passive immunization when indicated. Appropriate follow-up should confirm resolution.

Antiviral Therapy

With the exception of acute hepatitis C, antiviral therapy is not recommended for the treatment of acute hepatitis in immunocompetent hosts. Treatment has been advocated for immunocompromised children with acute hepatitis due to EBV or CMV infection. Acyclovir and ganciclovir have been used for the treatment of EBV infection, but only in the active and not the latent phase of infection. The antiviral effect of ganciclovir for EBV is believed to be more prolonged after withdrawal than that of acyclovir.[230] Ganciclovir has been used with success in newborns and immunocompromised children with active CMV. Induction therapy for 2 to 3 weeks is usually followed by prolonged maintenance therapy because viral excretion most usually recurs on cessation. CMV immune globulin derived from pooled plasma from adults selected for high CMV antibody titers has also been used in conjunction with an antiviral agent.

Treatment of Chronic Hepatitis

Chronic-Phase Supportive Care

Supportive care for the child with chronic hepatitis involves maintenance of long-term well-being, monitoring for the complications of chronic liver disease, and avoidance of any further hepatic injury. Many children with chronic hepatitis are diagnosed fortuitously and are asymptomatic. In these children there are no restrictions to activity and they may lead normal lives. Some children with stable disease and mild symptoms such as fatigue or poor appetite will require interventions commensurate with their disability, to maintain nutritional status and normal schooling. Other children, such as those with chronic AIH, may have labile disease, with frequent "flares" separated by disease-free periods of variable duration. These children will require early recognition of relapses with appropriate modification of therapy. Patients with advanced disease and manifestations such as ascites or coagulopathy require aggressive therapy directed at the specific sequelae of long-term liver disease.

Children with chronic hepatitis should avoid chronic high dosages of potentially hepatotoxic medications to avoid further aggravation of liver injury and should be immunized against hepatitis A and B if their serologic tests do not reveal adequate immunity. Exposure to all environmental hepatotoxic agents (e.g., organophosphates) should be avoided.

Specific therapies for the various type of chronic hepatitis have been discussed.

SUMMARY

Over the past 2 decades, much has been learned about childhood hepatitis. Early intervention in childhood may significantly improve longevity. Effective treatment regimens are available for HBV and HCV, and NAFLD has gained prominence as a major potential cause of morbidity. New directions for research include elucidation of appropriate patient selection for treatment, clinical trials of newer agents in children, and exploration of the molecular basis of liver injury in the various causes of hepatitis.

REFERENCES

4. Centers for Disease Control. Surveillance for acute viral hepatitis–United States, 2007. MMWR 2009;58(SS–3):1–27.
27. Centers for Disease Control. Prevention of hepatitis A through active or passive immunization. MMWR 2006;55(rr07):1–23.
80. Centers for Disease Control. A comprehensive immunization strategy to eliminate transmission of hepatitis B virus infection in the United States. MMWR 2005;54(RR16):1–23.
86. Bortolotti F, Cadrobbi P, Crivellaro C, et al. Long-term outcome of chronic type B hepatitis in patients who acquire hepatitis B virus infection in childhood. Gastroenterology 1990;99:805–810.
152. Goodman ZD, Makhlouf HR, Liu L, et al. Pathology of chronic hepatitis C in children: liver biopsy findings in the Peds-C Trial. Hepatology 2008;47:836–883.
157. González-Peralta R, Kelly DA, Haber B, et al. Interferon alfa-2b in combination with ribavirin for the treatment of chronic hepatitis C in children: efficacy, safety, and pharmacokinetics. Hepatology 2005;42:1010–1018.
160. Wirth S, Pieper-Boustani H, Lang T, et al. Peginterferon alfa-2b plus ribavirin treatment in children and adolescents with chronic hepatitis C. Hepatology 2005;41:1013–1018.
194. Wiegard C, Schramm C, Lohse AW. Scoring systems for the diagnosis of autoimmune hepatitis: past, present and future. Semin Liv Dis 2009;29:254–261.
200. Mieli-Vergani G, Vergani D. Autoimmune paediatric liver disease. World J Gastroenterol 2008;14:3360–3367.

See expertconsult.com for a complete list of references and the review questions for this chapter.

PORTAL HYPERTENSION

76

Naim Alkhouri • Charles G. Winans • Vera F. Hupertz

Portal hypertension and its complications during childhood remain important clinical problems that lead to significant morbidity and mortality. The most common causes of portal hypertension in children are biliary atresia and extrahepatic portal vein thrombosis. Evidence-based guidelines for the management of portal hypertension in adults have been published[1-3]; however, similar guidelines in children are lacking, and most recommendations are based on opinions by pediatric experts.[4] This chapter highlights the pathogenesis, clinical features, diagnosis, and therapy of portal hypertension in the pediatric population.

PATHOGENESIS OF PORTAL HYPERTENSION

The portal system drains the capillaries of the mesenteric and splenic veins and ends in the hepatic capillaries (Figure 76-1). The portal vein supplies partially oxygenated blood flow to the liver, supplementing the highly oxygenated blood flow of the hepatic artery to the liver. Blood flow to the liver is finely tuned such that any disturbance to flow in one of these vessels can be offset to a certain degree by increased flow through the other vessel. This is known as the hepatic arterial buffer response. Blood from both the portal venous system and the hepatic arterial system combines within the sinusoids.

Portal hypertension occurs when there is increased portal resistance or an increased portal blood flow (Figure 76-2). In general the portal venous system has a low baseline portal pressure of 7 to 10 mm Hg, and the hepatic venous pressure gradient (HVPG) ranges from 1 to 4 mm Hg. Portal hypertension is defined as a portal pressure greater than 10 mm Hg or a gradient greater than 4 mm Hg. Pressure gradients above 10 mm Hg have been associated with esophageal varices, and those above 12 mm Hg are associated with ascites and variceal bleeding in adult patients.[5] To obtain a measurement of the portal pressure gradient, a catheter can be wedged into the hepatic vein and a wedged hepatic venous pressure (WHVP) measurement made. The catheter is then retracted into a free-flowing hepatic vein and free hepatic venous pressure (FHVP) is measured. The HVPG is the difference between the WHVP and the FHVP. Causes of portal hypertension can be suggested by the HVPG. In presinusoidal obstruction, the HVPG is normal but the WHVP is slightly raised, whereas in cirrhosis both the WHVP and the HVPG are increased (Table 76-1).

Clinically, portal hypertension causes splenomegaly and the formation of collateral circulation. Collaterals develop in response to elevation of the portal pressure, and they form in the cardia of the stomach, the anus, the falciform ligament through remnants of the fetal umbilical circulation, and the retroperitoneum. In prehepatic obstruction, collaterals form to attempt to bypass the blockage and enter directly into the liver at the porta hepatis (cavernous transformation).

Despite the formation of a significant collateral network, portal hypertension persists as a result of increased cardiac output and decreased splanchnic arteriolar tone. Retention of sodium and water via a hepatorenal reflex increases the circulating blood volume. The production of vasodilatory factors cause arterial vasodilation of the splanchnic circulation. Several factors have been cited as possible mediators of splanchnic vasodilation, including glucagon, bile acids, nitric oxide (NO),[6] prostaglandins, and others. In cirrhosis, there is evidence for decreased endothelial nitric oxide synthetase (eNOS) activity in the liver (which leads to decreased NO production and intrahepatic vasoconstriction).[7-9] Increases in intrahepatic resistance could also be due to hepatocyte swelling, fibrosis, and inflammation within the portal tracts.

CLINICAL FEATURES

Gastrointestinal Bleeding

Hematemesis and melena are the most frequent presentation of portal hypertension, with variceal bleeding as the most common cause. Esophageal varices occur in the distal esophagus, which is supplied by the anterior branch of the left gastric vein. Valves in the penetrating veins of the distal esophagus become incompetent and allow blood to flow in a retrograde fashion into the deep intrinsic veins of the esophagus. The risk of first-time bleeding from pediatric studies in children with cirrhosis is 22%, but rises to 38% in children with known varices over a 5-year period. Bleeding occurs in 15 to 25% of patients with biliary atresia in long-term follow-up.[10,11] Age at bleeding is also dependent on the underlying cause of cirrhosis, with patients who have surgically corrected but progressive biliary atresia bleeding for the first time at a mean age of 3 years and those with cystic fibrosis at a mean age of 11.5 years.[12]

Gastric varices are fed by the short gastric veins. They may be isolated to the stomach (generally in the fundus, or in the antrum, corpus, or pylorus) without the presence of esophageal varices, or may extend from the esophagus into the stomach (either along the lesser curve or toward the fundus).[13] Primary gastric varices generally refer to the presence of gastric varices at initial examination in someone who has never had treatment for esophageal varices. Secondary gastric varices refer to the development of gastric varices after endoscopic therapy for esophageal varices. Gastric varices tend to lie deeper within the submucosa under the gastric mucosa, compared with the more superficial esophageal varices that form in the lamina propria and submucosa.

Rectal bleeding may occur as a result of inferior mesenteric-internal iliac venous collaterals. Hemorrhoids do not seem to be more common in patients with portal hypertension, but anorectal varices and portal colopathy are found more frequently.[14] Sites within the small intestine may also bleed[15,16] and may

829

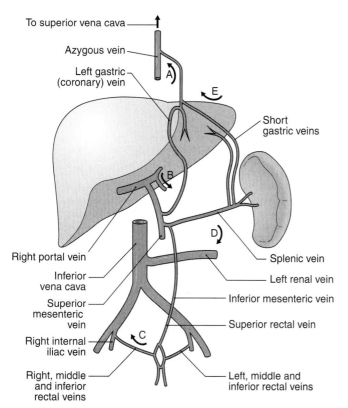

Figure 76-1. Diagram of portal circulation. The normal vascular anatomy and most common sites for the development of portal systemic collaterals are shown. A, Esophageal submucosal veins, which are supplied by the left gastric vein and drain into the superior vena cava via the azygous vein. B, Paraumbilical veins, which are supplied by the umbilical portion of the left portal vein and drain into the abdominal wall veins near the umbilicus. These veins may form a caput medusae. C, Rectal submucosal veins, which are supplied by the inferior mesenteric vein through the superior rectal vein and drain into the internal iliac veins through the middle rectal veins. D, Splenorenal shunts, which are created spontaneously or surgically. From Feldman et al., 2002, with permission.[146]

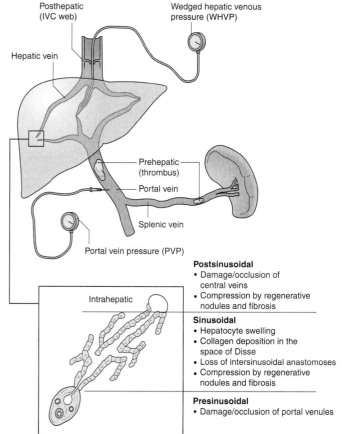

Figure 76-2. Sites of obstruction to portal venous flow and measurement of portal pressure, illustrating the major locations of extrahepatic (prehepatic and posthepatic) and intrahepatic (presinusoidal, sinusoidal and postsinusoidal) obstruction. A catheter tip is also shown wedged into a small hepatic vein (HV) for the measurement of the wedged hepatic venous pressure (WHVP). When the catheter tip is withdrawn into the hepatic vein the free hepatic vein pressure (FHVP) is obtained. Hepatic venous pressure gradient (HVPG) = WHPV − FHVP. Direct measurement of the portal venous pressure (PVP) is accomplished during surgery by catheterization of either the umbilical vein or the portal vein via the transjugular or transhepatic approach. IVC, inferior vena cava. From Feldman et al., 2002, with permission.[146]

respond only to surgical correction. Gallbladder varices seem to be more common in children with portal hypertension from extrahepatic portal vein obstruction (EHPVO). They can be easily diagnosed by ultrasonography of the biliary tract.[17]

Portal hypertensive gastropathy (PHG) can result in bleeding and is secondary to increased submucosal arteriovenous communications and increased gastric perfusion. PHG can appear as discrete cherry-red spots assuming a mosaic pattern, or may be more confluent, and can occur over large areas of the stomach. Gastric antral vascular ectasia may be seen as linear streaks (watermelon stomach).[18] Bleeding may be worsened by the ingestion of gastric irritants such as nonsteroidal anti-inflammatory drugs (NSAIDs). PHG can occur before variceal eradication but is more common in patients who have undergone variceal obliteration. Venous congestion may also occur in the small intestine, making the mucosa edematous and friable. Duodenal erosions are often seen in portal hypertensive duodenopathy.[19] Bleeding also occurs more frequently at sites of mucocutaneous junctions such as stomas. Bleeding distal to the esophagus may be increased after successful esophageal variceal sclerotherapy and may respond only to reducing portal pressure.

Patients with portal hypertension can bleed from other gastric lesions such as ulcers and gastritis not secondary to portal hypertension. Coagulation problems may exacerbate bleeding. Patients with cirrhosis may have abnormalities of the prothrombin time due to decreased factor production. Coagulation abnormalities similar to a mild disseminated intravascular coagulation picture have been reported in teenagers with extrahepatic portal venous obstruction and in adults with noncirrhotic portal fibrosis. Abnormality of the international normalized ratio (INR), decreased fibrinogen, and decreased platelet aggregation may be due to low circulating levels of endotoxin and increased cytokine activation.[20]

Variceal bleeding in children often follows an acute upper respiratory infection. The combination of factors including increased abdominal pressure from coughing or sneezing, increased cardiac output from fever, and possibly medications such as NSAIDs or aspirin contribute to the rupture of varices. Prolonged gastroesophageal reflux could also be associated with erosions over the varices that could lead to bleeding.

Esophageal varices can be graded[21]; the severity of the grading is considered to be a risk factor for bleeding:

- Grade I varices are flattened by insufflation.
- Grade II varices are not flattened by insufflation and are separated by areas of healthy mucosa.
- Grade III varices are confluent and not flattened by insufflation.

TABLE 76-1. **Hepatic Venous Pressure Gradients in Various Forms of Portal Hypertension**

	Hepatic Venous Pressure Gradient Measurements		
Cause of Portal Hypertension	**Wedged Hepatic Venous Pressure**	**Free Hepatic Venous Pressure**	**Hepatic Venous Pressure Gradient**
Intrahepatic: sinusoidal (cirrhosis)	Raised	Normal	Raised
Posthepatic: hepatic venous obstruction	Raised	Raised	Normal
Intrahepatic: presinusoidal	Mildly raised	Normal	Normal
Prehepatic: portal venous obstruction	Normal	Normal	Normal

Patients with no varices or grade I varices are significantly less likely to bleed than patients with grade II or III varices. Other signs of increased bleeding risk include red wale markings.[22]

The risk of esophageal variceal bleeding in children with portal vein obstruction was thought to decrease in adolescence because of the development of spontaneous portosystemic collaterals. Lykavieris et al.[14] followed 44 children from age 12 years for a mean of 8 years. At the time of diagnosis of portal venous obstruction, no child had abnormal liver enzymes or function. The actuarial probability of bleeding was 49% at age 16 years and 76% at age 24 years. If the child had bled before the age of 12 years, the probability of bleeding was higher than in those who had not bled. In addition, there was no variceal regression but rather progression of varices in the majority of children, suggesting a lack of *significant* collateral formation (Figure 76-3).[23]

Splenomegaly

The enlarged spleen may be picked up incidentally on routine physical examination or by laboratory work showing changes consistent with hypersplenism. Hypersplenism can result in anemia as well as leukopenia and thrombocytopenia. Thrombocytopenia could result in frequent nose bleeds or petechiae. Hypersplenism rarely requires surgical intervention, except when the symptoms of anemia or physical discomfort are severe.[24]

Abdominal Venous Patterning

Portal hypertension-induced collateral formation can reperfuse the umbilical veins and lead to increased abdominal venous markings, known as caput medusae. A caput medusae may have an audible venous hum, producing a Cruveilhier-Baumgarten murmur. If the level of obstruction is within the inferior vena cava, the flow in these vessels is cephalad. If the level of obstruction is not in the inferior vena cava, the flow is caudad in those vessels located below the umbilicus.

Ascites

Increased sodium retention and raised portal pressure may cause accumulation of fluid within the abdomen. Impaired lymphatic drainage may compound this. Treatment entails the use of diuretics. Albumin infusions can also be used to increase intravascular osmotic pressure. Paracentesis has been used safely in children when the ascites is difficult to control, though it may be associated with serious complications such as bacterial peritonitis and hypotension secondary to intravascular volume depletion.[25-27]

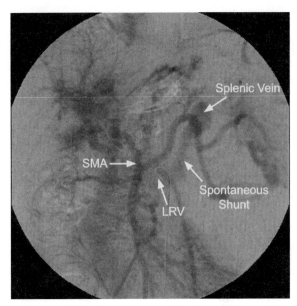

Figure 76-3. Angiogram from a 16-year-old patient with neonatal extrahepatic portal vein obstruction with persistent variceal bleeding despite the large patent spontaneous shunt shown above. LRV, left renal vein; SMA, superior mesenteric artery.

Cholangiopathy

In several series including children and adults with extrahepatic venous obstruction, biliary changes were reported in 80 to 100% of patients.[28-31] The common bile duct is most frequently affected, but changes may involve the intrahepatic bile ducts. The abnormalities include strictures, luminal irregularity, segmental dilation, ectasia, external compression by collateral veins, displacement of ducts, and pruning of the intrahepatic ducts. Some of these changes are reversible after shunt surgery, suggesting that the pathogenesis is due to compression by collaterals.[28] Other changes were not reversible, indicating that the lesions may have been due to ischemic changes, possibly secondary to venous thrombosis.

Pulmonary Complications

Hepatopulmonary syndrome (HPS) and portopulmonary hypertension are probably underdiagnosed in children. Barbe et al.[32] reported on the presence of HPS in 29 pediatric patients, 26 of whom had cirrhosis and 3 had extrahepatic causes of portal hypertension. HPS seems to progress more rapidly in patients with biliary atresia associated with polysplenia.[33] In an adult study of 31 noncirrhotic portal hypertensive patients compared with 46 patients with liver cirrhosis, HPS as diagnosed by contrast echocardiography and lung perfusion scans were equally common.[34] Patients with HPS have a higher incidence of dyspnea, cyanosis, platypnea (dyspnea that worsens in the upright position), clubbing, and spider nevi.[32,35,36] There are two forms of HPS. In type I, there is dilatation of pulmonary vessels decreasing red blood cell contact time with oxygen-rich alveoli. In type II HPS, the diffusion-perfusion mismatch is presumed to be due to arteriovenous communications completely bypassing alveoli.[37,38] HPS is thought to occur as a result of shunting of vasodilatory mediators from the mesentery away from the liver in portal hypertension. It is not related to the duration or severity of liver dysfunction. Liver transplantation may reverse HPS in more than 80% of patients, but if large shunts are present and the arterial partial pressure of oxygen is less than 50 mm Hg on 100% oxygen, a poorer outcome may be expected.

Portopulmonary syndrome eventually leads to right-sided heart failure. Histologically there is pulmonary arteriopathy with concentric laminar intimal fibrosis consistent with a vasoconstrictive etiology. Pediatric cases have been reported.[39,40] The condition is defined by a pulmonary arterial pressure greater than 25 mm Hg at rest and above 30 mm Hg with exercise, raised pulmonary vascular resistance with pulmonary arterial occlusion pressure, or a left-ventricular end-diastolic pressure of less than 15 mm Hg.[41] The most common symptom of portopulmonary hypertension is exertional dyspnea. Other symptoms may include fatigue, palpitations, syncope, or chest pains. Physical findings may include an accentuated second heart sound and systolic murmur of tricuspid regurgitation. Mild to moderate pulmonary hypertension may be reversible after liver transplantation.[42]

DISORDERS ASSOCIATED WITH PORTAL HYPERTENSION (TABLE 76-2)

Prehepatic Disorders

Most cases of portal hypertension in children are due to extrahepatic obstruction of the portal vein, although splenic vein thrombosis can also lead to segmental portal hypertension. Portal vein thrombosis is idiopathic in the majority of cases (65%),[23] but could be secondary to neonatal omphalitis and/ or catheterization of the umbilical vein (4.8%),[43] or pyelophlebitis secondary to appendicitis or other intra-abdominal infections in older children. Ando et al.[44] determined that many cases were caused by an embryologic malformation resulting in a tortuous, abnormal portal vein. Other associations include cartilage-hair hypoplasia syndrome, malignancies such as neuroblastoma, and non-Hodgkin's lymphoma.[45-47]

A prospective randomized study of 20 patients with EHPVO showed that, despite lower levels of protein C, protein S, and antithrombin III, there was no genetic basis, and it was hypothesized to be due to increased clearance of activated clotting factors or to passive adsorption on the endothelium.[48] Factor V Leiden mutation and an acquired JAK2 mutation (JAK2V617F) have been reported in adult patients with EHPVO[49-51]; however, in a large pediatric study from King's College Hospital, none of these mutations were found in children with EHPVO.[52]

Portal hypertension can result from increased portal flow. Causes include arteriovenous fistula and splenomegaly. Arteriovenous fistulas have resulted from blunt or penetrating

TABLE 76-2.   **Causes of Portal Hypertension in Children**

Prehepatic Disorders
Portal vein thrombosis
Arteriovenous fistula
Splenic vein thrombosis
Splenomegaly

Posthepatic Disorders
Budd-Chiari syndrome
Congestive heart failure
Inferior vena cava obstruction

Intrahepatic Disorders (Hepatocellular)
Autoimmune hepatitis
Hepatitis B
Hepatitis C
α_1-Antitrypsin deficiency
Wilson's disease
Steatohepatitis
Glycogen storage disease type IV
Toxins
   Methotrexate
   6-Mercaptopurine
   Valproate
   Phenytoin
   Vitamin A
   Arsenic
   Alcohol

Intrahepatic Disorders (Biliary)
Biliary atresia
Primary sclerosing cholangitis
Cystic fibrosis
Congenital hepatic fibrosis
Caroli's disease
Choledochal cyst
Familial cholestasis
   Progressive familial intrahepatic cholestasis type 1
   Alagille's syndrome
   Nonsyndromic paucity syndrome
Primary biliary cirrhosis

Intrahepatic Disorders (Other)
Veno-occlusive disease
Schistosomiasis
Gaucher's disease
Idiopathic portal hypertension
Peliosis hepatis
   Anabolic steroids
   Azathioprine

trauma to the liver (including diagnostic procedures such as liver biopsy and percutaneous cholangiography), hepatocellular carcinomas, hepatic artery aneurysms, and congenital malformations.[53] Diagnosis is based on aortoportography. Splenoportography is not helpful, as the flow in the portal vein is hepatofugal.

Posthepatic Disorders

Budd-Chiari syndrome results from obstruction of the hepatic venous outflow including the inferior vena cava and/or hepatic veins. This can be due to webs or thrombi in these vessels, although it has also been associated with pregnancy, contraceptive pills, myeloproliferative states, tumors, and hypercoagulable states.[54] Congestive heart failure can cause chronic congestion in the liver that can progress to cirrhosis. Liver biopsy may show centrizonal congestion and necrosis. Presenting symptoms usually include abdominal pain, distention, jaundice, and upper gastrointestinal bleeding. Hepatosplenomegaly, ascites, and pedal edema may be present.

Intrahepatic Disorders

In developed countries, intrahepatic causes are more frequent than extrahepatic causes of portal hypertension. Cirrhosis is the most common cause of intrahepatic portal hypertension and may develop as a hepatocellular or biliary process. Hepatocellular causes of cirrhosis include α_1-antitrypsin deficiency, autoimmune hepatitis, infectious hepatitis, metabolic disease, and toxins. Biliary causes include uncorrected or partially corrected biliary atresia, cystic fibrosis, primary sclerosing cholangitis, congenital hepatic fibrosis (CHF), Caroli's disease, and progressive familial intrahepatic cholestasis.

Portal hypertension has been reported to occur in 35 to 75% of patients with biliary atresia due to progressive cirrhosis.[55] Caroli's disease is due to faulty remodeling of the early ductal plate with the formation of saclike dilations of the larger intrahepatic bile ducts. These changes can generally be determined by ultrasonography.[56] CHF is due to a progressive necroinflammatory process of immature bile ducts causing presinusoidal intrahepatic portal hypertension from hepatic venule compression. It is often associated with autosomal recessive polycystic kidney disease, but has also been associated with medullary sponge kidney, Ivemark's familial dysplasia, vaginal atresia, Meckel's syndrome, and, rarely, adult polycystic kidney disease.[57]

Complications of portal hypertension can be especially severe in patients with cystic fibrosis, owing to a compromised pulmonary status. Meconium ileus or its equivalent in the newborn period has been associated with more severe liver disease and portal hypertension. Long-term therapy may include liver transplantation alone, or with lung transplantation if there is significant pulmonary disease. In cases where there is limited lung and liver failure, surgical portosystemic shunting may be appropriate and has been associated with long-term survival.[12]

Other miscellaneous causes of portal hypertension include veno-occlusive disease, Gaucher's disease, peliosis hepatis and idiopathic portal hypertension.[58] Veno-occlusive disease is often secondary to some toxic agent/process such as exposure to Jamaican bush tea, chemotherapy and radiotherapy in preparation of bone marrow transplantation, and after standard chemotherapy such as actinomycin D. Liver histology in veno-occlusive disease shows nonthrombotic hepatic venule occlusion by intimal proliferation and fibrosis along with centrilobular necrosis with portal sparing.[59] Idiopathic portal hypertension, also known as noncirrhotic portal fibrosis or hepatoportal sclerosis, is a rare entity that occurs primarily in adults in the Indian subcontinent and in east Asia.[60,61] Recently a report of a series of children with this disorder has been published from India.[62] Diagnosis of this disorder is based on the presence of a liver biopsy without cirrhosis, and fibrotic, sclerosed, and obliterated portal vein branches. Hepatomegaly in Gaucher's disease is associated with infiltration of the liver by macrophages. In general, this does not progress, but in some it can lead to portal hypertension and parenchymal liver failure.[63,64] Schistosomiasis is endemic in tropical and subtropical regions of Africa, Asia, the Caribbean, and South America and causes a granulomatous hepatic fibrosis.[57] It usually presents in adolescence or early adulthood, but has been reported in younger children.[65]

DIAGNOSIS

Portal hypertension should be considered in any patient presenting with hematemesis and unexplained splenomegaly. Evaluation should begin with careful examination of the child for signs of chronic liver disease, as well as for signs of other chronic organ dysfunction such as heart failure.

Ultrasonography of the liver can uncover venous blockage of the prehepatic or posthepatic venous system, collaterals, liver echotexture abnormalities, and ascites. Doppler ultrasonography is useful for measurement of flow and determining the direction of flow. Ascites may have many causes aside from portal hypertension, and measurement of the serum:ascites albumin gradient (SAAG: serum albumin minus ascitic fluid albumin concentration) is a helpful way to predict portal hypertension (Figure 76-4). A SAAG greater than or equal to 1.1 g/dL is consistent with portal hypertension. Cardiac causes can also cause raised gradients but are associated with increased ascitic fluid albumin levels (greater than 2.5 g/dL), compared with low ascitic fluid albumin levels in patients with cirrhosis.[66] Other causes of a high SAAG are alcoholic hepatitis, hepatocellular carcinoma, massive liver metastases, myxedema, acute fatty liver of pregnancy, and mixed ascites.[67] Other useful measurements done on ascites include the total white blood cell count, amylase, lactate dehydrogenase, glucose, total protein and triglycerides.

Esophagogastroduodenoscopy (EGD) can detect the presence of esophageal and gastric varices as well as other causes of acute hemorrhage such as portal gastropathy. Several adult studies have tried to identify patients with varices by noninvasive or minimally invasive methods including biochemical parameters, ultrasound parameters, and capsule endoscopy.[68-70] Two large multicenter trials have evaluated the role of capsule endoscopy as a minimally invasive tool for screening of esophageal varices.[71,72] They demonstrated reasonable performance characteristics of capsule endoscopy; however, it was somewhat inferior to EGD, though patient compliance with capsule screening may be improved, especially in adolescent patients. Endoscopic retrograde cholangiography is useful for identifying biliary causes of intrahepatic portal hypertension.

Transvenous insertion of a balloon catheter in the hepatic vein allows for measurement of the WHVP and FHVP. Risks include perforation and bleeding, but the procedure is fairly safe in experienced hands. Transient elastography is a novel and noninvasive method that measures liver tissue stiffness and has been shown to correlate strongly with HVPG.[73,74] If validated in pediatric studies, this technique could be used to noninvasively evaluate the portal pressure and select patients at higher risk of having esophageal varices.

Magnetic resonance imaging (MRI) and magnetic resonance angiography (MRA) are complementary techniques that can evaluate the hepatic vasculature. These investigations are less operator dependent than ultrasonography, and they are noninvasive. They can be useful to demonstrate congenital hepatic vascular anomalies, vascular supply, portal vein thrombosis, and hepatic tumor localization, and also in assessing the patency of surgical shunts.[75,76]

Testing for HPS includes contrast echocardiography, perfusion scans, oxygen saturation measurements with and without supplemental oxygen, transcutaneous hyperoxia testing,[77] and alveolar-arterial oxygen gradients. Simple echocardiography will show a normal heart. The injection of agitated saline (to introduce microbubbles) during echocardiography allows distinction between a person with no shunt, a cardiac shunt, or a pulmonary shunt. Macroaggregated albumin perfusion scanning is more specific and can confirm the diagnosis. Technetium-99-labeled microspheres (20 to 100 µm in diameter) are

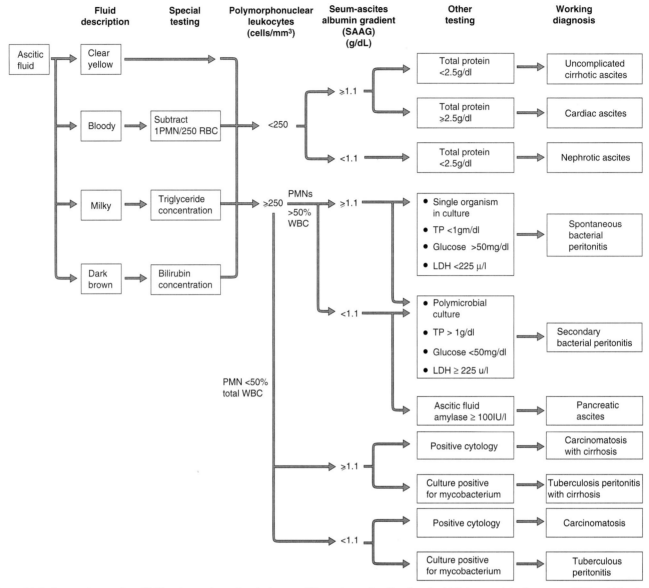

Figure 76-4. Approach to ascites. PMN, polymorphonuclear leukocytes; TP, total protein; alb, albumin; LDH, lactate dehydrogenase; RBC, red blood cells; SAAG, serum ascites:albumin gradient. Adapted from Feldman et al. (1998), with permission.[147]

injected intravenously and should be completely removed by the lungs. If radioactivity is detected in extrapulmonary tissue, pathologic shunts are present.[78]

Echocardiography is a noninvasive test for portopulmonary hypertension, producing estimates of pulmonary pressures. Right heart catheterization may be necessary in some unclear cases.[41]

THERAPY

Acute Variceal Hemorrhage

Gastrointestinal bleeding is the major cause of morbidity and/ or mortality in patients with portal hypertension. In adults, the mortality rate used to be as high as 50%,[79] with rebleeding rates as high as 47 to 84% in the 1 to 2 years following the first episode. However, mortality from variceal bleeding in adults has greatly decreased in the past two decades to 15 to 20% because of implementation of effective treatments (endoscopic and pharmacological) and improved general medical care.[80,81] Mortality

rates in children are lower (0 to 8%) because the majority of children with cirrhosis do not have comorbid pulmonary and cardiac disease, and many children with portal hypertension suffer from extrahepatic portal obstruction with normal liver function.[82-85] In children with biliary atresia, total bilirubin at the time of first variceal bleeding episode is the most relevant variable in predicting prognosis.[86]

Stabilization of the patient is the first step in management of gastrointestinal hemorrhage. Fluid resuscitation demands rapid placement of intravenous lines and the administration of either fluids (colloids or crystalloids) or blood with the goals of maintaining hemodynamic stability and a hemoglobin of approximately 8 g/dL[1] (Figure 76-5). It is important to avoid volume overload, as this would inadvertently increase the portal pressure and cause further bleeding. Vital signs need to be monitored closely and, if the airway is compromised, the patient should be intubated. Coagulopathy should be corrected with vitamin K, fresh frozen plasma (FFP), and possibly recombinant factor VIIa replacement.[87] Significant bleeding may predispose

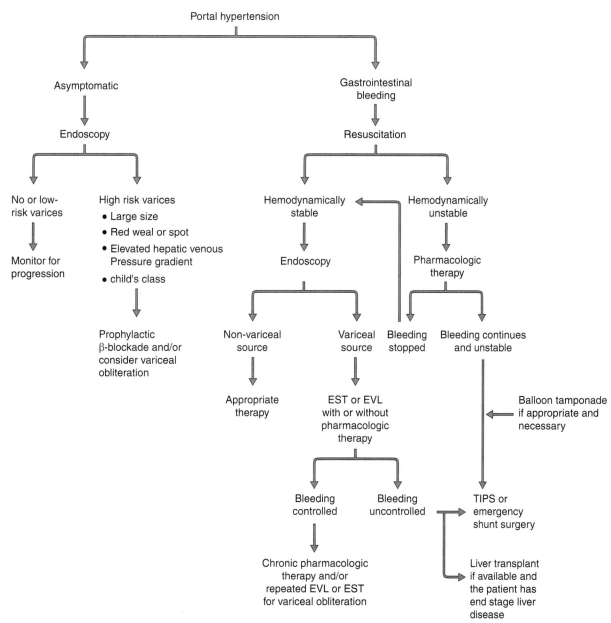

Figure 76-5. Management of portal hypertension in children. EST, esophageal sclerotherapy; EVL, esophageal variceal ligation; TIPS, transjugular intrahepatic portosystemic shunt.

to encephalopathy in patients with cirrhosis, and therapy may be needed. Placement of a nasogastric tube allows monitoring for ongoing bleeding as well as removing the blood from the gastrointestinal tract to prevent encephalopathy. Bleeding will stop spontaneously in 40 to 50% of patients, but rebleeding is common, thus requiring more definitive therapy if possible (Table 76-3).

If bleeding is thought to be due to varices, pharmacotherapy should be initiated while more definitive therapy and evaluation can be organized. Vasopressin has been used effectively in 53 to 85% of children to treat variceal bleeding and works by inducing splanchnic vasoconstriction.[88] The dosage is 0.3 units per kg per hour after a bolus of 0.3 U/kg over 20 min.[89] Higher doses (above 0.01 U/kg/min) have been associated with complications such as peripheral vasoconstriction, myocardial ischemia or infarction, arrhythmias, mesenteric ischemia, and cerebrovascular accidents. The addition of nitroglycerin,

a venous dilator, to vasopressin reduces vascular resistance in the portal venous system and decreases the systemic effects of vasopressin.

Somatostatin and its synthetic analogue, octreotide, cause splanchnic vasoconstriction and thus lower portal pressure and portal blood flow. This is caused by a direct effect on the mesenteric vascular smooth muscle and by glucagon reduction. Somatostatin has a much better side-effect profile than vasopressin and in adults is reported to be effective in 64 to 92%, of cases which was comparable to vasopressin, balloon tamponade, or endoscopic sclerotherapy for initial control of bleeding.[79] A pediatric dose of 3 to 5 µg per kg per hour has been used.[90] Octreotide has a longer half-life (1 to 2 hours) and can be given as a bolus (2 µg/kg) followed by continuous infusion (1 to 5 µg per kg per hour)[91] or as subcutaneous injections three times daily. Reported side effects of somatostatin and octreotide include abdominal pain, nausea, diarrhea,

TABLE 76-3. Major Types of Therapy for Acute Variceal Bleeding

Treatment	Mechanism of Action	Complications
Vasopressin	Constriction of splanchnic arterioles, decreasing flow to the gut and portal system	Coronary artery vasoconstriction, peripheral vasoconstriction
Somatostatin and analogues	Vasoconstriction of both splanchnic and systemic circulations	Altered glucose homeostasis, abdominal pain
Esophageal balloons	Direct tamponade	Pressure necrosis of the esophagus, rupture, aspiration, rebleeding (rarely used)
Sclerotherapy	Direct obliteration of esophageal varices	Esophageal ulcers, fever, bleeding
Variceal banding	Ligation of esophageal varices	Esophageal ulcers, bleeding
Surgical shunts	Establishes altered flow to lower portal pressure	Shunt thrombosis, rebleeding, encephalopathy

fat malabsorption, bradycardia, and disturbances in glucose homeostasis, but there is rarely a need to terminate the medication. In a study of 21 patients with portal hypertension, octreotide at a dose of 1 to 2 µg per kg per hour stopped the bleeding in 71% of patients.[92] Use of short-term prophylactic antibiotics is an integral part of therapy for adult patients presenting with variceal bleeding, as it has been shown not only to decrease the rate of bacterial infection but also to decrease variceal rebleeding and increase survival.[3,93,94] Cultures (blood, urine, and ascites) should be obtained, and antibiotic prophylaxis directed at intestinal flora (third-generation cephalosporin) should be started from admission.[4]

To establish the source of bleeding, an experienced endoscopist should perform endoscopy as soon as the patient is stable. If the bleeding is from esophageal varices, sclerotherapy or banding can be attempted. Technically, esophageal sclerotherapy (EST) may be easier than banding in the acute situation if there is significant bleeding. Sclerosant should be injected paravariceally or intravariceally. Intravariceal injections lead to thrombosis of the varix, whereas paravariceal injections lead to a local inflammatory response, thereby compressing the varix.[95] Varices close to the esophagogastric junction should be targeted. Long-term eradication of varices has been reported with this technique in children, with control of bleeding in 80%.[85,96] Up to 63% had no further bleeding after variceal obliteration. Rebleeding was managed with further sclerotherapy of esophageal varices, but if nonesophageal bleeding occurred as a result of portal hypertension (e.g., due to gastrointestinal varices or hypertensive gastropathy), more definitive therapy was indicated to relieve the portal hypertension. Complications of EST include ulceration, pain, perforation, and bacteremia. Long-term complications include strictures.

Owing to the complications associated with sclerotherapy, endoscopic variceal ligation (EVL) has been developed. Variceal banding draws a visible varix into the lumen of the ligator that is attached to the end of the endoscope, and a band is placed around the varix, crimping off the blood supply. The band and varix are sloughed off in approximately 5 to 7 days and may leave a small round ulcer. Special care should be taken in patients less than 3 years old because of the risk of entrapping the entire esophageal wall in the band, leading to necrosis and possible perforation. The effectiveness and safety of EVL were reported in a small study by Karrer et al.,[97] who reported on seven patients who underwent EVL following documented variceal bleeding. Most had already had sclerotherapy, without successful elimination of varices. The patients tolerated EVL without complications, and three of the seven patients had complete eradication of the varices. Others continued to require yearly esophagoscopy with banding, but had no further

bleeding episodes. One patient died from complications of liver transplantation. Zargar et al.[98] reported their experience of EVL in acute bleeding and in control of rebleeding, and compared it to EST in patients with EHPVO. EVL was just as effective as EST but was associated with fewer complications and faster obliteration of varices. This finding has been confirmed in larger adult studies showing that variceal band ligation had equal efficacy to variceal sclerotherapy in stopping active variceal bleeding, a faster time to variceal obliteration, and fewer endoscopic sessions.[99] Proton pump inhibitors may have a role in the healing of post-EST and post-EVL ulcerations, and their use is advisable in patients undergoing these procedures.[100,101]

Long-term drug therapy after an initial episode of bleeding is as effective as endoscopic therapy in adult patients[102,103] and may be associated with a lower complication rate.[104] Drug therapy with endoscopy was compared to endoscopy alone and showed that dual therapy provided better control of bleeding in adults.[105]

In adult European studies, gastric variceal bleeding was stopped by injecting the varices with n-butyl-2-cyanoacrylate, isobutyl-2-cyanoacrylate, or thrombin. This procedure is called endoscopic variceal obturation (EVO).[13] These substances are not easily washed away in the higher-flow gastric varices compared with other routine sclerosants. None of these agents is approved for use in gastric varices by the Food and Drug Administration in the United States. Side effects include pyrexia and abdominal pain, but more concerning is the risk of embolism to the brain, lungs, and liver, retroperitoneal abscesses,[106] and splenic infarction. Gastric variceal ligation with rubber bands or detachable snares has been used. Case studies have shown these methods to be safe, with hemostasis achieved in 83 to 100% of adult patients. In limited studies comparing variceal ligation with EVO for acute gastric variceal bleeding, EVO was superior and had a lower rebleeding rate.[107] Fibrin glue has also been used with some success, without the long-term risks associated with cyanoacrylate injection.[108] The study also included adolescent patients, who required one to four sessions.[108] Fuster et al.[109] reported success with the use of cyanoacrylate in two pediatric patients with gastric bleeding; no rebleeding was noted for 36 and 43 months. More recently, Rivet et al. reported on the use of cyanoacrylate glue in 8 young infants (2 years old or younger, 10 kg or less) with portal hypertension and gastroesophageal varices. Immediate control of bleeding was achieved in all cases and variceal eradication occurred after a mean of 1.4 sessions.[110] Currently, surgical shunting and transjugular intrahepatic portosystemic shunting (TIPS) are the treatments associated with long-term resolution. In one child, rectal varices were treated effectively with endoscopic ligation.[111]

Prophylaxis of Variceal Hemorrhage

Pre-primary prophylaxis is aimed at the prevention of formation and growth of varices. A large randomized placebo-controlled trial showed that nonselective beta-blockers are not effective in preventing the development of varices.[112] Thus, the use of beta blockers for pre-primary prophylaxis is not indicated for adult or pediatric patients. Surveillance endoscopies should be performed every 2 to 3 years in these patients.[113]

Primary prophylaxis in patients with varices attempts to stop the first bleeding episode from ever occurring. In patients with known portal hypertension, the family needs to be aware of the patient's risk of bleeding and need for rapid access to a medical center. Long-term reduction of splanchnic pressures may help to reduce the risk of bleeding. In adults, two therapies are currently accepted in the prevention of the first episode of variceal bleeding: nonselective beta-blockers and EVL.[3,114] Candidates for primary prophylaxis include patients with moderate to large variceal size, red wale marks on the varices, and advanced liver disease.

Most of the data regarding beta-blockade as primary prophylaxis come from adult studies. In meta-analyses,[79] beta-blockade resulted in a significant decrease in first-time bleeding and in some studies a possible reduction in the mortality rate.[115] Two non-placebo-controlled trials of propranolol in children with portal hypertension (primarily secondary to cirrhosis) as primary prophylaxis have been reported.[116,117] Use of propranolol, when treatment was adjusted to reduce the resting heart rate by 25%, was associated with a decreased risk of first-time bleeding of 15.6 to 19%. It was well tolerated with mild, transient side effects. Some of these side effects were eliminated by changing to long-acting preparations. Of the children who did bleed during therapy, compliance was an issue, as well as not being able to obtain a 25% reduction in heart rate. Twice-daily dosing was associated with bleeding more often than a three times a day dosing schedule, as were total daily doses of less than 1 mg/kg. Without large multicenter trials, there is not enough data to recommend the use of nonselective beta-blockers in children for primary prophylaxis.[4] Beta-blockade may inhibit the compensatory increase in heart rate due to hypovolemia and worsen the outcome from variceal hemorrhage, especially in young infants.[118] Using transvenous portal pressure measurements before and during therapy with beta-blockers, a reduction of 20% in the HVPG has been shown to be associated with a decreased risk of bleeding to 10% in adult patients. Dropping the HVPG to less than 12 mm Hg eliminated the risk of initial and recurrent variceal bleeding.[119]

There are few studies on the use of sclerotherapy in children to prevent first-time bleeding. Goncalves et al.[120] reported the long-term results of a prospective randomized controlled trial of sclerotherapy versus clinical monitoring. Prophylactic sclerotherapy significantly reduced the incidence of the first episode of esophageal variceal bleeding compared with that in controls without sclerotherapy (6% versus 42%, respectively) and did not result in any significant complications. It did not increase the incidence of gastric varices, but, when varices were present, patients with prophylactic sclerotherapy had a higher risk of bleeding. Congestive hypertensive gastropathy occurred at a higher rate in patients with prophylactic sclerotherapy and was associated with a higher risk of bleeding. This increase in congestive hypertensive gastropathy may be associated with higher morbidity in the prophylactic sclerotherapy group overall and

would possibly require beta-blockade as therapy. Prophylactic sclerotherapy does not affect the survival rate. A meta-analysis of 19 adult studies[79] showed conflicting results. Studies that demonstrated high bleeding rates in control groups receiving only medical therapy but no beta-blockade demonstrated benefit of sclerotherapy for both bleeding and death. Studies that had low bleeding rates among the control populations did not show any benefit for sclerotherapy. EST actually resulted in a higher mortality rate in one study, and higher bleeding rates in another study. With this information, sclerotherapy as primary prophylaxis does not seem warranted, although further studies need to be performed to evaluate variceal banding as an option.

Secondary prophylaxis against rebleeding is important, especially in extrahepatic portal hypertension. Variceal obliteration has been shown to limit the chance of rebleeding. Beta-blocker therapy along with nitrates has been shown to decrease the risk of rebleeding in adult studies. Beta-blockers lower portal pressure through β_2 blockade of the splanchnic vascular supply. α-Adrenergic stimulation is then unopposed and there is a net decrease in splanchnic and portal perfusion. Beta-blocker therapy may mask significant hypotension and is contraindicated in patients with asthma or heart block. Few studies have been performed in children, but those that have been done suggest that it is safe as well as effective.

Esophageal variceal sclerotherapy and band ligation have been used in children to avoid rebleeding after the initial bleeding episode. Repeated sessions every 2 to 4 weeks after the first episode has been shown to eradicate varices in 85 to 90% of patients, generally by five sessions (range 4.5 to 5.9).[43,82,121] In Poddar's large study of 207 children who underwent sclerotherapy for varices due to extrahepatic portal venous obstruction, complications included ulcers (17%), strictures (8%), and perforation (1.4%).[43] EVL may be associated with faster variceal eradication and fewer complications.[98,121] After sclerotherapy or band ligation, acid suppression or sucralfate should be instituted to promote ulcer healing. Follow-up endoscopy should be done yearly once variceal eradication has been achieved to reevaluate for recurrence of varices, which may occur in up to 17% of patients.[43] The addition of a beta-blocker to sclerotherapy shortened the time to variceal eradication but did not affect rebleeding significantly.[122]

Surgical management is rarely needed in the acute situation but may be useful in long-term management for the prevention of rebleeding. In patients with normal liver function, such as those with extrahepatic portal vein thrombosis, appropriate surgical shunting is associated with a low risk of encephalopathy and markedly improves the long-term morbidity and mortality of recurrent bleeding. In patients with intrinsic liver disease whose varices cannot be obliterated and continue to bleed, surgical shunting may be the best approach if liver transplantation is not expected to be necessary in the near future. Indications for shunting include bleeding gastric or other nonesophageal varices, severe hypersplenism, and continued acute bleeding despite the use of other nonsurgical methods.

Shunt Surgery

TIPS connects the portal vein with the hepatic vein via radiographic techniques. In adult studies it decreases the portal pressure by about 50%, and encephalopathy is a complication in only 20% of patients who have underlying severe liver disease. Occlusion rates for the shunts have improved with newer

TABLE 76-4.   TIPS: Indications and Effectiveness

Indication	Value
Prophylaxis of variceal bleeding	Effective
Refractory ascites in cirrhosis	Effective
Portal hypertensive gastropathy	Effective
Gastric antral vascular ectasia	Ineffective
Hepatic hydrothorax	Effective
Hypersplenism	Possibly effective
Acute hepatorenal syndrome	Possibly effective
Budd-Chiari syndrome	Effective
Chronic hepatorenal syndrome	Effective
Hepatopulmonary syndrome	Possibly effective
Veno-occlusive disease	Possibly effective

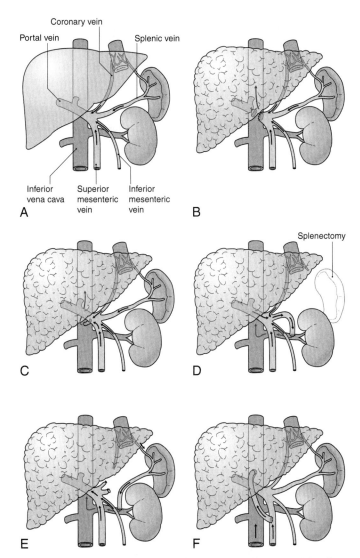

Figure 76-6. Types of portosystemic shunt. (**A**) Normal anatomy. (**B**) End-to-side portacaval shunt with ligation of portal vein at the liver. (**C**) Small-diameter portacaval H-graft. (**D**) Central splenorenal shunt requiring splenectomy. (**E**) Distal splenorenal shunt. (**F**) Superior mesenterico-left intrahepatic portal vein (Rex) shunt using the internal jugular as a graft.

polytetrafluoroethylene (PTFE)-covered stents. A multicenter randomized controlled trial showed much lower occlusion and reintervention rates with PTFE stents compared to bare stents without an increase in the incidence of hepatic encephalopathy,[123] but experience in children is limited.[4] Mortality from the procedure is low. Indications for the procedure in pediatric patients have included recurrent variceal bleeding not responsive to more conservative therapy, hypersplenism, ascites, Budd-Chiari syndrome,[124] hepatorenal syndrome, and hepatopulmonary syndrome (Table 76-4).[125-127] Rebleeding from esophageal varices post-TIPS was associated with shunt occlusion. Hypersplenism did not change significantly in the study by Huppert et al.[128] In veno-occlusive disease, early TIPS insertion led to a reduction in the portosystemic pressure gradient and improvement in arterial and majority portal flow to the liver, but the mortality rate remained extremely high from multiorgan system failure.[129,130] The procedure in pediatric patients may require general anesthesia, a longer procedure time, and modification of the equipment. Limitations for the procedure in pediatrics may be due to vascular anomalies, which may be a relative contraindication.[131] Biliary atresia may also lead to increased difficulty with TIPS placement due to periportal fibrosis and small portal veins.[128] Scheduled reevaluations of the shunts need to be carried out via physical examinations, laboratory testing, and Doppler ultrasonography. If necessary, shunt revision can be performed using the transjugular approach for balloon angioplasty and shunt replacement. Reinterventions may be necessary in more than 50% of patients before more definitive surgery such as liver transplantation or surgical shunt placement.[128,131] Long-term shunt patency has been achieved, reaching durations of up to 6 years. Complications with TIPS placement include portal vein leakage, encephalopathy, perforation, hemolysis, infection, and restenosis. Fever is common within the first 24 to 48 hours after the procedure. Serum aspartate aminotransferase and alanine aminotransferase levels may also rise immediately after the procedure and then return to baseline.[132]

TIPS has been proven very effective in acute refractory variceal bleeding because it is a minimally invasive radiologic intervention. If the TIPS fails or is not possible, a surgical shunt can be performed. The type of shunt selected should be determined by the prognosis of the underlying liver disease, likelihood of liver transplantation, anatomy, and surgical experience. Maintaining adequate hepatopetal flow following shunt surgery lowers the risk of encephalopathy and liver deterioration (Figure 76-6).

Hepatopetal flow has been maintained most consistently with a selective splenorenal shunt (distal splenorenal shunt; DSRS), or a partial small-caliber portacaval or mesocaval interposition shunt.[133] In the long term, surgical shunts achieve variceal hemorrhage control in more than 90% of patients. Surgical shunts are preferred in patients with noncirrhotic portal hypertension due to schistosomiasis, noncirrhotic portal fibrosis, idiopathic portal hypertension, CHF, EHPVO, Budd-Chiari syndrome, and veno-occlusive disease. In patients with noncirrhotic portal hypertension, a DSRS is optimal as the risk of encephalopathy is low and a splenectomy is not needed.

In pediatrics, shunts can be performed in any age with success rates greater than 90%.[83,134,135] Actuarial 15-year survival rates of 95% have been noted after shunt surgery.[23] Shunt thrombosis is related mostly to the caliber of the shunt. The type of shunt selected depends on the underlying pathology, the vascular anatomy present, and whether the shunt is intended to decompress the portal system permanently or to act as a bridge to transplant. Successful shunting alleviates the risk of variceal bleeding, over time decreases hypersplenism,[23,136] and improves growth parameters[134,137] and quality of life.

Splenectomy should not be used as a treatment for portal hypertensive hypersplenism in patients with a good long-term prognosis. Once splenectomy has been performed, the splenic vein cannot be used in any future shunt procedures,[138] and the patient is at risk of overwhelming sepsis. Partial splenic embolization has been performed in children for treatment of hypersplenism due to portal hypertension.[139,140] It was reported to result in improvement in the blood picture in more than 70% of the patients, although recurrences were seen in 30%. Embolization of 60 to 70% of the spleen was needed for adequate reduction of the symptoms of hypersplenism. Morbidity from fevers and abdominal pain could last for weeks, and the patients were at risk of abscess formation.[140] Further risk of recurrences and infection still needs to be studied. This type of procedure should be performed only on patients with normal liver function and before the spleen size is too massive. This procedure does not correct the underlying portal hypertension.

Rex Bypass

The Rex bypass (mesenteric-left portal vein bypass) is an option for children with EHPVO. It was originally developed to relive acute portal vein thrombosis occurring after liver transplantation[141] and was subsequently used in patients with EHPVO from different etiologies.[142] This bypass restores hepatopetal flow by using a jugular venous autograft between the intrahepatic left portal vein and the superior mesenteric vein. It requires an occlusion-free mesentericolienal confluence and flow in the left, unoccluded, central portal vein.[138] By restoring hepatopetal flow, encephalopathy is avoided; hypersplenism is reversed and varices are decompressed. HPS was relieved in one report.[138] Superina et al. reported their experience with a large group of children (n = 34) who underwent the Rex bypass and were followed for up to 7 years. The bypass was successful in 91% of all patients with complete relief from gastrointestinal bleeding, significant increase in platelet and leukocyte count, increased liver volume, and improvement in prothrombin time.[143] In another study, surgically restoring portal flow to the liver by the Rex bypass resulted in improved neurocognitive function in children with primary EHPVO.[144] One reported complication of the Rex bypass was pseudotumor cerebri secondary to reduced venous drainage which was successfully managed with acetazolamide until good cerebral collateralization had occurred.[138] The Rex bypass should be considered curative and is becoming the procedure of choice in children with EHPVO.[145]

REFERENCES

4. Shneider B, Emre S, Groszmann R, et al. Expert pediatric opinion on the Report of the Baveno IV Consensus Workshop on Methodology of Diagnosis and Therapy in Portal Hypertension. Pediatr Transplant 2006;10:893–907.

21. Lykavieris P, Gauthier F, Hadchouel P, et al. Risk of gastrointestinal bleeding during adolescence and early adulthood in children with portal vein obstruction. J Pediatr 2000;136:805–808.

88. Ryckman FC, Alonso MH. Causes and management of portal hypertension in the pediatric population. Clin Liver Dis 2001;5:789–818.

98. Zargar SA, Javid G, Khan BA, et al. Endoscopic ligation compared with sclerotherapy for bleeding esophageal varices in children with extrahepatic portal venous obstruction. Hepatology 2002;36:666–672.

112. Groszmann RJ, Garcia-Tsao G, Bosch J, et al. Beta-blockers to prevent gastroesophageal varices in patients with cirrhosis. N Engl J Med 2005;353:2254–2261.

120. Goncalves ME, Cardoso SR, Maksoud JG. Prophylactic sclerotherapy in children with esophageal varices: long-term results of a controlled prospective randomized trial. J Pediatr Surg 2000;35:401–405.

See expertconsult.com for a complete list of references and the review questions for this chapter.

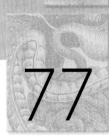

77

LIVER FAILURE

Deirdre Kelly

Pediatric liver disease is a significant cause of morbidity and mortality worldwide. Advances in diagnosis and treatment, particularly the successful development of transplantation, have dramatically improved the outcome of infants and children with liver disease so that many can now expect to grow into adult life.

Liver failure is a loss of the synthetic properties of the liver. It may occur as a result of the progression of chronic liver disease or acute hepatocellular necrosis in acute liver failure. Both are significant indications for liver transplantation. This chapter explores the etiology and pathogenesis of liver failure and links with Chapter 78, which describes the indications for and outcome of liver transplantation.

CHRONIC LIVER FAILURE

Chronic liver failure is associated with the development of cirrhosis and its complications such as malnutrition, portal hypertension, bleeding esophageal varices, ascites, encephalopathy, and hepatorenal syndrome.

Pathogenesis

Cirrhosis

Cirrhosis is characterized by diffuse hepatic fibrosis and nodule formation with regeneration and is the end result of many different liver diseases. Cholestasis, which is the accumulation of hydrophobic bile acids that are toxic to hepatocytes, is a major cause of cirrhosis, particularly in pediatric liver disease. [1]

The liver responds to injury in a similar way, irrespective of the type of injury. The critical steps are programmed cell death (apoptosis), cell necrosis, and fibrogenesis. Oxidant stress, the release of cytokines and other soluble growth factors, leads to activation of hepatic stellate cells and fibrosis. The subsequent formation of fibrotic and regenerative nodules develops vascular anastomoses that cause increased resistance to portal blood flow and the development of portal hypertension and portosystemic shunting.

Hepatic Fibrogenesis

Studies in animal models and histologic information from both adult and pediatric liver diseases[2,3] have shown that different mechanisms of hepatic damage lead to characteristic patterns of fibrosis. For instance, chronic viral hepatitis is associated with periportal fibrosis, whereas centrilobular fibrosis is common with toxic/metabolic damage. Biliary fibrosis is usual in congenital hepatic fibrosis and biliary atresia. It is now known that different cell types are involved in the development of hepatic fibrogenesis, because hepatic stellate cells are activated in hepatocellular damage whereas portal myofibroblasts and fibroblasts are activated in portal tract damage.

Much progress has been made in understanding the mechanisms of hepatic fibrosis.[4,5] It is known that hepatic stellate cells (HSCs) are the primary source of extracellular matrix in liver fibrosis and that the development of fibrosis is dependent on the effects of transforming growth factor beta and platelet-derived growth factor on HSCs, which leads to activation characterized by chemotaxis, proliferation, contraction, fibrogenesis, and extracellular matrix degradation.

In chronic liver injury, the extracellular matrix is constantly remodeled, leading to new collagen formation and deposition.[6] This is regulated by proteases, inhibitors, and growth factors. Matrix metalloproteinases (MMPs) and their tissue inhibitors (TIMPs) play a major role in matrix degradation, and there is now much interest in the reversal of hepatic fibrosis and the identification of apoptotic mediators in stellate cells and how they contribute to recovery from liver injury. Different platelet-derived growth factor and transforming growth factor beta inhibitors have been shown to effectively prevent liver fibrosis in animal models and represent promising therapeutic agents for humans.

In addition, it is possible that in the future MMPs and TIMPs may be of value as noninvasive serum markers for inflammation and fibrosis.

Portal Hypertension

Portal hypertension develops because of the combination of increased portal blood flow and increased portal resistance and is defined as a portal and hepatic-venous pressure gradient (the portal vein–vena cava pressure gradient) more than 10 to 12 mm Hg. In cirrhosis, there is an increase in intrahepatic resistance, followed by an increase in splanchnic blood flow that increases portal pressure, giving rise to a hyperdynamic circulation with increased cardiac and decreased splanchnic arteriolar tone, both of which further increase portal inflow. Intrahepatic resistance is responsible for many of the complications of cirrhosis, such as bleeding esophageal varices, renal dysfunction, encephalopathy, and ascites.[7,8]

Splenomegaly and hypersplenism rarely require specific intervention, as they do not significantly affect morbidity or mortality. There is often (unfounded) concern about traumatic splenic rupture, but this is extremely rare. The pancytopenia due to sequestration in the spleen likewise causes little or no morbidity, as the blood cells present, though lower in number, are highly functional.

Causes of Chronic Liver Failure

Chronic liver failure is the end-result of many different diseases discussed in previous chapters, many of which result in cirrhosis (Table 77-1), including reduced bile secretion or bile duct obstruction (cholestasis), infections, toxins, and metabolic, vascular, and nutritional disorders. Hepatic dysfunction and

TABLE 77-1.   Chronic Liver Failure

Cholestatic liver disease
   Biliary atresia
   Idiopathic neonatal hepatitis
   Alagille's syndrome
   Progressive familial intrahepatic cholestasis (1, 2, and 3)
Metabolic liver disease
   α_1-Antitrypsin deficiency
   Tyrosinemia type I
   Wilson's disease
   Cystic fibrosis
   Glycogen storage type IV
Chronic hepatitis
   Autoimmune
   Postviral (hepatitis B, C, other)
Cryptogenic cirrhosis
Fibropolycystic liver disease ± Caroli syndrome
Primary immunodeficiency with sclerosing cholangitis

cholestasis lead to malnutrition, impaired protein synthesis, coagulopathy, portal hypertension, hepatorenal and hepatopulmonary syndromes, encephalopathy, and ascites. Cholestasis is also associated with pruritus and malabsorption. Many children with chronic liver disease are immunosuppressed, with resulting bacterial infection. Hepatocellular carcinoma may complicate cirrhosis in childhood, particularly in chronic hepatitis B, tyrosinemia type I, and progressive fibrosing intrahepatic cholestasis.

Chronic liver disease may be either *compensated,* when there are no clinical or laboratory features of liver failure, or *decompensated,* at which time transplantation is required.

The pattern of progression to cirrhosis and decompensation is variable. In neonatal extrahepatic biliary atresia, the development of hepatic fibrosis is rapid, with cirrhosis occurring by 8 to 16 weeks of age, whereas in cystic fibrosis (CF)-associated focal biliary cirrhosis, liver function may be normal for many years. The importance of genetic modifiers on outcome and progression of chronic liver diseases is under investigation.[4] The cellular mechanisms and factors responsible for the development of liver fibrosis in most chronic liver diseases are similar (see earlier discussion). Activation of hepatic stellate cells and production of type I collagen have been documented in both biliary atresia[9] and CF.[10] Transforming growth factor (TGF)-β_1 is produced in biliary atresia by damaged hepatocytes and bile duct epithelial cells, whereas in cystic fibrosis liver disease, it is expressed in bile duct epithelium.

Clinical Presentation

In compensated liver disease, children are usually asymptomatic. The first indication of liver disease may be an incidental finding of hepatosplenomegaly, splenomegaly alone, or increased serum transaminases. The liver is enlarged, hard, or nodular in early cirrhosis, but becomes small and impalpable in advanced cirrhosis with splenomegaly. Cutaneous features such as spider angiomata, prominent periumbilical veins, and palmar erythema are a sign of chronic liver disease. Spider angiomata may also occur in healthy children under the age of 5 years, or in teenagers during puberty, but the appearance of new spider angiomata or more than five or six suggests liver disease. They are frequently observed in the vascular drainage of the superior vena cava and feature a central arteriole from which radiate numerous fine vessels, ranging from 2 to 5 mm

in diameter. The presence of prominent veins radiating from the umbilicus is an indication of portal hypertension. Other cutaneous features include easy bruising; fine telangiectasia on the face and upper back; white spots, most often on buttocks and arms; and clubbing of the fingers. On examination of the nasal membranes, prominent telangiectasia of Little's area is associated with recurrent epistaxis.

Some diseases, such as autoimmune hepatitis type 1, cystic fibrosis, and α_1-antitrypsin deficiency, may present with compensated cirrhosis without jaundice, and the first sign of liver disease may be hepatosplenomegaly, splenomegaly alone, increased hepatic transaminases, or increased alkaline phosphatase levels. In Wilson's disease, specific features include hemolytic anemia, subtle signs of encephalopathy such as slurred speech, personality changes, loss of memory or poor performance at school, and Kayser-Fleischer rings, which are best seen on slit-lamp examination.

In contrast, children with cholestatic liver disease have persisting jaundice and pruritus, as in biliary cirrhosis. The liver is usually enlarged, and xanthelasma, malnutrition, and deficiency of fat-soluble vitamins (particularly vitamins D and K) may be prominent features. Clubbing is more likely to occur in biliary cirrhosis, and malnutrition and decompensation occur earlier in this form of liver disease.

Decompensated liver disease is characterized by clinical and laboratory findings of liver synthetic failure, and the occurrence of complications such as malnutrition, ascites, peripheral edema, coagulopathy, gastrointestinal bleeding, and hepatic encephalopathy. Malnutrition with reduced lean tissue and fat stores and poor linear growth is an important sign of chronic liver disease in children.[1] Spontaneous bruising caused by reduced synthesis of clotting factors and thrombocytopenia due to hypersplenism is a sign of advanced disease. There may also be changes in the systemic and pulmonary circulations, with arteriolar vasodilation, increased blood volume, a hyperdynamic circulatory state, and cyanosis due to intrapulmonary shunting. Renal failure is a late but serious event. Laboratory investigations may reveal increased levels of alkaline phosphatase, bilirubin, hepatic transaminases, and ammonia, but in particular there is abnormal liver synthetic function, reflected by such findings as hypoalbuminemia and prolonged prothrombin time.

Diagnosis of Chronic Liver Disease

Diagnosis of chronic liver disease requires a multidisciplinary approach including clinical, laboratory, radiologic imaging, and pathologic investigations. It is usually based on clinical findings and the results of *liver biopsy* findings, which will confirm the extent of cirrhosis and possibly the cause of the liver disease.

Investigations

Biochemical Liver Function Tests. Biochemical liver function tests (Table 77-2) reflect the severity of hepatic dysfunction but rarely provide diagnostic information on individual diseases. The most useful tests of liver "function" are plasma albumin concentration and coagulation time. Low serum albumin indicates chronicity of liver disease, whereas abnormal coagulation indicates significant hepatic dysfunction, either acute or chronic. Fasting hypoglycemia in the absence of other causes (e.g., hypopituitarism or hyperinsulinism) indicates poor hepatic function and is a guide to prognosis in acute liver failure. Diagnostic tests are summarized in Table 77-3.

TABLE 77-2. Liver Function Tests

Reference Range of Test	Abnormality
Conjugated bilirubin < 20 mmol/L	Elevated: hepatocyte dysfunction or biliary obstruction
Aminotransferases Aspartate (AST) < 50 U/L Alanine (ALT) < 40 U/L	Elevated: hepatocyte inflammation or damage
Alkaline phosphatase (ALP) < 600 U/L (age dependent)	Elevated: biliary inflammation or obstruction
γ-Glutamyltransferase (GGT) < 30 U/L (age dependent)	Elevated in biliary obstruction/ enzyme induction Low in PFIC 1 and 2
Albumin 35-50 g/L	Reduced: chronic liver disease
Prothrombin time (PT) 12-15 s Partial thromboplastin time (PTT) 33-37 s	Prolonged: (i) Vitamin K deficiency (ii) Reduced hepatic synthesis
Ammonia < 50 mmol/L	Elevated: abnormal protein catabolism, urea cycle defect, or other inherited metabolic disease
Glucose > 4 mmol/L	Reduced: acute or chronic liver failure, metabolic disease, or hypopituitarism

PFIC, progressive familial intrahepatic cholestasis.

TABLE 77-3. Investigation of Chronic Liver Disease in Children

General
Bilirubin
Aminotransferases
γ-Glutamyl transferase
Alkaline phosphatase
Albumin
Cholesterol
Urea and creatinine
Ammonia
α-Fetoprotein
Full blood count
Prothrombin time
PELD or PHD score
Chest x-ray
Hepatobiliary and renal ultrasound
Upper gastrointestinal endoscopy
Electrocardiogram
Electroencephalogram
Liver biopsy

Specific (for diagnosis)
Viral serology (TORCH, hepatitis B, C, EBV)
Autoimmune antibodies, immunoglobulins
Liver copper or ceruloplasmin
Serum iron and ferritin

General/Metabolic
Urinary sugars, amino acids, organic acids, fatty acids
Blood sugar (fasting), lactate, pyruvate, urate
Serum amino acids, copper, ceruloplasmin, α₁-antitrypsin, iron ferritin, bile acids
Serum acylcarnitine profile
Sweat test, CF mutation studies
Protease inhibitor phenotype
Muscle biopsy, liver fibroblasts for specific enzymes

Vascular
Doppler images of hepatic venous blood flow
Digital subtraction angiography
Inferior venacavography

CF, cystic fibrosis; EBV, Epstein-Barr virus; PELD, Pediatric End-stage Liver Disease; PHD, Pediatric Hepatic Dependency; TORCH, toxoplasma, rubella, cytomegalovirus, herpes simplex.

Radiology. Several radiologic techniques provide valuable information in the investigation and diagnosis of pediatric liver disease. Chest x-rays may show skeletal abnormalities, for example, butterfly vertebrae in Alagille's syndrome or a dilated heart secondary to fluid overload in end-stage liver disease. Wrist and knee x-rays will demonstrate bone age and/or the development of osteopenia or rickets in chronic liver disease.

Ultrasound. Ultrasonic investigation of the abdomen provides information on the size and consistency of the liver, spleen, and portal and hepatic veins. Cirrhosis may be suggested if there is abnormal homogeneity of the liver architecture, and an irregular liver edge. Color-flow Doppler techniques permit rapid evaluation of vascular patency without the use of intravenous contrast material. It is particularly useful in pretransplant examinations to identify whether the portal vein, hepatic veins and artery, and splenic vessels are patent. Portal hypertension is suggested by the presence of ascites, splenomegaly, and splenic or gastric varices.

Computed Tomography. Computed tomographic (CT) scanning of the liver is usually not required for the diagnosis of chronic liver failure but may be useful for the identification and biopsy of hepatic tumors or regenerative nodules. Intravenous contrast medium causes enhancement of vascular lesions and the walls of abscesses, and it may be helpful in differentiating tumors from other solid masses. CT scans of the brain are helpful for the detection of cerebral edema in acute liver failure.

Endoscopic Ultrasound. Endoscopic ultrasound (EUS) is a new imaging modality that visualizes the lower biliary tree. The technique uses mini probes (external diameter 2.6 mm), which are small enough to be passed via the operating channel of conventional pediatric duodenoscopes. EUS has also proved useful in the diagnosis of submucosal esophageal and gastric varices.[11]

Angiography. Visualization of the celiac access and hepatic and splenic blood vessels is obtained by femoral artery catheterization and injection of radiologic contrast. This technique has two parts: (1) the arterial phase, which provides information on the celiac axis, hepatic and splenic artery abnormalities, vascularization and anatomy of hepatic tumors, hepatic hemangiomas, and detection of hepatic artery thrombosis; and (ii) the venous phase, which provides information about the patency of the portal, splenic, and superior mesenteric veins and the presence of portal hypertension by identification of mesenteric, esophageal, or gastric varices.

Splenoportography. This technique, in which the splenic and portal veins are visualized by the injection of radiologic contrast into the spleen, has largely been replaced by hepatic angiography. It may be useful for measuring splenic pulse pressures in the evaluation of portal hypertension but carries a small risk of splenic rupture.

Magnetic Resonance Imaging. Magnetic resonance imaging (MRI) scanning has now replaced hepatic angiography as the best way to stage or diagnose hepatic tumors or regenerative nodules and identify their vascular supply. It may provide valuable information about liver or brain consistency and storage of heavy metals, for example iron in hemochromatosis, copper in Wilson's disease, and cerebral edema in acute liver failure.[12]

Endoscopy. Upper gastrointestinal endoscopy (gastroscopy) using a flexible fiberoptic endoscope is the best way to diagnose esophageal and gastric varices secondary to portal hypertension. The technique is normally performed under sedation or general anesthetic. In children with hematemesis, gastroscopy not only provides rapid diagnosis but enables therapy with variceal banding or endoscopic sclerotherapy for bleeding varices or injection of bleeding ulcers with adrenaline or thrombin.

Neurophysiology. Electroencephalography is mostly used in the assessment of hepatic encephalopathy. It will identify abnormal rhythms secondary to encephalopathy due to either acute or chronic liver failure or drug toxicity such as posttransplant immunosuppression. It may also be of value in determining brain death: A flat electroencephalogram (EEG) in the absence of sedation is an indication for withdrawal of therapy. CT or MRI scans of the brain (see previous discussion) may identify cerebral edema, infarction, or hemorrhage.

Histopathology

The diagnosis of most liver diseases requires histologic confirmation; thus liver biopsies are a routine procedure in specialist centers. An aspiration technique, using a Menghini needle (or disposable variant), has a complication risk of 1:1000 liver biopsies and may be performed under sedation with local anesthesia. In fibrotic or cirrhotic livers, a Tru-cut needle, which removes a larger core, may be necessary. Transjugular liver biopsies, in which the liver is biopsied through a special catheter passed from the internal jugular vein into the hepatic veins, is now possible for children as small as 6 kg and is the only safe way to perform a biopsy if coagulation times remain abnormal despite support (prothrombin time (PT) more than 5 s prolonged over control value).[13] The complications of this potentially dangerous procedure are much reduced if it is performed in expert hands in specialized units under controlled conditions.[14]

Classically, cirrhosis is described as micronodular, macronodular, and mixed types. Micronodular cirrhosis is characterized by fibrous septa separating small (less than 3 mm) regeneration nodules of almost uniform size, present throughout the liver. Macronodular cirrhosis is characterized by nodules up to 5 cm in diameter, separated by irregular septa of varying widths. Regenerative nodules larger than 2 cm in diameter suggest that the cirrhotic process is long-standing. This pattern is usually seen in α_1-antitrypsin deficiency, autoimmune hepatitis, and Wilson's disease. Alternatively, cirrhosis is defined as postnecrotic, biliary (periportal), or hepatic venous outflow (cardiac) cirrhosis. Postnecrotic cirrhosis is seen in chronic hepatitis due to viruses, autoimmune factors, or drugs, or in neonatal hepatitis. Histologic features include piecemeal necrosis, bridging fibrosis, collapse of the hepatic lobules, and regeneration, with the development of macronodular cirrhosis. In biliary cirrhosis fibrosis develops from the portal tracts, extending into the parenchyma linking adjacent portal tracts with preservation of the lobular architecture. Bile duct proliferation is a feature of extrahepatic biliary atresia, and bile duct paucity or hypoplasia is a feature of intrahepatic cholestatic syndromes, such as Alagille's syndrome. Obstruction to hepatic venous outflow due to cardiac lesions with increased right atrial pressure or hepatic vein-occlusive disorders leads to centrilobular hemorrhagic necrosis, with fibrosis extending from central veins to portal tracts.

Percutaneous needle liver biopsy interpretation may be difficult because of fragmentation of the specimen or if the specimen

TABLE 77-4.   Complications of Cirrhosis in Children

Malnutrition and growth failure
Portal hypertension and variceal bleeding
Hypersplenism
Ascites
Encephalopathy
Coagulopathy
Hepatopulmonary syndrome
Hepatorenal syndrome
Bacterial infections, spontaneous bacterial peritonitis
Hepatocellular carcinoma

is taken from a macronodule, which may look almost normal, although there may be hyperplasia of the hepatocytes or a relative excess of hepatic vein branches.

Specific histologic patterns may be diagnostic such as a plasma cell or lymphocytic portal infiltrate with piecemeal necrosis and interface hepatitis in autoimmune hepatitis, Mallory's hyaline and copper deposition in Wilson's disease, and intracellular periodic acid-Schiff-positive, diastase-resistant inclusions in α_1-antitrypsin deficiency.

Management of Chronic Liver Disease

The primary aims of management are:
- To prevent progressive liver damage by treating the cause
- To prevent or control the complications (Table 77-4)
- To consider liver transplantation before irreversible disease

Diagnosis and Prevention of Progressive Liver Damage

In most circumstances, there is no specific therapy for the liver disease, and general supportive management is required.

Cholestatic Liver Disease. Biliary atresia is the commonest cause of cholestatic liver failure in children worldwide and is the main indication for liver transplantation[15] (see Table 77-1). It is a disease of unknown etiology in which there is destruction of the extrahepatic and intrahepatic biliary ducts leading to cholestasis, fibrosis, and cirrhosis. The clinical features include progressive obstructive jaundice and failure to thrive. The diagnosis is based on evidence of biliary obstruction and liver histology that demonstrates fibrosis, cholestasis, and proliferation of biliary ductules.

Surgical removal of the fibrosed biliary tree and formation of a Roux-en-Y anastomosis (Kasai portoenterostomy) is a palliative procedure, which achieves biliary drainage in 60% of infants. It is more likely to be successful if carried out in experienced pediatric units.[16] Medical management consists of prevention of cholangitis with low-dose oral antibiotics (e.g., amoxicillin, 125 mg/day; cephalosporin, 125 mg/day; or trimethoprim, 120 mg/day), and nutritional and family support (see later discussion). If surgery is unsuccessful, or recurrent cholangitis is a problem, chronic liver failure with the development of cirrhosis and portal hypertension is inevitable and an indication for liver transplantation.

There is no specific therapy for the remaining forms of cholestatic neonatal liver disease, but supportive and nutritional therapy is essential and may prevent the rapid progression of liver disease (see later discussion).[17]

The outcome of cholestatic liver diseases such as Alagille's syndrome and progressive familial intrahepatic cholestasis is variable. Many children have compensated liver disease for some time or are well maintained on supportive management. Liver transplantation is indicated when cirrhosis and portal hypertension develop, when malnutrition and growth failure are unresponsive to nutritional support, or when there is intractable pruritus that is resistant to maximal medical therapy or biliary diversion.

Cystic Fibrosis

As long-term survival improves in children with cystic fibrosis (CF), liver disease is recognized in over 20% of children, with a male preponderance.[18] Children usually present with hepatomegaly and/or splenomegaly. Early diagnosis is difficult, but is based on elevated hepatic transaminases (twice the upper limit of normal); abnormal liver ultrasound (demonstrating fatty infiltration, nodularity, and irregularity); and liver histology with steatosis, chemical cholangitis, focal biliary fibrosis, or cirrhosis.

Management is supportive and involves nutritional therapy, particularly vitamin A and E supplementation and ursodeoxycholic acid (20 mg/kg/day).[19] Hepatic decompensation is a late feature of CF liver disease, but portal hypertension is common and bleeding esophageal varices may be a serious recurrent problem, which requires standard therapy. Liver transplantation is indicated for children with hepatic decompensation (falling serum albumin, prolonged coagulation unresponsive to vitamin K), severe malnutrition, and portal hypertension unresponsive to medical management. Assessment of pulmonary function is required, because severe lung disease (loss of more than 50% of lung function) may indicate the necessity for a heart, lung, and liver transplant.[20]

Autoimmune Hepatitis

Autoimmune liver disease is the commonest liver disease in older children, particularly in teenaged girls. The clinical presentation is variable and includes both acute and chronic liver failure, but often the presentation is insidious with the discovery of hepatosplenomegaly in a child with a history of recurrent jaundice with lethargy, fatigue, and weight loss.[2,19]

The diagnosis is confirmed by identifying: elevated immunoglobulins, particularly IgG; reduced levels of complement (C3, C4); nonspecific autoantibodies (type I: anti-nuclear antibody (ANA) and anti-smooth muscle (SMA); type II: anti-liver kidney microsomal antibodies (LKM); liver histology with portal inflammation, bridging fibrosis, and interface hepatitis. Cirrhosis may be present at diagnosis. Therapy includes supportive management and initiating immunosuppression with prednisolone 2 mg/kg and azathioprine (0.5 to 1 mg/kg). Steroids should be limited to a maximum dose of 60 mg as they may exacerbate encephalopathy and induce obesity, which may be persistent in adolescent girls. Second line drugs such as cyclosporin A, tacrolimus, or mycophenolate mofetil may be required if there is a delayed response or relapse.

Liver transplantation[22] is indicated in about 25% of children who do not respond to immunosuppression, have intolerable side effects, or develop end-stage liver failure with jaundice, malnutrition, ascites, encephalopathy, and coagulopathy despite medical therapy.

Failure of medical treatment is more likely when established cirrhosis is present at diagnosis.

Wilson's Disease

Wilson's disease may present with acute or chronic liver failure. Biochemical liver function tests indicate chronic liver disease with low albumin (less than 3.5 g/dL or 35 g/L), minimal transaminitis, and a low alkaline phosphatase (less than 200 U/L). The diagnosis is established by detecting a low serum copper (less than 1 mmol/dL or 10 mmol/L); a low serum ceruloplasmin (less than 20 mg/dL or 200 mg/L); excess urine copper (above 1 mmol/24 hours), particularly after penicillamine treatment (20 mg/kg/day); and an elevated hepatic copper (more than 250 mg/g dry weight of liver). Approximately 25% of children may have a normal or borderline ceruloplasmin, as it is an acute-phase protein.[23]

Management is with a low copper diet and penicillamine (20 mg/kg/day), or trientine (triethylenetetramine) 25 mg/kg/day, in addition to oral zinc. In asymptomatic children or in those who have minimal hepatic dysfunction, the outlook is excellent, although fulminant hepatic failure with hemolysis may occur if treatment is discontinued. Liver transplantation is essential for children who present with subacute or fulminant hepatitis and in children with advanced cirrhosis and portal hypertension.[24,25]

Tyrosinemia Type I

Tyrosinemia type I may present with acute liver failure in infants between 1 and 6 months of age and chronic liver disease in older children. Biochemical liver function tests show an elevated bilirubin, transaminases, alkaline phosphatase, and a reduced albumin. Plasma amino acids indicate an increase in plasma tyrosine, phenylalanine, and methionine with grossly elevated α-fetoprotein levels. Urinary succinylacetone is a pathognomonic but not an invariable finding. The diagnosis is confirmed by measuring FAA activity in fibroblasts or lymphocytes.

Hepatic histology is nonspecific with steatosis, siderosis, and cirrhosis, which may be present in infancy. Hepatocyte dysplasia is associated with a risk of hepatocellular carcinoma.

Initial management is with a phenylalanine and tyrosine-restricted diet which may improve overall nutritional status and renal tubular function, but does not affect progression of liver disease. The discovery of 2-(2-nitrotrifluoromethylbenzoyl)-1,3-cyclohexenedione (NTBC) or nitisinone, which prevents the formation of toxic metabolites, has altered the natural history of this disease in childhood. There is rapid reduction of toxic metabolites, normalization of tubular function, prevention of porphyria-like crises, and improvement in both nutritional status and liver function, particularly in those who have acute liver failure. Liver transplantation is now only indicated for the development of acute or chronic liver failure unresponsive to NTBC, or suspicion of hepatocellular carcinoma.[26,27]

Viral Hepatitis

Chronic liver failure due to hepatitis B or C is unusual in childhood.

Therapy for hepatitis B is unsatisfactory The indications for treatment are persistently raised serum aminotransferases, presence of HBe antigen with detectable HBV DNA in serum, and features of chronic hepatitis on liver biopsy. Interferon-α (5 to 10 μ/m^2 thrice weekly) by subcutaneous injection for 6 months has a sustained clearance rate of 40 to 50%. Children who have active histology, low HBV DNA levels (less than 1000 pg/mL), high serum aminotransferase enzymes, and horizontal transmission are more likely to respond to interferon. Both lamivudine and adefovir have a 26% seroconversion rate after 12 months of treatment. Viral resistance is an issue, especially with lamivudine. Antivirals such as entecavir, telbivudine, and tenofovir are under evaluation.[28]

In contrast, therapy for hepatitis C is more satisfactory. Children who have persistent positivity of HCV RNA and evidence of liver disease should be selected for therapy that is best tolerated in younger children (3 to 5 years of age). The combination of pegylated interferon and ribavirin given for 12 months has a sustained viral response rate of 45% in genotype 1 and a 90% response rate in children with genotypes 2 and 3 when given for 6 months.[29]

Primary Immunodeficiency

As bone marrow transplantation for primary immunodeficiency becomes increasingly successful, it has been recognized that some children have associated liver disease and may die from liver failure. The most common immunodeficiency is CD40 ligand deficiency – hyperimmunoglobulin M (hyper-IgM) syndrome – in which recurrent cryptosporidial infection of the gut and biliary tree leads to sclerosing cholangitis. In this group of children it is important to consider bone marrow transplantation before the development of significant liver disease, or to consider combined liver and bone marrow transplantation.[30]

Supportive Therapy for Chronic Liver Failure

The liver has a central role in regulating fuel and metabolism, nutrient homeostasis, and the absorption of a number of nutrients; malnutrition is thus a common complication of chronic liver failure, particularly in infants, because of their higher energy and growth requirements.[31] A wide range of nutrient deficits occurs in most chronic liver diseases in children and may be reversed with intensive nutritional supplementation and fat-soluble vitamins (Table 77-5).

Nutritional Support

The main aim of nutritional support is to provide sufficient caloric intake to reverse or prevent fat malabsorption and protein malnutrition. An intensive approach to feeding is required,

TABLE 77-5. Management of Nutritional Deficiency in Pediatric Liver Failure

Deficit	Management
Energy	Increase calorie intake Achieve 130-150% EAR Nocturnal enteral nutrition Continuous enteral nutrition
Protein	Provide adequate protein (3-4 g/kg daily) BCAA-enriched protein (32%) Albumin infusion (if serum albumin < 25g/L)
Fat	Improve fat absorption (MCT/LCT) 50:50 Provide saturated fats high in EFA ?Supplement DHA
Fat-soluble vitamins	Light exposure Vitamin $D_1\alpha$ (50 ng/kg) Vitamin K (2.5-5 mg/day) Vitamin E (50-400 IU/day) (as TPGS) Vitamin A (5000-10, 000 IU/day)
Water-soluble minerals	Supplement vitamins Supplement as requested

AAA, aromatic amino acids; BCAA, branched-chain amino acids; DHA, docosahexaenoic acid; EAR, estimated average requirement; EFA, essential fatty acids; LCT, long-chain fatty acids; MCT, medium-chain fatty acids; PEM, protein-energy malnutrition; TPGS, tocopherol polyethyleneglycol-1000 succinate.

including nasogastric supplementation if oral feeding cannot meet caloric needs.[32] Increased energy expenditure is the main cause of malnutrition, but anorexia, behavioral feeding, and gastroesophageal reflux are additional reasons, particularly in Alagille's syndrome.

Infants with severe cholestatic jaundice require a calorie intake of 120-150% EAR (estimated average requirement) using either a standard infant formula with appropriate supplements or a modular feed in which individual constituents can be added. A formula containing medium-chain triglyceride (MCT), which can be absorbed regardless of luminal concentrations of bile acids, is useful. Caloric density can be increased by concentrating the formula or adding glucose polymer. Breastfeeding should be encouraged with supplementation with a high-calorie-density formula. There is no good evidence for adding increased amounts of branched chain amino acids.[33,34] Deficiency of essential fatty acids may occur with prolonged cholestasis after maternal stores are depleted, approximately 3 months after birth, or in infants fed high-MCT feeds.

Older children will require calorie supplements in addition to their normal diet, but nocturnal nasogastric enteral feeding may be necessary to provide the volume required. It may be difficult to achieve this intake in fluid-restricted children. If enteral feeding is not tolerated, because of ascites, variceal bleeding, or recurrent hepatic complications, parenteral nutrition in normal amounts is required.

Fat Soluble Vitamin Supplementation

Generous oral supplements of the fat-soluble vitamins are essential especially in cholestatic children[32] and should include:
- Vitamin A, 5 to 15,000 IU/day
- Vitamin D (alphacalcidol), 50 ng/kg/day
- Vitamin E, 50 to 200 mg/day
- Vitamin K, 2.5 to 5 mg/day

Metabolic bone disease may be severe with pathologic fractures. Treatment with infusions of bisphosphonates is beneficial.[35] Vitamin levels should be monitored to ensure adequate absorption and prevent toxicity.

Pruritus

Pruritus due to cholestasis interferes with quality of life. It is often difficult to treat; local measures such as nonperfumed skin cream may help. Medical therapy includes:
- Cholestyramine (1 to 4 g daily) is effective but unpalatable. The mechanism of action is to bind bile salts in the intestinal lumen, thus interrupting the enterohepatic circulation and reducing bile salt concentration. Side effects include malabsorption of fat-soluble vitamins and drugs, folic acid deficiency, constipation, and acidosis.
- Ursodeoxycholic acid (UDCA) may be effective when given in a dose of 20 to 30 mg/kg/day. It is thought to have a choleretic action but is not universally effective.
- Phenobarbitone (5 to 10 mg/kg/day) may stimulate bile salt-independent bile flow, decrease jaundice, and control pruritus.
- Rifampicin (5 to 10 mg/kg/day) relieves pruritus in at least 50%, producing a significant improvement in the remainder.[36] Results are variable. Side effects include hepatotoxicity in 5 to 10% and thrombocytopenia.
- Antihistamines are largely ineffective but, as they cause drowsiness, may be useful at night. Toxic side effects include cardiac dysrhythmias.

- Partial external biliary diversion, in which part of the jejunum is anastomosed to the gallbladder and brought to the surface of the abdominal wall, may relieve pruritus in some conditions, including PFIC and Alagille's syndrome.[37,38] The operation is most likely to be successful if performed before significant fibrosis has developed.
- The Molecular Adsorbent Recirculating System (MARS), which is a form of albumin dialysis, has produced relief of pruritus for 6 to 12 months.[39]

Portal Hypertension

Therapy with endoscopic sclerotherapy, band ligation, and prophylactic beta-blockade therapy is discussed elsewhere.[40-42] Insertion of a transjugular intrahepatic portosystemic stent (TIPS) may be useful in intractable bleeding.[43]

Fluid Balance and Circulatory Changes

Patients with chronic liver failure have fluid retention with ascites. This is managed with diuretics such as spironolactone or furosemide, with salt and water restriction. Peripheral vasodilation, dilation of the splanchnic vascular bed, and arteriovenous shunting are common, as is intravascular depletion. Vigorous diuretic administration or therapeutic paracentesis may further decrease the circulating plasma volume, reducing renal perfusion and increasing sodium retention.[44]

Electrolyte Changes and Renal Failure

Hypoglycemia (blood glucose level less than 40 mg/dL) is due to depletion of hepatic glycogen stores and impaired gluconeogenesis.[45] Contributing factors include raised serum insulin concentrations, as a result of decreased hepatic insulin catabolism, and abnormal levels of glucagon and growth hormone. Hyponatremia is frequently present because of decreased water excretion, increased renal sodium retention due to stimulation of the renin-angiotensin-aldosterone system, and decreased activity of the sodium-potassium pump.[46] Hypokalemia often accompanies hyponatremia and may be due to renal losses and hyperaldosteronism. With severe renal impairment, hyperkalemia may develop. Other electrolyte abnormalities include hypocalcemia and hypomagnesemia. Calcium levels should be corrected for corresponding albumin levels.

Renal excretion of sodium is significantly decreased in patients with well-established cirrhosis and is an important pathophysiologic cause of ascites formation.[46] In addition to the development of hepatorenal syndrome characterized by redistribution of blood flow away from the renal cortex, renal changes in cirrhosis include glomerular sclerosis and membranoproliferative glomerulonephritis.[47] Acute tubular necrosis is also seen in patients with cirrhosis and is distinguished by a higher fractional excretion of sodium than seen with hepatorenal syndrome. Ascites should be managed with diuretics such as spironolactone or furosemide, and restriction of salt and water. Intervention with hemodialysis and hemofiltration should be considered if acute renal failure or hepatorenal failure develops.[48]

Hepatic Encephalopathy

Chronic hepatic encephalopathy may be present in up to 50 to 70% of patients with cirrhosis.[49] Episodes of encephalopathy usually have a precipitating event such as gastrointestinal hemorrhage, infection, and hypokalemia, which increase ammonia production; systemic alkalosis, which increases diffusion of ammonia across the blood-brain barrier; or hypoxemia, hypotension, and dehydration. In addition, such episodes may be due to portosystemic shunting, for example after the insertion of a TIPS for the management of esophageal varices.[49] Of children without encephalopathy but with chronic liver disease, those with early-onset liver disease (initial symptoms in the first year of life) have reduced intelligence quotient scores when compared with children with chronic liver disease of later onset.[50] This may be due to the vulnerability of an infant's brain to the metabolic abnormalities accompanying liver disease or to poor nutritional status, including vitamin E deficiency in young children with chronic liver disease.[47]

Although ammonia levels are typically raised in patients with chronic hepatic encephalopathy, especially those with portosystemic shunting, they correlate poorly with the degree of encephalopathy and are therefore not helpful in following the progression of encephalopathy.[49]

Treatment is directed at identifying and treating precipitating factors, avoiding fasting and sedatives, and reducing protein intake. Although protein restriction may be beneficial in the short term, this may result in growth failure and nutritional depletion in children. Thus, restriction of dietary and/or intravenous protein to 1 to 2 g/kg should be used in only acute or very symptomatic encephalopathy, and protein may be reintroduced as the encephalopathy subsides. A reduction in intestinal protein load and bacterial flora in the gastrointestinal tract can be achieved by enemas, particularly if an acute episode of encephalopathy is secondary to gastrointestinal hemorrhage, or by lactulose.

Nutritional supplements enriched with branched-chain amino acids (BCAAs) may be useful in hepatic encephalopathy by reducing muscle protein breakdown and normalizing plasma amino acid profiles.[34]

Pulmonary Disease

Pulmonary arteriovenous shunting with hypoxemia (hepatopulmonary syndrome) may be present in children with chronic liver disease and portal hypertension, and it presents with dyspnea on exertion or with cyanosis. This condition is reversible after liver transplantation.[51]

Coagulopathy

The liver is responsible for the synthesis of factors II, V, VII, VIII, IX, and X. Reduced levels of these factors, and of other proteins important in coagulation, reflect abnormalities of protein synthesis and impaired posttranslational modification of vitamin K–dependent proteins (factors II, VII, IX, X; protein C, S) or malabsorption of vitamin K in cholestasis.. Patients with coagulopathy secondary to liver disease may be asymptomatic or may have bleeding from the gastrointestinal tract, nasopharynx, retroperitoneum, tracheobronchial tree, genitourinary tract, or subcutaneous tissues, or intracranial bleeding.[52] Petechiae from hypersplenism may cause epistaxis or exacerbate coagulopathy. Treatment consists of adequate vitamin K provision and use of fresh frozen plasma, cryoprecipitate, and platelets as required.[52]

Family and Psychologic Support

Specific attention to the child's developmental and psychologic needs is essential. Physiotherapy may improve gross motor development, especially in children who require frequent hospitalization. Family education and support are essential, particularly for children with progressive illness requiring liver transplantation.

Predicting Outcome

Because liver transplantation is the definitive therapy for many causes of chronic liver disease, assessment of prognosis and the progression of liver disease is essential in order to consider transplantation in a timely way (see Chapter 78).

Most available liver function tests have poor predictive value until liver decompensation has taken place and the development of complications such as gastrointestinal hemorrhage or encephalopathy is unpredictable. Bilirubin, international normalized ratio (INR), growth failure, and albumin were significant for poor outcome in all causes of end-stage disease in an analysis of data from the Studies of Pediatric Liver Transplantation (SPLIT) Consortium. This Pediatric End-Stage Liver Disease (PELD) score is used as the standard for organ sharing in the United States.[53] A similar, but more extensive scoring system for disease severity in children with mild to severe liver disease, the Pediatric Hepatology Dependency (PHD) score comprises 10 parameters (aspartate transaminase, prothrombin time, albumin, bilirubin, ascites, nutritional support, organ dysfunction, blood product support, sepsis, and intravenous access) and correlates with the PELD score for patients requiring transplantation, but also is a measure of dependency and disease severity in other groups of patients with liver disease.[54]

In previous studies,[55] malnutrition was an important independent risk factor, possibly because major nutritional deficits in energy, protein, lipids, vitamins, and minerals may independently compromise outcome and further compromise liver function per se. Quantitative dynamic liver function tests, such as monoethyl-glycinexylidide (MEGX) formation from lignocaine, and caffeine clearance, have also been evaluated as prognostic indicators of residual functional capacity of the liver but are no longer used.[56,57] In general, expert clinical evaluation using a range of modalities included in the PELD and/or PHD score (Table 77-6) is necessary in determining prognosis and predicting the need for transplantation.

ACUTE LIVER FAILURE

Fulminant hepatic failure (FHF) or acute liver failure (ALF) is a rare but fatal disease. It is a heterogeneous condition with many different etiologies in which the pathophysiology is unclear (Table 77-7).

The definition of FHF is the development of hepatic necrosis with hepatic encephalopathy and coagulopathy within 8 weeks of the onset of liver disease, and the absence of preexisting liver disease in any form.[58] This definition is not useful in children because encephalopathy is difficult to detect or may not be a feature in infants. Second, acute liver failure may be the first presentation of an unrecognized autoimmune or metabolic liver disease (e.g., Wilson's disease or tyrosinemia type I). Third, most hepatic failure in neonates is secondary to an inborn metabolic error or an intrauterine insult, which are preexisting liver diseases.

Pathology

The pathologic features of acute liver failure differ according to etiology. There are three basic lesions.

Hepatic Necrosis

Severe hepatic necrosis with loss of lobular architecture and collapse of the reticulin framework is the commonest lesion seen in either viral infection[59] or an idiosyncratic drug reaction. In viral hepatitis, necrosis tends to be panacinar in distribution, whereas in toxic injury it is zonal. Most acute liver failure is associated with massive confluent necrosis[60,61] and it is difficult to identify any viable hepatocytes. In non-A-E hepatitis or indeterminate hepatitis, there may be lymphoid aggregates around bile ducts with congestion of centrilobular sinusoids. In hepatitis B there is a minimal inflammatory infiltrate, whereas in Epstein-Barr viral hepatitis, centrilobular necrosis with bridging and collapse may be obvious with cholestasis and lymphoid "blast cells." In most cases, some evidence of regeneration can be found,[61] with proliferation of ductules. The degree and pattern of necrosis do not correlate with the development of encephalopathy or cerebral edema.[60-62]

Hepatocellular Degeneration

In ALF due to metabolic or toxic injuries in children, the prominent lesion is hepatocellular degeneration with diffuse fatty infiltration of hepatocytes.[63,64] There is minimal hepatocyte necrosis or inflammatory infiltrate. In Reye's syndrome, toxic

---

TABLE 77-6. Prognostic Factors in Children With Chronic Liver Disease

Risk Factors
Bilirubin > 300 mmol/L
Prolonged prothrombin time unresponsive to intravenous vitamin K
Partial thromboplastin time > 20 s
Malnutrition (Wt. SD score < 1.5)
Low plasma cholesterol
Ascites

PELD (Pediatric End-Stage Liver Disease)
Score for transplant waiting list mortality
An algorithm of five parameters
  Age, bilirubin, INR, growth failure, and albumin

PHD (Pediatric Hepatology Dependency)
Score for dependency and severity of chronic liver disease
An algorithm of 10 parameters
  Aspartate transaminase, prothrombin time, albumin, bilirubin, ascites, nutritional support, organ dysfunction, blood product support, sepsis, and intravenous access

---

TABLE 77-7. Causes of Acute Liver Failure in Children

Etiology	Disease
Neonates	
Infectious	Herpesviruses, echovirus, adenovirus, HBV
Metabolic	Galactosemia,* tyrosinemia,* neonatal hemochromatosis,* mitochondrial disease
Older children	
Infectious	HAV, HBV, NA-G, herpesviruses, sepsis,* other
Drugs	Valproate, isoniazid, acetaminophen, carbamazepine, halothane
Toxins	Amanita phalloides, carbon tetrachloride, phosphorus
Metabolic	Hereditary fructose intolerance,* Wilson's disease†
Autoimmune	Types 1 and 2

HAV, hepatitis A virus; HBV, hepatitis B virus; NA-G, non-A, non-G virus.
*Disease does not fulfill definition of FHF.
†Rare under 3 years of age.

injury (valproic acid, aspirin) and inborn errors of metabolism (disorders of fatty acid oxidation) intracellular fat is microvesicular and does not displace the nuclei. Rarely, macrovesicular steatosis is found with drug and toxic injury (hydrocarbon ingestion, amiodarone therapy). In ALF due to either tyrosinemia type 1 or Wilson's disease, the pathologic features will include preexisting cirrhosis.

Spontaneous recovery from ALF is usually associated with complete histologic recovery, even when extensive necrosis is present. Recovery from massive confluent necrosis is distinctly unusual, but when it occurs, postnecrotic cirrhosis often remains.[62,63]

Chemical Biochemistry

Serum aminotransferase levels (ALT, AST) are usually markedly elevated in children with acute liver failure. Levels are almost always above 1000 IU/L and may reach values above 10,000. Peak values tend to be higher in nonsurvivors, but aminotransferase values are not predictive of outcome.[42] Rapidly falling aminotransferase values signify "exhaustion" of the hepatocyte mass and terminal hepatic failure unless associated with evidence of functional recovery, such as improved coagulation and reduced encephalopathy.[65,66]

Marked jaundice is typically seen with severe hepatic necrosis.[65] Serum bilirubin concentrations typically range from 200 to 1200 μmol/L. The rate of increase in serum bilirubin often exceeds that expected with a normal rate of production and zero clearance. Increased production may result from catabolism of hepatic heme proteins or from hemolysis. Early in the course, most of the serum bilirubin is in the conjugated form, indicating excretory dysfunction of viable hepatocytes. Later, most of the bilirubin may be unconjugated, indicating loss of conjugating ability. Children with acetaminophen poisoning, fulminant hepatitis secondary to hepatitis B, and metabolic disease may be anicteric or only mildly jaundiced.[65]

Pathogenesis

Acute liver failure leads to multiorgan failure affecting the brain and kidney. The process leading to hepatic injury is multifactorial and dependent on the balance between the susceptibility of the host, for example, a neonate who develops fulminant HBV; the severity and nature of hepatic injury, such as a dose of acetaminophen; and the ability of the liver to regenerate.[52]

Liver Regeneration

The ability of the liver to regenerate is a crucial factor for survival. It is possible that failure of regeneration is due to prolonged viral injury and persistent viral replication with failure of eradication of the virus, as patients with ALF due to acetaminophen or other drug poisoning or hepatitis A have a better prognosis than those with indeterminate hepatitis (non-A-E hepatitis).[65,67]

Encephalopathy

Encephalopathy is a unique feature of ALF that occurs in the majority of children. It results from an indirect effect of hepatocyte failure on the function of the brain,[68-70] although the neuropharmacologic events that lead to clinical hepatic encephalopathy are complex and not understood. It is thought that in acute hepatocyte dysfunction the liver fails to produce neuroregulatory substances and/or fails to eliminate neurotoxins, which result in brain dysfunction. There have been many candidates

for potential neurotransmitters or neurotoxins such as ammonia, glutamine, short-chain fatty acids, amino acids, mercaptans, and octopamine, and more recently γ-aminobutyric acid (GABA). Acute hepatic encephalopathy is reversible unless complicated by ischemia or cerebral edema.[68]

Etiology

The etiology of acute liver failure varies depending on the age of the child (see Table 77-7). In neonates, an inborn error of metabolism or severe infection is likely, whereas viral hepatitis, autoimmune liver disease, or drug-induced liver failure are common in older children.

Clinical Presentation

The clinical presentation depends on the age of the patient and the etiology of acute liver failure, but the presentation may either be acute (within hours or days) or prolonged for up to 8 to 10 weeks, particularly if due to metabolic liver disease. The extent of jaundice and encephalopathy is variable in the early stages of acute liver failure, but all children have significant coagulopathy.[52]

In neonates, encephalopathy is particularly difficult to diagnose. Vomiting and poor feeding may be an indication of encephalopathy due to metabolic liver disease, whereas irritability and reversal of day/night sleep patterns indicates more established hepatic encephalopathy. In older children, encephalopathy may present with aggressive behavior or convulsions.[71]

Neonatal Acute Liver Failure

One of the common causes of acute liver failure in neonates is septicemia secondary to infection with *Escherichia coli*, *Staphylococcus aureus*, or herpes simplex. Other causes of hepatitis include adenovirus, echovirus, and Coxsackie virus. Acute liver failure secondary to hepatitis B usually presents at about 12 weeks of age, whereas hepatitis A is rare in neonates. Hepatitis C does not cause acute liver failure in neonates or infants.

Hepatitis B

Hepatitis B is vertically transmitted during pregnancy or delivery. The transmission rate is approximately 70% in mothers who are hepatitis B surface antigen (HBsAg) and hepatitis B e antigen (HBeAg) positive. Most infected infants become asymptomatic carriers. In contrast, infants born to mothers who are HBeAg negative have a high risk of developing fulminant hepatitis within the first 12 weeks of life unless successfully vaccinated.[72] The increased incidence of fulminant hepatitis B in these infants has now been demonstrated to be due to the transmission of a pre-core mutant hepatitis virus from mother to child.[73] Both the development of the carrier state and fulminant hepatitis B may be prevented by vaccination of all infants of hepatitis B carrier mothers, irrespective of their e antigen status.

Neonatal Hemochromatosis

Neonatal hemochromatosis is a rare disorder that is associated with iron accumulation in liver, pancreas, heart, and brain. It is now thought to be a maternal alloimmune disorder in which there is iron accumulation in the liver, pancreas, and brain of the fetus.[74] Clinical presentation may be within hours or weeks of birth with jaundice, hypoglycemia, and severe coagulopathy. Encephalopathy, although present, may not be obvious. The diagnosis is suggested by identifying raised ferritin levels (2000 to 3000 g/L) and is confirmed by demonstrating a high serum iron concentration with hypersaturation of iron-binding capacity (95 to 105%) and the demonstration of extrahepatic hemosiderosis. Because of the severe coagulopathy, liver biopsy is usually contraindicated, although extrahepatic siderosis may be demonstrated in salivary glands obtained by lip biopsy, or the accumulation of iron in the pancreas and brain on MRI. Intensive supportive management of the liver failure and the use of an antioxidant cocktail may be effective if begun within 24 to 48 hours of birth, but liver transplantation is usually required within the first weeks of life.[75,76] The disease is prevented by weekly immunoglobulin infusion in subsequent pregnancies.[77]

Tyrosinemia Type I

Infants between 1 and 6 months of age may present with acute liver failure with mild jaundice, hypoglycemia, coagulopathy, encephalopathy, ascites, and occasionally hyperinsulinism. The diagnosis is suggested by identifying increased plasma tyrosine, phenylalanine, and methionine levels and confirmed by identifying a toxic metabolite, succinylacetone, in the urine. Management includes supportive management of acute liver failure and with nitisinone, which prevents the formation of toxic metabolites and allows hepatic regeneration (see earlier discussion). Liver transplantation is required for children who fail to respond.[26,27]

Mitochondrial Disorders

Mitochondrial disorders present with acute liver failure in the context of multiorgan disease. There are many different clinical phenotypes with varying modes of inheritance including transmission through maternal DNA. The disorders include deficiencies of the electron transport chain enzymes or depletion of mitochondrial DNA and a number of genetic mutations have been recognized.[78] Neonates and infants may present with jaundice, coagulopathy and neurologic features very similar to those of hepatic encephalopathy. The diagnosis is suggested by evidence of multiorgan failure (cardiac, renal, bone marrow involvement). Infants usually have metabolic acidosis with a increased blood lactate level, but this may be intermittent or nonspecific. Other useful investigations are an increased plasma 3-hydroxybutyrate:acetoacetate ratio (>2) or detection of abnormal organic acids such as urinary 3-methylglutaconic acid. Evidence of multiorgan failure may be confirmed by muscle biopsy, which may demonstrate abnormal mitochondria; an increased lactate concentration in the cerebrospinal fluid (CSF) or the presence of cerebral atrophy on CT or MRI may confirm neurologic involvement. Liver histology demonstrates microvesicular fatty infiltration, hepatocyte degeneration, and micronodular cirrhosis. The diseases are fatal; liver transplantation is not indicated because of progressive neurologic disease and multiorgan failure.[79]

Familial Hemophagocytic Syndrome

Hemophagocytic syndrome is thought to be an autosomal recessive disorder due to a defect in immunomodulation. It may also be virally induced and the distinction may be difficult

to make in neonates. Infants present with multiorgan failure with jaundice, hepatosplenomegaly, fever, skin rash, and pancytopenia. The diagnosis is confirmed by the demonstration of erythrophagocytosis in bone marrow, liver, and occasionally CSF. Confirmatory investigations are raised plasma triglycerides and increased serum ferritin levels. Treatment includes supportive management of acute liver failure, etoposide, and corticosteroids. Cyclosporin and anti-T lymphocyte globulin have also been used with some effect in children who have achieved remission. Liver transplantation is not indicated, but bone marrow transplantation should be considered.[80]

Acute Liver Failure in Older Children

Viral Hepatitis

Hepatitis B is the commonest cause of fulminant hepatitis worldwide, but acute hepatitis A is more common in children and has a better prognosis. Hepatitis C and D rarely cause fulminant hepatic failure in childhood, whereas hepatitis E virus may be associated with fulminant hepatic failure, particularly in children returning from the Indian subcontinent. Viruses G and transfusion-transmitted virus (TTV), which are parentally transmitted viruses, have not been proven to cause liver disease. Hepatitis secondary to other viruses, such as Epstein-Barr virus (EBV) and parvovirus B19, occasionally lead to fulminant hepatitis. Approximately 50% of children with viral fulminant hepatic failure have no obvious etiology and are classified as having non-A, non-E hepatitis or indeterminate hepatitis.[67]

The survival associated with each type of infection varies; the highest spontaneous survival rates are found with acute hepatitis A infection, and lowest rates with non-A, non-E hepatitis.[81] The main causes of death are cerebral edema, renal failure, coagulopathy, and infection.[82] Survival rates without liver transplantation are 67% when cerebral edema or renal failure is absent, 50% in patients with isolated cerebral edema, and 30% in those with coexisting cerebral edema and renal impairment.[83]

The clinical presentation includes a prodromal illness with anorexia, vomiting, lethargy, gradual onset of jaundice, coagulopathy and encephalopathy. The history may vary from 48 hours to 6 to 8 weeks. The diagnosis is made by viral serology.[67]

Autoimmune Hepatitis

Both forms of autoimmune hepatitis (types I and II) may present with hepatic failure, although fulminant hepatitis is more common in type II. The clinical presentation is similar to that of viral hepatitis, or there may be a history of recurrent episodes of jaundice with lethargy, fatigue, and weight loss.[21]

The diagnosis is confirmed, as indicated previously, by identifying raised levels of immunoglobulins (particularly IgG), reduced levels of complement (C3, C4), and nonspecific autoantibodies (type I: ANA and anti-SMA; type II: anti-LKM). Therapy includes supportive management and initiating immunosuppression with prednisolone (2 mg/kg). Encephalopathy may be exacerbated by high doses of steroids, and caution is required; 60 mg is the maximum dose. Liver transplantation is indicated for children who do not respond quickly to immunosuppression.[22]

Drug-Induced Liver Failure

In pediatric series, toxin- or drug-induced liver injury represents 15 to 20% of cases of FHF[81,84] (see Table 77-3). Liver toxicity may be dose related, as seen with acetaminophen, aspirin, azathioprine, and cyclosporin, or may represent an idiosyncratic reaction seen with valproic acid, phenytoin, isoniazid, chlorpromazine, and halothane.[84,85] The most common cause of drug-related FHF in adolescents and young adults is intentional acetaminophen overdose,[86,87] with doses of more than 150 mg/kg. Maximal liver injury develops between 2 and 4 days after the overdose and may be associated with metabolic acidosis and renal failure. The risk of significant acute liver failure is associated with ingestion of other drugs (e.g., anticonvulsant therapy), recreational drugs such as ecstasy, or alcohol ingestion. Management includes estimation of serum acetaminophen levels and prompt treatment with intravenous N-acetylcysteine to prevent massive hepatic necrosis. The median survival after acetaminophen ingestion for patients who ultimately die is 6 to 7 days, with a range of 3 to 56 days.[83] Poor prognostic factors include the presence of cerebral edema, oliguric renal failure, and decompensated metabolic acidosis. The presence of cerebral edema alone decreases the survival rate to 71%; coexisting cerebral edema and renal failure decrease the survival rate to 53%. If decompensated metabolic acidosis is present, the survival rate decreases to 7%.[83]

The risk of acute liver failure with sodium valproate is particularly high in the first 3 years of life, but has been reported at any stage including adolescence and young adulthood. It may be the first presentation of an underlying metabolic disorder of fatty acid oxidation. The presentation may be atypical with jaundice, vomiting, and increased frequency of convulsions, followed by edema and encephalopathy. Treatment is supportive. Liver transplantation is usually contraindicated, because of either an underlying metabolic disorder or the presence of multiorgan disease.[88]

Anticonvulsant medication with carbamazepine usually produces a cholestatic hepatitis, but may rarely cause fulminant hepatitis.[84]

With some toxic reactions, damage may not resolve after medication withdrawal. Before the availability of liver transplantation, the survival rate for patients developing FHF with grade 3 or 4 encephalopathy due to idiosyncratic drug reactions or halothane hepatitis was 12.5%, compared with 53% for other causes.[83]

Metabolic Liver Disease

Wilson's disease is the commonest metabolic cause of fulminant hepatic failure in children over the age of 3 years. The presentation is variable and may be with features similar to those of viral hepatitis or hemolysis. The diagnosis (see earlier discussion) is suggested by demonstrating hemolysis on a blood film, a relatively low alkaline phosphatase level (less than 600 U/L), raised urinary copper concentration (before and after penicillamine challenge), and a low ceruloplasmin level. Kaiser-Fleisher rings may be absent, but there may be a response to D-penicillamine (20 mg/kg daily); liver transplantation is indicated for those who do not respond quickly or have advanced liver failure with severe coagulopathy and encephalopathy.[24]

Hepatoneurologic Deterioration

Alpers' disease causes cerebral degeneration and disordered hepatic function and may present with fulminant hepatic failure, which may be confused with primary hepatic failure if the characteristic neurologic symptoms are not obvious.[79] Disorders of fatty acid oxidation and of oxidative phosphorylation produce episodes of recurrent hepatic dysfunction and coma that may be confused with Reye's syndrome or severe hepatitis at any age.

Reye's Syndrome

Reye's syndrome is characterized by acute encephalopathy and hepatic dysfunction. The cause is unknown but is thought to be due to a disorder of mitochondrial function. There is a prodromal illness, which may be precipitated by influenza or varicella if this is followed by vomiting, irritability, listlessness, evidence of cerebral edema, and severe hepatic dysfunction. The administration of aspirin may play a role. Liver function abnormalities consist of markedly increased aminotransferase levels and prothrombin times, without a proportionate increase in serum bilirubin levels.[89] Ammonia levels may be increased and hypoglycemia may be present. Hepatomegaly may be found, and liver biopsy reveals a microvesicular steatosis, with swollen mitochondria on electron microscopy.[90] Management is directed to control of cerebral edema, while maintaining cerebral perfusion pressure.[91] There is a high case fatality rate due to cerebral herniation, and a high morbidity rate if the disorder is unrecognized and appropriate management is not initiated. Patients who survive show rapid improvement in liver function test results. Several inborn errors of metabolism such as medium and long-chain acyl coenzyme A dehydrogenase deficiency and organic acidemias mimic Reye's syndrome in presentation and may preclude liver transplantation.[92]

Diagnosis

The diagnosis may be clear from the clinical presentation, but it is important to establish a baseline by performing standard liver function tests and coagulation studies. Investigations will show a marked conjugated hyperbilirubinemia, raised aminotransferase levels (above 10,000 IU/L), raised plasma ammonia concentration (above 100 IU/L), and coagulopathy (prothrombin time greater than 40 s). Liver biopsy is contraindicated because of abnormal coagulation, but can be performed by the transjugular route if essential for diagnosis.

Prevention and Management of Complications of Acute Liver Failure

The clinical course is dominated by the complications of hepatic failure, and therapy should be focused on their prevention and management, which includes early consideration for liver transplantation.

Hypoglycemia

Hypoglycemia (blood glucose below 400 mg/L) develops in the majority of children. It may contribute to central nervous system impairment and other organ dysfunction. Factors contributing to hypoglycemia include[93,94]:

- Failure of hepatic glucose synthesis and release
- Hyperinsulinemia (due to failure of hepatic degradation)
- Increased glucose utilization

Regular monitoring of blood glucose concentrations and the intravenous administration of glucose (10 to 50% dextrose) to maintain a blood glucose level above 4 mmol/L (60 mg/dL) are required. Profound refractory hypoglycemia is a poor prognostic sign and may be preterminal.

Coagulopathy and Hemorrhage

The management of coagulopathy and hemorrhage is essential. Bleeding from needle puncture sites and line insertion is common, and pulmonary or intracranial hemorrhage may be terminal events. Major disturbances in hemostasis develop secondary to failure of hepatic synthesis of clotting factors and fibrinolytic factors, reduction in platelet numbers and function, or intravascular coagulation.[95] The coagulation factors synthesized by hepatocytes include factors I (fibrinogen), II (prothrombin), V, VII, IX, and X, and a reduction in synthesis leads to prolongation of prothrombin and partial thromboplastin times.

The prothrombin time is the most clinically useful measure of hepatic synthesis of clotting factors and determines the necessity for liver transplantation. Administration of parenteral vitamin K is important but may be ineffective.

Factor VII, which has a shorter half-life than other coagulation factors, is a sensitive indicator of hepatic function, as is factor V, which is vitamin K independent.[96] Fibrinogen concentrations are usually normal unless there is disseminated intravascular coagulation (DIC). The level of factor VIII may help differentiate between DIC and FHF, because factor VIII is synthesized by vascular endothelium and its concentration is normal or increased in FHF. Decreased levels of factor XIII may contribute to poor clot stabilization.

A reduction in platelet numbers (80×10^9/L) requires platelet transfusion and suggests hypersplenism, intravascular coagulation, or aplastic anemia.

Once the need for liver transplantation has been established, coagulopathy should be corrected with fresh frozen plasma (FFP), cryoprecipitate, and platelets as needed. Administration of recombinant factor VII (80 g/kg) reliably corrects the coagulation defect in patients with FHF for a period of 6 to 12 hours and may be useful in preparation for invasive procedures. Double-volume exchange transfusion may temporarily improve coagulation and DIC and control hemorrhage. Hemofiltration may be necessary to control fluid balance to allow adequate coagulation support.[52]

Prevention of Gastrointestinal Hemorrhage

Gastrointestinal tract hemorrhage due to gastritis or stress ulceration may be life-threatening. High-dose H_2 antagonists (ranitidine 1 to 3 mg/kg every 8h) or H-pump inhibitors (omeprazole 10 to 20 mg/kg daily) should be administered intravenously and sucralfate (1 to 2 g 4-hourly) may be given by nasogastric tube.[52]

Fluid Balance and Renal Function

Acute liver failure is associated with a hyperdynamic circulation: a high cardiac output and a decrease in systemic vascular resistance and mean arterial pressure.[73] Vasodilation may trigger activation of neurohumoral factors that result in sodium retention, extracellular fluid volume expansion, and the development of ascites.[97]

Renal failure is present in 40% of patients with acute liver failure and may be due to an imbalance among neurohumoral factors, renal vasoconstrictors, and vasodilators.[98] Patients have marked renal vasoconstriction despite systemic vasodilation. Plasma renin activity is typically increased and renal prostaglandin activity is decreased in patients with acute liver failure. Acid-base disturbances may be present in up to 60% of children with FHF.[98] Acute tubular necrosis is present at autopsy in some children with FHF, although others appear to have "functional renal failure" with normal histologic appearance.[99]

The aim of fluid balance is to maintain hydration and renal function while preventing cerebral edema. Maintenance fluids consist of 10% dextrose in 0.25 N saline, and intake should be 75% of normal maintenance requirements unless cerebral edema develops. A total sodium intake of 0.5 to 1 mmol/kg daily is usually adequate. Potassium requirements may be large, 3 to 6 mmol per kg per day, as guided by the serum concentration. As patients may become hypophosphatemic, intravenous phosphate may be given as potassium phosphate.[99]

Urinary output should be maintained using loop diuretics (furosemide at 1 to 3 mg/kg every 6 hours), dopamine (2 to 5 (g per kg per min), and colloid/FFP to maintain renal perfusion. Hemofiltration or dialysis may be required.

Cerebral Edema and Encephalopathy

Hepatic encephalopathy is graded from I to IV[100,101] (Table 77-8) and is variable in onset. Cerebral edema occurs in 45% or more of patients with FHF and is the major cause of morbidity and mortality. It may develop concurrently with other symptoms of hepatitis, or its development may be delayed.[102]

TABLE 77-8.   **Stages of Hepatic Encephalopathy**

Stage	Clinical Manifestations	Asterixis/Reflexes	Neurologic Signs	EEG Changes
Subclinical	None	Absent/normal	Abnormalities on psychometric testing and proton magnetic spectroscopy in older patients	Usually absent
I	Confused, mood changes, altered sleep habits, loss of spatial orientation, forgetfulness	Absent/normal	Tremor, apraxia, impaired handwriting	May be absent or diffuse, slowing to theta rhythm, triphasic waves
II	Drowsy, inappropriate behavior, decreased inhibitions	Present/hyperreflexive	Dysarthria, ataxia	Abnormal, generalized slowing, triphasic waves
III	Child is stuporous but obeys simple commands; infant is sleeping but arousable	Present/hyperreflexive with positive Babinski sign	Muscle rigidity	Abnormal, generalized slowing, triphasic waves
IV	Child is comatose but arousable by painful stimuli (IVa) or does not respond to stimuli (IVb)	Absent	Decerebrate or decorticate	Abnormal, very slow delta activity

Data from Rogers (1985)[100] and Devictor et al. (1995).[101]
EEG, electroencephalographic.

Cerebral blood flow adjusted for carbon dioxide levels (aCBF) correlates with cerebral swelling and mortality in patients with FHF. Patients with FHF may have hyperemia, normal flow, or decreased cerebral blood flow. Increased cerebral blood flow may be associated with cerebral swelling on CT, but CT changes occur late and are absent in the majority of patients with increased intracranial pressure (ICP) on epidural monitoring.[103]

A baseline electroencephalogram (EEG) is helpful to stage coma and provide information on prognosis. CT may provide information on cerebral edema or irreversible brain damage later in the disease. Frequent evaluation of neurologic function and blood ammonia is essential to follow the progress of hepatic encephalopathy. The role of ICP monitoring remains controversial as there are significant complications, including bleeding, in patients with severe coagulopathy, but it may provide information on changes in ICP and improve selection for liver transplantation.[104]

Other Therapy

The role of N-acetylcysteine (70 mg/kg 4-hourly) in the management of FHF other than acetaminophen poisoning is unproven, but anecdotal results suggest that it may have a role. A multicenter study, supported by the U.S. National Institutes of Health, of the role of N-acetylcysteine in the management of acute liver failure has just been completed and the results are awaited.

Antibiotic Therapy

The results of surveillance cultures can be used to guide antibiotic therapy in the event of suspected infection, but broad-spectrum antibiotics (amoxicillin, cefuroxime, metronidazole, and prophylactic fluconazole) are prescribed only if sepsis is suspected or liver transplantation is anticipated.[99]

Nutritional Support

The role of parenteral nutrition in the management of patients with acute liver failure is controversial. The main aims of therapy are to maintain blood glucose and ensure sufficient carbohydrate for energy metabolism, reduce protein intake to 1 to 2 g/kg daily and provide sufficient energy intake to reverse catabolism. Children who are mechanically ventilated should have parenteral nutrition, as it may be 7 to 10 days before full normal diet is resumed following transplantation.

Hepatic Support

Many different measures have been used to support the liver while awaiting regeneration or transplantation, including a variety of experimental drugs such as prostaglandin E, insulin, and glucagon, which have not been shown to be effective.

Methods to remove potential neuroactive toxins include double-volume exchange transfusion, plasmapheresis, charcoal hemoperfusion, liver assist devices containing chemical scrubbers[105] or cultured hepatocytes,[106] extracorporeal perfusion through human or animal livers,[107] and cross-circulation with animals. Although these therapeutic maneuvers may provide support during liver regeneration or while awaiting a donor, none has been shown to have any benefit with regard to survival.

Double-volume exchange transfusion (in children weighing less than 15 kg) and plasmapheresis in older children may produce a transient improvement in coagulopathy and neurologic state, but may contribute to hemodynamic instability.[108]

Artificial liver support, using either porcine hepatocytes or a hepatoma cell line, has shown some benefit in improving coagulopathy and reducing encephalopathy in adults, acting as a "bridge to transplantation," although long-term outcome and survival was not affected.[109] There is limited anecdotal experience in children.[110]

Molecular Adsorbent Recirculating System (MARS)

MARS is an alternative form of hemodialysis that uses a specific filter to remove toxic products, but not albumin. It has a role in the management of both acute liver failure and acute-on-chronic liver failure in adults.[111] Use of MARS in the management of children is anecdotal, but it may have a role to play in creating a "bridge to transplantation."

Hepatocyte Transplantation

Hepatocyte transplantation as therapy for acute liver failure using cell suspensions or synthetic constructs is at an early stage of research.[112]

SUMMARY

Much progress has been achieved in the etiology and management of acute and chronic liver failure that has been dependent on a multidisciplinary approach among basic scientists, physicians, and surgeons. Although the outcome for many children has improved dramatically, for many the chance of future life is related to the availability of liver transplantation.

REFERENCES

5. Consolo M, Amoroso A, Spandidos DA, et al. Matrix metalloproteinases and their inhibitors as markers of inflammation and fibrosis in chronic liver disease [Review]. Int J Mol Med 2009;24:143–152.
15. Davenport M, de Ville de Goyet J, Stringer MD, et al. Seamless management of biliary atresia in England and Wales (1999-2002). Lancet 2004;363:1354–1357.
28. Shah U, Kelly D, Chang MH, et al. Management of chronic hepatitis B in children. J Pediatr Gastroenterol Nutr 2009;48:399–404.
29. Mieli-Vergani G, Heller S, Jara P, et al. Autoimmune Hepatitis. JPGN 2009;49:158–164.
53. McDiarmid SV, Merion RM, Dykstra DM, et al. Selection of pediatric candidates under the PELD system. Liver Transplant 2004;10(10 Suppl. 2):S23–S30.
54. Cowley AD, Cummins C, Beath SV, et al. Paediatric Hepatology Dependency score (PHD score): an audit tool. J Pediatr Gastroenterol Nutr 2007;44:108–115.
67. Squires Jr RH. Acute liver failure in children. Semin Liver Dis 2008;28:153–166.

See expertconsult.com for a complete list of references and the review questions for this chapter.

LIVER TRANSPLANTATION IN CHILDREN

78

Bijan Eghtesad • Deirdre Kelly • John J. Fung

Orthotopic liver transplantation (LTX) has become an accepted means for the treatment of end-stage liver disease in both adults and children. The history of pediatric LTX starts with the first human attempt at transplantation by Dr. Starzl in 1963. The 3-year-old boy, who had biliary atresia, ultimately died of hemorrhage and coagulopathy.[1] The first successful LTX in 1967, in a 1-year-old patient with hepatoma, was followed by seven more transplants in children, with four of those patients surviving for more than 1 year.[2,3] Despite advances in surgical techniques, 1-year patient survival remained poor and around 30% throughout the1970s. The introduction of cyclosporine in 1980 resulted in marked improvements in graft and patient survival. Consequently, several centers in the United States and Europe started their experience in pediatric LTX in the early 1980s. At the first international symposium on pediatric liver transplantation, held in Brussels in 1986, larger transplant programs in the United States and Europe presented their experiences with 1-year patient survival rates ranging from 57 to 83%.[4,5]

Improvements in operative techniques, preoperative and postoperative management, organ preservation, donor management, and the availability of more potent and less toxic immunosuppressive drugs have contributed to better outcome in pediatric LTX in recent years. These improvements have led to 1-year survival rates of more than 90% and 5- and 10-year survival rates of 80%.[6-9] Paradoxically, improvements in survival have expanded the range of indications for LTX in children and led to a substantial increase in the number of children on the waiting list, resulting in a shortage of organs for this group of patients. The organ shortage, especially in the pediatric age group, has led to development of novel surgical techniques, such as reduced-size cadaveric allografts, cadaveric split-liver allografts, and more importantly adult-to-child live-donor allografts.[10-16] These innovations have dramatically decreased loss of pediatric patients on the waiting list, allowing these patients to be transplanted earlier in the course of their disease process with resultant better posttransplant survival.[17,18]

INDICATIONS FOR LIVER TRANSPLANTATION

The indications for liver transplantation in children are markedly different from those in their adult counterparts and are based on the diverse causes of liver disease in this group of patients (Tables 78-1 and 78-2). Primary liver diseases with progression to liver failure are the main indications for LTX in children with over 50% of the cases being done for biliary atresia.[19-22] Acute liver failure, metabolic disorders of the liver, hepatitis, inborn errors of metabolism, and certain hepatic tumors are other indications for transplantation.[23-33]

Indications for Liver Transplantation for Chronic Liver Failure

The presence of cirrhosis should not be considered an indication for liver transplantation, unless signs of hepatic failure are evident. Decompensated liver disease is characterized by clinical and laboratory findings of liver synthetic failure and the occurrence of complications such as malnutrition, ascites, peripheral edema, coagulopathy, gastrointestinal bleeding, and signs of portal hypertension and hepatic encephalopathy. Malnutrition with reduced lean tissue and fat stores and poor linear growth is an important sign of chronic liver disease in children. Spontaneous bruising, caused by reduced synthesis of clotting factors and thrombocytopenia due to hypersplenism, is a sign of advanced disease. There may also be changes in the systemic and pulmonary circulations, with arteriolar vasodilation, increased blood volume, hyperdynamic circulatory state, and cyanosis due to intrapulmonary shunting. Renal failure is a late but serious event. Laboratory investigations may reveal abnormalities in liver function tests and an increase in ammonia levels, but in particular there is abnormal liver synthetic function, reflected by such findings as hypoalbuminemia and prolonged prothrombin time. With the marked improvement in patient survival with resultant improvements in quality-of-life measures, the timing of liver transplantation with respect to other medical and surgical options is being constantly reassessed; however, effective alternative therapies should be attempted before referral for LTX.[34,35]

Timing of Liver Transplantation for Chronic Liver Failure

It may be difficult to plan the best time for LTX for children with chronic liver failure, as many children have compensated liver disease for years. The most useful guide to the timing of LTX is provided by a variety of parameters that include[36] (1) a persistent rise in total bilirubin concentration; (2) prolongation of prothrombin time and international normalized ratio (INR); and (3) a persistent fall in serum albumin concentration.

Serial evaluation of nutritional parameters is a useful guide to early hepatic decompensation.[37] Progressive reduction of fat (measured by triceps skinfold or subscapular skinfold) or protein stores (measured by midarm circumference or midarm muscle area) despite intensive nutritional support is a good guide to hepatic decompensation. The development of the PELD (Pediatric End-Stage Liver Disease) score has confirmed these observations. The PELD scoring system was developed based on the evaluation of data from the Studies of Pediatric

TABLE 78-1. Indications for Pediatric Liver Transplantation (Chronic Liver Disease)

Cholestatic Disease
Biliary atresia
Progressive familial intrahepatic cholestasis (Byler disease)
Idiopathic neonatal hepatitis
Alagille's syndrome (bile duct paucity syndrome)
Sclerosing cholangitis

Metabolic Liver Disease
Alpha1-antitrypsin deficiency
Wilson disease
Tyrosinemia type I
Cystic fibrosis
Glycogen storage disease types I, III, and IV
Cirrhosis secondary to prolonged total parenteral nutrition

Chronic Hepatitis
Autoimmune hepatitis
Chronic viral hepatitis (B and C)
Cryptogenic cirrhosis
Nonalcoholic steatohepatitis (NASH)

Miscellaneous
Budd-Chiari syndrome
Polycystic liver disease
Caroli's disease
Traumatic/postsurgical biliary tract diseases

Inborn Errors of Metabolism
Crigler-Najjar syndrome type I
Urea cycle defects
Primary hyperoxaluria
Organic acidemia
Familial hypercholesterolemia

Hepatic Tumors
Unresectable hepatoblastoma
Unresectable hepatocellular carcinoma
Unresectable large benign tumors (hemangioendothelioma)

TABLE 78-2. Causes of Acute Liver Failure in Children

Neonates	
Infectious	Herpesviruses, echovirus, adenovirus, HBV
Metabolic	Galactosemia,* tyrosinemia,* neonatal hemochromatosis,* mitochondrial disease
Older children	
Infectious	HAV, HBV, herpesviruses, sepsis,* other..
Drugs	Acetaminophen, valproate, isoniazid, carbamazepine, halothane, propylthiouracil....
Toxins	*Amanita phalloides*, carbon tetrachloride, phosphorus.
Metabolic	Wilson's disease, hereditary fructose intolerance
Autoimmune	Types 1 and 2
Other	Cryptogenic

*Disease does not fulfill definition of acute liver failure.
HAV, hepatitis A virus; HBV, hepatitis B virus.

management, should be referred for transplantation. In some children, hepatopulmonary syndrome secondary to pulmonary shunting develops and is an important indication for LTX.[43] It is essential that transplantation be performed before the development of severe pulmonary hypertension, as this might preclude successful LTX.[44,45] The patients with these complications are provided additional priority out of proportion to the degree of their biologic PELD score, recognizing that these complications are not factored into the PELD equation.

For children with chronic liver disease to benefit from transplantation, it is essential that this procedure be considered before the complications of liver disease adversely impair the quality of their life, and before their growth and development are irreversibly retarded (Chapter 77).

Liver Transplantation for Acute Liver Failure

Acute liver failure is rare, but associated with high mortality.[23,24,47] It is a heterogenous condition with many different etiologies (see Table 78-2).

The definition of acute liver failure is the development of hepatic necrosis with hepatic encephalopathy and coagulopathy within 8 weeks of the onset of liver disease, and the absence of preexisting liver disease in any form (the exception is Wilson's disease).[46] This definition is not useful in children, and especially the younger age group, because encephalopathy is difficult to detect or may not be a feature in infants. Second, acute liver failure may be the first manifestation of an unrecognized metabolic liver disease (e.g., Wilson's disease or tyrosinemia type 1). Third, most hepatic failure in neonates is secondary to an inborn error or an intrauterine insult, which are preexisting liver diseases.

The etiology of acute liver failure varies depending on the age of the child (see Table 78-2). In neonates, an inborn error of metabolism or severe infection is likely, whereas viral hepatitis, autoimmune liver disease, drug-induced liver failure, or Wilson's disease are common causes in older children.[23,24,48]

Prognosis of acute liver failure is worse in the younger ages. Severe coagulopathy, severe metabolic acidosis, cardiovascular instability, and renal failure are signs of a poor prognosis. Age less than 10 years, INR of more than 4, and cryptogenic nature of the disease carry a mortality of more than 80% without LTX.[49-53] In general, in addition to all the poor prognostic signs,

Liver Transplantation (SPLIT), a consortium of 29 U.S. and Canadian centers.[38-40] In the multivariate analysis, age, bilirubin, INR, growth failure, and albumin were significant factors for predicting outcome. This method has been in use for the past 7 years and is a useful tool for categorizing patients awaiting transplantation based on their disease severity and their waiting list mortality risk. The formula to determine the PELD score is:

PELD Score = 0.436 (Age (<1 year)) − 0.687 × log$_e$(albumin g/dL) + 0.480 × log$_e$(total bilirubin mg/dL) + 1.857 × Log$_e$ (INR) + 0.667 (Growth failure (<2 standard deviations present). Scores for patients listed for liver transplantation before the patient's first birthday continue to include the value assigned for age (<1 year until the patient reaches the age of 24 months) + 0.667 (if patient has growth failure of <−2 standard deviation).

In addition to these objective measures, another important consideration in the timing of LTX is psychosocial development. Children with chronic liver disease have both social and motor developmental delay that increases with time unless reversed after early LTX.[41,42]

Children with severe hepatic complications, such as chronic hepatic encephalopathy, refractory ascites, intractable pruritus, or recurrent variceal bleeding despite appropriate medical progression of encephalopathy to stage III in these patients is an indication for expedited LTX. One-year patient survival in this setting is inferior to that of LTX for chronic liver disease, being 75 to 80%.[24,54] The management of these patients, either supportive or as a bridge to LTX, is prevention of complications of acute liver failure. Treatment of coagulopathy, management of fluid and electrolyte balance, support of renal function, and prevention of infection, cerebral edema, and intracranial hypertension are the prime goals in management of these patients.[24,54]

Liver Transplantation for Hepatic Malignancies

Pediatric primary hepatic malignancies have an incidence of 1:1,000,000 and account for 0.5% to 2% of solid tumors in children.[55,56] The most common tumor is hepatoblastoma (HB) accounting for approximately 28% of all pediatric liver malignancies. Hepatocellular carcinoma (HCC) (18.9%) and infantile hemangioendotheliomas (16.5%) are other common malignant tumors of the liver in children.[55,56] Total excision with or without adjuvant chemotherapy is the treatment of choice for these tumors. However, in patients with unresectable and chemoresistant tumors, complete surgical excision in the form of total hepatectomy and LTX is a viable option.[57-59] The role of LTX in the treatment of hepatic malignancies in children is still to be evaluated. Post-LTX survival depends on the stage of the tumor and nature of the malignancy.[60-63]

GENERAL CONTRAINDICATIONS FOR LIVER TRANSPLANTATION IN CHILDREN

With increasing experience, there are fewer contraindications to LTX. Although historically considered difficult, in the era of reduced-size liver and living donor transplantation, candidate age below 1 year and weight of less than 10 kg are no longer considered contraindications for transplantation. Venous thrombosis and vascular abnormalities, such as absent inferior vena cava and hypovascular syndrome, are no longer considered contraindications. Although infection with human immunodeficiency virus (HIV) was previously a contraindication, the improvement in long-term prognosis and survival with antiretroviral agents has changed the pattern of the disease. In most situations, HIV can be controlled before and kept under control after transplantation.[64-67] There are few absolute contraindications to LTX, which include overwhelming sepsis due to bacterial, fungal, or viral infection outside the liver; severe cardiovascular disease; extrahepatic malignancies; and inherited diseases with multisystem involvement, such as mitochondrial disorders with advanced neurologic deficits. In some circumstances, a markedly dysfunctional psychosocial environment may require drastic interventions in order to render the child a candidate for LTX.

EVALUATION OF PEDIATRIC LIVER TRANSPLANT CANDIDATES

The pretransplant evaluation of the patient should include the following:
1. Confirmation of the diagnosis and assessment of the severity of the liver disease and the possibility of medical management
2. Consideration of any contraindications for transplantation
3. Psychologic preparation of the family and child

The severity of liver disease should be assessed by evaluating the following.

Hepatic Function

Listing for liver transplantation is based on evidence of deterioration in hepatic function as indicated by serum albumin concentration (less than 3.5 g/dL), coagulation time (INR more than 1.4), and cholestasis as evidenced by a rise in bilirubin concentration (more than 8 mg/dL). In children with chronic liver failure, the presence of portal hypertension should be determined by estimating the size of spleen and portal vein by ultrasonography, by determining low white blood cell count and platelet count as a result of hypersplenism, and by diagnosing esophageal and/or gastric varices by gastrointestinal endoscopy.

Renal Function

Children with acute or chronic liver failure have abnormalities of renal function in the form of primary renal disease or hepatorenal syndrome. Assessment of renal function is important to provide a baseline for the nephrotoxic effect of immunosuppressive drugs following transplantation and to consider the necessity for perioperative renal support, placement on renal-sparing immunosuppressive protocols, or in case of chronic renal insufficiency, listing for combined liver and kidney transplantation. In addition, children with fulminant liver failure may develop oliguria or anuria as a result of hepatorenal syndrome and may need renal replacement therapy.[68]

Hematology and Coagulation Profile

Baseline information on full blood count, platelets, and coagulation is obtained. Determination of blood group is essential for organ donor matching.

Serology

Previous evidence of varicella, measles, or infection with hepatitis A, B, or C viruses, cytomegalovirus (CMV), or Epstein-Barr virus (EBV) is important information for postoperative management and placement on prophylactic protocols.

Radiology

Successful liver transplantation requires thorough preoperative knowledge of hepatic vasculature, anatomy, patency, and possibly size. This is critical for surgical planning of revascularization of the new liver. Doppler sonography is performed routinely as surveillance preoperatively and provides information regarding the size and patency of the portal vein (PV), hepatic veins, inferior vena cava (IVC), and hepatic artery. Children with biliary atresia have an increased incidence of abnormal vasculature including the hypovascular syndrome, which consists of an absent IVC, preduodenal or absent PV, and hepatic outflow abnormalities.[69] Polysplenia in association with situs inversus and dextrocardia are other potential findings in these patients. Because these abnormalities may increase the technical risk associated with LTX, it is important to diagnose them before the procedure.[70] However, none of these are contraindications to LTX.

Cardiac and Respiratory Assessment

Liver transplantation is associated with significant hemodynamic changes during the operative and anhepatic phases, and information on both cardiac and respiratory function is needed. Electrocardiography, echocardiography, and oxygen saturation provide most of the necessary information for management of these hemodynamic changes. Children with biliary atresia have an increased incidence of congenital cardiac disease, particularly atrial and ventricular septal defects, whereas peripheral pulmonary stenosis is a known feature of Alagille's syndrome. Cardiomyopathy may develop secondary to tyrosinemia type I and organic acidemia, and children with malignant tumors who have received chemotherapy need particular cardiac assessment. Cardiac catheterization is required in some cases to determine whether cardiac function is adequate to sustain the hemodynamic effect of LTX, or whether cardiac surgery or other interventions may be required before transplantation. In some cases with large atrial septal defects, paradoxical cerebral vascular accident may occur, if a venous embolism should traverse the defect and embolize to the brain. If the cardiac defect is uncorrectable, LTX occasionally may be contraindicated.

The development of intrapulmonary shunts (hepatopulmonary syndrome) is detected by measuring serial arterial blood gases while breathing room air and 100% oxygen, or ^{99m}Tc-macroaggregated albumin scan and contrast echocardiography.[71,72]

Neurodevelopmental Assessment

Because the aim of LTX is to improve quality of life by restoring normal liver function, it is important to identify any preexisting neurologic or psychologic defects, not only to consider whether they would be reversible following transplantation, but also to evaluate the need for corrective management. This is particularly important in children with metabolic disorders such as urea cycle deficiencies, Wilson's disease, or acute liver failure, because irreversible advanced brain damage may be a contraindication for transplantation.[29,48]

Dental Assessment

Advanced liver disease has an adverse affect on all aspects of growth and development, including dentition. Pretransplant dental problems include hypoplasia with staining of the teeth and gingival hyperplasia. Because gingival hyperplasia is a significant side effect of cyclosporine, it is important to establish a good dental hygiene in the patient before transplantation.[73-75]

PREPARATION FOR LIVER TRANSPLANTATION

Immunization

Because it is generally a contradiction to use live attenuated vaccines after LTX, it is best to complete normal immunizations before transplantation. This includes diphtheria, tetanus, polio, and pneumococcal polysaccharide vaccine (Pneumovax) for protection from streptococcal pneumonia, and *Haemophilus influenzae* type b (HIB) vaccine for protection against *Haemophilus influenzae*. In children older than 6 months, measles, mumps, rubella, and varicella vaccinations should be offered in addition to hepatitis A and B vaccination. It should be noted that live vaccines and vaccination for measles, mumps, and rubella should not be given within 6 to 8 weeks of transplantation. Children with functional asplenia or multiple spleens should have Pneumovax and receive penicillin prophylaxis.

Management of Hepatic Complications

It is important to ensure that specific hepatic complications, related to either acute or chronic liver failure, are appropriately managed while the patient waits for transplantation. Sepsis, including ascending cholangitis, spontaneous bacterial peritonitis, and pneumonia, should be treated with broad-spectrum antibiotics. In children awaiting transplantation for acute liver failure, prophylactic antifungal therapy is essential.

Nutritional Support

The main purpose of nutritional therapy is to prevent or reverse catabolism and the malnutrition associated with either acute or chronic liver disease. High-calorie feeds (150 to 200% estimated average requirement) with adequate fat-soluble vitamin supplementation and appropriate protein content may be effective. It is possible to provide this high energy intake with standard feeds using caloric supplements, but a modular feed that can be adapted may be better for infants. Feeds are best given by nocturnal nasogastric enteral feeding or continuous enteral feeding. Occasionally, enteral feeding is not tolerated because of severe hepatic complications such as ascites and intractable variceal bleeding; in these circumstances, parenteral nutrition is necessary.[76]

Psychologic Preparation

Liver transplantation is a major undertaking for the child and family. Psychologic counseling, relaying information, and preparation of the child and family are crucial, using a skilled multidisciplinary team with play therapists, psychologists, and school teachers. Parents of children who develop acute liver failure maybe too stressed to appreciate fully the implications and consequences of LTX. In these families, counseling – in particular, counseling of the child – should continue after surgery.

Medical Management Challenges During the Waiting Period for Transplantation

With an increase in the number of patients listed for transplantation and as a result of organ shortage and a longer waiting period, the transplant candidates should be under close observation and follow-up. Aggressive medical management is required for the major complications caused by worsening liver failure. These could present as variceal bleeding, ascites, spontaneous bacterial peritonitis, encephalopathy, hepatorenal syndrome, severe electrolyte disturbances, or hepatopulmonary manifestations of liver failure (Chapter 77).

ORGAN ALLOCATION

Organ donation and recovery are handled regionally or nationally, depending on geographic variations, but most countries have a national network: United Network for Organ Sharing (UNOS) in the United States, United Kingdom Transplant Support Service Authority (UKTSSA) in the UK, and Eurotransplant in parts of Europe. Once patients have been evaluated and accepted by the transplant team, they are listed and prioritized according to the severity of liver disease. It is important to recognize that the priority system gives patients with acute liver failure the greatest priority. For staging children with chronic liver disease, no reliable set of criteria is available. The current method of allocation is based on a numeric system to calculate mortality risk in children with end-stage liver disease.[37,39] The PELD score system was developed to prioritize patients for LTX on the waiting list and is based on their mortality risk.[38]

The PELD scoring system cannot provide a numerical score for complications that increase the mortality risk in children with liver failure, such as gastrointestinal bleeding and refractory medical conditions such as ascites and encephalopathy. Patients who develop such complications may be prioritized on the waiting list by assessment of arbitrary PELD points or consideration of regional review boards.

In the United States, priority is given to critically ill children. Status 1 refers to patients in five allowable diagnostic groups: (i) fulminant liver failure; (ii) primary nonfunction; (iii) hepatic artery thrombosis; (iv) acute decompensated Wilson's disease; and (v) chronic liver disease, all defined as follows[77]:

(i)   Fulminant liver failure is defined as the onset of hepatic encephalopathy within 8 weeks of the first symptoms of liver disease. The absence of preexisting liver disease is critical to the diagnosis. One of three criteria below must be met to list a pediatric candidate with fulminant liver failure: (1) ventilator dependence, (2) dialysis requirement, or (3) INR above 2.0.

(ii) The diagnosis of primary nonfunction of a transplanted liver must be made within 7 days of implantation and include two of the following: ALT greater than or equal to 2000 IU/L, INR greater than or equal to 2.5, total bilirubin greater than or equal to 10 mg/dL, or acidosis, defined as having an arterial pH less than or equal to 7.30 or venous pH of 7.25 and/or lactate greater than or equal to 4 mmol/L.

(iii) The diagnosis of hepatic artery thrombosis must be made in a transplanted liver within 14 days of implantation.

(iv) Acute decompensated Wilson's disease.

(v)   Pediatric candidates with chronic liver disease and in the ICU can be listed at urgent if the candidate has a calculated PELD score above 25 or calculated MELD score above 25 for adolescent candidates (12 to 17 years) and one of the following criteria is met: (a) On a mechanical ventilator; or (b) gastrointestinal bleeding; or (c) renal failure or renal insufficiency defined as requiring dialysis; or (d) Glasgow coma score less than 10.

For patients with inherited metabolic diseases, arbitrary PELD assignment is given as follows: (a) candidates with a urea cycle disorder or organic acidemia are assigned a PELD (less than 12 years old) or MELD (12 to 17 years old) score of 30; (b) candidates with primary hyperoxaluria with alanine-glyoxylate aminotransferase (AGT) deficiency proven by liver biopsy (sample analysis and/or genetic analysis) and listed for a combined liver-kidney transplant are assigned an initial MELD score of 28/PELD score of 41. For patients with nonquantifiable chronic liver disease complications, PELD assignment for the more common complications are listed next: (a) candidates with a clinical evidence of portal hypertension, evidence of a shunt, and a PaO_2 less than 60 mm Hg on room air will be listed at a MELD score of 22, and (b) candidates with portopulmonary hypertension who have a response to treatment with a mean pulmonary artery pressure less than 35 mm Hg and pulmonary vascular resistance less than 400 dyn/s/cm⁻⁵ are eligible for a MELD/PELD exception score of 22 points.

For pediatric recipients with malignancies, consideration for PELD/MELD assignment is given as follows: (a) a pediatric candidate with nonmetastatic hepatoblastoma who is otherwise a suitable candidate for liver transplantation may be assigned a PELD (less than 12 years old) or MELD (12 to 17 years old) score of 30. If the candidate does not receive a transplant within 30 days of being listed with a MELD/PELD of 30, then the candidate may be listed as critically urgent.

LIVER TRANSPLANTATION SURGERY

Management during the transplant operation has been improved by increased knowledge of and experience with the anesthesia requirements in pediatric LTX, by better understanding of coagulation disorders, by improved monitoring, and by sophisticated hemostatic techniques that have reduced transfusion requirements and allowed for better hemodynamic stability. Constant monitoring of cardiopulmonary function, electrolytes, and blood gases, along with thromboelastography (to assess coagulation), is essential and allows adequate fluid and electrolyte resuscitation and supplementation of coagulation products and platelets.[78-80]

Surgical Technique

The recipient operation is a *tour de force* of general surgery, with the hepatectomy often being the most difficult step. Although the hepatectomy technique has been standardized to a large extent, no two transplants are exactly the same. This may be much harder in children who have undergone previous abdominal surgeries for a variety of indications such as for biliary atresia. This is true not only in LTX with full liver but with reduced-size, split, or living-donor livers as well. Full attention must be paid to do a meticulous dissection to prevent major blood loss in a small recipient and to preserve and protect all the liver vasculature and bile duct to be used at the time of implantation of the new liver. In children, especially smaller ones and infants, use of smaller grafts, left lateral segment from a living donor, or cadaveric split or reduced size liver is needed. Therefore, the continuity of the native IVC must be preserved.[18,81-83]

The principles of implantation, regardless of the type of organ used (full-size, reduced-size, split, or segmental living donor), is reconnection of the inflow vasculature, that is, the portal vein and hepatic artery, and establishment of outflow of the new liver, via the hepatic vein(s) and IVC, to the recipient's IVC.[81,84-88] These procedures have been done using variations of these principles, including the use of interposed vascular conduits. At the conclusion of the operation, biliary drainage is in the form of duct-to-duct anastomosis between the donor and recipient bile ducts (choledochocholedochostomy), or Roux en-Y hepaticojejunostomy between the donor bile duct and the recipient jejunum when the native bile duct is unsatisfactory for drainage (Figure 78-1). The decision to use a biliary stent is often program or surgeon specific, with pros and cons to their use.

Generally, organ size is the most important issue in LTX in children. The majority of children awaiting LTX are younger than 2 years of age. In contrast, most of the organ donors are older and, consequently, most pediatric livers are too large for

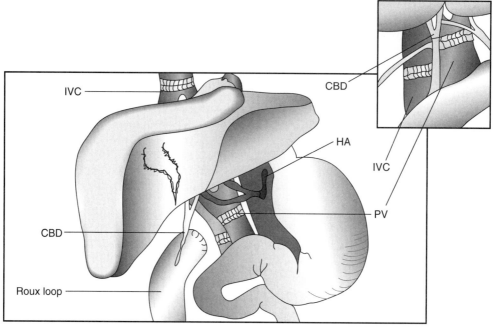

Figure 78-1. Standard implantation of the liver with vascular anastomoses and biliary reconstruction as hepaticojejunostomy (large box) or duct-to-duct (small box). CBD, common bile duct; HA, hepatic artery; IVC, inferior vena cava; PV, portal vein.

the typical pediatric recipients, resulting in an excessively long waiting time and correlating with increased mortality on the waiting list among these children. The development of technical variations of donor liver sizing options has been critical in providing timelier LTX to pediatric candidates on the waiting list.

Reduced-Size, Split, and Living-Donor Liver Transplantation

The growth of the pediatric waiting list and increased pretransplant patient losses prompted the transplant programs to develop innovative techniques to increase the number of organs and especially the number of organs for pediatric patients. The concept of the reduced-size liver transplantation technique was first described in France by Bismuth.[10] In this operation the donor liver, based on its segmental anatomy, is reduced in size to fit the recipient hepatic fossa, with great care to preserve the vascular and biliary system of the remnant to be used at the time of implantation. This procedure increased the number of grafts available to the pediatric population but did not increase the total number of grafts available to potential recipients.[11,89] Advances in this technique subsequently prompted the transplant surgeons to divide the cadaveric liver into two pieces (left lateral segment and remnant right tri-segment) with complete preservation of the vascular inflow and outflow and biliary system to each piece, for use in a pediatric and adult recipients, respectively.[12,13,90] These technical advances then ushered in the era of successful living donor liver transplantation.

The first report of the use of a left lateral segment was by Raia et al. in Brazil, in 1989.[14] Subsequently, Strong et al. in Australia reported the first successful use of left lateral segment in a pediatric LTX[15] (Figure 78-2). This was followed by the first case series of 20 living related LTX reported by Broelsch at the University of Chicago.[16] The success of living donor transplant

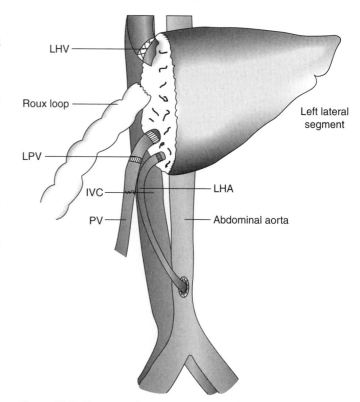

Figure 78-2. Liver transplantation using the left lateral segment (living donor or split). HA, hepatic artery; IVC, inferior vena cava; LHV, left hepatic vein; LPV, left portal vein; PV, portal vein.

rapidly expanded to the rest of the world. Indications for living donor liver transplantation are the same as those for cadaveric whole organ or split/reduced-size LTX. Its application varies dramatically around the world because of cultural, religious, and social differences. The procedure has become very common and the main source for liver transplantation in many Asian countries, whereas in Europe and the United States it accounts for less than 10% of all the liver transplants performed.[16,17,92-94]

The use of the left lateral segment is generally adaptable to most pediatric LTX recipients in the 10- to 25-kg weight range. Their use in small infants less than 5 kg may require further reduction to monosegments in order to allow for proper closure of the abdominal cavity.

POSTTRANSPLANT MANAGEMENT AND COMPLICATIONS

Immunosuppression

Primary baseline immunosuppression has varied over time according to the availability of newer drugs and ongoing protocols. The calcineurin inhibitors (CNIs) cyclosporine (CyA) and tacrolimus (Tac) are considered the backbone of immunosuppression in transplant recipients. Both drugs cause selective suppression of T cell–mediated responses by inhibition of the calcineurin mediated calcium dependent pathway of T cell activation with resultant inhibition of production of interleukin-2.

Pediatric patients eliminate CNI faster than adults and require larger doses, up to 50% to 100% more than adult doses on a per-kilogram basis. The initial dose of CyA ranges from 5 to 10 mg/kg/day divided in two doses with a goal to achieve a trough level between 250 and 350 ng/mL during the first month, 150 to 250 ng/mL during the first 6 months, and 100 to 200 ng/mL for the remainder of the first year, with a further drop after the first year based on patient condition and presence or absence of signs of toxicity or overimmunosuppression. Common CyA side effects are hypertension, renal dysfunction, hirsutism, gingival hypertrophy, hyperkalemia and hypomagnesemia, and dyslipidemia.[95-97]

Tac is another CNI, which is 100 times more potent than CyA on a weight-to-weight basis with a similar mechanism of action. The initial dosage of Tac is 0.1 to 0.15 mg/kg/day divided in two doses with the initial goal for blood levels of 10 to 15 ng/mL for the first month and gradual decrease in dosage to achieve a level between 6 and 10 ng/mL by 6 months after LTX. Compared to CyA, Tac is associated with more posttransplant new-onset diabetes but a lower incidence of dyslipidemia. Both drugs can cause renal dysfunction, hyperkalemia, hypomagnesemia, and a variety of neurologic manifestations. Because of the high potency of Tac, it can be used to reverse rejection and allow discontinuation of steroids shortly after LTX.[98-101] It should be kept in mind that both CyA and Tac are metabolized by the cytochrome p450-3A system, and drug interactions are common. Careful dose adjustment of CNIs is needed in this situation to prevent toxicity due to high levels or rejection secondary to low levels of the drugs with concomitantly administered drugs that interact with cytochrome p450.[102]

Corticosteroids have been the mainstay of immunosuppression from the early days of transplantation. Side effects are numerous and include hypertension, diabetes, osteoporosis, and dyslipidemia. The initial dosage is often in the range of 10 to 20 mg/kg of methylprednisolone as a single dose with gradual tapering of the daily dose. Because of the side effects, steroid-sparing protocols are becoming popular in transplant programs.[103-105]

Azathioprine (AZ) and mycophenolate mofetil (MMF) are both anti-metabolites and have been used in LTX. AZ was one of the first immunosuppressive agents used in transplantation. Currently it is rarely used in the United States because of its side effects which include severe myelosuppression and hepatotoxicity. MMF and mycophenolic acid (MPA), are the newer generation of antimetabolites. They inhibit *de novo* purine nucleotide synthesis and, as a result, block DNA replication and T and B lymphocyte proliferation. This action contributes to their side effects including anemia, leukopenia, and thrombocytopenia. Their other major side effect is gastric upset with nausea, vomiting, and diarrhea, which is generally dose dependent. These agents are used as an adjunct with CNI to increase immunosuppressive potency, thus allowing reduction of CNI dosing to reduce side effects.[106-108]

Sirolimus is structurally related to Tac, yet despite binding to the same family of intracellular binding proteins, it has a completely different mode of action. It blocks T-cell proliferation induced by IL-2. It has less renal toxicity than CNI; however, it has other side effects of its own, including leukopenia, thrombocytopenia, increased serum lipid profiles, anemia, pneumonitis, and defective wound healing.[109-111] The preliminary reports from multicenter trials of the use of sirolimus in liver transplantation showed higher rates of hepatic artery and portal vein thrombosis, which generated a black box warning for use as primary immunosuppression in liver transplantation. The drug interaction profile is similar to those of other CNIs.[106]

A variety of antibody induction protocols have been adopted by the transplant programs as a means of delaying the introduction of CNI, referred to as renal sparing protocols,[112-113] or avoidance of corticosteroids to reduce their long-term side effects in the posttransplant period.[103-106] Anti-thymocyte globulins and IL-2 receptor antibodies are the more common drugs used in these protocols.[105,106]

Tailoring immunosuppressive therapy in the transplant patient is an important concept. Today, with the availability of a variety of antirejection drugs, we are able to tailor for our patients a variety of different protocols that best fit their need, and to avoid specific complications after LTX. In many cases, pediatric recipients gradually self-wean their doses of CNI; as they grow, many practitioners do not increase their CNI doses accordingly.

Rejection

Acute cellular rejection is diagnosed in these patients based on clinical and biochemical evidence and confirmed by histologic examination of a liver biopsy. It may occur after the first week following the LTX and anytime afterward. The incidence is less than 20% in younger children but can be seen in up to 50% of older children and adults.[114,115] Rejection may present with fever, irritability, abdominal discomfort, and ascites, and in some cases patients may be completely asymptomatic. Elevation of bilirubin, alkaline phosphatase, and transaminases is diagnostic, but confirmation is based on liver biopsy demonstrating histologic evidence of rejection. All the clinical symptoms and abnormal blood tests suggestive of rejection can happen in conditions such as ischemic damage to the liver, in cases of hepatic artery thrombosis, or in patients with biliary disorders. Histologic changes suggestive of rejection are variable, too. Rejection can present with necrosis in the pericentral vein (zone III) and lymphocytic infiltration in the central vein as central venulitis, or lymphocytic infiltration in the portal zone either in bile ducts or portal vein as portal venulitis

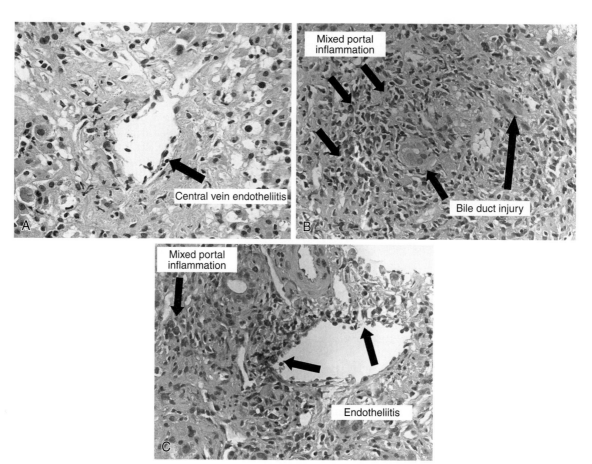

Figure 78-3. Histologic changes in acute liver allograft rejection. (**A**) Central venulitis, (**B**) interstitial infiltrate in the portal region with bile duct damage, (**C**) portal venulitis.

(Figure 78-3A,B,C). Involvement of vascular system is usually suggestive of more severe rejection.[25]

Treatment of acute cellular rejection in most transplant centers start with one to three boluses of 10 to 20 mg/kg/dose of methylprednisolone followed by a tapering cycle of steroids. In addition to steroid therapy, changes are made in the baseline immunosuppressive regimen. In cases of mild rejection, higher doses of Tac might be effective without the need for steroid therapy. Higher doses of Tac or CyA to achieve higher blood levels, and addition of a third agent, usually MMF, is the usual treatment protocol after the initial treatment. In cases of steroid-resistant rejection, use of antilymphocyte agents, such as anti-thymocyte globulin or monoclonal antibodies against lymphocytes, is indicated, but increases the risk for infectious complications.

Chronic rejection occurs in less than 10% of children after LTX. Since the introduction of Tac, the rate of chronic rejection has decreased. Clinical features include gradual onset of jaundice, pruritus, and at some point pale stools. The diagnosis is made by biochemical changes, that is, increases in bilirubin, alkaline phosphatase, and γ-glutamyl transpeptidase. Liver histology demonstrates extensive damage and loss to bile ducts (vanishing duct syndrome with arterial obliteration and fibrosis). Conversion from CyA to Tac and the addition of agents such as MMF may reverse the process if done early in the process (bilirubin less than 10 to 15 mg/dL). Lack of response to treatment requires retransplantation. Unlike kidney transplantation, because of the specific nature of the liver and excellent histologic recovery after an episode of rejection, chronic rejection is not a consequence of repeated episodes of acute rejection. Poor medication absorption due to increased gastrointestinal motility, such as diarrhea, and medication noncompliance are possible reasons for acute and chronic rejection.

Early Complications

Complications after LTX have a significant impact on outcome and the cost of the procedure. The postoperative course in these children ranges from straightforward to extremely complicated, and the outcome depends on the status of the recipient, the donor organ, and technical issues in the operation. Timely diagnosis of alterations in the normal postoperative course is the critical factor to minimize morbidity and mortality and to have better outcome.

Primary Nonfunction

Primary nonfunction (PNF) is characterized by encephalopathy, coagulopathy, minimal bile output, and progressive renal and multisystem failure with increasing serum lactate level and rapidly rising liver enzymes and histologic evidence of hepatocyte necrosis in the absence of any vascular complication. This can happen with whole organ, split-liver cadaveric grafts (4 to 10%), and less commonly in living-donor grafts (1-2%).[116-118]

Hepatic Artery Thrombosis/Stenosis

Angiographic evidence of greater that 50% reduction in the caliber of the lumen of the hepatic artery is defined as hepatic artery stenosis. This occurs in about 5% of the cases after LTX. Clinically these patients may show an increase in liver function tests or may be asymptomatic. Sonographically the presence of a low resistive index of less than 0.5 with increase in focal peak velocity is suggestive of vascular pathology. Hepatic artery stenosis can be revised by surgical intervention, especially early on after LTX. Percutaneous angioplasty is generally reserved for stenosis occurring several weeks after the transplant procedure with success rates over 90%.[119-121]

Complete thrombosis of the hepatic artery (HAT) is often secondary to technical issues, such as injury to the artery due to excessive handling of the artery in the donor or recipient. When this occurs suddenly, the presentation can be dramatic with acute, massive necrosis with markedly elevated transaminases, formation of central biloma secondary to intrahepatic duct necrosis, multiple biliary strictures, and/or intermittent bacteremia.[122-127] Occasionally, rarely in adults but more often in children, HAT can be asymptomatic. In this case the liver usually derives its arterial supply from the surrounding structures and through collateral circulation. According to the report by SPLIT (Studies of Pediatric Liver Transplantation), looking at the impact of graft type on outcome of pediatric LTX in more 2000 patients, HAT occurred in about 8% of the recipients of the whole liver, and in between 6 and 8% of recipients of reduced liver, split liver, and living-donor livers.[128] Angiography is the gold standard in diagnosis; with early identification of the problem, urgent revascularization may result in arterial patency.[124] However, a significant number of these patients may require retransplantation because of early graft failure or late biliary complications and sepsis.

Portal Vein Thrombosis

Portal vein thrombosis is an uncommon but significant complication after LTX in children. It can manifest as rapid graft dysfunction with resultant production of massive ascites. Ultrasonography or computed tomographic (CT) scan is usually diagnostic. Portal vein thrombosis can occur as a result of technical errors such as kinking or redundancy of the vein, poor mesenteric flow, or major anastomotic stricture. Treatment requires immediate surgical revascularization of the graft by thrombectomy and correction of the technical problem. Retransplantation maybe the only therapeutic option should revascularization fail. Portal vein thrombosis, based on the SPLIT data, is more common in live-donor, split, or reduced-size liver transplantation (8%), compared to whole liver transplantation (3.6%).[128-130] On occasion, the use of transhepatic portal vein stents may address the stenosis and restore portal vein patency.

Hepatic Outflow Obstruction

Hepatic outflow obstruction secondary to IVC anastomotic stenosis or hepatic vein anastomotic strictures in whole organ or segmental liver transplant is reported in between 2.5 and 4.5% of cases.[128] Depending on the site of narrowing and obstruction, this can present with liver dysfunction, ascites and lower extremity edema, and renal dysfunction. Diagnosis can be made by cavogram and measurements of the venous pressure gradients proximal and distal to the cava anastomosis or hepatic vein

anastomosis in segmental grafts.[130-133] Treatment is generally done by interventional radiology because these strictures are difficult to access once the liver is revascularized.

Biliary Complications

Biliary complications continue to be a major problem after LTX with an overall incidence of about 15 to 20%.[134-137] These complications range from early anastomotic leaks to late biliary stricture and obstruction, in either the intrahepatic or extrahepatic biliary system. SPLIT data show biliary complication rates of 15 to 19% in the recipients of segmental grafts, with the most common complication as leaks (15%), followed by anastomotic stricture (2 to 4%).[128] Anastomotic strictures are the result of either imperfect anastomotic technique or ischemia of the bile duct. Use of imaging modalities such as cholangiography, either transhepatic or endoscopic, to evaluate for the presence of strictures, obstruction or leak; ultrasonography, for detection of biliary dilatation; and radioisotope studies to evaluate anastomotic or cut surface leak are helpful in making an accurate diagnosis.[138-140] In cases of anastomotic stricture or obstruction, endoscopic or percutaneous balloon dilatation of the bile duct stricture and stenting has been successful. In cases with no response, revision of the choledochojejunostomy or conversion of a duct-to-duct anastomosis to choledochojejunostomy with a Roux-en-Y loop is the treatment of choice.[81]

Long-Term Complications of Immunosuppression

Infection

Many medical and technical conditions can predispose the LTX patient to infectious complications. These factors can be present before the transplant procedure, as a result of problems happening during the operation, shortly after, or in the long-term posttransplantation period. Pre-LTX infections can be secondary to the primary liver disease such as cases of cholangitis or spontaneous bacterial peritonitis. Intraoperative factors, such as spillage of bowel content, or leakage of abscesses in the liver or biliary system, prolonged operative time, and need for extensive blood transfusion at the time of surgery can predispose the patient to develop infection.[141-143] Technical problems and surgical complications, such as primary nonfunction or HAT leading to massive necrosis of the liver, exacerbated by immunosuppression and the presence of risk factors such as indwelling catheters or central intravenous lines, all predispose the patient to bacterial or fungal infections.[144-148]

The pattern of infections that develop after LTX is dependent on the susceptibility of the recipient and timing after transplantation. Depending on the type of infection, this can be divided into three intervals: early (up to 30 days), intermediate (up to 6 months), and late infection (more than 6 months). In general, early infections are caused by bacteria or yeast. They are usually due to reactivation of a pretransplant infection or secondary to complications of the transplant procedure. The majority of bacterial and fungal infections occur within the first 180 days after transplantation.

The most important infection in the intermediate period is CMV infection, in the form of either reactivation or primary disease as a result of transmission of the virus from a seropositive donor to a seronegative recipient. CMV infection is associated with increased risk of morbidity and mortality.[149,150] The use of CMV prophylaxis has been effective for prevention of the disease. CMV can present as simple viremia or tissue invasive disease involving gastrointestinal track, liver, or lungs. The diagnosis of CMV disease may be confirmed by CMV/DNA polymerase chain reaction (PCR), pp65 antigenemia assay, viral cultures from urine or bronchoalveolar lavage, or tissue obtained at the time of endoscopy, colonoscopy, or liver biopsy. Antiviral agents with activity against CMV have improved survival of these patients.[151]

Another infection with significant morbidity and mortality is infection due to EBV. As many as 80% of pediatric patients who are seronegative before LTX will develop a primary infection. However, only 30% of the patients will present with clinical symptoms.[150,152] The spectrum of clinical presentation of EBV infection includes nonspecific viral symptoms, mononucleosis, and posttransplant lymphoproliferative disorders (PTLDs). Measurement of EBV by PCR in blood can show the level of the virus and may aid in identifying patients who need further investigation to look for PTLD. Treatment with antivirals and lowering the immunosuppression is the first step in EBV management.

Other viral infections such as herpes virus, adenovirus, and community-acquired viruses can affect pediatric patients after LTX and are diagnosed based on clinical signs and symptoms and appropriate tests.[150] Opportunistic infections such as *Pneumocystis jirovecii*, tuberculosis, cryptococcosis, coccidiomycosis, and histoplasmosis, though uncommon, have been reported in posttransplant pediatric population.

Posttransplant Lymphoproliferative Disorders

The development of primary infection with EBV is a significant problem in pediatric transplantation.[152,153] As many as 80% of children who are EBV-seronegative before LTX will develop a primary EBV infection following this procedure; however, clinical disease develops in less than one third of these children.[152,154] There is a well-known association between primary EBV infection and subsequent development of PTLD. Historically, the prevalence of EBV infection in PTLD has been reported to be as high as 90 to 95%.[153,155] In a report from the University of Pittsburgh on 4000 liver transplants, which included 808 pediatric patients, 170 cases of PTLD were diagnosed. Of these, 78 (46%) were children.[156] The Canadian multicenter experience also reported that 42% of the cases of PTLD in 4280 liver transplants occurred in patients less than 18 years of age. Interestingly, only 15% of the total cohort was pediatric patients.[157] In another report from the Cincinnati Transplant Tumor Registry, PTLD comprised 52% of all the posttransplant tumors occurring in children, compared to only 15% in adults.[158] The clinical features are varied and include symptoms of infection, mononucleosis (tonsillitis, lymphadenopathy), isolated lymph node involvement, and EBV infiltration of the liver, gut, or brain, ranging from isolated organ involvement to systemic disease and malignant lymphoma.[159]

The diagnosis of EBV-associated PTLD is made on the basis of clinical, laboratory, and histopathologic examination. Patients with unexplained fever, exudative tonsillitis, and organomegaly, lymphadenopathy, and atypical lymphocytosis should be worked up for this possibility. Patients with gastrointestinal symptoms such as diarrhea, weight loss, fever, and malnutrition should also be evaluated for this possibility.[160-161] The measurement of EBV by PCR as an indicator

of viral load has gained wide acceptance. High levels of viral load, though sensitive for presence of the virus, lack specificity as it is elevated in asymptomatic patients as well. In cases of PTLD, in addition to histologic evaluation of the diseased organ, full radiologic evaluation of the patient by computed tomography of head and brain, chest, abdomen and pelvis is necessary. Endoscopic evaluation in patients with diarrhea is recommended.

Management of patients with PTLD is controversial. First line of management is reduction of immunosuppression. The role of antiviral agents in PTLD is not clear, and there have not been any formal studies in this regard.[162] Sixty-five percent of patients show complete response to reduction of immunosuppression and antivirals.[155,160-161] Two thirds of patients who fail to respond to withdrawal of immunosuppression will respond to a 4-week course of the anti-CD20 monoclonal agent rituximab.[163] Relapse rates of 20 to 25% have been reported in patients after complete initial response. Chemotherapy for patients with no response to initial treatment has been proposed.[164] Surgical intervention in the form of debulking or resection of the involved part of intestine is recommended.

Renal Dysfunction

Renal dysfunction, either acute or chronic, is a common sequela of LTX and is multifactorial. In most cases, this is a side effect of the CNIs administered postoperatively.[165-167] Long-term follow-up data in adult liver transplant recipients indicate that the incidence of progressive renal dysfunction increases over time, and by 10 years after LTX about 10% have developed end-stage renal disease. Data in children, though short-term, have shown that the glomerular filtration rate (GFR) falls abruptly within a month after LTX and remains suppressed during the first posttransplant year.[168-170] In one study on 117 pediatric patients who survived more than 3 years after LTX, 32% showed renal dysfunction. In this study, the risk factors identified for renal dysfunction were measured GFR at 1 year after transplant less than 70 mL/min/1.7m^2, cyclosporine immunosuppression, and length of time since transplant.[168] In another study of 12 pediatric patients after LTX on cyclosporine, calculated GFR at 2 years decreased significantly and by 10 years, 6 of 12 patients had chronic renal failure.[171] Interestingly, most of the studies show that renal function at the time of LTX is not a reliable predictor of subsequent renal function, whereas serum creatinine and measured GFR at 1 year posttransplant maybe a better predictor.[168,169] It is important to keep in mind that children may live long enough after LTX that they are at higher risk to progress from asymptomatic renal dysfunction to advanced end-stage renal disease.

Many transplant programs have adopted protocols to prevent or minimize CNI toxicities by three main CNI-sparing strategies: CNI reduction, CNI withdrawal, and complete avoidance of CNI. These strategies have been made possible by supplementation of non-CNI drugs, MMF, or sirolimus and use of antilymphocyte preparations.[172]

GROWTH AND DEVELOPMENT AND QUALITY OF LIFE

Children who survive LTX can expect to achieve a significantly improved lifestyle despite the necessity for continuous immunosuppressive management. An important aspect of achieving good quality of life is nutritional rehabilitation after LTX. Follow-up studies have demonstrated that, with appropriate nutritional support, 80% of survivors achieve normal growth patterns and habitus.[173-180] Growth patterns are better in children who received transplant before the age of 2 years; growth is impaired by chronic steroid use.[181]

An important aspect of long-term survival is the appropriate attainment of puberty. A long-term study from France has demonstrated that there are no differences between the sexes in attaining puberty and developing secondary sexual characteristics.[182] Girls develop menarche, and successful pregnancies have been reported for females receiving both CyA and Tac immunosuppression.[183]

Cognitive disorders are characteristic of chronic liver insufficiency and are more common in children who have received LTX than in the normal population. However, post-LTX children are far better than those with chronic liver disease. Controlled studies are lacking, and specific risk factors have not been defined.[184] LTX does not substantially affect schooling, and mental abilities tend to improve over time, but learning disabilities have been found in 26% of children.[184-186] Adverse psychologic reactions are shown in 50% or more of children after LTX.[187]

NONADHERENCE WITH IMMUNOSUPPRESSION

Noncompliance or nonadherence with immunosuppressive therapy in pediatric patients is most likely during their teenage years. The reality is that although LTX offers the hope of a cure in patients with a life-threatening illness, this is in exchange for another lifelong/chronic condition, which is lifelong adherence to medical care. Although it is not clear when noncompliance becomes a clinically important issue, it is quite clear that it is currently the leading cause of rejection and graft loss and death after transplantation in the pediatric age group.[188-190] This requires careful attention and education of patients, their parents, and other caregivers.

SURVIVAL AFTER LIVER TRANSPLANTATION

Current results from international centers indicate that the 1-year survival rate following LTX in children is in excess of 90% at experienced centers. The reports from larger centers such as UCLA with 657 patients,[9] University of Pittsburgh with 808 patients,[7] Kyoto University with 600 living donor transplants in 572 patients,[191] 555 LTX in 467 children from Catholic University of Louvain,[192] and 322 LTX in 280 pediatric patients from Hospital Bicette in Paris[8] show comparable results with 5- and 10-year patient survival of 81% and 78% and graft survival of 72% and 67% at the same time.

Many different factors influence survival.[193-198] Reduced-sized liver transplantation and live-donor liver transplantation have reduced the waiting-list mortality rate[128,199] and extended liver transplantation to infants, and have also demonstrated that equivalent survival may be achieved in infants transplanted under the age of 1 year and in older children.[200,201]

Protein malnutrition at the time of LTX has a significant influence on both morbidity and mortality. The degree of malnutrition, in addition to the severity of liver disease, has a significant effect on short-term survival. A number of studies have demonstrated improved survival for children with metabolic liver disease compared to those with chronic liver disease or fulminant liver failure.[195]

An important aspect contributing to improved survival has been the increase in surgical and medical experience, particularly with the development of innovative surgical techniques and better immunosuppressive drugs. As a result, there has been a reduction in the rate of retransplantation as well as a reduction in graft failure secondary to chronic rejection.

In some instances, survival maybe affected by recurrence of the original disease. Recurrence of hepatitis B has been dramatically reduced by therapy with the nucleoside analogues and the use of hepatitis B immunoglobulin. Hepatitis C, though very rare in children, still has a high recurrence rate after LTX in children.

The rate of recurrence of autoimmune hepatitis, both immunologically and histologically, is about 25% after LTX. The recurrence may be more severe than the original disease, and it is important to ensure that immunosuppression with steroids is continued in this group of patients.[202-204]

Several studies have documented the development of autoantibodies (ANA, SMA, and rarely LKM) following LTX in both pediatric and adult recipients who had no autoimmune disease before transplantation (i.e., *de novo* autoimmune hepatitis). The pathogenesis of the disease is unknown, but in some cases it may present with graft hepatitis and fibrosis.[205-208] Early diagnosis is crucial, because treatment with prednisone and azathioprine at the doses used for classical autoimmune hepatitis, if initiated promptly, is graft and life saving.[209] In some cases, it is thought that this may represent an atypical form of chronic rejection mediated via alloimmune humoral mediated rejection.

LIVER TRANSPLANTATION IN SPECIAL GROUPS

Combined Liver and Kidney Transplantation

Unlike adults, the most common indication for combined liver and kidney transplantation (LKTx) in children are liver-based metabolic abnormalities in which the liver is replaced at the time of kidney transplantation to correct the underlying enzymatic disorder as the cause of renal insufficiency.[210-213] Primary hyperoxaluria type I is the most common indication for this combined procedure. Despite the debate on concurrent versus sequential liver and kidney transplantation in these patients, the advantages of concurrent LKTx are the immediate correction of metabolic defect and renal failure. Other indications are metabolic diseases affecting both organs, such as glycogen storage disease type Ia, tyrosinemia, and congenital hepatic fibrosis with autosomal recessive polycystic kidney disease. There is also a potential long-term immunologic benefit, with kidneys from the same donor as the liver experiencing less acute and chronic rejection. Indeed, it has been shown that the protective effect of the liver in positive cross-matches will allow simultaneous liver/kidney transplants in sensitized patients.

Liver Transplantation for Hepatic Malignancies

A review based on the UNOS database of the outcome of 195 LTX for HB[152] and HCC[43] that were performed between 1987 and 2004 showed 1-, 5-, and 10-year survival of 79%, 69%, and 66% for HB and 86%, 63%, and 58% for HCC. The primary cause of death for both groups was metastatic or recurrent disease, accounting for 54% of deaths in the HB group and 86% in the HCC group.[59] In another study in 8 children with HB who received LTX followed by chemotherapy for stage III HB, 6 patients survived for 23 months to 9 years. Four of the survivors did not have any pre-LTX attempt at resection. The authors concluded that primary transplantation in patients with large HB has a better outcome than resection followed by LTX.[60] Several other reviews showed the same conclusion that despite the challenges of long-term immunosuppression, LTX is a life-saving procedure for selected children with hepatic malignancies.[55-58,61-63]

Liver Transplantation in Neonates

Acute liver failure is the main indication for LTX in neonates. They usually present in an extremely critical condition and, because of their size and their rapid deterioration of condition, have high rates of pretransplant, operative, and post-transplant complications and mortality.[214] The most common indication for LTX in this group of patients is giant cell hepatitis, which accounts for more than 50% of cases. Neonatal hemochromatosis; viral infections such as HBV, echovirus, and other retroviruses; and hemangioendotheliomatosis are considered as other indications for LTX in these patients. The patient and graft survival in these neonates is 57% and 38%, respectively. The high mortality rates in these patients are multifactorial and due to technical difficulties and operative complications such as vascular thrombosis, bleeding, and bile leak; higher rates of graft dysfunction; and the broad spectrum of bacterial, viral, and fungal infections that accounts for more than 50% of mortality in these patients.[201,202,215,216] The principal challenges in these patients are to support them until a timely liver transplant can be performed and to find an appropriately sized liver allograft, which may require technically challenging reduction of partial grafts as monosegment transplant grafts.

Retransplantation of the Liver in Children

Retransplantation of the liver happens in about 10 to 15% of pediatric recipients of a cadaveric whole organ transplant. The most common indications are vascular complications and primary nonfunction of the liver allograft, chronic rejection, and recurrent disease. Survival after retransplantation depends on the etiology of graft failure. The 1-year patient survival after liver retransplantation is approximately 60% for chronic rejection, 50% for HAT, and less than 30% for primary nonfunction.[217-219] The most common indication for retransplantation after segmental liver graft transplantation, including grafts from living donors, is vascular complications and especially HAT with 1-year survival of 47%.[220]

WITHDRAWAL OF IMMUNOSUPPRESSION AND TOLERANCE

Pediatric recipients are ideal candidates for immunosuppression withdrawal. The indications for LTX are generally not autoimmune in nature, they face a lifelong exposure to immunosuppression, and with living donor grafts, they share more HLA antigens than adult LTX recipients and cadaveric combinations. Pediatric patients tend to self-wean over time, as

many practitioners do not increase the dose of immunosuppression as the pediatric recipient grows. In several studies, the ability to wean patients from chronic immunosuppression is more successful in pediatric than adult recipients. In contrast to neonatal tolerance, where there is deletion of lymphocytes reacting toward a foreign antigen, in the clinical setting, operational tolerance is defined as the absence of immunologic injury to the allograft. In this setting, robust operational tolerance envisions indefinite graft survival with normal function in an immunosuppression-free, fully immunocompetent host. As the mechanism(s) whereby the allograft is maintained in an immunocompetent recipient are not clearly defined, the definition of operational tolerance becomes pragmatic – it does not mean complete unresponsiveness of the immune system toward donor antigens, but rather the lack of a destructive immune response toward the graft despite the presence of generalized immune competence.[221-223]

Although a small number of grafts are not rejected after total removal of immunosuppression, the deliberate withdrawal of immunosuppressive drugs must be done according to a strict protocol. In general, such attempts should be done only with stable patients under controlled situations. It is not suggested to do this in an unmonitored fashion, and it is probably not safe to do so for most patients. Until there are reliable markers that can predict the success of immunosuppression drug weaning and withdrawal, this should be done only under dire circumstances or under careful supervision.

In one Japanese study of 87 patients of whom 33 had complications of chronic immunosuppression, 54 underwent programmed withdrawal. Successful withdrawal was associated with presence of IL-10 producing $V\delta 1$ γ-δ T cells in blood.[224]

CONCLUSION

Thomas E. Starzl, in an article entitled "Evolution of Liver Transplantation," concluded with the following statement: "What was inconceivable yesterday, and barely achievable today, often becomes routine tomorrow."[205] Liver transplantation has proved to be the prime example.

Over a period of 50 years, the field of pediatric liver transplantation has continued to advance. To overcome the impact of organ shortage, more attention was paid to the improvement of organ allocation, decreasing death rate on the waiting list, and expanding the donor pool by innovative techniques such as the use of organs from live donors and split grafts, better organ preservation, and the use of organs from more marginal donors. Extensive effort in the prevention of disease recurrence in the transplanted liver continues. Newer immunosuppressive drugs and better protocols continue to change the pattern of rejection and to reduce the long-term complications of these agents, and, as a result, to increase patient and graft survival and improve quality of life. Xenotransplantation has continued to progress, and efforts to induce tolerance after organ transplantation have shown promising results.

REFERENCES

9. Farmer DG, Venick RS, McDiarmid S, et al. Predictors of outcomes after pediatric liver transplantation: an analysis of more than 800 cases performed at a single center. J Am Coll Surg 2007;204:904–916.
16. Broelsch CE, Whitington PF, Emond JC, et al. Liver transplantation in children from living related donors. Surgical techniques and results. Ann Surg 1991;214:428–437.

38. McDiarmid SV, Anand R, Lindbald AS. The Principal Investigators and Institutions of the Studies of Pediatric Liver Transplantation (SPLIT) Research Group. Development of a pediatric end-stage liver disease score to predict poor outcome in children awaiting liver transplantation. Transplantation 2002;74:173–181.

81. Eghtesad B, Kadry Z, Fung J. Technical considerations in liver transplantation: what hepatologist needs to know (and every surgeon should follow). Liver Transplant 2005;11:861–871.

106. Fung J, Kelly D, Kadry Z, et al. Immunosuppression in liver transplantation. Beyond calcineurin inhibitors. Liver Transplant 2005;11:267–280.

128. Diamond IR, Fecteau A, Millis M, et al. Impact of graft type on outcome in pediatric liver transplantation: a report from Studies of Pediatric Liver Transplantation (SPLIT). Ann Surg 2007;246:301–310.

156. Jain A, Nalesnik M, Reyes J, et al. Posttransplant lymphoproliferative disorders in liver transplantation: a 20-year experience. Ann Surg 2002;74:1721–1724.

See expertconsult.com for a complete list of references and the review questions for this chapter.

79 DISEASES OF THE GALLBLADDER

Douglas S. Fishman • Mark A. Gilger

Gallbladder disease in children has evolved over the past 20 years. Improved diagnostic modalities, such as abdominal ultrasound, have led to "incidental" or "silent" gallstones being detected more often in children, even in utero. Although hemolytic disease remains a common cause of cholelithiasis, obesity- and metabolic syndrome–related stones are increasing in frequency. Gallstones may also be found in patients with other conditions such as prematurity, necrotizing enterocolitis, congenital heart disease, cystic fibrosis, and conditions necessitating total parenteral nutrition (TPN).

EPIDEMIOLOGY OF GALLSTONE DISEASE

More than 20 million adults in the United States have gallstones and approximately 300,000 cholecystectomies are performed yearly with an estimated 1.8 million ambulatory visits.[1-3] Predominantly a disease of adulthood, gallstone disease ranges in prevalence from 4 to 11% in Western societies, with wide variations along racial and ethnic lines.[4-10] The incidence in adults is approximately 1 to 3%.[11] The incidence and prevalence of gallstone disease is influenced by age, sex, culture, ethnicity, and a variety of medical factors,[1,8,12-16] and it varies geographically. For instance, members of the Masai tribe of East Africa, whose bile is only half saturated with cholesterol, do not develop gallstones, whereas the Pima Indians of Arizona have an 80% prevalence.[7,17] Furthermore, epidemiologic studies suggest there is a strong heritable effect in gallstone formation.[18] Puppala et al. demonstrated a genome-wide link on chromosome 1p in a Mexican American cohort with gallstones.[19]

Investigations using a mouse model suggest that the Lith family of genes, such as Lith1 and Lith2, may determine susceptibility to cholesterol gallstone formation.[20] Apobec-1, an RNA-specific enzyme of ApoB, is linked to Lith6, and when down-regulated, there is decreased expression of 7-α-hydroxylase and increase in gallstones.[21] The nuclear receptor FXR, encoded by NR1H4, has been linked to Lith7 as a genetic factor in gallstone development.[22] MDR3/ABCB4 is the physiologic translocator of phospholipids across the canalicular membrane of the hepatocyte, and ABCB11 is responsible for bile salt export. Mutations of the gene ABCB4 have been described in adults with cholesterol gallstones and less often in young adults.[23, 24] Patients with mutations in ABCB11 are also at risk for gallstone development. Other genes with strong associations to gallstone formation include CYP7A1 and CCK1R.[25] Polymorphisms in hepatic uridine diphosphate (UDP)-glucuronosyltransferase (UGT1A1) have also been described in patients with hemolytic disease that predispose to increased gallstone formation rates.[26]

The earliest reported case of cholelithiasis in a child was by Gibson in 1737.[27] Attempts to estimate the frequency of childhood gallstones included an extensive review of 5037 cases in 1959, in which a prevalence of 0.15% in children younger than

16 years of age was noted.[28] The prevalence of gallbladder disease in children since the 1960s appears to be increasing.[29-37] For example, in a review in 1984, of 708 infants referred for cholestasis between 1970 and 1981, an incidence of 1.4% was found,[34] whereas a review in 2000 of 4200 children who underwent abdominal ultrasound between 1988 and 1998 estimated a prevalence of gallstones at 1.9%.[35] Other reports have noted that 4% of all cholecystectomies are performed in patients younger than 20 years of age.[38,39] In a review of 693 cases of childhood gallstones reported since 1968, early infancy and adolescence were the most common ages for diagnosis.[40] Infants younger than 6 months of age represented 10% of all cases in which the age was known. Children from 6 months to 10 years of age accounted for 21% and adolescents (mostly female) 11 to 21 years of age represented 69% of all cases.[40] Most gallstones in children have an underlying predisposing condition, such as hemolytic disease, pregnancy and TPN. Gallstones of infancy are typically found in "ill" infants receiving TPN. Stones found in children from the ages of 1 to 5 years are usually secondary to hemolysis, and stones found in adolescents are most likely associated with obesity, menarche, pregnancy, and the use of oral contraceptives.[23,40,41]

PATHOPHYSIOLOGY OF GALLSTONE DISEASE

Bile is composed of five major components: water, bilirubin, cholesterol, bile pigments, and phospholipids. The primary phospholipid is lecithin. Calcium salts and some proteins are minor components of bile. Stone formation occurs owing to the precipitation of the insoluble constituents of bile, which are cholesterol, bile pigments, and calcium salts. Gallstones are classically divided into either cholesterol stones or pigment stones (Table 79-1). Chemically pure gallstones are rare, and in any single stone the composition varies from the core to the crust. Most stones are "mixed" in composition, and the formation patterns of both cholesterol and pigment stones share many characteristics.

Cholesterol, the major sterol in bile, is nearly insoluble in water. It is made soluble in aqueous bile by aggregation with bile salts or lecithin. When cholesterol is no longer soluble, cholesterol monohydrate crystals precipitate from solution, a process known as *nucleation*.[42,43]

The interplay among the major bile components cholesterol, lecithin, and bile salts is depicted in Figure 79-1.[44] When the composition of bile lies in the micellar zone, the bile can solubilize additional cholesterol. As the cholesterol concentration continues to increase, the likelihood of cholesterol crystallization, and hence gallstone formation, increases. A decrease in bile salt concentration or lecithin also predisposes to gallstones.

Three primary conditions must be met to permit the formation of cholesterol gallstones.[45] First, the bile must be

TABLE 79-1. **Characteristics of Gallstones in Children**[25,59,60]

		Pigment Stones	
Characteristics	**Cholesterol Stones**	**Black**	**Brown**
Color	Yellow-white (often with dark core)	Black to brown	Brown to orange
Consistency	Hard	Hard, shiny	Soft, greasy, 50% amorphous; rest crystalline, inorganic salts
	Crystalline	Crystalline	
	Layered		
Number and morphology			
Multiple: 2-25 mm faceted, smooth	Multiple: <5 mm	Multiple: 10-30 mm	
	Solitary: 2-4 cm (~10%) round, smooth	Irregular or smooth	Round, smooth
Composition	Cholesterol monohydrate >50%	Bile pigment polymer ~40%	Calcium bilirubinate ~60%
	Glycoprotein	Calcium carbonate or phosphate salts ~15%	Calcium palmitate and stearate soaps ~15%
	Calcium salts	Cholesterol ~5%	Cholesterol ~15%
		Mucin glycoprotein ~20%	Mucin glycoprotein ~10%
Radiopaque	No	Yes, ~50%	No
Location	Gallbladder ± common bile duct	Gallbladder ± common bile duct	Common bile duct, intrahepatic ducts
Clinical associations	Hyperlipidemia	Hemolytic anemia	Bacterial infection (*Escherichia coli*)
	Obesity	Cirrhosis	Parasitic infection
	Clofibrate	Total parenteral nutrition	Bile duct anomaly
	Pregnancy	Ileal disease (after puberty) Ceftriaxone	Birth control pills
	Cystic fibrosis		
	Octreotide		
Recurrent	Yes	No	Yes
Sex	Female > male	No difference	No difference
Age	Pubertal; increases with age	Any; increases with age	Any; increases with age
Bacteria	No	No	Yes (consistently found at core)
Soluble	Yes	No	No (minimally)

supersaturated with cholesterol, which then acts as the driving force behind crystal precipitation. Second, bile kinetics must be such as to allow nucleation, the transition to solid cholesterol crystals. Finally, gallbladder stasis must exist to allow agglomeration of cholesterol crystals into stones.[46] Two secondary conditions also appear to be critical in lithogenesis: gallbladder hypersecretion of mucus and excess arachidonyl lecithin (Figure 79-2).[47-50]

Cholesterol supersaturation can result from the following conditions:

1. An increased delivery of cholesterol to the liver via increased lipoprotein (low-density lipoprotein and chylomicrons). Very low-density lipoprotein (VLDL) production and trafficking of bile acids are increased in gallstone patients and may be due to increased activity of hepatic microsomal triglyceride transfer protein (MTTP).[51] This can occur in women secondary to estrogen or oral contraceptive use or with increased dietary cholesterol intake.[47,52]

2. An increased endogenous cholesterol synthesis secondary to 3-hydroxy-3-methylglutaryl coenzyme A (HMG-CoA) reductase activity. Both obesity and hypertriglyceridemia are causes of increased HMG-CoA reductase activity.[53,54]

3. A decrease in 7-α-hydroxylase activity, thus decreasing the conversion of cholesterol to bile acids.[21,55] This defect occurs most commonly with increasing age.

4. A decrease in the conversion of cholesterol to cholesterol esters from inhibited acyl-CoA cholesterol acyltransferase activity (ACAT).[47] Progesterone, either pregnancy induced or exogenous, and clofibrate are examples of ACAT inhibitors.

The potential defects leading to cholesterol supersaturation are thus numerous and overlapping.

Figure 79-2 summarizes the current understanding of the formation of cholesterol gallstones and, perhaps, of any gallstone. The process must have a supersaturated solution (either cholesterol or bilirubin pigment); a "still" environment, or gallbladder stasis; and crystal agglomeration or nucleation. The initial nucleating event creates the core of the stone, from which a self-perpetuating process ensues. Nucleation is not as well understood as cholesterol supersaturation. Nucleation times are strikingly different between gallstone patients and control subjects. Gallbladder hypomotility seems to be involved in the crystallization process, because agitation prevents aggregation. Animal studies support hypomotility as an important causative factor.[56,57] Technetium-99m-dimethyl iminodiacetic acid gallbladder emptying studies in adult gallstone patients have documented diminished gallbladder emptying after meals.[58]

Biliary sludge, or tumefacient sludge, a collection of mucus, calcium bilirubinate, and cholesterol crystals, appears to precede the formation of gallstones in animal models.[42,43,59] However, some clinical studies in children do not support sludge as being a precursor of gallstones.[35] Mucin hypersecretion appears to be a primary event in sludge formation, and evidence suggests that prostanoids, such as arachidonyl lecithin, mediate the hypersecretion.[47-49] Mucin may serve as the nidus for nucleation and subsequent sludge formation owing to its hydrophobic domain, which binds phospholipid and cholesterol.[60]

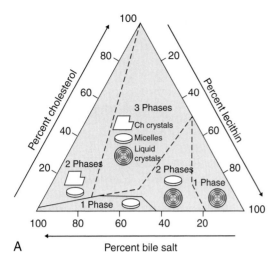

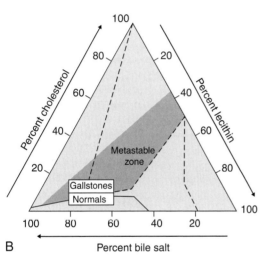

Figure 79-1. (**A**) Triangular phase diagram showing phases present at equilibrium in biles of differing compositions. In the micellar zone (the area in the lower left of the triangle), all the cholesterol is held in solution as micelles. Biles with a composition outside the micellar zone, if allowed to come to equilibrium, would form liquid and/or solid cholesterol crystals (as depicted schematically in each of the zones). The micellar zone is larger for gallbladder bile (a 10% lipid solution shown here) than for hepatic bile (a 3% lipid solution not shown). (**B**) Triangular phase diagram with schematic representations of ranges of lipid compositions found in gallbladder biles of normals and gallstone patients. Bile with a composition that falls in the metastable zone takes a prolonged time to come to equilibrium and thus appears to be stable. Excess cholesterol is "carried" in the metastable zone by cholesterol-rich unilamellar vesicles. The boundaries of the physiologically relevant metastable zone are approximate.[33] From Carey MC, Cohen DE. Biliary transport of cholesterol in micelles and liquid crystals. In: Paumgartner G, Stiehl A, Gerak W, eds. Bile Acids and the Liver. Lancaster: MTP Press; 1987:287-300, with permission.[44]

CHOLESTEROL STONES

Cholesterol gallstones are yellowish-white in appearance, hard, crystalline and layered. They frequently have a brownish core, with a variety of substances found there, including calcium salts. "Rings" of protein (glycoproteins) and calcium salts (calcium bilirubinate, calcium hydroxyapatite, and calcium carbonate) form around the core, resulting in the layered appearance. The cholesterol content is higher than 50%, with minimal calcium salt content. This composition is not radiopaque; thus, the stones are rarely seen on plain film radiographs. Cholesterol stones form within the gallbladder and are frequently multiple,

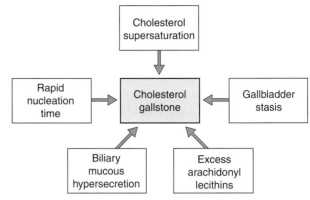

Figure 79-2. Current understanding of cholesterol gallstone formation. Cholesterol supersaturation is an essential prerequisite, which combined with a more rapid nucleation time and gallbladder stasis allows crystal formation. Excess biliary mucus provides a structural nidus for crystal growth, driven by increased dietary arachidonyl lecithins. Adapted from Hay DW, Carey MC. Pathophysiology and pathogenesis of cholesterol gallstone formation. Semin Liver Dis 1990; 10:159-170, with permission.[40]

ranging in size from approximately 2 to 25 mm in diameter. The presence of cholesterol stones in the biliary tree is the result of migration. Cholesterol gallstones account for approximately 70% of all stones found in Western populations.

There clearly are genetic influences, with high prevalence rates seen in both children and adult Native Americans. Studies of the Pimas of Arizona have demonstrated the development of lithogenic bile containing excess cholesterol during adolescence.[61] The prevalence of cholesterol gallstones in children is unknown, but increases slowly with age in both sexes.[62] Pubertal changes, in particular early menarche, cause a dramatic increase in the incidence of cholesterol gallstones.[61-63] This phenomenon has been attributed to the effect of estrogen and progesterone surges that occur during puberty; it has also been seen in pregnancy and with the use of oral contraceptives, although investigation suggests no relationship between oral contraceptives and gallstones.[64] Sex hormones appear to induce biliary stasis and cause cholesterol hypersecretion by the liver.[65] It remains unclear whether estrogen, the progestins, or a combination of both are responsible. Data from a high-risk Chilean population also suggest that insulin resistance plays a major role in gallstone formation.[66] Insulin resistance has also been shown to be a risk factor for gallstones and sludge during pregnancy independent of body mass index.[67]

The metabolic syndrome, a constellation of disorders linked to obesity and insulin dysregulation, now includes cholesterol gallstone disease.[68,69] In a mouse model, hepatic insulin resistance was found to directly promote cholesterol formation, when a liver-specific insulin receptor (Fox01) was downregulated.[70] In addition, high dietary carbohydrates have also been linked to diminished gallbladder volume and increased cholesterol crystal formation.[71] Obesity has also been shown to increase the likelihood of cholesterol gallstone formation, likely from excessive hepatic cholesterol secretion secondary to increased cholesterol synthesis.[72]

PIGMENT STONES

Pigment stones account for a much higher percentage of stones in prepubertal children, whereas cholesterol stones are predominant in adolescence and adulthood. Two types of pigment gallstones are found in children and are referred to as *black* and *brown*. In both black and brown stones, the pigment present is calcium bilirubinate, which interacts with mucin glycoproteins to form stones (see Table 79-1).[73]

Black pigment stones are black to dark brown in color and small (usually less than 5 mm), occur multiply, and are typically hard, shiny, and crystalline.[74] They are composed primarily of highly crosslinked polymers of bilirubin with mucin glycoproteins and calcium salts of phosphate and carbonate.[75,76] The high concentration of calcium salts (as compared with brown and cholesterol stones) accounts for the 50 to 75% radiopacity seen on plain radiographs. Black stones typically form within the gallbladder and do not recur after resection. They are usually associated with hemolytic diseases, of which sickle cell disease and hereditary spherocytosis are the most common. The duration of the hemolytic disease appears to be a significant risk factor for stone formation. Children younger than 10 years of age with sickle cell disease have a 14% prevalence of stones, whereas children 11 to 20 years of age have a 36% prevalence. Older adults with sickle cell disease have more than a 50% prevalence.[77,78] In a study from Houston, Texas, the median age of detecting gallstones in 458 patients with sickle cell disease was 10.5 years.[79] Other disease states, such as thalassemia, Wilson's disease, and mechanical shearing of erythrocytes associated with artificial heart valves, have all been associated with black pigment stones. Black pigment stones form within the gallbladder, and their presence in the common bile duct is the result of migration. Black stones are found in sterile bile and are not associated with infection.[80]

The formation of black stones results from altered gallbladder bile homeostasis and supersaturation of the bile. This process could occur by at least three mechanisms: an increase in bilirubin anions, an increase in unbound Ca^{2+}, and a decrease in factors that solubilize bilirubin and calcium.[74] An increase in bilirubin anions has been shown to occur secondary to hemolysis.[74,81] Increased unbound calcium could occur secondary to increased plasma ionized calcium or to a decrease in calcium-binding agents, such as micellar bile salts and lecithin-cholesterol vesicles.[81] The decrease in the bile salt pool secondary to an interruption of the enterohepatic circulation as seen in ileal resection or the nothing by mouth (NPO) status accompanying TPN could result in this phenomenon.

Brown pigment stones are brown to orange in color, soft, soap-like or greasy in texture, and commonly assume the shape of their origin, the common bile duct.[74] The stone color is derived from calcium bilirubinate, and their greasy texture results from a significant component of fat (calcium palmitate or stearate derived from lecithin).[82] The scarcity of calcium carbonate and phosphate accounts for their lack of opacity on radiography.[73] The cholesterol content ranges from 2 to 28%, which is higher than in black stones and allows in part for their increased solubility. The most distinct clinical feature of brown gallstones in both adults and children is the association with infection.[34,83] These stones are a major public health problem in rural areas of Asian countries, where they are found secondary to parasitic infestation with such organisms as *Opisthorchis sinensis* and *Ascaris lumbricoides*.[84] They are an uncommon type of stone in Western society and are typically found in the common bile duct after cholecystectomy when the bile is infected. Urinary tract infections may predispose to stone formation in early childhood.[85] In some 85% of cases, the bile grows *Escherichia coli*.[86] In children, especially infants, these stones can be seen in association with other organisms such as *Staphylococcus*, *Enterobacter*, *Citrobacter*,[83] and *Salmonella virchow*.[87] Infection with stasis results in excessive secretion of mucin, which may serve as the glycoprotein nidus for stone formation.[81] Bacteria also release beta-glucuronidase, phospholipase A_1, and conjugated bile salt hydrolase, which hydrolyze bilirubin glucuronides, lecithin, and conjugated bile salts, producing unconjugated bilirubin, free saturated fatty acids, lysolecithin, and free bile acids.[88] With the exception of lysolecithin, these products precipitate with calcium to form stones.[81] Duodenal diverticula and biliary tree abnormalities, such as stenosis, also may predispose to brown stone formation.

GALLSTONES IN INFANTS

Infants younger than 12 months of age may be predisposed to gallstone formation, as compared with older children[83] (Table 79-2). For example, the bile of infants is more dilute than that

TABLE 79-2. Gallstones in Infancy (<12 Months Old)

Author	Number of Infants	Spontaneous Resolution	Surgical Treatment*	Persistent Asymptomatic	Follow-up Data NA	Recurrence
Keller (1985)[78]	5	5				
Jacir (1986)[79]	4	3	1			
Jonas et al. (1990)[80]	7	2	5			
Ljung et al. (1992)[81]	5	1	1	3		
Debray et al. (1993)[77]	40	15	21	4		2
Roman et al. (1994)[82]	1	1				
Johart (1995)[83]	2	1		1		
Monnerie (1995)[84]	11					
Morad (1995)[76]	14	8			6	
Ishitani et al. (1996)[85]	1		1			
Stringer et al. (1996)[75]	3	2	1			
Klar et al. (2005)103a	16	8	2	6		
King et al. (2007)86a	1	1	1			
Totals	83	47 (56%)	33 (40%)	14 (17%)	6 (6%)	2 (2%)

*Includes therapeutic endoscopic retrograde cholangiopancreatography (ERCP).

of older children, with a lower bile salt concentration, a shorter nucleation time, and a higher cholesterol saturation index.[89] These factors may help explain the increased tendency of infants to produce sludge and gallstones.[40] Table 79-2 demonstrates the likelihood (nearly one half of reported cases) for spontaneous resolution of gallstones during infancy.[90-102] Such information deserves special consideration concerning therapeutic intervention in infants and suggests that, unless symptomatic, gallstones during infancy do not require surgical intervention and often resolve without treatment.[35]

TOTAL PARENTERAL NUTRITION–ASSOCIATED STONES

The association between TPN and cholelithiasis is clearly established.[103] Gallstone formation in premature infants and neonates receiving TPN appears to have four stages: decreased hepatobiliary flow due to immaturity, stasis within the biliary tree, sludge formation, and finally, stone formation. Cholestasis, which increases with decreasing gestational age, is found in at least 50% of infants with a birth weight less than 1000 g.[104] After 2 months on TPN, 80% of infants have cholestasis.[104] This predisposition to cholestasis in infancy is multifactorial. Bile acid transport, bile secretion, and basal and stimulated bile salt flow rates all are immature.[105,106] Bile salt–dependent and -independent flow are decreased, approximating only 50% of that in adults.[103,105] The absence of oral feeding reduces the enterohepatic circulation of bile acids.[103] Fasting also inhibits the release of gut and biliary tree hormones, such as cholecystokinin, gastrin, secretin, motilin, and glucagon. The formation of echogenic, thick, "molasses-like" biliary sludge within the gallbladder has been documented in both adults and children receiving TPN.[103,107,108] Serial ultrasound examinations of adults receiving continuous TPN infusion show sludge formation increasing from 6% of patients in the first week to 50% in the fourth week and 100% after 6 weeks.[109] Gallbladder enlargement may be the first physical sign of sludge formation in the infant. Stagnant bile in a dilated gallbladder provides an ideal milieu for the development of both acalculous cholecystitis and cholelithiasis. TPN-induced gallstones are pigment stones, typically black and usually found in the gallbladder. They often have a high calcium phosphate or carbonate content; however, stone analysis indicates that they are of a mixed bilirubin-cholesterol composition and perhaps belong to a special group of TPN-induced pigment stones.

CYSTIC FIBROSIS–ASSOCIATED GALLSTONES

Gallstones, gallbladder, and biliary tract abnormalities are frequently found in patients with cystic fibrosis and they increase with age.[110] "Microgallbladders" have been identified in as many as 16% of adult cystic fibrosis patients radiologically and in 30% of patients at autopsy.[111] Common bile duct stenosis has been identified in 96% of cystic fibrosis patients with liver disease, resulting in enlarged gallbladders and elevated serum bile acid levels, which may predispose to gallstone formation.[110] Gallstones in cystic fibrosis patients appear secondary to excessive bile acid loss resulting in a reduced bile acid pool. The bile composition becomes abnormal, with a relative excess of cholesterol associated with the decrease in bile salts, thus making the bile lithogenic. The bile acid malabsorption

and reduced bile salt pool respond to pancreatic enzyme therapy. Gallstones have not been found without pancreatic insufficiency.[112,113]

ILEAL DISEASE AND ILEAL RESECTION–ASSOCIATED STONES

The enterohepatic circulation constantly replenishes the bile acid pool, which in turn governs the rate of bile salt secretion. The terminal ileum serves as the site of nearly 98% of bile acid resorption. Terminal ileal disease, typically Crohn's disease, or surgical resection of the ileum can result in an interruption of this bile acid recycling. The bile salt pool is subsequently reduced, thus altering the balance of bile components and favoring cholesterol supersaturation and increased bile lithogenicity. The formation of gallstones secondary to ileal disease has been reported in both adults and children. However, it appears that ileal resection only increases the tendency to gallstone formation after puberty.[114] After puberty, cholesterol secretion increases, whereas bile salt secretion declines, predisposing to cholesterol supersaturation and, hence, stone formation.[114]

DRUG-ASSOCIATED STONES

The use of several drugs, furosemide, octreotide, ceftriaxone, cyclosporine, and tacrolimus, has been associated with an increased tendency to form gallstones. In reported cases associated with furosemide administration, numerous other contributing factors, such as prematurity, sepsis, and small bowel disease, were also noted. Whether furosemide alone contributes to gallstone formation remains unclear.[114-118]

Octreotide has a wide range of biologic activities, including several clinically useful applications such as treatment of upper gastrointestinal bleeding, secretory diarrhea, acromegaly, and gastroenteropancreatic endocrine tumors. Gallstone formation has been found in about half of patients who receive chronic octreotide therapy.[119-121] It is believed that this may be related to octreotide-induced gallbladder stasis or a direct effect of octreotide on gallbladder absorption.[122]

Ceftriaxone can induce gallbladder concretions. Ceftriaxone is excreted in bile and has the ability to displace bilirubin from albumin-binding sites. Reports in both adults and children have noted biliary echo densities or sludge often causing symptoms of cholecystitis with right upper quadrant pain, nausea, and vomiting. Analysis of the sludge reveals high concentrations of a calcium salt of ceftriaxone, with traces of bilirubinate and cholesterol, thus resembling pigment stone composition.[123] Fasting, dehydration, and age older than 24 months are risk factors associated with this so-called pseudolithiasis.[102,116,124] The process of bile concretion and the related symptoms are reversible when the drug is discontinued.[116,125]

Cyclosporine usage in children undergoing bone marrow and solid organ transplant has been implicated in gallstone formation, possibly related to elevated drug levels and hepatic toxicity.[126,127] However, underlying sepsis, total parenteral nutrition, and NPO status are also likely contributors. Heart transplant in infants under 3 months of age appears to confer the greatest risk of cholelithiasis,[128] substantially higher than that seen in kidney or liver graft recipients.[117] Children undergoing bone marrow transplant also have been reported to have a higher likelihood of cholelithiasis.[118]

DIAGNOSIS OF GALLSTONE DISEASE

The classic symptom complex of right upper quadrant pain and vomiting is usually associated with stones only in older children and adolescents. Younger children tend to present with nonspecific symptoms. Jaundice is frequently encountered in "symptomatic" infants.[40] The most likely age for silent stones is infancy through the preschool years. Intolerance to fatty food is rarely reported in children. Fever is an unusual finding at any age and, if present, indicates associated cholecystitis. Complications of gallstone disease include cholecystitis, choledocholithiasis, cholangitis, and gallbladder perforation, but these occur rarely in children. Pancreatitis has been identified in 8 to 27% of children with gallstone disease and may represent the most common complication in children.[129, 130]

Laboratory evaluation typically is nondiagnostic. Occasional patients will have a leukocytosis as well as mildly elevated aminotransaminase levels and GGT. Because black pigmented stones are more common in children than adults, plain-film radiography may be helpful and demonstrate radiopaque stones. Ultrasonography is the diagnostic procedure of choice, because it is noninvasive, sensitive, and specific. Ultrasonography also allows examination of the surrounding abdominal viscera, such as the pancreas and the biliary tree. Annual biliary ultrasonography has been suggested in children with known predisposition to gallstones, such as those with hereditary spherocytosis and sickle cell anemia.[131,132] Oral cholecystography has been largely replaced by ultrasound, but it can occasionally be useful in the evaluation of gallbladder function. Endoscopic retrograde cholangiopancreatography (ERCP) is particularly useful in the evaluation of ductal stones.[133] Percutaneous cholangiograms offer another approach, but are seldom used in children for this purpose.

TREATMENT OF GALLSTONE DISEASE

Observation may be the most prudent treatment in infants with asymptomatic gallstone disease (see Table 79-2). As the infant ages, the hepatobiliary enzyme systems mature and the potential for spontaneous stone dissolution exists. Spontaneous stone resolution also has been observed in TPN-induced gallstones. In children for whom the duration of TPN is expected to be limited and the stones are asymptomatic, observation is indicated. However, in children who are chronically dependent on TPN, such as those with pseudo-obstruction syndrome or short bowel syndrome, stones should be removed.[134]

Gallstones in older children should be removed, because spontaneous resolution seldom occurs. Cholecystostomy is indicated for acute drainage of the gallbladder and perhaps in seriously ill patients for whom only simple stone extraction is needed. Laparoscopic cholecystectomy has become the surgical procedure of choice, in both adults and children.[135-137]

Options for nonsurgical treatment of gallstone disease continue to proliferate. Despite the growing popularity of medical therapy for adults, there is no such approved medical treatment for gallstones in children (Table 79-3). Two bile acids currently exist for oral gallstone dissolution: chenodeoxycholic acid (chenodiol) and ursodeoxycholic acid (ursodiol). Both agents occur naturally and are present in bile. Chenodiol works by inhibiting HMG-CoA reductase, which suppresses hepatic cholesterol synthesis.[115,116] Side effects such as diarrhea and hepatotoxicity have limited its widespread use. The mechanism of action of

ursodiol is similar to chenodiol, inhibiting HMG-CoA reductase and additionally, blocking intestinal absorption of cholesterol.[138] Ursodeoxycholic acid also reduces lipid peroxidation and mucin secretagogue activity.[139] Diarrhea and hepatotoxicity are rare.[140] Combination use of both chenodiol and ursodiol appears more effective and allows a 50% reduction in dosage with fewer side effects.[141] Drawbacks to the use of such therapy include the long duration of therapy, recurrence after stopping, low success rate, and high cost. However, only cholesterol stones are amenable to this therapy. Animal studies may provide future treatment modalities. For example, ezetimibe, a cholesterol-lowering agent, has recently been shown in mice to prevent gallstone formation.[142] Another mouse model has demonstrated reduction of cholesterol gallstones using garlic and onion![143]

Extracorporeal shock-wave lithotripsy (ESWL) was first used successfully in humans to fragment renal calculi. ESWL generates high-amplitude pressure waves that are focused on the stone by computerized ultrasonography. Only symptomatic stones that are radiolucent can be treated with this method, again limiting its use in children. Best results are obtained with solitary stones, with success rates of 95 to 100% reported.[144] Oral dissolution therapy appears to be a rational addition to lithotripsy to achieve complete stone dissolution.[145] The two major complications of lithotripsy are cholecystitis and pancreatitis,

TABLE 79-3. Treatment Alternatives for Gallstones in Children and Adults

Type	Comments
Cholecystectomy	Method of choice in most cases
Cholecystostomy	Effective for acute gallbladder drainage (i.e., acalculous cholecystitis)
Laparoscopic cholecystectomy	Effective with severely ill patients, shortens hospitalization (e.g., cystic fibrosis)
ERCP	
Basket removal	Bile duct stone removal
Mechanical basket lithotripsy	Stone crushing within bile ducts
Electrohydraulic lithotripsy	Stone destruction within bile ducts
Laser lithotripsy	Stone destruction within bile ducts
ESWL	Limited experience (unpublished), only for cholesterol stones currently
Dissolution	
Oral	Ursodeoxycholic acid and chenodeoxycholic acid
	Blocks HMG-CoA reductase, decreases cholesterol synthesis
Contact	Methyl *tert*-butyl-ether (for cholesterol stones only)
	Bile acid EDTA (for pigment stones; experimental)
Preventive	
Enteral feeds	Even small amounts during TPN decrease stone risk
Weight loss	For obesity – gradual weight loss
Lovastatin and simvastatin	Block HMG-CoA reductase, decrease cholesterol synthesis (experimental)
Cholecystokinin	Stimulates gallbladder contraction while NPO (experimental)

EDTA, ethylenediaminetetraacetic acid; ERCP, endoscopic retrograde cholangiopancreatography; ESWL, extracorporeal shock-wave lithotripsy.

reported in 1 to 2% of patients.[118,119] Successful treatment of gallstones in children has been accomplished.[146,147]

Cholesterol gallstones can be dissolved using methyl *tert*-butyl ether (MTBE). The procedure first requires placement of a percutaneous transhepatic catheter into a contrast-enhanced gallbladder. A greater than 95% success rate in stone dissolution has been reported.[148] Complications include leakage of the MTBE, causing nausea, vomiting, and duodenitis and intravascular hemolysis if the MTBE enters the vascular system, which has limited its application in both adults and children.[148] Chemical dissolution of calcified cholesterol stones and brown pigment stones has been tried experimentally with bile acid ethylenediaminetetraacetic acid (EDTA), but has shown only limited success.

The prevention of gallstones in children entails recognition of risk factors and an understanding of the pathophysiology of stone disease. The use of limited enteral feedings during TPN therapy, for example, stimulates gallbladder contraction, thus decreasing gallbladder stasis. Early use of pancreatic enzyme supplements in patients with cystic fibrosis decreases the propensity to stone formation. Informed use of contraceptives other than birth control pills, particularly in women with known gallstone risk factors, would seem advisable. Weight control and physical activity in obese patients is advisable to decrease the risk of gallstone disease, but rapid weight loss programs in obese patients may actually promote gallstone formation secondary to increased bile cholesterol saturation and gallbladder stasis.[149,150] Medical therapy with cholesterol-lowering agents, such as lovastatin and simvastatin, may be considered in high-risk patients, although no data exist for the use of this therapy in children (see Table 79-3).

CHOLECYSTITIS

Cholecystitis is a disease that results from inflammation of the gallbladder, typically secondary to gallstone obstruction of the cystic duct. Cholecystitis may be acute or chronic. Most cholecystitis in children is chronic and is associated with gallstones. The presentation of "acute" cholecystitis in children most likely represents a significant episode of an ongoing process of gallbladder distention and mucosal damage that culminated in cholecystitis.

The pathophysiology of cholecystitis parallels that of gallstone formation, with gallbladder stasis as the initiating event. The stasis is usually secondary to obstruction of the cystic duct by a gallstone or to local edema secondary to a stone. Other causes include external compression of the cystic duct by swollen lymph nodes, torsion of the gallbladder, congenital ductal abnormalities, and trauma. The basis for the inflammation is unclear, although mechanical distention, ischemia, bacteria, and lysolecithins have been implicated.

The typical presenting symptom is right upper quadrant abdominal pain, occasionally radiating to the back and associated with vomiting. When distended and inflamed, the gallbladder lies on the anterior abdominal wall between the 9th and 10th costal cartilages, causing localized tenderness on palpation and giving rise to the diagnostic Murphy's sign. Jaundice and fever are seen in 25 to 30% of children and are more common in young infants. The onset of symptoms is usually over a period of 1 week, but lesser symptoms of biliary colic may occur over several years. The differential diagnosis should include hepatitis, hepatic abscess, tumor, gonococcal perihepatitis

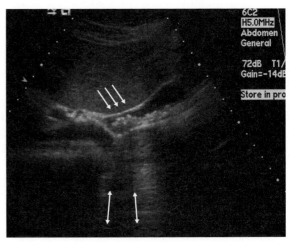

Figure 79-3. Ultrasound of gallstones within the gallbladder (single white arrows) showing acoustic shadowing (double white arrows).

(Fitz-Hugh-Curtis syndrome), pancreatitis, appendicitis, peptic ulcer disease, pneumonia, pyelonephritis, and kidney stones.

Laboratory evaluation should include a complete blood count with differential; total and conjugated bilirubin, alkaline phosphatase, γ-glutamyltransferase (GGT), serum aminotransferases, amylase, and lipase levels; and urinalysis. Leukocytosis is frequently found. Elevated aminotransferase levels and mild hyperbilirubinemia are seen in 20% of patients in the absence of obstruction. Elevated amylase levels are common even without pancreatitis. Marked elevation of the bilirubin, alkaline phosphatase, or GGT levels may indicate choledocholithiasis (stones in the bile duct). The characteristic ultrasound finding is a discrete echo density indicating a stone, usually occupying a dependent position in the gallbladder, which changes or moves when the patient is moved and is associated with acoustic shadowing (Figure 79-3). Gallbladder dilation, a thickened gallbladder wall, the presence of sludge, and biliary tree anomalies also may be seen. Cholescintigraphy can be helpful to evaluate gallbladder function, revealing normal hepatic uptake, but nonvisualization of the gallbladder at 1 hour.[151] False-positive results may occur with prolonged fasting, TPN, and hepatocellular disease. Oral cholecystography is used less frequently, owing to several inherent drawbacks, such as failure to concentrate the dye (particularly if hyperbilirubinemia exists), a 6 to 8% false-negative rate, hypersensitivity to the dye, and radiation exposure.

Hospitalization with institution of intravenous fluids, cessation of oral feeding, gastric decompression, and analgesics is appropriate. Antibiotics are not needed in simple cases, but indicated for persistent fever, clinical worsening, or concern for obstruction. Cefoxitin or piperacillin/tazobactam are often used to cover enteric organisms and provide good biliary excretion.

Cholecystectomy is the procedure of choice in calculous cholecystitis. In children with sickle cell disease, a combination of packed red blood cell transfusion, exchange transfusion, and adequate hydration with dextrose-containing intravenous fluids is typical. Children with certain medical disorders, such as congenital heart disease, appear to have an increased risk of death after urgent cholecystectomy, and elective cholecystectomy may be advisable.[152] Cholecystostomy with stone removal can be done in those patients for whom a functioning gallbladder is important, such as in patients with Crohn's disease. Table 79-3 lists the possible treatment options in children.

Most cases of cholecystitis usually resolve over several days. Complications occur in 30% of cases and include gallbladder perforation, abscess, or empyema formation. When fever persists or exceeds 102° F and pain or tenderness worsens, perforation is likely. Such perforations typically occur in the fundus of the gallbladder. A local perforation may wall off as an abscess, extend into the peritoneum as peritonitis, or lead to a cholecystoenteric fistula. Surgical evaluation with appropriate antibiotic support is essential.

Chronic obstruction of the cystic duct may lead to the interesting finding of the "milk of calcium" gallbladder or "limy bile" syndrome. In this situation, complete obstruction of the cystic duct leads to a hydropic gallbladder. Bile pigments are deconjugated to colorless compounds and excess calcium is secreted, opacifying the bile to a white appearance both visually and radiographically. Calcium accumulating in the wall of the gallbladder secondary to chronic cystic duct obstruction may produce the "porcelain gallbladder." This condition appears secondary to chronic cholecystitis and in adults leads to carcinoma in as many as 50% of cases.[153] Courvoisier's gallbladder is a markedly enlarged gallbladder secondary to chronic, often malignant obstruction of the common bile duct.[154] This condition is unusual in adults and has not been reported in children.

CHOLEDOCHOLITHIASIS (COMMON BILE DUCT STONES)

Once considered rare, common bile duct stones have become more common in children.[130] Most ductal stones in children are black pigment or cholesterol stones. Both of these types of stones originate from the gallbladder. Less common are brown pigment stones, which form within the common bile duct secondary to infection.[83] Chronic stone passage can lead to papillary stenosis, although stones can be trapped within the common bile duct because of congenital narrowing or stenosis.[155] The usual clinical presentation of common bile duct stones in children is jaundice, with or without pain, and can progress to symptoms similar to those of cholecystitis. Right upper quadrant pain with fever is common. Pancreatitis is also possible, as the distal common bile duct traverses through the head of the pancreas, and a stone in the bile duct can obstruct the pancreatic duct.

Laboratory evaluation may reveal leukocytosis, elevated aminotransferase levels, and specific elevations of biliary tract enzymes such as alkaline phosphatase and GGT. If fever is present, blood cultures may be positive and require broad-spectrum antibiotic coverage, as with cholecystitis. Abdominal ultrasound is indicated to detect the presence of stones or ductal dilation. The bile duct diameter varies by age with a normal adult bile duct of 5 mm, less than 1.6 mm in children less than 1 year of age, and less than 3.3 mm in early adolescence.[156-159] When present, stones or sludge may be visualized in the distal common bile duct. Magnetic resonance cholangiopancreatography (MRCP) is a useful diagnostic tool for viewing lithiasis in the pancreaticobiliary tree and does not require contrast; however, sedation may be necessary (Figure 79-4). MRCP is especially useful if suspected stones are not detected by ultrasound.[160-163] Endoscopic ultrasound (EUS) is another diagnostic tool used with increasing frequency in children, which can give a description of both gallstones and choledocholithiasis as well as pancreatic parenchymal and ductal abnormalities.

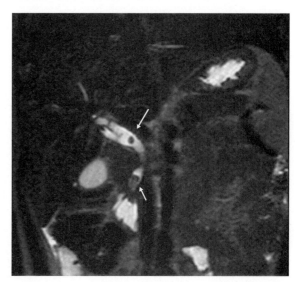

Figure 79-4. T2 axial MRCP of a 5-year-old male with pancreatitis and jaundice demonstrating two filling defects (white arrows). ERCP confirmed lithiasis.

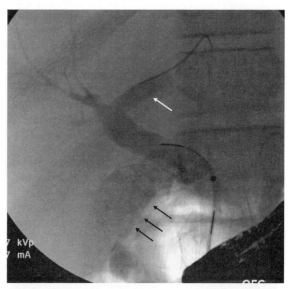

Figure 79-5. Fluoroscopic view during an ERCP of a patient with dilated bile duct and multiple intraductal stones. Left hepatic duct stone (white arrow) and gallbladder (black arrows) filled with gallstones.

ERCP is an excellent tool for both diagnosis and therapy, including sphincterotomy, stone removal, dilation of a stenosis, or stent placement. The use of ERCP has become much more common in children, even infants[133,164-166] (Figures 79-5 through 79-8). For choledocholithiasis not removed by standard methods, stent therapy may be a temporary solution to decompress the biliary system along with antibiotics until definitive therapy can be performed. Alternatively, choledochoscopy with intraductal lithotripsy (electrohydraulic or holmium laser) can be performed for large or difficult stones (Figure 79-9A,B). Although biliary stones can pass without intervention, a dilated biliary tree with accompanying fever necessitates prompt endoscopic or surgical intervention, with drainage and stone removal. Other relative indications for ERCP in choledocholithiasis include persistent conjugated hyperbilirubinemia,

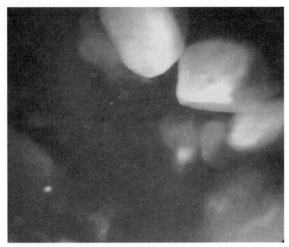

Figure 79-6. Endoscopic view of multiple large cholesterol stones in a morbidly obese teenager. *(See plate section for color.)*

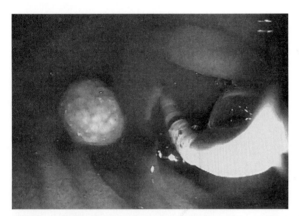

Figure 79-7. Endoscopic view of a spherical gallstone in a patient with Duchenne's muscular dystrophy. *(See plate section for color.)*

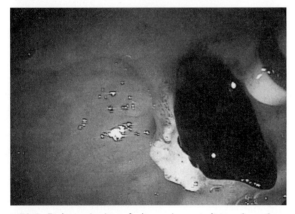

Figure 79-8. Endoscopic view of a large pigmented stone in an 8-year-old with autoimmune hemolytic anemia. *(See plate section for color.)*

pancreatitis with obstructing stone, or markedly dilated bile duct with or without pain or other biochemical abnormalities. ERCP can be performed precholecystectomy, or alternatively, intraoperative cholangiogram (IOC) may be performed at time of cholecystectomy. If a filling defect is visualized or failure of contrast excretion from the bile duct to the duodenum, ERCP can be performed.

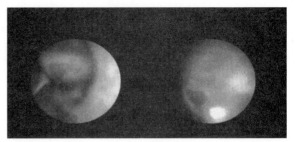

Figure 79-9. Choledochoscopy views of common bile duct stone. Image on right is before holmium YAG laser lithotripsy. *(See plate section for color.)* Courtesy Dr. Isaac Raijman.

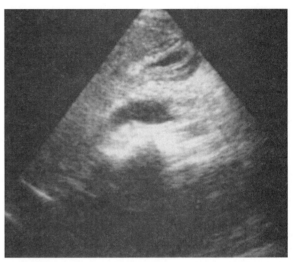

Figure 79-10. Ultrasound of dilated gallbladder with a thickened wall. Courtesy Dr. Robert V. Dutton.

ACALCULOUS CHOLECYSTITIS

Cholecystitis can occur without the presence of gallstones. This condition is rare in adults, but occurs with surprising frequency in pediatrics, the acute form usually in extremely ill children. The cause is not known but is associated with the immediate postoperative state, trauma, or burns. Sepsis from a variety of organisms, including *Leptospira*, group A beta-hemolytic streptococci, *Shigella*, *Salmonella*, and *E. coli*, has been associated with this condition, although no organism has emerged as the definitive cause.[167] A variety of other conditions are also associated with acalculous cholecystitis, including congestive heart failure, diabetes, malignant disease, and systemic vasculitis.[168,169] Because no obstructing stone is present, gallbladder stasis likely plays an important role and, although controversial, may be found with sludge. The stasis may be due to fever, dehydration, prolonged fasting, ileus, or TPN, which are common in the severely ill child.[167]

The clinical findings are usually fever, abdominal pain, and jaundice. Physical examination reveals a palpable abdominal mass, quite tender to touch. Laboratory studies are usually not helpful, but may reveal leukocytosis and elevated bilirubin levels. Diagnosis is aided by ultrasound identification of a large, distended gallbladder with a thickened wall (Figure 79-10) and tenderness during the procedure (ultrasonographic Murphy's sign). Biliary scintigraphy also is accurate, revealing normal liver uptake but no visualization of the gallbladder. Unfortunately, false-negative results of both ultrasound and scintigraphy occur in as many as 20% of cases when no stone is seen.[170]

Along with treatment of causative disease process, the treatment is either cholecystectomy or cholecystostomy. Because the incidence of gallbladder gangrene is rare in children as compared with adults, simple drainage is appropriate. If gangrene is suspected on inspection of the gallbladder at laparotomy, resection is necessary.

ACUTE HYDROPS OF THE GALLBLADDER

Hydrops of the gallbladder is characterized by distention without inflammation. The distinction between acalculous cholecystitis and hydrops is therefore one of histology. Clinically, the differentiation of these two entities may be difficult. Most cases of acalculous cholecystitis are in severely ill patients, whereas hydrops tends to occur in a more benign setting, frequently involving a systemic vasculitis. Kawasaki syndrome (mucocutaneous lymph node syndrome) is the most common cause of gallbladder hydrops.[171] Hydrops also has been associated with other vascular disorders, such as Sjögren's disease, systemic sclerosis, and Henoch-Schönlein purpura, as well as nephrotic syndrome, familial Mediterranean fever, mesenteric adenitis, leptospirosis, Epstein-Barr virus, and bacterial infection with *Staphylococcus* and *Streptococcus*.[167,172,173] The cause is unknown, although local lymph node enlargement around the cystic duct and local vasculitis causing gallbladder ischemia are potential mechanisms.

The clinical presentation is acute right upper quadrant abdominal pain, nausea, and vomiting. Examination reveals upper abdominal tenderness, often with a palpable mass. Diagnosis is aided by ultrasound findings of a distended gallbladder with a thin or normal wall and no echo densities. Biochemical studies are usually indistinguishable from other biliary diseases. Medical management is supportive, but surgical consultation should be obtained in all cases of suspected hydrops, although surgical intervention is rarely indicated. The development of fever or an increasingly tender abdomen suggests perforation and requires surgery. Most cases show steady resolution over about 2 weeks, without known long-term sequelae.

UNUSUAL DISEASES OF THE GALLBLADDER

Carcinoma of the gallbladder has been reported in children, but is rare.[174] In adults, gallbladder carcinoma is usually associated with gallstones. Although commoner than gallbladder carcinoma in children, benign gallbladder tumors also are rare. Adenomatous polyps have been described associated with Peutz-Jeghers syndrome.[175]

Adenomyomatosis, or hyperplastic gallbladder, denotes hyperplasia of the mucous membrane, thickening of the muscularis, and deep diverticular formations known as *Rokitansky-Aschoff sinuses*.[72] Odd deformities of the gallbladder, such as the phrygian cap, fish-hook anomaly, and Hartmann's pouch, are associated with adenomyomatosis of the gallbladder.[3] The cause

of the hyperplasia is unknown, although increased intraluminal gallbladder pressure has been implicated. No specific symptoms have ever been attributed to this condition; therefore, no specific therapy is advised. Duplications of both the gallbladder and common bile duct have also been described.[176,177]

Cholesterolosis is characterized by accumulation of cholesterol esters in the mucosa and submucosa of the gallbladder. After resection, these areas are visible as yellow spots on a red mucosal background, giving the appearance of a strawberry; hence the term *strawberry gallbladder*. Occasionally, these areas enlarge and become polypoid, leading to cystic duct obstruction. Typically, though, no symptoms are directly attributed to this condition and thus no therapy is indicated. If symptoms do occur, cholecystectomy is indicated.

Metachromatic leukodystrophy, or sulfatide lipidosis, is an autosomal recessive disorder of sphingolipid metabolism. The biochemical defect is the absence or deficiency of the lysosomal enzyme arylsulfatase A disorder and the inability to degrade sphingolipid sulfatide or galactose-3 sulfate ceramide. This results in the accumulation of sulfatide in both neural and nonneural tissues, in particular the gallbladder. Gallstones have been reported in association with this disorder and may be related to gallbladder hypomotility secondary to sulfatide accumulation in the wall of the gallbladder or sulfatide granules serving as "seeds" for gallstone formation.[178]

Polypoid gastric heterotopia in the gallbladder is extremely rare in children, consisting of polyps within the gallbladder with ectopic gastric mucosa.[179] Gallbladder polyps are usually asymptomatic and occur in association with other diseases such as Crohn's disease, Peutz-Jeghers syndrome, or leukodystrophy.[180,181] The presence of ectopic gastric mucosa may allow acid secretion, causing mucosal inflammation leading to cholecystitis.

Gallstones have been noted in pseudohypoaldosteronism,[182] presumed secondary to dehydration and electrolyte abnormalities. Wildervanck's syndrome (cervico-oculo-acoustic syndrome) also has been found to include gallstones,[183] although the cause is unknown.

REFERENCES

2. Everhart JE, Ruhl CE. Burden of digestive diseases in the United States Part III: Liver, biliary tract and pancreas. Gastroenterology 2009;136:1134–1144.
25. Lammert F, Sauerbruch T. Mechanisms of disease: the genetic epidemiology of gallbladder stones. Nat Clin Pract Gastroenterol Hepatol 2005;2:423–433.
40. Friesen CA, Roberts CC. Cholelithiasis: clinical characteristics in children, case analysis and literature review. Clin Pediatr 1989;28:294.
50. Hay DW, Carey MC. Pathophysiology and pathogenesis of cholesterol gallstone formation. Semin Liver Dis 1990;10:159–170.
70. Biddinger SB, Haas JT, Yu BB, et al. Hepatic insulin resistance directly promotes formation of cholesterol gallstones. Nat Med 2008;14:778–782.

See expertconsult.com for a complete list of references and the review questions for this chapter.

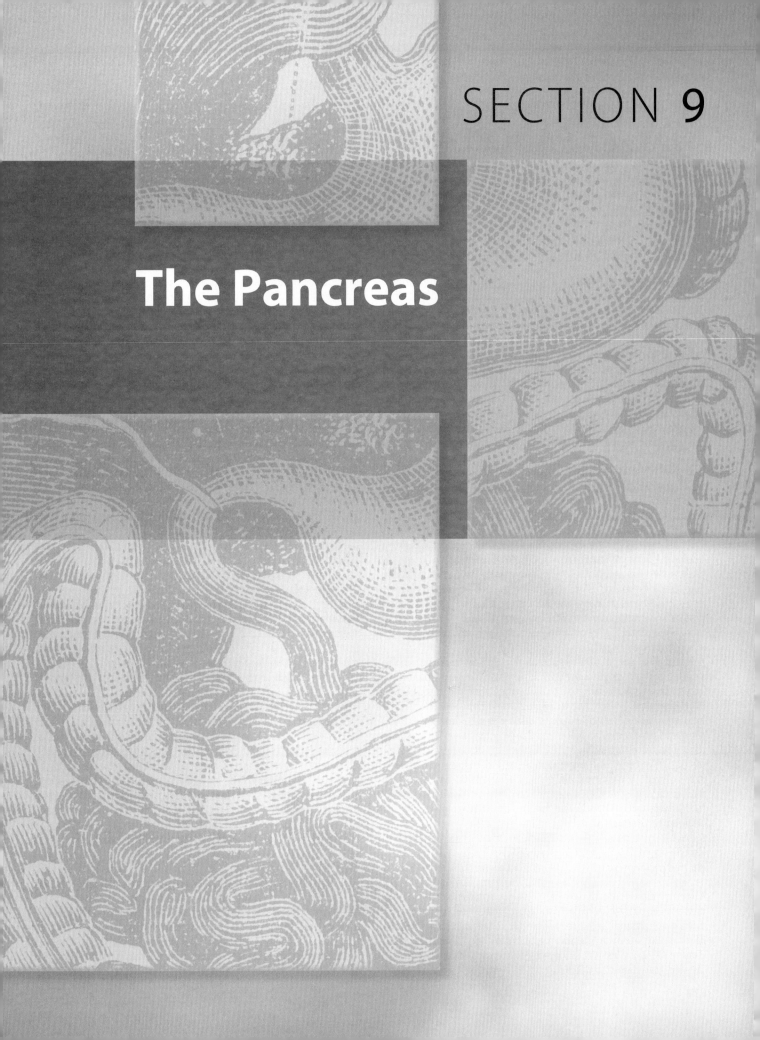

SECTION 9

The Pancreas

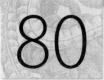

80 PANCREATIC DEVELOPMENT

Aaron Turkish • Sohail Z. Husain

BUDS FORM AND FUSE

The pancreas arises during mid-gestation from posterior foregut endoderm.[1] Morphologically, two buds, a dorsal and ventral, form, then migrate toward one another, and eventually fuse. At day 26 of gestation, the foregut evaginates into a condensation of overlying mesenchyme to form the first morphologic evidence of the dorsal bud; 6 days later, a ventral bud forms. Both buds undergo elongation of a stalk region and branched morphogenesis of the apical portions. At 37 to 42 days, the ventral pancreas rotates around the duodenum and fuses with the dorsal pancreas (see Figure 81-4).

DUCTAL SYSTEM FORMS

The dorsal pancreas forms the tail, body, and superior portion of the pancreatic head along with the distal portion of the main pancreatic duct (of Wirsung) and all of the minor accessory duct (of Santorini) (Figure 80-1). The ventral pancreas forms the uncinate process and the inferior part of the head. It also contributes the proximal portion of the main pancreatic duct. The two duct systems corresponding to the ventral and dorsal buds fail to fuse in 5 to 10% of the general population; these data come primarily from autopsy reports.[2] In this situation, termed *pancreas divisum*, the accessory duct functions as the main conduit for drainage of pancreatic juice. The possible pathologic significance of pancreas divisum is discussed further in Chapter 82.

Failure of the ventral pancreas to fully rotate around the duodenum can lead to the development of annular pancreas, in which a ring of pancreatic tissue constricts the duodenum. The condition presents with high-grade small bowel obstruction in roughly half of patients during the neonatal period.[3] An alternative hypothesis for annular pancreas formation is that the pancreas abnormally hypertrophies around the duodenum during development.[4] For example, mice lacking the signaling molecule Indian hedgehog (Ihh) develop increased ventral pancreatic mass, and just under half form an annulus around the duodenum.[5] The clinical features of annular pancreas are detailed in Chapter 82.

DIFFERENTIATION OF PANCREATIC PROGENITORS

After the pancreatic buds fuse, the cellular architecture of the pancreas rapidly expands. Notably, all three functionally distinct parenchymal cell types – acinar, duct, and islet cells – differentiate from a common pancreatic progenitor lineage (Figure 80-2). Classical studies by Rutter and colleagues have divided pancreatic differentiation into two distinct phases.[6]

The first, termed the primary transition, is defined as the conversion of predifferentiated cells to a protodifferentiated state in which low levels of pancreas-specific proteins are present. The second phase, or the secondary transition, is marked by a dramatic rise in pancreatic cell number and pancreas-specific protein synthesis, as well as an acceleration in both exocrine and endocrine differentiation. Ultrastructurally, acinar cells at this stage develop their characteristic abundance of endoplasmic reticulum and dense apically localized zymogen granules.[7] Although the dorsal pancreas arises before the ventral, both appear to exhibit simultaneous exocrine differentiation according to the two phases.[8]

In the ontogeny of endocrine cells in mouse, glucagon-positive alpha cells initially predominate.[9] After the secondary transition, however, insulin-positive beta cells outnumber all other endocrine cell types. In addition, a remarkable morphologic transformation occurs in the endocrine lineage. Although they start off as epithelial cells, it is thought that at this point in development, instead of dividing parallel to the basement membrane, they begin to divide perpendicular to it.[7] The newly oriented cell descendants lose their tight junctions and connections to the lumen. The process causes the endocrine lineage to undergo epithelial-to-mesenchymal transformation.[1]

The sequence and signaling factors that guide pancreatic development appear to be strikingly similar across vertebrate species, differing mostly in the time to organ formation.[10] Indeed, much of our knowledge base is derived from the manipulation of the mouse genome.[11] However, there are three notable differences in endocrine pancreas development between mice and humans.[12] First, in contrast to the scenario in mice, beta cells in humans appear before alpha cells. Second, the first identifiable human endocrine cells arise much later in the relative frame of development. Third, however, human islets are fully formed before the second trimester (by 12 to 13 weeks of gestation[12]), whereas islets assemble just before term in the mouse. Although the significance of these differences is unclear, they remind us of the need to confirm findings from animal models.

PROGRAMMED DEVELOPMENT BY HIERARCHICAL SIGNALS

The morphologic changes in the pancreas and the cellular growth, expansion, and differentiation of pancreatic progenitors are orchestrated by hierarchical signals from two distinct sources: (1) from within the genome of the pancreas, notably by a host of transcription factors,[13] and (2) from tissues and structures adjacent to the forming pancreas. Each will be discussed later.

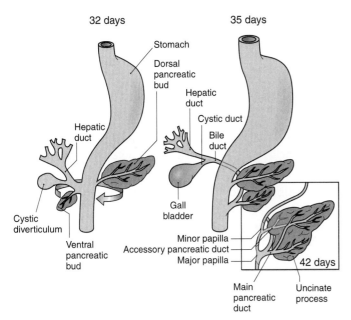

Figure 80-1. Development of the pancreas and its duct systems. The ventral pancreatic bud rotates around the duodenum to fuse with the dorsal bud. Contributing pancreatic structures from each of the buds are denoted. Adapted from Larson (2001), with permission.[208]

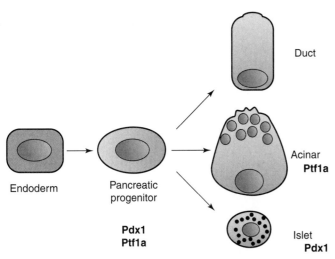

Figure 80-2. A single pancreatic progenitor gives rise to all three pancreatic lineages.

Transcriptional Factors Mediate Pancreatic Development

Transcriptions factors are proteins that bind to specific DNA sequences.[14] They function to either activate or suppress the recruitment of RNA polymerase, required for transcription. Transcription factors are classified according to their DNA binding domains. Recent genetic tools have utilized transcription factors to determine lineage relationships between populations of progenitor cells and their descendants during organogenesis.[15] The principle is to permanently tag a cell that expresses a transcription factor, even transiently, by recombinase-based fate mapping, in order to follow its progeny. Briefly, the DNA sequence binding to a transcription factor of interest is inserted into the genome along with the sequence for a recombinase

enzyme (e.g., Cre- or Flp-recombinase). Another sequence containing a ubiquitous promoter, followed by recombinase target sites and a reporter gene, is also inserted. The latter sequence does not lead to expression of the reporter because a "STOP" cassette is engineered between the recombinase targets. However, endogenous expression of the transcription factor triggers a chain of events in which first the recombinase is expressed. It then binds to its target sites and excises the intervening sequence containing the "STOP" cassette, thus allowing reporter gene expression in the cell. Because the excision event modifies genomic DNA, the recombined allele is stably inherited by progeny cells. The result is that all cell lineages derived from the progenitor express the reporter. Based on this genetic lineage analysis, the role of a large array of transcription factors was delineated. A summary of a few key factors is provided next.

Pdx1

Pancreatic and duodenal homeobox 1 (Pdx1), also known as insulin promoter factor 1 (Ipf1) or islet/duodenum homeobox 1 (IDX1), is the earliest pancreas-specific transcription factor, detected at 5 weeks of development, before bud formation.[12,16] Thus Pdx1 is used as a marker of early pancreatic progenitors. Studies on pancreatic development frequently target the Pdx1 gene as a promoter for pancreas gene-specific events. Deletion of Pdx1 in mice[17] and humans[18] leads to pancreatic agenesis, highlighting its importance in morphogenesis. The first reported human case was homozygous for an inactivating single nucleotide mutation in PDX1. She was small for gestational age and presented with neonatal diabetes mellitus along with pancreatic exocrine insufficiency. Notably though, her heterozygote parents had subtle findings; her father had adult-onset diabetes, and her mother was diagnosed with gestational diabetes. Indeed, Pdx1 has been identified as the MODY4 gene, a defect contributing to maturity onset diabetes of the young (MODY).[19] Pdx1-deficiency prevents the pancreatic epithelium from responding to mesenchymal growth-promoting signals.[20]

Pdx1 is itself regulated by several upstream transcription factors. The winged-helix transcription factors Foxa1 and Foxa2 co-occupy multiple regulatory domains on the Pdx1 gene and are essential in controlling the expansion and differentiation of the pancreatic primordium.[21] Mice with compound, conditional ablation of both Foxa1 and Foxa2 resulted in loss of Pdx1 expression, severely disrupted acinar and islet development, and neonatal death. During adulthood, Pdx1 expression becomes largely confined to the beta cells, where it binds to and activates the insulin promoter.[16] Conditional inactivation of Pdx1 in adult mouse beta cells results in diabetes.[22] Thus Pdx1 is required for proper pancreas development as well as beta cell function.

Ptf1a

The alpha subunit of pancreas-specific transcription factor 1 (Ptf1a), also known as p48, is a basic helix-loop-helix protein that functions as part of a trimeric protein complex in the regulation of exocrine gene expression.[23] It is initially coexpressed with Pdx1 and supports the specification of all three pancreatic cell type precursors, but later becomes confined to acinar cells.[24,25] The temporal shift in expression pattern of Ptf1a can be explained by the finding that during embryonic development a 2.3-kb autoregulatory enhancer region initiates expression of Ptf1a in the early precursor epithelium and then superinduces expression in nascent acinar cells.[26] In mature acinar cells, the enhancer, along with the active trimeric form of Ptf1a, establishes an autoregulatory loop that reinforces and maintains Ptf1a expression.

Ptf1a deficiency in mice results in pancreatic agenesis with complete absence of exocrine development, but ectopic endocrine cells can still be found.[27] In a human pedigree, a truncating single nucleotide mutation in Ptf1a led to pancreatic and cerebellar agenesis.[28]

Hlxb9

Human homeobox gene 9 (Hlxb9) is expressed as early as the eighth somite stage in the notochord and pancreatic endoderm. Hlxb9-deficient mice have complete agenesis of the dorsal pancreas, but only minimal defects of the ventral portion.[29,30] However, persistent Hlxb9 expression under the control of Pdx1 leads to impaired pancreas development.[31] The dual results with Hlxb9 highlight a common theme in development, which is that a delicate temporal and spatial balance of transcription factor expression is essential for proper pancreas development. Postdevelopment, Hlxb9 expression within the pancreas is maintained only in beta cells.[29,30]

Ngn-3

Neurogenin3 (Ngn3) is a basic helix-loop-helix transcription factor that heralds the differentiation of Pdx1-expressing progenitor cells into an endocrine lineage.[32] Interestingly, Ngn3 expression is down-regulated after endocrine differentiation initiates. Mice completely deficient in Ngn3 lack pancreatic endocrine cells.[33] However, patients with a hypomorphic mutation in Ngn3 develop a profound congenital diarrhea, but not neonatal diabetes.[34] Taken together, the results suggest that low levels of Ngn3 expression are required for endocrine differentiation.[35]

Additional transcriptions factors involved in endocrine specification include Mafa, Isl1, Brn-4, NeuroD, Nkx6.1, Nkx2.2, Pax4, Pax6, and Arx.[10]

Signals from Adjacent Structures and Tissues

In addition to the critical role of transcription factors expressed from within the developing pancreas, fluctuating levels of signaling proteins from adjacent tissues and structures also control pancreatic development. Early on, pancreas specification from endoderm requires that suppression of Wnt and fibroblast growth factor 4 (FGF4) signaling from adjacent mesoderm.[36,37] In addition, mesodermal retinoic acid signals refine the anterior-posterior position in which the pancreas can develop.[38-40]

The relation of dorsal and ventral pancreas to their respective structures allows for them to be specified differently. Early in embryonic development, the notochord is in direct contact with the dorsal pancreas and controls its development. Removal of the notochord prevents expression of pancreatic exocrine and endocrine markers from the dorsal bud, whereas coculture of notochord with endoderm initiates and maintains pancreatic gene expression.[41] Signals from the notochord permit dorsal pancreas specification by suppressing the expression of the anti-pancreatic factor sonic hedgehog (Shh).[42,43] In contrast, development of the ventral pancreas is dependent on withdrawal of FGF signaling from adjacent cardiac mesenchyme.[44] The expression of factors from nascent organs adjacent to the pancreas, such as notochord and heart, also regulates pancreatic development.

Endothelial Cells

At a later period, endothelial tissue, such as dorsal aorta and the vitelline veins, influences pancreatic development.[45,46] For example, dorsal aorta could induce in isolated endoderm Pdx1 and insulin expression.[46] In addition to points of endodermal-endothelial contact, sphingosine-1-phosphate secreted by endothelial cells in circulation promotes dorsal pancreatic budding.[47]

Pancreatic Mesenchyme and Stroma

Growth factors secreted by pancreatic mesenchymal cells also appear to be important to development of the endodermal primordium.[48] The presence of mesenchyme shifts the growth state of pancreatic progenitors from differentiation to proliferation. Notably, the mesenchymal factor FGF-10 promotes proliferation. FGF-10 deficient mice exhibit severe growth retardation of the pancreas.[49] On the other hand, overexpression of FGF-10 controlled by the Pdx1 promoter results in sustained proliferation over differentiation.[50,51] FGF-10 signaling causes activation of the Notch pathway.[50-52] Mice deficient in various Notch signaling components show accelerated differentiation and less proliferation, resulting in pancreas hypoplasia.[32,53-55] Overexpression of Notch1 in pancreatic epithelium prevents endocrine and exocrine differentiation.[56-58] The Notch target gene Hes1 may be preventing p57-mediated cell cycle exit, required for differentiation during early stages of pancreas formation.[59] The importance of ensuring pancreatic progenitor proliferation is underscored by the finding that the final size of the pancreas is determined by the original number of progenitor cells present at an early embryonic stage.[60] Stromal components also influence the pancreas during development. For example, neural crest cells that migrate into the pancreas influence beta cell number.[61] Finally, it is also likely that the pancreas contributes instructive signals to its adjacent tissues; however, the postulate has not been well characterized.

Epigenetic Control

The epigenetic modification of chromatin by either loosening or compacting its structure via histone acetylation or deacetylation, respectively, constitutes an important mode of guiding pancreatic development. Both expression and activity of histone deacetylase (HDAC) are reduced over embryonic life into adulthood in the rat.[62] Using an in vitro embryonic culture method of the pancreas, pharmacologic inhibition of HDAC classes I and II abolishes acinar cell differentiation but enhances ductal and beta cell pools. The results indicate a role for histone modification in determining pancreatic cell fate.

Bioelectric Theory

Finally, an additional signaling mechanism for embryonic development is based on what has been termed the "bioelectric" theory.[63] Ion transporters are differentially expressed in developing embryonic cells to generate pH and voltage gradients. The resulting ion flux regulates in certain developmental systems critical functions such as left-right patterning or limb growth.[64] In the adult state, these biophysical signals can trigger regenerative potential. Although not yet confirmed, it is

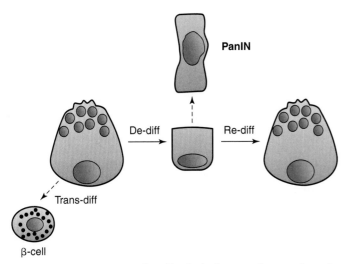

Figure 80-3. Mature acinar cell are "facultative" pancreatic progenitor cells. They have the capacity to regenerate, transdifferentiate, or undergo neoplastic change.

plausible that bioelectric gradients might play an important role in shaping pancreatic development as well.

REGENERATIVE CAPACITY OF THE PANCREAS

The importance of understanding early pancreatic development is underscored by recent work showing that in certain conditions, various aspects of pancreatic development reemerge. This reemergence is not simply an epiphenomenon, but is necessary for the regenerative component of recovery. Regeneration can occur to varying degrees in the pancreas during pregnancy,[65] partial pancreatectomy,[66] or pancreatitis.[67,68]

Regenerative Capacity after Pancreatitis

A prime example of this regenerative potential occurs after the injury of pancreatitis. Pancreatitis induced in mice by intraperitoneal administration over a 2-day period with high concentrations of a cholecystokinin analogue results in about a 50% dropout of acinar cells.[68] However, 7 days after the injury, the exocrine gland is almost completely restored. In response to the injury, the pancreas activates regenerative processes to maintain tissue homeostasis. Although there are differing views, the prevailing notion is that after injury, acinar cells might dedifferentiate into a ductal epithelium that expresses early developmental factors. These "facultative" progenitor cells would then redifferentiate into mature acinar cells[69,70] (Figure 80-3).

Reemergence of Embryonic Transcriptional Factors

Acinar cells that survive pancreatic injury induce genes normally associated with early embryonic progenitor cells, including Pdx1 and Notch pathway components such as Notch1, Notch2, Jagged2, and Hes1.[68] In addition, beta-catenin is expressed, a marker that is normally found in undifferentiated proliferating exocrine progenitor cells.[71,72] Reactivation of the Notch signaling pathway during injury from cerulein-induced pancreatitis is required for acinar cell regeneration.[73] Mice

that were either chemically treated with a gamma-secretase inhibitor to block Notch receptor cleavage or conditionally deficient in Notch1 had fewer mature acinar cells after acute pancreatitis.

In addition, embryonic signaling by Hedgehog is upregulated in acinar cells after cerulein-induced pancreatitis.[74] Hedgehog blockade, either pharmacologically or genetically using Pdx1- or Elastase-Cre recombinase, allows the formation of a ductal epithelium from acinar cells, but it does not permit redifferentiation into acini. Intriguingly, it was suggested that the "redifferentiation arrest" might provide a link between pancreatitis injury and subsequent neoplasia. The results also underscore the capacity of the acinar cell to revert to an earlier progenitor state in response to injury.

Significance of Pancreatic Development on Postnatal Pancreatic Disorders

The degree to which regeneration of the pancreas occurs after pancreatitis may turn out to be as important in determining the outcome of the disease as the level of inflammation induced by the injury. Thus, these and other studies might in the near future be utilized to enhance the recovery phase after pancreatitis and thus perhaps cause net improvement in pancreatitis outcome.

Another intriguing aspect to the balance between pancreatic regeneration/recovery and injury is that a reduced regenerative response might explain why certain patients are predisposed to pancreatitis. For example, as mentioned earlier, HDACs exert epigenetic control over pancreatic development. Treatment of developing mouse embryos in vitro with the HDAC class 1 inhibitor valproic acid (VPA) reduces acinar cell differentiation and leads to the development of cystic structures in the pancreas.[62] Interestingly, VPA use is highly associated with pancreatitis.[75,76] Thus medications like VPA, which inhibit acinar cell development during embryonic development, might also prevent the necessary regeneration that mimics development after pancreatitis.

The pluripotential of the pancreas has recently been utilized to cause transdifferentiation of acinar cells to beta cells that can secrete insulin. Adenoviral vectors expressing early progenitor and islet transcription factors Pdx1, Neurogenin3, and Mafa were directly injected into the tail of the pancreas in vivo.[77] They primarily infected acinar cells, and within days, greater than 20% of former acinar cells, evidenced by genetic lineage tracing, began to express insulin and assumed beta cell morphology. The results confirm the potential of the acinar cell to undergo forced transdifferentiation. They also offer the prospect of an endogenous pancreatic source of beta cells to treat diabetes. By borrowing genetic cues from a basic understanding of pancreatic development, this ingenious approach might provide a new paradigm to rescue type 1 diabetes using a large acinar cell reserve.

Reemergence of Embryonic Transcriptional Factors or Their Forced Expression Can Result in Metaplasia

The change of acinar cells to either a progenitor-like state or another cell type, however, runs the risk of malignant transformation. Mounting evidence suggests that pancreatic ductal adenocarcinoma (PDAC) and it noninvasive precursor lesions known as pancreatic intraepithelial neoplasia (PanIN) are the result of acinar cell metaplasia to a ductal cell form. Conditional expression of oncogenic Kras along with Notch using Pdx1 Cre-recombinase synergistically causes mature acinar cells to convert to PanIN lesions.[78] The study further supports the theory that PDAC can arise from acinar or acinar-like cells when early embryonic factors reemerge.

SUMMARY ON PANCREATIC DEVELOPMENT

In summary, the pancreas is formed from the fusion of ventral and dorsal endodermal buds. All three pancreatic parenchymal cells arise from common pancreatic progenitor cell. Pancreatic development is delicately controlled by the temporal expression of various transcriptional factors. Adjacent tissues secrete factors that also control pancreatic development. Factors observed primarily during embryonic development may reemerge during situations requiring pancreatic cells to assume a pluripotential state in order to regenerate the pancreas, such as in response to injury after pancreatitis. Harnessing the pluripotent capacity of the pancreas may yield future therapies aimed at augmenting cell types, such as beta cells in the setting of diabetes. Thus, an improved understanding of pancreatic development may provide crucial translational tools to treat pancreatic disorders in both children and adults.

PANCREATIC SECRETION AND EXOCRINE FUNCTION

Overview of Pancreatic Physiology

The pancreas is a vital endocrine and exocrine organ responsible for the release of hormones and the secretion of fluid, electrolytes, and various enzymes that are intricately involved in the digestion of food. Although pancreatic secretion has traditionally thought to be under distinct hormonal and neuronal regulation, there is increasing evidence that its regulation is mediated by a complex neuroendocrinologic interplay.[79] Within this milieu, a variety of stimulatory and inhibitory factors regulate pancreatic secretion.

Functional Anatomy of the Exocrine Pancreas

More than 80% of the exocrine pancreas is composed of clusters of acini lobules within a network of connective tissue[79-81] (Figure 80-4). The acinus, a spherical or tubular group of pyramidal cells arranged with their apices toward its center, synthesizes, stores, and releases pancreatic digestive enzymes.[79] The basal region of the acinar cell contains the nucleus and endoplasmic reticulum, where proteins and digestive enzymes are synthesized.[80,82] The rate of synthesis is 10 million enzyme molecules per acinar cell per minute.[83] These enzymes are then sorted and packaged into secretory (zymogen) granules in the Golgi complex, transported, and stored in the apical region of the cell until their release via exocytosis.[80] The entire process from enzymatic synthesis to the point at which enzymes are ready for secretion is about 50 minutes.[83]

There are several proteins thought to be involved with the intracellular transport of zymogen granules to the apical pole of the acinar cell. Muclin, a sulfated membrane mucin-like glycoprotein, and GP-2 are two proteins known to be involved with this process.[84] Several recent studies identified many of the

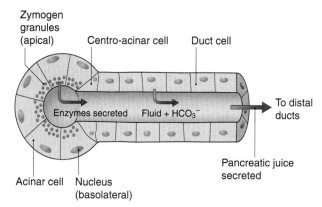

Figure 80-4. The acinus and cross-sectional appearance of the pancreatic ductule.

proteins localized to the zymogen granule membrane.[85,86] The most abundant are the monomeric G proteins, including the Rab proteins, which mediate intracellular transport. Recently there has been increasing evidence that the soluble N-ethylmaleimide-sensitive factor attachment protein receptor (SNARE) proteins play an important role in zymogen granule fusion with the apical membrane and exocytosis,[85,87,88] but their mechanism of action remains unclear.

The basolateral membrane of the acinar cell harbors multiple receptors for secretagogues such as cholecystokinin (CCK) and for neurotransmitters such as acetylcholine and vasoactive intestinal peptide (VIP).[79] Centroacinar (proximal ductular) cells that extend into the acinar lumen and pancreatic duct cells modify pancreatic juice by secretion of water and bicarbonate (HCO_3^-).[79,83] Intercalated ducts that empty into intralobular ducts drain these cells. Intralobular ducts drain into extralobular ducts that eventually drain into the main pancreatic duct, which, in combination with the common bile duct, enters the duodenum.

The endocrine cells of the pancreas are distributed within the islets of Langerhans. They are composed of A-cells, which produce glucagon; B-cells, which produce insulin; D-cells, which secrete the largely inhibitory hormone somatostatin; and F-cells, which secrete pancreatic polypeptide[79] in response to vagal stimulation. Acinar cells are exposed to endocrine secretions (in a reciprocal relationship) via cell-to-cell contact between exocrine and endocrine tissue as well as direct capillary connections between the islets and acini within the insulinoacinar portal system.[89,90] Islet cell hormones enter the systemic circulation via pancreatic blood flow. The pancreas also falls under the influence of a complex neuronal network composed of parasympathetic (vagal), sympathetic, peptidergic, and sensory innervates of glandular cells and vessels. The pancreas also has its own intrinsic nerve plexus, comparable to the enteric nervous system.[91]

Formation of Pancreatic Juice

About 1 liter of pancreatic juice is secreted into the small intestine per day[81,92]; it is a clear, isotonic, and colorless alkaline fluid composed of water, electrolytes, and enzymes important in the digestion of protein, fat, and starch.[93] The centroacinar and ductal cells are responsible for secretion of the HCO_3^- rich fluid that transports the digestive enzymes synthesized and secreted by the acinar cells into the small intestine (Figure 80-5).

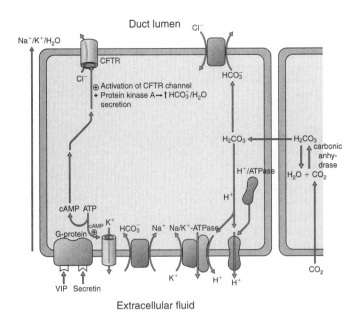

Figure 80-5. Model of fluid and bicarbonate secretion in a pancreatic duct cell. ATP, adenosine triphosphate; cAMP, cyclic adenosine monophosphate; CFTR, cystic fibrosis transmembrane conductance regulator; VIP, vasoactive intestinal peptide.

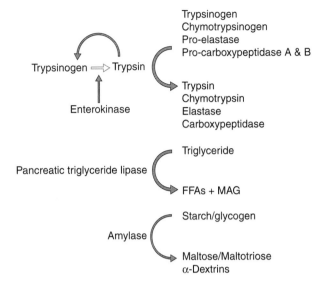

Figure 80-6. Digestive enzymes secreted by the pancreas. FFA, free fatty acids; MAG, monoacylglycerol.

Fluid and Electrolytes

Utilizing an osmotic gradient created by the active secretion of electrolytes such as sodium (Na^+), potassium (K^+), bicarbonate (HCO_3^-) and chloride (Cl^-), water enters pancreatic juice via passive diffusion[81] into the pancreatic duct lumen. There are two means by which HCO_3^- enters the cell: (1) The Na^+-HCO_3^- cotransporter on the basolateral membrane[94,95]; and (2) CO_2 is produced in the cell as a metabolic product or enters the cell via diffusion from the extracellular fluid by the action of H^+ on plasma HCO_3^-. Carbonic anhydrase hydrates CO_2 and produces carbonic acid (H_2CO_3), which then dissociates into HCO_3^- and H^+.[81]

There are several channels, transporters and exchangers on the basolateral membrane responsible for creating the pH and ionic gradients that drive HCO_3^- into the cell. Some animal studies have shown that the Na^+ gradient created by the Na^+, K^+-ATPase pump greatly contributes to HCO_3^- influx via the Na^+-HCO_3^- cotransporter.[96] Other evidence has revealed that an H^+-ATPase actively moves H^+ out of the cell, driving HCO_3^- back into the cell.[97] This vacuolar ATPase merges with the basolateral membrane via exocytosis in response to secretin. A Na^+-H^+ exchanger appears to play a minor role in H^+ efflux–induced HCO_3^- entry into the cell.[97] The gastrointestinal hormone secretin binds to its receptor on the basolateral membrane and activates adenylate cyclase to produce cyclic adenosine monophosphate (cAMP). A rise in cAMP activates the CFTR Cl^- channel on the luminal membrane, resulting in increased Cl^- secretion into the duct lumen.[98,99] This, in turn, induces an increase in HCO_3^- efflux into the lumen via the Cl-HCO_3^- exchanger. The resulting net luminal electronegative potential pulls Na^+ and K^+ into the lumen intercellularly, with a burst of water following this osmotic gradient.[81] HCO_3^- in pancreatic juice can then provide the necessary pH for digestion and absorption of protein, lipids and carbohydrates within the small intestine.

At rest, pancreatic juice is secreted at 0.2 mL/min and the bicarbonate concentration equals that of plasma. During secretin-induced stimulation, the rate of secretion increases to about 4.0 mL/min, and bicarbonate concentration increases asymptotically to a maximum of 140 mEq/L, creating a pH of about 8.2 in pancreatic juice.[92,93] The sum of Cl^- and HCO_3^- concentrations remains constant as the Cl^- concentration falls with increasing secretion rates. Pancreatic juice also contains calcium (Ca^{2+}) and small amounts of magnesium (Mg^{2+}), zinc (Zn^{2+}), phosphate (HPO_4^{2-}), and sulfate (SO_4^{2-}).[81]

Pancreatic Enzymes

Of pancreatic juice, 0.7 to 10% is composed of various proteins synthesized and secreted by the pancreas, including the digestive enzymes and proenzymes, plasma proteins, trypsin inhibitors, and mucoproteins.[81]

The digestive enzymes secreted by the pancreas are responsible for about half of overall digestion of nutrients in the gastrointestinal tract[79,81] and are composed of proteolytic, lipolytic, and amylolytic enzymes (Figure 80-6). Many are synthesized and stored in zymogen granules as inactive proenzymes before secretion in pancreatic juice and must be activated in the duodenum in order to possess activity. This also provides a degree of autoprotection by preventing pancreatic autodigestion by these proteins. Enzymes within the zymogen granules are in a solid form and solubilize once they enter the alkaline environment in the pancreatic ducts. In turn, these acid-sensitive enzymes are protected by the bicarbonate-rich pancreatic fluid in which they are transported.[82,92,100,101]

The proteolytic enzymes account for most enzymes in pancreatic juice and are secreted as inactive precursor enzymes.[81] Trypsinogen is a proenzyme that undergoes hydrolysis of its amino-terminal fragment via enterokinase at the intestinal brush border and is activated by its conversion to trypsin. Trypsin makes up about 19% of the protein and is the most abundant of all the pancreatic enzymes in pancreatic juice.[102] Several forms of trypsin with similar genetic and amino acid sequence have been identified, termed cationic trypsinogen (or PRSS1), anionic trypsinogen (PRSS2), mesotrypsinogen

(PRSS3), and, most recently, pancreasin.[102,103] Trypsin then catalyzes the activation of other proteolytic enzymes such as chymotrypsinogen, proelastase, procarboxypeptidase A and B, and trypsinogen itself. Carboxypeptidase cleaves peptide bonds at the carboxy-terminal ends of proteins. Trypsin cleaves interior peptide bonds involving basic amino acids. Chymotrypsin acts on interior peptide bonds involving aromatic amino acids, leucine, glutamine, and methionine. Elastase cleaves peptide bonds at neutral aliphatic amino acids, and it is the measurement of the inactive fragments of elastase in stool that is increasingly being used to determine sufficiency of exocrine pancreatic function.[102,104] The combined action of gastric pepsin and pancreatic proteases digests proteins into oligopeptides and amino acids, which are further digested by intestinal brush border enzymes before absorption.[92,100,105] There is significant overlap in the function of several of these proteases, highlighting the importance of adequate amino acid availability for growth and stability of an organism.[102] Trypsinogen activation within the acinar cell may be regulated by several factors including low calcium levels and protein compartmentalization.[102] The pancreas also secretes pancreatic secretory trypsin inhibitor, SPINK1, which acts as a first line of defense against pancreatic autodigestion by small amounts of active trypsin by binding to and inactivating 20% of trypsin.[106,107]

The intestinal epithelium is only able to absorb carbohydrates as monosaccharides, and depends on α-amylase to hydrolyze dietary starch into glucose. α-Amylase is secreted by the salivary glands and the pancreatic acinus in its active form, and digests dietary starch from plants and glycogen from animal sources. The major dietary starches are amylose, a straight-chained α-1,4-linked glucose polymer, and amylopectin, which has α-1,4-glucose linkages and α-1,6 linked branches. α-Amylase hydrolyzes α-1,4-glucose linkages but not α-1,6 linkages or terminal glucose residues of starch and glycogen. The products of amylase digestion are short-chain α-1,6-linked polysaccharides termed α-limit dextrins, composed of maltose (an α-1,4-linked glucose dimer), maltotriose (a trimer of α-1, 4-linked glucose molecules), and branched oligosaccharides with α-1,4 and α-1,6 linkages. Sucrase, glycoamylase, and isomaltase complete the digestion of dextrins at the intestinal brush border, allowing for glucose absorption by intestinal epithelial cells.[1]

Triglycerides account for the overwhelming majority of dietary lipid[108] and must be digested into fatty acids and monoacylglycerols before absorption by the intestine. Following emulsification of dietary lipids, gastric lipase secreted by chief cells begins the process and cleaves 15 to 20% of the fatty acids.[109,110] Several pancreatic lipases are secreted into pancreatic juice in their active forms[81,92] and complete the digestion of triglyceride in the upper small intestine via hydrolysis. When the pancreatic function fails, it is fat malabsorption that appears before protein and carbohydrate loss.[111] Although animal studies do not support its role in phospholipid digestion,[112] phospholipase A2 is able to hydrolyze phospholipids such as phosphatidylcholine at its sn-2 position to lysophosphatidyl choline and a free fatty acid.[92] Although its precise role in lipid digestion also remains unclear, carboxylesterase has a wide spectrum of substrate specificity,[113] including cholesterol esters, fat-soluble vitamin esters, tri-, di-, and monoacylglycerides, ceramides, and phospholipids.

Pancreatic triglyceride lipase (PTL) is the predominant enzyme responsible for triglyceride hydrolysis[114] at the sn-1

TABLE 80-1. Pancreatic Stimulatory and Inhibitory Factors

Stimulatory
Cholecystokinin (CCK)
Secretin
Vasoactive intestinal peptide (VIP)
Gastrin-releasing peptide (GRP)
Insulin
Gastrin
Nitric oxide
Serotonin
Substance P
Pancreatic phospholipase A$_2$
Natriuretic peptides (ANP, CNP)
Melatonin
Adenosine

Inhibitory
Somatostatin
Pancreatic polypeptide (PP)
Peptide YY
Neuropeptide Y
Calcitonin gene-related peptide (CGRP)
Glucagon
Serotonin
Enkephalins
Leptin
Ghrelin

and sn-3 positions, producing fatty acids and 2-monoacylglycerols that are absorbed by the intestinal epithelium. Interestingly, mice lacking PTL are capable of absorbing triglyceride but have markedly delayed and decreased cholesterol absorption.[115] Thus, other lipases must account for triglyceride absorption. The pancreas synthesizes two proteins with a high degree of sequence and structural homology to PTL, temporarily termed pancreatic lipase related proteins 1 and 2 (PLPR 1 and 2).[114,116] The function of PLPR1 remains undetermined. Human PLPR2 is a galactolipase and likely plays a major role in the digestion of plant lipids.[117] It is also capable of hydrolyzing retinyl palmitate and thus may play a role in the metabolism of vitamin A.[118] Because bile salts, dietary proteins, and phospholipids in the small intestine inhibit PTL, a pancreatic protein, colipase, is required for the full activity of PTL.[114,119,120] In concert with bile acids, which emulsify triglyceride droplets into smaller particles, colipase forms a 1:1 complex with PTL to greatly increase the surface area on which PTL can act.[92,114]

Regulation of Pancreatic Secretion

Regulation of pancreatic secretion is mediated by a complex interplay of several stimulatory and inhibitory gastrointestinal hormones and neuronal pathways (Table 80-1). There is an increasing body of evidence that other novel regulatory peptide hormones and neurotransmitters are also involved in pancreatic secretion. Pancreatic juice is secreted during basal, fasting states (the interdigestive period) and the postprandial (digestive) period.

Interdigestive Pancreatic Secretion

The interdigestive phase is cyclic and closely follows the pattern of the migrating myoelectric complex (MMC) in the intestine.[79,92] Phase I of the MMC is characterized by a lack of motility, with phases II and III possessing increasingly more activity. During phase I, pancreatic secretion of enzymes and bicarbonate is at its nadir (about 10% and 2% of maximum rates, respectively).[81] Every 60 to 120 minutes, there is a surge in intestinal motility associated with phases II and III of the MMC in the duodenum and a progressive increase in gastric acid, bile, and pancreatic secretion.[101,121,122] It is thought that this cyclic secretion of pancreatic juice is important in digestion of residual food, cellular debris, and pathogens in the duodenum during the interdigestive period. Although the mechanism of this process remains to be determined, it appears that the gastrointestinal hormones motilin and pancreatic polypeptide, as well as the autonomic nervous system, are involved with the regulation of MMC cycling.[79,121,123-125] Administration of motilin prematurely activates the MMC and shortens the frequency between peaks.[125] It appears that pancreatic polypeptide is an inhibitory hormone in this process. MMC blockade following the administration of atropine implicate a vagal cholinergic stimulatory role during the interdigestive period.[81]

Postprandial Pancreatic Secretion

Exocrine pancreatic secretion begins almost immediately after ingestion of a meal and is associated with an increase in the concentration of several pancreatic stimulatory and inhibitory hormones in plasma as well as neural stimulation via the vagus nerve. Postprandial pancreatic secretion is divided into three phases: the cephalic, gastric, and intestinal phases, which contribute 20%, 10%, and 70%, respectively, to the overall postprandial response.[126]

The cephalic phase is mediated by the vagus nerve in response to sight, smell, taste, and thought of food and accounts for a significant amount of pancreatic enzyme secretion and a smaller portion of HCO_3^- secretion.[79,81] This is accompanied by a rise in plasma gastrin and CCK, a minor rise in plasma secretin, and elevation of the inhibitory hormones pancreatic polypeptide and leptin.[79,127] Sham feeding studies in which subjects smell, taste, and chew but do not swallow food suggest that direct vagal stimulation of acinar cells is the major stimulant during the cephalic phase.[128] Because subjects with achlorhydria continue to secrete pancreatic juice during sham feeding, it is now thought that gastric acid secretion does not contribute substantially to the cephalic phase.[81] Sham feeding experiments that revealed an incomplete block of pancreatic secretion during atropine administration suggest that peptidergic neurons from the vagus nerve may directly activate acinar cells via release of stimulatory peptides such as vasoactive intestinal peptide (VIP) and gastrin-releasing peptide (GRP).[92] VIP is known to stimulate acinar cells and duct epithelial cells.[92,129]

The gastric phase begins when food enters the stomach, increasing the rate of pancreatic secretion of enzymes as the stomach distends.[130-132] Stimulation of mechanoreceptors in the body of the stomach activates the vagovagal cholinergic reflex that leads to a low-volume, enzyme-rich secretion from the pancreas.[92] The precise contribution of the gastric phase in postprandial pancreatic secretion has not been determined.

When gastric juice and food in the form of chyme enters the duodenum, the most important and final phase of postprandial pancreatic secretion, the intestinal phase, begins. The intestinal phase is neurohormonally regulated and produces the largest contribution to pancreatic secretion, with increases in both acinar and ductal secretions.[79,81] The major hormonal mediators of the intestinal phase are secretin and CCK. A vasovagal cholinergic neural input also contributes to secretion during this phase.[91]

Secretin

The proximal intestine plays an important role in pancreatic secretion by releasing secretin, the most potent stimulant of pancreatic fluid and HCO_3^-. Secretin is an intestinal hormone synthesized by S-type enteroendocrine cells in the proximal small intestine and is released in the presence of duodenal acidification, bile, and the products of protein and fat digestion.[79,81] The pH in the duodenum is the primary regulator of secretin release; the threshold for release of secretin and pancreatic HCO_3^- secretion is a pH of 4.5.[133,134] The means by which HCl stimulates secretin release has yet to be determined. Animal studies suggest a role for an uncharacterized secretin-releasing peptide and pancreatic phospholipase A_2 as a secretin-releasing peptide.[135,136] The release of secretin may also be augmented by nonacid factors such as fatty acids and other products of fat and protein digestion, as well as by the presence of bile in the upper intestinal tract.[92,137,138] It remains unclear whether secretin stimulates the pancreatic acinus directly via secretin-binding sites and/or via action on vagal afferents that directly stimulate pancreatic secretion. It has been proposed that secretin binds to the amino terminus of its receptor, revealing a previously concealed portion of the receptor that can bind to the core of the receptor.[139] Although CCK alone does not stimulate bicarbonate release, clearly it has a synergistic role in enhancing the secretin response.[140] When secretin is given simultaneously with vagal stimulation, the response is also highly augmented, suggesting that there is a cholinergic influence on pancreatic secretion.[141,142]

Cholecystokinin

CCK is the other major gastrointestinal hormone with a large influence on pancreatic secretion, primarily during the gastric and intestinal phases of digestion. It is secreted primarily by intestinal I cells in response to products of protein and fat digestion in the duodenum and stimulates pancreatic enzyme secretion.[79,81,92] Although intact protein and fat do not stimulate release of CCK, their digested products in the form of peptides, amino acids, fatty acids, and monoacylglycerol are potent promoters of its release.[143-146] Carbohydrate digestive products have little effect on CCK release.[92]

The CCK response to fatty acids differs based on chain length (C18 > C12 > C8), degree of saturation, concentration, and total amount of exposure in the gut.[147] The exact mechanism behind CCK release has yet to be determined. It is thought that an enterocyte secreted trypsin-sensitive peptide, CCK-releasing peptide (CCKRP), stimulates enterocytes to release CCK in response to exposure to digestive products.[92,148] During fasting periods, CCKRP is inactive because it is digested by free trypsin in the small intestine. During the postprandial phase, a duodenal protein load binds trypsin, and much more CCKRP becomes free to stimulate CCK release from enterocytes with subsequent pancreatic secretion.[79,92] A second, monitor peptide has been partially characterized as a promoter of CCK release with actions similar to those of CCKRP. Both proteins appears to be under vagal-cholinergic and somatostatin control.[79,92] Several other CCK-releasing peptides are being studied in animal models.

It appears that CCK exerts its effect primarily through extrapancreatic, cholinergic pathways via neural reflexes, rather than direct endocrine effects on acinar cells.[91,149-152] Several bodies of evidence support this concept of pancreatic secretion. CCK is known to stimulate CCK_A receptors at sensory nerve terminals in the gastrointestinal tract,[149,150] activating vagovagal reflexes that mediate relaxation of the proximal stomach, and increase antral and pyloric contraction, duodenal motility, gallbladder contraction, and relaxation of the sphincter of Oddi.[79] Animal studies found that pancreatic secretion is inhibited when atropine is administered in the presence of CCK stimulants such as amino acids and CCK itself.[153-156] In rats, physiologic doses of CCK act via stimulation of vagal afferents originating in the upper small intestine, but supraphysiologic plasma CCK levels act on intrapancreatic neurons and to a lesser extent, pancreatic acinar cells.[140] In dogs, CCK acts via humoral and paracrine routes.[157] Human studies also found inhibition of pancreatic enzyme secretion in the presence of anticholinergics during the postprandial phase, and infusing CCK to plasma levels similar to the postprandial state stimulates pancreatic secretion in an atropine-sensitive manner.[155] In addition, pancreatic enzyme secretion appears to be mediated by stimulation of CCK_A receptors on the vagus nerve under physiologic conditions.[149] The cloning of the CCK receptor gene, and the discovery that it is not expressed in the pancreas and that pancreatic acinar cells do not respond to CCK receptor agonists, provides evidence that CCK acts outside of the pancreas.[158] Thus, under physiologic conditions in humans, CCK stimulates pancreatic secretion entirely via the cholinergic pathway via vagovagal and enteropancreatic reflexes stimulating the release of neurotransmitters such as acetylcholine, and neuropeptides such as GRP and VIP.[79] There may also be more central input effects, such as from the brainstem, on these cholinergic pathways.[159] Clearly, the mechanism by which CCK acts is species-specific.[160]

Serotonin

Serotonin (5-hydroxytryptamine; 5-HT) is found in intestinal enterochromaffin cells and also plays a role in postprandial pancreatic secretion. It is released in response to several stimuli such as duodenal acidification and vagal and mechanical stimulation.[81] Serotonin may stimulate the vagovagal reflex, leading to pancreatic secretion.[161] A recent study showed that not only CCK, but serotonin also mediates pancreatic secretion by activating CCK_1 and $5-HT_3$ receptors on dorsal vagal afferents.[162] CCK, however, is incapable of activating $5-HT_3$ receptors. Administering $5-HT_3$ antagonists greatly inhibits pancreatic secretion in rats, suggesting that this is a significant non-CCK-mediated pathway of pancreatic secretion.[163] Serotonin also appears to regulate acid-induced pancreatic secretion of fluid and HCO_3^- by effecting the release and action of secretin.[164,165] The precise role of serotonin in pancreatic secretion remains to be determined.

Other Stimulatory Factors

Although secretin, CCK, and serotonin are the predominant hormones involved in pancreatic secretion, recent studies support an increasingly apparent role for other factors such as insulin, GRP, and nitric oxide. The physiologic significance of these hormones and factors is still unclear.

Previous studies using several different experimental methods revealed that insulin plays a role in the potentiation of the secretory response to CCK, secretin, and acetylcholine.[163,166-176] Reports on the effects of insulin alone, however, have been conflicting. In vivo studies have found an increase in secretion[167,175,177,178] or no stimulatory effects[166,168,176] in response to insulin. Other studies have shown that insulin inhibits secretin-induced bicarbonate secretion.[179,180]

Gastrin releasing peptide, also known as bombesin, is a polypeptide secreted in the intestinal tract that is able to greatly stimulate pancreatic enzyme secretion, and to a smaller extent, HCO_3^-.[181-183] It is unclear whether it exerts its effect by promoting the release of CCK from the small intestine,[184] by direct activation of at acinar GRP receptors, or via cholinergic pathways whereby GRP-containing nerves stimulate acetylcholine release from postganglionic cholinergic fibers.[91]

Nitric oxide (NO) is produced in the epithelium, endothelium, and macrophages of the intestinal tract and is abundant in the ducts, neurons, and vascular endothelium of the pancreas.[185] Nitric oxide inhibitors such as nitric oxide synthase inhibitor and N-(G)-nitro-L-arginine (L-NNA) are effective in reducing pancreatic secretion, suggesting an important role of NO in exocrine pancreatic function.[79,91,186] It is suspected that NO affects pancreatic secretion by altering the blood perfusion of the pancreas.[187-189] Thus, NO may have a role in the prevention of pancreatitis by increasing perfusion through the pancreas.

There has also been increased interest in the role of natriuretic peptides on pancreatic secretion. Although atrial natriuretic peptide (ANP) and C-type natriuretic peptide (CNP) are classically known for their role in blood pressure regulation, they also stimulate pancreatic fluid and protein secretion.[190] Both are capable of modifying bicarbonate and chloride secretions in pancreatic fluid and CNP is capable of stimulating amylase release.[190] ANP and CNP bind to the natriuretic peptide receptor C on the pancreatic acinar cells, which activates phospholipase C and initiates the intracellular signaling pathway leading to secretion.[191] CNP also exerts itself through vagovagal reflexes at the pancreatic acinus.[190]

Although melatonin is known for its role in maintaining the circadian rhythm, its receptors are located on pancreatic exocrine and endocrine cells, and it is known to stimulate pancreatic enzyme release.[192] It may play a role in maintaining intracellular calcium stores and act as an antioxidant in the pancreas.[193,194]

Finally, adenosine may also play a role in secretion by stimulating the opening of Cl^- channels. This is supported by the recent discovery of A2 adenosine receptors in human duct cell lines.[195]

Neural Regulation

For the most part, the parasympathetic nervous system innervates the pancreas through the vagus nerve, with the majority of its preganglionic fibers terminating on the pancreatic ganglia.[91] As previously mentioned, cholinergic effects of the vagus nerve have a tremendous influence from the cephalic phase through the postprandial phase of pancreatic secretion of fluid, electrolytes, and enzymes (Figure 80-7). It remains to be determined which neurotransmitters are involved in these processes. Adrenergic innervation of the pancreas occurs through postganglionic neurons whose cell bodies are in the celiac and superior mesenteric ganglia, and is distributed primarily amongst the pancreatic vasculature.[91] Inhibition of fluid and bicarbonate secretion

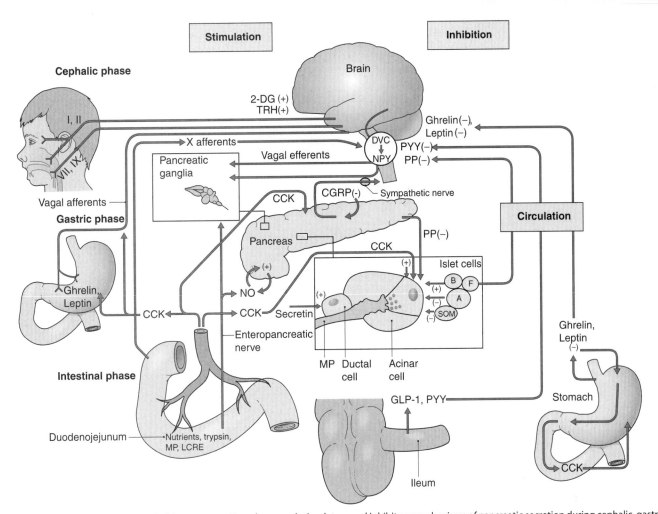

Figure 80-7. Neurohormonal control of the pancreas. Neurohormonal stimulatory and inhibitory mechanisms of pancreatic secretion during cephalic, gastric, and intestinal phases involving lone vagovagal and short enteropancreatic reflexes activated by cholecystokinin (CCK) acting on sensory receptors on afferent nerves. Various hormonal and humoral substances stimulate or inhibit the pancreatic secretion, acting either through the central nervous system or directly on the exocrine pancreas. A, A cells; B, B cells; CGRP, calcitonin gene-related peptide; 2-DG, 2-diacylglycerol; DVC, dorsal vagal complex; F, F cells; GLP, glucagon-like peptide; 1, luminal cholecystokinin releasing factor; 2, monitor peptide NO, nitric oxide; NPY, neuropeptide Y; PP, pancreatic polypeptide; PYY, peptide YY; SOM, somatostatin; TRH, thyrotropin-releasing hormone. Adapted from Konturek SJ, Zabielski R, Kanturek JW, Czarnecki J. Neuroendocrinology of the pancreas; role of the brain-gut axis in pancreatic secretion. Eur J Pharmacol 2003; 481:1-14, with permission.[209]

is achieved by sympathetic stimulation and subsequent pancreatic vasoconstriction.[81] Neurons in ganglia from the myenteric plexuses of the upper gastrointestinal tract also innervate the pancreas, and have cholinergic and serotoninergic characteristics.[196,197] Neurons containing VIP are the most common of the pancreatic peptidergic nervous system. VIP released from vagal neurons can stimulate both acinar cells to secrete enzymes, and ductal cells to secrete fluid and HCO_3^-.[81] Other peptidergic neurotransmitters with possible roles in pancreatic secretion include GRP,[181-183] substance P,[198] neuropeptide Y,[79] enkephalins,[92] and calcitonin gene-related peptide.[199,200] Similar to the enteric nervous system, the pancreas has its own intrinsic innervation whose precise physiologic function has yet to be clarified.[91]

Cellular Regulation of Pancreatic Secretion

There are generally two pathways in the intracellular regulation of pancreatic secretion (Figure 80-8). VIP and secretin bind to their respective receptors on the pancreatic acinus, which then couple to a G protein. This coupling leads to the activation of

adenylate cyclase, production of cAMP, and subsequent activation of protein kinase A. Protein kinase A alters the phosphorylation of several proteins, leading to pancreatic bicarbonate and fluid secretion. The second intracellular pathway begins with the binding of gastrin-releasing protein, CCK, and acetylcholine to their respective receptors, leading to coupling with G proteins and activation of phospholipase C. Phospholipase C then hydrolyzes phosphatidylinositol 4,5-bisphosphate (PI-P2) to inositol 1,4,5-trisphosphate (IP_3) and diacylglycerol (DAG). IP_3 releases Ca^{2+} from endoplasmic reticulum stores and ushers in a Ca^{2+} influx into the cell through activated plasma membrane Ca^{2+} channels. Ca^{2+} binds to calmodulin (CAM), which activates several protein kinases and one protein phosphatase. DAG, in combination with Ca^{2+}, activates protein kinase C. These protein kinases and phosphatases also alter the phosphorylation of several proteins and induce secretion of pancreatic enzymes via the exocytosis and fusion of zymogen granules with the apical membrane of the acinus.[81,92,201] It appears that muscarinic cholinergic receptors are more important than CCK in initiating IP_3 production.[202] CCK activates the production of nicotinic acid adenine dinucleotide phosphate (NAADP), which

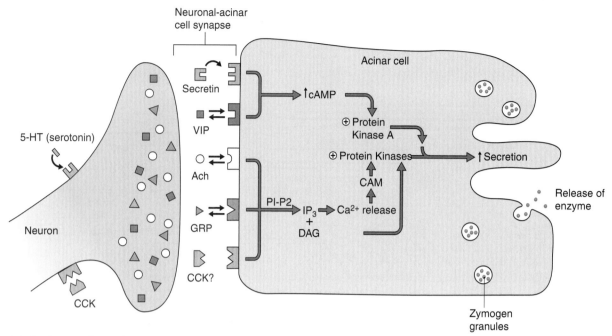

Figure 80-8. Mechanism of intracellular regulation of secretion in acinar cells. Ach, acetylcholine; CAM, calmodulin; cAMP cyclic adenosine monophosphate; CCK, cholecystokinin; DAG, diacylglycerol; GRP, gastrin-releasing peptide; IP$_3$, inositol 1,4,5-trisphosphate; PI-P2, phosphatidylinositol 4,5-bisphosphate; VIP, vasoactive intestinal peptide.

leads to the release of Ca^{2+} from a lysosome-related organelle.[84] CCK and muscarinic receptors also lead to an increase of cyclic ADP-ribose (cADPR), which can also mobilize Ca^{2+} from both the endoplasmic reticulum and the lysosome. Ca^{2+} is also released from the endoplasmic reticulum via ryanodine receptors, which open in response to a rise in Ca^{2+}.[202]

A recent study suggests that multiple Ca^{2+}-releasing messengers determine specific agonist-elicited Ca^{2+} signatures by controlling the balance among different acidic Ca^{2+} stores, endocytosis, and the ER.[203] It revealed that Ca^{2+} spikes in the apical region of the acinus cell require Ca^{2+} originating from both the lysosome as well as the endoplasmic reticulum in various proportions.[203] CCK and ACh recruit Ca^{2+} from lysosomes and from zymogen granules through different mechanisms; CCK uses NAADP and cADPR, respectively, and ACh uses Ca^{2+} and IP$_3$, respectively. In addition, endocytosis is important for the generation of repetitive local Ca^{2+} spikes evoked by the agonists and by NAADP and IP$_3$. cADPR-evoked repetitive local Ca^{2+} spikes are particularly dependent on the endoplasmic reticulum.[203]

Pancreatic Secretion Inhibitors

Much less is known about the mechanisms of pancreatic secretory inhibition, although there are several known peptides, hormones, and neural regulators involved in this process. It is likely that pancreatic exocrine secretion can be negatively regulated by the presence of active pancreatic proteases in the gut lumen via hydrolysis of CCK and secretin-releasing factors, as well as other peptides in the pancreatic juice.[204] However, there are other gut hormones and components of bile that also are involved in secretion inhibition.[204] It appears that the hormones and neurotransmitters involved do not act directly on pancreatic acinar cells, but modulate cholinergic influences on pancreatic secretion.[81,91]

Somatostatin is a pancreatic hormone produced in the gastric and duodenal mucosa as well as the D cells in the islets of Langerhans.[92,121] Its release is stimulated by cholinergic activation in response to exposure to fat and amino acids in the intestinal tract.[92,121] Somatostatin may act directly on pancreatic acinar cells, but the prevailing thought is that it inhibits pancreatic secretion through a cholinergic mechanism in the central nervous system.[205]

Pancreatic polypeptide (PP) is a peptide hormone found in the islets of Langerhans and between the acinar cells that inhibits pancreatic secretion of fluid, bicarbonate, and enzymes.[81,92] Plasma levels of PP increase after sham feeding, eating and after duodenal acidification.[92] Although vagal cholinergic activation is the most powerful stimulant to PP secretion,[206] exposure to CCK, secretin, VIP, gastrin, and GRP also results in its release.[92] PP probably modulates cholinergic transmission to the pancreas by interfering with acetylcholine release by presynaptic neurons in the pancreas.[207] The discovery of PP receptors within the central nervous system suggests a central target of PP in the negative feedback of pancreatic secretion.[81]

Peptide YY is a small peptide predominantly released in response to fat in the distal ileum and colon; it significantly attenuates HCO$_3^-$ and enzyme secretion by decreasing pancreatic responses to CCK and secretin.[121] Peptide YY likely inhibits release of acetylcholine and mucosal CCK as its primary mechanism of action.[92]

Although its mechanism of action is still unknown, pancreatic glucagon inhibits pancreatic secretion stimulated by CCK, secretin, or both, to decrease fluid, bicarbonate, and enzyme release.[81] It appears that other hormones and peptides, such as pancreastatin, calcitonin gene-related peptide, and enkephalins, inhibit pancreatic secretion by modulation of cholinergic stimulation at central vagal sites.[81,92] Ghrelin and leptin also appear to neurohormonally inhibit pancreatic secretion, but this mechanism of action remains to be determined.[204]

REFERENCES

84. Williams JA. Receptor-mediated signal transduction pathways and the regulation of pancreatic acinar cell function. Curr Opin Gastroenterol 2008;24:573–579.
102. Whitcomb DC, Lowe ME. Human pancreatic digestive enzymes. Dig Dis Sci 2007;52:1–17.
192. Chandra R, Liddle RA. Neural and hormonal regulation of pancreatic secretion. Curr Opin Gastroenterol 2009;25:441–446.

209. Konturek SJ, Zabielski R, Konturek JW, Czarnecki J. Neuroendocrinology of the pancreas; role of brain-gut axis in pancreatic secretion. Eur J Pharmacol 2003;481:1–14.

See expertconsult.com for a complete list of references and the review questions for this chapter.

CYSTIC FIBROSIS AND CONGENITAL ANOMALIES OF THE EXOCRINE PANCREAS

Arthur B. Atlas • Joel R. Rosh

CYSTIC FIBROSIS

Cystic fibrosis (CF) is the most common inherited life-shortening disease in whites. It is a disease that affects pancreatic exocrine gland function, involves numerous organs, and presents with varied clinical symptoms. Even though pulmonary disease is the major cause of morbidity and mortality, most patients have pancreatic insufficiency and suffer from gastrointestinal symptoms. The majority of patients are currently diagnosed soon after birth because of newborn screening programs, which are now available in every state in the United States. Failure to thrive, chronic diarrhea, and recurrent respiratory symptoms used to be the typical symptoms associated with diagnosing CF in infancy. These signs and symptoms are now rare at presentation, because most infants are diagnosed through screening, before symptoms develop. A positive newborn screening test requires a follow-up sweat test. Diagnosis of CF is confirmed by an elevated sweat chloride, or the identification of two abnormal mutations of the CF gene. Early diagnosis is associated with better growth and improved outcomes. The current average life expectancy is approximately 37 years, but is significantly higher in patients with sufficient pancreatic function.

Cystic Fibrosis Transmembrane Regulator

CF is an autosomal recessive disorder caused by mutations found on both alleles of a 250,000- base-pair gene found on the long arm of chromosome 7 (7q31 region). This gene, the cystic fibrosis transmembrane regulator (CFTR), codes for a single-chain polypeptide of 1480 amino acids called the CFTR protein.[1] CFTR is a cyclic adenosine monophosphate (cAMP)-regulated chloride channel, which also regulates other ion channels. It is a member of a family of proteins called ATP-binding cassette (ABC) proteins, which are involved with ATP hydrolysis-mediated solute transport.[2] CFTR contains two membrane-spanning domains (MSD1 and MSD2), two nucleotide-binding domains (NBD1 and NBD2), and a central intracellular regulatory domain, or R region, with multiple phosphorylation sites (Figure 81-1).[1,3] The MSDs form the channel pore, and ATP hydrolysis by NBDs controls gating through the pore.[3] Phosphorylation of the R domain determines channel activity.

CF mutations can be divided into five or six major classifications reflecting the location of the protein processing defect (Figure 81-2).[4] Class I mutations have little or no protein synthesis because of premature termination signals. Class II mutations are characterized by defective processing or trafficking of CFTR protein. ΔF508,

a class II mutation – and the most common CF mutation – has a three-nucleotide deletion of phenylalanine, which prevents normal glycosylation. The partially glycosylated protein is retained in the endoplasmic reticulum, where it is degraded, instead of being transported and inserted into the apical cellular membrane.[5] In class III mutations, proteins are processed properly, but the chloride channel lacks sensitivity to stimulation of intracellular cAMP due to the defect in the NBD region. Class IV mutations are characterized by alterations of conductance and have reduced cAMP-regulated currents in the chloride channel. Class V mutations affect splicing of mRNA, producing extra or skipped exons, which affects stability of the protein and mRNA. Class VI mutations share accelerated turnover from the cell surface and may also affect the regulatory function of CFTR on other ion channels. Individual mutations can have characteristics of more than one class.[6]

Class I, II, and III mutations are associated with more severe pulmonary disease and pancreatic insufficiency. Class IV and V are associated with milder disease, or no symptoms of disease. Polymorphisms, especially the truncated polythymidine tract called 5T, can affect CFTR function, either when found on two alleles, or in combination with a deleterious mutation on the opposite allele. 5T defects are usually associated with congenital bilateral absence of the vas deferens (CBAVD), either without other clinical symptoms of CF, or with mild CF symptoms.

ΔF508 is the most common mutation of CFTR, found in 70% of chromosomes in American whites with CF. There are ethnic and regional variations of CFTR mutations. ΔF508 is found in approximately 45% of the chromosomes of African Americans,[7] approximately 30% of Ashkenazi Jews,[8] and in less than 5% of Native Americans.[9] Currently, more than 1600 mutations of CFTR have been identified (http://www.genet.sickkids.on.ca/cftr), accounting for 95 to 97% of abnormalities in CF.

The CFTR protein has variable expression and probably functions differently in the epithelium of different organs. There is clinical variability among patients with the same CFTR genotype, suggesting that environmental and hereditary factors can modify the disease phenotype. Evidence is accumulating that phenotypic heterogeneity is influenced by genes at one or more unlinked loci in the human genome, which act as modifier genes of CFTR.[10-12]

CFTR Function in the Pancreas

In the pancreas, CFTR is found predominantly in the cell membrane of centroacinar and intralobular duct epithelium,[13] which is responsible for secreting fluid with a high concentration of sodium bicarbonate. Normally, chloride excreted into the lumen is exchanged for bicarbonate, with sodium and water following. In CF, the abnormal CFTR limits this exchange, and also limits apical trafficking of zymogen, resulting in a more viscous sodium bicarbonate-depleted fluid.[14] The viscous fluid contributing to ductal inspissation is unable to carry pancreatic enzymes adequately and efficiently from the pancreas to the duodenum, where normal digestion occurs.[15]

There are progressive histologic findings in the CF pancreas, correlating to the severity and age of the patient. Initially, focal intraluminal eosinophilic concentrations with dilation of pancreatic ducts are present. There is progression of acinar atrophy, and fibrosis with ductal ectasia. Late in the disease there is total loss of acinar tissue and ductal obliteration. Islets of Langerhans are diminished, but not totally destroyed.[16] The preserved islets have decreased glucagon-secreting α cells, insulin-secreting β cells, and pancreatic polypeptide-secreting cells.[17] Autopsy studies show that pancreatic nesidioblastosis is common in children with CF, but not in adolescents and adults.[18] With

age there is increased loss of β cells, increasing the prevalence of diabetes, which is rare in young children with CF, possibly because of children's ability to form new islets.

Pancreatic Sufficiency

Approximately 15% of patients with CF retain enough residual pancreatic secretion for normal digestion, and are termed pancreatic sufficient. The CFTR genotype-phenotype relationship has its strongest correlation with pancreatic function. Mutations that are associated with pancreatic sufficiency are considered "mild" mutations. Patients who have one or two mild mutations are typically pancreatic sufficient and typically have a class IV or V CFTR abnormality. Patients who remain pancreatic sufficient have less enzyme secretion and lower concentrations of bicarbonate in pancreatic fluid compared with normals.[15] Their growth is usually normal or close to normal, and therefore, as a group they were diagnosed with CF later than patients with pancreatic insufficiency, until routine CF newborn screening was instituted. In general, pancreatic-sufficient patients have less severe disease and lower sweat chloride levels, and their life expectancy is substantially longer than that of pancreatic-insufficient patients.

Pancreatic Insufficiency

"Severe mutations" identify genotypes specifically associated with pancreatic insufficiency and do not necessarily correlate with severity of lung function or disease. Mutations associated with pancreatic insufficiency are usually class I-III defects, which affect CFTR function more severely. Clinical signs of pancreatic insufficiency develop when less than 10% of normal pancreatic enzyme activity is present in the duodenum.[19]

CF is the major cause of pancreatic exocrine failure in children. Approximately 85% of patients with CF are pancreatic insufficient. At birth approximately 65% of infants with CF are pancreatic insufficient (PI). Of the remaining pancreatic-sufficient (PS) infants, approximately 15 to 20% will have progressive loss of pancreatic function by 3 years of age.[20] CF was typically diagnosed before 6 months of age in

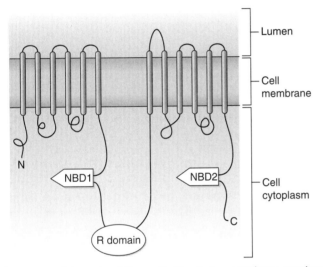

Figure 81-1. Schematic of the cystic fibrosis transmembrane regulator protein. NBD, nucleotide-binding domain; R domain, regulatory domain. (Redrawn from http://www.tripod.com/cellbiology).

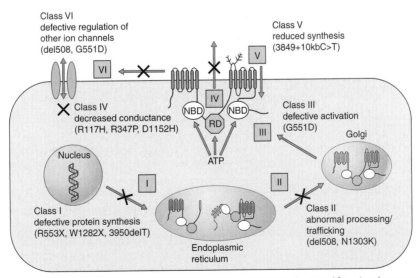

Figure 81-2. Classes I-VI of *CFTR* mutation. The subdivision reflects the known or predicted biosynthetic and functional consequences. ATP, adenosine triphosphate; NBD, nucleotide-binding domain; RD, regulatory domain. Redrawn from Witt (2003).[216]

pancreatic-insufficient infants, because of failure to thrive and malnutrition, before newborn screening was instituted. The calorie and protein losses in the stool prevent normal weight gain, growth, and development and can be associated with hypoalbuminemia, edema, and normochromic, normocytic anemia.[21]

Pancreatic Function Testing

Even though most infants and children with CF have pancreatic insufficiency, pancreatic function testing (Table 81-1) should be obtained before beginning replacement pancreatic enzymes. The best method for measuring pancreatic exocrine function is direct stimulation of pancreatic secretions. The pancreas is stimulated with exogenous hormones, secretin/cholecystokinin, or endogenous nutrients that stimulate pancreatic secretions, and the secretions are collected through a tube placed at the ligament of Treitz and analyzed for pH, bicarbonate, chymotrypsin, trypsin, lipase, colipase, amylase, and carboxypeptidase output.[22] Although this is the best test for evaluating pancreatic function, because of the invasive nature and expense, it is seldom used in clinical CF practice. Advances in radiographic imaging may replace the invasive endoscopic retrograde cholangiopancreatography (ERCP). Secretin-stimulated diffusion-weighted magnetic resonance (SS-DW-MRI) discriminates patients with mild, moderate, and severe exocrine insufficiency.[23] Indirect analysis of pancreatic function is less accurate, but more practical clinically. A 72-hour quantitative fecal fat collection evaluates the amount of fat ingested compared to the amount excreted. The percentage of fat absorbed correlates with the degree of pancreatic function. Fat absorption less than 85% is abnormal in children younger than 3 months, and in older children and adults less than 93% is abnormal.[24] The 72-hour stool fecal fat collection is a noninvasive test, but is laborious and unpleasant for patients, parents, and staff.

Detection of fecal enzymes is an easier test for determining pancreatic function and does not require prolonged stool collections. Fecal enzyme levels can be influenced by supplemental pancreatic enzyme replacement, with the exception of fecal elastase, which is not found in pancreatic enzyme supplements.

TABLE 81-1. Testing of Pancreatic Function[22,24]

Direct Stimulation of Pancreatic Secretions
Pancreozymin-secretin test
Lundh test

Fecal Studies
Titrimetric method
Fat absorption coefficient
Steatocrit method
Microscopic examination using Sudan III staining
Near-infrared reflectance spectroscopy

Fecal Enzyme Studies
Fecal chymotrypsin
Fecal elastase
Fecal immunoreactive lipase
Stool nitrogen excretion

Breath Test
Mixed triglyceride
Cholesteryl octanoate

Blood Levels
Immunoreactive trypsin (IRT)
Pancreatitis-associated protein

Fecal immunoreactive lipase and fecal elastase measurements have a high level of sensitivity and specificity for pancreatic insufficiency.[25,26] Fecal elastase concentration is currently the simplest and most reliable indirect method of accessing pancreatic exocrine function.[24] The mixed triglyceride breath test is also sensitive for detection of pancreatic function. It is expensive and time consuming, and results are influenced by supplemental pancreatic enzyme replacement.[24]

Serum immunoreactive trypsin (IRT) is elevated in infants with CF, but the level falls sharply in the first few years of life in PI infants and is typically subnormal at 7 years. Under the age of 7, IRT fails to distinguish PI from PS patients.[24] IRT is not as sensitive or specific as the fecal enzyme studies, but because its levels are elevated in CF infants, it is used as the standard test for CF newborn screening programs. Most state newborn CF screening programs, using a blood spot on a Guthrie filter card, measure IRT levels and CFTR DNA mutation screening to improve specificity.

Pancreatic Enzyme Replacement Therapy

Pancreatic insufficiency in CF is treated with oral exogenous pancreatic enzyme replacement therapy derived from processed porcine pancreas. The original powdered supplemental enzymes improved fat absorption, but many patients continued to have steatorrhea or needed numerous capsules per meal. Skin and mucous membrane irritation secondary to contact with the enzymatic powder was common, and hyperuricosemia and hyperuricosuria frequently occurred because of the high purine content in the powdered enzymes.[27,28] IgE-mediated hypersensitivity has been reported rarely in individuals exposed to powdered and enteric-coated pancreatic preparations.[29,30] Gelatin capsules with enteric-coated enzyme beads, or microspheres, encased in an acid-resistant coating are the current standard and have essentially replaced powdered enzymes. Enteric preparations have improved fat and protein absorption, with fewer side effects and easier administration of the enzymes. The capsules can be swallowed whole or opened and the beads sprinkled on nonalkaline foods. Once the beads have been swallowed, the coating dissolves at a pH above 5.5, allowing enzyme activation to occur in the proximal small bowel. With appropriate enzyme replacement, fat absorption improves, and abdominal complaints decrease for most patients. Bioengineered enzymes are being developed, which will likely replace porcine-derived products in the near future. They are likely to improve fat and protein absorption, with fewer pills and fewer side effects, compared to current products.

Pancreatic enzyme replacement therapy is initiated once pancreatic insufficiency has been diagnosed. In infants, preparations with the smallest microspheres either mixed in a small amount of fruit or applied to the tongue just before offering the bottle or breast works well. In infants, dosing of enzymes can be based on food intake, but for the older child weight-based dosing in combination to fat/protein intake is better. The National Cystic Fibrosis Foundation guidelines on pancreatic enzyme dosing (Table 81-2) should be used when starting or adjusting therapy. The goals of therapy are to promote weight gain, growth, and development and limit abdominal symptoms. There is a wide individual variation in response to supplemental enzyme dosing. The lower range of the recommended dosage should be started and adjusted upward based on stool pattern and weight gain. To decrease the risk of fibrosing colonopathy,

TABLE 81-2. Current Recommended Pancreatic Enzyme Dosing in Cystic Fibrosis[33]

Age	Recommended dose
Infant	2000-4000 lipase units per 4 oz formula or per breast-feed
4 years and younger	1000 lipase units per kg per meal 500 lipase units per kg per snack
4 years and older	500 lipase units per kg per meal 250 lipase units per kg per snack
Adolescents and adults	Lower enzyme doses can be tried as intake of fat/kg declines with age

In general, patients need 500-4000 U lipase per gram of fat ingested per day. There is individual patient variability with enzyme dosing. These recommended doses for enzyme replacement should be used as a starting point and adjustments made as necessary to control signs and symptoms of malabsorption. Doses greater than 2500 lipase units per kg per meal should be used with caution, and only if there is documented improved fat absorption by 72-hour fecal fat measurement. Doses greater than 6000 lipase units per kg per meal have been associated with colonic stricture in children aged less than 12 years.[33]

TABLE 81-3. Factors That Can Reduce the Effects of Supplemental Pancreatic Enzymes

Nonadherence to prescribed dosing
Expired enzymes
Inactivated enzymes due to prolonged exposure to heat
Highly acidic small intestinal environment
Prolonged exposure of microspheres to alkaline foods
Taking enzymes after eating
"Grazing"
Generic enzymes with lower potency
Chewed or crushed microspheres
Inadequate dose of enzymes reaching the small intestine
Glycine-conjugated bile acids limiting micelle formation

TABLE 81-4. Potential Confounding Gastrointestinal Conditions in Cystic Fibrosis

Causing Steatorrhea
Hepatobiliary disease with portal hypertension
Cholestatic liver disease
Celiac disease
Giardiasis
Short gut syndrome
Bacterial overgrowth of small intestine

Without Steatorrhea
Recurrent abdominal pain
Inflammatory bowel disease
Irritable bowel syndrome
Lactose intolerance
Infectious enteritis
Esophagitis
Gastroesophageal reflux
Fibrosing colonopathy
Eating disorders
Digestive tract cancers

enzyme doses should be less than 2500 lipase units/kg per meal, or less than 4000 lipase units/g fat per day.[31]

Once adequate dosing of pancreatic enzyme replacement is established, a rapid improvement in the degree of steatorrhea should be seen, with decreased stool frequency, abdominal pain and bloating, and reduced appetite with improved weight gain. Because the absorption and digestion of fats is complex and requires pancreatic enzymes, bile salts, and a normal intestinal mucosa and milieu, some patients continue to be symptomatic with abnormal fat absorption, despite taking appropriate amounts of enzymes. Many of these patients benefit with the addition of H_2-receptor antagonists or proton pump inhibitor, which optimizes the intraluminal action of the supplemental enzymes by reducing the gastric acidic environment.[32] Other common causes of diminished response to enzyme replacement include nonadherence, lack of synchronized delivery with meals, and decreased enzyme potency as a result of either exposure to heat or use past the expiry date (Table 81-3). There is a tendency for clinicians to continue to increase the enzyme dose when a patient complains of increased abdominal symptoms. However, patients on high-dose enzymes and acid suppression therapy who continue to have persistent abdominal symptoms require a fecal fat absorption study and evaluation for other causes of steatorrhea or abdominal pain, including celiac disease, Crohn's disease, lactose intolerance, parasitic disease, and bacterial overgrowth (Table 81-4).

Fibrosing Colonopathy

Fibrosing colonopathy is a potentially significant complication of pancreatic enzyme replacement therapy and is associated with prolonged use of greater than 6000 units lipase per kg per meal.[31,33] Symptoms include abdominal pain, vomiting, bloody or persistent diarrhea, and poor weight gain or weight loss. Thickening of the bowel wall can be seen by ultrasonography and predates stricture formation.[34] Barium enema can show focal or generalized narrowing, with the ascending colon most frequently affected, although total colonic involvement has been reported.[35] Many patients show clinical improvement with decreasing supplemental enzymes and parenteral nutrition, but some require surgical resection of the narrowed

section of colon. The pathophysiology of the colonic damage in fibrosing colonopathy is not clear, but is associated with high-dose supplemental pancreatic enzymes, even though there are reports of it occurring before initiation of supplemental enzymes in CF.[36] The association of high-dose enzyme use with fibrosing colonopathy led to a commercial recall of very high-potency enzymes. Since the recall there has been a decreased incidence of fibrosing colonopathy. Because of the association with high doses of enzymes, The Cystic Fibrosis Foundation recommends enzyme doses be less than 2500 lipase units per kg per meal, or less than 4000 lipase units per gram of fat per day.[31,33]

Meconium Ileus

Meconium ileus (MI) is the earliest clinical manifestation of CF. Infants with CF are at risk for delayed passage of meconium, intestinal plugging with meconium, and meconium ileus. In CF, meconium has an increased concentration of albumin, and decreased water and mineral concentrations, resulting in a thicker, more viscous texture.[37,38] Increased mucus production from goblet cell secretions, combined with gelatinous meconium, contributes to inspissation of meconium, resulting in partial or total intestinal obstruction. MI occurs almost exclusively in patients with pancreatic insufficiency and occurs in between 10% and 18% of those patients. Modifier genes found on chromosome 19 determine susceptibility to MI, but do not influence the likelihood of intestinal obstruction later in life.[12,39] When an infant with CF develops MI, the occurrence

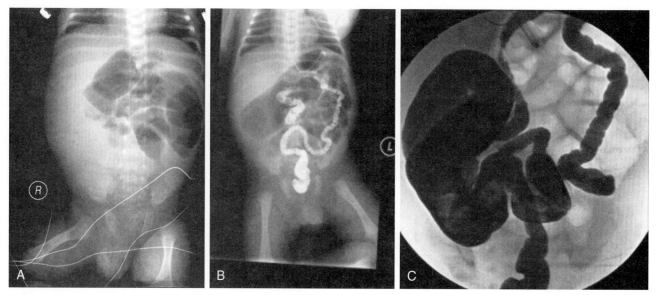

Figure 81-3. (A) Abdominal radiograph of meconium ileus with a "bubbly" fullness in the right lower quadrant and dilated proximal small bowel loops. (B) Contrast enema in meconium ileus with dilated small bowel and unused microcolon. (C) Contrast enema in meconium ileus showing a huge dilated distal ileum with filling defects due to inspissated meconium. Dilated loops of small bowel and unused microcolon can also be seen. Courtesy of Robin C. Murphy, MD.

rate significantly increases in subsequent siblings with CF.[40-42] The vast majority of infants with MI are diagnosed with CF, but there are reports of rare exceptions.[41,43] Neonatal intestinal obstruction can be diagnosed with prenatal ultrasonography. A hyperechoic pattern with dilated bowel, with or without ascites, has a high specificity for CF.[44]

Clinical symptoms of intestinal obstruction from MI are present at birth, or soon after birth, with absence of passage of meconium in the first 48 hours. Abdominal radiographs show distended bowel loops, usually without air-fluid levels, with a bubbly ground-glass density at the terminal ileum (Figure 81-3A). Contrast enema is diagnostic, showing an unused microcolon and filling defects from inspissated meconium in the distal small bowel (Figure 81-3B,C). Hyperosmolar contrast enema successfully relieves the obstruction in 50 to 90% of uncomplicated cases.[44,45] Approximately 50% of cases of MI are complicated by intestinal perforation, peritonitis, necrosis, volvulus, meconium cysts, or intestinal atresia and require laparotomy.[44] Intraoperative bowel infusion with acetylcysteine, or hyperosmolar contrast, has been shown to decrease the need for surgical resection.[45,46] If intraoperative infusions are unsuccessful, or there are complications, resection of the affected bowel with primary anastomosis or side-by-side enterostomy is performed.[44]

Current surgical and nutritional modalities have significantly decreased the formerly high mortality rate in infants with MI.[46] However, MI in CF is associated with a higher mortality rate when diagnosed late or skilled care is delayed.[47] Children with CF who are born with MI have similar nutritional outcomes but go on to have more clinically significant pulmonary disease[48] and a shorter life expectancy[49] than those without neonatal MI.

Other abnormalities due to the abnormal meconium besides MI can occur in CF. Meconium plug syndrome (MPS) is seen in infants with CF as well as those with Hirschsprung's disease, hypotonia, and prematurity. The presenting signs and symptoms of MPS are similar to those of MI, but there is distal obstruction at the level of the colon rather than the ileum. A contrast enema shows a normal-caliber colon with filling defects from

inspissated meconium and is usually diagnostic and therapeutic. Surgical intervention is usually not indicated.[43]

Distal Intestinal Obstruction Syndrome

Distal intestinal obstruction syndrome (DIOS), once called meconium ileus equivalent, occurs at all ages but is more common in adolescents and adults. It is seen almost exclusively in patients with pancreatic insufficiency, but has been reported in pancreatic sufficient patients.[50] Patients with prior MI may be at increased risk for DIOS,[51] and DIOS may be a risk factor for developing liver disease.[52] The exact incidence varies considerably and has been reported between 4 and 40%.[51,53] Since the introduction of enteric-coated microsphere preparations of pancreatic enzymes, the frequency of DIOS has decreased.[53] DIOS is believed to result from a combination of retained stool, abnormal intestinal secretions, and abnormal intestinal motility leading to impaction of stool in the terminal ileum, cecum, and proximal colon.[54,55] Precipitating causes of DIOS are frequently not identified, but noncompliance with supplemental pancreatic enzyme, dehydration, change in diet, opiates, and anticholinergics have all been implicated. Symptoms include crampy lower abdominal pain, abdominal distention, vomiting, and anorexia. A palpable mass in the lower right quadrant can be felt on physical examination. During episodes of DIOS, normal stool patterns may continue, but progression to complete obstruction, intussusception, or volvulus can occur.[16] A diagnosis of DIOS is made by the history and physical examination. Abdominal radiography shows retained stool in the ileum and cecum, which can appear as "bubbly" granular opacities. Air-fluid levels can be seen. The differential diagnosis includes intussusception, volvulus, pancreatitis, gallbladder disease, appendicitis, peptic ulcer disease, and esophagitis.

In the absence of complete bowel obstruction, the preferred treatment is gastrointestinal lavage with a balanced isotonic solution containing polyethylene glycol administered orally or through a nasogastric tube.[54] The endpoint of therapy is to relieve the partial obstruction, which is determined by passage of stool, resolution of pain, and resolution of the palpable lower right quadrant mass. Follow-up radiography may be helpful in documenting resolution. Therapeutic enemas using water-soluble contrast containing N-acetylcysteine under radiologic control are used less frequently because of the success of antegrade intestinal lavage. Once the acute episode of DIOS has been managed, dose optimization or improved compliance with pancreatic enzymes, increasing fluid intake, and additional dietary fiber help to prevent recurrence. Osmotic laxatives including lactulose and chronic polyethylene glycol may decrease the risk of recurrence.

Rectal Prolapse

The most common cause of rectal prolapse in children is severe constipation. However, rectal prolapse can be a presenting sign of CF, and sweat testing should therefore be considered. Rectal prolapse occurs in up to 20% of patients with CF, usually between 6 months and 2 years of age.[55] It is uncommon in patients with CF diagnosed and treated with pancreatic enzymes before 3 months of age. Rectal prolapse may become even less common because infants are treated earlier as a result of newborn screening. Constipation, malnutrition, chronic cough, and pelvic muscle weakness increase the risk of rectal prolapse.

Rectal prolapse initially starts as intussusception of the rectum, and then progresses.[56] The prolapse can involve just the mucosa (mucosal prolapse) or all layers of the rectum – a complete prolapse or procidentia. Rectal prolapse is frequently recurrent in CF and initially noticed by the parents. Usually it can easily be reduced and does not require medical intervention, but rarely surgical intervention is required. Recurrence of rectal prolapse is minimized by improved nutrition, and decreased malabsorption with appropriate use of pancreatic enzyme supplementation.

Pancreatitis

Approximately 15% of pancreatic-sufficient patients with CF develop pancreatitis in their lifetime. Pancreatitis in CF occurs almost exclusively in older pancreatic sufficient patients, but has been described in PI patients and infants and can be the presenting symptom of CF.[57,58] Pancreatitis can occur in patients with severe CF mutations, before the complete loss of pancreatic function. The progression from PS to PI due to recurrent pancreatitis may be more common in patients with the R117H mutation of CFTR.[59] The exact pathophysiology of pancreatitis in patients with CF is not clear, but some preservation of acinar tissue function is required.

The CFTR protein is found at the apical cell membrane of the ductal epithelial cells and maintains normal pancreatic secretions by controlling the movement of chloride and water into the duct, which alkalizes and dilutes the fluid as it flows through the pancreatic duct. In CF, abnormal CFTR causes low acinar luminal pH, which inhibits endocytosis of secretory granule proteins and reduces the solubility of the concentrated fluid.[60] Therefore, patients with CF have pancreatic secretions that are highly concentrated and proteinaceous. Physical obstruction of the pancreatic ducts from proteinaceous plugs, or alteration of acinar function, develops from the concentrated pancreatic secretions. Pancreatic proteolytic enzymes are subsequently activated, leading to pancreatic autodigestion.[16,60] Early destruction of functional acinar tissue leading to acinar atrophy presumably protects pancreatic insufficient patients from pancreatic autodigestion and pancreatitis. The natural history of pancreatitis in CF is characterized by the onset of acute pancreatitis that recurs and over time can develop into chronic pancreatitis.[61]

CFTR compound heterozygote genotypes, containing one severe mutation and one mild-variable mutation of CFTR, are at greatest risk for CF-related pancreatitis. The 5T polymorphism on intron 8, which causes inefficient splicing of exon 10, producing nonfunctional copies of CFTR, is frequently found in patients with CF and pancreatitis.[62] The pancreatic secretory trypsin inhibitor (PSTI) gene is a Kazal type 1 serine protease inhibitor (SPINK1). PSTI is the first line of protection that inactivates some trypsin activity if trypsinogen is accidentally converted to trypsin in the acinar cells.[63] The cationic trypsinogen, serine protease 1 gene (PRSS1) encodes cationic trypsinogen. CF patients with genetic mutations of PRSS1 are strongly associated with chronic pancreatitis and reoccurring acute pancreatitis, whereas defects in PST1/SPINK1 are associated with pancreatitis to a lesser degree.[64] Patients may also be at increased risk of progression from acute to chronic pancreatitis, with abnormalities of both genes.[65] The risk for recurrent pancreatitis is increased in CF, with the presence of pancreas divisum.[66]

Patients with pancreatitis develop severe or progressive abdominal pain, with vomiting, and epigastric tenderness. Serum and urinary amylase and serum lipase levels are elevated. Imaging studies may be normal, but narrowing of the pancreatic duct on pancreatography, peripancreatic edema on abdominal computed tomography, and increased pancreatic echogenicity on ultrasonography have been described.[67,57] Acute episodes of pancreatitis can be precipitated by alcohol ingestion, tetracycline, or fatty meals, but most episodes appear to occur spontaneously. Recurrent acute episodes are typical, but pseudocyst and systemic complications of CF-related pancreatitis are unusual. Because patients with recurrent acute episodes may eventually develop pancreatic insufficiency, pancreatic function should be monitored closely. Treatment for CF-related pancreatitis consists of intravenous fluids, nutritional support, and analgesics. Supplemental pancreatic enzymes may provide a negative feedback to the pancreas by limiting endogenous enzyme secretions, thereby decreasing pancreatic autodigestion and pain. In patients with frequent attacks, supplemental enzymes may prevent or increase the interval between episodes.

Abdominal Pain

Abdominal pain is a frequent complaint in patients with CF, especially if malabsorption is not well controlled. Besides the obvious causes of abdominal pain associated with conditions described earlier, intra-abdominal pain from causes that occur in non-CF also needs to be considered. Intussusception occurs in 1% of CF patients and is caused by inspissated secretions, enlarged lymphoid follicles, or a distended appendix creating the pathological lead point. Ultrasound may show the typical "donut" sign, but in some cases has failed to be diagnostic. Therefore, contrast enema can be diagnostic and therapeutic. There are reports of chronic intussusception in CF.[68,69]

The diameter of the appendix is enlarged in CF because of luminal mucus distention; therefore, diagnosing acute appendicitis radiographically can be challenging. Acute appendicitis occurs less frequently in CF patients than in the general public, but the diagnosis is often delayed, leading to increased incidence of appendiceal abscesses and perforation.[68,69] Because imaging studies can be misleading in the diagnosis of acute appendicitis, clinical signs of increasing or persistent local tenderness in the right iliac fossa remains an important clinical clue for early diagnosis.

Gastroesophageal reflux disease (GERD) is reported to occur in between 20 and 100% of CF patients, depending on age and patient selection. Chronic cough, worsening lung function, increased abdominal pressure, and frequent chest physiotherapy contribute to the high incidence.[70] Besides frequent abdominal pain, GERD can exacerbate lung disease through aspiration and bronchospasm, worsening lung function and chest x-ray findings.[71,72] Long-standing GERD may predispose to Barrett's metaplasia and esophageal adenocarcinoma.[73]

Cystic Fibrosis–Related Diabetes Mellitus

Diabetes mellitus is a well recognized complication of CF. In CF, the total pancreatic mass decreases due to progressive fibrosis of the pancreas, producing a decrease in glucagon-secreting α cells and insulin-secreting β cells. As the proportion of β cells decreases, glucose intolerance increases and diabetes mellitus may develop. Pancreatic insufficiency is a prerequisite for CF-related diabetes (CFRD). Glucose intolerance is present in a substantial number of young children with CF,[74] and approximately 75% of adults with CF have some degree of glucose intolerance.[75] CFRD rarely develops before the age of 10 years, and average onset is at approximately 20 years, with prevalence increasing with age. Females may be more susceptible and develop diabetes at a younger age.[76] A significant deterioration in lung function and growth may occur years before CFRD is diagnosed.[77,78] Development of CFRD was believed to increase the mortality rate by as much as sixfold.[77,79] With increased awareness and aggressive therapy, the gap between mortality of CF with and without CFRD has greatly narrowed.[80]

In CFRD, along with loss of insulin-secreting β cells, there is impaired hepatic response to the antigluconeogenic effects of insulin, and impaired insulin sensitivity.[81] It is likely that insulin sensitivity increases initially, but insulin resistance ensues as glucose tolerance deteriorates.[82] Insulin resistance increases with glucocorticosteroid use, pregnancy, and acute infections. CFRD is not autoimmune mediated and is rarely associated with ketoacidosis. Microvascular complications may be seen in CFRD, usually after 10 years' duration, but macrovascular complications have not been reported.[82]

Patients untreated for CFRD complain of lethargy and have difficulty maintaining weight. There is calorie loss from glycosuria, with subsequent loss of weight and muscle mass. Lung function typically deteriorates, and there is an increased risk of pulmonary infection due to immune system impairment. In spite of adequate diabetes control, lung function is worse in CF patients with CFRD, as compared to those without CFRD.[80] The progression from glucose intolerance to diabetes is a slow, indolent process, and there is no way to predict which patients with glucose intolerance will develop CFRD. Monitoring hemoglobin A_{1c} is not useful as a screening test for CFRD owing to shortened erythrocyte survival, but can be used to monitor diabetes control.[82] Adolescent patients with CF should be screened with annual oral glucose tolerance testing. Patients younger than 10 years who demonstrate unexplained lung function deterioration or weight loss should also be considered for oral

glucose tolerance testing. The goal of treatment for CFRD is maintenance of glucose homeostasis, normal growth, and good nutrition. Carbohydrates are not restricted, but foods and drinks with concentrated simple sugars are discouraged. Fats are encouraged as an important source of calories, and calories typically are not restricted. Although insulin remains the standard of care for treating CFRD in those with fasting hyperglycemia, oral therapies are being used with increased frequency and efficacy.[81] Insulin may be needed intermittently with acute infections in patients with glucose intolerance.

Nutrition

Malnutrition and growth retardation are common problems in children with CF. Malnutrition results from a combination of increased energy expenditure, decreased caloric intake, chronic infection and inflammation, and caloric and nutrient losses due to malabsorption in pancreatic-insufficient patients. Optimal dietary intake is an essential component of CF care. The nutritional recommended daily allowance (RDA) is 120 to 140% of that of healthy children. Most patients with CF obtain only 80 to 100% of the RDA. Patients with CF often require 35 to 40% of calories from fat, and 15% of calories from protein, which are higher than the levels recommended for the healthy population.[83] There is a negative correlation between the degree of malnutrition and the degree of illness, pulmonary function, and survival. Prolonged malnutrition in young children with CF is associated with decreased cognitive function.[84]

Pancreatic function has a direct influence on nutritional status and is a strong predictor of outcome. However, obtaining full predicted height potential is a strong indicator of nutritional status. Growth, pulmonary function, and survival is better in cohorts of patients in higher height and weight percentiles, compared with those in lower percentiles.[85] When nutrition improves, height and weight percentiles increase, and the differences between the two groups disappear.[86] Early nutritional intervention in patients diagnosed by neonatal CF screening results in a sustained improvement in growth parameters.[87]

Nutritional deficiencies in CF affect body stores of fat-soluble vitamins, essential fatty acids, prealbumin, albumin, triglycerides, cholesterol and some trace metals. All water-soluble vitamins are well absorbed, except vitamin B_{12}, which is absorbed normally with adequate pancreatic enzyme supplementation.[88] However, even with appropriate pancreatic enzyme replacement and supplemental fat-soluble vitamins (Table 81-5), serum vitamin levels may remain decreased.

Vitamin A

Vitamin A is required for normal vision, immunity, and epithelial cell integrity and proliferation. Pancreatic lipase is needed for absorption of retinyl esters, placing pancreatic-insufficient patients at risk for vitamin A deficiency. Decreased vitamin A levels are associated with decreased retinol-binding protein, due to decreased vitamin A absorption from the gut.[89] In spite of vitamin A and pancreatic enzyme replacement, low serum vitamin A levels are common, although clinical signs of deficiency are rare. However, dark-field adaptation deficits have been described in as many as 18% of adolescent and adult patients with CF. This risk is greatest in patients with liver disease and those noncompliant with enzyme and vitamin supplementation.[90] A normal ratio of serum vitamin A to retinol-binding protein is the goal to ensure adequate levels. Because vitamin A is an

TABLE 81-5. **Recommendations for Vitamin Supplementation and Calcium Intake in Cystic Fibrosis**

	0-12 Months	1-3 Years	>8 Years	Adults
Vitamin A (IU)	1500	5000	5000-10000	10 000
Vitamin E (IU)	40-50	80-150	100-200	200-400
Vitamin D (IU)	400	400-800	400-800	400-800
Vitamin K (mg)	At least 0.3 mg/day	At least 0.3mg/day	At least 0.3mg/day	2.5-5 mg/week
Calcium (mg/day)	0-6months: 210 7-12months: 270	500	800	1300

acute-phase reactant and can be negatively influenced by infections, serum levels can be misleading during hospitalization for acute illness.[91]

Vitamin D

Vitamin D has physiologic effects beyond bone health and calcium homeostasis. There is increasing evidence that vitamin D plays a beneficial role in lung health and the prevention of a wide range of diseases. In the lungs, it inhibits pulmonary inflammation by enhancing innate defense mechanisms against respiratory pathogens and may be involved in remodeling and lung function.[92,93] Vitamin D deficiency is seen in 10 to 40% of patients with CF and is more common in the very ill and in patients living in northern latitudes.[94] Studies of biochemical markers of bone turnover suggest that bone reabsorption exceeds bone formation in CF, which contributes to decreased bone mineral density (BMD). [95] The prevalence of bone disease increases with severity of lung disease and malnutrition, but decreased BMD is probably multifactorial, and related to a combination of nutrition, pancreatic insufficiency, chronic infection, activity level, sunlight exposure, and effects of the various medications used in CF care. [96] The risk of osteoporosis and fractures increases with age, and these are more problematic in adult CF.

The consensus group on osteoporosis recommends that children with CF older than 1 year receive 800 IU/day of oral ergocalciferol (vitamin D_2), to maintain a serum level of 25-hydroxyvitamin D (OHD) above 30 ng/mL (greater than 75 nmol/L) for optimal bone health. If serum 25-OHD levels remain below 30 ng/mL, aggressive stepwise supplementation with high-dose oral ergocalciferol is recommended. Calcitriol or phototherapy can be considered for persistent serum 25-OHD levels below 30 ng/mL.[96] There is increasing evidence that the original recommended doses of 25-OHD is too low to maintain an adequate serum level above 30 ng/mL, and doses as high as 10,000 IU/day are suggested.[97,98] There is also increasing evidence of a relationship of decreased bone health and vitamin K defieciency.[99]

Vitamin E

Vitamin E (α-tocopherol) is an antioxidant that has been shown to act as a free radical scavenger and to have positive effects on immune function. Vitamin E deficiency develops early in life in pancreatic-insufficient patients. Vitamin E deficiency is present in almost all PI patients with CF not receiving tocopherol supplementation,[100] and 5 to 10% of patients continue to have low serum levels of vitamin E, even with presumed adequate supplementation.[101]

Supplementation with multivitamins and pancreatic enzymes in infants diagnosed with CF more easily corrects levels of vitamin A and D than of vitamin E. Most infants with vitamin E deficiency continue to be deficient for prolonged periods of time.[94] Despite supplementation, sporadic or recurrent deficiencies of all fat-soluble vitamins occur in childhood, but are seen more frequently with vitamin E. Plasma levels of α-tocopherol below 300 mg/dL are associated with cell membrane instability, erythrocyte destruction, and risk of hemolytic anemia.[84] Neurologic findings associated with vitamin E deficiency include decreased vibratory sensation and proprioception, decreased deep tendon reflexes, muscle weakness, and ataxia. Neurodevelopment and cognitive function are significantly reduced in vitamin E–deficient patients with CF, as compared with those with normal vitamin E levels.[84]

Vitamin K

Vitamin K is a fat-soluble nutrient, absorbed in the presence of bile salts and pancreatic lipase from the gut. Vitamin K is required for the biosynthesis of clotting factors. Risk of deficiency is greater in PI patients, and deficiency is uncommon in patients with CF who are supplemented with pancreatic enzymes[102]; however, there have been reports of vitamin K deficiency in CF.[103,104] Patients with liver disease are at greatest risk for deficiency, which can be corrected with higher doses of vitamin K.[105] It is widely believed that chronic antibiotic use reduces vitamin K levels because of disruption of the enteric flora. However, Beker et al.[106] were unable to find significant changes of serum levels with antibiotic use. PIVKA-II (protein induced by vitamin K absence or antagonism) concentration is a sensitive assay for the measurement of vitamin K deficiency, but is not practical because of the lack of clinical availability.[101] Therefore, prothrombin time is used as an indirect and probably insensitive measure, and when prolonged, it is a late indicator of vitamin K deficiency. There remains controversy regarding the extent of vitamin K deficiency in CF and the appropriateness of the current recommendations of 0.3 to 0.5 mg/day supplementation. Because subclinical deficiency is probably common in CF, and because oral vitamin K_1 is very safe, the standard of CF care includes daily vitamin K supplementation. Further studies are needed to clarify the need for and the appropriate amount of oral supplementation.[104]

Calcium

There is a high prevalence of osteopenia and osteoporosis, and an increased risk of fractures in patients with CF. Bone calcium deposition rates in female CF patients during early and late puberty can be insufficient to retain adequate amounts of bone calcium. Besides vitamin D, bone calcium deposition rates are related to dietary intake of calcium, serum leptin concentrations, and serum osteocalcin concentrations.[107] It is important to emphasis the need to achieve optimal intakes of calcium, to maximize bone calcium deposition in children with CF. Bone mineral density decreases with advancing age in CF because of chronic inflammation, inactivity, steroid use, and chronic malabsorption of vitamin D and calcium. Calcium absorption is augmented by pancreatic enzyme supplementation, but calcium supplementation (see Table 81-5) is frequently needed to improve bone density. The CF Foundation recommends dual-energy x-ray absorptiometry (DEXA) as the preferred method of measuring BMD in CF patients.[96] Its use is still limited by lack of standardized normal data in children and is not indicated in children under 8 years.

Iron

The prevalence of iron deficiency anemia in CF increases with age. Serum ferritin is frequently used to monitor iron status. Because ferritin is an acute-phase reactant and can be affected by acute inflammation, interpretation of serum ferritin levels can be misleading during an acute pulmonary exacerbation. Serum transferrin receptors are not affected by inflammation and may be a more reliable indicator of iron deficiency, but are of limited use in clinical practice, because they are not readily commercially available.[108] Annual hemoglobin and hematocrit levels are often used to monitor iron status, even though they are less sensitive.

Trace Metals

Normal zinc metabolism is critical for normal growth and immune function. Approximately 30% of young infants diagnosed with CF by newborn screening have been shown to have low plasma zinc levels, which significantly improve with pancreatic enzyme supplementation.[109] Zinc homeostasis is dependent on the absorption of exogenous zinc, and the secretion and excretion of endogenous zinc through the gastrointestinal tract. Endogenous zinc is found in pancreatic secretions. Zinc absorption from the gastrointestinal tract is influenced by physiologic demand, zinc load, and the presence of dietary enhancers including human milk and animal proteins.[110] Zinc deficiency can affect vitamin A status, and supplementation with zinc should be considered in patients with suboptimal vitamin A levels.[110] Severe zinc deficiency is more common in malnutrition and can be associated with an acrodermatitis enteropathica-like rash. Plasma zinc concentration is used to monitor zinc status, but is not a sensitive marker. The best assessment of zinc status is the response to a trial of approximately 1 mg elemental zinc per kg per day. A plasma zinc concentration of less than 80 mg/dL has been used as a predictor for a significant growth response to zinc supplementation.[110]

Malabsorption of magnesium can occur in CF, but symptomatic hypomagnesemia is usually due to exogenous factors. Paresthesias, muscle weakness, carpopedal spasms, and other symptoms of hypomagnesemia should be treated with magnesium replacement.

Copper deficiency occurs in CF, possibly because of abnormal copper metabolism. The exact mechanism is not clear, but may be related to low activity levels of superoxide dismutase and plasma diamine oxidase, enzymes involved in copper metabolism. Zinc deficiency can have a negative impact on copper status. Copper supplementation does not readily correct the deficiency, even in conjunction with zinc supplementation.[111] Ceruloplasmin is an acute-phase reactant, and its concentration may be raised in CF.[112]

Selenium serum levels in CF are frequently decreased, and CF PI patients are at increased risk to develop symptoms of subclinical or clinical selenium deficiency. There is a strong correlation between selenium concentration and red blood cell (RBC) glutathione peroxidase activity, and a negative correlation between plasma selenium and 24-hour fecal fat excretion.[113] Clinical symptoms are rare, but erythrocyte macrocytosis, loss of skin and hair pigmentation,[114] and muscle disorders occur with selenium deficiency. Oxidative stress appears to play a role in development of symptoms, because many people with decreased levels are asymptomatic.[115]

Essential Fatty Acids

Essential fatty acid deficiency in CF is well described, and until recently was thought to be due to malabsorption.[116] Studies support the hypothesis that essential fatty acid abnormalities in CF may be due to CFTR dysfunction, because CFTR has a potential role in cellular fatty acid metabolism.[117,118] Chronic inflammation affects fatty acid metabolism, but CFTR-regulated tissue levels may not reflect plasma fatty acid levels.[118] Linoleic acid and docosahexaenoic acid levels are decreased in CF, and eicosatrienoic acid concentration is increased.[116,117] Linoleic and arachidonic acid (a metabolite of eicosatrienoic acid) are n-6 fatty acids, and docosahexaenoic acid is an n-3 fatty acid. The biologic effects of fatty acids depend not only on the absolute levels, but also on the ratio of n-6 to n-3 fatty acids. In CF there is an increased ratio of arachidonic to docosahexaenoic acid. Metabolites of arachidonic acid are proinflammatory agents, and metabolites of docosahexaenoic acid are potent anti-inflammatory agents. The altered ratio may play a role in increased inflammation in CF. Recent studies, however, suggest that linoleic acid concentration is a more clinically relevant biomarker of essential fatty acid status than the triene:tetraene ratio in children with CF and PI.[119] High doses of docosahexaenoic acid fed to CF-knockout mice not only correct the fatty acid deficiency, but also reverse the histologic inflammatory changes in the pancreas and ileum.[118,120]

Nutritional Management

In spite of all the improvements in CF care, undernutrition and malnutrition continue to be problematic in patients with CF and to influence morbidity and mortality. There are numerous factors that contribute to the nutritional status in CF, and numerous studies have shown the value of improved nutrition for longevity and lung health, but maintaining optimal nutrients and calories is not easy.[85,121,122] Patients with CF have increased basal metabolic rates and total daily energy expenditures. Chronic coughing, posttussive emesis, and tachypnea increase caloric needs, but also increase anorexia. Calorie and nutrient losses from malabsorption, and losses due to CFRD, further contribute to malnutrition.[123,124] Even when aggressive dietary intervention is used, maintenance of the required high calorie levels may not be met.[122,125]

Growth may also be affected by factors unrelated to energy absorption and requirements. Chronic inflammation results in increased levels of interleukin 6 (IL-6), which can decrease levels of insulin-like growth factor 1 (IGF-1) and interfere with growth.[126] Synthetic growth hormone increases IGF-1, decreases protein degradation, and improves growth and nutritional status in CF.[126,127] Reduced stores of essential fatty acids result in increased eicosanoid synthesis in CF, which increases inflammation. Administration of essential fatty acids, and n-3 fatty acids in particular, decreases inflammation and can also improve nutrition and growth.[128,129] Chronic respiratory infections have been the assumed culprit for chronic inflammation seen in CF. Improved airway clearance and antibiotics are the cornerstone of care for pulmonary infections, which has a positive effect on nutritional status. However, the pathophysiology of growth disturbance in chronic inflammatory states such as CF continues to be poorly understood and requires further research.

Stunting of growth occurs when malnutrition exists for at least 4 months.[126] Early detection of suboptimal growth with early evaluation and intervention is one benefit of CF newborn screening. To detect early signs of nutritional failure, growth and nutritional status should be monitored routinely at 3-month intervals. Accurate sequential measurements for height, length, weight, and head circumference are obtained and plotted on the 2000 NCHS/CDC growth chart. Assessment of "weight for height proportions," using ideal body weight (IBW) by the Moore method, [101] is also plotted as a percentile on NCHS/CDC growth charts. Patients can have early signs of nutritional failure even if their percentage IBW is 90% or higher, but demonstrate a plateau of weight or loss of weight. If a child's height is below the predicted genetic potential, or the weight for length is below the 25th percentile, evaluation should be considered, because the patient is at risk for nutritional failure. Children whose height is below the fifth percentile for age, or weight for height is below the 10th percentile, or below the 10th percentile for ideal body weight (IBW), are considered as having nutritional failure.[101]

Body mass index (BMI) is an estimate of body fat, which remains fairly constant throughout adulthood, but varies in childhood. Therefore, BMI percentiles, also available on a CDC growth chart, may be an early indicator of nutritional problems when there is variation from a consistent percentile. For children under the age of 2 years, weight for length percentiles are used, because percentiles for BMI are not available. Children with CF are at risk for nutritional failure when their BMI is below the 25th percentile and are exhibiting nutritional failure if they fall below the 10th percentile.[101]

Children with CF are frequently unable to consume the volume of food needed consistently to obtain their energy requirements. Their appetite decreases with acute exacerbations of infections, when energy requirements increase. In infants with CF, breast-feeding is preferred, although commercial formulas can be used. When additional calories are needed to maintain optimal growth, fortification of breast milk, concentrating formula, or adding oil or carbohydrates to the fluid increases the number of calories without significantly changing the volume. Solid foods should be introduced according to the recommendations of the American Academy of Pediatrics. Carbohydrate polymers, vegetable oil, or medium-chain triglyceride oil can provide additional calories without significantly affecting taste or volume. In older children, calorie-dense foods and liquid supplements are added to a balanced diet to boost energy intake. High-calorie snack bars are useful in school and for active children "on the run" who do not find the time for between-meal snacks. The ability or desire to maintain a consistently high-calorie diet with oral supplementation is limited. Nasogastric or gastrostomy tube feedings are the most effective method of providing consistent nutritional supplementation. Percutaneous placement of a gastrostomy tube reduces morbidity but can affect body image in the older child. Continuous nighttime feedings allow for a normal daytime lifestyle and eating pattern. Gastrostomy tube feedings also remove the battles that frequently develop over constant prodding to eat more.

If there is limited response to nutritional supplementation, further evaluation for the etiology of growth failure needs to be considered. Behavioral feeding issues are more common in early childhood, but may be present at any age. School-aged children and adolescents may try to hide their disease from peers and not take enzymes in school. Adolescents are at greatest risk for eating disorders and also are the most resistant to gastrostomy tubes, because of body image issues. When adequate calories are being consumed, but weight loss persists, other causes need to be considered. The older patient with CF is at a greater risk than the general population for intestinal cancer,[130] which can contribute to weight loss or nutritional failure. If other causes of anorexia or malnutrition have been excluded, and decreased food intake secondary to inadequate appetite is the principal cause of the malnutrition, appetite stimulants should be considered.[131]

Hepatobiliary Complications of Cystic Fibrosis

Hepatobiliary complications of CF are a well recognized aspect of the disease (Table 81-6). Although the majority of CF patients will have liver involvement at some point in their lifetime, clinically significant hepatobiliary disease is far less common.[132] Recognition of liver disease in CF has led to increased surveillance with a possible increase in its diagnosis. In addition, improved longevity in patients with CF has served to increase the prevalence of this usually slow-moving process.[133] Although several studies have shown significant liver disease to occur in 15 to 20% of adult CF patients, fatal hepatobiliary disease is relatively rare.[134]

Pathophysiology

CF-associated liver disease begins in the biliary tree. The CFTR protein is not found in hepatocytes but, as is the case with other secretory and absorptive epithelial cells, CFTR is located at the apical portion of the biliary epithelial cell as well as in the bile ducts and gallbladder.[135] It is thought that in CF the impaired secretory function of the biliary epithelium affects water and solute composition of the bile.[136] The adverse effects on bile flow and its alkalinization allow for cholestasis, bile plugging in small biliary radicals, and damage to the biliary tree by cytotoxins and bacteria.[137] In addition to biliary obstruction and defective ion transport, the effect of defective bile salts in some patients can lead to periportal fibrosis.[138] Over many years, this can progress toward bridging fibrosis, and ultimately focal biliary followed by multilobular cirrhosis with portal hypertension.

Unlike CF-associated pancreatic disease, a solid genotype-phenotype relationship has not yet been established in CF-associated liver disease.[132] Recent studies have suggested that the clinical expression of liver disease in CF is likely influenced by a combination of factors, including severe CFTR genotypes, modifier genes, and environmental factors such as nutritional status.[139] Potential disease-modifying genes have included the

TABLE 81-6. Manifestations of Cystic Fibrosis-Associated Liver Disease

Neonatal cholestasis
Hepatomegaly
Raised levels of liver enzymes
Hepatic steatosis
Focal biliary cirrhosis
Multilobular cirrhosis with portal hypertension

histocompatibility complex (HLA), raising the possibility that the immune response may be playing a role in the development of liver disease in CF.[140] Patients who are heterozygotes for specific α_1-antitrypsin mutations may also have an increased risk of developing hepatic complications.[141]

Clinical Evaluation and Diagnosis

The definition and identification of hepatobiliary involvement in CF can be problematic, with some patients not demonstrating clinical disease until the development of multilobular cirrhosis and portal hypertension.[132] Clinical evaluation can be challenging because physical findings may be absent, or may include only hepatomegaly, which might be dismissed in the light of pulmonary hyperinflation. Liver chemistries, especially alanine aminotransferase and γ-glutamyltranspeptidase, are used to look for hepatic and biliary damage, although it has long been recognized that liver chemistries may not be fully reliable indicators even in cases of documented cirrhosis.[142] Percutaneous liver biopsy can show the underlying pathology but has also been shown to be subject to sampling error and false-negative results.[143] There has been recent evidence that ultrasonography may be a useful modality for the screening and staging of liver involvement in CF.[144] These clinically important issues have been addressed by a consensus statement from the Cystic Fibrosis Foundation that recommends screening for liver involvement through yearly physical examination and determination of liver chemistries. Further liver evaluation such as ultrasonography or possibly biopsy is recommended for persistent or marked (three times normal) increases in liver chemistries.[143]

Spectrum of Disease

The most common pathologic change seen in the liver of patients with CF is hepatic steatosis.[145] Fatty change probably occurs in more than one third of patients with CF and can be seen independent of nutritional status and body habitus. The etiology of hepatic steatosis in CF is not fully known. It is as common early in life as in older patients. The relationship between steatosis and the development of fibrosis and cirrhosis in CF is unknown. The pathognomonic CF liver lesion is focal biliary cirrhosis with inspissated, granular eosinophilic material within the bile ducts.[132] Focal biliary cirrhosis can progress to multilobular cirrhosis, predisposing to portal hypertension. Although rare, this can be associated with variceal bleeding and liver failure, requiring liver transplantation.

TABLE 81-7. Biliary Complications of Cystic Fibrosis

Asymptomatic cholelithiasis
Cholecystitis – acute and chronic
Micro or absent gallbladder
Biliary strictures (primary sclerosing cholangitis–like)
Biliary atresia

TABLE 81-8. Treatment of Cystic Fibrosis–Associated Liver Disease

Avoid potential toxic medications, herbs, etc.
Hepatitis A and B immunizations
Optimize nutrition
Ursodeoxycholic acid therapy

Neonatal cholestasis is certainly one of the more obvious modes of presentation of CF-associated liver disease.[146] It is estimated that as many as 5% of patients with CF suffer from this complication. Many authors have questioned whether neonatal cholestasis can lead to a higher incidence of cirrhosis, although one study has not supported this concern.[132]

Extrahepatic biliary complications are also seen in patients with CF (Table 81-7). Asymptomatic gallbladder abnormalities can be seen on imaging of the biliary system.[147] Microgallbladder and absence of the gallbladder can also been seen in biliary atresia that has been diagnosed in patients with CF.[132] Cholelithiasis is seen in as many as 10% of patients with CF, but is often asymptomatic. The gallstones are composed primarily calcium bilirubinate and are not responsive to medical treatment with ursodeoxycholic acid.[148] Extrahepatic strictures, including a beading of the extrahepatic ducts reminiscent of primary sclerosing cholangitis (PSC), has been reported. This is of interest because patients with PSC have an increased incidence of CFTR mutations.[149]

Treatment

As described earlier, there is a potential progression from steatosis to multilobular cirrhosis with portal hypertension. Treatment is designed to attempt to slow and even prevent this progression.[150] Nutritional rehabilitation and maintenance of adequate nutrition remains the cornerstone of therapy. In addition, potential toxins such as herbal agents and hepatotoxic medications should be avoided in CF patients demonstrating liver involvement. As with any chronic liver disease, immunization to hepatitis A and B should be confirmed by titer. Ursodeoxycholic acid (urso) therapy is choleretic and cytoprotective and has been shown to have an immunomodulatory effect.[151] In CF, improvement in liver chemistries has been shown with urso therapy, especially at increased doses of 20 mg/kg daily.[152] Although it is not clear whether this treatment has an effect on the long-term outcome and progression of liver involvement, a 10-year study has suggested improvement in ultrasonographic findings.[153] The recommendation of the Cystic Fibrosis Foundation consensus statement is to use such therapy in the presence of liver disease[143] (Table 81-8).

Varices and portal hypertension are treated in the usual manner, with endoscopic band ligation or sclerotherapy. Beta-blockade may be problematic because of its effect on pulmonary bronchoconstriction. Cirrhosis can lead to end-stage liver failure and the need for liver transplantation. Liver transplantation is rarely indicated, although good results are possible in patients without severe pulmonary compromise who are nutritionally replete and in whom careful attention has been paid to colonization with potential infectious pathogens.[154]

STRUCTURAL ABNORMALITIES OF THE PANCREAS

Structural abnormalities of the pancreas originate from the complex embryologic development of the gland. Failure of normal pancreatic development in utero can result in anomalies of the pancreatic duct system as well as the parenchyma of the gland. The resultant congenital anomalies can then be classified in terms of ductal abnormalities, abnormalities in location (migration) of pancreatic tissue, and abnormalities in the amount of pancreatic tissue (Table 81-9).

TABLE 81-9. Congenital Pancreatic Abnormalities

Ductal Abnormalities
Pancreas divisum
Anomalous pancreaticobiliary union

Defects in Pancreatic Migration
Ectopic pancreas
Annular pancreas

Fatty Replacement of Pancreatic Tissue
Shwachman-Diamond syndrome
Johanson-Blizzard syndrome

Pancreatic Fibrosis
Pearson's marrow-pancreas syndrome
Jeune's syndrome

Abnormalities in Pancreatic Volume
Pancreatic hypoplasia
Pancreatic agenesis

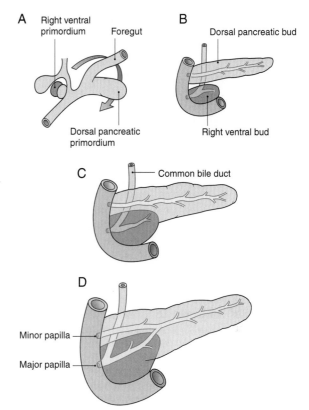

Figure 81-4. Embryologic development of the pancreas. (**A**) 4 weeks' gestation: formation of the dorsal and ventral pancreatic buds. (**B**) 6 weeks' gestation: rotation of the ventral bud bringing it alongside the dorsal bud. (**C**) 7-8 weeks' gestation: fusion of the dorsal and ventral pancreatic buds. (**D**) Final arrangement of the pancreatic ducts with the accessory duct draining part of the head of the pancreas via the minor papilla (above). The common bile duct meets the main pancreatic duct, which drains the majority of the pancreas via the main papilla (below).

Embryology

By the end of the first month of gestation, two outpouchings, one dorsal and the other ventral, arise from the caudal aspect of the embryonic foregut.[155] The dorsal primordium arises from the posterior wall of the duodenum and becomes the tail, body, and part of the head of the pancreas. The ventral bud develops from the hepatic diverticulum and commonly has a bilobed origin. The right and left lobes of the ventral portion later fuse to form the uncinate process and remaining portion of the head of the pancreas (Figure 81-4).[156,157]

A critical aspect of normal pancreatic development occurs by the end of the second month of gestation when the ventral bud rotates in a clockwise manner and comes to lie in an inferior and posterior location, where it then joins the dorsal bud. There are separate ducts associated with the dorsal and ventral portions of the embryonic pancreas. These independent ducts undergo subsequent division and merge to become the drainage system of the mature pancreas.

The dorsal duct arises from the duodenum along with the dorsal tissue. The proximal portion of this duct becomes the accessory duct, or duct of Santorini. The accessory duct drains a portion of the head of the pancreas and enters the duodenum via the minor papilla in 70% of individuals.[158] The distal portion of the embryonic dorsal duct merges with the duct from the ventral bud of the pancreas. This merged structure becomes the duct of Wirsung, or main pancreatic duct. The main duct drains the tail, body, and remaining head of the pancreas and enters the duodenum via the ampulla of Vater in the main papilla. It should be noted that the common bile duct shares this entrance. Therefore, the common entrance into the duodenum of the common bile duct and the duct of Wirsung results from the hepatic origins of the ventral pancreatic bud and its associated duct.[156,159]

Ductal Abnormalities

Various abnormalities in the anatomy of the pancreatic ducts can occur; these find their roots in the complex embryology just described. Pancreas divisum, for example, results when the embryonic dorsal and ventral ducts do not merge.[160]

Pancreas Divisum

More than 90% of individuals undergo normal development of the main pancreatic duct via fusion of the ducts associated with the dorsal and ventral pancreatic buds. When the ducts fail to fuse in utero, the result is two separate drainage systems known as pancreas divisum.[158,161-166] In individuals with pancreas divisum, the head of the pancreas drains independently through the major papilla. The minor papilla then drains the body and tail, which is the majority of the pancreatic tissue. It is postulated that the flow of a relatively high volume of pancreatic secretions through this smaller opening can allow pancreatic enzymes to inflame the papilla, leading to stasis, stenosis, and recurrent pancreatitis.[166]

Diagnosis of pancreas divisum is most commonly made by means of ERCP.[164-166] There are now reports demonstrating that this anomaly can be diagnosed using endoscopic ultrasonography, as well as magnetic resonance cholangiopancreatography (MRCP) (Figure 81-5).[167] Administration of secretin has been shown to increase the potential yield of such an MRCP examination by increasing the secretions in the ducts, thereby allowing clearer delineation of the anatomy.[168-170]

It remains controversial whether pancreas divisum is simply a normal anatomic variant[171,172] or whether it increases the risk of recurrent pancreatitis.[166,173-175] Successful therapeutic trials are usually used as evidence for the argument that pancreas divisum is a cause of recurrent pancreatitis. There are studies

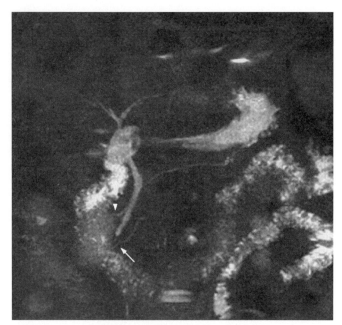

Figure 81-5. Magnetic resonance cholangiopancreatogram showing the separate ventral duct (arrow) and dorsal duct (arrowhead) of pancreas divisum. Courtesy of Brian Herts, MD.

looking at surgical[176-178] and endoscopic[179-182] interventions, including sphincterotomy and stent placement across the minor papilla. Many experts point out potential selection bias in these studies and urge caution in interpreting the results.[183]

Anomalous Pancreaticobiliary Union

Anomalous pancreaticobiliary union (APBU) describes an abnormality in the junction between the common bile duct and the main pancreatic duct. In APBU, this confluence occurs outside the duodenal wall, forming a channel more than 15 mm in length.[184] It is believed that APBU arises from an uneven proliferation of bile duct epithelium during fetal development,[185] perhaps explaining the development of some choledochal cysts. APBU interferes with normal flow of pancreatic and biliary secretions, possibly causing recurrent pancreatitis,[186,187] and may increase the risk of cholangiocarcinoma. When associated with a choledochal cyst, treatment includes removal of the cyst with Roux-en-Y reconstruction of the remaining biliary tree. When there is no cyst, prophylactic cholecystectomy is recommended in light of the increased risk of cholangiocarcinoma.[188]

Abnormalities of Migration

As already described, embryologic development of the pancreas requires migration of parenchymal tissue to the site of the gland's normal anatomic location. There are several recognized congenital abnormalities in the location, volume, and structure of the pancreatic parenchyma that can result from a disordered progression of this aspect of pancreatic development.

Ectopic Pancreas

Ectopic pancreatic tissue is most commonly referred to as a pancreatic rest. Other terms in the literature include heterotopic, aberrant, and accessory pancreatic tissue. Consistent with its embryologic origins, the majority of ectopic pancreatic tissue is found in the foregut, with 75% being found in the

stomach, including the prepyloric gastric antrum.[189,190] Duodenal and proximal jejunal sites have also been reported. Ectopic pancreatic tissue has also been seen in the ileum, Meckel's diverticulum, gallbladder, common bile duct, splenic hilum, umbilicus, and lung, and in perigastric and periduodenal tissue.[191] In autopsy series, the average frequency of ectopic pancreas is between 1% and 2% (range 0.55 to 13%).[192]

By definition, such tissue has no physical or vascular continuity with the pancreatic gland. Pancreatic rests are frequently functional but are usually asymptomatic and discovered as an incidental finding on upper gastrointestinal contrast study.[193] Upper endoscopy can also demonstrate these lesions, which appear as a round, smooth, submucosal mass with a central umbilication, most commonly found in the antrum and gastric outlet.

There have been reports of clinical symptoms associated with large (more than 1.5 cm) pancreatic rests.[194] The most common symptoms were abdominal pain, dyspepsia, and gastrointestinal bleeding. Biliary and pyloric obstruction may occur.[195] Pancreatitis in the ectopic tissue has also been described, and there are reported cases of cancer occurring in the ectopic pancreas.[196] Because ectopic pancreatic tissue is usually asymptomatic, management is usually observational with operative treatment reserved for complicated cases.[197] The submucosal location of pancreatic rests makes endoscopic removal unattractive, owing to the perforation risk.

Annular Pancreas

During its migration in the second month of gestation, the ventral portion of the pancreas can become misaligned, encircle the second portion of the duodenal sweep, and then fuse with the dorsal aspect of the developing pancreas.[198] This anatomy is known as annular pancreas (Figure 81-6). The most common clinical presentation of annular pancreas is a neonatal bowel obstruction proximal to the ampulla of Vater. This anatomic abnormality can occur in isolation or together with other congenital malformations. The most commonly associated malformations are usually gastrointestinal, including intestinal malrotation, duodenal abnormalities such as web, stenosis, and atresia, tracheoesophageal fistula, imperforate anus, and Hirschsprung's disease. Annular pancreas can occur with congenital heart disease and has an increased incidence in patients with trisomy 21.[199]

Annular pancreas has a variety of clinical presentations. In infancy, it can present as upper gastrointestinal obstruction with a classic "double bubble" sign on abdominal radiography. It may be asymptomatic or present in adulthood with duodenal obstruction, chronic pancreatitis, or ulceration. Because duodenal malformation frequently accompanies annular pancreas, the treatment of choice is surgical bypass of the lesion, usually with a duodenoduodenostomy.

Abnormalities in Volume

Both pancreatic agenesis and hypoplasia have been reported in isolation and with other congenital abnormalities.[200] Endocrine and exocrine insufficiency may occur, and appropriate hormone and enzyme replacement therapy can lead to improved survival if diagnosed in a timely manner. Intrauterine growth retardation can be a consequence of lack of fetal insulin in utero. Hypoplasia may result from agenesis of the dorsal bud of the pancreas, which normally supplies 90% of the pancreatic

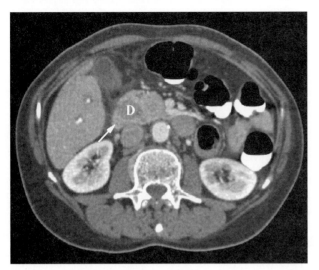

Figure 81-6. Annular pancreas. Contrast-enhanced axial computed tomogram showing pancreatic tissue (arrow) lateral to and surrounding the duodenum (D). Courtesy Brian Herts, MD.

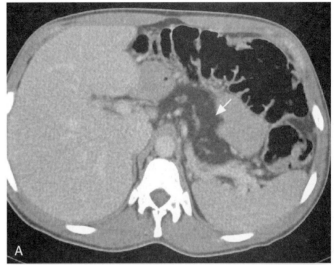

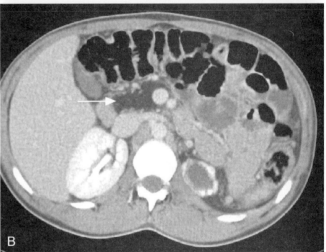

Figure 81-7. Shwachman-Diamond syndrome. Contrast-enhanced axial computed tomograms through (**A**) the body and (**B**) the head of the pancreas showing complete fatty replacement of the gland (arrows). Courtesy Brian Herts, MD.

tissue.[201] Such a short gland has been reported to occur with other congenital abnormalities, including polysplenia.[202] Fatty replacement of the gland has also been reported and can be considered a form of pancreatic hypoplasia.[203]

Epithelium-lined congenital pancreatic cysts have also been described. The mode of presentation of these rare cysts includes gastrointestinal obstruction, biliary obstruction, and the finding of an asymptomatic mass. Treatment is by surgical excision.

FUNCTIONAL ABNORMALITIES OF THE PANCREAS

Several syndromes have been described that include congenital exocrine pancreatic insufficiency and other anomalies, including the bone marrow and skeletal systems. In these syndromes pancreatic insufficiency results from an inadequate volume of acinar cells due to fibrosis or fatty replacement of parenchymal tissue. The most common of these is the Shwachman-Diamond syndrome (SDS).

Shwachman-Diamond Syndrome

SDS is the second most common inherited cause of pancreatic insufficiency. This autosomal recessive syndrome is characterized by exocrine pancreatic insufficiency, bone marrow dysfunction and skeletal abnormalities.[204]

The pathogenesis of pancreatic insufficiency in SDS probably results from the failure of normal development of acinar tissue in utero. The normal tissue is replaced with fatty deposition (Figure 81-7).[205] Pancreatic lipomatosis accounts for the distinctive appearance of the pancreas on abdominal ultrasonography. Computed tomography can be even more sensitive and is a useful test to establish the diagnosis of SDS.[206] Clinically, pancreatic insufficiency that results in steatorrhea is most prominent early in life. Subsequent malabsorption, calorie loss, and failure to thrive are treated with appropriate dietary intervention, including pancreatic enzyme and fat-soluble vitamin supplementation. Unlike cystic fibrosis, which leads to obstruction and damage to the pancreatic ducts, SDS affects the acinar tissue, and the ductal elements remain intact. Over time,

pancreatic hypoplasia is reversed, and there is an increase in normal pancreatic tissue volume. Improved pancreatic function has been reported in several series of patients with SDS. Approximately half of patients can establish pancreatic sufficiency by 4 years of age.[207,208] In managing patients with SDS, potential improvement in pancreatic function over time should be kept in mind. Accordingly, pancreatic function and clinical tests of fat absorption are followed serially, and pancreatic enzyme replacement therapy adjusted accordingly.

Bone marrow dysfunction is another hallmark component of SDS. Persistent or noncyclic but recurrent neutropenia is the most common abnormality seen. Infectious complications, especially in young patients with neutropenia, become a clinical concern leading to significant morbidity and mortality in some patients.[207] Prophylactic antibiotics have been a mainstay of therapy, but successful use of bone marrow transplantation has been reported.[209] The advent of human granulocyte colony-stimulating factor has improved the treatment of neutropenia in patients with SDS.[210] In addition to neutropenia, both the red cell and platelet lines can be affected separately or in combination. Patients with SDS also have an increased risk of developing myelodysplasia and a variety of leukemias that may be treatment resistant.[207] Bone marrow surveillance is prudent in these patients.

Skeletal abnormalities are also seen in patients with SDS. Progressive long-bone dysostosis or metaphyseal chondrodysplasia is the most common finding seen over time in approximately half of patients with SDS. Abnormalities of the thoracic cage are seen in as many as one-third of patients.[207]

Research into the genetics of SDS has focused on a region on chromosome 7. In 2003, Boocock et al.[210] reported their genetic findings after studying 156 unrelated patients with SDS. Some 89% of these patients had mutations in a previously uncharacterized gene mapped to chromosome 7q11, which the authors labeled the *SDS* (Shwachman-Diamond) or *SBDS* (Shwachman-Bodian-Diamond syndrome) gene. This genetic breakthrough should help further the understanding of the pathogenesis of SDS. Genetic testing will also aid in the diagnosis of SDS. Because the diagnosis of SDS continues to be made clinically, this can prove to be challenging in light of the variable clinical manifestations that can be seen with this syndrome.

Johanson-Blizzard Syndrome

This is a syndrome of exocrine pancreatic insufficiency with multiple congenital anomalies including deafness, imperforate anus, urogenital malformations, and dental anomalies.[211] As with SDS, pancreatic insufficiency results from fatty replacement of the gland. Multiple endocrine abnormalities have been associated with Johanson-Blizzard syndrome, including hypothyroidism, growth hormone deficiency, diabetes, and panhypopituitarism.[212]

The syndrome is characterized by typical facies including nasal hypoplasia leading to a "beak-shaped" appearance, small or misshapen teeth, and sparse, dry hair.

Pearson's Marrow-Pancreas Syndrome

Similar to SDS, Pearson's syndrome involves the bone marrow and pancreas and results from deletions in mitochondrial DNA.[213,214] Patients with Pearson's syndrome present with a profound and frequently refractory sideroblastic anemia. The bone marrow examination is distinctive, showing vacuolization of bone marrow precursors and ringed sideroblasts. Ultimately other blood cell lines may be involved. There is pancreatic exocrine insufficiency, and autopsy data have demonstrated significant pancreatic fibrosis. As a mitochondrial disease there is a resultant defect in oxidative phosphorylation, explaining the often persistent and even fatal lactic acidosis that has been reported in patients with Pearson's syndrome. Ultimately, there can be renal, endocrine, and other multiorgan involvement and failure. Death frequently ensues in infancy or early childhood as a result of sepsis or metabolic disarray.

Jeune's Syndrome

This rare syndrome is characterized by pancreatic insufficiency and fibrosis with anomalies of the skeletal structure of the upper thorax that lead to respiratory compromise.[215]

REFERENCES

24. Walkowiak J, Nousia-Arvanitakis S, Henker J, et al. Indirect pancreatic function testing in children. J Pediatr Gastrenterol Nutr 2005;40: 107–114.
49. Lai HJ, Cheng Y, Cho H, et al. Association between initial disease presentation, lung disease outcomes and survival in patients with cystic fibrosis. Am J Epidemiol 2004;159:537–546.
58. De Boeck K, Weren M, Proesmans M, Kerem E. Pancreatitis among patients with cystic fibrosis: Correlation with pancreatic status and genotype. Pediatrics 2005;115:463–469.
64. Sobczynska-Tomaszewska A, Bak D, Oralewska B, et al. Analysis of CFTR, SPINK1, PRSS1 and AAT mutations in children with acute or chronic pancreatitis. J Pediatr Gastroenterol Nutr 2006;43:299–306.
80. Moran A, Dunitz J, Nathan B, et al. Cystic fibrosis-related diabetes: current trends in prevalence, incidence, and mortality. Diabetes Care 2009;3:1626–1631.
84. Koscik RL, Farrell PM, Kosorok MR, et al. Cognitive function of children with cystic fibrosis: deleterious effect of early malnutrition. Pediatrics 2004;113:1549–1558.
118. Freedman SD, Blanco PG, Zaman MM, et al. Association of cystic fibrosis with abnormalities in fatty acid metabolism. N Engl J Med 2004;350: 560–569.
132. Moyer K, Balistreri W. Hepatobiliary disease in patients with cystic fibrosis. Curr Opin Gastroenterol 2009;25:272–278.
141. Bartlett JR, Friedman KJ, Ling SC, et al. Genetic modifiers of liver disease in cystic fibrosis. JAMA 2009;302(10):1076–1083.
216. Witt H. Chronic pancreatitis and cystic fibrosis. Gut 2003;52(Suppl 2): ii31-ii41.

See expertconsult.com for a complete list of references and the review questions for this chapter.

PANCREATITIS 82

Mark E. Lowe

ACUTE AND CHRONIC PANCREATITIS

Pancreatitis is more prevalent in children than previously believed. The diagnosis of pancreatitis has increased over the past decade and large children's hospitals treat 100 to 150 children a year for pancreatitis.[1-4] Most patients have acute pancreatitis, and 10% or fewer have chronic pancreatitis. Greater physician awareness likely accounts for the increase in the diagnosis of acute pancreatitis in childhood.[2] The etiologies of acute pancreatitis differ between children and adults, in whom gallstone- and alcohol-associated pancreatitis are predominant. In children, systemic illness, biliary disease, medications, and trauma encompass the majority of children with an identifiable etiology. A large portion of patients have no identifiable cause.[5] Similarly, many patients have no identifiable cause for their chronic pancreatitis. Despite advances in understanding the pathophysiology of pancreatitis, care remains supportive. Fortunately, most children have a benign clinical course. Some develop complications, with fluid collections being the most common problem. A small group will have recurrent episodes of acute pancreatitis.

Definition and Classification

Over the years, the classification of inflammatory disorders of the pancreas has changed, but two broad categories have remained constant: acute and chronic. Acute pancreatitis is a reversible process with no lasting effects on the pancreatic parenchyma or function. Chronic pancreatitis is an irreversible process leading to changes in the parenchyma and function of the pancreas. Clinical criteria define both diagnoses. The diagnosis of acute pancreatitis requires two of three criteria: (1) appropriate clinical symptoms, (2) elevations of serum amylase or lipase above three times the upper reference limit (URL) and (3) radiographic evidence of pancreatitis, generally by transabdominal ultrasound or by contrast-enhanced computed tomography (CECT). Acute pancreatitis can be further separated into two types, interstitial and necrotizing pancreatitis. Interstitial pancreatitis is most common and generally follows a benign clinical course, whereas necrotizing pancreatitis often heralds a severe clinical course with complications.

The diagnosis of chronic pancreatitis requires the demonstration of typical histologic and morphologic changes in the pancreas or evidence of decreased digestive function. Radiologic methods and rarely biopsy can demonstrate changes in the structure of the pancreas. Typically, most radiologic methods detect advanced disease. Detection of early changes has proven difficult and makes the identification of patients in the early stages of chronic pancreatitis almost impossible. Both direct and indirect measures of pancreatic function can help establish the presence of pancreatic insufficiency, but most cannot detect losses in function that do not result in maldigestion.

ACUTE PANCREATITIS

Pathophysiology

The development of pancreatitis can be modeled into three phases.[6] First, an event triggers the process (Figure 82-1). Obstruction of the pancreatic duct from gallstones and ethanol ingestion commonly incites pancreatitis in adults. Common triggers in children include systemic illness, medications, trauma, and bile or pancreatic duct disease secondary to gallstones or congenital abnormalities. The triggering event stresses the pancreatic acinar cells through mechanisms that remain speculative.[7]

This stress, likely metabolic or oxidative, initiates the second phase of acute pancreatitis, acinar cell injury. Ever since Chiari proposed that pancreatitis results from autodigestion by digestive enzymes, the premature activation of digestive enzymes, in particular trypsinogen, has been central to theories on the mechanism of acinar cell injury.[8] Under this scheme, trypsinogen is prematurely activated to trypsin inside the acinar cell. To this day, the mechanism of activation remains obscure. Because an early event in experimental pancreatitis is the colocalization of digestive enzymes and lysosomal enzymes in vacuoles, many theories of pathogenesis speculate that activation of trypsinogen occurs in the vacuoles through the action of lysosomal enzymes, in particular cathepsin B.[9] Although some studies have implicated cathepsin B in the intracellular activation of trypsinogen, other studies do not support this theory, and the relevance to human disease has not been established.[10]

Premature activation of digestive enzymes may not be the dominant event in the pathogenesis of pancreatitis. Other mechanisms may contribute to acinar cell injury. For instance, some have proposed that reactive oxygen species may produce injury by increasing lipid peroxidation. Or, alterations in the microcirculation of the pancreas may produce area of hypoperfusion and subsequent hypoxic damage to acinar cells. The observed changes in cell membrane permeability may lead to pathologic increases in cellular calcium, another early event in experimental pancreatitis, or the leak of proteins from the cells. Impairments in autophagy, a cytoprotective mechanism for maintaining homeostasis of cellular functions such as organelle and protein turnover, likely contributes to the pathogenesis of cell injury.[11] The formation of autophagosomes is an early event in experimental pancreatitis. Some have proposed that autophagy contributes to trypsinogen activation within the acinar cells.[12] Finally, the role of the endoplasmic reticulum (ER) stress response in acute pancreatitis has been recently appreciated.[13-16] One of the major triggers of the ER stress response is an imbalance in the ER protein folding capacity. Increases in the concentration of unfolded proteins in the ER set off a series of pathways known as the unfolded protein

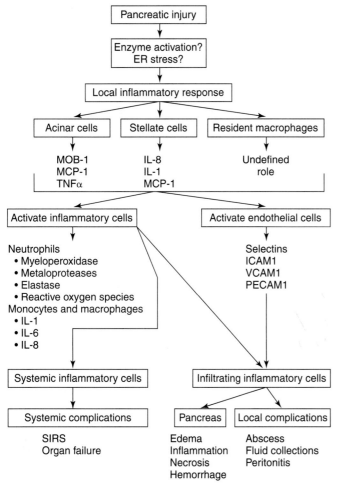

Figure 82-1. Pathophysiology of pancreatitis. ICAM, intercellular adhesion molecule; IL, interleukin; MCP, monocyte chemoattractant protein; MOB, Mps one binder; PECAM, platelet/endothelial cell adhesion molecule; TNF, tumor necrosis factor; VCAM, vascular cell adhesion molecule.

Pathology

The histology of interstitial pancreatitis shows relatively minimal changes. The prominent feature is interstitial edema. The inflammatory infiltrate is minimal and includes neutrophils, monocytes, macrophages, and lymphocytes.[23] The leukocyte migration is triggered by chemokines released from resident macrophages, acinar cells, and, likely, stellate cells. The inflammatory response results in little cell death, mostly through apoptosis, although small areas of acinar cell necrosis may be present. Additionally, focal areas of fat necrosis may be present within the gland or adjacent to the gland. In the more severe necrotizing pancreatitis, the areas of necrosis are extensive and include acinar, ductal, and islet cells. Erosion into blood vessels produces hemorrhage into the parenchyma. Areas of fat necrosis adjacent to the pancreas can also be extensive. Grossly, the pancreas contains areas of red-black hemorrhagic necrosis and foci of yellow-white fat necrosis.

Etiology

A wide array of factors can trigger acute pancreatitis in children (Table 82-1).[5] The prevalence of any specific etiology is not well established, because there is wide variation in reported prevalence among published studies. The variation stems from the retrospective nature of the studies, the bias or experience of the clinicians at a particular institute, the lack of thorough investigations for the etiology in many patients, and the recognition of new etiologies in the time between reports. All reports include a sizable number of patients with no identifiable etiology. Of those with an identifiable etiology, several broad categories, systemic illness, biliary disease, trauma, and medications, stand out as causing the majority.

The reported proportion of patients with acute pancreatitis in the setting of a systemic illness has varied considerably, 3.5% to 48%, with more recent reports finding the higher rates. Although acute pancreatitis can occur with a number of different systemic illnesses, hemolytic uremic syndrome has been reported most often in association with acute pancreatitis.[4,24,25] The mechanism of pancreatitis in this illness is unknown and probably multifactorial. Both uremia and hemolysis are risk factors for acute pancreatitis and acute pancreatitis should be considered in every child with hemolytic uremic syndrome.[26,27]

Biliary disease includes both gallstones and congenital anomalies of the biliary tree. Gallstone pancreatitis is likely more common in pediatric patients than previously believed. Solid data on the incidence are lacking, but it clearly occurs at all ages. Almost 30% of 56 patients in a Korean study had gallstone pancreatitis.[28] In a study of infants and toddlers, nearly 10% had gallstone pancreatitis.[25] Congenital anomalies include pancreas divisum, choledochal cysts, and choledochoceles. Pancreas divisum is the most common anomaly, occurring in up to 10% of the population. Its role in acute pancreatitis remains controversial and most people with pancreas divisum do not develop pancreatitis. The subgroup that develops pancreatitis may have another risk factor such as dysfunction of the cystic fibrosis transmembrane conductance regulator protein (CFTR).[29]

A variety of medications associate with acute pancreatitis.[30-32] Valproic acid has the highest rate reported in series of children with acute pancreatitis.[4,24] Because the incidence of pancreatitis in children taking valproic acid is quite low, another factor may be involved. Consequently, the possibility of an underlying

response. Prolonged activation of the unfolded protein response leads to programmed cell death. Interestingly, misfolding of a human trypsinogen mutant, which is associated with human disease, activated the ER stress response in transfected tissue culture cells, thereby implicating the ER stress response in the disease mechanism of pancreatitis.[17]

Whatever the mechanism, acinar cell injury is followed by a local inflammatory process that sets off the final stage of pancreatitis, the inflammatory response. The transcription factor NF-κB is central to this response. NF-κB regulates genes encoding cytokines, chemokines, adhesion molecules, and proteins in cell death pathways among other gene products. In experimental models of pancreatitis, NF-κB is activated in the early stages.[18-20] Moreover direct activation of NF-κB results in pancreatic inflammation and a systemic inflammatory response.[21] The subsequent release of cytokines and chemokines mediates a systemic inflammatory response. The clinical severity of pancreatitis depends largely on the vigor of the inflammatory response.[22] A brisk response leads to pancreatic necrosis and inflammation of adjacent and distant organs. Clearly, the systemic complications of acute pancreatitis result from the activated immune response in distant organs and not from the circulating pancreatic digestive enzymes.

TABLE 82-1. Etiologies of Acute Pancreatitis in Children

Biliary
  Cholelithiasis
  Choledochal cyst
  Biliary sludge
Anatomic
  Pancreas divisum
  Anomalous junction of the biliary and pancreatic ducts
  Annular pancreas
  Ampullary obstruction
  Crohn's disease
  Diverticulum
  Cyst
  Ulcer
  Tumor
Drugs
  L-Asparaginase
  Valproate
  Metronidazole
  Mercaptopurine
  Azathioprine
  Tetracycline
  Pentamidine
  Didanosine
Genetic
  PRSS1 mutations
  CFTR mutations
  Systemic disease
  Sepsis
  Hemolytic uremic syndrome
  Diabetic ketoacidosis
  Collagen vascular disease
  Kawasaki disease
  Organ transplantation
  Sickle cell disease
  Anorexia nervosa
  Shock
  Inflammatory bowel disease
Trauma
  Blunt injury
  Duodenal hematoma
  Child abuse
  Post-ERCP
Metabolic
  Hyperlipidemia
  Hypercalcemia
  Glycogen storage disease
  Organic acidemias
  Malnutrition (refeeding)
Postoperative
  Spinal surgery
  Cardiothoracic surgery
  Autoimmune pancreatitis
Indeterminate

ERCP, endoscopic retrograde cholangiopancreatography.

TABLE 82-2. Signs and Symptoms of Acute Pancreatitis

	Common	Uncommon
Symptoms	Abdominal pain	Back pain
	Irritability (infants)	Jaundice
	Nausea	Fever
	Vomiting	Feeding Intolerance
	Anorexia	Respiratory distress
Signs	Abdominal tenderness	Turner's sign
	Abdominal distention	Cullen's sign
	Evidence of dehydration	Evidence of ascites
		Evidence of pleural effusion

Clinical Presentation

The symptoms and signs of acute pancreatitis are nonspecific and vary with age (Table 82-2). Upper abdominal pain and vomiting are the most common symptoms. Abdominal pain is present in 68 to 95% of patients in various series.[4,33,34] Some of the variation may reflect the age distribution of patients in the studies. Only 29% of patients younger than 3 years of age had abdominal pain, and even if irritability was considered a surrogate for pain, the percentage of patients was still only 46%.[25] Vomiting is present in 45 to 85% of reported cases. In younger patients, vomiting is the most common symptoms. Less common symptoms and signs include abdominal tenderness or distention, tachycardia, fever, hypotension, jaundice, and back pain. Ecchymoses of the flank (Turner's sign) or blue discoloration of the umbilicus (Cullen's sign) are unusual in children. Acute pancreatitis should be considered when a hospitalized patient has worsening of clinical status or feeding intolerance.

Diagnosis

Because the signs and symptoms of acute pancreatitis are nonspecific, the physician must consider acute pancreatitis in any child with gastrointestinal complaints. The accepted clinical definition of acute pancreatitis in adults requires two of the following: (1) abdominal pain consistent with pancreatitis; (2) serum amylase or lipase levels at least three times the URL; and (3) radiologic evidence of acute pancreatitis. Although most pediatric patients with acute pancreatitis will fulfill these criteria, a number of children may not complain of abdominal pain.

Laboratory Studies

Although there is no gold standard for the diagnosis of acute pancreatitis, in practice serum amylase and lipase levels are measured to screen for pancreatitis. The reliability of these measurements to diagnose acute pancreatitis is uncertain. Several studies have attempted to define the sensitivity and specific city of serum amylase and lipase for acute pancreatitis, but all suffer from the lack of a method to separately and definitively diagnose acute pancreatitis. Furthermore, both can be normal when there is clear clinical and radiologic evidence of acute pancreatitis or both can be elevated in other conditions where there is no other evidence for acute pancreatitis. Finally, a significant fraction of patients will have a selective elevation of either amylase or lipase at presentation. Consequently, both amylase and lipase should be measured in patients suspected of having acute pancreatitis.

inborn error of metabolism, particularly of fatty acid metabolism, should be considered. The next most commonly associated medication is L-asparaginase.

Trauma remains a common cause of acute pancreatitis in children. Usually the trauma is blunt and accidental, but child abuse should be considered. Cutaneous findings of trauma may not be present. The injury can vary from a small hematoma to rupture of the main pancreatic duct. In the latter case, endoscopic or surgical intervention may be required.

Despite increased awareness of pancreatitis and potential etiologies, no cause is found in about one fifth of patients. As genetic testing and better radiologic testing become more widely available and new etiologies are recognized, the proportion of children with indeterminate pancreatitis will fall.

Infants present a theoretical problem with the use of amylase and lipase to diagnose acute pancreatitis.[5] Expression of both pancreatic amylase and lipase are low at birth. Amylase may not reach adult levels until adolescence, and lipase may not reach adult levels until 1 year of age. The clinical significance of these developmental patterns of expression is unknown, but should be kept in mind when considering acute pancreatitis in infants.

Other conditions such as renal failure rarely increase serum amylase or lipase levels more than three times the URL. Two exceptions can increase serum enzyme levels considerably more than three times the upper reference limit. Both are benign, and their recognition prevents unnecessary testing and treatment. In general, they cause confusion in patients who have a laboratory panel done that includes amylase for reasons unrelated to symptoms of pancreatitis or in patients who have abdominal pain but normal radiographs. In each case, the serum enzyme elevations persist even in the absence of symptoms. First, either lipase or amylase can complex with a larger molecule, often an immunoglobulin, to form macroenzymes called macroamylase or macrolipase.[35,36] Because the complex does not clear the serum as rapidly as unbound enzyme, the enzyme accumulates to higher than normal levels in the bloodstream. At present, there is a commercially available test for macroamylasemia but not for macrolipasemia. Second, some patients have elevations of pancreatic enzymes in the serum without any clinical or radiographic evidence of pancreatitis or of macroenzymes.[37,38] Typically, lipase or amylase is detected, but all pancreatic enzymes are elevated in most patients. The levels fluctuate from normal to many times the URL. Other family members may have benign elevations of pancreatic enzymes. The mechanism is unclear and may involve alterations in the normal secretory pathways with shunting of more enzymes to basolateral secretion as happens in acute pancreatitis.

Imaging

No studies have investigated the utility of imaging studies in children with suspected acute pancreatitis. In patients with abdominal pain and elevated amylase or lipase, imaging may not be necessary unless there are systemic signs of severe disease or suspicion of biliary pancreatitis. If there are clinical symptoms of acute pancreatitis and the serum enzyme levels are not above three times the URL, imaging may help make the diagnosis. Transabdominal ultrasonography represents a good initial choice for the radiographic evaluation of children.

Ultrasonography is widely available and less expensive than other options (Figure 82-2A). Typical findings are pancreatic hypertrophy, decreased echogenicity, dilated pancreatic duct, and peripancreatic fluid. Also, ultrasound can detect gallstones. Obesity or the presence of bowel gas may limit the ability of ultrasound to provide useful information.

Contrast-enhanced computed tomography is another option. CECT is probably the best imaging modality for the overall assessment of the pancreas and complications (Figure 82-2B). Information about the presence of pancreatic inflammation, the presence of gallstones, possible etiologies, and complications such as pancreatic necrosis or fluid collections can be obtained. Animal studies raised concern that intravenous contrast may increase the severity of pancreatitis, but this concern has not held for humans.[39]

The prevalence of gallstone pancreatitis in childhood, particularly adolescence, provides the best argument for imaging studies early in the course of acute pancreatitis. Clearly, elevations of serum transaminases or bilirubin should prompt investigations for gallstone pancreatitis. Although ultrasound and CECT can detect gallstones, studies in adults suggest that endoscopic ultrasound (EUS) or magnetic resonance cholangiopancreatography (MRCP) may be better options (Figure 82-3).[40,41] No studies have been done in pediatrics.

In addition to gallstones, MRCP can reveal other pancreaticobiliary disorders. Choledochal cysts, pancreas divisum, and anomalous junction between the pancreatic and biliary ducts can be identified. MRCP performs well in children of all ages and does not require ionizing radiation.[42-44] The major limitation of MRCP is the need for sedation or general anesthesia in many pediatric patients. In most centers, MRCP has replaced endoscopic retrograde cholangiopancreatography (ERCP) in the diagnosis of pancreaticobiliary disease. ERCP is now primarily utilized for therapy of gallstones or duct anomalies.

In adults, EUS increases the diagnostic yield for gallstones and microlithiasis.[45] The size of EUS endoscopes and the reluctance of trained EUS endoscopists, primarily adult gastroenterologists, to perform procedures on young patients have limited EUS in pediatric patients. Still, experience with EUS in children is accumulating.[46,47] As happened with ERCP, smaller endoscopes will become available and the comfort of the endoscopists with pediatric patients will increase. Eventually the role of EUS in children with pancreatitis will be defined.

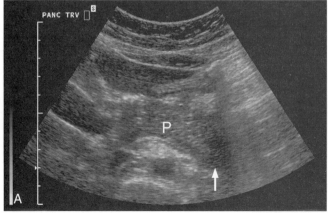
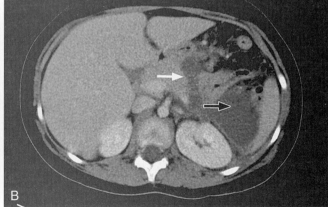

Figure 82-2. Necrotizing pancreatitis. (**A**) Transverse ultrasonography of a 9-year-old patient with necrotizing pancreatitis of the distal body and tail (marked by letter "P"). The arrow is pointing to the developing pseudocyst. (**B**) Computed tomogram of the patient in (**A**) showing necrosis of the distal body and tail (white arrow) and pseudocyst (black arrow). Courtesy Dr. Janet Reid.

Investigations of Etiology

Clinical judgment should determine which testing is necessary to identify the etiology for a patient's first episode of acute pancreatitis. Systematic consideration of probable, possible, and rare causes based on history and physical exam findings should limit unnecessary testing. For instance, patients who develop acute pancreatitis associated with a systemic illness may not require additional studies. History can identify drugs that may cause pancreatitis or suggest trauma as the cause. CECT, ERCP, or MRCP can provide evidence of duct rupture (Figure 82-4). A family history of pancreatitis should prompt genetic testing. Jaundice should prompt an investigation into biliary causes of pancreatitis. Serum calcium and triglycerides should be measured in all patients. Although hypercalcemia and hypertriglyceridemia are uncommon in pediatrics, they can be treated and future episodes of acute pancreatitis can be prevented.

In the 10% of patients who have a second episode of acute pancreatitis, a more thorough investigation for etiology is necessary. A complete evaluation for structural anomalies of the pancreaticobiliary tree and upper gastrointestinal tract should

be pursued. MRCP is the choice for ductal abnormalities in children of all ages. CECT or an upper gastrointestinal series can identify duplication cysts of the stomach or duodenum and congenital cysts in the pancreas. Duodenal ulcers, duodenal Crohn's disease, and tumors of the papilla can be found by esophagogastroduodenoscopy. Genetic testing for *PRSS1* (cationic trypsinogen gene) and *CFTR* mutations should considered.[48] Testing for *SPINK1* (serine protease inhibitor Kazal type 1) mutations is probably not helpful, because heterozygous mutations are not associated with disease, and even though homozygous mutations associate with chronic pancreatitis, they modify the disease course rather than cause the disease primarily.[49,50] Knowing a patient has a *SPINK1* mutation does not help in advising the family about the disease course.

Management

Treatment, as it always has, relies on supportive care to provide adequate intravenous hydration, to control pain, and to monitor for complications. Pancreatic rest or nothing by mouth is still practiced but should be limited.

Fluid Management

In recent years, the importance of fluid resuscitation at presentation of acute pancreatitis has had much discussion.[51] Animal models and retrospective studies in humans indicate that early fluid resuscitation may improve outcome and prevent severe disease, and aggressive intravenous (IV) fluid replacement was recommended in the American College of Gastroenterology practice guidelines for acute pancreatitis without defining what aggressive means.[52] Recommendations in the literature on adults range from 250 to 1000 mL/hour depending on initial volume status. Gradually replacing fluid deficits (5 to 10 mL/kg/hour) may give better outcomes than more rapid fluid infusions (10 to 15 mL/kg/hour).[53] There are no studies of pediatric patients to guide fluid management. Without clear guidelines, it seems reasonable to provide intravenous fluids at a rate that exceeds basal requirements and to give additional fluids determined by the patient's hemodynamic status.

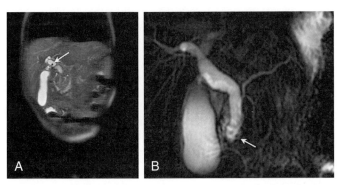

Figure 82-3. MRCP (T2-wieghted image reconstruction) of two patients with dilated common bile duct and gallstones. (**A**) The common bile duct is dilated, and a gallstone is revealed as a filling defect (white arrow). This patient had an anomalous junction of the common bile duct and main pancreatic duct (not shown). (**B**) Another dilated common bile duct with gallstones impacted in the distal duct (white arrow).

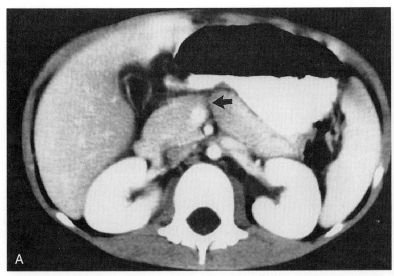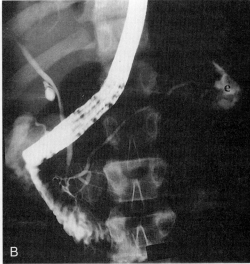

Figure 82-4. Ruptured duct. (**A**) Computed tomogram showing enlarged linear low-attenuation area at the neck of the pancreas (arrow) compatible with a pancreatic laceration. (**B**) ERCP examination showing extravasation at the pancreatic duct tail compatible with pancreatic duct lacerations (shown by letter **e**).

Pain Control

Patients with pain should be treated with parenteral narcotics. Some centers avoid morphine in the belief that morphine may increase sphincter of Oddi pressure and worsen the course of pancreatitis. Frequently, meperidine is given. In truth, all opiates, including meperidine, can increase sphincter pressure, and no clinical evidence indicates poorer outcome when morphine is used in acute pancreatitis.[54] Morphine has the advantage over meperidine in that it has a longer half-life and fewer side effects. Regardless of the choice for analgesia, adequate pain relief should be provided. Dosing of pain medications should be monitored regularly and the daily dose adjusted as required.

Nutritional Therapy

Pancreatic rest, starvation, has long been a mainstay of care in patients with acute pancreatitis. Now, experimental and clinical evidence strongly supports early feeding of patients with pancreatitis, and nutritional support is considered an active and beneficial intervention.[55] Enteral nutrition should start within 24 hours of admission after fluid resuscitation and pain control are implemented.

Patients with mild acute pancreatitis can be safely allowed to eat and drink as tolerated without a period of fasting.[56] In this study, patients who were fed advanced to solid foods faster and had a shorter hospital stay than fasted, control patients. In another study, patients with mild acute pancreatitis were randomized to a low-fat diet or a clear liquid diet.[57] The reoccurrence of pain and the need to stop oral intake did not differ between the groups. Because patients with mild acute pancreatitis generally tolerate oral intake early in their course, fasting until symptoms resolve or until serum amylase or lipase return to normal is not necessary.

Patients with severe pancreatitis can also be fed shortly after they have been stabilized. In fact, early enteral feeds may provide more benefit and cause fewer complications than parenteral nutrition.[58] Various studies support the safety and tolerance of both nasogastric and nasojejunal feeds. Delivery of nutrients beyond the ligament of Treitz has theoretical advantages over gastric feeds. It avoids the stomach in a group of patients with a high prevalence of abnormal gastric emptying, and modern jejunal feeding tubes allow simultaneous decompression of the stomach. In addition, jejunal feeding causes less stimulation of the exocrine pancreas.[59,60] Presently, the choice of route is institution specific.

The final consideration is what type of diet to provide. Standard practice in most centers is to start with a low-fat diet or formula, although there is no evidence that a low-fat diet offers any advantage over a regular diet. Immunomodulating diets supplemented with glutamine, arginine, omega-3 fatty acids, or antioxidants are controversial in critically ill patients. Their use in severe acute pancreatitis is not indicated currently.

Outcome

In most cases, children and adolescents have a mild course of acute pancreatitis and their symptoms resolve without complications. However, the average length of hospital stay can exceed 2 weeks. The mean length of hospital stay before 1999 was 13.2 ± 2.4 days.[33] Recently, two studies reported 24 and 25.7 days as the mean length of stay.[4,34] In one, the median hospital stay was 8 days, and the authors suggested that the presence of comorbid conditions strongly influenced the length of stay.[4] Another study focusing on infants and toddlers supports that contention.[25] The median length of stay for all subjects was 19.5 days, whereas patients admitted with only acute pancreatitis had a median length of stay of 8.5 days. Overall about one fifth of children will have prolonged courses with persistent symptoms or complications.[24,25,33] Many of these patients may have another illness when they develop acute pancreatitis, and it is likely these conditions rather than pancreatitis contribute to many of the more significant complications like shock or renal failure.

Children have the same local and systemic complications of acute pancreatitis that occur in adults (Table 82-3). Peripancreatic fluid collections and pseudocysts occur the most often and can be found in about 15% of patients (Figure 82-5).[4,33,34] Age may influence the rate of fluid collection, because only 1 of 79 patients under age 3 years developed a fluid collection.[25] Limited data suggest that most fluid collections resolve without therapy, although some cause persistent symptoms and require intervention. Surgical, endoscopic, and interventional radiologic approaches have all been employed in children.[61] Some children develop pancreatic necrosis. Reliable data about the rate are not available, but pancreatic necrosis appears to be uncommon with only 1 case out of 380 subjects from seven centers.[4,24] The diagnosis is made when CECT shows a segment of the pancreas without perfusion (see Figure 82-2B).

TABLE 82-3. Complications of Acute Pancreatitis in Children

Local	Systemic
Inflammation	Shock/vascular leak syndrome
Edema	Pulmonary edema
Pancreatic necrosis	Pleural effusions
Fat necrosis	Coagulopathy
Fluid collections/pseudocyst	Acute renal failure
Phlegmon	Dehydration
Abscess	Sepsis
Hemorrhage	Distant fat necrosis
Pancreatic duct rupture	Multiorgan system failure
Extension to nearby organs and vessels	Hypocalcemia
	Hyperglycemia

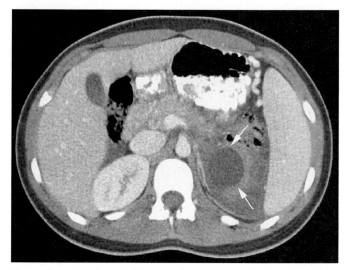

Figure 82-5. Pseudocyst (white arrows) near the distal body and tail of the pancreas in a 14-year-old girl with pancreatitis.

Infected necrosis, a rare event in children, should be suspected if abdominal pain worsens, leukocytosis develops, or a fever appears. These patients should have antibiotics added to their care. Typically, the necrosis will liquefy and wall off with conservative therapy, and surgical debridement is rarely indicated. Deaths do occur in children and rates from 2% to 11% have been reported.[3,4,24,25,33] Two series found that all deaths occurred in patients with complications of systemic illness and not from complications clearly related to acute pancreatitis.[4,25] Most likely, death from complications of acute pancreatitis is uncommon in children, but better data are required to definitively determine the death rate.

CHRONIC PANCREATITIS

Pathophysiology

Chronic pancreatitis results from the sequelae of long-standing pancreatic injury. Early in the course, patients with chronic pancreatitis behave like patients with recurrent acute pancreatitis. Eventually, the continued inflammation leads to enough irreversible destruction of acinar cells and fibrosis that the diagnosis becomes apparent. The inability to diagnose chronic pancreatitis early in its course has hampered investigations into the pathophysiology of the disease, and investigators have speculated freely about theories to explain the development of chronic changes in the pancreas. The sentinel acute pancreatitis event (SAPE) hypothesis was proposed in 1999 to explain the observations that chronic pancreatitis begins with an episode of acute pancreatitis followed by ongoing chronic or recurrent inflammation to produce fibrosis.[62] According to the SAPE hypothesis, a metabolic or oxidative stress triggers the sentinel episode of acute pancreatitis. During this episode, activated lymphocytes, macrophages, and stellate cells infiltrate the pancreas and produce cytokines and deposit small amounts of collagen. Most patients recover uneventfully, but in some patients the inflammatory cells and stellate cells remain active and ultimately lead to fibrosis of the gland. Because everyone is exposed to environmental factors that can stress the pancreas, patients who develop chronic changes must have a predisposition to developing fibrosis. This concept has led to the theory that patients who develop chronic pancreatitis must have a genetic predisposition for ongoing inflammation. The description of several genes that associate with chronic pancreatitis, including *PRSS1*, *CFTR*, and *SPINK1*, supports this theory.

Pathology

Although the pathology may vary according to etiology, in general fibrosis is patchy in the early stages of chronic pancreatitis.[63] The cut surface of the gland may show lobulation or nodular scarring. Ducts embedded in fibrotic tissue are irregular and may contain calculi. Pseudocysts are relatively common. Over time, the pancreas develops a firm consistency and an irregular contour from diffuse fibrosis. The main pancreatic duct is distorted by strictures and dilation. The lumens of interlobular ducts fill with protein plugs and calculi. Duct epithelium disappears and may be replaced by inflammatory cells. Islets may form large aggregates with reduced numbers of beta cells. These changes occur in chronic pancreatitis of all etiologies, although some changes may be more prominent in some etiologies than in others.

TABLE 82-4. Etiologies of Chronic Pancreatitis in Children

Toxic-metabolic
  Medications (see Table 82-1)
  Hypercalcemia
  Hyperlipidemia
  Post graft-versus-host disease
  Toxins
  Organic compounds
Genetic
  Autosomal dominant
  PRSS1 mutations
  Autosomal recessive/modifiers
  CFTR mutations
  SPINK1 mutations
Autoimmune
  Isolated autoimmune pancreatitis
  Syndromic autoimmune pancreatitis
  Inflammatory bowel disease associated
Anatomic
  See Table 82-1
  Severe acute pancreatitis
  Postnecrotic
  Vascular disease/ischemic
  Postirradiation
Indeterminate

Etiology

As with acute pancreatitis, the frequency of various etiologies for chronic pancreatitis remains uncertain (Table 82-4).[64] Most cases remain indeterminate. Of the identifiable causes, autosomal dominant hereditary pancreatitis and autosomal recessive familial pancreatitis form a large group.[48] Some cases are associated with drugs, inborn errors of metabolism, or chronic obstruction.

Clinical Presentation

Early in the course, recurrent episodes of acute pancreatitis may predominate. The signs and symptoms are the same as described for acute pancreatitis. Whenever patients have multiple episodes of acute pancreatitis, chronic pancreatitis should be considered. In some patients, mild to intense upper abdominal pain may be the only presenting symptom. The frequency can range from intermittent to persistent. Older children may describe the pain as deep and penetrating with radiation to the back. Eating may aggravate the pain. Often the patients have had frequent physician visits for abdominal pain. The source of the pain varies according to the etiology and length of symptoms. At first, acute inflammation may contribute substantially to pain. Later, increased ductal or parenchymal pressure, tissue acidosis, or perineural inflammation may dominant the pathophysiology of pain. Rarely, patients may present with symptoms secondary to malabsorption, typically weight loss, fatty stools, or diarrhea, although physicians need to remember that significant steatorrhea can occur without diarrhea. Even fewer present with jaundice resulting from extrahepatic biliary obstruction from fibrosis in the head of the pancreas or from a pseudocyst. An occasional patient may present with an upper gastrointestinal hemorrhage from venous thrombosis, generally of the splenic vein. Because diabetes develops late in the course of chronic pancreatitis, patients seldom, if ever, present with symptoms of diabetes mellitus.

Diagnosis

The diagnosis of chronic pancreatitis requires histologic or morphologic evidence or a combination of morphologic, functional, and clinical findings. Functional abnormalities alone do not differentiate between chronic pancreatitis and pancreatic insufficiency without pancreatitis and cannot be used to make the diagnosis of chronic pancreatitis without other evidence.[65] For instance, patients with Shwachman-Diamond syndrome can have pancreatic insufficiency without evidence of pancreatitis.

Imaging

In most patients, imaging studies provide evidence of morphologic change, and histologic evidence is rarely obtained. Transabdominal ultrasound, CECT, MRCP, ERCP, and EUS are all employed in evaluating pancreatic morphology. ERCP has been considered the standard for evaluating the pancreatic ducts. ERCP shows main pancreatic duct dilation, ductal stones, and changes in main duct branches and in small ducts (Figure 82-6). CECT has poor sensitivity compared to ERCP, but can reliably detect the calcification, gland atrophy, fat replacement, and ductal dilation found in advanced chronic pancreatitis, giving CECT high specificity for the diagnosis (Figure 82-7). In addition, CECT can also demonstrate other pancreatic pathology and other pathology that might explain the patient's pain. MRCP is excellent for evaluating the main pancreatic duct, but is not suitable for evaluating subtle side-branch abnormalities (Figure 82-8). In adults, EUS is rapidly gaining acceptance as the preferred imaging study to evaluate the pancreas for chronic changes. A recent consensus conference proposed EUS standards for the diagnosis of chronic pancreatitis.[66] If the recommendations are validated, they will provide a framework for various investigators to study the role of EUS in adults and children being evaluated for chronic pancreatitis.

Pancreatic Insufficiency

Pancreatic function testing can support the diagnosis of chronic pancreatitis by identifying pancreatic insufficiency and can serve as a basis for rational therapy as chronic pancreatitis progresses.[67] Duodenal intubation with secretin-cerulein stimulation remains the standard for the diagnosis of pancreatic insufficiency. Importantly, the test can detect decreases in enzyme production before there is detectable maldigestion. In practice, it is rarely performed. Few centers have the expertise and volume to reliably do the test, in large part because the test is time-consuming and labor-intensive to perform. Consequently, some physicians substitute suction of duodenal fluids at endoscopy for the intubation test. This approach likely underestimates pancreatic secretion and leads to incorrect classification in a large number of patients.[68]

Over the years, a number of noninvasive tests of pancreatic function have been developed as replacements for the intubation test. Alternatives include fecal elastase or chymotrypsin, the pancreolauryl test, the bentiromide test, and breath tests with labeled triglycerides. Each only detects patients with advanced chronic pancreatitis. With mild to moderate loss of exocrine function, the tests all have poor sensitivity. Of these tests, fecal elastase is the most readily available. A spot stool sample is required, and patients can remain on pancreatic enzyme supplements. Watery stools present a problem because they dilute the pancreatic elastase and produce a false positive result.

Once a routine part of the evaluation for suspected malabsorption, the 72-hour fecal fat collection has fallen out of favor despite the fact it remains the best test for steatorrhea. The test is not specific for pancreatic disease, because diseases of the intestinal mucosa can produce steatorrhea. Additionally, the test is difficult to administer. Families do not like to collect and store the stool and may not keep the required food diet accurately. Some patients may have problems adhering to the prescribed diet. Performance of the test in a metabolic lab can

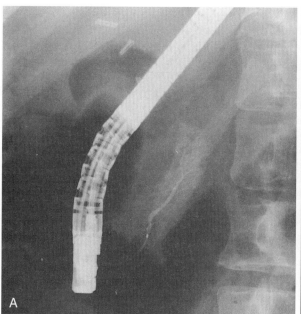
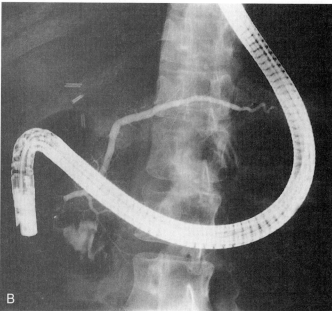

Figure 82-6. ERCP in pancreas divisum. (**A**) Injection into the major papilla (Wirsung) fills only the ventral pancreas. (**B**) In the same patient, injection into the minor papilla (Santorini) fills the dorsal pancreatic duct.

overcome some of these issues, but this is impractical for clinical practice. As with other noninvasive tests, the 72-hour fecal fat collection is only abnormal in the face of advanced disease.

Genetic Testing

The discovery of gene mutations that associate with chronic pancreatitis advanced our understanding of this disease more than any other finding before or since. Mutations in the cationic trypsinogen gene, *PRSS1*, were initially described in families with hereditary pancreatitis.[69] Subsequently, *CFTR* and *SPINK1* mutations were found to be associated with chronic pancreatitis in many patients.[48] As a result, genetic testing is frequently offered to patients with chronic pancreatitis or recurrent acute pancreatitis. Genetic testing for *PRSS1* mutations should be offered patients with unexplained chronic pancreatitis or with a family history of pancreatitis in a first- or second-degree relative. Whether to test for *CFTR* and *SPINK1* mutations is less

clear. Some would argue that the presence of two alleles with *CFTR* mutations is an adequate explanation for chronic pancreatitis and will prevent further unnecessary testing. Others are less certain that this explanation is adequate in all patients. If *CFTR* testing is done, the complete sequence of the gene should be ordered because many patients have rare mutations in one or both alleles that will not be detected in standard panels, which are set up to diagnose classic cystic fibrosis. The question is even murkier for *SPINK1* mutations because, with one exception, they appear to modify the risk of developing chronic pancreatitis and alone are not sufficient for causing disease. Before any genetic testing is ordered, the family should be counseled about why the test is being suggested, the implications of finding a mutation for the health and medical care of the patient, who will communicate the results, who else has access to the results, the pancreatic cancer risk, possible adverse effects on health and life insurance, and the implications of a positive test for relatives. Additional counseling should be provided after the test result is returned.[48]

Management

The stage and etiology of chronic pancreatitis dictates the treatment. During the early phases when discrete episodes of acute pancreatitis reoccur, the management is identical to that for acute pancreatitis. As the disease advances, therapy is mostly directed toward complications that arise such as chronic pain, pancreatic insufficiency, or diabetes mellitus.

Pain Relief

Persistent, unrelenting pain dominates the clinical symptoms in many patients.[70] The prevalence of chronic pain in children is not known. Furthermore, therapeutic trials of pain management have not been done in both adults and children. Consequently, pain management is guided by local practices and expert opinion. Typically analgesia starts slowly with acetaminophen but usually advances quickly to narcotics. Patient comfort must take precedence over concerns for addiction,

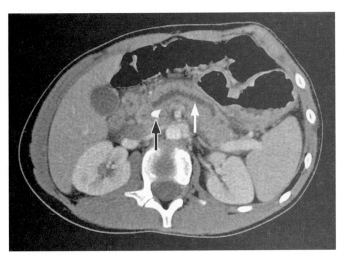

Figure 82-7. Chronic pancreatitis. Computed tomography shows calcification in the head of the pancreas (black arrow) and dilated pancreatic duct (white arrow) in a 12-year-old patient. Courtesy Dr. Janet Reid.

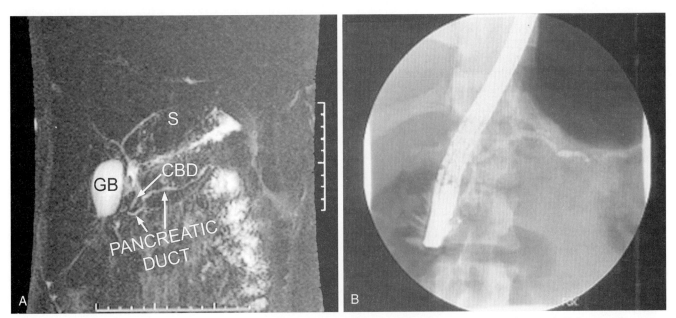

Figure 82-8. Chronic pancreatitis. (**A**) MRCP (T2-weighted image reconstruction) showing dilated, irregular pancreatic duct. (**B**) ERCP showing dilated, irregular pancreatic duct.

although it is important that a side effect of chronic narcotic use is abdominal pain, the narcotic bowel syndrome.[71,72]

Many centers also prescribe pancreatic enzyme supplementation based on the theory that this will reduce the cholecystokinin-mediated secretion of pancreatic enzymes. A handful of trials have tried to determine if enzyme supplementation effects chronic pain. Only two reported efficacy, and they both employed non-enteric-coated enzymes, whereas the other studies used enteric-coated preparations. Some have interpreted the studies to suggest that enzyme supplementation is most effective in patients with some pancreatic function and predominantly small-duct disease.[70] Frequently a therapeutic trial of pancreatic enzyme replacement is started in patients with chronic pain. A proton inhibitor should also be prescribed if non-enteric-coated enzymes are given.

Based on the belief that oxidation plays a role in the pathophysiology of pancreatitis, physicians have prescribed antioxidant therapy to patients with chronic pancreatitis. Investigators have tested the efficacy of antioxidants in reducing pain. The results have not been convincing, and all studies suffer from methodologic flaws. A recent report of adults randomized to placebo or antioxidant therapy (selenium, ascorbic acid, β-carotene, α-tocopherol, and methionine) reported improved pain relief in the treatment group.[73] Further studies are required to fully understand the efficacy of antioxidant therapy. Still, a therapeutic trial is often done as empiric therapy for persistent pain in chronic pancreatitis.

Invasive therapies have also been tried in the treatment of pain.[70] Endoscopic, surgical, and nerve block therapies are all reported, but clinical trials do not support the efficacy of these methods. Nerve blocks and neurolysis have been more effective in patients with pancreatic cancer than in those with chronic pancreatitis. They are rarely performed in chronic pancreatitis. Although frequently done, endoscopic sphincterotomy with stent placement is not supported by evidence of efficacy. The long-term effects of sphincterotomy in children are not known. The individual anatomy guides surgical approaches. If the main duct is dilated, operations aimed at drainage or decompression of the duct are done. Patients with more severe, localized disease may benefit from partial pancreatic resection. Multiple centers now offer total pancreatectomy with islet cell autotransplantation. After the procedure, many patients have pain relief and some have no insulin requirement. Interestingly, some of these patients have continued pain.[74] The timing of total pancreatectomy is an issue with this therapy, because islet cell yield decreases with advanced disease, and the numbers of islet cells are a major determinant of outcome.

Pancreatic Insufficiency

The treatment of pancreatic insufficiency currently depends on the use of pancreatic replacement therapy with extracts of porcine pancreas. The goal is to restore digestive function as much as possible. There are no studies of dose range in pediatric patients with chronic pancreatitis, and doses are based on the current recommendations for treating patients with cystic fibrosis. In children or young adults with CF, pancreatic enzymes are given by units of lipase/kg/meal or in units of lipase/g of fat ingested. This translates into approximately 500 to 2000 units of lipase/kg/meal, or 500 to 4000 units of lipase/g of fat. Doses exceeding 10,000 units/kg/day are not recommended, and doses in excess of 6000 units/kg/meal have been associated with colonic strictures in children younger than 12 years.[75] Generally, enteric-coated enzyme formulations are preferred. The timing of the dose has been the subject of some disagreement. Some contend that the enzymes should be given before, during, and after the meal, whereas others argue that before and during, or during and after, the meal is sufficient. A recent trial found that administration of enzymes was most effective when given during or after the meal.[76] In children, the goal is to maintain normal weight and height gain.

REFERENCES

1. Lopez MJ. The changing incidence of acute pancreatitis in children: a single-institution perspective. J Pediatr 2002;140:622–624.
3. Nydegger A, Heine RG, Ranuh R, et al. Changing incidence of acute pancreatitis: 10-year experience at the Royal Children's Hospital, Melbourne. J Gastroenterol Hepatol 2007;22:1313–1316.
4. Werlin SL, Kugathasan S, Frautschy BC. Pancreatitis in children. J Pediatr Gastroenterol Nutr 2003;37:591–595.
58. Marik PE, Zaloga GP. Meta-analysis of parenteral nutrition versus enteral nutrition in patients with acute pancreatitis. BMJ 2004;328:1407.
69. Whitcomb DC, Gorry MC, Preston RA, et al. Hereditary pancreatitis is caused by a mutation in the cationic trypsinogen gene. Nat Genet 1996;14:141–145.
74. Blondet JJ, Carlson AM, Kobayashi T, et al. The role of total pancreatectomy and islet autotransplantation for chronic pancreatitis. Surg Clin North Am 2007;87:1477–1501; x.

See expertconsult.com for a complete list of references and the review questions for this chapter.

83

TOTAL PANCREATECTOMY WITH AUTOISLET TRANSPLANTATION, AND PANCREATIC ALLOTRANSPLANTATION

R. Matthew Walsh • Charles G. Winans

TOTAL PANCREATECTOMY WITH AUTOISLET TRANSPLANTATION (TP-AIT)

Chronic pancreatitis is associated with irreversible morphologic and functional changes in the pancreas as a result of persistent or recurrent inflammation. Fortunately, it is particularly uncommon in childhood and adolescence, perhaps occurring in 1 of 50,000 children, which is nearly half the prevalence in adults.[1] The general concepts regarding presentation and management are well covered in Chapter 82. The clinical presentation and course of chronic pancreatitis is similar to that seen in adults. Thus, the presentation in younger years is also one of abdominal pain, and definitive management focuses on elimination of pain to improve quality of life.

An important consideration in management should focus on causes of pancreatitis that can be eliminated to avoid ongoing inflammation. The etiology of pancreatitis is of particular interest when considering the differences between adult and pediatric patients. In adults the principal causes are alcohol and biliary tract disease, whereas in children hereditary and idiopathic causes predominate.[2] The natural history of chronic pancreatitis would be of great interest in the pediatric population. The conflicting outcome variables of possible interest would include eventual relief of pain, so-called burn-out, versus risk of developing narcotic dependence and irreversible exocrine and endocrine insufficiency during the period of medical management. These competing outcomes are expected to likely play out over the course of a longer life expectancy in children than in the adult population. Natural history data for chronic pancreatitis are available only for adults and are illustrative in their shortcomings. Some European centers have tried to investigate the long-term success of complete pain relief with medical management alone, which has not been confirmed elsewhere. Data from these centers suggest that any sustained pain relief for chronic pancreatitis requires decades to achieve, requires removal of the initiators of pancreatitis (alcohol in adults), is likely dependent on the type of pancreatic pain experienced (type A versus type B), and will predominantly occur at the expense of addiction and complete functional insufficiency.[3,4] This has not led to a groundswell to treat adults with medical therapy alone.[5] The differences in etiologies are of importance when considering the natural history. In adults the major causes of chronic pancreatitis are potentially mutable, especially the elimination of alcohol.

In the pediatric population, the most common causes of chronic pancreatitis cannot be altered, because they include idiopathic and hereditary etiologies. Chronic idiopathic pancreatitis when it develops in juveniles may be more likely associated with early onset of severe pain but with better preservation of pancreatic function over time compared to adults.[6] Hereditary pancreatitis is better characterized and is of greater concern for long-term consequences. Multiple germline mutations have been determined to cause pancreatitis, with the most common being a mutation in the cationic trypsinogen gene (*PRSS1*), which has a penetrance of over 90%. The median age of symptom onset in hereditary pancreatitis is 10 years, yet the median age at diagnosis is 19 years. There are no clinical or morphologic differences in patients with hereditary chronic pancreatitis, but half will ultimately die from pancreatic adenocarcinoma.[7]

There are numerous surgical options available to treat patients who have failed medical management of chronic pancreatitis. The plethora of surgical options should highlight the need to tailor the appropriate operation for each patient, and not be a reflection of uncertainty as to how to surgically manage the disease, including in children.[8] All surgical options available in adults are options for the pediatric population and entail one of two categories: resection or drainage. The drainage procedures are aimed at decompressing the ductal system by either ablation of any sphincter obstruction or surgical bypass to the duct directly. Surgical procedures of the sphincter include procedures for both the minor and major ampullae. The former is classically associated with pancreas divisum, and the latter with sphincter of Oddi dysfunction. Endoscopic sphincterotomy has substantially reduced the frequency of surgical sphincteroplasty,[9,10] although surgery may still be necessary for recurrent stenosis post endoscopic drainage, or when the orifice is too small to allow access for endoscopic therapy. Paramount in determining whether a patient is a candidate for surgical therapy directed at a sphincter is the character of the pancreatic duct and the length of sphincter stenosis. Multiple strictures in the main duct will not respond to sphincter-directed procedures alone, and the length of obstruction at the sphincter must be short. The length of obstruction and diameter of the dorsal duct are critically important for therapy directed at the minor sphincter where it enters the duodenum at a right angle, making entry difficult without coring out the pancreatic head. The maximal size of the opening cannot be made larger

915

than the diameter of the duct. In properly selected patients, the results of surgical sphincteroplasty are acceptable, making it an appropriate initial operative approach for some pediatric patients with pancreas divisum.[11] Decompression by suturing the main pancreatic duct, with or without incorporation of a chronic pseudocyst, is more commonly done and includes lateral longitudinal pancreaticojejunostomy (Partington-Rochelle modification of the Puestow procedure). The modified Puestow procedure is the most frequently done decompressive procedure, including in children, and is applicable to patients with firm fibrotic glands with a dilated duct due to multiple strictures without an inflammatory mass.[12] Initial results from this operation in children are good, but long-term pain control is difficult to assess because of both poor and unbiased follow-up. In some series follow-up is absent in half the cohort of operated patients.[13] At best, pain relief is achieved in 50 to 80% of patients; this result is better than what can be achieved in comparable patients managed with endoscopic therapy.[14] In pediatric patients, endoscopic treatment is associated with more admissions for recurrent pancreatitis, with comparable pain response compared to a tailored surgical approach.[15]

Resectional treatment inherently includes a component of ductal decompression, but some component of parenchymal loss is required. These procedures involve a proportional loss of the body and tail of the gland, or the pancreatic head. The most limited type of pancreatic resection is the DuVal procedure, where a small portion of the tail is removed and the remaining gland is sutured to a defunctionalized limb of jejunum principally for ductal drainage. This procedure is infrequently done, but may be indicated for distal outflow obstruction where the duct is uniformly dilated and a sphincteroplasty is not technically achievable. Distal pancreatectomy up to and including subtotal pancreatectomy can be considered for focal pancreatitis of the distal portion of the gland. Focal pancreatitis is not a common indication for distal pancreatectomy. In one series only 12% of patients undergoing distal pancreatectomy had the procedure for that indication, which can result in substantial loss of gland volume.[16] A 50 to 55% loss of insulin secretion is expected for major resections of the pancreas, of either the body or the head.[17] Pancreatic head resections involve complex operations that either preserve the duodenum (Beger, Bern, or Frey procedures) or remove the duodenum and distal bile duct (Whipple procedure). All remove an inflammatory head mass, considered to be the location responsible for the elicitation of pain, the "pancreatic pain pacemaker." They all achieve excellent pain relief in patients with head-centric disease, and the Whipple procedure removes areas secondarily affected such as duodenal and biliary strictures.[18] These procedures have been used in appropriately selected children with chronic pancreatitis.[13,15,19]

The ultimate option for management of pancreatic pain in chronic pancreatitis is total pancreatectomy. This has the advantage of completely removing the offending source of pain and leaves no potential for recurrent disease. Clearly irrevocable, it has immediate and long-term consequences. Fortunately, the operative consequences of total pancreatectomy have improved so that it is comparable to pancreaticoduodenectomy (Whipple procedure),[20] but the long-term metabolic consequences of metabolic bone disease and exocrine and endocrine insufficiency appropriately caution its application. The major resultant complication, endocrine insufficiency, that is, diabetes mellitus, in the setting of no islet cell mass can be ameliorated

by the use of autoislet beta cell transplantation. Although the clear indication for total pancreatectomy and autoislet transplantation is to improve quality of life through pain reduction and return to normal activity, this is supplemented by return of islet cell mass that may prevent the onset of diabetes or improve glucose control by providing some insulin production.

Paramount in importance is proper patient selection, particularly in afflicted children with chronic pancreatitis where the long-term success of decisions regarding the medical management of chronic pancreatitis and durability of islet cell function are incompletely known. A multidisciplinary team assessment of prospective candidates is ideal, and at our center this includes involvement of the primary treating physician or pediatrician, a gastroenterologist, a surgeon, a clinical psychologist specializing in chronic pain, and an endocrinologist. A decision to proceed with TP-AIT must involve consensus by all members of the team as well as the patient and family. Although the chief indication is for pain relief, it is important to realize that degree of symptoms does not clearly correlate with morphologic changes in the pancreas. Indeed, some patients who are candidates for this procedure have "minimal change pancreatitis" causing incapacitation and frequent hospitalizations despite a clear lack of radiologic abnormalities.[21] Minimal change pancreatitis can therefore be difficult to diagnose and requires an appreciation of the entity, as well as investigational tests beyond endoscopic retrograde cholangiopancreatography (ERCP), magnetic resonance cholangiopancreatography (MRCP), and computed tomographic (CT) imaging, which may not be commonly available, and includes tests such as endoscopic ultrasound (EUS) and pancreatic function testing. EUS allows the identification of specific parameters used to grade the extent of chronic pancreatitis in a reproducible manner and is less dependent on subjective interpretation. These EUS findings include hyperechoic parenchymal foci, strands, hypoechoic lobules, cysts, main duct irregularity, ductal dilation, hyperechoic duct walls, visible side branches, and calcifications. The standard diagnosis of chronic pancreatitis is made when five of these nine features are found.[22] Some authors believe a better sensitivity to specificity balance to diagnose minimal change chronic pancreatitis may require finding only three of the nine features.[23] Pancreatic function testing is aimed at quantifying pancreatic bicarbonate secretion into the duodenum with secretin stimulation. This has progressed at our institution to endoscopic duodenal aspiration, and a bicarbonate level of <80 mg/L is suggestive of exocrine dysfunction.[24,25] Supportive objective data are valuable in making the diagnosis of minimal change chronic pancreatitis that must also be supported by clinical features of chronic pancreatic-type pain. This might be difficult in the pediatric population where the incidence of chronic pancreatitis is low and familiarity with the disease is uncommon. The indications for TP-AIT for chronic pancreatitis are the same in children as in adults, with pain being responsible for all reported cases. There is a heightened need to correctly identify pediatric patients for consideration of all available surgical options, because the associated narcotic dependence can impair normal growth and development as well as important childhood activities such as school attendance. It is difficult to know what time frame before surgical intervention is appropriate, but the reported median time to surgical intervention in pediatric patients is 4 years.[2] Patients who have failed prior surgical treatment are candidates for TP-AIT understanding that the islet yield is less than that for an unaltered gland. A key factor in selecting patients for TP-AIT is assessing the extent of islet dysfunction. Diabetic patients are not candidates for the operation, but most patients with only an abnormal oral glucose tolerance test will be acceptable, under the presumption that their beta cell mass will result in improved glucose utilization.[26-28]

Surgical Procedure of Total Pancreatectomy

There have been various approaches to pancreatectomy for TP-AIT that primarily deal with the extent of pancreatic resection and length of duodenum removed. Initial enthusiasm to preserve a small rim of pancreatic head has been supplanted at most centers with complete gland removal and resection of some portion of the duodenum. This ensures no possibility of recurrent symptoms and does not compromise the perfusion of the duodenum, which is interrupted with division of the pancreaticoduodenal arterial arcade.[29] To reduce the length of warm ischemia time, the gland is mobilized completely without dividing any of the major blood supply (Figure 83-1). Thus, the division of the uncinate process and division of the gastroduodenal and splenic arteries constitute the final steps of the resection. Precise hemostasis must be achieved throughout the resection, because full heparinization will be necessary at the time of reinfusion of the islet cells. Some centers have favored a limited resection of the duodenum to preserve local endocrine interactions, whereas most have performed complete duodenal resection with or without maintaining the pylorus. Splenic preservation has not been a common feature of the operation, but it may be of greater importance in pediatric patients. The main splenic artery and vein are often densely adherent to the pancreas in advanced forms of chronic pancreatitis and therefore are not often able to be safely removed for the gland. The need to avoid prolonged warm ischemia may also limit the enthusiasm for the tedious dissection of small vessels from the pancreatic body and tail. Preservation of the spleen is therefore typically done where the main vessels are sacrificed at the hilum and the spleen is meant to survive on

the short gastric vessels.[30] This can lead to immediate ischemia requiring removal or delayed complications such as gastric varices and splenic abscesses. Reconstruction following resection requires reconstitution of the gastrointestinal tract by advancement of the jejunum to the duodenum or stomach, and a bile-duct-to-jejunum anastomosis. Feeding tube access is favored by most groups because many of these patients have nutritional deficiencies and altered motility.

Islet Isolation and Reintroduction

Islet purification must be performed in a U.S. Food and Drug Administration (FDA)-approved biolaboratory under sterile conditions and quality control measures for processing of human tissues. The pancreas undergoes both enzymatic and mechanical digestion to yield islet isolates. Enzymatic digestion is the first step, with collagenase infused under pressure into the main pancreatic duct (Figure 83-2). This initiates tissue digestion and dissolution of the intact gland.[31,32] This process is continued in an isolation chamber until the islets are separated from acinar tissue as detected by *dithizone* staining (Figure 83-3). The extent of islet purification is imprecise. A balance must be achieved between purifying the islets away from surrounding tissue to reduce the volume of the infusate and lessen the thrombogenic particulate matter versus reducing the

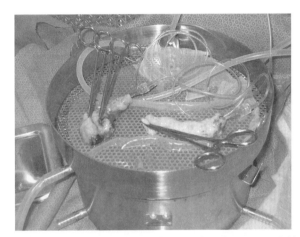

Figure 83-2. Explanted pancreas perfused with collagenase to initiated digestion.

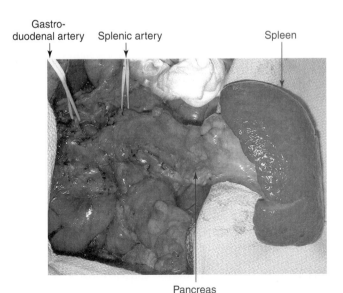

Gastro-
duodenal artery   Splenic artery   Spleen

Pancreas

Figure 83-1. Total pancreatectomy specimen with splenectomy. The splenic artery and gastroduodenal artery are looped and will be divided last to minimize warm ischemia time.

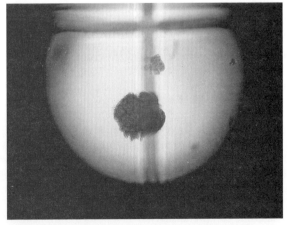

Figure 83-3. Detail of a stained islet of approximately 150 μm diameter.

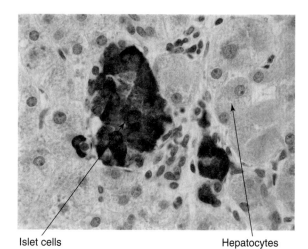

Islet cells   Hepatocytes

Figure 83-4. Liver biopsy showing normal hepatocytes and viable transplanted islet (chromogranin stain).

TABLE 83-1. Operative Variables and Perioperative Morbidity/Mortality of TP-AIT in Adults by Center

Center	Minnesota	Leicester	Cincinnati
Operative duration (hrs)	Mean 9 ± 1-1.5	Median 8 (4-11)	Mean 9 (5-12)
Blood loss (ml)	Median 2000	Median 400	Mean 563
Length of stay (days)	Median 25 (9-82)	Median 20 (8-144)	Mean 15 (5-40)
Major complication (%)	25	15	18
Mortality (%)	2	4	4
References:	38	37 71	36, 40

absolute number of islets with successive purification cycles.[33] Up to 40% of islet cell mass can be lost during purification, which tempers the enthusiasm for extended purification.[28] Most centers further purify the islet preparation if the crude tissue digest exceeds 15 mL.[33] Before transplantation, islet preparations are suspended in a 50:50 solution of 20% human serum albumin and transplant media, and antibiotics are added.

Islets preparations are currently introduced into the liver via the portal venous system to achieve islet engraftment (Figure 83-4). The major complications of this route of access are portal hypertension, venous thrombosis, and infarction. Intrasplenic, renal capsule, peritoneal cavity, and omental transplantation were attempted experimentally to reduce the incidence of these complications, but have not been successful in humans.[34] The current methods to reduce these complications include limiting the volume and rate of infusion, and transient heparinization (70 mg/kg). There are multiple routes to access the portal system, which include catheterization of the splenic vein, mesenteric vein, or umbilical vein in the falciform ligament and transhepatic direct portal puncture. Most centers, including our own, favor portal reinfusion via a major portal branch at the time of laparotomy, during either the same or a subsequent operation depending on the time of islet purification and transport. The portal pressures must be monitored periodically throughout the infusion and should not exceed 25 to 30 cm H$_2$O.

Results of Autoislet Transplantation

Total pancreatectomy and autoislet transplantation was first successfully performed at the University of Minnesota in 1977 for a patient with chronic pancreatitis.[35] The patient recovered from the operation and lived a pain-free, insulin-independent life for 6 years, which spurred interest in the procedure as well as the outcomes. Outcomes of interest include surgical morbidity, islet graft function, and pain improvement. Operative mortality of 0 to 4% has been reported for TP-AIT,[36,37] and long-term patient survival rates of 95% at 1 year and 85% at 5 years and 10 years are reported from the Minnesota group.[38] Most series report a major operative complication rate of between 15 and 25%, and one comprehensive series reports a complication rate of 56% in 27 patients, but no perioperative mortality.[39] This

would be similar to large patient series of patients undergoing pancreaticoduodenectomy for any indication where operative mortality is rare, but complications frequent even at high-volume centers. Notable operative variables and results of TP-AIT are summarized in Table 83-1.

Autotransplantation of islets recovered from the resected pancreas aims to preserve a proportion of beta cell mass and result in endogenous insulin production. The success and durability of the transplanted islets is therefore of great interest. It would appear intuitive that a higher number of islets transplanted correlates with insulin independence, and this indeed is generally found.[40,38] This correlation is not straightforward or linear, because long-term insulin independence has been demonstrated in patients who received at few as 882 IEQ islets/kg body weight.[41] Although not as high as what can be achieved by harvesting alloislets, the islet yields for autoislets are robust and the current median transfused islets transplanted across multiple sites range from 2245 to 6635 IEQ/kg (Table 83-2). The largest experience from the University of Minnesota showed that islet function as defined by partial or total insulin independence was significantly correlated with islet yield (p less than 0.05). Recipients with fewer than 2500 IEQ/kg showed islet function at 1 year in 32%, those with 2501-5000 IEQ/kg showed islet function in 79%, and those with greater than 5000 IEQ/kg showed function in 86%.[38] As suspected, insulin independence also correlated with stimulated C-peptide levels at 3 to 12 months posttransplant, with mean levels of 3.9 ± 1.5 ng/mL in insulin independent subjects and 2.7 ± 1.3 ng/mL in those with partial graft function (p = 0.017). Overall, up to 65% of transplanted patients are expected to have autoislet function, with 32% of all patients being independent of exogenous insulin. The durability of islet performance is of great concern especially when considering application to the pediatric population, and these data are lacking. The best follow-up data from the Minnesota program indicate that 85% of patients will have some islet function at 2 years. Can we expect similar results in pediatric recipients? At a median follow-up of 2.5 years in 18 of 24 pediatric patients who underwent TP-AIT, 56% were insulin independent and 22% had partial function requiring once-daily exogenous insulin.[2]

The ability to achieve relief of chronic pain is a critical outcome variable. There are many factors that can affect this outcome measure, such as duration and etiology of disease, etiology of pain in chronic pancreatitis, and confounding opioid-induced hyperalgesia.[42] Objective measures of pain response are often poorly studied in retrospective series of surgical patients treated for chronic

TABLE 83-2. **Islet Yield and Glucose Control Following TP-AIT**

Center	Minnesota	Leicester	Cincinnati
Patient Number	173	50	45
Islet yield (median IEQ/kg)	**1977-1990***: 1375 (49-12470) **1990-2007***: 3588 (23-17035)	2245 (405-20385)	Insulin independent: 6635 ± 229 Insulin dependent 3799 ± 629
Glucose control	Insulin independence 32% Partial dependence 33%	Insulin independence: 24% C-peptide positive: 100%	Insulin independence 40%
Factors influencing outcome	Islet function correlates with islet mass (IEQ/kg) P<0.05	Nonsignificant trend for increase insulin requirement over time	Higher IEQ/kg islet shows insulin independence p=0.04
References	38	37 31	36

*=data period

TABLE 83-3. **Pain Control Following TP-AIT**

Center	Minnesota	Leicester	Cincinnati
Patient Number	112	50	45
Opiate requirement	40% pain resolved 32% improved 12% no change 16% lost to follow-up	16% require opiates at 60 months	Morphine equivalent: (mean) Preop: 206 mg Post-op: 90 mg P = 0.005
Pain score: mean ± SD	Pain score (N=48) Pre-op 9.6 ± 0.9 Post-op 3.8 ± 1.5 P < 0.05	Pain score Pre-op 10 Post-op 3 P < 0.05	Pain rating index Pre-op 37 Post-op 11 P < 0.01
References	72, 73	37	36

pancreatitis. Common parameters studied that can give some measure of success include opiate requirements and pain scores. These results are summarized in Table 83-3. Fortunately, improvement in pain, whether measured as a global assessment, mean morphine equivalents required, or by pain scales, show improvement across multiple sites. Improvement in pain results was seen in the Cincinnati group to be associated with time from surgery; patients were likely to require at least 6 months to wean from their narcotics.[36] Objective pain scale measurements all show significant reductions in pain. In pediatric patients undergoing TP-AIT, 61% had discontinued all narcotic pain medication, with 67% reporting no pain symptoms and 27% with pain improvement postoperatively. Additionally, 80% were able to attend school or work, and 73% reported their overall quality of life as excellent or good.[2]

It appears apparent that total pancreatectomy with autoislet transplantation is an appropriate treatment for highly selected patients with chronic pancreatitis. This similarly appears appropriate in pediatric patients with chronic pancreatitis, although the data are preliminary. Total pancreatectomy is effective in reducing pain and dependence on opioid analgesia in patients with chronic pancreatitis. The addition of an islet cell transplant results in reduction in exogenous insulin requirements, as well as potentially achieving insulin independence.

WHOLE-ORGAN PANCREAS ALLOTRANSPLANTATION

Although whole-organ and isolated islet allotransplantation remain theoretical options for the child with either type 1 diabetes mellitus or acquired insulin-dependent diabetes mellitus secondary to chronic pancreatitis or other diseases, complications and limited success of both these therapies continue to restrict their use. Both therapies subject the patient to the potential risks of long-term immunosuppression, and although the former can provide long-term insulin independence with relative normoglycemia in the adult, the isolation of islets of Langerhans in adequate quantities to achieve either of these therapeutic goals remains elusive and expensive.

Indications for pancreas transplantation in adults include end-stage renal disease (ESRD), hypoglycemic unawareness, diabetic neuropathy and retinopathy, gastroparesis, and labile blood sugars. Although these diabetic complications may occur in children, only the latter occurs with frequency in this population, who have not had the disease as long. Also, ESRD in children often is due to hemolytic-uremic syndrome (HUS), glomerulonephritis, or congenital urologic conditions rather than diabetic nephropathy.[44] Only 43 kidney pancreas transplants and 389 pancreas transplants alone had been done in children as of the end of 2009 in the United States (based on OPTN data as of January 15, 2010). The goals of pancreas transplantation are to normalize glucose metabolism and to halt or reverse secondary diabetic complications. An additional goal of pancreas transplant alone (PTA) is to preemptively halt the progression of diabetic nephropathy and eliminate the need for a future kidney transplant, thereby freeing scarce kidneys allografts for allocation to patients with nondiabetic causes of renal failure.

Whether intended for whole organ or islet transplantation, donor pancreata are procured in a standard fashion. At the donor hospital, a total, en bloc, pancreatectomy and splenectomy is performed, leaving the duodenum and proximal jejunum attached to the graft. The spleen is generally left attached during the procurement operation to minimize the risk of injury to the tail of the pancreas and risk of intraoperative hemorrhage from the spleen. This could result in hemodynamic instability and threaten the suitability of the pancreas and other organs for transplantation. The duodenum is transected, generally with a stapler, just distal to the pylorus, and the proximal jejunum and small bowel mesentery are transected with a stapler in the area of the first superior mesenteric branch. After transport to the recipient hospital, the pancreas is prepared for whole-organ transplantation on a sterile "back table" in a basin containing chilled sterile preservative solution. The jejunum and a variable amount of distal duodenum are resected. The spleen is usually removed also at this point, because the splenic vessels can now be carefully dissected and ligated with good visibility and low risk of injury to the pancreas allograft (Figure 83-5). Routinely in the past, however, and currently according to surgeon preference, the spleen may be left attached until the graft is implanted, reperfused, and warmed, theoretically serving as a low-resistance vascular sink to minimize the risk of acute graft thrombosis.

The whole-organ implantation operation proceeds transabdominally through a midline laparotomy or retroperitoneally through a lateral lower quadrant incision parallel to the iliac crest similar to the incision for a kidney transplant. Ultimately the pancreas is implanted heterotopically (i.e., in a different location than the native organ, as in a kidney transplant, as opposed to orthotopically as in heart, lung, and liver transplantation). Its artery is sewn to a recipient artery, its portal vein to a recipient vein, and its duodenum to the recipient bowel or bladder for exocrine drainage. The pancreas is implanted typically in one of three ways named for the type of venous and exocrine drainage: systemic-bladder; systemic-enteric; or porto-enteric.

In the first, the graft artery and vein are sewn to the recipient external iliac vessels (so secreted insulin is drained through the graft portal vein into the systemic venous circulation) and the graft duodenum is sewn to the recipient bladder (Figure 83-6).[46] This was the first routinely successful technique. It allows measurement of urinary amylase and lipase to monitor for rejection, evidenced by a fall in the concentration of these enzymes, and avoids the life-threatening complications of

enteric leak or pancreatic fistula (leak from the pancreatic duct into the abdomen or out through the incision). In this case the graft is positioned in a so-called head-down position, with the head of the pancreas directed inferiorly into the pelvis and the tail superiorly into the mid-abdomen.

In systemic-enteric drainage, the arterial inflow is via the recipient external or common iliac artery, and the venous drainage is to a systemic vein of the recipient (either the external or common iliac vein, or the inferior vena cava) with the graft lying in a "head-down" or "head-up" (head of the pancreas directed superiorly into the mid-abdomen and the tail inferiorly into the pelvis) orientation. The graft duodenum is then sewn or stapled to a Roux limb of recipient jejunum, a loop of recipient jejunum, or, more recently (and our preferred approach for the past 2 years) the recipient duodenum.

Finally, using the porto-enteric technique (Figure 83-7), the portal vein of the graft is sewn to a major tributary to the superior mesenteric vein in the small bowel mesentery just inferior to the transverse mesocolon. The arterial inflow to the pancreas comes from the recipient common iliac artery to which a segment of donor iliac artery, brought back with the organ from the donor, is sewn. This so-called donor conduit is then sewn to the graft's arteries after being tunneled up through the small bowel mesentery to the graft from the recipient common iliac artery in the retroperitoneum. The exocrine drainage passes from the graft duodenum, which, as for the systemic-enteric technique, is sewn to a Roux limb or loop of recipient jejunum. The graft lies in a "head-up" orientation.

Advantages of the systemic bladder drainage are ease of implantation because it requires less dissection, an excellent

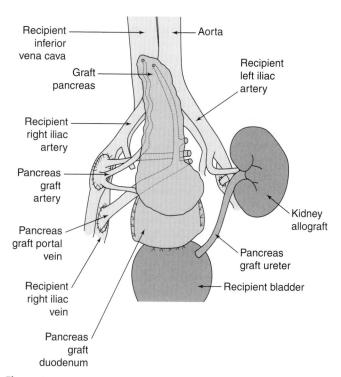

Figure 83-6. Systemic-bladder drained pancreas transplant. The kidney transplant is sewn to the left external iliac vessels with the ureter draining to the bladder. The pancreas transplant blood vessels are sewn to the right external iliac vessels. The tail of the pancreas is superior, overlying the aortic bifurcation in the figure; the head of the pancreas transplant and associated graft duodenum is directed inferiorly and sewn to the bladder. Adapted from Nghiem and Corry (1987).[46]

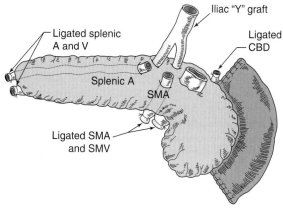

Figure 83-5. Prepared whole-organ pancreas allograft. A, artery; CBD, common bile duct; SMA, superior mesenteric artery; SMV, superior mesenteric vein; V, vein. Adapted from Sollinger et al. (1998).[51]

source of arterial inflow and low-resistance venous outflow in the iliac vessels or vena cava, safety of exocrine drainage because leaks from recipient bowel cannot occur, and the ability to measure urinary amylase and lipase to monitor for rejection (with decreased concentration of these enzymes in the urine suggesting rejection). The problems with this technique include dehydration and other metabolic derangements from the loss of pancreatic exocrine secretions from the patient's system into the urine (at times requiring chronic intravenous hydration), hemorrhagic cystitis, urethritis, urethral stricture, urinary tract infection, and reflux pancreatitis.[47] These complications often result in the need for reoperation to convert from bladder exocrine drainage to enteric exocrine drainage.[48] Advantages of the systemic-enteric technique are ease of implantation and elimination of the risk of dehydration and urologic complications associated with the bladder-drained technique. The disadvantage of intestinal leak has diminished over time. Although the porto-enteric method is technically more challenging, it may confer some immunologic advantage in limiting rejection because shed graft antigen may be cleared by the liver, and it avoids the hyperinsulinemia of systemic venous drainage and the associated hyperlipidemia.[49]

Immunosuppression for pancreas transplantation generally parallels that of kidney transplantation. An induction agent is given at the time of transplant, often in the operating room, to create a state of immediate "immunoparalysis" to promote early acceptance of the graft. During the postoperative hospitalization a maintenance regimen is instituted, typically a triple-drug regimen including a steroid (intravenous methylprednisolone in the immediate postoperative period followed by oral prednisone), a calcineurin inhibitor (cyclosporine or tacrolimus), and an antimetabolite (azathioprine or mycophenolate mofetil). Although use of three drugs is most common, some double-drug or steroid-free regimens may be employed successfully, avoiding exposure to steroids. Sirolimus, an mTOR (mammalian target of rapamycin) immunosuppressant, is also occasionally used in pancreas transplantation for its kidney-sparing effect. The great variety of specific induction, two-drug and three-drug maintenance regimens is demonstrated in Tables 83-4 and 83-5, taken from the OPTN 2008 Annual Report.[45]

Both short- and long-term complications remain significant in pancreas transplantation. Immediate graft thrombosis in the operating room or within 24 to 48 hours occurs in about 1% of cases. Although this results in graft loss and need for removal, its early recognition usually results in minimal morbidity. Therefore, hourly or every other hour glucose testing is done during the first day or two postoperatively. An abrupt rise in glucose level from normal, which is generally achieved in the first few postoperative hours, mandates either surgical reexploration or duplex ultrasonography of the graft to assess the presence or absence of blood flow in the graft. Exocrine and enteric leaks can occur if there is hemodynamic instability or imperfect technique in making the anastomosis between the graft duodenum and the recipient bladder or bowel. Postoperative bleeding can occur with imperfect vascular anastomotic technique or imperfect preparation of the graft after removing it from the donor, especially if a patient is uremic or on antiplatelet drugs as many adult recipients are, because of concomitant cardiovascular disease. Wound infection and intra-abdominal abscess can occur, as well as pneumonia. Acute cellular rejection can occur at any time posttransplant and is usually managed with any of the anti-T-cell antibody medications used for induction therapy; for less severe rejections, boluses and tapered dose cycles of intravenous methylprednisolone can be used. Chronic rejection can occur as well. It probably progresses gradually without any clinically apparent abnormality until hyperglycemia develops and becomes symptomatic. The exact evolution of graft loss outside of episodes of acute graft thrombosis is not well understood. Other delayed complications such a pseudoaneurysm, ruptured pseudoaneurysm, and adhesive bowel obstruction also can occur. Perhaps the most important complications limiting the use of pancreas transplantation in children are the potentially nefarious side effects of long-term exposure to immunosuppression. These include renal failure (up to 15% of recipients requiring dialysis or kidney transplantation at 5 years), *de novo* solid organ malignancy, and posttransplant lymphoproliferative disorder (an immunosuppression-driven lymphoma). PTA should only therefore be done in patients with a serum creatinine less than 1.5 mg/dL at the time of transplant.[51]

Patient survival is generally greater than 90% at 1 year and greater than 80% at 5 years posttransplant at some large centers.[52] The common causes of death are infection, cardiocerebrovascular, hemorrhage, Posttransplantation lymphoproliferative disorder (PTLD), and graft-versus-host disease (GVHD) in decreasing order, with the first two constituting the great majority. One- and 5-year graft survival rates are lower, at 75% and 50%, respectively. U.S. Organ Procurement and Transplantation Network (OPTN) Scientific Registry of Transplant Recipients (SRTR) data for all centers combined are shown in Tables 83-6 and 83-7. The relative mortality risk between recipients of PTA and patients on the waiting list is debatable,[53] and questions have been raised about the utility of transplantation even in diabetics suffering from hypoglycemic unawareness.[54]

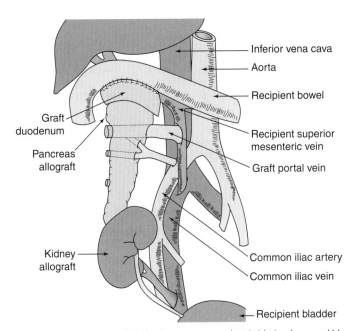

Inferior vena cava
Aorta
Recipient bowel
Recipient superior mesenteric vein
Graft portal vein
Common iliac artery
Common iliac vein
Recipient bladder

Graft duodenum
Pancreas allograft
Kidney allograft

Figure 83-7. Porto-enteric drained pancreas transplant (with simultaneous kidney transplant shown below). The kidney transplant is sewn to the right external iliac vessels with its ureter draining into the bladder. The pancreas transplant has its tail directed inferiorly with the head and associated graft duodenum directed superiorly. The graft duodenum is sewn side-to-side to a loop of recipient bowel. Adapted from Nghiem DD. Ipsilateral portal enteric drained pancreas-kidney transplantation: a novel technique. Transplant Proc 2008; 40: 1555-1556.

TABLE 83-4. US OPTN Data for Maintenance Immunosuppression Used for Pancreas Transplant Alone

	Transplant Year									
	1998	1999	2000	2001	2002	2003	2004	2005	2006	2007
Function Graft at Discharge	**73**	**127**	**113**	**151**	**169**	**141**	**171**	**180**	**153**	**197**
With Immunosuppression Info	66	126	113	150	169	139	167	180	152	182
Tac	1.5%	25.4%	16.8%	19.3%	22.5%	17.3%	13.2%	17.8%	10.5%	6.0%
--- + MMF/MPA	0.0%	0.0%	0.0%	0.0%	0.6%	11.5%	19.8%	2.8%	0.0%	0.0%
CyA + MMF/MPA	1.5%	0.0%	0.0%	0.7%	1.2%	0.7%	0.6%	0.0%	0.7%	1.1%
Tac + MMF/MPA	0.0%	2.4%	0.9%	0.0%	1.2%	5.0%	8.4%	17.2%	18.4%	20.3%
--- + Siro/Evero	0.0%	0.0%	0.0%	0.7%	0.0%	0.0%	0.0%	0.0%	0.0%	0.0%
CyA + Siro/Evero	0.0%	0.0%	0.0%	0.0%	0.6%	0.7%	0.6%	0.0%	0.0%	0.0%
Tac + Siro/Evero	0.0%	0.0%	0.0%	0.0%	0.0%	0.0%	0.0%	0.0%	0.7%	0.0%
--- + MMF/MPA + Siro/Evero	0.0%	0.8%	1.8%	1.3%	1.8%	10.8%	7.2%	6.7%	3.9%	1.6%
CyA + MMF/MPA + Siro/Evero	0.0%	0.0%	0.0%	0.0%	0.0%	0.7%	0.0%	0.6%	0.0%	0.0%
Tac + MMF/MPA + Siro/Evero	0.0%	0.0%	0.0%	0.0%	0.0%	0.0%	0.0%	0.0%	0.0%	0.5%
--- + Steroids	0.0%	0.0%	0.0%	0.7%	3.0%	0.0%	1.25	3.3%	12.5%	12.1%
Tac + Steroids	0.0%	0.0%	0.9%	0.0%	0.6%	0.7%	1.8%	3.3%	0.7%	1.6%
--- + MMF/MPA + Steroids	9.1%	8.7%	4.4%	12.0%	7.1%	7.9%	15.6%	10.6%	21.7%	28.6%
CyA + MMF/MPA + Steroids	4.5%	2.4%	0.0%	0.0%	0.0%	0.7%	0.6%	0.0%	0.0%	1.1%
Tac + MMF/MPA + Steroids	1.5%	2.4%	3.5%	3.3%	1.2%	0.7%	0.0%	0.0%	0.7%	0.5%
Tac + OtherAntimet + Steroids	71.2%	57.1%	61.9%	54.0%	49.1%	38.1%	27.5%	33.3%	20.4%	22.0%
--- + Siro/Evero + Steroids	4.5%	0.0%	1.8%	0.7%	0.6%	0.0%	1.2%	0.0%	0.0%	1.15%
CyA + Siro/Evero +Steroids	0.0%	0.0%	0.0%	0.7%	0.0%	0.7%	0.6%	0.6%	0.7%	0.0%
Tac + Siro/Evero + Steroids	0.0%	0.0%	0.9%	0.0%	0.6%	0.7%	0.6%	0.0%	0.0%	0.0%
Other Regimen	0.0%	0.8%	4.4%	4.7%	7.1%	1.4%	0.6%	3.3%	6.6%	2.7%
	6.1%	0.0%	2.7%	2.0%	3.0%	2.2%	0.6%	0.6%	2.6%	0.5%

Tac = tacrolimus; MMF = mycophenolate mofetil; MPA = mycophenolic acid; CyA = cyclosporine A; antimet = antimetabolite; Siro = sirolimus; Evero = everolimus (Data from 2008 Annual Report of the U.S. Organ Procurement and Transplantation Network and the Scientific Registry of Transplant Recipients: Transplant Data 1994-2003. Department of Health and Human Services, Health Resources and Services Administration, Healthcare Systems Bureau, Division of Transplantation, Rockville, MD; United Network for Organ Sharing, Richmond, VA; University Renal Research and Education Association, Ann Arbor, MI.)

TABLE 83-5. US OPTN Data for Induction Immunosuppression Used for Pancreas Transplant Alone

	Discharge Regimen (w/or w/o Steroids Use)								
	Tac	CyA+MMF	Tac+MMF	Tac+Aza	Siro+MMF	CyA+Siro	Tac+Siro	Other	All
Functioning Graft with Immunosuppression Info at Discharge	246	8	347	4	3	3	72	37	820
% of All Regimens	30.0%	1.0%	42.3%	0.5%	0.4%	0.4%	8.8%	16.7%	100.0%
Induction Drug									
Atgam/NRATG/NRATS	0.0%	0.0%	2.3%	0.0%	0.0%	0.0%	0.0%	0.7%	1.1%
OKT3	5.7%	0.0%	2.3%	0.0%	0.0%	0.0%	2.8%	3.6%	3.5%
Thymoglobulin	15.9%	87.5%	58.8%	25.0%	66.7%	66.7%	23.6%	97.8%	49.5%
Zenapex	16.3%	12.5%	3.7%	0.0%	0.0%	0.0%	6.9%	9.5%	8.8%
Simulect	0.8%	12.5%	4.6%	0.0%	0.0%	0.0%	0.0%	4.4%	3.0%
Campath	30.9%	25.0%	16.1%	50.0%	33.3%	0.0%	48.6%	60.6%	31.1%
No Induction Drugs Recorded	37.0%	0.0%	18.2%	25.0%	33.3%	33.3%	26.4%	8.8%	22.9%

Tac = tacrolimus; CyA = cyclosporine A; MMF = Mycophenolate Mofetil; Siro = sirolimus; AZA = azathioprine; NRATG = non-rabbit anti-thymocyte globulin; NRATS = non-rabbit anti-thymocyte serum; OKT3 = mouse anti-human CD3 antibody (Data from 2008 Annual Report of the U.S. Organ Procurement and Transplantation Network and the Scientific Registry of Transplant Recipients: Transplant Data 1994-2003. Department of Health and Human Services, Health Resources and Services Administration, Healthcare Systems Bureau, Division of Transplantation, Rockville, MD; United Network for Organ Sharing, Richmond, VA; University Renal Research and Education Association, Ann Arbor, MI.)

Patients are usually monitored for graft dysfunction with blood tests including drug levels of immunosuppressive medications, chemistries, and amylase and lipase. However, these are not sensitive or specific for rejection, and a high index of suspicion of this complication is required. Symptoms such as pain, nausea, or vomiting usually occur late in rejection and often signal acute graft thrombosis. Biopsy is the only way to confirm the diagnosis when rejection is suspected. An excellent update of this issue was published by Drachenberg et al.[55] Normal biopsies demonstrate no inflammation or inactive septal inflammation not involving veins, arteries, or ducts. Biopsies that are indeterminate may demonstrate active septal inflammation without features satisfying the criteria for mild rejection. Acute cell-mediated rejection is characterized by activated

TABLE 83-6. US OPTN Data for Pancreas Transplant Alone Patient Survival

Trans-plant Year	# Trans-plants	3 Months		1 Year		3 Years		5 Years		10 Years	
		Surv.	Std. Err.	Surv.	Std. Err.	Surv.	Std. Err.	Surv.	Std. Err.	Surv.	Std. Err.
1987	5	60.0%	21.9%	40.0%	21.9%	40.0%	21.9%	40.0%	21.9%	0.0%	0.0%
1988	30	76.7%	7.7%	53.3%	9.1%	40.0%	8.9%	23.3%	7.75%	23.3%	7.7%
1989	28	75.0%	8.2%	46.4%	9.4%	27.1%	8.6%	15.5%	7.1%	3.9%	38%
1990	18	66.7%	11.1%	44.4%	11.7%	22.2%	9.8%	22.2%	9.8%	11.1%	7.4%
1991	35	80.0%	6.8%	51.4%	8.4%	30.8%	7.9%	30.8%	7.9%	12.3%	5.7%
1992	29	89.7%	5.7%	72.4%	8.3%	54.1%	9.4%	37.7%	9.5%	20.9%	8.2%
1993	42	73.8%	6.8%	44.6%	7.8%	36.2%	7.7%	30.7%	7.4%	22.3%	6.8%
1994	36	86.1%	5.8%	66.0%	8.0%	59.4%	8.4%	39.6%	8.7%	19.8%	7.25
1995	36	86.1%	5.8%	63.9%	8.0%	44.4%	8.3%	23.7%	7.2%	15.8%	6.6%
1996	42	85.6%	5.4%	71.0%	7.1%	34.6%	7.9%	31.4%	7.8%	17.6%	6.9%
1997	63	76.0%	5.4%	67.9%	5.9%	53.1%	6.4%	39.4%	6.3%	15.1%	4.9%
1998	69	87.3%	4.2%	77.8%	5.2%	59.6%	6.3%	47.1%	6.5%	+	+
1999	98	91.8%	2.8%	82.5%	3.9%	65.8%	4.9%	57.2%	5.3%	+	+
2000	99	80.8%	4.0%	74.5%	4.4%	59.3%	5.0%	53.5%	5.2%	+	+
2001	109	88.9%	3.0%	77.6%	4.0%	60.2%	4.8%	54.2%	4.9%	+	+
2002	128	93.0%	2.3%	80.0%	3.6%	61.1%	4.5%	52.7%	4.6%	+	+
2003	104	81.7%	3.8%	68.1%	4.6%	47.3%	4.9%	+	+	+	+
2004	120	90.8%	2.7%	74.6%	4.0%	54.2%	4.7%	+	+	+	+
2005	127	89.7%	2.7%	85.7%	3.1%	+	+	+	+	+	+
2006	94	85.1%	3.7%	75.3%	4.5%	+	+	+	+	+	+

Surv. = % survival; Std. Err. = Standard Error (Data from 2008 Annual Report of the U.S. Organ Procurement and Transplantation Network and the Scientific Registry of Transplant Recipients: Transplant Data 1994-2003. Department of Health and Human Services, Health Resources and Services Administration, Healthcare Systems Bureau, Division of Transplantation, Rockville, MD; United Network for Organ Sharing, Richmond, VA; University Renal Research and Education Association, Ann Arbor, MI.)

TABLE 83-7. US OPTN Data for Pancreas Transplant Alone Graft Survival

Trans-Plant Year	# Trans-plants	3 Months		1 Year		3 Years		5 Years		10 Years	
		Surv.	Std. Err.	Surv.	Std. Err.	Surv.	Std. Err.	Surv.	Std. Err.	Surv.	Std. Err.
1987	4	75.0%	21.7%	75.0%	21.7%	75.0%	21.7%	75.0%	21.7%	50.0%	25.0%
1988	28	96.4%	3.5%	89.3%	5.8%	85.7%	6.6%	71.4%	8.5%	64.3%	9.1%
1989	19	89.5%	7.0%	89.5%	7.0%	63.2%	11.1%	52.6%	11.5%	31.6%	10.7%
1990	15	100.0%	0.0%	86.7%	8.8%	73.3%	11.4%	66.7%	12.2%	60.0%	12.6%
1991	34	94.1%	4.0%	88.2%	5.5%	82.4%	7.1%	82.4%	6.5%	61.8%	8.3%
1992	26	100.0%	0.0%	92.3%	5.2%	84.6%	5.8%	80.8%	7.7%	61.5%	9.5%
1993	32	100.0%	0.0%	87.5%	5.8%	87.5%	6.4%	78.1%	7.3%	68.8%	8.2%
1994	29	100.0%	0.0%	93.1%	4.7%	86.2%	6.1%	82.8%	7.0%	58.6%	9.1%
1995	34	97.1%	2.9%	91.2%	4.9%	85.3%	5.4%	4.7%	8.2%	52.9%	8.6%
1996	35	100.0%	0.0%	100.0%	0.0%	88.6%	5.1%	85.7%	5.9%	68.6%	7.8%
1997	58	93.1%	3.3%	91.4%	3.7%	81.0%	3.9%	74.1%	5.7%	56.9%	6.5%
1998	54	100.0%	0.0%	98.1%	18%	90.7%	2.9%	87.0%	4.6%	+	+
1999	86	100.0%	0.0%	96.5%	2.0%	91.9%	1.5%	90.7%	3.1%	+	+
2000	92	100.0%	0.05	100.0%	0.0%	97.8%	3.0%	94.6%	2.4%	+	+
2001	101	100.0%	0.0%	97.0%	1.7%	90.1%	2.4%	87.1%	3.3%	+	+
2002	115	99.1%	0.9%	97.4%	1.5%	93.0%	3.0%	88.7%	3.0%	+	+
2003	96	96.9%	1.8%	93.8%	2.5%	90.6%	2.6%	+	+	+	+
2004	98	99.0%	1.0%	94.9%	2.2%	92.9%	+	+	+	+	+
2005	11	99.1%	0.9%	98.2%	1.3%	+	+	+	+	+	+
2006	84	98.8%	1.2%	97.6%	1.7%	+	+	+	+	+	+

Surv. = % survival; Std. Err. = Standard Error (Data from 2008 Annual Report of the U.S. Organ Procurement and Transplantation Network and the Scientific Registry of Transplant Recipients: Transplant Data 1994-2003. Department of Health and Human Services, Health Resources and Services Administration, Healthcare Systems Bureau, Division of Transplantation, Rockville, MD; United Network for Organ Sharing, Richmond, VA; University Renal Research and Education Association, Ann Arbor, MI.)

blastic lymphocytes and/or eosinophils causing septal inflammation, venulitis, arteritis, or ductitis marked by inflammatory cells lifting endothelial or epithelial cells off the basement membrane or frankly disrupting the endothelial/epithelial layer. Foci of inflammatory cells in acini also progress with increasing severity of rejection. Necrosis is present in severe rejection. Severity is graded as I mild, II moderate, III severe in accordance with the likelihood of responding to treatment (90%, 71 to 85%, rare, respectively). Chronic active cell-mediated rejection is characterized by arterial intimal fibrosis with mononuclear field infiltrates. The less well defined entity of antibody-mediated rejection is identified histologically by C4d (a classical pathway complement degradation product) positive immunostaining and supported by the presence of donor-specific antibodies (DSAs) in recipient serum. Hyperglycemia, generally absent except in the late stages of graft failure from cell-mediated rejection, may be present in antibody-mediated rejection, possibly due to involvement of the islet microvasculature. Hyperacute antibody-mediated rejection usually occurs at the time of reperfusion due to preformed antibodies. Accelerated antibody-mediated rejection (or "delayed hyperacute rejection") is a fulminant process like hyperacute rejection but progresses more slowly over hours to days. Acute antibody-mediated rejection is demonstrated by positive C4d staining without evidence of fibrosis, and histologic changes ranging from none to diffuse thrombosis and necrosis. Graft dysfunction is often present, and DSA is detected in the recipient's serum. Chronic active antibody-mediated rejection is marked histologically by graft sclerosis and C4d positively staining capillaries. The presence of DSA is required for diagnosis. Finally, chronic allograft rejection or graft sclerosis is staged as mild when less than 30% of the biopsy is fibrotic; moderate with 30 to 60% fibrosis; and severe with greater than 60% fibrosis. Treatment of mild cell-mediated rejection may be with intravenous steroids, usually methylprednisolone. Moderate or severe acute cell-mediated rejection requires using anti-lymphocyte antibody therapy, such as OKT3 (mouse anti-human CD3 antibody), ATGAM (horse anti-human T cell antibody), or thymoglobulin (rabbit anti-human T cell antibody). Severe rejection is rarely salvageable. Acute humoral rejection has been treated with anti-lymphocyte immune globulin, intravenous immune globulin (IVIG), and/or plasmapheresis.

Several other factors make pancreas transplantation an attractive approach, however. First, no form of insulin therapy currently available can match the consistent level of normoglycemia offered by a functioning pancreas transplant. Diabetics' perceptions of quality of life, identified by surveys, is highest for recipients of pancreas transplants even if the transplants are no longer functioning.[56] There is a moderate amount of evidence that pancreas transplantation can halt and in some cases reverse the complications of diabetes, including diabetic nephropathy,[57,58] retinopathy,[59] and cardiovascular disease.[60] Finally, unlike other solid organ transplants, there is an abundant supply of acceptable donor organs with underutilization remaining a persistent problem.

Selection criteria for whole-organ pancreas transplantation vary widely. Allografts from healthy, young adult donors, with a normal body mass index (BMI) and without a history of pancreatitis or diabetes, and who have no evidence of injury to the pancreas or pancreatitis are generally believed to have the best chance of success. In addition, a short transport time from the donor to recipient hospital is also associated with

improved success rates. The relative risks of different donor parameters for adverse short- and long-term outcomes are not well quantified.[61,62] Although series of living donor pancreas transplantation have been reported, the risks of the donor operation and subsequent diabetes in the donor as well as the technical challenges of implanting the partial graft have limited its applicability. Indications include a highly sensitized patient for whom a suitable living donor is identified and a recipient with a suitable kidney living donor who also needs a pancreas but does not want two operations.[63] Whole pancreas grafts from Donation after Cardiac Death donors appear to be suitable for successful pancreas transplantation.[64]

PANCREATIC ISLET ALLOTRANSPLANTATION

Although islet transplantation is an attractive appearing therapy with its promise of being minimally invasive and free of surgical complications, it is far from being a standard and routine treatment for diabetes mellitus, in particular in children. Islets of Langerhans are isolated from whole pancreata by enzymatically digesting the exocrine pancreas and its supporting structure with a collagenase and then centrifuging the cellular component on a density gradient, allowing the islet layer to be isolated, and sometimes cultured.[65] Specifically, a whole-organ pancreas is obtained from a cadaveric brain-dead organ donor by total pancreatectomy with in situ arterial flush with a preservation solution, typically University of Wisconsin, in an identical manner to the whole-organ graft. After transport to the recipient transplant center in cold storage at 4° C, the duodenum is removed from the pancreas and the gland is injected with collagenase via a cannula inserted through the ampulla of Vater into the main duct. The pancreas is then placed in culture medium containing collagenase and placed in a Ricordi chamber containing marbles to gently disrupt the tissue and a screen to retain indigestible particulate matter from the cellular component. The chamber is attached to a circuit (Figure 83-8) through which the culture medium–collagenase solution carrying the cellular material is pumped. The chamber is shaken, and intermittently the fluid is sampled, stained, and examined under the microscope to assess for dissociation of the islets from the exocrine tissue. The digestion process is then quenched and the solution is centrifuged. The cellular pellet is aspirated and loaded onto a density gradient and centrifuged. The islet layer is then aspirated and washed to remove the toxic gradient solution. The islets are resuspended in culture medium and either directly transplanted or incubated. The yield of islets is measured in islet equivalents.

Currently most islet transplants are performed in radiology by a percutaneous transhepatic approach as for biliary drainage under fluoroscopic and ultrasonographic guidance. This provides access to the portal vein. The islets are then slowly embolized into other branches of the portal vein while portal venous pressure is assessed. A hemostatic sealant is deposited in the tract while removing the access device in order to minimize the risk of bleeding. In addition to bleeding, complications of portal hypertension or portal vein thrombosis can occur. Anticoagulation is therefore used often for several days after islet infusion to minimize the risk of major thrombosis and in theory promote survival of the dispersed graft tissue by minimizing thrombosis at the sites of implantation.[66]

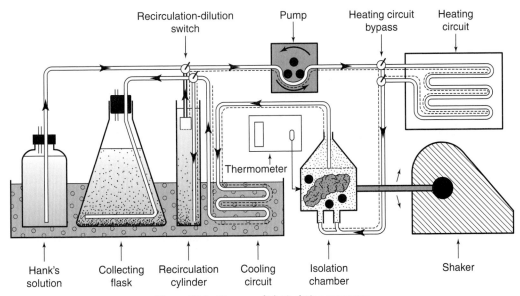

Figure 83-8. Diagram of islet isolation apparatus.

Enthusiasm in the promise of clinically applicable islet transplantation was catalyzed by the report from the University of Alberta of greater success than previously achieved using a new approach to immunosuppression. The so-called Edmonton protocol[66] involves a steroid-free regimen including lower target levels of the current mainstay maintenance drug, tacrolimus, along with sirolimus. Limiting exposure to the calcineurin inhibitor tacrolimus, which is diabetogenic and nephrotoxic, and avoiding the hyperglycemic effects of steroids gave hope of having effective but safe immunosuppression to go along with the elimination of need for an open surgical procedure. The possibility of potentially culturing the isolated islets was also attractive in opening the possibility of matching donors and recipients electively and performing daytime, nonemergent implantations with islets that had demonstrated good function. At a mean follow-up of 11.9 months, all 7 recipients were insulin independent, although 6 required islets from two donors and 1 from three. There were no episodes of rejection, although rejection was assessed by glycemic control, serum insulin, and C-peptide. No patient had any hypoglycemic unawareness. Portal pressure did not change, and liver function tests remained normal. Patients had normal glycosylated hemoglobin and detectable C-peptide. Oral glucose tolerance tests were normal. No patients developed cytomegalovirus infection.[66]

The encouraging initial results have had a lasting effect on the appeal of this method. Unfortunately the long-term results have been poor compared to whole-organ transplantation. One of the greatest challenges is isolating an adequate number of quality islets to permit transplantation. In their 5-year follow-up report,[67] the Edmonton group reported results of transplants in 65 patients. Five patients had insulin independence after one transplant, 52 after transplant of two pancreata, and 11 after transplant of three organs' worth of islets. At 5 years, 80% still had detectable C-peptide, but only 10% remained insulin independent. On average, the patients who did require insulin required about half as much as pretransplant, had much less labile blood sugars, fewer episodes of hypoglycemia, and, most importantly, much improved hypoglycemic awareness. Adverse effects included bleeding in 15 of 128 implantation procedures, and portal vein thrombosis in 5 recipients.

Complications of immunosuppression included mouth ulcers, diarrhea, and anemia. The need for antihypertensive medication increased from 6 to 42%, and the rate of therapy for hyperlipidemia increased from 23 to 83%. In fact, even early after transplantation, the response of islets to stimuli of insulin secretion is low, and even a normal fasting glucose is rare, all pointing to a relatively low rate of engraftment from the outset. It is surmised that alloimmune and autoimmune as well as toxic effects of immunosuppression contribute to the waning function of engrafted islets over time.

Although the islet isolation and transplantation process is conceptually simple in schematic form, biochemically it is fraught with obstacles. First, a highly purified blend of enzymes including class I and class II collagenases and neutral proteases is required for successful digestion of the whole gland to dissociate the islets from the exocrine tissue. Second, each of these enzymes suffers from high lot-to-lot variability and is subject to progressive degradation even when stored at $-80°$ C.[68] This requires expending enzyme supplies and available donor pancreata to optimize isolation conditions for obtaining adequate yields of quality islets when an organ intended for transplantation becomes available. Development of recombinant enzymes with more predictable activity and durability to permit more efficient use of resources and reproducibility is underway. Third, separation of the islets from other liberated cellular components, which make up more than 95% of the whole-organ tissue, requires centrifugation on a density gradient, which yields several layers of islets of varying purity. Fourth, despite moving from Ficoll-based gradients to iodixanol-based gradients, islets still suffer from the toxicity of these materials and the digestion process. Release of tissue factor and macrophage chemoattractant protein-1, along with activation of NF-κB, result in worse outcomes in clinical islet transplantation. Culture techniques have evolved aiming to promote recovery of islets from these insults and have permitted long-distance shipping of isolated islets to remote areas for implantation resulting in similar transplant outcomes to those at the isolation center. Despite testing isolated islets for viability (by DNA-binding dye exclusion), purity (by dithizone staining) and function with in vitro glucose-stimulated insulin release, it is not possible to predict reliably which isolations will have good function and which will have no function after implantation.

Furthermore, managing islet transplants is even more difficult than managing whole organ transplants. Unlike whole organs, which have exocrine tissue and therefore secrete amylase and lipase, which can be measured in the blood or urine, islets can only be monitored by glucose levels and glucose tolerance tests. Nor is there any way currently to reliably biopsy the islets. This leads to more immunosuppression being used for maintenance therapy to minimize the risk of rejection, thereby subjecting recipients to a higher risk of the side effects of gastrointestinal dysfunction, infection, neutropenia, anemia, and nephrotoxicity.[69] The reverse reflex in response to complications or poor graft function of reducing or discontinuing immunosuppression in the usual setting of HLA mismatches predisposes the recipient to developing anti-donor specific and cross-reacting anti-HLA antibodies, resulting in significant sensitization and potentially precluding future islet, pancreas, or kidney transplants.[69]

The early success of the Edmonton protocol with a steroid-free immunosuppression regimen based on sirolimus with lowered levels of tacrolimus led to its use in many clinical trials of islet transplantation. The combination is not, however, without its own adverse effects. These include hypertension, hypercholesterolemia, oral mucosal ulceration, anemia, neutropenia, diarrhea or constipation, and peripheral edema. Replacing sirolimus with mycophenolate mofetil has been required on occasion, and adjustments of drugs and dosing is as in many recipients of different solid organ transplants. Investigations therefore into humanized OKT3 (to minimize the cytokine release syndrome of the murine antibody product), rabbit anti-human T cell immune globulin, anti-CD52 T-cell depleting antibody, or anti-CD20 (rituximab) may be included in alternative regimens to improve islet allograft outcomes.

For all of these reasons, despite the many significant advances in islet isolation and immunotherapy, clinical islet transplantation continues to be an experimental therapy limited to difficult to control type 1 diabetics with severe hypoglycemic unawareness despite expert medical management using the latest exogenous insulin therapies and optimized glucose monitoring. Although islet transplantation results in prolonged C-peptide secretion, stabilization (but not normalization) of blood glucose levels, and elimination of hypoglycemic unawareness, low islet isolation yields, poor long-term graft survival, rare insulin independence, and inability to monitor the graft and optimize immunosuppression continue to limit its implementation. There is no doubt after the Diabetes Control and Complications Trial (DCCT) that normalization of blood sugars with intensive insulin therapy limits the onset and progression of microvascular complications in adults and adolescents with type I diabetes mellitus. Improvements in insulin pumps and continuous glucose monitoring systems offer some hope of providing a technological approach to this goal. Functioning whole-organ pancreas allografts and islet allografts offer that reality for many patients currently in the adult population. Their limitations in long-term function however, the consequences of graft loss, and the toxicity of immunosuppression medications limit their broad applicability in the pediatric population at this time. In addition to development of designer insulin and new methods for beta-cell generation, finding ways to predict who is likely to develop diabetes-related microvascular complications will help to reduce morbidity and mortality in children with diabetes and allow physicians to choose which risks of which therapies are most appropriate to take for achieving a good outcome.[70]

REFERENCES

2. Bellin MD, Carlson AM, Kobayashi T, et al. Outcome after pancreatectomy and islet autotransplantation in a pediatric population. J Pediatr Gastroenterol Nutr 2008;47:37–44.

36. Ahmad SA, Lowy AM, Wray CJ, et al. Factors associated with insulin and narcotic independence after islet autotransplantation in patients with severe chronic pancreatitis. J Am Coll Surg 2005;201:680–687.

37. Garcea G, Weaver J, Phillips J, et al. Total pancreatectomy with and without islet cell transplantation for chronic pancreatitis. A series of 85 consecutive patients. Pancreas 2009;38:1–7.

38. Sutherland DE, Gruessner AC, Carlson AM, et al. Islet autotransplant outcomes after total pancreatectomy: a contrast to islet allograft outcomes. Transplantation 2008;86:1799–1802.

See expertconsult.com for a complete list of references and the review questions for this chapter.

SECRETORY NEOPLASMS OF THE PANCREAS

84

Hillel Naon • Daniel W. Thomas

Pancreatic neoplasms are exceedingly rare in children. The majority of childhood pancreatic tumors are benign endocrine neoplasms that secrete hormonally active peptides.[1,2] A case of insulinoma was first described in 1927 by Wilder et al.[3] in an adult with a metastatic islet cell carcinoma and profound hypoglycemia. Islet cell adenoma in a neonate was described by Sherman[4] in 1947 and was the first reported case of a secretory type of pancreatic neoplasm in pediatrics. The focus in this chapter is on functioning neoplasms of the pancreas occurring in childhood.

Functioning pancreatic neoplasms are composed primarily of islet cells that elaborate various endocrine secretory products. More than 50% of pancreatic endocrine neoplasms are multihormonal. However, clinical manifestations are nearly always derived primarily from hypersecretion of only one of the hormones that is produced.[5-8] The diagnosis of pancreatic islet cell neoplasms with excessive hormone production depends on the recognition of clinical syndromes associated with autonomous endocrine product secretion. The pancreatic islet A cells secrete glucagon; the B cells secrete insulin; the D cells secrete somatostatin; the F cells secrete vasoactive intestinal polypeptide (VIP), substance P, and secretin; and the G cells secrete gastrin.[7-9]

Great progress has been made regarding our understanding of congenital hyperinsulinism, formerly known as nesidioblastosis. The development of highly specific and sensitive radioimmunoassays for detection of circulating peptides in the blood has facilitated the recognition and diagnosis of hormone-secreting neuroendocrine tumors and their associated syndromes. In children, the most common secretory pancreatic neoplasm comparatively is insulinoma associated with islet B-cell adenoma, which is a benign tumor, or hyperplasia. Zollinger-Ellison syndrome (ZES) associated with gastrinoma, VIPoma (Verner-Morrison syndrome), and multiple endocrine neoplasia (MEN) have been described in children and are often malignant.[10] Glucagonoma and somatostatinoma have not been reported in children.[11] Table 84-1 lists these tumors and their characteristics.

MULTIPLE ENDOCRINE NEOPLASIA

Three distinct types of multiple endocrine neoplasms have been identified (MEN-I, MEN-IIA and MEN-IIB).[12] MEN-I, or Wermer's syndrome, is associated with islet cell tumors of the pancreas, hyperparathyroidism, and nonfunctional adenomas of the pituitary. The MEN-II syndromes are not associated with pancreatic tumors but include thyroid (medullary carcinoma) and adrenal (pheochromocytoma) tumors. MEN-IIA, or Sipple's syndrome, is distinguished by its association with parathyroid hyperplasia, and MEN-IIB is associated with multiple mucosal and alimentary tract neuromas. Each of these syndromes has autosomal dominant inheritance. MEN-I and -IIA usually occur in adults, whereas MEN-IIB may present in childhood. MEN-I rarely presents in childhood. Both sexes are affected with equal frequency.[10,13] The disorder is inherited in a dominant mode with a high degree of penetrance.[14,15] The *MENI* gene has been mapped to chromosome 11q13,[16] and more than 1300 mutations were reported in the first decade following identification of the gene.[17,18] The *MENII* gene has been mapped to chromosome 10.[19] Evidence suggests that tumor formation is associated with loss of a specific gene, which possibly unmasks a recessive mutation at this locus.

The clinical manifestations of MEN-I are heterogeneous and depend on the endocrine organ involved and the functional nature of the secretory neoplasm. An extensive review of 88 patients, only seven of whom were pediatric patients, by Ballard et al.[10] provided much of the early knowledge concerning the various features of MEN-I. These include parathyroid gland hyperfunction (84%), pituitary neoplasms (65%), adenomas and hyperplasia of the adrenal cortex (38%), thyroid disease (19%) (thyrotoxicosis, thyroid carcinoma, and nonfunctioning adenomas) and peptic ulcers (58%). Ulcers were multifocal in more than half of the patients. Some patients had watery diarrhea or bronchial carcinoids. Pancreatic neoplasms were found in more than 75% of all the patients with MEN-I. These neoplasms were almost always multiple and consisted of both B cells, giving rise to insulinoma, and non-B cells, resulting in ZES. Other associated neoplasms included glucagonoma, VIPoma, and somatostatinoma. Genetic counseling, confirmatory genetic testing,[20] and screening of family members with careful follow-up are important aspects in the management of patients with MEN-I. Treatment of pancreatic neoplasms associated with MEN-I is discussed later in the section dealing with insulinoma.

Children with MEN-IIB may have a distinctive phenotype with a marfanoid habitus, muscle wasting, growth failure, everted eyelids, thick lips, and multiple mucosal neuromas. Thickened lips and everted eyelids are secondary to the development of neuromas and tend to be more prominent over time.[21] The importance of recognizing MEN-IIB early is in the detection of medullary carcinoma of the thyroid, which tends to occur early in patients with MEN-IIB, with rapid metastasis.

The gastrointestinal manifestations of MEN-IIB range from mild constipation to symptoms mimicking Hirschsprung's disease or episodes of pseudo-obstruction. Histologic examination of intestinal biopsies demonstrates diffuse proliferation of

TABLE 84-1. **Secretory Neoplasms of the Pancreas**

Neoplasm	Hormone Secreted	Islet Cell Type	Major Clinical Features	Malignant (%)	Treatment
Insulinoma (adenoma, hyperplasia, congenital hyperinsulinism)	Insulin	B	Hypoglycemia	10	Diazoxide combined with frequent feedings, octreotide acetate, surgery
Gastrinoma	Gastrin	G	Peptic ulcers, diarrhea, excessive acid secretion	65	Gastric acid antagonists/blockers, surgery
VIPoma	VIP	F	Secretory diarrhea, hypokalemia, hypochlorhydria	50	Fluid and electrolyte replacement, octreotide acetate, corticosteroids, surgery
Glucagonoma	Glucagon	A	Rash, stomatitis, diabetes	75	Octreotide acetate, surgery

VIP, vasoactive intestinal peptide.

nerves and ganglion cells throughout the small and large intestine. In children who have growth failure or physical stigmata of MEN-IIB, rectal suction biopsy often demonstrates hyperplasia of nerve fibers. Abnormally high serum calcitonin levels confirm the diagnosis.

INSULINOMA

Insulinomas, although rare, are by far the most common form of hormone-secreting tumors of the pancreas in children and adults.[22] They are discrete pancreatic endocrine neoplasms composed mainly or exclusively of islet B cells. Insulinomas have been recognized as a cause of inappropriate insulin secretion for more than half a century. Whipple[23] described the typical triad of symptoms associated with this syndrome: insulin shock with fasting, a fasting blood sugar level less than half the normal value, and relief of symptoms with the administration of glucose. More than 100 cases of insulinoma, including islet B-cell adenoma and hyperplasia, were compiled by Tudor in the Childhood Disease Registry.[24] The number of reports has increased considerably since a radioimmunoassay for insulin became available for clinical use. Published cases of insulinoma indicate that an islet cell adenoma or hyperplasia may become manifest at any age during childhood, but there are two periods of peak incidence: (1) the neonatal period through the first year of life, and (2) after age 4 years, with a peak from age 8 to 13 years.[13] Insulinomas are more frequent in females.[24,25] Eighty percent are solitary neoplasms, and more than 90% are benign.[24,26] Malignant insulinomas are exceedingly rare in children.[2] Patients with insulinomas and the MEN-I syndrome often have multiple insulinomas and are usually diagnosed at 15 to 25 years of age.[13] They account for about 10% of adult patients with insulinoma. In neonates, diffuse islet adenomatosis is frequently the cause of hyperinsulinemia.[27]

Insulinomas vary in size from lesions that are difficult to find even under dissection to huge tumors that weigh more than 1500 g.[25] Ninety percent of insulinomas are less than 20 mm in diameter. Solitary tumors that are smaller than 5 mm in diameter are seldom associated with hypoglycemia.[25] They are usually encapsulated, firm, yellow-brown nodules that are composed histologically of cords and nests of well-differentiated B islet cells. Regardless of their size, insulinomas can be located anywhere in the pancreas and are rarely found outside the pancreas. Distinction between a benign or malignant insulinoma is difficult on the basis of histologic appearance alone. Because MEN-I is the most common condition associated with multiple

benign insulinomas, the presence of genetic markers for MEN-I may alert the physician to the possibility of multiple insulinomas.[16] The α chain of human chorionic gonadotropin (hCG-a) has been reported as a marker for malignancy in functioning endocrine neoplasms, including insulinomas.[28]

Symptoms of hypoglycemia such as headaches, visual disturbances, confusion, weakness, sweating, and palpitations are characteristic; convulsions and coma are features of significant sustained hypoglycemia. Most symptoms occur after fasting and are often confused with neurologic or psychiatric disease. The finding of hypoglycemia that can be provoked with fasting remains the keystone in the recognition of the possibility of an insulinoma. Significant hypoglycemia can be demonstrated after a 12-hour overnight fast in more than 90% of patients with proven insulinoma.[25] Plasma insulin levels are inappropriately raised during hypoglycemia. Patients with insulinoma have insulin-connecting peptide (C-peptide) concentrations that parallel the increased plasma insulin levels. Normally when insulin is cleared from its precursor proinsulin, the C-peptide is released into the portal vein in a 1:1 ratio with insulin. Because insulinoma cells often process proinsulin incompletely, the serum often has a high ratio of proinsulin to insulin.[25] In normal subjects, serum insulin concentrations decrease to less than 5 μU/mL when the blood sugar level falls to 40 mg/dL or lower, and the ratio of plasma insulin concentration (μU/mL) to serum glucose concentration (mg/dL) remains less than 0.3. In patients with insulinomas, this ratio is usually greater than 0.4 and increases with fasting.[26] Hypoglycemia in the absence of urinary ketones and the presence of low plasma β-hydroxybutyrate is consistent with the diagnosis of insulinoma.

It is often difficult to localize insulinomas once the diagnosis has been made on clinical and laboratory grounds. Noninvasive studies, such as computed tomography, ultrasonography, and magnetic resonance imaging, are usually helpful when the insulinoma is greater than 2 cm in diameter. Insulinomas that are less than 2 cm in diameter can sometimes be visualized before surgery by endoscopic ultrasonography.[29,30] The sensitivity of somatostatin receptor scintigraphy is less than 60% for insulinomas that express the somatostatin receptor subtype that can be recognized by the current radionuclide-labeled somatostatin analogue.[31,32] Selective arteriography is usually performed if the noninvasive studies are negative. A hypervascular insulinoma can be detected by selective arteriography in 50 to 80% of cases.[33] In patients with negative noninvasive studies and nondiagnostic arteriography, portal venous sampling of blood for insulin is performed before surgery. Tumors that cannot be identified before surgery can be either palpated during surgery or detected by intraoperative ultrasonography.[34,35] Selective intra-arterial calcium injection of the major pancreatic arteries with hepatic venous sampling (calcium arterial stimulation, CaStim) was demonstrated to be superior to abdominal ultrasound, computed tomography, or magnetic resonance imaging as a preoperative localizing tool for insulinomas.[36]

The treatment of choice for insulinoma is surgical ablation, which carries an excellent prognosis in most infants and children. At surgery, the islet cell tumor is often pink and firmer than the surrounding gland. The tumor is usually discrete and well encapsulated. The majority of these neoplasms can be simply enucleated. If the neoplasm cannot be localized, distal pancreatectomy with careful examination of sequential frozen sections of the gland is advisable. Resection of more than 80% of the gland is rarely required.[11]

In patients with MEN-I syndrome who have extensive pancreatic microadenomatosis, a 95% subtotal pancreatectomy is needed to achieve a cure.[1] The residual pancreatic tissue mass is usually sufficient to maintain normal exocrine and endocrine function. Transient hyperglycemia is frequent in the immediate postoperative period.[37,38] Diabetes mellitus with refractory hyperglycemia and ketonemia may develop immediately after massive subtotal pancreatectomy,[38,39] but may occur years after subtotal pancreatectomy.[40] Improved medical treatment has facilitated postponement of blind pancreatectomy until the tumor can be identified. Regularly scheduled feedings combined with diazoxide therapy can be used to manage some patients for a prolonged period of time. Octreotide acetate (Sandostatin; Novartis Pharmaceuticals) is an eight-amino-acid synthetic peptide that possesses pharmacologic effects similar to those of the native hormone somatostatin but has much longer duration of action. Octreotide has an apparent elimination half-life of 1.7 hours in plasma, compared with 1-3 minutes for the natural hormone somatostatin. The duration of action of subcutaneously administered Sandostatin is variable, but extends up to 12 hours, necessitating multiple daily doses. Sandostatin LAR Depot is long acting and designed to be injected intramuscularly once every 4 weeks. Lanreotide (Somatuline Depot) is a depot formulation of somatostatin receptor-specific peptide that can be administered once weekly. Octreotide effectively suppresses insulin release in approximately half the patients with insulinoma.[41] The agent most frequently used in the chemotherapy of malignant insulinoma is streptozotocin.[25,42]

CONGENITAL HYPERINSULINISM

Congenital hyperinsulinism, formerly termed nesidioblastosis, or diffuse proliferation of nesidioblasts, was first described and named by Laidlaw in 1938.[43] Infants with congenital hyperinsulinism present in the neonatal period with symptomatic hypoglycemia, which may cause seizures or permanent brain damage. In the past, these infants were believed to have a disturbance in pancreatic development associated with persistence of the fetal pattern of islet cell formation, termed nesidioblastosis.[44] This concept of congenital hyperinsulinism has been discarded, owing to the recognition in many infants of specific genetic defects in the regulation of insulin secretion. The recessive mutations of sulfonylurea receptor 1 (SUR1) and potassium inward rectifier, the two adjacent genes on chromosome 11p that comprise the islet B cell plasma membrane

ATP-sensitive potassium channels, are responsible for the most common form of this congenital hyperinsulinism.[44,45] Dominant hyperinsulinism mutations have been identified in the gene for glucokinase on 7p and the gene for glutamate dehydrogenase on 10q. In addition, some infants with congenital hyperinsulinism were found to have isolated focal lesions of islet adenomatosis.[44,45] Affected infants have the same broad spectrum of clinical manifestations as described for insulinoma and are equally refractory to medical therapy. They have a relatively high plasma insulin:glucose ratio.

The treatment of choice has been 95% pancreatectomy, which is successful in 80 to 90% of infants with this disorder.[44] Recent imaging advances using fluorine-18 dihydroxyphenylalanine positron emission tomography (^{18}F-DOPA-PET) for differentiation between focal and diffuse congenital hyperinsulinism allows the surgeon to perform a curative limited resection of a focus without the risk of long-term diabetes.[46,47]

Medical therapy with diazoxide or octreotide is used for preoperative management, as well as in infants who fail surgery.[41,44] Providing permanent brain damage from hypoglycemia has not occurred, the prognosis of congenital hyperinsulinism is good.

GASTRINOMA: ZOLLINGER-ELLISON SYNDROME

In 1955, Zollinger and Ellison[48] described one adult patient and a 16-year-old girl who presented with the triad of gastric hypersecretion, fulminant and intractable peptic ulcer disease, and a non-B-cell neoplasm of the pancreas. The hormone produced by the pancreatic tumor in this syndrome was recognized as gastrin more than 10 years later.[49,50] Tumors producing gastrin may be associated with symptoms other than those of ZES, such as diarrhea, steatorrhea, and malabsorption.[51] Gastrinomas can originate in organs other than the pancreas, but they occur in the pancreas more often than any other site. The duodenum is the second most common site of origin.[52,53]

There are at least four major peptide forms of gastrin that differ in the length of their polypeptide chains but have identical C-terminal peptide amides. The C-terminal tetrapeptide amide has been shown to constitute the physiologically active site of the gastrin molecule.[54] Each of the peptide forms of the gastrin molecule exists in sulfated and nonsulfated forms; this appears to confer no differences in physiologic activity or potency of the molecule. The principal form of gastrin in gastrinoma is a heptadecapeptide (G-17), which contains 17 amino acid residues.[55,56]

ZES can develop at any age. It occurs most frequently, however, between the ages of 35 and 65 years and is more common in men than in women. Forty-six cases of childhood gastrinomas have been reported in the Childhood Disease Registry,[24] 43 of which occurred in boys. The youngest patient reported was a 5-year-old girl who also had Marden-Walker syndrome.[57] The age range of ZES reported in children is 5 to 16 years. Thirty-seven children had documented neoplasms, and hyperplasia was observed in six. Sixty-five percent of the tumors were malignant. This is similar to the findings in adults, in whom 60% are malignant, and most patients have liver metastases at the time of diagnosis.[58] Twelve cases of gastrinoma in childhood were associated with islet cell carcinoma.[24] Although many adult patients with ZES have accompanying diseases, especially MEN-I syndrome,[59] similar cases have not been reported in the pediatric age group.[11]

Symptoms in ZES are due to the high circulating serum gastrin levels, which cause proliferation of the gastric parietal cell mass and stimulation of excessive gastric acid secretion. Children with ZES invariably have volumes of gastric secretions ranging from 600 to 2000 mL/day or more, with total acid production of 23 to 164 mEq/L.[60] Abdominal pain due to peptic ulcer disease is the most common clinical finding. Ulcers usually occur in the first portion of the duodenum or in the stomach. The ulcers are usually single but can be multiple. When multiple ulcers occur, they are frequently located not only in the first portion of the duodenum but also in the remainder of the duodenum, or even the jejunum. Diarrhea is a frequent problem; it may precede ulceration in some patients or occur without ulcers in others. The diarrhea is due to the excessive amount of hydrochloric acid released into the duodenum. In addition to an osmotic diarrhea, the increased amounts of acid and pepsin entering the small bowel produce inflammatory changes of the intestinal mucosa. Steatorrhea is less common than diarrhea. Acidity of the duodenum and small intestine causes inactivation of pancreatic lipase, reduction of conjugated bile acids, and the previously mentioned mucosal damage.

The diagnosis of ZES is based on the presence of gastric acid hypersecretion and hypergastrinemia.[61] Raised fasting serum gastrin levels can also occur with massive small intestinal resection, pernicious anemia with gastric achlorhydria, renal failure, chronic gastritis, peptic ulcer disease, and antral G-cell hyperplasia. Basal acid output greater than 15 mEq/hour in the unoperated patient should prompt suspicion of gastrinoma. There is a smaller increase between basal acid output and pentagastrin-stimulated gastric acid secretion in patients with gastrinoma. This test by itself cannot establish or exclude the diagnosis of ZES because of the overlap in values with normal and peptic ulcer patients. Acid output is difficult to measure after ulcer surgery because it is difficult to recover all the acid, and because bile and pancreatic juice often reflux into the stomach. Therefore, decreased acid secretion after partial gastric resection does not exclude the diagnosis of ZES.

Using radioimmunoassay for gastrin, the upper limit of normal is 100 to 150 pg/mL. Gastrin levels greater than 500 pg/mL in a patient with acid hypersecretion are diagnostic of gastrinoma.[61] Several provocative tests have been used to evaluate patients with possible gastrinoma, especially those who do not exhibit serum gastrin levels higher than 500 pg/mL. These tests use measurements of serum gastrin levels in response to intravenous secretin, calcium infusion, or ingestion of a standard meal. The secretin stimulation test is by far the most valuable provocative test in identifying patients with ZES.[61] Secretin, at a dose of 1 to 2 units per kg bodyweight, is given intravenously over 30 to 60 seconds. Gastrin is measured in serum samples obtained before the injection of secretin and at 5-minute intervals thereafter for 30 minutes. In normal individuals and patients with peptic ulcer disease, achlorhydria or antral G-cell hyperplasia, the infused secretin has little effect. In patients with ZES, intravenous secretin induces a substantial and prompt increase of serum gastrin by at least 200 pg/mL, usually at 5 minutes, gradually returning to basal levels by 30 minutes. In patients with gastrinoma, intravenous calcium infusion produces an increase in serum gastrin concentration of more than 400 pg/mL above the basal serum concentration. However, because this test does not add to the sensitivity or specificity of the secretin stimulation test and calcium infusion is potentially more hazardous, this test is not recommended.

The third provocation test involves the feeding of a meal. In patients with gastrinoma, serum gastrin levels increase little or not at all after a meal, but an increase in serum gastrin level of more than 200% is observed in individuals with antral G-cell hyperplasia.

Gastrinomas are difficult to localize. In almost half of the patients with clinical and laboratory evidence, the tumor cannot be identified at surgery.[53] Upper gastrointestinal series, computed tomography, magnetic resonance imaging, duodenography, selective angiography, and transhepatic portal venous sampling have been used to locate gastrinomas before surgery. It has been recommended that somatostatin receptor scintigraphy should be the initial imaging study of choice in patients with gastrinomas because of the test's high sensitivity and specificity, and the results may affect clinical management[62] (Figure 84-1). Endoscopic ultrasonography is highly effective in localizing gastrinomas.[63]

Treatment of ZES centers on control of the effects of hypergastrinemia, in particular peptic ulcer disease, as well as surgical

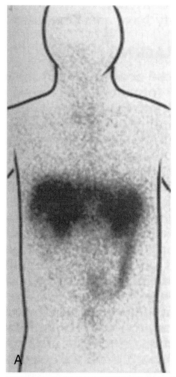

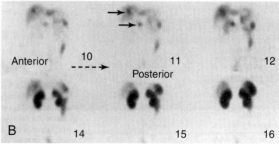

Figure 84-1. Gastrinoma. (**A**) Anterior view obtained at 24 hours on an indium-111-labeled octreotide (somatostatin) scan does not demonstrate any obvious abnormalities. Hepatobiliary excretion into the bowel and renal activity limit interpretation. (**B**) Multiple coronal single-photon emission computed tomography (SPECT) images from anterior to posterior clearly demonstrate an intrahepatic lesion as well as an anterior lesion in the region of the epigastrium (arrows). From Mettler and Guiberteau (1998), with permission.[112]

treatment of the tumor, which is often malignant. Treatment should be individualized. In selecting the best therapy, the biologic behavior of these neoplasms and the clinical manifestations in each patient must be taken into consideration. A high dose of proton pump inhibitors given twice daily is the most effective way to reduce gastric acid secretion and induce ulcer healing in patients with ZES.[64-66] Massive doses of oral histamine (H$_2$)-receptor antagonists must be used every 4 to 6 hours to control acid hypersecretion in patients with ZES[10,61,64,67] and should be restricted to the intravenous form in fasting patients. However, in ZES an intravenous proton pump inhibitor (pantoprazole or lansoprazole) may be more effective.[68,69] The dose of H$_2$-receptor antagonist or proton pump inhibitor that is required to maintain a satisfactory reduction in gastric acid secretion can be assessed by measuring the basal gastric acid output during the hour immediately before the next scheduled dose. The goal is to reduce gastric acid output to less than 10 mEq/hour during this interval.[61] This approach is based on endoscopic evidence that duodenitis and ulceration are absent when acid secretion is kept below 10 mEq/hour.[65] Data demonstrate that medically induced achlorhydria may lead to malabsorption of vitamin B$_{12}$ and iron, both of which require acid for optimal absorption.[70] In one study, researchers reported that 3% of patients with ZES receiving long-term treatment with a proton pump inhibitor developed low serum vitamin B$_{12}$ levels.[71]

Complete surgical resection of the tumor should be performed when possible. Full surgical removal of gastrinoma with cure has been achieved in approximately 30% of all patients with ZES.[72-75] Forty percent of patients with sporadic gastrinoma who have no evidence of metastatic disease have occult neoplasms, which are found most often in the duodenal wall and are frequently no greater than 2 mm in diameter.[54] These microgastrinomas can be detected only after duodenotomy and intraluminal exploration.[53] Pancreatic gastrinomas are not completely resectable in most cases. When a metastatic or irresectable gastrinoma is present, control of the ulcer disease may be accomplished in most cases by treatment with acid production inhibitors, in conjunction with parietal cell vagotomy,[76] and in some patients by total gastrectomy.[58,77,78] Total gastrectomy is not a preferred option in the management of gastric hypersecretion in patients with ZES, except in the minority of patients who are noncompliant or unable to take medication.[79] There is no convincing evidence that tumor progression is influenced by gastrectomy.[80] The routine use of selective parietal cell vagotomy at the time of surgical exploration has been recommended, whereas aggressive resections such as the Whipple resection are not advised.[81] Success with chemotherapy using streptozotocin, 5-fluorouracil and doxorubicin is limited.[75] Patients with metastatic liver disease given interferon-α and octreotide in combination with chemotherapy showed an improved outcome.[82,83]

VIPOMA

Pancreatic cholera,[84] also called watery diarrhea, hypokalemia, and achlorhydria (WDHA) syndrome or Verner-Morrison syndrome,[85] is a secretory diarrheal disorder associated with pancreatic neoplasms. Secretory diarrhea in conjunction with a pancreatic islet non-B-cell tumor in adults was first described by Verner and Morrison in 1958.[86] One of the patients they reported was a 19-year-old woman. It is now widely accepted that VIP is the principal mediator involved in the pathogenesis of the diarrhea.[87] In adults, about 50% of VIP-producing

tumors are malignant and the remainder are due to pancreatic adenomas, hyperplasia, or nonpancreatic ganglioneuromas.[88] Most VIP-producing neoplasms in children are of neurogenic origin and include ganglioneuroblastomas, ganglioneuromas, and neuroblastomas.[24,89,90] Rare occurrences have been reported in association with neurofibromatosis and pheochromocytoma.[24] Sixty-four cases of childhood VIPoma have been reported.[24] Primary pancreatic islet cell lesions were evident in only two of these children. In 1979, Ghishan et al.[91] were the first to report on the association between sustained watery diarrhea and increased levels of plasma VIP and pancreatic islet non-B-cell hyperplasia. Their patient was a 3-month-old infant presenting with secretory diarrhea beginning at 2 weeks of age. After a 95% pancreatectomy, plasma VIP levels returned to normal. Brenner et al.[92] described a 15-year-old girl with massive watery and protein-losing diarrhea who was found to have an islet cell tumor secreting high levels of VIP. A subtotal pancreatectomy was required to remove the tumor. There was no recurrence for up to 6 years later.

VIP is composed of 28 amino acids. Because the amino acid sequence of VIP is similar to that of secretin and glucagon,[93] VIP has endocrine functions similar to secretin, such as increased pancreatic bicarbonate excretion and inhibition of gastric acid secretion stimulated by pentagastrin and histamine. VIP also has a glucagon-like action of abnormal glucose tolerance. It stimulates cyclic adenosine monophosphate in intestinal epithelial cells, resulting in increased secretion of water and electrolytes into the small bowel that exceeds the normal reabsorptive capacity of the colon.[94] General physiologic effects of VIP include vasodilation in the systemic and splanchnic vascular beds, bronchodilation, immunosuppression, hormonal secretion, and increased gastric motility. VIP has pivotal roles in the regulation of sleep, circadian rhythm, and neuroendocrine control of the hypothalamic-pituitary-adrenal axis.[95] Localization of VIP is widespread throughout the body, it being found normally in the ganglion cells of the autonomic nervous system, adrenal medulla, brain, bladder, and predominantly in the gastrointestinal tract.[96] Since the first cloning of the VIP gene[97] and chromosomal localization,[98] many important advances in the understanding of the molecular biology of VIP have been made, including gene regulation by innervation and hormonal control, splicing mechanisms, and newly discovered regulatory sites.

Clinically, the most prominent features of VIPoma are profuse diarrhea, hypochlorhydria, hypokalemia, and metabolic acidosis. Other described features include spontaneous cutaneous flushing, hypokalemic renal failure, reduced or absent gastric acid secretion, diabetes mellitus, hypomagnesemia, hypercalcemia, and excessive tearing.[96]

Diagnosis of VIPoma is made based on the clinical picture associated with increased plasma concentrations of VIP by radioimmunoassay. Confirmatory laboratory findings include hypokalemic acidosis, prerenal azotemia, and decreased gastric secretion. Table 84-2 summarizes the symptoms and laboratory findings in VIPoma. Catecholamine levels should be obtained. Once the diagnosis of VIPoma has been confirmed, it is necessary to determine whether the tumor is situated in the pancreas or in another location such as a paraspinal ganglioneuroma. Computed tomography and somatostatin receptor scintigraphy are indicated in the evaluation (Figure 84-2). If the pancreas is the suspected organ of origin, selective arteriography may localize the tumor. Transhepatic portal venous sampling for VIP may help localize the tumor before surgery.[99] Surgical exploration is often necessary for diagnostic purposes. Confirmation of the diagnosis is made by the immunocytochemical detection of neuron-specific enolase, VIP in the neoplasm, and electron microscopy for secretory granules.[1,88]

TABLE 84-2. Symptoms and Laboratory Findings in VIPomas

Symptom or Laboratory Finding	Frequency (%)
Watery diarrhea	100 (31/31)
Dehydration	100 (31/31)
Weight loss	100 (31/31)
Flushing	33 (9/27)
Flaccid paralysis	20 (5/25)
Acidosis	35 (9/26)
Skin rash (chest, back, upper limb)	3 (1/31)
Multiple adenomatous polyps of colon	32 (1/31)
Hypokalemia	68 (21/31)
Achlorhydria	64 (16/25)
Hyperglycemia	28 (7/25)
Vasoactive intestinal peptide	100 (15/15)
Pancreatic peptide	50 (1/2)
Calcitonin	50 (1/2)
Somatostatin	100 (2/2)
5-Hydroxytryptamine	0 (0/3)
Human chorionic gonadotropin	67 (2/3)

From Peng et al. (2004), with permission.[114]

It is important that dehydration and electrolyte imbalance be corrected before surgery. Many palliative agents for symptomatic relief have been used with some success (Table 84-3) and may allow time for further diagnostic studies to localize the tumor. The most potent pharmacologic antagonist of VIPomas is the long-acting somatostatin analogue octreotide acetate. This drug has been given successfully to patients with VIPoma to suppress peptide secretion and watery diarrhea.[41,87] The mechanism of action of this somatostatin analogue is to inhibit the release of VIP from the tumor and to inhibit intestinal secretion at the level of the enterocyte. The plasma concentrations of VIP in patients treated with octreotide acetate usually decline, but normalize in only 30% of treated patients.[100] Although all patients treated with octreotide acetate responded initially with an improvement in diarrhea and lower VIP plasma levels, some patients have had a short-term effect. In other cases, a rebound situation was observed for the diarrhea as well as VIP levels.[100] In such cases, increased dosage of octreotide acetate in combination with corticosteroids has proved to be helpful. Indomethacin may be useful in cases of VIPoma associated with raised prostaglandin E_2 levels.[101] Other pharmacologic agents, including clonidine, phenothiazine, lithium carbonate, propranolol, and interferon, may be helpful in selected patients in whom other therapies have failed.

The most definitive treatment of VIPoma is surgery. Because most VIPomas in children are of neurogenic origin, they are usually found in the adrenals or retroperitoneal area. Removal

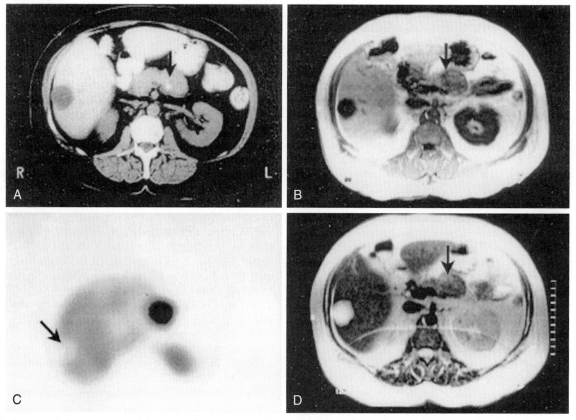

Figure 84-2. VIPoma. **(A)** On a noncontrasted computed tomogram, a 4.5-cm mass with a solitary calcification is seen in the midline (arrow). This mass is in the inferior portion of the pancreas and corresponds to the lesion seen on the magnetic resonance imaging (MRI) and somatostatin receptor scintigraphy (SRS) scans. A poorly characterized lesion in the right lobe of the liver is also visible. On MRI, T1 gradient echo **(B)** and T2 **(C)** images show an approximately 5-cm pancreatic mass that is partially exophytic and corresponds to the results of the nuclear medicine study (arrow). A cystlike density is seen again in the right lobe of the liver and is low signal on T1 and high signal on T2. **(D)** With SRS, an axial SPECT image shows an area of intense accumulation of octreotide in the anterior aspect of the pancreas. No accumulation of the radiopharmaceutical was seen in the region of the liver or adrenal glands. Note the small photopenic area in the right lobe of the liver, now clearly representing a cyst rather than metastatic disease (arrow). From Thomason et al. (2000), with permission.[113]

TABLE 84-3. **Treatment Regimens for VIPoma Syndromes**

Modality	Comment
Acute Supportive	
Intravenous fluids	May require >6 L/day
Correct hypokalemia, metabolic acidosis	350 mEq K⁺/day often required
Peptide/Peptidomimetic	
Octreotide	First-line symptomatic therapy
	Octreotide acetate is effective in the symptomatic improvement of watery diarrhea syndrome in more than 90% of patients with VIPoma
Pharmacotherapy	
Corticosteroids	All enhance absorption; corticosteroids most effective. All inhibit secretion; lithium carbonate and phenothiazines may be slightly more effective. All are effective only transiently
α₂ agonists	
Angiotensin II	
Indomethacin	
Lithium carbonate	
Phenothiazines	
Opiates	
Propranolol	
Calcium channel blockers	
Adenylate cyclase inhibitors	
Surgery	
	Considered as both definitive therapy and, when possible, debulking therapy
Chemotherapy	
Streptozotocin	Combination therapy is useful but does not produce permanent remission
5-Fluorouracil	Renal impairment can be very serious and is usually drug limiting
Chlorozotocin	
Dacarbazine (DTIC)	
Interferon-α with chemotherapy	

Modified from O'Dorisio et al. (1989), with permission.[87]

of the tumor with or without adjunctive chemotherapy is indicated. The infant with VIPoma reported by Ghishan et al.[91] died from sepsis after a 95% pancreatectomy. Histopathologic examination revealed non-B islet cell hyperplasia. The 15-year-old girl with VIPoma described by Brenner et al.[92] was found to have a large tumor of the body and tail of the pancreas. Microscopic examination revealed a tumor of islet cells. Because the tumor was found in 1 of 25 perisplenic lymph nodes and also in a small pancreatic vein, the diagnosis was islet cell carcinoma. An 85% distal pancreatectomy achieved complete cure in this patient. Because the experience with primary pancreatic VIPoma is extremely limited in children, information concerning this type of pancreatic neoplasm is derived from the adult literature. This type of secretory neoplasm is usually found in the distal two thirds of the pancreas. Isolated, single tumors have been reported in 80% of the patients. About half of all VIPomas are benign. Twenty-five percent of the tumors consist of islet cell hyperplasia.[96] A complete cure can be expected

with subtotal (85%) pancreatectomy for biopsy-proven islet cell hyperplasia.[1,96] Excision of the primary malignancy even in the presence of liver metastasis, is indicated to reduce the bulk of the tumor for subsequent chemotherapy. The combination of 5-fluorouracil, streptozotocin, and interferon-α is reported to have a response rate of more than 65%.[82,83,102]

OTHER TUMORS

Glucagonoma and somatostatinoma have been reported only in adults. Glucagonoma is associated with increased levels of glucagon due to islet A cell tumors of the pancreas. Mallinson et al.[103] reported nine patients with pancreatic tumors who had a clinical complex consisting of diabetes mellitus, stomatitis, anemia, weight loss, diarrhea, and rash. Although the rash is not always present, it is the most characteristic feature of a glucagonoma. The rash is described as necrolytic with migratory erythema that most commonly involves the trunk, perineum, and thighs, but may also involve the face and legs. As the erythematous rash spreads, central necrosis and scales appear. The etiology of the rash is uncertain but is directly related to the hyperglucagonemia. It is possible that the panhypoaminoacidemia induced by chronic hyperglucagonemia may be the cause of the dermatologic findings. Long-term use of intermittent infusions of amino acids and fatty acids has been reported to produce resolution of the rash.[104] The youngest patient reported with glucagonoma was a 19-year-old woman[105]; the average age of patients with glucagonoma is 56 years.[106,107] Localization of the tumor is attempted by computed tomography, ultrasonography, liver sulfur colloid scan, transhepatic portal venous sampling for glucagon, and arteriography if knowledge of the tumor vascular supply is desired before surgery. Somatostatin receptor scintigraphy is the best technique to visualize the tumor preoperatively. The majority of the tumors are found in the body and tail of the pancreas, are at least 3 cm in diameter, and have distinctive characteristics.[107] Surgery is the treatment of choice. Chemotherapy for metastatic glucagonomas includes streptozotocin, with or without 5-fluorouracil. Occasionally, dacarbazine (DTIC) is used.[108]

Somatostatinoma has been designated the "inhibitory syndrome" because of its physiologic and pharmacologic effects of suppression of insulin, glucagon, gastrin, and cholecystokinin release.[1] Clinical findings include diabetes, cholelithiasis, steatorrhea, indigestion, hypochlorhydria, and, occasionally, anemia.[109] The majority of tumors are found coincidentally at the time of cholecystectomy for cholelithiasis. However, the appearance of gallstones and steatorrhea in a diabetic patient should alert the physician to the remote possibility of a somatostatinoma, necessitating exploration of the foregut organs for a tumor during cholecystectomy. When found, the tumor is usually single, although it may metastasize to the liver. The diagnosis can be confirmed by radioimmunoassay for an increased plasma concentration of somatostatin. Treatment is surgical removal of the tumor. Chemotherapy consists of streptozotocin and 5-fluorouracil.[1]

SUMMARY

Endocrine pancreatic tumors in children are rare. The dominant peptide they secrete and the resulting clinical syndromes have determined classification of these tumors. Most, because they are insulinomas, are benign, tend to grow slowly, and are difficult to localize. Resection of a localized tumor is usually curative, and a variety of potent drugs facilitates medical management in advanced cases. More advanced diagnostic techniques will make the diagnosis of such tumors much easier once the condition is suspected. The application of a somatostatin receptor scanning technique using a labeled analogue of octreotide as a radionuclide for the imaging of most somatostatin receptor-positive tumors and their metastases has proved to be highly successful.[31,32,62,110,111] This technique is based on evidence that the majority of endocrine neoplasms responding to octreotide therapy do so because they have abundant somatostatin receptors. Positron emission tomography scanning holds great promise and may be the optimal method to visualize these tumors.

With improved technology in the field of cancer genetics, such as large-scale sequencing of entire tumor genomes, it is possible that significant advancements will occur in the understanding of endocrine pancreatic tumors. Further studies of gene function may lead to development of novel therapeutic modalities.

REFERENCES

8. Oberg K, Eriksson B. Endocrine tumors of the pancreas. Best Pract Res Clin Gastroenterol 2005;19:753–781.
18. Lemos MC, Thakker RV. Multiple endocrine neoplasia type 1 (MEN1): analysis of 1336 mutations reported in the first decade following the identification of the gene. Hum Mutat 2008;29:22–32.
46. Hardy OT, Hernandez-Pampaloni M, Saffer JR, et al. Diagnosis and localization of focal congenital hyperinsulinism by ^{18}F-fluorodopa PET scan. J Pediatr 2007;150:140–145.
61. Ellison EC, Sparks J, Verducci JS, et al. 50-year appraisal of gastrinoma: recommendations for staging and treatment. J Am Coll Surg 2006;202:897–905.
69. Metz DC, Forsmark C, Lew EA, et al. Replacement of oral proton pump inhibitors with intravenous pantoprazole to effectively control gastric acid hypersecretion in patients with Zollinger-Ellison syndrome. Am J Gastroenterol 2001;96:3274–3280.

See expertconsult.com for a complete list of references and the review questions for this chapter.

INFANT AND TODDLER NUTRITION

Robert D. Baker • Susan S. Baker

Infancy, considered as the time of birth until erect posture is assumed, is a highly vulnerable period of life, especially when nutrition is considered. Infants have high nutrient requirements, are unable to secure food for themselves, and have immature digestive and absorptive functions. In the narrow sense, the focus of nutrition is on meeting nutritional needs to ensure health of the infant. In fact, growth is well recognized as a sensitive, but not specific, indicator of the overall health and nutritional status of infants. It is likely, however, that infant nutrition has long-term health effects. Some parameters that may be affected by nutrition in infancy include cardiovascular health, blood pressure, bone mineralization, low-density lipoprotein cholesterol, split proinsulin,[1] and cognitive development.[2,3] Although these observations are tantalizing, they are only observations: a causal relationship has not been established. It is likely that genetic and environmental factors also have an effect on health parameters, but present knowledge does not permit us to understand the relative importance of these factors or how they might interact. This chapter uses the definition of a nutrient requirement enunciated by Fomon,[4] "that because of practical difficulties in determining the influence of diet on the achievement of optimal health, the requirement for a nutrient usually is defined in a much more limited context: the quantity of the nutrient that will prevent all evidences of under nutrition attributable to the deficiency of the nutrient." Even this limited definition is problematic, because it is not always possible to factor out influences of the environment, genetics, nutrient-nutrient interactions, or nutrient-infant/child interactions.

Several approaches have been used to determine nutritional requirements. These include direct experimental evidence, extrapolation from experimental evidence relating to human subjects of other ages, analogy with the breast-fed infant, metabolic balance studies, clinical observations, and theoretically based calculations. Most recently, in setting the dietary reference intakes, the Institute of Medicine (IOM)[5] relied heavily on clinical trials including dose-response, balance, depletion-repletion, prospective observational, case-control studies, and clinical observations in humans. Greater emphasis was placed on studies that measured actual dietary and supplement intake than those that depended on self-reported food and supplement intake. All studies were published in peer-reviewed journals. Nevertheless, for some nutrients the available data did not provide a basis for proposing different requirements for various life stages or gender groups, most notably children less than 6 months of age. For infants of 0 to 6 months, only Adequate Intakes (AI) (Table 85-1) exist. The AI[6] is based on the reported intake of human milk (780 mL/day), determined by test-weighing of full-term infants in three studies[7-9] and by the reported average human milk concentration of a specified

nutrient after 1 month of lactation. Although this is an intuitively logical approach, it provides information only for breast-fed infants. Human milk is a matrix of interacting factors, and each factor may be more or less biologically available in this matrix compared with the biologic availability of the factor when not in the human milk matrix. This means that there are no reference values applicable to non-breast-fed infants (Tables 85-2 and 85-3). The AIs, based solely on estimates of nutrients in human milk, will result in frank deficiency for some nutrients if those nutrients are fed to non-breast-fed infants at the level of AI. Further, this approach assumes that the mother has no nutrient deficiency, that all events surrounding the birth were optimal (cord clamping, etc.), and that the mother's milk has at least the average amount of nutrients. If any of these is not optimal and the infant is not supplemented, nutrient deficiency can occur.

GROWTH

Growth within the first year is remarkable for its velocity, variations in the velocity, and demand for nutrients. The first 6 months of life are marked by the most rapid changes in physical growth, cognitive development, and nutrient intake. Overall health is intimately associated with growth. In fact, physical growth has been used as a marker of overall health. During the first 6 months of life, growth is more rapid than at any other time. Table 85-4 shows the increase in weight in the first 12 months of life. A substantial proportion of nutrient intake is allocated for growth – accretion of body mass. Over time, less and less of dietary intake is used for growth.

The source of nutrients – human milk or formula – may have an effect on the rate of weight gain. For example, in a pooled analysis of 453 breast-fed infants from seven longitudinal observational studies of infant growth in North America and northern Europe, Dewey et al.[10] showed that breast-fed infants grow more rapidly in the first 2 months and less rapidly from 3 to 12 months of age than formula-fed infants. A longer duration of breast-feeding was associated with a greater decline in weight for age and weight for length, but not in length for age. The only randomized study of breast-feeding and growth included 17,046 mother-infant pairs and, like the Dewey study, showed that breast-fed infants gained more weight in the first 3 months of life than formula-fed infants.[11] Unlike the Dewey study, however, Kramer et al.[11] showed there was no detectable deficit at 12 months. It is unclear whether human milk offers a true biologic value that results in different growth compared with formula-fed infants, or that human milk is limiting in calories and/or other nutrients after 4 to 6 months of age. For example, using an oxygen-18 dilution technique to estimate lean body mass and body fat

TABLE 85-1. Dietary Reference Intakes

Term	Abbreviation	Definition
Estimated Average Requirement	EAR	The average daily nutrient intake level estimated to meet the requirement of half the healthy individuals in a particular life stage and gender group
Recommended Dietary Allowance	RDA	Average daily nutrient intake level sufficient to meet the nutrient requirement of nearly all (97-98%) healthy individuals in a particular life stage and gender group
Adequate Intake	AI	Recommended average daily nutrient intake level based on observed or experimentally determined approximations or estimates of nutrient intake by a group (or groups) of apparently healthy people that are assumed to be adequate – used when an RDA cannot be determined
Tolerable Upper Intake Level	UL	The highest average daily nutrient intake level likely to pose no risk of adverse health effects to almost all individuals in the general population. As intake increases above the UL, the potential risk of adverse effects increases
Acceptable Macronutrient Distribution Range	AMDR	Range of macronutrient intakes for a particular energy source that are associated with reduced risk of chronic disease while providing adequate intakes of essential nutrients

TABLE 85-2. Estimated Energy Requirements for Infants Aged 0 Through 2 Years (kcal/day)

Age (months)	5th Percentile	50th Percentile	95th Percentile
Males			
0	306	395	467
4	437	561	686
7	572	670	830
13	703	830	1041
25	899	1059	1291
35	988	1184	1451
Females			
0	252	378	520
4	401	508	686
7	518	616	759
13	650	792	952
25	846	1006	1237
35	944	1148	1433

EER = TEE + Energy Deposition
0-3 months (89 × Weight (kg) − 100) + 175 (kcal for ED)
4-6 months (89 × Weight (kg) − 100) + 56 (kcal for ED)
7-12 months (89 × Weight (kg) − 100) + 22 (kcal for ED)
13-25 months (89 × Weight (kg) − 100) + 20 (kcal for ED)
Where:
TEE (kcal/day) = 89 (± SE 3) × Weight of the child (kg) − 100 (± SE 56)
EER = Estimated Energy Requirements
TEE = Total Energy Expenditure
ED = Energy Deposition

in breast-fed and formula-fed infants, Motil et al.[12] showed that length and weight gains and lean body mass and body fat accretion during the first 24 weeks of life were similar between the two groups despite significantly higher nitrogen and energy intakes in the formula-fed group. This suggests that human infants can adapt to achieve normal growth despite variability of nutrient intake. Most investigators believe there is a difference in growth between formula-fed and breast-fed infants, and some believe that the weight gain in formula-fed infants is excessive. In 2006 the World Health Organization (WHO) published growth curves (www.who.int/childgrowth) that are described as growth standards for children from 2 to 71 months of age. The curves are based on cross-sectional data from 6697 children and longitudinal data for 1743 children from middle to upper socioeconomic status families from 6 countries. For inclusion, infants had to rely on breast milk as the predominant source of nourishment, but could also have sweetened beverages, vitamins, minerals, medicines, and ritual fluids. The introduction of complementary foods was as close as possible to 6 months. However, when the WHO curves are plotted against the curves from the U.S. Centers for Disease Control and Prevention (CDC), there is very little difference,[13] and it is unlikely that the choice of curves has any clinical significance.

Charts used to describe the growth of infants in the United States are based on data collected by the NCHS and published in 2000.[14] These data were designed specifically to address concerns of the previous growth charts and thus represent a cross-section of children and breast-fed children (approximately 30% for at least 3 months), and match the national distribution for birth weights. The data were smoothed. Nevertheless, this sampling of children contained few breast-fed infants, especially older than 6 months.

BREAST-FEEDING

Breast-feeding is strongly recommended as the preferred feeding for all infants, including premature newborns, by many health organizations including the American Academy of Pediatrics (AAP), the Canadian Paediatric Society (CPS), the WHO, the IOM, and the U.S. Department of Health and Human Services.[15] There are many medical, nutritional, health, and social reasons for this recommendation. Initial studies on the health benefits of breast-feeding were criticized for failings in study design and data analysis. More recent research has been rigorous, and studies performed in developed countries show that breast-feeding provides benefits for infants. Infants who are exclusively breast-fed have fewer episodes of infections, such as otitis media,[16-21] lower rates of respiratory tract illness,[22] fewer gastrointestinal illnesses during the first year of life,[23] and fewer urinary tract infections,[24,25] and human milk may confer protection against specific infectious agents, such as *Haemophilus influenzae* type b[26,27] and botulism.[28]

Human milk is dynamic. Nutrient concentrations vary over time (months, and within a single day), within a single feed, and among women. The tremendous variability of human milk contents makes it difficult to assume average nutrient content,

TABLE 85-3. **Dietary Reference Intakes**

Nutrient	Age	RDA	AI	UL
Carbohydrate (g/day)	0-6 months		60	
Total digestible; acceptable macronutrient distribution range: 45-65	7-12 months	130	95	Sugars ≤ 25% of calories
	1-3 years	130		
	4-8 years			
Total fiber (g/day)	0-6 months	ND		
	7-12 months	ND	19	
	1-3 years		25	
	4-8 years			
Total fat (g/day)	0-6 months		31	
	7-12 months	30-40	30	
	1-3 years	25-35		
	4-8 years			
n-6 PUFAs (g/day) (linoleic acid)	0-6 months	ND	4.4	
	7-12 months	ND	4.6	
	1-3 years	5-10	7	
	4-8 years	5-10	10	
n-3 PUFAs (g/day) (α-linolenic acid)	0-6 months	ND	0.5	
	7-12 months	ND	0.5	
	1-3 years	0.6-1.2	0.7	
	4-8 years			
Saturated and trans fatty acids, and cholesterol	0-6 months	ND		
	7-12 months	ND		
	1-3 years			
	4-8 years			
Protein (g/day)	0-6 months	ND	9.1	
	7-12 months	13.5		
	1-3 years	13		
	4-8 years	19		
Biotin (µg/day)	0-6 months		5	
	7-12 months		6	
	1-3 years		8	
	4-8 years		12	
Choline (mg/day)	0-6 months		125	ND
	7-12 months		150	ND
	1-3 years		200	1000
	4-8 years		250	1000
				2000
Folate (µg/day)	0-6 months		65	ND
	7-12 months	150	80	ND
	1-3 years	200		300
	4-8 years			400
Niacin (mg/day)	0-6 months		2	ND
	7-12 months	6	4	ND
	1-3 years	8		10
	4-8 years			
Pantothenic acid (mg/day)	0-6 months		1.7	
	7-12 months		1.8	
	1-3 years		2	
	4-8 years		3	
Riboflavin (mg/day) (vitamin B$_2$)	0-6 months		0.3	
	7-12 months	0.5	0.4	
	1-3 years	0.6		
	4-8 years			

Nutrient	Age	RDA	AI	UL
Thiamin (mg/day) (vitamin B$_1$)	0-6 months		0.2	
	7-12 months	0.5	0.3	
	1-3 years	0.6		
	4-8 years			
Vitamin A (µg/day)	0-6 months		400	600
	7-12 months	300	500	600
	1-3 years	400		600
	4-8 years			900
Vitamin B$_6$ (mg/day) (pyridoxine)	0-6 months		0.1	ND
	7-12 months	0.5	0.3	ND
	1-3 years	0.6		30
	4-8 years			40
Vitamin B$_{12}$ (µg/day) (cobalamin)	0-6 months		0.4	
	7-12 months	0.9	0.5	
	1-3 years	1.2		
	4-8 years			
Vitamin C (mg/day) (ascorbic acid)	0-6 months		5	25
	7-12 months		5	25
	1-3 years		5	50
	4-8 years		5	50
Vitamin D (µg/day) (calciferol) 1 µg calciferol = 40 IU vitamin D	0-6 months		5	25
	7-12 months		5	25
	1-3 years		5	50
	4-8 years		5	50
Arsenic	0-6 months	ND	ND	
	7-12 months	ND	ND	
	1-3 years	ND	ND	
	4-8 years	ND	ND	
Boron (mg/day)	0-6 months	ND	ND	ND
	7-12 months	ND	ND	ND
	1-3 years	ND	ND	3
	4-8 years	ND	ND	6
Calcium (mg/day)	0-6 months		210	ND
	7-12 months		270	ND
	1-3 years		500	2500
	4-8 years		800	2500
Chromium (µg/day)	0-6 months		0.2	
	7-12 months		5.5	
	1-3 years		11	
	4-8 years		15	
Copper (µg/day)	0-6 months		200	ND
	7-12 months	340	220	ND
	1-3 years	440		1000
	4-8 years	1300		3000
Fluoride (mg/day)	0-6 months		0.01	0.7
	7-12 months		0.5	0.9
	1-3 years		0.7	1.3
	4-8 years		1	2.2
Iodine (µg/day)	0-6 months		110	ND
	7-12 months	90	130	ND
	1-3 years	90		200
	4-8 years			300
Iron (mg/day)	0-6 months		0.27	40
	7-12 months	11		40
	1-3 years	7		40
	4-8 years	10		

Continued

TABLE 85-3. **Dietary Reference Intakes**—cont'd

Nutrient	Age	RDA	AI	UL	Nutrient	Age	RDA	AI	UL
Magnesium (mg/day)	0-6 months		30	ND	Selenium (µg/day)	0-6 months		15	45
	7-12 months	80	75	ND		7-12 months	20	20	60
	1-3 years	130		65		1-3 years	30		90
	4-8 years			110		4-8 years			150
Manganese (mg/day)	0-6 months		0.003	ND	Silicon	0-6 months	ND	ND	
	7-12 months		0.6	ND		7-12 months	ND	ND	
	1-3 years		1.2	2		1-3 years	ND	ND	
	4-8 years		1.5	3		4-8 years	ND	ND	
Molybdenum (µg/day)	0-6 months		2	ND	Vanadium (mg/day)	0-6 months	ND	ND	
	7-12 months	17	3	ND		7-12 months	ND	ND	
	1-3 years	22		300		1-3 years	ND	ND	
	4-8 years			600		4-8 years	ND	ND	
Nickel (mg/day)	0-6 months	ND	ND	ND	Zinc (mg/day)	0-6 months		2	4
	7-12 months	ND	ND	ND		7-12 months	3		5
	1-3 years	ND	ND	0.2		1-3 years	3		7
	4-8 years	ND		0.3		4-8 years	5		12
Phosphorus (mg/day)	0-6 months		100	ND					
	7-12 months	460	275	ND					
	1-3 years	500		3000					
	4-8 years			3000					

ND, not determined; PUFA, polyunsaturated fatty acid.

TABLE 85-4. **Growth in Weight for an Infant Born at the 50th Percentile and Growing at the 50th Percentile**

		Age (months)											
	At Birth	1	2	3	4	5	6	7	8	9	10	11	12
Weight (kg)	3.6	4.4	5.2	6.0	6.8	7.4	8.0	8.4	8.8	9.2	9.6	10.0	10.4
Weight increase (kg)	0.8	0.8	0.8	0.8	0.8	0.6	0.6	0.4	0.4	0.4	0.4	0.4	0.4
% increase		22	18	15	13	9	7.5	4.7	4.4	4.3	4.2	4	3.8

as the IOM has in establishing AI for nutrients.[29] Human milk is generally considered as colostrum, transitional milk, and mature milk.

Colostrum is the fluid secreted by the mammary gland for the first 7 days after birth. The volume varies from 2 to 20 mL per feeding, and colostrum consists of a mixture of mammary duct contents, newly secreted milk, and immunologically active cells.[30] Colostrum is recognized by its intense yellow color, due to a high concentration of carotenoids, α-carotene, β-carotene, β-cryptoxanthin, lutein, and xeaxanthin[31]; its high levels of vitamin E, protein and immunoglobulin, especially IgA[32]; and its low fat levels.[29]

Transition milk is produced between colostrum and mature milk, from about 7 to 10 days postpartum. Its nutrient content gradually changes from that of colostrum to mature milk. The protein, immunoglobulin, and fat-soluble vitamin content decreases, while the lactose, water-soluble vitamin, fat, and total caloric content increases. Interestingly, the total fat content may have predictive value, as 90% of women whose milk contained 20 g or more fat per feeding on the seventh day of lactation successfully breast-fed for at least 3 months, whereas those whose milk contained 5 to 10 g of fat had an 80% dropout rate by 3 months.[33]

In general, mature human milk is a reliable source of all nutrients for healthy, term infants, except for vitamin D[34] (and some argue iron[35]) for the first 4 to 6 months. Exclusively breast-fed infants must be supplemented with vitamin D to prevent rickets,[34] and infants of vegan mothers must be supplemented with vitamin B_{12}.

At 4 to 6 months, the concentrations of calories, iron, and zinc may become limiting. The WHO and UNICEF recommend exclusive breast-feeding for the first 6 months of life. The AAP supports exclusive breast-feeding for approximately 6 months, but recognizes that infants are developmentally ready to accept complementary foods between 4 and 6 months and that some infants may require complementary foods as early as 4 months.[36] A systematic review of the literature examining the length of time for which exclusive breast-feeding can provide the nutritional needs of infants was published[37] and reviewed.[38]

There are few contraindications to breast-feeding. The AAP lists the following contraindications: galactosemia, women with human immunodeficiency virus (HIV) and T-cell lymphotrophic virus (TCLV) infection in developed countries, herpetic lesions on the breast (not the vagina), untreated miliary tuberculosis, women receiving antimetabolite drugs, and those using drugs of abuse.[39]

Human milk is not without risks, however. The fifth edition of the AAP's *Nutrition Handbook*,[40] Tables B-1 through B-7, lists medications and environmental agents that may have an effect on human milk, are excreted in human milk, or may have an effect on infants. The impact of environmental factors on human milk is discussed in depth by the AAP[41] and the National Research Council.[42]

The Centers for Disease Control maintains a website (http://www.cdc.gov/breastfeeding/) that contains information on breast-feeding promotion, support for breast-feeding activities and national policies on breast-feeding.

FORMULA FEEDING

Infant formulas are liquids or reconstituted powders fed to infants and young children to serve as substitutes for human milk. They are safe and efficacious complete foods. No vitamin or mineral supplementation is necessary for healthy infants who are solely formula-fed. Ready-to-feed preparations are produced with defluorinated water, and fluoride is not specifically added during manufacturing. For formula-fed infants over 6 months of age the amount of fluoride in the family's drinking water determines if fluoride supplements are necessary.[43] Infant formulas are regulated under the Federal Food, Drug and Cosmetic Act of 1938, the Federal Meat Inspection Act of 1907, and the Poultry Products Inspection Act of 1957. The U.S. Food and Drug Administration (FDA), an agency in the Department of Health and Human Services, regulates infant formulas and evaluates the safety of food and color additives. This information is outlined and updated on a regular basis.[44]

Formula feeding is indicated if the infant or mother has a medical problem (e.g. galactosemia, HIV infection), the family chooses not to breast-feed, or the infant fails to thrive on exclusive breast-feeding. For breast-fed infants who develop failure to thrive, infant formula should be provided as a supplement and not a replacement for human milk. It is important to note, however, that if formula replaces breast-feeding, the mother's milk supply will decrease, making it likely that complete cessation of breast-feeding will occur. If an infant is formula-fed, the formula should be provided to the infant for the full first year to avoid malnutrition.[45]

Infant formulas have undergone considerable changes in the recent past, and they continue to be reevaluated and reformulated in the light of new knowledge. Although the makers of infant formulas have sought to replicate the content of human milk in their formulas, more recently infant formula makers have sought to replicate the *performance* of human milk. In making this concept shift, they have recognized that it is not possible to replicate all the contents of human milk; moreover, it is not possible to reconstruct the complex matrix in which nutrients and other factors interact to alter absorption, bioavailability, and function.

Formulas can be grouped according to protein, carbohydrate, or fat content.[46] With respect to protein, there are four types of formula: cow's milk based, soy, hydrolyzed cow's milk, and chemically defined. Only cow's milk formula is available with low iron content, and no indication exists for its use.[47] Formulas are produced with and without lactose; with sucrose, hydrolyzed cornstarch, and glucose polymers; and with and without fiber, tapioca, and maltodextrins. Formulas can contain more or less medium-chain triglycerides, soybean oil, safflower oil, sunflower oil, canola oil, lecithin, corn oil, coconut oil, and structured lipids.

Standard, iron fortified, cow's milk formula is the formula of choice when breast-feeding is not used or is stopped before 1 year of age. The AAP *Nutrition Handbook* notes that cow's milk formulas from different producers have similarities, but differ substantially from one another in the quality and quantity of nutrients. Although manufacturers offer rationales for the composition of their formulas, the AAP notes that physiologically significant differences have not been clearly demonstrated among the various products. Appendices G, H, and I of the AAP handbook list the formulas and their composition as of 2009.[46] It is important to note that the content of infant formulas is in constant flux, and for up-to-date information it is best to contact the formula maker.

Soy formulas were developed during the 1960s for infants who could not tolerate milk proteins or lactose. Currently soy formulas constitute about 25% of the sales of all infant formulas in the United States. Soy formulas support growth and development equivalent to that of breast-fed and cow's milk–based formula-fed infants.[48-50] Soy formulas have added methionine to compensate for the low concentration of this essential amino acid in soy protein, and a trypsin inhibitor is added. Soy formulas have sucrose, cornstarch hydrolysates, or mixtures as the carbohydrate source, and palm olein, soy, coconut, and high-oleic safflower oils as the fat source. Minerals and vitamins are added, as are taurine and carnitine. Soy formulas contain phytoestrogens that have physiologic activity in rodents, but to date no significant effects have been found on growth or pubertal development in humans.[51] The AAP recommends the use of soy formulas for term infants whose nutritional needs are not met from breast milk, term infants with galactosemia or hereditary lactase deficiency, term infants with documented transient lactase deficiency, infants with documented IgE-associated allergy to cow's milk, and parents who wish to feed a vegetarian diet to their term infant.[52] Soy formulas are contraindicated for preterm infants with birth weights of less than 1800 g, for infants with cow's milk protein-induced enterocolitis or enteropathy, or for the prevention of colic or allergy.[52]

Protein hydrolysate formulas were developed for infants who could not digest or were intolerant to intact cow's milk protein and are recommended for infants intolerant to cow's milk and soy proteins and for those with significant malabsorption due to gastrointestinal or hepatobiliary disease such as cystic fibrosis, short gut, biliary atresia, cholestasis, or protracted diarrhea. The hydrolysates have the disadvantage of poor taste due to the presence of sulfated amino acids, high cost, and high osmolality. There are several protein hydrolysates available.[46] To produce the hydrolysate, either casein or whey is heat-treated and enzymatically hydrolyzed. The resulting hydrolysate consists of free amino acids and peptides of various lengths. In some instance the peptides are so small that they are incapable of eliciting an immunologic response in infants. The formula is then fortified with amino acids to compensate for the amino acids lost in the manufacturing process. The various products contain differing amounts of peptides of various chain lengths. These formulas are free of lactose and contain sucrose, tapioca starch, corn syrup solids, and cornstarch as the carbohydrate source. The formulas contain varying amounts of medium-chain triglycerides and polyunsaturated vegetable oil to supply essential fatty acids.

Chemically defined formulas are those produced from single amino acids and formulated specifically for infants with extreme protein hypersensitivity whose symptoms persist on hydrolyzed protein formulas.

There are no definitive in vitro tests that quantify the allergenicity of a formula. Studies of allergenicity in animals are not indicative of allergenicity in human infants. The only way to test the allergenicity accurately is in studies in infants.

Long-chain polyunsaturated fatty acids, those with a chain length of more than 18 carbons and two or more double bonds, particularly arachidonic acid (AA) and docosahexaenoic acid (DHA), are found in breast milk. Some studies on cognitive development in term babies have suggested that there might be a difference in development between infants fed formulas supplemented with AA and DHA, and those who were not supplemented; other studies have shown no differences.[53-56] For these reasons, the AAP has no official position on the supplementation of term infant formulas with AA and DHA. DHA and AA supplements offer an advantage to premature infants.[57]

Cow's milk, full-fat, skim, 1%, 2% fat, goat milk, evaporated milk, and other "milks" not specifically formulated to meet infant nutritional requirements are not recommended for use during the first 12 months of life.[58] Infants fed these milks are at risk of iron deficiency anemia because of low iron concentration, low bioavailability of iron, and possible intestinal blood loss.[59,60] These milks also contain higher protein, sodium, potassium, and chloride concentrations and increase renal solute load.[61] The essential fatty acids, vitamin E, and zinc are so low that deficiency may result. Low-fat milks may cause the infant to consume excessive amounts of protein to satisfy caloric needs.[62]

COMPLEMENTARY FEEDING

The American Academy of Pediatrics supports exclusive breast-feeding for a minimum of 4 but preferably 6 months,[36] but recognizes that some infants have unique needs or feeding problems that require complementary foods be introduced as early as 4 months or as late as 8 months. Longer exclusive breast-feeding protects against the exposure to potentially contaminated and/or low-nutrient-density foods that put infants at risk for diarrhea and malnutrition. If a safe supply of water and complementary foods exists, then the focus for the timing of introduction of complementary foods is on nutrients themselves. Exclusively breast-fed infants are at risk of developing iron, zinc, and calorie deficiency after 4 to 6 months of age and may benefit from the introduction of complementary feedings at that time. There is no evidence that prolonged exclusive breast-feeding protects against allergy. There are no studies that compare neurocognitive development or behavior in exclusively breast-fed infants and those on mixed feedings. No information exists on the optimal time at which to introduce complementary foods for formula-fed infants. Developmentally, infants are ready to receive complementary foods when they have some hand-eye coordination and the extrusion reflex abates (Table 85-5).

As breast-fed infants are at risk of developing iron and zinc deficiency, complementary foods high in these minerals, such

TABLE 85-5. **Development and Eating Skills in Infants and Toddlers**

	Newborn	Head Up	Supported Sitter	Independent Sitter	Crawler	Beginning to Walk	Independent Toddler
Physical skills	Needs head support	More skillful head control with support emerging	Sits with help or support On tummy, pushes up on arms with straight elbows	Sits independently Can pick up and hold small object in hand Leans toward food or spoon	Learns to crawl May pull self to stand	Pulls self to stand Stands alone Takes early steps	Walks well alone Runs
Eating skills	Baby establishes a suck-swallow-breathe pattern during breast- or bottle-feeding	Breast- or bottle-feeds Tongue moves forward and back to suck	May push food out of mouth with tongue; this gradually decreases with age Moves puréed food forward and backward in mouth with tongue to swallow Recognizes spoon and holds mouth open as spoon approaches	Learns to keep thick purées in mouth Pulls head downward and presses upper lip to draw food from spoon Tries to rake foods toward self into fist Can transfer food from one hand to the other Can drink from a cup held by feeder	Learns to move tongue from side to side to transfer food around mouth and push food to the side of the mouth so food can be mashed Begins to use jaw and tongue to mash food Plays with spoon at mealtime, may bring it to mouth, but does not use it for self-feeding yet Can feed self finger foods Holds cup independently Holds small foods between thumb and first finger	Feeds self easily with fingers Can drink from a straw Can hold cup with two hands and take swallows More skillful at chewing Dips spoon in food rather than scooping Demands to spoon-feed self Bites through a variety of textures	Chews and swallows firmer foods skillfully Learns to use a fork for spearing Uses spoon with less spilling Can hold cup in one hand and set it down skillfully

TABLE 85-5. Development and Eating Skills in Infants and Toddlers—cont'd

	Newborn	Head Up	Supported Sitter	Independent Sitter	Crawler	Beginning to Walk	Independent Toddler
Baby's hunger and fullness cues	Cries or fusses to show hunger Gazes at caregiver; opens mouth during feeding indicating desire to continue Spits out nipple or falls asleep when full Stops sucking when full	Cries or fusses to show hunger Smiles, gazes at caregiver, or coos during feeding to indicate desire to continue Spits out nipple or falls asleep when full Stops sucking when full	Moves head forward to reach spoon when hungry May swipe the food toward the mouth when hungry Turns head away from spoon when full May be distracted or notice surroundings more when full	Reaches for spoon or food when hungry Points to food when hungry Slows down in eating when full Clenches mouth shut or pushes food away when full	Reaches for food when hungry Points to food when hungry Shows excitement when food is presented when hungry Pushes food away when full Slows down in eating when full	Expresses desire for specific foods with words or sounds Shakes head to say "no more" when full	Combines phrases with gestures, such as "want that" and pointing Can lead parent to refrigerator and point to a desired food or drink Uses words like "all done" and "get down" Plays with food or throws food when full
Appropriate foods and textures	Breast milk or infant formula	Breast milk or infant formula	Breast milk or infant formula Infant cereals Thin puréed foods	Breast milk or infant formula Infant cereals Thin puréed baby foods Thicker puréed baby foods Soft mashed foods without lumps 100% juice	Breast milk or infant formula 100% juice Infant cereals Puréed foods Ground or soft mashed foods with tiny soft noticeable lumps Foods with soft texture Crunchy foods that dissolve (such as baby biscuits or crackers) Increase variety of flavors offered	Breast milk, infant formula, or whole milk 100% juice Coarsely chopped foods, including foods with noticeable pieces Foods with soft to moderate texture Toddler foods Bite-sized pieces of foods Bites through a variety of textures	Whole milk 100% juice Coarsely chopped foods Toddler foods Bite-sized pieces of foods Becomes efficient at eating foods of varying textures and taking controlled bites of soft solids, hard solids, or crunchy foods by 2 years

Butte N, Cobb K, Dwyer J. The healthy feeding guidelines for infants and toddlers. Journal of the American Dietetic Association 1994; 104:452 with permission from the American Dietetic Association.

as meats, should be introduced as the first food. Iron-fortified infant cereal is often recommended as the initial solid food; however, the absorption and bioavailability of iron from fortified cereals is uncertain,[33,63] and they do not provide zinc.

Juice is sometimes recommended in the first year of life, and parents often provide it without consulting their doctors. Historically, pediatricians recommended fruit juice as a source of vitamin C when scurvy was a serious concern for infants. Fruit juice is marketed as a healthy, natural source of vitamins and, in some instances, calcium. Because juice tastes good, children readily accept it. There is no nutritional indication to feed juice to infants younger than 6 months of age. Offering juice before solid foods are introduced into the diet could risk having juice replace breast milk or infant formula in the diet. This can result in reduced intake of protein, fat, vitamins, and minerals such as iron, calcium, and zinc.[64] Malnutrition has been associated with excessive consumption of juice.[65]

Because foods high in iron are recommended as weaning foods, beverages that contain vitamin C do not offer a nutritional advantage for iron-sufficient individuals. The AAP recommends that juice not be offered to infants younger than 6 months and for those older than 1 year that it be provided in limited amounts.[66]

SUPPLEMENTS

As noted previously, exclusively breast-fed infants require supplementation with vitamin D to prevent rickets. Breast milk is a poor source of iron. Iron deficiency and iron deficiency anemia can be prevented by supplementing exclusively breast-fed infants starting at four months of age and continuing through 12 months of age. Exclusively breast-fed infants of vegan mothers require supplementation with vitamin B_{12}. Healthy, term, formula-fed infants do not require vitamin or mineral supplements as all of the formulas, except the low-iron formulas, are complete foods. Infants aged 6 months or more may benefit from fluoride supplementation if their water is not fluoridated.[43] No information is available on the fluoride content of bottled water.

TODDLERS

There is no widely accepted definition of *toddler*. The term is taken from the wide-based gait seen in children who are just learning to walk. It is generally agreed that "toddlerhood" begins at the age of 12 months; the upper boundary of this age bracket is poorly defined. In this discussion it is assumed that toddlerhood ends at 36 months. Thus, a child aged less than 12 months is an infant and after 36 months a toddler becomes a "preschooler." Because many of the data in the literature are given for children aged 2 to 5 years, preschoolers are often included in the discussion.

Growth and therefore nutritional requirements peak during the first year of life. Growth rate during the second 12 months of life continues to be high. The second year of life is one of transition from an infant diet to a modified adult diet, yet there are a paucity of studies and guidelines on toddlers' nutrition. There are a number of studies that describe what toddlers eat.[67-72] There have been studies documenting change in eating patterns of toddlers[73,74] and reports on the psychologic and behavioral aspects of toddler nutrition.[75-77] However, few studies have been performed to determine the nutritional requirements of toddlers.[78,79] There are also few published guidelines,[80,81] and those that are available often use data extrapolated from other age groups.

Barker Hypothesis

This hypothesis proposes that "a baby's nourishment before birth and during infancy" programs the development of blood pressure, fibrinogen concentration, factor VIII concentration, and glucose tolerance, and so is an important determinant of future coronary artery disease.[82,83] The Barker hypothesis, as originally stated, was limited to fetal and infant nutrition and the subsequent development of coronary artery disease. The hypothesis has been broadened to include any adult ailment that may have its beginning during childhood, such as osteoporosis and renal disease. The Barker hypothesis continues to be debated, but to the extent that it proves true, early nutrition gains tremendous importance. It is during toddler years that dietary patterns are established for life.[84]

DESCRIPTIVE INFORMATION

A number of cross-sectional national studies as well as some longitudinal studies are presently available for analysis. The major national cross-sectional studies are the National Health and Nutrition Examination Survey (NHANES I, II and III) and the present continuous NHANES study. There are four Continuing Survey of Food Intake by Individuals studies (CSFII, 1998; 1994-1996; 1989-1991; 1985-1986). Data on toddlers are also available from the National Food Consumption Survey (1977-1978). In addition, there is one recent industry-sponsored survey addressing toddler nutrition, the Feeding Infants and Toddlers Study (FITS) conducted and supported by Gerber Products.[85] The FITS data include 3022 infants and toddlers

aged from 4 to 24 months. FITS does not provide information on the older toddler. All of these studies point to consistency in energy intake and in the relative proportions of macronutrients across the country, across racial and ethnic groups, and over the years. This consistency lends support to the long-held notion that toddlers, when presented with adequate nutrition, self-regulate their intake to a remarkable extent.[86-88] In counterdistinction to this consistency, a number of trends in toddler nutrition have been documented over the past 30 years. As with other segments of the population, in children less than 5 years of age there has been an increased prevalence of overweight from 7.2% in the NHANES II to 10.4% in the NHANES III survey[89] (Figure 85-1). Snacking has always been an important source of nutrition for toddlers. Recent surveys have shown an increase in the importance of snacking as a component of toddlers' diets. Snacks now represent 24% of total caloric intake by 2- to 5-year-olds (Figure 85-2).[73] The change is attributed to an increase in the number of snacks (rather than larger portion size) and a shift to higher-calorie, higher-fat snacks.

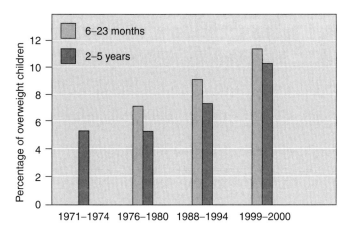

Figure 85-1. Percentage of overweight children aged 6 to 60 months, as reported by the National Health and Nutrition Examination Surveys (NHANES).

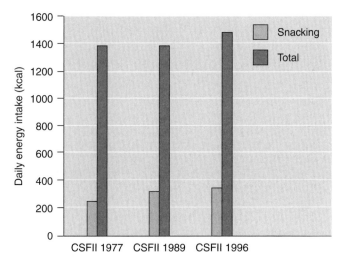

Figure 85-2. Contribution of snacking to total energy intake by 2- to 5-year-old children, as reported by Continuous Survey of Food Intakes by Individuals (CSFII).

EXPERIMENTAL INFORMATION

Energy

Energy needs are variable in toddlers, as they are for other age groups, and depend on basal metabolic rate, rate of growth, physical activity and body size. Energy requirements also depend on whether the child is over-weight or underfed. The reader is directed to the most recent Dietary Reference Intakes (DRIs) for a thorough discussion of the various factors that influence energy requirements.[6,90-94]

Energy needs can be determined experimentally in a number of ways: indirect calorimetry, doubly labeled water, and the factorial method. Of these, doubly labeled water, the most accurate method, has the advantage of measuring energy consumption in a free-living individual over a prolonged period of time. Its disadvantages are expense and lack of availability. Indirect calorimetry determines oxygen consumed and carbon dioxide produced by careful measurement of inspired and expired gases. Accurate measurements are difficult in the toddler age range. The factorial method sums the contributions of basal metabolic rate, physical activity, thermic effect of food, growth, and any known losses. The factorial method is the least accurate, but was the method most frequently used in the past.

It is now generally believed that previous estimates of toddlers' energy needs were erroneously high. The 10th edition of the Recommended Dietary Allowances (RDAs) set the energy requirements of 1- to 3-year-olds at 103 kcal per kg body weight per day.[94]

Prentice et al.,[95] using doubly labeled water, determined the energy expenditure of children aged 12, 24, and 36 months at 83, 84, and 85 kcal per kg per day, respectively. The most recent DRIs, depending on doubly labeled water measurements, set the estimated energy requirement for 12-month-old boys at 844 kcal/day and that for 12-month-old girls at 768 kcal/day. The estimated energy requirements of boys aged 24 months are 1050 kcal/day and those for girls 997 kcal/day. For 35-month-old boys, the estimated energy requirement is 1184 kcal/day and for girls, 1139 kcal/day. Assuming a weight at the 50th percentile for age, these numbers translate into 81.2 kcal/kg daily for 12-month-old boys and 80.6 kcal/kg daily for girls, and 82.7 and 83.1 kcal/kg daily for 24-month-old boys and girls, respectively. For 35-month-old boys, the estimated energy requirement is 84.0 kcal/kg daily and that for girls is 83.8 kcal/kg daily. The new DRIs are in line with the measurements of Prentice et al.[95] and significantly lower than the previous RDAs.

Fats

The principle of any diet for children must be that it adequately supports growth and development. Particularly with fats, this principle has led to controversy. Limiting fat intake should not jeopardize a toddler's growth and neurologic development, but excess fat might lead to obesity and future atherosclerotic disease. The AAP recommends that fat not be limited in the diet of toddlers until 24 months of age. It is feared that a fat-restricted diet might be deficient in energy or other nutrients. Between 24 months and 18 years of age, the recommendation calls for a child to be taking not more than 30% but not less than 20% of calories from fat; of this, not more than 10% should be from saturated fats. The recommendations say that average daily cholesterol intake should be less than 300 mg.[96] With emphasis on decreasing the amount of fat in the diet of adults, there has been a steady decline in the amount of fat that toddlers consume: the latest FITS reports that fat intake for many toddlers is less than that recommended.[97]

Essential Fatty Acids

For humans, α-linoleic acid, an omega-6 polyunsaturated fatty acid, and linolenic acid of the omega-3 series of polyunsaturated fatty acids are essential fatty acids (EFAs). Approximately 1 to 2% of dietary calories must come from these two EFAs to avoid deficiencies. α-Linoleic acid is a precursor of arachidonic acid, whereas linolenic acid is metabolized to docosahexaenoic acid. AA and DHA are prominent fatty acids of neural tissue, and DHA is found in high concentration in the retina. Humans can synthesize both AA and DHA, but recent studies have suggested that premature infants and possibly full-term infants may synthesize inadequate quantities of these fatty acids (conditionally essential). AA and DHA are present in human milk and have been added to infant formulas. Whether the addition of these fatty acids to infant formulas will improve vision and cognition, as claimed, is the subject of a number of studies with diverse results.[53,56,57,98,99] Nevertheless, this debate over AA and DHA for infants has led to speculation as to whether AA and DHA are required by toddlers. Toddlers continue to lay down significant amounts of neural tissue and, hence, DHA. Whether toddlers synthesize adequate amounts of AA and DHA from precursors is not known. Improvement with administration of DHA has been reported in children known to have illnesses associated with disordered fat metabolism, such as cystic fibrosis[100] and peroxisomal disease.[101] Low levels of red blood cell DHA have been demonstrated in malnourished Pakistani children.[102,103]

Trans-Fats

In an unsaturated fatty acid, the carbon atoms on either side of the double bond can be in either a cis or a trans configuration. The higher the concentration of trans fatty acids, the more solid the fat. So oils are generally high in cis fatty acids, and margarine and lard are high in trans fatty acids. Fatty acids can be changed from the cis to the trans form by processes such as heating, baking, and frying. Trans fatty acids are implicated in cardiovascular disease in adults.[104] The importance of cis versus trans fatty acids for toddlers is entirely unknown, but, by extrapolation from adult data and invoking the extended Barker hypothesis, it is important to study this question carefully.

Proteins

Proteins are essential for all metabolic functions in the body and serve as the main structural element of the body, as biochemical catalysts, and as regulators of gene expression. Proteins are complex, and their function is influenced by energy and nutrients, such as minerals, vitamins, and trace elements. Proteins consist of amino acids that have been categorized as essential (or indispensable) and nonessential (or dispensable). The nine essential amino acids cannot be synthesized from precursors and hence must be provided. However, as more information on protein and intermediary metabolism is understood, the definition of essential becomes blurred. Laidlaw and Kopple[105] propose adding a third category of amino acid: conditionally indispensable. Conditionally indispensable amino acids are those that are synthesized from other amino acids in limiting quantities or that have limited synthesis under special physiologic conditions.[105-107] Protein quality is determined by digestibility and the indispensable amino acid composition of the protein. If the content of a single indispensable amino acid is less than the requirement, that amino acid limits the utilization of other amino acids, preventing normal rates of protein synthesis even when the total nitrogen is adequate.

Unlike energy and other nutrients, the body has little in the way of protein that can be mobilized during times of insufficient intake. In a 70-kg adult the "reservoir" of labile protein is estimated at about 1% of total body protein. More than half of the body protein is present as skeletal muscle, skin, and blood. The liver and kidney are metabolically active tissues that contain about 10% of total body protein. Brain, heart, lung, and bone account for about 15% of whole-body protein. The distribution of protein among these organs varies with age. The toddler has proportionately more brain and visceral tissue and less muscle. When exogenous protein is inadequate, functional body proteins are used. The body can adapt to a wide range of protein intakes; however, pathologic conditions such as infection or trauma can cause substantial protein loss, either as demand for amino acids increases or as amino acid carbon skeletons are used to meet energy demands. If these extra needs are not met, a serious depletion of body protein mass occurs. Skeletal muscle is the largest single contributor to protein loss.

Protein requirements are based on the assumptions that adequate energy is provided, so that the carbon skeletons of amino acids are not needed as an energy source and the protein quality is high. Estimates of protein requirements for toddlers range from 0.88 g/kg daily[90] to 1.2 g/kg daily.[108] Proposed amino acid requirements of the nine indispensable amino for children and adults have been reviewed.[109]

The most reliable method to assess the adequacy of dietary protein is nitrogen balance: the difference between nitrogen intake and the amount excreted in urine, feces, skin, and sweat. This measurement is not practical clinically, especially for children. There is no reliable clinical measure of protein nutritional status. Failure to gain weight or length can be used to assess the overall nutritional adequacy of a diet, and failure to gain length occurs with borderline inadequate protein intake.[110] Other anthropometrics are less sensitive. The most commonly used clinical tools for assessing protein status are albumin and prealbumin.

Most individuals can tolerate a wide range of protein intakes. The vast majority of well toddlers in the developed world have a diet adequate in protein.[97] Diets high in protein are associated with an increase in renal solute load, a potential safety concern for water balance.

Carbohydrates

As with the other macronutrients, carbohydrate can no longer be considered a single category. Not only are there sugars, starches, and fiber, but in addition carbohydrates are assigned different "glycemic indices."[111] The glycemic index of an individual food is the effect on blood sugar of 50 g of available carbohydrate compared with 50 g of a control food. From the glycemic indices, the glycemic load of a diet can be calculated. Glycemic load has been shown to be an independent risk factor for type 2 diabetes,[112,113] for cancer,[114] and for cardiovascular disease in women.[115] Relatively few studies have been done to determine glycemic load in children.[116] There are no recommendations for carbohydrate intake in toddlers;

however, carbohydrate accounts for 52% of the energy intake of children aged 1 to 5 years.[94,117] Fiber and nonabsorbable starch are important carbohydrate components of the diet. They change the viscosity of the small bowel content, thus altering transit time and the absorption of nutrients. After entering the large intestine, these substances are not "inert" but regulate colonic bacterial bulk as well as changing the composition of the flora. Bacteria use fiber to produce short-chain fatty acids through fermentation. These short-chain fatty acids are used for fuel by colonocytes, but are also absorbed into the circulation. These actions of fiber and nonabsorbable starch promote defecation, a desirable effect, as constipation is a major problem among toddlers.[118] Toddlers in the United States ingest a mean of 8.5 g fiber per day.[97] The Institute of Medicine recommends that toddlers have 19 g fiber daily.[90]

SPECIFIC NUTRIENT DEFICITS

Iron

Despite a demonstrable decline in prevalence, iron deficiency anemia remains the most common cause of anemia in young children.[119] However, perhaps more important than anemia itself is the suggestion that iron deficiency alters long-term development and behavior, and that some of these effects may not be reversible. There have been an overwhelming number of studies linking iron deficiency with neurodevelopmental and motor delays and indicating the benefits of iron supplementation. These studies are the subject of a Cochrane Database Review.[120] The conclusion of the review was that there was no firm evidence for a short-term (2 weeks) beneficial effect of iron supplementation on neurologic and motor development, but there did appear to be a long-term (3 months) effect. McCann and Ames have reviewed the evidence for a causal relationship between iron deficiency/iron deficiency anemia and deficits in cognitive and behavioral function. They concluded that although evidence of causality existed, it was insufficient at this time to establish unequivocally a cause and effect relationship between iron deficiency/iron deficiency anemia and neurodevelopmental delays.[121] Even more concerning than the evidence that iron deficiency is adversely affecting development is that these adverse effects can be documented 10 years or more after the deficiency has been corrected, and so are likely permanent.[3]

Iron is present in the body in association with hemoglobin and myoglobin and as a cofactor for enzymes (functional iron), or as a part of ferritin and hemosiderin (stored iron).

Depleted Iron Stores

If there is a negative iron balance, iron stores are depleted and serum ferritin levels decrease. Because ferritin levels are affected by mechanisms other than iron depletion, such as inflammation, ferritin alone cannot be used to determine iron status. Measured levels of serum transferrin receptors (TfRs) increase early with depletion of iron stores. TfR levels are not affected by inflammation, but experience with this measurement in children is limited.[122]

Iron Deficiency Without Anemia

As iron stores become more limiting, there is disordered erythropoiesis leading to increased erythrocyte protoporphyrin and decreased transferrin saturation.

Iron Deficiency Anemia

When hemoglobin levels and the hematocrit begin to decrease, iron deficiency anemia is present. There are a number of conditions that mimic iron deficiency anemia, such as anemia of chronic disease, lead poisoning, thalassemia minor, or other mild hereditary anemias. These other conditions need to be considered and excluded. The WHO recently recommended using hemoglobin, ferritin, and transferrin receptor levels to identify iron deficiency anemia, and hemoglobin, ferritin, and C-reactive protein to monitor anemia.[123]

Comparison of the NHANES III and the present NHANES data suggests that the prevalence of iron deficiency and iron deficiency anemia have decreased. National data place the prevalence of iron deficiency at 9% and iron deficiency anemia at 3% of toddlers.[124] Looking at disadvantaged areas, the prevalence is reported to be as high as 24% for iron deficiency and 11% for iron deficiency anemia.[125] Presently, two types of screening programs are recommended: universal and selective screening. Universal screening at 9 to 12 and 15 to 18 months of age is used in communities with a high incidence of iron deficiency. In communities where iron deficiency is not common, selective screening uses the same schedule, but screens only children thought to be at risk. At-risk children include preterm babies, those with a low birth weight, those not receiving iron-fortified formula, and breast-fed children over the age of 6 months not consuming a diet with adequate iron. Confirmation of a positive screen with a second test will eliminate most false positives.[126]

There are a number of possible approaches to dealing with the problem of iron deficiency in the toddler years: selective treatment, universal supplementation, and food fortification. At present, selective treatment based on the screening programs outlined above is recommended. Oral supplementation (3 to 6 mg/kg daily of elemental iron) is given for 4 weeks, and hemoglobin and hematocrit are then remeasured. An appropriate rise in the hemoglobin concentration (1 g/dL) confirms iron deficiency anemia. An insufficient rise should trigger further investigations, including adherence, blood loss, hemoglobinopathy, and lead poisoning. This selective treatment approach is certain to miss a proportion of children with iron deficiency and iron deficiency anemia. In view of the long-term sequelae associated with iron deficiency, including behavioral and developmental changes, we may want to consider another approach.

Zinc

Zinc is essential for growth. It is involved in chromosome replication, regulation of the translation of genetic information, provides structure for "zinc-finger" proteins, stabilizes ribosomes and membranes, and is a component of a number of enzymes.[127] Zinc deficiency in humans impairs cell-mediated immunity. Signs of zinc deficiency include dermatitis, alopecia, diarrhea, and immune deficiency. Severe, parenteral nutrition-associated zinc deficiency mimics acrodermatitis enteropathica.[128,129] With zinc deficiency, relatively more fat accrues than lean tissue.[130] Zinc status is difficult to monitor. Stress, infections, and trauma all alter circulating zinc levels. Despite these shortcomings, serum zinc is commonly used to monitor zinc nutriture. Zinc is lost from the body through urine, sweat, and stool. Zinc status should be assessed and corrected, if necessary, in the face of extra losses – as in the case of diarrhea or high ostomy output. Studies using the RDAs from 1989 found the zinc intake of toddlers to be too low[131]; however, using the new DRI recommendations, the FITS found that the majority of toddlers achieved the recommended intakes.[97] Whether the new standards are too low needs to be monitored carefully.

Vitamin E

Vitamin E deficiency has been associated with spinocerebellar disorders.[132] As an antioxidant, vitamin E has an unsubstantiated but potential role in the long-term prevention of oxidative damage, including cardiovascular disease, osteoarthritis, and others. The vitamin E status of toddlers is of concern. A number of studies have documented intakes of vitamin E less than the recommendations.[80,97] However, none of these studies has identified any signs or symptoms of vitamin E deficiency.

TODDLERS' NUTRITON AND STOOLING

Toddlers are going through a time of transition. As the diet changes from a predominantly milk-based one to a modified adult diet, the colonic flora also changes from an infant-type to more adult flora. Eating behavior is also in transition, going from being fed to self-feeding. All of these factors lead to extreme variation in stooling patterns. Many toddlers suffer from constipation, sometimes made worse by withholding behavior.[118] Some toddlers have diarrhea and some alternate between the two. Toddlers tend not to chew their food well, and it is not uncommon for food particles to appear in the feces apparently unchanged.

Diarrhea

Toddler's diarrhea is defined as diarrhea in a toddler who is otherwise healthy and for whom no other cause of diarrhea can be identified. Experience shows that this type of diarrhea eventually resolves.[133] Merely normalizing the toddler's diet and following the recommendations of the AAP to limit the quantity of juice result in resolution or improvement.[66]

Constipation

There is general agreement that functional constipation is extremely common among toddlers. The exact prevalence, however, is not known. Toddlers with constipation account for 3% of visits to the general pediatrician and for 25% of visits to pediatric gastroenterologists.[134] At least a part of the reason for the high prevalence of constipation among toddlers may be the low-fiber content of their diet. Toddlers consume an average of 8.5 g fiber a day, whereas the IOM recommends 19 g per day. There is little experimental evidence that increasing the fiber intake improves symptoms of constipation, except in those with developmental disabilities.[135,136]

PSYCHOLOGY OF TODDLERS' NUTRITION

The parent-child interaction around eating behavior is extremely complex and varies with the special needs of the child and the parents. The family makeup and economic, social, ethnic, and other factors influence this relationship. No rigid rules can be given, but some general principles apply. Structure and consistency are all important. Parents should identify what is acceptable to them and contrive ways to stay within the acceptable limits. Power struggles are to be avoided. Although a parent may win the battle ("You will not leave the table until every bit of broccoli is gone from your plate"), the war will probably be lost because the child may develop a lifelong loathing of broccoli. Bribery, especially with food, is not a good idea.

Eating the Right Amount

The toddler years are marked by transition to an adult-like diet. Although growth remains high, this is a time of decelerating growth and growth velocity. Toddlers are also becoming increasingly independent in their feeding skills and vocal in their likes and dislikes. There is often a perception that toddlers do not eat enough and are "picky eaters."[137] The FITS reports that by 24 months of age 50% of children are identified as picky eaters by their caregivers. However, the study found that picky eaters were no more likely than nonpicky eaters to have inadequate diets. Further, the study found that picky eaters were less likely to be overweight.[138]

Toddlers frequently exhibit "food neophobia," that is, a reluctance to try new foods. Sullivan and Birch[76] found that repeated exposures (5 to 10) to a new food increased the likelihood of a toddler accepting it. However, parents and caregivers questioned in the FITS identified a food as not liked by their toddler if refused an average of three times.

Meals and Snacks

For the toddler, both meals and snacks are important opportunities for nutrition. They are also a time to learn skills and values and to interact with others. For all toddlers, but especially for the younger toddler aged 12 to 24 months, all meals and snacks should be supervised. The danger of choking on small, hard foods is significant throughout toddlerhood. By 12 months of age the pattern of breakfast, lunch, and dinner plus snacks is well established. In the FITS, toddlers ate an average of seven times per day. Snacks provided 25% of the toddlers' energy intake. Snacks tended to be of lower nutritional quality compared with meals.[139] Snacking, as a component of the toddler's diet, has increased over time. In 1977, the average number of snacks per day consumed by children aged 2 to 5 years was 1.7. By 1996, the average had increased to 2.3. During the same time frame, the energy provided by snacking increased by 100 kcal/day.[73] Snacks, like meals, should be a planned part of the toddler's nutrition.

REFERENCES

2. Algarin C, Peirano P, Garrido M, et al. Iron deficiency anemia in infancy: long-lasting effects on auditory and visual system functioning. Pediatr Res 2003;53:217–223.
6. Institute of Medicine. Dietary Reference Intakes for Calcium, Phosphorus, Magnesium. Vitamin D and Fluoride. Washington, DC: National Academies Press; 1997.
13. de Onis M, Garza C, Onyango AW, Borghi E. Comparison of the WHO child growth standards and the CDC 2000 growth charts. J Nutr 2007;137: 144–148.
15. Kleinman RE, editor. Nutrition Handbook. Elk Grove Village, IL: American Academy of Pediatrics; 2004. p. 55.
37. Kramer MS, Kakuma R. Optimal duration of exclusive breastfeeding. Cochrane Database Syst Rev 2002(1):CD003517.
66. American Academy of Pediatrics. Committee on Nutrition. The use and misuse of fruit juice in pediatrics. Pediatrics 2001;107:1210–1213.
85. Feeding Infants and Toddlers Study (FITS). J Am Diet Assoc 2004;104 (Suppl 1):S1–S79.

See expertconsult.com for a complete list of references and the review questions for this chapter.

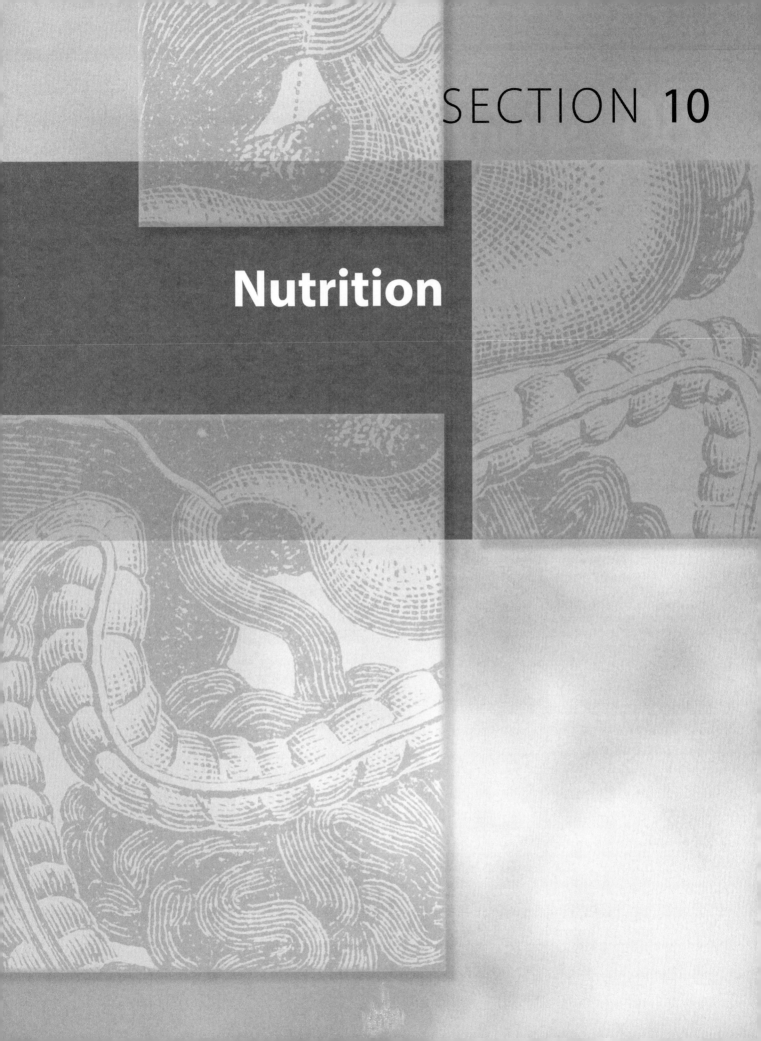

SECTION **10**

Nutrition

86 NUTRITIONAL ASSESSMENT

Kathleen J. Motil • Sarah M. Phillips • Claudia Conkin

Nutritional assessment is an essential component of the history and physical examination of children with gastrointestinal disorders. An understanding of the patterns of growth and the changes in body composition during childhood, as well as a working knowledge of the methods used to assess the nutritional status of the child, is important for the care of children with gastrointestinal disease.

EPIDEMIOLOGY OF NUTRITIONAL DISORDERS IN PEDIATRIC PATIENTS

Undernutrition, growth failure, overweight, and micronutrient deficiencies are seen frequently in the practice of pediatric gastroenterology. Forty-four percent of all children admitted to Texas Children's Hospital (n = 655) during a 2-week survey period had evidence of altered nutritional status. Twenty percent were acutely undernourished, 13% were overweight, and 31% were chronically undernourished. Acute undernutrition and overweight were found most frequently among adolescents, whereas chronic undernutrition was distributed evenly across all age groups. Children hospitalized with general pediatric problems were at greatest risk for acute undernutrition, whereas children diagnosed with gastrointestinal disease were at greatest risk for chronic undernutrition.

Undernutrition and growth failure occur as a consequence of poor dietary intake due to loss of appetite or abdominal symptoms, increased intestinal losses secondary to diarrhea or malabsorption, and increased nutrient requirements associated with inflammatory or infectious complications of gastrointestinal diseases. Overweight may be identified in children who use medications such as corticosteroids, which are prescribed for specific gastrointestinal disorders.

CLINICAL SIGNIFICANCE OF NUTRITIONAL ASSESSMENT

Nutritional assessment is useful to characterize the change in growth and body composition of the child in response to altered dietary intake (Figure 86-1). During periods of food deprivation in infancy, body weight loss is progressive.[1] Total body fat, as well as the proportion of body fat that composes body weight, decreases markedly. Body protein stores also decrease, although their proportion relative to body weight is unchanged. A loss of 40% or more of body weight is associated with an increased risk of morbidity and mortality.

Nutritional assessment also demonstrates the changes in growth and body composition that occur in response to infectious or inflammatory diseases. A febrile illness promptly initiates a catabolic response that results in negative body nitrogen balance because of increased urinary losses (Figure 86-2).[2] Negative nitrogen balance persists until the fever resolves. The cumulative loss of urinary nitrogen is significant and continues well beyond the period of the acute febrile illness. The recovery process may require as long as 3 weeks to replenish depleted body stores. Failure to pay attention to brief episodes of nutritional depletion leads to a vicious cycle in which the nutritional status of the child worsens with each repeated illness and becomes a factor contributing to morbidity or mortality.

CLINICAL FEATURES OF NORMAL GROWTH AND BODY COMPOSITION IN CHILDREN

Normal Patterns of Growth in Children

Growth is most rapid in healthy children during early infancy and adolescence (Table 86-1).[3] Length velocity averages 25 cm during the first year of life, declines abruptly to 11 cm during the second and third years, then slows to 6 cm per year in the preschool- and school-age child. Weight velocity averages 7 kg during the first year of life and declines abruptly to 2.5 kg in toddlers and school-age children. During adolescence, peak weight velocities average 3 kg, but may be as high as 6 to 7 kg per 6 months. Estimates of height and weight velocities are important because these measurements predict the energy needs for normal growth. If the average energy cost of tissue deposition is 5.5 kcal/g and the composition of newly deposited tissue is 75% lean and 25% fat, then an additional 15,200 kcal/year is required to support growth in the preschool- and school-age child.[4]

Normal Patterns of Body Composition in Children

The clinical features of body composition are more difficult to characterize because of the biologic complexity of the human body. From a theoretical perspective, the body can be divided into multiple compartments.[5] In a two-compartment model, the body is divided into the fat and fat-free mass (FFM) (Figure 86-3). The fat mass is composed entirely of fat, as opposed to adipose tissue, which contains body fat and the supporting cellular and extracellular tissues. The FFM is composed of the lean body mass (LBM) plus the nonfat components of adipose tissue. In clinical practice, the two-compartment model is useful because of the ease with which body fat and FFM can be measured by anthropometry and the simplicity with which their changes during health and disease can be assessed. However, the two-compartment model is subject to error because the methods used to measure body fat and FFM are based on the assumption that the chemical composition of these tissue stores remains constant across a broad range of ages and disease states.

Multi-compartment models of body composition have been developed to reduce the errors inherent in the two-compartment

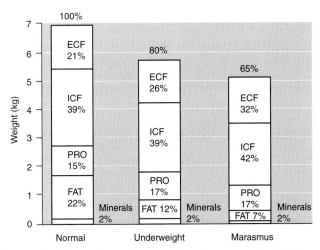

Figure 86-1. Changes in body composition during starvation in infancy. Adapted from Viteri (1981), with permission.[1]

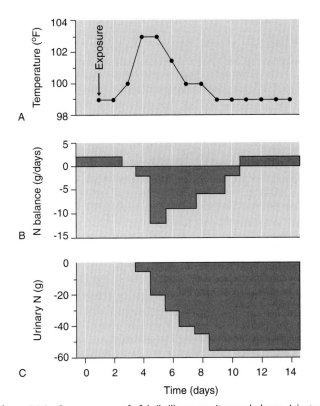

Figure 86-2. Consequences of a febrile illness on nitrogen balance. Adapted from Beisel (1972), with permission.[2]

TABLE 86-1. Normal Growth Rates in Children

Age Group	Height Velocity	Weight Velocity
Infant (1st y)	25 cm/y	7 kg/y
Toddler (2nd/3rd y)	11 cm/y	2.2 kg/y
Preschool/school age child	6 cm/y	2.8 kg/y
Adolescent	3-4 cm/6 mo	6-7 kg/6 mo

increase with increasing age throughout childhood, but vary at any given age depending on gender and race or ethnicity. These estimates serve as reference values for healthy children and may be useful comparative indices to assess the degree of nutritional deficits of children with gastrointestinal disorders.

Methods to Measure Body Composition

Anthropometry may be used to characterize body composition in the clinical setting. A metal tape measure and calibrated skinfold calipers are the only instruments needed. The upper-arm muscle circumference (or area) serves as a measure of body protein stores because it can be compared with reference standards to determine the degree of muscle wasting in children.[9] The triceps skinfold thickness is most frequently selected as a measure of body fat because it can be compared with reference standards to determine the degree of overweight in children.[9] No single skinfold site is entirely representative of the combined subcutaneous and deep fat stores of the body. A method that uses multiple skinfold thickness measurements, such as biceps, triceps, subscapular, and suprailiac sites, may provide a better estimate of body fat and its regional distribution.[10,11] Accurate estimates of body fat using anthropometry are difficult to obtain in morbidly overweight children or in children with generalized edema because of altered relationships between body tissue water and fat in these conditions. Waist circumference[12] and waist-for-height[13] may serve as alternative indicators of adiposity because these measure correlate with truncal fat and obesity-related comorbidities.[14,15]

Body fat and lean body mass can be measured by densitometry or derived from total body water. Underwater weighing is a density technique based on the individual's actual weight and the weight lost while under water. Air displacement plethysmography is a density technique that measures body composition from body mass and volume within an air-filled chamber.[16,17] Total body water can be measured directly by isotope dilution using the stable isotopes of hydrogen (^2H_2O) or oxygen ($H_2{}^{18}O$)[18] and indirectly by total body electrical conductance[19] or bioelectrical impedance analysis.[20]

Total body potassium counting, a method that measures the natural abundance of radioactive potassium (^{40}K) in the body, assesses lean body mass based on the assumption that the potassium content of the FFM is proportional to tissue nitrogen content.[21] Neutron activation analysis, a method that generates a known amount of radioactivity within a given mass from a defined dose of neutrons, characterizes the elemental composition of the body.[22] The particular element being examined, such as nitrogen, can be identified by the characteristic energy of the electromagnetic radiation it emits and its decay rate. Ultrasonography, computerized axial tomography, and nuclear magnetic resonance imaging display a visual image of body fat and fat-free mass throughout the body, but the inaccuracy of some of these methods, the high level of radiation exposure, and the

model (see Figure 86-3).[5] The elemental model describes body composition in terms of the most common elements of the body (oxygen, carbon, hydrogen, nitrogen, calcium, phosphorus, sodium, potassium, chloride). The chemical model characterizes body composition on the basis of its water, mineral (osseous, nonosseous), and organic (protein, glycogen, fat) components. The cellular model describes the body on the basis of its cell mass and body water compartments. The tissue model integrates the elemental, chemical, and cellular aspects of body composition into functional units that can be measured in the clinical setting.

The body composition of children from birth to 16 years of age, derived from a multicompartment model, is summarized in Table 86-2.[6-8] Estimates of lean body mass and body fat

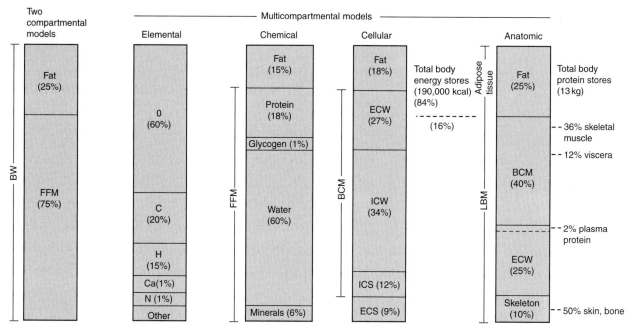

Figure 86-3. Multicompartment models of body composition. FFM, fat-free mass; BCM, body cell mass; ICW, intracellular water; ECW, extracellular water; ICS, intracellular solids; ECS, extracellular solids. Adapted from Wang et al. (1992),[5] with permission; and Heymsfield SB, Waki M. Body composition in humans: advances in the development of multicompartment clinical models. Nutr Rev 1991; 49:97-108, with permission.

cost and maintenance of the equipment preclude their use in children.[23]

Dual-energy x-ray absorptiometry (DXA) can be used to estimate FFM, body fat, and bone mineral content of the whole body or regions such as the spine and hip.[24] In this method, the child is scanned with an x-ray source of two different energy levels, the difference in the absorption being proportional to the type of tissue scanned. This technique is considered to be safe because the average radiation dose to the skin is only 1 to 3 mrem per scan. Because of their overall performance, DXA scans are accepted as a standard procedure in clinical practice.[25]

Two potential errors in interpreting the DXA scans of children are the use of bone mineral density (BMD) or T-scores to report loss of bone mineral content.[26,27] DXA instruments measure the mass of mineral within a bone, that is, bone mineral content (BMC), and bone area (BA), then calculate the ratio of these terms as bone mineral density (BMD). BMD is a misnomer because the measurement is a two-dimensional, rather than a three-dimensional, unit that does not distinguish which of the two components of bone mass is being assessed, bone size (volume) or density. BMD is affected by the person's size and tends to underestimate the concentration of minerals in bone in small individuals and overestimate it in larger individuals. Because consensus on the most appropriate way to report DXA results corrected for bone size has not been achieved, the mass of mineral within the bones of children commonly is reported as BMC and should be interpreted as Z-score values or standard deviation scores based on the child's body (bone) size, pubertal stage, pubertal tempo, age, gender, and racial or ethnic group.[25] In contrast, T-score values represent standard deviation scores calculated for young adults, which cannot be applied to children because there is no adjustment for their smaller size.

Other methods used to measure bone mineral mass and density include quantitative computed tomography, which has the disadvantage of a high radiation dose, and peripheral quantitative computed tomography, which provides a three-dimensional assessment of the appendicular skeleton using less radiation. Ultrasound techniques that measure the speed and attenuation of sound through appendicular bone have been developed, but have not been tested systematically in children.[28]

INDICATIONS FOR NUTRITIONAL ASSESSMENT

A nutritional assessment is warranted if a child with newly diagnosed gastrointestinal disease is at risk for developing undernutrition, growth failure, or overweight (Table 86-3). As a general guideline: (1) any child whose height-for-age is less than the 10th percentile is at risk for chronic undernutrition; (2) any child younger than 2 years of age whose weight-for-height is less than the 10th percentile or any child age 2 years or older whose body mass index (BMI) is less than the 10th percentile is at risk for acute undernutrition; and (3) any child age 2 years or older whose BMI is greater than the 85th percentile is overweight. These screening criteria imply that the child whose growth measurements plot at the extremes of the growth curves merits closer scrutiny to determine whether nutritional deficits or excesses truly are present.

Serial height and weight measurements provide additional information to evaluate nutritional risk. A nutritional assessment is warranted if a child older than 2 years fails to demonstrate appropriate linear or ponderal gains during a 6-month to 1-year interval. A height velocity less than 5 cm/year after 2 years of age may be consistent with linear stunting or chronic undernutrition. A prepubertal weight velocity less than 1 kg/year or a pubertal peak weight velocity less than 1 kg every 6 months may be consistent with acute undernutrition. Growth velocity measurements may be the most sensitive factors for elucidating which children with gastrointestinal diseases are at risk for nutritional disorders.[29]

TABLE 86-2. **Body Composition of Healthy Children**

Gender	Race/Ethnicity	Age (y)	Height (cm)	Weight (kg)	Lean Body Mass (kg)	Fat Mass (kg)
Female	Multiracial	Birth	50	3.3	2.8	0.5
		0.5	66	7	5.1	1.9
		1	74	9	6.8	2.2
		2	85	12	9.6	2.4
	Caucasian	4	107	18	14	4
		8	127	28	20	7
		12	151	44	30	12
		16	164	56	38	15
	African American	4	106	18	14	4
		8	133	33	23	9
		12	157	54	36	16
		16	162	63	40	21
	Hispanic	4	106	19	14	4
		8	124	30	19	8
		12	153	57	32	17
		16	161	67	39	25
Male	Multiracial	Birth	52	3.5	3.0	0.5
		0.5	68	8	6.0	2.0
		1	76	10	7.8	2.2
		2	87	13	10.5	2.5
	Caucasian	4	103	17	13	3
		8	126	26	20	5
		12	157	52	38	12
		16	174	67	54	10
	African American	4	105	18	15	2
		8	127	29	23	4
		12	161	60	46	13
		16	176	83	66	8
	Hispanic	4	99	16	12	1
		8	127	30	21	4
		12	158	56	39	9
		16	172	69	54	6

Adapted from Refs. 6-8.

COMPONENTS OF NUTRITIONAL ASSESSMENT

Nutritional assessment is defined as a comprehensive approach to characterizing quantitatively the nutritional status of the child.[30-32] A comprehensive nutritional assessment has four components: (1) dietary, medical, and medication history; (2) physical examination; (3) growth and anthropometric measurements; and (4) laboratory tests.

Dietary History

A dietary history that determines the quality and quantity of the child's pattern of food consumption and the eating behaviors and beliefs of the family is important to assess. The physician should ask about the type of food given to the child, the number of meals and snacks consumed per day, the use of a special diet, the consistency with which vitamin and mineral supplements are given, food allergies, food intolerances or avoidances, and unusual feeding behaviors. A review of the child's dietary history by 24-hour recall frequently is misleading because it

TABLE 86-3. **Indications for Nutritional Assessment**

Risk Criteria (NCHS, CDC)	Risk
HT-for-AGE < 10th percentile	Chronic malnutrition
HT velocity < 5 cm/y after age 2 years	
WT-for-HT < 10th percentile before age 2 years	Acute malnutrition
BMI < 10th percentile after age 2 years	
WT velocity <1 kg/y (prepubertal)	
WT velocity (peak) <1 kg/6 mo (prepubertal)	
BMI > 85th percentile after age 2 years	Obesity

NCHS, National Center for Health Statistics; CDC, Centers for Disease Control and Prevention; HT, height; WT, weight; BMI, body mass index

may not represent habitual patterns of food consumption, particularly when illness intervenes. A 3-day food record is a more valid tool to quantify dietary intake,[33] but its accuracy may be doubtful because parents tend to overestimate or underestimate the child's food consumption depending on the nature of the illness. The pattern of food consumption also may differ from usual, particularly in the hospital setting. If food records are obtained, a registered dietitian can estimate the energy content of the diet using the Atwater conversion factors (1 g of protein, carbohydrate, and fat equals 4, 4, and 9 kcal/g, respectively) or the nutrient composition of the diet using a computerized nutrient database. The energy and nutrient composition of the diet should be compared with age- and gender-specific Dietary Reference Intakes,[34] with the caveat that these standards meet the nutrient needs of healthy children, but do not account for the nutrient needs of children with acute or chronic illness. Indirect calorimetry may be more appropriate to assess the metabolic nutritional needs of the acutely ill hospitalized child.[35]

The assessment of the dietary intake of infants with gastrointestinal illness should be rigorous because of the rapidity with which failure to thrive may develop in this age group. The adequacy of the infant's intake can be estimated from the frequency and duration of nursing (8 to 12 times per day, 5 to 15 minutes per breast), the frequency of formula feeding, the volume of milk consumed (150 to 180 mL/kg per day), the energy density of the formula, and an expected average weight gain of 30 g/day during the first 6 months of life.[3] In the presence of nutritional deficits, daily energy intakes in the range of 150 to 180 kcal/kg per day and higher weight gains of 50 to 60 g/day should be anticipated to reverse the adverse nutritional consequences associated with gastrointestinal disorders.

The assessment of the dietary intake of children 2 years of age or older should follow the Dietary Guidelines for Americans.[36] Total daily fat intake should comprise 20 to 35% of total daily energy intake, with most fats derived from sources of polyunsaturated and monounsaturated fatty acids (fish, nuts, vegetable oils). Saturated fats should comprise less than 10% of total daily energy intakes. Cholesterol intake should be limited to 300 mg/day. Trans-fatty acid consumption should be as low as possible. Carbohydrate intake should consist of fiber-rich fruits, vegetables, and whole grains with little added sugars or caloric sweeteners. A high-fiber diet should be encouraged. A useful guideline is the child's age in years plus 5 equals the grams of fiber per day, where one serving of fruit, vegetable, or cereal each contains 2 to 3 g of fiber.[37] Less than 1 tsp of table salt should be consumed daily. The diet should be nutritionally complete, include a variety of nutrient-dense foods and beverages within

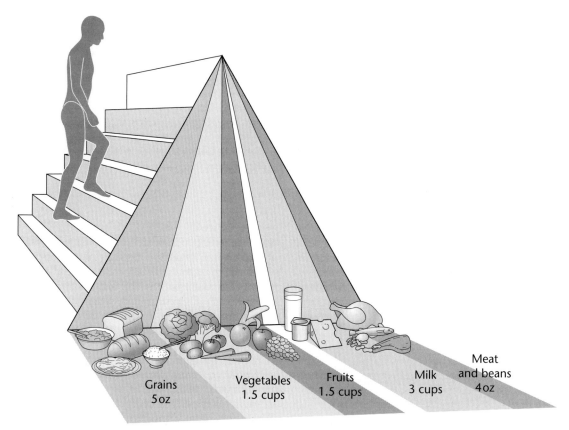

Figure 86-4. U.S. Department of Agriculture. Food Guide Pyramid. Available at http://www.mypryamid.gov (accessed on September 1, 2009).

and among the basic food groups, and be adequate for normal growth and physical activity. In conditions where dietary modifications may be necessary to ameliorate gastrointestinal symptoms, careful attention to appropriate nutrient substitutes or supplements should be given to prevent specific nutrient deficiencies, imbalances, or toxicities. MyPyramid, published by the U.S. Department of Agriculture, is the practical tool to assess dietary intakes across all age groups (Figure 86-4).[38] The specific kinds and amounts of food that should be consumed daily can be determined for any individual based on age, gender, and physical activity by connecting to the website.

Physical Examination

Undernutrition includes two entities: marasmus and kwashiorkor. Marasmus is characterized by the wasting of muscle mass and the depletion of body fat stores, whereas kwashiorkor is characterized by generalized edema (anasarca) and flaky, peeling skin rashes. Children with undernutrition may manifest a broad spectrum of clinical features (Table 86-4). However, it is uncommon to find many of the signs of severe undernutrition in children with acute or chronic gastrointestinal illnesses. A combination of wasting and peripheral edema, signifying a combination of marasmus and kwashiorkor, is found most commonly. The clinician should have a high index of suspicion for micronutrient deficiencies in the presence of these findings, particularly in children with malabsorptive or inflammatory disorders.

Overweight is characterized by increased deposition of truncal and peripheral body fat. Increased body fat is associated with several effects on growth including increased lean body mass,

increased height, advanced bone age, and the early onset of menarche. Overweight children may be hypertensive and often display dysfunctional behaviors because of poor self-esteem. Morbid overweight is associated with metabolic complications, such as diabetes mellitus and hyperlipidemia, hepatic steatosis, cholelithiasis, orthopedic disorders including slipped capital femoral epiphysis or bowing of the tibia and femur, and cardiopulmonary problems including congestive heart failure and obstructive sleep apnea. Whereas simple, exogenous overweight is a national epidemic, the type of overweight that occurs in conjunction with medications such as prednisone is more difficult to manage because these drugs ameliorate inflammatory conditions but lead to voracious appetites.

Growth and Anthropometric Measurements

Growth measurements are the most important components of the nutritional assessment because normal growth patterns are the gold standard by which physicians assess the health and well-being of the child. The physician should be able to convert the growth measurements to relative standards to interpret correctly the information provided by these measurements.[3] A normal growth pattern is not a guarantee of overall health, but the child with an atypical growth pattern is more likely to manifest the nutritional complications of gastrointestinal disease. Altered growth patterns are a relatively late consequence of nutritional insult. Thus, surveillance is an important component of the nutritional assessment of the child with gastrointestinal disease.

Height and weight measurements are the mainstay of the nutritional assessment of the child. The appropriate way to measure length or height is to use a flat, horizontal or vertical

TABLE 86-4. **Clinical Features of Nutritional Deficiencies**

Nutritional Deficiency	Clinical Features
Protein-energy malnutrition	Irritability, apathy
Kwashiorkor	Flag sign (loss of hair color)
Vitamin A	Follicular hyperkeratosis, night blindness
Thiamine (vitamin B$_1$)	Weakness of the leg muscles, pedal edema, tachycardia, congestive heart failure, aphonic cry, seizures (beriberi)
Riboflavin (vitamin B$_2$)	Angular stomatitis, chelosis, seborrheic dermatitis of the lips and nose
Niacin	Dry, cracked skin in areas exposed to sunlight, including neck, hands, feet (pellagra)
Pyridoxine (vitamin B$_6$)	Weakness, nervousness, insomnia, hypochromic, microcytic anemia, seizures
Folate	Macrocytic anemia
Cobalamin (vitamin B$_{12}$)	Peripheral neuropathy including loss of vibratory sensation and proprioception, paresthesias, motor weakness, macrocytic anemia
Vitamin C	Petechiae, ecchymoses, hyperkeratotic hair follicles with red hemorrhagic halos, bleeding gums, painful, subperiosteal bleeding of lower extremities
Vitamin D	Bone abnormalities including craniotabes, frontal bossing of skull, rib cage beading (rachitic rosary), tibial bowing, radial widening of wrists
Iron	Smooth tongue, spooning and pallor of nail beds, microcytic, hypochromic anemia
Calcium	Tetany, Chvostek, Trousseau, or Erb signs
Magnesium	Personality changes, muscle spasms, seizures
Zinc	Diarrhea, alopecia, dermatitis localized to perioral and perianal areas, short stature

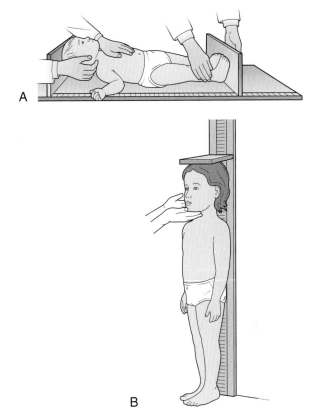

Figure 86-5. Technique for measuring (**A**) recumbent length or (**B**) height. From Jelliffe (1966), with permission.[39]

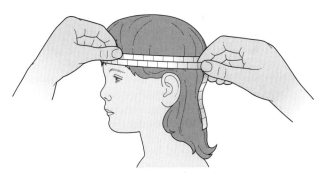

Figure 86-6. Technique for measuring head circumference. From Jelliffe (1966), with permission.[39]

surface with perpendicular surfaces at each end (Figure 86-5).[39] Weight measurements should be obtained on a scale that has been calibrated properly. The head circumference should be measured at the maximum diameter through the glabella and occiput (Figure 86-6).[39] Growth measurements, including length or height, weight, and head circumference, should be plotted on growth charts from the National Center for Health Statistics, which can be accessed readily from the website for the Centers for Disease Control and Prevention.[3] Any length, height, or weight measurement that falls below the 5th percentile, is greater than the 95th percentile, or crosses two major growth channels is considered to represent an abnormal growth pattern. Serial measurements should be obtained to determine if the growth pattern is truly abnormal or if these findings merely represent constitutional short stature or the rechanneling of normal growth curves. Radiographic studies of bone age may help to clarify the presence of abnormal growth patterns because chronic undernutrition is one of the causes of delayed bone maturation, and hence, delayed linear growth.[40]

Incremental growth measurements that characterize height and weight velocities over a 6-month interval may be valuable in assessing the growth response of children with chronic illness.[41] Height velocity measurements may be the most sensitive measure to detect growth abnormalities early in the course of chronic gastrointestinal illnesses.[29] Any child older than 2 years whose height velocity is less than 5 cm/year should be monitored carefully for progressive nutritional deficits. A prepubertal child with a weight velocity less than 1 kg/year, or a pubertal child with a peak weight velocity less than 1 kg every 6 months, may be at risk for the nutritional complications of chronic illness.

Height and weight measurements may be converted to Z-scores, or values that represent standard deviations from the median height and weight values for age. Any child whose height or weight Z-score is less than –1.64 (i.e., less than the 5th percentile) is considered to have an abnormal growth pattern; height and weight Z-scores more than 2 standard deviations below the median are considered to represent significant nutritional deficits.

The BMI is an anthropometric measure used to screen for altered nutritional status because it best characterizes the proportionality of the body mass and body size of the child.[42] The BMI can be determined from the equation:

$$BMI\ (kg/m^2) = weight\ (kg) / [height\ (cm) / 100\ (cm/m)]^2$$

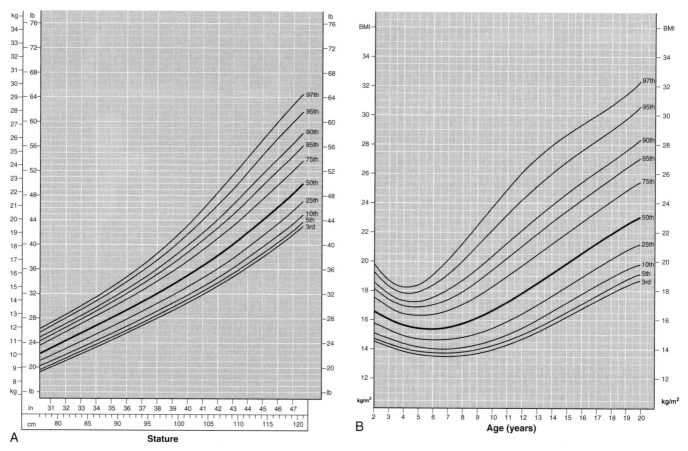

Figure 86-7. Centers for Disease Control and Prevention United States Growth Charts Body Mass Index (BMI) (**A**) for girls: 2 to 20 years, (**B**) for boys: 2 to 20 years. Available at http://www.cdc.gov/growthcharts (accessed on September 1, 2009).

The BMI should be plotted on gender-appropriate BMI charts from the National Center for Health Statistics (Figure 86-7), which can be accessed readily from the website for the Centers for Disease Control and Prevention.[3] Although the BMI is an indirect measure of body fatness, it correlates well with other more direct measures of body composition such as those obtained by underwater weighing and DXA.[43] The BMI is gender- and age-specific for children[44] and increases in a nonlinear fashion with increasing age. Consequently, BMI-for-age is the measure that relates BMI values in childhood to those obtained in adults. For children older than 6 years, BMI-for-age predicts underweight and overweight better than weight-for-height measurements.[45] For children younger than 6 years, BMI-for-age and weight-for-height estimates equally predict discrepancies in body fatness. The BMI is useful because it can be used to track body size throughout the life cycle and correlates well with the risk factors for cardiovascular disease in adulthood, including hyperlipidemia, hyperinsulinemia, and hypertension.[46] BMI-for-age in adolescence is associated directly with the risk of developing these chronic diseases in adulthood.[47]

The Centers for Disease Control and Prevention recommend that (1) BMI-for-age be used routinely to screen children for overweight and underweight, and (2) children be classified as underweight if their BMI is less than the 5th percentile, overweight if their BMI-for-age is the 85th to less than the 95th percentile, and obese if their BMI-for-age is equal to or greater than the 95th percentile.[3] The significance of these estimates is that they serve as a useful guideline for the approach to

dietary modification or intervention. For example, aggressive nutritional intervention such as nasogastric or gastrostomy tube feedings may be indicated if the BMI is less than 11 to 13 kg/m² because of the increased risk of morbidity and mortality associated with these low values.[48] An energy-deficit diet can be implemented in the child with moderate overweight (e.g., BMI above 30 kg/m²), whereas a more restrictive diet, such as the protein-sparing modified fast, may be necessary for morbid obesity (e.g., BMI above 40 kg/m).[49]

Laboratory Tests

Selected laboratory tests may be useful to assess the nutritional status of the child with gastrointestinal disease (Table 86-5). However, laboratory tests have limited usefulness over and above the clinical findings determined from growth measurements. Laboratory tests may identify deficiencies before clinical findings are evident, may confirm the presence of selected nutrient deficiencies that are commonly associated with specific gastrointestinal entities, or may be helpful to monitor the clinical recovery from undernutrition when it occurs as a complicating feature of gastrointestinal diseases.

Undernutrition is associated with global nutrient deficits, but these deficiencies generally are not severe enough to be reflected in blood plasma or serum values. Iron deficiency anemia is the most common nutritional anemia associated with chronic gastrointestinal diseases and should be assessed routinely. Hypochromic, microcytic red cell morphology suggests

TABLE 86-5. **Biochemical Measurements of Nutritional Status: Normal Values**

Tests	Neonate Birth-1 mo	Infant 1-12 mo	Child 1-9 y	Child 9-18 y
	Age and Sex Group			
Protein				
Blood				
Serum albumin (g/dL)	≥2.5	≥3	≥3.5	≥3.5
Retinol-binding protein (mg/dL)	2-3	2-3	2-3	3-6
Blood urea nitrogen (mg/dL)	7-22	7-22	7-22	7-22
Thyroxine-binding protein (mg/dL)	20-50	20-50	20-50	20-50
Transferrin (mg/dL)	170-250	170-250	170-250	170-250
Fibronectin (mg/dL)	30-40	30-40	30-40	30-40
Urine				
Creatinine/height index	>0.9	>0.9	>0.9	>0.9
3-Methylhistidine (μmol/kg)	4.2 ± 1.3	-	-	3.2 ± 0.6
3-Methylhistidine (μmol/kg creatinine)	253 ±78	-	-	126 ± 32
Hydroxyproline index	>2	>2	>2	>2
Vitamin A				
Plasma retinol (μg/dL)	≥30	≥30	≥30	≥30
Plasma retinol-binding protein (mg/dL)	2-3	2-3	2-3	2-3
Vitamin D				
25-OH-D_3 (ng/mL)	≥30	≥30	≥30	≥30
Riboflavin				
Red cell glutathione reductase stimulation effect (%)	<20	>20	>20	<20
Vitamin B_6				
Red cell transaminases	Not readily available, not practical in children younger than 9 years of age			
Plasma pyridoxal phosphate				
Xanthurenic acid excretion				
Folacin				
Serum folate (ng/mL)	>6	>6	>6	>6
Red blood cell folate (ng/mL)	>160	>160	>160	>160
Vitamin K				
Prothrombin time (seconds)	11-15	11-15	11-15	11-15
Vitamin E				
Plasma alpha-tocopherol (mg/dL)	≥0.7	≥0.7	≥0.7	≥0.7
Red blood cell hemolysis test (%)	≤10	≤10	≤10	≤10
Vitamin C				
Plasma (mg/dL)	>0.2	>0.2	>0.2	>0.2
Leukocyte (μg/108 cells)	Difficult to perform on infants and children owing to sample requirements			
Thiamine				
Red blood cell transketolase stimulation effect (%)	>15	>15	>15	>15
Vitamin B_{12}				
Serum vitamin B_{12} (pg/mL)	≥200	≥200	≥200	≥200
Absorption test	Excretion of more than 7.5% of the orally ingested labeled vitamin B_{12}			
Iron				
Hematocrit (%)	31	33	36	36
Hemoglobin (g/dL)	12	12	13	13
Serum ferritin (ng/mL)	>10	>10	>10	>10
Serum iron (μg/dL)	>30	>40	>50	>60
Serum total iron-binding capacity (μg/dL)	350-400	350-400	350-400	350-400
Serum transferrin saturation (%)	>12	>12	>15	>16
Serum transferrin (mg/dL)	170-250	170-250	170-250	170-250
Erythrocyte protoporphyrin (μg/dL red blood cells)	<80	<75	<70	<70
Zinc				
Serum zinc (μg/dL)	80-120	80-120	80-120	80-120
Erythrocyte zinc	Erythrocytes contain approximately 10 times more zinc than does plasma			

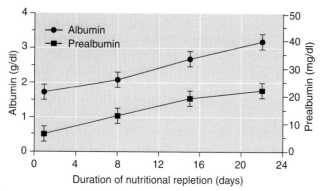

Figure 86-8. Response of serum albumin and prealbumin to refeeding in malnourished children. Data from Helms et al. (1986)[50] and Ingenbleek Y, De Visscher M, De Nayer P. Measurement of prealbumin as index of protein-calorie malnutrition. Lancet 1972; 2:106-109.

iron deficiency anemia. Serum ferritin is the most sensitive measure of the adequacy of body iron stores, but may be falsely elevated with increased inflammatory activity. Depressed serum folate levels may be the consequences of drug-nutrient interactions (e.g., sulfasalazine) or diffuse inflammation of the gastrointestinal tract. Low serum vitamin B_{12} levels occur in response to localized disease of the terminal ileum. Potassium and phosphorus are labile serum minerals that should be monitored carefully early in the course of nutritional rehabilitation of children with undernutrition. Serum potassium and phosphorus levels may decline rapidly during the early refeeding period (refeeding syndrome) because of intracellular ion shifts and can lead to unwanted complications such as cardiac arrhythmias. Transthyretin, a rapidly turning-over protein with a half-life of 2 days, is a good predictor of the adequacy of the diet and serves to corroborate the details of the diet history obtained from the parent. If dietary intakes have been poor, serum transthyretin levels fall rapidly.[50] If adequate refeeding has been instituted, serum transthyretin levels will rise to low normal levels within 10 days after initiating nutritional therapy, whereas serum albumin, a slowly turning-over protein, may not be restored to normal levels for at least 3 weeks (Figure 86-8).[50] On the other hand, the serum albumin level serves as a good predictor of gastrointestinal tolerance to enteral feedings,[51] with the likelihood that higher protein and energy intakes can be provided when serum albumin levels are greater than 30 g/L. Serum albumin also is a good predictor of morbidity and mortality; when serum albumin levels fall below 10 to 15 g/L, the mortality rate of undernourished children approximates 40%.[52]

The assessment of specific nutrient deficiencies may be necessary in gastrointestinal diseases in which malabsorption or inflammation is a prominent feature of the clinical course. Magnesium or zinc deficiencies may be found in chronic diarrheal illnesses. Fat-soluble vitamin (A, D, E, K) levels should be monitored at 6-month to yearly intervals in children with fat malabsorption disorders of the gastrointestinal tract. Low serum vitamin A, E, and 25-hydroxyvitamin D levels or a prolonged prothrombin time indicate the need for supplemental therapy. Serum folate and vitamin B_{12} levels should be monitored at similar time intervals in gastrointestinal disorders associated with inflammatory processes of the terminal ileum. Although

water-soluble vitamin deficiencies have been described, the subclinical abnormalities that occur in children with chronic gastrointestinal diseases remain difficult to diagnose and are of questionable value. Elevated serum cholesterol and triglyceride levels, impaired glucose tolerance, increased insulin levels, and altered liver function tests may occur in conjunction with overweight.

SUMMARY

Nutritional assessment is an essential component of the evaluation of children with gastrointestinal diseases because their clinical course frequently is complicated by undernutrition, growth failure, overweight, and micronutrient deficiencies. Although a complete nutritional assessment includes a review of the diet history, physical examination, growth and anthropometric measurements, and selected laboratory testing, accurate height and weight measurements and their transformation to relative indices of undernutrition or overnutrition serve as the mainstay of the nutritional assessment of the child with gastrointestinal disorders. The maintenance of a favorable nutritional status is essential to minimize disease-associated morbidity and maximize the child's quality of life.

ACKNOWLEDGMENTS

The authors thank V. Moore for secretarial support and A. Gillum for illustrations. This chapter is a publication of the USDA/ARS Children's Nutrition Research Center, Department of pediatrics, Baylor College of Medicine, Houston, TX, and has been funded in part with federal funds from the U.S. Department of Agriculture, Agricultural Research Service, under Cooperative Agreement Number 58-6250-1-003. The contents of herein do not necessarily reflect the views or policies of the U.S. Department of Agriculture, nor does mention of trade names, commercial products, or organizations imply endorsement by the U.S. government.

REFERENCES

12. Fernandez JR, Redden DT, Pietrobelli A, et al. Waist circumference percentiles in nationally representative samples of African-American, European, and Mexican-American children and adolescents. J Pediatr 2004;145: 439–444.

34. Institute of Medicine. Dietary Reference Intakes Charts. Available at http://www.iom.edu/Object.File/Master/21/372/0.pdf (accessed on September 1, 2009).

35. Mehta NM, Compher C. ASPEN Board of Directors. ASPEN Clinical Guidelines: nutrition support of the critically ill child. J Parenter Enteral Nutr 2009;33:260–276.

36. United States Department of Health and Human Services and United States Department of Agriculture. Dietary Guidelines for Americans 2005. Available at http://www.healthierus.gov/dietarygidelines (accessed on September 1, 2009).

38. United States Department of Agriculture. Food Guide Pyramid. Available at http://www.mypyramid.gov (accessed on September 1, 2009).

42. Dietz WH, Story M, Leviton LC, editors. Issues and implications of screening, surveillance, and reporting of children's body mass index. Pediatrics 2009;124(Suppl. 1):S1–S101.

See expertconsult.com for a complete list of references and the review questions for this chapter.

TUBES FOR ENTERIC ACCESS 87

Donald E. George • Maryanne L. Dokler

There are a multitude of tubes available to allow access to the gastrointestinal tract, but only two reasons for using them: to remove or add contents. Decompression with suction is required when there is obstruction, ileus, or pernicious vomiting. Nasogastric tubes also are used to remove stomach contents after ingestion of a toxic substance or to examine the contents, for example, gastric aspirate for blood. These tubes are generally larger in diameter and stiffer, and they do not collapse when suction is applied. Tubes suitable for aspiration of gastric contents may have a second lumen for venting. Continuous suction may be applied, and the venting lumen will prevent suction of mucosa into the lumen of the tube. If the tube has a single lumen, intermittent suction is used to prevent aspiration of gastric mucosa into the tube. Tubes also may be used to introduce content, usually nutrients or medications, into the gastrointestinal tract. There are numerous tubes made with a myriad of differences, all based on the desired route and use. Of greatest interest are the tubes for feeding.

Ideally all patients receive nutrition by mouth. However, when a child is unable to eat normally or when oral intake fails to meet nutritional needs for any reason, alternative modes of nutrient delivery are considered. When gut failure is present, intravenous routes are used. Conversely, it is axiomatic that "if the gut works, use it." Enteral feedings by tube have multiple advantages in maintaining gut function, promoting mucosal integrity and reducing infection.[1] There are clear advantages in terms of cost and ease of use. However, it should not be assumed that enteral nutrition is safer than parenteral nutrition in all patients.[2-4]

The ancient Egyptians used nutrient enemas. Silver, leather, and rubber tubes placed in the stomach were used in the 17th and 18th centuries.[5] Use of tubes for gavage feeding of pediatric patients was first described in the late 1800s. Over the past two decades a multitude of formulas, supplements, tubes, and other enteral access devices have been developed to allow delivery of enteral nutrition to neonates, infants, and children.[6] Many different techniques have been described, all with particular indications, advantages, and disadvantages.

EVALUATION

The decision to use an enteric tube requires a thoughtful analysis of the clinical situation, nutritional needs, and prognosis (Figure 87-1). The indications, risks, potential benefits, and possible alternatives should be reviewed for each patient. Several parameters should be assessed including nutritional status, etiology, and prognosis of the underlying disease and respiratory status. All patients should have an evaluation to document ability to protect the airway. Other factors to be considered include size of the patient, medical condition, surgical history,

presence of gastroesophageal reflux disease, and potential risk of aspiration. The probable duration of treatment and proposed type of feed should also be considered. Attention must be paid to the child's developmental abilities, social situation, and growth potential (Table 87-1). The evaluation is enhanced when a team of professionals is available to assess the child. The team may include oromotor specialists, dietitians, nurses, and social workers as well as gastroenterologists, surgeons, and the child's primary doctor. If the tube feedings are to be relatively short term and take place while the child is in the hospital, the issues are often straightforward. If tube feedings are to be longer in duration and used at home or an alternative site, the issues may be more complex. It is crucial to include the parents (and the patient, if appropriate) in the decision process.[7]

In pediatrics, the provision of enteral feedings is often required because of an inability to swallow or progressive dysphagia. Some common indications and contraindications are noted in Tables 87-2 and 87-3, respectively. Patients with neurologic and neuromuscular disorders, head and neck malignancy, major trauma, or congenital anomalies often have normal gastrointestinal tracts, but are unable to take adequate feeds orally.[8] Supplemental enteral feeding may also be needed when the patient is unable to consume adequate nutrition orally because of illness or choice. Gastrostomy tube feeds provide a means of delivering continuous feedings or unpalatable diets, which may be needed in a wide variety of disorders including cystic fibrosis,[9] short bowel syndrome, severe gastrointestinal allergy, metabolic disorders, anorexia associated with malignancy,[10] chronic diarrhea, intestinal hypomotility, chronic renal failure, intestinal lymphangiomatosis, Crohn's disease,[11,12] chronic cholestasis,[13] or congenital heart disease.[14] Feedings by tube pose risks to the child (Table 87-4), and the potential benefits of nutrition must be evaluated in each patient. Careful patient selection and evaluation will minimize complications.

Selection of enteral tubes is guided by patient comfort and tube performance. Multiple tubes are available, and the choice is often influenced by product availability and cost. Tubes vary by composition, inner and outer diameter, presence or absence of weighted tip, tip size and shape, and location and number of access ports and egress ports. Some tubes have a stylet to aid insertion (Figures 87-2 and 87-3). Feeding tubes may be placed into the stomach or advanced beyond the pylorus. Transpyloric feeds are suggested when there is vomiting, gastroparesis, or a risk of aspiration.

The anticipated duration of need for the tube is another consideration in selecting the route and type of enteral tube (Table 87-5). Tubes can be divided arbitrarily into those best suited for short-term and those for long-term use. For short-term feedings, tubes are most often passed through the nose into the gastrointestinal tract. In special situations, orally placed tubes are

958 PEDIATRIC GASTROINTESTINAL AND LIVER DISEASE

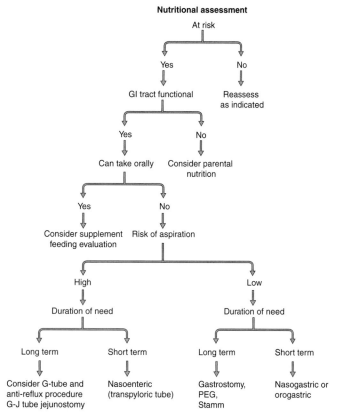

Figure 87-1. Algorithm for enteric feeding.

TABLE 87-1. Considerations in Enteral Feeding

Underlying condition and reason for feeding
Comorbidities (e.g., craniofacial defects, vomiting, aspiration, cardiac defects)
Age and size of patient
Nutritional needs and volume of feeding
Ease of administration and location of care (home, hospital)
Projected duration of support (for how long will it be needed?)
Patient activity, cooperation, and comfort
Tube composition (polyvinyl chloride, polyurethane, Silastic)
Tube length, diameter, style, weighted tip, end or side port

TABLE 87-2. Indications for Enteral Feeds

Condition	Indication
Dysphagia	
Anatomic	ENT abnormalities
	Pierre-Robin sequence
	Cleft lip and/or cleft palate
Neurologic	Head trauma, cerebral palsy
	Hypoxic encephalopathy
Esophageal disease	Atresia, stricture
	Caustic ingestion
	Eosinophilic esophagitis (elemental diet)
Failure to grow	Cholestasis, chronic liver disease
	AIDS, chronic renal failure
	Food refusal, chronic diarrhea, malignancy
	Congenital heart disease
	Cystic fibrosis, bronchopulmonary dysphasia
Bowel disease	Short bowel syndrome, intestinal dysmotility
	Inflammatory bowel disease, eosinophilic gastroenteritis,
	Malabsorption
Inability to eat for other reasons	Trauma, burns, prematurity, chemotherapy, bone marrow transplant
Special nutrient needs	Inborn errors of metabolism

AIDS, acquired immunodeficiency syndrome; ENT, ear, nose, and throat.

TABLE 87-3. Relative Contraindications to Enteral Feeds

Ileus
Bowel obstruction
Peritonitis or intra-abdominal sepsis
Necrotizing pancreatitis
High-output gastrointestinal fistulas

TABLE 87-4. Complications of Tube Feedings

Mechanical
  Tracheobronchial intubation
  Erosive tissue damage
  Tube occlusion
Metabolic
  Increased blood glucose level
  Electrolyte abnormality
  Refeeding syndrome
Pulmonary
  Aspiration
  Cough
Gastrointestinal
  Nausea and vomiting
  Diarrhea
  Abdominal pain
  Bowel necrosis

also used. They are readily available and do not require surgery to place them. They are relatively easy to place, less invasive, and less costly than surgically placed tubes. However, they are easily displaced and must be positioned and monitored carefully.[15,16] If long-term use is anticipated – percutaneous endoscopic gastrostomy (PEG), gastrostomy, jejunostomy, and so on – a more permanent enterostomal tube is preferred. These are generally placed through the skin into the desired area of the gastrointestinal tract; a surgical procedure is required for placement. There is no consensus as to what is long term versus short term, although most agree that less than 4 weeks is short term and more than 8 to 12 weeks long term.[1,17,18]

CONSIDERATIONS FOR SHORT-TERM ACCESS

The placement of a soft, small-diameter tube is the simplest technique for tube feeding. The nasogastric route is generally the preferred route. Orogastric tubes are sometimes used in preterm infants, though there is little evidence of advantage.[64] Gastric feeding allows normal mixing of nutrients with bile and pancreatic secretions and maintains the physiologic digestive process. Feeding into the stomach allows bolus feedings and the use of hypertonic formulas. In patients with a high risk of aspiration or gastroparesis, or after some gastric surgical procedures, postpyloric feeding is indicated.

The size of the tube influences both performance and tolerability. Tube length is determined by the size of the patient and whether it is positioned in the stomach, duodenum, or jejunum. Tube diameter is measured in French (1 Fr = 0.33 mm), and both inner and outer diameters are important. Large-bore tubes are used for decompression or suction. For patient comfort, the smallest diameter tube that allows flow of formula is used for feeding. Smaller-diameter tubes, 5 to 8 Fr, can be used with most commercially available formulas. Larger-diameter tubes may be needed for more viscous formulas or those containing

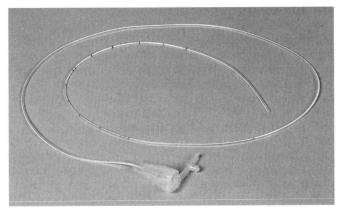

Figure 87-2. Typical "fine-bore" nasoenteric tube without stylus. The single-lumen marking helps to assess placement.

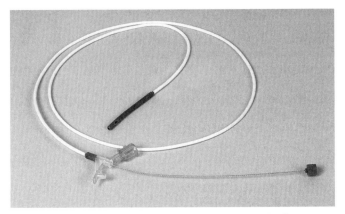

Figure 87-3. Nasoenteric tube with stylet and weighted tip.

fiber. Smaller-diameter tubes can easily be misplaced into the tracheobronchial tree, especially in a patient who is obtunded or has a poor gag or cough reflex; therefore, it is important to ensure correct placement. Multiple techniques are suggested to ensure correct positioning of these tubes, such a measuring pH or bile content of aspirated material, auscultation of injected air, and measurement of tube length. All have been shown to somewhat inaccurate, and confirmation of position by x-ray remains the most accurate method to confirm placement.[63] Smaller-diameter tubes may decrease the risk of reflux because of lower esophageal sphincter compromise or reduced gagging.[19-21] In addition, smaller and softer tubes are less likely to affect swallowing.

Smaller-diameter tubes have a greater risk of clogging. Tube occlusion can be treated by using a small-volume (10 mL) syringe to flush warm water through the tube. Powdered pancreatic enzymes (not enteric-coated beads) dissolved in water have also been used. Of note, the pressure that can be generated is sufficient to rupture the tube. There are commercial products available that either dissolve or mechanically remove the obstruction.[22]

The most commonly available tubes are made of polyvinyl chloride (PVC), polyurethane, or silicone polymers (Table 87-6). PVC is rather firm and becomes less flexible and more brittle with exposure to gastric acid. The walls are not easily compressed or collapsed, and gastric content can be easily aspirated. PVC tubes are not recommended for tube feedings and are most often used for gastric decompression and drainage. Straight drainage tubes have a single lumen and multiple distal ports. They can be left open for venting or attached to intermittent suction. "Sump type" (Figure 87-4) tubes are used specifically for decompression and have a second lumen that allows air in during suction and thus prevents the gastric mucosa from being pulled into the tube ports. They are best used with continuous suction.

Polyurethane does not stiffen or discolor and permits a thinner wall construction. Polyurethane tubes can be used for

TABLE 87-5. **Enteral Feeding Routes**

	Indications	Benefits	Considerations
Orogastric	Used mainly in premature infants or patients with no nasal access	Relatively inexpensive, easy to place, generally available	Risk of pulmonary aspiration due to misplacement or GER. Impaired swallowing
Nasogastric	Short-term feedings in patients without vomiting or failure to protect airway	As for orogastric	Visible on face; irritation to nares, sinusitis. May interfere with oromotor development. Impairs patient mobility
Nasoenteric (beyond pylorus)	Useful when aspiration, GER, and/or gastroparesis are present. Short-term feedings	Reduces vomiting and aspiration risk. NJ feed may allow earlier feeds in pancreatitis or early after surgery	Visible on face. Requires continuous rather than bolus feeds. Requires a pump. Placement more cumbersome and time consuming. Frequently dislodged. Risk of perforation or necrosis of intestine
Gastrostomy (Stamm or PEG)	Useful for long-term feedings	Less likely to dislodge. Greater patient comfort and mobility. No tube visible during day	Relatively more expensive and requires a procedure for placement. Stoma care needed. Risk of pulmonary aspiration or GER; stomal infection; scar
G-J	Placed when there is a high risk of aspiration	Allow drainage of stomach and enteral feeds. Useful when stomach function is impaired	May dislodge or migrate to stomach. Small-bore tubes clog. Requires monitoring and continuous infusion. Requires fluoroscopic or endoscopic placement. Risk of perforation
Jejunostomy	Useful for long-term feeds	Allows drainage of stomach and enteral feeds. Useful when stomach function is impaired. Usually stable and less likely to dislodge	May dislodge or migrate to stomach. Small-bore tubes clog. Requires monitoring and continuous infusion. Requires fluoroscopic or endoscopic placement. Increased risk of perforation. Requires surgery

GER, gastroesophageal reflux; G-J, gastrojejunostomy; NJ, nasojejunal; PEG, percutaneous endoscopic gastrostomy.

TABLE 87-6. Tube Composition

Material	Comments
Polyvinyl chloride	Stiff, and gets stiffer with long-term placement. Useful for aspiration of stomach
Polyurethane	Thinner walled. Large internal diameter. Can aspirate without collapsing the tube
Silicone	Very flexible and soft. Collapses with suction. Often requires a stylet for positioning

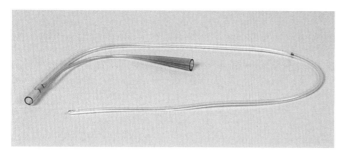

Figure 87-4. Tube for nasogastric suction. Note the thick wall and "sump" port.

TABLE 87-7. Complications of Gastrostomy Placement

		Early	Late
Major complications		Pneumoperitoneum, Bleeding, Enteroenteric fistula, External migration, Perforation, Aspiration, Buried or extruded tube, Gastric ulceration	Enteroenteric fistulas, Enterocutaneous fistula, Tube migration, Volvulus, gastric ulceration, Intestinal obstruction, Cutaneous necrosis
Minor complications		Stomal infection, Neuralgia, Diarrhea, Bleeding	Stomal infection, Granulation tissue, Displacement, leakage, Tube obstruction, Gastric prolapse

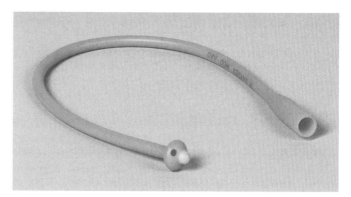

Figure 87-5. Gastrostomy tube with mushroom tip. These tubes are placed at operation.

aspiration without collapsing. Silicone or silicone elastomer tubes are very soft and generally collapse when suction is used. They frequently require a stylet to facilitate placement.

Many nasoenteric tubes have weights on the distal tip (see Figure 87-3). They come in several sizes, styles, and materials. Weighted tips are thought to be advantageous when advancing a tube past the pylorus, but similar rates of passage are achieved using unweighted tubes.[23] Further, it is not clear whether weighted tubes stay in place longer than unweighted tubes.[24]

Unless a nasogastric or nasoenteric feeding tube has been placed under direct vision endoscopically or with fluoroscopic guidance, there is a risk of misplacement into the bronchial tree. This is especially important when using fine-bore tubes for feeding. Patients who are obtunded or in whom the gag reflex is inadequate are at greater risk for both aspiration and tube misplacement. Neonates and very young patients are at particular risk.[60] Tip position cannot be ensured by auscultation of air injected through the tube. Radiographic confirmation of distal tip placement must be obtained before initiating feedings because of the severe consequences of aspiration or feeding into the lungs. Checking the pH of aspirate has been recommended to confirm tube position between feedings,[15] but radiography remains the most accurate method.[14] If available, positioning may be both facilitated and monitored with an electromagnetic guidance device.[61]

CONSIDERATIONS FOR LONG-TERM ACCESS

Tubes suitable for short-term use are usually not used for long-term access because of patient comfort, complications (e.g., sinusitis), malposition, or mechanical failure. Further, they require careful monitoring because of the risk of inadvertent displacement[63] and need to be replaced frequently. Percutaneous enteral access confers many advantages including stability, patient acceptance, and ease of care. Many techniques for placement of more stable and longer-lasting tubes are available:

laparotomy, laparoscopy, endoscopy, radiography, or any combination. All require particular skills and experience to accomplish safely, and expertise and facilities for each may not be available in all institutions. Gastrostomy and jejunostomy are most often done by surgeons, usually at the time of laparotomy for another reason. Endoscopic, laparoscopic, and radiologic techniques are considered less invasive, although morbidity and complication rates are similar[25, 26] (Table 87-7).

Gastrostomy, the operative creation of a fistulous tract between the stomach and the abdominal surface, is a common way of providing enteral access for patients. The Stamm gastrostomy is the most common surgical gastrostomy. A tube is inserted through the abdominal wall into the stomach and secured to the wall of the stomach with a purse-string suture. Many types of catheter can be used, including dePezzar, Melecot, and Foley catheters. All have a balloon or mushroom tip to hold the stomach to the anterior abdominal wall (Figure 87-5). It is important that the tube be anchored to the abdominal wall (external bolster) to prevent it from migrating into the small bowel and causing obstruction. Latex catheters erode with prolonged exposure to gastric juices; silicone or PVC catheters last longer. Gastrostomy tubes can be used for feeding or decompression.[27]

The percutaneous endoscopic gastrostomy was developed by Gauderer and Ponsky utilizing the idea of sutureless approximation of the stomach to the abdominal wall with a catheter.[28] Over time, adhesions develop between the stomach and the peritoneum around the tract of the catheter. PEG has been used extensively in both adults and children to provide long-term enteral nutrition in a wide variety of clinical conditions. Currently more than 200,000 PEGs are performed in the United States annually,[29] and approximately 5000 of these procedures are done in children. PEGs are now widely available and have become a commonly used method of enteral access. Indeed, PEGs now represent the most utilized technique for long-term enteral access.

A PEG may be used for feeding, decompression, combined feeding and decompression, gastric access for esophageal dilation or medication administration, management of gastric volvulus, and multiple portals for intragastric surgical interventions.[27]

Contraindications to the placement of a PEG include the inability to perform upper endoscopy safely and to bring the anterior gastric wall in apposition to the abdominal wall. The inability to juxtapose the anterior gastric and abdominal walls should be considered in patients with ascites, hepatomegaly, or obesity. Failure to identify transabdominal illumination or to visualize the indentation of the finger on the stomach wall should suggest this problem. A PEG should not be used for nutrition when obstruction of the gastrointestinal tract is present, although it may be used for decompression in some circumstances. The presence of gastric varices, although not an absolute contraindication, may make placement of any gastrostomy device more concerning. Depending on severity, relative contraindications to PEG placement include coagulopathy, inflammatory or infiltrative disease of the gastric or abdominal walls, and intra-abdominal infection. Young age and low weight are not contraindications to PEG.[28,30]

At times the transverse colon may lie across the desired placement site. Concomitant fluoroscopy at the time of the PEG may identify the transverse colon, facilitating placement.

Except for gastric resection, prior abdominal surgical procedures are not an absolute contraindication to PEG placement.[31] Placement could be more difficult because of disruption of the normal anatomy by adhesions, and careful attention to preoperative contrast studies and intraoperative technique is important. Morbidity and types of complication following PEG are similar in previously operated and nonoperated patients.[32] Also, these complication may also occur after any type of gastrostomy.[58] Elective placement of a PEG in patients with existing ventriculoperitoneal shunts has been accepted by neurosurgeons, although simultaneous placement of a shunt and PEG should be avoided.[33] PEG is not associated with a higher risk of infection than open gastrostomy and may be associated with less morbidity. Careful attention should be paid to infection, and an intraoperative antibiotic is recommended (see later discussion). Common alternatives to PEG are nasogastric or orogastric feeds, open gastrostomy, gastrostomy with antireflux procedure, and percutaneous endoscopic or open jejunostomy.

Several techniques have been described for the placement of a PEG. They share several basic elements (Table 87-8), and the published outcomes are similar.[34,35]

Laparoscopic guided placement of a gastrostomy tube is also an accepted method of providing enteral access. The laparoscopic approach is advantageous in children with craniofacial anomalies, esophageal abnormalities, distorted gastric anatomy, or prior abdominal surgery. It can be done as an isolated procedure or in conjunction with another abdominal procedure.[55]

Nonendoscopic, radiologically controlled insertion of a gastrostomy tube has been described in adults but has not been

TABLE 87-8. **Basic Elements of PEG Placement Common to All Techniques**

Adequate gastric insufflation to bring gastric wall in apposition to abdominal wall
Placement of cannula into stomach
Passage of guidewire
Placement of tube/button
Verification of position
Perioperative antibiotic

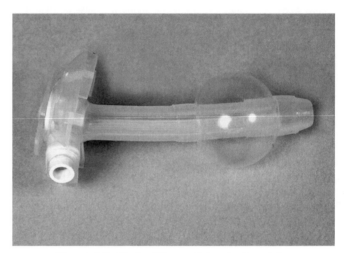

Figure 87-6. Skin-level (low profile) gastrostomy tube.

widely adopted in children, because of the risk of pushing the stomach away from the abdominal wall and the small size of the catheters utilized. Gastrostomies can also be placed percutaneously utilizing a "push" technique under laparoscopic guidance in conjunction with other abdominal procedures. A variety of percutaneous gastrostomy tubes are available. The original procedure utilized a dePezzer catheter threaded onto a tapered Medicut sheath. Similar tubes are now available made of Silastic and in a variety of sizes.

Because the tubes pass through the mouth, PEG procedures carry a substantial risk of infection, generally stomal infections with either oropharyngeal or cutaneous bacteria; in addition, bacteremia may occur. Systemic antimicrobial prophylaxis at time of PEG placement reduces the incidence of peristomal infections.[57] Therefore, a single preoperative or postoperative dose of antibiotic is recommended to minimize the incidence of infection in uncomplicated procedures.[36,37] Cefazolin or cefotaxime is often used. Prophylaxis for subacute bacterial endocarditis, recommended by the American Heart Association, is utilized for patients at risk owing to certain types of congenital heart disease or implanted vascular devices. The duration of antibiotic therapy has not yet been defined; patients may receive one to several doses. Antibiotics are continued for a minimum of 24 hours for patients with ventriculoperitoneal shunts.

In 1982, the gastrostomy button was introduced. This is a skin-level device with a one-way valve at the gastric opening of the shaft to prevent reflux of gastric contents externally (Figure 87-6). Some 2 to 3 months after placing a long gastrostomy tube percutaneously, the tube can be removed and replaced with a gastrostomy button. The low-profile devices are preferred by many patients and their parents because they are less obtrusive. They are not as effective for decompression. Some centers use

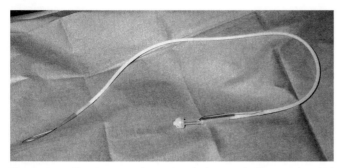

Figure 87-7. The "one-step button" technique is similar to other PEG techniques.

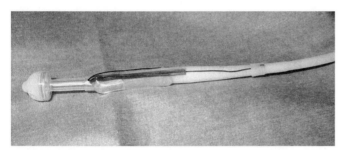

Figure 87-8. "One-step button". The button is released from the rest of the tube.

the one-step button (Figures 87-7 and 87-8).[38] Complications of catheter removal and replacement are reduced. The one-step button can be placed as the initial gastric tube, allowing families to use a low-profile device immediately for feedings.[27,39] This obviates the need to change the long tube for a button at a later date, and training caregivers and obtaining supplies is somewhat easier. The PEG buttons are less likely to become dislodged, and rates of infection are not different. [62] Use of a long gastrostomy tube is reserved for very small infants (less than 3 kg) or for very large patients where a low-profile device of adequate length is not available. The low-profile gastrostomy device has additional advantages. Because it is skin level, inadvertent displacement is less likely. The shorter shaft of the tube results in less clogging from feeds and less tube movement, which minimizes leakage around the tube. Tube migration with potential for obstruction or perforation, seen with the use of Foley catheters as gastrostomy tubes, rarely occurs. As all the gastrostomy buttons are made with silicone rubber, there is often less granulation tissue.

GASTROESOPHAGEAL REFLUX AND TUBES

Conditions for which feeding tubes are considered in children are frequently associated with a high rate of gastroesophageal reflux (GER). This can be manifested as recurrent vomiting, malnutrition, esophagitis, or recurrent aspiration pneumonia. Nasoenteric tubes are known to exacerbate GER.[19-21] Further, it is well accepted that Stamm-type open gastrostomy is associated with development of GER.[40,41] This finding has led many to propose antireflux surgery for all neurologically disabled children who need a feeding gastrostomy.[42] The recognition that antireflux surgery has both early and late complications (such as dumping syndrome, retching, aerophagia, and gas bloat), and a significant rate of recurrence of GER, has caused

a rethinking of this approach.[43,44] No single preoperative study can reliably identify all the children who need an antireflux procedure.

The unmasking of GER may be less pronounced after PEG compared with operative gastrostomy. However, contradictory data exist about the effect of PEG on GER and the need for antireflux procedures.[45-47] The development or worsening of GER, or the need for subsequent conversion to an antireflux procedure, percutaneous gastrojejunostomy (PEJ), or jejunostomy is considered a complication of a PEG. Much attention has been paid to the role of PEG placement in the child with GER, and the possibility that the PEG procedure might promote reflux. Several factors may contribute to worsening of reflux, including volume of feeding, method of feeding (continuous or bolus), and type of formula. Malnutrition has a deleterious effect on GER, and nutritional rehabilitation may lessen vomiting attributed to GER.[48]

It is recommended that all children be evaluated clinically to determine the presence of GER and whether the GER can be controlled medically. If GER is absent or can be controlled by medical treatment, including proton pump inhibitors and/or prokinetic agents, PEG should be performed. In the presence of severe GER, especially with impaired pulmonary function, or the inability to tolerate nasogastric feeds, an antireflux procedure with gastrostomy, jejunostomy, or gastrojejunostomy (G-J tube) may be appropriate. As a previous PEG does not make subsequent fundoplication more risky, it seems reasonable to suggest a trial of feedings via PEG in patients with mild symptoms or symptoms controlled by medication before embarking on a more extensive procedure.[49,50] Although both are beneficial, neither fundoplication nor gastrojejunal feeding completely protect against aspiration, and the rates of aspiration with each are similar.[59]

Feedings into the jejunum are used to reduce the risk of aspiration, or in patients with severe GER or those with a nonfunctioning stomach. Even though the risk of aspiration is reduced with jejunal feedings when compared to gastric feedings, it is important to note that aspiration is not completely avoidable. For temporary transpyloric feeds or in small infants, placement of a combined gastrostomy tube/jejunostomy tube (GT/JT) is appropriate. A low-profile GT/JT is available. If a jejunostomy tube is felt to be needed long term, surgical placement is most commonly done. Surgically placed jejunostomy tubes are somewhat more stable and require fewer adjustments than the combined GT/JT tubes.[56] Multiple techniques using surgery, laparoscopy, endoscopy, and radiology are available.[1,26] They are all operator dependent, and the choice is based on experience and expertise available within an institution.

Complications of jejunal feedings are related to the small bowel location. Jejunal tubes are difficult to anchor and prone to dislodgment. Gastrointestinal complaints are common including abdominal distention, pain and diarrhea. Bolus feeds cannot be used, and continuous feeds are often cumbersome. Small bowel ischemia and necrosis have been described.[26,51]

PEJ may be an alternative to surgery in selected cases (Figure 87-9). This involves the placement of a jejunal feeding tube through a previously created gastrostomy tube, most often using fluoroscopy or endoscopy. Several systems are available commercially. Experience with PEJ in children is limited.[52] The initial enthusiasm to convert PEG to PEJ has waned as high rates of dysfunction without elimination of aspiration have been. There seems to be a tendency for the jejunal arm to migrate

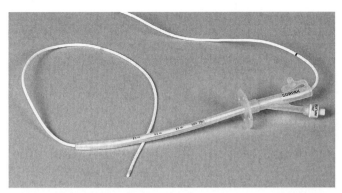

Figure 87-9. Gastrostomy tube with jejunal extender (PEJ). The smaller internal tube is placed into the jejunum either endoscopically or fluoroscopically through the gastrostomy.

back into the stomach, and careful monitoring is essential. Further, these tubes are of small diameter and tend to clog.[53] Direct placement of a PEJ tube into the jejunum is described in adults, but has not been studied in children. The technique is similar to PEG, and the need for careful transillumination and visualization of the fingertip indentation on the wall of the intestine is emphasized.

SUMMARY

A wide variety of tubes are available to allow intubation of the gastrointestinal tract. These can be used for decompression (suction) or for feeding. Newer techniques of endoscopic tube placement have reduced the need for surgery and improved tolerance in many patients. They allow the delivery of enteral nutrition; however, the contribution of GER to morbidity and mortality remains considerable. Careful patient selection and scrupulous attention to technique can minimize complications and improve outcomes.

REFERENCES

20. Peter CS, Beichers C, Bohwhorst B, et al. Influence of nasogastric tubes on gastroesophageal reflux in preterm infants: a multiple intraluminal impedence study. J Pediatr 2002;141:277–279.
29. Gauderer MW. Percutaneous endoscopic gastrostomy – 20 years later: a historical perspective. J Pediatr Surg 2001;36:217–219.
36. American Society for Gastrointestinal Endoscopy Standards of Practice Committee. Antibiotic prophylaxis for gastrointestinal endoscopy. Gastrointest Endosc 2008;67:791–798.
57. Lipp A, Lusardi G. Systemic antimicrobial prophylaxis for percutaneous endoscopic gastrostomy. Cochrane Database of Systematic Reviews 2006; Issue 4 Art No. CD005571 DOI:10.1002/14651858 CD005571.pub2.
59. Srivastava R, Downey EC, O'Gorman M, et al. Impact of fundoplication versus gastrojejunal feeding tubes on mortality and in preventing aspiration pneumonia in young children with neurologic impairment who have gastroesophageal reflux disease. Pediatrics 2009;123:338–345.

See expertconsult.com for a complete list of references and the review questions for this chapter.

88 PARENTERAL NUTRITION

Maria R. Mascarenhas • Elizabeth C. Wallace

Parenteral nutrition (PN) is the intravenous administration of nutrients necessary for the maintenance of life. The nutrient components of PN include dextrose, amino acids, fat, electrolytes, multivitamins, and trace elements. Clinicians caring for infants and children should pay close attention to the changing nutrient requirements with age; specialized needs of children; vascular access; and the sometimes limited ability of infants, children, and the critically ill to handle large amounts of fluid, protein, fat, and carbohydrates.[1] In the 1960s, Dudrick and Wilmore showed that beagle puppies and subsequently an infant could be successfully nourished with the use of PN solutions and central venous access.[1,2] Since that time, research has promoted substantial advancement in the fields of intravenous access and PN solution components, as well as an improved understanding of the needs of patients with various illnesses to provide individualized care across the spectrum of life. Normal growth and development have been shown in patients exclusively fed by PN.

INDICATIONS

PN may be used as primary, adjunctive, or supportive therapy. The enteral route is the preferred choice when the clinician is deciding how to provide nourishment for any patient. It is only when a patient cannot receive adequate nutrition enterally for an extended period of time that the parenteral route should be used. When the patient's tolerance for enteral feeds improves, every attempt should be made to start and advance the delivery of enteral nutrition. PN is therefore used in patients who cannot be fed enterally for 5 or more days and should be used to support the patient until recovery from the underlying condition has occurred. In the very low-birth-weight (VLBW) or malnourished infant with limited nutritional reserves, PN should begin no later than the third day of life, but preferably earlier.[3] In some neonatal intensive care units, a protein- and glucose-containing solution is started on the first day of life. Appropriate indications for initiating PN include compromised gut integrity (resection, high-output fistulas, complete obstruction, paralytic ileus, ischemia), malabsorption, severe short bowel syndrome, intractable vomiting or diarrhea, or inability to obtain enteral access (Table 88-1). PN is especially important in the patient with preexisting malnutrition or with a chronic disease. It may be used to supplement enteral intake in patients who have increased needs (e.g., patients with chronic diarrhea, malabsorption, short bowel syndrome, or cystic fibrosis) or those who are unable to tolerate adequate enteral feeds to support themselves nutritionally. Most patients with 25 cm of small bowel and an ileocecal valve will be able to ultimately tolerate enteral feeds and be able to discontinue PN.[2] The use of supplemental PN should also be considered when slow advancement of enteral feeds is anticipated. In addition to a supportive role, PN may be used to treat an underlying condition (e.g., chylothorax).

ROUTE OF ADMINISTRATION

Parenteral nutrition can be administered via a central or peripheral venous route depending on the available access and the composition of the PN solution. Peripheral PN is generally used for patients whose anticipated period of inadequate enteral feedings is less than 1 week and who have normal fluid requirements.[4] It is often difficult to maintain peripheral access for longer than 1 to 2 weeks or to deliver adequate calories with solutions containing 10% or 12.5% dextrose. When hyperosmolar solutions with dextrose concentrations higher than 12.5% are administered through a peripheral intravenous line, there is a risk of phlebitis and thrombosis. Though institution dependent, limiting the infusion of a peripheral solution to a maximum osmolarity of 850 to 1000 mmol is a typical standard of practice.[5] Solutions with high dextrose (more than 12.5% dextrose) and calcium concentrations may have increased risk for phlebitis. The concomitant administration of intravenous fat may help decrease phlebitis in a peripheral vein. Depending on the size of the vein, it may not be possible to infuse large volumes or run PN at a high rate.

The central venous route is used for the administration of large fluid volumes at high infusion rates, for hypertonic solutions, and for prolonged administration of PN solutions more than 4 to 6 weeks.[5,6] PN may be administered via a peripherally inserted central catheter (PICC), a tunneled central venous catheter (CVC, e.g., Broviac), or an implantable port (e.g., Port-a-Cath). It is recommended the tip of the catheter be placed at the junction of the superior vena cava and right atrium. The best place for a line associated with the least amount of complications is the right internal jugular vein with the tip of the catheter high in the superior vena cava.[5,6] This position, corresponding to the level of thoracic vertebra level-T6, is at the level of the right mainstem bronchus and the junction of the right atrium and superior vena cava. When femoral lines or umbilical venous catheters are used, the tip of the catheter should be placed above the level of the diaphragm in the inferior vena cava. Though these two specific catheters are adequate for central infusion, both have increased risk of infection due to the contamination at the exit site.[5] Malpositioned catheters, such as those at the level of the renal vessels and those in the liver, should not be used for PN administration because of the risk of thrombosis. It is not recommended that PN be administered via umbilical arterial catheters because of the risk of sepsis. The incidence of peripheral venous access and thrombosis has been well described.[7] Measures to prevent thrombosis of vessels include making sure the vessel is not traumatized during insertion of the catheter, using correct tip placement, avoiding

TABLE 88-1. Indications for Parenteral Nutrition

Primary	Gut failure, necrotizing enterocolitis, severe motility disorders, inability to obtain enteral access
Supportive	Postoperative patients, burns, liver failure, renal failure, severe viral gastroenteritis, oncology and bone marrow transplant recipients, inflammatory bowel disease, trauma
Supplemental	Nutritional failure, feeding intolerance

the subclavian and femoral veins, always using the smallest catheter possible, using the smallest vein possible, and using an appropriately sized catheter for the vein.[8] Other measures utilized to prevent thrombosis include administering PN into a larger vessel, using ultrasound guidance at the time of insertion, removing the CVC as soon as possible, treating CVC blockages early, preventing and treating all infections and venous occlusions, reusing previous access sites for CVC placement, and not placing the CVC into a fibrin sheath. In a patient with poor access, the following sites for placing a CVC may need to be considered: translumbar inferior vena cava, recannulation of the central vein, transhepatic intravenous catheter, use of collateral veins, azygous and hemi-azygous veins, intercostal veins, and putting the line directly into the right atrium. Long lines or PICC lines are threaded into the heart through a large peripheral vein like the antecubital fossa. The success of placement is dependent on the patency of the vein chosen, the presence of valves, and the experience of the person placing the line. PICC lines have been used for over 20 years and are now quite popular because there are few limitations regarding their use related to age, gender, or diagnosis. There is a low incidence of complications with PICC lines, less than 1% for infection, central vein thrombosis, and catheter malposition, as long as their use is limited to 6 to 8 weeks. In addition, significant cost savings are associated with the use of this type of catheter. Contraindications to the placement of PICC lines include dermatitis, cellulitis, burns at or near the insertion site, and previous ipsilateral venous thrombosis.

Patients receiving chronic PN benefit from the placement of a permanent CVC or tunneled silicone elastomer (Silastic) catheter (e.g., Broviac, Hickman and Groshong) and subcutaneous portacaths.[9-11] A surgeon or an interventional radiologist using general anesthesia or conscious sedation generally places these catheters. Tunneled catheters can be placed either via a cutdown or percutaneously and have a Dacron cuff located on the midportion of the catheter. This cuff stimulates the formation of dense fibrous adhesions, which anchor the catheter subcutaneously, to prevent dislodgment of the catheter. The cuff also acts as a barrier to bacteria migrating subcutaneously along the catheter surface. Sutures are needed to anchor the catheter at the exit site for several weeks after insertion to allow time for the formation of fibrous adhesions to the Dacron cuff.

Implantable ports are made of plastic or titanium with a compressed silicon disk designed for 1000 to 2000 insertions with a non-coring needle. They are inserted percutaneously into the jugular, subclavian, or cephalic vein and placed in a subcutaneous pocket over the upper chest wall. There are smaller ports available that are primarily used for arm placement and for children. These ports are generally used in situations in which the catheter is only periodically accessed. Patients at high risk for thrombosis of their catheter are those with cancer, those with infections, and those receiving chemotherapeutic agents or PN.

PN can also be delivered via peritoneal or hemodialysis catheters. Intradialytic PN is the administration of PN during dialysis and has been shown to be useful in those patients with end-stage renal disease who do not respond to oral nutritional intervention.[12] PN can also be administered to patients who are on extracorporeal membrane oxygenation (ECMO). The dextrose/amino acid solution is administered through the ECMO circuit and intravenous fat is given through a peripheral line to avoid occlusion of the ECMO circuit.[13]

PARENTERAL NUTRITION COMPONENTS AND REQUIREMENTS

Energy

A patient's enteral requirements are 5 to 10% higher than their parenteral requirements to account for the thermic effect of food and for the loss of some nutrients in the stool during the process of digestion and absorption. There are several ways to estimate energy requirements: the World Health Organization (WHO) equation, Dietary Reference Intakes (DRIs), and prediction equations such as the Schofield height/weight equation and those developed by Duro et al. and Pierro et al.[14-16] Demonstration of adequate weight gain in the absence of edema and normalization of certain nutritional markers (e.g., prealbumin) is the best way to determine if a patient's energy requirements have been accurately assessed. This response is sometimes hard to assess in the critically ill patient, in patients with edema or renal failure, or in those on corticosteroids. It is also unclear whether one should expect normal rates of growth in the critically ill patient or just provide enough energy to prevent catabolism. The reader is referred to an excellent discussion of about energy requirements in patients on PN.[17] Recent data documents the occurrence of under- or overfeeding in the critically ill population as the result of using predictive equations to determine energy needs.[18] Indirect calorimetry (IC) measures oxygen consumption and carbon dioxide production during respiratory gas exchange, providing the most accurate measurement of resting energy expenditure (REE). IC is increasingly available and is often helpful to determine the caloric requirements of patients who are nutritionally at risk such as infants and children with failure to thrive, those who are dependent on PN or enteral tube feeds, obese patients, and critically ill patients. It was previously thought that measurement of mechanically ventilated patients was not accurately calculated by IC; however, current literature supports the use of IC with this population to prevent energy imbalance.[18]

Infants and children have higher per-kilogram caloric requirements compared with adults, because of growth and development requirements.[19] For infants up to 1 year of age, a per-kilogram caloric requirement that decreases with age is used.[19] This is based on their energy requirements and the need for catch-up growth. We use the WHO equation for determining the needs of children older than 1 year of age.[20] This equation, which provides an estimate of REE, is based on data from several thousand children and has been found to be accurate in children older than 1 year of age. Total energy needs may then be determined by multiplying the REE by a factor determined by the severity of underlying disease, the activity level of the patient, and the need for catch-up growth (Tables 88-2 and 88-3).

The energy needs of obese patients are best determined by the Schofield height-weight equation.[21] Caloric needs and

TABLE 88-2. **Estimated Daily Resting Energy Expenditure (kcal)**[*]

Age (years)	Male	Female
1-3	60.9 wt−54	61.0 wt−51
3-10	22.7 wt+495	22.5 wt+499
10-18	17.5 wt+651	12.2 wt+746
18-30	15.3 wt+679	14.7 wt+496

Adapted from World Health Organization: Energy and protein requirements. Technical Report Series No. 734. Geneva: World Health Organization; 1985.[20]
[*]Estimated daily energy requirements = REE × disease activity/stress factor. wt, weight in kilograms.

TABLE 88-3. **Disease Activity/Stress Factors**[*]

1.1-1.3	Well-nourished child at rest with mild to moderate stress or after minor surgery
1.3-1.5	Normal active child with mild-to-moderate stress, inactive child with severe stress (trauma, cancer, extensive surgery), or malnourished child requiring catch-up growth or with severe stress
1.5-1.7	Active child requiring catch-up growth or with severe stress

[*]Estimated daily energy requirements = REE × disease activity/stress factor.

energy intake may be increased in a patient with head injury or sepsis. The paralyzed patient on a ventilator will have no physical activity and has lower energy needs. Often the "stressed" patient will be given additional calories, but it is not clear whether this practice should be endorsed. Various studies have shown that the increased demands of illness are often counterbalanced by decreased physical activity, which keeps total energy expenditure the same whether the patient is well or sick.[22] Although a major concern is to provide adequate energy to prevent catabolism, it is equally important to not overfeed the patient. Providing energy in excess increases the risk of complications including hyperglycemia, azotemia, immunosuppression, and hepatic steatosis.[23] Some research in adults suggests the approach of permissive underfeeding to prevent complications from overfeeding in the obese population. A large body of evidence supports the use of a reduced energy PN formulation to provide similar nitrogen balance as a eucaloric regimen, without the negative effects just noted. Research in the pediatric population will be important to determine if hypocaloric feeding regimens can maintain adequate nitrogen balance while promoting growth.

It is necessary to provide not only calories but also protein in adequate amounts so the patient is in positive nitrogen balance; otherwise the patient will utilize protein for energy.

Protein

The protein source in PN is provided by crystalline amino acids, which provides approximately 4 cal/g of protein.[24] Protein usually provides 10 to 20% of total PN calorie needs. Since the advent of these purer forms of amino acids, the incidence of hyperammonemia and metabolic acidosis has been rare. It has also been shown that nitrogen retention is better with amino acid formulations when compared with protein hydrolysates. There are a variety of protein solutions available for use in children and adults and in patients with hepatic disease, renal disease, and metabolic disease. An example of a protein solution used in a metabolic disorder is the parenteral protein solution

that has been designed for use in methylmalonic acidemia. In this instance, the amounts of certain amino acids can be dosed based on daily blood amino acid levels. The compositions of protein solutions for infants, including preterm, are different than those used in children and adults. Infant amino acid formulations, such as TrophAmine (B. Braun), provide essential amino acids such as cysteine, histidine, and tyrosine that are not found in adult formulations.[25] TrophAmine also contains taurine, which is important for brain and retinal growth, and deficiency of this amino acid is associated with cholestasis.[26,27] The plasma amino acid pattern seen in infants receiving TrophAmine resembles normal 2-hour postprandial levels seen in 1-month-old healthy full-term breast-fed infants.[28] The low pH of TrophAmine allows for large amounts of calcium and phosphorus to be added to the PN solution without precipitation.[29] TrophAmine also contains a higher concentration of branched-chain amino acids. Branched-chain amino acids have been shown to improve nitrogen balance, protein synthesis, and immunocompetence in septic or trauma patients.[24] TrophAmine is a better choice of protein for the neonate than Freamine III or Aminosyn PF. Improved weight gain and nitrogen retention and better amino acid profiles have been seen in patients receiving TrophAmine as their protein source.[29] TrophAmine is used in patients under 6 months of age, and an adult amino acid preparation is used in patients over 6 months of age. TrophAmine can be used for patients with end-stage liver disease and cholestasis because of its branched chain amino acid profile. Aminosyn-PF is another amino acid formulation designed for neonates, and it has similar beneficial properties for neonates when compared to the adult amino acid preparations. Novamine (Clintec Nutrition, Chicago) is a standard protein formulation given to patients older than 6 months of age. It is available in 1% to 15% solutions. The 15% solution is particularly useful in fluid-restricted patients. Specialized amino acid formulations are available for certain disease states (renal and hepatic failure). These solutions are expensive, and studies have not demonstrated a clear beneficial survival effect when these solutions have been used in patients with renal and hepatic failure. The amino acid formulation designed for use in patients with severe liver failure and hepatic encephalopathy contains increased amounts of branched-chain amino acids and reduced amounts of methionine and aromatic amino acids. However, study results using this formulation are mixed and have not demonstrated a clear beneficial survival effect in these patients.[30,31] Specialized formulations for renal failure have also been developed, but their use is not widespread in renal failure due to a lack of clear benefit (Table 88-4).[32,33]

There is question as to the benefit of adding albumin to the PN solution in patients with hypoproteinemia. This practice is generally not recommended, because albumin has a short half-life and no nutritional value. Endogenous albumin has a half-life of 21 days, but exogenous albumin does not stay in circulation very long, and its purpose is to increase oncotic pressure. There is a significant amount of aluminum and sodium present in albumin solutions, which can be detrimental to the patient with sensitive fluid status. There is also a concern that albumin may increase sepsis.[34]

In addition to providing calories to patients, it is also important to include protein in adequate amounts. The most commonly used method for determining the protein needs of full-term infants less than 1 year of age and older children is the Recommended Dietary Allowances (RDAs) or Dietary Reference Intakes (DRIs)

TABLE 88-4. **Composition of Crystalline Amino Acid Solutions (mg amino acid/g protein)**

	TrophAmine	Aminosyn	Novamine	HepatAmine	Aminosyn RF
Essential Amino Acids					
L-Isoleucine	82	72	50	113	88
L-Leucine	140	94	69	138	139
L-Lysine	82	72	79	76	102
L-Methionine	34	40	50	13	139
L-Phenylalanine	48	44	69	13	139
L-Threonine	42	52	50	56	63
L-Tryptophan	20	16	17	8	31
L-Valine	78	80	64	105	101
Nonessential Amino Acids					
L-Alanine	54	128	145	96	-
L-Arginine	120	98	98	75	115
L-Aspartic acid	32	-	29	-	-
L-Glutamic acid	50	-	50	-	-
L-Glycine	36	128	69	113	-
L-Histidine	48	30	60	30	82
L-Proline	68	86	60	100	-
L-Serine	38	42	39	63	-
L-Taurine	2.5	-	-	-	-
L-Tyrosine	24	44	3	-	-
% Branched chain amino acids	30	-	-	36	33
% Essential amino acids	53	47	45	52	80
% Nonessential amino acids	47	53	55	48	20

Adapted from The Children's Hospital of Philadelphia Pharmacy Handbook and Formulary 2006-2007. Department of Pharmacy Services. Hudson, OH: Lexi-Comp; 2006.[33]

for age and gender.[35] The protein recommendations are derived from the minimum amount of protein intake required to maintain nitrogen balance. The protein needs for premature infants or children with chronic disease may be higher than the RDA.

Protein needs decline progressively with age. The protein needs of infants and children are higher than those of adults because of differing growth rates.[19] The amount of protein required to enhance protein accretion is higher in sick patients. Increased protein needs may be found in conditions such as protein-losing enteropathy, protein-calorie malnutrition, sepsis, burns, patients on ECMO, or inflammatory gastrointestinal conditions. Infants need a 25% increase in protein intake during the postsurgical period and a 100% increase if they have sepsis or are on extracorporeal membrane oxygenation (ECMO).[36-38] Protein can be safely administered on the first or second day of life in preterm infants. Protein is typically started at 2.0 g/kg of amino acids per day the first day PN is used and then increased to 3.0 g/kg on day 2, in most preterm infants.[39] Some preterm infants may need as much as 4 g/kg per day.[40] Exceptions to this rule may be in VLBW infants, critically ill patients with hepatic or renal insufficiency (not on dialysis), and patients with disorders of protein metabolism (Table 88-5).[41] Older children and adolescents require protein intakes of 1 to 2 g/kg per day. At our institution, we use a maximum of 150 g protein/day. Unless the patient has hepatic or renal failure, or a disorder of protein metabolism is suspected, there is no evidence to suggest that starting protein at the low amount, then advancing it to goal at a slow rate is beneficial. The practice only results in a delay of adequate nutrition. Protein needs in infants, children, and adolescents vary from 0.75 g/kg per day to 2.5 g/kg per day.[42-44] Blood urea nitrogen (BUN) is a useful measure of adequate or excessive protein intake if nutritional status and hydration are within normal limits.

TABLE 88-5. **Guidelines for Dosing Intravenous Protein (g/kg per day)**

Infants 0-5 kg	3-3.5
Children 5-20 kg	2-3
Children 20-40 kg	1-2
Children/adults > 40 kg	0.8-2*

*A maximum of 150 g protein/day is recommended.

Cysteine is a conditionally essential amino acid in neonates and infants. Improved nitrogen retention has been seen with the administration of cysteine to PN solutions.[45] However, it is not present in significant amounts in amino acid solutions due to instability. Cysteine can be added to TrophAmine to reduce the pH of the PN, which allows for increased phosphorus and calcium solubility. Cysteine should not be added to the PN solution if the infant is acidotic, because cysteine may exacerbate metabolic acidosis. The recommended dose for cysteine is 40 mg/g of PN protein. Taurine can also be found in infant amino acid formulations and plays an integral role in brain and retinal membrane development as well as bile acid conjugation.[46] Some evidence suggests that parenteral supplementation of taurine can prevent cholestatic liver disease.[27] Parenteral supplementation has improved plasma levels and transaminase concentrations in adults with short bowel syndrome, but has not been studied in children.[47] Glutamine was originally classified as a nonessential amino acid but is currently classified as a conditionally essential amino acid.[48] Studies have shown that supplementation with glutamine has improved nitrogen balance and immunocompetence, decreased sepsis, and maintained protein synthesis in postoperative patients. Other studies have shown a beneficial effect of PN supplemented with glutamine in patients with short bowel syndrome or trauma, patients who have undergone bone marrow transplantation, and critically ill burn patients.[49-52] The current standard of practice in Canada and Europe is to provide parenteral glutamine in adult trauma and burn patients.[53-57] Beneficial effects from supplementation include decreased incidence of bacteremia, improved nitrogen balance, decreased duration of hospital stay, reduced incidence of severe mucositis and veno-occlusive disease, and a decrease in drug toxicity. Glutamine has also been found to be safe for use with preterm infants, but there has been no significant effect on morbidity or mortality.[58] Intravenous glutamine is not readily available in the United States at this time.

Carnitine is synthesized in the body from two essential amino acids, lysine and methionine, and is required for the transport of long-chain fatty acids into the mitochondria.[59] Neonates and infants are unable to produce carnitine endogenously and need an exogenous supply. Serum and tissue carnitine levels may be depleted in patients who are exclusively on PN for an extended period of time.[60] Inadequate carnitine may reduce fatty acid transport, limiting oxidation and energy production. Carnitine supplementation in PN solutions in premature infants has been suggested to correct low free and acylcarnitine levels. Although hereditary carnitine deficiency responds to carnitine supplementation, it is not clear whether the low levels seen in premature infants and patients with short bowel syndrome represent a true deficiency and need to be supplemented.[61] Indeed, while there have been studies showing improved levels, fat tolerance and some increase in growth and nitrogen retention, other studies have failed to show any significant effect or have shown a negative effect with high doses.[62-64] An intravenous form of L-carnitine is available and may be added to PN formulations. The recommended dose for L-carnitine in pediatrics is 10 to 20 mg/kg per day.[65] It has been suggested that intravenous carnitine be added to the PN of VLBW infants to assist with triglyceride beta-oxidation, if triglyceride levels increase over 200 g/dL.[66] However, this practice is not widespread and has not been found to be beneficial in the short term.[67-69] Though no overwhelming evidence supports supplementation, a typical standard of practice is to provide carnitine parenterally if PN is the only source of nutrition for more than 2 weeks, if the patient has hypertriglyceridemia, or if low serum carnitine levels are present.

Choline is a precursor of acetylcholine and phosphatidylcholine, is required for the synthesis on very low-density lipoproteins (VLDL) and triacylglycerol (TAG) export. Choline deficiency has been suggested as a contributing factor of hepatic steatosis due to the impairment of hepatic TAG secretion.[70-72] The premature infant and the patient on long-term PN without sufficient enteral feeds is at risk for choline deficiency. Buchman et al. showed a reduction in hepatic steatosis and increased plasma free choline levels after administration of a choline supplemented PN solution for 6 weeks.[73] Buchman et al. also showed lower than normal plasma free choline levels in patients on home TPN. This observation was made in about 80% of home PN patients. The provision of oral lecithin caused increased plasma free choline levels as well as decreased hepatic steatosis.[74] Buchman was also able to show that low choline status was associated with fatty liver and elevated transaminases. In addition, in a pilot study Buchman et al. showed that choline-supplemented PN reversed hepatic abnormalities in four patients.[73] In another trial, 15 patients were randomized to receive standard PN or PN supplemented with 2 g of

choline. An improvement in liver function tests was noted in the choline-supplemented group. After the choline supplementation was stopped, there was a recurrence of steatosis.[75]

Carbohydrates

The majority of calories in PN are provided by the intravenous monohydrate form of dextrose, which provides 3.4 kcal/g, different from the 4 kcal/g provided by the enteral form of carbohydrates. Carbohydrates usually provide 50 to 60% of total calorie intake. PN given through a peripheral vein should have a maximum concentration of 10% dextrose because more concentrated dextrose solutions can result in osmolalities greater than 900 mmol/L and an increased risk of phlebitis.[7] In special circumstances, a 12.5% dextrose solution may be used peripherally with caution, but it should not be used in neonates and infants because of the increased risk of extravasation and phlebitis. PN given through a centrally placed line allows for the infusion of solutions with higher dextrose concentrations and osmolalities greater than 900 mmol/L and is typically appropriate for patients requiring PN for more than 7 to 10 days.

It is important to calculate glucose delivery or glucose infusion rate (GIR) in patients who receive PN. The GIR allows the practitioner to determine whether glucose delivery will exceed glucose utilization rates. The GIR is expressed in mg/kg of body weight/minute. The recommended GIR for infants is between 5 and 12 mg/kg per min. Glucose utilization is known to decrease when the GIR exceeds 14 mg/kg per min.[76] If the GIR is higher than recommended, greater amounts of insulin are released. Insulin hypersecretion stimulates hepatic lipogenesis, producing aglycerol from glucose, and inhibits mitochondrial fatty acid oxidation.[77] These concurrent processes promote a buildup of TAG within hepatocytes. The initial rate of dextrose infusion should be approximately 5 mg/kg per min in infants. The GIR can then be increased by 2 to 5 mg/kg per minute daily or 5 to 10% per day. In older children, the recommended GIR is between 2 and 5 mg/kg per minute. Urine should be monitored for glucose when PN is started and after changes in GIR. Serum glucose levels should be checked if a patient has glucosuria, and the GIR should be reduced as appropriate. LBW infants, malnourished infants, and children with small glycogen stores are at increased risk of hypoglycemia when parenteral glucose is abruptly stopped.[78] It is commonly recommended to taper down the rate of the PN solution when cycling PN with a dextrose concentration greater than 10% to decrease the risk of rebound hypoglycemia, but a small study in pediatric patients found that abrupt discontinuation on PN was not a concern in children greater than 2 years of age.[79] Cycling PN in stable patients over the course of 16 hours may prevent or delay the onset of hepatic steatosis.[80,81]

Hyperglycemia in critically ill patients on PN has been associated with increased mortality and morbidity. Increases in energy expenditure and respiratory quotient have been seen with regimens with high glucose infusion rates.[82,83] Serum glucose levels should be maintained in the normal range for age. Patients receiving PN who have significant hyperglycemia may require an insulin infusion to help achieve and maintain euglycemia. Hyperglycemia is common in the stressed LBW and VLBW infant soon after birth. Insulin can be used to maintain serum glucose levels in the normal range and may be considered as an alternative to the use of a hypocaloric regimen.[84] It is preferable to run the insulin as a separate infusion as opposed

TABLE 88-6. Composition of Intralipid Emulsions (per liter)

	Intralipid 10%	Intralipid 20%	Intralipid 30%
Purified soybean oil (g)	100	200	300
Purified egg phospholipids (g)	12	12	12
Glycerol (g)	22	22	16.7
Osmolality (mmol/L)	300	350	310
kcal/mL	1.1	2	3

TABLE 88-7. Guidelines for Dosing Intravenous Fat (g/kg per day)

	0-5 kg Infants	5-20 kg Children	20-40 kg Children	>40 kg Children/Adults
Initial dose	1-1.5	1-1.5	1-1.5	0.5-1
Dose increase	0.5-1	1	1	0.5-1
Standard dose*	3	3	1.5-2	0.5-1

*Percentage of calories from fat should not exceed 60% of total caloric intake.

to adding it to the PN solution, because the insulin may adhere to the tubing, resulting in lower amounts being delivered to the patient. It is also difficult to adjust the rate of the insulin infusion without affecting calorie intake and glucose homeostasis when insulin is mixed with the PN solution.

Lipids

Fat provides a concentrated form of both calories and essential fatty acids, which are required for prostaglandin and membrane lipid synthesis, brain and somatic growth, immune function, skin integrity, and wound healing. Intravenous fat emulsions available in the United States are composed entirely of long-chain triglycerides, usually from soybean and safflower oils. There are two product types available: a 100% soy-based emulsion (Intralipid, Liposyn III) or a 50% soy and 50% safflower oil-based emulsion (Liposyn II). Intralipid is a commonly used intravenous fat and is available in 10%, 20%, and 30% emulsions (Table 88-6).[85] The 20% emulsion is preferred because of its lower phospholipid content and improved triglyceride clearance.[86-88] The 10% solution may result in hyperlipidemia because of its high phospholipid:triglyceride ratio and is infrequently used. Phospholipids are thought to inhibit lipoprotein lipase, the main enzyme responsible for intravenous fat clearance. The 30% emulsion can only be used in a total nutrient admixture and cannot be infused alone into a peripheral vein.

A greater variety of lipid solutions are commonly used in Europe. Structured lipids (long-chain triglycerides [LCT] and medium-chain triglycerides [MCT] attached to a glycerol backbone); MCT emulsions; mixtures of MCT and LCT emulsions; olive oil-containing emulsions; mixtures of soybean oil, MCT, olive oil, and fish oil; and mixtures of MCT, LCT, and fish oil have been developed to prevent complications seen with conventional fat emulsions.[89-94] These emulsions have been studied in hospitalized patients as well as in home PN patients. The advantages of MCT-containing lipid emulsions are that they are more soluble, are rapidly hydrolyzed by lipases, are quickly eliminated from the circulation, and are taken up by the peripheral tissue. They are not stored by the body, are ketogenic, and are oxidized more rapidly than LCT. There is less elevation of liver enzymes with these emulsions. Emulsions containing MCT and LCT are more efficient and have less of a negative effect on the liver, immune system and reticuloendothelial system when compared with LCT containing intravenous fat emulsions. They produce a similar amount of prostaglandins and have been shown to be useful in patients with systemic inflammatory response syndrome. Structured lipids have been studied in the pediatric age group.[95,96] Studies in infants have been performed showing improved lipid levels in those receiving a mixture of MCT and LCT.[97] However, these new formulations

are not readily available in the United States. Currently there is interest in a fish oil-containing lipid emulsion called Omegaven, which is available in Europe but is not approved for use in the United States. Improvement in PN-associated cholestasis has been shown with use of this emulsion, especially in premature infants.[98]

The total daily dose of intravenous fat is usually delivered over 24 hours, except when the PN is cycled. However, continuous 24-hour infusions are better tolerated than intermittent infusions. There is a concern about the growth of bacteria in intravenous fat solutions when these solutions have been hung for more than 12 hours. It has been suggested the hang time be 12 hours or less and that unit doses be used so the bottle is only entered once in order to decrease the incidence of sepsis.[99] Intravenous fat is usually started at an initial dosage and increased over 1 to 3 days, if triglyceride clearance is within normal limits (Table 88-7). There are no clearly defined acceptable values for serum triglycerides during PN administration for hypertriglyceridemia. Although some authors have suggested that in neonates, intravenous lipids should be decreased if triglyceride levels are above 200 mg/dL, we accept triglyceride levels up to 300 mg/dL in infants and young children. A rising triglyceride value in the face of sepsis would be a reason to decrease intravenous fat administration. In adults, triglyceride levels greater than 400 mg/dL have been suggested as a cutoff value above which the intravenous fat dose should be decreased.[100] Triglyceride levels depend on the rate of clearance of the infused fat. This in turn is affected by nutritional status, degree of malnutrition, concurrent administration of medications, and the clinical situation (stress, organ dysfunction, and infection).[101] The impact of intravenous fat administration on lung function has been well discussed in two review articles.[102,103]

In general, when formulating a PN regimen, the fat percentage should provide 25 to 35% of total calories. There are some exceptions to this rule where fat percentage may be higher, but it should never exceed 60% of total calories. The maximum dose of intravenous fat in infants is 3 g/kg per day. The dosage of intravenous fat decreases with age. Patients requiring 100% of their caloric needs from PN need to receive intravenous fat in order to prevent essential fatty acid deficiency (EFAD). In the extremely LBW infant, EFAD can develop within 48 to 72 hours if no intravenous fat is provided.[104] Preterm infants on PN without intravenous fat and enteral feeds can develop EFAD biochemically within 7 days.[105] Clinical signs of EFAD include growth failure, flaky dry skin, alopecia, thrombocytopenia, increased infections, and impaired wound healing. EFAD can be diagnosed by a triene-to-tetraene ratio above 0.4. Some literature suggests that only 0.3 to 0.56% of total energy intake from linoleic acid is required to prevent EFAD, as opposed to

TABLE 88-8. **Intravenous Requirements (Daily) for Electrolytes**

	Infants 0-5 kg	Children 5-20 kg	20-40 kg	Adolescents/Adults >40 kg
Sodium	2-5 mEq/kg	2-6 mEq/kg	2-3 mEq/kg	80-150 mEq/day
Potassium	1-4 mEq/kg	2-3 mEq/kg	1.5-2.5 mEq/kg	40-60 mEq/day
Phosphorus	2-4 mEq/kg	1-2 mEq/kg	1-1.5 mEq/kg	30-60 mEq/day
Chloride	2-5 mEq/kg	2-5 mEq/kg	2-3 mEq/kg	80-150 mEq/day
Acetate	Balance	Balance	Balance	Balance
Calcium	1-4 mEq/kg	0.5-1 mEq/kg	10-25 mEq/day	10-20 mEq/day
Magnesium	0.3-0.5 mEq/kg	0.3-0.5 mEq/kg	0.3-0.5 mEq/kg	10-30 mEq/day

Initiate dose at lower end of range and increase based on individual needs. Dose ranges are suggested guidelines only. Specific clinical situations may require doses outside of these ranges. Use laboratory tests to adjust electrolyte dosing. (Adapted from The Children's Hospital of Philadelphia Pharmacy Handbook and Formulary 2006-2007. Department of Pharmacy Services. Hudson, OH: Lexi-Comp Inc; 2006.[33])

previous information stating the need of 2 to 4% (0.5 to 1.0 g/kg/day) of total calories needed from fat.

Electrolytes and Minerals

Electrolyte requirements vary with age and are added to the PN solution in maintenance concentrations.[106,107] These requirements are derived from the RDAs with allowances made for the efficiency of absorption (Table 88-8). These include sodium, potassium, calcium, magnesium, and phosphorus. Chloride and acetate are used to balance the PN solutions. It is recommended to obtain baseline serum electrolytes before ordering the PN solution and then add electrolytes accordingly. Periodic monitoring of serum electrolytes is required, especially in the critically ill and malnourished patient. In neonates and children with high calcium and phosphorus needs, the amounts added to a PN solution may be limited because of solubility issues. Increasing the amount of protein and adding cysteine (30 to 40 mg cysteine/g amino acid), thereby lowering the pH of the solution, can allow the addition of higher amounts of calcium and phosphorus to the PN solution without causing precipitation. In instances where the patient's calcium and phosphorus requirements cannot be met via the PN solution, a separate infusion of calcium or phosphorus may need to be given. Patients with high calcium needs and those who cannot get all the calcium in their PN may benefit from enteral calcium administration if tolerated. It should be noted that in patients with hypocalcemia and hypomagnesemia, magnesium status needs to be normalized before calcium levels will respond to calcium supplementation.

Vitamins

Though specific parenteral vitamin dosages for pediatrics in the United States have not been updated since 1988, the ESPEN/ESPGHAN/ESPR recommendations from 2005 do not suggest any changes.[107-109] There are currently two types of multivitamin preparations (Infuvite Adult, Infuvite Pediatric, M.V.I.-12, M.V.I. Adult) used in the United States: pediatric and adult formulations. The pediatric MVI was designed to meet the needs of preterm and term infants and children up to 10 years of age.[107,110] It is dosed on a per-kilogram basis, and preterm infants receive 40% of a vial/kg of body weight. The adult and pediatric MVI preparations differ in the concentration of the different vitamins per milliliter. In general, the adult MVI has a greater concentration of vitamins, except it contains less vitamin

D and has no vitamin K compared with the pediatric formulation. In children older than 10 years of age, the adult MVI is used with the addition of vitamin K. The new recommendation is for adult multivitamin preparations to contain vitamin K (Table 88-9). The dosing recommendations for vitamins take into account the losses associated with administration. Some vitamins may adhere to the intravenous tubing, whereas others may be affected by light exposure while the PN solution is being administered.[111] It is recommended that the adult multivitamin preparation not be used for children because it contains propylene glycol and polysorbate additives that may be toxic to the premature infant.[112,113]

Vitamin A is an important mediator of cell differentiation and repair in the lung and other organs. Greene et al. demonstrated a higher incidence of BPD and low plasma retinol levels in VLBW infants with a birth weight less than 1000 g who were on PN for 1 month. These levels progressively decreased over time.[114] This was subsequently confirmed in seven infants (450 to 1360 g) who were receiving standard multivitamin supplements and, despite parenteral vitamin A supplementation, all infants did not have complete normalization of retinol levels.[115] Shenai et al. showed that treatment with 400 to 450 µg/kg per day intermuscularly of vitamin A resulted in improved levels as well as decreased BPD.[116] Subsequently, it was shown that vitamin A supplementation resulted in a modest reduction in chronic lung disease, and the recommendation was made to routinely supplement vitamin A in all infants weighing less than 1000 g who require respiratory support on the first day of life. Vitamin A can adhere to tubing and can be destroyed by the effect of light and may result in decreased administration to the patient.

One recent study evaluated the need for thiamine in postoperative pediatric patients receiving parenteral nutrition.[117] The results from this small study demonstrated an increased requirement for thiamine after abdominal surgery. Further evaluation of the need for increasing the amount of parenteral thiamine is necessary before any changes can be made to current therapy.

Trace Elements

In addition to the previously discussed components, iron, zinc, copper, chromium, manganese, selenium, and molybdenum are to be added to make the PN solution complete. However, molybdenum is not routinely added to PN solutions. These trace elements are dosed according to published guidelines.[107,108] There are no parenteral requirements for fluoride and iodine. The latter trace element is present as a contaminant

TABLE 88-9. **Intravenous Vitamin Requirement Recommendations (Daily) and Products**

	Preterm infants/kg	Term Infants and Children >1 year	MVI Pediatric (5 mL)	MVI-12* (5 mL)
Biotin (μg)	8	20	20	60
Folate (μg)	56	140	140	400
Niacin (mg)	4-6.8	17	17	40
Pantothenic acid (mg)	1-2	5	5	15
Riboflavin (mg)	0.15-0.2	1.4	1.4	3.6
Thiamine (mg)	0.2-0.35	1.2	1.2	3
Vitamin A (retinol) (IU)	700-1500	2300	2300	3300
Vitamin B^6 (mg)	0.15-0.2	1	1	4
Vitamin B^{12} (μg)	0.3	1	1	5
Vitamin C (mg)	15-25	80	80	100
Vitamin D (IU)	40-160	400	400	200
Vitamin E (tocopherol) (IU)	3.5	7	7	10
Vitamin K (mg)	0.3	0.2	0.2	a

*Patients receiving MVI-12 will get 0.2 mg/day of vitamin K. (Adapted from The Children's Hospital of Philadelphia Pharmacy Handbook and Formulary 2006-2007. Department of Pharmacy Services. Hudson, OH: Lexi-Comp Inc; 2006.[33])

in many trace element preparations and in other products used in association with PN solutions. Copper and manganese are excreted in the bile and selenium, molybdenum, and chromium are excreted in urine. Increased copper losses occur in burns and increased zinc losses occur in diarrhea. Trace elements may need to be adjusted in patients with organ dysfunction because of altered elimination of certain trace elements (e.g., copper and manganese). Serum levels of trace elements eliminated from the PN solution need to be monitored. Trace elements such as zinc, copper, manganese, and selenium can also be present as contaminants of the components of PN.

There is some controversy as to whether iron should be routinely added to PN solutions as well as some controversy regarding the methods of administration of iron in PN solutions. Some practitioners give iron to all patients on PN, whereas others argue that it should be administered on a weekly basis in a separate bag of intravenous fluids only in patients who receive PN for more than 3 months.[118-120] There are currently three forms of intravenous iron available: iron dextran, sodium ferric gluconate, and iron sucrose. The greatest experience of iron in PN solutions is with iron dextran. There is concern about compatibility issues of iron and PN solutions especially with total nutrient admixture (TNA) solutions.[121] At our institution we give all patients maintenance doses of iron (0.1 mg/kg per day) after 2 months of age, with the exception of chronically transfused patients (e.g., those with inherited anemia, malignancies, and bone marrow transplant recipients). Iron-deficient patients may receive additional amounts based on results of iron studies. Parenteral iron may be contraindicated in patients with sepsis as there has been a documented increase in morbidity when provided during that time.[122]

Additional zinc may be required in patients with zinc deficiency. As zinc is lost primarily through the gastrointestinal (GI) tract, patients with increased GI losses may need additional zinc supplementation. In addition, patients with poor wound healing and/or decubitus ulcers should have zinc status evaluated. Low serum alkaline phosphatase levels may be suggestive of zinc deficiency.

Copper and manganese are excreted in bile and so may need to be removed from the PN solutions of patients with cholestatic liver disease and/or liver failure to prevent toxicity.[123] A recent study documented hypercupremia in pediatric patients receiving PN independent of cholestasis. If copper is removed from the PN solution secondary to cholestasis, levels should be monitored. Copper deficiency can develop in adult patients who receive PN.[124] Symptoms of copper deficiency include anemia, neutropenia, hypercholesterolemia, osteopenia, and pigmentary changes in hair. The presence of high blood manganese levels in patients on PN supplementation has been associated with psychosis and extrapyramidal symptoms. Manganese deposition in the basal ganglia has been seen in head magnetic resonance imaging (MRI) studies and confirmed in patients on long-term PN.[125] This improved when manganese was removed from the PN solution. There is a broad range of recommendations for manganese dosage ranging from 1 μg/kg/day to 100 μg/kg/day.[108] Current literature advises that these may be too high and encourages reformulation of multi–trace element doses.[126] Similar to copper, manganese is commonly removed with conjugated bilirubin values above 2 mg/dL, but this is not the only criterion for removal.[127] Manganese deficiency has not been reported in pediatric patients receiving TPN, but whole blood values should be monitored in long-term PN patients and adjusted as necessary.

Glomerular filtration rate needs to be monitored annually when chromium is added to PN solutions. It has been suggested that chromium and selenium be used with caution in patients with significant renal dysfunction because they are excreted in the urine. Molybdenum deficiency is extremely rare and need not be supplemented except in adolescent patients who receive 80% or more of their caloric requirements from PN for 3 to 6 months. Molybdenum is also excreted in the urine. Iodine is not added to PN solutions because patients usually receive adequate amounts of iodine from unavoidable contamination of PN solutions and from topical administration of iodine-containing antiseptic solutions.

Additives

Commonly used medications such as ranitidine may be added to the PN solution if they are compatible with the PN solution. When medications can be added to PN solutions, this can result in ease of care as well as a reduction of intravenous fluids, which is beneficial to the fluid-restricted patient. Certain drugs are not compatible with PN and therefore cannot be run concurrently. See Table 88-10 for some commonly used medications and their compatibility with PN and intravenous lipids.

TABLE 88-10. Compatibility of Parenteral Nutrition, Intravenous Lipid, and Commonly Used Intravenous Medications

Drug	Parenteral Nutrition	Intravenous Lipid
Albumin	Compatible	Incompatible
Amikacin	Compatible	Incompatible
Amphotericin B	Incompatible	Incompatible
Ampicillin	Incompatible	Compatible at Y-site
Ciprofloxacin	No information (NR)	No information (NR)
Cyclosporin	Incompatible	Compatible
Furosemide	Compatible up to 4 h	Compatible up to 4 h
Gentamicin	Compatible	Compatible at Y-site
Imipenem	Compatible up to 4 h	Compatible
Iron dextran	Compatible	No information-not recommended
Oxacillin	Compatible	Compatible up to 4 h
Penicillin	Compatible	Compatible up to 4 h
Phenobarbital	Compatible	Incompatible
Phenytoin	Incompatible	Incompatible
Propofol	Compatible up to 4 h	No information(NR)
Ranitidine	Compatible	Compatible
Ticarcillin	Compatible	Compatible
Tobramycin	Compatible	Compatible up to 4 h
Vancomycin	Compatible	Compatible

Adapted from The Children's Hospital of Philadelphia Pharmacy Handbook and Formulary 2008-2009. Department of Pharmacy Services. Hudson, OH: Lexi-Comp; 2009.[33]
NR, not recommended.

TABLE 88-11. Monitoring of Patients Receiving Parenteral Nutrition

Laboratory Tests*	
Baseline	Complete blood cell count, serum electrolytes, triglycerides, calcium, magnesium, phosphorus, alkaline phosphatase, total protein, albumin, blood urea nitrogen, creatinine, liver functions tests, iron studies, total bilirubin, and prealbumin
Weekly	Serum electrolytes, triglycerides, calcium, magnesium, phosphorus, alkaline phosphatase, total protein, albumin, blood urea nitrogen, creatinine, liver functions tests, total bilirubin, and prealbumin
Monthly	Complete blood cell count, reticulocyte count, iron studies
Bi-annually	Serum selenium, chromium, zinc, vitamin A, E, D (25-hydroxy), copper, ceruloplasmin, manganese, carnitine, prothrombin time or PIVKA II level
Growth measurement	
Baseline	Weight, height/length, head circumference (patients <3 years), arm anthropometrics
Daily	Weight (patients <2 years)
Weekly	Weight (patients >2 years and adolescents, height/length (<2 years)
Monthly	Height/length (>2 years), head circumference (patients <3 years), arm anthropometrics

*Serum electrolytes, calcium, magnesium, phosphorus, blood urea nitrogen should be monitored daily until goal regimen is reached.

Patients born with inborn errors of metabolism may need additional amounts of specific amino acids added to their PN. Hydrochloric acid may be added to PN solutions given to patients on ECMO to correct severe alkalosis. This has to be done through central access. When the patient comes off ECMO and PN is provided via peripheral access, the hydrochloric acid must be discontinued. Insulin may also be added to PN solutions to assist with blood glucose control. The addition of albumin has previously been discussed. Heparin is added to all PN solutions which results in less thrombosis formation, less fibrin sheath formation, reduced incidence of sepsis, and enhanced triglyceride clearance by stimulating lipoprotein lipase release.[128,129]

MONITORING

Monitoring patients on PN is very important. This consists of monitoring the appropriateness of the regimen using serum chemistries and growth parameters (Table 88-11). Typically, a baseline nutritional assessment and check of serum chemistries should be completed before starting PN. Daily laboratory values should be obtained and the PN regimen adjusted accordingly until goal regimen is achieved. Laboratory values should be obtained after any changes in the PN regimen. Most patients in the hospital can have weekly laboratory blood tests to assess response to the PN regimen once a stable regimen is achieved. Growth monitoring is based on the age of the patient. Malnourished patients at risk for refeeding syndrome must be closely monitored until they are on a stable PN regimen and have stable electrolyte (potassium, calcium, magnesium, and glucose) values. Patients on long-term PN solutions, those with increased losses or increased needs, may need to have trace element and vitamin levels checked periodically.

COMPLICATIONS

Complications related to the use of PN can be divided into three main categories: mechanical, infectious, and metabolic. With careful use of PN, these complications can be avoided or minimized.[130,131]

Mechanical Complications

Mechanical complications seen with the use of PN include those associated with the initial insertion of a CVC and subsequent use of the catheter. These include arrhythmias, hemomediastinum, air embolism, pneumothorax, hemothorax, hydrothorax, intravascular and extravascular malpositioning, brachial plexus injury, arterial injury, catheter embolism, superior vena cava syndrome, perforation of the heart or pericardium, and thrombosis formation.[132,133] Introduction of an air embolus can occur at the time of CVC insertion, with defective catheters, and with catheters with faulty connections. Symptoms of air embolism include shortness of breath, hypoxia, tachycardia, hypotension, and neurologic changes. Pneumothorax, hydrothorax, and hemothorax can occur at the time of CVC placement or as a result of delayed catheter perforation due to erosion of the blood vessel. Intravascular malpositioning refers to coiled catheters, and those in the right atrium or ventricle. If the catheter tip is positioned in the right atrium, arrhythmias can occur as a result of irritation of the myocardium. Extravascular malpositioning results when the catheter becomes lodged in the pleural space, in the mediastinum, or outside the vascular space.

Catheter breakage and occlusion can occur with chronic use of CVC. Small tears, pinholes, or breakage may occur in the silicone elastomer material of the catheter. Damage to the septum of the implantable port may occur if an inappropriate needle is used, resulting in leakage of fluid into the surrounding tissue. Extravasation of fluid can also occur with tunneled catheters with fluid leaking into the surrounding tissue. The complication rate for any line placement should be less than 8%.[134] Catheter occlusion can occur as a result of an intramural thrombus, extraluminal fibrin sleeve, mural thrombosis, development of a biofilm, or a buildup of precipitate from drugs or components of the PN solution. The occlusion can range from a withdrawal problem such as an inability to aspirate blood but fluids infuse without difficulty to a complete occlusion when nothing can be infused through the catheter. The development of thrombi may occur as a result of a vascular injury during the catheter placement or from contact with the tip of the catheter. These thrombi can develop either within the catheter (intramural thrombi) or at the site of the vascular injury (mural thrombi). Over time, mural thrombi can become large veno-occlusive thrombi. Fibrin sleeves also develop from the catheter's contact with blood. As with the development of a thrombus, platelets and fibrin adhere to the catheter, causing a "sleeve" to form that encapsulates the catheter.

Solutions used to flush the catheter are intended to maintain catheter patency and include heparin and normal saline. The results of prophylactic heparin therapy preventing occlusion in PN solutions remain questionable. The risk of potential adverse effects and optimal dosage regimen are unclear. Currently, a dose of 0.5 U/mL PN solution is recommended for neonates under 1500 g and 1 U/mL of PN solution for neonates over 1500 g, infants, children, and adolescents. With intraluminal blockages, tissue plasminogen activator (t-PA), ethanol, hydrochloric acid, and sodium bicarbonate may be instilled in the catheter. Urokinase is not used as much because of potential allergy. Occasionally, a combination of fibrinolytic agents and guidewire manipulation is needed to restore patency. Embolization of occluding compounds may occur in such settings. Warfarin or other anticoagulants may need to be used.[135]

Infectious Complications

The use of CVC is frequently complicated by local or systemic infections. These include sepsis (bacterial and fungal), line contamination, and infective thrombophlebitis. Though central line–associated bloodstream infection (CLABSI) incidence has decreased from 7.8 per 100 central line days to 3.7 in pediatric ICUs in the past 10 years, it continues to be a major problem within the health care system.[136] Common infectious agents in patients receiving PN are coagulase-negative staphylococci, *Staphylococcus aureus*, *Klebsiella pneumoniae*, *Acinetobacter*, and *Candida albicans*.[137] Children with abnormal gastrointestinal tracts such as in short bowel syndrome have a significant incidence of gram-negative infection, presumably by blood invasion of bowel bacteria. Other risk factors include age, underlying disease, site of the CVC, environmental factors, length of use and frequency of line entry for blood drawing.[138] Some bloodstream infections (BSIs) probably arise from a bacterial biofilm (bacteria embedded within an extracellular matrix consisting of polysaccharide) that develops on the catheter surface. In conditions of stress the bacteria break off resulting in bacteremia.[139] The majority (70 to 85%) of infections can be treated safely without line removal. Management of BSI consists of preventing initial contamination by using aseptic technique and minimizing biofilm development. Treatment consists of initial antibiotic therapy to cover common organisms pending cultures.[140] Once the organism has been identified, the appropriate antibiotic course is chosen depending on the clinical situation. Persistent fevers, positive blood cultures, and tunnel infections may require removal of the line. Minimizing duration of catheter placement; use of antimicrobial-coated catheters, and use of ethanol in a catheter-lock solution are additional measures that can be used.[140] The ethanol lock technique has been used for prevention as well as treatment of persistent catheter-related infections in pediatric patients.[141,142] The reader is referred to recommendations from the Centers for Disease Control and Prevention and the European Society of Parenteral and Enteral Nutrition for further guidelines on CVC treatment with parenteral nutrition.[5,143]

Metabolic Complications

Metabolic complications related to PN solution include electrolyte and mineral imbalances, hyperammonemia, hyperglycemia, hypertriglyceridemia, hypoglycemia, bone disease, and cholestasis.[145] Hyperammonemia was initially reported in infants who received casein hydrolysate–containing PN solutions and is no longer noted with the currently available amino acid solutions. Hyperglycemia can occur with high infusion rates, especially in the presence of sepsis, trauma, surgery and the use of corticosteroids. Hypoglycemia may occur when total parenteral nutrition (TPN) is abruptly stopped in infants and young children.

Hyponatremia can result from inadequate sodium intake, excessive free water, excess sodium loss, and renal disease. Hypernatremia can occur with excessive sodium intake and fluid restriction. Hyperkalemia may be noted with excessive intake and renal disease. Hypokalemia may result from increased losses, from inadequate replacement, or from increased requirements, as is seen with refeeding syndrome. Hypocalcemia occurs with osteopenia of prematurity, diuretics, excessive phosphate intake, severe vitamin D deficiency, inadequate calcium intake, and magnesium deficiency. Hypophosphatemia can result with refeeding syndrome, inadequate intake, certain antifungal medications (amphotericin B), hypomagnesemia, and increased renal excretion of phosphorus. Hypomagnesemia occurs with decreased intake, increased losses as seen with diarrhea and renal disease, and use of certain drugs including antifungals and immunosuppressive medications (cyclosporine and tacrolimus).

Rapid infusions of intravenous fat can result in hypertriglyceridemia and elevated free fatty acid levels due to saturation of lipoprotein lipase and subsequent accumulation of atypical lipoproteins. Hypertriglyceridemia occurs when there is decreased triglyceride clearance and is seen with excessive intravenous fat intake, sepsis, and overfeeding. Fat overload syndrome occurs with extremely high fat infusions over a short period. This is characterized by a decrease in oxygenation, thrombocytopenia, and tachypnea. If PN solutions without intravenous fat are administered, essential fatty acid deficiency can occur with deleterious effects on energy metabolism, membrane structure, prostaglandin synthesis, and fat tissue storage. There has been evidence suggesting an association between intravenous fat administration and the incidence of chronic lung disease and death in neonates, but a meta-analysis did not find any significant effect on death or chronic lung disease.[146-149] The oxidation of intravenous fat by phototherapy and ambient lights results in the formation of lipid hydroperoxides. Decreased hydroperoxide levels have been shown when intravenous fat emulsions were protected from light.[150,151] These hydroperoxides lead to the formation of free radicals and injury in various organs. There is increasing evidence suggesting that the currently available lipid formulations in the United States increase the development of parenteral nutrition-associated liver disease.[81] Replacing the soybean oil content with monounsaturated fatty acids or medium-chain triglycerides had been shown to decrease the risk of PN-associated cholestasis. Allergy to intravenous fat is rare,[152,153] but patients allergic to eggs, soy, peas, and peanuts may have a reaction to the contents of current intravenous fat emulsions. It is recommended that patients with potential allergies be given a test dose of 0.1 g/kg of intravenous fat over 1 hour after appropriate skin testing has been performed. An allergy consultation may be valuable in these cases.

PN-related bone disease can occur in up to 3% of adult patients on long-term PN. It is also seen in children receiving home PN.[154-156] It is characterized by bone pain, pathologic fractures, and hypercalcuria. Symptoms usually improve after discontinuation of PN. The exact etiology is unknown, but possible factors include abnormal vitamin D metabolism, aluminum toxicity, hypercalcuria, inadequate phosphate administration, and abnormal calcium-to-phosphorus ratio.[157,158] Premature infants are at high risk for developing osteopenia. Care must be taken to administer adequate calcium and phosphorus intake as well as to maintain an optimal calcium-to-phosphorus ratio.[159]

Aluminum contamination of PN solutions is a well-known complication. On July 26, 2004, the U.S. Food and Drug Administration (FDA) is issued a new safety mandate regarding aluminum content in large-volume parenterals (LVPs), small-volume parenterals (SVPs), and pharmacy bulk packaging (PBPs).[160,161] Some LVPs include amino acids, concentrated dextrose, and parenteral lipids, and some SVPs include calcium, potassium, and sodium. The FDA is recommending aluminum exposure in intravenous solutions not exceed 5 μg/kg per day. Pediatric populations are particularly at risk for developing aluminum toxicity, including metabolic bone disease, encephalopathy, and impaired neurologic development. The pediatric patients most at risk are premature infants, patients with renal disorders, and those on long-term PN.[162] Bishop et al. showed that neonates in a neonatal intensive care unit in the UK who were given an aluminum-depleted PN solution had a higher Bayley mental development index.[163] For those infants who did not have neuromotor impairment, increasing aluminum exposure reduced Bayley mental development index by 1 point for each day of PN.[163,164] Impaired neurologic development and decreased bone density are among the toxic effects of increased aluminum levels. The FDA mandate requires manufacturers to state the aluminum content on the labels of all LVPs, SVPs, and PBPs and has determined that the safe upper limit for aluminum in all LVPs, SVPs, and PBPs is 25 μg/L or less.

Refeeding syndrome occurs when malnourished patients receive aggressive nutritional rehabilitation via the enteral or parenteral route.[165] Patients with protein-calorie malnutrition commonly maintain normal serum electrolyte levels in the presence of intracellular depletion of these same electrolytes. Administration of carbohydrate calories results in the stimulation of insulin secretion, which mobilizes phosphorus and potassium into the cell, with resultant hypokalemia, hypophosphatemia, and hypomagnesemia. Vitamin deficiency and abnormalities in glucose metabolism can occur in certain types of patients. Increased metabolic rate and anabolism further decrease potassium and phosphorus levels and also induce hypomagnesemia. Refeeding syndrome can be fatal if not recognized and treated appropriately. In patients with risk of refeeding syndrome, it is prudent to start calories at 75% of a patient's REE or at a previously tolerated level of calories. Calories should then be increased by 10 to 20% per day provided serum electrolyte levels are normal and congestive heart failure or significant edema is not evident.[166]

Hepatobiliary complications are associated with PN and can occur as early as 2 weeks after the initiation of PN.[167-170] The earliest signs are elevated serum γ-glutamyltransferase and cholylglycine levels. The exact incidence is not known, but may vary from 7.4 to 84%. The highest incidence occurs in the LBW premature infant with necrotizing enterocolitis, short bowel syndrome, multiple bouts of sepsis, or multiple periods of not being fed. The etiology is unknown, but the following factors have been implicated: source of intravenous fat; excessive protein and carbohydrate intake; amino acid composition; relative carbohydrate-to-nitrogen imbalance; carnitine, taurine, or serine deficiency; excessive phytosterol intake; EFAD; bacterial overgrowth; lack of enteral stimulation; alteration in canalicular membrane transport proteins; effects of ambient light and photo-oxidation on PN constituents; and continuous delivery of PN.[81,171-173] Adults on chronic PN appear to get steatosis, whereas neonates and children develop cholestasis, cirrhosis, and portal hypertension. Acalculous cholecystitis, biliary sludge, and gallstones can also be seen in patients on chronic PN. Ursodeoxycholic acid has been used to treat this hepatobiliary damage, but there have been no controlled trials demonstrating efficacy. Prevention of PN-associated liver disease consists of the following measures: avoiding overfeeding and excessive protein and carbohydrate intake, using an alternative form of lipid emulsion, decreasing soy-based lipid products to 1 g/kg/day, cycling of PN, using an appropriate amino acid solution, and initiating enteral feeds as soon as possible. Copper and manganese should be decreased or discontinued from the PN solution, and copper, ceruloplasmin, and manganese levels should subsequently be monitored. All episodes of sepsis should be treated promptly.[174,175]

TOTAL NUTRIENT ADMIXTURES

PN admixtures may be administered in one of two forms: (1) a 2-in-1 solution in which the dextrose and amino acid solution is delivered in one bag and the intravenous fat is administered separately as a piggyback infusion, or (2) a 3-in-1 solution or total nutrient admixture where the intravenous fat is added directly to the dextrose and amino acid solution. This obviates the need for separate infusion lines and pumps. TNAs simplify PN administration and are particularly useful in the pediatric home PN patient. In 1995, the Food and Drug Administration issued a safety alert after the death of two patients related to microvascular pulmonary thrombi containing calcium phosphate precipitates.[176] Several recommendations were made regarding the amount of calcium and phosphorus added to the PN solution, the order in which the components of the PN are added when the solution is mixed, and the use of a filter.[177-179] With a TNA, it is difficult to meet the high calcium and phosphorus needs of neonates without resulting precipitation of the solution. The emulsion may also separate out with high electrolyte concentrations. TNAs are associated with a possible increased risk of thrombosis, pulmonary emboli, shorter catheter life and infection, because a standard 0.2-μm filter cannot be used. In addition, precipitates may not be noticed in a TNA because it is an opaque or cloudy solution. The advantages of a TNA solution is that it costs less, is easier to use because only one pump is required both at home, and requires less tubing. Other advantages of TNAs are less risk of contamination and growth of bacteria because there is only one system and it requires less nursing time and pharmacy preparation time. Disadvantages are that it is difficult to see particulate material because the solution is opaque, there could be more growth of bacteria, and the stability of the intravenous fat may be affected when high concentrations of electrolytes are used. Typically water-soluble additives are added first, the fat-soluble vitamins are then added to the intravenous fat, and finally the two are mixed together. All TNA solutions need to be refrigerated similar to the 2-in-1 solutions. An inline filter of 1.2 μm has to be used with a TNA, and this is different from the 0.22-μm filter that is used for the 2-in-1 solution.[177] It is recommended that TNA solutions not be used in neonates and infants.[180] In our institution we do not use TNA for hospitalized patients. Some patients on home PN are provided with TNAs for ease of care. If home PN patients are on solutions that contain high electrolyte concentrations and a TNA will result in precipitation, then the patient is prescribed a 2-in-1 solution.

FORMULATING A REGIMEN

Once the decision has been made to start the patient on PN, it is important to determine whether the patient will require central or peripheral PN. The patient who will require PN for a short time, who has low to average energy, protein and electrolyte needs and has adequate nutritional status should be given PN administered through a peripheral intravenous catheter, called peripheral PN (PPN). The patient with increased fluid, caloric, protein, and energy needs who is malnourished and who will need PN for more than 1 week should be given PN that is administered through a central line. Maintenance fluid requirements can be calculated using body weight or surface area. Fluid needs are not only influenced by age and weight, but also by insensible losses, as well as the underlying medical condition or disease state. Allowances will need to be made for ongoing losses. Some patients with renal failure or fluid overload, as well as neonates with bronchopulmonary dysplasia or patent ductus arteriosus or who are receiving high-volume intravenous medications, may require fluid restriction and smaller volumes of concentrated PN. PN should not be used as a replacement solution for the patient with excessive fluid losses, because this will result in the excessive delivery of some nutrients. In these circumstances, we recommend using specifically designated replacement solutions. A common method for determining fluid requirements is as follows: 100 mL/kg for each of the first 10 kg of body weight, then an additional 50 mL/kg for the each of the next 10 kg of body weight, up to 20 kg. Patients whose weight is above 20 kg have an additional 20 mL/kg for every kilogram over 20 kg. Alternatively, 1600 mL/m^2 can be used if body surface area

can be determined. Whatever the method chosen, the patient should always be examined for excessive or inadequate fluid intake by evaluating fluid intake and output data, weight, and urine specific gravity and by physical examination. The next step in formulating a PN regimen is to determine the goal for the patient's caloric and protein needs. Depending on the current nutritional status, a patient can usually receive calories equaling the REE or 75 to 85% of goal calories and then be increased to goal calories incrementally over the next 2 to 3 days. Patients at risk for refeeding syndrome should have their PN regimen advanced more slowly. A dextrose solution of 10% is used initially; if it is tolerated and central access is present, a more concentrated dextrose solution of up to 30 to 35% can be used if needed. Most patients receive dextrose concentrations of less than 20%. Once the fat and protein calories have been calculated, the balance of calories is provided as intravenous carbohydrate. It is important to make sure the final PN solution is balanced to prevent complications of overfeeding as well as excessive administration of any macronutrient. Current literature suggests am macronutrient mixture of 50 to 60% carbohydrate, 10 to 20% protein, and 20 to 30% fat to reduce the risk of parenteral nutrition associated liver disease (PNALD).[81]

It is also important to calculate the GIR and make sure that it does not exceed the recommended ranges. After a baseline chemistry panel is reviewed, appropriate amounts of electrolytes and minerals are added. Serum electrolyte levels should initially be monitored daily, until a stable regimen has been reached. A triglyceride level should be checked whenever intravenous fat intake is increased. In addition, patients with sepsis may have problems with triglyceride clearance and need to have values checked periodically. A weekly measurement of prealbumin may be a is a useful test of protein status and the caloric adequacy of the PN regimen, if C-reactive protein is less than 1 mg/L and the patient is not on steroids.

CYCLIC PARENTERAL NUTRITION

The administration of cyclic PN allows for the provision of PN over a specified period of time each day.[181] Cycling allows for a more normal daytime routine and increased mobility of the patient. Cycling is not usually initiated until a patient is on a stable PN regimen and/or can tolerate a large volume of fluid and nutrients over a short period of time. PN can be cycled from 24 hours/day to as low as 8 hours/day, but most cycled TPN runs for 10 to 12 hours in children over 4 to 6 months of age. Reductions in the number of hours a patient is receiving PN can be done in 4- to 6-hour increments. Infants under 4 to 6 months of age who receive all their nutrition parenterally may only be able to tolerate being off of PN for up to 4 hours.[182]

There are many benefits to cycling PN. Cycling PN may help to decrease the risk of PN-associated steatosis by allowing time for the mobilization of hepatic fat stores.[19,182] When cycling PN, the rate is commonly cut in half during the last 1 to 2 hours of the infusion to prevent hypoglycemia.[8,20] More recent data indicated that abrupt discontinuation on PN was not a concern in children greater than 2 years of age.[79] It is important to monitor for the presence of glucosuria during the PN cycle, because this may be indicative of a lack of tolerance to the regimen. There is the occasional patient who does not tolerate cycling and develops nausea and vomiting. Lengthening the cycle usually allows for improvement of these symptoms. An easy way to calculate the cycling rate is to divide the total volume of PN to be infused by the number of hours the PN will run, minus one-half hour, and then half the rate for the last half hour. (Fore example, a total PN volume of 1500 mL is to be infused over 12 hours. 1500/11.5 = 130.4 mL/hour for 11 hours and 65.2 mL/hour for the last hour.) Some institutions also start the PN infusion at half the goal rate for the first half hour.

HOME PARENTERAL NUTRITION

Home PN may be required in patients who are unable to transition to adequate enteral nutrition regimens and do not otherwise need to be hospitalized. Patients may receive a combination of enteral and parenteral feeds, and every attempt is made to increase enteral feeds and wean PN, but sometimes this is not possible and the patient will remain on PN for months to years. Home PN patients have central access and are usually on cycled PN for ease of care, for the achievement of a more normal lifestyle, and to decrease long-term complications of PN. Patients who fail to tolerate sufficient enteral regimens and wean off PN in the hospital are often sent home on PN. Common patient diagnoses include the patient with short bowel syndrome following surgical resection; oncology patients with vomiting and poor oral intake who cannot tolerate tube feeds; patients with significant small bowel damage from villous atrophy, intestinal pseudo-obstruction, and other motility disorders; and patients with severe pancreatitis with pseudocyst formation. It is important to make sure the patient, parent, or guardian receives adequate training and is selected carefully. In order for home PN to be successful, a thorough evaluation of the home environment (water source, electricity, refrigeration, cleanliness, safety/mobility), family/psychosocial support, and insurance coverage must be completed before discharge.

A nutrition support team is recommended for the management of home PN patients. This includes a physician, nurse practitioner, dietitian, social worker, pharmacist, and psychologist. Members of the home PN team assist with determining the eligibility for home PN, training, developing the home regimen before discharge, and education with the family. They also meet with the inpatient team and primary care physician and discuss objectives and goals for the patient, and are responsible for adjustments and monitoring at home. Parents and guardians need to document competency with line care and PN setup, as well as an understanding of pumps and infusion rates and addition of vitamins and other additives to the PN solution. A nurse from the home care company usually visits the family the first night the PN is infused at home to assist the family with the setup and technique. It is essential the patient have long-term central access. The patient's PN may be cycled for 8 to16 hours, depending on the individual's needs, tolerance, and size.

Complications are similar to those described in the earlier section on metabolic complications. Common complications include line sepsis, line malfunction including occlusion, tunnel infections, PN-associated liver disease, bone disease, and abnormal micronutrient status: either deficiency or excessive levels depending on the patient and underlying disease state.*

---

*References 73,155,156,169,182,183.

TABLE 88-12. Home Parenteral Nutrition Laboratory Monitoring

Monthly-quarterly	Serum electrolytes, liver function tests, bilirubin (total, unconjugated, conjugated), complete blood cell count, reticulocyte count, iron studies
Biannually	Serum selenium, chromium, zinc, vitamin A, E, D (25-hydroxy), copper, ceruloplasmin, manganese, carnitine, prothrombin time or PIVKA II level
Yearly	Dual-energy x-ray absorptiometry scan

Sepsis can be a difficult complication to manage in certain home PN patients. All patients with possible line sepsis need to be evaluated and blood cultures obtained from the line as well as from a peripheral vein. In addition, patients need to have their line site examined and other possible sources of infection excluded. Other laboratory tests that need to be performed include complete blood count with differential, clotting function, comprehensive metabolic panel, triglyceride level, and evaluation for disseminated intravascular coagulation. Most line infections can be treated through the line, but in the case of persistent bacterial or fungal sepsis, the line may need to be removed. Once the sepsis has been cleared, the line will need to be replaced. Catheter-related thrombosis and occlusion of vessels in patients on home PN have been described.[184]

MONITORING THE HOME PN PATIENT

All home PN patients need to be monitored closely for growth and nutritional status, advancement of enteral feeds, and laboratory status. Guidelines have been developed, and laboratory values are usually obtained weekly after discharge until a stable regimen has been achieved.[41,185] Thereafter the frequency of laboratory testing is gradually decreased to once per month. Vitamin, trace element, and carnitine levels are checked every 3 to 6 months. Bone densitometry evaluations should be obtained at the initiation of PN and then every 1 to 2 years depending on the presence and severity of bone disease. Table 88-12 provides an example of laboratory monitoring guidelines.[186]

Normal long-term growth can be achieved in patients on home PN who receive enteral and parenteral nutrition. Those whose primary source of nutrition is parenteral may not grow as well.[186] Improved growth has been seen with correction of essential fatty acid and trace element deficiency, correction of a coexisting endocrine disorder, and supplementation of α-ketoglutarate deficiency.[187] Some studies have shown normal developmental function in patients on home PN and defects in perceptual motor function, but overall normal functioning can be achieved.[188,189]

SUMMARY

There have been significant developments in the field of parenteral nutrition for neonatal and pediatric patients to provide safer and more appropriate nutritional regimens. Continuing efforts need to focus on the development of more concrete parenteral nutrition guidelines for both macronutrient and micronutrient needs in chronic disease, as well as determining the effectiveness of parenteral nutrients and additives.

REFERENCES

3. Price PT. Parenteral nutrition: administering and monitoring. In: Groh-Wargo S, Thompson M, Cox J, editors. Nutritional Care for High-Risk Newborns. 3rd ed. Chicago: Precept Press; 2000. p. 91–108.

5. Pittiruti M, Hamilton H, Biffi R, et al. ESPEN guidelines on parenteral nutrition: central venous catheters (access, care, diagnosis of complications). Clin Nutr 2009;28:365–377.

100. Koretz RL, Lipman TO, Klein S. AGA Technical Review on parenteral nutrition. Gastroenterology 2001;121:970–1001.

101. Shulman RJ, Phillips S. Parenteral Nutrition in infants and children. J Pediatr Gastroenterol Nutr 2003;36:421–441.

107. Greene HL, Hambidge M, Schanler R, Tsang RC. Guidelines for the use of vitamins, trace elements, calcium, magnesium and phosphorus in infants and children receiving total parenteral nutrition: report of the Subcommittee on Pediatric Parenteral Nutrient Requirements from the Committee on Clinical Practice Issues of the American Society for Clinical Nutrition. Am J Clin Nutr 1988;48:1324–1342.

See expertconsult.com for a complete list of references and the review questions for this chapter.

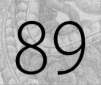

89

ENTERAL NUTRITION

Lesley Smith • Jennifer Garcia

The normal route of entry for nutrients into the body is via the gastrointestinal tract. When it is not possible to maintain adequate growth and nutritional status by oral feeding alone, supplemental or sole feeding by the enteral route is preferred over the use of parenteral feeding when the gut is intact (and even sometimes when it is compromised).[1] Use of the gastrointestinal tract maintains gut integrity, utilizes and induces the specialized transport systems available for nutrients, and increases intestinal cell mass.[2,3] Enteral feeding stimulates pancreatic enzymes and intestinal disaccharidases and promotes physiologic neurohumoral mechanisms important in enhancing gut and hepatobiliary function including motility.[4-6] Enteral feeding also avoids the complications associated with total parenteral nutrition (TPN) including cholestasis, sepsis, and thrombosis and is considerably less expensive and time-consuming to administer.[7,8] Enteral feeding provides trophic nutrients such as glutamine, trace elements, short-chain fatty acids, and fiber and stimulates epithelial growth factor and glucagon-like peptide II production, which are usually not present in TPN.[9] The addition of prebiotics such as oligosaccharides (to positively influence colonic flora) and fish oils (to reduce inflammation by prostaglandin modulation) to defined formulas is also currently of interest.[10-14] The goal of enteral feeding should be to support and maintain growth and development in the face of the metabolic challenges faced by children with acute or chronic disease who are unable or unwilling to maintain an adequate oral intake.

This chapter summarizes the indications for enteral nutrition support in childhood disease; the appropriate nutritional care of the hospitalized malnourished child; the types of enteral feeding available and their specific uses; the composition of enteral feeds for the preterm and term neonate, infant, child, and adolescent; practical issues of enteral feeding; complications pertaining to its use and the method of delivery; and enteral nutrition support in the community.

MALNUTRITION IN THE HOSPITAL SETTING

Malnutrition in hospitalized children is recognized as common even in the developed world.[15] Malnutrition may occur quite rapidly in the face of acute disease necessitating hospital admission and is particularly of concern in critically ill patients nursed in the pediatric intensive care unit, in postsurgical patients facing unforeseen complications, in traumatized patients with increased metabolic needs, on oncology units during and following chemotherapy or bone marrow transplantation, and in the burn unit. Malnutrition may also occur on a chronic basis in patients who are hospitalized for weeks or months, often following a bout of critical illness. The significant occurrence of malnutrition in children in hospital has led to the concept

of risk assessment at admission and on an ongoing basis during the hospital stay (see Chapter 86 for more on nutritional assessment).[16]

The global severity of this problem is addressed by the World Health Organization (WHO) in its manual for physicians and other senior health workers, which provides a protocolized management tool for severely malnourished children, but deals mainly with the issue of primary malnutrition.[17] Malnutrition in hospitalized children in the developed world is usually of a secondary nature and contributes significantly to mortality in a variety of severe acute and chronic diseases of childhood, interferes with recovery from surgery, and is economically costly.[18,19] It has been recommended that patients hospitalized with malnutrition not be discharged until the attainment of 90% of the median WHO/National Center for Health Statistics (NCHS) reference values for weight-for-height, a goal that is often difficult to achieve in the developed world with hospital bed pressures and that is often not practical or economically feasible in developing countries. Despite this, acknowledgment of the issue and the development of nutrition support teams within hospitals have influenced the incidence and prognosis of the condition.[20] The prevalence of malnutrition in hospitalized patients globally seems to have been consistently as high as 30% over the past 20 years.[21,22] Hendricks et al. showed that the incidence of acute malnutrition in hospitalized children fell from 33 to 25% from 1979 to 1995 and chronic malnutrition from 55 to 27%.[23] Despite the improvement, the issue of malnutrition in the hospital remains significant. The early institution of enteral feeding in the face of inadequate oral intake in the hospital has consistently been shown to improve outcomes following acute and chronic illnesses. Increasingly, community care teams (often called home enteral feeding teams) are being utilized to successfully care for children with a need for nutritional support in their own homes on a chronic basis.

INDICATIONS FOR ENTERAL FEEDING (TABLE 89-1)

Inadequate Intake

Inadequate intake may be caused by any disease that disrupts the normal oral phase of ingestion for anatomical or functional reasons, chronic diseases that elaborate anorexia-inducing cytokines, and psychogenic states causing food aversion. Severe head, neck, and oral trauma may make it impossible to achieve significant oral intake, and head and neck tumors, particularly those that affect the nasopharynx or mouth, may interfere with ingestion. Lesions affecting the brainstem may significantly impair mastication and swallowing mechanisms, and chemotherapy or radiotherapy may induce severe

TABLE 89-1. Indications for Enteral Feeding

Inadequate Intake
Severe head and neck trauma
Tumors of the oropharynx, head, and neck
Severe mucositis
Brainstem injury or neoplasm
Caustic injury to mouth and esophagus
Cleft lip and palate
Tracheoesophageal fistula
Other congenital and acquired disorders of oropharyngeal function
Anorexia of chronic disease
Psychogenic food aversion
Anorexia nervosa

Gastrointestinal Dysfunction, Hepatobiliary Disease, and Malabsorption
Short bowel syndrome
Chronic intestinal pseudo-obstruction
Inflammatory bowel disease
Autoimmune enteropathy
Allergic enteropathy
Intractable diarrhea
Celiac disease
Severe gastroesophageal reflux
Acute pancreatitis
Chronic cholestasis and liver transplantation

Critical Illness

Growth Failure Associated with Chronic Disease
Cardiac disease
  Cyanotic congenital heart disease with pulmonary hypertension
Respiratory disease
  BPD
  Cystic fibrosis
  Pulmonary disorders requiring lung transplantation
Renal failure
  Chronic peritoneal dialysis
Neurologic disease
  Acute neurologic dysfunction
  Cerebral palsy
  Neuromuscular disease
  Degenerative disease
Oncologic disease and bone marrow transplantation
Hypermetabolic states
  HIV/AIDS
  Head injury, trauma, and surgery
  Burns
Metabolic disease
  Glycogen storage disease type 1

AIDS, acquired immunodeficiency syndrome; BPD, bronchopulmonary dysplasia; HIV, human immunodeficiency virus

mucositis. Caustic injuries to the mouth and esophagus may also acutely impair intake, although sufficiently severe injury causing stricture may require long-term feeding by nasogastric tube, or gastrostomy feeding. Congenital disorders of the palate, pharynx, larynx, and esophagus may also impair ingestion and swallowing mechanisms. Children with cleft lip and palate and those with tracheoesophageal fistula are particularly at risk. The latter frequently have esophageal strictures and esophageal motility disorders and are prone to gastroesophageal reflux. In general, such patients require relatively short-term support. Infants with swallowing dysfunction where no anatomical lesion or chronic neurologic condition have been identified may also require temporary nutritional support while normal physiologic mechanisms mature. Depending on the severity of the problem and the likely length of support required, this may be provided by means of nasogastric or gastrostomy feeding, or, if there is a significant risk of aspiration, by jejunal feeding.

Many children with chronic systemic disease, particularly if these involve significant inflammation, may develop impaired intake that is largely due to the presence of circulating cytokines that are anorexigenic, such as tumor necrosis factor α (TNF-α). Lastly, but important, anorexia nervosa in adolescents and food aversion states of a psychogenic nature that may occur in infancy or early childhood may also require supplemental enteral feeding, in some cases to preserve life. The care of such patients is often difficult and the intervention poorly tolerated by anorexic patients, who may be noncompliant and controlling. Multidisciplinary care teams, inpatient care, and intensive community support are essential in the usually long-term management of children and adolescents with these disorders.

Gastrointestinal Disease, Malabsorption, and Hepatobiliary Disease

Short bowel syndrome occurring as a result of surgical treatment for congenital disorders of the gastrointestinal (GI) tract in infancy (e.g., gastroschisis, intestinal atresias, Hirschsprung's disease), acquired disease (e.g., volvulus, necrotizing enterocolitis), or intestinal failure caused by congenital disorders of absorption or chronic intestinal pseudo-obstruction (e.g., microvillus inclusion disease, megacystis-microcolon hypoperistalsis syndrome) usually require nutritional support. Initially this support may need to be provided by the parenteral route, but gradually enteral feeding is introduced to the maximum tolerated, as this has been shown to promote intestinal adaptation and reduce TPN-associated cholestasis and sepsis. Careful attention must be paid to fluid and electrolyte balance, because these patients may have significant vomiting, stomal losses, or diarrhea, and the choice of feeding in terms of its macronutrient composition and osmolality is important in management of these challenges. In general, long-chain triglycerides promote intestinal adaptation, and thus defined formulas that include hydrolyzed protein, low-osmolality glucose polymers, and long-chain fat may optimize gut function.[24] However, limited absorptive capacity may make a formula containing a significant proportion of fat in the form of medium-chain triglyceride a more rational choice, especially if there is significant hepatobiliary dysfunction as a result of TPN-associated cholestasis. Cycling of TPN in association with continuous and then intermittent enteral feeding is associated with a lower risk of TPN-associated liver failure. The period required for adaptation and thus nutritional support is highly variable depending on the length and function of the remaining bowel, but may be months or years.

Inflammatory bowel diseases such as Crohn's disease and ulcerative colitis often result in a requirement for supplemental nutrition.[25] Because Crohn's disease may involve the small bowel, where significant nutrient absorption takes place, it more frequently requires nutrition support on a long-term basis.[26] Sole enteral feeding by nasogastric tube in Crohn's disease may be used to induce remission in mild to moderately active disease, thus avoiding the systemic side effects of steroids, and both polymeric whole-protein and defined formula diets ("elemental" formulas) have been shown to have beneficial effects on acute inflammatory parameters and to promote weight gain and growth. Recent confirmation of the utility of this approach continues to accumulate from Europe and

Australia, but this modality has not found much support or practice in North America.[27,28] Inflammatory parameters may decrease much earlier (3 days) than the simple improvement in nutrition afforded by the use of enteral nutrition.[29] Continuation of supplementation of calories by nocturnal enteral feeding after induction of remission may be associated with prolongation of remission. Children with small bowel disease seem to do better than those with colonic disease. Supplemental enteral feeding may be used during acute exacerbations to reverse catabolism and may be used chronically by nocturnal feeding via nasogastric tube or gastrostomy to reverse growth failure.[30] Supplemental enteral feeding can be useful in promoting anabolism in children with ulcerative colitis undergoing exacerbation or awaiting colectomy. However, modulation of the disease itself by using elemental enteral feeding does not occur with ulcerative colitis patients.[28]

Children with autoimmune or allergic enteropathy may also require enteral nutrition to achieve appropriate weight gain, and those with allergic disorders may need formulas that contain hydrolyzed protein.[31] In some cases, severe allergic enteropathy may require a peptide- or amino acid–based formula. Depending on the severity of the mucosal injury, the fat may be provided in the form of long-chain triglycerides (LCT) to promote repair or a mix of MCT and LCT to promote absorption in the face of severe loss of villous surface area. When the prognosis is good for eventual reversal of the condition, as in cow's milk protein hypersensitivity or where food elimination diets are effective, this support is only likely to be required in the short term. However, patients with severe enteropathy that is poorly controlled may require extensive and prolonged support that can usually be provided in the home. Patients with severe, intractable diarrhea who do not respond to a food elimination diet may recover more quickly if fed enterally compared with parenteral feeding, although severe monosaccharide intolerance may preclude this route of feeding. In such cases, an elemental feed is usually required, and the protein may need to be fully hydrolyzed to amino acids. Enteral feeding supports a more rapid return of intestinal disaccharidase function.

In celiac disease, it is rare to require enteral feeding once a gluten-free diet has been instituted. However, from time to time and usually in infancy, nasogastric feeding with a lactose-free polymeric formula may be necessary for nutritional rehabilitation. Infants with severe gastroesophageal reflux and growth failure may also require enteral nutrition supplementation until their disease comes under control with medication or surgery.

Acute pancreatitis has been shown to increase the rate of protein catabolism by 80% and energy expenditure by 20%.[32] The standard of care for patients with acute pancreatitis requiring nutritional support is enteral rather than parenteral feeding, and early support is advocated, safe, and effective.[33] There are very few pediatric, but a wealth of adult, data to support this assertion. Evidence from meta-analyses and randomized, controlled clinical trials in adults shows that enteral feeding, if provided distal to the ligament of Treitz, is superior to parenteral feeding in acute pancreatitis. Jejunal feeding has been associated with a significantly lower incidence of infections, reduced surgical interventions to control pancreatitis, lower metabolic complication rate, improved gut barrier function, reduced oxidative stress, and decreased length of hospital stay and is significantly less costly when compared to parenteral feeding.[34] Enteral feeding is safe even in instances of severe necrosis and is best provided early in the case of moderate to severe pancreatitis, although no specific benefits in terms of survival have been demonstrated. Supplementation of calories by jejunal feeding in chronic pancreatitis has also been found to be helpful, especially when surgery or transplantation is contemplated. This is an uncommon condition in pediatric patients, and there are no data presently available in children to support this practice.[35]

Malnutrition associated with chronic cholestasis is common in children and is especially important in infancy, when it can be associated with poor neurodevelopmental outcomes and with decreased survival following liver transplantation.[36,37] Specific micronutrient deficiencies, especially of fat-soluble vitamins and essential fatty acids, may occur.[38] Both nasogastric and gastrostomy feeding have been shown to be safe and effective in promoting catch-up growth, improving body composition, anthropometric parameters, and weight gain without an effect specifically on growth factors such as insulinlike growth factor 1 (IGF-1) and IGF-binding proteins.[39-41] Enteral feeding does not result in an increase in ammonia concentration or the development of encephalopathy in such patients.[42] Severe portal hypertension has been felt to be a relative contraindication to the placement of percutaneous endoscopic or radiologic gastrostomy tubes, particularly if there is hypersplenism and severe thrombocytopenia, because of the risk of bleeding and organ trauma. Transplant surgeons should be consulted before a gastrostomy is placed, because this may provide a challenge during the transplant operation with further upper abdominal adhesions.

Critical Illness

Patients with critical illness in the pediatric intensive care unit (PICU) face significant metabolic stress as a result of shock, sepsis, trauma, burns, severe inflammation, organ failure, or other extensive tissue injury and elaborate cytokines that increase the resting energy expenditure by as much as 30% in mild to moderate stress and 50% in severe stress.[43] Pharmacologic neuromuscular paralysis and sedation may reduce this requirement. Despite this significant hypermetabolism, caloric intake is often limited in the early stages of illness because of fluid management and medications, and paralysis may make enteral feeding difficult. Enteral nutrition during critical illness helps to maintain gastrointestinal form and function, enhances immunocompetence, and attenuates the metabolic consequences of the stress response. Interestingly, however, the use of formulas designed to be immunomodulatory has not been shown to improve outcomes in patients admitted in septic shock or who develop infections in the unit.[44] Clinical studies have shown that early institution of enteral feeding within 24-48 hours of hospital admission is beneficial in improving patient outcome and survival. Transpyloric feeding may be of benefit in the ventilated patient, especially if pharmacologic paralysis can be weaned, and jejunal tubes can usually be placed by a simple bedside insufflation technique and, failing that, endoscopically.[45,46] However, there are several studies that show that intragastric feeding is usually possible in the intubated and ventilated PICU patient and should usually be tried before using the transpyloric route.[47,48] Once the patient is extubated and if the aspiration risk is deemed to be minimal, then nasogastric feeding and progression to bolus feeding can usually be achieved provided gastrointestinal function has not been compromised by the illness or its treatment.[49] Indeed, studies have shown that there is no significant difference between continuous and bolus feeding (in terms of tolerance) in the PICU patient.[50,51] However, achieving early enteral feeding goals is challenging in terms of calories, because frequent feeding interruptions (usually for procedures) can reduce the caloric intake to around 50% of the desired level.[52,53] The introduction of enteral feeding protocols within the unit has been successful in improving the attainment of these goals.[54,55]

GROWTH FAILURE ASSOCIATED WITH CHRONIC DISEASE

Cardiac Disease

Children and especially infants with chronic cardiac disease, either congenital or acquired, often require supplemental nutrition during acute exacerbations of their disease, such as heart failure or infection that increase their energy needs.[56] Growth impairment may occur also because of the nature of the hemodynamic lesion, especially if there is chronic heart failure, tissue hypoxia, acidosis and increased metabolic needs due to stress, impaired intake due to dyspnea or associated gastroesophageal reflux, and malabsorption due to lymphangiectasia or bowel edema. Cyanotic patients with pulmonary hypertension appear to be the most at risk for adverse nutritional outcomes.[57] The impaired intake may be improved by supplemental nasogastric feeding, but because of limitations on fluid intake, the formula may need to be concentrated initially to 24 kcal/oz and sometimes as much as 30 kcal/oz. Judicious use of enteral feeding can promote anabolism in the infant with congenital heart disease awaiting surgery (where resting energy expenditures are often high) and improve surgical outcomes.[58] Continuous enteral feeding appears to be the most efficacious means of provision.[59] Care in the concentration of formulas may be required so as not to provide too high a renal solute load in the face of fluid restriction and use of diuretics. These children may also have impaired gastric motility and delayed gastric emptying, which may decrease intake and increase gastroesophageal reflux. Gastrostomy feeding may be helpful if nutritional support is required on a chronic basis, and continuous nocturnal feeding is the preferred means of provision, with children taking intermittent bolus feeding by mouth or by tube during the day.[60] Lymphangiectasia (which may be relatively common following the Fontan procedure) and chylous ascites/pleural effusion following surgery may require the use of formulas containing a large proportion of medium-chain triglyceride (such as Pregestimil or Portagen) for prolonged periods of support.

Respiratory Illness

Preterm infants with bronchopulmonary dysplasia may have growth failure for a variety of reasons, including poor sucking and swallowing mechanisms, poor intake due to circulating inflammatory cytokines, increased work of breathing, hypoxia and oxygen dependence, hypercapnia, and recurrent vomiting due to gastric emptying and reflux.[61] They may require hypercaloric supplementation up to 30 kcal/oz, best achieved by a mix of fat and carbohydrate modulars in equal amounts.[62] However, overzealous carbohydrate supplementation may aggravate existing hypercapnia, and attention must be paid to electrolytes, particularly if diuretics are required for associated heart failure.

Children with cystic fibrosis (CF) have elevated caloric needs due to the increased work of breathing and resting energy expenditures. They also frequently have decreased intake as a result of circulating cytokines from the chronic inflammatory processes in their lungs and increased caloric losses due to maldigestion and absorption from chronic pancreatic insufficiency and hepatobiliary dysfunction.[63] For this reason, early institution of a high-calorie diet is an important component of the care of such children, and supplementary enteral nutrition by nasogastric feeding may be required during acute exacerbations of pulmonary disease. However, the chronic nutritional care of children with CF is important in maintaining a positive energy balance, preventing respiratory muscle fatigue, and preventing micronutrient deficiencies such as fat-soluble vitamin and essential fatty acid deficiency. Oral supplementation with a high-calorie polymeric product is advocated first, and if patients are still unable to ingest sufficient calories to maintain desirable growth parameters, then supplemental nutrition with polymeric or defined enteral formulas by nasogastric tube (often provided nocturnally) may be instituted and on a short-term basis has proved very beneficial. The long-term use of nasogastric (NG) feeding often leads to noncompliance, however, and if supplemental nutrition is still required on a chronic basis, then consideration of placement of an enterostomy tube should be undertaken. Nocturnal gastrostomy or jejunostomy feeding of a long-term nature is being undertaken with benefit more frequently in malnourished patients with cystic fibrosis.[64] Gastrostomy tube feeding post double lung transplant for cystic fibrosis is associated with better weight gain than oral intake alone in the first year posttransplant.[65]

Children with other severe chronic pulmonary diseases, and especially those awaiting lung transplantation, also require close nutritional observation and early institution of supplemental feeding by the enteral route if required.[66] Avoidance of parenteral nutrition is preferred because of the additional risks of sepsis and the contribution of highly concentrated intravenous glucose sources to hypercapnia. Maintenance of a positive energy balance pretransplant is important in the clinical outcome of children following lung transplantation.[67]

Renal Disease

Children with renal failure, particularly those in whom the disease was congenital or acquired in infancy, frequently exhibit impaired nutritional status and developmental delay. This may occur because of metabolic acidosis, chronic electrolyte disturbances, protein-calorie malnutrition, endocrine abnormalities, osteodystrophy, gastroesophageal reflux, and delayed gastric emptying. Nutritional supplementation during peritoneal dialysis (PD) and nasogastric or gastrostomy feeding have been safe and associated with improved outcomes including neurologic development.[68-70] Gastrostomy tubes have often been placed at the same time as Tenckhoff catheter insertion for PD and need to be placed before cycling PD is started; percutaneous endoscopic gastrostomy (PEG) placement during PD is unsafe.[71] Gastrostomy buttons may be placed safely as early as 4 weeks post PEG insertion,[72] though many clinicians prefer to wait longer (8 to 12 weeks). Nocturnal nasogastric feeding for up to 12 hours a day has resulted in catch-up growth and normalization of weight parameters, especially if started before the age of 2 years.[73] The importance of early preventive intervention must be emphasized, because it can be difficult to repair chronic deficits later.

Neurologic Disease

The nutritional impact of neurologic disease is variable and depends on the severity and distribution of the disability involved. Determinants include the ability to orally feed and swallow, hyper- or hypotonia, mobility, severity of impairment, cognitive ability, and gastrointestinal complications of neurologic dysfunction including gastroesophageal reflux, delayed gastric emptying, and constipation.[74] In the acute phase of spinal injury, early enteral feeding has been associated with improved nutritional outcomes and appears to be safe. Most patients can be fed by NG tube, although occasionally nasojejunal (NJ) feeding may be required if there are high gastric residuals.[75] Children with cerebral palsy involving spastic quadriparesis and cognitive delay frequently are unable to achieve sufficient caloric intake to maintain growth and development and will thus require chronic enteral feeding via a permanent enterostomy.[76,77] Recent publications have emphasized the need for new methods of assessing resting energy expenditure in nonambulatory tube-fed patients with severe neurodevelopmental disabilities and have led to a downward assessment of energy needs.[78] However, increased energy needs may be seen in the face of choreoathetosis or with severe contractures. Chronic, progressive neurologic diseases, especially of a degenerative nature, usually also require nutritional intervention and support for the duration of life. Feeding in these severe cases usually occurs via continuous nocturnal gastrostomy feeding with bolus supplements if tolerated in the daytime. The risk of aspiration from above due to swallowing dysfunction and from below due to gastroesophageal reflux disease (GERD) will determine the choice of feeding route. Considerations with regard to the composition of feeding include fluid intake (because often not enough free water is provided), caloric density, osmolality, and fiber intake in such children. If it is anticipated that a transition to oral feeding may occur, then adequate oral stimulation, even of a nonnutritive nature, should be provided.

Oncologic Disease and Bone Marrow Transplantation

The systemic effects of malignant disease, the side effects of necessary treatment involving chemotherapy and radiotherapy, and complications such as sepsis contribute to malnutrition in the pediatric oncology patient.[79] Cachexia with significant weight loss and growth failure may occur as a result of increased metabolic rate and circulating cytokines (TNF-α, interleukin-1, and interleukin-6) inducing anorexia, increased whole-body protein breakdown, increased lipolysis, and increased gluconeogenesis. Food intake may be reduced as a consequence of nausea, vomiting, dysgeusia, mucositis, and xerostomia. Acute illnesses such as neutropenic fever and infections place further nutritional stress on the child with oncologic disease by increasing metabolic rate and catabolism. Some children may suffer palatal and pharyngeal dysfunction with subsequent swallowing difficulties as a result of radiotherapy to the head and neck. Children with intestinal lymphomas and other intestinal tumors may suffer malabsorption and subacute obstruction, which can often still be supported with enteral nutrition. Emphasis is now being placed on "room service" for patients at

significant risk, with good nutritional choices of whole foods available in a "just-in-time" fashion on the oncology unit itself and where possible the fresh food itself is cooked locally rather than centrally. Nutritional difficulties often stress the child and parents from a psychologic perspective, and a multidisciplinary approach to the support of the family is required, with careful preparation for supplemental enteral feeding by the nasal or enterostomal approach. PEG for chronic nutritional support is effective and safe if performed in oncology patients when they are not neutropenic, thrombocytopenic, or septic.[80]

Nutritional insult after bone marrow transplantation is common because the conditioning and treatment regimes cause considerable gastrointestinal disturbance, nausea, and vomiting, and mucositis may be severe. Enteral feeding is both cheaper and easier to provide than parenteral nutrition and avoids venous catheter-related complications.[81,82] Intense multidisciplinary counseling is necessary to ensure success, because tubes may need to be replaced and mucositis may cause significant pain, requiring morphine infusion. Children undergoing bone marrow transplantation benefit from early enteral feeding with improved weight gain and anthropometric parameters, and this route of caloric supplementation is preferred over TPN, decreasing the incidence of graft-versus-host disease and decreasing mortality from infection.[83,84] Interestingly, diarrhea does not seem to be more of a problem with enteral feeding compared with TPN, and common micronutrient deficiencies such as hypomagnesemia, hypophosphatemia, and zinc and selenium deficiency are not different between enterally and parenterally fed children.

HYPERMETABOLIC STATES

HIV/AIDS

Pediatric patients with human immunodeficiency virus infection/acquired immunodeficiency syndrome (HIV/AIDS) are often at risk nutritionally because inflammatory processes and sepsis associated with the condition elevate metabolic rate and the side effects of the drugs required for management of the disease often give rise to nausea, vomiting, and diarrhea, limiting intake. Protein-calorie malnutrition and malabsorption are relatively common in children with established AIDS and often require nutritional support via nasogastric or gastrostomy feeding.[85] In addition, such tubes may be required to administer the drugs because children frequently find them unpalatable. Malnutrition itself may further impair immune function. Deficiencies of micronutrients including zinc, iron, selenium, B_2, B_6, B_{12}, carnitine, vitamin A, vitamin D, and essential fatty acids may occur, and vitamin B_{12} and vitamin A deficiency may influence the rate of mother-to-infant transmission of the disease in developing countries.[86] Micronutrient repletion may slow progression of the disease, increasing growth and T lymphocyte function in the case of zinc. Energy repletion may increase the CD4 count.[87] Antiviral treatment with protease inhibitors is important, as decreased viral load correlates with a positive outcome in nutritional support.[88]

Head Injury, Trauma, and Surgery

Children with uncomplicated severe, closed head injuries have been demonstrated to have resting energy expenditures similar to patients with burns and require appropriate enteral support, usually given via NJ tube in the ICU while ventilated, and by

NG tube on the ward once stable from a cardiorespiratory point of view, or by gastrostomy feeding if the duration is likely to exceed 2 months. In the surgical patient, postoperative enteral feeding has been associated with reduced sepsis, improved wound healing, enhanced gut mucosal barrier function, and increased mass of gut-associated lymphoid tissue (GALT) as well as prevention of bacterial translocation. Posttrauma surgical patients may benefit with improved nitrogen balance and nutritional status if fed early in the postoperative phase via the enteral route, although the choice of route and type of feeding is determined by the operative intervention. Early provision of enteral nutrition even in the face of gut resection by transpyloric and transanastomotic routes has been advocated for the neonate (premature or otherwise) undergoing gut resection for necrotizing enterocolitis, volvulus, or congenital malformation.[89] The child undergoing orthopedic spinal manipulation is at risk for superior mesenteric artery syndrome, which may be obviated by feeding distal to the relative obstruction. Any child expected to have limited oral intake of greater than 5 days' duration or sooner if at nutritional risk before surgery should have supplemental enteral nutrition provided as soon as feasible postoperatively.

Burns

Early enteral nutritional support is believed to improve gastrointestinal, immunologic, nutritional, and metabolic responses to critical injury in burned patients.[90] Enteral feeding has been shown to reduce caloric deficits and promote insulin secretion and protein retention.[91] Gut-derived endotoxemia and increased intestinal permeability are also improved by early feeding after thermal injury and reduce the rate of enterogenic sepsis.[92] Indeed, intolerance to enteral feeding has been seen as an early marker preceding overt sepsis.[93] In adult studies, early successful enteral feeding after burn injury has been associated with significantly decreased mortality. In very young children with mild to moderate burns (8 to 25% of body surface area [BSA]) who nevertheless had hypermetabolism with resting energy expenditures (REEs) averaging 130% of normal, early enteral feeding normalized protein status and significantly increased energy intake.[94] Immediate enteral feeding following burn injury even in ventilated patients has been shown to be safe and effective without an increase in aspiration through the judicious use of nasojejunal and nasogastric feeding.[95] Some children with moderate burn injury, but who are not in shock, may be resuscitated using enteral feeding safely, ameliorating the hormonal stress response and improving outcomes.[96] Most severely burned children require frequent surgery for wound debridement and skin grafts, and the promotion of enteral feeding through the extensive perioperative period has been associated with a reduction in caloric deficits, wound infections, and requirement for exogenous albumin supplementation.[97] Early in the postburn period, a hydrolyzed defined formula may be helpful if a polymeric formula is not well tolerated, with emphasis on a high-protein, high-calorie intake.

Metabolic Disease

Glycogen storage disease type 1 usually requires the institution of nocturnal supplementation, usually with cornstarch, to prevent hypoglycemia and to reduce hypertriglyceridemia. Other metabolic syndromes require specialized formulas to treat the disease and avoid the effects of accumulated toxic substrates. A team approach to the management of these children is advocated with strong input from the nutrition support service.

CHOICE OF ENTERAL FEEDING ROUTE

Oral Feeding

The choice of feeding route depends on the functional status of the child.[98] Even when adequate intake cannot be achieved in total by mouth, preservation of this route of feeding for even partial nutrition is recommended because it preserves normal physiology and function and is psychologically satisfying for the child and family. Coma, ventilation, head and neck trauma or tumors, severe mucositis following chemotherapy, impaired swallowing mechanisms, and risk for aspiration may preclude this route of feeding.

Enteral Feeding

Once the requirement has been established, enteral feeding may be provided for the patient with short-term needs, for example, after trauma or during a bout of severe pancreatitis. It may be necessary to continue nutrition support for prolonged periods of time such as with chronic renal or liver disease or indefinitely in the case of patients with chronic neurologic dysfunction. The type of feeding required and the route by which it is provided depend on the individual circumstances of the child, but in general the use of nasoenteric tubes is preferred where the time required for nutritional support is likely to be short (less than 8 weeks), and enterostomy tubes are preferred for long-term use. The gastric route is preferred over delivery into the jejunum to maintain gastric barrier function and the normal pulsatile delivery of nutrients to the small bowel. However, patients in coma, requiring ventilatory support and pharmacologically paralyzed, at risk of aspiration, with severe gastroesophageal reflux or delayed gastric emptying, or with pancreatitis may require jejunal feeding, which must be given continuously to avoid overdistention and the metabolic equivalent of dumping syndrome. Long-term jejunal feeding is difficult from a practical perspective, especially at home, where tubes may be frequently dislodged accidentally. An algorithm for the choice of enteral feeding route is found in Figure 89-1.

Polyvinyl nasogastric tubes may only be used for a few days before they become stiff and traumatizing to the nares and thus should only be used for very short-term feeding, or should be changed frequently. Tubes made of silicone or polyurethane can be used for prolonged periods and are soft, comfortable, and flexible.[99] Polyurethane tubes have a greater internal diameter than silicone tubes for the same external diameter and therefore may block less easily. Evidence is accumulating that the durability of polyurethane tubes is significantly greater than that of silicone tubes, and polyurethane tubes should therefore be used when it is likely that they will required for prolonged periods of time.[100] Such NG tubes often have weighted tips, theoretically to allow for easier onward passage into the duodenum or jejunum and to prevent easy dislodgement. However, studies have shown that such weighting is probably unnecessary and some weights may be too large to allow easy passage into the small bowel.[101] Tube sizes between 5 and 8 Fr are appropriate for most pediatric indications and with patients and caregivers trained in their placement. With appropriate psychologic support, even very young children can be trained to place their own tubes.

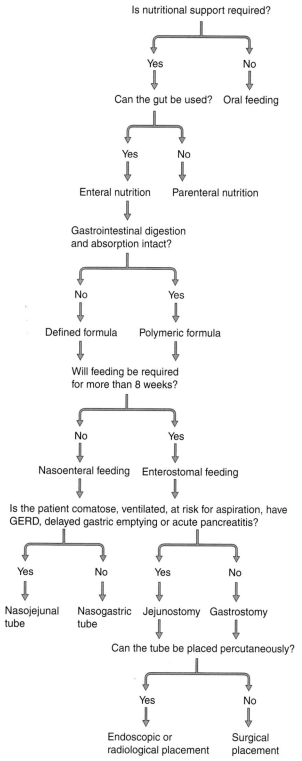

Figure 89.1. Algorithm for enteral feeding.

appears to be as safe as endoscopic placement using the most common pull technique and has a similar complication rate.[104] Care should be exercised in patients with ventriculoperitoneal shunts, and PEG should probably only be performed if the shunt is placed in the right side of the abdomen. PEG is also contraindicated when the patient has already started peritoneal dialysis, because of a high rate of complications such as peritonitis, but may be placed safely before the dialysis is commenced.[71] Percutaneous gastrostomy placement may be contraindicated in patients who have had previous upper abdominal surgery; have significant ascites, portal hypertension, or hepatosplenomegaly; in the presence of an abdominal tumor; or in obesity. The main complication of cellulitis occurring after PEG placement can be prevented by a single dose of intravenous broad-spectrum antibiotic given at the time of placement and avoidance of tension on the outer bolster. However, confirmation of the tube in the stomach, preferably endoscopically, should occur before it is used. To prevent the complication of bowel interpolation between the abdominal wall and the stomach, approaches using localization by endoscopic ultrasound or by laparoscopic visualization have been advocated but are not routinely used.[105,106] Mechanical irritation of the stomach may occur with any tube, and intermittent blockage of the pylorus may occur in those that can migrate such as Malechot or Foley catheters placed surgically.

Gastrostomy buttons may be placed usually 6 to 8 weeks after primary tube placement, sometimes without anesthesia if the tube is traction-removable. The time interval should probably be longer, up to 12 weeks, in patients who are significantly immunocompromised and may have poor wound healing. Button gastrostomies are preferred by most families because they lie flush to the skin and therefore cannot be easily pulled out, and tubing is just attached by a locking method at the time of feeding. Those with inflatable internal bolsters are less traumatic to place and remove but are more prone to breakage than those with deformable internal bolsters, which may tear, disrupt the tract, or cause perforation (2%). The durability of button gastrostomies is 5 to 6 months, usually requiring removal and replacement because of internal rupture of the gastric balloon.[107] Some children at significant risk of aspiration due to GERD, particularly those with neurologic impairment, may require a surgical antireflux procedure with or without a pyloroplasty for delayed gastric emptying and a surgically placed gastrostomy.[108] Such patients might also be successfully managed by placement of a gastrojejunal tube, but this is usually difficult to sustain on a long-term basis. However, unless the symptoms of GERD are severe or aspiration has already occurred, or both, it is preferred to assess the patients first by way of a trial of nasogastric feeding. If this is tolerated, it is likely that fundoplication is not required at that time, although it may be in the future.

Jejunal tubes may be placed nasally, via a gastrostomy, or directly into the jejunum by a percutaneous or surgical approach. Surgical approaches have been both open and direct, but laparoscopic and Roux-en-Y approaches to surgical jejunostomies have also been suggested as both safe and effective.[109,110] The nasojejunal route is preferred for short-term feeding, but tubes are easily dislodged and difficult to replace. Placement of jejunal tubes through existing gastrostomy tubes is feasible either endoscopically or radiologically, but there are few products suitable for use in children, and the jejunal tubes to fit within existing gastrostomy tubes are often too long without any easy

Children with a chronic requirement for enteral nutrition support beyond two months should be considered for placement of a gastrostomy tube.[102] In most cases this may be achieved by placement of a percutaneous gastrostomy tube endoscopically (PEG) or radiologically, and both types are generally associated with fewer complications than surgically placed tubes.[103] Radiologic placement using a push technique method for shortening.[111] However, with sufficient ingenuity a solution can usually be fashioned. For long-term use, a surgically placed jejunostomy tube may be a good alternative.

CHOICE OF FEEDING METHOD (CONTINUOUS, NOCTURNAL, OR BOLUS FEEDING)

In general, intermittent bolus feeding is preferred to continuous feeding, as it is more practical, is more physiologic in providing a pulsatile delivery of nutrients to the GI tract, and requires much less in the way of supplies. The feed is usually delivered over 15 to 20 minutes as if the food were being delivered orally, and feeds may be given at increasing time intervals as the volume of each feed is increased. It is also not unusual in transitional states to have the child continually fed nocturnally and to have bolus feeding or even oral feeding in the daytime, again mainly for practical reasons. Many studies have shown that patients often can tolerate bolus feeding more readily than appreciated, and several studies in premature infants, in critically ill children, and in those who have undergone surgery have suggested that it is as well tolerated as continuous feeding without a significant difference in outcomes. Thus, bolus feeding should be attempted early and only abandoned if it is met with intolerance (vomiting, retching, increased gastric residuals, aspiration).

Continuous feeding is required for those patients who are intolerant of bolus feeding, or who may be transitioning from parenteral or jejunal feeding. Nocturnal continuous nasogastric feeding is frequently used for the patient with a requirement for chronic nutritional support as it may free the patient for oral or bolus feeding in the daytime. It is particularly useful for patients with significant intestinal dysfunction and malabsorption and those with protracted diarrhea. Patients on jejunal feeds also require continuous feeding as mentioned earlier. Continuous feeding requires more supplies in terms of feeding tubes, and pumps for the delivery of the feed are more technologically demanding on the family and the nutrition support team. Care must be taken to ensure adequate support for families using pumps, because failures almost inevitably happen on nights or weekends. Continuous feeding is therefore both more resource-intensive and expensive than bolus feeding. The specifics of formula choice under different circumstances are covered in the next section.

ENTERAL NUTRITION IN THE NEONATE

With the development of neonatal care over the past 30 years, increasing attention is being paid to the role of adequate nutrition on both short- and long-term outcomes. Enteral nutrition support is an important tool in the neonatal intensive care unit, delivering nutrients to the gastrointestinal tract when oral feeding is limited by prematurity or illness.[112-115]

Minimal Enteral Nutrition

The approach to enteral nutrition will vary depending on the gestational age and clinical status of the individual infant. Infants deemed too ill to begin regular, progressively increased feeds may receive "priming" or "minimal enteral feeds." In this approach, infants receive very small volumes of milk – usually 10 to 20 mL/kg per day – either continuously or intermittently. Although these volumes contribute minimally to energy and macronutrient intake, they appear to be beneficial in improving later feeding tolerance and gut function.[116-118] This may be based on the maintenance of more normal mucosal architecture, motility, or mucosal function. If an infant is unstable and unable to increase feeds, these low-volume feeds may be maintained until clinical status improves. Early trophic feeding of very low-birth-weight infants in the neonatal intensive care unit (NICU) has been studied using a meta-analysis approach in the Cochrane database, and it was concluded that there was, as yet, no statistically significant beneficial or adverse effect apparent in terms of tolerance, growth rates, or induction of necrotizing enterocolitis. It was felt that much larger randomized studies would be required in order to confirm or refute the benefits of such feeding.[119]

Progression of Enteral Nutrition

Once the infant attains cardiorespiratory stability, enteral feeds are incrementally advanced by 10 to 50 mL/kg per day, depending on the birth weight of the infant, tolerance, and clinical status.[120] In general, approximately 150 mL/kg per day will provide adequate energy and nutrients to support appropriate growth, but this is variable depending on the clinical status of the individual infant.[121]

Continuous Versus Bolus Feeds

Although both methods of administration may effectively deliver formula to the growing premature infant, theory and evidence exist to support each as the superior approach. Continuous feeds offer the advantage of using the smallest possible volume, resulting in less gastric and abdominal distention and, potentially, less pulmonary compromise. Despite this potential benefit, some studies have demonstrated no adverse effects on pulmonary parameters during bolus feeds.[122] It has been postulated that episodes of apnea and bradycardia may be reduced during continuous compared with bolus feeds, but evidence is inconsistent.[123] It has also been argued that bolus feeds trigger a more physiologic series of events by stimulating hormonal responses that increase motility, gallbladder contraction, and pancreatic enzyme release.[124,125] It is possible that this sequence of events results in more effective digestion and absorption of nutrients and may minimize the effects of complications such as neonatal cholestasis.[126] Although these issues have been examined by systematic review, the evidence was insufficient to support the benefits of one approach over the other.[123] Practice varies between neonatal units and may be based on experience within the unit and the clinical evaluation of individual infants. If continuous feeds are used for a prolonged period of time, the transition to bolus feeds may be achieved by gradually shortening the infusion time and lengthening the time between feeds. This may be useful in supporting a gradual increase in gastric volume and lessening the risk of intolerance, but this has not been scientifically evaluated.[127]

Choice of Feeding

All neonatal units strongly support the use of expressed mother's milk as the food of choice for all neonates.[128] Mothers are encouraged and supported to begin milk expression as soon as possible after delivery. Milk may be used fresh, or may be refrigerated or frozen for later use. Mother's milk presents some unique challenges when it is delivered by tube. Fat separates readily and may adhere to syringes and tubing, decreasing the amount that reaches the baby.[129] Positioning the syringe with the tip directed upward and limiting the frequency of syringe and tubing changes (while maintaining standards consistent with bacteriologic safety) may be useful in decreasing fat loss, but optimal practice to maximize fat delivery has not yet been clarified.

Human Milk Fortifiers

Despite the many benefits of mother's milk, particularly to the vulnerable premature infant, it is clear that mother's milk alone is insufficient to meet the extremely high needs of the growing premature infant. In particular, protein, calcium and phosphorus, and sodium needs exceed the availability in mother's milk at usual intakes. Human milk fortifiers have been developed to address this issue and, when added to expressed milk, support improved growth compared with that attained with unsupplemented mother's milk.[130,131] All preparations currently available are cow's milk based and may be liquid or powdered formulations. Although either preparation is acceptable, recently reported deaths due to infection related to use of powdered products have raised concerns regarding handling and administration procedures when using these products.[132] Initially, mother's milk alone is used to begin enteral feeding. Once the infant has become established at or near full-volume feeds, fortifier is added in a gradual fashion.

Formulas

If mother's milk is unavailable, infants will receive infant formula (Table 89-2). In addition to the standard infant formulas described, specially designed premature formulas that provide increased protein, calcium, phosphorus, sodium, and variable micronutrients support superior growth outcomes in premature infants compared with standard term formula (Table 89-3). A summary of available formulas with their protein, carbohydrate, and fat sources is found in Table 89-4. Furthermore, this improvement in growth may be accompanied by improved neurodevelopmental outcomes.[133-135] There is some evidence that feeding a formula with hydrolyzed protein may accelerate the gastrointestinal response to feeding in very low-birth-weight infants, but currently there is not enough evidence to change standard practice.[136,137] Standard infant formula and premature formula are compared later.

Transition to Oral Feeds

For the ill term infant in the neonatal intensive care unit, the transition to oral feeds will be directed by the clinical status of the infant. In order to initiate oral feeds, cardiorespiratory stability is mandatory. The infant must tolerate the handling associated with feeds without compromising this stability. Although infants may feed safely while receiving supplemental oxygen, it may be hazardous to do so if continuous positive airway pressure or high-flow oxygen are necessary to maintain oxygen saturations. These methods of respiratory support may compromise the ability of the infant to coordinate sucking, swallowing, and breathing and increase the risk of pulmonary aspiration. Bolus feeds must be established before beginning oral feeds, and the baby must demonstrate appropriate sucking behavior, be neurologically alert, and ideally demonstrate appropriate hunger cues. Initial feedings in particular must be carefully observed by an experienced caregiver to determine the safety and efficacy of oral feeding.

Premature infants will most often be unable to begin oral feeds before approximately 32 to 34 weeks' gestational age, because of immature coordination of sucking, swallowing, and breathing. After that, the determination of feeding readiness will be based on clinical criteria as described earlier. The introduction of "kangaroo care" (skin-to-skin handling between mother and infant) and nuzzling at a pumped breast may be useful in supporting successful breast-feeding and can begin whenever the infant can tolerate these activities.[138] Initially breast-feeding or bottle feeding must be introduced gradually (initially once or twice per day) to prevent exhaustion of the infant and facilitate progressive success. Once a significant volume of mother's milk or formula is consumed orally, enteral feeding may be reduced by a corresponding amount. Similarly, if the infant is unable to consume the expected volume orally, the remainder of the volume may be provided enterally to ensure sufficient energy intake to maintain growth.

TABLE 89-2. Comparison of Macronutrient Concentration of Term Formulas, Premature 20 kcal/oz Formulas, and Premature 24 kcal/oz Formulas Expressed as Mean Value (Range)

Formula Type	Protein (g/L)	Carbohydrate (g/L)	Fat (g/L)
Term infant formula	17.8 (14-21)	71.6 (67-78)	35 (30-37)
Premature 20 kcal/oz formula	19 (18-20)	72.5 (72-73)	35.5 (34-37)
Premature 24 kcal/oz formula	23 (22-24)	86.5 (86-87)	42 (40-44)

TABLE 89-3. Comparison of Micronutrient Concentration of Term Formulas, Premature 20 kcal/oz Formulas and Premature 24 kcal/oz Formulas Expressed as Mean Value (Range)

Formula Type	Na (mEq/L)	K (mEq/L)	Ca (mg/L)	PO_4 (mg/L)	Mg (mg/L)	Vitamin D (IU/L)	Vitamin A (IU/L)	Fe (mg/L)
Term infant formula	11 (7-14)	20 (7-27)	664 (435-827)	457 (245-624)	65 (48-83)	395 (300-580)	2057 (1200-2727)	11.8 (10.2-12)
Premature 20 kcal/oz formula	15 (13-17)	19.5 (17-22)	1158 (1100-1216)	615 (553-676)	70 (60-80)	1307 (1014-1600)	8389 (8333-8445)	12.1 (12-12.2)
Premature 24 kcal/oz formula	17.5 (15-20)	23.5 (20-27)	1391 (1320-1463)	738 (664-813)	97 (96-98)	1569 (1219-1920)	10,082 (10,000-10,163)	14.5 (14-15)

TABLE 89-4. **Infant Formula Summary**

Infant Formulas	Manufacturer	Protein Source	CHO Source	Fat Source	Osmolality	Caloric Distribution	Available forms
Whole protein							
Enfamil LIPIL	Mead Johnson	Reduced minerals whey, nonfat milk (liq) Whey protein, nonfat milk (pwd)	Lactose	Palm olein, soy oil, coconut oil, and high oleic sunflower oil, rich in DHA and ARA	300	8.5% PRO 43.5% CHO 48% FAT	Available 20 cal and 24 cal/oz; available lactose free and Enfagrow Next Step for 9-24 mo
Similac Advance	Abbott	Whey protein concentrate and nonfat milk	Lactose	High oleic safflower oil, soy oil and coconut oil, rich in DHA and ARA	300	8% PRO 43% CHO 49% FAT	Available in organic form, Lactose Free and Similac Go and Grow for 9-24 mo
Goodstart	Nestle	Whey protein	Lactose, corn maltodextrin	Palm olein, soy oil, coconut oil, high oleic sunflower and sunflower oil, rich in DHA and ARA	265	9% PRO 45% CHO 46% FAT	Available with *Bifidus* probiotic; available in Goodstart 2 for age 9-24 mo
Enfamil ProSoBee	Mead Johnson	Soy protein isolate, L-methionine	Corn syrup solids	Palm olein, soy oil, coconut oil and high oleic sunflower oil, rich in DHA and ARA	170	10% PRO 42% CHO 48% FAT	Available in Enfagrow Soy Next Step for 9-24 mo
Similac Isomil Advance	Abbott	Soy protein isolate, L-methionine	Corn syrup solids, sucrose	High oleic safflower oil, soy oil and coconut oil, rich in DHA and ARA	200	10% PRO 41% CHO 49% FAT	Available with Fiber (DF) and Similac Go and Grow for 9-24 mo
Goodstart Soy	Nestle	Hydrolyzed soy protein isolate	Corn maltodextrin, sucrose	Palm olein, soy oil, coconut oil, high oleic sunflower and sunflower oil, rich in DHA and ARA	265	10% PRO 44% CHO 46% FAT	Available in GoodstartSoy 2 for age 9-24 mo
Enfamil Enfacare Lipil (Enfamil 22 kcal/oz)	Mead Johnson	Whey protein concentrate and nonfat milk	Maltodextrin, lactose (liq) Corn syrup solids, lactose (pwd)	High oleic vegetable oil, soy oil, MCT oil (20%) and coconut oils, rich in DHA and ARA	250(liq) 300(pwd)	11% PRO 42% CHO 47% FAT	Available in Lactose Free
Enfamil Premature Lipil	Mead Johnson	Nonfat milk, whey protein concentrate	Corn syrup solids, Lactose	MCT oil (40%), soy oil and high oleic vegetable oils, rich in DHA and ARA	240	12% PRO 44% CHO 44% FAT	Available with Low Iron or Iron Fortified, 20 and 24 kcal/oz
Similac Neosure (22 kcal/oz)	Abbott	Nonfat milk, whey protein concentrate	Lactose, Corn syrup solids	Soy oil, coconut oil, MCT (25%), soy lecithin and monoglycerides	250	11% PRO 40% CHO 49% FAT	
Similac Special Care	Abbott	Nonfat milk, whey protein concentrate	Corn syrup solids, lactose	MCT oil (50%), soy oil and coconut oil, rich in DHA and ARA	235	12% PRO 41% CHO 47% FAT	Available with Low Iron or Iron Fortified, 20, 24, and 30 kcal/oz and 24 kcal/oz High Protein
Partially hydrolyzed							
Nutramigen LIPIL	Mead Johnson	Casein hydrolysate, L-cysteine, L-tyrosine, L-tryptophan	Corn syrup solids, modified cornstarch	Palm olein, soy oil, coconut oil and high oleic sunflower oil, rich in DHA and ARA	260-320	11% PRO 41% CHO 48% FAT	Available with probiotic LGG (Enflora)
Pregestimil LIPIL	Mead Johnson	Casein hydrolysate, L-cysteine, L-tyrosine, L-tryptophan	Corn syrup solids, dextrose, modified cornstarch	MCT oil (55%), soy oil and high oleic safflower oil, rich in DHA and ARA	290-320	11% PRO 41% CHO 48% FAT	Available in 20 and 24 kcal/oz

Continued

TABLE 89-4. **Infant Formula Summary**—cont'd

Infant Formulas	Manufacturer	Protein Source	CHO Source	Fat Source	Osmolality	Caloric Distribution	Available forms
Similac Alimentum	Abbott	Casein hydrolysate	Sucrose, modified tapioca starch (liq) Corn maltodextrin, sucrose (pwd)	High oleic safflower oil, MCT oil (33%), soy oil	370	11% PRO 41% CHO 48% FAT	
Amino acids							
Elecare	Abbott	Free L-Amino Acids	Corn syrup solids	High oleic safflower oil, MCT (33%), soy oil	350	15% PRO 43% CHO 42% FAT	
Neocate	Nutricia	L-Amino Acids	Corn syrup solids	Soy oil, coconut oil, high oleic safflower oil, MCT (5%)	375	12% PRO 47% CHO 41% FAT	
Nutramigen AA LIPIL	Mead Johnson	Free amino acids	Corn syrup solids, modified tapioca starch	Palm olein, soy oil, coconut oil and high oleic sunflower oil, rich in DHA and ARA	350	11% PRO 41% CHO 48% FAT	
Special indications							
Enfamil A.R.	Mead Johnson	Nonfat milk	Lactose, Pregelanized rice starch, Dextrin	Palm olein, soy oil, coconut oil and high oleic sunflower oil, rich in DHA and ARA	240 (liq)230 (pwd)	10% PRO 44% CHO 46% FAT	GER
Similac Sensitive R.S.	Abbott	Milk protein isolate	Corn syrup, rice starch, sucrose	High oleic safflower oil, soy oil and coconut oil, rich in DHA and ARA	180	9% PRO 43% CHO 49% FAT	GER
Enfaport Lipil (30cal/oz)	Mead Johnson	Calcium and sodium caseinates	Corn syrup solids	MCT (84%), soy oil, rich in DHA and ARA	280	14% PRO 41% CHO 45% FAT	For chylothorax, LCHAD
Similac PM 60/40	Abbott	Whey protein concentrate, sodium caseinate	Lactose	High oleic safflower oil, soy oil and coconut oil	280	9% PRO 41% CHO 50% FAT	For lowered mineral intake; Renal dysfunction

ARA, arachidonic acid; CHO, carbohydrate; DHA, docosahexaenoic acid; FAT, fat; liq, liquid; PRO, protein; pwd, powdered.

ENTERAL FEEDING IN THE INFANT AND CHILD

One of the more challenging tasks in providing enteral nutrition support is to select from an ever-increasing variety of products those best suited to the needs of individual patients. The choice of enteral formulas should be the result of a systematic, detailed assessment of patient requirements based as much as possible on objective information. A thorough knowledge of available formulas is essential to facilitate a formula choice that most closely matches requirements. Additional modifications may be made when required to meet specialized requirements. This process can be approached in a stepwise fashion, as outlined next.

Patient Evaluation

In order to provide appropriate enteral nutrition support, it is critical to begin with an analysis of the needs of the individual patient and goals of therapy. Although nutritional evaluation has previously been described in detail in Chapter 86, it is worthwhile emphasizing two specific aspects relevant to enteral nutrition support. First, quantitative needs for energy, macro- and micronutrients, and fluid must be estimated as accurately as possible to minimize the risks of under- or over-nutrition. Second, the patient's ability to digest and absorb nutrients must be determined in order to determine qualitative nutrient requirements and minimize the risk of adverse events related to enteral feeding.

Selecting the Formula Category to Meet Quantitative Requirements

Formulas suitable for enteral feeding are categorized as infant, pediatric, or adult. The first step in selecting a formula is to identify the formula category that most closely approximates the patient's needs. Infant formulas are intended to meet normal requirements of infants to 1 year of age, pediatric formulas are generally suitable for children from 1-10 years and adult formulas may be utilized thereafter. However, while these age ranges provide a useful guide for formula selection, they should not be rigidly adhered to. The most appropriate formula will be that which most closely meets the estimated needs of the individual patient, regardless of age.[139]

Within the infant and pediatric categories, the composition of formulas is quantitatively very similar across products. Much greater variation occurs among adult formulas, in order to meet the specialized needs of various patient groups. In general, progression from infant to adult formulas results in increasing protein and carbohydrate content and decreasing fat content, consistent with recommended dietary intakes across the lifespan. While this generalization holds true for "standard" adult formulas, many exceptions occur within this category such as "high protein" or low carbohydrate (and thus higher fat) "diabetic" formulas. Caloric density is generally greater in formulas intended for pediatric or adult patients than in infant formulas and this results in a corresponding increase in osmolality. As caloric density increases, nutritional requirements may be met with smaller volumes of formula. While this may be a distinct advantage where fluid intake is restricted, it may also result in the need for additional fluids to be provided to meet daily fluid requirements. A recent study suggested that keeping the nutrient density low (at 1 kcal/mL versus 1.5 kcal/mL), and therefore using a greater volume to achieve caloric goals, stimulated oral intake but this effect was seen in boys only.[140] Composition of formulas may change rapidly and without notice, and the reader is advised to consult the product monograph or manufacturer's website for precise details. Table 89-5 compares average energy density, macronutrient content, and osmolalities of infant, pediatric, and standard adult formulas as well as some specialty adult formulas. Tables 89-6 and 89-7 summarize the different formulas currently available for children and adolescents in North America, their protein, carbohydrate, and fat sources, and their overall composition.

Selecting the Formula Category to Meet Qualitative Requirements

Enteral nutrition support in its simplest form is merely a delivery system to overcome limitations of oral intake. This implies that all other gastrointestinal functions, that is, digestion, absorption, motility, and elimination, are intact and will function normally when nutrients are delivered into the stomach. In fact, derangements of any or all of the listed functions are extremely common in children requiring enteral nutrition support, and these abnormalities may have implications for formula selection. In addition, allergy or other adverse reaction may require that formula be selected to eliminate the suspected trigger. The most significant differences between formulas suitable for

enteral administration are among the forms in which macronutrients are provided.

Protein

Formulas may provide nitrogen in any of three forms: intact protein, peptides of varying chain length, or free amino acids.

Intact Protein

Often referred to as "polymeric," these formulas contain large intact protein molecules, which require digestion before absorption by the small intestine. Infant and adult formulas may be based on either cow's milk protein or soy protein. All currently available pediatric products are cow's milk–based. Because plant protein is partly contained within cell walls resistant to digestion by human digestive enzymes, soy protein bioavailability is reduced compared with that of cow's milk protein. For this reason, the protein content of soy-based formulas is slightly higher than that of cow's milk formulas to provide equivalent utilizable protein. This is most evident when comparing infant formulas, where there is otherwise little variability in protein content between products. Cow's milk is modified for use in all products and is often provided as calcium or sodium caseinates. Whey protein concentrate may also be included or may be the primary protein source. The inclusion of whey in infant formulas makes them more closely resemble the protein profile found in human milk. In addition, whey-based formulas may enhance gastric emptying to a moderate degree.[141,142] Although whey protein is partially hydrolyzed, whey protein–based formulas contain significant concentrations of intact cow's milk protein and have provoked serious reactions in many allergic infants.[143] Partially hydrolyzed whey-based formulas should therefore not be used in infants with documented cow's milk protein allergy.

Protein Hydrolysates

Protein may also be provided in a "partially digested" form consisting entirely or mainly of peptides. These formulas are referred to as "extensively hydrolyzed" and contain small peptides of less than 1500 Da, equivalent to approximately 8 to 12 amino acid residues. These formulas meet established clinical criteria for hypoallergenicity and are appropriate for most children with cow's milk allergy. However, even these short peptides require digestion by pancreatic carboxypeptidases and/or mucosal aminopeptidases to produce free amino acids

TABLE 89-5. Summary of Macronutrient Content, Energy Content and Osmolality Within Categories of Formulas Suitable for Enteral Feeding Expressed as Mean Value (Range)

Category	Protein (g/L)	Fat (g/L)	Carbohydrate (g/L)	Energy (kcal/100ml)	Osmolality (mmol/kg H₂O)
Infant	17.7 (14-28)	35 (30-37)	71.5 (67-78)	67	294 (200-375)
Pediatric	29.8 (24-38)	41.1 (24-50)	127.5 (104-146)	100 (80-106)	448 (290-820)
Standard adult	45 (34-56)	35.8 (17-46)	152.9 (135-170)	109 (100-120)	383 (270-600)
Adult low fat	44 (38-63)	17 (2.8-39)	173 (105-220)	101 (100-106)	493 (270-650)
Adult high calorie	70.7 (60-90)	64.9 (22.8-106)	188.7 (150-220)	159.8 (128-200)	567.2 (385-790)
Adult pulmonary	62.7 (62.4-63)	93.3 (92.8-93.7)	106 (105.5-106.4)	150	490
Adult diabetes	53 (42-64)	51 (47-55)	96 (95-97)	103 (100-106)	412.5 (375-450)
Adult renal	72 (70-74)	98 (96-100)	210 (200-220)	200	652 (665-700)

TABLE 89-6. **Pediatric Summary Table**

Pediatric Formulas (1-10 years)	Manufacturer	Protein Source	CHO Source	Fat Source	Osmolality	Caloric Distribution	Available Forms
Whole protein							
Boost Kids Essentials	Nestle	Sodium caseinate, whey protein isolate	Maldodextrin, sucrose	High oleic sunflower oil, soybean oil, MCT (20%), soy lecithin	390-440	12% PRO 44% CHO 44% FAT	Available 1.5 kcal, 1.5 kcal with Fiber, and with Probiotic Straw
Bright Beginnings	Bright Beginnings	Soy protein isolate	Sucrose, corn maltodextrin	High-oleic safflower oil, soy oil, coconut oil, mono- and diglycerides	—	12% PRO 44% CHO 44% FAT	
Ensure (> 4 years old)	Abbott	Milk protein concentrate, soy protein isolate	Sucrose, corn maltodextrin, scFOS	Soy oil, canola oil, corn oil, soy lecithin	620-640	14.4% PRO 64% CHO 21.5% FAT	Available 1.5 kcal, Fiber. and High Protein
Carnation Instant Breakfast Junior	Nestle	Nonfat milk	Sucrose	Soybean oil	—	13% PRO 43% CHO 44% FAT	
Compleat Pediatric	Nestle	Sodium caseinate milk, chicken, pea puree	Corn syrup	Canola oil, MCT (20%)	380	15% PRO 50% CHO 35% FAT	Contains Benefiber
Nutren Junior	Nestle	Milk and whey (50%) protein concentrate	Maltodextrin and sucrose	Soybean oil, canola oil, and MCT (21%)	350	12% PRO 44% CHO 44% FAT	Available with Fiber
Pediasure	Abbott	Milk protein concentrate, whey protein concentrate, soy protein isolate	Corn maltodextrin, sucrose, and dextrose	High-oleic safflower, soy, MCT (15%), lecithin mono and diglycerides	345	12% PRO 53% CHO 35% FAT	Available with Fiber, and with Fiber and FOS
NutriPals (0.6 kcal/mL)	Abbott	Milk protein concentrate	Sucrose, dextrose, sucralose	Soy oil, soy lecithin, and monoglycerides	—	19% PRO 51% CHO 30% FAT	
Partially hydrolyzed							
Peptamen Junior	Nestle	Enzymatically hydrolyzed whey	Maltodextrin and cornstarch	MCT (60%), soy and canola oil, soy lecithin	260	12% PRO 55% CHO 35% FAT	Available in 1.5 kcal, with Fiber, and with Prebio
Vital Junior	Abbott	Whey protein hydrolysate, sodium caseinate	Corn maltodextrin, sucrose, sucralose, scFOS	Structure lipid- canola oil and MCT (50%), soy lecithin	390	12% PRO 53% CHO 35% FAT	
Peptide Junior	Nutricia	Hydrolyzed pork and soy protein, free L-amino acids	Corn syrup solids	Coconut oil, canola oil, high-oleic safflower oil, MCT (35%), mono- and diglycerides	430-440	12% PRO 42% CHO 46% FAT	
Amino acids							
Elecare	Abbott	Free L-amino acids	Corn syrup solids	High-oleic safflower oil, MCT (33%), soy oil	350	15% PRO 43% CHO 42% FAT	
Neocate One+	Nutricia	Free L-amino acids	Corn syrup solids	Coconut oil, canola oil, high-oleic safflower oil, MCT (35%), mono- and diglycerides	610	10% PRO 58% CHO 32% FAT	
Neocate Junior	Nutricia	Free L-amino acids	Corn syrup solids	Coconut oil, canola oil, high oleic safflower oil, MCT (35%), mono and diglycerides	590-700	13% PRO 42% CHO 45% FAT	Contain extra vitamins and minerals

TABLE 89-6. **Pediatric Summary Table**—cont'd

Pediatric Formulas (1-10 years)	Manufacturer	Protein Source	CHO Source	Fat Source	Osmolality	Caloric Distribution	Available Forms
Amino acids							
E028 Splash	Nutricia	Free L-amino acids	Sucrose	Coconut oil, canola oil, high oleic safflower oil, MCT (35%)	820	10% PRO 58% CHO 32% FAT	Fruit flavors
Vivonex Pediatric	Nestle	L-Amino acids	Maltodextrin and modified starch	MCT (68%) and soy oils	360	12% PRO 63% CHO 25% FAT	
Special indications							
Monogen (22 kcal/oz)	Nutriticia	Whey protein concentrate	Corn syrup solids	MCT (90%), coconut oil, walnut oil, mono- and diglycerides	250	10.8% PRO 64.2% CHO 25% FAT	For chylothorax; also available in 30 kcal/oz
KetoCal	Nutriticia	Milk protein	Lactose	Palm oil, soy oil	180	8.8% PRO 4.1% CHO 87% FAT	For intractable epilepsy
Portagen	Mead Johnson	Sodium caseinate	Corn syrup, sucrose	MCT (87%), corn oil	350	14% PRO 46% CHO 40% FAT	For chylothorax

TABLE 89-7. **Adolescent Summary Table**

Adolescent Formulas (>10 years)	Manufacturer	Protein Source	CHO Source	Fat Source	Osmolality	Caloric Distribution	Available Forms
Whole protein							
Boost	Nestle	Milk protein concentrate	Sucrose, corn syrup solids	Canola oil, high-oleic safflower oil, corn oil, soy lecithin	625	17% PRO 67% CHO 16% FAT	Available High Protein, Plus, and Glucose Control
Carnation Instant Breakfast	Nestle	Nonfat milk	Maltodextrin, sucrose, lactose	N/A	—	25% PRO 75% CHO 2% FAT	Available Lactose free (1.0, 1.5, and 2.25 kcal), Ready to Drink, No Sugar added, Juice drink.
Compleat	Nestle	Sodium caseinate milk, chicken	Corn syrup, Maltodextrin	Canola oil	340	18% PRO 48% CHO 34% FAT	Contains Benefiber
Ensure	Abbott	Milk and soy protein concentrate	Sucrose, corn maltodextrin	Soy oil, canola oil, corn oil, soy lecithin	620-640	14.4% PRO 64% CHO 21.5% FAT	Available 1.5 kcal, High Calcium, High Protein, with Fiber
Jevity	Abbott	Sodium and Ca Caseinate, soy protein isolate	Corn maltodextrin, corn syrup solids	Canola oil, corn oil, MCT (19%), soy lecithin	300	16.7% PRO 54.3% CHO 29% FAT	Available 1.2 kcal and 1.5 kcal
Nutren	Nestle	Ca-K Caseinate	Maltodextrin, corn syrup solids	MCT (25%), canola oil, corn oil, and soy lecithin	315-370	16% PRO 51% CHO 33% FAT	Available 1.5 kcal, 2.0 kcal, with Fiber and Glytrol
IsoSource HN (1.2cal/mL)	Nestle	Soy protein isolate	Corn syrup, Maltodextrin	Canola oil, MCT (20%)	490	18% PRO 53% CHO 29% FAT	Available with Benefiber (FibersourceHN) and 1.5cal
Osmolite	Abbott	Sodium-calcium caseinate, soy protein isolate	Corn maltodextrin, corn syrup solids	Canola oil, corn oil, MCT (20%), soy lecithin	300	16.7% PRO 54.3% CHO 29% FAT	Available 1.2cal and 1.5cal

Continued

TABLE 89-7. **Adolescent Summary Table** —cont'd

Adolescent Formulas (>10 years)	Manufacturer	Protein Source	CHO Source	Fat Source	Osmolality	Caloric Distribution	Available Forms
Whole protein							
Promote	Abbott	Sodium-calcium caseinate, soy protein isolate	Corn maltodextrin, sucrose, oat fiber, soy fiber	Soy oil, MCT (19%), safflower oil, soy lecithin	380	25% PRO 50% CHO 25% FAT	Available with Fiber
TwoCal HN (2.0)	Abbott	Sodium-calcium caseinate	Corn syrup solids, corn maltodextrin, sucrose, scFOS	High-oleic safflower oil, MCT (19%), canola oil, soy lecithin	725	16.7% PRO 43.1% CHO 40.1% FAT	
Partially hydrolyzed							
Peptamen	Nestle	Enzymatically hydrolyzed whey protein	Maltodextrin	MCT (70%), soybean oil, soy lecithin	270-380	16% PRO 51% CHO 33% FAT	Available in 1.5cal, High Protein (AF), and with Prebio
Vital HN	Abbott	Partially hydrolyzed protein (soy and collagen), whey protein concentrate and hydrolysate, free amino acids	Corn maltodextrin, sucrose	Safflower oil, MCT (45%),soy lecithin, monoglycerides	500	16.7% PRO 73.8% CHO 9.5% FAT	
Amino acids							
Elecare	Abbott						
Vivonex	Nestle	Free amino acids	Maltodextrin, food starch modified	Safflower oil	550	15% PRO 82% CHO 3% FAT	Available RTF, TEN, and Plus
Tolerex	Nestle	Free amino acids	Maltodextrin, food starch modified	Safflower oil	550	8.2% PRO 90.5% CHO 1.3% FAT	
Special indications							
Modulen	Nestle	Casein	Corn syrup, sucrose	MCT (25%), corn oil, and soy lecithin	370	14% PRO 44% CHO 42% FAT	For Crohn's disease
Glucerna	Abbott	Sodium and calcium caseinate	Corn maltodextrin, soy fiber, fructose	High-oleic safflower oil, canola oil, soy lecithin	355	16.7% PRO 34.3% CHO 49% FAT	For diabetes; available 1.2 kcal and 1.5 kcal
DiabeticSourceAC (1.2 kcal/mL)	Nestle	Soy protein, L-arginine	Corn syrup, fructose, tapioca dextrin	Canola oil, refined menhaden oil (fish)	450	20% PRO 36% CHO 44% FAT	For diabetes
Nepro with Carb Steady	Abbott	Caseinates (Na, Ca, Mg), milk protein isolate	Corn syrup solids, sucrose, corn maltodextrin, FOS	High-oleic safflower oil, canola oil, soy lecithin	585	18% PRO 34% CHO 48% FAT	For renal failure
Suplena with Carb Steady (1.8 kcal/mL)	Abbott	Milk protein isolate, sodium caseinate	Corn maltodextrin, sucrose, scFOS	High-oleic safflower oil, canola oil, soy lecithin	600	10% PRO 42% CHO 48% FAT	For renal disease
NutrenRenal (2.0 kcal/mL)	Nestle	Calcium-potassium caseinate	Corn syrup solids, maltodextrin	MCT (50%), canola oil	650	14% PRO 40% CHO 46% FAT	For renal disease
RenalCal (2.0 kcal/mL)	Nestle	Whey protein, amino acid blend	Maltodextrin, cornstarch	MCT (70%), canola oil, corn oil, soy lecithin	600	7% PRO 58% CHO 35% FAT	For acute renal failure; electrolyte sensitivity
NutriHep (1.5 kcal/mL)	Nestle	Crystalline L-amino acids, whey protein concentrate	Maltodextrin	MCT (70%)	790	11% PRO 77% CHO 12% FAT	For hepatic failure with encephalopathy

TABLE 89-7. **Adolescent Summary Table**—cont'd

Adolescent Formulas (>10 years)	Manufacturer	Protein Source	CHO Source	Fat Source	Osmolality	Caloric Distribution	Available Forms
NutrenPulmonary (1.5cal/mL)	Nestle	Calcium-potassium caseinate	Maltodextrin	MCT (40%), canola oil	330-450	18% PRO 27% CHO 55% FAT	For pulmonary disease
Oxepa	Abbott	Sodium-calcium caseinate	Sucrose, Corn maltodextrin	Canola oil, MCT (25%), marine oil	535	16.7% PRO 28.1% CHO 55.2% FAT	For pulmonary disease
Pulmocare (1.5 kcal/mL)	Abbott	Sodium-calcium caseinate	Sucrose, Corn maltodextrin	Canola oil, MCT (20%), corn oil, high oleic safflower oil, soy lecithin	475	16.2% PRO 28.1% CHO 55% FAT	For pulmonary disease
NutrenReplete	Nestle	Calcium-potassium caseinate	Maltodextrin	Canola oil, MCT (25%),	300-350	25% PRO 45% CHO 30% FAT	For surgery and burn patients, wound healing; available with Fiber
Impact	Nestle	Sodium and calcium caseinate, L-arginine	Maltodextrin	Palm kernel oil, refined menhaden (fish) oil, safflower oil, soy lecithin	375	22% PRO 53% CHO 25% FAT	For surgery and trauma patients; Available 1.5 kcal, with Glutamine, and with Fiber
Perative (1.3 kcal/mL)	Abbott	Partially hydrolyzed sodium caseinate, whey protein hydrolysate, L-arginine	Corn maltodextrin, FOS	Canola oil, MCT (40%), corn oil, soy lecithin	460	20.5% PRO 54.5% CHO 25% FAT	For surgery and trauma patients
Pivot (1.5 kcal/mL)	Abbott	Partially hydrolyzed sodium caseinate, whey protein hydrolysate, L-arginine	Corn maltodextrin, scFOS	Structured Lipid, MCT (20%), soybean oil, canola oil, soy lecithin	595	25% PRO 45% CHO 30% FAT	For critically ill patients (immune support), wound healing
Crucial (1.5 kcal/mL)	Nestle	Enzymatically hydrolyzed casein, L-arginine	Maltodextrin, cornstarch	MCT (50%), fish oil, soybean oil, soy lecithin	490	25% PRO 36% CHO 39% FAT	For critically ill patients (immune support), wound healing
Optimental	Abbott	Whey protein hydrolysate, partially hydrolyzed sodium caseinate, L-arginine	Corn maltodextrin, sucrose, scFOS	Structured Lipid, canola oil, soybean oil, MCT (28%)	585	20.5% PRO 54.5% CHO 25% FAT	For critically ill patients (immune support), wound healing
Portagen	Mead Johnson	Sodium caseinate	Corn syrup, sucrose	MCT (87%), corn oil	350	14% PRO 46% CHO 40% FAT	For Chylothorax

and di- and tripeptides, which can then be transported into the enterocyte.

Free Amino Acid

These formulas contain only free amino acids and require no digestion before intestinal absorption. In addition, the absence of intact protein and peptides eliminates the possibility of allergic reaction in those children with cow's milk protein allergy.

Carbohydrate

Carbohydrate may be provided in formula as complex carbohydrate (starch), disaccharides, or simple sugars (glucose or glucose polymers).

Complex Carbohydrate (Starch)

Complex carbohydrate may be included in formulas in a digestible form as a source of energy, or in a largely nondigestible form as a source of fiber. Digestible carbohydrates will most often be identified as starch (often cornstarch) or as maltodextrin, which is a modified starch with enhanced solubility and digestibility. These products will require the action of pancreatic amylase for initial digestion and mucosal oligosaccharidases for final digestion before absorption.

Nondigestible Carbohydrates

Nondigestible carbohydrates in a variety of forms may be added to formulas primarily for their effect on intestinal motility. Fiber that is soluble and viscous in nature will form a gel within the stomach and will effectively delay gastric emptying and nutrient absorption, effects that may be used to advantage in various clinical settings. The fiber then passes undigested into the colon, but there is fermented by colonic bacteria to various short-chain fatty acids. These can be either used as an energy source locally by colonic cells, or transported for use elsewhere in the body. Thus soluble fiber, although classified as nondigestible carbohydrate, does make a small contribution to the energy provided by carbohydrate. Fiber that behaves in this way will be most commonly identified as a gum or pectin or soy fiber. Recently, formulas containing fructo-oligosaccharides (FOS) and/or gum arabic (a soluble but nonviscous fiber) have become available. These compounds have no significant effect on gastric motility, but their presence in the colon influences the composition of colonic flora.[10] As bifidobacteria and lactobacilli possess the enzymes to utilize these compounds, their growth is promoted,[144] whereas the growth of *Escherichia coli* and *Clostridium perfringens* (which do not possess these enzymes) is suppressed. It is postulated that these additives may protect against gastrointestinal infection or enhance recovery from antibiotic-associated diarrhea, as has been shown in an animal model.[145] Insoluble fiber has no significant effect on upper intestinal motility, but exerts its most significant effect in the colon. Because it is resistant to digestion by colonic bacteria, it remains intact during its passage through the colon. This contributes bulk to the stools, but also increases their water content. These effects result in decreased colonic transit time and improvement in constipation.[146] Because insoluble fiber remains undigested, it makes no contribution to the energy content of formula. Fiber that acts in this way is most often identified as cellulose, lignin, or hemicellulose. Many enteral products include a combination of soluble and insoluble fiber.

Fat

All fat included in formula is provided in the form of triglyceride and will be identifiable on product labels as oils. The oils most commonly found in formulas include high-oleic sunflower, soybean, canola, corn, safflower, and palm olein. All of these oils provide triglyceride composed of long-chain fatty acids and are a source of essential fatty acids. Although the specific fatty acid composition differs among the oils, these differences are not clinically significant. In addition, formulas may contain coconut oil or MCT (medium-chain triglyceride) oil, as a variable proportion of the total fat content. These oils are preferentially digested by pancreatic lipase, and the resulting fatty acids are readily absorbed without the need for micellar solubilization. In addition, MCT may also be absorbed intact into the enterocyte, subsequently undergoing hydrolysis intracellularly. Thus MCT is utilized more effectively than long-chain fat in the setting of pancreatic insufficiency and/or cholestasis. It must be recognized that essential fatty acid requirements cannot be met by MCT oil alone, as essential fatty acids are all of long chain length. A source of long-chain fat must be included in order to prevent essential fatty acid deficiency. A recent development in infant formula production in North America has been the inclusion of *Crypthecodinium cohnii* oil and *Mortierella alpina* oil. These oils are sources of docosahexaenoic acid (DHA) and arachidonic acid (ARA), respectively. Although these fatty acids may be produced endogenously in older children and adults by elongation and desaturation of alpha linolenic and linoleic acids, their presence in human milk prompted questions as to

the efficiency of this process in infants. Several studies have now demonstrated small but significant gains in developmental scores and visual acuity in infants receiving formula supplemented with DHA and ARA.[147-149]

Modular Products

Despite the wide range of products currently available, it is sometimes useful to modify existing formulas to tailor them more specifically to individual patient requirements. Modular products – preparations of fat, carbohydrate or protein alone – are designed for this purpose. It should be emphasized that modular products are not nutritionally complete formulas, but merely provide an additional source of an individual macronutrient to be added to a complete formula. Protein modulars may contain intact protein as found in complete formulas, or free amino acids only. Amino acid preparations may contain either a full complement of amino acids, or essential amino acids alone. The amino acids arginine and glutamine are also available, either individually or in combination, although the clinical indications for their use remain to be clarified. Carbohydrate modulars may be used to increase the caloric density of formulas and consist mainly of glucose polymers. In addition, either soluble or insoluble fiber may be added for specific clinical effects as described earlier. Additional fat may be provided by the addition of MCT oil or oils containing long-chain fatty acids. Although a specialized preparation of safflower oil is available for tube feeding, formulas may also be supplemented with readily available cooking oils such as canola oil. The addition of these products to formulas may allow very precise adaptation of enteral nutrition to patient needs; however, they should be used judiciously to ensure that the additional cost and labor required for preparation and administration are justified by patient outcome. Table 89-8 summarizes some of the currently available modular products and their constituents.

PRACTICAL ISSUES OF ENTERAL NUTRITION

Calculating Formula Needs

A thorough nutritional assessment of children who require enteral feeding should be performed by a pediatric registered dietitian along with a medical evaluation by the health care team.[150] Energy, protein, and nutrient needs must first be determined. Energy and protein are required for maintenance of body metabolism as well as for growth in children. Caloric requirements in children may be calculated in various ways, including a modification of the Harris-Benedict equation,[151,152] using the Dietary Reference Intakes (DRIs)[153,154] or FAO/WHO tables.[155,156]

Estimated energy and protein needs of infants and older children are shown in Tables 89-9 and 89-10. Other conditions that may alter the child's nutritional status must be taken into account, such as cardiac, renal, and pulmonary diseases and activity level. Often the initial goal of nutrition therapy is "catch-up growth," but this will need to be monitored so that children starting out as underweight do not become overweight.[150] A pediatric formula will often meet nutrient needs based on the DRI for age in children.[153,154]

Children with decreased energy needs may need a lower volume of formula with supplemental protein, vitamins, and minerals, using the DRI as a guide. Children with developmental disabilities are at risk for malnutrition as a result of

TABLE 89-8. **Modular Formula/Additive Summary**

Modular Formulas	Manufacturer	Protein Source	CHO Source	Fat Source	Osmolality	CaloricDistribution	Available Forms
Pro-Phree	Abbott	N/A	Corn syrup solids	High-oleic safflower, coconut and soy oil	205	0% PRO 51% CHO 49% FAT	Protein-free powder
Duocal	Nutricia	N/A	Hydrolyzed cornstarch	Corn oil, coconut oil, MCT, mono and diglycerides	310	0% PRO 59% CHO 41% FAT	1 Tbsp = 42 kcal
ProViMin	Abbott	Casein, L-amino acids	N/A	Coconut oil	–	93% PRO 4% CHO 3% FAT	CHO-free powder
RCF	Abbott	Soy protein isolate, L-methionine	N/A	High-oleic safflower oil, coconut oil, soy oil	90	20% PRO 0% CHO 80% FAT	
Product 3232A	Mead Johnson	Casein hydrolysate, L-cysteine, tyrosine, tryptophan, carnitine	Modified tapioca starch	MCT (85%), corn oil	250	18% PRO 27% CHO 55% FAT	Mono- and disaccharide-free powder
Modular additives							
Polycal	Nutricia	N/A	Maltodextrin	N/A	–	0% PRO 100% CHO 0% FAT	1 scoop = 5 g = 20 kcal
Polycose	Abbott	N/A	Glucose polymers	N/A	247	0% PRO 100% CHO 0% FAT	1tsp = 2g = 8 kcal
Resource Benefiber	Nestle	N/A	Partially hydrolyzed guar gum	N/A	–	0% PRO 100% CHO 0% FAT	1 Tbsp = 4 g CHO = 16 kcal
MCT oil	Nestle	N/A	N/A	Coconut oil-MCT (100%)	–	0% PRO 0% CHO 100% FAT	7.7 kcal/mL
Microlipid	Nestle	N/A	N/A	Safflower oil, soy lecithin	62	0% PRO 0% CHO 100% FAT	4.5 kcal/mL
Protifar	Nutricia	Milk protein concentrate	N/A	Soy lecithin		100% PRO 0% CHO 0% FAT	1 scoop = 2.2 g = 4 kcal
Complete Amino Acid mix	Nutricia	Free L-amino acid	N/A	N/A	360	100% PRO 0% CHO 0% FAT	1 Tbsp = 9.5 g Ptn = 38 cal
Enfamil Human Milk Fortifier	Mead Johnson	Milk protein isolate, whey protein isolate	Mineral salts, corn syrup solids	MCT (70%), soy oil	35	32% PRO 5% CHO 63% FAT	4 packets = 14 kcal and 1.1 g Ptn
Similac Human Milk Fortifier	Abbott	Nonfat milk, whey protein isolate	Corn syrup solids	MCT, soy lecithin		30% PRO 24% CHO 46% FAT	4 packets = 14 kcal and 1 g Ptn
Resource Benecalorie	Nestle	Calcium caseinate	N/A	High-oleic safflower oil, mono and diglycerides	–	9% PRO 0% CHO 91% FAT	1.5 oz = 330 kcal
Resource Beneprotein	Nestle	Whey protein isolate	N/A	N/A	–	100% PRO 0% CHO 0% FAT	1 scoop (1½Tbsp) = 7 g Ptn = 25 kcal
Promod	Abbott	Hydrolyzed beef collagen	Glycerin	N/A	–	40% PRO 60% CHO 0% FAT	1 oz = 100 kcal and 10 g Ptn

Continued

TABLE 89-8. **Modular Formula/Additive Summary**—cont'd

Modular Formulas	Manufacturer	Protein Source	CHO Source	Fat Source	Osmolality	CaloricDistribution	Available Forms
Oral Supplements							
Ensure Enlive! (>4 years old)	Abbott	Whey protein isolate	Corn maltodextrin, sucrose	N/A	–	14.4% PRO 85.6% CHO 0% FAT	Apple, Mixed Berry
Resource Breeze	Nestle	Whey protein isolate	Corn syrup	N/A		14% PRO 86% CHO 0% FAT	Orange, Peach, Wild Berry

TABLE 89-9. **Estimated Energy Needs of Infants and Older Children**

Age (years)	kcal/kg Body Weight
0-1	90-120
1-7	75-90
7-12	60-75
12-18	30-60
>18	25-30

Data from ASPEN Board of Directors and the Clinical Guidelines Task Force. Guidelines for the use of parenteral and enteral nutrition in adult and pediatric patients. JPEN J Parenter Enteral Nutr 2002; 26(Suppl 1):1SA-138SA.[156]

TABLE 89-10. **Estimated Protein Needs of Infants and Older Children**

Age	g Protein/kg Body Weight
Low birth weight	3-4
Full term	2-3
1-10 years	1-1.2
Adolescent boy	0.9
Adolescent girl	0.8
Critically ill child/adolescent	1.5

Data from ASPEN Board of Directors and the Clinical Guidelines Task Force. Guidelines for the use of parenteral and enteral nutrition in adult and pediatric patients. JPEN J Parenter Enteral Nutr 2002; 26(Suppl 1):1SA-138SA.[156]

TABLE 89-11. **Calculating Fluid Requirements in Children**

Weight	Baseline Daily Fluid Requirement
1-10 kg	100 mL/kg
11-20 kg	1000 mL + 50 mL/kg for each kg >10 kg
Over 20 kg	1500 mL + 20 mL/kg for each kg >20 kg

Adapted from Holliday MA, Segar WE. The maintenance need for water in parenteral fluid therapy. Pediatrics 1957; 19:823.[158]

oropharyngeal dysphagia, interactions between nutrients and medications, altered energy and nutrient requirements, and their reliance on others to feed them. A variety of proprietary formulas have been developed to provide these patients with nutritional support. The nutritional requirements of patients with developmental delay in general and cerebral palsy in particular are poorly understood. Studies using indirect calorimetry confirm that energy requirements are often much lower than standard predictive equations suggest. This has been hypothesized to be a result of decreased energy due to inactivity, decreased muscle tone, or lowered growth potential. As a result, the amount of energy provided in tube feedings is often reduced to match energy needs and this can be as low as 50% of the usual age-based recommended DRIs for energy.

Most formulas designed for children aged 1 to 10 years meet the DRIs for micronutrients when volumes between 980 mL/day and 1100 mL/day are given. Amino acid–based formulas generally have a lower concentration of micronutrients, and therefore more volume must be given to meet the DRI. For children aged 4 to 10 years, this amount can be as high as 1400 mL/day to 2000 mL/day. When patients receive less than the DRI for energy, their micronutrient intake may be inadequate. Vitamin A, C, and zinc deficiencies have been reported in such instances.[157]

Calculating Fluid Requirements

Free water requirements may be altered by cardiac and renal dysfunction, drainage tubes and insensible water losses. Fluid requirements may be higher than the formula volume. Fluid requirements in children are based on body weight according to the Holliday-Segar method[158] as seen in Table 89-11. All formulas provide water, but the level of free water varies based on the osmolality of each individual product. To calculate the additional free water required, the sodium-free water content of the tube feeding must be known. This varies from product to product and

ranges from 600 to 923 mL free water/1000-mL tube feeding. Values can be found in the product literature. Otherwise, these guidelines are frequently used to calculate free water: approximately 90% of infant formula volume, approximately 85% of most other formula volume, and approximately 72% for pediatric formulas providing 1.5 kcal/mL.[150] If the patient has no other source of hydration (i.e., intravenous fluids or medications), then the additional free water can be supplied as "flushes" through the feeding tube that also serve to facilitate tube patency.[159] It can also be given in between feeds if larger bolus feeds are not well tolerated, or it can be mixed in to the formula.

Feeding Schedules and Mode of Administration

Children starting on tube feedings may be started at full strength formula given at low volumes. Children should be fed with head elevated 30 to 45° during feeding and for 1 hour afterwards to limit risk of aspiration. The following is a sample schedule to initiate enteral feedings:

Infants under 10 kg	10 mL/hour
Children 10 to 20 kg	20 mL/hour
Children 20 to 40 kg	30 mL/hour
Children over 40 kg	50 mL/hour

The rate should be advanced as tolerated to meet the nutrition goal. The volume should then be increased every 4 to

12 hours, monitoring for tolerance. Tolerance is defined as absence of diarrhea, abdominal distention, vomiting, or gagging. If the formula is not tolerated, the formula volume or strength can be decreased and the child given a longer time to adjust. After the child tolerates the formula and becomes accustomed to the volume, gradual adjustments to feeding schedule may be made to fit with the family lifestyle.[150] The method of delivery will depend on a variety of factors such as tolerance, volume requirements, safety, and the family schedule. A schedule that works well in a hospital (with 24-hour-per-day nursing care) may be impractical and exhausting for a parent to do at home.[160]

When possible, increments of formula should be delivered in user-friendly volumes. For example, if a can of formula can be used at one time, this is easier for the caregiver and left-overs are less of a problem. If syringe feeding, increments easy to measure in the syringe should be used, such as 60 mL rather than 63 mL. Portable pumps can make life easier for caregivers, particularly when a child requires continuous feeds.[160] Viscosity, temperature, and feeding tube size affect flow rate. The former two can be improved by diluting with free water and warming the formula.

Enteral pumps are accurate to plus or minus 10%. The more additives, that is, protein, carbohydrate or fat powders/liquids, the less accurate the infusion. Caregivers should be instructed to give total prescribed volume versus rate calculated volume.[160] Children who suffer significant regurgitation, pulmonary gastroesophageal reflux disease (GERD), or bolus feeding–induced retching may benefit from continuous feeds given over 12 to 24 hours.[160,161]

Medications

Medications should never be added directly into the formula, because drug-nutrient interactions and incompatibility with enteral feeds may occur.[160] For instance, iron added to a formula results in almost complete degradation of vitamin C if hung at room temperature for 12 hours. This has led to scurvy in clinical situations.[162] Other recognized drug-nutrient interactions include vitamin C and phenobarbital.[157]

SAFETY OF ENTERAL FEEDS

Closed Versus Open Systems

Bacterial contamination may occur at any stage of preparation and infusion. For open systems, 27% are contaminated at the start and 67% by the end of an infusion. Coliforms, *Enterococcus* spp., and mesophilic aerobic organisms have been cultured.[163] Adding new formula to a bag already in use or adding modular components amplifies this risk. Closed systems that require only spiking onto the infusion system greatly reduce bacterial contamination risk.[164-166] Antimicrobial agents have been added to formula by some manufacturers, but the long-term effects of these requires careful study in children.

Bacterial Contamination of Feeds

There is a growing body of information pertaining to *Enterobacter sakazakii* infections in premature infants and those with underlying medical conditions fed milk-based powdered infant formulas from various manufacturers and different countries.[167] The majority of cases of *E. sakazakii* infection occur in neonates. Sepsis, meningitis, and necrotizing enterocolitis have been

reported with a case fatality rate as high as 33%. The pathogen is also a rare cause of bacteremia and osteomyelitis in adults. Powdered infant formulas are not guaranteed to be sterile. Powdered milk-based infant formulas are heat-treated during processing but, unlike liquid formula products, are not subjected to high temperature for sufficient time to guarantee sterility. A substantial percentage of premature neonates in neonatal intensive care units are fed powdered infant formula. In light of the epidemiologic findings, the FDA has recommended that powdered infant formulas should not be used in neonatal intensive care settings, unless there is no alternative available.[168,169] If the only option available to address the nutritional needs of a particular infant is a powdered formula, the risk of infection in a tube-fed infant can be reduced by preparing only a small amount of reconstituted formula for each feeding to reduce the quantity and time that formula is held at room temperature for consumption, minimizing the holding time, whether at room temperature or while under refrigeration, before the formula is fed and minimizing the hang time (i.e., the amount of time a formula is at room temperature in the feeding bag and accompanying lines during enteral tube feeding), with no hang time exceeding 4 hours.[170] Longer times should be avoided because of the potential for significant microbial growth in reconstituted infant formula.[168] An outbreak of *Salmonella enterica* Saintpaul in a children's hospital was traced to contaminated enteral feeding formula.[171] Implementation of Hazard Analysis Critical Control Points systems has shown an improvement in the quality of feeds. Blenders used in reconstituting feeds may be a source of bacterial contamination.[163] Enteral feeding tubes and feeding sets represent another potential hazard in terms of bacterial contamination.[172-175]

Tubing

Safety with tubing is a concern for children who are active in their crib or bed. Some hospitals now have a device that encases the tubing, making it rigid and less able to become a strangling device. Also, guiding the tubing through the bottom of a child's pajamas directs the tubing away from the neck.[156]

COMPLICATIONS

Complications of enteral tube feeding can largely be anticipated and prevented. If they occur, most are capable of being solved without stopping enteral nutrition. Complications can be dependent on the underlying disease state, the access to the intestinal tract (e.g., nasoenteric versus percutaneous-gastric versus small bowel), the feeding technique (e.g., type of formula, gravity versus pump feeding) and the metabolic state (e.g., anabolism, catabolism, postoperative stress). The reported frequency of these complications varies greatly. Gastrointestinal side effects (including diarrhea) are most frequent. Individual assignment of feeding regimens to each patient and close monitoring are the best means of prevention, with monitoring by a specialist team. Awareness of the existence, frequency, and etiologic factors of complications represents the most important means of preventing them (Table 89-12).[176]

Diarrhea

Diarrhea (unformed stool, usually increased in number and changed from the usual stool habit of that person) may occur in a child receiving enteral nutrition. Because enteral feeding

TABLE 89-12. **Complications of Enteral Feeding**

Gastrointestinal
  Diarrhea
  Nausea and vomiting
  Constipation
  Aspiration
  Bloating/gas
Metabolic
  Dehydration or overhydration
  Hyperkalemia
  Hypokalemia
  Hypernatremia
  Hypophosphatemia
  Hypoglycemia
  Refeeding syndrome
Microbial
  Bacterial contamination of feed
  Bacterial contamination of administration sets
Developmental
  Food aversion due to inadequate oral stimulation
Mechanical
  Perforation
  Disruption of tract
  Burial of bolster in stomach wall
  Fistula formation
  Pyloric obstruction
  Leakage
  Nasal/esophageal erosion
  Tube blockage
  Strangling with tubing
  Equipment malfunction

formulas are frequently low in residue, stool consistency is normally looser than with a normal full oral diet. A sudden onset of diarrheal stool requires investigation of all possibilities, including enteric infection (e.g., *Clostridium difficile,* nosocomial viral infection), bacterial contamination of the feed, lactose content, enteral medications, systemic illness, maldigestion or malabsorption of the feed, and anatomic peculiarities of the bowel. Enteral nutrition itself should not be cited as the cause of diarrhea without evidence and should be continued until the cause is identified.[177,178]

Nausea and Vomiting

Nausea and vomiting often impede successful enteral nutrition. However, effective antiemetics and prokinetic agents (e.g., metoclopramide or low-dose erythromycin) may be used before turning to TPN.[179-181] The rate of feeding can be decreased until nausea subsides, then gradually returned to full volume. Whey-based formulas induce faster gastric emptying than casein-based formulas. These are helpful for children who have poor weight gain secondary to volume intolerance as manifested by gagging, discomfort, or emesis following bolus feeds.[182] Persistent true vomiting (as opposed to gastroesophageal reflux) may indicate a gastric motility disorder and may require intestinal rather than gastric feeding.

Constipation

Constipation may be related to inadequate fluid or fiber intake, side effects of medications, inactivity, gastrointestinal dysmotility, or bowel obstruction. A prophylactic bowel regimen should be discussed with a physician and dietitian ensuring adequate fluid and fiber intake and/or use of a stool softener or laxative.

Where possible, regular exercise is encouraged and the physician should review the medications for possible constipating side effects. This is a particular problem for children with cerebral palsy or neuromuscular disorders.

Metabolic Complications

Care must be taken with the composition and reconstitution of enteral feeds. Underhydration is relatively common if insufficient free water is provided, or if the formula is overconcentrated. Overhydration may occur if large volumes are provided, or large volumes of water are used to flush the tube. Both hypo- and hyperkalemia may occur, particular if the patients have diarrhea or renal compromise. Hypoglycemia may occur if bolus feeding with too long a period between feeds after continuous feeding or TPN have preceded boluses, or attempted bolus feeding into the jejunum, occurs. Refeeding syndrome has rarely been reported with enteral feeding and usually takes the form of profound hypophosphatemia.[183]

Mechanical Complications

Perforation may occur at the time of placement or due to erosion of the tube through the bowel wall. Disruption of the tract most commonly occurs when button gastrostomy tubes with deformable internal bolsters are changed. It is also possible for an internal bolster to become buried in the stomach wall, often when the tube is cinched too tightly, usually requiring surgical removal. Pyloric obstruction occurs with migrating Foley and Malechot catheters, especially if tubes are mistakenly placed in the antrum. Leakage may occur because of infection in the tract or surrounding skin or granuloma formation at the tract, or because cinching too tightly causes necrosis and skin breakdown. Nasal, esophageal, and stomach irritation may occur as a result of movement or pulling on the tube. Equipment malfunction can occur at any time, but seems to have a predilection for nights, weekends, and holidays.

Tube Clogging

Tube clogging is a common complication, especially in long, small-bore feeding tubes used frequently in acute care settings. Nasally placed gastric and jejunal tubes tend to clog more readily than gastrostomy tubes because of length and the smaller internal diameter. Minimizing the incidence of tube clogging decreases time off feeds, time and expense of reinsertion, radiography, and child/parent frustration and trauma.[184] Feeding tubes can clog for a variety of reasons that include formation of a formula precipitate from contact with an acidic fluid, stagnant formula, feeding tube properties, contaminated formula, and improper medication administration. Crushed insoluble medication (e.g., metronidazole) is particularly likely to clog a tube.

Formula Contact With Gastric Acid

Acid precipitates protein at its pK. For milk proteins, this is about pH 4.5. A feeding tube with intact casein containing formula will clog within seconds with the addition of acid at pH below 4.6. The normal fasting gastric pH is 1.5 to 2.0. Any maneuver that increases the exposure of the formula within the tube to gastric acid will increase the risk of tube clogging. This includes checking for gastric residuals, disconnecting the tube, and allowing siphoning and stopping feeds without flushing the tube. Formulas with only amino acids and dipeptides greatly reduce the risk of clogging. Jejunal feeding tubes have the advantage of no exposure to acid, but the disadvantage of a longer tube.

Stagnant Formula

Nutritional formulas can easily precipitate when they are infusing at slow rates, or paused without a water flush. This occurs because nutrition formulas are suspensions and the larger particles (sodium, calcium caseinate, soy protein) will settle in the tube if the flow rate is too slow or stops. Calorically dense or fiber-containing formulas are more viscous and further increase the risk for clogging. Feeding tubes should be flushed routinely with about 5 to 30 mL of water at least every 4 hours during continuous feedings, and at least a 5 to 30 mL water flush should be done after each intermittent or bolus feeding. The amount depends on the size of the child and the internal diameter and length of the tube. Enteral infusion pumps should be used when slow infusion rates are ordered. The formula container should not be allowed to run dry, and pump alarms should be responded to promptly.

Contaminated Formula

A formula clog may be caused by significant bacterial contamination (bacterial count above 10^7 cfu/mL). Proper handwashing and clean technique should be used when preparing and administering the formula to minimize contamination. Manufacturers' recommendations should be followed regarding formula hang times and proper use of the enteral delivery sets.[146] Undesirable levels of bacterial contamination of enteral feeding sets have been confirmed at 48 hours, and evidence suggests that this may be largely due to contamination of the hub connector. However, although the contamination is evident, the patients do not appear to suffer the consequences of infection.[185,186]

Solutions for Feeding Tube Flushes

Various solutions have been used to flush feeding tubes. These include water, carbonated beverages, and cranberry juice. Cranberry juice (pH 2.6) has consistently been shown to be inferior to water in preventing tube clogging.[184] Coca-Cola showed no advantage over water. Water is the preferred solution for feeding tube flushes because it is easily obtainable at low cost and has a low neutral pH, and because no solution has been shown to be superior in maintaining tube patency.

Medication Clogs

Tube clogging can be caused by inadequately crushed pills, congealed medications, formation of precipitate from medication with formula, or medication-medication interactions. Medications should not be mixed together or mixed with the nutritional formula, unless approved by a pharmacist. Feeding tubes should be flushed with at least 5 mL water before and after medication administration, and medications should be administered separately with at least a 5-mL water flush between each one. Whenever possible, liquid medications should be used. Elixirs or suspensions are less likely to cause clogging compared with syrups that tend to be acidic. Pharmacies may be able to formulate a liquid solution or suspension from powders or tablets. If not, tablets should be crushed into a fine powder and dispersed well in warm water. A crushed tablet can be placed into a 60-mL syringe, 30 mL of warm water drawn up, and the

diluted medication administered through the feeding tube. It is wise to test administration through a similar tube first to check for obstruction risk. Enteric coated or timed-release tablets or capsules should be not be crushed.

The use of crushed tablets should be discouraged wherever possible, as they are more likely to clog tubes, especially jejunal tubes, which are often smaller in caliber. The resultant clogs are also more difficult to clear than those caused by formula.[187] The administration of bulk-forming agents such as soluble fiber (e.g., psyllium) through feeding tubes should be avoided, because these agents quickly congeal when combined with water. Some fiber sources, such as Unifiber by Novartis, have instructions for tube feeding administration. Some formulas already contain insoluble fiber or a blend of soluble and insoluble fibers. These formulas should be shaken vigorously before administration to ensure that the fiber remains in solution.

Tube Unclogging

Proper tube feeding administration and handling, medication administration, and water flushes should minimize the incidence of tube clogging. In instances where it would be difficult to replace a clogged tube (e.g., newly placed jejunostomy tube, or gastrojejunal tube), a solution of Viokase in bicarbonate solution may be used (Viokase: 1 tablet crushed or ¼ tsp powder; sodium bicarbonate 324 mg tablet or ⅛ tsp baking soda in 5 mL tap water). The solution is injected into the tube and clamped for 30 min, then flushed well with water. This is done at home once or twice weekly for nasoenteric and gastrojejunal tubes. This practice successfully resolves sluggish infusions and prevents tube occlusions, possibly by clearing any residue buildup in the tube lumen. It frequently allows parents to unclog tubes at home without coming to the hospital. Tubes should be unclogged as soon as the obstruction is identified.

Aspiration

Children on tube feedings may aspirate oral secretions, formula, and/or gastric contents. Pulmonary damage may be due to nutritional (e.g., lipid) or microbiologic factors. Pulmonary aspiration may occur if the child has poor airway protection, usually associated with incoordinate swallowing, significant gastroesophageal reflux, delayed gastric emptying, or oral positioning of the feeding tube itself. Gastric acid suppression increases the risk of bacterial overgrowth and bacterial aspiration pneumonia. Fundoplication and jejunal tube feeding (beyond the ligament of Treitz) may reduce the risk of aspiration of formula if gastroesophageal reflux is severe, and the latter reduces gastric and duodenal secretions.[188] The progression from an aspiration event to aspiration pneumonia is very difficult to predict, and several studies support oropharyngeal bacteria as a more significant factor in aspiration, or even the key factor, rather than colonization of gastric contents.[164] Body position can make a significant difference in the risk of aspiration. The head of the bed should be elevated at 20 to 30°.

Monitoring

Initial monitoring parameters for a child on enteral feedings should include daily intake of calories, protein and electrolytes, fluid intake and output and the weight of the patient.

Appropriate laboratory investigations, including but not limited to electrolytes, albumin or prealbumin, blood urea nitrogen (BUN), and glucose, are done daily to weekly until stable. Vitamin, mineral, and trace element intake should be evaluated at regular intervals. Once the formula feeding is tolerated and any complications managed, then growth can be monitored by weekly weight measurement. Once expected growth is realized, then review for tolerance, tube problems, and growth (weight, length, and head circumference) can be decreased to approximately monthly. In addition, laboratory monitoring will decrease concomitantly. Trace elements and vitamin assays should be performed twice annually and supplements provided if required.[157] When children are discharged home on tube feeding, the child and family should be seen again within 10 days to troubleshoot and to provide support. The frequency of subsequent visits will depend on the abilities of the family, their needs, and the complexity of the case.

As the child grows, enteral feedings need to be adjusted. At each outpatient visit, the indications for and goals of enteral feeding should be reevaluated, techniques of problem solving reinforced, and signs and symptoms of complications identified.[189] Formula volume should be modified based on a child's rate of growth. For this reason, it is important to monitor a child's growth regularly. Changes in weight and height should be monitored at least every 3 to 6 months for a child who is tube-fed. This is especially important during periods of transitional feeding, such as when transitioning from fully tube feeding to oral feeding or from fully oral feeding to supplemental feeds.

Routine monitoring should include the following:
1. Weight measurement, length, and head circumference
2. Intake (including enteral and oral)
3. Review of current medications for drug-nutrient interactions
4. Laboratory parameters
5. Psychologic status: changes in lifestyle, home environment
6. Assessment of relevant organ function to evaluate feasibility of transitional feeding

The frequency of monitoring children on home enteral nutrition depends on the needs of the family and the complexity of the case.[190] Many decisions require health professionals' input, documentation, or support. A team including a physician, nurse, occupational or speech therapist, and dietitian works best for the child and family.[150]

Oral Stimulation

Patients who have no contraindications to oral feeding should be encouraged to feed by mouth.[189] Feeding time is important to children and parents. It should be an enjoyable and relaxing time. This does not have to change while children are being tube-fed. Caretakers can hold, talk to, and play with children during feeding. All children on tube feeding require oral stimulation for development of feeding skills. If the child is unable to take foods orally, some type of oral stimulation is needed such as offering a pacifier. This will help children develop the skills necessary to begin eating by mouth. For infants, the denial of oral stimulatory experiences because of gastrointestinal dysfunction may have significant deleterious side effects such as appetite suppression, inability to distinguish hunger and satiety, food aversion, inadequate and uncoordinated sucking and

swallowing, poor mother-child bonding, and developmental delays in language and gross motor skills. The goal is to have children associate sucking or chewing with satiety in order to ease transition from tube to oral feeds. A speech language pathologist or occupation therapist with experience in feeding/swallowing disorders can outline an oral motor program to follow during feedings.[150]

TRANSITION FROM PARENTERAL TO ENTERAL/ORAL NUTRITION

As soon as the gut can be accessed and fluid safely infused, then enteral feeding should be started. Enteral feeding promotes bowel growth. Initial enteral feeding may be minute (1 to 2 mL/hour) but should be gradually advanced as tolerated. When 20% of required nutrients can be absorbed from the bowel, parenteral nutrition can start to be weaned. If oral feeds are progressing, parenteral nutrition may be given solely at night until no longer required.

Tube Removal

Parents are often anxious to know when the tube can be removed. For nasoenteric tubes, the tube is removed as soon as oral feeding is fully adequate.[165] The tube can be replaced as required. For gastrostomy or gastrojejunal feeding tubes, a general rule of thumb (established only by expert opinion) is that if the tube has not been used for 90 days and the child continues to thrive, the tube can be removed. Some physicians prefer to also see if the child can manage to get through an illness without having to rely on the tube for feeds, oral rehydration therapy, or medications.[131]

Home Enteral Nutrition

Home enteral feeding should be considered for any patient whose sole reason for hospitalization is to receive enteral support.[191] The decision to provide enteral feeding in the patient's home must take into account medical needs as well as social, psychologic, and financial factors.[192] Enteral feeding offers a safe and cost-effective alternative to parenteral nutrition and can usually be carried out at home, preferably under the supervision of a nutritional care team.[193] The provision of nutritional support at home allows for a return to a comfortable environment, avoidance of the negative emotional effects of hospitalization, reduction of the risk of infection, and reduction in costs.[189]

Home enteral nutrition is appropriate for children with diagnoses falling into several broad categories but that all relate to the child being unable to safely and voluntarily ingest adequate nutrition by mouth.[194] Enteral feeding has usually been started in the hospital and is continued at home. However, when used as a supplement or primary therapy for conditions such as Crohn's disease, enteral feeding may be started in the outpatient clinic. Enteral feeding is started with the agreement of the parents, with whom the objectives of treatment must be fully discussed. It is important that parents do not see tube feeding as a failure, but rather as a positive step that will free them from the worries of maintaining an adequate nutritional intake and allow them to devote more time to their child with activities that are less stressful and more rewarding than feeding.

An important element of home enteral nutrition is continuous parental support and regular follow-up of the patients by both the nutritional care team of the base hospital and the community medical and nursing staff.[195] It is apparent in studies of the follow-up of such patients at home that there are many obstacles facing families of children cared for at home, both in the month following hospital discharge and in the long term. Problems such as delivery of formula, feeding pumps, training in the use of the pumps, dislodgement and clogging of tubes, accidental removal of the tube, and stress levels induced in families are all significant complications in home delivery of enteral nutrition and over a 10-month period have resulted in at least five calls or visits to the enteral feeding base program.[196-200] Home-based care has been increasingly practiced in the care of children. It requires a multidisciplinary team that includes physicians, a dietitian, and nurses as well as occupational therapists, speech-language pathologists, physiotherapists, and social workers and allows many children with multiple handicaps to be cared for at home.

SUMMARY

Enteral feeding provides the best solution to the nutritional support of the child with acute or chronic disease who is unable to maintain adequate growth and development with oral feeding alone, where the gut is intact and functional (and sometimes even when it is not). The malnourished, hospitalized child is a particular challenge, but children with a chronic need for nutritional support can often have it provided in the safety and comfort of their own homes. A variety of disease states may give rise to a requirement for nutritional supplementation by the enteral route, including disorders that impair intake, gastrointestinal dysfunction and malabsorption, hepatobiliary disease, critical illness, chronic system-based disorders that impair growth, and hypermetabolic states. Enteral feeding may be provided by nasoenteral or enterostomal approaches depending on individual circumstances, and the choice of formula to be used, whether polymeric or defined, will depend on the digestive and absorptive capabilities of the child and the metabolic stressors involved at the time of provision of nutritional support. The complications of enteral feeding can largely be anticipated and avoided with appropriate care and monitoring of the patient. The nutritional care of the hospitalized patient may be transitioned appropriately into the community, to continue rehabilitation or long-term nutritional support. The importance of a multidisciplinary team-based approach to the care of children requiring enteral feeding, with appropriate psychosocial support, cannot be overemphasized.

REFERENCES

27. Day AS, Whitten KE, Lemberg DA, et al. Exclusive enteral feeding as primary therapy for Crohn's disease in Australian children and adolescents: a feasible and effective approach. J Gastroenterol Hepatol 2006;21: 1609–1614.
29. Bannerjee K, Camacho-Hubner C, Babinska K, et al. Anti-inflammatory and growth-stimulating effects precede nutritional restitution during enteral feeding in Crohn's disease. J Pediatr Gastroenterol Nutr 2004;38: 239-241.
33. Marik PE, Zaloga GP. Meta-analysis of parenteral versus enteral nutrition in patients with acute pancreatitis. BMJ 2004;328:1407.
47. Mehta NM. Approach to enteral feeding in the PICU. Nutr Clin Pract 2009;24: 377-387.
114. Newell SJ. Enteral feeding of the micropremie. Clin Perinatol 2000;27:221–234.
165. Papadopoulou A, Booth I. Home enteral nutrition in infants and children. In: Preedy H, Grimble G, Watson R, editors. Nutrition in the Infant – Problems and Practical Procedures. London: Greenwich Medical Media; 2001. p. 69–78.

See expertconsult.com for a complete list of references and the review questions for this chapter.

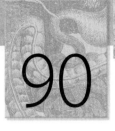

90

MANAGEMENT OF DIARRHEA

Bhupinder Sandhu • David Devadason

Hippocrates was the first to define the term *diarrhea* literally from the Greek *rhea* ("to flow") and *dia* ("through"). Diarrhea is classified as acute or chronic (lasting greater than 2 weeks). Infectious diarrhea, commonly referred to as gastroenteritis, is the commonest cause of acute diarrhea. Etiologic agents may vary in different countries. Other causes of acute diarrhea are listed in Table 90-1.

The World Health Organization (WHO) estimates that diarrheal disease causes around 17% of deaths in children under 5 years worldwide.[1] Diarrhea remains a leading cause of childhood death, although on a global scale diarrheal deaths have decreased from 5 million annually in 1980 to 2.2 million in 1999.[1,2] Such a dramatic decrease in mortality rate has largely occurred as a direct result of the increasing use of the oral rehydration solution (ORS).[2,3] In developed countries, death due to acute diarrhea is fortunately rare, but gastroenteritis is associated with enormous costs either directly (medical expenses) or indirectly (loss of working days by the parents of ill children) because of the frequency of disease.[4] In the United States, incidence rates for diarrhea have been estimated at 1 to 2.5 episodes per child per year resulting in, annually, 38 million cases, 2 million to 3.7 million physician visits, 320,000 hospitalizations, and 325 to 425 deaths.[5] Diarrhea may be associated with up to 9% of all hospitalizations of children less than 5 years of age.[6]

MANAGEMENT OF ACUTE DIARRHEA

Pathophysiology of Diarrhea and the Evolution of ORS

Intestinal mucosa actively absorbs large quantities of sodium, chloride, bicarbonate, and solutes. It also secretes chloride and hydrogen ions. Water passively follows net solute transport. In the villus cell, sodium potassium adenosine triphosphatase (Na,K-ATPase) maintains low intracellular sodium, which allows the entry of sodium coupled to chloride and nutrients (glucose/amino acids). Absorptive processes in the villus cell exceed the minor secretory activity in the crypt, and therefore the net result is absorption of nutrients and electrolytes and water. Under pathologic influences (for example, exposure to enterotoxins giving rise to increase in cyclic adenosine monophosphate [AMP] or cyclic guanosine monophosphate [GMP]), chloride channels open up in the luminal membrane of crypt cells, causing the leak of chloride and hence sodium, which follows along with water, and this shift of ions moves the equilibrium from net absorption to net secretion. Diarrhea ensues when there is a derangement in the absorptive-secretory

processes. The reversal of the net absorptive status can be either the result of suboptimal absorption ensuing in an osmotic force acting in the lumen that drives water across the tight junctions from the serosa into the lumen (for example, in lactose malabsorption) or the result of an active secretory state induced in the crypt cells (for example, in enterotoxin-induced diarrhea). In many disease states, both mechanisms coexist (Figure 90-1).

Fluid losses from the gastrointestinal tract can be profound and lead to devastating effects, particularly in infants and young children. The discovery that in cholera, sodium-glucose coupled transport remains intact although sodium chloride transport is inhibited[7] and that oral administration of a sugar-salt solution can rehydrate and maintain hydration in patients with infective diarrhea[8] remains one of the greatest scientific advances in the past 50 years. The use of ORS in the management of gastroenteritis has been associated with a dramatic fall in mortality, not only in developing countries but also in the developed world. In the UK, for instance, the mortality fell from 300 deaths annually in the 1970s to 25 in the 1980s.[9] Hypernatremic dehydration, a major cause of mortality in acute gastroenteritis, has also become much less common.[10] Although controversy continues about the ideal composition of ORS, there is consensus about the scientific rationale for its use. The sodium concentration of the standard WHO-ORS, 90 mmol/L, was in part based on the fecal sodium concentration in adults with cholera.[11] This product, with an osmolarity of 311 mmol/L, has been used worldwide and has contributed substantially to the global reduction in mortality from diarrheal disease. Concerns that this solution, which is slightly hyperosmolar when compared to plasma, may cause hypernatremia[12] in well-nourished children with noncholera diarrhea in the developed world resulted in the proliferation of ORS formulations with a range of sodium concentrations (30 to 60 mmol/L). Stools in children infected with rotavirus, the commonest infective pathogen, particularly in the developed world, have a lower concentration of sodium.[13] In the 1980s, the American Academy of Pediatrics (AAP) recommended a solution containing 45 mmol/L sodium for American children for the correction of dehydration. In 1992, a working group on Acute Diarrhoea of the European Society of Paediatric Gastroenterology, Hepatology and Nutrition (ESPGHAN) considered the scientific evidence and published "Recommendations for the composition of ORS for the children of Europe."[14] ESPGHAN recommended a solution containing 60 mmol/L sodium and 70 to 110 mmol/L glucose with an osmolarity of 225 to 260 mmol/L. Various manufacturers of ORS adopted the recommendations, and this solution has gradually replaced other solutions in Europe.

Super ORS

During the past 20 years there have been attempts to develop a super ORS by using rice powder, amino acids, glucose polymers, and so forth, instead of glucose. Laboratory studies were encouraging, but in a clinical setting, results were disappointing for amino acids[15] and harmful using a glucose polymer.[16] The initial results using rice powder and other cereals were more encouraging.[17] However, a meta-analysis in a well-conducted systematic review, evaluating 22 hospital-based randomized controlled trials (RCTs) of rice-based ORS, concluded that the benefit of rice-based ORS is sufficient to warrant use in patients with cholera but is considerably smaller in noncholera diarrhea.[18] Furthermore, a study by Santhosham et al. showed that treatment with standard ORS and simultaneous feeding with boiled rice produced similar results to using rice-based ORS.[19]

Hypo-osmolar ORS

In vitro experiments have shown that water absorption is increased from hypotonic ORS when compared to isotonic ORS.[20,21] Clinical trials have shown that in both the developing world and the developed world, hypotonic ORSs with a sodium concentration of 50 to 70 mmol/L are safe and effective for rehydration and maintenance therapy of mild to severe dehydration from noncholera diarrhea.[22,23] In vitro and in vivo data suggest that low osmolarity may be the key for enhancing the clinical effectiveness of ORS.[24] A meta-analysis of randomized trials of reduced osmolarity ORS versus standard WHO ORS in children with noncholera diarrhea[25] concluded that the use of a reduced osmolarity ORS was associated with (a) a reduction in the need for unscheduled intravenous (IV) fluids (defined as the clinical requirement for intravenous fluids once oral rehydration has commenced), (b) a trend toward reduced stool output (about 20%), and (c) reduction in the incidence of vomiting (about 30%). The incidence of hyponatremia (serum sodium 130 mEq/L at 24 hours) was higher, but this difference was not statistically significant. The accumulating evidence on its greater efficacy of hypo-osmolar ORS has resulted in an expert consultation on ORS formulation by the WHO/UNICEF. This concluded that the efficacy of glucose-based ORS for treatment of children with acute noncholera diarrhea is significantly improved by reducing the sodium content to 60 to 75 mEq/L, glucose to 75 to 90 mmol/L, and total osmolarity to 215 to 260 mmol/L.[26] The composition of the new hypo-osmolar WHO ORS (2002) is listed with the other ORSs in Table 90-2. It preserves the 1:1 molar ratio of sodium to glucose that is critical for the efficient cotransport of sodium. Citrate content allows for a longer premixed shelf life.

TABLE 90-1. Causes of Acute Diarrhea

Gastrointestinal infection
  Viruses (60-70% of gastroenteritis)
    Rotavirus, Norovirus, enteric adenoviruses
  Bacteria (around 10%)
    Salmonella, Shigella, Campylobacter, Yersinia, Escherichia coli,
    Clostridium difficile, toxigenic bacteria
  Parasites
    Giardia lamblia, Cryptosporidium, Entamoeba
  Pathogen unidentified (20%)
Systemic infection
  E.g., urinary tract infection
Drugs
  E.g., antibiotics, laxatives
Food intolerance/allergies
  Cow's milk, fish, egg, soy
Malabsorption syndromes
  E.g., lactose intolerance, sorbitol
Surgical causes
  Intussusception, appendicitis, necrotizing enterocolitis

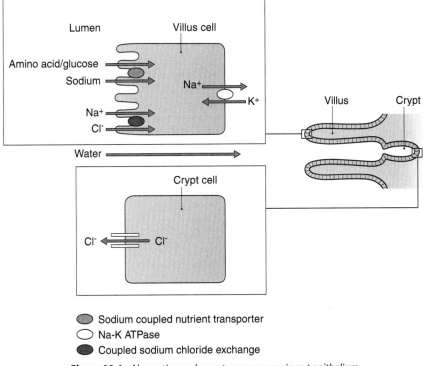

Sodium coupled nutrient transporter
Na-K ATPase
Coupled sodium chloride exchange

Figure 90-1. Absorptive and secretory processes in gut epithelium.

TABLE 90-2.   The Evolution of the Oral Rehydration Solution (Composition of WHO, AAP, ESPGHAN, and 2002 WHO-ORS)

Component	Old WHO ORS	AAP ORS	ESPGHAN ORS	New Hypo-osmolar WHO ORS
Sodium (mmol/L)	90	45	60	75
Glucose (mmol/L)	111	138	74-111	75
Osmolarity (mmol/L)	311	250	225-260	245
Chloride (mmol/L)	80	60	60	65
Potassium (mmol/L)	20	20	20	20
Citrate (mmol/L)	10	10	10	10

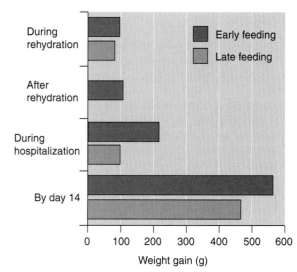

Figure 90-2. ESPGHAN study on early feeding. Comparison of weight gain between early feeding group and late feeding group.

Oral therapy remains the mainstay of the WHO efforts to reduce the morbidity and mortality caused by acute diarrheal disease. In the developing world, the uptake is still suboptimal. Simultaneous uptake of ORS in industrialized countries has been slow, despite many clinical trials documenting the safety and efficacy of this form of therapy. A major barrier to the wider uptake of ORS is that it is not perceived to be a medication. A WHO report estimates that fewer than 50% of acute diarrheal episodes are treated with ORS.[27] An American study that looked at practices compared with AAP recommendations found that fewer than 30% of responding physicians used a recommended solution to treat dehydration.[28] Another study showed that in the United States, several barriers among pediatricians exist to the use of oral rehydration, including its lack of convenience, the need for additional training for support staff, and the discrepancy in reimbursement for intravenous versus oral rehydration.[29] Similar problems exist in Europe. A recent ESPGHAN survey reported that one in six doctors in Europe would not prescribe ORS.[30]

Early Feeding

The primary goals in treating acute diarrhea are preventing and reversing ongoing dehydration and minimizing the nutritional consequences of mucosal injury. Diarrhea, malnutrition, and intestinal integrity have a close complex relationship. Malnutrition leads to an increased susceptibility to gastrointestinal (GI) infections, and this vicious cycle leads to thousands of children dying every day worldwide. It has been observed in animal models that starvation alters mucosal barrier function. In addition to the development of ORS, one other milestone has been the advent of early feeding and the avoidance of the so-called intestinal rest.

Historical review of published literature reveals that introduction of a period of starvation dates back to 1926 when Powers wrote his treatise on treatment of diarrhea.[31] There was no scientific basis for the recommendation of this practice. Following this, children were routinely starved during diarrhea and then gradually graded from quarter-strength formula to full-strength formula over 2 to 4 days. A study in 1948 showing that there was no scientific rationale for grading was ignored.[32] In 1979, Rees and Brook,[33] and later Dugdale et al.[34] and Placzek and Walker-Smith,[35] showed that gradual grading of feed to full strength was not needed. In 1985, a study by Khin-Maung[36]

showed that continued breast-feeding at the time of acute diarrhea was of benefit. Isolauri et al., in 1986, showed that in children older than 6 months after initial oral rehydration therapy, full feeding appropriate for age (including milk) is well tolerated with no adverse effects.[37] Brown et al. then published studies clearly showing advantages of continued feeding for clinical and nutritional outcomes.[38,39]

A community-based study in the UK[40] and an Eastern European study[41] involving infants from birth to 1 year of age further suggested that early feeding was safe, with no increase in lactose intolerance or vomiting, and resulted in better weight gain.

The ESPGHAN Working Group on acute diarrhea conducted a large multicenter study that compared the effect of ORS and early or late feeding on the duration and severity of diarrhea, weight gain, and complications (carbohydrate intolerance and vomiting) in weaned European infants and has made recommendations based on this.[42]

The conclusions of this study were as follows:
1. Complete resumption of a child's normal feeding including lactose containing formula after 4 hours of rehydration with glucose ORS (ESPGHAN recommended composition) led to significantly higher weight gain after rehydration and during hospitalization (Figure 90-2).
2. There was no worsening of diarrhea, no prolongation of diarrhea and no increased vomiting or lactose intolerance in the early-feeding group compared with the late feeding group (Figures 90-3 and 90-4).

In malnourished children, the nutritional benefits of early feeding have been clearly established.[38] This study, involving a range of hospitals from around Europe, lends further credence to this practice and suggests that there are benefits for children who are not necessarily nutritionally compromised. Theoretical benefits of continuing feeding are minimizing protein loss and energy deficits and reduced functional hypotrophy associated with starving.[43] There is indirect evidence to support the strategy of early feeding, based on studies revealing the positive effects of luminal nutrition on regeneration and mucosal growth as seen in short bowel syndrome. Early refeeding reduces the abnormal increase in intestinal permeability that occurs in acute gastroenteritis and may promote recovery of the

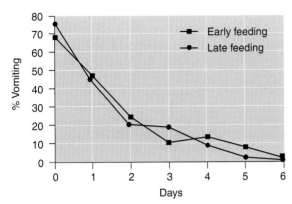

Figure 90-3. Frequency of vomiting between early feeding group and late feeding group (ESPGHAN study).

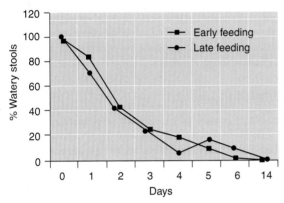

Figure 90-4. Frequency of watery stools between early feeding group and late feeding group (ESPGHAN study).

brush border membrane disaccharidase.[44,45] Early resumption of feeding is now recommended by ESPGHAN,[43] the AAP,[46] and WHO.

Treatment Strategies and Practical Guidelines

There is now general consensus among pediatric gastroenterologists that the optimum management of acute diarrhea of mild to moderately dehydrated children should consist of the following "Six Pillars of Good Practice"[30,46-49]:

1. The use of ORS to correct dehydration in the initial 4 hours of management
2. The use of the hypo-osmolar solution (60 mmol/L sodium, 74 to 111 mmol/L glucose)
3. Continuation of breast-feeding throughout
4. Early refeeding, that is, resumption of a normal diet once rehydration is complete
5. Prevention of further dehydration by supplementing maintenance fluids with ORS (10 mL/kg ORS for every watery stool)
6. Avoidance of the routine use of medication

Clinical Signs and Symptoms

A range of symptoms and signs have traditionally been considered useful in the detection of dehydration. It is important for caretakers and health care professionals to be familiar with these symptoms and signs, particularly those signs that suggest worsening of dehydration. Irritability, sunken eyes, and reduced urine output have been shown to have good correlation with dehydration and therefore should be part of the systemic inquiry process. It should be remembered that infants with acute diarrhea are more prone to dehydration than are older children because they have a higher ratio of body surface area to weight.

History and examination should guide the clinician to the severity of dehydration. The severity of dehydration is most accurately assessed in terms of weight loss as a percentage of total body weight. The reference standard used for assessing dehydration is the percentage of volume lost calculated as the difference between rehydration weight (posthydration weight) and the acute (prehydration) weight. This is the gold standard against which other tests are measured.[48] In the absence of weight, clinical markers may be used to approximate the degree of dehydration (Tables 90-3 and 90-4). Previous studies have suggested that prolonged skin retraction time and deep breathing may be reliable indicators of dehydration[50] and have pointed out a good correlation between capillary refill and fluid deficit.[51] These observations have been corroborated in a systematic review that suggests that specific signs are associated with dehydration (prolonged capillary refill time, abnormal skin turgor, and abnormal respiratory pattern).[52] However, all studies were conducted in secondary care settings where children with more severe dehydration are managed, and therefore there may not necessarily be the same degree of correlation with lesser degrees of dehydration. If dehydration is less than 5%, the child can be managed at home. Indications for hospital admission include (a) the child is more than 5% dehydrated; (b) parents are unable to manage oral rehydration at home; (c) the child does not tolerate oral rehydration (severe vomiting, insufficient intake); (d) failure of treatment, worsening diarrhea, and/or dehydration despite oral rehydration treatment; and (e) other concerns, such as uncertain diagnosis, potential for surgery, child "at risk," irritable or drowsy, or a child younger than 2 months.

Recently published guidelines from the National Institute for Health and Clinical Excellence (NICE) in the United Kingdom adopt a new and even simpler clinical assessment scheme. Patients are merely classified as follows: "no clinically detectable dehydration," "clinical dehydration" and "clinical shock." The guideline acknowledges that this simplified scheme does not imply that the degree of dehydration is uniform.[53] The NICE guidelines highlight that the presence of red flag symptoms and signs should alert the clinician to a risk of progression to shock. These symptoms and signs are altered responsiveness (lethargy, irritability), sunken eyes, tachycardia, tachypnea, and reduced skin turgor. Children with such signs need close monitoring.

Work-up and Laboratory Studies

Most children with acute gastroenteritis do not need any laboratory work-up. The development group for the NICE guidelines found that there was a lack of satisfactory evidence with regard to the incidence of clinically important biochemical disturbances in children with gastroenteritis in the UK.[53] Nevertheless, the guidelines recommend measuring plasma sodium, potassium, urea, creatinine, and glucose concentrations if IV fluid therapy is required or there are symptoms and signs that suggest hypernatremia, and measuring venous blood acid-base

TABLE 90-3. Assessment of Dehydration

Signs and Symptoms	General Condition	Eyes	Tears	Mouth and Tongue	Thirst	Skin	Percentage Body Weight Loss	Estimated Fluid Deficit (mL/kg)
No signs of dehydration	Well, alert	Normal	Present	Moist	Drinks normally, not thirsty	Pinch retracts immediately	<5	<50
Some dehydration	Restless, irritable	Sunken	Absent	Dry	Thirsty, drinks eagerly	Pinch retracts slowly	5–10	50–100
Severe dehydration	Lethargic, unconscious, floppy and dry	Very sunken	Absent	Very dry	Unable to drink	Pinch retracts very slowly	>10	>100

From Sandhu BK. Practical guidelines for the management of acute gastroenteritis in children. J Pediatr Gastroenterol Nutr 2001; 33:S36-S39.[49]

TABLE 90-4. Classification of Dehydration Severity by WHO*

No Dehydration	Some Dehydration	Severe Dehydration
Not enough signs to classify as some or severe dehydration	Two or more of the following signs: • Restlessness, irritability • Sunken eyes • Drinks eagerly, thirsty • Skin pinch goes back slowly	Two or more of the following signs: • Lethargy/unconsciousness • Sunken eyes • Unable to drink or drinks poorly • Skin pinch goes back very slowly (>2 seconds)

*World Health Organization. Pocket Book of Hospital Care for Children: Guidelines for the Management of Common Illnesses with Limited Resources. Geneva: WHO; 2005.

status and chloride concentration if shock is suspected or confirmed.

Stool microscopy and culture and electron microscopy or enzyme-linked immunosorbent assay (ELISA) for rotavirus may be useful for etiologic information but usually have little influence on immediate management. Microscopy for leukocytes in the stool and Gram staining of the stools may help in differentiating bacterial from nonbacterial diarrhea. Stool cultures are indicated for patients who have bloody diarrhea. There may be circumstances in which identification would be important because of the significance of pathogens. For example, amebic dysentery would require antibiotics, and *Escherichia coli* 0157:H7 is associated with hemolytic uremic syndrome (HUS) – a serious and potentially fatal disorder.

Management in the Home Setting (Prehospital Care)

Ideally, management of acute diarrhea should begin at home, because early intervention can reduce complications. The child should be rehydrated using ORS. Effective teaching of the parent or guardian about procedures for administering the solution and instructions about when to bring the child back for reassessment are absolutely crucial. The use of "clear fluids" (water alone, cola, or fruit juice) is inappropriate and may be dangerous because these fluids lack adequate sodium. Fruit juices and cola can potentially worsen diarrhea because they have a high osmolar load.

The calculated fluid deficit is replaced over 4 hours. Thus, in a 10-kg child with 5% dehydration, the deficit is 5% of 10 kg, which equals 500 mL. This is given as ORS over 4 hours. It is vital to emphasize the importance of adequate hydration with clear instructions to make up the ORS. If the child is breast-fed, this should continue. Ideally, a child should be reassessed 4 hours after rehydration, and if the child is fully hydrated, normal feeding should be commenced. Ongoing fluid losses in the form of vomiting or diarrhea should be made up in addition to maintenance fluid requirements, by administering ORS 10 mL/kg for every loose stool or vomitus.

Hospital Management

An accurate estimate of the degree of dehydration should be made ideally by using current and previous weights (when available). Rehydration with oral rehydration therapy is usually carried out over a period of 4 hours. A reasonable approach in a child presenting with clinical manifestations of dehydration is to assume 5% dehydration at the outset. Based on that assumption, rehydration should be attempted by giving 50 mL/kg over the initial 4-hour rehydration period. However, one must be aware that in other more severely dehydrated children, 50 mL/kg may be insufficient. It would therefore be important to regularly reassess the child's state of hydration and when necessary to increase the final volume of replacement fluid administered.

The child should be fully assessed in order to exclude other causes of acute diarrhea. If the patient does not tolerate oral rehydration (refuses, vomits profusely, or takes inadequate amounts), a nasogastric tube can be used to give ORS. The patient should be reviewed after 4 hours and if sufficiently hydrated, a normal diet should be commenced and maintenance fluids continued (100 mL/kg per day for the first 10 kg, plus 50 mL/kg per day for the next 10 kg, plus 20 mL/kg per day for the remainder of weight over 20 kg). Supplement ORS, 10 mL/kg for every watery stool, should be continued to make up for ongoing losses. If dehydration persists, the degree of dehydration should be reassessed and the fluid deficit corrected with ORS over the following 4 hours. If the child is moderately or severely dehydrated, investigations should include plasma urea and electrolytes, and a stool analysis for viruses and bacteria.

Intravenous Therapy

A high-quality Cochrane review compares the effectiveness of ORS with IV therapy for the treatment of dehydration due to gastroenteritis in children.[54] A systematic review of 17 trials that compared an IV therapy arm with one or more ORS arms (oral or nasogastric) did not find any significant difference in the incidences of hyponatremia and hypernatremia, the duration of diarrhea, weight gain, or total fluid intake in children treated with ORS compared with IV therapy. Dehydrated children treated with ORS had a significantly shorter stay in the hospital, and those receiving IV therapy had a higher risk of phlebitis.

Intravenous therapy is only indicated if the estimate of dehydration is 10% or more, if the child is in shock, or if there is failure of oral replacement therapy. If the child is shocked, he should be first resuscitated with 20 mL/kg of normal saline. Deficits should be replaced with isotonic solutions (0.9% saline or 0.9% saline in 5% dextrose) and calculations based on uncorrected weight. Once dehydration is corrected, *maintenance fluids should be continued*, oral feeding commenced, and ongoing stool losses replaced with ORS (10 mL/kg per watery stool). Early and gradual reintroduction of oral rehydration solution during IV therapy is recommended with the aim of continuing rehydration with ORS, if this is then tolerated.

Although many experts now support rapid intravenous rehydration (4 to 8 hours), rehydration with intravenous fluid therapy has traditionally been undertaken slowly – over 24 hours. WHO recommends that intravenous rehydration should be completed in 3 to 6 hours. However, instances of hypernatremia have led the National Patient Safety Agency (NPSA) in the UK to advise that intravenous fluid replacement should be over 24 hours or longer. The NPSA patient safety alert highlights the importance of both measuring electrolytes at the start of IV fluids and regularly monitoring sodium concentrations thereafter.[55] Randomized controlled trials are needed to examine the safety of the practice of rapid intravenous rehydration.

Hypernatremic Dehydration

The recent NICE guidelines did not find any evidence for the often-mentioned "doughy skin" as a sign of hypernatremic dehydration but do highlight the increased frequency under 6 months of age. Children with hypernatremic dehydration have an increased frequency of central nervous system manifestations such as jitteriness, altered conscious levels, or convulsions.[53] A child with hypernatremia (i.e., sodium greater than 150 mmol/L) needs careful monitoring with frequent reassessment. Oral rehydration or nasogastric rehydration is by far the safest method. If this fails, resuscitation with IV fluids should be carried out slowly, because the aim is a gradual reduction in the sodium as a sudden fall can be dangerous and lead to cerebral edema and convulsions. The calculated deficit should be replaced with 0.9% saline in 5% dextrose over 48 hours, with careful monitoring of the plasma sodium until the child becomes normonatremic. The rate of fall of serum sodium should not exceed 0.5 mmol/L per hour. The management should then be as for nonhypernatremic dehydration.

Complications

If diarrhea continues for more than 10 days, parents should be advised to return with the child for a reassessment, and the stool should be checked for persistent infection. The recurrence of diarrhea each time with reintroduction of milk should alert the physician to the possibility that the child may have developed lactose intolerance. The stool pH should be checked and the stool reducing substances measured. This can be done at the bedside using Clinitest or carried out by the laboratory. If the reducing substances are present at 1% or more, it is considered diagnostic of lactose malabsorption, and the child should be placed on a lactose-free diet for a 2-week period and then reassessed. Most lactose intolerance is temporary and caused by patchy villous damage, and once the gut villi regenerate, lactase and other disaccharidase levels normalize. If the stool is negative to reducing substances and the diarrhea is related to milk protein intake, the child may have developed cow's milk protein intolerance and may require a protein hydrolysate formula.

Antimicrobial Therapy

Because viral agents are the predominant cause of acute diarrhea, antibiotics play a limited role in its management. Treatment with appropriate antibiotics is indicated if there is evidence of systemic bacterial infection. Predisposing factors include a history of recent travel, immunodeficiency, and history of recent antibiotic use (in which case *Clostridium difficile* should be suspected). Appropriate antibiotics have been shown to be effective in the treatment of shigellosis, *C. difficile*, and *Campylobacter*. Randomized control trials have shown that in shigellosis, appropriate antibiotic therapy shortens the duration of diarrhea by 2.4 days, decreases the duration of fever, and reduces the excretion of infectious organisms.[56,57] Ciprofloxacin has been shown to be safe and effective in children with shigellosis.[58] Nontyphoidal *Salmonella* gastroenteritis is usually self-limiting, and studies have failed to show any benefit from antibiotic treatment.[59] Protozoal pathogens associated with diarrhea that persists for more than 7 to 10 days are *Giardia lamblia* and *Cryptosporidium*. Metronidazole or tinidazole is used for treating proven *Giardia* infection, whereas nitazoxanide, which was recently approved by the U.S. Food and Drug Administration (FDA) for use in children,[60] is effective against *Cryptosporidium*. Regardless of the causative agent, initial therapy should include rehydration.

Probiotics

In recent years there has been a growing interest in probiotics as a potential method of changing intestinal bacterial flora. Probiotics may potentiate host gastrointestinal defenses and stimulate nonspecific host resistance to microbial pathogens. They may protect by increasing nonimmunologic defenses. The exact mechanisms by which probiotics carry this out are not yet known, although the possible mechanisms include the synthesis of antimicrobial substances and competition at the substrate level.

Lactobacillus rhamnosus strain GG (ATCC 53103) has been the most common bacterial species used to counteract intestinal infections. It has been shown in trial settings to have a number of potentially beneficial effects in preventing and treating acute diarrhea.[61-64] A multicenter trial to evaluate the efficacy of *Lactobacillus* GG administered in the oral rehydration solution in children aged 1 month to 3 years with acute-onset diarrhea of all causes was conducted by the ESPGHAN Working Group on acute diarrhea.[65] This showed that in rotavirus-positive children, diarrhea lasted longer in children in the placebo arm of the trial, and the risk of having diarrhea for more than 1 week was reduced nearly fourfold in the *Lactobacillus*-treated group. The study showed no benefit in children who were more likely to have had a bacterial cause of diarrhea. This is in concordance with previous reports.[66,67]

A systematic review of published randomized, double-blind, placebo-controlled trials reviewed 13 studies carried out between 1974 and 2000.[68] The outcome measures that were considered included duration of diarrhea, number of watery stools per day, risk of diarrhea lasting more than 7 days, duration of hospitalization, and weight gain. The meta-analysis concluded that the use of probiotics was associated with a significant reduced risk of diarrhea lasting more than 3 days. This observation was limited to *Lactobacillus GG*, and no adverse outcome measures were seen. However, based on WHO recommendations of using stool output rather than duration of diarrhea as a primary outcome measure when evaluating diarrhea treatment, no firm conclusions could be drawn on the effect of probiotics on stool output in acute diarrhea.[68] A systematic review, published in 2003, was conducted to examine the effectiveness of probiotics compared with control in the treatment of infectious diarrhea. This review included 23 randomized controlled trials published between 1981 and 2002. Fourteen of these studies were carried out in developing countries. The meta-analysis showed that those receiving probiotics were less likely to have diarrhea lasting 3 days or more. However, there was significant variation with regard to the specific probiotic, therapeutic regimes, and methods used.[69]

Antidiarrheal Agents

Table 90-5 summarizes the evaluation of safety and efficacy of various antidiarrheal drugs. Antidiarrheal agents are not indicated in the management of acute diarrhea. Opioids have an antimotility effect that may mask the severity of diarrhea. They can also have serious side effects. Very few over-the-counter antidiarrheal products have been demonstrated to be effective in randomized, controlled trials. Because antimotility agents have been implicated in hemolytic-uremic syndrome in children infected with Shiga toxin–producing *E. coli*,[70] these agents should be avoided in children with bloody diarrhea. There are insufficient data to support the routine use of adsorbents such as kaolin-pectin, activated charcoal, and attapulgite. Despite the fact that pediatric guidelines discourage the use of antidiarrheal drugs in children,[46,49,71] various studies have highlighted the widespread use of drugs by caregivers in treating children with diarrhea. Easy availability of antidiarrheal drugs is an important factor in perpetuating their misuse.[72] The key strategy in regulating therapy would be to make antidiarrheal agents unacceptable to caregivers and physicians through appropriate education and training. Caregivers and physicians must realize that such drugs are not only unnecessary, but also potentially harmful. Simultaneously, confidence in ORS needs to be boosted.

Although a recent meta-analysis performed in a systematic review[73] showed that children receiving loperamide experienced less stool output and had a reduction of the duration of diarrhea when compared with children who did not receive the drug, it was noted that serious adverse effects such as drowsiness, abdominal distention, and ileus occurred only in the treated groups, and therefore the use of loperamide is not recommended by the Guideline Development Group that drew up the NICE guidelines for the management of acute gastroenteritis.[53]

In theory an antisecretory agent without antimotility effect or significant side effects may have a role. Racecadotril (acetorphan) has been proposed as such an agent. Unlike loperamide and other opioids, it is said to have only antisecretory properties. A placebo-controlled trial from Peru showed that with racecadotril there was a 46% reduction in stool output and reduction in the duration of diarrhea, with only minor adverse effects.[74] Similar evidence for its effectiveness comes from a European RCT conducted in 13 centers in France.[75] However, its antisecretory selectivity has been questioned,[76] and much further research is needed before reliable conclusions can be drawn on the role of racecadotril in the treatment of acute diarrhea.

There has been a recent systematic review of trials comparing smectite with placebo or no treatment for diarrhea in children. This review showed that smectite resulted in a reduction in the frequency and duration of diarrhea, higher resolution of diarrhea by day 3, and a decreased likelihood of diarrhea lasting more than 7 days. Equally, the review showed no statistically significant differences between the smectite and control groups in the number of episodes or duration of vomiting or in the resolution of diarrhea by day 5.[77]

In 1995, a study from India was the first among many to report significant clinical benefit from zinc therapy in gastroenteritis.[78] A Cochrane review was recently undertaken that included 18 trials in total and did not find a statistically significant reduction in diarrhea.[79] The use of zinc might be beneficial in patient groups with similar population characteristics as in studies where a benefit from zinc was confirmed. WHO recommends zinc in the management of diarrhea in developing countries at a dose of 20 mg elemental zinc for 10 to 14 days during a diarrheal episode (10 mg under 6 months of age).[80]

Prevention

Acute diarrhea is a preventable disease, and properly applied measures aimed at decreasing its incidence lead to a considerable decrease in infant mortality and morbidity. This is particularly challenging in the developing nations. The obvious measures are improvement in sanitation, provision of clean

Table 90-5. Status of Antidiarrheal Drugs in Children

Drug	Available Evidence	Status
Loperamide (Imodium)	Well-designed trials have shown some benefit in reducing stool volume and duration of diarrhea. Effects are statistically significant but not clinically significant. Unacceptably high rate of side effects, e.g., lethargy, ileus	Not recommended
Other opiates	Hardly any data supporting use. High potential for toxicity including respiratory depression, paralytic ileus	Not recommended
Anticholinergics	High toxicity especially in infants and children	Not recommended
Bismuth subsalicylate	No conclusive evidence to demonstrate decreased duration or frequency of diarrhea	Not recommended

From: American Academy of Pediatrics. Provisional Committee on Quality Improvement, Subcommittee on Acute Gastroenteritis. Practice parameter: the management of acute gastroenteritis in young children. Pediatrics 1996; 97:424-435.[46]

drinking water, sewerage systems and garbage disposal, adequate housing, promotion of breast-feeding and safe weaning practices, and education about basic principles of hygiene.

Recommendations on preventing primary spread of diarrhea (and vomiting) should form part of the advice that parents, children, and caregivers receive. This advice includes washing hands with soap in warm running water and careful drying, washing of hands after going to the toilet or changing diapers, and washing of hands before preparing, serving, or eating food. Children should not attend school or other child care facilities while they have diarrhea caused by gastroenteritis, and children should not swim in swimming pools for 2 weeks after the last episode of diarrhea.[81]

Vaccines

Over the past few years, efforts have been put into the development, trial, and production of vaccines against different causes of infectious diarrhea such as cholera, typhoid, *Shigella*, and rotavirus. Major factors that interfere with the massive utilization of vaccines are variability in antigenic determinants and the high cost of manufacturing. Rhesus-based rotavirus tetravalent vaccine was withdrawn voluntarily from the market in 1999 because of concerns about an increase in cases of intussusception. A Cochrane database systematic review of 64 trials on efficacy and safety of three main types of rotavirus vaccines recently concluded that the rhesus rotavirus vaccine (particularly RRV-TV) and the human rotavirus vaccine 89-12 are effective in preventing diarrhea caused by rotavirus and all causes of diarrhea.[82] Two new live, oral, attenuated rotavirus vaccines were licensed in 2006: the monovalent human rotavirus vaccine (Rotarix) and the pentavalent bovine-human, reassortant vaccine (Rotateq). Both vaccines have demonstrated very good safety and efficacy profiles in large clinical trials in Western industrialized countries and in Latin America. In general they provide about 90 to 100% protection against severe rotavirus disease and about 74 to 85% protection against rotavirus diarrhea of any severity. The Global Advisory Committee on Vaccine Safety (GACVS) concluded that the prelicensing safety profiles of the current rotavirus vaccines were reassuring, and in June 2007 GACVS stated that to date, careful postlicensure surveillance did not indicate any increased risk of intussusception or other serious side effects with either vaccine. In June 2009, WHO recommended that rotavirus vaccine be included in all national immunization programs where appropriate infrastructure exists to sustain vaccine uptake.[83]

Conclusion

In the past three decades, the development and use of scientifically based ORS has dramatically improved the management of children with acute diarrhea, although uptake is still suboptimal. The benefits of early feeding following rehydration have been well recognized and are gaining wider acceptance. This combination of oral rehydration therapy and early feeding should be the mainstay of management of acute diarrhea. Introduction of safe vaccines, improvement in public health, further optimization of ORS, and perhaps development of safe antisecretory agents and probiotics may help further combat one of the most common public health problems in children worldwide.

MANAGEMENT OF CHRONIC DIARRHEA

Chronic diarrhea is defined as passing four or more watery stools per day for a period of 2 weeks or more. The etiology varies (Table 90-6), and a systematic approach to assessment, investigation, and management is needed. It is important to consider the child's age when establishing a differential diagnosis, because particular conditions manifest for the first time at certain ages. A history of onset in the neonatal period, after excluding infection, suggests cow's milk protein enterocolitis, Hirschsprung's disease, cystic fibrosis, adrenogenital syndrome, lymphangiectasia, congenital microvillus atrophy, and inherited transport defects such as congenital chloridorrhea. Bloody diarrhea suggests necrotizing enterocolitis in the neonatal period and inflammatory bowel disease in the older child. In the age group 6 months to 2 years, the conditions to be considered are toddler diarrhea, postenteritis syndrome, and celiac disease. Associated recurrent respiratory tract infection may suggest cystic fibrosis or immunologic deficiency. In countries where there is a high prevalence of human immunodeficiency virus (HIV), this needs to be considered early. Clinical examination is important and may give clues to the diagnosis: for example, an abdominal mass in pheochromocytoma and erythema

Table 90-6. Possible Causes of Chronic Diarrhea

Chronic intestinal infections	Viruses, bacteria, giardiasis, *Cryptosporidium* Postenteritis syndrome
Carbohydrate intolerance	Lactase deficiency: primary, secondary Glucose: galactose malabsorption Sucrase: isomaltase deficiency
Protein intolerance	Celiac disease Cow's milk protein intolerance Cow's milk colitis
Nonspecific functional diarrhea	Toddler diarrhea Irritable bowel syndrome
Inflammatory bowel disease	Ulcerative colitis Crohn's disease
Surgical	Necrotizing enterocolitis Short gut syndrome Hirschsprung's disease
Pancreatic insufficiency	Cystic fibrosis Shwachman-Diamond syndrome Chronic pancreatitis
Immunodeficiency syndromes	HIV/acquired immunodeficiency syndrome IgA deficiency Severe combined immunodeficiency Hypogammaglobinemia
Tumors	Pheochromocytoma Vasointestinal peptide secreting tumors Lymphoma Histiocytosis X
Endocrine causes	Adrenogenital syndrome Thyrotoxicosis
Inborn errors of transport and severe protracted diarrhea of infancy	Congenital chloridorrhoea Autoimmune enteropathy Congenital microvillus atrophy Abetalipoproteinemia, hypobetalipoproteinemia Lymphangiectasia Primary hypomagnesemia
Drug related	Chemotherapy Antibiotics
Other causes	Dysmotility, Munchausen's by proxy

nodosum in Crohn's disease. Investigation, such as endoscopy and biopsy for celiac disease and inflammatory bowel disease, will help make a definite diagnosis. Treatment will depend on specific cause. It is beyond the scope of this chapter to deal with every specific cause of chronic diarrhea. Many of these specific causes are dealt with separately in detail in other parts of the text.

Chronic Infectious Diarrhea

Chronic infectious diarrhea remains the most common cause of prolonged diarrhea across all pediatric age groups including infancy. Stool samples are required for microscopy in order to detect pathogens, including ameba and parasites. Often more than one sample of stool is required; for instance, in giardial infection, three stool specimens on three separate days will identify around 75% of cases. Electron microscopy is needed to detect viruses.

With improvement in mortality associated with acute infectious diarrhea, persistent diarrhea and its nutritional consequences is still a major cause of childhood mortality in developing countries. Risk factors to the development of persistent diarrhea include young age, malnutrition, lack of breast-feeding, impaired immune function, and previous antibiotic use.[84,85]

Postenteritis Syndrome (or Persistent Diarrhea)

Postenteritis syndrome (or persistent diarrhea) is the term used to describe diarrhea that continues even after the offending infective organism has been cleared. It is multifactorial and related to pathogens causing diffuse mucosal injury of the gastrointestinal tract, resulting in persisting symptoms. Postenteritis syndrome is associated with malabsorption and malnutrition. It should be considered in any child who presents with continuing diarrhea following acute gastroenteritis. Postenteritis syndrome may involve lactose, other disaccharides, or protein intolerance. Treatment with protein hydrolysate may be necessary.

It has been postulated that the persistence of diarrhea may be related to nutritional deficiencies such as zinc. Recent studies have evaluated the impact of zinc supplementation on the clinical course of persistent diarrhea. In a trial carried out in Bangladesh, zinc supplementation resulted in shortening the duration of diarrhea by 33%, less reduction in the mean body weight, and a decrease in mortality.[86] In another study from South America, there was also a significant reduction in the duration of persistent diarrhea in zinc-supplemented children.[87]

Carbohydrate Intolerance

Carbohydrate intolerance can follow acute gastroenteritis. The most common form is lactose intolerance (secondary lactose intolerance). The reduction in disaccharidase activity is dependent on the degree of mucosal injury.[88] Although lactase activity decreases with age, primary lactase deficiency is rare. Lactose intolerance is diagnosed by the presence of more than 0.5% reducing sugars in the stool and by stool sugar chromatography. Treatment is by excluding lactose in the diet.

Protein Intolerance

Cow's milk protein intolerance should be considered in the differential of prolonged diarrhea in the infant.[89] Clues to the diagnosis may be obtained from history of exposure to cow's milk, positive skin prick test, and positive radioallergosorbent (RAST) tests for cow's milk. Treatment includes exclusion of dairy in the mother's diet for the child who is breast-fed, excluding cow's milk, or introducing a protein hydrolysate.

Any child with chronic diarrhea should be investigated for celiac disease, as the estimated incidence of this condition is 0.5 to 1% with particular at-risk groups such as diabetes mellitus and IgA deficiency. Treatment is lifelong gluten-free diet with careful monitoring of compliance.

Nonspecific Functional Diarrhea

Toddler Diarrhea

Toddler diarrhea is the commonest cause of chronic diarrhea in otherwise well children referred to pediatricians in the developed world. It is characterized by normal growth and examination and the absence of weight loss or bleeding per rectum. Rapid transit times, dietary factors such as excessive fiber and low fat, and ingestion of large amounts of osmotically active carbohydrates such as apple juice have all been implicated. Studies have also suggested abnormality of motility with a disordered major motor complex that may be prostaglandin mediated.[90,91] Despite the rapid transit, absorption is not affected and the child continues to thrive. A reduction in fiber and osmotically active carbohydrate and increasing dietary fat is often helpful.[92,93] If this fails and the diarrhea is affecting quality of life, an antidiarrheal agent such as loperamide may be used on an as-required basis.

Irritable Bowel Syndrome

Irritable bowel syndrome in the older child may present as chronic diarrhea, although it is usually characterized by alternating diarrhea and constipation, increased flatulence, and/or abdominal bloating. It may be the commonest cause of functional abdominal pain in childhood.[94] Symptomatic treatment can be tried with improved fiber intake and antispasmodics. This aspect is discussed elsewhere in this book.

Inflammatory Bowel Disease

Diarrhea with bleeding PR, once infection has been excluded, suggests a colitic process and is an indication for upper and lower gastrointestinal endoscopy with biopsies. Diagnosis is by histology. Inflammatory bowel disease (IBD) comprises Crohn's disease, ulcerative colitis, and indeterminate colitis. Treatment options include steroids, elemental diet, 5-aminosalicylates, and surgery; these are fully discussed elsewhere in the book.

Pancreatic Insufficiency

Pancreatic insufficiency may present as chronic diarrhea and failure to gain weight in infancy. Causes include cystic fibrosis and Shwachman-Diamond syndrome, and treatment consists of pancreatic enzyme supplements.

Immunodeficiency Syndromes

Immune deficiency can present with protracted diarrhea, but is usually accompanied with a history of recurrent infections, faltering growth and abnormalities in the white cell count. On a global scale, HIV/acquired immunodeficiency syndrome (AIDS) is the commonest cause. Congenital forms of immune deficiency include IgA deficiency, IgG subclass deficiency, and, rarely, severe combined immunodeficiency and hypogammaglobulinemia. Treatment in the last group includes regular intravenous immunoglobulins and appropriate antibiotics.

Severe and Protracted Diarrhea (Intractable Diarrhea) of Infancy

This rare but potentially serious condition, often requiring parenteral nutrition, presents with protracted diarrhea in infancy. Arriving at a specific diagnosis is not always possible,[95] but known causes include congenital defects in gut morphology and function. Application of small bowel biopsy and electron microscopy has identified a number of newer entities such as microvillus inclusion disease, "tufting" enteropathy and epithelial dysplasia, and autoimmune enteropathy.[96] Congenital microvillus atrophy (microvillus inclusion disease) is characterized by hypoplastic atrophy of the villi.[97] There remains a group with unexplained small intestinal enteropathy where newer conditions with a genetic basis are being discovered, such as the phenotypic diarrheas of infancy and others with an autoimmune basis such as the IPEX (immune dysregulation, polyendocrinopathy, enteropathy, X-linked) syndrome. Many infants with severe protracted diarrhea of infancy will have anti-enterocyte antibodies, up to 50% in some series.[98,99] The prognosis of this group of conditions is poor, with an overall 50 to 85% mortality.[100] The successful use of long-term hospital and home-based parenteral nutrition has allowed survival and aided the identification of these conditions in patients who would otherwise not have survived.

Expert nutritional management, appropriate stimulation of the various secretions, improving intestinal motility, control of bacterial proliferation, and the use of hypoallergenic protein sources such as comminuted chicken[101] or elemental feeding may all have a role. Parenteral nutrition used in complement reduces stool volume, lowers fecal organic levels, and results in weight gain and hence a recovery of the nutritional status.[102] While on parenteral nutrition, these infants should also receive some oral feeds, because intraluminal substrates exert a trophic effect on the small intestinal mucosa. Despite aggressive nutritional management, many of these infants do poorly, develop liver disease, and require a small bowel or combined liver and small bowel transplant. In a recent retrospective study, of 20 children receiving some form of intestinal transplant, 8 were for intractable diarrhea of infancy.[103]

Congenital Chloridorrhea

Congenital chloridorrhea is caused by a defect in the intestinal brush border chloride/bicarbonate exchange mechanism. This impedes sodium-chloride exchange and leads to secretory diarrhea characterized by voluminous watery stools containing an excess of chloride present from a few weeks of age. A stool chloride content that exceeds the sum of fecal sodium and potassium confirms diagnosis. Serum electrolytes in these patients show hyponatremia, hypokalemia, hypochloremia, and metabolic alkalosis.[104] Treatment involves ensuring a high intake of chloride and careful monitoring of dietary intake and serum electrolyte concentrations. Suppression of gastric chloride secretion by a proton pump inhibitor has been shown to reduce fecal electrolyte losses.[105] Use of proton pump inhibitors may be useful as an adjunct in the treatment of these children.

Conclusion

Identifying a specific cause for chronic diarrhea by a logical systematic approach is important in order to provide specific appropriate therapy and prognosis. Protracted diarrhea of infancy often needs parenteral nutrition and carries a significant mortality risk. Advances in small bowel transplantation are offering improving prognosis. Endorphin-based medications such as racecadotril may have a role to play in protracted diarrhea of childhood, and further research is needed in this area.

REFERENCES

1. Bryce J, Boschi-Pinto C, Shibuya K, Black R. WHO Child Health Epidemiology Reference Group. WHO estimates of the causes of death in children. Lancet 2005;365:1147–1152.
42. Walker-Smith J, Sandhu BK, Isolauri E, et al. Recommendations for feeding in childhood gastroenteritis. Medical position paper on behalf of ESP-GHAN. J Pediatr Gastroenterol Nutr 1997;24:619–620.
49. Sandhu BK. Practical guidelines for the management of gastroenteritis in children. J Pediatr Gastroenterol Nutr 2001;33:S36–S39.
53. Guidelines for the Management of Acute Gastroenteritis under 5 Years of Age. National Institute for Clinical Excellence (NICE); April 2009.
78. Sazawal S, Black RE, Bhan MK, et al. Zinc supplementation in young children with acute diarrhea in India. N Engl J Med 1995;333:839–844.
83. WHO. Meeting of the immunization strategic advisory group of experts,April 2009-conclusions and recommendation. Weekly Epidemiol Rec 2009;23:213–236.

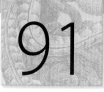

91 EFFECTS OF DIGESTIVE DISEASES ON BONE METABOLISM

Francisco A. Sylvester

Bone has a variety of functions, including mechanically supporting organs and soft tissues, hematopoiesis, acid-base buffering, and serving as the largest reservoir for calcium and phosphate in the body. In this chapter we focus on the effects of chronic digestive diseases on skeletal mass and structure. Bone mass, the most important determinant of bone strength, is regulated by the activities of bone-forming cells (osteoblasts) and bone-resorbing cells (osteoclasts). Bone is formed when bone formation outpaces bone resorption. Bone loss and structural deterioration occur when osteoclast activity predominates over bone formation. Both osteoblasts and osteoclasts can respond to systemic and local signals, and their function can be altered in disease states. Therefore, it is not surprising that many gastrointestinal and liver diseases have an impact on bone mass. Because growing children have actively remodeling bones, they may be particularly vulnerable to the effects of disease on the skeleton. However, restoration of health in children offers the hope of skeletal reconstitution, a characteristic that may be unique to pediatric patients. Current knowledge indicates that the response of children's bone metabolism to both disease and therapy is different than in adults. Therefore, similar to other fields in pediatrics, observations on the impact of gastrointestinal and liver disease on the adult skeleton should not be directly extrapolated to children. This chapter points out differences in how digestive diseases affect bone in children and in adults. To achieve this goal, we first review basic bone biology, then the assessment of bone mass and bone metabolic activity; we then review current knowledge on the effects of digestive diseases on bone metabolism and bone mass in children, and available therapies to enhance bone mass. The reader is referred to excellent recent reviews on this subject that focus on the impact of these diseases on skeletal health of adult patients.[1-4]

BONE BIOLOGY IN CHILDREN

Growing children increase the size of their bones ("bone modeling") until they reach pubertal maturity, when their growth plate closes and their linear growth ceases. This normal physiologic process is regulated by an array of endocrine and paracrine factors.[5] These systems act on osteoblasts, cells derived from mesenchymal precursors, and osteoclasts, which develop from hematologic precursors (Figure 91-1). Osteoblasts go through a sequence of developmental events controlled by hormones and transcriptional factors that ensure the proper expression of their mature phenotype and functional properties. The main function of osteoblasts is to form a protein matrix that is rich in type I collagen. Under normal circumstances, this matrix becomes mineralized with calcium phosphate crystals to form

mature bone tissue. Some osteoblasts become embedded in the mineralized matrix and become osteocytes. Osteocytes develop radiating processes that form a network that senses mechanical stress, which induces bone adaptation.[6] Other osteoblasts die by apoptosis, and others form lining cells over newly repaired bone. These lining cells can become active osteoblasts when needed. The protein matrix is embedded with many other proteins besides type I collagen, some of which have regulatory functions, such as transforming growth factor β, osteonectin, and osteopontin.[7] Osteoblasts can respond to a variety of cytokines that are produced in the inflamed intestine and may reach the bone microenvironment.[5,8,9]

Osteoclasts require receptor activator of nuclear factor κB-ligand (RANKL) to differentiate and become active. RANKL is produced by osteoblasts and other cells, such as stromal cells and activated T cells, and serves as the final common mediator by which other factors affect osteoclast development.[10,11] RANKL can be bound to the osteoblast surface, or released into the extracellular fluid in a soluble form. RANKL binds to its receptor RANK on the osteoclast precursor surface, stimulating its proliferation, differentiation, and activity. Mice lacking RANKL or RANK have abnormally dense bones because of lack of osteoclasts. These mice also fail to develop lymph nodes, establishing a link between the immune system and bone cell biology.[11] Interestingly, cytokines associated with inflammation such as tumor necrosis factor (TNF)-α can increase osteoclast formation by stimulating RANKL synthesis, and interleukin (IL)-17 stimulates osteoclastogenesis directly.[12-14] On the other hand, interferon (IFN)-γ, IL-4, and IL-12 are potent inhibitors of osteoclast formation by inhibiting RANKL function.[15-17]

During bone remodeling the activities of osteoblasts and osteoclasts are normally coupled (Figure 91-2) so that increased osteoblast activity leads to activation of osteoclastogenesis and vice versa. Therefore, diseases that decrease osteoblast activity eventually result in decreased bone resorption, a state referred to as *low bone turnover*. In this state, bone mass is lost primarily because of a decrease in osteoblast function. Conversely, when bone resorption is increased, osteoblast activity is induced. However, because bone formation is slower than bone resorption, this will result in loss of bone mass. This remodeling state is known as *high bone turnover*. In some diseases, the function of osteoblasts and osteoclasts can be uncoupled; for example, in adults with Crohn's disease, decreased bone formation can be associated with increased bone resorption.[18] Digestive diseases in children in general tend to induce a state of growth arrest, decrease bone modeling, and low bone turnover,[19,20] rather than increased bone resorption, which is common in adult patients. This has important implications for the optimization

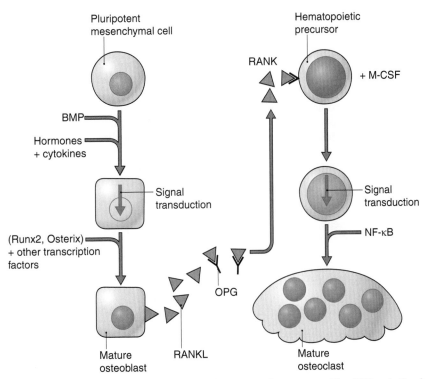

Figure 91-1. Osteoblasts are derived from pluripotent mesenchymal precursors present in bone marrow. Wnt, BMP, and other factors stimulate specific signal transduction pathways in stromal cells that lead to the transactivation of critical transcription factors (Cbfa1/runx2). These regulate the expression of appropriate genes to direct the differentiation of immature cells into osteoblasts. RANKL produced by osteoblasts can then stimulate osteoclastogenesis and osteoclast activation. RANKL activity can be blocked by a soluble decoy receptor osteoprotegerin (OPG).

of bone mass in children with digestive and liver diseases (see later discussion).

Structurally, bone tissue can either be compact or trabecular. Compact bone, which forms the shafts of long bones, constitutes approximately 80% of the bone mass. It is formed by an array of tightly packed mineralized cylinders, each with an axis formed by a nourishing blood vessel that runs parallel to the long axis of the bone. Each cylinder is made of concentric layers of mineralized matrix in which there are embedded osteocytes. On the other hand, trabecular bone is made by interconnecting mineralized elements (trabeculae), resembling the structure of a sponge, and is well represented in the epiphyses of long bones, vertebral bodies, and ribs. Each trabecula is made of mineralized matrix containing osteocytes, and lined by osteoblasts and osteoclasts. Trabecular bone is intimately associated with the bone marrow. It is the most metabolically active bone tissue, accounting for 80% of its metabolic activity. Therefore, chronic diseases may preferentially affect trabecular bone.

PEAK BONE MASS

Bone mass is the major determinant of bone strength over the life of the individual. Rapid gain of bone mass occurs throughout childhood, especially during puberty when bones grow rapidly in longitude, volume, and strength. Eventually, newly formed matrix becomes fully mineralized, signaling the end of bone mass accretion, usually early in the third decade of life. At this time, an individual has finished bone modeling and has gained the maximum of bone tissue, called *peak bone mass*.[21,22] Peak bone mass is achieved earlier in women than in men because women complete their sexual maturation earlier. After

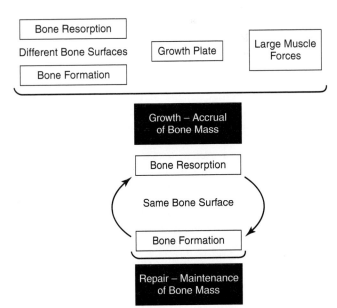

Figure 91-2. After birth, the period of most rapid accrual of bone mass is puberty. This rapid acquisition of bone mass occurs in parallel to linear growth (which depends on the cartilaginous growth plate). Osteoclasts and osteoblasts act on different bone surfaces at the same time to expand the medullary cavity and the periosteal envelope, and to reshape the metaphyses of long bones. Large muscle forces stimulate bone accrual. These processes are collectively known as *bone modeling* and are susceptible to effects of digestive and liver diseases in children. Bone mass is maintained by the coordinated activities of osteoblasts and osteoclasts. This is known as *bone remodeling*. Bone formation lags behind bone resorption, which can result in microarchitectural bone damage and propensity to fractures. In adults with digestive and liver diseases, bone remodeling can be subverted.

late adolescence (around 20 years of age), bone is remodeled and lost at a steady rate for the rest of the person's life, predominantly at the expense of trabecular bone. Eventually, in some individuals the remaining bone may be unable to sustain the stresses of daily living or trauma, fail structurally, and fracture with ordinary physical activity. Therefore, the amount of bone that a child has built is the most important determinant of life-long skeletal health. Peak bone mass is primarily determined by heredity. A family history of osteoporosis and fractures is a major risk factor risk for decreased bone mass. Other factors that influence bone mass include body weight, physical activity, diet, and ethnicity.[23,24] There is a narrow, fixed window of opportunity during puberty and early adulthood when peak bone mass can be acquired. If this time passes, the individual may not attain genetically programmed peak bone mass.[25] This has important practical implications for children with gastrointestinal and liver diseases in whom delayed puberty is common. Every effort should be made to minimize the impact of the underlying disease on pubertal maturation.

MEASUREMENT OF BONE METABOLISM AND BONE MASS IN CHILDREN

Bone biopsy can be used to assess bone remodeling and diagnose bone metabolic disease in both children and adults. Although it is considered the "gold standard," a major disadvantage of bone biopsy for routine pediatric use is its invasive nature. Bone biopsy is usually done in the iliac crest after timed administration of oral tetracycline to label the mineralizing front in the bone, so bone formation rates can be calculated. Ward et al. recently published a bone biopsy study in children with Crohn's disease at diagnosis that suggests that bone turnover is low in these patients.[26]

Several indirect markers of bone metabolism that can be measured in serum and urine are used to assess bone formation and bone resorption. However, their interpretation in children is difficult because they depend on multiple factors including age, pubertal stage, growth velocity, nutritional status, circadian variation, day-to-day variation, and specificity for bone tissue.[27-29] For bone formation, available biomarkers include serum osteocalcin, a protein secreted by mature osteoblasts; bone-derived alkaline phosphatase, a marker of osteoblast activity; and procollagen I extension peptides. For bone resorption, the products of type I collagen degradation N- and C-terminal telopeptides (NTx and CTx), and collagen crosslinks (urinary deoxypyridinoline) are measured. At this point, these markers are most often used in the research setting.

There are several methods to determine bone mineral mass, but in children two methods are most commonly used. One is dual x-ray absorptiometry (DXA), and the is other quantitative computed tomography (qCT). In DXA, an x-ray source generates fan beams of two different energies, which are differentially attenuated by bone and soft tissues. After traversing the body, the residual x-ray energy is measured by an array of detectors placed on a wand that scans the patient from head to toe in a C-arm configuration. A computer analyzes the data and reports them as bone mineral content (BMC, in grams) and bone mineral density (BMD in g/cm^2). BMD is a calculated value (BMC divided by bone area). In addition, information on body composition (percent fat and lean tissue) can be collected. Newer instruments can reconstruct an image of the lateral spine and analyze vertebral bodies for compression fractures (vertebral fracture analysis). DXA involves minimal radiation and time and is reproducible; its use has been validated in children, and there are adequate reference data, at least for some instruments.[28,30] DXA in children should be performed in the total body (minus head) and lumbar spine. DXA scanners are not interchangeable, so longitudinal measurements should be performed in the same instrument when possible, using the same software package. A key concept in DXA scanning is that it is a two-dimensional projection of a three-dimensional object. DXA does not measure the dimension of depth of bone. Bone density by DXA will appear to increase in growing bones, even if the true volumetric density remains constant. Therefore, special caution needs to be taken to properly interpret DXA measurements in children with growth retardation and/or delayed puberty,[28] a common complication of gastrointestinal and liver diseases in children. DXA tends to underestimate BMD in children who are small for their age, whereas it tends to overestimate BMD in children with larger skeletons. To overcome this limitation, the volumetric bone density can be calculated using geometrical assumptions to generate a value called the bone *apparent* mineral density (BAMD).[31] In children who have not yet reached peak bone mass, BMD should be expressed as a Z score, which measures the deviation of the observed BMD from normative values (Z score = Observed BMD – BMD for age, sex, and race/standard deviation). For children with short stature or pubertal retardation, it may be more appropriate to use adjustments for height Z-score to interpret DXA results.[32] In adults, BMD is expressed as a T score, which measures the variance from mean BMD values from young, healthy adults. T scores should never be used in children. In addition to bone density, other properties of bone are important to determine bone strength, including bone geometry, bone quality, and material properties that are not examined by DXA. For example, an equal amount of bone mineral distributed across a larger diameter will confer increased bone strength. We have an incomplete understanding of how childhood illness affects these properties.[33]

Quantitative CT (qCT) can measure true volumetric bone density, but it involves considerably more ionizing radiation and time. On the other hand, peripheral qCT devices involve minimal radiation exposure (comparable to DXA) and measure volumetric bone density, differentiate compact from trabecular bone, and directly visualize limb muscle compartments. This technology is promising for use in children and may be adapted more widely with standardization of measurements at different skeletal sites, improved precision, and generation of normative data.[33]

Measurement of BMD should be considered in children with chronic inflammatory diseases at diagnosis, especially if their disease is severe, they have growth retardation, or their body mass index is low. In addition, BMD should be measured in children on chronic corticosteroid therapy, those with poorly controlled chronic disease, and those who have radiographic evidence of bone demineralization or who have recurrent low impact fractures.

DEFINITION OF OSTEOPOROSIS IN CHILDREN

Based on epidemiologic data in postmenopausal women, the World Health Organization established DXA BMD T score definitions for normal bone mass, mild-to-moderate (osteopenia), and severe demineralization (osteoporosis) *for postmenopausal women*.[34] Accordingly, a T score less than –1 is normal; less than –1 but greater than –2.5 is osteopenia; and less than –2.5

is osteoporosis. Besides the BMD T score, other risk factors for fracture are older age, visual impairment, and low body mass index. There is no "cutoff" value for fracture risk; instead, there is a continuous increase in fracture risk with each decrease in T score. Although the WHO definitions were originally intended to be used in population studies, they are now widely applied to individual postmenopausal women and elderly men to establish the need for therapy. These definitions should not be directly extrapolated to children, and low BMD should not be the sole reason to start a therapeutic intervention in a child. A panel of experts convened by the International Society for Clinical Densitometry suggests that in children low BMD should be described as mild or severe depending on their Z score. A Z score less than −2 should be reported descriptively as "low bone density for chronological age,"[28] without using the terms *osteopenia* or *osteoporosis*. In healthy children, a relationship between low BMD and fracture risk is emerging from longitudinal studies. For example, a study in preadolescent children (average age of 9 years) showed that bone size relative to body size and humeral volumetric BMD are inversely correlated with fracture risk, irrespective of whether fractures followed slight or moderate/severe trauma.[35] In another study, BMD at the total body and spine measured at 8 years of age was a strong predictor of fracture (especially upper limb) during puberty.[36] In addition, there appears to be a period of relative bone fragility during the pubertal growth spurt, when long bone area expands more rapidly that it can mineralize.[37] The implications of these findings in children with chronic digestive disorders are not known.

COMMON MECHANISMS BY WHICH DIGESTIVE DISEASES AFFECT BONE MASS

Puberty is characterized by rapid longitudinal bone growth, volumetric expansion, and bone mineralization.[21] These events require many endocrine and paracrine systems working in harmony. Chronic gastrointestinal and liver diseases can affect normal bone development by affecting these systems. For example, malnutrition due to lack of intake and/or malabsorption is common in children with these diseases. Protein malnutrition is associated with suboptimal bone development.[38,39] Malabsorption of luminal fatty acids in cholestatic states or enteropathies can bind calcium and prevent its absorption. In addition, it is possible that the inflamed intestine may leak calcium into the lumen and be lost in the stool. This can affect the pool of calcium available to mineralize bone. Moreover, malabsorption of fat-soluble vitamins such as vitamin D and vitamin K can adversely affect bone metabolism. Vitamin D insufficiency can result in rickets. Children who are ill may spend more time indoors and limit their exposure to sunlight, thereby decreasing the cutaneous synthesis of vitamin D.[40] They may also limit their intake of vitamin D–fortified dairy products because of primary or secondary lactose intolerance, which will also decrease their calcium intake. In rodent models of colitis, vitamin D supplementation ameliorates inflammation[41] and the lack of vitamin D receptor exacerbates it.[42] However, it is not known if vitamin D supplementation changes clinical outcomes in humans. Vitamin K may play a role in normal bone mineralization, as a cofactor in the γ-carboxylation of glutamic acid to form γ-carboxyglutamic acid residues that can bind calcium. Deficient osteocalcin carboxylation due to vitamin K deficiency leads to markedly decreased affinity of osteocalcin for calcium. The presence of elevated serum uncarboxylated osteocalcin is a sensitive indicator of vitamin K deficiency, before changes in prothrombin time occur. Subclinical vitamin K deficiency has been reported in Crohn's disease[43] and cystic fibrosis.[44] Despite significant changes in BMD, high-dose vitamin K supplementation reduces fracture risk in postmenopausal women.[45]

Delayed puberty is often a feature of chronic digestive diseases and can permanently affect the attainment of peak bone mass.[25] Estrogen is critical in maintaining bone mass in both males and females.[46,47] A relative estrogen deficiency, as seen in children with delayed sexual maturation, may therefore affect bone mass in growing children. Normal bone development is stimulated by weight-bearing exercise. Children with chronic disease may have limitations in their endurance and prefer more sedentary activities. This can potentially decrease bone strength over time.

During puberty there is a marked increase in the magnitude and frequency of growth hormone release. This induces the expression of insulinlike growth factor (IGF)-1 in the liver and other tissues, including the skeleton. IGF-1 is a potent growth factor for bone. It stimulates longitudinal growth by chondrocytes and expansion of the outer cortical layer by periosteal osteoblasts. In the trabecular bone compartment, IGF-1 promotes the recruitment of undifferentiated stromal cells into cells of the osteoblast lineage.[48,49] IGF-1 also is essential for the activation of 1,25-dihydroxyvitamin D.[50] Active chronic diseases in childhood are frequently associated with decreased serum IGF-1, probably as a result of a combination of cytokine effects and nutritional deficiencies (e.g., protein and zinc). Serum IGF-1 tends to increase in parallel with clinical improvement, which helps to reestablish normal skeletal homeostasis.[51-53]

Cytokines and other factors released by inflamed tissues can influence the function of bone cells, and bone cells can secrete cytokines conventionally associated with inflammation. For example, IL-6 is an acute-phase reactant commonly elevated systemically in inflammatory diseases.[54] IL-6 can activate bone resorption by osteoclasts and can also inhibit some aspects of osteoblast function[55] but activate others.[56,57] IFN-γ, a product of activated Th$_1$ CD4$^+$ cells found in inflamed tissues, can inhibit both osteoclastogenesis and osteoblast function.[15,58-61] TNF-α inhibits osteoblast differentiation[62] and can directly (but modestly) induce osteoclast formation.[63,64] RANKL, a member of the TNF family and a potent stimulus for osteoclast differentiation and activity, is synthesized by activated T cells.[65] The specific role of these and other factors in the regulation of bone mass is the subject of intense study.

Medications used to treat digestive disorders can also affect bone cell function. Corticosteroids decrease BMD and increase the risk of fractures in adults, an effect that occurs early in the course of therapy and can be observed even with small doses.[66] A large case-control study involving children who received four or more courses of oral corticosteroids (mean duration 6.4 days), found an increased risk of fracture among children who received the medication as compared with controls.[67] Corticosteroids affect both osteoblasts and osteoclasts, although their initial effect is primarily on bone formation. They can directly inhibit osteoblast function and decrease osteoblast number. In addition, they can affect osteoblasts indirectly by decreasing the synthesis of anabolic sex steroids. Corticosteroids can also inhibit the activity of vitamin D and stimulate parathyroid hormone (PTH) activity, thus stimulating bone resorption. Increased PTH also impairs intestinal calcium absorption and promotes renal elimination of calcium and phosphate. However, it is difficult to dissect the impact of corticosteroids on skeletal mass from the underlying disease in individuals with chronic inflammation.[68] The calcium-binding phosphatase calcineurin regulates osteoblast function,[69-71] and its substrate nuclear factor of activated T cells (NF-AT) is critically important in osteoblast and osteoclast differentiation.[72] Calcineurin inhibitors such as cyclosporin and tacrolimus can inhibit osteoblasts.[73-76] However, under certain conditions cyclosporin and tacrolimus may induce osteoblast differentiation from mesenchymal precursors.[77] Limited information on IFN-α suggests that it decreases the proliferation of human osteoblast precursors,[78] and treatment of chronic hepatitis C with IFN-α and ribavirin may result in bone loss.[79] Ribavarin in vitro up-regulates osteoclast differentiation[80] and reduces osteoblast formation.[81] These effects have not been confirmed in vivo to date. Cholestyramine used to treat pruritus from cholestasis or diarrhea due to unconjugated bile acids can adsorb vitamin D and prevent its absorption from the intestinal lumen. Loop diuretics for treatment of ascites can increase urinary calcium loss.

SELECTED GASTROINTESTINAL DISEASES ASSOCIATED WITH DECREASED BMD

Inflammatory Bowel Diseases

Both Crohn's disease and ulcerative colitis are associated with decreased bone mass. In adults with IBD, bone mass deficits are present in 0 to 65%, depending on the population studied and the method used to determine bone mass; most large studies report a prevalence of low BMD of about 15%.[2] Some studies suggest that patients with Crohn's disease may be affected more severely than patients with ulcerative colitis.[82-84] Children with IBD can also have decreased BMD,[85-87] even at the time of diagnosis, before corticosteroid use.[19,33] Nontraumatic fractures have been reported in both adults and children with IBD, especially at sites rich in trabecular bone.[84,88-96] Several large studies have been conducted to estimate the risk of fracture in adults with IBD. In a retrospective population-based cohort study, Bernstein et al. reported that Canadian patients with IBD had a 41% greater risk of fractures compared to the general population, with similar increases for Crohn's disease and ulcerative colitis.[97] A case-control study in patients recruited from the Danish Colitis/Crohn's Association found a 2.5-fold increase of fracture only in females with Crohn's disease.[84] A subsequent study using a hospital discharge registry by the same group reported a modest increase in fracture risk in Crohn's patients, but not in those with ulcerative colitis.[98] Using a primary care-based nested case-control approach, a study from the United Kingdom showed that the risk of fracture was higher in IBD patients than in controls, especially for subjects with Crohn's disease in the hip.[93] On the other hand, Loftus et al. did not detect an overall increased risk of fracture in adults with Crohn's disease or ulcerative colitis.[99,100] However, the true prevalence of fractures in IBD patients may be underestimated, because a minority of vertebral fractures come to clinical attention.[91,92] In fact, several studies show a high prevalence of asymptomatic vertebral deformities and fractures in adults with IBD.[95,96] The only available study in children evaluated appendicular fractures with a recall questionnaire and found that fracture rates were similar in patients and their unaffected siblings.[101] Additional studies are needed to determine the prevalence of long bone and vertebral fractures in children.

The pathogenesis of bone loss in IBD, as in other digestive disorders, is likely multifactorial, with roles for protein-calorie malnutrition,[86] vitamin deficiencies (e.g., D[40] and possibly K[43]),

malabsorption, inactivity, hypogonadism,[102] corticosteroid use,[103-105] and systemic inflammation.[106] Interestingly, endogenous overproduction of active vitamin D has been reported in Crohn's disease, suggesting up-regulation of 1-α-hydroxylase and vitamin D paracrine effects in inflamed intestinal mucosa.[107,108] Children with Crohn's disease have persistent deficits in lean body mass and skeletal muscle,[109,110] which result in reduced mechanical strain and decreased bone formation.[111]

Biochemical markers of bone metabolism suggest that bone formation is reduced in both adults and children with long-standing Crohn's disease,[18,89,112,113] whereas bone resorption is increased in adults but not in children.[18,19,112,113] In patients newly diagnosed with Crohn's disease, recently published bone biopsy data also suggest a state of low bone turnover, with decreased bone formation and resorption.[26] In animal models of colitis, which mimic the physiologic situation in a growing child, bone loss occurs primarily due to decreased bone formation.[114] Using an in vitro model of intact bone, Hyams et al. showed that serum from newly diagnosed children with Crohn's disease decreases bone weight and calcium incorporation, with no increase in bone resorption. Serum of children with ulcerative colitis had no effect.[115] Antibody neutralization of serum IL-6 in part reverses the effects of Crohn's serum in this model.[55] Similar studies using primary osteoblast cultures showed that osteoblast function is impaired by serum from newly diagnosed, untreated children with Crohn's disease.[116] These data suggest important differences in the pathogenesis of osteopenia between Crohn's disease and ulcerative colitis, and between children and adults with IBD, which have implications for how these children should be treated.

Inflammation is thought to play an important role in inducing bone loss in these patients. Specific cytokines have been implicated in the osteopenia associated with IBD. For example, Pollak et al. observed that high serum IL-6 was associated with osteoporosis (spine or hip BMD T score less than −2.5) in a cohort of adult patients with Crohn's disease and ulcerative colitis.[117] In the skeleton, IL-1β stimulates bone resorption by increasing osteoclast activity. Nemetz et al. found that an IL-1β polymorphism that confers a phenotype of increased IL-1β secretion, is associated with decreased BMD in adult IBD patients compared to healthy controls.[118] Schulte et al. observed that noncarriage of the 240-base pair allele of the IL-1 receptor antagonist gene and carriage of the 130-base pair of the IL-6 gene were independently associated with increased bone loss.[119] Thayu et al. reported that treatment with infliximab, a TNF-α antibody, is associated with a dramatic increase in biomarkers of bone turnover, especially bone formation.[20] These studies emphasize the need to adequately control inflammation to promote skeletal reconstitution in patients with IBD.

A rare skeletal complication associated with IBD is chronic recurrent multifocal osteomyelitis. This condition is associated with sterile inflammation of the clavicles, vertebrae, and long bones, and it usually appears years before the onset of gastrointestinal symptoms. It is not specific to IBD, as it can occur in other chronic inflammatory diseases. It responds to treatment of the underlying disease.[120,121]

Celiac Disease

Loss of bone mass can occur in patients with celiac disease, even in patients who do not present with classic symptoms.[122,123] In adults, the prevalence of bone mass deficits at the spine is

28% and at the hip 15%.[124-126] The risk of fracture in adults with celiac disease appears to be increased,[127,128] especially in subjects with high concentrations of tTG antibodies and typical symptoms.[129,130] In a large population-based cohort study of middle-aged patients, West et al. observed a modest increase in the overall risk ratio for any fracture of 1.30 (95% confidence interval 1.16 to 1.46). The most commonly affected sites were the hip, ulna, and radius.[131] In a cross-sectional, case-control study, patients with "classic" symptoms of celiac disease had a higher prevalence of fractures than patients with subclinical or "silent" disease,[129] with fractures more common in the peripheral skeleton.[132] However, other studies have failed to detect an increase in the risk of fractures in these patients.[98,133] These apparent discrepancies may be due to patient selection and degree of compliance with a gluten-free diet (GFD).[125] The risk of hip fracture in children may also be increased,[134] but children who follow a GFD strictly have an excellent chance of full skeletal repair 1 year after diagnosis.[135-137] There are reports of osteopenia in adolescents following a gluten-free diet long-term,[138,139] which may reflect low adherence to the diet in this age group and decreased skeletal plasticity in these older children.

The pathogenesis of bone loss in celiac disease is not well understood. Studies in children suggest that bone formation is reduced at the time of diagnosis, as judged by decreased serum osteocalcin and carboxy-terminal peptide of type I collagen (PICP).[140] Bone remodeling becomes significantly more active after the initiation of a GFD, as determined by biochemical indices of bone turnover.[135,140] Bone turnover may be inhibited by inflammation in untreated children. For example, elevated serum IL-6 a marker of active inflammation, and reduced IL-1ra, an anti-inflammatory factor, correlate with decreased BMD in celiac disease at diagnosis.[141] Malnutrition could also adversely affect bone metabolism in celiac disease, but bone mineral deficits occur in well-nourished individuals with celiac disease. Calcium may bind to unabsorbed fatty acids and form indigestible soaps, but this has not been proven. Malabsorption of vitamin D can further impair intestinal calcium absorption and lead to secondary hyperparathyroidism and phosphaturia.[142-144] Clinical vitamin K deficiency with prolongation of prothrombin time has been observed in patients with celiac disease.[145] Vitamin K deficiency may also affect the posttranslational γ-carboxylation of osteocalcin, a matrix protein that plays a role in bone calcification. Magnesium deficiency has been detected by sensitive methods in patients with celiac disease, but others have reported normal levels.[146] Magnesium deficiency can decrease bone turnover and contribute to osteopenia.[139,147]

It is probably not helpful to perform bone density scanning in children with celiac disease. This would be justified if children who strictly avoid gluten were at an increased risk of fracture. This scenario is unlikely because children rapidly accrue bone mass in response to a GFD. The question of screening for bone mass deficits in adults with celiac disease who have idiopathic osteoporosis has not yet been resolved.[133,148-153]

LIVER DISEASES

Cholestatic Liver Disease

Cholestatic liver disease is associated with decreased BMD in both children and adults. In adults, primary biliary cirrhosis (PBC) is the major cholestatic disease, which rarely (if ever) occurs in children.[154] Therefore, studies that examined patients with PBC are not discussed here, as the mechanisms by which it affects bone metabolism may be different than in childhood cholestatic disorders. The reader is referred to recent excellent reviews on bone loss associated with PBC for more information.[1,155,156] Studies in children with cholestatic diseases such as extrahepatic biliary atresia and Alagille syndrome have shown that osteopenia is prevalent, as judged by DXA.[157-162]

In a rat model of cholestasis (bile duct ligation), bone histomorphometry shows signs of reduced bone volume and bone formation, a decreased osteoblast pool, and increased bone fragility.[163,164] The nature of bone disease in children with cholestasis is not precisely known. In adults with cholestasis, bone histomorphometry suggests decreased bone formation and osteoblast activity, consistent with a low bone turnover state,[165] although in women there may be uncoupling of bone remodeling with increased bone resorption.[166] In these patients, osteoporosis is more common than osteomalacia.[167] Such studies have not been conducted in children. Indirect biochemical markers of bone metabolism suggest decreased bone formation.[168,169] Although fragility fractures occur in cholestatic children,[170-173] their precise increase in fracture risk is not known.

The pathogenesis of bone loss in cholestatic liver disease probably involves multiple factors. Vitamin D malabsorption is common and serum concentration of 25-hydroxyvitamin D, which reflects vitamin D stores, needs to be followed carefully.[174-178] Radiologic changes of rickets are typically not present.[159,177] Adequacy of vitamin D stores can be difficult to ensure in children with cholestasis. Coadministration of vitamin D with an amphipathic form of vitamin E (D-α-tocopheryl polyethylene glycol-1000 succinate or TPGS) can increase its absorption.[179] Plasma protein induced in vitamin K absence II (PIVKA-II), an indicator of vitamin K stores, is often reduced in children with cholestasis. This potentially can affect the γ-carboxylation of osteocalcin and bone mineralization.[180] Calcium absorption is normal in cholestatic patients who have normal serum vitamin D.[181] The precursor for the formation of vitamin D in the presence of UV light (7-dehydrocholesterol) is present in normal concentration in the skin of cholestatic patients, so skin photoconversion of vitamin D is probably normal.[182] IGF-1 is a potent anabolic agent for bone growth. Interestingly, growth hormone (GH) concentration is elevated in children with cholestasis, while serum IGF-1 and its binding protein 3 are both low. This suggests that in chronic cholestasis there is peripheral resistance to GH and decreased production of IGF-1 in the liver and other tissues.[53,183] Unconjugated bilirubin has direct negative effects on osteoblast proliferation and function in vitro, whereas the role of bile acids is not clear.[184] In addition, specific genetic defects associated with Alagille syndrome in the Notch pathway[185,186] may affect osteoblast differentiation and skeletal maturation.[187] Lastly, children with cholestatic liver disease who are receiving parenteral nutrition can develop hypercalcemia of unknown cause. Intravenous pamidronate, a bisphosphonate, has been used successfully to control this metabolic abnormality.[188]

Liver Transplantation

The most common indication for liver transplantation in children is biliary atresia, and most of these children are transplanted in infancy. This is in contrast to adults who require liver transplantation for chronic viral hepatitis, cancer and alcoholic liver disease. Consequently, there are significant differences in the posttransplantation effects on bone cells between children and adults. In adults there is a rapid decline in bone mass and increased fracture risk after surgery, especially in the early postoperative period.[189-191] Histomorphometry of dual tetracycline-labeled bone biopsies obtained at the time of transplantation and 4 months later shows loss of bone volume and increased bone resorption at baseline and an increase in bone formation but continued high resorption after transplantation, with a net decrease in bone mass.[192] Low bone turnover (decreased bone formation and resorption) has also been reported.[193] Pretransplantation bisphosphonates, which mainly inhibit bone resorption, can decrease bone loss in adults,[194-197] but they may not prevent fractures.[198] Contrary to adults, liver transplantation appears to have an anabolic effect on bone in children, with a significant increase in bone mass by 3 months after transplantation.[161,199] BMD becomes normal approximately 1 year after transplantation,[200,201] which may be due in part to increases in bone size associated with catch-up growth. These data suggest that restoration of normal liver function, with consequent improvement in nutrient intake, absorption, and physical activity, may outweigh the negative effects of immunosuppressive therapy on bone metabolism in these children. Although fragility fractures have been reported after liver transplantation,[202] more studies are needed to examine their precise risk, especially in the context of more refined posttransplantation medical therapy that reduces steroid exposure. In addition, some patients receive liver grafts from living-related donors, which allow for earlier surgery and may prevent long-term complications from end-stage liver disease such as bone loss.

CYSTIC FIBROSIS

Low Bone Mass

Bone loss and fractures have been reported both in adults and children with cystic fibrosis. Fractured ribs can make it more difficult to cough effectively and to perform chest physiotherapy, and chest deformities from kyphosis can further restrict lung capacity.[203] Approximately one third of patients with CF have a significant decrease in bone mineral mass.[204-209] Low BMD by DXA correlated with decreased lung function and mortality in an Irish pediatric cohort.[209] However, the precise prevalence of osteopenia in children is debated, because of methodologic limitations of studies (small sample sizes, mixed age groups, inclusion of severely ill adults) and because patients with CF can be short for their age, so their bone density can be underestimated by DXA.[32,210,211] It is also possible that there are regional differences in BMD in patients with cystic fibrosis, depending on their content of trabecular or cortical bone. Fractures tend to occur in skeletal sites that are rich in trabecular bone.[203] Louis et al. reported normal radius BMD measured by pQCT in well-nourished young adults with cystic fibrosis, but reduced cortical thickness,[212] whereas Gronowitz et al. using similar methodology observed an increase in endosteal surface.[213] This could affect the biomechanical properties of long bones such as resistance to bending and make them more prone to fracture. In studies measuring bone density of the lumbar spine by quantitative computed tomography (which measures volumetric BMD), Gibbens et al. showed a statistically significant decrease in mineral density in 57 patients under 21 years of age with CF compared to healthy controls,[214] but Haworth et al. reported only mild bone mineral deficits in 151 adult

patients using the same method.[215] On the other hand, Buntain et al reported normal BMD measured by DXA in well-nourished prepubertal children with CF, but decreased bone density after the onset of adolescence.[216] This suggests that increased longevity in CF patients may convey a higher risk of bone loss.

The pathogenesis of bone loss in CF is not precisely known. Histomorphometry data are very limited. A 25-year-old male with cystic fibrosis who sustained a fragility fracture of the femoral neck and was treated with an oral bisphosphonate had severe cortical and trabecular osteopenia with no osteomalacia.[217] Serum osteocalcin is low in young patients with CF, suggesting decreased osteoblast activity and bone formation.[218-220] A longitudinal study of patients with cystic fibrosis that included both children and adults showed failure to gain bone mineral at the expected rate.[221] As judged by balance studies using stable isotopes of calcium, rates of calcium deposition into bone are decreased despite normal calcium absorption in clinically stable females with cystic fibrosis.[222] Calcium absorption is not augmented by supplemental vitamin D and calcium.[223] Therefore, bone formation may be compromised in young individuals with cystic fibrosis due to unknown mechanisms. The specific contribution of the disease versus the impact of age, malnutrition, severity of lung disease, underlying inflammation, gonadal function, physical activity and corticosteroid use is not clear.[210] Interestingly, levels of undercarboxylated osteocalcin and plasma prothrombin in vitamin K absence (PIVKA-II) are increased in CF, indicating subclinical vitamin K deficiency[44,224,225] that may negatively affect calcium balance. Vitamin D can be normal[226] or low,[227,228] so serum 25-hydroxyvitamin D should be monitored periodically and supplemented. Recent calcium balance data suggest that excessive fecal losses of calcium occur in girls with cystic fibrosis, in spite of normal calcium absorption, suggesting that calcium is abnormally leaked back into the intestinal lumen.[222] Hardin et al. have reported that recombinant growth hormone improves general health in patients with cystic fibrosis and bone mineral content.[229,230]

Hypertrophic Pulmonary Osteoarthropathy

Patients with CF with advanced lung disease may develop joint swelling, pain, and morning stiffness.[231] The etiology of this complication is not understood. It is usually controlled with nonsteroidal anti-inflammatories, physiotherapy, and sometimes corticosteroids. IV pamidronate, a bisphosphonate that inhibits bone resorption, has also been used.[232,233]

TREATMENT

In the vast majority of children with digestive diseases, measures that improve general well-being may promote bone health as well. For example, optimal nutrition (including adequate caloric and protein intake, vitamins D and K, calcium, and magnesium), encouraging weight-bearing physical activities, control of the underlying inflammatory activity of the disease, and judicious use of medications that can affect bone metabolism such as corticosteroids should be considered in all children, regardless of their diagnosis. Clinical experience has demonstrated the potential for complete skeletal reconstitution in children treated for digestive diseases, a feature that may be unique to patients who have not yet achieved skeletal maturity. As physicians we have a responsibility to take advantage of this opportunity to optimize lifelong bone health.

In the absence of pediatric data, it is common to extrapolate indications and results obtained with therapeutic agents in adults. We need to be aware of the potential dangers of this assumption, given important physiologic differences. This principle is important to consider when deciding whom to treat for decreased bone mineral mass. We cannot assume that drugs used to treat osteoporosis in adults are appropriate for use in children. Although there is strong evidence suggesting that decreased bone mass (as defined by reduced BMD) is common in pediatric gastrointestinal disorders, it is critical to remember that the important clinical endpoint for decreased bone mass is fracture. Therefore, reduced BMD alone should never be used as the sole criterion to start therapy in a child. In children in whom a fracture(s) have occurred, risk factors for osteoporosis should be identified and, if possible, corrected. These children should probably be considered for pharmacologic therapy to try to prevent future fractures and alleviate bone pain.

Therapeutic options for children with decreased bone mass and fractures are limited. Bisphosphonates are derivatives of pyrophosphate that have been shown to increase BMD and decrease the risk of new fractures in postmenopausal women and in patients receiving long-term corticosteroids. These drugs are potent antiresorptive agents. Although oral forms are poorly absorbed, they accumulate in bone tissue where they can remain for several years. There is very limited published experience with these agents in patients who have digestive diseases and decreased bone mass and most experience in children is with intravenous pamidronate.[234,235] Before treatment with bisphosphonates can be recommended, it is important to remember that no trials have been conducted in this group of patients using reduced fracture risk as an endpoint, but rather increases in BMD. Increases in BMD do not necessarily result in decreased fracture risk. In addition, these agents have neither been licensed for use nor adequately studied in children. Although observational studies suggest that pamidronate reduces fractures and increases bone mineral density in children, there are no randomized, controlled trials to establish the safety, efficacy, and optimal dose of bisphosphonates for use in children.[234] Also, one needs to consider that digestive diseases in children appear in general to retard bone formation rather than increasing bone resorption, suggesting that bisphosphonates may have a limited role. The administration of bisphosphonates should be done in conjunction with by a pediatric endocrinologist with experience in bone diseases.

Anabolic agents are being developed to promote osteoblast function. Teriparatide (a new recombinant human parathyroid hormone, hPTH (1-34)), is the first U.S. FDA-approved anabolic growth agent for bone, but its use is contraindicated in individuals whose growth plate is not fused because of the theoretical concern of promoting the development of osteosarcoma.[236] Other agents, such as intranasal calcitonin, have seen limited use in children.

Low-intensity vibration is a promising treatment modality aimed at mechanically stimulating bone formation. It is currently being tested in children with Crohn's disease and cystic fibrosis.[237]

REFERENCES

19. Sylvester FA, Wyzga N, Hyams JS, et al. Natural history of bone metabolism and bone mineral density in children with inflammatory bowel disease. Inflamm Bowel Dis 2007;13:42–50.
28. Lewiecki EM, Gordon CM, Baim S, et al. International Society for Clinical Densitometry 2007 Adult and Pediatric Official Positions. Bone 2008;43:1115–1121.
33. Dubner SE, Shults J, Baldassano RN, et al. Longitudinal assessment of bone density and structure in an incident cohort of children with Crohn's disease. Gastroenterology 2009;136:123–130.
67. van Staa TP, Cooper C, Leufkens HG, Bishop N. Children and the risk of fractures caused by oral corticosteroids. J Bone Miner Res 2003;18: 913–918.
68. Leonard MB. Glucocorticoid-induced osteoporosis in children: impact of the underlying disease. Pediatrics 2007;119(Suppl. 2):S166–S174.
106. Harris L, Senagore P, Young VB, McCabe LR. Inflammatory bowel disease causes reversible suppression of osteoblast and chondrocyte function in mice. Am J Physiol Gastrointest Liver Physiol 2009;296:G1020–G1029.
110. Sylvester FA, Leopold S, Lincoln M, et al. A two-year longitudinal study of persistent lean tissue deficits in children with Crohn's disease. Clin Gastroenterol Hepatol 2009;7:452–455.
122. Mora S. Celiac disease in children: impact on bone health. Rev Endocr Metab Disord 2008;9:123–130.
179. Argao EA, Heubi JE, Hollis BW, Tsang RC. D-Alpha-tocopheryl polyethylene glycol-1000 succinate enhances the absorption of vitamin D in chronic cholestatic liver disease of infancy and childhood. Pediatr Res 1992;31:146–150.
220. Schulze KJ, O'Brien KO, Germain-Lee EL, et al. Calcium kinetics are altered in clinically stable girls with cystic fibrosis. J Clin Endocrinol Metab 2004;89:3385–3391.
234. Ward L, Tricco AC, Phuong P, et al. Bisphosphonate therapy for children and adolescents with secondary osteoporosis. Cochrane Database Syst Rev 2007(4):CD005324.

See expertconsult.com for a complete list of references and the review questions for this chapter.

NUTRITION AND FEEDING FOR CHILDREN WITH DEVELOPMENTAL DISABILITIES

Stanley A. Cohen • Aruna S. Navathe

Although the primary problems for individuals with developmental disabilities are physical and mental incapacities, these individuals are more likely to have problems with feeding and nutrition, which may then be reflected in growth and nutrition disorders. As many as 60 to 90% of children with developmental disabilities have feeding problems, based on parental report,[1] observation,[2] and videofluoroscopy.[3] Often, feeding difficulties may precede and in fact herald the diagnosis of cerebral palsy in 60% of children whose mothers note poor sucking, vomiting, and choking.[2,4] Many individuals with developmental disabilities may have significant oral motor dysfunction with medical sequelae such as retching, choking, and aspiration and subsequent behavioral factors[5-7] that have a further impact on their nutritional status.[2] Moreover, the lack of self-feeding skill was associated with a sixfold risk of mortality in 12,000 young children less than 3.5 years of age with cerebral palsy compared to the 1.4- to 3-fold risk associated with low birth weight, the severity of their retardation, and their underlying disease.[8]

NUTRITIONAL GOALS AND RISKS

The nutritional goals for the individual with developmental disabilities may appear obvious and implicit: adequate nutritional substrate to maintain the individual's metabolic and fluid requirements, sufficient energy intake to perform those metabolic tasks, additional energy stores to withstand stress (e.g., infections) and optimize growth, rehabilitation of malnutrition, and the correction and prevention of nutrient deficiencies. The challenges that arise at the practical level are:

- How do we assess the individual's status and best estimate his or her real needs (e.g., what is optimal growth for a patient with developmental disabilities)?
- How do we account for those needs and the caregiver's abilities to deliver the appropriate nutrition?
- How do we involve the individual's family and caregivers in the decision making and delivery of those services?
- How do we modify the feedings to lessen potential risks and problems (e.g., aspiration and constipation)?
- How can we best transition medical and nutritional care and these services as the individual reaches adulthood?

Historically, severe malnutrition was accepted as a concomitant of these disabilities,[9] and aspiration pneumonia was often the expected mode of death.[10] Poor nutritional state was often marked by linear growth failure, decreased lean body mass, and diminished fat stores.[11] Over the past two to three decades, enteral feedings and surgical intervention to protect the airway and provide these feedings have significantly improved the outcome for individuals with severe disabilities.[12] In addition, recognition of the complex interplay of gastroesophageal, oropharyngeal, and neurobehavioral factors has driven the development of multidisciplinary feeding programs that provide comprehensive evaluation and treatment of feeding disorders in children with developmental disabilities, thereby improving nutritional status and reducing the hospitalization rate.[13]

The periods of greatest nutritional risk are in early infancy during the phase of rapid physical growth and brain development, and in the second decade of life when nutritional needs increase as a result of increasing size – with feeding time needing to increase concomitantly to meet caloric and nutritional needs. Oral feeding difficulties can result in decreased feeding efficiency and may become more problematic as the child grows, requiring increased oral intake[14] and skill as foods of greater complexity (variously textured solids and cupped liquids) are presented. Moreover, children with developmental disabilities seem to have a slow convalescence from illnesses because of their inability to increase their energy consumption during or following illness.

Studies on small groups of children with developmental disabilities have demonstrated that increased nutrient intake can improve weight for height, muscle mass, subcutaneous energy stores, peripheral circulation, the healing of decubitus ulcers, and general well-being, while decreasing irritability and spasticity.[15-17] The weight gain is both lean body mass (15%) and body fat (85%). More important, earlier initiation of nutritional intervention leads to a significantly improved outcome.[16] However, this improved nutritional status may not translate into an increase in height or improved function. Children with mild cerebral palsy, who are not malnourished and able to walk, are still below average for height.[18] Even those receiving improved nutrition do not necessarily attain commensurate linear growth.[19] As a result these children are smaller in height and weight than their peers.[20] Because they may also have a late and longer puberty,[21] and because subnormal growth hormone levels were present in 60% of the 10 patients studied, abnormalities in growth hormone secretion may play a role.[22]

VARIABILITY IN NEEDS

Those individuals with cerebral palsy who have the highest level of physical functioning and are fully ambulatory have growth centiles close to the general population, whereas those with lower accomplished functionality lag substantially behind.[23]

Growth is affected not only by a greater degree of motor impairment, but by nutritional status as well. When examined by dietary recall with home visits and a 3-day diet record, the predominant nutritional deficit is in energy intake, with only 20% of these children regularly ingesting 100% of their estimated average requirement, while protein intake was normal. Half of the children with severe disabilities consumed less than 81% of the reference nutrient intake for copper, iron, magnesium, and zinc, with that influenced by their large consumption of milk. Those in the mild and moderately impaired groups had deficiencies of folate, niacin, selenium, and vitamin A.[24] Even among those children with cerebral palsy receiving nutritional supplements, intake of calcium, iron, folate, niacin, vitamin A, and vitamin E may be low, with low concentrations of folate, α-tocopherol, ferritin, and pyridoxal 5-phosphate not uncommon.[25] Tube feeding and use of supplements resulted in greater weight gain[23] and higher concentrations of micronutrients in blood and serum.[25]

These deficiencies and nutritional issues are of particular importance in this population because trabecular bone architecture appears underdeveloped in the distal femurs of children with cerebral palsy,[26] and the fracture rate in children with moderate or severe cerebral palsy is increased, with those who have greater body fat, gastrostomy feedings, and a previous history of fracture at highest risk.[27] Similarly, nutritional status affects health care utilization and social participation. Each increase in standard deviation for triceps skinfold correlated with a 50% reduction in hospitalization, 20% reduction in physician visits, 22% reduction in days missed from school, and 33% reduction in missed activities for the family in the preceding 4 to 8 weeks.[28] Those children with best overall growth, a compilation of linear growth, body mass, fat mass, and lean tissue mass, required fewer days of health care and were able to participate in more days of their usual activities.[29]

At the other end of the spectrum, children with some genetic disorders that are often accompanied by low muscle tone, such as Down, Prader-Willi, Rubenstein-Taybi, and Turner syndromes, may have lower energy needs, as do children with limited gross motor activity. These children are at risk for overfeeding, for many of the same reason as normal children: lack of physical exercise, increased hours in front of the television and computers, and deleterious family food habits. But certain medications with a side effect of increased appetite or sedation and the family's sympathy expressed by increased feeding to please or quiet the child can also contribute to the risk of obesity. Moreover, moderately or severely impaired children can receive overnutrition through gastrostomy feedings because of their low energy expenditure.[30]

Children with autism spectrum disorders (including pervasive developmental disorder, childhood disintegrative disorder, and Asperger's syndrome) are often perceived to have different nutritional needs. These needs are based on a perceived increase in gastrointestinal disorders in this population that often extend to feeding issues and food selectivity[31,32] and on the concept of intestinal permeability ("leaky gut") with penetration of proteins through the intestinal mucosa with subsequent crossing of the blood-brain barrier, affecting the endogenous opiate systems and neurotransmission, creating neurochemical changes that affect behavior. As a result many children with these disorders are placed on gluten- and casein-restricted diets.[33] Although few studies have been performed to evaluate the efficacy of the diet, and despite the risk of nutritional deficiency,[34] some parents elect to continue.[35] Similarly relying on anecdotal reports generating hope for response, families may seek behavioral improvement with a polypharmacy of dietary supplements, probiotics, and nutraceuticals, other restrictive diets, and chelation therapy.[33]

Data on nutritional factors for adults with developmental disorders are equally limited, despite the fact that increased survival of low-birth-weight infants and increased longevity results in 65 to 90% of children with developmental disabilities surviving into adulthood, depending on the age at which survival is calculated.[36] In a study of 86 adult men and women recruited through a cerebral palsy center or participating in regional games sponsored by the U.S. Cerebral Palsy Association, 40% had heights below the 5th percentile, although their body mass indices and mean body fat were within normal range compared with healthy individuals.[37] In a comparative study of 14 adults and 8 adolescents receiving enteral feedings, both groups had decreased body weight and height, although the adolescents were significantly more so (body weight 26.9 ± 4.9 versus 37.8 ± 10.5 kg, and height 120 ± 12 versus 149 ± 11 cm). However, the calculated percentage of body fat and measured resting energy expenditures were similar for both groups.[38] These data suggest that these individuals do not necessarily "grow out of" their feeding problems. That is, caloric intake may not improve with time, and intervention may be necessary to achieve adequate nutritional status if feeding problems are manifested early.

CONTRIBUTING FACTORS

In the child or adolescent with developmental delay, the interconnectedness of malnutrition, growth impairment, and physical/motor function is intuitively obvious and increasing in recognition. The scientific evidence, recognition of other contributing factors, and efforts to interrupt this cycle have resulted in improvements and increased survival over the past 20 years.[39] Gastrostomy feedings are often recommended to supplement or replace oral feedings in patients with dysphagia, aspiration pneumonia, or inadequate weight gain, or where normal dietary intake is insufficient to meet nutritional needs, and it has become a reliable, effective intervention to achieve improved results with lessened feeding time for those with moderate and severe incapacity, benefiting the child and the family,[40] though parents often have initial resistance and oral feed are regarded as optimal.[41]

However, multiple factors may complicate the ability of individuals with developmental disabilities to feed normally and obtain nutritional sufficiency by mouth.[42] Historically the classification of feeding was assigned to an organic or nonorganic cause, with nonorganic causes reflecting social and environmental antecedents[43-45] and comprising the majority of children hospitalized for failure to thrive.[46] More recent classification recognizes the complex overlap of these parameters with physical features and concurrent, often consequential, behavioral elements.[6] Gastrointestinal abnormalities,[47,48] neurologic conditions, structural/oromotor disorders, and behavioral issues often contribute to aberrant eating dysfunction.[6,49]

A model to evaluate undernutrition (Figure 92-1) can assist in understanding the issues involved in order to direct the assessment and approach the treatment of individuals with developmental disabilities who have feeding problems and/or potential nutritional deficiency or impairment.

The *historical perspectives* include the genetic endowment provided by the biologic parents as well as any mutations that may modify the inherent potential growth of the individual. The model then accounts for the child's or adult's underlying illness. For example, not only may a cardiorespiratory problem with tachypnea increase caloric expenditure and need, but the rate of breathing may also complicate the issue of oral coordination and ability. Metabolic dysfunctions, such as phenylketonuria or fructose intolerance, may cause growth disturbances and vomiting if not recognized and appropriately treated. A multicenter study[48] of 14 children with lifelong feeding aversion, retching or vomiting, 11 of whom had cerebral palsy, demonstrated motility and sensory abnormalities of the gastrointestinal abnormalities that responded to treatment in 80% of the children involved.

Neurodevelopmental status logically has the largest impact on children and adults with neurologic impairments. Knowledge of the natural history of the specific disease involvement is imperative in order to understand whether the individual's condition is degenerative, static, or temporary, as this knowledge will guide therapy and nutritional counseling with the family. The degree of disability correlates with risk of malnutrition,[50] with lower nutrient levels associated more with the degree of mental retardation and learning of self-help skills than the motor handicaps imposed by cerebral palsy.[51]

As indicated earlier, *oral motor dysfunction* is a frequent concomitant and often one of the first signs of neuromuscular impairment.[1-3] In addition, anatomic abnormalities such as cleft palate, laryngeal clefts, and tracheoesophageal fistula may accompany neurologic deficits as part of a congenital or genetic syndrome. These problems often manifest with difficult or unsuccessful feeding, nasopharyngeal regurgitation, aspiration, choking, persistent drooling, recurrent respiratory tract infections, and/or poor weight gain.[1-3]

Normal feeding and swallowing are complex, sequential processes often taken for granted. Motor and/or sensory problems[52] may initiate a disturbance in any of these functional phases (Table 92-1), resulting in dysphagia.[48,53] Children with hypotonia or hypertonia may have difficulty using the tongue to move a food bolus through the mouth; others with motor problems may have choking or aspiration with incoordination of the larynx, as the vocal cords close to protect the airway and pharyngeal muscles propel food to the esophagus.[48]

These motor-based dysphagias often demonstrate greater difficulty with thin liquids, such as juice or water; difficulty with chewing; choking or gagging during or immediately after meals, with the meals often prolonged; gurgly vocal quality after meals; or respiratory compromise.[35]

Individuals with sensory-based problems often have more problems with foods that require chewing, and may separate foods of thicker texture and pocket them in their mouths. They often have a sensory integration defect with the texture and perhaps the taste of foods. This may be localized and associated with gastroesophageal reflux (GER), which may result in lessened sensitivity in the hypopharynx from inflammation, or it may be more global, associated with other with sensory problems involving light, touch, and noise.[54]

Intercurrent illnesses, with events as mundane as an upper respiratory infection, may temporarily affect feeding function, with more prolonged infections, such as respiratory syncytial virus bronchiolitis, interfering with nutrition for considerably longer, by increasing caloric needs and impairing efficient and effective feeding. Children with feeding impairment have a slower convalescence from illness because of their inability to increase their energy consumption.[55]

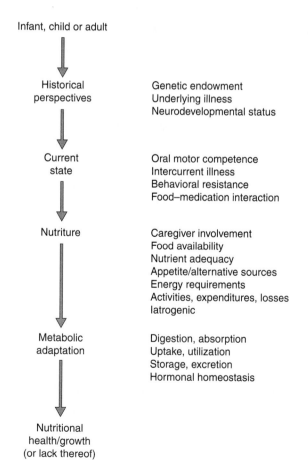

Figure 92-1. Conceptual model of the etiology of feeding disorders and undernutrition in children and adults with developmental disabilities. Adapted from Cohen SA. The Underweight Infant, Child, and Adolescent. New York: Appleton, Century, Crofts; 1986:xvi.

TABLE 92-1. **Phases of Normal Feeding**

Phase	Description
Pre-oral	Appropriate food provided and presented Food introduced into oral cavity
Oral	Suck or mastication prepares bolus Passage of bolus into pharynx
Pharyngeal	Respiration ceases Elevation of larynx; glottic closure Opening of upper esophageal sphincter Pharyngeal peristalsis with clearance of pharynx
Esophageal	Esophageal peristalsis Opening of lower esophageal sphincter
Gastrointestinal	Receptive relaxation allows storage of food in stomach Controlled emptying of nutrients into small intestine Mixing with digestive enzymes and secretions Intestinal digestion and absorption of nutrients

Adapted from Rudolph and Link (2002).[49]

Concurrent, acute, and chronic disorders such as food allergies, malabsorption, GER, delayed gastric emptying, metabolic anomalies, or congenital defects of the gastrointestinal tract may add another layer of complexity to ensuring nutritional adequacy for those who also have neurologic impairment. These medical problems may cause eating to be painful, either directly (as in the case of GER) or indirectly (when illness causes general malaise or nausea, which becomes associated with eating). Again, the association of the presentation of food with pain may produce aversions to food. Temperature of food and texture sensitivity can play a big role in acceptance of food.

It appears that nausea in particular plays an important role in the development of aversions to food.[56] When nausea is paired with eating, aversions to tastes may develop after only one or a few trials and may generalize to many foods. In addition, studies on conditioned food aversions show that when these aversions develop, they can be long-lasting. Children with a complex medical history also miss early critical experiences with feeding. These early opportunities to feed are important for the development of appropriate oral motor skills such as tongue lateralization and elevation.

Studies on hospitalized children indicate that recurrent or chronic hospitalization may have a negative impact on behavior.[57]

Negative behaviors such as crying infants with a complex medical history also are subjected to numerous invasive diagnostic tests and procedures, which may involve manipulation of the face and mouth (e.g., laryngoscope, nasogastric tubes). However, even noninvasive caregiving activities can result in negative, distressed behaviors such as crying that are likely to carry over into the feeding situation in children with a history of hospitalization.[58] From the child's perspective, a spoon may not appear to be substantially different from a laryngoscope or other devices that are used during invasive tests and procedures. Therefore, the child may associate the presentation of objects to the face and mouth (e.g., a spoon) with these early negative experiences and exhibit behaviors such as crying, batting, and head turning when objects are presented to the face and mouth. Parents of hospitalized and medically fragile children often report "oral aversions" that affect feeding and other behaviors associated with the face and mouth (e.g., tooth brushing, face washing).

Although these food aversions and biobehavioral resistances to feeding may result from underlying medical problems, their presence can evolve into a dominant issue. In a study of 103 children referred to an interdisciplinary feeding team, 85% had a behavioral component to their feeding dysfunction irrespective of the underlying medical disorder, with only 12% having an isolated behavioral issue.[6]

The parents' or *caregiver's involvement* is important throughout the entire range of events surrounding feeding. This obvious statement extends beyond a parent's normal expectation of parenthood. Unless ultrasonography or amniocentesis indicates a problem with the fetus prenatally, parents are often ill prepared to raise a child who may not be completely healthy. Feeding often becomes the quintessential embodiment of their parenting and nurturing. In addition to learning the basics of infant feeding, they need to recognize problems quickly and carry out a plan to solve or ameliorate any problems. The caretakers' active involvement and competence is absolutely necessary, but may require considerable support and education. The living situation can be important as well. Children moved to a residential facility are older on average than those living at home and have significantly greater height, weight, skinfold thickness, and midarm muscle area, after controlling for functional level and gastrostomy feedings.[56]

Problems for the teenager with a developmental disability emanate from the increased quantity of nutrients and calories needed because of increased body size. The same may be true for adults, depending on their feeding skills and access to repletional fluids and calories. Decreased feeding efficiency occurs in individuals with cerebral palsy: chewing and swallowing that takes 12 to 15 times longer than in normal controls translates into extended mealtimes. Even then, longer feeding times may not be sufficient to compensate for caloric and nutritional needs,[59] with caregivers often overestimating the individual's caloric intake and the time spent feeding their child with a developmental disability.[60] For those who are not self-feeders, feeding can be further compromised by an oral aversion that develops because of the times that the caregiver must approach the mouth with distasteful medications and foods that are difficult for the child to handle because of delayed oral motor skills.

The combined issues of nutriture become complex because most individuals with developmental disabilities have somewhat *different nutritional requirements*. Body composition is leaner, with eventual height shorter.[20,61] Those who also have oral motor dysfunction have lower Z scores for weight, height, and weight-for-height.[62] Physical activity, intake, and often energy needs are less.[63,64] In addition, a decreased ability to communicate can make it difficult for the caregiver to appreciate hunger or satiety. When oral feedings are supplemented or replaced by nasogastric or gastrostomy feedings, the issues of oral resistance, interpretation of hunger signals, and feeding time are largely obviated, with rapid[65] and sustained[15-17] weight gain and small increments of height growth achieved. (Please refer to the sections on physical assessment and enteral feedings for a more detailed discussion.)

Proper nutriture assumes that nutritious foods are available and provided, and that nutrient needs are adequately met. However, with our still limited knowledge of specific nutrient needs for the individual with neurologic impairment, and with costs high and insurance reimbursement low for medically necessary nutrition, nutrient sufficiency cannot be assumed for any given individual. Indeed, individual metabolic variation and physical activity may be different from one individual to another, and even at different points in time (with increased seizure activity or change in neurologic status with an intercurrent or concurrent illness). Feeding time may also need to change for a particular child or adult based on oral consumption or the schedule for enteral feedings.

Each of the etiologic factors in Figure 92-1 can be seen with its own dynamic continuum affecting and interrelating with the other factors. For example, a child's oral aversion may at times be greater than at others, perhaps affected by, and then further affecting, the parent or caregiver's efforts and abilities (in a bidirectional biofeedback loop). Underlying this could be the degree to which the child's GER is active, which might be exacerbated by a meal containing acidic foods or spicy food such as tomato sauce, or the position in which the child was fed. Thus, an understanding of the nutritional consequences of feeding for the child or adult with developmental disabilities requires a broad understanding of the numerous factors that inform each other and continue to change.

PRESENTATION AND EVALUATION

The complex etiology of feeding problems necessitates an interdisciplinary approach to assessment and treatment. The purpose of a thorough medical and nutritional evaluation is:

- To recognize the patient with, or at risk for, chronic malnutrition and/or specific nutrient deficiencies
- To assess the extent of those problems or potential issues
- To identify underlying, contributory, or resultant conditions and behaviors
- To determine the sufficiency of current intake

This information will allow the medical and therapeutic team to recommend continuation or modifications in the nutritional approach (including the food to be offered, the mechanics of delivery, and any therapies or behavioral changes that may improve of both these), with a plan for ongoing reassessment.

Thus, the medical evaluation (Table 92-2) should document the full context and evolving *history of the underlying illness*, its resulting impairments, and associated conditions. Because prematurity can delay acquisition of oral motor skills and prolonged neonatal hospitalization can further contribute to oral defensiveness, as noted previously, obtaining a careful medical history is essential. The child's medications should be noted in detail, because as many as 25% of nonambulatory patients who receive anticonvulsants may have rickets.[66-68] Impairment or associated conditions should be noted, because these conditions may require specific medical, nutritional, or other types of intervention (e.g., a child with VACTERL may have a ventriculoseptal defect requiring fluid limitations or additional calories, or may have had anorectal surgery necessitating nutritional attention to bowel habits and delayed oropharyngeal skills and tracheoesophageal fistulas that would dictate the amount, texture, and delivery of foods needed). Furthermore, the presence of feeding problems may be significant diagnostically, as indicated earlier.[2]

Specific focus on the *development of oral motor skills* will help to recognize those with malnutrition[69] or feeding dysfunction. The acquisition of feedings skills seems to parallel speech abilities as concurrent oral motor activities, with delayed or anomalous speech patterns often indicative of pervasive oral dysfunction.[70] Refusal to eat contributes further to the child's failure to develop appropriate oral motor skills and to gain weight. The *individual's level of function* and oral motor skill should be assessed carefully. The parent should be queried about the time required to feed the child, their own desire and ability to continue, and the quality of the interaction. If there are other caretakers at home or school, the success of those feedings should be discussed as well. The less skilled the child is in terms of oral competency, the more likely the child is to refuse food and fail to gain weight. In children with cerebral palsy, failure to thrive is contributory to poor feeding skills, because undernourished children have lower feeding competency than children who are adequately nourished.[69] A cycle then develops in which the child refuses food, fails to learn that eating is no longer painful, misses opportunities to practice and develop oral motor skills, and fails to gain weight, which then further reduces the child's motivation to eat.[69]

Dietary history, including a 3-day food record, should document the child's actual food and fluid intake and schedule, as well as any food intolerances, preferences, and supplements. Past and current medications should be noted in detail, because as many as 25% of nonambulatory patients who receive anticonvulsants may have osteomalacia or rickets. The patient or parents also should be asked about any herbal, nutraceutical, or other formulations they are administering, and whether these have been recommended or self-prescribed. They may be reluctant initially to admit to alternative therapies, but use of these may alert the physician to the degree of the parents' frustration with their child's medical progress and to possible interactions of these substances with other foods or medications. Any changes in appetite, intake, oral function, weight, or activity should be addressed as part of an expanded systems review. The patient's bowel habits and urine output may have an important relation to the feedings and should be noted.

This family-centered history should include:

- Degree of self-feeding and tube feedings, as well as the timing and duration of each – occasionally the timing of tube feedings or the parents' efforts to get their child "to eat anything" may be counterproductive and interfere with the child developing hunger; the duration may be overly long and fatigue a child's efforts; dependent feeders have a higher risk of aspiration.[71]
- Textures, types, and amounts of foods offered and consumed – children with a developmental disability often do not consume nearly the volume that is offered. Taste, temperature, and texture may change the acceptance of a given food.
- Presentation of food, the setting and circumstances – distraction by ambient television may lessen or increase the food consumed. Children with oral defensiveness may suck a bottle

TABLE 92-2. Medical Evaluation for Nutritional Abnormalities

History

Illness, level of function
Development and acquisition of oral motor skills
Medications, associated conditions
Bowel habits
Dietary/feeding history
    Appetite, intake, schedule
    Allergies, intolerances, preferences
    Nutritional, vitamin, and mineral supplements
    Changes in activity, weight, appetite, function
    Dysfunction with feeding, swallowing, reflux

Physical (in Addition to Routine)

Height, weight, triceps skinfold thickness, vital signs
Observation and general impression
Abdomen for constipation
Spine for kyphoscoliosis, sacral anomalies
Neurologic for tone and level of function
Oral for gag, swallow, seal, drooling, mucosal problems
Signs of deficiency state or chronic illness (clubbing or ridging of nails, skin turgor and texture, bruises, decubitus)

Laboratory (When Indicated)

Complete blood count – hemoglobin, red blood cell indices, lymphocyte population
Electrolytes with urea nitrogen
Proteins – albumin, prealbumin, transferrin
Calcium, phosphorus, alkaline phosphatase
Vitamin, mineral levels (rarely needed)
Anticonvulsant levels
Thyroid function
Radiography
    Radiography of hand for osteomalacia, bone age
    Ultrasonography or scan of head for hydrocephalus
    Technetium-99m milk scan
    Upper gastrointestinal series (upper GI)
    Oropharyngeal motility study (modified barium swallow)
Videofluoroscopy
pH esophagram

better when first falling asleep or may feed better as they imitate others.

- The individual's position – arched extensor tone, common in individuals with cerebral palsy, can increase the risk for aspiration.[72] In addition, adults with developmental disability who are tube-fed in a horizontal position have a lower life expectancy.[73]
- Troublesome aspects of the feedings (e.g., choking, gagging, change in respiration, regurgitation, feeding refusal) and the stage at which these occur – problems later in the feedings often appear to have a greater correlation with medical issues such as cardiopulmonary problems, dysphagia, or GER, whereas problems at the onset may relate to positioning, parent-child interaction, or oral defensiveness.[72]
- Interaction with the different caregivers, and the amounts consumed with each – different feeding patterns and techniques are often seen with specific caregivers. Those forcing feedings may find an inability to achieve optimal feeding.

Anthropometrics will corroborate and amplify the physician's general clinical impression about the individual's nutritional status. Height and weight should be measured when possible. Specific growth charts are available for patients with Down syndrome[74] and cerebral palsy.[75] The latter uses single leg lengths to achieve better approximation of expected growth, as children and adults with developmental disabilities often have contractures or severe spasticity, countering any attempts at obtaining an accurate measurement of height or length. However, an estimate to use for standard growth charts can be calculated by multiplying the tibial length (measured from the medial popliteal line to the bottom of the medial malleolus) by a constant of 3.26 and adding 30.8 cm:

$$Stature = 3.26 \times tibial\ length + 30.8\ cm$$

Similarly, upper arm measures can be utilized in patients with myelomeningocele to assess their growth on normalized curves.[76]

We must rely on measures that evaluate growth and malnutrition in terms of calculations based on body weight and height for other neurodevelopmental conditions. Height and weight measurements in former premature infants must be adjusted for the months of prematurity in the first 3 years of life, with the expectation that those with 32-week gestations will catch up by 2 years of age and those with gestations of shorter duration may take 3 years to achieve their genetic growth potential. Body mass index (BMI) establishes a ratio between weight and height with comparative percentiles for the general population. Although easily calculated, this measure has not been tested adequately in those at different ages and levels of developmental disability. A single study in adults evaluated 44 men and 33 women with cerebral palsy. At a mean age of 27 years they had a mean ± SD BMI of 22.6 ± 3.6 and 23.6 ± 7.2, respectively, with the percentage of body fat at 13.5 ± 6.0% and 23.2 ± 7.4%.[21]

A weight for height should be obtained by first finding the patient's height age (the age at which the patient's current length would be at the 50th percentile on the appropriate CDC growth chart). The ideal weight is traditionally the 50th percentile weight at that height. However, this may overestimate the ideal weight for those with neurodevelopmental impairment. The 25th percentile, or lower perhaps, is more appropriate. The patient's actual weight as a percentage of the ideal weight for height then can be used to assess the stage of wasting from malnutrition according to Waterlow criteria[77] (Table 92-3).

The limitations of this calculation, resulting from an individual's genetic and ethnic background, must be recognized. Discrepancies within the height age that may not have been reflected by the previous National Center for Health Statistics (NCHS) editions should now be corrected by the more heterogeneous populations that were used to standardize the current Centers for Disease Control and Prevention (CDC) version. However, attempts to use height measures as a valid measure of stunting are fraught with difficulty in patients with developmental disabilities because of contractures and scoliosis.

More sophisticated measurements, using midarm circumference and triceps or subscapular skinfold thickness, may be worthwhile as a measure of muscle mass and energy stores, especially if they are used to monitor a patient's progress. A study of 69 children with cerebral palsy demonstrated that body fat (derived from skinfold thickness) and percentage weight compared to height age (calculated from upper arm length) differentiated children with malnutrition from those with seemingly sufficient energy stores and better growth.[77]

Physical examination is useful in detecting dehydration, malnutrition, or specific nutritional deficiencies. Thus, as part of a comprehensive evaluation, the examiner should document the individual's skin turgor, subcutaneous tissue, and muscle mass carefully, noting any bruising, pressure-induced ulcers, clubbing, edema, or rashes (these may be the result of specific nutrient deficiency states). If a feeding tube is in place, the site should be examined for erythema, edema, granulation tissue, purulence, herniation, or the satellite lesions of a cutaneous yeast infection.

The physical examination also should focus on the sufficiency of oral motor skills as well as posture, tone, and neurodevelopmental function. Arching, spasticity, and neck position should be noted. Respiratory signs including stridor or wheezing are important indicators of the potential for aspiration. The characteristics of an infant's cry may allude to intrinsic laryngeal abnormalities or those that are secondary to GER. Specific anomalies may cause disordered swallowing, which may preclude safe oral feeding. Particular attention to swallowing dysfunction is necessary in muscular dystrophy and similar myopathic disorders. Drooling, mouth closure, and pocketing of food in the mouth during meals are all factors that require careful consideration as feeding therapy is planned, because these may be indicators of oral motor dysfunction. Any evidence of regurgitation, choking or possible aspiration should be evaluated. Well-trained members of the team may observe the individual eating for a better understanding of his or her oral motor competencies.

If the individual's ability to swallow is questioned, or if he or she appears to aspirate, an oropharyngeal motility study (known in some institutions as a modified barium swallow) fluoroscopically evaluates oral/laryngeal mechanisms and protection of the airway. While the patient is normally seated, different textures (at specific temperatures) are offered to the individual while fluoroscopic images are viewed, allowing visualization of

TABLE 92-3. Stages of Wasting From Malnutrition

	% Ideal Weight
Mild malnutrition	<90
Moderate	<80
Severe	<70

Actual weight as a percentage of ideal weight for height (see text).

chewing and swallowing mechanics (Figure 92-2). In addition, the parent-child interaction while feeding can be observed to evaluate behavioral aspects of feeding. If recorded, this can be jointly reviewed by a team of therapists, dietitian, physician, and behavioral specialist so that conjoint goals and therapy can be achieved.

Infants, children and adolescents with the primary diagnosis of severe spastic cerebral palsy who were slow, inefficient eaters demonstrated severe dysphagia on videofluorographic swallow studies, and a significant number (68.2%) had significant silent aspiration during videofluorographic swallow study.[14] Decreased or poorly coordinated pharyngeal motility was predictive of silent aspiration, whereas moderately to severely impaired oral-motor coordination was indicative of severity of feeding complications. Furthermore, the data on the 22 individuals evaluated suggested that early diagnostic work-up, including baseline and comparative videofluoroscopic swallow studies, could be helpful in managing the feeding difficulties in these children and preventing chronic aspiration, malnutrition, and unpleasant lengthy mealtimes.[14]

Biochemical studies, such as determination of serum zinc or vitamin B_{12} levels, have limited use for nutritional evaluation in these individuals, unless they have concomitant problems with malabsorption. Blood tests primarily measure the quality of the diet, whereas they are insensitive to quantitative insufficiencies, which are more frequent problems for these individuals.[54] Protein status is usually normal, when reflected by albumin, transferrin, or prealbumin levels (their half-lives reflecting protein status in the preceding 20 to 30 days, 10 to 14 days, and 3 to 7 days, respectively). Hemoglobin can screen for iron deficiency anemia, which is common. A hand or limb radiograph may indicate the presence of osteopenia or osteomalacia, particularly in the non-weight-bearing individual, as a more sensitive measure than chemical analysis for calcium, phosphorus, or alkaline phosphatase levels. Radiography also can approximate a child's bone age. Anticonvulsant levels and liver and renal function tests may be obtained when indicated.

Currently, bone densitometry may not be cost-effective, as many non-weight-bearing patients can be presumed to develop osteopenia eventually. Bone mineral content and density are reduced in nutritionally adequate children with spastic cerebral palsy, with an even greater reduction in nonindependent ambulators.[19] Hair and nail analyses have not proven useful

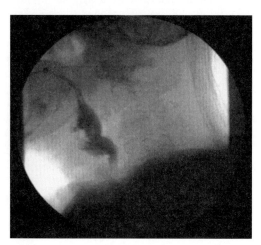

Figure 92-2. Laryngeal penetration demonstrated on oral pharyngeal motility study.

clinically in most cases, although they remain available, but expensive.

GER may be assessed with a 24-hour pH esophagram. A technetium-99m milk scan may quantify reflux in a child unable to complete 24-hour esophagram and may differentially diagnose pulmonary aspiration from the feeding itself or from GER if an image taken 2 to 4 hours later is stained over the lungs. An upper gastrointestinal barium study may be used to assess the suspicion of an anatomic abnormality (but does not diagnose or denote the presence of GER). Gastroesophageal reflux disease may not become obvious until children who have not been fed for prolonged periods actually commence oral food intake during the treatment process.

INTERVENTION

A regimen for feeding the child or adult with a developmental disability must provide adequate nutritional substrates and sufficient energy intake to maintain the individual's metabolic and fluid requirements, with additional energy and micronutrient stores to withstand stressful events, such as infection. Malnutrition and nutrient deficiencies should be corrected and prevented. Each child with a developmental disability, at whatever level, should be able to optimize his or her growth. The question is: how much growth is optimal? In the context of achievable height, children with neurologic impairment historically have been smaller.[11,19,79] Short-term studies with aggressive nutritional regimens have been able to increase weight, but not height.[9,12,16,17] In addition, optimal size for a bed-bound, bedridden child or adult who is severely impaired and requires assistance to move from bed to wheelchair to toilet is perhaps more of an ethical or pragmatic concern. The ease and practicality of providing care for that child or adult may determine the quality of his or her care and the length of time the caregiver can continue to manage that individual's needs in the home setting. Normal weight for height is at the 50th percentile for those with normal activity, the 25th percentile for those able to perform independent transfers, and the 10th percentile for those who are bedridden, with the exception that those under 3 years of age who should be maintained at the 25th to 50th percentile to ensure sufficient growth.[80]

Thus, the goals for nutritional management and rehabilitation (Table 92-4) must be considered, with attention to physiologic function as well as the ethics and practical factors in the delivery of care. More important, an individual must be medically monitored to adjust for changes in his or her physical condition and for the caregiver's status as well.[9,11,12,16,17]

Focus is usually directed toward caloric requirements, because other macro- and micronutrient requirements have not been well established for children with developmental disabilities though

TABLE 92-4. Goals of Intervention

Physiologic maintenance
Rehabilitation of malnutrition
Prevention or correction of nutritional deficiencies
Assist ease of care
Support caregivers in their efforts
When possible:
    Tailor weight/growth to home care need
    Treat feeding problems and behaviors
    Assist development of self-feeding skills
    Regulate bowel habits

TABLE 92-5. Caloric Requirements for Specific Disabilities[74]

Condition	kcal/cm Height
Cerebral palsy (5-11 years)	13.9 if mild-moderate activity 11.1 if severely restricted
Down's syndrome (5-12 years)	16.1 males 14.3 females
Myelomeningocele (over 8 years)	7 to achieve weight loss 9-11 for maintenance
Prader–Willi syndrome	10-11 for maintenance 8.5 for weight loss

TABLE 92-6. Increased Calorie Concentrations of Standard 20-kcal/oz Infant Formulas

	20 kcal/oz	22 kcal/oz*	24 kcal/oz	26 kcal/oz
Powder[†]	4 scoops	4½ scoops	4¾ scoops	5¼ scoops
Water to make	8 oz	8 oz	8 oz	8 oz
Powder[†]	1 cup	1 cup	1 cup	1 cup
Add	29 oz	26 oz	24 oz	21.5 oz
Concentrate	13 oz	13 oz	13 oz	13 oz
Water	13 oz	10½ oz	8½ oz	7 oz

*Concentrations are approximate, and useful for parental instruction.
[†]Scoops (equivalent to 1 tablespoon) and cups should be level, not pressed or packed.

they may differ from those for the nondisabled child, where other requirements generally parallel energy needs. Because of the disproportion between weight and height, calculations are usually conceived in terms of body surface area or height. These can be modified for activity level (or lack thereof) and weight repletion. Normally growing children with spastic quadriplegic cerebral palsy have an energy intake of 60 ± 15% of the recommended dietary allowance (RDA) for sex and age, and 103 ± 32% of that for weight, when exclusively gastrostomy fed.[45] Patients who are nonambulatory require an average of 75% of the calories needed by ambulatory patients of comparable height.[63]

Total energy expenditure is reduced relative to resting metabolic rate because both fat-free mass and activity are decreased, even in patients with spastic, quadriplegic cerebral palsy.[60] Resting energy expenditure (REE) correlates poorly with body cell mass in patients with spastic quadriplegia. Accretion of fat-free mass is significantly reduced in these patients. Moreover, the range of REE in adults extends from 16 to 39 kcal per kg per day when measured and is significantly less than would be predicted by Harris-Benedict and World Health Organization (WHO) equations.[37] Total energy needs for children with spastic quadriplegic cerebral palsy (1.1 × measured REE)[64] are considerably less than the 1.5 to 1.6 × calculated REE suggested by WHO standards.[50] Should REE be used to calculate patient needs, it must be modified by factors that address muscle tone (increasing 10% for hypertonicity; decreasing 10% for hypotonicity), activity (increasing 15% for those bedridden, and 30% for those ambulating), and growth.[80]

Even though measurement of each individual's REE by indirect calorimetry or bioelectrical impedance might be optimal, repeated measurements may be impractical or at least difficult. Initially, at least, the primary physician or practitioner can calculate caloric needs based on height in centimeters[81] (Table 92-5) and add 5 kcal per gram of weight repletion needed divided by the time of acceptable accretion (e.g., 30 to 90 days). Another technique[82] uses a calculation based on height with modifications: 11.1 kcal/cm for nonambulatory children with motor dysfunction, 13.9 kcal/cm in those who are ambulatory without motor dysfunction, and 14.7 kcal/cm for children without motor dysfunction. Estimations can also encompass basal metabolic rate and growth, with variations applied for muscle tone and activity.[75]

ORAL FEEDING

The technique of feeding and the food provided are interrelated. Standard, grocery-shelved foodstuffs are the cheapest and simplest means of providing oral feedings. Moreover, the social and emotional pleasures and the expectations of mealtimes often

are important for the caregiver, even if only a portion of the individual's nutrient needs can be delivered by mouth. Taste and texture can be varied if the child or adult is identified as a safe oral feeder. Children and adults who can swallow safely but cannot chew effectively may be able to receive the same foods blenderized into a puree or acceptable consistency. Those who can tolerate solids but not liquids can have commercial thickeners added to their fluids. It is important in these children and adults that optimal feeding posture and appropriate food temperature be maintained, as these subtle nuances can make a real difference in feeding tolerance and the prevention of aspiration.

For infants, breast-feeding should be encouraged for its various benefits. Human milk fortifier or proprietary formulas, when used, can be concentrated an additional 10 to 50% by decreasing free water for children whose nutritional status is compromised (Table 92-6). This allows feedings to lessen critical feeding rates and volumes, with some infants and children unable to sustain growth on standard 20-kcal/oz products because of their volume sensitivity. Small quantities of carbohydrate polymers, cereal or lipids (as long- or medium-chain triglycerides) may be added progressively to either breast milk or formula (Table 92-7), titrating to increase caloric density to 30 kcal or more,[83] while carefully monitoring the child for tolerance to ensure adequate urination and to avoid diarrhea, vomiting, and/or feeding refusal.

Numerous proprietary products are now available as liquids or puddings to supplement calories, protein, and various nutrients. A particular product can be chosen based on the patient's need for fiber in regulating bowel movements and the patient's tolerance of the product's components and taste. Other methods of calorie loading include modification of the foods added to a milk or soy base, which can be adapted for calories, fluid and fiber content, vitamin and mineral requirements, and allergy restrictions according to the child's needs. Potentially, these modular feedings or "homebrews" (the technique is provided in Table 92-8) are less expensive and offer caregivers the perception of providing their child "real food" and "hands-on care."

The modular feedings are easily adapted to enteral needs, where taste fatigue will not become an issue. Milk, soy milk, or formula can be used as the base ingredient for "homebrew" feeding. Various calorie-strength recipes can be prepared according to a child's nutritional needs (see Table 92-6). For those children who are volume sensitive, nutrient-dense formulations may be appropriate. Others with relative gastroparesis may need to meet their fluid and nutritional requirements from less dense, lower-fat formulations.

A variety of foods can be blended finely together to make the homebrew nutritionally balanced to meet the child's individual

TABLE 92-7. **Modular High-Calorie Additions**

	kcal/g	kcal/Tbs	Nutrient Source
Human milk fortifier		3.5 per packet	Whey, sodium caseinate, corn syrup solids, lactose
Promod Liquid Protein	4.7	18	Glycerine, hydrolyzed beef collagen, water, malic acid, citric acid, L-tryptophan, potassium sorbate, sodium benzoate
Beneprotein	3.6	17	Whey protein isolate (milk) soy lecithin
Formula powder*	5-5.2	40	Variable
Nonfat dry milk	8.7	27	Milk
MCT oil	8.2	115	Medium-chain triglycerides
Vegetable oil	8.9	124	Variable
Polycose	3.8	23	Glucose polymer
Polycal	3.8	29	Maltodextrin
Duocal	4.9	42	Hydrolyzed corn starch, refined vegetable oils, fractionated coconut oil
Additions	5.2	43	Sodium caseinate, whey protein
Benecalorie (liquid)	7 kcal/mL	110	High-oleic sunflower oil, calcium caseinates, sodium ascorbate, polysorbate, zinc, etc.
Rice cereal	4.4	15	Rice flour, soy oil, barley malt
Corn syrup	2.9	61	Corn syrup, sugar

*20 cal/oz infant formula. Tbs, tablespoon.

TABLE 92-8. **Directions for Preparation of Home Tube-Feeding**

1. Measure all ingredients carefully, using measuring cups
2. Pour ingredients into a large mixing bowl and stir contents to combine
3. Mix well, using blender or mixer method
   Blender method: Blend at medium speed for 3 minutes or until mixed thoroughly
   Mixer method: Mix at medium speed for 5 minutes or until mixed thoroughly
4. There should be no lumps in the formula
5. If the mixture is thick, thin it with water as recommended by dietitian
6. Pour formula into a clean container or individual jars. Cover and refrigerate immediately
7. The refrigerated formula may be safely used within 24-36 hours
8. Before each feeding, the amount of formula needed should be measured into a separate container, covered and warmed slightly before use
9. To warm formula: place the container with one feeding into a pan of hot water for 15 to 20 minutes, or use a microwave oven on a low setting for approximately 1 minute
10. Do not overheat the formula
11. Shake the formula or stir it to avoid hotspots
12. Do not use formula that has been heated or removed from the refrigerator for more than 2 hours. Discard immediately
13. Flush tube with 15 to 30 mL water, or as recommended
14. If any problems are noted (intolerance to formula, diarrhea, thickness of formula), please review with registered dietitian

Note: Once you know your child is tolerating this recipe, it may be helpful to "stock up" on all of the ingredients, because each one is *important*. The simple omission of one ingredient could have a serious impact, so call your dietitian if you have any questions or concerns about this recipe before changing it.
Courtesy Aruna Navathe, Children's Healthcare of Atlanta.

TABLE 92-9. **Modular Formula Instructions for Parents**

For: .... Date: ....
Home Tube-Feeding Recipe
'Home Brew'
The feeding formula should be prepared fresh daily. To prepare this formula safely, you must always:
1 Wash your hands
2 Use clean mixing bowls, equipment and utensils
3 Sanitize the blender or mixer bowl by filling with boiling water. Allow to stand for 3 minutes and then discard water

Recipe:
In a large clean mixing bowl or blender combine the following ingredients:
___ ounces or _____ cups of milk or formula
___ teaspoon(s) vegetable oil
___ tablespoon(s) cereal ({1/4} cup)
___ packet Carnation Instant Breakfast
___ table salt
Strained baby food:
___ jar(s) fruit (4 oz)
___ jar(s) vegetable (4 oz)
___ jar(s) meat (2.5 oz)
Note: You may vary the selection of strained baby foods daily.

Volume:	oz	
Calories:	cal/recipe	Per ounce: cal/oz
Protein:	g/recipe	Per ounce: g/oz
Fat:	g/recipe	
Carbohydrate:	g/recipe	
kcal distribution:	% protein,% fat,% carbohydrate	
Rate:	mL/h	
Flushes:	20–30 mL water	
Vitamins/minerals:	This will meet RDA for all nutrients.	

Courtesy Aruna Navathe, Children's Healthcare of Atlanta.

needs (Tables 92-7, 92-8, and 92-9). Mixing the foods in a blender and/or straining results in a smooth, thin consistency that will avoid clogging a gastrostomy (G) or nasogastric (NG) tube. Vitamin and mineral supplement may be needed to ensure adequate nutritional status. The feeding tube should be flushed with tap water before and after delivering feedings and medication.

Because homebrew feedings may be thicker than commercial formulas, a large feeding tube may be necessary. Bolus feedings may work better for homebrew tube feedings than a continuous drip because of the thicker consistency and increased risk of bacterial contamination without refrigeration. As always, aseptic techniques, proper handling of utensils, and hand-washing should be used to prepare formula to avoid cross-contamination and ensure food safety.

Assessment of nutritional status and determination of an optimal nutritional plan to meet the child's needs should be done initially, with reassessments of formulation and nutritional needs at 1-, 3-, 6-, and 12-month intervals as needed.

If a currently available proprietary formula is used, the physician must recognize that these have fixed nutrient/energy ratios, so that reducing the prescribed calories proportionate to the debilitated patient's needs based on height also may reduce that individual's intake of all other nutrients significantly below the dietary reference intake (DRI) for age. The potential reduction in calcium, phosphorus, and vitamin D poses risks of bone disease in these individuals, with other vitamin and mineral deficiencies possible as well, although many vitamin and mineral needs do parallel caloric requirements. In a study of children with cerebral palsy, most nutrient levels exceeded two thirds of the DRI, but the serum level for calcium was decreased below normal levels.[84] Another study demonstrated increased alkaline phosphatase levels in institutionalized children and adolescents on anticonvulsants.[85] Thus, intervention with maintenance doses of vitamin D and calcium may be prudent as the individual ages, if he or she is not at particular risk for nephrolithiasis.

Tube feeding may be indicated even in the child who is able to eat, if the volume of fluids or feeding required is beyond the capacities and/or oral abilities of the child or caretaker to meet these needs.

ORAL FEEDING PROBLEMS

Oral feeding is an option when the child or adult is identified as a safe oral feeder. A primary consideration in treatment of children with feeding problems is that the child with food refusal has a different history or experience of food than the typically eating child, with the problems often persisting and worsening over time.[86] Therefore, the techniques or recommendations that are used for typically eating children may not apply to children with food refusal.

As indicated earlier, the first step is a comprehensive evaluation. Specificity of diagnosis allows targeted therapy. GER, renal disorders, and brain tumors may create a loss of intake, vomiting, or weight loss, with GER-induced esophagitis potentially diminishing intake as well. Moreover, Zangen et al.[48] have demonstrated that 43% of medically fragile toddlers (most of whom had cerebral palsy) responded to medication, using nifedipine and dicycloverine for diffuse esophageal spasm; dicycloverine for continuous duodenal contractions; imipramine or amitriptyline and/or gabapentin and/or ondansetron for raising the gastric pain threshold; octreotide or erythromycin for inducing phase three migrating motor complexes; and cyproheptadine for increasing appetite. In addition, attention should focus on the amount of enteral feeding, as large volumes may satiate the child, and the protein predominance of the formula. Whey-based formulas markedly reduce gastric emptying time and decrease the frequency of emesis in gastrostomy-fed children with spastic quadriplegia.[87]

Effective, empirically supported interventions in the treatment of complex feeding problems are those contingency management treatments that include positive reinforcement of appropriate feeding responses and ignoring or guiding inappropriate responses.[88]

Oral competency and painful feedings have great impact on nutritional status in a cyclical devolution, unless the cycle can be interrupted. Poor oral motor feeding skills result in an inability to eat, subsequent inadequate weight gain, and failure to thrive. This leads to lessened motivation and ability to learn these skills (J. Fagan and A. Navathe, unpublished observations).

Thus the main goals of oral feeding are:
- To increase oral intake
- To meet the child's nutritional needs
- To decrease G-tube dependence
- To increase the texture
- To increase the variety of foods
- To decrease bottle dependence
- To increase self-feeding
- To decrease inappropriate behaviors
- To support parental nurturance of the child
- To maintain family stability

Initially, treatment for children with total food refusal and inappropriate mealtime behavior (e.g., crying, head turning, batting at the spoon, refusal to open the mouth) should focus on reducing these inappropriate behaviors and increasing more appropriate eating-related behaviors (e.g., opening the mouth) to establish that eating is no longer painful.[89,90] Meals should be time limited and focus on a specific end goal (e.g., having the child taste one bite of food[91]). It is also important to understand what additional gains the child may achieve by avoiding food or engaging in inappropriate mealtime behavior. Adaptive feeding utensils; changing the texture, temperature, and variety of presented food; and altering the child's feeding posture may be helpful in furthering oral feeding, particularly for the mildly impaired child.

Sensorimotor interventions focusing on oral motor skills may also be helpful for this population and those with moderate impairments.[92] Appetite enhancement with cyproheptadine can be used and continued when effective. Olfactory stimulation with black pepper oil has been effective to facilitate swallowing and increase feeding in a small study of selected patients, though severe cerebral tissue loss and intractable seizures seem to reduce efficacy.[93]

Where the etiology of difficult feeding problems is multidetermined, treatment should focus on all of the components (physiologic, oral motor, and psychologic), combining the services of a psychologist, occupational therapist, speech therapist, dietitian, and pediatric gastroenterologist. Often the programs provide a continuum of services (evaluation, outpatient therapy, day treatment, and hospitalization), based on the patient's individual needs.[13,94,95] Rapid (2 to 3 weeks) success has been described with inpatient care, specifically selected candidates, and a consistent approach to overcoming the child's resistance.[96]

Successful treatment of feeding problems should include measurable goals developed by the interdisciplinary team and caregivers. Feeding behaviors (e.g., amounts consumed, acceptance of bites of food) should be assessed regularly throughout the duration of treatment in order to establish feeding patterns that can be maintained by the caregivers. Thus, caregiver training should be an essential component to the success of the program.

Preliminary analysis of the outcome measures for one program with approximately 50 children, half of whom had been diagnosed with a developmental disability,[96] indicated that over 87% of the goals for treatment were met by the time of discharge. All of the children met their goals for increasing texture, decreasing bottle dependence, increasing self-feeding skills, and increasing variety of foods consumed. When increases in oral calories were the goal of treatment, 70% of the children reached their goal for caloric intake. When increases in liquid intake (for children who did not consume liquids by mouth) were the goal of treatment, 80% of the children reached their goal for oral liquid intake. All others increased solid or liquid intake over baseline levels, but did not reach their final goal during the day treatment admission. Even though not all of the children reached their goal for oral intake, the mean percentage of the PO goal met was 82%, suggesting that even when children did not reach 100% of their oral intake goal, their levels of oral intake were increased substantially and within 20% of the goal. Progress toward increasing oral intake continued during outpatient follow-up.[96]

Levels of enteral feedings were decreased for all children who entered the program receiving nutritional supplementation via tube, and 70% of children met their goals for decreases in enteral feedings. Children who entered the program with an NG tube either left the program without the tube (75%) or the tube was removed shortly after discharge (100%). Thus, surgical placement of a gastric (G) tube was avoided for 100% of children who entered the program as candidates for G tubes as a result of the presence of failure to thrive and an NG tube at admission. The goals for decreasing inappropriate mealtime behaviors were met for 97% of the children. Some 88% of caregivers were trained to implement the treatment protocols with greater than 90% accuracy, and the treatment was transferred successfully to the home and community in 100% of cases.

Preliminary analysis of follow-up data indicates that the majority of children (87%) continue to be followed after discharge from the day treatment program. Of those who are currently followed, 85% have continued to make progress toward age-typical feeding, which included further volume increases, further G-tube decreases and G-tube removal, increases in the variety of foods consumed, texture advances, initiation of cup drinking, and initiation of self-feeding.

In addition, structured diagnosis-specific treatment has resulted in increased tissue stores and decreased hospitalization.[13] When combined with pharmacotherapy to treat esophageal spasm and duodenal dysmotility, to reduce gastric pain threshold, and/or to increase appetite, 80% had improved emotional health, with 43% able to eat orally.[48]

ENTERAL DELIVERY

When necessary, proprietary and homemade supplemental formulas can be delivered via nonoral means. An NG tube may be used in the infant needing a brief (less than 2 months) infusion to allow acquisition of feeding skills. Similarly, a child needing perioperative intervention to prevent negative nitrogen balance may benefit from a short-term infusion by NG tube. Any enteral therapy that is expected to extend for a longer duration (greater than 2 to 3 months) should use a tube placed directly into the stomach or intestine. In most situations, a G tube will function well for the delivery of nutrition and medication. The tube can be converted to a "button" device with internal bolsters to decrease traction and any interference with the child's activity and therapies. Gastrostomy placement has been shown to reduce feeding time, food-related choking episodes, frequency of chest infections, and family stress, and to improve weight

gain and nutritional status significantly in children with severe neurologic impairment.[12,17]

However, percutaneous gastrostomy (PEG) is not without complications or concerns. In a review of a 10-year experience with 220 children, Gauderer[97] reported four minor catheter infections and 13 more significant complications. This included two deaths with underlying cardiac disease. In another series, perforation occurred with 15% of the tubes.[12] Population-based data compiled from the roles of the California Department of Developmental Services[72,98,99] and elsewhere[100] reveal that feeding tubes in severely disabled children with a tracheostomy reduce the risk of mortality, but significantly shorten survival in adults and increase mortality risk by 2.1 in children without a tracheostomy.

Use of the feeding tube is not necessarily causal, as factors such as immobility, malnutrition, oral motor dysfunction, and recurrent aspiration that require the use of an alternative nutritional method may contribute to the patient's morbidity. However, the protection offered by a tracheostomy does suggest that the potential for aspiration in patients with gastrostomy devices is considerable; even though quality of life may be improved with the use of enteral feedings through a gastrostomy, the length of survival may be lessened.

Therefore, the anatomy and function of the stomach should be evaluated before the placement of the feeding tube. The coexistence of GER may require a simultaneous fundoplication, and delayed gastric emptying must necessitate pyloroplasty or duodenal placement of the distal portion of the tube. Of importance, symptomatic GER may be recognized only after gastrostomy placement, even though it is not demonstrated initially.[101-103] In children with recurrent aspiration, fundoplication and gastrostomy are not able to lower the rate of postoperative aspiration.[104,105] Moreover, recurrent GER can occur after fundoplication and may be increased in children with profound neurologic disability.[106-109] Attempts to identify the risk factors that increase morbidity and mortality include stratifying the disabled population by degree of impairment[110,111] and using serum albumin[112] to predict at least early survival after PEG placement.

Physiologically designed formulas of increased caloric and protein density can be used for gastric and nasogastric infusion, as palatability is no longer an issue. Modifications must be made for osmolality and speed of delivery with a feeding tube in the duodenum or jejunum. Lower osmotic or predigested formulas are needed for duodenal or jejunal infusions and must be delivered by a slow drip to avoid dumping or discomfort. Bolus or cyclic drip feedings may be chosen for the patient with a G or NG tube. The choice between bolus and drip may depend on esophagogastric function, the volume to be delivered, or the home care needs of the child and his or her caregivers. Often nocturnal drip feedings can provide 30 to 50% of the child's nutrient needs, so that daytime meals can be offered orally without the pressure and large blocks of time that have to be devoted when all requirements need to be met by three or four daily meals.

Gastric emptying has been shown to be delayed in children with cerebral palsy and contributes to GER, which in itself contributes to recurrent vomiting, with the most common manometric abnormality being a reduction in lower esophageal pressure.[113] Whey-based formulas do lessen that impact, however, by decreasing gastric emptying time and reducing the frequency of emesis in gastrostomy-fed children with spastic quadriplegia.[87] The choice of formula may be less of an issue than the volume delivered to children and adults with developmental disabilities with these assistive feedings. The amount ingested is no longer defined by appetite, but determined by caregivers and medical providers. Pectin liquid added to the formula can reduce cough, with a higher pectin diet (enteral formula: pectin liquid = 2:1 by volume) also reducing vomiting episodes and GER as evaluated by pH esophagram in a small study in children with cerebral palsy.[114]

Long-term overnutrition presents as much risk as undernutrition. Hypertension and obesity can increase cardiovascular concerns in these patients, especially those with neuromuscular disorders. Moreover, overweight and obese children or adults with developmental disabilities present increased problems for caretakers, who have to risk their own health in lifting or assisting movement. Therefore, calculations must approximate a patient's need for calories and nutrients.

As these prescriptions for volume may overestimate or underestimate actual requirements, and because growing children increase their nutritional needs as they age and grow, reevaluation at appropriate intervals for serial examination and measurement with the calculations revisited is perhaps more important than any individual prescription.

When safety of oral feeding is not an issue, these enteral techniques can merely supplement the child's own nutrition, with the caregivers continuing to feed the child actively. This dual feeding method often provides great satisfaction to parents and caregivers, because the mealtime interaction is improved when there is no longer any need for force-feeding of medication or nourishment. However, the risk of satiation (i.e., that the patient will not be motivated to feed orally) must be considered in conjunction with the schedule of feedings. Even overnight tube feedings may produce satiation and unwillingness of the child to orally feed concomitant with NG- or G-tube feedings.

Many parents are apprehensive about feeding and ensuring adequate nutrition for their children. Understandably, caregivers for children with a developmental disability may be even more anxious. Based on the method of delivery, the caregivers should be trained carefully in the preparation and delivery of the feeding. Parents should be reassured and provided with information about medical, nutritional, and home-care agencies that can serve as resources. They should be informed that success may be most dependent on appropriate follow-up visits to assess the patient's progress and adjust the feeding regimens. Moreover, social service agencies and/or medical care facilities should be encouraged to facilitate these efforts. In one study,[115] a hospital providing high-calorie, ready-to-feed nutritional supplementation at cost improved compliance with dietary recommendations. Such a policy has the potential to increase the effectiveness of nutrition intervention.

SUMMARY

Children with chronic illnesses often are debilitated further as a result of secondary nutritional problems that require the attention of their primary care physicians and subspecialists. Recent advancements in understanding and meeting the nutritional needs of children and adults with developmental disabilities have resulted in an improved quality and length of life.

The delivery of nutrient and energy sources should be based on the child's neurologic function, oral motor skills, and the presence of GER or other superimposed conditions. The use of proprietary formulas with fixed nutrient/energy ratios may provide sufficient calories, but also have the potential for specific nutrient deficiencies, most notably calcium, phosphorus, and vitamin D.

The complex etiology of feeding problems requires a multidisciplinary approach for successful treatment. Goals for treatment should be specified in measurable terms, and outcomes should be tracked during treatment and over time. Caregivers must bee adequately instructed, trained, and reassured and appropriate follow-up arranged to assess the patient's progress and adjust the regimen to achieve an optimal outcome.

REFERENCES

1. Dahl M, Thommessen M, Rasmussen M, Selberg T. Feeding and nutritional characteristics in children with moderate or severe cerebral palsy. Acta Paediatr 1996;6:697–701.
11. Stallings VA, Cronk CE, Zemel BS, Charney EB. Body composition in children with spastic quadriplegic cerebral palsy. J Pediatr 1995;126:833–839.
28. Samson-Fang L, Fung E, Stallings VA, et al. Relationship of nutritional status to health and social participation in children with cerebral palsy. J Pediatr 2002;141:637–643.
31. Ibrahim SH, Voigt RG, Katusic SK, et al. Incidence of gastrointestinal symptoms in children with autism: a population based study. Pediatrics 2009;124:680–686.
39. Kuperminc MN, Stevenson RD. Growth and nutrition disorders in children with cerebral palsy. Dev Disabil Res Rev 2008;14:137–146.
42. Cohen SA, Navathe AS. Feeding the developmentally delayed child. J Med Assoc Georgia 1999;88:71–76.
92. Gisel E. Interventions and outcomes for children with dysphagia. Dev Disabil Res Rev 2008;14:165–173.

See expertconsult.com for a complete list of references and the review questions for this chapter.

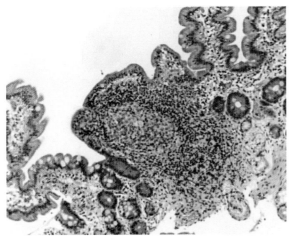

Figure 6-3. An organized lymphoid follicle in the duodenum. Large numbers of dark-staining intraepithelial lymphocytes may be seen in the epithelium overlying the follicle.

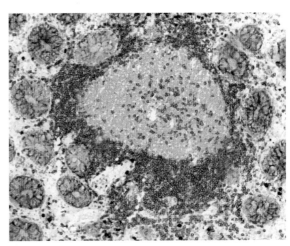

Figure 6-4. CD3+ T cells (showing brown surface staining) clustered in the cortex of an inflammatory colonic follicle). Individual T cells may also be seen within the medulla.

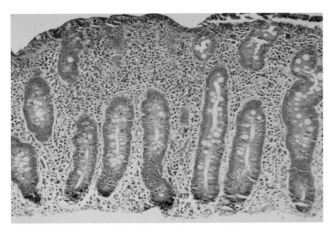

Figure 10-1. Small bowel biopsy from patient with celiac disease demonstrating villous atrophy and increased number of intraepithelial lymphocytes.

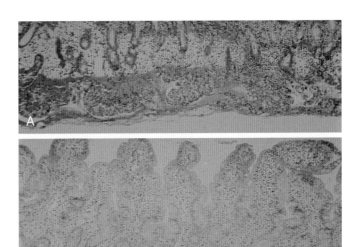

Figure 10-2. Small bowel biopsy before (**A**) and after (**B**) soy challenge in child with soy allergy. After the challenge, the epithelium is damaged: villi are destroyed and the mucosa is invaded by a dense cellular infiltrate.

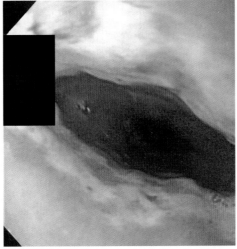

Figure 19-1. "Pill esophagitis" in a teenage girl on doxycycline.

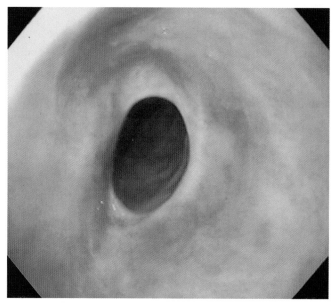

Figure 19-2. Esophageal stenosis in a toddler resulting from ingestion of oven cleaner.

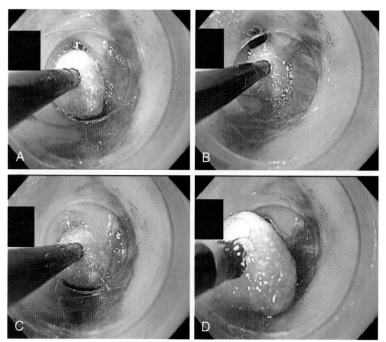

Figure 19-3. Application of mitomycin C to dilated, stenotic lesion in the esophagus. (**A**) Dry pledget is advanced from clear plastic hood on endoscope. (**B**) Mitomycin C is injected down forceps sheath onto pledget. (**C**) Pledget is held on mucosa at site of dilation. (**D**) Pledget is withdrawn into hood for safe removal.

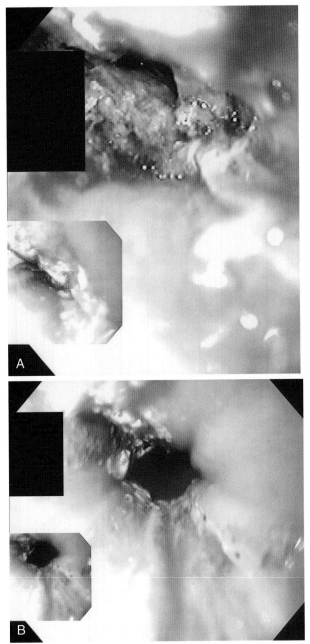

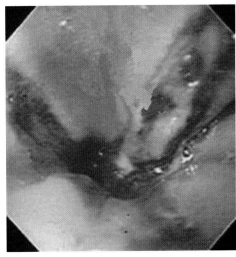

Figure 20-11. Endoscopic view of the distal esophagus revealing thickened folds resulting from edema, often a sign of chronic esophagitis.

Figure 19-7. (**A**) Disk battery in the esophagus with necrotic debris at the burn site. (**B**) Typical bilateral esophageal burn after removal of a disk battery.

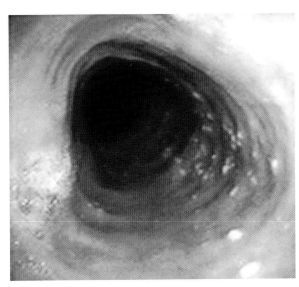

Figure 20-12. Endoscopic view of the distal esophagus revealing circumferential furrows, a sign of eosinophilic esophagitis.

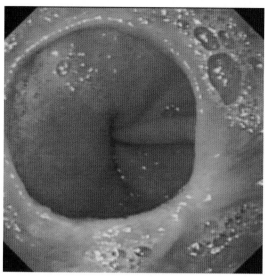

Figure 20-14. Endoscopic view of the distal esophagus revealing a Schatzki ring.

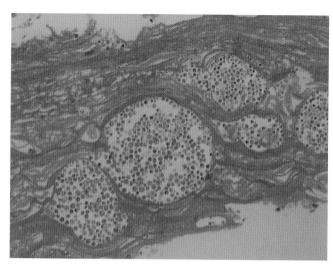

Figure 24-1. Invasive *Candida* esophagitis. The mucosa is necrotic, and the yeasts are within the mucosa (H&E, ×132). Courtesy David R. Kelly, MD, Children's Hospital of Alabama and University of Alabama.

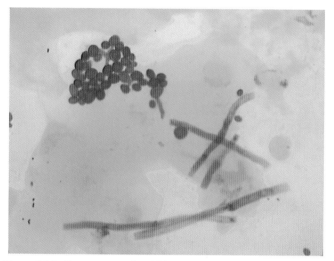

Figure 24-2. Yeasts, germ tubes (chlamydospores), and pseudohyphae of *Candida* in esophageal brushing specimen (GMS, ×330). Courtesy David R. Kelly, MD, Children's Hospital of Alabama and University of Alabama.

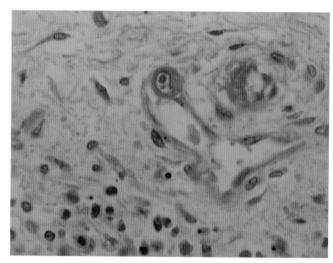

Figure 24-3. CMV esophagitis. This virus typically is characterized by a prominent eosinophilic intranuclear inclusion and displays vascular tropism (H&E, ×330). Courtesy David R. Kelly, MD, Children's Hospital of Alabama and University of Alabama.

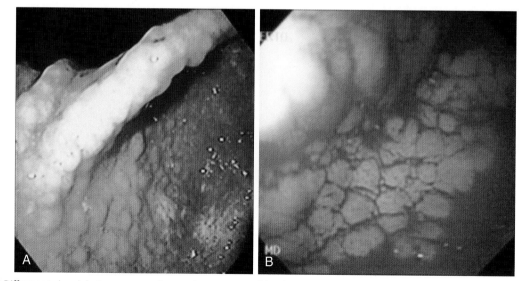

Figure 27-2. (**A**) Diffuse antral nodularity seen on endoscopy in a teenager with epigastric pain. (**B**) Following biopsy, blood acts as a "vital" stain to highlight the nodules. This is particularly useful when nodules are not so apparent. Histologic examination demonstrated *H. pylori* infection with chronic active pangastritis. The patient responded well to anti–*H. pylori* therapy.

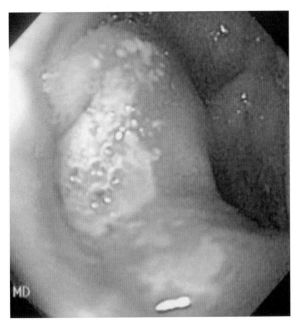

Figure 27-3. A chronic punched-out duodenal ulcer with overlying exudate, surrounded by swollen erythematous mucosa. This picture was from a 14-year-old boy with epigastric pain and nausea. He was positive for *H. pylori* infection.

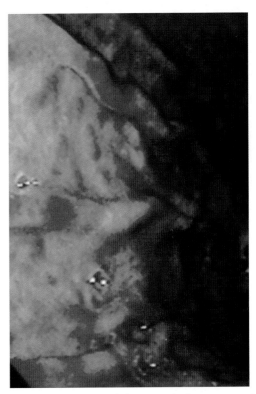

Figure 27-4. Endoscopic view of the stomach demonstrates cherry-red spots overlying a mildly swollen erythematous gastric body mucosa in a patient with portal hypertensive gastropathy and esophageal varices secondary to biliary atresia.

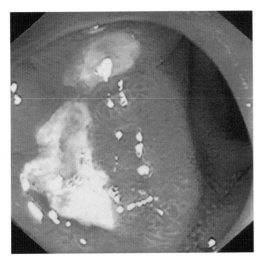

Figure 27-6. Ulcer in the duodenal bulb in a 12-year-old patient who presented with abdominal pain and loss of appetite with early satiety. His gastric biopsies were normal, and no *H. pylori* was present. He had no history of use of NSAIDs, and no antibiotics in the prior 6 months. He had true *H. pylori*–negative duodenal ulcer disease.

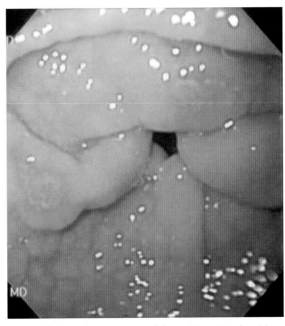

Figure 27-7. Endoscopic appearance of the gastric antrum in a 14-year-old Vietnamese boy with chronic abdominal pain. Multiple gastric antral erosions with surrounding erythema and nodularity are seen. *H. pylori* infection was confirmed on biopsy. There was no history of NSAID use.

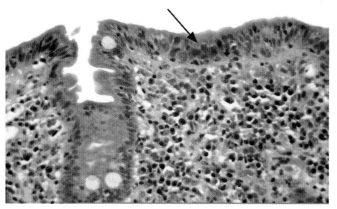

Figure 33-2. Villous atrophy in a patient with autoimmune enteropathy due to IPEX syndrome. Despite the dense increase in T cells within the lamina propria, there is minimal increase in intracellular lymphocyte numbers (arrow). This finding provides contrast to the high density of intraepithelial lymphocytes in celiac disease.

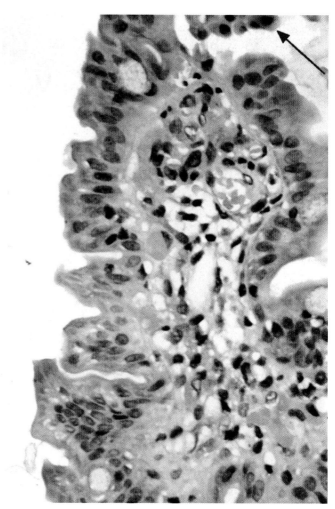

Figure 33-3. Shedding of surface epithelium at villus tip (arrow) in a patient with tufting enteropathy.

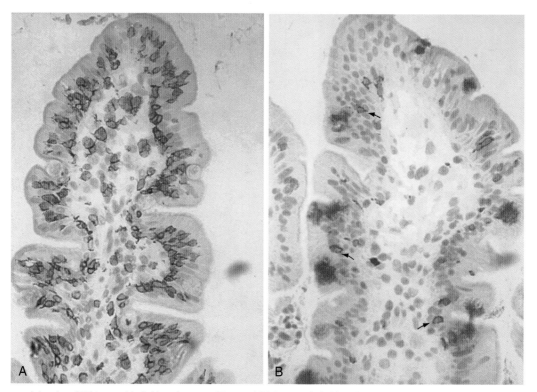

Figure 35-3. Increased density of (**A**) intraepithelial lymphocytes CD3+ and (**B**) intraepithelial lymphocytes expressing the gamma/delta T-cell receptor, in a celiac patient with serum positive antiendomysial antibodies, but normal jejunal architecture.

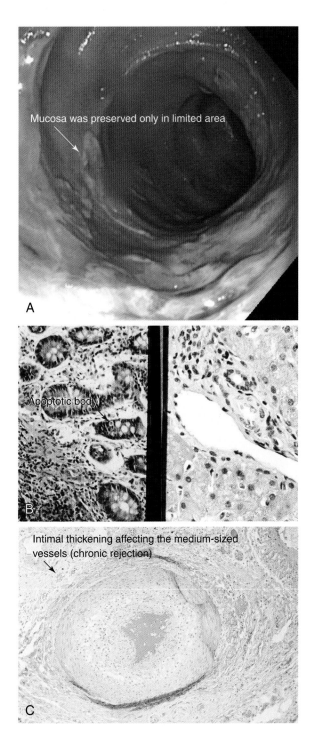

A

Mucosa was preserved only in limited area

Apoptotic body

B

Intimal thickening affecting the medium-sized vessels (chronic rejection)

C

Figure 37-3. (**A**) Endoscopic picture of severe acute rejection of the intestinal allograft with extensive loss of intestinal mucosa. (**B**) Photomicrograph of an H&E-stained section of a mucosal biopsy from an intestinal allograft. Acute cellular rejection is objectively defined as more than six apoptotic cells per 10 consecutive crypts with accompanying enterocyte injury, characterized by mucin depletion, cytoplasmic basophilia, and nuclear hyperchromasia. (**C**) Although not as well defined as acute cellular rejection, this photomicrograph of an H&E-stained section demonstrates obliterative arteriopathy that is characteristic of chronic allograft rejection. These vascular changes are usually only encountered at the time of explant.

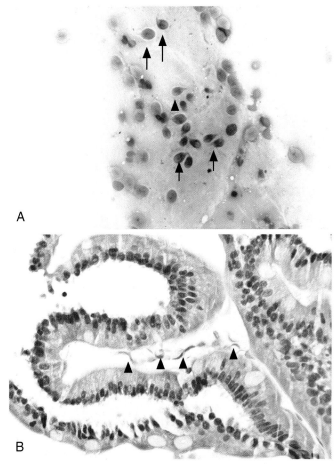

A

B

Figure 40-1. Trophozoites (arrows) of *Giardia lamblia* from small bowel biopsy. (**A**) Giemsa stain of touch prep. (**B**) Routine section (hematoxylin and eosin). *Courtesy Drs. Gerald Berry and Terry Longacre.*

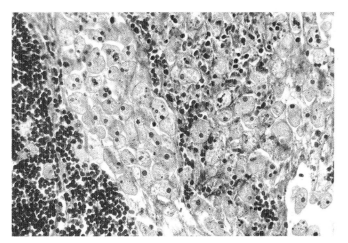

Figure 40-2. *Entamoeba histolytica* trophozoites in a colonic biopsy. *Courtesy Drs. Gerald Berry and Terry Longacre.*

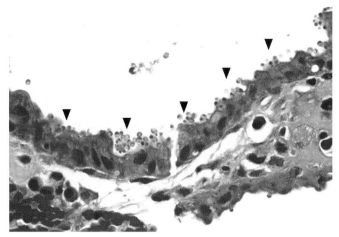

Figure 40-3. Cryptosporidia on the surface of a small intestinal biopsy. Courtesy Drs. Gerald Berry and Terry Longacre.

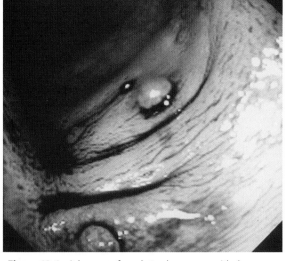

Figure 43-4. Adenomas found at colonoscopy with dye spray.

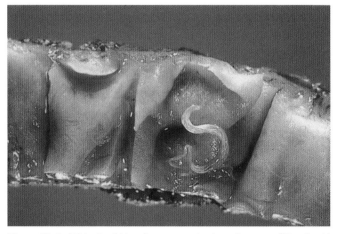

Figure 40-4. *Trichuris trichiura* in a resected colon. Courtesy of Drs. Gerald Berry and Terry Longacre.

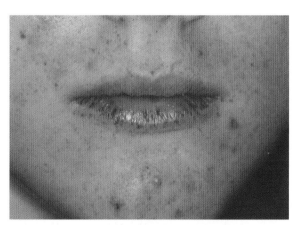

Figure 43-7. Typical mucocutaneous pigmentation seen in PJS.

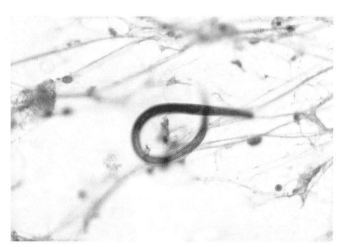

Figure 40-5. *Strongyloides stercoralis* (adult form). Courtesy Drs. Gerald Berry and Terry Longacre.

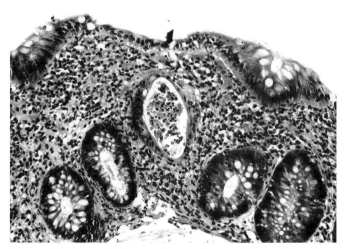

Figure 44-8. Neutrophilic crypt abscess and crypt architectural distortion.

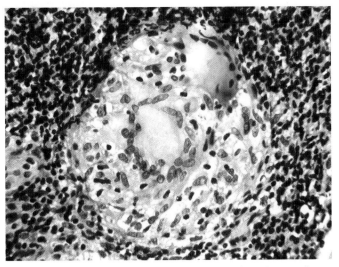

Figure 44-9. Epithelioid granuloma with multinucleated giant cells.

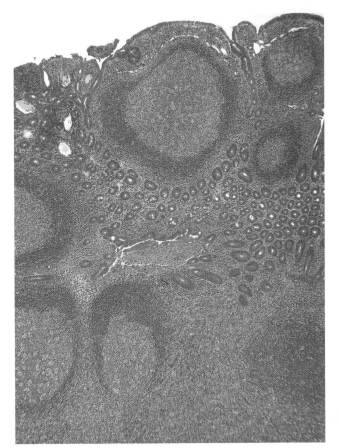

Figure 49-1. Lymphonodular hyperplasia. Numerous reactive germinal centers distort the normal villous architecture of the small bowel.

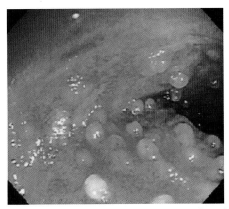

Figure 44-14. Marked lymphoid hyperplasia in Crohn's disease.

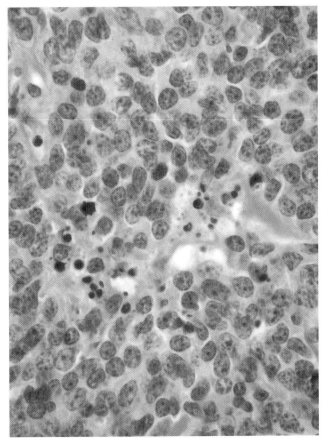

Figure 49-2. Burkitt's lymphoma. Sheets of monotonous intermediate-sized lymphoid cells have nondiscrete nucleoli. Abundant apoptotic nuclear debris is present centrally.

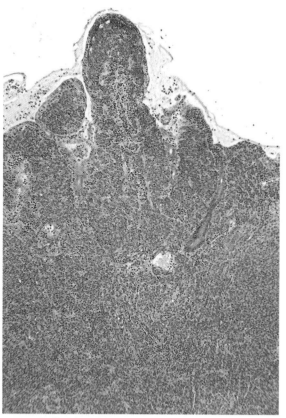

Figure 49-3. Burkitt's lymphoma. The neoplastic lymphoid cells diffusely infiltrate the mucosa, overrunning the epithelium. Contrast with the benign lymphoid reaction in Figure 49-1.

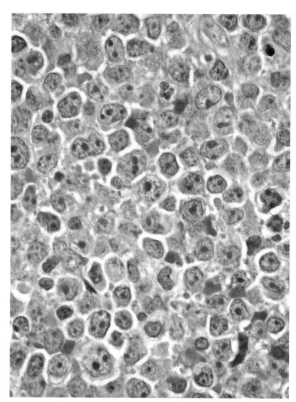

Figure 49-4. Diffuse large-cell lymphoma. Sheets of large, immunoblastic cells have prominent nucleoli; the tumor cells can diffusely infiltrate the bowel wall, similarly to Burkitt's lymphoma.

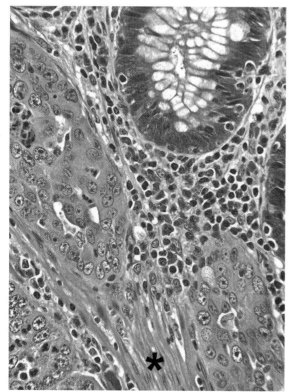

Figure 49-5. Adenocarcinoma, well differentiated. Malignant glands with complex architecture invade the muscularis (*) and are composed of crowded large epithelial cells with prominent nucleoli. By contrast, the overlying normal glands have a regimented nuclear polarization and obvious goblet cells.

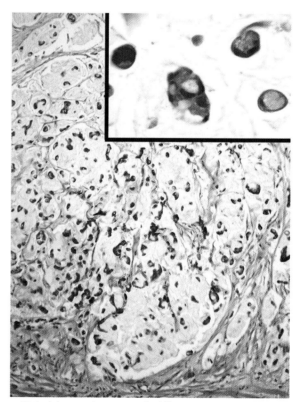

Figure 49-6. Adenocarcinoma, poorly differentiated (signet-ring cell carcinoma). Malignant epithelial cells float in pools of mucin. A "signet-ring" cell is created by a large mucin vacuole that fills the cytoplasm and displaces the nucleus (inset).

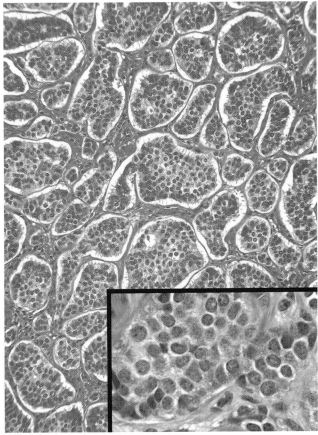

Figure 49-7. Carcinoid tumor. Fibrous stroma surrounds numerous well-demarcated islands of tumor cells. Uniform cells with faintly granular cytoplasm and round, bland nuclei that contain finely stippled chromatin are characteristic features of endocrine cell neoplasms (inset).

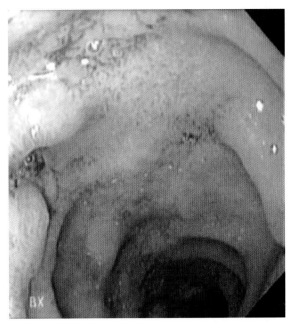

Figure 49-8. Intestinal vascular lesion. Endoscopic view of the duodenum with diffuse infiltration by a vascular lesion, composed of interdigitating capillary-sized vessels, in a 14-year-old boy who presented with gastrointestinal bleeding.

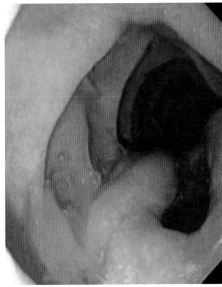

Figure 49-9. Primitive neuroectodermal tumor of the duodenum, endoscopic view.

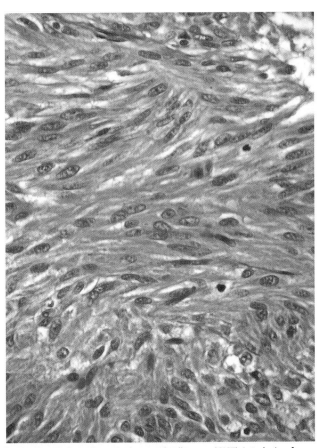

Figure 49-10. Gastrointestinal stromal cell tumor (GIST). Interlacing fascicles of plump cigar-shaped cells with tapered ends form the spindle cell GIST.

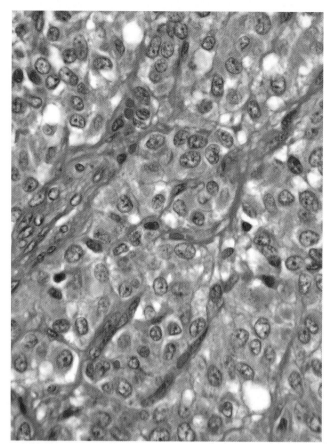

Figure 49-11. Gastrointestinal stromal cell tumor (GIST). Nests of medium-sized epithelioid cells with a moderate amount of eosinophilic cytoplasm form the epithelioid GIST.

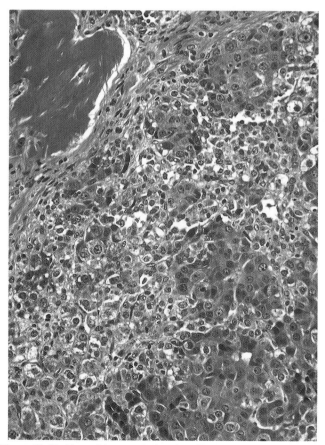

Figure 49-12. Hepatoblastoma. Trabeculae of hepatocyte-like cells resembling the fetal liver (lower right) mingle with the smaller "embryonal" cells (center); this biphasic pattern helps distinguish a primary liver tumor as hepatoblastoma. Homogenous eosinophilic osteoid-like material is a common mesenchymal element (top left).

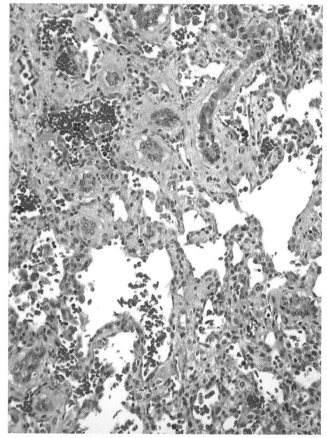

Figure 49-13. Hepatic hemangioma. Slightly ectatic vascular spaces are lined by plump endothelial cells and contain erythrocytes. Scattered hepatocytes and bile ducts may be entrapped (top).

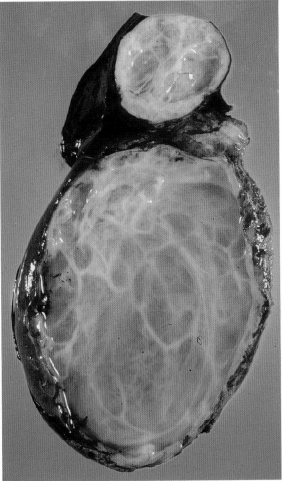

Figure 49-14. Mesenchymal hamartoma. The bisected multiloculated mass has fibrous septa dividing the lesion into cysts that contain viscous clear fluid. A thin rim of liver parenchyma is noted (upper left).

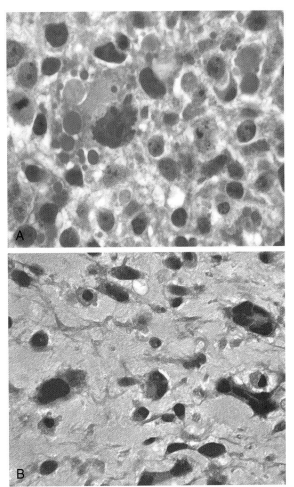

Figure 49-15. Undifferentiated embryonal sarcoma. Marked pleomorphism is characteristic, and cellular density is variable. Scattered atypical hyperchromatic multinucleated cells are sporadically distributed within abundant myxoid stroma (bottom). Another more cellular tumor has abundant eosinophilic hyaline globules (top).

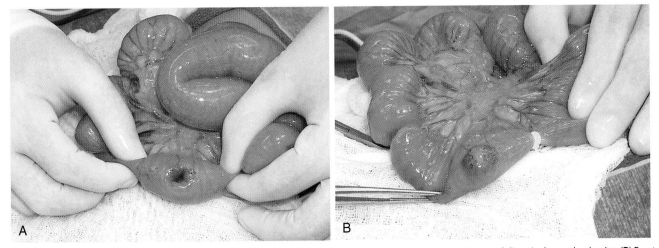

Figure 52-1. Surgically reduced ileocolic intussusception secondary to Meckel's diverticulum as lead point. (**A**) Inverted diverticulum as lead point. (**B**) Everted diverticulum in normal orientation.

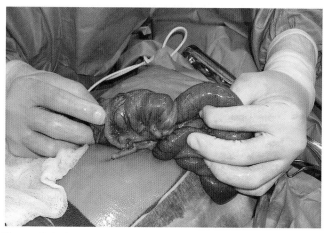

Figure 52-8. Intraoperative photograph of an ileocolic intussusception through the ileocecal valve. The absence of ischemic changes predicts successful manual reduction.

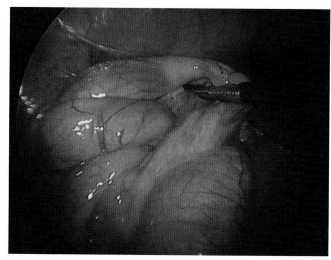

Figure 52-9. Laparoscopic reduction of ileocolic intussusception.

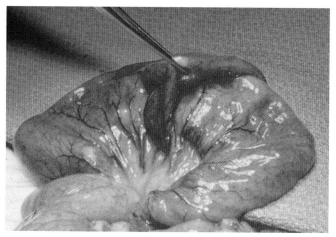

Figure 52-10. Small intestinal (enteroenteric) intussusception.

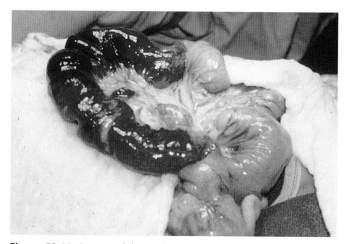

Figure 52-11. Intramural hemorrhage in small intestine secondary to Henoch-Schönlein purpura.

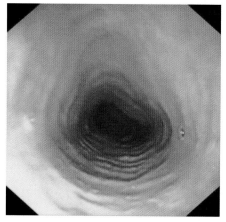

Figure 61-6. Rings of the proximal and midesophagus in a patient with eosinophilic esophagitis.

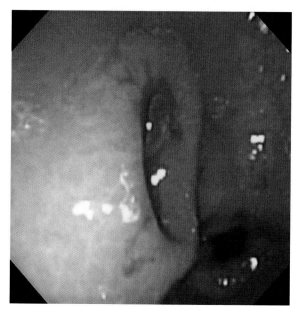

Figure 61-7. Endoscopic appearance of gastric PTLD in a 1-year-old following liver transplantation on tacrolimus immunosuppression. Note the large characteristic raised lesion with central umbilication proximal to the pylorus. The lesion was positive for Epstein-Barr virus (EBV) by in-situ hybridization.

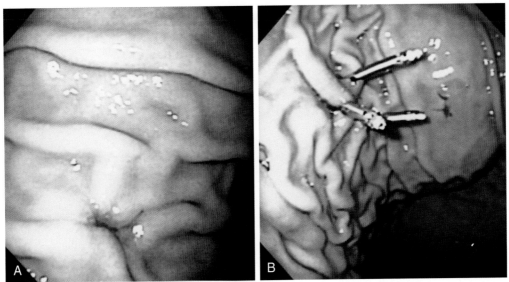

Figure 61-10. Endoscopic clipping of a gastric Dieulafoy lesion in a teenage patient following cardiac surgery on aspirin and antiplatelet therapy. The patient presented with a massive upper GI bleed with ongoing hemodynamic instability despite transfusion. (**A**) The clips were applied sequentially to approximate the edges of the lesion which terminated the bleeding episode. (**B**)

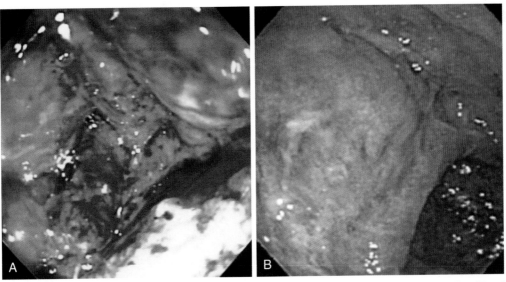

Figure 62-1. Endoscopic appearance of the colonic mucosa in a pediatric patient with acute infectious colitis due to *Escherichia coli* O157:H7 infection (**A**) compared to the mucosal appearance of ulcerative colitis (**B**). Although both are characterized by marked friability, hemorrhage, and superficial erosions, the infectious process lacks some of the typical features seen in chronic IBD. In addition to clinical and laboratory features, endoscopic biopsy may help to distinguish the two conditions.

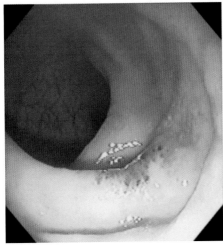

Figure 62-2. Endoscopic appearance of the rectum in a patient with mucosal prolapse. Note localized friability due to repetitive prolapse with an otherwise normal mucosal appearance.

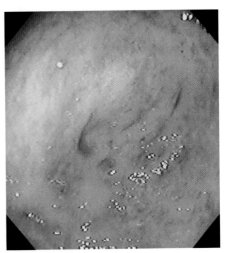

Figure 62-4. Typical appearance of the appendiceal orifice at colonoscopy.

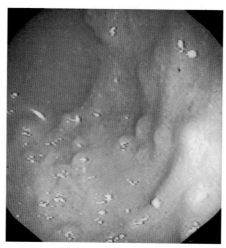

Figure 62-5. Lymphonodular hyperplasia of the terminal ileum. Note glistening mucosa and nodularity without erosions, which is characteristic.

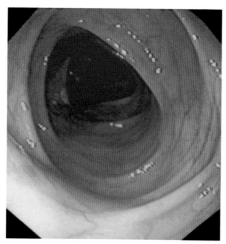

Figure 62-12. Normal colonic mucosal appearance of the transverse colon. Triangular shape of the folds is typical of this area.

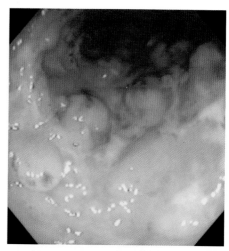

Figure 62-14. Endoscopic appearance of Crohn's colitis involving the transverse colon. Note marked nodularity, mucosal erosions, and overlying exudate in contrast to the appearance in Figure 62-12.

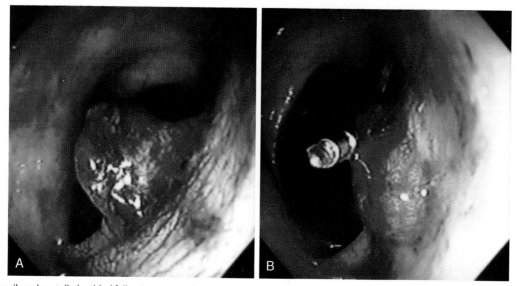

Figure 62-17. Juvenile polyp stalk that bled following snare polypectomy. Stalk was initially injected with epinephrine to achieve hemostasis (**A**) and clip was then applied to stalk after injection to achieve permanent hemostasis. (**B**)

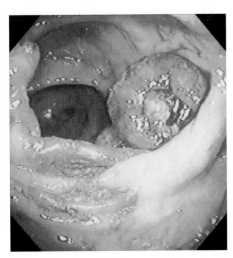

Figure 62-19. Head of a resected and coagulated juvenile polyp. Note the whitish area in the center of the polyp representing the area of coagulation.

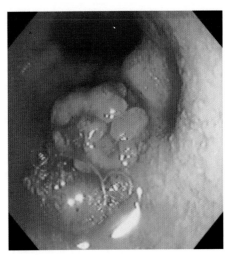

Figure 62-20. Large right-sided sessile polyp in a patient with long-standing Crohn's disease.

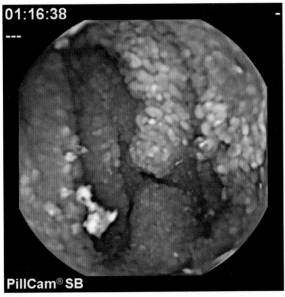

Figure 64-2. Dilated lacteals and focal bleeding in the mid small bowel seen on capsule endoscopy of an 8-year-old girl with protein-losing enteropathy and edema.

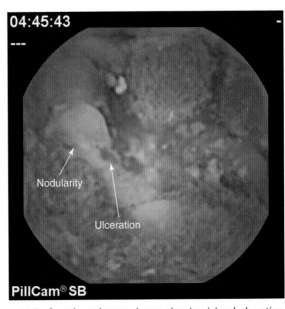

Figure 64-3. Capsule endoscopy image showing jejunal ulceration, exudates, and nodularity in a child with Crohn's disease.

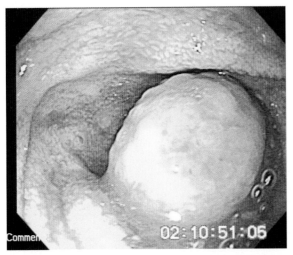

Figure 64-6. Ileal polyp before snare resection using single-balloon enteroscopy in a 14-year-old girl with juvenile polyposis syndrome.

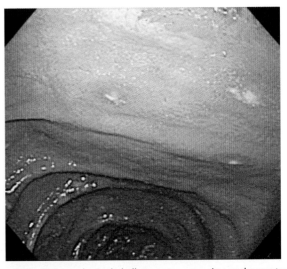

Figure 64-8. Retrograde single-balloon enteroscopy image demonstrating scattered, focal, aphthous ulcers in the proximal ileum of a child with Crohn's disease.

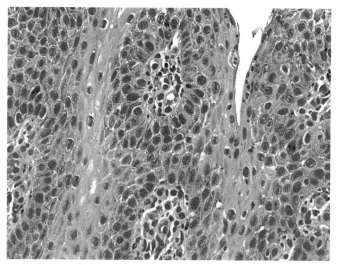

Figure 66-1. Esophageal squamous epithelial changes of reflux. In addition to papillomatosis, an increase in the squamous basal cell layer, and increased intraepithelial lymphocytes and eosinophils, surface neutrophils are also present.

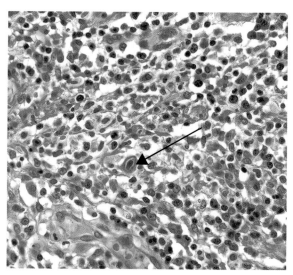

Figure 66-2. Cytomegalovirus inclusion found in ulcer base (center). The infected mesenchymal cell shows cellular enlargement. The nucleus contains a large basophilic inclusion body with surrounding halo and preservation of the nucleolus.

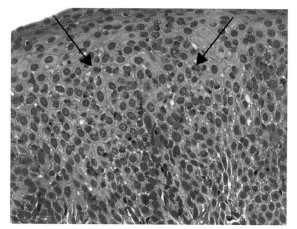

Figure 66-3. Eosinophilic esophagitis. Sections show squamous papillomatosis, a marked increase in the squamous epithelial basal cell layer, and numerous intraepithelial eosinophils leukocytes.

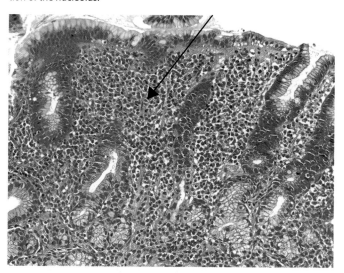

Figure 66-4. *Helicobacter pylori*–associated gastritis. Sections show a dense chronic inflammatory cell infiltrate of the lamina propria associated with some acute inflammation.

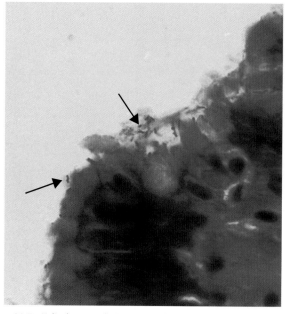

Figure 66-5. *Helicobacter pylori*–associated gastritis, Giemsa stain. Note the curved bacilli within the mucous layer.

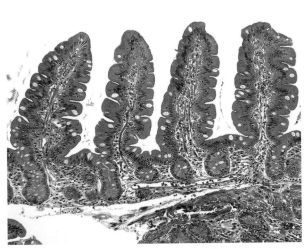

Figure 66-6. Normal small-bowel mucosa. The villi are long and slender. The ratio of villus:crypt length is approximately 4:1. Enterocyte nuclei are basilar in location and evenly aligned. Occasional intraepithelial lymphocytes are present.

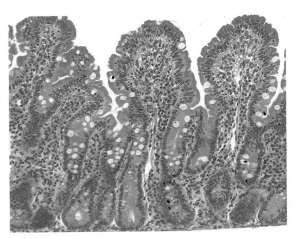

Figure 66-7. Severe villous abnormality typical of celiac sprue. The villus:crypt length is less than 1:1. Inflammatory cells are increased within the lamina propria. Numerous intraepithelial lymphocytes are also present.

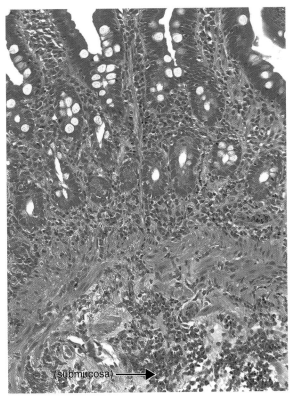

Figure 66-8. Small bowel with eosinophilic gastroenteritis. Note the large collection of eosinophils within the submucosa with lesser numbers infiltrating the muscularis mucosae and lamina propria.

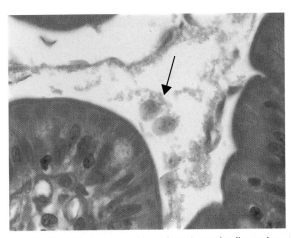

Figure 66-9. Giardiasis. In this small bowel specimen, the diagnosis rests on demonstration of the trophozoite in tissue section. Seen *en face*, *Giardia lamblia* is pear-shaped and demonstrates prominent paired nuclei.

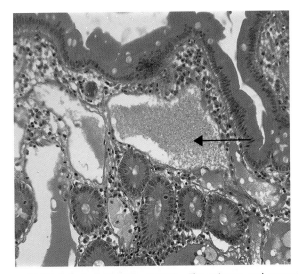

Figure 66-10. Intestinal lymphangiectasia. The primary and secondary forms appear identical in histologic sections, demonstrating dilated lymphatics located in otherwise normal mucosa.

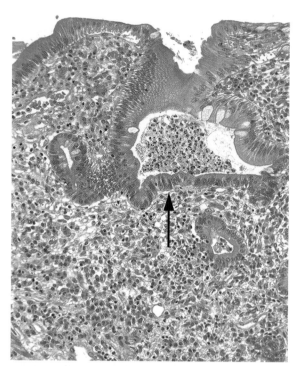

Figure 66-11. Ulcerative colitis in an active phase. Sections show diffuse architectural change, prominent lamina proprial plasmacytosis, and crypt abscess formation (arrow).

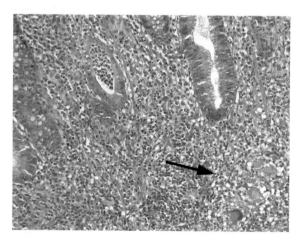

Figure 66-12. Colonic Crohn's disease showing focal active colitis with an intramucosal nonnecrotizing granuloma (arrow).

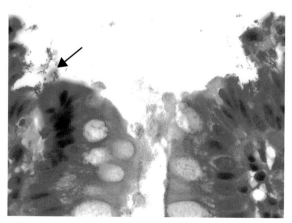

Figure 66-13. Enteroadherent *Escherichia coli.* Note the surface epithelial changes with adherent rod-shaped bacteria.

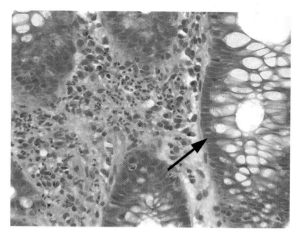

Figure 66-14. Infectious-type focal active colitis pattern of injury from a patient with culture-proved *E. coli* O157:H7 infection. Sections show a collection of lamina proprial neutrophils adjacent to a relatively normal colonic crypt (arrow).

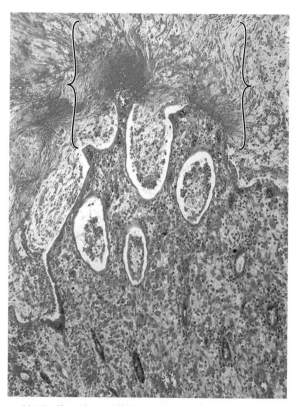

Figure 66-15. *Clostridium difficile*–associated pseudomembranous colitis. An inflammatory pseudomembrane exudes from dilated degenerating crypts in an erosive fashion. The karyorrhectic debris and neutrophils within the pseudomembrane tend to align in a linear configuration within the mucus.

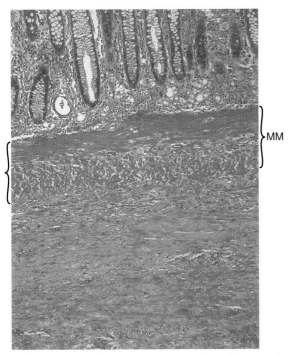

MM

Figure 66-16. Biopsy specimen from patient with Hirschsprung's disease illustrating an absence of ganglion cells associated with marked hypertrophy of the muscularis mucosae.

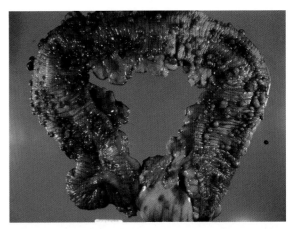

Figure 66-17. Resected colonic resection specimen from a patient with familial adenomatous polyposis.

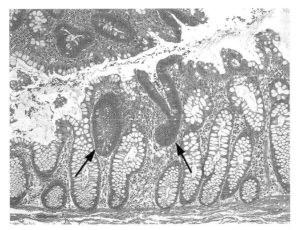

Figure 66-18. Familial adenomatous polyposis. Sections show tubular adenomas including one-gland adenomas (arrow) typical for the syndrome.

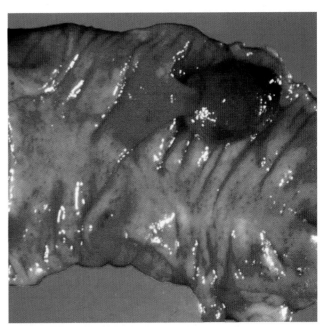

Figure 66-19. Resected colonic juvenile polyp. Note the spherical red polyp attached by an elongate pedicle.

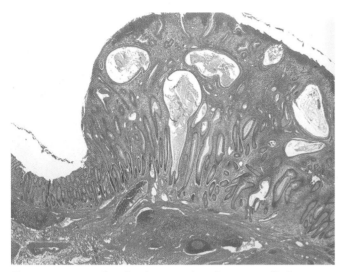

Figure 66-20. Juvenile polyp demonstrating edematous and inflammatory expansion of the lamina propria with colonic mucosal epithelial microcyst formation.

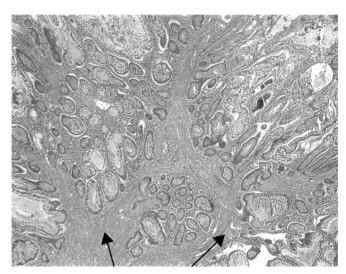

Figure 66-21. Peutz-Jeghers polyp composed of fairly normal epithelium and lamina propria lining an abnormal arborizing overgrowth of the smooth muscle of the muscularis mucosae.

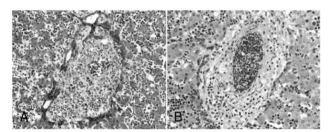

Figure 67-6. Human fetal liver tissue at weeks 16 (**A**) and 20 (**B**). (**A**) Remodeling of the ductal plate. (**B**) Remodeling is almost complete.

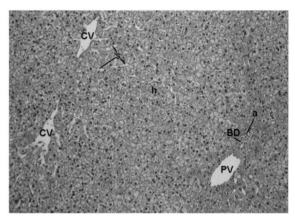

Figure 67-10. Microscopic functional unit of the liver: the liver lobule, from a mature child. a, Arteriole; BD, bile duct; CV, central vein; h, hepatocytes; PV, portal vein; s, sinusoids.

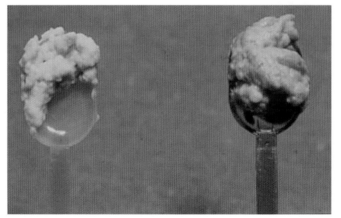

Figure 69-1. Acholic stool (left) strongly suggestive of a surgical problem during neonatal period. Children with biliary atresia can, however, have initially pigmented stools (right). Reproduced from Francavilla R, Mieli-Vergani G. Liver and biliary disease in infancy. Medicine 2002; 30:45-47, with permission from The Medicine Publishing Company, Abingdon.

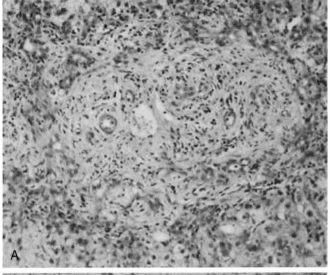

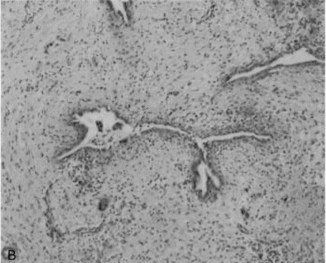

Figure 69-2. Histologic appearance of biliary atresia. (**A**) Liver biopsy showing typical changes – edematous portal tract with increased fibrosis, duplicating bile ducts, and cholestatic plugs (hematoxylin-eosin stain, ×250). (**B**) Bile duct remnant obtained at Kasai portoenterostomy showing fibrosis and occlusion of extrahepatic bile ducts (hematoxylin-eosin stain, ×125). Reproduced from Francavilla R, Mieli-Vergani G. Liver and biliary disease in infancy. Medicine 2002; 30:45–47, with permission from The Medicine Publishing Company, Abingdon.

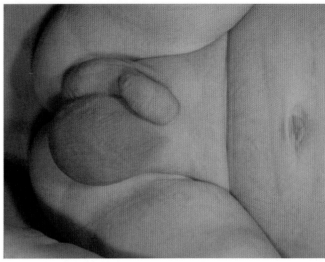

Figure 69-6. Green-yellow discoloration of scrotum and umbilicus due to intra-abdominal presence of bile following spontaneous perforation of the bile duct.

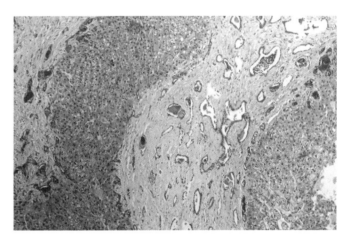

Figure 69-10. Liver biopsy in the ductal plate malformation; loose fibrous tissue containing small irregular bile ducts, some of them dilated and containing bile (hematoxylin-eosin stain, ×125).

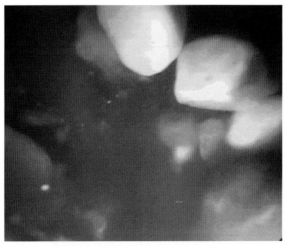

Figure 79-6. Endoscopic view of multiple large cholesterol stones in a morbidly obese teenager.

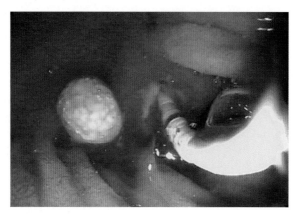

Figure 79-7. Endoscopic view of a spherical gallstone in a patient with Duchenne's muscular dystrophy.

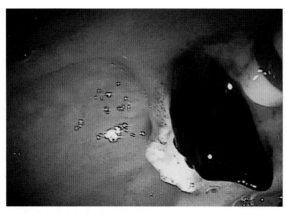

Figure 79-8. Endoscopic view of a large pigmented stone in an 8-year-old with autoimmune hemolytic anemia.

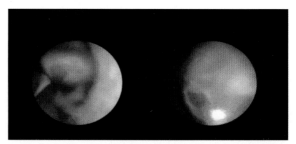

Figure 79-9. Choledochoscopy views of common bile duct stone. Image on right is before holmium YAG laser lithotripsy. Courtesy Dr. Isaac Raijman.

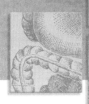
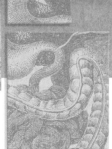

INDEX

Page numbers followed by *b* indicate boxes; *f*, figures; *t*, tables.

		DATE DUE		